SIXTH EDITION

Physical Rehabilitation

SIXTH EDITION

Physical Rehabilitation

Susan B. O'Sullivan, PT, EdD
Professor Emerita
Department of Physical Therapy
School of Health and Environment
University of Massachusetts Lowell
Lowell, Massachusetts

Thomas J. Schmitz, PT, PhD
Professor Emeritus
Department of Physical Therapy
School of Health Professions
Long Island University
Brooklyn Campus
Brooklyn, New York

George D. Fulk, PT, PhD
Chair and Associate Professor
Department of Physical Therapy
Clarkson University
Potsdam, New York

 F.A. Davis Company • Philadelphia

F.A. Davis Company
1915 Arch Street
Philadelphia, PA 19103
www.fadavis.com

Printed in the United States of America

Last digit indicates print number: 10 9 8 7 6 5 4 3 2

Editor-in-Chief: Margaret M. Biblis
Senior Acquisitions Editor: Melissa A. Duffield
Manager of Content Development: George W. Lang
Senior Developmental Editor: Jennifer A. Pine
Art and Design Manager: Carolyn O'Brien

As new scientific information becomes available through basic and clinical research, recommended treatments and drug therapies undergo changes. The author(s) and publisher have done everything possible to make this book accurate, up to date, and in accord with accepted standards at the time of publication. The author(s), editors, and publisher are not responsible for errors or omissions or for consequences from application of the book, and make no warranty, expressed or implied, in regard to the contents of the book. Any practice described in this book should be applied by the reader in accordance with professional standards of care used in regard to the unique circumstances that may apply in each situation. The reader is advised always to check product information (package inserts) for changes and new information regarding dose and contraindications before administering any drug. Caution is especially urged when using new or infrequently ordered drugs.

Library of Congress Cataloging-in-Publication Data

Physical rehabilitation / [edited by] Susan B. O'Sullivan, Thomas J. Schmitz, George D. Fulk. — 6th ed.
   p. ; cm.
Includes bibliographical references and index.
ISBN 978-0-8036-2579-2
I. O'Sullivan, Susan B. II. Schmitz, Thomas J. III. Fulk, George D.
[DNLM: 1. Physical Therapy Modalities. 2. Disability Evaluation. 3. Orthopedic Equipment. 4. Physical Examination. WB 460]
   RM700
   615.8′2—dc23
                                                              2013015288

With the sixth edition of *Physical Rehabilitation*, we continue a tradition of striving for excellence that began more than 25 years ago. We are gratified by the continuing wide acceptance of *Physical Rehabilitation* by both faculty and students.

The text is designed to provide a comprehensive approach to the rehabilitation management of adult patients. As such, it is intended to serve as a primary textbook for professional-level physical therapy students, and as an important resource for practicing therapists as well as for other rehabilitation professionals. The sixth edition recognizes the continuing growth of the profession and integrates basic and applied clinical research to guide and inform evidence-based clinical practice. It also integrates terminology, practice patterns, specific tests and measures, and interventions presented in the American Physical Therapy Association's *Guide to Physical Therapist Practice* and the World Health Organization's *International Classification of Functioning, Disability, and Health* (ICF).

Physical Rehabilitation is organized into three sections. Section One (Chapters 1–9) includes chapters on clinical decision making and examination of basic systems, as well as examination of functional status and the environment. Section Two (Chapters 10–29) addresses many of the diseases, disorders, and conditions commonly seen in the rehabilitation setting. Appropriate examination and intervention strategies are discussed for related body structure/function impairments, activity limitations, and restrictions in social participation. Health promotion and wellness strategies are also considered. Emphasis is placed on parameters of learning critical to ensuring the patient/client can achieve anticipated goals and expected outcomes. The final section, Section Three (Chapters 30–32), includes orthotics, prosthetics, and the prescriptive wheelchair.

A central element of the text is a strong pedagogical format designed to facilitate and reinforce the learning of key concepts. Each chapter of *Physical Rehabilitation* includes an initial content outline, learning objectives, an introduction and summary, review questions for self-assessment, and extensive references. Additional supplemental readings and recommended resources are also provided. Key terms are bolded throughout each chapter indicating their inclusion in a master glossary toward the end of the text. Application of important concepts is promoted through end-of-chapter case study examples and guiding questions designed to enhance clinical decision making skills. Disability-focused chapters contain *Evidence Summary Boxes* that summarize and critically appraise research focused on a particular topic or intervention relevant to the chapter content. Our hope is that the boxes may provide a model for readers to continue to critically examine clinical practice using validated clinical methodologies. We also hope it will inspire enthusiasm about the importance of continuous, lifelong, self-directed learning.

The visuals have been substantially enhanced with the addition of many new illustrations and photographs. Changes in design and the introduction of a full-color format provide a reader-friendly environment, as well as augment understanding of content. New to the sixth edition are 13 online case studies with accompanying video segments illustrating aspects of the initial examination, interventions, and outcomes for patients undergoing active rehabilitation. The cases were authored by practicing therapists from various parts of the country who were directly involved in the care of the case study patient participant. The case studies include patients with chronic obstructive pulmonary disease and respiratory distress syndrome, burns, amputation, spinal cord injury, Parkinson's disease, traumatic brain injury, stroke, and vestibular dysfunction. Questions are posed that address key elements in developing the plan of care for each patient. All case study materials (patient history, examination data, video segments, answers to guiding questions for student feedback) are available online at Davis*Plus*.

Also new to this edition are sample examination questions consistent with the format of the National Physical Therapy Examination. In separate files, answers to the questions are provided for student feedback that are also available at Davis*Plus*.

As we have noted in previous editions, our greatest asset and inspiration in preparing the sixth edition of *Physical Rehabilitation* has been an outstanding group of contributing authors. We are most fortunate to have this group of talented individuals whose breadth and scope of professional knowledge and experience seems unparalleled. These individuals are recognized experts from a variety of specialty areas who have graciously shared their knowledge and clinical practice expertise by providing relevant, up-to-date, and practical information within their respective content areas. To our group of contributors, we enthusiastically welcome the many talented, dedicated clinicians whose knowledge and clinical skills are well represented in the online case study materials that accompany the text. To the sixth edition, a welcome is also extended to George D. Fulk as a new contributing editor.

The sixth edition has also benefited from the input of numerous individuals engaged in both academic and clinical practice settings who have used and reviewed the content. We are grateful for their constructive feedback and have instituted many of their suggestions and changes. As always, we welcome suggestions for improvements from our colleagues and students.

As physical therapists continue to take on more and greater professional responsibilities and challenges, the very nature of this text makes it a perpetual "work in progress." We are grateful for the opportunity to contribute to the academic literature in physical therapy, as well as to the professional development of those preparing to enter a career devoted to improving the quality of life of those we serve.

We acknowledge the very important contributions that physical therapists make in the lives of their patients. This book is dedicated to those therapists—past, present, and future—who guide and challenge their patients to lead a successful and independent life.

—SUSAN B. O'SULLIVAN
THOMAS J. SCHMITZ
GEORGE D. FULK

Case Study and Multimedia Editor

Edward W. Bezkor, PT, DPT, OCS, MTC
University of California, San Diego Health System
Perlman Clinic, Rehabilitation Services
La Jolla, California

New York University Langone Medical Center
Rusk Institute of Rehabilitation Medicine
New York, New York

Test Bank Editor

Evangelos Pappas, PT, PhD, OCS
Senior Lecturer
Department of Physiotherapy
Faculty of Health Sciences
University of Sydney
Lidcombe, NSW 2127

Andrea L. Behrman, PT, PhD, FAPTA
Professor
Department of Neurological Surgery
University of Louisville
Louisville, Kentucky

Edward W. Bezkor, PT, DPT, OCS, MTC
University of California, San Diego Health System
Perlman Clinic, Rehabilitation Services
La Jolla, California

New York University Langone Medical Center
Rusk Institute of Rehabilitation Medicine
New York, New York

Janet R. Bezner, PT, PhD
Vice President
Education and Governance and Administration
American Physical Therapy Association
Alexandria, Virginia

Beth Black, PT, DSc
Assistant Professor
Physical Therapy Program
School of Health Sciences
Oakland University
Rochester, Michigan

Judith M. Burnfield, PT, PhD
Director, Institute for Rehabilitation Science and Engineering
Institute for Rehabilitation Science and Engineering
Madonna Rehabilitation Hospital
Lincoln, Nebraska

Kevin K. Chui, PT, DPT, PhD, GCS, OCS
Associate Professor
Department of Physical Therapy
Program in Geriatric Health and Wellness
College of Health Professions
Sacred Heart University
Fairfield, Connecticut

Vanina Dal Bello-Haas, PT, PhD
Associate Professor
Assistant Dean, Physiotherapy Program
School of Rehabilitation Science
McMaster University
Hamilton, Ontario
Canada

Konrad J. Dias, PT, DPT, CCS
Associate Professor
Program in Physical Therapy
Maryville University of St. Louis
St. Louis, Missouri

Joan E. Edelstein, PT, MA, FISPO, CPed
Special Lecturer
Program in Physical Therapy
Columbia University
New York, New York

George D. Fulk, PT, PhD
Chair and Associate Professor
Department of Physical Therapy
Clarkson University
Potsdam, New York

Jessica Galgano, PhD, CCC-SLP
Associate Research Scientist
Department of Rehabilitation Medicine
School of Medicine
New York University
New York, New York

Maura Daly Iversen, PT, DPT, SD, MPH
Professor and Chairperson
Department of Physical Therapy
School of Health Professions
Bouve College of Health Sciences
Northeastern University
Boston, Massachusetts

Clinical Epidemiologist
Division of Rheumatology, Immunology and Allergy
Brigham and Women's Hospital
Harvard Medical School
Boston, Massachusetts

Deborah Graffis Kelly, PT, DPT, MSEd
Associate Professor
Division of Physical Therapy
Department of Rehabilitation Sciences
College of Health Sciences
University of Kentucky
Lexington, Kentucky

Bella J. May, PT, EdD, FAPTA, CEEAA
Professor Emerita
Georgia Health Science University
August, Georgia

Adjunct Professor of Physical Therapy
California State University Sacramento
Sacramento, California

Coby D. Nirider, PT, DPT
Area Director of Therapy Services
Touchstone Neurorecovery Center
Conroe, Texas

Cynthia C. Norkin, PT, EdD
Former Director and Associate Professor
School of Physical Therapy
Ohio University
Athens, Ohio

Susan B. O'Sullivan, PT, EdD
Professor Emerita
Department of Physical Therapy
School of Health and Environment
University of Massachusetts Lowell
Lowell, Massachusetts

Leslie G. Portney, PT, DPT, PhD, FAPTA
Professor and Dean
School of Health and Rehabilitation Sciences
MGH Institute of Health Professions
Boston, Massachusetts

Pat Precin, MS, OTR/L, LP
Assistant Professor
Occupational Therapy Program
School of Health Sciences
Touro College
New York, New York

Licensed Psychoanalyst
Private Practice
New York, New York

Reginald L. Richard, PT, MS
Clinical Research Coordinator Burn Rehabilitation
U. S. Army Institute of Surgical Research
Fort Sam Houston, Texas

Leslie N. Russek, PT, DPT, PhD, OCS
Associate Professor
Department of Physical Therapy
Clarkson University
Potsdam, New York

Martha Taylor Sarno, MA, MD (hon), CCC-SLP, BC-ANCDS
Research Professor
Department of Rehabilitation Medicine
School of Medicine
New York University
New York, New York

Faith Saftler Savage, PT, ATP
Seating Specialist
The Boston Home
Boston, Massachusetts

David A. Scalzitti, PT, PhD, OCS
Associate Editor, Evidence-Based Resources
American Physical Therapy Association
Alexandria, Virginia

Thomas J. Schmitz, PT, PhD
Professor Emeritus
Department of Physical Therapy
School of Health Professions
Long Island University
Brooklyn Campus
Brooklyn, New York

Robert J. Schreyer, PT, DPT, NCS, MSCS, CSCS
Assistant Professor
Department of Physical Therapy
Touro College
New York, New York

Physical Therapist, Owner
Aspire Center for Health + Wellness
New York, New York

Michael C. Schubert, PT, PhD
Associate Professor
Otolaryngology Head and Neck Surgery
Laboratory of Vestibular Neurophysiology
School of Medicine
Johns Hopkins University
Baltimore, Maryland

Julie Ann Starr, PT, DPT, CCS
Clinical Associate Professor
Department of Physical Therapy
Sargent College
Boston University
Boston, Massachusetts

Carolyn Unsworth, OTR, PhD
Professor, Research and Higher Degrees Coordinator
Department of Occupational Therapy
Faculty of Health Sciences
La Trobe University
Bundoora, Victoria
Australia

R. Scott Ward, PT, PhD
Professor and Chair
Department of Physical Therapy
University of Utah
Salt Lake City, Utah

Marie D. Westby, PT, PhD
Physical Therapy Teaching Supervisor
Mary Pack Arthritis Program
Vancouver Coastal Health
Vancouver, British Columbia

D. Joyce White, PT, DSc, MS
Associate Professor
Department of Physical Therapy
University of Massachusetts Lowell
Lowell, Massachusetts

Christopher Kevin Wong, PT, PhD, OCS
*Assistant Professor of Clinical Rehabilitative and
    Regenerative Medicine*
Program in Physical Therapy
Columbia University
New York, New York

Edward W. Bezkor, PT, DPT, OCS, MTC
University of California, San Diego Health System
Perlman Clinic, Rehabilitation Services
La Jolla, California

New York University Langone Medical Center
Rusk Institute of Rehabilitation Medicine
New York, New York

Faye Bronstein PT, DPT, NCS
New York University Langone Medical Center
Rusk Institute of Rehabilitation Medicine
New York, New York

Alicia Esposito, PT, DPT, NCS
New York University Langone Medical Center
Rusk Institute of Rehabilitation Medicine
New York, New York

Alex Eubank, PT, DPT
Dodd Hall Rehabilitation Services
Wexner Medical Center at The Ohio State University
Columbus, Ohio

Michelle Farella-Accurso, PT, DPT
New York Institute of Technology
College of Osteopathic Medicine
Adele Smithers Parkinson's Disease Research and
    Treatment Center
Department of Physical Therapy
Old Westbury, New York

Greg Hartley, PT, DPT, GCS
St. Catherine's Rehabilitation Hospital
North Miami, Florida

Bryan Hujsak, PT, DPT, NCS
New York Eye and Ear Infirmary
Vestibular Rehabilitation
New York, New York

Karen J. Lagares, PT, DPT, GCS
St. Catherine's Rehabilitation Hospital
North Miami, Florida

Patricia Laverty, PT, DPT
New York University Langone Medical Center
Rusk Institute of Rehabilitation Medicine
New York, New York

Hendrika Lietz, PT, DPT, NCS
University of Michigan Hospital
Ann Arbor, Michigan

Gemma Longfellow, PT, MSPT, GCS
St. Catherine's Rehabilitation Hospital
North Miami, Florida

Sophie Manning, PT, BSc
University of Michigan Hospital
Ann Arbor, Michigan

Bhavesh Patel, MD, FRCP(C), RDMS
Department of Critical Care
Mayo Clinic Arizona
Scottsdale, Arizona

Laura Pink-Baker, PT, DPT
University of Michigan Hospital
Ann Arbor, Michigan

Jill Quarles, PT, MS
University of Michigan Hospital
Ann Arbor, Michigan

Kim Stover Rosso, PT, MSPT
University of Michigan Hospital
Ann Arbor, Michigan

Kate Rough, PT, DPT
University of Washington Medical Center
Rehabilitation Medicine
Seattle, Washington

Victoria Stevens, PT, NCS
University of Washington Medical Center
Rehabilitation Medicine
Seattle, Washington

Sally M. Taylor, PT, DPT
Rehabilitation Institute of Chicago
Chicago, Illinois

University of Michigan Hospital
Ann Arbor, Michigan

James Tompkins, PT, DPT
Department of Physical Medicine and Rehabilitation
Mayo Clinic Arizona
Scottsdale, Arizona

Joseph L. Verheijde, PhD, MBA, PT
Department of Physical Medicine and Rehabilitation
Mayo Clinic Arizona
Scottsdale, Arizona

Maria Julia Vila, PT, MPT
New York University Langone Medical Center
Rusk Institute of Rehabilitation Medicine
New York, New York

Airelle Hunter-Giordano, PT, DPT, OCS, SCS, CSCS
Sports Residency Director, Assistant Professor
University of Delaware
Newark, DE 19716

Phyllis Guarrera-Bowlby, PT, Ed.D., PCS
Associate Professor
University of Medicine and Dentistry in NJ, Doctoral
    Programs in Physical Therapy
Newark, NJ

Cindy Flom-Meland, PT, PhD, NCS
Associate Professor
University of North Dakota
Grand Forks, ND

Matthew B. Dodson, OTD, OTR/L
Supervisor, Traumatic Brain Injury
Department of Occupational Therapy
Directorate of Rehabilitation
Walter Reed National Military Medical Center
Bethesda, MD
and
President
Braintrust Performance Services
Rockville, Maryland

Cristiana Kahl Collins, PT, PhD, CFMT, NCS
Assistant Professor
Long Island University
Brooklyn, NY

Jodie A. McClelland, PT, PhD
Lecturer and Research Fellow
La Trobe University
Melbourne, Victoria

William Culbertson, PhD
Professor
Northern Arizona University
Flagstaff, Arizona

Ingrid S. Parry MS, PT
Shriners Hospital for Children, Northern California
Sacramento, CA 95817

Alan Taylor PT, MSc, MCSP
University of Nottingham (UK)
Nottingham, Nottinghamshire, UK

Sarah Steffensmeier PT, DPT
Adjunct Assistant Professor
Long Island University
Brooklyn, NY

James Gurley, PT, DPT, NCS
Assistant Professor
Mercy College
Dobbs Ferry, NY

Donna Wang, PhD, LMSW
Assistant Professor, Chair of the Social Work Department
Long Island University-Brooklyn
1 University Plaza
Brooklyn, NY 11201

Michael Wong DPT OCS FAAOMPT
Associate Professor
Azusa Pacific University
Azusa, CA

Robyn Gisbert PT, DPT
Senior Instructor
University of Colorado –School of Medicine
Department of Physical Therapy
Aurora, CO 80045

Mary Lou Galantino, PT, MS, PhD, MSCE
Professor of Physical Therapy
Holistic Health Minor Coordinator
School of Health Sciences Office: G-233
The Richard Stockton College of New Jersey
101 Vera King Farris Drive
Galloway, NJ 08025

Herb Karpatkin, PT, DSc, NCS, MSCS
Hunter College
Program in Physical Therapy
New York

Carol A. Courtney PT, PhD, ATC
Fellow, American Academy of Orthopedic Manual Physical Therapy
Clinical Associate Professor
Department of Physical Therapy
University of Illinois at Chicago
1919 W. Taylor Street, 4th floor
Chicago IL 60612

Elizabeth Dylke, PT
Associate Lecturer
University of Sydney
Sydney, NSW

Shari McDowell, PT, DPT
Director, Spinal Cord Injury Program
Shepherd Center
Atlanta, GA

Julie Redfern, PhD, BAppSc (Physiotherapy Hons 1), BSc
Associate Professor
The George Institute for Global Health, University of Sydney
PO Box M201, Missenden Road, Camperdown, NSW,
    AUSTRALIA 2050

Evangelos Pappas PT, PhD, OCS
Associate Professor
Long Island University-Brooklyn Campus
Department of Physical Therapy
1 University Plaza
Brooklyn, NY 11201

Zoe McKeough, BAppSc(Physiotherapy), PhD
Senior Lecturer
The University of Sydney
Sydney, NSW

The ongoing development of *Physical Rehabilitation* has been in all aspects a collaborative venture. Its fruition has been made possible only through the expertise and gracious contributions of many talented individuals. Our appreciation is considerable.

Heartfelt thanks are extended to our contributing authors. Each has brought a unique body of knowledge, as well as distinct clinical practice expertise, to their respective chapters. Their commitment to physical therapist education is collectively displayed in content presentations that carefully reflect the scope of knowledge and skills required of a dynamic, evolving physical therapy practice environment. We are extremely grateful to each of our contributors and heartened by the excellence they bring to the sixth edition.

Heartfelt thanks are also extended to the practicing clinicians who prepared the case studies and video segments. Their contributions expertly move text content to clinical practice and significantly add to the development of clinical reasoning skills of our readers. We would like to thank Edward W. Bezkor, who served tirelessly as Case Study and Multimedia Editor and effectively coordinated case study contributions, as well as many production elements. Thanks also to Yvonne Gillam, Freelance Editor and Media Consultant, and Liz Schaeffer, Developmental Editor/Electronic Products Coordinator, for their work in editing the patient videos.

A note of special thanks is extended to the following individuals for their assistance with filming the online video case studies: Jan BenDor, Producer and Videographer, Christine Flynn, New York College of Osteopathic Medicine of New York Institute of Technology, Don Packard, University of Michigan Hospital, Robert Price, University of Washington Medical Center, and Sarah Zaluski, New York University Langone Medical Center.

Many of the new patient photographs were possible owing to the efforts of Edward W. Bezkor and Robert J. Schreyer, and the photography expertise of Jason Torres, J. Torres Photography. We thank also those individuals and companies who contributed new photographs to the individual chapters and to those patients/clients who allowed their photographs to be used throughout the text.

We would like to thank Evangelos Pappas, Test Bank Editor, for his expertise and efforts in developing guidelines for questions consistent with the National Physical Therapy Examination format and soliciting expert item writers for the test bank of examination questions. Our hope is that the test bank will become a valuable resource for both faculty and students who use our book.

Our appreciation goes to the dedicated professionals at F.A. Davis Company, Philadelphia, PA: Margaret M. Biblis, Editor-in-Chief, Melissa Duffield, Senior Acquisitions Editor, Jennifer A. Pine, Senior Developmental Editor, Liz Schaeffer, Developmental Editor/Electronic Products Coordinator, Sharon Lee, Production Manager, and Paul Marone, Marketing Manager. These individuals are recognized for their continued support, encouragement, and unwavering commitment to excellence. Thanks also are extended to Cassie Carey, Senior Production Editor, and Rose Boul, Senior Art Coordinator, at Graphic World Publishing Services.

We wish to thank the numerous students, faculty, and clinicians who over the years have used *Physical Rehabilitation* and provided us with meaningful and constructive comments that have greatly enhanced this edition. It is our sincere hope that this feedback will continue.

Finally, we are grateful for our continuing strong and productive working relationship that has allowed us to complete a project of this scope through six editions.

—SUSAN B. O'SULLIVAN
THOMAS J. SCHMITZ
GEORGE D. FULK

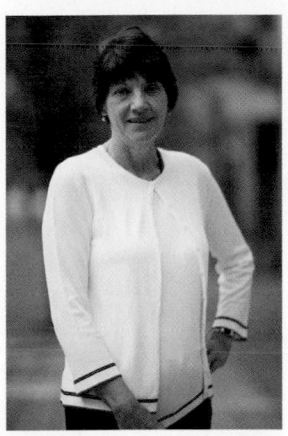

Dr. Susan B. O'Sullivan is Professor Emerita, Department of Physical Therapy, University of Massachusetts Lowell. She holds an EdD in Human Development from the School of Education and Master of Science and Bachelor of Science degrees from Sargent College at Boston University. Dr. O'Sullivan's research, teaching, and clinical experience is in the area of adult neurological rehabilitation. She has also held academic appointments at Boston University. In 2012 the APTA Neurology Section honored Dr. O'Sullivan with the Award for Excellence in Neurologic Education. She is also the recipient of the University of Massachusetts Lowell Award for Teaching Excellence. She is the co-author of *Physical Rehabilitation,* now in its sixth edition, *Improving Functional Outcomes in Physical Rehabilitation,* and Therapy Ed's *National Physical Therapy Examination Review and Study Guide.*

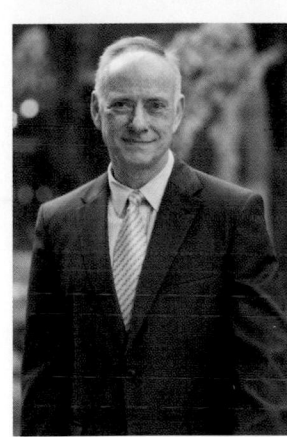

Dr. Thomas J. Schmitz is Professor Emeritus, Department of Physical Therapy, Long Island University. He is coeditor and contributing author of *Physical Rehabilitation* and *Improving Functional Outcomes in Physical Rehabilitation.* He holds a PhD from New York University, a Master of Science degree from Boston University, and a Bachelor of Science degree from SUNY at Buffalo. His primary clinical experience is in the area of adult neurological rehabilitation. Dr. Schmitz is the recipient of Long Island University's David Newton Award for Excellence in Teaching and the Trustees Award for Scholarly Achievement. He has also held academic appointments at Boston University, Sargent College, and Columbia University, College of Physicians and Surgeons.

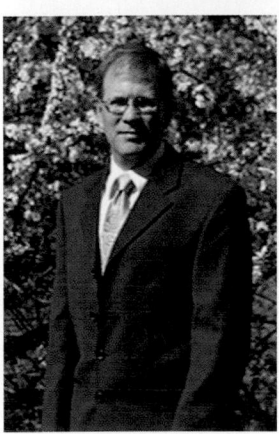

Dr. George D. Fulk is Associate Professor and Chair, Clarkson University. He received his entry-level physical therapy degree from the University of Massachusetts at Lowell and his PhD from Nova Southeastern University. Dr. Fulk's research, teaching, and clinical expertise are in the areas of enhancing motor recovery and quality of life in people with neurological involvement. He has also held a faculty appointment at Notre Dame College in Manchester, New Hampshire.

Dr. Fulk's research has focused on measuring and improving locomotor capability in people with stroke and he has authored numerous journal articles, conference papers, and textbook chapters in these areas. He is also the Digital Media Editor and an Associate Editor for the *Journal of Neurological Physical Therapy,* is on the Editorial Board for *PTNow,* and serves as a reviewer for many peer-reviewed journals.

CONTENTS

SECTION THREE: # Orthotics, Prosthetics, and Prescriptive Wheelchairs

Clinical Decision Making and Examination

Clinical Decision Making

Susan B. O'Sullivan, PT, EdD   Chapter **1**

LEARNING OBJECTIVES

1. Define *clinical reasoning* and identify factors that affect clinical decision making.
2. Describe the key steps in the patient/client management process.
3. Define the major responsibilities of the physical therapist in planning effective treatments.
4. Identify potential problems that could adversely affect the physical therapist's clinical reasoning.
5. Discuss strategies to ensure patient participation in the plan of care (POC).
6. Identify key elements of physical therapy documentation.
7. Differentiate between the clinical decision making approaches used by the expert versus novice physical therapist.
8. Discuss the importance of evidence-based practice in developing the POC.
9. Analyze and interpret patient/client data, formulate realistic goals and outcomes, and develop a POC when presented with a clinical case study.

■ CLINICAL REASONING/ CLINICAL DECISION MAKING

Clinical reasoning is a multidimensional process that involves a wide range of cognitive skills physical therapists use to process information, reach decisions, and determine actions. Reasoning can be viewed as an internal dialogue that therapists continuously employ while meeting the challenges of clinical practice. *Clinical decisions* are the outcomes of the clinical reasoning process and form the basis of patient/client management. A number of factors influence decision making, including the clinician's goals, values and beliefs, psychosocial skills, knowledge base and expertise, problem-solving strategies, and procedural skills. Many of these factors are the focus of discussion in later chapters in this text. Decision making is also influenced by patient/client characteristics (goals, values and beliefs, and physical, psychosocial, educational, and cultural factors) as well as environmental factors (clinical practice environment, overall resources, time, level of financial support, level of social support).

Decision making frameworks, such as algorithms, have been developed by experienced practitioners to guide clinicians in their reasoning processes. For example, Rothstein and Echternach developed the Hypothesis-Oriented Algorithm for Clinicians II (HOAC).[1] An algorithm is a graphically represented step-by-step guide designed to assist clinicians in problem solving by considering several possible solutions. It is based on specific clinical problems and identifies the decision steps and possible choices for remediation of a problem. A series of questions are posed, typically in yes/no format, addressing whether the measurements met testing criteria, the hypotheses generated were viable, goals were met, strategies were appropriate, and tactics were implemented correctly.

Hypotheses are defined as the underlying reasons for the patient's problems, representing the therapist's conjecture as to the cause. Problems are defined in terms of activity limitations. A "no" response to any of the questions posed in an algorithm is an indication for reevaluation of the viability of the hypotheses generated and reconsideration of the decisions made. In using HOAC II as a model for clinical decision making, the therapist also distinguishes between existing problems and anticipated problems, defined as deficits that are likely to occur if an intervention is not used for prevention. The value of an algorithm is that it guides the therapist's decisions and provides an outline of the decisions made. See Chapter 17, Figures 17.7 and 17.8, for examples of problem-centered algorithms.

Physical therapists today practice in complex environments and are called upon to reach increasingly complex decisions under significant practice constraints. For example, a therapist may be required to determine a POC for the complicated patient with multiple co-morbidities within 72 hours of admission to a rehabilitation facility. Reduced levels of treatment authorization with shorter and shorter stays in rehabilitation also complicate the decision making process. Novice practitioners can easily become overwhelmed. This chapter introduces a framework for clinical decision making and patient/client management that can assist in organizing and prioritizing data and in planning effective treatments compatible with the needs and goals of the patient/client and members of the health care team.

■ INTERNATIONAL CLASSIFICATION OF FUNCTIONING, DISABILITY, AND HEALTH (ICF)

The World Health Organization's (WHO's) *International Classification of Functioning, Disability, and Health (ICF) model* provides an important framework of terminology for understanding and categorizing health conditions and patient problems by clearly defining health condition, impairment, activity limitation, and participation restriction.[2] The American Physical Therapy Association (APT) has joined the WHO, the World Confederation for Physical Therapy (WCPT), the American Therapeutic Recreation Association (ATRA), and other international professional organizations in endorsing the ICF classification. Figure 1.1 presents the ICF model of disability.

Impairments are the problems an individual may have in body function (physiological functions of body systems) or structure (anatomical parts of the body). The resulting significant deviation or loss is the direct result of the **health condition**, a disease, disorder, injury, or trauma, or other circumstance, such as aging, stress, congenital anomaly, or genetic predisposition. For example, a patient with stroke may present with sensory loss, paresis, dyspraxia, and hemianopsia *(direct impairments)*. Impairments may be mild, moderate, severe, or complete and may be permanent or resolving as recovery progresses. Impairments may also be *indirect* (secondary), the sequelae or complications that

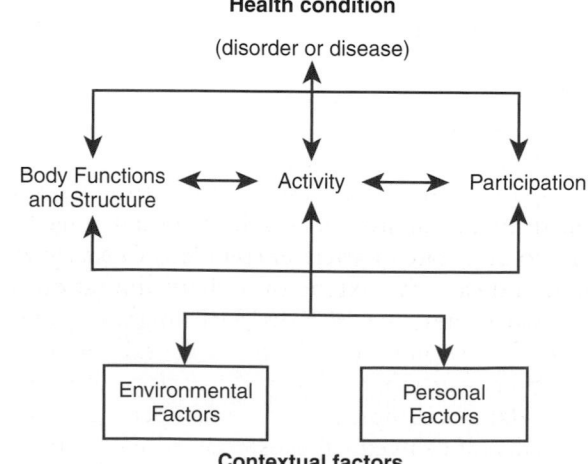

Figure 1.1 ICF Model of Disability. The WHO classification of functioning, disability and health (ICF). World Health Organization. ICF: International Classification of Functioning, Disability, and Health. 2002. Geneva, Switzerland, p 18, with permission. *(Form for request for permission available at www.who.int/about/licensing/copyright_form/en/index.html.)*

originate from other systems. They can result from pre-existing impairments or the expanding multisystem dysfunction that occurs with prolonged bedrest and inactivity, an ineffective POC, or lack of rehabilitation intervention. Examples of indirect impairments include decreased vital capacity and endurance, disuse atrophy and weakness, contractures, decubitus ulcers, deep venous thrombosis, renal calculi, urinary tract infections, pneumonia, and depression. The term *composite impairment* refers to impairments that are the result of multiple underlying origins, the combined effects of both direct and indirect impairments (e.g., balance deficits, gait deficits).

Activity limitations are difficulties an individual may have in executing tasks or actions. Activity limitations can include limitations in the performance of cognitive and learning skills, communication skills, *functional mobility skills* (FMS) (such as transfers, walking, lifting or carrying objects), and *activities of daily living* (ADL). *Basic activities of daily living* (BADL) include self-care activities of toileting, hygiene, bathing, dressing, eating, drinking, and social (interpersonal) interactions. The person with stroke may demonstrate difficulties in all of the above areas and be unable to perform the actions, tasks, and activities that constitute the "usual activities" for this individual.

Participation restrictions are problems an individual may experience in involvement in life situations and societal interactions. Categories of life roles include home management, work (job/school/play), and community/leisure. These include *instrumental activities of daily living* (IADL) such as housecleaning, preparing meals, shopping, telephoning, and managing finances, as well as work and leisure activities (e.g., sports, recreation, trips). Thus, the individual with stroke is unable to resume societal roles such as working, parenting, attending church, or traveling.

Performance qualifiers indicate the extent of participation restriction (difficulty) in performing tasks or actions in an individual's current real-life environment. All aspects of the physical, social, and attitudinal world constitute the environment. Difficulty can range from mild to moderate to severe or complete. *Capacity qualifiers* indicate the extent of activity limitation and are used to describe an individual's highest probable level of functioning (ability to do the task or action). Qualifiers can range from the assistance of a device (e.g., adaptive equipment) or another person (minimal to moderate to maximal assistance) or environmental modification (home, workplace). Thus, the patient with stroke may demonstrate moderate difficulty in locomotion in the home environment (performance qualifiers) and require the use of an ankle-foot orthosis, small-based quad cane, and moderate assistance of one (capacity qualifiers).

Environmental factors make up the physical, social, and attitudinal environment in which people live and function. Factors range from products and technology (for personal use in daily living, mobility and transportation, communication) and physical factors (home environment, terrain, climate) to social support and relationships (family, friends, personal care providers), attitudes (individual and societal), and institutions and laws (housing, communication, transportation, legal, financial services, and policies). Qualifiers include factors that serve as barriers (disablement risk factors) or facilitators (assets). Barriers can range from mild to moderate to severe to complete. Facilitators can also range from mild to moderate to substantial to complete.

Box 1.1 summarizes ICF disablement terminology. The ICF Checklist (Version 2.1a, Clinician Form for the International Classification of Functioning, Disability, and Health) is a practical tool to elicit and record information on functioning and disability of an individual.[3]

■ PATIENT/CLIENT MANAGEMENT

Steps in patient/client management include (1) examination of the patient; (2) evaluation of the data and identification of problems; (3) determination of the physical therapy diagnosis; (4) determination of the prognosis and POC; (5) implementation of the POC; and (6) reexamination of the patient and evaluation of treatment outcomes (Fig. 1.2).[4]

Examination

Examination involves identifying and defining the patient's problem(s) and the resources available to determine appropriate intervention. It consists of three components: the patient history, systems review, and tests and measures. Examination begins with patient referral or initial entry (direct access) and continues as an ongoing process throughout the episode of care. Ongoing reexamination allows the therapist to evaluate progress and modify interventions as appropriate.

History

Information about the patient's past history and current health status is obtained from review of the medical record and interviews (patient, family, caregivers). The medical record provides detailed reports from members of the health care team; processing these reports requires an understanding of disease and injury, medical terminology, differential diagnosis, laboratory and other diagnostic tests, and medical management. The use of resource material or professional consultation can assist the novice clinician. The types of data that may be generated from a patient history are presented in Figure 1.3.[4]

The interview is an important tool used to obtain information and gain understanding directly from the patient. The therapist asks the patient a series of questions regarding general health, past and present medical conditions/complications, and treatment. Specifically

Box 1.1   Terminology: Functioning, Disability, and Health

Health condition is an umbrella term for disease, disorder, injury, or trauma and may also include other circumstances, such as aging, stress, congenital anomaly, or genetic predisposition. It may also include information about pathogeneses and/or etiology.

Body functions are physiological functions of body systems (including psychological functions).

Body structures are anatomical parts of the body such as organs, limbs, and their components.

Impairments are problems in body function or structure such as a significant deviation or loss.

Activity is the execution of a task or action by an individual.

Activity limitations are difficulties an individual may have in executing activities.

Participation is involvement in a life situation.

Participation restrictions are problems an individual may experience in involvement in life situations.

Contextual factors represent the entire background of an individual's life and living situation.

• **Environmental factors** make up the physical, social, and attitudinal environment in which people live and conduct their lives, including social attitudes, architectural characteristics, and legal and social structures.

• **Personal factors** are the particular background of an individual's life, including gender, age, coping styles, social background, education, profession, past and current experience, overall behavior pattern, character, and other factors that influence how disability is experienced by an individual.

Performance qualifier describes what an individual does in his or her current environment. (The current environment includes assistive devices or personal assistance, whenever the individual uses them to perform actions or tasks.)

Capacity qualifier describes an individual's ability to execute a task or an action (highest probable level of functioning in a given domain at a given moment).

From World Health Organization (WHO): *International Classification of Functioning, Disability and Health* (ICF).[3]

the patient is asked to describe the current problems, primary complaint (reason for seeking physical therapy), and anticipated goals/expected outcomes for the episode of care. The patient will often describe his or her difficulties in terms of activity limitations or participation restrictions (what he or she can or cannot do). The patient is then asked a series of questions designed to explore the nature and history of the current problems/primary complaint. General questions about functional activities and participation should be directed toward delineating the difference between *capacity* and *performance*. For example, "Since your stroke, how much difficulty do you have walking long distances?" "How does this compare to before you had the stroke?" (capacity). Questions directed toward examining performance can include "How much of a problem do you have in walking long distances?" "Is this problem with walking made worse or better with the use of an assistive device?" Questions are also posed regarding the patient's social and physical environment, vocation, recreational interests, health habits (e.g., smoking history, alcohol use), exercise likes and dislikes, and frequency and intensity of regular activity. Sample interview questions are included in Box 1.2.[4, 5]

Pertinent information can also be obtained from the patient's family or caregiver. For example, patients with central nervous system (CNS) involvement and severe cognitive and/or communication impairments and younger pediatric patients will be unable to accurately communicate their existing problems. The family member/caregiver then assumes the primary role of assisting the therapist in identifying problems and providing relevant aspects of the history. The perceived needs of the family member or caregiver can also be determined during the interview.

The therapist should be sensitive to differences in culture and ethnicity that may influence how the patient or family member responds during the interview or examination process. Different beliefs and attitudes toward health care may influence how cooperative the patient will be. During the interview, the therapist should listen carefully to what the patient says. The patient should be observed for any physical manifestations that reveal emotional context, such as slumped body posture, grimacing, and poor eye contact. Finally, the interview is used to establish rapport, effective communication, and mutual trust. Ensuring effective communication with the patient and cooperation serves to make the therapist's observations more valid and becomes crucial to the success of the POC.

Systems Review

The use of a brief *screening examination* allows the therapist to quickly scan the patient's body systems and determine areas of intact function and dysfunction in each of the following systems: cardiovascular/pulmonary, integumentary, musculoskeletal, and neuromuscular. Information is also obtained about cognitive functions, communication, learning style, and emotional status. Areas of deficit together with an accurate knowledge of the main health condition (disorder or disease) (1) confirm the need for further or more detailed examination; (2) rule out or differentiate specific system involvement; (3) determine if referral to another health care professional is warranted (triage); and (4) focus

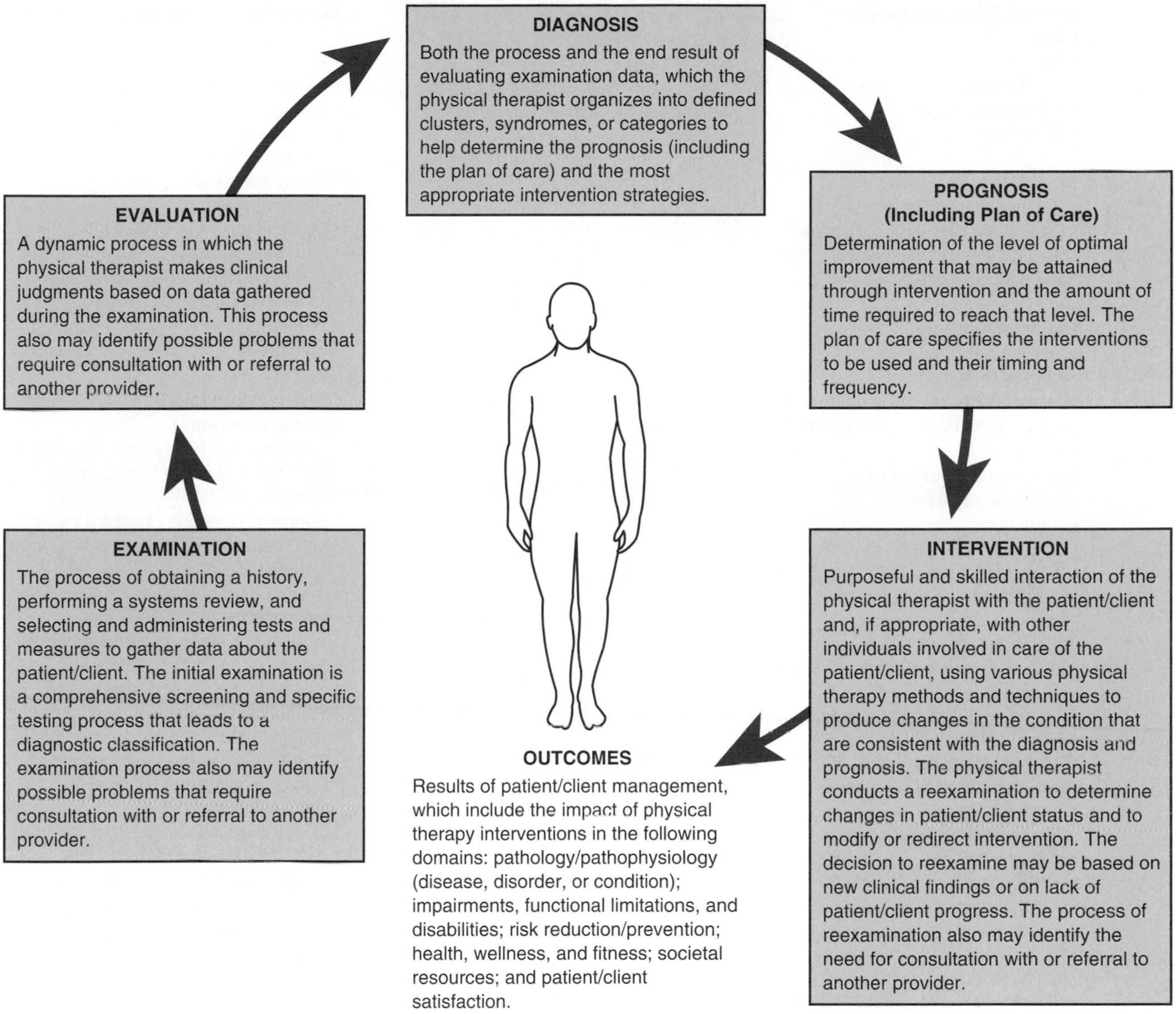

DIAGNOSIS
Both the process and the end result of evaluating examination data, which the physical therapist organizes into defined clusters, syndromes, or categories to help determine the prognosis (including the plan of care) and the most appropriate intervention strategies.

EVALUATION
A dynamic process in which the physical therapist makes clinical judgments based on data gathered during the examination. This process also may identify possible problems that require consultation with or referral to another provider.

PROGNOSIS
(Including Plan of Care)
Determination of the level of optimal improvement that may be attained through intervention and the amount of time required to reach that level. The plan of care specifies the interventions to be used and their timing and frequency.

EXAMINATION
The process of obtaining a history, performing a systems review, and selecting and administering tests and measures to gather data about the patient/client. The initial examination is a comprehensive screening and specific testing process that leads to a diagnostic classification. The examination process also may identify possible problems that require consultation with or referral to another provider.

OUTCOMES
Results of patient/client management, which include the impact of physical therapy interventions in the following domains: pathology/pathophysiology (disease, disorder, or condition); impairments, functional limitations, and disabilities; risk reduction/prevention; health, wellness, and fitness; societal resources; and patient/client satisfaction.

INTERVENTION
Purposeful and skilled interaction of the physical therapist with the patient/client and, if appropriate, with other individuals involved in care of the patient/client, using various physical therapy methods and techniques to produce changes in the condition that are consistent with the diagnosis and prognosis. The physical therapist conducts a reexamination to determine changes in patient/client status and to modify or redirect intervention. The decision to reexamine may be based on new clinical findings or on lack of patient/client progress. The process of reexamination also may identify the need for consultation with or referral to another provider.

Figure 1.2 Elements of patient management leading to optimal outcomes. *(From APTA* Guide to Physical Therapist Practice *[4, p. 35] with permission.)*

the search of the origin of symptoms to a specific location or body part. An important starting point for identification of areas to be screened is consideration of all potential (possible) factors contributing to an observed activity limitation or participation restriction. Consultation is appropriate if the needs of the patient/client are outside the scope of the expertise of the therapist assigned to the case. For example, a patient recovering from stroke is referred to a dysphagia clinic for a detailed examination of swallowing function by a dysphagia specialist (speech-language pathologist).

Screening examinations are also used for healthy populations. For example, the physical therapist can screen individuals to identify risk factors for disease such as decreased activity levels, stress, and obesity. Screening is also conducted for specific populations such as pediatric clients (e.g., for scoliosis), geriatric clients (e.g., to identify fall risk factors), athletes (e.g., in pre-performance examinations), and working adults (e.g., to identify the risk of musculoskeletal injuries in the workplace). These

screens may involve observation, chart review, oral history, and/or a brief examination. Additional screening examinations may be mandated by institutional settings. For example, in a long-term care facility, the therapist may be asked to review the chart for indications of changes in functional status or need for physical therapy. The therapist then makes a determination of the need for further physical therapy services based on completing a screening examination.

Tests and Measures

More definitive tests and measures are used to provide objective data to accurately determine the degree of specific function and dysfunction. Examination begins at the level of impairments, for example, diminished muscle strength (manual muscle test [MMT]) and impaired range of motion (ROM) (goniometric measurements), and progresses to functional activities (6-minute Walk Test, Timed Up and Go, Berg Balance Test). Alternatively,

General Demographics
- Age
- Sex
- Race/ethnicity
- Primary language
- Education

Social History
- Cultural beliefs and behaviors
- Family and caregiver resources
- Social interactions, social activities, and support system

Employment/Work (Job/School/Play)
- Current and prior work (job/school/play), community, and leisure actions, tasks, or activities

Growth and Development
- Developmental history
- Hand dominance

Living Environment
- Devices and equipment (eg., assistive, adaptive, orthotic, protective, supportive, prosthetic)
- Living environment and community characteristics
- Projected discharge destinations

General Health Status (Self-Report, Family Report, Caregiver Report)
- General health perception
- Physical function (eg., mobility, sleep patterns, restricted bed days)
- Psychological function (eg., memory, reasoning ability, depression, anxiety)
- Role function (eg., community, leisure, social, work)
- Social function (eg., social activity, social interaction, social support)

Social/Health Habits (Past and Current)
- General health perception
- Physical function (eg., mobility, sleep patterns, restricted bed days)
- Psychological function (eg., memory, reasoning ability, depression, anxiety)
- Role function (eg., community, leisure, social, work)
- Social function (eg., social activity, social interaction, social support)

Family History
- Familial health risks

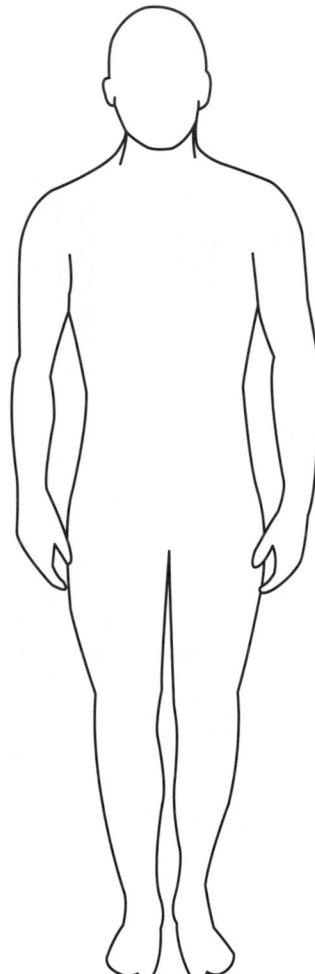

Medical/Surgical History
- Cardiovascular
- Endocrine/metabolic
- Gastrointestinal
- Genitourinary
- Gynecological
- Integumentary
- Musculoskeletal
- Neuromuscular
- Obstetrical
- Prior hospitalizations, surgeries, and preexisting medical and other health related conditions
- Psychological
- Pulmonary

Current Condtion(s)/ Chief Complaint(s)
- Concerns that led the patient/client to seek the services of a physical therapist
- Concerns or needs of patient/client who requires the services of a physical therapist
- Current therapeutic interventions
- Mechanisms of injury or disease, including date of onset and course of events
- Onset and patterns of symptoms
- Patient/client, family, significant other, and caregiver expectations and goals for the therapeutic intervention
- Previous occurrence of chief complaint(s)
- Prior therapeutic interventions

Functional Status and Activity Level
- Current and prior functional status in self-care and home management, including activities of daily living (ADL) and instrumental activities of daily living (IADL)
- Current and prior functional status in work (job/school/play), community, and leisure actions, tasks, or activities

Medications
- Medications for current condition
- Medications previously taken for current condition
- Medications for other conditions

Other Clinical Tests
- Laboratory and diagnostic tests
- Review of available records (eg., medical, education, surgical)
- Review of other clinical findings (eg., nutrition and hydration)

Figure 1.3 Types of data that may be generated from patient history. *(From APTA Guide to Physical Therapist Practice [4, p. 36] with permission.)*

the therapist may begin with an examination of functional performance, during which the therapist analyzes the differences between the patient's performance and the "typical" or expected performance of a task. For example, the patient with stroke is asked to transfer from bed to wheelchair. The therapist observes the performance and determines that the patient lacks postural support (stability), adequate lower extremity (LE) extensor strength to reach the full upright position, and adequate ROM in ankle dorsiflexors. The therapist then progresses

Box 1.2 Sample Interview Questions

I. Interview questions designed to identify the nature and history of the current problem(s):

What problems bring you to therapy?

When did the problem(s) begin?

What happened to precipitate the problem(s)?

How long has the problem(s) existed?

How are you taking care of the problem(s)?

What makes the problem(s) better?

What makes the problem(s) worse?

What are your goals and expectations for physical therapy?

Are you seeing anyone else for the problem(s)?

II. Interview questions designed to identify desired outcomes in terms of essential functional activities include the following:

What activities do you normally do at home/work/school?

What activities are you unable to do?

What activities are done differently and how are they different (i.e., extra time, extra effort, different strategy)?

What activities do you need help to perform that you would rather do yourself?

What leisure activities are important to you?

How can I help you be more independent?

III. Interview questions designed to identify environmental conditions in which patient activities typically occur include the following:

Describe your home/school/work environment.

How do you move around/access areas in the home (i.e., bathroom, bedroom, entering and exiting the home)? How safe do you feel?

How do you move around/access areas in the community (i.e., workplace, school, grocery store, shopping center, community center, stairs, curbs, ramps)? How safe do you feel?

IV. Interview questions designed to identify available social supports include the following:

Who lives with you?

Who assists in your care (i.e., basic activities of daily living [BADL], instrumental activities of daily living [IADL])?

Who helps you with the activities you want to do (i.e., walking, stairs, transfers)?

Are there activities you have difficulty with that would benefit from additional assistance?

V. Interview questions designed to identify the patient's knowledge of potential disablement risk factors include the following:

What problems might be anticipated in the future?

What can you do to eliminate or reduce the likelihood of that happening?

Sources: Section I: from the Documentation Template for Physical Therapist Patient/Client Management in the *Guide to Physical Therapist Practice* (4, pp. 707–712); Sections II–IV adapted from Randall (5, p. 1,200).

---

to a detailed examination of impairments. The decision as to which approach to use is based on the results of the screening examination and the therapist's knowledge of the health condition. Key information to obtain during an examination of function is the level of independence or dependence, as well as the need for physical assistance, external devices, or environmental modifications.

Adequate training and skill in performing specific tests and measures are crucial in ensuring both validity and reliability of the tests. Failure to correctly perform an examination procedure can lead to the gathering of inaccurate data and the formation of an inappropriate POC. Later chapters focus on specific tests and measures and discuss issues of validity and reliability. The use of disability-specific standardized instruments (e.g., for individuals with stroke, the Fugl-Meyer Assessment of Physical Performance) can facilitate the examination process but may not always be appropriate for each individual patient. The therapist needs to carefully review the unique problems of the patient to determine the appropriateness and sensitivity of an instrument. Box 1.3 presents the categories for tests and measures identified in the *Guide to Physical Therapist Practice*.[4]

Novice therapists should resist the tendency to gather excessive and extraneous data in the mistaken belief that more information is better. Unnecessary data will only confuse the picture, rendering clinical decision making more difficult and unnecessarily raising the cost of care. If problems arise that are not initially identified in the history or systems review, or if the data obtained are inconsistent, additional tests or measures may be indicated. Consultation with an experienced therapist can provide an important means of clarifying inconsistencies and determining the appropriateness of specific tests and measures.

Evaluation

Data gathered from the initial examination must then be organized and analyzed. The therapist identifies and prioritizes the patient's impairments, activity limitations, and participation restrictions and develops a *problem list*. It is important to accurately recognize those clinical problems associated with the primary disorder and those associated with co-morbid conditions. Table 1.1 presents a sample prioritized problem list.

Impairments, activity limitations, and participation restrictions must be analyzed to identify causal relationships. For example, shoulder pain in the patient with hemiplegia may be due to several factors, including hypotonicity and loss of voluntary movement, which are direct impairments, or soft tissue damage/trauma from improper transfers, which is an indirect impairment, resulting from an activity. Determining the causative

---

Box 1.3   Categories for Tests and Measures

Aerobic Capacity/Endurance
Anthropometric Characteristics
Arousal, Attention, and Cognition
Assistive and Adaptive Devices
Circulation (Arterial, Venous, Lymphatic)
Cranial and Peripheral Nerve Integrity
Environmental, Home, and Work (Job/School/Play) Barriers
Ergonomics and Body Mechanics
Gait, Locomotion, and Balance
Integumentary Integrity
Joint Integrity and Mobility
Motor Function (Motor Control and Motor Learning)
Muscle Performance (Including Strength, Power, and Endurance)
Neuromotor Development and Sensory Integration
Orthotic, Protective, and Supportive Devices
Pain
Posture
Prosthetic Requirements
Range of Motion (Including Muscle Length)
Reflex Integrity
Self-Care and Home Management (Including Activities of Daily Living and Instrumental Activities of Daily Living)
Sensory Integrity
Ventilation and Respiration/Gas Exchange
Work (Job/School/Play), Community, and Leisure Integration or Reintegration (Including Instrumental Activities of Daily Living)

Adapted from APTA *Guide to Physical Therapist Practice.*[4]

---

factors is a difficult yet critical step in determining appropriate treatment interventions and resolving the patient's pain.

The skilled clinician is able to identify the role barriers and facilitators in the patient's environment in order to incorporate measures to minimize or maximize these factors into the POC. A POC that emphasizes and reinforces facilitators enhances function and the patient's ability to experience success. Improved motivation and engagement are the natural outcomes of reinforcement of facilitators. For example, the patient with stroke may have intact communication skills, cognitive skills, and good function of the uninvolved extremities. Facilitators can also include supportive and knowledgeable family members/caregivers and an appropriate living environment.

Diagnosis

A *medical diagnosis* refers to the identification of a disease, disorder, or condition (pathology/pathophysiology) by evaluating the presenting signs, symptoms, history, laboratory test results, and procedures. It is identified primarily at the cellular level. Physical therapists use the term **diagnosis** to "identify the impact of a condition on function at the level of the system (especially the movement system) and at the level of the whole person."[4] Thus, the term is used to clarify the professional body of knowledge as well as the role of physical therapists in health care. For example:

Medical diagnosis: Cerebrovascular accident (CVA)
Physical therapy diagnosis: Impaired motor function and sensory integrity associated with nonprogressive disorders of the central nervous system—acquired in adolescence or adulthood[4, p. 365]
Medical diagnosis: Spinal cord injury (SCI)
Physical therapy diagnosis: Impaired motor function, peripheral nerve integrity, and sensory integrity associated with nonprogressive disorders of the spinal cord[4, p. 437]

The diagnostic process includes integrating and evaluating the data obtained during the examination to describe the patient/client condition in terms that will guide the prognosis and selection of intervention strategies during the development of the POC. The *Guide to Physical Therapist Practice* organizes diagnostic categories specific to physical therapy by *preferred practice patterns.*[4] There are four main categories of conditions: Musculoskeletal, Neuromuscular, Cardiovascular/Pulmonary, and Integumentary, with preferred practice patterns identified in each (see Appendix 1.A). The patterns are described fully according to the five elements of patient/client management (i.e., examination, evaluation, diagnosis, prognosis, and intervention). Each pattern also includes reexamination to evaluate progress, global outcomes, and criteria for termination of physical therapy services. Inclusion and exclusion criteria for each practice pattern and criteria for multiple-pattern classification are also presented. The patterns represent the collaborative effort of experienced physical therapists who detailed the broad categories of problems commonly seen by physical therapists within the scope of their knowledge, experience, and expertise. Expert consensus was thus used to develop and define the diagnostic categories and preferred practice patterns. Given the central role of physical therapists as movement specialists, the therapist will need to focus the diagnosis on the results of activity analysis and movement problems identified during the examination when formulating the prognosis and POC.

The use of diagnostic categories specific to physical therapy, as Sarhman points out, (1) allows for successful communication with colleagues and patients/caregivers about the conditions that require the physical therapist's expertise, (2) provides an appropriate classification for establishing standards of examination and treatment, and (3) directs examination of treatment effectiveness, thereby enhancing evidence-based practice.[6] Physical therapy diagnostic categories also facilitate successful reimbursement when linked to functional outcomes and enhance direct access of physical therapy services.

Table 1.1	Sample Prioritized Problem List for a Patient With Stroke			
Direct Impairments	Indirect Impairments	Composite Impairments	Activity Limitations	Participation Restrictions
R hemiparesis RUE > RLE	R shoulder subluxation	Balance deficits Standing > sitting	Dep bed mobility: minA	Dec community mobility
	Dec ROM R shoulder	Gait deficits	Dep BADL: min/mod A	IADL: unable
Hypotonicity RUE	Kyphosis, forward head	Dec endurance	Dep transfers: modA X 1	Dec ability to perform social roles: husband
Spasticity RLE: knee ext, plantiflexors			Dep locomotion: modA X 1	
Synergy patterns RLE > RUE			Stairs: unable	
Mild dysarthria			Inc fall risk	
Mild cognitive deficits: dec STM				
Dec motor planning ability				
CO-MORBIDITIES:	Diabetic Peripheral Neuropathy			
Dec sensation both feet		Dec balance	Inc fall risk	
Small ulcer L foot (5th toe)		Dec endurance		
		Gait deficits: requires special shoes		Dec community mobility

Contextual factors: physical, social, attitudinal
One-level ranch house; entry with 2 steps, no handrails
Highly motivated
Personal factors: individual's life and living situation
Spouse is primary caregiver; has osteoporosis and decreased vision (bilateral cataracts).
Has 2 involved sons living within 30 mile radius.
Key: BADL: basic activities of daily living; Dec: decreased; Dep: dependent; IADL: instrumental activities of daily living; Inc: increased; minA: minimal assistance; modA: moderate assistance; RLE: right lower extremity; RUE: right upper extremity; STM: short term memory.

Prognosis

The term **prognosis** refers to "the predicted optimal level of improvement in function and amount of time needed to reach that level."[4, p. 46] An accurate prognosis may be determined at the onset of treatment for some patients. For other patients with more complicated conditions such as severe traumatic brain injury (TBI) accompanied by extensive disability and multisystem involvement, a prognosis or prediction of level of improvement can be determined only at various increments during the course of rehabilitation. Knowledge of recovery patterns (stage of disorder) is sometimes useful to guide decision making. The amount of time needed to reach optimal recovery is an important determination, one that is required by Medicare and many other insurance providers. Predicting optimal levels of recovery and time frames can be a challenging process for the novice therapist. Use of experienced, expert staff as resources and mentors can facilitate this step in the decision making process. For each preferred practice pattern, the *Guide to Physical Therapist Practice* includes a broad range of expected number of visits per episode of care.[4]

Plan of Care

The **plan of care (POC)** outlines anticipated patient management. The therapist evaluates and integrates data obtained from the patient/client history, the systems review, and tests and measures within the context of other factors, including the patient's overall health, availability of social support systems, living environment, and potential discharge destination. Multisystem involvement, severe impairment and functional loss, extended time of involvement (chronicity), multiple co-morbid conditions, and medical stability of the patient are important parameters that increase the complexity of the decision making process.

A major focus of the POC is producing meaningful changes at the personal/social level by reducing activity limitations and participation restrictions. Achieving independence in locomotion or activities of daily living (ADL), return to work, or participation in recreational activities is important to the patient/client in terms of improving **quality of life (QOL)**.[7] QOL is defined as the sense of total well-being that encompasses both physical and psychosocial aspects of the patient/client's life. Finally, not all impairments can be remediated by physical therapy. Some impairments are permanent or progressive, the direct result of unrelenting pathology such as amyotrophic lateral sclerosis (ALS). In this example, a primary emphasis on reducing the number and severity of indirect impairments and activity limitations is appropriate.

Essential components of the POC include (1) anticipated goals and expected outcomes; (2) the predicted level of optimal improvement; (3) the specific interventions to be used, including type, duration, and frequency; and (4) criteria for discharge.

Goals and Expected Outcomes

An important first step in the development of the POC is the determination of anticipated **goals** and **expected outcomes**, the intended results of patient/client management. Goal and outcome statements address patient-identified priorities and predicted changes in impairments, activity limitations, and participation restrictions. They also address predicted changes in overall health, risk reduction and prevention, wellness and fitness, and optimization of patient/client satisfaction. The difference is in terms of time frame. Outcomes define the patient's expected level at the conclusion of the episode of care or rehabilitation stay, whereas goals define the interim steps that are necessary to achieve expected outcomes.[4]

Goal and outcome statements should be realistic, objective, measurable, and time limited. There are four essential elements:

- *Individual:* Who will perform the specific behavior or activity required or aspect of care? Goals and outcomes are focused on the *patient/client*. This includes individuals who receive direct care physical therapy services and/or individuals who benefit from consultation and advice, or services focused on promoting, health, wellness, and fitness. Goals can also be focused on family members or caregivers, for example, the parent of a child with a developmental disability.
- *Behavior/Activity:* What is the specific behavior or activity the patient/client will demonstrate? Goals and outcomes include changes in impairments (e.g., ROM, strength, balance) and changes in activity limitations (e.g., transfers, ambulation, ADL) or participation restrictions (e.g., community mobility, return to school or work).
- *Condition:* What are the conditions under which the patient/client's behavior is measured? The

goal or outcome statement specifies the specific conditions or measures required for successful achievement, for example, distance achieved, required time to perform the activity, the specific number of successful attempts out of a specific number of trials. Statements focused on functional changes should include a description of the conditions required for acceptable performance. For example, the functional levels of performance in the Functional Independence Measure (FIM) are used in the majority of rehabilitation centers in the United States. This instrument grades levels from No Helper/Independence (grade 7) to No Helper/Modified Independence (grade 6; device), to Helper/Modified Dependence (grades 5, 4, and 3; supervision, minimal, moderate, assistance), to Helper/Complete Dependence (grades 2 and 1; maximal, total assistance) (see Chapter 8 and Figure 8.5 for a complete description of this instrument).[8] The type of environment required for a successful outcome of the behavior should also be specified: clinic environment (e.g., quiet room, level floor surface, physical therapy gym), home (e.g., one flight of eight stairs, carpeted surfaces), and community (e.g., uneven grassy surfaces, curbs, ramps).

- *Time:* How long will it take to achieve the stated goal or outcome? Goals can be expressed as *short-term* (generally considered to be 2 to 3 weeks) and *long-term* (longer than 3 weeks). Outcomes describe the expected level of functional performance attained at the end of the episode of care or rehabilitation stay. In instances of severe disability and incomplete recovery, for example, the patient with traumatic brain injury, the therapist, and team members may have difficulty determining the expected outcomes at the beginning of rehabilitation. Long-term goals can be used that focus on the expectations for a specific stage of recovery (e.g., minimally conscious states, confusional states). Goals and outcomes can also be modified following a significant change in patient status.

Each POC has multiple goals and outcomes. Goals may be linked to the successful attainment of more than one outcome. For example, attaining ROM in dorsiflexion is critical to the functional outcomes of independence in transfers and locomotion. The successful attainment of an outcome is also dependent on achieving a number of different goals. For example, independent locomotion (the outcome) is dependent on increasing strength, ROM, and balance skills. In formulating a POC, the therapist accurately identifies the relationship between and among goals and sequences them appropriately. Box 1.4 presents examples of outcome and goal statements.

In rehabilitation settings, the POC also includes a statement regarding the patient's overall *rehabilitation*

Box 1.4 Examples of Outcome and Goal Statements

The following are examples of expected outcomes, all to be achieved within the anticipated rehab stay:

The patient will be independent and safe in ambulation using an ankle-foot orthosis and a quad cane on level surfaces for unlimited community distances and for all daily activities within 8 weeks.

The patient will demonstrate modified dependence with close supervision in wheelchair propulsion for limited household distances (up to 50 feet) within 8 weeks.

The patient will demonstrate modified dependence with minimum assistance of one person for all transfer activities in the home environment within 6 weeks.

The patient will demonstrate independence in basic activities of daily living (BADL) with minimal setup and equipment (use of a reacher) within 6 weeks.

The patient and family will demonstrate enhanced decision making skills regarding the health of the patient and use of health care resources within 6 weeks.

The following are examples of anticipated goals with variable time frames:

Short-Term Goals

The patient will increase strength in shoulder depressor muscles and elbow extensor muscles in both upper extremities from good to normal within 3 weeks.

The patient will increase ROM 10 degrees in knee extension bilaterally to within normal limits within 3 weeks.

The patient will be independent in the application of lower extremity orthoses within 1 week.

The patient and family will recognize personal and environmental factors associated with falls during ambulation within 2 weeks.

The patient will attend to task for 5 min out of a 30-min treatment session within 3 weeks.

Long-Term Goals

The patient will independently perform transfers from wheelchair to car within 4 weeks.

The patient will ambulate with bilateral knee-ankle-foot orthoses (KAFOs) and crutches using a swing-through gait and close supervision for 50 feet within 5 weeks.

The patient will maintain static balance in sitting with centered, symmetrical weight-bearing and no upper extremity support or loss of balance for up to 5 minutes within 4 weeks.

The patient will sequence a three- to five-step routine task with minimum assistance within 5 weeks.

---

potential. This is typically a one-word statement: *excellent, good, fair,* or *poor.* The therapist considers multiple factors when determining rehabilitation potential, such as the patient's condition and onset date, co-morbidity, mechanism of injury, and baseline data.

Interventions

The next step is to determine the **intervention**, defined as the purposeful interaction of the physical therapist with the patient/client and, when appropriate, other individuals involved in the care of the patient/client, using various physical therapy procedures and techniques to produce changes in the condition. Components of physical therapy intervention include coordination, communication, and documentation; patient/client-related instruction; and procedural interventions (Fig. 1.4).[4]

Coordination and Communication

Case management requires therapists to be able to communicate effectively with all members of the rehabilitation team, directly or indirectly. For example, the therapist communicates directly with other professionals at case conferences, team meetings, or rounds or indirectly through documentation in the medical record.

Effective communication enhances collaboration and understanding.

Therapists are also responsible for coordinating care at many different levels. The therapist delegates appropriate aspects of treatment to physical therapy assistants and oversees the responsibilities of physical therapy aides. The therapist coordinates care with other professionals, family, or caregivers regarding a specific treatment approach or intervention. For example, for early transfer training to be effective, consistency in how everyone transfers the patient is important. The therapist also coordinates discharge planning with the patient and family and other interested persons. Therapists may be involved in providing POC recommendations to other facilities such as restorative nursing facilities.

Patient/Client-Related Instruction

In an era of managed care and shorter time allocations for an episode of care, effective patient/client-related instruction is critical to ensuring optimal care and successful rehabilitation. Communication strategies are developed within the context of the patient/client's age, cultural backgrounds, language skills, and educational level, and

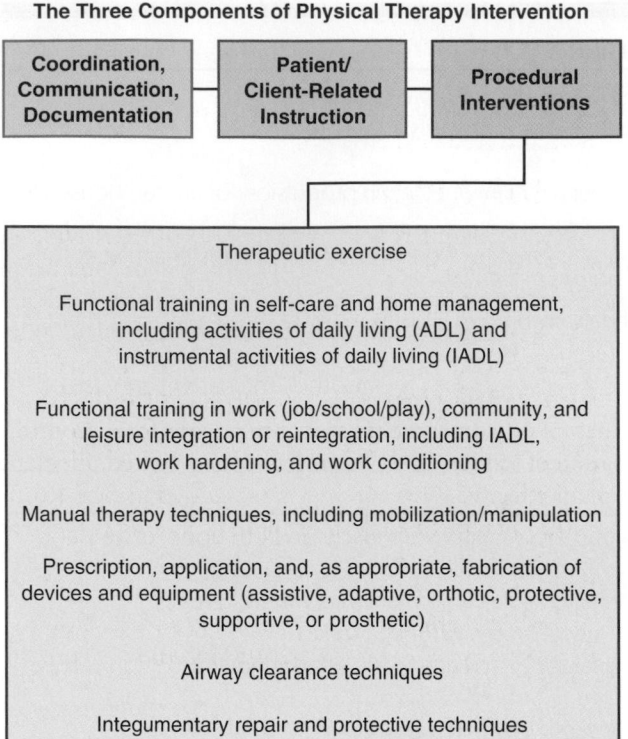

The Three Components of Physical Therapy Intervention

Coordination, Communication, Documentation — Patient/Client-Related Instruction — Procedural Interventions

Therapeutic exercise

Functional training in self-care and home management, including activities of daily living (ADL) and instrumental activities of daily living (IADL)

Functional training in work (job/school/play), community, and leisure integration or reintegration, including IADL, work hardening, and work conditioning

Manual therapy techniques, including mobilization/manipulation

Prescription, application, and, as appropriate, fabrication of devices and equipment (assistive, adaptive, orthotic, protective, supportive, or prosthetic)

Airway clearance techniques

Integumentary repair and protective techniques

Electrotherapeutic modalities

Physical agents and mechanical modalities

Figure 1.4 The three components of physical therapy intervention. *(From APTA* Guide to Physical Therapist Practice [4, p. 98] *with permission.)*

the presence of specific communication or cognition impairments. Therapists may provide direct one-on-one instruction to a variety of individuals, including patients, clients, families, caregivers, and other interested persons. Additional strategies can include group discussions or classes, or instruction through printed or audiovisual materials. Educational interventions are directed toward ensuring an understanding of the patient's condition, training in specific activities and exercises, determining the relevance of interventions to improve function, and achieving an expected course. In addition, educational interventions are directed toward ensuring a successful transition to the home environment (instruction in home exercise programs [HEP]), returning to work (ergonomic instruction), or resuming social activities in the community (environmental access). It is important to document what was taught, who participated, when the instruction occurred, and overall effectiveness. The need for repetition and reinforcement of educational content should also be documented in the medical record.

Procedural Interventions

Skilled physical therapy includes a wide variety of procedural interventions, which can be broadly classified into three main groups. **Restorative interventions** are directed toward remediating or improving the patient's status in terms of impairments, activity limitations, participation restrictions, and recovery of function. The involved segments are targeted for intervention. This approach assumes an existing potential for change (e.g., neuroplasticity of brain and spinal cord function; potential for muscle strengthening or improving aerobic endurance). For example, the patient with incomplete spinal cord injury (SCI) undergoes locomotor training using body weight support and a treadmill (BWSTT). Patients with chronic progressive pathology (e.g., the patient with Parkinson's disease) may not respond to restorative interventions aimed at resolving direct impairments; interventions aimed at restoring or optimizing function and modifying indirect impairments can, however, have a positive outcome.

Compensatory interventions are directed toward promoting optimal function using residual abilities. The activity (task) is adapted (changed) in order to achieve function. The uninvolved or less involved segments are targeted for intervention. For example, the patient with left hemiplegia learns to dress using the right upper extremity (UE); the patient with complete T1 paraplegia learns to roll using upper extremities (UEs) and momentum. Environmental adaptations are also used to facilitate relearning of functional skills and optimal performance. For example, the patient with TBI is able to dress by selecting clothing from color-coded drawers. Compensatory interventions can be used in conjunction with restorative interventions to maximize function or when restorative interventions are unrealistic or unsuccessful.

Preventative interventions are directed toward minimizing potential problems (e.g., anticipated indirect impairments, activity limitations, and participation restrictions) and maintaining health. For example, early resumption of upright standing using a tilt table minimizes the risk of pneumonia, bone loss, and renal calculi in the patient with SCI. A successful educational program for frequent skin inspection can prevent the development of pressure ulcers in that same patient with SCI.

Interventions are chosen based on the medical diagnosis, the evaluation of examination, the physical therapy diagnosis, the prognosis, and the anticipated goals and expected outcomes. The therapist relies on knowledge of foundational science and interventions (e.g., principles of motor learning, motor control, muscle performance, task-specific training, and cardiovascular conditioning) in order to determine those interventions that are likely to achieve successful outcomes. It is important to identify all possible interventions early in the process, to carefully weigh those alternatives, and then to decide on the interventions that have the best probability of success. Narrowly adhering to one treatment approach reduces the available options and may limit or preclude successful outcomes. Use of a protocol (e.g., predetermined exercises for the patient with hip fracture) standardizes some aspects of care but may not meet the individual needs of the patient. Protocols can foster a separation of examination/evaluation findings from the selection of treatments.

Watts suggests that clinical judgment is clearly an elegant mixture of art and science.[9] Professional consultation with expert clinicians and mentors is an effective means of helping the novice sort through the complex issues involved in decision making, especially when complicating factors intervene. For example, a consultation would be beneficial for the inexperienced therapist who is treating a patient that is chronically ill, has multiple co-morbidities or complications, impaired cognition, inadequate social supports, and severe activity limitations.

A general outline of the POC is constructed. Schema can be used to present a framework for approaching a specific aspect of treatment and assist the therapist in organizing essential intervention elements of the plan. One such commonly used schema for exercise intervention is the *FITT equation (frequency-intensity-time-type)*, presented in Box 1.5.

The therapist should ideally choose interventions that accomplish more than one goal and are linked to the expected outcomes. The interventions should be effectively sequenced to address key impairments first and to achieve optimum motivational effect, interspacing the more difficult or uncomfortable procedures with easier ones. The therapist should include tasks that ensure success during the treatment session and, whenever possible, should end each session on a positive note. This helps the patient retain a positive feeling of success and look forward to the next treatment.

Discharge Planning

Discharge planning is initiated early in the rehabilitation process during the data collection phase and intensifies as goals and expected outcomes are close to being reached. Discharge planning may also be initiated if the patient refuses further treatment or becomes medically or psychologically unstable. If the patient is discharged before outcomes are reached, the reasons for discontinuation of services must be carefully documented. Elements of an effective *discharge plan* are included in Box 1.6.

The therapist should also include the *discharge prognosis,* typically a one-word response such as *excellent, good, fair, or poor.* It reflects the therapist's judgment of the patient's ability to maintain the level of function achieved at the end of rehabilitation without continued skilled intervention.

Implementation of the Plan of Care

The therapist must take into account a number of factors in structuring an effective treatment session. The patient's comfort and optimal performance should be a priority. The environment should be structured appropriately to

---

Box 1.5 The FITT Equation for Exercise Intervention

Frequency: How often will the patient receive skilled care?

This is typically defined in terms of the number of times per week treatment will be given (e.g., daily or three times per week), or the number of visits before a specific date.

Intensity: What is the prescribed intensity of exercises or activity training?

For example, the POC includes sit-to-stand repetitions, 3 sets of 5 reps each, progressing from high seat to low.

Time (duration): How long will the patient receive skilled care?

This is typically defined in terms of days or weeks (e.g., three times per week for 6 weeks). The duration of an anticipated individual treatment session should also be defined (e.g., 30- or 60-minute sessions).

Type of intervention: What are the specific exercise strategies or procedural interventions used?

Necessary components that should be identified include the following:

- **Posture and activity:** a description of the specific posture and activity the patient must perform (e.g., sitting, weight shifting or standing, modified plantigrade, reaching).
- **Techniques used:** mode of therapist action or intervention used (e.g., guided, active-assisted, or resisted movement), or specific technique (e.g., rhythmic stabilization, dynamic reversals).
- **Motor learning strategies used:** strategies specific to type of feedback (e.g., knowledge of results, knowledge of performance) and scheduling of feedback (e.g., constant or variable), practice schedule (e.g., blocked, serial, or random order), and environment (e.g., closed/structured or open/variable).
- **Additional required elements:** those elements necessary to assist the patient in the exercise or activity (e.g., verbal cues, manual contacts) or equipment (e.g., elastic band resistance, therapy ball, body weight support system with motorized treadmill).

Box 1.6   Elements of the Discharge Plan

Patient, family, or caregiver education: instruction includes information regarding the following:

- Current condition (pathology), impairments, activity limitations, and participation restrictions
- Ways to reduce risk factors for recurrence of condition and developing complications, indirect impairments, activity limitations, and participation restrictions
- Ways to maintain/enhance performance and functional independence
- Ways to foster healthy habits, wellness, and prevention
- Ways to assist in transition to a new setting (e.g., home, skilled nursing facility)
- Ways to assist in transition to new roles

Plans for follow-up care or referral to another agency: patient/caregiver is provided with the following:

- Information regarding follow-up visit to rehabilitation center or referral to another agency (e.g., home care agency, outpatient facility) as needed
- Information regarding community support group and community fitness center as appropriate

Instruction in a home exercise plan (HEP): patient/caregiver instruction regarding the following:

- Home exercises, activity training, ADL training
- Use of adaptive equipment (e.g., assistive devices, orthoses, wheelchairs)

Evaluation/modification of the home environment:

- Planning regarding the home environment and modifications needed to assist the patient in the home (e.g., installation of ramps and rails, bathroom equipment such as tub seats, raised toilet seats, bathroom rails, furniture rearrangement or removal to ease functional mobility)
- All essential equipment and renovations should be in place before discharge

reduce distractions and focus the patient's attention on the task. Patient privacy should be respected, with adequate draping and positioning. The therapist should consider good body mechanics, effective use of gravity and position, and correct application of techniques and modalities. Any equipment should be gathered prior to treatment and be in good working order. All safety precautions must be observed.

The patient's pretreatment level of function or initial state should be carefully examined. General state organization of the CNS and homeostatic balance of the somatic and autonomic nervous systems are important determinants of how a patient may respond to intervention.

A wide range of influences, from emotional to cognitive to organic, may affect how a patient reacts to a particular treatment. Patients who are overly stressed may demonstrate altered homeostatic responses. For example, the patient with TBI who presents with high arousal and agitated behaviors can be expected to react to treatment in unpredictable ways, characterized by "fight or flight" responses. Similarly, patients with TBI who are lethargic may be difficult to arouse and demonstrate limited ability to participate in therapy sessions. Responses to treatment should be carefully monitored throughout the episode of care, and treatment modifications should be implemented as soon as needed to ensure successful performance. Therapists develop the "art of clinical practice" by learning to adjust their input (e.g., verbal commands and manual contacts) in response to the patient. Treatment thus becomes a dynamic and interactive process between patient and therapist. Shaping of behavior can be further enhanced by careful orientation to the purpose of the tasks and how they meet the patient's needs, thereby ensuring optimal cooperation and motivation.[10]

Reexamination of the Patient and Evaluation of Expected Outcomes

This last step is ongoing and involves continuous reexamination of the patient and a determination of the efficacy of treatment. Reexamination data are evaluated within the context of the patient's progress toward anticipated goals and expected outcomes set forth in the POC. A determination is made whether the goals and outcomes are reasonable given the patient's diagnosis and progress. If the patient attains the desired level of competence for the stated goals, revisions in the POC are indicated. If the patient attains the desired level of competence for the expected outcomes, discharge is considered. If the patient fails to achieve the stated goals or outcomes, the therapist must determine why. Were the goals and outcomes realistic given the clinical problems and database? Were the interventions selected at an appropriate level to challenge the patient, or were they too easy or too difficult? Were facilitators appropriately identified and the patient sufficiently motivated? Were intervening and constraining factors (barriers) identified? If the interventions were not appropriate, additional information is sought, goals modified, and different treatment interventions selected. Revision in the POC is also indicated if the patient progresses more rapidly or slowly than expected. Each modification must be evaluated in terms of its overall impact on the POC. Thus, the plan becomes a fluid statement of how the patient is progressing and what goals and outcomes are achievable. Its overall success depends on the therapist's ongoing clinical decision making skills and on engaging the patient's cooperation and motivation. Patient involvement in the development and monitoring of the POC should be documented.

■ PATIENT PARTICIPATION IN PLANNING

A *patient-centered approach* that involves the patient in collaborative planning and evaluation of outcomes is important in a successful POC. The patient is viewed as an active participant and partner who can make informed choices and assume responsibility for his or her own health care. Therapists who place strong emphasis on communicating effectively; educating their patients, families, and caregivers; and teaching self-management skills are able to successfully empower patients. The natural outcomes of this approach are improved therapy outcomes and overall satisfaction with care.[11] Some rehabilitation plans have failed miserably simply because the therapist did not fully involve the patient in the planning process, producing goals or outcomes that were not meaningful to the patient (e.g., for the patient with incomplete SCI, independent wheelchair mobility). That same patient may have established a very different set of personal goals and expectations (e.g., return to walking). For many patients for whom complete recovery is not expected, the overall "goal of any rehabilitation program must be to increase the ability of individuals to manage their lives in the context of ongoing disability, to the greatest extent possible."[11, p. 7] This cannot be effectively done if the therapist assumes the role of expert and sole planner, establishing the rules, regulations, and instructions for rehabilitation. Rather, it is critical to engage the patient in collaborative problem solving and promote lifelong skills in health management. The patient's ability and motivation to participate in planning do vary. The more ill the patient, the more anxiety, and the less likely that he or she will want to be actively involved in planning. As the illness resolves and the patient begins to improve, the more likely he or she will be to want to be engaged in planning the treatment. Also the more difficult the problems encountered, the more likely patients are to put their trust in "the experts" and the less likely they are to trust their own abilities to reach effective decisions. The therapist needs to guard against promoting dependence on the expert (the "my therapist syndrome") to the exclusion of the patient's listening to his or her own thoughts and feelings. The patient's feelings of perceived helplessness are increased while the patient's ability to utilize his or her own decision making abilities is delayed or restricted.

Ozer et al[11] address these issues in an excellent reference titled *Treatment Planning for Rehabilitation—A Patient-Centered Approach.* The authors suggest asking the patient a series of *probing questions* to engage patients in the treatment planning process (Box 1.7). The level of participation in this process may start out limited but can be expected to expand as the collaborative process is continued. A *Levels of Participation Scale* can be used to evaluate and document patient participation in the planning process (Box 1.8). In determining the patient's level

---

Box 1.7 Questions Designed to Engage the Patient in the Treatment Planning Process

1. What are your concerns?
2. What is your greatest concern?
3. What would you like to see happen? What would make you feel that you are making progress in dealing with your chief concern? What are your goals?
4. What is your specific goal?
5. What results have you achieved?
6. What problems do you have? What questions do you have?
7. What would you like to see accomplished that would make you feel that you are making some progress in dealing with your greatest concern?

From Ozer, M, Payton, O, and Nelson, C: Treatment Planning for Rehabilitation—A Patient-Centered Approach. McGraw-Hill, New York, 2000, pp. 37 and 60, with permission.

Box 1.8 Levels of Participation Scale

A = FREE CHOICE: The therapist asks an open-ended question. The patient explores and selects the answer (what) and further specifies where? and to what degree?

B = MULTIPLE CHOICE: The therapist asks questions, provides suggestions (three options). The patient selects one choice from the alternatives presented.

C = CONFIRMED CHOICE: The therapist asks questions, provides a recommendation (one choice), and asks for agreement. The patient puts into own words what has been selected.

D = FORCED CHOICE: The therapist asks questions, provides a recommendation (one option); the patient agrees (or disagrees) with what has been selected.

E = NO CHOICE: The therapist prescribes, does not ask; the patient is compliant (or noncompliant).

From Ozer, M, Payton, O, and Nelson, C: Treatment Planning for Rehabilitation—A Patient-Centered Approach. McGraw-Hill, New York, 2000, p. 44, with permission.

---

of functioning, the therapist starts at the upper end of the scale (free choice) and moves down the scale as necessary. The lowest level of participation is recorded. For most patients, the lowest level of participation is optimally Level B Multiple Choice. Patients with significant cognitive or communication deficits (e.g., the patient with TBI) typically will require lower levels of participation. The goal as the patient recovers and progresses in rehabilitation is to increasingly involve the patient in the planning process, to whatever extent possible. In these situations, the therapist can document improving levels of participation as evidence of meeting a goal of improving self-efficacy and self-management.

■ DOCUMENTATION

Documentation is an essential requirement for timely reimbursement of services and communication among the rehabilitation team members. Written documentation is formally done at the time of admission and discharge, and at periodic intervals during the course of rehabilitation (interim or progress notes). Many facilities require documentation for every treatment session. The format and timing of notes will vary according to the regulatory requirements specified by institutional policy and third-party payers. Data included in the medical record should be meaningful (important, not just nice to have), complete and accurate (valid and reliable), timely (recorded promptly), and systematic (regularly recorded). All handwritten entries should be in ink, legible, and signed with a legal signature. Written charting errors should be corrected by a single line through the error and initialing and dating directly above the error. See Appendix 1.B: Defensible Documentation—General Documentation Guidelines from APTA (American Physical Therapy Association), practice-dept@apta.org.

In the United States, all health care facilities must adhere to the *ICD-9-CM Official Guidelines for Coding and Reporting*.[12] These codes are developed by the Centers for Medicare and Medicaid Services (CMS) and the National Center for Health Statistics (NCHS) and based on the *International Classification of Diseases, 9th Revision, Clinical Modification (ICD-9-CM)*. Adherence to these guidelines is required under the Health Insurance Portability and Accountability Act (HIPAA). Typical billing codes related to the preferred practice patterns are listed in the *Guide to Physical Therapist Practice*.[4]

Electronic Documentation

There is increasing emphasis on using electronic documentation in physical therapy, which can provide a fully integrated and completely paperless workflow for managing patient care. This includes managing referrals, initial intake data, progress and discharge notes, scheduling, and billing. Advantages of electronic documentation include standardization of data entry, increased speed of access to data, and integration of data that can be used for a wide variety of applications (e.g., clinical management of patients, quality control, clinical research). Therapists no longer have to track down medical records to review or input data, because information is readily available from any computer or electronic device with Internet access. Therapists also can receive notification of when the patient arrives or checks in, what notes are due, and scheduled evaluations and POC updates. Software programs typically do not allow notes be filed unless all the required elements are completed. Overall efficiency of practice management is increased with decreased errors in documentation and improved accuracy of reimbursements.

Many different companies provide software programs for physical therapy that focus on specific practice settings (e.g., outpatient rehabilitation therapy, home care, private practice). Therapists using documentation software for electronic entry of patient data should ensure that programs comply with appropriate provisions for security and confidentiality.

■ CLINICAL DECISION MAKING: EXPERT VERSUS NOVICE

There is an accumulating body of evidence on expertise in physical therapy practice, spearheaded by the pivotal work of Jenson and colleagues.[13-15] These researchers have shown that the knowledge, skills, and decision making abilities used by expert clinicians can be identified, nurtured, and taught. Embrey et al[16] suggest that the novice therapist may benefit from a period of active mentoring by expert clinicians early in clinical practice (e.g., clinical residency). This information has important implications for novice therapists and for educators involved in teaching clinical decision making.

Experienced clinicians utilize a *forward reasoning process* (reasoning from data to hypothesis) in which the clinician is able to recognize patient cues and patterns as being similar to previously identified cases. Decisions are formulated based on higher-order (metacognitive) skills and reflective processes. Hypothesis testing is not typically verbalized. Thus, actions are based on a rich experience-based clinical knowledge and pattern recognition. In contrast, a *backward reasoning process* (also termed *hypothetico-deductive process*) involves identifying cues from the patient, proposing a hypothesis (reasoning from hypothesis to data), gathering supporting data for cue interpretation and evaluating the hypothesis, and determining appropriate actions. Experts may use hypothesis-testing methods when routine problem recognition fails (e.g., for an unfamiliar problem) or when they are practicing out of their area of expertise.[15, 17]

Decision making is influenced by knowledge and experience. Experts have more knowledge and experience and are able to organize, integrate, and shape information into a usable format. Their knowledge base is multidimensional; their clinical reasoning is reflective and focused; and they demonstrate increased confidence in evaluating patients and problem solving.[15] Organization of knowledge is specific and highly dependent on the mastery of a particular practice area. Content domains in physical therapy take the form of the specialty areas (orthopedic, neurological, pediatric, and so forth). As expertise increases, master clinicians increase their abilities to categorize information, improving in both mastery of depth and complexity of content. They are able to use collegial knowledge effectively, seeking out mentors and readily consulting their peers on practice issues. Novice therapists, on the other hand, collect data, but do not always recognize important data. Simple review of data and use of book-learned, declarative knowledge do not allow the novice to recognize meaningful relationships and generate accurate hypotheses within a realistic time frame. New therapists also tend to be rigidly governed by rules for decision making. For example, they adhere to standardized frameworks (protocols), whereas experts easily adapt and refocus their approach if a different direction is indicated. Experts also demonstrate improved intervention skills that are well integrated with their mastery of knowledge and clinical reasoning. Improved skills and expertise are developed through intense, focused, and deliberate practice. Jensen et al point out that experts are highly motivated and are constantly striving to improve their skills, demonstrating a strong inner drive for lifelong learning.[18] The APTA recognizes expertise in a board-certification process for clinical specialists.

The therapist who utilizes a *receptive/systematic data-gathering style* generally suspends judgment until all possible data are gathered. The data are analyzed individually and collectively before a final determination is made of how to organize and use them. A contrasting style is perceptive and intuitive. The individual who utilizes a *perceptive data-gathering style* will seek and respond to ongoing cues and patterns, defining and organizing clinical problems early. Information processing is largely intuitive. Thus, these clinicians are able to respond to a large number of stimuli as they occur and consider initiation of early treatment options.[15] Research suggests that styles may differ by expert group. May and Dennis[19] and Jensen et al[18] found that clinicians with expertise in orthopedics tended to utilize a receptive/systematic style, generating hypotheses only after a methodical and ordered search of data. Embrey et al[16, 20] found that expert clinicians working in pediatric settings tended to utilize a perceptive data-gathering style and process information intuitively. Thus, they responded rapidly to cues and patterns (movement scripts) and changes that occurred within the treatment session. May and Dennis[19] reported that practitioners experienced in cardiopulmonary and neurological physical therapy also tended to respond more favorably to the perceptive/intuitive style. Thus, the differences noted in terms of the types of cognitive strategies reported appear to be evoked by specific problem structure and domain.

Important differences exist between expert and novice clinicians in the area of self-monitoring. Expert clinicians are able to frequently and effectively utilize self-assessment to modify and redefine their clinical decisions. This reflective aspect of practice results in improved improvisational performance, the actions that occur when therapists are actually treating patients. They are better able to control the treatment situation (i.e., constant interruptions, the demands of many scheduled patients, and multiple tasks) and the time allotted. Conversely, novice therapists demonstrate self-monitoring, but are less able to utilize the information effectively to control the situation. They react more to external stimuli and the confusion of competing demands and are less able to offer alternate intervention strategies. Self-monitoring is viewed as a positive experience by the experts twice as often as by novice therapists, an indication that the inexperienced therapists are sensitive to their limitations. The experts are also more willing to take risks and to admit when they did not know something.[15, 21]

Expert clinicians provide patient-centered care. They spend more time with their patients, gathering and evaluating information and involving their patients in collaborative problem solving. Experts maintain as a central goal of care the empowerment of their patients to make autonomous decisions. They affirm the importance of patient education in assisting patients to resolve problems and assume control over their own health care. Teaching strategies therefore focus on maintaining health and preventing the development of indirect impairments, activity limitations, and restrictions to participation. The therapist assumes active roles as coach and teacher.[10] In an era of cost containment and limited services, this is an important value and one that is essential for ensuring successful long-term outcomes. Novice therapists, on the other hand, demonstrate greater interest in mastering hands-on skills and in ensuring the success of their treatments.[17]

Expert clinicians are able to maintain focus on the patient during treatment, as evidenced in their verbal and nonverbal communications. They are able to consistently demonstrate a sense of commitment and caring toward their patients. The experts demonstrate a smooth interplay of hands-on treatment with effective communication that is responsive to the needs of each individual patient.[10, 15] Conversely, novice therapists are influenced by the demands of full-time clinical practice and experience increased challenges in finding adequate time to listen and talk with their patients. They report increased difficulties communicating with "difficult" and "unmotivated" patients.[22] Psychosocial sensitivity is a key factor in directing experienced clinicians during the physical therapy sessions. Novice therapists maintain their focus more on the problems and the mechanics of treatment rather than on the psychosocial needs of the patient.[22]

■ EVIDENCE-BASED PRACTICE

The analysis of research evidence paired with the physical therapist's experience and expertise provides a powerful tool to guide clinical decision making. There are areas of practice in physical therapy that lack rigorous examination and evidence. Therapists may employ some interventions simply because they are in widespread use. Therapists may also elect to use interventions because they are new and different or because they are the focus of "anecdotal testimonials" in continuing education courses. Harris points out, "The responsibility to deliver evidence-based treatment techniques rests with *all* physical therapists."[23, p. 176] To that end, the APTA developed a *Clinical Research*

Agenda designed to support, explain, and enhance physical therapy clinical practice.[24] The *Research Agenda* was revised in 2011 to be reflective of the rapid changes in health care and in rehabilitation.[25] It identifies broad categories of research and is consistent with the ICF. The APTA's *Hooked on Evidence* project provides links to *Evidence in Practice* (www.ptjournal.org) and provides training programs to assist individuals in this process.

Evidence-based medicine (EBM) is defined as "the integration of best research evidence with our clinical expertise and our patient's unique values and circumstances."[26, p. 1] The term **evidence-based practice (EBP)** encompasses a broader range of health professions.

The essential steps of EBP[26] are as follows:

Step 1: A clinical problem is identified and an answerable question is formulated.

Step 2: A systematic literature review is conducted and evidence collected.

Step 3: The research evidence is critically analyzed for its validity (closeness to the truth), impact (size of the effect), and applicability (usefulness in clinical practice).

Step 4: The critical appraisal is synthesized and integrated with the clinician's expertise and the patient's unique biology, values, and circumstances.

Step 5: The effectiveness and efficiency of the steps in the evidence-based process are evaluated.

A well-built *research question* contains three elements: (1) a specific patient/client group or population, (2) the specific interventions or exposures to be studied, and (3) the outcomes achieved. For example, one study examined interventions commonly applied for low back pain (therapeutic exercise, transcutaneous electrical nerve stimulation [TENS], thermotherapy, ultrasound, massage, E-stim system, traction) using outcomes identified as being important to the patient (pain, function, patient global assessment, QOL, and return to work).[27]

Systematic review (SR) is a comprehensive examination of the literature. The researcher determines key resources to provide the evidence. These include (1) peer-reviewed and evidence-based journals, (2) online services (e.g., Cochrane Reviews, APTA Open Door, PEDro), and (3) search engines (e.g., PubMed). Box 1.9 provides a brief list of electronic medical databases. Specific criteria are developed for the inclusion and exclusion of the research studies selected for review. Studies employing different designs may be analyzed individually or compared qualitatively; studies of similar design may be combined quantitatively (e.g., meta-analysis).

Critical analysis of research findings involves detailed examination of methodology, results, and conclusions. The clinician should be able to answer the following questions: (1) What is the level of evidence? (2) Is the evidence valid? and (3) Are the results important and clinically relevant? Thus, interpretation and synthesis of the evidence must be considered within the context of the specific patient/client problem. Examination begins with the purpose of the study, which should be clearly stated, and the review of literature, which should be relevant in terms of the specific question asked. The

---

Box 1.9   Evidence-Based Practice: Electronic Medical Databases

www.ncbi.nlm.nih.gov/PubMed	PubMEd—U.S. National Library of Medicine (NLM): search service to Medline and Pre-Medline (database of medical and biomedical research), free public access
www.hookedonevidence.com	APTA Open Door—Hooked on Evidence: database of evidence-based physical therapy practice, members only
www.pedro.org.au/	Physiotherapy Evidence Database (PEDro) of physical therapy: RCTs, systematic reviews, and evidence-based clinical practice
www.cochrane.org/reviews	Cochrane Database of Systematic Reviews (Cochrane Reviews); primary source for clinical effectiveness information
http://hiru.mcmaster.ca/cochrane/centers/Canadian	Canadian Cochrane Center
www.cinahl.com	CINAHL: database of nursing and allied health research
www.york.ac.uk/inst/crd/crddatabases.htm	DARE: database of abstracts of evidence reviews from medical journals
www.naric.com/research	RehabDATA: database of disability and rehabilitation research
www.cirrie.buffalo.edu?	Center for International Rehabilitation Research Information and Exchange: database of rehabilitation research
www.ovid.com	Ovid: database of health and life science research

methods/design should be closely examined. Research design varies and can be evaluated in terms of levels of evidence, with grades of recommendation in order of most to least rigorous (Table 1.2). Although a randomized clinical trial (RCT) provides the most rigorous design, there are times when other designs are indicated. For example, there may be ethical issues involving control groups that receive no treatment when treatment is clearly beneficial. In addition, when outcomes are not clearly understood or defined (e.g., quality-of-life issues), designs such as single-case studies may be indicated. The reader is referred to Appendix 1-C: Overview of Evidence-Based Practice Concepts for additional discussion.

Critical Appraisal Tools (CATs) are available to assist the inexperienced clinician in the evaluation of research (see Law, Appendix A: Critical Review Form, Quantitative Studies[28, p. 331]; and Jewell, Appendix B: Evidence Appraisal Worksheets).[29, p. 427] Clinicians also need to utilize effective strategies to organize and store the data and to update data on a regular basis. Reference management systems such as *Endnote* and *Reference Manager* (ISI ResearchSoft, 800 Jones Street, Berkeley, CA 94710) are available to assist the therapist.

Evidence-based clinical practice guidelines (EBCPGs) are defined by the Institute of Medicine as systematically developed statements to assist practitioner and patient decisions about appropriate health care for specific clinical circumstances.[30] They are developed through a combination of (1) expert consensus (e.g., the *Guide to Physical Therapist Practice*[5]); (2) systematic reviews and meta-analysis; and (3) analysis of patient preferences combined with outcome-based guidelines. For example, the *Philadelphia Panel* is a multidisciplinary, international panel of rehabilitation experts comprising a group of Clinical Specialty Experts from the United States and the Ottawa Methods Group from Canada. This panel developed a structured and rigorous methodology to formulate evidence-based practice guidelines.[31] For example, the panel analyzed the evidence following a structured and rigorous review of selected interventions for low back pain.[27] The evidence was then translated into EBCPGs by reviewing key outcomes and deciding whether the intervention had clinical benefit. Categories of absolute and relative benefit were used. The panel established a clinical improvement of 15% or more relative to the control as an acceptable level of evidence. Recommendations were graded based on levels (methodological quality) of the studies. Grade A or B recommendations were required to demonstrate clinically important changes and statistical significance. The panel's positive recommendations were then sent to 324 clinical practitioners for their feedback. The panel reviewed practitioners' feedback and revised their recommendations accordingly. In the low back pain study, the panel recommended the following EBCPGs: (1) the use of therapeutic exercises for chronic, subacute, and post-surgery low back pain and (2) continuation of normal activities for acute low back pain. The panel found lack of evidence regarding efficacy for the use of other interventions (e.g., thermotherapy, therapeutic ultrasound, massage, electrical stimulation). EBCPGs have

Table 1.2	Levels of Evidence for Treatment Effectiveness
Level 1	SR[a] of a number of RCTs[b] of studies (meta-analysis) that substantially agree (do not have significant statistical variation)
Level 2	Individual RCT with narrow confidence window (size of treatment effect precisely defined) Observational study with dramatic effect[c]
Level 3	Nonrandomized controlled cohort study[d]
Level 4	Case-control,[e] case-series,[f] or historically controlled studies
Level 5	Mechanism-based reasoning (expert opinion)

a. SR, systematic review: a review in which the primary studies are summarized, critically appraised, and statistically combined; usually quantitative in nature with specific inclusion/exclusion criteria.

b. RCT, randomized controlled trial: an experimental study in which participants are randomly assigned to either an experimental or control group to receive different interventions or a placebo; the most rigorous study design.

c. All-or-none study: a study in which treatment produces a dramatic change in outcomes; all patients die before treatment; none die after treatment.

d. Cohort study: a prospective (forward-in-time) study; a group of participants (cohort) with a similar condition receives an intervention and is followed over time and outcome evaluated; comparison is made to a matched group who do receive the intervention (quasi-experimental with no randomization).

e. Case-control study: a retrospective study in which a group of subjects with a condition of interest are identified for research after outcomes are achieved; e.g., studying the impact of an intervention on level of participation; a comparison group is used.

f. Case series: clinical outcomes are evaluated of a single group of patients with a similar condition.

Adapted from OCEBM Levels of Evidence Working Group—Jeremy Howick, Iain Chalmers (James Lind Library), Paul Glasziou, Trish Greenhalgh, Carl Heneghan, Alessandro Liberati, Ivan Moschetti, Bob Phillips, Hazel Thornton, Olive Goddard, and Mary Hodgkinson: The Oxford 2011 Levels of Evidence. Oxford Centre for Evidence-Based Medicine. Retrieved from www.cebm.net/index.aspx?o=5653.

been published for rehabilitation of patients with the following conditions:

- Low back pain[27]
- Knee pain[32]
- Knee pain and mobility impairments: meniscal and articular cartilage lesions[33]
- Hip pain and mobility impairments: osteoarthritis[34]
- Heel pain: plantar fasciitis[35]
- Neck pain[36]
- Shoulder pain[37]
- Fibromyalgia[38, 39]

According to Rothstein, these studies are clinically important in that they "are not telling us what is known and what is not known, but what is supported by evidence and what is not supported by evidence."[40, p. 1,620] The guidelines provide a summation of best possible evidence for use in clinical practice.

SUMMARY

An organized process of clinical decision making allows the therapist to systematically plan effective treatments. The steps identified in the patient/client management process are (1) examine the patient, and collect data through history, systems review, and tests and measures; (2) evaluate the data and identify problems; (3) determine the diagnosis; (4) determine the prognosis and POC; (5) implement the POC; and (6) reexamine the patient and evaluate treatment outcomes. Patient participation in planning is essential in ensuring successful outcomes. Evidence-based practice allows the therapist to select interventions that have been shown to provide meaningful change in patient's lives. Inherent to the therapist's success in this process are an appropriate knowledge base and experience, cognitive processing strategies, self-monitoring strategies, and communication and teaching skills. Documentation is an essential requirement for effective communication among the rehabilitation team members and for timely reimbursement of services.

Questions for Review

1. What are the key steps in patient/client management?
2. Differentiate between impairments, activity limitations, and participation restrictions. Define and give an example of each.
3. What are the essential elements of goal and outcome statements? Write two examples of each.
4. Differentiate between restorative and compensatory interventions. Give an example of each.
5. What is the FITT equation? Give an example of how is it used in formulating interventions for a POC.
6. What are the advantages of electronic documentation systems? Disadvantages?
7. What are the elements of a well-built research question? Give an example. What is the highest level of evidence available for evidence-based clinical practice guidelines?

CASE STUDY

PRESENT HISTORY

The patient is a 78-year-old woman who tripped and fell at home ascending the stairs outside the front door. She was admitted to the hospital after sustaining a transcervical, intracapsular fracture of the right femur. The patient had an open reduction and internal fixation (ORIF) procedure of the right lower extremity (RLE) to reduce and pin the fracture. After 2 weeks of acute hospital admission, the patient is at home and referred for home care physical therapy.

PAST MEDICAL HISTORY

Patient is a very thin woman (98 pounds) with long-standing problems with osteoporosis (on medication for 5 years). She has a history of falls, three in the last year alone. Approximately 3 years ago she had a myocardial infarction and presented with third-degree heart block, requiring implantation of a permanent pacemaker. She underwent cataract surgery with lens implantation in the right eye 2 years ago; the left eye is scheduled for similar surgery within the next few months.

MEDICAL DIAGNOSES

Coronary artery disease (CAD), hypertension (HTN), mitral valve prolapse, s/p permanent heart pacer, s/p right cataract with implant, osteoporosis (moderate to severe in the spine, hips, and pelvis), osteoarthritis with mild pain in right knee, s/p left elbow fracture (1 year ago), left ankle fracture (2 years ago), urinary stress incontinence.

MEDICATIONS

Fosamax 70 mg weekly
Atenolol 24 mg PO qd
MVI (multivitamin concentrate) with Fe tab PO qd
Metamucil 1 tbs prn PO qd, Colace 100 mg PO bid
Tylenol No. 3 tab prn/mild pain

SOCIAL SUPPORT/ENVIRONMENT

The patient is a retired schoolteacher who was recently widowed after 48 years of marriage. She has two sons, one daughter, and four grandchildren; all live within an hour's driving distance. One of her children visits every weekend. She has a rambunctious black Labrador puppy that is 8 months old and was given to her "for company" at the time her husband died. She was walking the dog at the time of the accident. She is an active participant in a garden club, which meets twice a month, and in weekly events at the local senior center. Previously she was driving her car for all community activities.

   She lives alone in a large old New England farmhouse. Her home has an entry with four stairs and no rail. Inside there are 14 rooms on two floors. The downstairs living area has a step down into the family room with no rail. There are 14 stairs to the second floor, with rails on either side. The upstairs sleeping area is cluttered with large, heavy furniture. The second floor bathroom is small, with a high old tub with pedestal feet and a lip. There is no added equipment.

PHYSICAL THERAPY EXAMINATION

1. Mental status

   Alert and oriented × 3

   Pleasant, cooperative, articulate

   No apparent memory deficits

   Good problem solving and safety awareness about hip precautions

2. Cardiopulmonary status

   Pulse 74; BP 110/75

   Endurance: good; min SOB with 20 min of activity

3. Sensation

   Vision: wears glasses; cloudy vision L eye; impaired depth perception

   Hearing: WFL

   Sensation: BLEs intact

4. Skin

   Incision is healed and well approximated

   Wears bilateral TEDs q a.m. × 6 wks

5. ROM

   LLE, BUEs: WFL

   Affected RLE:

   Flex 0° to 85°

   Ext NT

   Abd 0° to 20°

   Add NT

   IR, ER NT

   Right knee and ankle WFL

6. Strength

LLE, BUEs: WFL

Affected RLE:

Hip flex NT (not tested)

Hip ext NT

Hip abd NT

Knee ext 4/5

Ankle DF 4/5, PF 4/5

7. Posture

Flexed, stooped posture: moderate kyphosis, flexed hips and knees

$1/_2$-inch leg length shortening on RLE; uses wedge when sitting

Mild resting head tremor

8. Balance

Sitting balance: WFL

Standing balance:

Eyes open: good; leans slightly to left side

Eyes closed: unsteady, begins to fall

Arises from chair without help, some initial unsteadiness; sitting down: safe, smooth motion

Uses 2-inch foam cushions to elevate seat of kitchen chair and living room chair

9. Functional status

Patient was completely independent (I) before her fall.

Results of functional examination:

I bed mobility

I transfers; unable to do tub transfers at present

I ambulation with standard walker × 200 feet on level surfaces, partial weight-bearing RLE
Increased flexion of knees and dorsal spine

I one flight of stairs with rail and SBQC

I dressing; requires minimal assist (MinA) of home health aide for sponge baths

Requires moderate assistance (ModA) of home health aide for homemaker activities

10. Patient is highly motivated

"I want to get my life back together, get my dog home again so I can take care of him."

PRIMARY INSURANCE

Medicare

Guiding Questions

1. Develop a prioritized problem list for this patient's POC. Identify and categorize the patient's impairments (direct, indirect, composite). Identify her activity limitations and participation restrictions.

2. What information is available about her functional status within the home in terms of performance versus capacity qualifiers?

3. What is her rehabilitation prognosis?

4. Write two expected outcome and two goal statements to direct her POC.

5. Identify two treatment interventions for her POC.

6. What precautions should be observed?

7. What tests and measures can be used to determine successful attainment of outcomes?

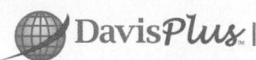 **DavisPlus** | For additional resources, including answers to the questions for review and case study guiding questions, please visit **http://davisplus.fadavis.com**

References

1. Rothstein, JM, Echternach, JL, and Riddle, DL: The hypothesis-oriented algorithm for clinicians II (HOAC II): A guide for patient management. Phys Ther 83:455, 2003.
2. World Health Organization (WHO): ICF: Towards a Common Language for Functioning, Disability, and Health. Geneva, Switzerland, 2002. Retrieved March 4, 2011, from www.who.int/classifications/en.
3. World Health Organization (WHO): ICF CHECKLIST, Version 2.1a, Clinician Form for International Classification of Functioning, Disability and Health. Geneva, Switzerland, 2003. Retrieved March 4, 2011, from www.who.int/classifications/icf/training/icfchecklist.pdf.
4. American Physical Therapy Association: Guide to physical therapist practice. Phys Ther 81:1, 2001.
5. Randall, KE, and McEwen, IR: Writing patient-centered functional goals. Phys Ther 80:1197, 2000.
6. Sarhman, SA: Diagnosis by the physical therapist—a special communication. Phys Ther 68:1703, 1988.
7. Rothstein, J: Disability and our identity. Phys Ther 74:375, 1994.
8. Guide for the Uniform Data Set for Medical Rehabilitation (including the FIM instrument), Version 5.0. State University of New York, Buffalo, 1996.
9. Watts, N: Decision analysis: A tool for improving physical therapy education. In Wolf, S (ed): Clinical Decision Making in Physical Therapy. FA Davis, Philadelphia, 1985, p 8.
10. Resnik, L, and Jensen, G: Using clinical outcomes to explore the theory of expert practice in physical therapy. Phys Ther 83:1090, 2003.
11. Ozer, M, Payton, O, and Nelson, C: Treatment Planning for Rehabilitation—A Patient-Centered Approach. McGraw-Hill, New York, 2000.
12. World Health Organization: International Classification of Diseases, Ninth Revision, Clinical Modification (ICD-9-CM) (Volumes 1, 2, 3, and Guidelines). Distributed by the National Center for Health Statistics (NCHS) and the Centers for Medicare and Medicaid Services (CMS). Retrieved March 4, 2011, from www.cdc.gov/nchs/icd/icd9cm.htm.
13. Jensen, GM, Shepard, KF, and Hack, LM: The novice versus the experienced clinician: Insights into the work of the physical therapist. Phys Ther 70:314, 1990.
14. Jensen, GM, Gwyer J, Shepard KF, et al: Expert practice in physical therapy. Phys Ther 80:28–51, 2000.
15. Jensen, GM, Gwyer, JM, Hack, LM, et al: Expertise in Physical Therapy Practice, ed 2. Saunders Elsevier, St. Louis, 2006.
16. Embrey, DG, Guthrie, MR, White, OR, et al: Clinical decision making by experienced and inexperienced pediatric physical therapists for children with diplegic cerebral palsy. Phys Ther 76:20, 1996.
17. Edwards, I, Jones, M, Carr, J, et al: Clinical reasoning strategies in physical therapy. Phys Ther 84:312, 2004.
18. Jensen, GM, et al: Attribute dimensions that distinguish master and novice physical therapy clinicians in orthopedic settings. Phys Ther 72:711, 1992.
19. May, BJ, and Dennis, JK: Expert decision making in physical therapy: A survey of practitioners. Phys Ther 71:190, 1991.
20. Embrey, DG: Clinical applications of decision making in pediatric physical therapy: Overview. Pediatr Phys Ther 8:2, 1996.
21. Embrey, DG, and Yates, L: Clinical applications of self-monitoring by experienced and novice pediatric physical therapists. Pediatr Phys Ther 8:3, 1996.
22. Greenfield, BH, Anderson, A, Cox, B, et al: Meaning of caring to 7 novice physical therapists during their first year of clinical practice. Phys Ther 88:1154, 2008.
23. Harris, S: How should treatments be critiqued for scientific merit? Phys Ther 76:175–181, 1996.
24. Guccione, A, Goldstein, M, and Elliott, S: Clinical research agenda for physical therapy. Phys Ther 80:499–513, 2000.
25. Goldstein, M, Scalzitti, D, Craik, R, et al: The revised research agenda for physical therapy. Phys Ther 91:165–174, 2011.
26. Staus, S, Glasziou, P, Richardson, W, et al: Evidence-Based Medicine: How to Practice and Teach EBM, ed 4. Churchill-Livingstone-Elsevier, New York, 2011.
27. Philadelphia Panel: Evidence-based clinical practice guidelines on selected rehabilitation interventions for low back pain. Phys Ther 81:1641, 2001.
28. Law, M, and MacDermid, J (eds): Evidence-Based Rehabilitation, ed 2. Slack Inc., Thorofare, NJ, 2008.
29. Jewell D: Guide to Evidence-Based Physical Therapy Practice. Jones & Bartlett, Boston, 2008.
30. Scalzitti, D: Evidence-based guidelines: Application to clinical practice. Phys Ther 81:1622, 2001.
31. Philadelphia Panel: Evidence-based clinical practice guidelines on selected rehabilitation interventions: Overview and methodology. Phys Ther 81:1629, 2001.
32. Philadelphia Panel: Evidence-based clinical practice guidelines on selected rehabilitation interventions for knee pain. Phys Ther 81:1675, 2001.
33. Orthopedic section, APTA: Knee pain and mobility impairments: Meniscal and articular cartilage lesions clinical practice guidelines linked to the International Classification of Functioning, Disability, and Health. JOSPT 40(6):A30, 2010.
34. Orthopedic section, APTA: Hip pain and mobility impairments—hip osteoarthritis: Clinical practice guidelines linked to the International Classification of Functioning, Disability, and Health. JOSPT 39(4):A18, 2009.
35. Orthopedic section, APTA: Heel pain—plantar fasciitis: Clinical practice guidelines linked to the International Classification of Functioning, Disability, and Health. JOSPT 40(6):A30, 2010.
36. Orthopedic section, APTA: Neck pain: Clinical practice guidelines linked to the International Classification of Functioning, Disability, and Health. JOSPT 40(6):A30, 2010.
37. Philadelphia Panel: Evidence-based clinical practice guidelines on selected rehabilitation interventions for shoulder pain. Phys Ther 81:1719, 2001.
38. Ottawa Panel: Ottawa Panel evidence-based clinical practice guidelines for aerobic fitness exercises in the management of fibromyalgia: Part 1. Phys Ther 88:857, 2008.
39. Ottawa Panel: Ottawa Panel evidence-based clinical practice guidelines for strengthening exercises in the management of fibromyalgia: Part 2. Phys Ther 88:873, 2008.
40. Rothstein, J: Autonomous practice or autonomous ignorance? Phys Ther 81:1620, 2001.

Preferred Practice Patterns: APTA *Guide to Physical Therapist Practice* [4]

■ MUSCULOSKELETAL

Pattern A: Primary Prevention/Risk Reduction for Skeletal Demineralization

Pattern B: Impaired Posture

Pattern C: Impaired Muscle Performance

Pattern D: Impaired Joint Mobility, Motor Function, Muscle Performance, and Range of Motion Associated With Connective Tissue Dysfunction

Pattern E: Impaired Joint Mobility, Motor Function, Muscle Performance, and Range of Motion Associated With Localized Inflammation

Pattern F: Impaired Joint Mobility, Motor Function, Muscle Performance, Range of Motion, and Reflex Integrity Associated With Spinal Disorders

Pattern G: Impaired Joint Mobility, Motor Function, Muscle Performance, Range of Motion Associated With Fracture

Pattern H: Impaired Joint Mobility, Motor Function, Muscle Performance, Range of Motion Associated With Joint Arthroplasty

Pattern I: Impaired Joint Mobility, Motor Function, Muscle Performance, Range of Motion Associated With Bony or Soft Tissue Surgery

Pattern J: Impaired Motor Function, Muscle Performance, Range of Motion, Gait, Locomotion, and Balance Associated With Amputation

■ NEUROMUSCULAR

Pattern A: Primary Prevention/Risk Reduction for Loss of Balance and Falling

Pattern B: Impaired Neuromotor Development

Pattern C: Impaired Motor Function and Sensory Integrity Associated With Nonprogressive Disorders of the Central Nervous System—Congenital Origin or Acquired in Infancy or Childhood

Pattern D: Impaired Motor Function and Sensory Integrity Associated With Nonprogressive Disorders of the Central Nervous System—Acquired in Adolescence or Adulthood

Pattern E: Impaired Motor Function and Sensory Integrity Associated With Progressive Disorders of the Central Nervous System

Pattern F: Impaired Peripheral Nerve Integrity and Muscle Performance Associated With Peripheral Nerve Injury

Pattern G: Impaired Motor Function and Sensory Integrity Associated With Acute or Chronic Polyneuropathies

Pattern H: Impaired Motor Function, Peripheral Nerve Integrity, and Sensory Integrity Associated With Nonprogressive Disorders of the Spinal Cord

Pattern I: Impaired Arousal, Range of Motion, and Motor Control Associated With Coma, Near Coma, or Vegetative State

■ CARDIOVASCULAR/ PULMONARY

Pattern A: Primary Prevention/Risk Reduction for Cardiovascular/Pulmonary Disorders

Pattern B: Impaired Aerobic Capacity/Endurance Associated With Deconditioning

Pattern C: Impaired Ventilation, Respiration/Gas Exchange, and Aerobic Capacity/Endurance Associated With Airway Clearance Dysfunction

Pattern D: Impaired Aerobic Capacity/Endurance Associated With Cardiovascular Pump Dysfunction or Failure

Pattern E: Impaired Ventilation, Respiration/Gas Exchange Associated With Ventilatory Pump Dysfunction or Failure

Pattern F: Impaired Ventilation, Respiration/Gas Exchange Associated With Respiratory Failure

Pattern G: Impaired Ventilation, Respiration/Gas Exchange, and Aerobic Capacity/Endurance Associated With Respiratory Failure in the Neonate

Pattern H: Impaired Circulation and Anthropometric Dimensions Associated With Lymphatic System Disorders

■ INTEGUMENTARY

Pattern A: Primary Prevention/Risk Reduction for Integumentary Disorders

Pattern B: Impaired Integumentary Integrity Associated With Superficial Skin Involvement

Pattern C: Impaired Integumentary Integrity Associated With Partial-Thickness Skin Involvement and Scar Formation

Pattern D: Impaired Integumentary Integrity Associated With Full-Thickness Skin Involvement and Scar Formation

Pattern E: Impaired Integumentary Integrity Associated With Skin

Defensible Documentation— General Documentation Guidelines From APTA

Documentation is required for every visit/encounter.

Documentation should include indication of a patient/client's cancellations of appointments and/or refusal of treatment.

All documentation must comply with the applicable jurisdictional/regulatory requirements.

All handwritten entries shall be made in ink, dated, and properly authenticated. Legibility is critical in clinical documentation. If an entry cannot be read, it cannot be understood.

Electronic entries are made with appropriate security and confidentiality provisions.

Documentation must include adequate identification of the patient/client, the physical therapist, and/or physical therapist assistant:

- The patient/client's full name and identification number, if applicable, must be included on all official documents.
- All entries must be dated and authenticated with the provider's full name and appropriate designation (license number and printed name if required by state law).

Charting errors should be corrected by drawing a single line through the error and initialing and dating the error or through the appropriate mechanism for electronic documentation that clearly indicates that a change was made without deletion of the original record. *Example:* Pain in the right shoulder will decrease to 2/10 VAS within 5 4ABD 11/2/06 visits.

Documentation of examination, evaluation, diagnosis, prognosis, plan of care, progress report, and discharge summary must be authenticated by the physical therapist who provided the service.

Documentation of physical therapist service in pediatrics is aligned with family-centered care.

Documentation should emphasize the functional abilities of the child rather than highlight the deficits and should be written in a respectful manner. Therapists often collaborate with the family, child, and other team members on the documentation and record their involvement in the physical therapy services.

Abbreviations should be minimized.

Documentation must be clear about who is providing the service whether it is the physical therapist (PT), the physical therapist assistant (PTA), or both when the PT may perform mobilization and the PTA may perform therapeutic exercises with the same patient/client.

Documentation of intervention in visit/encounter notes must be authenticated by the PT or PTA who provided the service. Medicare requires handwritten signatures or electronic signatures only. Stamp signatures are not acceptable.

Documentation by PTs, PTA graduates, or others pending receipt of an unrestricted license shall be authenticated by a licensed physical therapist, or, when permissible by state law; documentation by PTA graduates may be authenticated by a PTA.

Documentation by students (SPT/SPTA) in PT or PTA programs must be additionally authenticated by the PT or, when permissible by state law, documentation by PTA students may be authenticated by a PTA. The following link provides information regarding student documentation/billing requirements: www.apta.org/Payment/Medicare/Supervision.

Documentation should include the referral mechanism by which physical therapy services are initiated. Examples include the following:

- Direct access when permissible by state law.
- Request for consultation from another practitioner.
- Referral from practitioner authorized to refer per Medicare regulations or state practice act.

From American Physical Therapy Association, with permission. Retrieved November 7, 2011, from www.apta.org/Documentation/DefensibleDocumentation. Last updated March 10, 2011.

Overview of Evidence-Based Practice Concepts

Prepared by Kevin K. Chui, PT, PhD, GCS, OCS

1. Sensitivity and Specificity

As evidence-based diagnosticians, physical therapists need to consider the accuracy of diagnostic tests.[1] When establishing the accuracy (clinometric properties) of a novel diagnostic test against a reference standard (i.e., the best available examination, which may be a laboratory or clinical test), there are four possible outcomes:

		Reference Standard	
		Positive	Negative
Novel Diagnostic Test	Positive	True Positive	False Positive
	Negative	False Negative	True Negative

- A *true positive (TP),* in which the diagnostic test and the reference standard are both positive
- A *false negative (FN),* in which the diagnostic test is negative and the reference standard is positive
- A *true negative (TN),* in which the diagnostic test and the reference standard are both negative
- A *false positive (FP),* in which the diagnostic test is positive and the reference standard is negative

These outcomes are then used to calculate the probability that test results are correct, that is, the sensitivity and specificity of a diagnostic test.

The *sensitivity*, or the TP rate (= TP/TP + FN), refers to the ability of a diagnostic test to identify the condition when it is present. Based on the formula used to calculate sensitivity, there is an inverse relationship between the TP and FN rates. That is, as the TP rate increases (i.e., sensitivity increases), the FN rate will decrease. Therefore, a test that is highly sensitive will have a high TP rate and a low FN rate and can be used to rule out the condition when the test result is negative.

In contrast, the *specificity,* or the TN rate (= TN/TN + FP), refers to the ability of a diagnostic test to identify when the condition is absent. Based on the formula used to calculate specificity, there is an inverse relationship between the TN and FP rates. That is, as the TN rate increases (i.e., specificity increases), the FP rate will decrease. Therefore, a test that is highly specific will have a high TN rate and a low FP rate and can be used to rule in the condition when the test result is positive.

To assist practitioners when selecting and using diagnostic tests, Sackett et al[2] suggested the acronyms "SnNout" and "SpPin." For a highly sensitive (Sn) diagnostic test, a negative (N) finding can be used to rule out (out) the condition, hence SnNout. And for a highly specific (Sp) diagnostic test, a positive (P) finding can be used to rule in (in) the condition, hence SpPin.

2. Likelihood Ratios

The sensitivity and specificity values (i.e., the probability that test results are correct) of a diagnostic test can then be used to calculate likelihood ratios, which quantify the shift in pre-test probability (estimated from other examination findings or prevalence data) to post-test probability that the patient has the condition. Given a positive diagnostic test result, a *positive likelihood ratio* (= sensitivity/1 − specificity) quantifies the increase in pre-test to post-test probability that the patient has the condition. On the other hand, given a negative diagnostic test result, a *negative likelihood ratio* (= 1 − sensitivity/specificity) quantifies the decrease in pre-test to post-test probability that the patient has the condition.

To be clear, whether the diagnostic test is positive or negative and the corresponding positive or negative likelihood ratio is used, the likelihood ratio helps to quantify the probability that the patient has the condition. A likelihood ratio of 1 results in no shift in pre-test to post-test probability (i.e., the probability that the patient has the condition remains the same). As positive likelihood ratios start to exceed 1, the shift in pre-test to post-test probability increases (i.e., the probability that the patient has the condition increases). As negative likelihood ratios start to approach 0, the shift in pre-test to post-test probability decreases (i.e., the probability that the patient has the condition decreases).

Guyatt and Rennie[3] suggest useful guidelines for interpreting likelihood ratios:

- Likelihood ratios >10 or <0.1 result in large and often conclusive shifts in pre-test to post-test probabilities.

- Likelihood ratios of 5–10 or 0.1–0.2 result in moderate shifts in pre-test to post-test probabilities.
- Likelihood ratios of 2–5 or 0.5–0.2 result in small shifts in pre-test to post-test probabilities.
- Likelihood ratios of 1–2 or 0.5–1 result in shifts in pre-test to post-test probabilities that are rarely important.

The nomogram by Fagan[4] can assist practitioners in calculating the post-test probability with knowledge of the pre-test probability and the likelihood ratio.

For example, a study by Wainner et al[5] developed a clinical prediction rule to diagnose cervical radiculopathy. The corresponding positive likelihood ratio for a patient that tested positive on three out of the four items from the cluster is 6.1. Given a pre-test probability of 23% and a positive likelihood ratio of 6.1, the nomogram is then used to calculate a post-test probability of 65% for having cervical radiculopathy.

3. Clinical Decision or Prediction Rules

Clinical prediction (or decision) rules are tools designed to help practitioners with diagnosis and prognosis.[6] These tools identify a parsimonious list of predictor variables from the examination (e.g., history, systems review, and tests and measures) to diagnose a condition or prognosticate which patients are likely to recover, respond to treatment, or become chronic. For example, there are clinical prediction rules to help practitioners identify those at risk for lower and upper extremity deep vein thrombosis, those likely to respond to exercise, and those likely to develop persistent shoulder pain.[7] Furthermore, these clinical prediction rules have documented sensitivity, specificity, and likelihood values to assist the practitioner in interpreting results.

One frequently cited clinical prediction rule, the Wells Clinical Prediction Rule for Lower Extremity Deep Vein Thrombosis, has undergone extensive validation testing and impact analysis.[8,9] For this clinical prediction rule, there are nine criteria:

1. Active cancer (within 6 months of diagnosis or palliative care)
2. Paralysis, paresis, or recent plaster immobilization of lower extremity
3. Recently bedridden 3 days or major surgery within 4 weeks of application of clinical decision rule
4. Localized tenderness along distribution of the deep venous system
5. Entire lower-extremity swelling
6. Calf swelling by 3 cm compared with asymptomatic lower extremity
7. Pitting edema (greater in the symptomatic lower extremity)
8. Collateral superficial veins (non-varicose)
9. Alternative diagnosis as likely or greater than that of deep vein thrombosis

One point is added to the total score for each of the first eight criteria present, and 2 points are deducted from the total score if the ninth criterion is applicable. Low, moderate, and high risks for lower extremity deep vein thrombosis correspond to scores of ≤ 0, 1–2 points, and ≥ 3 points, respectively.

4. Outcome Measures

Outcome measures are standardized tests, measures, or instruments used to measure various aspects of a patient's health status.[10] Results from outcome measures can be used for patient care decisions, research, and quality assurance. Despite the growing body of evidence to support their use, outcome measures remain underutilized by physical therapists.[11,12] What follows is a review of considerations that the evidence-based practitioner must evaluate when selecting an appropriate outcome measure for their patient. These considerations include dimension, type, format, reliability, validity, responsiveness, and feasibility.[13,14]

Dimension

The *dimension* of an outcome measure refers to different aspects of health status, such as body structure and function, activity, and participation, which are examined by the outcome measure. Some outcome measures examine multiple dimensions, whereas others may focus on a particular dimension. Also, many *types* of outcome measures have been developed, such as those that are region specific (e.g., Lower Extremity Functional Scale),[15] disease, or condition specific (e.g., Western Ontario and McMaster Universities Arthritis Index),[16] patient specific (e.g., Patient Specific Functional Scale),[17] or global (e.g., Global Rating of Change).[18]

Format

The *format* of an outcome measure can be either self-reported or performance-based. For self-reported outcome measures, patients respond verbally or in writing about their self-perception of some aspect of their health status. For example, the SF-36 is a questionnaire that includes items addressing physical function, social function, role function, mental health, energy/fatigue, pain, and general health perception.[19] In contrast, performance-based measures require patients to perform a task that is graded by the physical therapist. One example of a performance-based outcome measure is the Functional Independence Measure,[20] which requires the patient to demonstrate self-care activities, transfers, locomotion, and bowel and bladder function.

Reliability

The *reliability* of an outcome measure refers to its consistency or reproducibility.[21] As the reliability increases, the amount of error inherent in the measurement decreases. There are different types of reliability that affect outcome measures. *Test-retest* refers to the stability of measurements over time. Assuming that the patient's health status has not changed, repeated administrations of an outcome measure should result in the same score. *Intratester* and *intertester* reliability refers to consistency of repeated measures obtained by the same practitioner or between two practitioners, respectively. The test-retest, intratester, and intertester reliability of continuous level data is calculated using *intraclass correlation coefficients,* whereas the *kappa coefficient* is used for categorical level data. Last, the *internal consistency* refers to the degree in which similar items on an outcome measure yield similar scores and is represented by *Chronbach's alpha.*

Validity

Validity, in the context of outcome measures, is the degree to which an outcome measure is measuring what it purports to measure,[21] for example, the degree to which the Berg Balance Scale[22] is actually measuring balance. There are four basic types of validity: face, content, criterion-related, and construct. If the instrument appears to reasonably measure what it purports to measure and makes sense to the patient and practitioner, it is said to have *face validity*. *Content validity* refers to the degree to which items on an outcome measure reflect the relevant dimensions of what is being measured. *Criterion-related validity* refers to the relationship between an outcome measure and a criterion test (i.e., another measure that has already been demonstrated to

be valid), both of which should be measuring the same thing. *Construct validity* refers to the degree to which a theoretical concept is measured by an outcome measure.

The *responsiveness* of an outcome measure refers to its ability to accurately detect a change or difference when it has occurred.[23,24] Commonly reported indexes of responsiveness include the *standard error of the measurement (SEM), minimal detectable change (MDC), and minimal clinically important difference (MCID).*[25] The SEM is a measure of response stability and is related to measurement error. The SEM is used to calculate the MDC, which is the smallest amount of change that is not likely to be due to error in the measurement. The MCID is the smallest amount of change in an outcome measure that the patient perceives to be beneficial. Practitioners should use these indexes of responsiveness when determining if meaningful change occurred on an outcome measure.

Another important consideration when selecting an outcome measure is its *feasibility*.[13,14] Physical therapists must consider the time, space, equipment, training required, cost (e.g., proprietary issues), and accessibility, among other considerations, associated with administering an outcome measure. Furthermore, practitioners should consider the ease with which scores are calculated for an outcome measure.

In this brief review, evidence-based concepts important to the clinical decision making process and progression through the steps of patient management have been discussed. The concepts of specificity, sensitivity, and likelihood ratios have been explained. Both diagnosis and prognosis can be informed by clinical prediction rules, and outcome measures can be used to measure the health status of patients and the effectiveness of physical therapy interventions.

References

1. Simoneau, GG, and Allison, SC: Physical therapists as evidenced-based diagnosticians. JOSPT 40:603, 2010.
2. Sackett, DL, et al: Clinical Epidemiology: A Basic Science for Clinical Medicine, ed 2. Little, Brown, Boston, 1992.
3. Guyatt, G, and Rennie, D: User's Guide to the Medical Literature: A Manual for Evidence-Based Clinical Practice. AMA Press, Chicago, 2002.
4. Fagan, TJ: Nomogram for Bayes's theorem. N Engl J Med 293: 257, 1975.
5. Wainner, RS, et al: Reliability and diagnostic accuracy of the clinical examination and patient self-report measures for cervical radiculopathy. Spine 28:52, 2003.
6. Childs, JD, and Cleland, JA: Development and application of clinical prediction rules to improve decision making in physical therapist practice. Phys Ther 86:122, 2006.
7. Glynn, PE, and Weisbach, PC: Clinical Prediction Rules: A Physical Therapy Reference Manual. Jones & Bartlett, Boston, 2011.
8. Wells, PR, et al: A simple clinical model for the diagnosis of deep-vein thrombosis combined with impedance plethysmography: Potential for an improvement in the diagnosis process. J Intern Med 243:15, 1998.
9. Riddle, DL, and Wells, PS: Diagnosis of lower-extremity deep vein thrombosis in outpatients. Phys Ther 84:729, 2004.
10. Finch, E, et al: Physical Rehabilitation Outcome Measures: A Guide to Enhanced Clinical Decision Making. Lippincott Williams & Wilkins, Hamilton, Ontario, 2002.
11. Copeland, JM, et al: Factors influencing the use of outcome measures for patients with low back pain: A survey of New Zealand physical therapists. Phys Ther 88:1492, 2008.
12. Jette, DU, et al: Use of standardized outcome measures in physical therapist practice: Perceptions and applications. Phys Ther 89:125, 2009.
13. Beattie, P: Measurement of health outcomes in the clinical setting: Applications to physiotherapy. Physiotherapy Theory and Practice 17:173, 2001.
14. Potter, K, et al: Outcome measures in neurologic physical therapy practice: Part 1. Making sound decisions. JNPT 35:57, 2011.
15. Binkley, JM, et al: The Lower Extremity Functional Scale (LEFS): Scale development, measurement properties, and clinical application. Phys Ther 79:383, 1999.
16. Bellamy, N, et al: Validation study of WOMAC: A health status instrument for measuring clinically important patient relevant outcomes to antirheumatic drug therapy in patients with osteoarthritis of the hip or knee. J Rheumatol 15:1833, 1998.
17. Stratford, P, et al: Assessing disability and change on individual patients: A report of a patient specific measure. Physiotherapy Canada 47:258, 1995.

18. Jaeschke, R, et al: Measurement of health status: Ascertaining the minimal clinically important difference. Controlled Clin Trials 10:407, 1989.

19. Ware, JE, and Sherbourne, CD: The MOS 36-item short-form health status survey (SF-36). 1. Conceptual framework and item selection. Med Care 30:473, 1992.

20. Ravaud, JF, et al: Construct validity of the Functional Independence Measure (FIM): Questioning the unidimensionality of the scale and the "value" of FIM scores. Scand J Rehabil Med 31: 31, 1999.

21. Portney, LG, and Watkins, MP: Foundations of Clinical Research: Applications to Practice, ed 3. Pearson Education Inc, Upper Saddle River, NJ, 2009.

22. Berg, K, et al: Measuring balance in the elderly: Preliminary development of an instrument. Physiother Can 41:304, 1989.

23. Beaton, DE, et al: Looking for important changes/differences in studies of responsiveness. J Rheumatol 28:405, 2001.

24. Beninato, M, and Portney, LG: Applying concepts of responsiveness to patient management in neurologic physical therapy. JNPT 35:75, 2011.

25. Haley, SM, and Fragala-Pinkham, MA: Interpreting change scores of tests and measures used in physical therapy. Phys Ther 86:735, 2006.

Chapter 2

Examination of Vital Signs

Thomas J. Schmitz, PT, PhD

LEARNING OBJECTIVES

1. Discuss the rationale for including vital sign measures in the patient examination.
2. Explain the relevance of vital signs data to assigning a diagnostic label, determining the prognosis, and establishing a plan of care.
3. Recognize the importance of vital signs data in determining physiological response to treatment and evaluating patient progress.
4. Describe the procedure for monitoring temperature, pulse, respiration, blood pressure, and hemoglobin oxygenation.
5. Differentiate between normal and abnormal values or ranges for each vital sign.
6. Identify the normative variations in vital signs and the factors that influence these changes.
7. Explain the rationale for using pulse oximetry in the presence of unstable hemoglobin oxygenation levels.
8. Describe the recommended elements for documentation of vital signs data.

CHAPTER OUTLINE

Examination of body temperature, heart (pulse) rate (HR), respiratory rate (RR), and blood pressure (BP) provides the physical therapist with important data about the status of the cardiovascular/pulmonary system. Owing to their importance as indicators of the body's physiological status and response to physical activity, environmental conditions, and emotional stressors, they are collectively referred to as **vital signs.** Because many important clinical decisions are based in part on these measures, accuracy is essential.

The *Guide to Physical Therapist Practice* includes examination of vital signs (HR, RR, and BP) in the cardiovascular/pulmonary systems review for each of the four major categories of practice patterns. Vital signs are also identified among the tests and measures used to characterize or quantify circulatory status. Pulse oximetry is included in the ventilation and respiration/gas exchange category of tests and measures for each of the cardiovascular/pulmonary practice patterns.[1] Although not considered a primary vital sign, **pulse oximetry** is an important related measure that provides information on arterial blood (hemoglobin) oxygen saturation levels. Pulse oximetry data allow the therapist to screen and monitor for *hypoxemia* (decreased oxygen concentrations of atrial blood). Hypoxemia is often associated with pulmonary disorders that impair ventilation of the lungs (e.g., pneumonia, chronic obstructive pulmonary disease [COPD], anemia, respiratory muscle weakness, and circulatory impairments).

Also referred to as *cardinal signs,* vital signs provide quantitative measures of the status of the cardiovascular/pulmonary system and reflect the function of internal organs. Variations in vital signs are a clear indicator that some change in the patient's physiological status has occurred. Taken at rest and during and after exercise, these measures also provide important data on aerobic capacity and endurance. Together with other examination data, vital sign measures assist the physical therapist in making clinical judgments to do the following:[1]

1. Assign a diagnostic label and classify patient findings within a specific practice pattern.
2. Determine the prognosis and plan of care (POC), including identification of anticipated goals and expected outcomes, and selection of specific interventions.
3. Evaluate patient progress through reexamination at periodic intervals during an episode of care.
4. Evaluate the effectiveness of selected interventions in achieving anticipated goals and expected outcomes (changes in impairment, activity limitations, and disabilities and changes in health, wellness, and fitness).
5. Determine if a referral to another practitioner is warranted.

The physical therapist's clinical decision making will determine which vital signs should be measured and the frequency of measurement for an individual patient within a specific context (e.g., self-paced ambulation on level surfaces vs. stair climbing). Although taking vital sign measures may be delegated to a physical therapist assistant (PTA) or other support personnel, the physical therapist will evaluate and determine the significance of the data.

■ NORMATIVE VITAL SIGN DATA

Multiple resources provide normal vital signs values across age groups. Normative data are typically presented as averages or as a range of values for the age group from which they were derived; using a range reflects the variability of values designated as normal. Tables 2.1 and 2.2 are examples of normative vital signs data presented by age using ranges (Table 2.1) and a combination of averages and ranges (Table 2.2).[2,3]

Table 2.1 Comparison of Normal Vital Signs for Various Ages Reported as Ranges

Age	Temperature °F (°C)	Pulse Rate	Respiratory Rate	Blood Pressure (mm Hg)
Newborn	98.6-99.8 (37-37.7)	120-160	30-80	Systolic: 50-52 Diastolic: 25-30 Mean: 35-40
3 yr	98.5-99.5 (36.9-37.5)	80-125	20-30	Systolic: 78-114 Diastolic: 46-78
10 yr	97.5-98.6 (36.3-37)	70-110	16-22	Systolic: 90-132 Diastolic: 5-86
16 yr	97.6-98.8 (36.4-37.1)	55-100	15-20	Systolic: 104-108 Diastolic: 60-92
Adult	96.8-99.5 (36-37.5)	60-100	12-20	Systolic: <120 Diastolic: <80
Older adult	96.5-97.5 (35.9-36.3)	60-100	15-25	Systolic: <120 Diastolic: <80

From Dillon,[2] with permission.

Table 2.2 Comparison of Normal Vital Signs for Various Ages Reported Using a Combination of Averages and Ranges

Age	Temperature Average °F (°C)	Pulse Average (Range) beats per min	Respirations Range breaths per min	Blood Pressure Average mm Hg
Newborn	98.2 (36.8) axillary	120 (70-170)	40-90	80/40
1 to 3 years	99.9 (37.7) rectal	110 (80-130)	20-40	98/64
6 to 8 years	98.6 (37.0) oral	95 (70-110)	20-25	120/56
10 years	98.6 (37.0) oral	90 (70-100)	17-22	110/58
Teen	98.6 (37.0) oral	80 (55-105)	15-20	110/70
Adult	98.6 (37.0) oral	80 (60-100)	12-20	<120/80
Adult older than 70 years	96.8 (36.0) oral	80 (60-100)	12-20	120/80, up to 160/95

From Wilkinson and Van Leuven,[3] with permission.

Clinical Note: Normative vital sign data provide the physical therapist with a *general reference* for comparison during evaluation of clinical findings. It is important to remember that normative values should be used cautiously because some discrepancy exists about the boundaries of normal values.

Normative BP and resting HR data are available from the National Center for Health Statistics (NCHS) Division of Health and Nutrition Examination Surveys (DHNES), part of the Centers for Disease Control and Prevention (CDC), which conducts annual National Health and Nutrition Examination Surveys (NHANES) on various health topics.[4] The NHANES 2001–2008 survey provides data on mean BP for 19,921 adults aged 18 and over.[5] Means of systolic blood pressure (SBP) and diastolic blood pressure (DBP) were reported for adults by multiple variables, including sex and hypertension status (normal, treated, and untreated). Data on mean BP values from this analysis are presented in Figure 2.1 for males and in Figure 2.2 for females. Based on the NHANES 1999–2008 survey data, mean resting HR values are also available, reported by several variables including sex and age using a sample of 35,302 people.[6] These resting pulse rate estimates are presented in Table 2.3 for males and Table 2.4 for females.

It is important to note that *normal* values are specific to an individual. Some individuals typically display values different from those represented by normative data. This illustrates the importance of monitoring vital signs as a sequential process for each patient. Vital sign measurements yield the most useful information when performed and recorded at *periodic intervals over time* as opposed to a single measurement taken at a given point in time. Serial recording allows changes in patient status or response to treatment to be monitored over time and can indicate an acute change in physiological status at a specific point in time (e.g., response to an exercise test).

On examination, initial vital sign measures may be well within normal ranges. In these circumstances, Wilkinson and Treas suggest that one should "not become complacent when a client's vital signs are within normal limits. Although stable vital signs *indicate* physiologic well-being, they do not *guarantee* it. Vital signs alone are limited in detecting some important physiologic changes; for example, vital signs may sometimes remain stable in the presence of moderately large blood loss. Vital signs must be evaluated in the context of your overall assessment of the client."[7, p. 305]

At times, an abnormally high or low value for a vital sign may be obtained. In such situations, it is important to maintain a calm professional demeanor and not adversely react to the information. As discussed later in this chapter, multiple factors can alter vital sign values, including those that are patient related (emotion, stress, excessive caffeine ingestion) and/or practitioner related (e.g., faulty positioning and measurement, incorrect blood pressure cuff size). Any abnormal values should be investigated and, if deemed appropriate, repeated to confirm accuracy.

If repeated measures are required, calmly explain to the patient that you want to verify the values obtained. Alfaro-LeFevre[8, p. 75] offers the following guidelines for validating questionable data:

- Double-check information that is extremely abnormal or inconsistent with patient cues.
- Double-check that equipment is functioning correctly.
- Recheck data obtained (e.g., take BP in opposite arm or 10 minutes later).
- Examine for factors that may alter accuracy (e.g., determine if someone with an elevated temperature and no other symptoms has just had a hot cup of coffee).
- When uncertain, ask a more experienced therapist to recheck a vital sign measure.

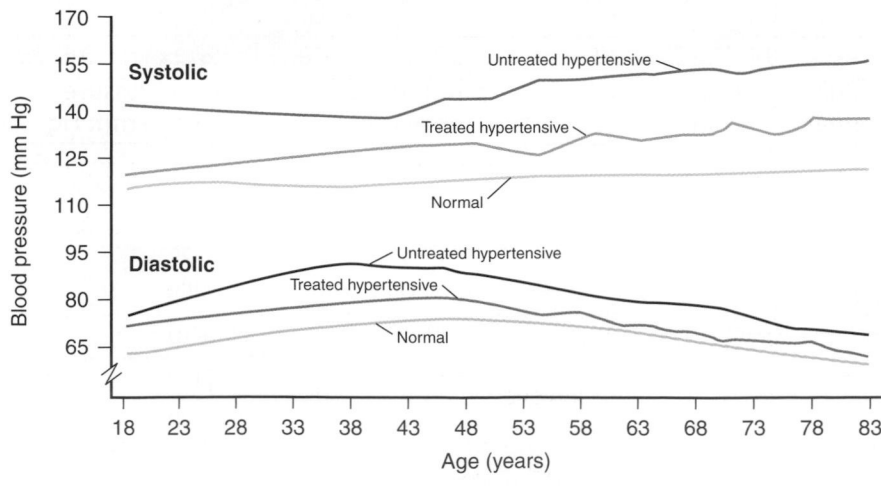

Source: CDC/NCHS, National Health and Nutrition Examination Survey, 2001–2008.

Figure 2.1 Mean systolic and diastolic pressure for men aged 18 years and over, by age and hypertension status. *(From Wright et al.[5])*

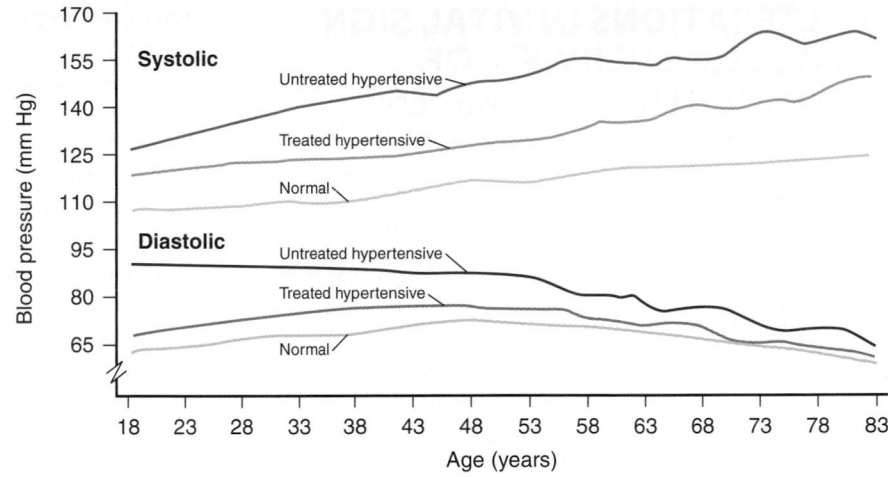

Figure 2.2 Mean systolic and diastolic pressure for women aged 18 years and over, by age and hypertension status. *(From Wright et al.[5])*

Source: CDC/NCHS, National Health and Nutrition Examination Survey, 2001–2008.

• Make a comparison of subjective and objective data to determine if what the patient *states* is consistent with *data obtained* (e.g., compare actual pulse rate with the patient's subjective perceptions of a "racing heart").

Although not a new idea, a *fifth* or even a *sixth* vital sign has been proposed. Perhaps the most common suggestion is adding pain intensity as a fifth vital sign. The American Pain Society (APS) advocates examination of "pain as a fifth vital sign" as a way to increase awareness, to emphasize that pain status is as important as the standard vital signs, and to focus attention on improved management strategies.[9] As part of its National Pain

Management Strategy, the Veterans Health Administration (VHA) has embraced the concept of "pain as the fifth vital sign."[10] The principal goal of this strategy is to provide a single, system-wide standard level of care to minimize suffering from preventable pain, thus moving pain management to a top priority within the system. To raise awareness about critical issues, often for specific populations, the designation "5th or 6th vital sign or *newest vital sign*" has also been applied to various lifestyle factors, patient characteristics, and specific tests and measures, such as emotional stress,[11-13] pulse oximetry,[14,15] health literacy,[16,17] functional status,[18] walking speed,[19] dyspnea,[20] smoking status,[21] and continence.[22]

Table 2.3	Resting Pulse Rate Estimates for U.S. Males, by Age Group National Health and Nutrition Examination Survey, 1999–2008		
Age Group (years)	*n*	Mean	SE Mean
Under 1	972	128	1.1
1	712	116	0.8
2-3	1,148	106	0.4
4-5	864	94	0.6
6-8	1,212	86	0.5
9-11	1,130	80	0.5
12-15	2,190	77	0.4
16-19	2,411	72	0.4
20-39	3,445	71	0.3
40-59	2,559	71	0.3
60-79	1,147	70	0.5
80 and over	197	71	1.1

n = sample size for each age category; SE: standard error. Data exclude persons with a current medical condition or medication use that would affect the resting pulse rate.

Table 2.4	Resting Pulse Rate Estimates for U.S. Females, by Age Group National Health and Nutrition Examination Survey, 1999–2008		
Age Group (years)	*n*	Mean	SE Mean
Under 1	931	130	1
1	633	119	0.8
2-3	1,107	108	0.5
4-5	900	97	0.6
6-8	1,264	88	0.5
9-11	1,236	85	0.5
12-15	2,310	80	0.4
16-19	2,082	79	0.4
20-39	3,061	76	0.3
40-59	2,409	73	0.3
60-79	1,163	73	0.4
80 and over	219	73	0.9

n = sample size for each age category; SE: standard error. Data exclude persons with a current medical condition or medication use that would affect the resting pulse rate.

ALTERATIONS IN VITAL SIGN VALUES: OVERVIEW OF INFLUENTIAL VARIABLES

Lifestyle Patterns and Patient Characteristics

Several lifestyle patterns (modifiable) and patient characteristics (non-modifiable) influence vital sign measures. Lifestyle patterns include, but are not limited to, caffeine intake, tobacco use, diet, alcohol consumption, response to stress, obesity, physical activity level, medications, and use of illegal drugs. Patient characteristics include hormonal status, age, sex, and family history. Other variables that affect vital sign measures include time of day, time of the month (menstrual cycle), general health status, emotional distress, and pain. Information about lifestyle patterns and patient characteristics is gathered from the patient history, the systems review, and tests and measures. Factors identified as modifiable become the focus of patient-related instruction (e.g., current condition, risk factor reduction) and/or health promotion and wellness strategies. Specific factors influencing each vital sign are addressed in greater detail later in the chapter.

Culture and Ethnicity

As with any physical therapy test or measure, the influence of culture and ethnicity on vital sign measures can vary from subtle to marked. For example, a patient who appears anxious or hostile during examination of vital signs may be displaying a response to stress typically shared by others who have a deep-seated distrust of American health care practices. Another example might be a Muslim female patient who exhibits a stress reaction to being examined by a male therapist. These situations can clearly affect the accuracy of the vital sign measures. *Culture* refers to an integration of learned behaviors (not biologically inherited), norms, and symbols characteristic of a society that are passed from generation to generation.[23] It is a set of shared behavioral standards that includes fundamental values, beliefs, attitudes, and customs, including those related to health care and illness.[24-26] *Ethnicity* is defined as an affiliation with a group of people who share a common cultural origin or background, or common racial, national, religious, linguistic, or cultural characteristics.[25] Culture and ethnicity directly affect the attitudes held by an individual toward health care.[27]

Cultural competency in health care can be defined as having the appropriate knowledge and skills to deliver care consistent with a patient's cultural beliefs and practices.[26] Emphasizing the overarching importance of cultural competence, Leavitt proposes that "for physical therapy practitioners, cultural competence is an essential element in making effective and efficient examination, evaluation, diagnosis, prognosis, and intervention

possible. Developing rapport, collecting and synthesizing patient data, recognizing personal functional concerns, and developing the plan of care for a particular patient requires cultural competence."[23, p. 4]

Recent demographic changes in the United States have created greater societal diversity and have heightened the need for culturally competent physical therapists. Data from the 2010 Census demonstrate the evolving diversity of cultures and ethnicities that comprise the U.S. population (Table 2.5).[28] Several salient elements of the data report include the following:

- All major race groups increased in population size between 2000 and 2010, but they grew at different rates.
- The Asian population grew faster than any other major race group between 2000 and 2010.
- More than half the growth in the total population of the United States between 2000 and 2010 was due to an increase in the Hispanic population.
- The only major race group to experience a decrease in its proportion of the total population was the "white alone" population (i.e., those reporting only one race). This group's share of the total population fell from 75% in 2000 to 72% in 2010.

Reflective of the importance of cultural competence in understanding and responding effectively to the cultural needs of patients in health care settings, the U.S. Department of Health and Human Service (USDHHS) Office of Minority Health (OMH) published *Recommended Standards for Culturally and Linguistically Appropriate Health Care Services* with input from a national advisory committee. The proposed standards are offered as guidelines for providers, policymakers, accreditation and credentialing agencies, purchasers of health benefits (including labor unions), patients, and advocates (e.g., local and national ethnic, immigrant, and other community-focused organizations), as well as educators and other members of the health care community.[29]

The American Physical Therapy Association (APTA) has addressed cultural competence in a variety of important documents, including the *Blueprint for Teaching Cultural Competence in Physical Therapy Education*;[30] in the evaluative criteria for accreditation of education programs for the preparation of physical therapists[31] and physical therapist assistant[32] education (Commission on Accreditation of Physical Therapy Education [CAPTE]); and in *A Normative Model of Physical Therapist Professional Education*[33] and *A Normative Model of Physical Therapist Assistant Education.*[34]

Burton and Ludwig[35] offer the following suggestions for interaction with a culturally diverse population:

- Address the patient using his or her surname with appropriate title (Mr., Mrs., Ms., or Miss). First names should be used only with the patient's invitation to do so.

Table 2.5	Population by Hispanic or Latino Origin and by Race for the United States: 2000 and 2010		
Hispanic or Latino Origin and Race	2000 Number (% of Total Population)	2010 Number (% of Total Population)	Change, 2000 to 2010 Number (%)
Total population	281,421,906 (100.0)	308,745,538 (100)	27,323,632 (9.7)
Hispanic or Latino	35,305,818 (12.5)	50,477,594 (16.3)	15,171,776 (43.0)
Not Hispanic or Latino	246,116,088 (87.5)	258,267,944 (83.7)	12,151,856 (4.9)
• White alone	194,552,774 (69.1)	196,817,552 (63.7)	2,264,778 (1.2)
Race			
Total population	281,421,906 (100.0)	308,745,538 (100)	27,323,632 (9.7)
One race	274,595,678 (97.6)	299,736,465 (97.1)	25,140,787 (9.2)
• White	211,460,626 (75.1)	223,553,265 (72.4)	12,092,639 (5.7)
• Black or African American	34,658,190 (12.3)	38,929,319 (12.6)	4,271,129 (12.3)
• American Indian and Alaska Native	2,475,956 (0.9)	2,932,248 (0.9)	456,292 (18.4)
• Asian	10,242,998 (3.6)	14,674,252 (4.8)	4,431,254 (43.3)
• Native Hawaiian and other Pacific Islander	398,835 (0.1)	540,013 (0.2)	141,178 (35.4)
• Some Other Race	15,359,073 (5.5)	19,107,368 (6.2)	3,748,295 (24.4)
Two or More Races*	6,826,228 (2.4)	9,009,073 (2.9)	2,182,845 (32.0)

From U.S. Census Bureau.[28]

*In Census 2000, an error in data processing resulted in an overstatement of the Two or More Races population by about 1 million people (about 15%) nationally, which almost entirely affected race combinations involving Some Other Race. Therefore, data users should assess observed changes in the Two or More Races population and race combinations involving Some Other Race between Census 2000 and the 2010 Census with caution. Changes in specific race combinations not involving Some Other Race, such as White *and* Black or African American or White *and* Asian, generally should be more comparable. (For information on confidentiality protection, nonsampling error, and definitions, see www.census.gov/prod/cen2010/doc/pl94-171.pdf.)

Sources: U.S. Census Bureau, *Census 2000 Redistricting Data (Public Law 94-171) Summary File,* Tables PL1 and PL2, and *2010 Census Redistricting Data (Public Law 94-171) Summary File,* Tables P1 and P2.

• Respect the individual's beliefs and attitudes regarding health care, traditions, and religion.
• Use common proper English; slang terms should be avoided.
• If a language barrier exists, an interpreter should be used (preferably not a family member).
• Eye contact should be used cautiously; some cultures perceive eye contact as disrespectful or a challenge to authority.
• Direct attention to the patient's facial expressions and nonverbal communication, because this may provide clues that your communication is not being understood.
• Seek clarification if you do not understand something that the patient has said.

Cultural competency is addressed in an expanding body of literature. For further examination of the impact of cultural diversity in health care, the reader is referred to the work of Leavitt,[23] Spector,[27] Purnell and Paulanka,[26,36] Galanti,[37] Perez and Luquis,[38] Srivastava,[39] and Kosoko-Lasaki, Cook, and O'Brien.[40]

■ PATIENT OBSERVATION

Observation refers to the deliberate use of the senses (vision, hearing, smell) to gather information about the patient.[7,8] Observation alone will not provide definitive diagnostic information, nor will it allow one to draw conclusions or inferences[35]; however, observation may provide clues to underlying problems,[2] inform development of well-structured impairment-specific questions during history taking, guide selection of screening examinations, and assist with prioritizing tests and measurements.[41]

Using a logical, consistent sequence will create a systematic approach to observation (e.g., first facial expression and overall appearance, then any immediate signs of pain or distress, skin condition, and so forth). This will improve efficiency, conserve time, and help ensure that no areas are overlooked. Several examples follow of the types of information and/or clues to underlying problems that may be gathered via observation.

- Signs of immediate patient distress or discomfort (e.g., pain, grimacing, difficulty breathing) are typically evident by observation of facial expressions, use of accessory muscles for breathing, an irregular or labored breathing pattern, and frequent positional changes. Use of accessory muscles of breathing may be indicative of cardiac or pulmonary impairments.
- Obesity or the presence of **cachexia** (a state of ill health), the appearance of malnutrition, or wasting associated with many chronic diseases may indicate clues about nutritional status. Central obesity (trunk and face) and fat pads near the collarbone and the back of the neck may be associated with Cushing's syndrome.
- *Diaphoresis* (profuse perspiration) may indicate that the body is working to compensate for a reduced cardiac output. It is associated with a variety of potential causes, including myocardial infarct, **hypotension,** and shock; it may also be associated with hyperthermia (e.g., faulty thermoregulation), thyroid hyperactivity, anxiety, and overactive sweat glands. Excessive sweating may also be related to environmental conditions or patient participation in strenuous physical activity prior to visit. The term *hyperhidrosis* also refers to abnormally increased perspiration.
- A disagreeable body odor may suggest poor hygiene (e.g., impaired self-care abilities or lack of resources) or the presence of a wound (e.g., infected drainage) or underlying disease[7]; a fruity breath smell may be suggestive of high blood glucose or diabetic ketoacidosis.[41]
- Various sounds of respiration may be heard, such as wheezing, crackles, or sighs (discussed later in this chapter and in Chapter 12: Chronic Pulmonary Dysfunction). Potential considerations include a narrowed airway (e.g., asthma, congestive heart failure [CHF], tracheal stenosis), COPD, presence of foreign object, or secretions partially blocking an airway.
- The presence of a cough may be caused by a relatively benign airway irritant (e.g., dust particles) or may indicate the presence of a disease such as asthma, bronchitis, COPD, lung cancer, or pneumonia. An acute cough typically resolves within 3 weeks or less (e.g., upper respiratory tract infection). A chronic or persistent cough lasts more than 8 weeks.[42]
- Asymmetry of body parts at rest and during movement may suggest atrophy, hypertrophy, impaired motor function, or underlying disease (e.g., cerebral vascular accident [CVA]). Facial features should also be observed for symmetry.[2,43]

- The skin is the largest organ of the body; observation of skin color provides important preliminary data about the efficiency of the cardiovascular/pulmonary system and may be an indicator of disease, inflammation, and infection.[35,41] **Cyanosis** is a bluish-gray discoloration associated with inadequate oxygenation of the blood (i.e., hemoglobin does not contain normal levels of oxygen). **Central cyanosis** causes diffuse skin color changes in "central" aspects of the body (e.g., trunk, head) as well as color changes in the mucous membranes.[44] These membranes are normally pink and shiny irrespective of skin color. Central cyanosis indicates marked arterial desaturation and occurs when oxygen saturation is less than 80% (normal is 95% to 100%).[2] It is associated with diseases of the cardiovascular/pulmonary system and carbon monoxide poisoning. **Peripheral cyanosis** causes color changes in the nail beds and lips owing to decreased cardiac output, exposure to cold (vasoconstriction), or arterial or venous obstruction. It is frequently transient and is often relieved by warming the area. Common skin color changes with associated causes are presented in Box 2.1.
- The skin should also be observed for changes in texture and hair growth. Patients with diabetes mellitus or atherosclerosis typically lack hair growth on the legs and display thickening of the nails of the fingers and toes. Skin texture also varies with age and poor nutritional status. Skin lesions may be indicative of pathological changes or trauma.
- The color and appearance of fingernails should be noted. With normal circulation and oxygen supply, they should be pink (or light brown in dark-skinned individuals) and free of irregularities. Examples of pathological changes in nails include the following:
  - *Beau's lines* are deep grooved (indented) transverse lines across the nail resulting from disruption of nail growth caused by trauma or disorders such as Raynaud's disease (decreased blood flow to fingers), psoriasis, or infection around the nail plate.
  - *Black nails* are caused by blood under the nail; usually the result of trauma.
  - *Clubbing* is a bulbous swelling of fingertips accompanied by a loss of the normal angle between the nail bed and the skin (Fig. 2.3); nails appear bluish-gray (cyanotic) and become soft and boggy (spongy). Clubbing develops gradually over time and is associated with diagnoses imposing long-standing **hypoxia,** such as congenital heart defects and cardiopulmonary diseases.
  - *Half-and-half nails* (also called *Lindsay's nails*) are seen with renal failure; the distal portion of the nail turns red, pink, or brown; there is a distinct line of demarcation between the two halves.
  - *Onycholysis* is detachment of the nail from the nail bed; associated with trauma, fungal infections, psoriasis, and overactive thyroid gland.

Box 2.1   Common Skin Color Changes

- **Cyanosis:** Bluish-gray discoloration of the skin and mucous membranes.
  - **Central cyanosis:** Caused by hypoxia and results in color changes in central aspects of body and mucous membranes; associated with diseases of the cardiovascular/pulmonary system.
  - **Peripheral cyanosis:** Caused by hypoxia with color changes in the nail beds and lips; associated with decreased cardiac output and exposure to cold (extreme vasoconstriction).
- **Ecchymosis:** Caused by bruising (bleeding under the skin) and may be seen anywhere on the body; new bruises appear *bluish-purple* while older bruises are *greenish-yellow*; often caused by trauma (e.g., falls, sports injury, physical abuse); patients on blood thinning agents (e.g., Coumadin) tend to bruise more easily.
- **Erythema:** Reddened area of skin caused by increased blood flow (hyperemia); associated with skin irritation or injury, infection, and inflammation; redness over a bony prominence warns of the potential development of a decubitus ulcer.
- **Flushing:** Diffuse redness of face; may involve other body areas; related to emotions (embarrassment, anger), physical exertion, fever, and increased temperature of environment.
- **Jaundice:** Caused by impaired liver function (e.g., hepatitis, liver cancer), the skin takes on a yellow-orange hue; it is best observed in the sclera, mucous membranes, and palm of hands and sole of the feet.
- **Pallor (pale):** The skin takes on a lighter tone (more white with decreased pink hue) than normal for the individual (a normally "fair" skin color should be ruled out); for darker skin, pallor is apparent by loss of red tones; associated with anemia (low hemoglobin) and impaired circulation; observed in the face, palms, mucous membranes, and nail beds.
- **Petechiae:** Tiny red or purple hemorrhagic spots caused by capillary bleeding with subsequent leakage of blood into the skin; tend to appear in clusters and often seen on the ankles and feet but can occur anywhere on body; may be a sign of thrombocytopenia (low platelet count); as platelets play a critical role in clotting, reduced counts impair clotting and increase the risk of bleeding; low platelet counts are associated with a variety of medications (e.g., anticoagulants, aspirin, steroids, and chemotherapy drugs) and disorders (e.g., acute and chronic infections, leukemia, systemic lupus erythematosus, and scleroderma).

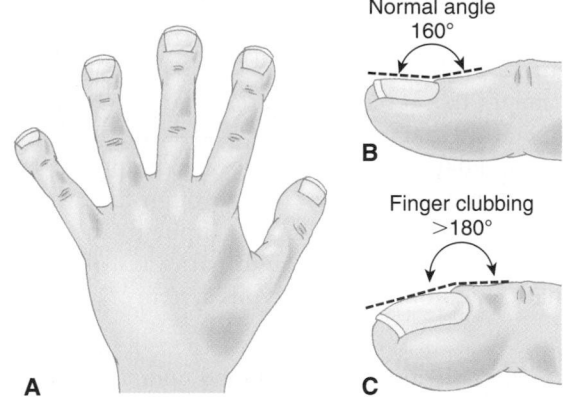

Figure 2.3 (A) Clubbing of fingertips is associated with long-term hypoxic states; **(B)** normal nail plate angle of 160°; **(C)** a nail plate angle of 180° or more occurs with clubbing.

- *Mee's lines* are transverse white lines across the breadth of the nail associated with systemic diseases such as renal failure, Hodgkin's disease, malaria, and sickle cell anemia; classically associated with arsenic poisoning.
- *Pitting* is characterized by tiny punctate depressions in the nail caused by systemic diseases such as Reiter's syndrome, psoriasis, and eczema.
- *Splinter hemorrhages* are tiny hemorrhages creating reddish lines of blood under the nail (appears as if a "splinter" is lodged under nail) associated with bacterial endocarditis and trauma.
- Abnormal sitting postures may be suggestive of pain or structural abnormalities of the pelvis (pelvic obliquity), pectoral, or vertebral regions that may also interfere with respiratory patterns.
- Edema may be associated with CHF, liver failure, lymphedema, or venous insufficiency; localized edema may result from varicose veins, thrombophlebitis, or trauma.

■ TEMPERATURE

Body temperature represents a balance between the heat produced or acquired by the body and the amount lost. Because humans are warm blooded, or *homoiothermic*, body temperature remains relatively constant despite changes in the external environment. This is in contrast to cold-blooded, or *poikilothermic*, animals (such as reptiles), in which body temperature varies with that of their environment.

Thermoregulatory System

The purpose of the thermoregulatory system is to maintain a relatively constant internal body temperature. This system monitors and acts to maintain temperatures that are optimal for normal cellular and vital organ function. The thermoregulatory system consists of three primary components: the thermoreceptors, the regulating center, and the effector organs (Fig. 2.4).[45,46]

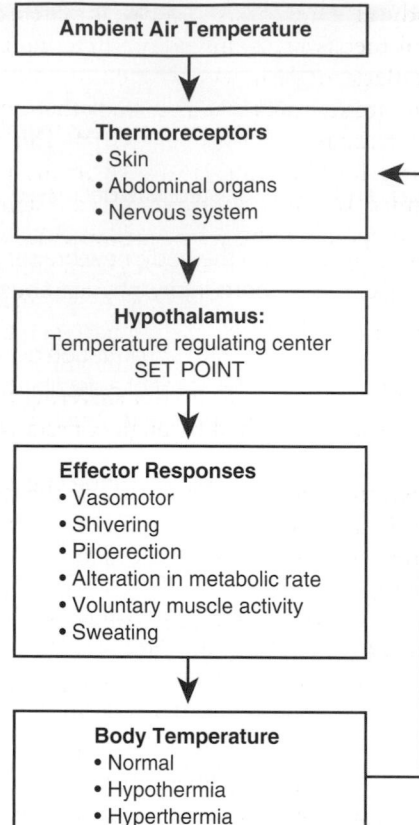

Figure 2.4 Thermoregulatory responses. The thermoreceptors provide input regarding changes in body temperature that signal the preoptic nucleus of the hypothalamus. This physiological thermostat compares incoming signals of actual body temperature with the set point value. If body temperature is lower than the set point value, heat gain mechanisms are implemented. If body temperature is higher than the set point value, heat loss mechanisms are implemented.[45,46]

Thermoreceptors

The thermoreceptors provide input to the temperature-regulating center located in the hypothalamus. The regulating center is dependent on information from thermoreceptors to achieve constant temperatures. Once this information reaches the regulatory center, it is compared with a "set point" standard or optimal temperature value. Depending on the contrast between the "set" value and incoming information, mechanisms may be activated either to conserve or to dissipate heat.[47]

Peripheral and central thermoreceptors provide afferent temperature input to the regulating center. The peripheral receptors (skin temperature), composed primarily of free nerve endings, have a high distribution in the skin. Central thermoreceptors (core temperature) are located in the deep tissues (e.g., abdominal organs), nervous system, and the hypothalamus itself.[47,48] The thermoreceptors located in the hypothalamus are sensitive to temperature changes

in blood perfusing the hypothalamus. These cells also can initiate responses to either conserve or dissipate heat. They are particularly sensitive to core temperature changes and monitoring body warmth.[45] The thermoreceptors permit *feed forward* responses to expected changes in core temperature (e.g., change in environmental temperature).

The cutaneous peripheral thermoreceptors demonstrate a larger distribution of cold receptors than warmth receptors and are sensitive to rapid changes in temperature.[45] Signals from these receptors enter the spinal cord through afferent nerves and travel to the hypothalamus via the lateral spinothalamic tract.

Regulating Center

The temperature-regulating center of the body is located in the hypothalamus. The hypothalamus coordinates the heat production and loss processes, much like a thermostat, ensuring an essentially constant, stable body temperature. By influencing the effector organs, the hypothalamus achieves a relatively precise balance between heat production and heat loss. In a healthy individual, the hypothalamic thermostat is set and carefully maintained at 98.6° ± 1.8°F (37° ± 1°C).[45] In situations in which input from thermoreceptors indicates a drop in temperature below the "set" value, mechanisms are activated to conserve heat. Conversely, a rise in temperature will activate mechanisms to dissipate heat. Mechanisms to dissipate heat are particularly important during strenuous exercise. Figure 2.5 summarizes the primary physiological adjustments to exercise or increases in environmental temperature that occur during heat acclimation (physiological adaptations to improve tolerance to heat). These responses are activated through hypothalamic control of the effector organs. Input to the effector organs is transmitted through pathways of both the somatic and autonomic nervous systems.[45,46,49,50]

Effector Organs

The effector organs respond to both increases and decreases in temperature. The primary effector systems include vascular, metabolic, skeletal muscle (shivering), and sweating. These effector systems function either to increase or to dissipate body heat.

Conservation and Production of Body Heat

When body temperature is lowered, mechanisms are activated to conserve heat and increase heat production. The following are descriptions of heat conservation and production mechanisms:

- *Vasoconstriction of Blood Vessels:* The hypothalamus activates sympathetic nerves, an action that results in vasoconstriction of cutaneous vessels throughout the body. This significantly reduces the lumen of the vessels and decreases blood flow near the surface of

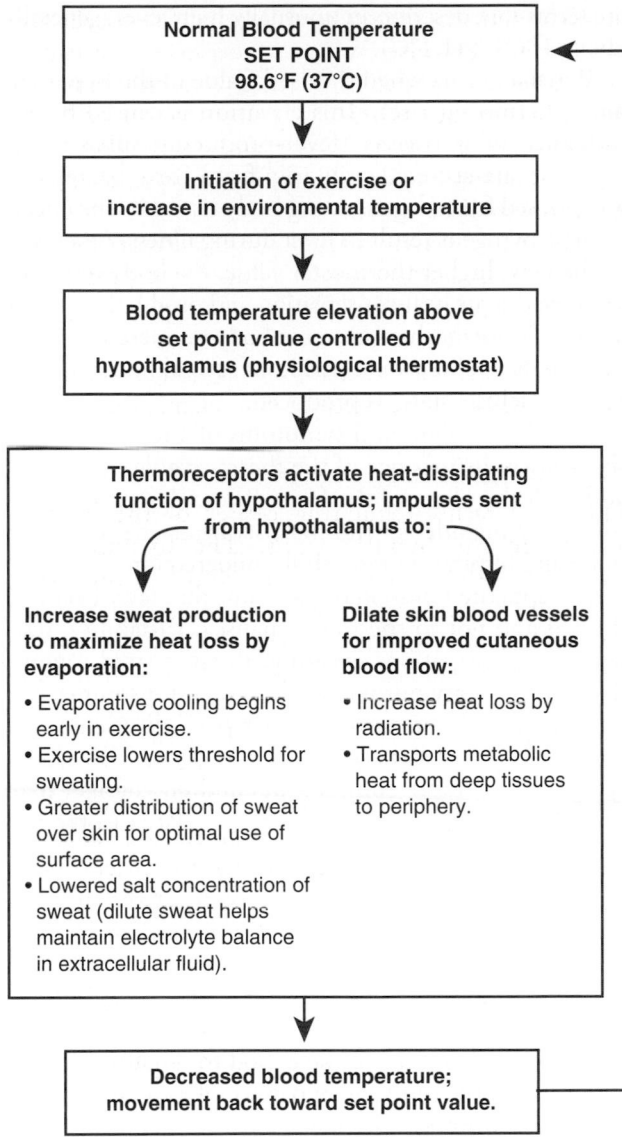

```
┌─────────────────────────────┐
│   Normal Blood Temperature   │ ◄──────┐
│        SET POINT             │         │
│      98.6°F (37°C)           │         │
└─────────────────────────────┘         │
              │                          │
              ▼                          │
┌─────────────────────────────┐         │
│   Initiation of exercise or  │         │
│ increase in environmental    │         │
│      temperature             │         │
└─────────────────────────────┘         │
              │                          │
              ▼                          │
┌─────────────────────────────┐         │
│ Blood temperature elevation  │         │
│   above set point value      │         │
│  controlled by hypothalamus  │         │
│ (physiological thermostat)   │         │
└─────────────────────────────┘         │
              │                          │
              ▼                          │
┌───────────────────────────────────┐   │
│ Thermoreceptors activate heat-     │   │
│ dissipating function of            │   │
│ hypothalamus; impulses sent        │   │
│        from hypothalamus to:       │   │
│   ┌───────┘         └───────┐      │   │
│   ▼                         ▼      │   │
│ Increase sweat          Dilate skin│   │
│ production to           blood      │   │
│ maximize heat           vessels for│   │
│ loss by                 improved   │   │
│ evaporation:            cutaneous  │   │
│                         blood flow:│   │
│ • Evaporative           • Increase │   │
│   cooling begins          heat loss│   │
│   early in exercise.      by       │   │
│ • Exercise lowers         radiation.│  │
│   threshold for         • Transports│  │
│   sweating.               metabolic │  │
│ • Greater distribution    heat from │  │
│   of sweat over skin      deep      │  │
│   for optimal use of      tissues to│  │
│   surface area.           periphery.│  │
│ • Lowered salt                      │  │
│   concentration of sweat            │  │
│   (dilute sweat helps               │  │
│   maintain electrolyte              │  │
│   balance in extracellular          │  │
│   fluid).                           │  │
└───────────────────────────────────┘   │
              │                          │
              ▼                          │
┌─────────────────────────────┐         │
│ Decreased blood temperature; │─────────┘
│ movement back toward set     │
│      point value.            │
└─────────────────────────────┘
```

Figure 2.5 Physiological adjustments during heat acclimation. Increased body temperature activities heat (loss) dissipation to maintain normal body temperature.

the skin, where the blood would normally be cooled. Thus, the amount of heat lost to the environment is decreased.

- *Decrease (or Absence) of Sweat Gland Activity:* To reduce or to prevent heat loss by evaporation, sweat gland activity is diminished. Sweating is totally abolished with cooling of the hypothalamic thermostat below approximately 98.6°F (37°C).[45,51]
- *Cutis Anserina or Piloerection*: Also a response to cooling of the hypothalamus, this heat conservation mechanism is commonly described as "gooseflesh." The term *piloerection* means "hairs standing on end." Although of less significance in humans, this mechanism functions to trap a layer of insulating air near the skin and decrease heat loss in lower mammals with greater hair covering.

The body also responds to decreased temperature with several mechanisms, including shivering and hormonal regulation, designed to produce heat. These mechanisms are activated when the body thermostat falls below approximately 98.6°F (37°C).[51] The primary motor center for shivering is located in the posterior hypothalamus. This area is activated by cold signals from the skin and spinal cord. In response to cold, impulses from the hypothalamus activate the efferent somatic nervous system, causing increased tone of skeletal muscles. As the tone gradually increases to a certain threshold level, *shivering* (involuntary muscle contraction) is initiated, and heat is produced. This shivering reflex can be at least partially inhibited through conscious cortical control.[51]

The function of hormonal influence in thermal regulation is to increase cellular metabolism, which subsequently increases body heat. Increased metabolism occurs through circulation of two hormones from the adrenal medulla: *norepinephrine* and *epinephrine*. Circulating levels of these hormones, however, are of greater significance in maintaining body temperature in infants than in adults. Heat production by these hormones can be increased in an infant by as much as 100%, as opposed to 10% to 15% in an adult.[51]

A second form of hormonal regulation involves increased output of *thyroxine* by the thyroid gland. Thyroxine increases the rate of cellular metabolism throughout the body. This response, however, occurs only as a result of prolonged cooling, and heat production is not immediate.[45] The thyroid gland requires several weeks to hypertrophy before increased demands for thyroxine can be achieved.

Loss of Body Heat

Excess heat is dissipated from the body through four primary methods: radiation, conduction, convection, and evaporation.

- *Radiation:* The transfer of heat by electromagnetic waves from one object to another is accomplished by radiation. This heat transfer occurs through the air between objects that are not in direct contact. Heat is lost to surrounding objects that are colder than the body (e.g., a wall or surrounding objects in the room).
- *Conduction:* The transfer of heat from one object to another through a liquid, solid, or gas takes place by conduction. This type of heat transfer requires direct molecular contact between two objects, as when a person is sitting on a cold surface, or when heat is lost in a cool swimming pool. Heat is also lost by conduction to air.
- *Convection:* The transfer of heat by movement of air or liquid (water) is achieved by convection. This form of heat loss is accomplished *secondary to conduction*. Once the heat is conducted to the air, the air is then moved away from the body by convection currents. Use of a fan or a cool breeze

provides convection currents. Heat loss by convection is most effective when the air or liquid surrounding the body is continually moved away and replaced.

- *Evaporation:* Dissipation of body heat by the conversion of a liquid to a vapor occurs by evaporation. This form of heat loss occurs on a continual basis through the respiratory tract and through perspiration from the skin. Evaporation provides the major mechanism of heat loss during heavy exercise. Profuse sweating provides a significant cooling effect on the skin as it evaporates. In addition, this cooling of the skin functions to further cool the blood as it is shunted from internal structures to cutaneous areas. Figure 2.6 illustrates the mechanisms of heat dissipation from the body.

Abnormalities in Body Temperature
Increased Body Temperature

An elevation in body temperature is generally believed to assist the body in fighting disease or infection. *Pyrexia* is the elevation of normal body temperature, more commonly referred to as fever. *Hyperpyrexia* and *hyperthermia*

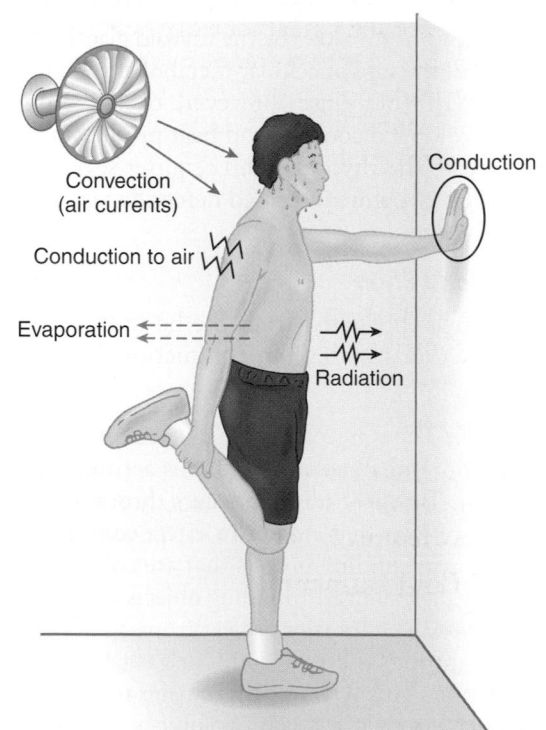

Figure 2.6 Mechanisms of heat dissipation from body. *Conduction* is the transfer of heat by direct contact between two objects (hand on wall), *radiation* occurs through electromagnetic waves between objects not in direct contact with each other (subject's body and wall), heat loss by *convection* is accomplished via air currents (wall fan) after the heat is conducted to air, *evaporation* converts liquid (perspiration) to a vapor.

Labels in figure: Convection (air currents); Conduction to air; Evaporation; Conduction; Radiation

are terms that describe an unusually high fever, generally above 106°F (41.1°C).[51]

Pyrexia occurs when the "set" value of the hypothalamic thermostat rises. This elevation is caused by the influence of **pyrogens** (fever-producing substances). Pyrogens are secreted primarily from toxic bacteria or are released from degenerating body tissue.[46] The effects of these pyrogens result in fever during illness. As a result of the new, higher thermostat value, the body responds by activating its heat conservation and production mechanisms. These mechanisms raise body temperature to the new, higher value over a period of several hours. Thus a fever, or febrile state, is produced.

The clinical signs and symptoms of a fever vary with the level of disturbance of the thermoregulatory center, and with the phase of the fever. These signs and symptoms may include general malaise, headache, increased pulse and respiratory rate, chills, piloerection, shivering, loss of appetite (**anorexia**), pale skin that later becomes flushed and hot to the touch, nausea, irritability, restlessness, constipation, sweating, thirst, coated tongue, decreased urinary output, weakness, and insomnia.[35,52] With higher elevations in temperature, disorientation, confusion, convulsions, or coma may occur. These latter symptoms are more common in children younger than 5 years of age and are believed to be related to the immaturity of the nervous system.

The *prodromal phase* is the period just prior to onset of fever; nonspecific symptoms may be experienced, such as a slight headache, muscles aches, general malaise, or loss of appetite. Three phases (stages) have been identified to describe a fever, as follows:

- *Phase 1—Onset:* This is the period from either gradual or sudden rise until the maximum temperature is reached; symptoms include chills, shivering, and pale appearance of skin. As body temperature is raised (e.g., in response to infection), cutaneous vasoconstriction moves blood to the interior of the body to retain heat. The skin becomes cool, and shivering is initiated to produce more heat. Attempts to preserve and produce heat continue until a new, higher temperature is reached.
- *Phase 2—Course:* This is the point of highest elevation of the fever. Once the new higher temperature is reached, it remains relatively stable (fever is sustained); heat production and heat loss are equal and shivering stops; skin may be warm and appear flushed.
- *Phase 3—Termination (defervescence):* This is the period during which the fever subsides and temperatures lower and move toward normal. Cutaneous vasodilation occurs, and sweating is initiated to help cool the body.

Several types of fevers present unique characteristics that are named based on their distinguishing clinical feature: *intermittent, remittent, relapsing,* or *constant* (Box 2.2).

Box 2.2 Types of Fever

Intermittent: Body temperature alternates at regular intervals between periods of fever and periods of normal temperatures.
Remittent: Elevated body temperature that fluctuates more than 3.6°F (2°C) within a 24-hour period but remains above normal.
Relapsing: Periods of fever are interspersed with normal temperatures; each last at least one day; also called *recurrent* fever.
Constant: Body temperature may fluctuate slightly but is constantly elevated above normal.

Decreased Body Temperature

Exposure to extreme cold produces a lowered body temperature called **hypothermia**. With prolonged exposure to cold, there is a decrease in metabolic rate, and body temperature gradually falls. As cooling of the brain occurs, there is a depression of the thermoregulatory center. The function of the thermoregulatory center becomes seriously impaired when body temperature falls below approximately 94°F (34.4°C) and is completely lost with temperatures below 85°F (29.4°C).[47] Therefore, the body's heat regulatory and protection mechanism is lost. Symptoms of hypothermia include decreased HR and RR, cold and pale skin, cyanosis, decreased cutaneous sensation, depression of mental and muscular responses, and drowsiness, which may eventually lead to coma. If hypothermia is left untreated, the progression of these symptoms may lead to death.

Factors Influencing Body Temperature

A statistical average or normal temperature of 98.6°F (37°C) taken orally has been established for body temperature in an adult population. However, a range of values is more representative of normal body temperature because certain everyday circumstances (e.g., time of day) or activities (e.g., exercise) influence the body's temperature. In addition, some individuals typically run a *slightly higher* or *lower* body temperature than the statistical average. Therefore, deviations from the average will be apparent from individual to individual, as well as between measures taken from the same person under varying circumstances.

Time of Day

The term **circadian rhythm** describes a 24-hour cycle of normal variations in body temperature. Certain predictable and regular changes in temperature occur on a daily basis. Body temperature tends to be lowest between 4 and 6 a.m., and highest between 4 and 8 p.m. Both digestive processes and the level of skeletal muscle activity influence these regular changes in body temperature significantly. For individuals who work at night, this pattern is usually inverted.[45,47]

Age

Compared with adults, infants demonstrate a higher normal temperature owing to the immaturity of the thermoregulatory system. Infants are particularly susceptible to environmental temperature changes, and their body temperature will fluctuate accordingly. Young children also average higher normal temperatures because of the heat production associated with increased metabolic rate and high physical activity levels. Elderly populations tend to demonstrate lower than average body temperatures, owing to a variety of factors, including lower metabolic rates, decreased subcutaneous tissue mass (which normally insulates the body against heat loss), decreased physical activity levels, and inadequate diet.

Emotions/Stress

Stimulation of the sympathetic nervous system causes increased production of epinephrine and norepinephrine with a subsequent increase in metabolic rate.

Exercise

The effects of exercise on body temperature are an important consideration for physical therapists. Strenuous exercise significantly increases body temperature because of an increase in metabolic rate. Active muscle contractions are an important and potent source of heat production. During exercise, body temperature increases are proportional to the relative intensity of the workload. Vigorous exercise can increase the metabolic rate by as much as 20 to 25 times that of the basal level.[45]

Menstrual Cycle

Increased levels of progesterone during ovulation cause body temperature to rise 0.5° to 0.9°F (0.3° to 0.5°C). This slight elevation is maintained until just prior to the initiation of menstruation, at which time it returns to normal levels.

Pregnancy

Because of increased metabolic activity, body temperature remains elevated by approximately 0.9°F (0.5°C). Temperature returns to normal after parturition.

External Environment

Generally, warm weather tends to increase body temperature, and cold weather decreases body temperature. Environmental conditions influence the body's ability to maintain constant temperatures. For example, in hot, humid environments the effectiveness of evaporative cooling is severely diminished because the air is already heavily moisture laden. Other forms of heat dissipation are also dependent on environmental factors such as movement of air currents (convection). Clothing also can be an important external consideration because it can function either to conserve and to facilitate release of body heat. The amount and type of clothing is important. To dissipate heat, absorbent, loose-fitting, light-colored clothing is most effective. To conserve heat, several layers of lightweight clothing to trap air and to insulate the body are recommended.

Measurement Site

Body temperatures vary among body parts. Rectal and tympanic (ear) membrane temperatures are from 0.5° to 0.9°F (0.3° to 0.5°C) higher than oral temperatures; axillary temperatures are approximately 1.1°F (0.6°C) lower than oral temperatures. The normative value for oral temperature in a healthy adult population is generally considered to be 98.6°F (37.0°C), and for rectal and tympanic membrane temperatures the value is 99.5°F (37.5°C). Being an external measure, the axillary normative value is somewhat lower at 97.6°F (36.5°C).

Ingestion of Warm or Cold Foods

Oral temperatures will be affected by oral intake, including smoking. Patients should refrain from smoking or eating for at least 15 minutes (preferably 30 minutes) prior to an oral temperature reading.

Types of Thermometers

Glass Mercury Thermometers

Traditionally, temperatures have been taken using a glass thermometer, which consists of a glass tube with a bulbous tip filled with mercury. Once the bulb is in contact with body heat, the mercury expands and rises in the glass column to register body temperature. A narrowing of the base prevents reflux of mercury down the tube. The device must be shaken vigorously to return the mercury to the bulb before the next use.

Glass thermometers are calibrated in centigrade (Celsius [C]) scale, Fahrenheit (F) scale, or both. The range is from approximately 93° to 108°F (34° to 42.2°C), with slight variations among different manufacturers. The calibrations are in degrees and tenths of a degree. As such, each long line represents a full degree, and each short line indicates 0.1° on the centigrade thermometer and 0.2° on the Fahrenheit thermometer. When recording temperatures, it is common practice to round the fractions of degrees to the nearest whole number (one tenth of a degree on the Fahrenheit scale). If a situation occurs that requires changing a temperature reading from one scale to the other, a conversion formula can be used. To convert centigrade into Fahrenheit, multiply the centigrade value by 9/5 and add 32 (F = [9/5 × C°] + 32°). To change from Fahrenheit into centigrade, subtract 32 from the Fahrenheit value and multiply by 5/9 (C = [F − 32°] × 5/9). Figure 2.7 presents a comparison of Fahrenheit and centigrade temperature values with ranges of normal and altered body temperature.

The distal tip (bulb) of the glass mercury thermometer is used for insertion and is long and slender or has a more blunt, round shape (Fig. 2.8). The long slender shape is used for oral temperatures and is designed with a larger surface area to maximize tissue contact with the oral mucosa. The more blunted, round bulb is used for

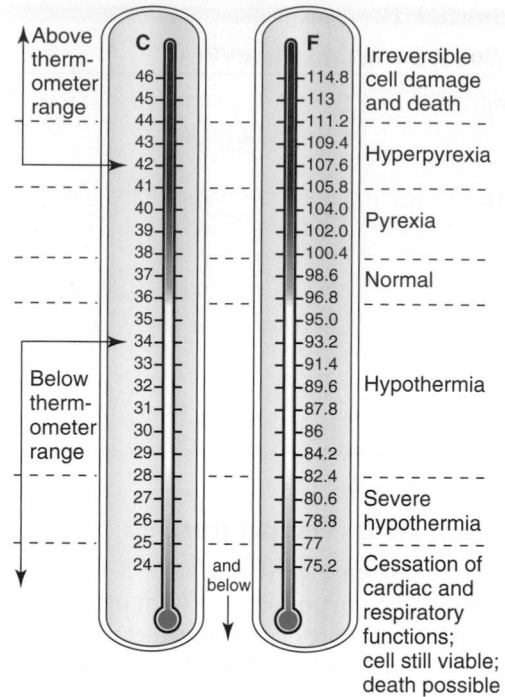

Figure 2.7 Comparison of Fahrenheit and Centigrade scales indicating ranges of normal and altered body temperature. *(From Wilkinson and Treas,[7 p. 319], with permission.)*

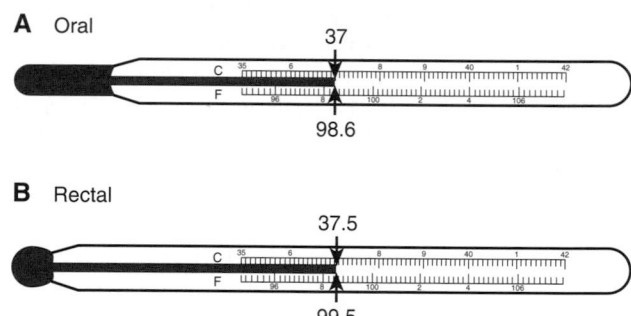

Figure 2.8 Shape of tips (bulbs) on mercury glass thermometers. The long slender shape **(A)** is for oral use and the blunt round shape **(B)** is for rectal measures.

rectal temperatures and is designed to minimize trauma to the rectal mucosa. The oral thermometer can also be used for axillary temperatures. The tips of mercury glass thermometers may also be color coded (*blue* for oral and *red* for rectal).

Although glass mercury thermometers may remain in use in the home care setting, automated (electronic) thermometers have largely replaced their use in patient care settings owing to environmental concerns of mercury pollution from breakage and medical waste disposal systems.[43] The U.S. Environmental Protection Agency (EPA) warns against use of mercury thermometers and encourages replacement with non-mercury thermometers wherever possible. Some states have laws restricting the manufacture and sale of mercury thermometers. Many areas also offer collection/exchange programs for mercury-containing devices.[53]

Automated Thermometers

Automated thermometers are widely used in patient care settings. They provide a rapid (several seconds), highly accurate measure of body temperature. Standard clinical automated thermometers consist of a portable battery-operated unit, an attached probe, and plastic disposable probe covers (Fig. 2.9A). The units provide a digital display of body temperature. An important advantage of these thermometers is the low chance of cross-infection, so long as the probe covers are used only once. Other automated devices are designed to monitor more than one vital sign and interface directly with the electronic medical record (EMR), reducing the potential for error associated with manual documentation (Fig. 2.9B).

Oral Thermometers

Handheld automated oral thermometers are readily available commercially. These units are typically about

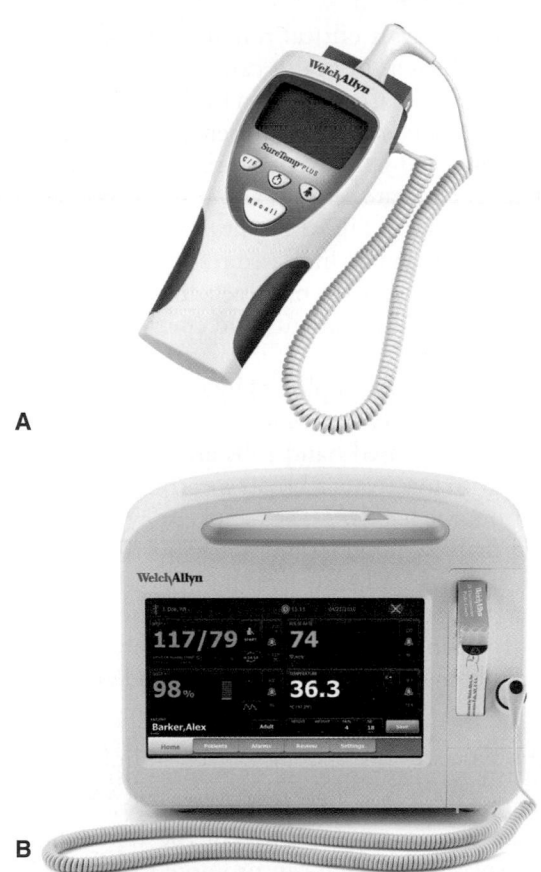

Figure 2.9 (A) Hand-held electronic thermometer with disposable probe covers reduces the risk of cross-contamination. **(B)** This device interfaces with the electronic medical record (EMR). By scanning the patient's hospital identification bracelet, two-way wireless communication links ID numbers to patient names for positive identification at the bedside. The unit measures temperature, blood pressure, and oxygen saturation levels (pulse oximetry). The device reduces time required and potential errors of manual documentation as data are relayed directly to the EMR. Manual data may also be entered (e.g., respiratory rate). *(Courtesy of Welch Allyn, Skaneateles Falls, NY 13153-0220.)*

5 inches in length with a tapered design (Fig. 2.10). One end of the device has a narrow tip and serves as the probe; in some models the tip is flexible. The opposite end is broad and houses the battery. These thermometers also provide a flashed, digital display of body temperature; most models have memory capabilities. Typically these devices are used for a single patient; however, many models allow use with disposable probe covers.

Tympanic Thermometer

Another type of automated thermometer is the tympanic (ear) infrared thermometer. These thermometers measure body temperature through a sensor probe placed in the ear that detects infrared radiation from the tympanic membrane.[54,55] This location provides an important reflection of core temperature because the tympanic membrane receives its blood supply from a tributary of the internal carotid artery, which supplies the hypothalamus (temperature-regulating center). These handheld portable thermometers include an ear probe (used with a single-use disposable cover) and provide a digital display of body temperature within several seconds (Fig. 2.11A). They are particularly useful with infants older than 2 months and children who may have difficulty remaining still during other types of monitoring and in emergency situations where rapid temperature values are required. A tympanic thermometer should never be used in the presence of a draining or infected ear.[55]

Temporal Artery Thermometer

Noninvasive temporal artery thermometers measure body temperature by sliding a probe from the center of the forehead, across the temporal artery area to the hairline (Fig. 2.11B). It detects heat emitting from the skin surface over the temporal artery. The probe can be cleaned with an alcohol swab or used with disposable probe caps. Temporal artery measures have been found to be more precise and more accurate than axillary or ear-based measures.

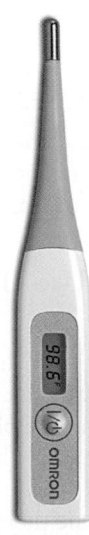

Figure 2.10 Hand-held automated oral thermometer. *(Courtesy of Omron, Inc., Lake Forest, IL 60045.)*

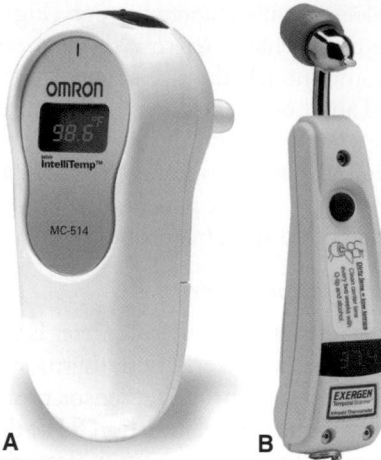

Figure 2.11 (A) Tympanic (ear) thermometer. This thermometer incorporates a sensor that detects infrared radiation from the tympanic membrane (eardrum) and converts the warmth into a digital temperature reading. *(Courtesy of Omron, Inc., Lake Forest, IL 60045.)* **(B)** Temporal artery thermometer. As a measurement site, the temporal artery is easily accessible and poses low risk of injury as there is no contact with mucous membranes. *(Courtesy of Exergen Corporation, Watertown, MA 02472.)*

Box 2.3 Evidence Summary presents studies examining the reliability and validity of measuring body temperature.

Other variations of automated thermometers place the sensor in earlobe clips, finger sleeves, or finger clips, and still others are noncontact. Infrared (IR) noncontact thermometers measure temperature using a surface area, typically the forehead. Because these thermometers do not touch the patient, there is no risk of contamination. Based on manufacturer's specifications, IR thermometers are held several inches from the forehead and provide a body temperature reading with approximately 0.3-degree accuracy. They are frequently used with infants and children and for initial fever screenings. However, their usefulness for fever screening of outpatients has been called into question because the gradient between surface and core temperature is considerably influenced by the patient's age and environmental factors.[56] Some IR thermometers are calibrated to convert the forehead measure into internal (core) temperature. Digital nipple-shaped pacifier designs are also available for monitoring oral temperatures of infants.

Disposable Single-Use Thermometers
Oral Thermometers
These devices are used in a similar fashion to the glass mercury thermometer because they are placed under the tongue. They consist of a thin plastic with a series of raised calibrated dots impregnated with a temperature-sensitive chemical (Fig. 2.12). The dots change color to indicate the temperature. After the thermometer is removed from the mouth, the dots are examined for color changes to determine the temperature reading (Fig 2.13). They are available in both Fahrenheit and Celsius scales and are disposed of after use. Although most commonly used for oral temperatures, disposable thermometers can also be used to obtain axillary temperatures, and some are available with covers (sheaths) containing semirigid stays that allow use for rectal measurements.

Skin Surface Thermometers
Heat-sensitive strips (tape, patches, or disks) provide a general measure of body surface temperature. They also respond to body temperature by changing color and are more frequently used with children. They must be applied to dry skin. The forehead and abdomen are common placement sites. The temperature readings are nonspecific and are usually confirmed with a more precise measuring instrument if deviations are noted.

Hand Hygiene
Hand hygiene plays a critical role in preventing transmission of pathogens in health care settings. According to the World Health Organization (WHO), *health care–associated infection (HCAI)* represents a major patient safety concern, and its prevention should be a top priority in all patient care settings and institutions. WHO states, "The impact of HCAI implies prolonged hospital stay, long-term disability, increased resistance of microorganisms to antimicrobials, massive additional financial burden, high costs for patients and their families, and excess deaths."[57, p. 6]

Hand hygiene is accomplished by *hand washing* using soap and water or *hand rubbing* using an alcohol-based formula. Alcohol-based hand rubs are an efficient and effective way to inactivate a broad spectrum of microorganisms from the hands.[57] The factors on which WHO has based its recommendations for hand rubs are presented in Box 2.4. When using an alcohol-based hand rub, enough product should be used to cover all hand surfaces. The hands are then rubbed together until dry. The hand rubbing technique is illustrated in Figure 2.14.

When one is using soap and water, enough product should be used to cover all hand surfaces. Clean running water assists with removal of microorganisms, and a warm temperature removes less protective oil from the hands than hot water. The force of the water should not cause splashing, which can promote the transfer of microorganisms. Care should be taken not to lean against the sink to avoid contact with a potentially contaminated area. The technique for hand washing is presented in Figure 2.15.

To draw attention to the indications for hand hygiene and its practical application, WHO has developed "My Five Moments for Hand Hygiene." The five moments are (1) before touching the patient; (2) before a clean/aseptic procedure; (3) after body fluid exposure risk; (4) after touching a patient; and (5) after touching patient surroundings.[57]

Box 2.3 Evidence Summary   Studies Examining the Reliability and Validity of Measuring Body Temperature

Reference	Method(s)	Subjects/Design	Results	Conclusions/Comments
Rubia-Rubia et al (2011)	To compare the axilla (using Gallium-in-glass[a]), reactive strip, compact electronic, electronic with probe, ear-based (infrared), and frontal forehead scan (infrared) to the pulmonary artery core temperature (Temp) using a Swan-Ganz catheter[b]	Older adults in an intensive care unit (ICU) (n = 201). All Temp methods were compared to the core Temp simultaneously.	The Gallium-in-glass in the axilla for 5 and 12 minutes, compact digital, digital with probe and ear-based (infrared, core equivalency) were among the most valid methods. The Gallium-in-glass in the right axilla for 5 and 12 minutes were the most reliable methods. The reactive strip, compact digital, and digital probe were the most accurate methods.	When methods were ranked based on validity, reliability, accuracy, and external influence the Gallium-in-glass in the axilla for 12 minutes attained the highest score. When also considering waste, ease-of-use, speed, durability, security, comfort and cost the compact digital and digital with probe, both in the axilla, scored the highest.
Kelechi et al (2011)	To compare skin Temp 8 cm above the right malleolus using the infrared contact thermometer[c] and the thermistor-type thermometer[d]	Healthy adults (n = 17). Temp was taken three times with 10 minutes between each recording.	Strong correlations between the infrared contact thermometer and thermistor-type thermometer were found at baseline ($r = 0.95$), after 10 minutes of rest ($r = 0.97$), and after 10 minutes of cold provocation ($r = 0.87$). There was a reasonable level of agreement between methods at baseline and after 10 minutes of rest, but not after cold provocation.	In summary, the results suggest better agreement between infrared contact and thermistor-type thermometers than within each method except after cold provocation.
Smitz et al (2009)	To compare and correlate two different infrared ear thermometers with a rectal Temp (electronic probe)	Older adult inpatients (n = 100). The order of thermometer type and side (right vs. left) used were randomized. Two measures taken for each device and each side. The highest ear Temp from each device used for analysis.	For both infrared ear thermometers: • The mean Temp was significantly higher than the rectal Temp. • There was a high correlation between both ear Temps and the rectal Temp ($r = 0.84-0.91$).	Either infrared thermometer can be used to predict rectal Temps in inpatients who are normothermic and febrile.

Continued

Box 2.3 Evidence Summary   Studies Examining the Reliability and Validity of Measuring Body Temperature—cont'd

Reference	Method(s)	Subjects/Design	Results	Conclusions/Comments
Duncan et al (2008)	To compare oral and core Temps (temp-sensing urinary catheter) to infrared over the patient's forehead	Adult patients in the emergency department (ED) (oral) ($n = 74$) and ICU (core Temp) ($n = 19$). The three Temps were taken within 2 minutes.	High correlation ($r = 0.94$) between first and second infrared measurements. Between the infrared and oral methods, there was a poor correlation ($r = 0.26$), poor agreement (mean difference between pairs = 0.87°C), and significant difference. Between the infrared and core methods, there was a high correlation ($r = 0.83$); there was also poor agreement and a significant difference between methods.	The infrared method was reliable and easy to use. There was poor agreement between the infrared method and (a) oral and (b) core methods. The infrared method provided lower readings than the oral and core methods.
Giantin et al (2008)	Gallium-in-glass under axilla without nurse assistance was compared to the axilla (electronic thermometer), tympanic (infrared) and Gallium-in-glass under axilla methods with nurse assistance.	Hospitalized older adults ($n = 107$). All temps were taken by the same nurse. All temps were taken at least three times daily at different times and on different days.	There were significant differences between the Gallium-in-glass under axilla with nurse assistance method and Gallium-in-glass under axilla without nurse assistance and tympanic (infrared) methods. There was no significant difference between Gallium-in-glass under axilla with nurse assistance and the tympanic methods and extremely narrow limits of agreement.	The Gallium-in-glass under axilla without nurse assistance method is inadequate for older adults. The tympanic method, however, provides adequate accuracy in this population.
Lawson et al (2007)	To compare oral (electronic), ear-based (infrared tympanic), temporal (infrared scanner), and axillary (electronic) to pulmonary artery (Swan-Ganz catheter[a])	Adult patients in the ICU ($n = 60$). Temps taken in random order within 1 minute. Temp was taken three times every 20 minutes.	Mean (SD) offset with pulmonary artery Temp and confidence limits: • Oral = 0.09°C (0.43°C) and -0.75°C to 0.93°C • Ear-based = -0.36°C (0.56°C) and -1.46° to 0.74°C • Temporal = -0.02°C (0.47°C) and -0.92° to 0.88°C • Axillary = 0.23°C (0.44°C) and -0.64° to 1.12°C	Oral and temporal methods were most precise and accurate. Axillary measurements underestimated pulmonary artery Temp. Ear-based measurements were the least accurate and precise.

Box 2.3 Evidence Summary   Studies Examining the Reliability and Validity of Measuring Body Temperature—cont'd

Reference	Method(s)	Subjects/Design	Results	Conclusions/Comments
Moran et al (2007)	To compare tympanic (infrared), urinary (Temp-sensing catheter), and axillary (glass mercury thermometer) to pulmonary artery core Temp (Swan-Ganz catheter)	Older adults in an ICU ($n = 110$). The Temp was measured every 4 hours for the first 72 hours and then every 6 hours for an additional 48 hours.	Concordance of pulmonary artery Temps with tympanic, urinary, and axillary Temps was 0.77, 0.92, and 0.83, respectively.	In critically ill patients, measuring core Temp using a urinary catheter is the most reasonable alternative to the pulmonary artery method.
Fountain et al (2008)	To compare an oral disposable thermometer, tympanic thermometer, and temporal (infrared) thermometer to an oral electronic thermometer	Adults in an inpatient oncology unit ($n = 60$). The order of the oral disposable thermometer, tympanic thermometer, and temporal (infrared) thermometer was randomized. The oral electronic device was always last.	Bias (and precision) was reported as 0.39 (1.01) for the tympanic device, 0.00 (0.92) for the disposable oral device, and 0.68 (0.99) for the temporal artery. Significant differences were found between the oral electronic device and the tympanic and temporal artery devices. No difference was found between the oral electronic and oral disposable thermometers.	Since Temp results are fairly similar, oral disposable thermometers can be used when oral electronic thermometer use is not feasible.

Prepared by Kevin K. Chui, PT, PhD, GCS, OCS.

[a]Gallium-in-glass thermometer: These thermometers are like the mercury thermometers, but have replaced the mercury with galinstan, a liquid alloy of gallium, indium, and tin.

[b]Swan-Ganz catheter: A flexible catheter inserted in the pulmonary artery to measure temperature as well as other hemodynamic characteristics.

[c]Infrared contact thermometer: Is used to detect the energy emitted from the body part.

[d]Thermistor-type thermometer: Is a semiconductor device used to measure temperature.

Rubia-Rubia, J, Arias, A, and Aguirre-Jaime, A: Measurement of body temperature in adult patients: Comparative study of accuracy, reliability and validity of different devices. Int J Nurs Stud 48:872, 2011.

Kelechi, TJ, Good, A, and Mueller, M: Agreement and repeatability of an infrared thermometer. J Nurs Meas 19:55, 2011.

Smitz, S, Van de Winckel, A, and Smitz MF: Reliability of infrared ear thermometry in the prediction of rectal temperature in older patients. J Clin Nurs 18:451, 2009.

Duncan, AL, Bell, AJ, Chu, K, Greenslade, JH: Can a non-contact infrared thermometer be used interchangeably with other thermometers in an adult Emergency Department? AENJ 11(3):130, 2008.

Giantin, V, Toffanello, ED, Enzi G, et al: Reliability of body temperature measurements in hospitalised older patients. Journal of Clinical Nursing 17:1518, 2008.

Lawson, L, Bridges, EJ, Ballou, I, et al: Accuracy and precision of noninvasive temperature measurement in adult intensive care patients. Am J Crit Care 16:485, 2007.

Moran, JL, Peter, JV, Solomon, PJ, et al: Tympanic temperature measurements: Are they reliable in the critically ill? A clinical study of measurements of agreement. Crit Care Med 35:155, 2007.

Fountain, C, Goins, L, Hartman, M, Phelps, N, Scoles, D, Hays, V, et al: Evaluating the accuracy of four temperature instruments on an adult inpatient oncology unit. Clin J Oncol Nurs 12:983, 2008.

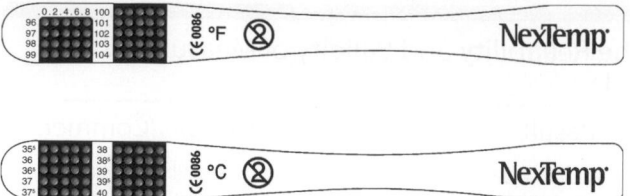

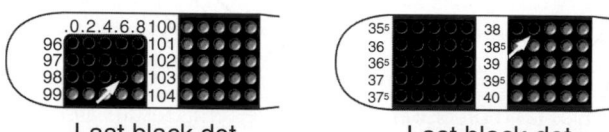

Last black dot
shows 98.6°F

Last black dot
shows 38.1°C

Figure 2.12 Disposable single-use thermometer in Fahrenheit *(top)* and Centigrade *(bottom)* scales. *(Courtesy of Medical Indicators, Inc., Pennington, NJ 08534.)*

Figure 2.13 The chemical dots on the disposable single-use thermometers change color from green to black to reflect the temperature (Fahrenheit, *left,* and Centigrade, *right*). The green dots turn black from left to right. The last dot to turn black indicates the temperature. Note there are two grids of dots on each scale (*left* and *right*). Values that fall in the right grid indicate fever is present. In the example on the right, 38.1°C (100.5°F) represents fever. *(Courtesy of Medical Indicators, Inc., Pennington, NJ 08534.)*

Box 2.4 Factors Considered by WHO in Recommending Hand Rubs

WHO recommends alcohol-based hand rubs based on the following factors:

1. Evidence-based, intrinsic advantages of fast-acting and broad-spectrum microbicidal activity with a minimal risk of generating resistance to antimicrobial agents
2. Suitability for use in resource-limited or remote areas with lack of accessibility to sinks or other facilities for hand hygiene (including clean water, towels, and so forth)
3. Capacity to promote improved compliance with hand hygiene by making the process faster and more convenient
4. Economic benefit by reducing annual costs for hand hygiene, representing approximately 1% of extra costs generated by health care–associated infection (HCAI)
5. Minimization of risks from adverse events because of increased safety associated with better acceptability and tolerance than other products

From WHO,[57] p. 57, with permission.

Clinical Note: Before a vital sign measure is taken, the procedure and its rationale should be explained in terms appropriate to the patient's understanding and confirmation made of patient safety, comfort, and understanding.

Measuring Body Temperature

For purposes of establishing baseline data and determining response to treatment, physical therapists generally use oral monitoring. Oral temperatures are contraindicated for patients with *dyspnea* or who are mouth breathers, have had oral surgery, or have a history of epilepsy or are prone to seizures. They also should not be used with infants or small children or patients who are irrational, unconscious, or uncooperative. In situations in which oral temperatures may be contraindicated and an automated unit with an alternative sensor (e.g., earlobe clip, finger sleeve) is unavailable, an axillary measurement may be substituted.

Measuring Oral Temperature: Automated Thermometer

A. Assemble equipment.
  1. An automated thermometer with disposable probe covers or sheaths. Oral temperature can also be taken with a glass mercury thermometer (Appendix 2.A) or a disposable single-use thermometer.
     Note: Hand-held automated oral thermometers are self-contained with an internal battery; the proximal end houses the digital display and battery, and the distal end serves as the temperature probe.
  2. Watch (or wall clock).
B. Wash hands.
C. Procedure.
  1. Turn on the power.
  2. Grasp the proximal aspect of the thermometer with the thumb and forefinger and attach the disposable cover over the distal probe tip until it snaps or locks in place. (Some units have a proximal button that releases the probe cover after temperature reading is complete.) For a small handheld automated unit, the probe covers are designed as a plastic sheath.
  3. Ask patient to open his or her mouth, and place the covered probe at the posterior base of the tongue to the right or left of the frenulum in the sublingual pocket. This placement positions the tip of the thermometer over superficial blood vessels that reflect core body temperature. Instruct the patient to close the lips (not teeth) around the thermometer. Continue to hold the

Hand Hygiene Technique with Alcohol-Based Formulation

🕐 **Duration of the entire procedure:** 20-30 seconds

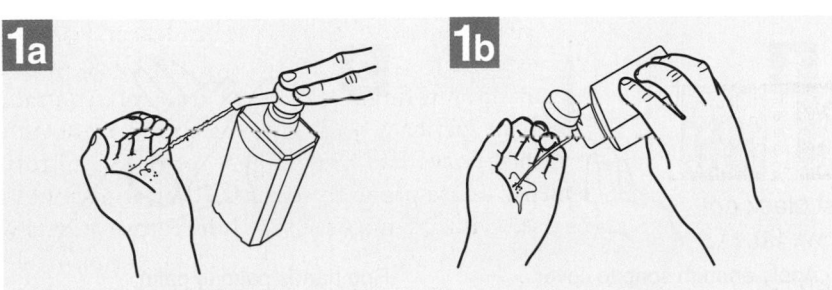

Apply a palmful of the product in a cupped hand, covering all surfaces;

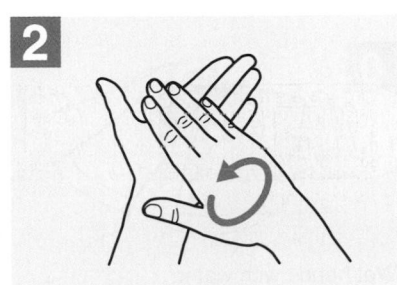

Rub hands palm to palm;

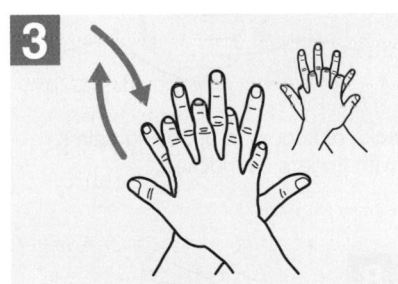

Right palm over left dorsum with interlaced fingers and vice versa;

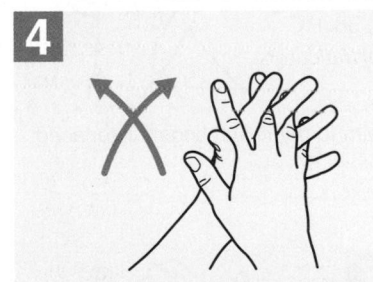

Palm to palm with fingers interlaced;

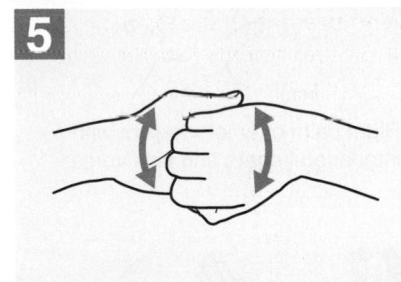

Backs of fingers to opposing palms with fingers interlocked;

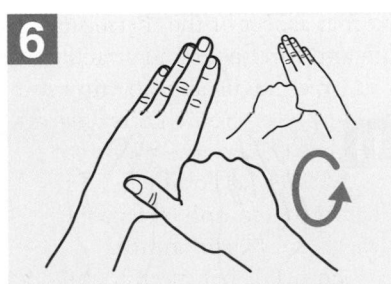

Rotational rubbing of left thumb clasped in right palm and vice versa;

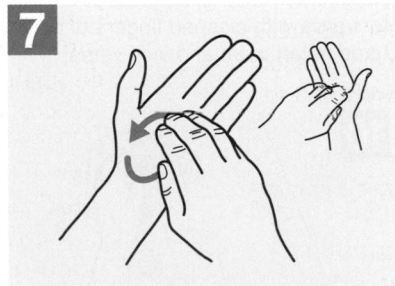

Rotational rubbing, backwards and forwards with clasped fingers of right hand in left palm and vice versa;

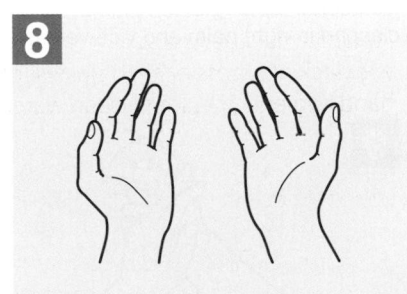

Once dry, your hands are safe.

Figure 2.14 Hand rubbing technique. *(From WHO,[57 p. 155], with permission.)*

Hand Hygiene Technique with Soap and Water

🕐 **Duration of the entire procedure: 40-60 seconds**

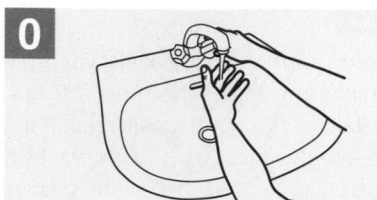

Wet hands with water;

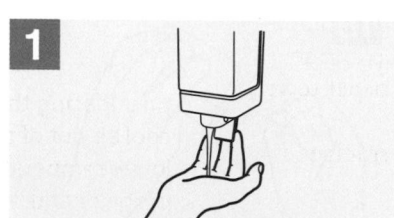

Apply enough soap to cover all hand surfaces;

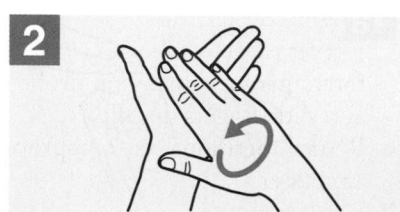

Rub hands palm to palm;

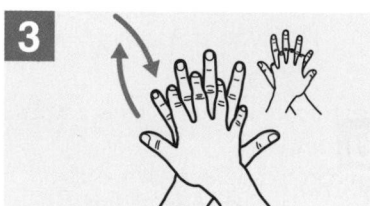

Right palm over left dorsum with interlaced fingers and vice versa;

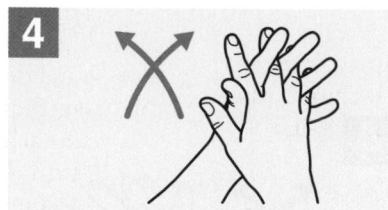

Palm to palm with fingers interlaced;

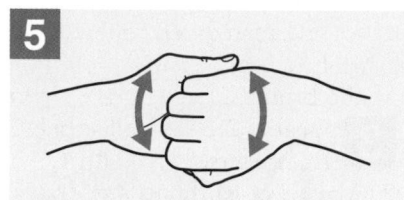

Backs of fingers to opposing palms with fingers interlocked;

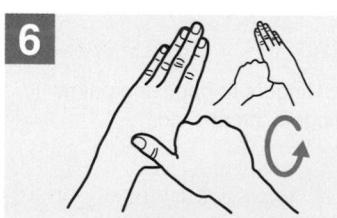

Rotational rubbing of left thumb clasped in right palm and vice versa;

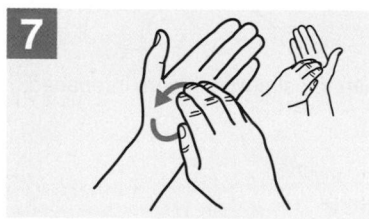

Rotational rubbing, backwards and forwards with clasped fingers of right hand in left palm and vice versa;

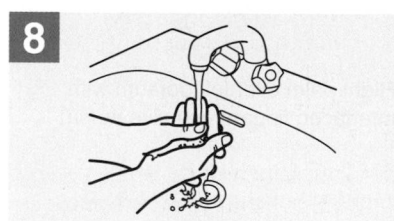

Rinse hands with water;

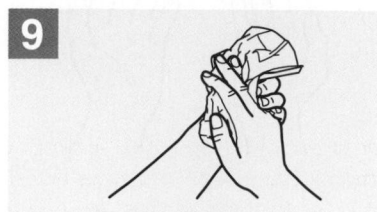

Dry hands thoroughly with a single use towel;

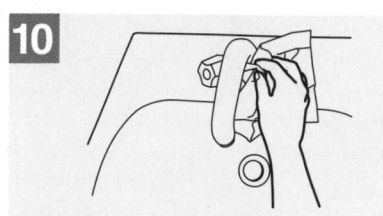

Use towel to turn off faucet;

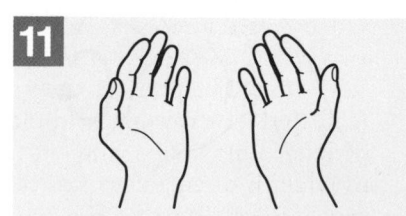

Your hands are now safe.

Figure 2.15 Hand washing technique. *(From WHO,[57 p. 156], with permission.)*

probe in place, because the weight of the probe may displace it from the sublingual pocket.

4. Hold the probe in the sublingual pocket until an audible beep is heard (several seconds). The beep indicates maximum temperature has been reached. Remove the probe from the patient's mouth and note the temperature reading on the digital display for recording.

5. Remove the probe cover over a waste receptacle for disposal. If available on the unit, use the probe release mechanism; if a plastic sheath cover is used, use a clean paper towel for removal. (Cover sheath with paper towel, place thumb and forefinger proximally on probe over paper towel, and slide fingers distally.)

6. Return thermometer to appropriate storage container.

7. Wash hands.

Measuring Axillary Temperature: Automated Thermometer

A. Assemble equipment.

1. An automated thermometer with disposable probe covers or sheaths. Axillary temperatures can also be measured with glass mercury thermometers (Appendix 2.B) as well as disposable single-use thermometers.

2. A towel or gauze pads to dry axillary region. (Moisture will conduct heat.)

3. Watch (or wall clock).

B. Wash hands.

C. Procedure.

1. Expose the axilla, and ensure that area is dry. If any moisture is present, the area should be gently towel dried with a patting motion. (Vigorous rubbing will increase temperature of the area.)

2. Turn on the power.

3. Grasp the proximal aspect of the thermometer with the thumb and forefinger, and attach the disposable cover or sheath over the distal probe tip.

4. With the patient in supine position, place the tip of the thermometer in the center of the axillary region between the trunk and upper arm (Fig. 2.16). The patient's upper extremity (UE) should be placed tightly across the chest to keep the thermometer in place. (Asking the patient to move the hand toward the opposite shoulder is often a useful direction.) If the patient is disoriented or very young, the thermometer must be held in place. Axillary temperature can also be taken in a sitting position, but this carries the risk of the thermometer dropping to the floor.

5. The thermometer is left in place until an audible beep is heard (several seconds). The beep indicates that maximum temperature has been

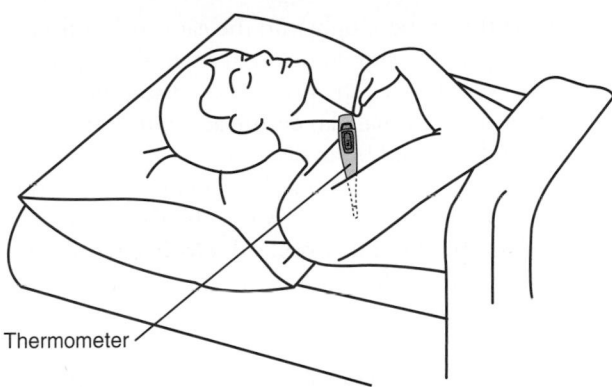

Thermometer

Figure 2.16 Positioning for monitoring axillary temperature. Placing the patient's arm across the chest forces cool air out of the axilla that could potentially result in a lower temperature value. This positioning also places the probe near the vascular supply to the axilla. The proximal portion of the thermometer should be angle toward the patient's head.

reached. Remove the probe from the patient's axilla, and note the temperature reading on the digital display for recording.

6. Remove the probe cover or sheath over a waste receptacle for disposal.

7. Return thermometer to appropriate storage container.

8. Wash hands.

Note: Generally, a temperature reading is assumed to be an oral measure unless otherwise noted. Axillary values are designated by a circled A after the temperature or the designation "AT" for *axillary temperature* (e.g., 95°F AT). Similarly, the designation RT (*rectal temperature*) or a circled R after the value indicates a rectal measure (e.g., 99°F ®).

Measuring Tympanic Membrane Temperature: Automated (Ear) Thermometer

A. Assemble equipment.

1. Tympanic (infrared) thermometer. (Many units include a storage base and a protective cap that fits over the probe tip.)

2. Disposable probe covers.

B. Wash hands.

C. Procedure.

1. Attach the disposable cover to the probe, holding it with the thumb and forefinger. (Ensure that the firm circular collar of the cover engages with the base by gently pushing it down; do not touch the plastic film of the probe cover.)

2. Turn the patient's head to one side. For adults, pulling on the pinna (auricle) may help straighten the ear canal and provide better access. For an adult, the pinna is pulled up and back; for a child, it is pulled down and back.[35,55]

3. Insert the probe snugly into the ear canal. A firm gentle pressure should be used; avoid forcing the probe too deeply. The probe should seal the opening of the ear canal. To ensure accurate reading, the probe should be angled anteriorly toward the jawline, as if approaching the patient from behind.
4. Press the button that activates the thermometer. The temperature is displayed within several seconds. Many units emit an audible beep or flashing light when the maximum temperature is reached.
5. Gently remove the probe from the ear. Eject or remove the probe cover over a waste receptacle for disposal. Manual removal of the probe cover should be done using a clean paper towel or tissue.
6. Return tympanic thermometer to protective case.
7. Wash hands.

■ PULSE

The *pulse* is the wave of blood in the artery created by contraction of the left ventricle during a cardiac cycle (one complete cycle of cardiac muscle contraction and relaxation). With each contraction, blood is pumped into an already full aorta. The inherent elasticity of the aortic walls allows expansion and acceptance of the new supply. The blood is then forced out and surges through the systemic arteries. It is this wave or surge of blood that is felt as the pulse. The strength or amplitude of the pulse reflects the amount of blood ejected with each myocardial contraction (stroke volume).

Peripheral pulses are those located in the periphery of the body that can be felt by palpating an artery over a bony prominence or other firm surface. Examples of peripheral pulses include the radial, carotid, and popliteal pulses. The *apical pulse* is a central pulse located at the apex of the heart that is monitored using a stethoscope.

Pressure changes in the large arteries during the cardiac cycle are reflected in the relatively smooth and rounded appearance of the normal arterial waveform (Fig. 2.17 [top]). The lowest point of pressure occurs during ventricular **diastole,** while the highest point occurs during ventricular systole (peak ejection). The notch on the descending slope of the pulse wave represents closure of the aortic valve and is not palpable.[58] A healthy adult heart beats an average of 70 times per minute, a rate that provides continuous circulation of approximately 5 to 6 liters of blood through the body. The pulse can be palpated wherever a superficial artery can be stabilized over a bony surface. In monitoring the pulse, specific attention is directed toward determining three parameters: *rate, rhythm,* and *quality*.

Rate

The HR is the number of pulsations (peripheral pulse waves) or frequency per minute. **Bradycardia** is an abnormally slow HR, less than 60 beats per minute. **Tachycardia** is an excessively high HR, greater than 100 beats per minute. *Palpitation* refers to the sensation of a rapid or irregular HR perceived by the patient without actually palpating a peripheral pulse. Multiple factors influence the HR, including age, sex, emotional status, stress, and physical activity level. Body size and stature also influence HR. Tall, thin individuals generally have a slower HR than those who are obese or have stout frames.

Rhythm

The pulse *rhythm* is the pattern of pulsations and the intervals between them. In a healthy individual, the rhythm is regular and indicates that the time intervals between pulse beats are essentially equal. *Arrhythmia* or *dysrhythmia* refers to an irregular rhythm in which pulses are not evenly spaced. An irregular rhythm may present as premature, late, or missed pulse beats, or random, irregular beats in either a predictable or an unpredictable pattern.[59] Irregular rhythms are often associated with conduction abnormalities or an impulse originating from a site other than the sinoatrial node.[60] See Chapter 13: Heart Disease, for further discussion.

Quality

The *quality* (force, volume) of the pulse refers to the amount of force created by the ejected blood volume against the arterial wall during each ventricular contraction. In examining the quality of the pulse, the therapist is determining the feel of the blood as it passes through a vessel. The quantity (volume) of blood within the vessel produces the force of the pulse. Normally, the pulse volume of each beat is the same. The force of the pulse is greater with a higher blood volume, and weaker with a lower blood volume. The volume is examined by noting how easily the pulse can be obliterated. A normal pulse is described as full or strong and can be palpated using moderate pressure of the fingers over a bony landmark. With lower volumes, the pulse is *small,* is easily obliterated, and is termed *weak* or *thready*. With increased volume, the pulse is *large,* is difficult to obliterate, and is termed a *bounding* (or *full*) pulse; a feeling of high tension is noted. A numerical scale is often used to document the quality (strength) of the pulse (Table 2.6).

In addition to rate, rhythm, and quality, the feel of the arterial wall under the examiner's fingertips should be determined. Normally, a vessel will feel smooth, elastic, soft, flexible, and relatively straight. With advancing age, vessels may demonstrate sclerotic changes. These changes frequently cause the vessels to feel twisted, hard, or cordlike, with decreased elasticity and smoothness.

Several other important terms are used to describe variations in pulse. The term *bigeminal* is used to describe an abnormality in pulse rhythm where two beats occur in rapid succession (double systolic peak). *Pulsus alterans* (alternating pulse) is marked by a fluctuation

Description	Possible Cause

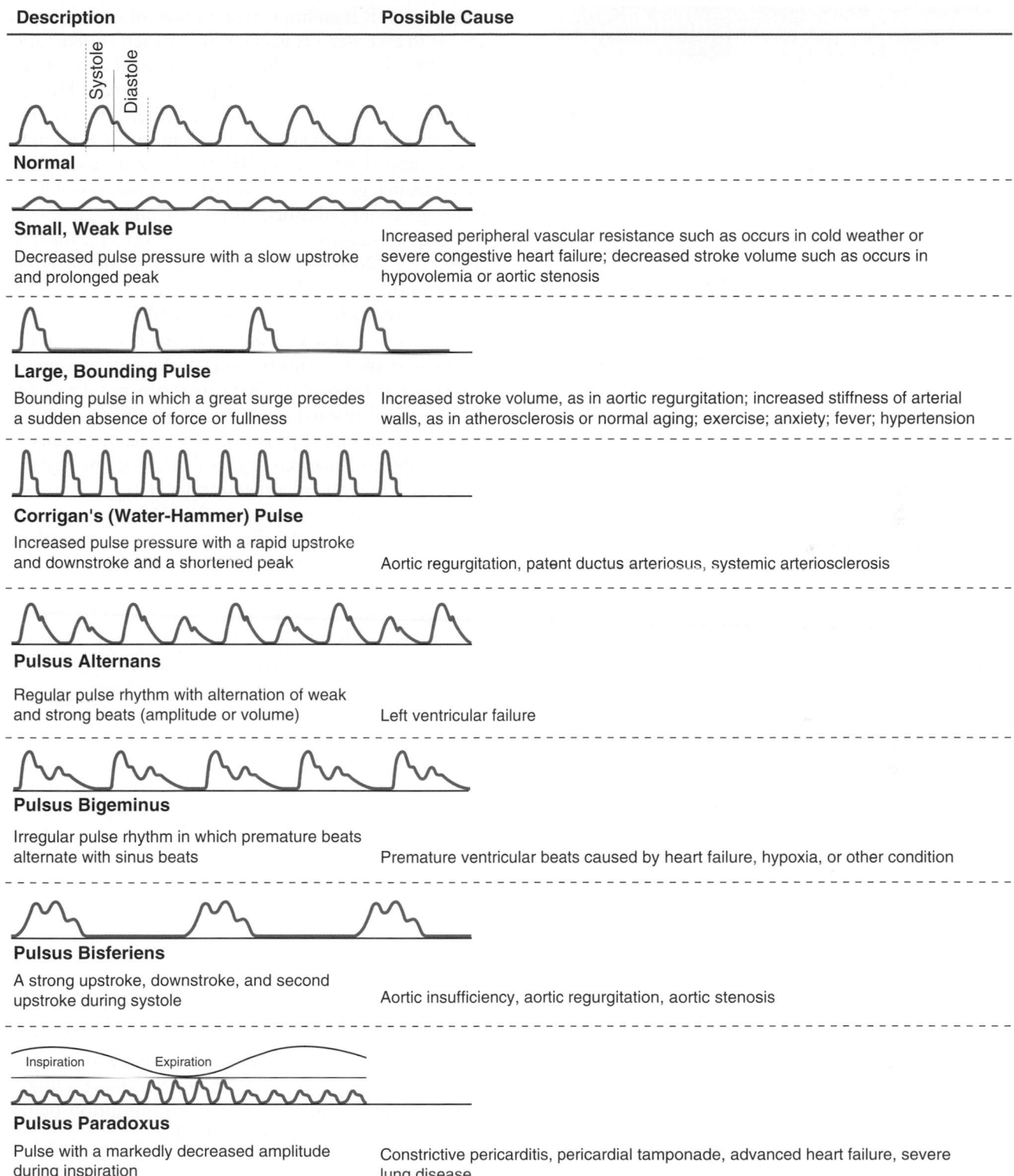

Normal

Small, Weak Pulse

Decreased pulse pressure with a slow upstroke and prolonged peak

Increased peripheral vascular resistance such as occurs in cold weather or severe congestive heart failure; decreased stroke volume such as occurs in hypovolemia or aortic stenosis

Large, Bounding Pulse

Bounding pulse in which a great surge precedes a sudden absence of force or fullness

Increased stroke volume, as in aortic regurgitation; increased stiffness of arterial walls, as in atherosclerosis or normal aging; exercise; anxiety; fever; hypertension

Corrigan's (Water-Hammer) Pulse

Increased pulse pressure with a rapid upstroke and downstroke and a shortened peak

Aortic regurgitation, patent ductus arteriosus, systemic arteriosclerosis

Pulsus Alternans

Regular pulse rhythm with alternation of weak and strong beats (amplitude or volume)

Left ventricular failure

Pulsus Bigeminus

Irregular pulse rhythm in which premature beats alternate with sinus beats

Premature ventricular beats caused by heart failure, hypoxia, or other condition

Pulsus Bisferiens

A strong upstroke, downstroke, and second upstroke during systole

Aortic insufficiency, aortic regurgitation, aortic stenosis

Pulsus Paradoxus

Pulse with a markedly decreased amplitude during inspiration

Constrictive pericarditis, pericardial tamponade, advanced heart failure, severe lung disease

Figure 2.17 Normal (*top*) and abnormal pulses, as reflected in arterial waveforms. *(From Dillon,[2 p. 477], with permission.)*

in amplitude between beats (a weak and a strong), with minimal change in overall rhythm. A normal pulse beat is followed by a premature beat of diminished amplitude. A *paradoxical* pulse (pulsus paradoxus) is decreased amplitude of the pressure wave detected during quiet inspiration with a return to full amplitude on expiration; it is often associated with obstructive lung disease. Figure 2.17 provides a schematic illustration of normal (top) and common alterations in arterial pulse waveforms.

Table 2.6	Numerical Scale for Grading Pulse Quality (Strength)	
Grade	Pulse	Description
0	Absent	No perceptible pulse even with maximum pressure
1+	Thready	Barely perceptible; easily obliterated with slight pressure; fades in and out
2+	Weak	Difficult to palpate; slightly stronger than thready; can be obliterated with light pressure
3+	Normal	Easy to palpate; requires moderate pressure to obliterate
4+	Bounding	Very strong; hyperactive; is not obliterated with moderate pressure

Factors Influencing Heart Rate

Essentially, any factor that alters the metabolic rate will also influence HR. Several factors are of particular importance when considering HR.

Age

Fetal HR averages 120 to 160 beats per minute. The HR for a newborn ranges between 70 and 170, with an average of 120 beats per minute. HR gradually decreases with age until it stabilizes in adulthood (see Tables 2.1 and 2.2). The adult HR range is generally considered to be between 60 and 100 beats per minute; however, in highly trained athletes, the resting value may be considerably lower. This lowered resting value occurs because the effectiveness of each cardiac contraction is 40% to 50% greater in the trained versus untrained individual.[46]

Sex

Men and boys typically have slightly lower HR than women and girls.

Emotions/Stress

Responses to a variety of emotions (e.g., grief, fear, anger, excitement, anxiety, or pain) activate the sympathetic nervous system, with a resultant increase in HR. The stress-inducing effects of moderate to severe pain will also elevate HR.

Exercise

Oxygen demands of skeletal muscles are significantly increased during physical activity. At rest, only 20% to 25% of the available muscle capillaries are open.[45,47] During vigorous exercise, extensive vasodilation causes all capillaries to open. The HR increases to provide additional blood flow to muscles and to meet the increased oxygen requirement. For physical therapists, monitoring a patient's HR is an important method of evaluating response to exercise. Typically, HR will increase as a function of the intensity of the activity (termed *chronotropic competence*). A linear relationship exists between HR and intensity of workload. To use the HR effectively, both the patient's resting and predicted maximal HRs must be determined. Maximum HR values can be determined by a maximal graded exercise test, whenever possible, or by using various published formulas. Common examples are the age-adjusted HR formula (maximum HR [HR_{max}] = 220 minus age), Karvonen formula (target HR = [($HR_{max} - HR_{rest}$) × % intensity] + HR_{rest}), and Inbar[61] formula (HR_{max} = 205.8 – [0.685 × age]). However, the age-adjusted HR formula has been called into question. In their discussion of the history of the formula, Robergs and Landwehr[62] indicate it was not developed from original research "but resulted from observation based on data from approximately 11 references consisting of published research or unpublished scientific compilations. Consequently, the formula HR_{max} = 220 – age has no scientific merit for use in exercise physiology and related fields."[62, p. 1] The authors suggest that there is currently no acceptable method to estimate HR_{max}, and, if a determination is needed, population-specific formulas should be used.

Generally, HR during a 15- to 30-minute therapeutic exercise program for a healthy individual should not exceed 60% to 90% of predicted HR_{max}. Lower exercise intensities are indicated for individuals with low fitness levels.[45]

In examining HR response to exercise, level of aerobic fitness also must be considered. Both resting HR and submaximal exercise HR are typically lower in trained individuals. In response to identical exercise intensity, a sedentary person's HR will demonstrate greater acceleration when compared with a trained individual. Although the metabolic requirements of an activity are the same, the lower HR response in a trained individual occurs as a result of a more efficient (increased) stroke volume (SV) owing to greater cardiac strength and efficiency. The linear relationship between HR and workload exists for both trained and untrained individuals. However, the rate of rise will differ. When compared with a sedentary person, the trained individual will achieve a higher work output and greater oxygen consumption before reaching a specified submaximal HR.

Medications

The impact of medications on HR is particularly important for patients with cardiac disease or hypertension. Beta blockers (beta-adrenergic blocking agents) are a category of drugs that blocks the sympathetic beta receptors and decreases both resting HR and HR response to exercise.[45] They are commonly used in the treatment of angina pectoris, arrhythmias, hypertension, and the acute phase of myocardial infarction. Examples of prescribed beta blockers include acebutolol, atenolol, bisoprolol, metoprolol, nadolol, nebivolol, and propranolol. Patients taking beta blockers typically experience early fatigue with exercise; an alternative to HR monitoring, such as Ratings of Perceived Exertion (RPE scale), should be considered to monitor exercise intensity.[63]

Systemic or Local Heat

During periods of fever, HR will increase. The body will attempt to dissipate heat by vasodilation of peripheral vessels. HR will increase to shunt blood flow to cutaneous areas for cooling. Local applications of thermal modalities (such as a hot pack) may also elevate HR to increase blood flow to cutaneous areas secondary to arteriolar and capillary dilation.

Pulse Sites

A peripheral pulse can be monitored at a variety of sites on the body. A superficial artery located over a bone or other firm surface is easiest to palpate. Table 2.7 identifies common peripheral pulse sites, their locations, and some general indications for their use.[59,60,64] Pulse sites are illustrated in Figure 2.18.

Considered the most accurate,[7] the apical (central) pulse is monitored by auscultation (listening), using a stethoscope directly over the apex (lower portion pointing to the left) of the heart or by placing the hand over the chest to feel the pulsations. In infants, the apical pulse can be felt with the fingertips. Apical pulses are used for weak heartbeats that are imperceptible peripherally when other sites are either inaccessible (e.g., because of medical or surgical contraindications) or difficult to locate and palpate. The apical pulse is typically used to monitor the effects of cardiac medications designed to alter HR and rhythm.[54] Box 2.5 Evidence Summary presents studies examining the reliability and validity of pulse and HR monitoring.

Monitoring Pulse

Peripheral pulses are monitored by palpation using the index and third finger or the first three fingers of one hand.[60] The thumb should not be used because it has

Table 2.7	Pulse Sites, Locations, and Indications for Use	
Pulse Site	**Location**	**Indication for Use**
Temporal	Over temporal bone; superior and lateral to the eye.	When radial pulse inaccessible; often used with infants; used by anesthesiologists for monitoring during surgical interventions.
Carotid	On either side of the lower neck, below the jaw, fingers over thyroid cartilage between the trachea and medial border of sternocleidomastoid; pressure should not be applied bilaterally or high on the neck to avoid stimulation of the carotid sinus and a subsequent reflex drop in pulse rate.	During shock or cardiac arrest, often used with infants; used to monitor cranial circulation; easily accessible if other peripheral pulses difficult or too weak to locate.
Brachial	Distal medial aspect of the humerus, the biceps can be gently pushed laterally during palpation, or medially in the antecubital fossa; elbow should be slightly flexed and supported to avoid contraction of biceps.	During cardiac arrest; used routinely to monitor blood pressure.
Radial	Distal radius at base of the thumb, lateral to tendon of the flexor carpi radialis.	Most common site for peripheral pulse monitoring; easy to locate and easily accessible.
Femoral	Inferior to the inguinal ligament, midway between the anterior superior iliac spine and the symphysis pubis; typically monitored in supine.	During cardiac arrest; used to monitor lower extremity circulation.
Popliteal	Inferior aspect of popliteal fossa; popliteal artery is deep and at times may be difficult to palpate; typically monitored in prone with knee flexed to relax hamstrings and popliteal fascia; can also be accomplished in supine.	Used to monitor lower extremity circulation; weak or absent popliteal pulse may indicate impaired flow or blockage in femoral artery.
Pedal (dorsalis pedis)	Dorsal, medial aspect of foot, lateral to the tendon of the extensor hallicus longus; ankle should be slightly dorsiflexed; some individuals have congenitally nonpalpable pedal pulses.	Used to monitor circulation to feet; weak or absent pulse may be indicative of arterial disease or occlusion.

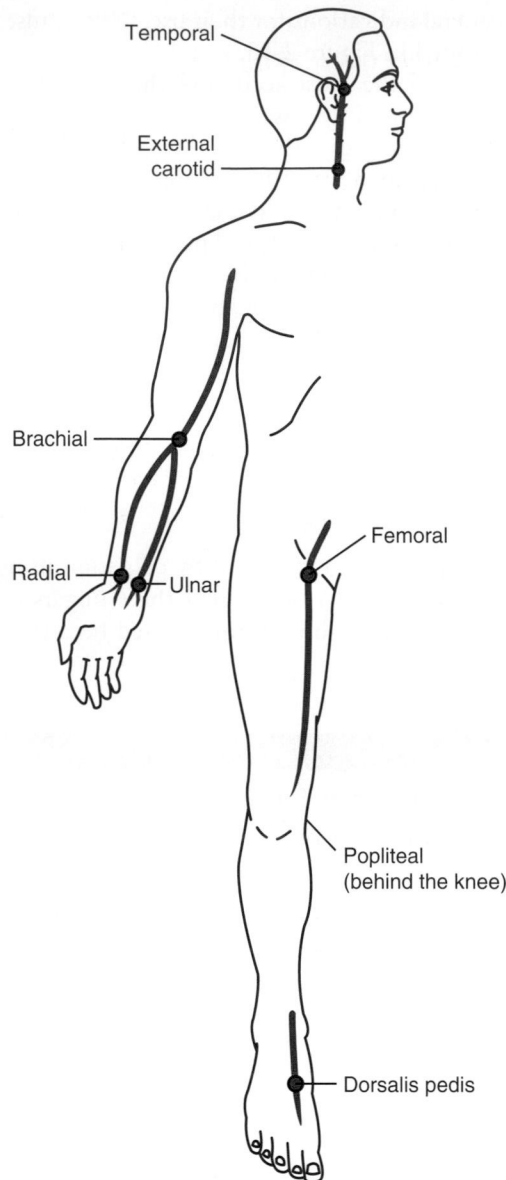

Figure 2.18 Common sites for monitoring peripheral pulses.

its own pulse, which will interfere with monitoring. Generally, a light pressure is used initially to locate the pulse, and then more firm pressure is used when determining the rate, rhythm, and quality. The fingertips should be moved gently over the selected site until the strongest pulsation is found. To monitor resting values, the patient should be resting quietly for at least 5 minutes prior to the pulse measurement.

The radial artery is the most common site for measuring the pulse. With few modifications, the same procedure can be followed for monitoring at other pulse sites.

Measuring Radial Pulse

A. Assemble equipment.
  1. Watch (or wall clock) with a second hand.
B. Wash hands.
C. Procedure.
  1. Explain procedure and rationale in terms appropriate to the patient's understanding.
  2. Ensure patient understanding, safety, and comfort.
  3. Place the patient's wrist in a neutral position relative to flexion and extension, and support the forearm in pronation. If measuring from a supine position, the forearm can be supported across the patient's chest or at his or her side with partial flexion of the elbow. From a sitting position, the forearm can rest across the patient's thigh, supported by a pillow or the therapist's arm. This relaxed positioning of the UE generally facilitates artery palpation.
  4. Place the fingers squarely and firmly over the radial pulse; use only enough pressure to feel the pulse accurately. If the pressure is too great, it will occlude the artery.
  5. Once the strongest pulsation is located, note the position of the second hand on the watch or clock. The first pulsation should be counted as zero to avoid overestimating.[60] Determine the *rate* (number of beats per minute [bpm]) by counting the

Box 2.5 Evidence Summary		Studies Examining the Reliability and Validity of Pulse and Heart Rate Monitoring		
Reference	Methods	Subjects/Design	Results	Conclusion/Comments
Senduran et al (2011)	Examined the safety and feasibility of early physical therapy in the intensive care unit (ICU).	Case study of a 41-year old male patient in the ICU following implantation of a biventricular assist device. Monitored vital signs before, immediately after, and 5 minutes after treatment.	Data from 15 sessions of physical therapy showed significant differences in pretreatment, immediately after treatment, and 5 minutes after treatment for heart rate (HR) and respiratory rate (RR) only. HR significantly	The findings highlight the importance of monitoring vital signs, such as HR, in order to observe the physiological response of the patient to physical therapy in the ICU.

Box 2.5 Evidence Summary   Studies Examining the Reliability and Validity of Pulse and Heart Rate Monitoring—cont'd

Reference	Methods	Subjects/Design	Results	Conclusion/Comments
			increased immediately after treatment and returned to baseline (before) values within 5 minutes.	
Lee et al (2011)	Examined the accuracy of using an infrared light-emitting diode (LED) device to measure HR. Compared HR from an infrared device to electrocardiogram (ECG).	Examined 46 healthy adults (mean age 24.8 ± 5.6 years). Subjects engaged in 4-minute periods of standing (0 mph), walking at 2.0 mph and 3.5 mph, jogging at 4.5 mph, and running at 6.0 mph.	HR measurements from the infrared device and ECG were highly correlated (ICC values provided with 90% confidence interval in parentheses). • 0 mph the ICC = 0.95 (0.94-0.96) • 2.0 mph the ICC = 0.95 (0.94-0.96) • 3.5 mph the ICC = 0.94 (0.92-0.95) • 4.5 mph the ICC = 0.92 (0.90-0.94) • 6.0 mph the ICC = 0.85 (0.81-0.88)	The infrared device used to measure HR was valid for monitoring HR at rest and lower exercise intensities. It becomes less accurate as exercise intensity (speed) increases.
Alexis (2009)	Reviews monitoring pulse rate.	This is a narrative review paper.	Defines pulse and rationales for measuring pulse. Discusses: • Assessment of pulses • Pulse sites • Conditions associated with pulse measurement • Factors influencing the pulse • Reference values • Equipment • Measuring pulses pregnant women, children, and older adults	Accurately measuring, recording, and interpreting pulse rate is critical for assessing the patient's condition and cardiovascular status.
Rawlings-Anderson et al (2008)	Reviews monitoring pulse rate.	This is a narrative review paper.	Defines pulse rate, rhythm, and amplitude. Provides reference values and reasons for tachycardia and bradycardia. Discusses indications, preparing the patient, procedures, and interpreting the results.	Accurately measuring, recording, and interpreting pulse rate is critical for assessing the patient's condition and cardiovascular status.

Continued

Box 2.5 Evidence Summary   Studies Examining the Reliability and Validity of Pulse and Heart Rate Monitoring—cont'd

Reference	Methods	Subjects/Design	Results	Conclusion/Comments
John et al (2007)	Compared post exercise pulse palpation with electronic (HR) monitoring. Examine the contribution of movement artifact and measurement delay to underestimations of postexercise pulse rate.	Examined 54 female subjects (mean age of 19.9 ± 1.6 years). Subjects palpated their pulse at the midpoint and end point of an exercise period.	It took 17-20 seconds for subjects to obtain their palpated pulse rate after exercise. The palpated pulse rate underestimated HR by 20-27 beats (nearly 20%). The authors calculated and provided correction factors.	Pulse palpation requires teaching and practice. After exercise, applying a correction factor to pulse palpation is recommended.
Lockwood et al (2004)	Examined the best available evidence related to monitoring vital signs, including: • Purpose • Limitations • Optimal measurement frequency • What measures should be considered vital signs	Narrative, systematic review of vital signs. Updated review of Evans et al (2001). Included 124 studies on neonatal, pediatric, and adult patient populations.	There is limited research on pulse rate measurements and its ability to detect serious physiological changes. Measuring pulse rate over 15 seconds will most likely reduce the accuracy.	Pulse rate should be assessed over 30 or 60 seconds. When the pulse rate is rapid or difficult to palpate, the HR should be measured apically using a stethoscope.
Evans et al (2001)	Examined the best available evidence related to monitoring vital signs including: • Measurements that constitute vital signs • Optimal measurement frequency • Limitations of vital signs	Narrative, systematic review of vital signs. Included 69 studies on neonatal, pediatric, and adult patient populations.	There is limited low-level evidence on the frequency with which vital signs should be monitored. There is little research on pulse rate measurement.	Much of current practice of vital sign measurement is not based on research but on tradition and expert opinion.

Prepared by Kevin K. Chui, PT, PhD, GCS, OCS.

Senduran, M, Malkoc, M, and Oto, O: Physical therapy in the intensive care unit in a patient with biventricular assist device. Cardiopulm Phys Ther J 22:31, 2011.
Lee, CM, Gorelick, M, and Mendoza, A: Accuracy of an infrared LED device to measure heart rate and energy expenditure during rest and exercise. J Sports Sci 29:1645, 2011.
Alexis, O: Providing best practice in manual pulse measurement. Br J Nurs 19:410, 2009.
Rawlings-Anderson, K, and Hunter, J: Monitoring pulse rate. Nurs Stand 22:41, 2008.
John, D, Sforzo, GA, and Swensen, T: Monitoring exercise heart rate using manual palpation. ACSM's Health & Fitness Journal 11(6):14, 2007.
Lockwood, C, Conroy-Hiller, T, and Page, T: Systematic review: Vital signs. JBI Reports 2:207, 2004.
Evans, D, Hodgkinson, B, and Berry, J: Vital signs in hospital patients: A systematic review. Int J Nurs Stud 38:643, 2001.

pulse for 30 seconds and multiplying by 2; if any irregularities are noted, a full 60-second count should be taken to improve accuracy. Note the *rhythm* (time intervals between pulse beats) and the *quality* (force) of the pulse.

   6. Wash hands.

Measuring Apical Pulse

A. Assemble equipment.

   1. Watch (or wall clock) with a second hand.

   2. Stethoscope.

   3. Antiseptic wipes for cleaning earpieces and diaphragm of stethoscope before and after use.

B. Wash hands.

C. Procedure.

   1. Explain the procedure and rationale in terms appropriate to the patient's level of understanding. Indicate that there will be a request to remain quiet during monitoring to avoid interference with auscultation.

2. Ensure patient understanding, safety, and comfort. Apical pulses are typically monitored with the patient either supine or sitting.
3. Use an antiseptic wipe to clean the earpieces and diaphragm of the stethoscope.
4. Expose the sternum and chest.
5. Locate the site where pulse will be monitored; the apical pulse is located approximately 3.5 inches (8.9 cm) to the left of the midsternum, in the fifth intercostal space, within an inch of the midclavicular line drawn parallel to the sternum (Fig 2.19). These landmarks are guides to locating the apical pulse. In some individuals, a stronger pulse may be noted by altering placement of the stethoscope (e.g., placement in the fourth or sixth intercostal space).
6. Place the earpieces of the stethoscope (tilting slightly forward) into the ears. The tubes of the stethoscope should not be crossed and should hang freely.
7. Place the flat disk diaphragm of the stethoscope over the apex of heart and locate the point where the apical pulse is heard most clearly. This is called the *point of maximal impulse (PMI)*. If the rhythm is regular, count the pulse for 30 seconds and multiply by 2. If any irregularities are noted, a full 60-second count should be taken. The pulse will be heard as a "lub-dub." The "lub" represents closure of the atrioventricular (tricuspid and mitral) valves. The "dub" represents closure of the semilunar (aortic and pulmonic) valves.
8. Wash hands and clean the stethoscope. If the same examiner is using the stethoscope again, it is not necessary to clean the earpieces; the diaphragm should always be cleaned.

Measuring Apical–Radial Pulse

Monitoring the apical–radial pulse involves two examiners simultaneously measuring the pulse at two separate locations: (1) the apical pulse at the apex of the heart; and (2) the radial pulse at the wrist. The values from the two different sites are then compared. Typically, the apical and radial pulse values are the same. However, in some situations (e.g., variations in SV or vascular occlusion), blood pumped from the heart may not be reaching the distal site, causing a weak or imperceptible radial pulse. For example, if the heart contracts prematurely, the ventricles have insufficient time to fill, resulting in a diminished stroke volume and creating an imperceptible pulse in the radial artery.[46] On the other hand, SV may be normal with a weak or imperceptible radial pulse, suggesting a more peripheral problem such as impaired flow or blockage within a vessel. In either situation, there is a deficit in the number of radial pulses when compared with the number of apical pulses.[46] This is called a **pulse deficit,** defined as the difference between the rate of radial and apical pulses. The value of this measure is that it provides important information about the cardiovascular system's ability to perfuse the body.

Automated Heart Rate Monitoring

Advances are continual in the design, features, accuracy, waterproofing, information storage capacity, and computer, tablet, and smartphone interface capabilities of heart rate monitors (HRMs). In addition to monitoring HR, some HRMs provide data on HR variability (calculation of the time between pulses), real-time display of percentage of maximum HR, and estimates of maximal oxygen uptake (VO_{2max}). HRMs with interface capabilities allow data to be downloaded to a computer (tablet or smartphone) for analysis and storage using HR

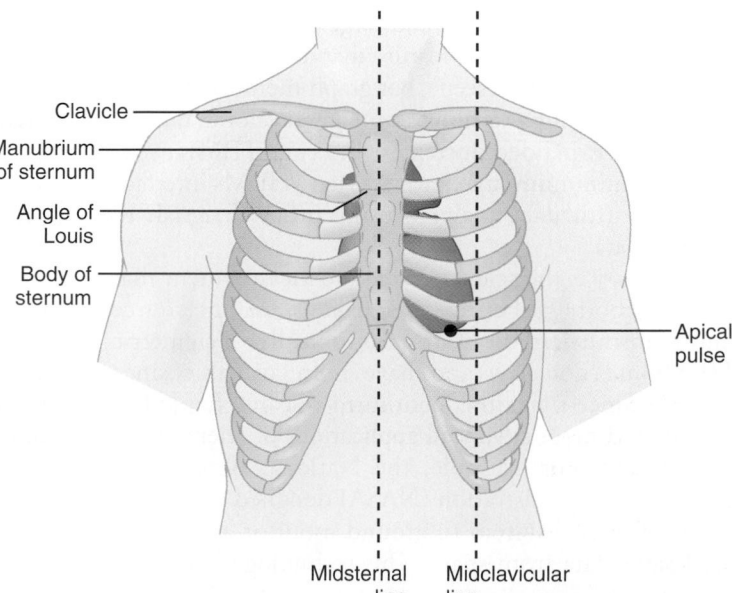

Figure 2.19 The apical pulse is located approximately 3.5 inches to the left of the midsternum, in the fifth intercostal space.

software programs. This provides a permanent record and sequential data on exercise performance. Most models allow programming of a prescribed exercise HR range with an audible and visible warning when the HR is outside the predetermined range. Some models include a talking feature that "speaks" HR information. Memory capabilities allow storage of exercise information over a variable number of exercise sessions.

HRMs consist of two basic elements: (1) a sensor that transmits data; and (2) a monitor that incorporates a receiver, microprocessor, and display. Many HRMs integrate sensors into a chest strap that provides wireless transmission of signals to a monitor worn as a wristwatch (Fig. 2.20A). Another style of HRM replaces the chest strap with fingertip sensors directly on the wristwatch (Fig. 2.20B) or a monitor that is worn around the neck (Fig 2.20C). HR data are recorded when a fingertip is placed in contact with the sensor. On some models, the bezel (ring surrounding the display dial) serves as the sensor. Wireless pulse monitors are available that interface with smartphones (Fig 2.20D) and tablets. HRMs are also available as finger rings. Still other HRMs incorporate a lead wire with a distal sensor housed in an earlobe clip, fingertip cover, or finger sleeve (Fig. 2.20E to H). Some HRMs are equipped with more than one type of sensor. This feature allows selection of the sensor that is most appropriate for the activity and the user.

HRMs are frequently used in prescribed exercise and training programs because they provide a practical, accurate method of pulse monitoring and are lightweight, comfortable, and easy to use. In recent years, many types of exercise training devices (e.g., treadmills, Stair-Climbers, bicycles, elliptical machines) incorporate HRMs directly into the unit design by means of a metal handgrip sensor device.

Other HRM features are available and differ with the model and manufacturer. Among the more common features are multifunction wrist monitors (consisting of a watch, stopwatch, alarm clock, lap timer, calendar, and data storage), illuminated and large-number LCD displays (some with a zoom feature that doubles the size of information on the screen), bar graph memory displays of previous training sessions, estimates of calories burned and energy expended during exercise, and HR statistics (average, minimum, maximum). Many HRMs interface wirelessly (for data analysis) using infrared signals to transfer data.

Telemetry is the science of remote measurement that includes both gathering data from a distant source and transmitting the data electronically. Telemetric HRMs are not new and have been available since 1983.[65] Since that time, continued research has led to greater and more advanced applications of telemetry in health care. For example, the National Aeronautics and Space Administration (NASA) designed a sophisticated telemetry system to ground monitor astronauts' vital signs data from space. This technology led to the development of the *Patient Monitoring System,* in which the patient continuously wears a small, portable, wireless transmitter that delivers real-time vital sign data to a central location that can monitor multiple patients simultaneously.[45] The Federal Communications Commission (FCC) defines *wireless medical telemetry* as "the measurement and recording of physiological parameters and other patient-related information via radiated bi- or unidirectional electromagnetic signals."[66, p. 1] In 2000, the FCC established the Wireless Medical Telemetry Service (WMTS) by allocating 14 MHz of spectrum for wireless medical telemetry. This networking infrastructure (available in specific geographical areas) was established owing to interference issues created by digital television and protects medical telemetry from interference by other in-band radio-frequency (RF) sources.[66] The FCC has designated the American Society for Healthcare Engineering of the American Hospital Association (ASHE/AHA) as the frequency coordinator for the WMTS.[67]

Gandsas et al[68] applied telemetric technology to examine the efficacy of using a low-cost approach to transmitting vital sign data from an aircraft to a medical ground facility. During an in-flight simulated medical emergency, vital sign data were collected with a monitoring device and transmitted using a laptop computer, an airline seat-back telephone, and the Internet. All data were received without corruption with a maximum delay of 1 second. The authors suggest that during an actual in-flight emergency, patient data could potentially be delivered to an assigned medical facility as well as to the physician's desktop computer anywhere in the world, irrespective of the geographical location of the aircraft.[68] Another area of research involves developing uniform standards of communication for transmission of data from vital sign monitoring equipment directly to clinical information systems currently in use in health care settings.

Doppler Ultrasound and Pulse Oximetry

Doppler Ultrasound

Doppler ultrasound (DUS) is a noninvasive instrument used to examine pulses that are extremely weak or faint or that are obliterated by even slight pressure, or when arterial flow is severely compromised. DUS is based on the principle that high-frequency ultrasound waves directed at a moving interface (i.e., blood flowing through a vessel) will cause a change in the wave frequency reflective of the velocity of the moving interface (called the *Doppler effect*). In essence, the DUS measures how sound waves are reflected off moving blood cells. The resultant frequency change caused by the movement alters the pitch of the sound waves as they are reflected back to the examiner; the pulse is heard as a swooshing sound.[69] The change in pitch heard by the examiner provides important information about the blood flow through a vessel.

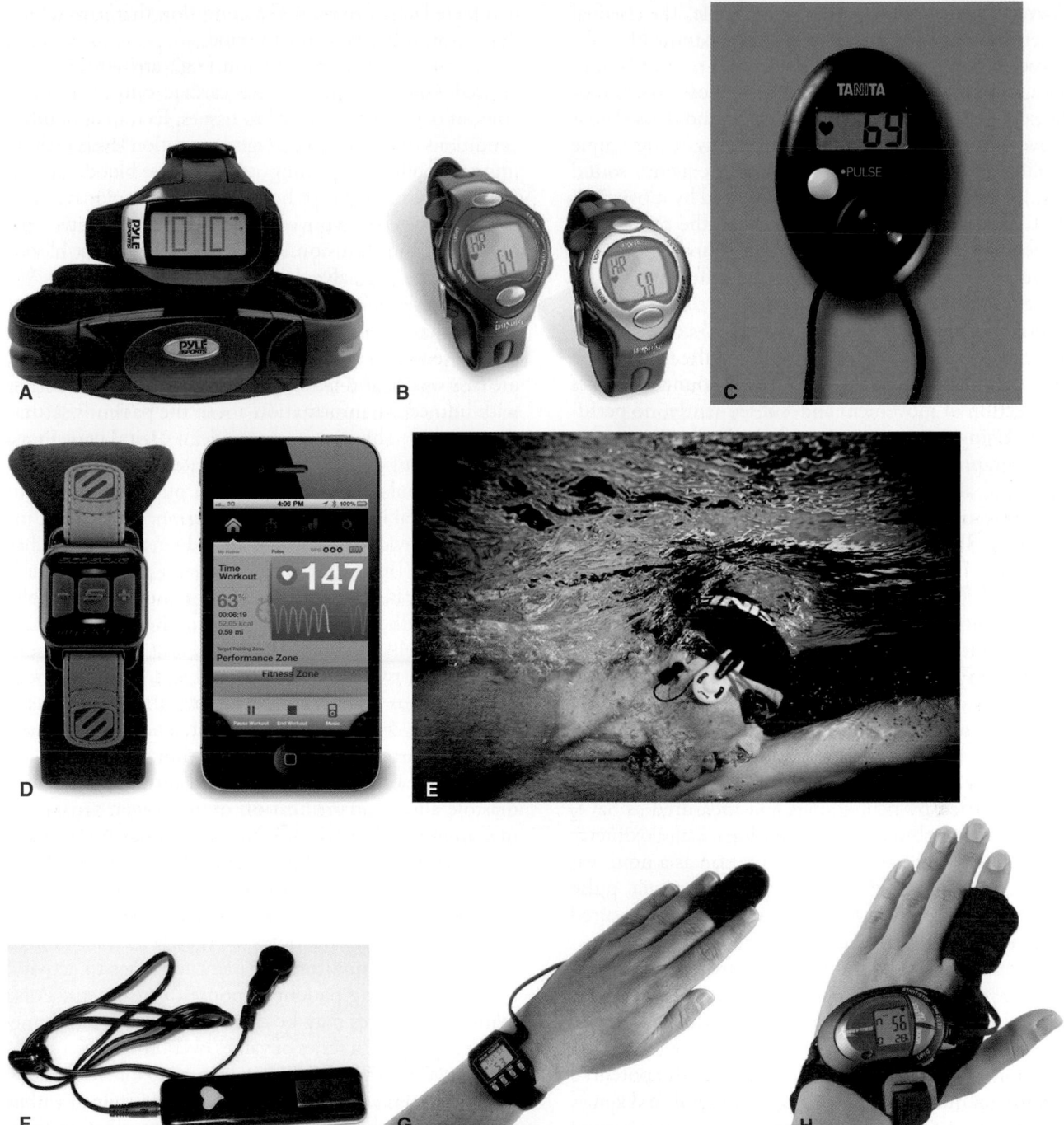

Figure 2.20 Heart rate monitors (HRMs). **(A)** Wrist monitor with chest strap transmitter worn directly on the skin and positioned at heart level. *(Courtesy of Pyle Audio, Inc., Brooklyn, NY 11204.)* **(B)** Example of wrist monitors with two fingertip sensors above and below LCD; the index and middle finger are placed on contact points to obtain HR. *(Courtesy of Sports Beat, Inc., Deer Park, NY 11729.)* **(C)** Monitor with neck strap and fingertip sensor. *(Courtesy of Tanita Corporation of America, Arlington Heights, IL 60005.)* **(D)** This monitor is worn on the forearm to wirelessly connect with an application downloaded to the smartphone. *(Courtesy of Scosche Industries Inc., Oxnard, CA, 93033.)* **(E)** Tucked under the goggle strap, this waterproof HRM has an earlobe clip with infrared sensor and verbally announces heart rate at time intervals preselected by the user. *(Courtesy of FINIS, Inc., Livermore, CA 94551.)* **(F)** HRM with earlobe clip sensor that has an integrated USB interface. *(Courtesy of Kyto Electronic Co., Ltd., Dongguan City, Guangdong, China.)* **(G)** Wrist monitor with lead wire and fingertip sensor. *(Courtesy of Mark of Fitness, Inc., Shrewsbury, NJ 07702.)* **(H)** HRM worn on dorsum of hand with finger sleeve. *(Courtesy of Mark of Fitness, Inc., Shrewsbury, NJ 07702.)*

Several models of DUS units are available. The essential elements include the ultrasound unit, a handheld probe (piezoelectric crystal) that transmits and receives sound waves, and earpieces that look similar to those on a stethoscope or a small speaker to amplify the sound. Passed gently over the skin surface above an artery using ample coupling gel, the probe transmits high-frequency sound waves to an artery. The waves are disturbed by movement of the red blood cells, reflected back to the probe, and transformed into an amplified audible sound.[70]

The audible sound represents the difference in frequency between the waves directed at the vessel and those reflected back by motion of blood cells; the frequency is proportional to the velocity of the moving red blood cells. The absence of an audible sound indicates no detection of movement and, subsequently, no perfusion.[69] Using a computer interface, the flow measures can be graphically displayed and stored. It should be noted that although the specific characteristics of the reflected sounds are not diagnostic, they can assist in identifying abnormal flow.[71]

Pulse Oximetry

Pulse oximetry provides a measure of arterial blood oxygenation that is updated with each pulse wave.[72] Oxygen is carried in the blood in two forms: (1) dissolved in arterial plasma; and (2) combined with hemoglobin.[45] Arterial plasma transports only about 3% of the oxygen in blood and is measured as PaO_2 (partial pressure of oxygen). The greater amount of oxygen (approximately 97%) is carried by hemoglobin and measured as SaO_2 (arterial hemoglobin oxygen saturation). Pulse oximetry measures arterial blood oxygen saturation as a noninvasive intervention.[73,74] Oxygen saturation via pulse oximetry is reported as SpO_2[75,76] and can be measured at any adequately perfused peripheral pulse.

Normal oxygen saturation levels are between 96% and 100%. In general, saturation levels below 90% are considered significant and warrant additional testing beyond the data provided by pulse oximetry (e.g., arterial blood gas analysis), as well as marking the potential need for administration of supplemental oxygen.[77] *Hypoxemia* is a term used to describe deficient oxygenation of the blood. *Hypoxia* is a diminished supply of oxygen available to body tissues, and *anoxia* is the complete lack of oxygen,[47] a condition that can be sustained for only a very brief period.

Alterations in heart function (e.g., arrhythmias, decreased HR) typically reduce cardiac output and the amount of oxygen delivered to tissues. Examples of other conditions that can affect oxygen saturation levels include impaired ability of the lungs to oxygenate blood, anemia (reduction in number of hemoglobin molecules available to carry oxygen), hypoventilation (e.g., bronchitis, emphysema), and diffusion impairments that affect blood-gas exchange (e.g., alveolar fibrosis, interstitial fluid).[76]

The pulse oximeter provides data on the percent of oxygen that is combined with hemoglobin (SpO_2). The automated units are relatively small (Fig. 2.21A and B), are easy to use and transport, and provide the therapist with immediate information about the patient's saturation levels.[76] The monitor provides a digital percentage of the amount of hemoglobin saturated with oxygen and displays a pulsatile waveform and pulse rate, with an audible signal indicating each pulsation. The patient interface is provided by a lead wire and sensor that attaches to the unit. The sensor is placed over a pulsating arteriolar vascular bed.[75] Several types of sensors are available, including adhesive fingertip and forehead (Fig. 2.22A and B) as well as nasal, earlobe, and foot styles. The sensors contain two light sources (red and infrared) and a photodetector (Fig. 2.23). The dual light source is used because oxygenated and deoxygenated hemoglobin have different patterns of light absorption.[78] The ratio of the amount of each light absorbed during systole and diastole allows quantification of an oxygen saturation measurement (SpO_2).[75-78] Nail polish has been found to interfere with oximetry and should be removed before monitoring.[79] Artificial acrylic fingernails may also interfere with oxygen saturation measurement.[80]

Pulse oximetry contributes to (1) early identification of hypoxemia; (2) monitoring patient tolerance to activity; and (3) evaluating patient response to treatment. Pulse oximetry measures may be done continuously, intermittently to generate a series of values over time, or as a single measure at a given point in time (e.g., as an initial screening tool). The measurement pattern will be determined within the context of the patient history and examination findings. Telemetry oximetry monitoring allows continuous communication of SpO_2 data from remote locations.[75]

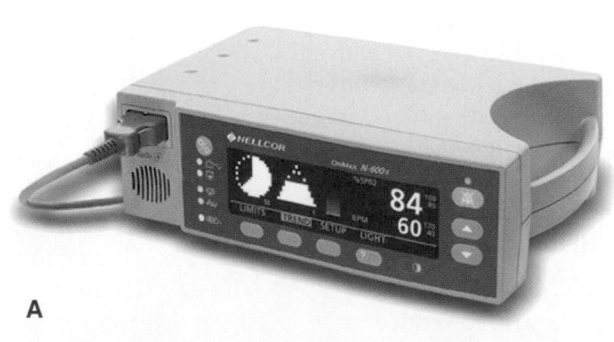

A

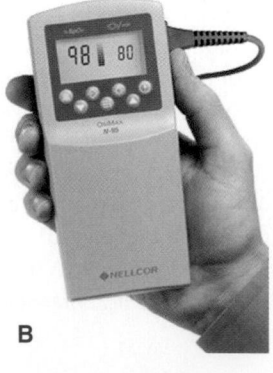

B

Figure 2.21 Pulse oximeters provide data on arterial blood oxygen saturation as well as pulse rate. **(A)** Standard pulse oximetry unit. **(B)** Portable hand-held pulse oximeter. *(Courtesy of Nellcor Puritan Bennett, LLC, Boulder, CO 80301, doing business as Covidien.)*

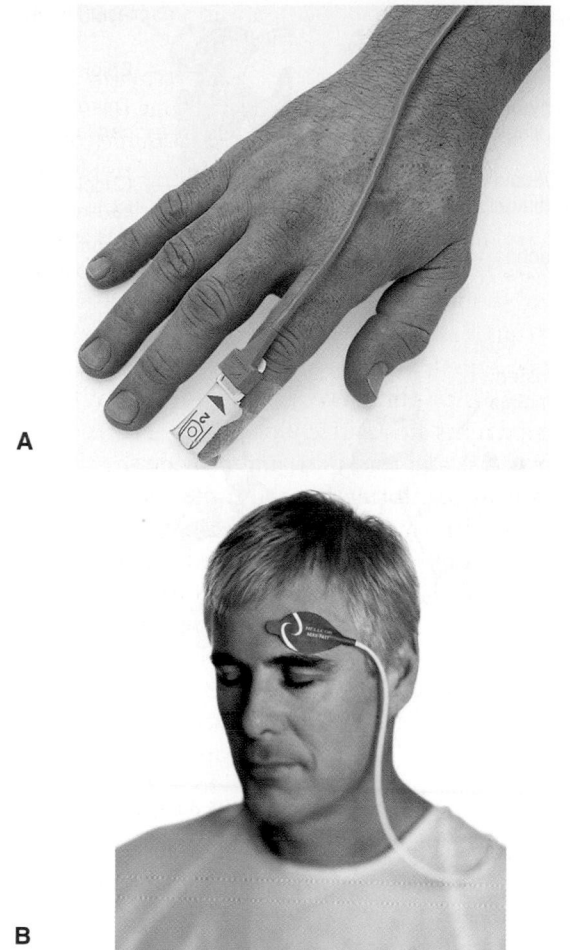

A

B

Figure 2.22 Oximetry sensors. **(A)** The fingertip (transmission) sensor and **(B)** forehead (reflectance) sensor. *(Courtesy of Nellcor Puritan Bennett, LLC, Boulder, CO 80301, doing business as Covidien.)*

RESPIRATION

The primary function of respiration (movement of air into and out of the lungs) is to supply the body with oxygen for metabolic activity and to remove carbon dioxide. The respiratory system consists of a series of branching tubes and brings atmospheric oxygen into contact with the gas exchange membrane of the lungs in the alveoli. Oxygen is then transported throughout the body via the cardiovascular system. *External respiration* is the exchange of oxygen and carbon dioxide between the lungs and the environment. *Internal respiration* is the exchange of oxygen and carbon dioxide between the circulating blood and body tissues.

Respiratory System

The entire pathway that transports air from the environment extends from the mouth and nose down to the alveolar sacs. Figure 2.24 illustrates the structures of the respiratory system. The upper respiratory airways include the nose, mouth, pharynx, and larynx. Air enters the body by way of the nose and mouth and is then moved to the

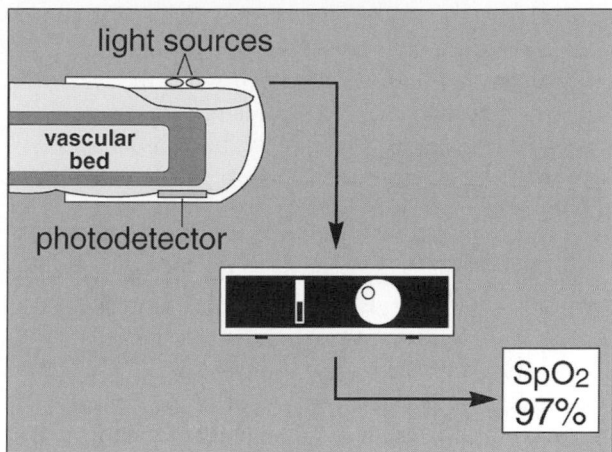

Figure 2.23 Cross-sectional drawing of a fingertip oximetry sensor illustrating the dual light sources, photodetector, schematic connection to oximeter and hypothetical oxygen saturation measurement output. *Note:* In the fingertip (transmission) sensors, the light sources are positioned opposite the photodetector. In the forehead (reflectance) sensors, the light sources and photodetector are positioned on one side of the sensor. *(Courtesy of Nellcor Puritan Bennett, LLC, Boulder, CO 80301, doing business as Covidien.)*

pharynx, where it is warmed, filtered, and humidified. The pharynx serves as a common pathway for both air and food. Inspired air is then moved to the larynx, which contains the epiglottis, vocal cords, and cartilaginous structures. The anatomical arrangement of the larynx and pharyngeal muscles provides the critical function of protecting the lungs from entry of foreign particles, as well as assisting with phonation (production of vocal sounds) and coughing, which is the primary physiological mechanism for clearing the airways. The *laryngopharynx* is the area where solid and liquid food intake is separated from inspired air. It is also the site of bifurcation into the larynx and esophagus. The pharyngeal muscles close the glottis during swallowing to protect the lungs from aspiration. If a foreign body passes the glottis and enters the tracheobronchial tree, the cough reflex is initiated to clear the air passage. Immediately below the thyroid cartilage of the larynx ("Adam's apple") is the site for emergency opening to the tracheal air pathway (*tracheostomy*).[47,76,81,82]

The trachea is approximately 4 to 5 inches (11 to 13 cm) long and continues from the cartilaginous structures of the neck into the thorax. At the level of the carina (Fig. 2.25), the trachea divides into two mainstem bronchi. The carina contains the majority of cough receptors and is located approximately between the sternum and manubrium at the second intercostal space. The right and left mainstem bronchi are asymmetrical in size and shape and continue into the lower respiratory tract, further subdividing into the respiratory bronchioles, where gas exchange begins. However, gas exchange primarily occurs in the alveolar ducts and the large surface area provided by the alveoli. The respiratory

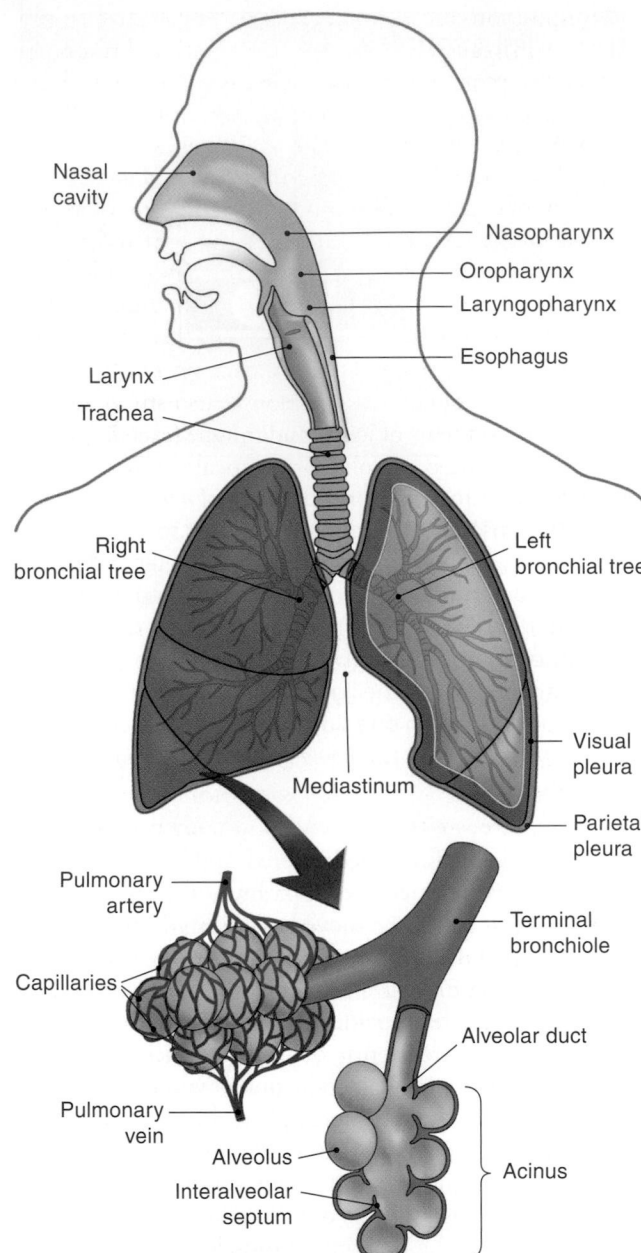

Figure 2.24 Structures of the respiratory system. *(From Dillon,[2 p. 394] with permission.)*

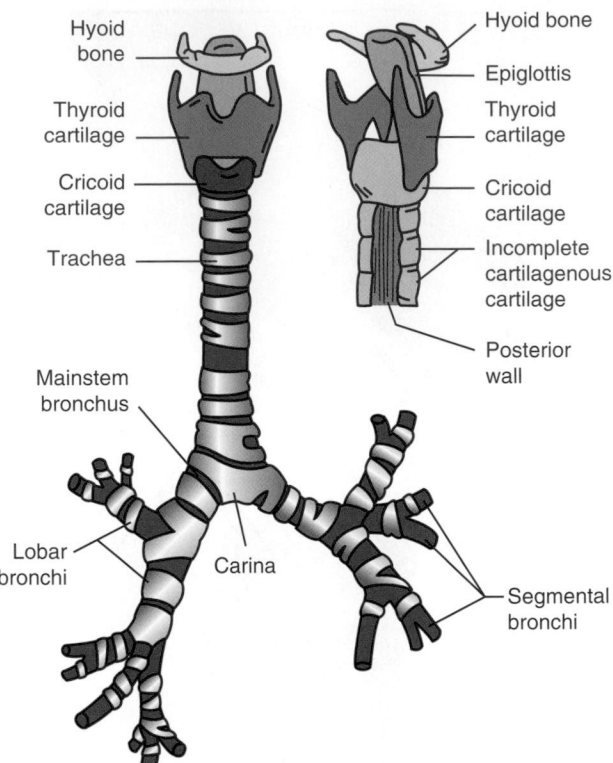

Figure 2.25 Structure of cartilaginous airways, including the trachea and major bronchi. *(From Henderson,[82 p. 388] with permission.)*

bronchioles, alveolar ducts, and alveoli (alveolar sacs) comprise the *respiratory zone* for gas exchange (Fig. 2.26). The *conductive zone* (trachea, bronchi, and terminal bronchioles) provides for continuous movement of air into and out of the lungs; these areas do not contribute to gas exchange.[47,76,78,81]

Inspiration

Inspiration is initiated by contraction of the diaphragm and intercostal muscles. During contraction of these muscles, the diaphragm moves downward and the intercostals lift the ribs and sternum up and outward. The thoracic cavity is thus increased in size and allows for lung expansion. Normal inspiration lasts 1 to 1.5 seconds.[59]

Expiration

During relaxed breathing, expiration is essentially a passive process. Once the respiratory muscles relax, the thorax returns to its resting position, and the lungs recoil. This ability to recoil occurs because of the inherent elastic properties of the lungs. Normal expiration lasts 2 to 3 seconds.[59]

Regulatory Mechanisms

Regulation of respiratory function involves multiple components of both neural and chemical control and is closely integrated with the cardiovascular system. Breathing is controlled by the respiratory center, which lies bilaterally in the pons and medulla. Motor nerves whose cell bodies are located in this area control the respiratory muscles. The respiratory center provides control of both the *rate* and the *depth* of breathing in response to the metabolic needs of the body.[83]

Both *central* and *peripheral* chemoreceptors influence respiration. *Central* chemoreceptors located in the respiratory center are sensitive to changes in either carbon dioxide or hydrogen ion levels of arterial blood. An increase in either carbon dioxide levels or hydrogen ions will stimulate breathing.[46] *Peripheral* chemoreceptors are

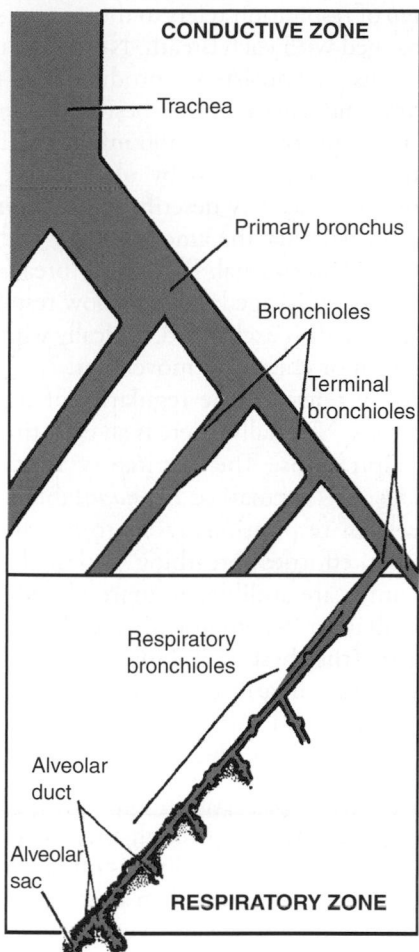

CONDUCTIVE ZONE
- Trachea
- Primary bronchus
- Bronchioles
- Terminal bronchioles

- Respiratory bronchioles
- Alveolar duct
- Alveolar sac

RESPIRATORY ZONE

Figure 2.26 Schematic illustration of the functional zones of the respiratory tract. The top area from the trachea to the terminal bronchioles is called the "conductive zone" because these airways transport (conduct) inhaled air to and from the respiratory zone. The bottom area of the illustration represents the areas where air exchange takes place. The air exchange occurs in progressively increasing increments in the respiratory bronchioles, alveolar ducts, and alveolar sacs. Collectively these areas constitute the "respiratory zone." *(From Henderson,[82 p. 389], with permission.)*

located at the bifurcation of the carotid arteries (carotid bodies) and in the arch of the aorta (aortic bodies). These receptors are sensitive to the partial pressure of oxygen (PaO_2) in the arterial blood. When PaO_2 levels in arterial blood drop, afferent impulses carry this information to the respiratory center. Motor neurons to the respiratory muscles are stimulated to increase **tidal volume** (amount of air exchanged with each breath) or, with very low oxygen levels, to increase the respiratory rate as well. These peripheral chemoreceptors cause an increase in respiration only when PaO_2 levels fall to approximately 60 mm Hg (from a normal level of about 90 to 100 mm Hg). This is because the receptors are sensitive only to PaO_2 levels in plasma and not to the total oxygen in blood.[46,83]

Respiration also is influenced by a protective stretch mechanism called the *Hering-Breuer reflex*. Pulmonary stretch receptors throughout the walls of the lungs detect the amount of stretch imposed by entering air.[84] When overstretched, these receptors send impulses to the respiratory center to inhibit further inspiration and increase the duration of expiration. Impulses stop at the end of expiration so that another inspiration can be initiated.[46,76] In adults, this reflex is rarely demonstrated and would likely not be activated until tidal volume reached higher than 1.5 liters.[46] However, evidence suggests that the Hering-Breuer reflex has a significant impact on the breathing pattern of neonates.[85] Respiration is also stimulated by vigorous movements of joints and muscle (exercise) and is strongly influenced by voluntary cortical control.

Factors Influencing Respiration

Multiple factors can alter normal, relaxed, effortless respiration. As with temperature and pulse, any influence that increases the metabolic rate also will increase RR. Increased metabolism and subsequent demand for oxygen will stimulate increased respiration. Conversely, as metabolic demands diminish, respirations also will decrease. Several influencing factors are of particular importance when examining respiration. These include age, body size, stature, exercise, and body position.

Age

The RR of a newborn is between 30 and 90 breaths per minute. The rate gradually slows until adulthood, when it ranges between 12 and 20 breaths per minute. In elderly individuals, the RR increases owing to decreased elasticity of the lungs and decreased efficiency of gas exchange. Other factors associated with normal aging that affect respiratory function include weakening of respiratory muscles, deterioration of alveolar walls, decreased thoracic mobility, and decreased lung volumes.[86]

Body Size and Stature

Men generally have a larger vital capacity than women, adults larger than adolescents and children. Tall, thin individuals generally have a larger vital capacity than stout or obese individuals. With larger lung capacity there is also a lower RR.

Exercise

Respiratory rate and depth will increase with exercise as a result of increased oxygen demand and carbon dioxide production.

Body Position

The recumbent position can significantly affect respiration and predispose the patient to stasis of fluids. Among the influential factors that limit normal lung expansion when lying down are compression of the chest against the supporting surface and pressure from abdominal organs against the diaphragm. Both of these factors cause increased resistance to breathing. Difficult recumbent breathing is common during the late stages of pregnancy as the fetus shifts the diaphragm upward.[60] Patients with congestive heart failure (CHF) also experience labored breathing when lying flat, which improves when standing or sitting up.

Environment

Exposure to pollutants such as gas and particle emissions, asbestos, chemical waste products, or coal dust can diminish the ability to transport oxygen. Other common offending pollutants include high ozone concentrations, sulfur dioxide, and carbon monoxide.[50] These respiratory irritants typically increase mucus production. High altitudes also affect the respiratory system owing to reduced air mass (i.e., the partial pressure of oxygen in inspired air is low). This means fewer oxygen molecules per liter of air, causing a reduction in arterial blood oxygen levels and triggering shortness of breath (*dyspnea*) and reduced tolerance to activity. Hyperventilation, tachycardia, and pulmonary edema (accumulation of fluid in alveolar walls) can also occur at high altitudes.[50,60,87,88]

Emotions/Stress

Stress as well as emotions can result in an increased rate and depth of respirations owing to stimulation of the sympathetic nervous system.

Pharmacological Agents

Essentially any drug that depresses central nervous system (CNS) function will result in respiratory depression. Narcotic agents (e.g., opioids [morphine], meperidine hydrochloride [Demerol]) will decrease the rate and depth of respirations. Other categories of CNS depressant agents include barbiturates (e.g., phenobarbitol [Nembutal], secobarbital [Seconal]), benzodiazepines (e.g., lorazepam [Ativan], midazolam [generic], diazepam [Valium]), neuroleptics (e.g., chlorpromazine [Thorazine], haloperidol [Haldol], clozapine [generic]) muscle relaxants, tricyclic antidepressants, and anticonvulsants. Conversely, bronchodilators decrease airway resistance and residual volume with a resultant increase in vital capacity and airflow. Common bronchodilator medications include albuterol (AccuNeb, Ventolin, Proventil), bitolterol (Tornalate), epinephrine (EpiPen), formoterol (Foradil), isoproterenol (Isuprel), metaproterenol (Alupent), and terbutaline (generic).[89,90]

Parameters of Respiration

In examining respiration, four parameters are considered: rate, depth, rhythm, and sound. The *rate* is the number of breaths per minute. Either inspirations or expirations are counted, but not both. The normal adult RR is 12 to 20 per minute. The rate should be counted for 30 seconds and multiplied by 2. If any irregularities are noted, a full 60-second count is indicated.

The *depth* of respiration refers to the amount (volume) of air exchanged with each breath. Normally, the depth of respirations is consistent, producing a relatively even, uniform movement of the chest. The normal adult tidal volume is approximately 500 mL of air. The depth of respiration is determined by observation of chest movements and is usually described as *deep* or *shallow*, depending on whether the amount of air exchanged is greater or less than normal. With deep breaths, a large volume of air is exchanged; with shallow respirations, a small amount of air is exchanged, typically with minimal lung expansion or chest wall movement.

The *rhythm* refers to the regularity of inspirations and expirations. Normally, there is an even time interval between respirations. The respiratory rhythm is described as *regular* (normal) or *irregular* (abnormal).

The *sound* of respirations refers to deviations from normal, quiet, effortless breathing. Although some respiratory sounds are audible, accurate identification requires auscultation (listening with a stethoscope placed directly against the chest wall). Normal (*vesicular*) breath sounds are heard primarily during inspiration and sound relatively smooth and soft.[78] Common abnormal (*adventitious*) sounds of breathing include the following:

- **Wheeze** *(Wheezing):* A continuous whistling sound produced by air passing through a narrowed airway such as a bronchi or bronchiole; is often compared to the whistling produced when stretching the neck of a balloon and allowing air to escape slowly through the narrowed passageway. It may be heard on both inspiration and expiration but is more prominent on expiration. Wheezing is a common symptom of asthma, is also seen in CHF, and can result from an airway obstruction.
- **Stridor:** A harsh, high-pitched crowing sound that occurs with upper airway obstructions resulting in narrowing of the glottis or trachea. It is apparent in patients with tracheal stenosis or presence of a foreign object.
- **Crackles** (also called *rales*): Rattling or bubbling sounds that occur owing to secretions in the air passages of the respiratory tract. The sound is often compared to that of rustling a cellophane bag. Crackles may be heard with the ear but are most accurately determined using a stethoscope. Crackles are apparent in patients with CHF.
- **Sigh:** A deep inspiration followed by a prolonged, audible expiration. Occasional sighs are normal and function to expand alveoli; frequent sighs are abnormal and may be indicative of emotional stress.
- **Stertor:** A snoring sound owing to partial obstruction (e.g., secretions) in the upper airway (e.g., trachea, large bronchi).

Patterns of Respiration

Examination of the rate, rhythm, and depth allows the therapist to determine the *pattern* of respiration. Not all patients will present with a distinct pattern of respiration. However, several patterns occur with sufficient frequency that uniform terminology has been developed for their identification. Common respiratory patterns are presented in Figure 2.27.

Eupnea is the term used to describe a normal breathing pattern of 12 to 20 times per minute in an adult. **Hyperventilation** is an abnormally fast rate and depth of respiration often associated with anxiety, emotional stress, and panic disorders. A common response to an acute episode is to have the patient rebreathe into a paper bag, which replaces some of the lost carbon dioxide (**hypocapnia**). CNS or pulmonary disorders may cause prolonged hyperventilation. **Hypoventilation** is a reduction in the rate and depth of respirations. This decrease in the amount of air entering the lungs causes an increase in arterial carbon dioxide levels.

Difficult or labored breathing is called **dyspnea**. Patients with dyspnea require increased, noticeable effort to breathe, and often appear as if struggling to get air into the lungs. In an effort to increase effectiveness of respiration, accessory muscles such as the intercostals and abdominals are often active. The intercostals assist in raising the ribs to expand the thoracic cavity; the abdominals assist function of the diaphragm. Additional muscles that may provide accessory functions in respiration are the sternocleidomastoid, pectoralis major and minor, scalenes, and subclavius. Use of accessory muscles to breathe is referred to as **costal** or **thoracic breathing**. Pain and nasal flaring sometimes accompany dyspnea

(to bring in more oxygen). Acute episodes may be brought on by blockage of an air passage, infection of the respiratory tract, or trauma to the thorax. Long-standing dyspnea is a hallmark of COPD, such as asthma or bronchitis. Therapists often teach patients with COPD a breathing technique called *pursed-lip breathing* to help prevent small airway collapse. In this technique, air is inhaled slowly through the nose and slowly exhaled through pursed lips.

Orthopnea is difficult or labored breathing (dyspnea) when the patient is lying down that is relieved by moving to a sitting or standing position. The change in positioning causes gravity to lower abdominal organs, allowing increased room for chest expansion. Orthopnea is a characteristic symptom of CHF and also may be seen with asthma, advanced emphysema, and pulmonary edema. **Tachypnea** is an abnormally fast RR, usually greater than 24 breaths per minute. This pattern is seen with respiratory insufficiency and fever as the body attempts to rid itself of excess heat. During fever, RR may increase as much as 4 per minute with each 1°F (0.6°C) increase in temperature.[54] **Bradypnea** is an abnormally slow RR, usually 10 breaths or fewer per minute. Bradypnea is associated with impairment of the respiratory control center, as may occur with increased intracranial pressure (tumor), drug intake (narcotics), or metabolic disorder. **Apnea** is the absence of respirations and is usually transient. If sustained for longer than several minutes, brain damage and death may occur. **Cheyne-Stokes respiration** is characterized by a period of apnea lasting 10 to 60 seconds, followed by gradually increasing depth

TYPE	DESCRIPTION	ILLUSTRATION
Eupnea	Normal respirations, with equal rate and depth, 12–20 breaths/min	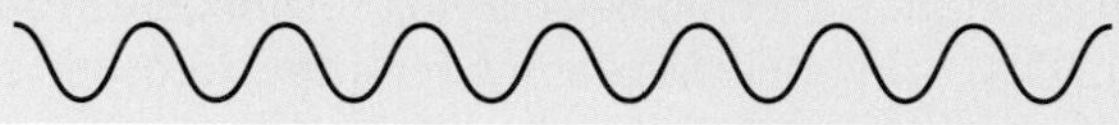
Bradypnea	Slow respirations, <10 breaths/min	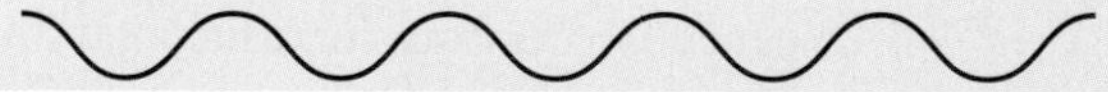
Tachypnea	Fast respirations, < 24 breaths/min, usually shallow	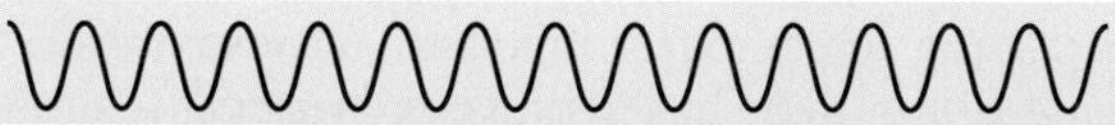
Kussmaul's Respirations	Respirations that are regular but abnormally deep and increased in rate	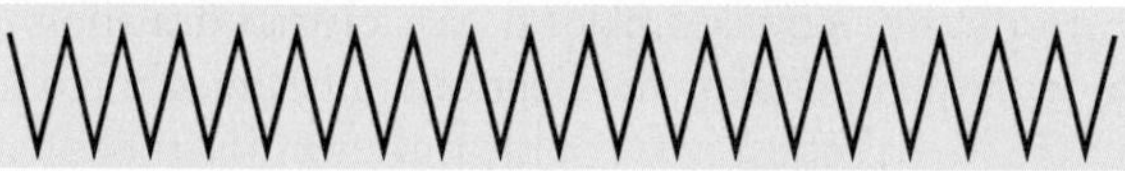
Biot's Respirations	Irregular respirations of variable depth (usually shallow), alternating with periods of apnea (absence of breathing)	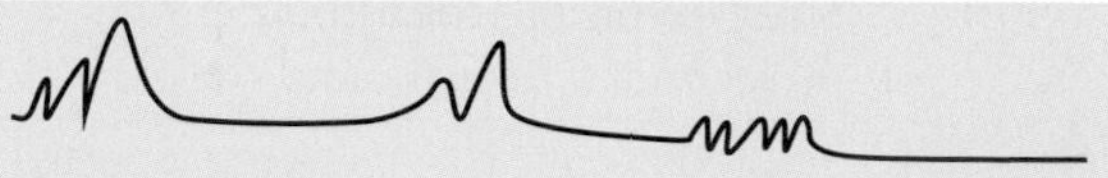
Cheyne-Strokes Respirations	Gradual increase in depth of respirations followed by gradual decrease and then a period of apnea	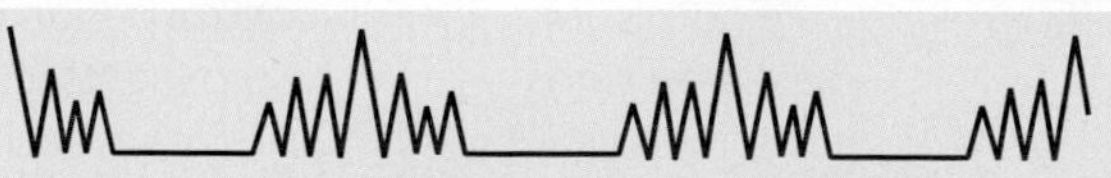
Apnea	Absence of breathing	

Figure 2.27 Normal (*top*) and abnormal respiratory patterns. When examining respiratory patterns, consider the *rate, rhythm,* and *depth* of breathing and describe what is observed using these terms. (*From Wilkinson and Treas,[7] [p. 339], with permission.*)

and frequency of respirations (hyperventilation). It occurs with depression of the cerebral hemispheres (e.g., coma), in basal ganglia disease, and occasionally in CHF. It is associated with a poor prognosis. Box 2.6 Evidence Summary includes studies examining the reliability and validity of measuring respiratory rate.

Respiratory Examination

Because respiration is under both voluntary (cortical) and involuntary control, it is important that the patient is unaware that respiration is being examined. Once aware of the examination, characteristics of the breathing pattern will likely be altered. This is a normal reaction to being observed. It is often recommended that respirations be observed immediately after taking the pulse. After monitoring the pulse, the fingers can remain in place at the pulse site, and respirations can be monitored without drawing the patient's conscious attention to his or her breathing pattern. Ideally, respiration should be examined with the chest exposed. If this is not possible, or if respirations cannot be easily observed through clothing, maintain fingers on the radial pulse site and place the patient's forearm across the chest. This will allow limited palpation without drawing conscious input from the patient. Chapter 12: Chronic Pulmonary Dysfunction, provides a more thorough discussion of the respiratory examination.

Monitoring Respiration

A. Assemble equipment.
   1. Watch (or wall clock) with a second hand.
B. Wash hands.
C. Procedure.
   1. Ensure patient safety and comfort. Respirations are typically monitored with the patient either supine or sitting.
      Note: The patient should be in a quiet resting position for at least 5 minutes prior to monitoring respirations.
   2. Expose chest area; if area cannot be exposed and respirations are not readily observable, place patient's forearm across chest and keep fingers positioned as if continuing to monitor the radial pulse.
   3. As the patient breathes, observe the rise and fall of the chest; note the amount of effort required or audible sounds produced during breathing. (Normally, respiration is effortless and silent.)
   4. Using the second hand of a watch or clock, determine the rate by counting respirations (either inspirations or expirations, but not both) for 30 seconds and multiply by 2.
   5. Identify the rhythm (regularity of inspirations and expirations); note deviations from normal

Box 2.6 Evidence Summary	Studies Examining the Reliability and Validity of Measuring Respiratory Rate			
Reference	Methods	Subjects/Design	Results	Conclusion/Comments
Smith et al (2011)	To compare an electronic respiratory rate (RR) monitor with the manual counting method. The manual method required the same health professional to place a hand on the patient's chest and count chest excursions for 60 seconds.	A total of 220 patients who required post-operative oxygen via an adult-sized mask were included. RR was measured using the electronic monitor and the manual method simultaneously.	There was a significant correlation ($r = 0.84$) between the two methods for measuring RR. The mean manual RR was 14.32 and the mean monitor RR was 13.46. The mean difference between RR methods was 0.86.	This study showed that the electronic RR monitor was easy to use and safe. In addition, the electronic monitor can provide continuous monitoring, which the manual method cannot provide. The greatest difference between methods was observed in unstable patient populations.
Considine et al (2009)	To predict critical care admissions based on signs (including vital signs) and symptoms.	A retrospective case control design of 386 patients (193 patients in each group). Groups were matched based on age, sex, emergency department diagnosis, and triage category.	Cases (32.3%) had a higher incidence of abnormal RR when compared to controls (22.3%). In fact, RR abnormalities at first nursing assessment (odds ratio = 1.66, 95% CI = 1.05-2.06) increased the odds of critical care admission.	This study indicates factors that may predict critical care admission, such as abnormal RR.

Box 2.6 Evidence Summary Studies Examining the Reliability and Validity of Measuring Respiratory Rate—cont'd

Reference	Methods	Subjects/Design	Results	Conclusion/Comments
Chaboyer et al (2008)	To predict adverse events within 72 hours of discharge from an intensive care unit (ICU). Predictors examined included demographic and clinical characteristics, including vital signs.	This study examined 300 patients admitted to the ICU, of which 208 (69.3%) had no adverse event, 92 (30.7%) had any adverse event, and 17 (5.7%) had a major adverse event.	Based on univariate analyses, an RR < 10 or ≥ 25 was a predictor for: Any adverse event (odds ratio = 4.23, 95% CI = 2.12-8.45) A major adverse event (odds ratio = 5.82, 95% CI = 2.03-16.68) Based on multivariate analysis, an RR < 10 or ≥ 25 was the stronger predictor of any adverse event (odds ratio = 3.22, 95% CI = 1.56-6.66).	Abnormal RR and high HR are commonly used in risk assessment after discharge from an ICU. Both RR and HR are independent predictors of adverse events, with RR being the strongest predictor based on univariate and multivariate analyses.
Lockwood et al (2004)	To examine the best available evidence related to monitoring vital signs, including: • Purpose • Limitations • Optimal measurement frequency • What measures should considered vital signs	Narrative, systematic review of vital signs. Updated review of Evans et al (2001). Included 124 studies on neonatal, pediatric, and adult patient populations.	There is limited research on RR measurements. Studies found focused on accuracy of measuring RR and RR as a marker for dysfunction.	Clinicians should not use RR alone as an indicator of deteriorating physiological function. In children, RR should not be used alone as a measure of serious illness. When measuring RR, count for 60 seconds, use a stethoscope for children and neonates when the RR is rapid, and assess the RR when the patient is at rest. In acute situations, an increasing RR may indicate respiratory dysfunction.
Evans et al (2001)	To examine the best available evidence related to monitoring vital signs, including: • Measurements that constitute vital signs • Optimal measurement frequency • Limitations of vital signs	Narrative systematic review of vital signs. Included 69 studies on neonatal, pediatric, and adult patient populations.	There is limited low-level evidence on the frequency with which vital signs should be monitored. There is little research on RR measurement.	Much of current practice of vital sign measurement is not based on research but on tradition and expert opinion. Several studies have reported inaccurate RR measurements as a function of the technique used. There is also evidence to support the use of pulse oximetry to detect deterioration in physiologic function.

Prepared by Kevin K. Chui, PT, PhD, GCS, OCS.

Smith, I, et al: Respiratory rate measurement: A comparison of methods. British Journal of Healthcare Assistants 15:18, 2011.

Considine, J, Thomas, S, and Potter, R: Predictors of critical care admission in emergency department patients triaged as low to moderate urgency. J Adv Nurs 65:818, 2009.

Chaboyer, W, et al: Predictors of adverse events in patients after discharge from the intensive care unit. Am J Crit Care 17:255, 2008.

Lockwood, C, Conroy-Hiller, T, and Page, T: Systematic review: Vital signs. JBI Reports 2:207, 2004.

Evans, D, Hodgkinson, B, and Berry, J: Vital signs in hospital patients: A systematic review. Int J Nurs Stud 38:643, 2001.

uninterrupted, even spacing. If any irregularities are noted, count for a full 60 seconds to accommodate the fluctuations and ensure an accurate count.

6. Observe the depth of respiration; determine if a small, large, or approximately normal volume of air is inspired. Observe involvement of accessory muscles, which suggests weakness in the primary muscles of breathing (diaphragm and external intercostal muscles); if difficult to observe, palpation of chest wall excursion can be used to identify depth of respiration. Record as shallow, deep, or normal.

   Note: Chest wall excursion can also be determined by circumferential chest measures using a tape measure at specific bony landmarks. Three common landmarks for circumferential chest measures are (1) the sternal angle of Luis; (2) the xiphoid process; and (3) midway between the xiphoid process and the umbilicus.

7. If indicated, determine the sound of breathing using a stethoscope.

8. Return clothing if chest has been exposed.

9. Wash hands.

■ BLOOD PRESSURE

Blood pressure refers to the force the blood exerts against a vessel wall. It is measured in millimeters of mercury (mm Hg) and recorded in the form of a fraction (e.g., 119/79). The top number indicates systolic pressure, and the bottom indicates diastolic pressure. Because liquid flows only from a higher to a lower pressure, the pressure is highest in the arteries, lower in the capillaries, and lowest in veins.[45,47]

Inasmuch as the heart is an intermittent pulsatile pump, pressure is measured at both the highest and lowest points of the pulse. These points represent the systolic (ventricular contraction) and diastolic (ventricular relaxation) pressures. The **systolic pressure** is the highest pressure exerted by the blood against the arterial walls. The **diastolic pressure** (which is constantly present) is the lowest pressure. The elastic properties of the arterial walls allow for expansion and recoil in response to the changing volume of circulating blood during the cardiac cycle. The mathematical difference between the systolic and diastolic pressures is called the **pulse pressure**. For example, a systolic pressure of 119 mm Hg and a diastolic pressure of 79 mm Hg result in a pulse pressure of 40 mm Hg.

BP is a function of two primary elements: (1) cardiac output (amount of blood flow, CO); and (2) peripheral resistance (impediment to blood flow within a vessel, R) that the heart must overcome. The relationship between BP, CO, and R is expressed in the equation: BP = CO × R. Additional factors that contribute to this relationship include the diameter and elasticity of vessel walls, blood volume, and blood viscosity.[91]

Blood Pressure Regulation

The *vasomotor center* is located bilaterally in the lower pons and upper medulla. It transmits impulses through sympathetic nerves to all vessels of the body. The vasomotor center is tonically active, producing a slow, continual firing in all vasoconstrictor nerve fibers. It is this slow, continual firing that maintains a partial state of contraction of the blood vessels and provides normal *vasomotor tone.*[49] The vasomotor center assists in providing the stable arterial pressure required to maintain blood flow to body tissue and organs. This occurs because of its close connection to the cardiac controlling center in the medulla (because changes in cardiac output will influence BP). In addition, the vasomotor and cardiac controlling centers require input from afferent receptors.

Afferent input regarding BP is provided primarily by *baroreceptors* and *chemoreceptors.* The *baroreceptors* (pressoreceptors) are stimulated by stretch of the vessel wall from alterations in pressure. These receptors have a high concentration in the walls of the internal carotid arteries above the carotid bifurcation and in the walls of the arch of the aorta. Baroreceptors located in the *carotid sinuses* of the carotid arteries monitor BP to the brain. Baroreceptors in the *aortic sinuses* of the aortic arch are responsible for monitoring BP throughout the body.

In response to an increase in BP, the baroreceptor input to the vasomotor center results in an inhibition of the vasoconstrictor center of the medulla and excitation of the vagal center.[47] This results in a decreased HR, decreased force of cardiac contraction, and vasodilation, with a subsequent drop in BP. The baroreceptor input during a lowering of BP would produce the opposite effects.

The *chemoreceptors* are stimulated by reduced arterial oxygen concentrations, increases in carbon dioxide tension, and increased hydrogen ion concentrations. These receptors lie close to the baroreceptors. Those located in the carotid artery are called *carotid bodies,* and on the aortic arch they are termed *aortic bodies.* Impulses from these receptors travel to the brain (cardioregulatory and vasomotor centers) via afferent pathways in the vagus and glossopharyngeal nerves. Efferent impulses from these centers, in response to alterations in BP, will alter HR, strength of cardiac contractions, and size of blood vessels.[46]

Factors Influencing Blood Pressure

Many factors influence pressure. As with all vital signs, BP is represented by a range of normal values and will yield the most useful data when monitored over a period of time. Important influences to be considered when examining BP include blood volume, diameter and elasticity of arteries, cardiac output, age, exercise, and arm position.

Blood Volume

The amount of circulating blood in the body directly affects pressure. Blood loss (e.g., hemorrhage) will cause pressure to drop, and can result in **hypovolemic shock** from inadequate tissue perfusion. Conversely, an increase in the amount of circulating blood (e.g., blood transfusion) will cause the pressure to rise. Reduced fluid volume, as may occur with diarrhea or inadequate oral intake (dehydration), will also lower BP; excess fluid, as occurs with CHF, will increase pressure.[60] Essentially, any situation causing a shift (increase or decrease) in body fluids (intravascular, interstitial, or intracellular) will alter BP.[60] Bladder distention can also contribute to BP elevation.

Diameter and Elasticity of Arteries

The diameter (size) of the vessel lumen will provide either *increased peripheral resistance* (vasoconstriction) or *decreased resistance* (vasodilation) to cardiac output. The elasticity of the vessel wall also influences resistance. Normally, the expansion and recoil properties of the arterial walls provide a continuous, smooth flow of blood into the capillaries and veins between heartbeats. With age, these properties are diminished; arterial stiffness decreases vessel wall compliance. Thus, there is a higher resistance to blood flow with resultant *increase* in BP.

A characteristic feature of arteriosclerosis is reduced vessel wall compliance in response to fluctuations in pressure. For older adults, elevated BP is often associated with the degenerative effects of arteriosclerosis. As the disease progresses, small arteries and arterioles lose elasticity, the walls become thick and hard and unable to yield to pressure exerted by blood flow, and the lumen gradually narrows and may eventually become blocked. Multiple factors may contribute to hypertension in elders (e.g., smoking, activity level, obesity, diet, comorbidities such as cardiac or vascular disease). In her extensive literature review, Pinto states, "The increase in BP with age is most likely due to complex and varied factors moulded [molded] and influenced by the individual environment and lifestyle."[92, p. 110]

Cardiac Output

When increased amounts of blood are pumped into the arteries, the walls of the vessels distend, resulting in a higher BP. With lower cardiac output, less blood is pushed into the vessel, and there is a subsequent drop in pressure.

Age

BP varies with age. It normally rises gradually after birth and reaches a peak during puberty. By late adolescence (18 to 19 years), adult BP is reached. For many years, the normal adult BP was considered 120/80 mm Hg. New BP guidelines were presented in the Seventh Report of the Joint National Committee (JNC) on Prevention, Detection, Evaluation, and Treatment of High Blood Pressure: The JNC 7 Report (Table 2.8).[93] The new recommendations recognize the high prevalence of hypertension that affects millions of individuals in the United States and people worldwide. Hypertension (equal to or greater than 140/90) is a primary risk factor

Table 2.8	Classification of Blood Pressure for Adults Ages 18 Years and Older	
BP Classification	**Systolic BP (mm Hg)**	**Diastolic BP (mm Hg)**
Normal	<120	<80
Prehypertension	120–139	80–89
Hypertension		
• Stage 1	140–159	90–99
• Stage 2	≥160	≥100

From Chobanian et al,[93] with permission.

for myocardial infarct, heart failure, stroke, and kidney disease. The former normal adult BP value of 120/80 mm Hg now falls into the new category of prehypertension (systolic pressure: 120 to 139; diastolic pressure: 80 to 89). "Prehypertension is not a disease category. Rather, it is a designation chosen to identify individuals at high risk of developing hypertension, so that both patients and clinicians are alerted to this risk and encouraged to intervene and prevent or delay the disease from developing."[93, p. 12] A BP value of 119/79 mm Hg or below is the new normal adult standard. The JNC 7 Report recommends implementation of measures to prevent further increases in the prevalence of hypertension.[93]

Clinical Note: Seen more frequently with elders is *white coat hypertension* or *nonsustained hypertension*. This occurs in individuals whose blood pressure is higher in a clinical setting than outside the clinic; it is believed to be associated with the stress and anxiety of seeing a doctor (the "white coat").

Exercise

Physical activity increases cardiac output, with a consequent linear increase in BP. Greater increases are noted in systolic pressure owing to proportional changes in pressure gradient of peripheral vessels. This means that although cardiac output during exercise is high, vasodilation reduces peripheral resistance to maintain a relatively lower diastolic pressure. BP increases are proportional to the intensity of the workload. A drop in SBP of 10 mm Hg or more with increasing exercise intensity is an indication for stopping exercise (per American College of Sports Medicine guidelines).

Valsalva Maneuver

The **Valsalva maneuver** is an attempt to exhale forcibly with the glottis, nose, and mouth closed. It causes an increase in intrathoracic pressure with an accompanying collapse of the veins of the chest wall. There is a subsequent decrease in blood flow to the heart, a decreased venous return, and a drop in BP. This maneuver serves to internally stabilize the abdominal and chest wall during periods of rapid and maximum exertion such as lifting a heavy object. When the breath is released, the intrathoracic pressure decreases, and venous return is suddenly reestablished as an "overshoot" mechanism to compensate for the drop in BP. In turn, there is a marked increase in HR and BP. This rapid rise in arterial pressure causes vagal slowing of the HR (bradycardia). Although the Valsalva maneuver can temporarily enhance muscle function via internal stabilization, it has an indirect undesirable effect of increasing BP and should be avoided by individuals with cardiac impairment and hypertension.[45,49]

Clinical Note: A common misconception concerning the Valsalva maneuver is that it directly increases HR and BP. As described earlier, it is the body's recovery mechanism of suddenly increasing venous return that causes this increase. The subsequent drop in BP due to the Valsalva maneuver may result in seeing "black dots" and the feeling of dizziness that often accompanies straining while lifting a heavy object.

Orthostatic Hypotension

Associated with prolonged immobility and periods of bedrest, **orthostatic** or **postural hypotension** is a sudden drop in BP that occurs when movement to upright postures (sitting or standing) is initiated. The positional change causes gravitational blood pooling in the lower extremity (LE) veins. Venous return and cardiac outputs are reduced, with resultant cerebral hypoperfusion. This can trigger an episode of light-headedness, dizziness, or even loss of consciousness (syncope). In response to positional changes under normal circumstances, BP is maintained by reflex vasoconstriction (via baroreceptors), which increases HR. After a period of inactivity, postural hypotension should be anticipated; it requires a gradual acclimation to the upright position until normal reflex control returns. Other predisposing factors for postural hypotension include exercise, drugs such as antihypertensives and vasodilators, reduction in baroreceptor response with aging, the Valsalva maneuver, and **hypovolemia** (abnormally low volume of circulating blood).[94,95] Patients with CNS involvement of the autonomic nervous system (e.g., patients with acute cervical spinal cord injury or Parkinson's disease) typically exhibit episodes of orthostatic hypotension with position changes. As a useful precaution, any patient restricted to a recumbent position for even short periods should be considered at risk for postural hypotension. These events can be minimized by use of external pressure supports such as abdominal binders and support or full-length elastic stockings (elastic bandages can also be used effectively) and a very gradual acclimation to upright postures. Should postural hypotension occur during treatment, the patient should be reclined from upright with the legs elevated.

Arm Position

BP may vary as much as 20 mm Hg by altering arm position. For consistency of measurements, the patient should be sitting with the arm in a horizontal supported position at heart level. If patient condition or the type of activity precludes these positions, alterations should be carefully documented. As with other vital signs, factors such as fear, anxiety, or emotional stress also will cause an increase in BP.

Risk Factors

High BP is also associated with a large number of risk factors, including high sodium intake, obesity and being overweight, a sedentary lifestyle, heavy alcohol consumption, pregnancy, sex, and age. In the United States, approximately 76.4 million people aged 20 or older have high BP.[96] Projections suggest that by 2030, another 27 million people could have high BP. Until age 45 years, a greater percentage of men than women have high BP; between 45 and 64 years of age, the percentage of men and women is comparable; and after that a much higher percentage of women than men have high BP.[96] African Americans are at greater risk for high BP than Caucasians. The rate of hypertension among this group is 44%, among the highest in the world.[97] Heredity (parental history of high BP) also places the individual at greater risk. Globally, high systolic BP is seen in 51% of patients with stroke and in 45% of patients with ischemic heart disease.[98]

In addition, some medications can either increase BP or interfere with antihypertensive drugs. These drugs include steroids, nonsteroidal anti-inflammatory agents, diet pills, cyclosporine, erythropoietin, tricyclic antidepressants, monoamine oxidase inhibitors, and some oral contraceptives.

Equipment Requirements

A noninvasive or *indirect* measure of BP is used by physical therapists. In critical care settings, invasive or *direct* measures of BP are obtained by placing a thin catheter directly into an artery. The equipment required for taking BP using the more common noninvasive auscultatory (listening) method includes a *sphygmomanometer* and a *stethoscope*. The sphygmomanometer (frequently referred to as a *blood pressure cuff*) consists of a flat, airtight, inflatable latex bladder. The bladder is covered with a cotton or nylon sleeve that extends beyond the length of the bladder. There are two tubes that extend from the cuff. One is attached to a rubber bulb that has a valve to maintain or to release air from the cuff. The second tube is attached to a pressure manometer (portion of sphygmomanometer that registers the pressure reading). In patient care settings, sphygmomanometers may be wall mounted (Fig 2.28A) or placed on a mobile stand with a wheeled base (Fig 2.28B). Box 2.7 Evidence Summary presents studies examining the reliability and validity of blood pressure measurements.

Box 2.7 Evidence Summary   Studies Examining the Reliability and Validity of Blood Pressure Measurements

Reference	Method(s)	Subjects/Design	Results	Conclusions/Comments
Frese et al (2011)	Provide blood pressure (BP) measurement guidelines for physical therapists and physical therapist assistants.	This is a narrative review paper.	Provides information on classification of hypertension, common sources of error, recommended cuff sizes, reference data, and considerations for special situations.	Accurately measuring BP is critical for physical therapists.
Verrij et al (2009)	Examined the effect of elevating the arm overhead for 30 seconds (sec) on the amplitudes of Korotkoff's sounds.	This study examined 46 patients (mean age of 54 years). Compared the amplitudes of Korotkoff's sounds after overhead and usual arm positions.	The amplitude of the first Korotkoff's sound with the arm overhead was significantly (1.82 times) greater than the amplitude of the first Korotkoff's sound with the arm at its usual position.	Korotkoff's sounds can be increased by positioning the arm overhead for 30 sec and then bringing the arm to its usual position before taking BP; positioning the arm overhead does not affect BP.
Scisney-Matlock et al (2009)	Examined the reliability and reproducibility of clinic (manual sphygmomanometer) and home (automated) BP. Compared clinic and home BPs to 24 hour ambulatory BP monitoring.	Middle-aged, racially diverse women ($n = 161$). The mean of the two clinic BPs and the higher of the two home BPs was used.	The correlation between systolic home BP measurements and systolic ambulatory BP monitoring was much stronger for white women than for African-American women.	For both African American and white women, home (automated) BP measurements are reliable when compared to 24-hour ambulatory BP monitoring.
Heinemann et al (2008)	Compared an automated blood pressure (BP) unit with manual sphygmomanometer.	Patients from different departments of a large regional hospital ($n = 63$). BPs taken concurrently using both devices.	There were significant differences between methods. The manual systolic BP (SBP) and diastolic BP (DBP) were significantly higher than the automated SBP and DBP.	The automated machine consistently under-read BPs. The automated machine can be used with some confidence to measure SBP, but caution should be used when measuring DBP.
Nelson et al (2008)	To compare the aneroid manometer, automatic arm monitor, and automatic wrist monitor with the mercury column manometer (used as the gold standard).	A total of 83 participants (age range 19-92 years) participated. Measurements were taken on the left arm with 5 minutes between measurements.	The SBP significantly increased with age but not by device. There was also a significant interaction between age and device.	Difference among monitors depends on the age of the person. The automatic wrist monitors were the most unreliable. The aneroid manometer, automatic arm monitor, and automatic wrist monitor are less accurate than the mercury column manometer.
Eser et al (2006)	Compared the effect of four different body positions on BP:	Measurements were taken on 157 healthy female students, aged 18-24 years. BP was taken on the	For all positions, there was no significant difference in DBP. The SBP in supine was significantly greater than in	The SBP and DBP was the highest in the supine position. There was a significant difference in SBP by posi-

Continued

Box 2.7 Evidence Summary Studies Examining the Reliability and Validity of Blood Pressure Measurements—cont'd

Reference	Method(s)	Subjects/Design	Results	Conclusions/Comments
	(1) sitting, (2) standing, (3) supine, and (4) supine with legs crossed. BP was measured using an automatic arm monitor.	left arm. Measurements were taken in the same order (sitting, standing, supine, and then supine with legs crossed).	the other positions. All changes in SBP between positions were significant except supine and supine with legs crossed.	tion, but not DBP. All of the changes in position significantly changed SBP except for supine and supine with legs crossed.
Fonseca-Reyes et al (2003)	Examined the effect of using a standard cuff on BP in patients with obese arms. Both a standard and large cuff were used.	In this study, 120 individuals with a mean age of 43.1 years and mean arm circumference of 37.9 cm (14.9 inches) were examined. The order of the cuff size used was randomized.	Both the SBP and DBP were significantly greater when the standard cuff size was used.	Using a standard cuff size on an obese arm will overestimate BP. Given the prevalence of obesity, clinics should have different size cuffs for taking BP.

Prepared by Kevin K. Chui, PT, PhD, GCS, OCS.

Frese, EM, Fick, A, and Sadowsky, HS: Blood pressure measurement guidelines for physical therapists. Cardiopulm Phys Ther J 22:5, 2011.

Verrij, EA, Nieuwenhuizen, L, and Bos WJ: Raising the arm before cuff inflation increases the loudness of Korotkoff sounds. Blood Press Monit 14(6):268, 2009.

Scisney-Matlock, M, et al: Reliability and reproducibility of clinic and home blood pressure measurements in hypertensive women according to age and ethnicity. Blood Press Monit 14:49, 2009.

Heinemann, M, et al: Automated versus manual blood pressure measurement: A randomized crossover trial. Int J Nurs Pract 14:296, 2008.

Nelson, D, et al: Accuracy of automated blood pressure monitors. J Dent Hyg 82:1, 2008.

Eser, I, et al: The effect of different body positions on blood pressure. J Clin Nurs 16:137, 2006.

Fonseca-Reyes, S, et al: Effects of standard cuff on blood pressure readings in patients with obese arms. How frequent are arms of "large circumference"? Blood Press Monit 8:101, 2003.

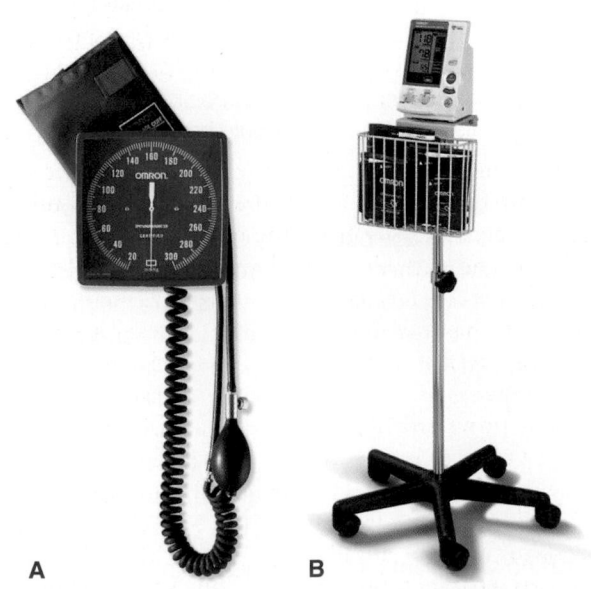

A   **B**

Figure 2.28 In clinical settings, sphygmomanometers may be **(A)** wall-mounted or **(B)** placed on a mobile stand. (*Courtesy of Omron, Inc., Lake Forest, IL, 60045.*)

BP cuffs are typically secured on the patient's extremity by a hook and loop closure. They come in a variety of sizes. In adults, the width of the bladder should be approximately 40% of the arm circumference, and bladder length should be enough to encircle at least 80% of arm circumference.[92,99] Obtaining a cuff of appropriate size is important. Cuffs that are too narrow will show inaccurately high readings; cuffs that are too wide will show inaccurately low readings.[93]

The manometer registers the BP reading. Manometers are either *mercury* or *aneroid* (Fig. 2.29A and B). The mercury manometer registers BP on a mercury-filled calibrated cylinder. At the uppermost portion of the mercury column is a convex curve called the *meniscus*. A reading is obtained by viewing the meniscus at *eye level*. If not observed directly at eye level, an inaccurate reading will be obtained. The aneroid manometer registers BP by way of a circular calibrated dial and needle; automated PB units provide a digital LCD. Owing to environmental concerns, aneroid manometers and automated displays have largely replaced mercury manometers in a majority of patient care settings.

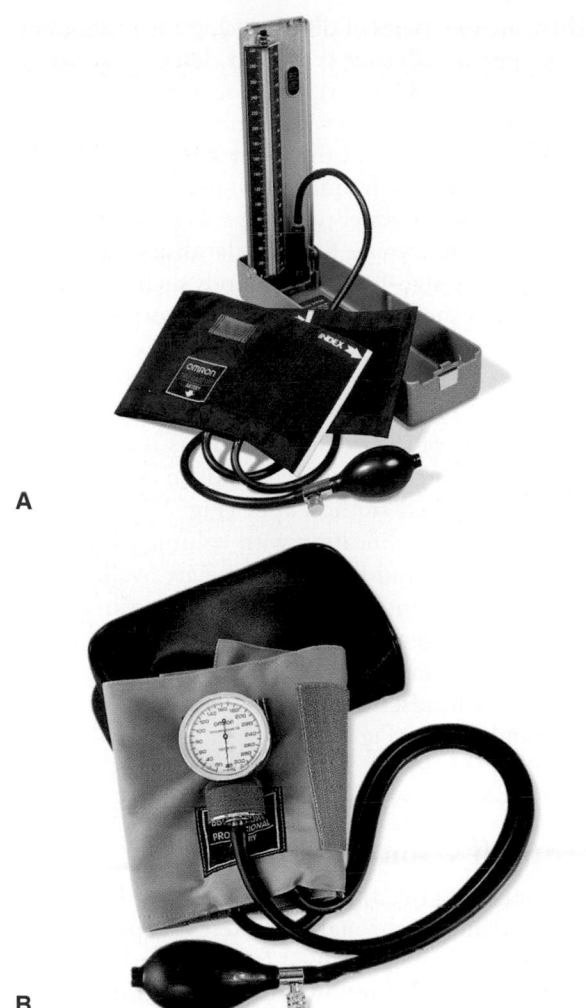

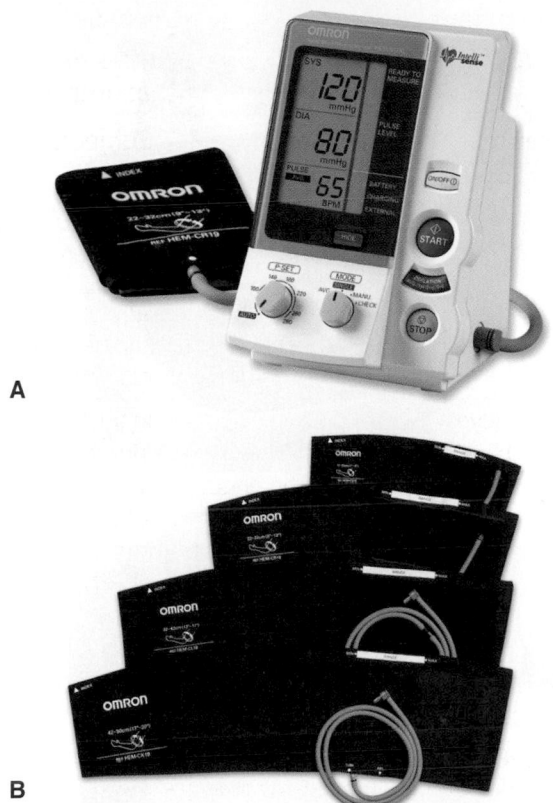

Figure 2.30 **(A)** Automated clinical sphygmomanometer with **(B)** differently sized cuffs. *(Courtesy of Omron, Inc., Lake Forest, IL 60045.)*

Figure 2.29 Sphygmomanometers. **(A)** Mercury gauge manometers have a vertical glass tube containing liquid mercury with a 300 mm Hg scale marked in 2-mm increments. **(B)** Aneroid manometers consist of a circular glass-covered 300 mm Hg gauge in 2-mm increments with needle marker. *(Courtesy of Omron, Inc., Lake Forest, IL 60045.)*

Automated sphygmomanometers (Fig. 2.30A) are self-inflating battery (rechargeable) or electrically powered units; many battery-powered models are also equipped with an AC adapter. Some include the "average mode" feature that performs two or three readings and then averages the total. Devices designed for clinical use often include several cuff sizes (e.g., small, medium, large, and extra-large) (Fig 2.30B).

Personal-sized automated sphygmomanometers are particularly useful and practical for patients requiring frequent self-monitoring. They provide a rapid digital display, monitor pulse (in most cases), allow data storage, and are easy to use. (Place cuff and activate start button.) Automated sphygmomanometers do not require a stethoscope; during automated inflation and deflation, the diastolic and systolic pressures are recorded. These devices monitor BP at the traditional arm location

(Fig. 2.31A) or at the wrist (Fig. 2.31B). For both types of cuffs, patients should be instructed that the UE should be supported at heart level.

To monitor BP with a mercury or aneroid sphygmomanometer, an acoustic stethoscope is used to listen to the sounds over the artery as pressure is released from the cuff. By a combination of listening through the stethoscope and watching the manometer, the BP reading is obtained. A stethoscope amplifies and carries body sounds to the examiner's ears. Proximally, it consists of two rubber or plastic earpieces attached to narrow metal tubing that projects laterally from the earpieces about 1 inch (2.5 cm) and then downward about 6 inches (15 cm). The tubes are connected by a flexible, semicircular metal spring mechanism; the total length of a stethoscope is approximately 30 inches. These metal tubes are referred to as *binaurals* (designed for use in both ears). The semicircular spring provides tension to maintain the position of the earpieces in the examiner's ears during use. The metal tubes then either (1) insert into fork-shaped rubber or plastic tubing that joins to form a single lumen and attach to the head distally (Fig. 2.32, left); or (2) insert into two separate rubber or plastic tubes that do not join (Fig. 2.32, right) and lead individually directly to the head of the stethoscope. (The two tubes are held together with small metal clasps.)

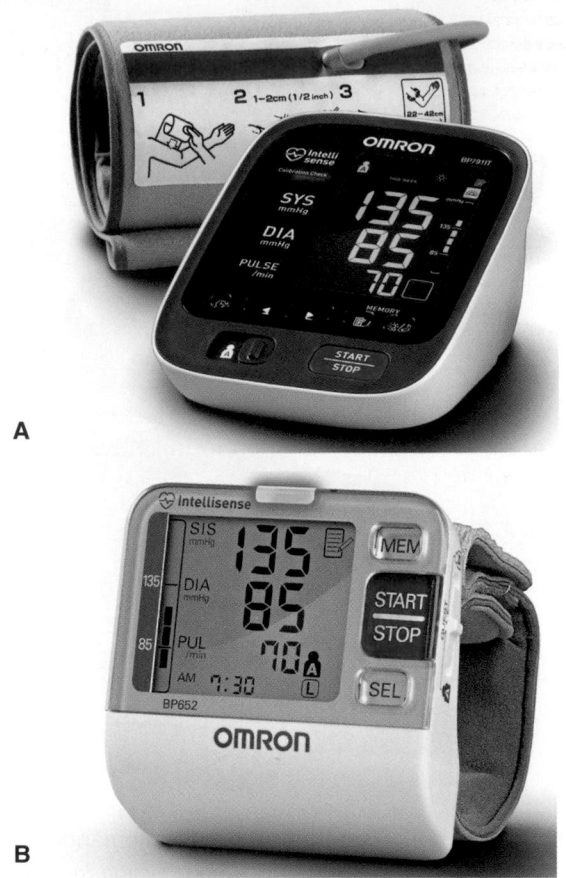

A

B

Figure 2.31 Personal-size automated sphygmomanometers **(A)** arm cuff and **(B)** wrist cuff. *(Courtesy of Omron, Inc., Lake Forest, IL 60045.)*

There are two types of distal sensing microphones on stethoscopes: a *bell-shape* (Fig. 2.33, left) and a *flat disk diaphragm* (Fig. 2.33, right). Stethoscopes may have only one type of head; others have a combination design with one side bell-shaped and the other a flat disk. The bell shape amplifies low-frequency sounds such as those produced in blood vessels; this type is generally recommended for determining BP. The flat disk diaphragm is more useful for high-frequency sounds such as heart and lung sounds. Another type of sensor incorporates both high- and low-frequency capabilities of the two shapes into a single-sided unit that eliminates the need to turn the head over. To hear low-frequency sound (bell-shape), lighter pressure of the examiner's fingers is used; firmer pressure allows high-frequency sounds to be heard.

Battery-powered stethoscopes (Fig 2.34A) provide higher levels of amplification with volume control, and dual-frequency sound filtering; some are available with interchangeable removable heads. A design variation for prehospital emergency medical service (EMS) personnel provides higher amplification levels by replacing the earpieces with a headset designed to block out noise in a moving ambulance (Fig 2.34B). Disposable stethoscopes are also available for use in high-risk settings where minimizing the risk of cross-infection is essential.

Korotkoff's Sounds

When measuring BP, a series of sounds called **Korotkoff's sounds** are heard through the stethoscope. The bell side of the stethoscope is used for auscultation because Korotkoff's sounds are low frequency. Initially when pressure is applied through the cuff around the patient's arm, the blood flow is occluded and no sound is heard

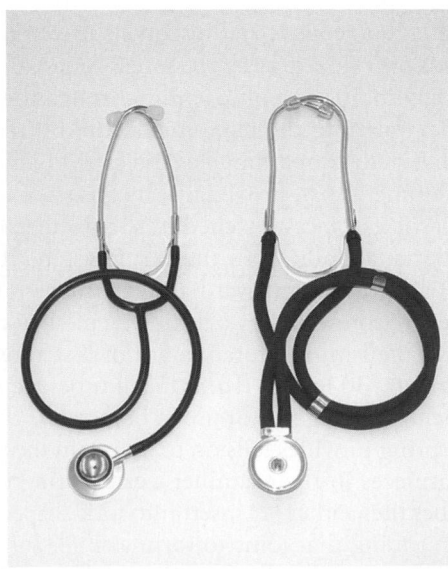

Figure 2.32 Stethoscopes. Standard acoustic stethoscope with a single tube leading to diaphragm (*left*) and Sprague Rappaport type stethoscope with two separate tubes leading to diaphragm (*right*).

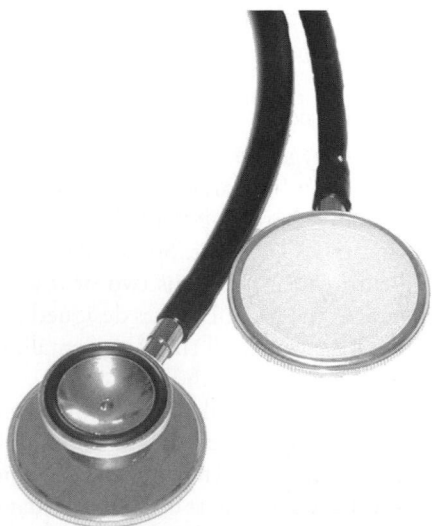

Figure 2.33 Combination design stethoscope head with one side bell-shaped (*left*) to auscultate low-frequency sounds and the opposite side a flat disk diaphragm (*right*) for high-frequency sounds.

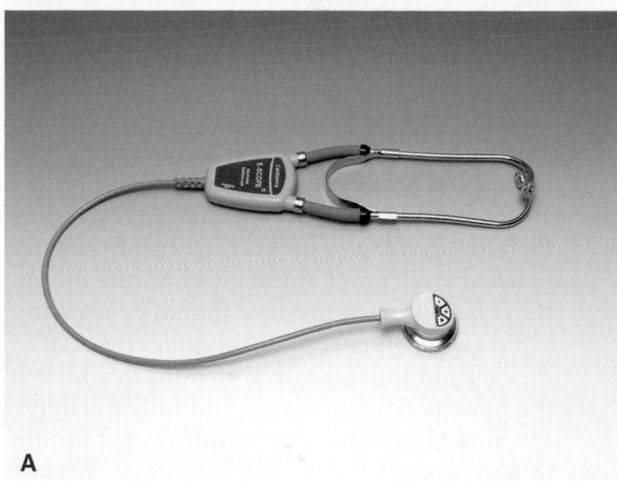

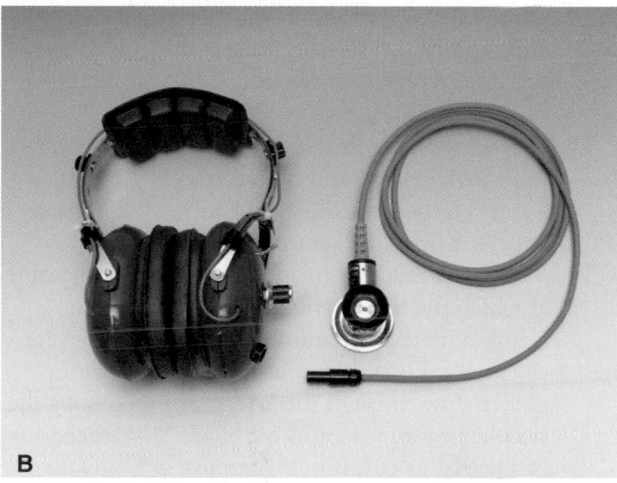

Figure 2.34 Automated stethoscopes. **(A)** Standard automated stethoscope and **(B)** automated stethoscope with headset to block out environmental noise designed for use by emergency medical service (EMS) personnel. *(Courtesy of Cardionics, Inc., Webster, TX 77598.)*

through the stethoscope. As the pressure is gradually released, a series of five phases of sounds can be identified.

The therapist should be alert for the presence of **auscultatory gap**, especially in patients with BP above normal values (hypertension). An auscultatory gap is the temporary disappearance of sound normally heard over the brachial artery between phase 1 and 2 and may cover a range of as much as 40 mm Hg. Not identifying this gap may lead to an underestimation of systolic pressure and overestimation of diastolic pressure.

1. Phase I: The first clear, faint, rhythmic tapping sound, which gradually increases in intensity, is heard. The period when blood initially flows through the artery is recorded as *systolic pressure*. This represents the highest pressure in the arterial system during ventricular contraction. *Be alert for an auscultatory gap.*

2. Phase II: A murmur or swishing sound is heard as artery widens and more blood flows through artery.

3. Phase III: Sounds become crisp, more intense, and louder; blood is now flowing relatively unobstructed.

4. Phase IV: Sound is distinct, with abrupt muffling; soft blowing quality.

5. Phase V: Last sound is heard; recorded as *diastolic pressure* in adults.

A BP reading with a systolic pressure of 117 and a second diastolic reading of 76 would be recorded as 117/76. An important consideration in determining BP is that it should be done in a minimal amount of time. The BP cuff acts as a tourniquet. As such, venous pooling and considerable discomfort to the patient will occur if the cuff is left in place too long. The brachial artery is the most common site for BP monitoring. A description for monitoring LE BP is also presented.

Measuring Brachial Blood Pressure

A. Assemble equipment.
   1. A stethoscope. A bell-shaped head is preferred.
   2. A sphygmomanometer with a bladder size appropriate for the arm. In adults, the width of the bladder should be about 40% of the arm circumference (measurement can be made using a tape measure midway between the acromion and olecranon processes), and bladder length should be enough to encircle at least 80% of arm circumference.[92,99] In children, the bladder should be long enough to completely encircle the entire arm.[92]
   3. Antiseptic wipes for cleaning earpieces and the head of the stethoscope before and after use.
B. Wash hands.
C. Procedure.
   1. Explain procedure and rationale in terms appropriate to the patient's understanding. Indicate that there will be a request to remain quiet during monitoring to avoid interference with auscultation.

   Note: As with other vital sign measures, BP is monitored after the patient has been in a relaxed quiet setting for a period of time because activity or physical exertion will cause an elevation in measurements.
   2. Guide the patient to the desired position. The sitting position is recommended with the back supported, the legs uncrossed, and feet flat on floor. Placing the chair next to a treatment table will facilitate UE positioning. The UE should be free of clothing. (Rolling up a garment sleeve is not acceptable owing to the tourniquet effect produced and interference with cuff positioning.) The midpoint of the arm should be at heart level with the elbow slightly flexed and the palm up. This can be effectively accomplished by supporting the UE on a treatment table. (If needed, pillows can be used to further adjust height.)

   Note: If a supine position is used, the arm should be at the patient's side and slightly elevated to the middle of the trunk. If measuring BP in standing position (e.g., monitoring postural hypotension), ensure that the arm is supported at heart level.

3. Ensure patient understanding, safety, and comfort.

4. Use antiseptic wipes to clean the earpieces and head of stethoscope.

5. Wrap the deflated cuff snugly and evenly around the patient's bare arm approximately 1 inch (2.5 cm) above the antecubital fossa; the center of the cuff should be in line with the brachial artery (Fig. 2.35). Some cuffs have markers to guide positioning over the artery.

6. Ensure that the aneroid gauge is easily visible. (A mercury manometer must be on a level surface at eye level.) Check that the sphygmomanometer registers zero.

    Note: The first time a patient's BP is measured, an estimation of the systolic pressure should be made. This will ensure that during the actual measure, an adequate level of cuff inflation is used. The procedure is as follows:

    a. Locate and palpate the radial artery on the distal forearm of the cuffed arm.

    b. Close the valve of the BP cuff (turn clockwise).

    c. While continuing to monitor the pulse, rapidly inflate the BP cuff to 30 mm Hg above the level at which the radial pulse is extinguished.

    d. Note the pressure value on the gauge. (This is the estimate of maximum pressure required to measure systolic pressure for the individual patient.)

    e. Allow air to release quickly.

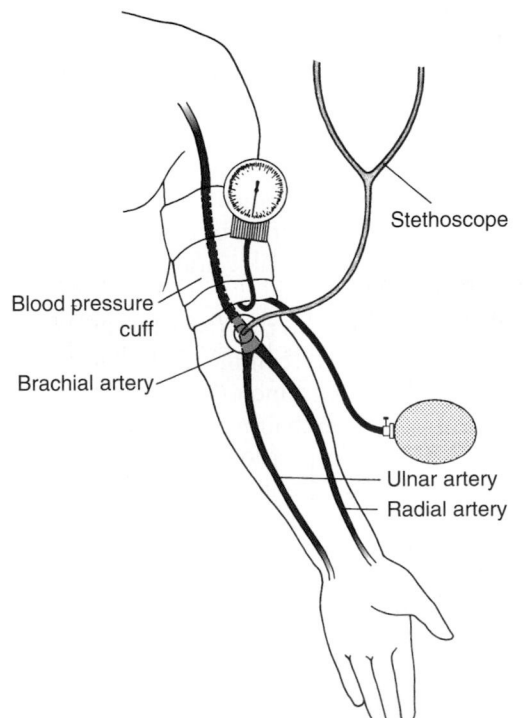

Figure 2.35 Placement of blood pressure cuff and stethoscope for monitoring brachial artery blood pressure.

7. Place the earpieces of the stethoscope (tilting slightly forward) into the ear canals; the tubes of the stethoscope should not be crossed or in contact with each other and should hang freely; use the low-frequency bell side of stethoscope.

8. Locate and palpate the brachial artery slightly above and medial to the antecubital fossa. Place the bell of the stethoscope firmly over the brachial pulse point at the lower border of the BP cuff. Sufficient pressure should be used to avoid gapping between the circumference of the bell and the skin. (In situations in which the pulse is extremely weak and undetectable, Doppler ultrasound may be substituted for use of stethoscope.)

9. Close the valve of the BP cuff (turn clockwise), and rapidly and steadily inflate the cuff to approximately 30 mm Hg above the estimated systolic pressure.

10. Release the thumb valve carefully, allowing air out slowly; air should be released at a rate of 2 mm Hg per heartbeat. Listen for the appearance of Korotkoff's sounds.

11. Watch the manometer closely and note the point at which the first rhythmic tapping sound is heard (a mercury manometer must be viewed at eye level); this is the point when blood first begins to flow through the artery and represents the systolic pressure (Korotkoff phase 1). Deflections in the dial or column of mercury will now be noted.

12. Continue to release air carefully at a rate of 2 mm Hg per heartbeat. Note when the sound first becomes muffled (Korotkoff phase 4) because quickly thereafter the sound will disappear (Korotkoff phase 5); this is recorded as the diastolic pressure.

13. Allow remainder of air to release quickly.

14. Clean the head and earpieces of the stethoscope with antiseptic wipes. If the same examiner is using the stethoscope again, it is not necessary to clean the earpieces. However, the head of the stethoscope should always be cleaned between patients.

15. Wash hands.

Note: It is recommended that at least two BP measurements be taken and the values averaged.[92] At least a 1-minute interval should elapse between repeated measures.

Measuring Popliteal (Thigh) Blood Pressure

Measurement of popliteal BP is indicated in situations in which comparisons between the UE and LE are warranted, such as peripheral vascular disease. They also are used when UE pressures are contraindicated, such as after trauma or surgery. In comparison to the brachial artery, the popliteal artery normally yields a higher systolic pressure; diastolic values are approximately the same. Essentially, the procedure is the same as that for determining pressure at the brachial artery, with the following variations:

1. The patient is in a prone position; alternatively, the supine position may be used. Expose the LE using appropriate draping procedures.
2. Locate the pulse by palpation in the popliteal fossa. Flexing the knee slightly facilitates pulse location as the artery is deep within the posterior knee. Knee flexion also facilitates stethoscope placement. Because the popliteal pulse is deep, it is often useful to initially palpate it using the first two or three fingers of each hand on either side of the posterior knee. Once a pulse is perceived, attention is then directed to locating the strongest pulse point.
3. Wrap the deflated cuff snugly and evenly around the patient's midthigh. (A wide cuff is used; use guidelines for cuff size described for brachial BP.) The center of the bladder should be directly over the popliteal artery.
    Note: As described for brachial BP, a palpatory estimate of maximum pressure required to measure systolic pressure can be made using the popliteal or dorsalis pedis artery.
4. Proceed with auscultating the pressure as for the brachial artery.

Recording Results

For purposes of physical therapy documentation, many therapists include vital sign data directly within the narrative portion of the note. An important element in recording this information is that it allows easy comparison from one entry to the next. The date, time of day, patient position, examiner's name, and equipment used should all be clearly indicated. Any deviations from standard BP measurement protocol should be documented.

The nursing section of the medical record is an important source of vital sign data and should be checked regularly. Here, data are typically provided in graph form, with time represented on the horizontal axis and the measured values on the vertical axis. Some medical record software programs automatically create graphs from numerical data entries. The visual record allows easy identification of data trends reflective of normal variations or a response to disease or therapeutic intervention.[60] For the therapist practicing in facilities where such forms are used, familiarity with the specific recording system is important. Several methods are used to differentiate vital sign entry; they generally include some variation of open and closed circles, connecting lines, color codes, or other symbols to discriminate among temperature, HR, RR, and BP data.

■ RESOURCES

Multiple Internet resources are available to enhance patient understanding of the implications of altered vital sign values and the importance of maintaining values within normal ranges, in addition to presenting strategies to prevent, detect, and obtain treatment for the precipitating causes. Many organizations provide a rich source of online information and education for patients and families as well as clinical guidelines and resource materials for health professionals. Several examples are provided in Appendix 2.C: Resources for Patients, Families, and Clinicians.

SUMMARY

Values obtained from monitoring vital signs provide the physical therapist with important information about the patient's physiological status. Results from these measures assist in establishing and maintaining a database of values for an individual patient. They also assist in formulating clinical judgments for determining the diagnosis and prognosis, designing the POC, and establishing and evaluating effectiveness of selected treatment interventions.

The procedure for measuring each vital sign has been presented. Because multiple factors influence vital signs, the most useful data are obtained when measures are taken at periodic intervals rather than as a single measure in time. Sequential measures allow changes in patient status or response to treatment to be monitored over time, as well as indicating an acute change in status at a specific point in time.

For purposes of physical therapy documentation, vital sign data are typically included within the narrative format of the note. Regardless of the system of documentation selected, of critical importance is that it allows easy comparison of serial entries over time.

Questions for Review

1. In monitoring a patient's blood pressure, you obtain values that are markedly higher from those documented by another therapist yesterday. How would you respond to this situation?

2. Prior to a vital signs examination, what preliminary data can be obtained by a careful systematic observation of the patient?

3. Together with other examination data, vital sign measures assist the physical therapist in making clinical decisions about what aspects of patient care?

4. Provide examples of lifestyle patterns (modifiable) and patient characteristics (nonmodifiable) that may influence vital sign measures.

5. What are the mechanisms by which the body conserves and produces heat?

6. What methods are used to dissipate excess heat from the body? Provide a description of each.

7. Hand hygiene plays a critical role in preventing transmission of pathogens. What are the five moments of hand hygiene developed by the World Health Organization to draw attention to its importance and practical application?

8. What is the procedure for measuring oral temperature using a hand-held battery-powered thermometer?

9. What three pulse parameters (characteristics) are considered during monitoring? Describe each.

10. Where is the stethoscope placed to monitor apical pulse?

11. What is a pulse deficit and how is it derived?

12. What medical conditions would alert the therapist to the potential need for monitoring oxygen saturation levels using pulse oximetry?

13. What parameters (characteristics) are considered in examining respiration? Describe each.

14. What is the procedure for measuring brachial blood pressure using a stethoscope and aneroid sphygmomanometer?

CASE STUDY

EMERGENCY ROOM ADMISSION

A 24-year-old man was separated from his skiing group due to an unexpected and violent snowstorm. His being in an unfamiliar area without electronic communication complicated the situation. A 2-day helicopter search located him after approximately 48 hours of exposure to temperatures that ranged between 10° and 20°F (−12.22°C and −6.67°C). The emergency team initiated intravenous fluid replacement (to help restore fluid and electrolyte balance) en route to the hospital.

HISTORY

As reported by his parents, medical history is unremarkable except for the usual childhood diseases. He had recently relocated to the area because of a desire to be a competitive skier (an activity he has enjoyed all his life). He works as an accountant for a local investment firm.

ADMITTING DIAGNOSIS

Hypothermia and frostbite of the toes, thumb, and index and middle fingers, bilaterally.
• **Blood pressure:** Systolic pressure is 45 mm Hg; diastolic not perceptible.
• **Pulse:** Decreased rate, small, weak carotid pulse (12 bpm); peripheral pulses not perceptible.
• **Respiratory rate:** 6 breaths per minute; respirations barely perceptible.
• **Temperature:** 82°F (27.78°C) (rectal).
• **Cognition:** Depressed, unresponsive.
• **Deep tendon reflexes:** Absent.
• **Motor function:** No spontaneous movement.
• **Cutaneous sensation:** Unresponsive to all sensory modalities, including pain.
• **Integument:** Pale, cold on palpation; bluish gray appearance of nail beds and lips.

PHYSICAL THERAPY

The patient is now in the intensive care unit (ICU) and a referral has been made to physical therapy requesting "examination and treatment."

GUIDING QUESTIONS

1. Describe the body system responses to hypothermia.

2. What symptoms of hypothermia are presented by the patient?

3. During the early portion of the patient being stranded, input from thermoreceptors would have indicated a drop in temperature below the "set" temperature value. What mechanisms would have been activated to conserve heat?

4. Considering this patient is unresponsive and cyanotic, what is the most appropriate pulse to monitor? Why?

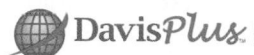 **DavisPlus** | For additional resources, including answers to the questions for review and case study guiding questions, please visit **http://davisplus.fadavis.com**

References

1. American Physical Therapy Association (APTA): Guide to Physical Therapist Practice, ed 2. APTA, Alexandria, Virginia, 2001.
2. Dillon, PM: Nursing Health Assessment, ed 2. FA Davis, Philadelphia, 2007.
3. Wilkinson, JM, and Van Leuven, K: Fundamentals of Nursing, Electronic Study Guide. FA Davis, Philadelphia, 2007.
4. Centers for Disease Control and Prevention (CDC): National Health and Nutrition Examination Survey. CDC, Atlanta, GA. Retrieved March 29, 2012, from www.cdc.gov/nchs/nhanes.htm.
5. Wright, JD, et al: Mean systolic and diastolic blood pressure in adults aged 18 and over in the United States, 2001–2008, National Health Statistics Reports; Number 35. National Center for Health Statistics, Hyattsville, MD, 2011. Retrieved March 29, 2012, from www.cdc.gov/nchs/products/nhsr.htm.
6. Ostchega, Y, Porter, KS, Hughes, J, et al: Resting pulse rate reference data for children, adolescents, and adults: United States, 1999–2008, National Health Statistics Reports; Number 41. National Center for Health Statistics, Hyattsville, MD, 2011. Retrieved March 5, 2012, from: www.cdc.gov/nchs/products/nhsr.htm.
7. Wilkinson, JM, and Treas, LS: Fundamentals of Nursing, ed 2, vol 1. FA Davis, Philadelphia, 2011.
8. Alfaro-LeFevre, R: Applying Nursing Process: A Tool for Critical Thinking, ed 7. Wolters Kluwer/Lippincott Williams & Wilkins, Philadelphia, 2010.
9. Dahl, JL, and Gordon, DB: Joint Commission pain standards: A progress report. APS Bull 12(6), 2002. Retrieved March 20, 2012, from www.ampainsoc.org/library/bulletin/nov02/poli1.htm.
10. Kerns, RD, et al: Veterans Health Administration national pain management strategy: Update and future directions. APS Bull 16(1), 2006. Retrieved March 20, 2012, from www.ampainsoc.org/library/bulletin/win06/inno1.htm.
11. Howell, D, and Olsen, K: Distress—the 6th vital sign. Curr Oncol 18(5):208–210, 2011.
12. Bultz, BD, et al: Implementing screening for distress, the 6th vital sign: A Canadian strategy for changing practice. Psychooncology 20(5):463, 2011.
13. Thomas, BC, and Bultz, BD: The future in psychosocial oncology: Screening for emotional distress—the sixth vital sign. Future Oncol 4(6):779, 2008.
14. Mower, WR, et al: Pulse oximetry as a fifth vital sign in emergency geriatric assessment. Acad Emerg Med 5(9):858, 1998.
15. Mower, WR, et al: Pulse oximetry as a fifth pediatric vital sign. Pediatrics 99(5):681, 1997.
16. Patel, PJ, et al: Testing the utility of the Newest Vital Sign (NVS) health literacy assessment tool in older African-American patients. Patient Educ Couns 85(3):505, 2011.
17. Welch, VL, VanGeest, JB, and Caskey, R: Time, costs, and clinical utilization of screening for health literacy: A case study using the Newest Vital Sign (NVS) instrument. J Am Board Fam Med 24(3):281, 2011.
18. Bierman, AS: Functional status: The sixth vital sign. J Gen Intern Med 16(11):785, 2001.
19. Fritz, S, and Lusardi, M: White paper: Walking speed: The sixth vital sign. J Geriatr Phys Ther 32(2):2, 2009.
20. Registered Nurses' Association of Ontario: Nursing care of dyspnea: The 6th vital sign in individuals with chronic obstructive pulmonary disease (COPD). Registered Nurses' Association of Ontario, Toronto, Canada, 2005. Retrieved March 14, 2012, from www.rnao.org/Storage/11/604_BPG_COPD.pdf.
21. Boyle, R, and Solberg, LI: Is making smoking status a vital sign sufficient to increase cessation support actions in clinical practice? Ann Fam Med 2(1):22, 2004.
22. Joseph, AC: Viewpoint: Continence: The sixth vital sign? AJN 103(7):11, 2003.
23. Leavitt, R (ed): Cultural Competence: A Lifelong Journey to Cultural Proficiency. Slack, Thorofare, NJ, 2010.
24. Tripp-Reimer, T, Johnson, R, and Sorofman, B: Cultural dimensions. In Stanley, M, Blair, KA, and Beare, PG (eds): Gerontological Nursing: Promoting Successful Aging with Older Adults, ed 3. FA Davis, Philadelphia, 2005, p 25.
25. Tseng, W, and Streltzer, J: Cultural Competence in Health Care: A Guide for Professionals. Springer Science and Business Media, New York, 2008.
26. Purnell, LD, and Paulanka, BJ (eds): Transcultural Health Care: A Culturally Competent Approach, ed 3. FA Davis, Philadelphia, 2008.
27. Spector, RE: Cultural Diversity in Health and Illness, ed 7. Pearson Education, Upper Saddle River, NJ, 2008.
28. US Census Bureau: Overview of Race and Hispanic Origin: 2010 Census Briefs. US Department of Commerce, Economics and Statistics Administration, Washington, DC, 2011. Retrieved December 17, 2011, from www.census.gov/prod/cen2010/briefs/c2010br-02.pdf.
29. Fortier, JP, et al: Assuring Cultural Competence in Health Care: Recommendations for National Standards and an Outcomes-Focused Research Agenda. US Department of Health and Human Service Office of Minority Health, Washington, DC, 1999. Retrieved March 29, 2012, from http://minorityhealth.hhs.gov/Assets/pdf/checked/Assuring_Cultural_Competence_in_Health_Care-1999.pdf.
30. American Physical Therapy Association (APTA) Committee on Cultural Competence: Blueprint for Teaching Cultural Competence in Physical Therapy. APTA, Alexandria, VA, 2008. Retrieved March 25, 2012, from www.apta.org/Educators/Curriculum/APTA/CulturalCompetence/.
31. Commission on Accreditation in Physical Therapy Education (CAPTE): Evaluative Criteria PT Programs Accreditation Handbook. APTA, Alexandria, VA, 2011. Retrieved March 25, 2012, from www.capteonline.org/AccreditationHandbook/.
32. Commission on Accreditation in Physical Therapy Education (CAPTE): Evaluative Criteria for Accreditation of Education Programs for the Preparation of Physical Therapist Assistants. APTA, Alexandria, VA, 2011. Retrieved March 16, 2012, from www.capteonline.org/AccreditationHandbook/.
33. American Physical Therapy Association (APTA): A Normative Model of Physical Therapist Professional Education: Version 2004. APTA, Alexandria, VA, 2004.
34. American Physical Therapy Association (APTA): A Normative Model of Physical Therapist Assistant Education: Version 2007. APTA, Alexandria, VA, 2007.
35. Burton, M, and Ludwig, LJM: Fundamentals of Nursing Care. FA Davis, Philadelphia, 2011.
36. Purnell, LD, and Paulanka, BJ: Guide to Culturally Competent Health Care, ed 2. FA Davis, Philadelphia, 2009.
37. Galanti, G: Caring for Patients from Different Cultures, ed 4. University of Pennsylvania Press, Philadelphia, 2008.
38. Perez, MA, and Luquis, RR (eds): Cultural Competence in Health Education and Health Promotion. Jossey-Bass/A Wiley Imprint, San Francisco, 2008.

39. Srivastava, R: The Healthcare Professional's Guide to Clinical Cultural Competence. Mosby/Elsevier, St Louis, 2006.

40. Kosoko-Lasaki, S, Cook, CT, and O'Brien, RL (eds): Cultural Proficiency in Addressing Health Disparities. Jones and Bartlett, Sudbury, MA, 2009.

41. Campbell, L, Gilbert, MA, and Laustsen, GR: Clinical Coach for Nursing Excellence. FA Davis, Philadelphia, 2010.

42. Chapman, S, et al: Oxford Handbook of Respiratory Medicine, ed 2. Oxford University Press, New York, 2009.

43. Jarvis, C: Physical Examination and Health Assessment, ed 6. Elsevier/Saunders, St Louis, 2012.

44. Wilkins, RL: Fundamentals of physical examination. In Wilkins, RL, Dexter, JR, and Heuer, AJ (eds): Clinical Assessment in Respiratory Care, ed 6. Mosby/Elsevier, St Louis, 2010, p 68.

45. McArdle, WD, Katch, FI, and Katch, VL: Exercise Physiology: Nutrition, Energy, and Human Performance, ed 7. Lippincott Williams & Wilkins, Philadelphia, 2009.

46. Hall, JE: Guyton and Hall Textbook of Medical Physiology, ed 12. Saunders/Elsevier, Philadelphia, 2011.

47. Barrett, KE, et al: Ganong's Review of Medical Physiology, ed 23. McGraw Hill/Lange, New York, 2010.

48. Sherwood, L: Human Physiology: From Cells to Systems, ed 7. Brooks/Cole (Cengage Learning), Belmont, CA, 2010.

49. McArdle, WD, Katch, FI, and Katch, VL: Essentials of Exercise Physiology, ed 4. Wolters Kluwer/Lippincott Williams and Wilkins, Philadelphia, 2010.

50. Powers, SK, and Howley, ET: Exercise Physiology, ed 5. McGraw-Hill, New York, 2004.

51. Guyton, AC, and Hall, JE: Human Physiology and Mechanisms of Disease, ed 6. WB Saunders, Philadelphia, 1997.

52. Goodman, CC, and Peterson, C: Infectious disease. In Goodman, CC, and Fuller, KS (eds): Pathology: Implications for the Physical Therapist, ed 3. Saunders/Elsevier, Philadelphia, 2009, p 298.

53. United States Environmental Protection Agency (EPA): Thermometers. EPA, Washington, DC, 2011. Retrieved February 1, 2012, from www.epa.gov/hg/thermometer-main.html.

54. Taylor, C, et al: Fundamentals of Nursing: The Art and Science of Nursing Care, ed 7. Wolters Kluwer/Lippincott Williams & Wilkins, Philadelphia, 2008.

55. Smith, SF, Duell, DJ, and Martin, BC: Clinical Nursing Skills: Basic to Advanced Skills, ed 7. Prentice Hall Health, Upper Saddle River, NJ, 2008.

56. Hausfater, P, et al: Cutaneous infrared thermometry for detecting febrile patients. Emerg Infect Dis 14(8):1255, 2008.

57. World Health Organization (WHO): WHO Guidelines on Hand Hygiene in Health Care. WHO, Geneva, Switzerland, 2009. Retrieved February 14, 2012, from http://whqlibdoc.who.int/publications/2009/9789241597906_eng.pdf.

58. Hogan-Quigley, B, Palm, ML, and Bickley, LS: Bates' Nursing Guide to Physical Examination and History Taking. Wolters Kluwer/Lippincott Williams & Wilkins, Philadelphia, 2011.

59. Berman, AJ, et al: Kozier and Erb's Fundamentals of Nursing: Concepts, Process, and Practice, ed 8. Prentice Hall, Upper Saddle River, NJ, 2007.

60. Craven, RF, and Hirnle, CJ (eds): Fundamentals of Nursing: Human Health and Function, ed 6. Lippincott Williams & Wilkins, New York, 2008.

61. Inbar, O, et al: Normal cardiopulmonary responses during incremental exercise in 20–70-yr-old men. Med Sci Sport Exerc 26(5): 538–546, 1994.

62. Robergs, RA, and Landwehr, R: The surprising history of the "HRmax=220-age" equation. JEPonline 5(2):1–10, 2002. Retrieved February 16, 2012, from http://faculty.css.edu/tboone2/asep/Robergs2.pdf.

63. Stevens, J, and MacAuley, D: Older exercise participants. In Kolt, GS, and Snyder-Mackler, L (eds): Physical Therapies in Sport and Exercise, ed 2. Churchill Livingstone/Elsevier, Philadelphia, 2007, p 484.

64. Moore, KL, Dalley, AF, and Agur, AMR: Clinically Oriented Anatomy, ed 6. Wolters Kluwer/Lippincott Williams & Wilkins, Philadelphia, 2009.

65. Laukkanen, RMT, and Virtanen, PK: Heart rate monitors: State of the art. J Sports Sci 16:S3, 1998.

66. US Food and Drug Administration (FDA): Radiation-Emitting Products: About Wireless Medical Telemetry. FDA, Silver Spring, MD, 2009. Retrieved February 20, 2012, from www.fda.gov/Radiation-EmittingProducts/RadiationSafety/Electromagnetic-CompatibilityEMC/ucm116574.htm#2.

67. Federal Communications Commission (FCC): Wireless Medical Telemetry Service (WMTS). FCC, Washington, DC (undated). Retrieved February 20, 2012, from www.fcc.gov/encyclopedia/wireless-medical-telemetry-service-wmts.

68. Gandsas, A, et al: In-flight continuous vital signs telemetry via the Internet. Aviat Space Envir Md 71(1):68, 2000.

69. Myers, BA: Wound Management: Principles and Practice, ed 2. Prentice Hall, Upper Saddle River, NJ, 2008.

70. Patterson, GK: Vascular evaluation. In Sussman, C, and Bates-Jensen, BM (eds): Wound Care: A Collaborative Practice Manual for Health Professionals, ed 3. Wolters Kluwer/Lippincott Williams & Wilkins, Philadelphia, 2007, p 180.

71. Rees, S: Vascular assessment. In Merriman, LM, and Turner, W (eds): Merriman's Assessment of the Lower Limb, ed 3. Churchill Livingstone/Elsevier, Philadelphia, 2009, p 75.

72. Howell, M: Pulse oximetry: An audit of nursing and medical staff understanding. Br J Nurs 11(3):191, 2002.

73. Vines, DL: Respiratory monitoring in the intensive care unit. In Wilkins, RL, Dexter, JR, and Heuer, AJ: Clinical Assessment in Respiratory Care. Mosby/Elsevier, St Louis, 2010, p 286.

74. McMahon, MD: Pulse oximetry and carbon monoxide oximetry. In Proehl, JA (ed): Emergency Nursing Procedures, ed 4. Saunders/Elsevier, St Louis, 2009, p 87.

75. Clinical Monograph: Monitoring Oxygen Saturation with Pulse Oximetry. Nellcor, Pleasanton, CA, 2001. Retrieved February 20, 2012, from http://macomb-rspt.com/FILES/RSPT1050/MODULE%20G/Pulse_Oximetry_Monograph.pdf.

76. Cottrell, GP: Cardiopulmonary Anatomy and Physiology for Respiratory Care Practitioners. FA Davis, Philadelphia, 2001.

77. Cahalin, LP, and Buck, LA: Physical therapy associated with cardiovascular pump dysfunction and failure. In DeTurk, WE, and Cahalin, LP (eds): Cardiovascular and Pulmonary Physical Therapy: An Evidence-Based Approach, ed 2. McGraw-Hill, New York, 2011, p 529.

78. Weinberger, SE, Cockrill, BA, and Mandel, J: Principles of Pulmonary Medicine, ed 5. WB Saunders/Elsevier, Philadelphia, 2008.

79. Coté, CJ, et al: The effect of nail polish on pulse oximetry. Anesth Analg 67(7):683, 1988.

80. Hinkelbein, J, et al: Artificial acrylic finger nails may alter pulse oximetry measurement. Resuscitation 74(1):75, 2007.

81. Collins, SM, and Cocanour, B: Anatomy of the cardiopulmonary system. In DeTurk, WE, and Cahalin, LP (eds): Cardiovascular and Pulmonary Physical Therapy: An Evidence-Based Approach, ed 2. McGraw-Hill, New York, 2011, p 85.

82. Henderson, BS: Anatomy and physiology of the respiratory system. In Ruppert, SD, et al (eds): Dolan's Critical Care Nursing: Clinical Management Through the Nursing Process, ed 2. FA Davis, Philadelphia, 1996, p 387.

83. Ikeda, B, and Goodman, CC: The respiratory system. In Goodman, CC, and Fuller, KS (eds): Pathology: Implications for the Physical Therapist, ed 3. WB Saunders, Philadelphia, 2009, p 742.

84. Schelegle, ES, and Green, JF: An overview of the anatomy and physiology of slowly adapting pulmonary stretch receptors. Respir Physiol 125:17, 2001.

85. Hassan, A, et al: Volume activation of the Hering Breuer inflation reflex in the newborn infant. J Appl Physiol 90:763, 2001.

86. Certo, C: Cardiopulmonary Rehabilitation of the Geriatric Patient and Client. In Lewis, CB: Aging: The Health-Care Challenge, ed 4. FA Davis, Philadelphia, 2002, p 143.

87. Robergs, RA, and Keteyian, SJ: Fundamentals of Exercise Physiology for Fitness, Performance, and Health. McGraw-Hill, New York, 2003.

88. Prentice, WE: Arnheim's Principles of Athletic Training: A Competency-Based Approach, ed 13. McGraw-Hill, New York, 2009.

89. Woo, TM: Drugs Affecting the Respiratory System. In Wynne, AL, Woo, TM, and Millard, M: Pharmacotherapeutics for Nurse Practitioner Prescribers. FA Davis, Philadelphia, 2002, p 311.

90. Ciccone, CD: Medications. In DeTurk, WE, and Cahalin, LP (eds): Cardiovascular and Pulmonary Physical Therapy: An Evidence-Based Approach, ed 2. McGraw-Hill, New York, 2011, p. 209.

91. Perry, AG, and Potter, PA: Clinical Nursing Skills and Techniques, ed 7. Mosby/Elsevier, St Louis, 2010.

92. Pinto, E: Blood pressure and ageing. Postgrad Med J 83:109, 2007. Retrieved February 23, 2012, from www.ncbi.nlm.nih.gov/pmc/articles/PMC2805932/pdf/109.pdf.

93. Chobanian, AV, Bakris GL, Black HR, et al: Seventh report of the Joint National Committee on Prevention, Detection, Evaluation, and Treatment of High Blood Pressure: The JNC 7 report. JAMA 289(19):2560, 2003.
94. Smirnova, IV, and Goodman, CC: The cardiovascular system. In Goodman, CC, and Fuller, KS (eds): Pathology: Implications for the Physical Therapist, ed 3. WB Saunders, Philadelphia, 2009, p 519.
95. Gould, BE, and Dyer, RM: Pathophysiology for the Health Professions, ed 4. Saunders/Elsevier, St Louis, 2011.
96. American Heart Association: High Blood Pressure Statistical Fact Sheet—2012 Update. American Heart Association, Dallas, TX. Retrieved February 24, 2012, from www.heart.org/idc/groups/heart-public/@wcm/@sop/@smd/documents/downloadable/ucm_319587.pdf.
97. American Heart Association: Heart Disease and Stroke Statistics—2012 Update. American Heart Association, Dallas, TX Retrieved. February 24, 2012, from http://circ.ahajournals.org/content/early/2011/12/15/CIR.0b013e31823ac046.
98. World Health Organization (WHO): Global Health Risks: Mortality and Burden of Disease Attributable to Selected Major Risks. WHO, Geneva, Switzerland, 2009. Retrieved February 24, 2012, from www.who.int/healthinfo/global_burden_disease/GlobalHealthRisks_report_full.pdf.
99. National Health and Nutrition Examination Survey (NHANES): Health Tech/Blood Pressure Procedures Manual. Centers for Disease Control and Prevention, Atlanta, GA, 2009. Retrieved February 26, 2012, from www.cdc.gov/nchs/data/nhanes/nhanes_09_10/BP.pdf.

Supplemental Readings

Aronow, WS, Fleg, JL, Pepine, CJ, et al: ACCF/AHA 2011 Expert Consensus Document on Hypertension in the Elderly: A Report of the American College of Cardiology Foundation Task Force on Clinical Expert Consensus Documents. Circulation 123(21):2434, 2011. Retrieved February 27, 2012, from http://circ.ahajournals.org/content/123/21/2434.full.pdf.
Frese, EM, Fick, A, and Sadowsky, HS: Blood pressure measurement guidelines for physical therapists. Cardiopulm Phys Ther J 22(2):5, 2011.
Gillespie, C, Kuklina, EV, Briss, PA, et al: Vital signs: Prevalence, treatment, and control of hypertension—United States, 1999–2002 and 2005–2008. MMWR 60(4):103, 2011. Retrieved December 6, 2010, from www.cdc.gov/mmwr/preview/mmwrhtml/mm6004a4.htm?s_cid=mm6004a4_w.
Hsia, J, et al: Women's Health Initiative Research Group. Resting heart rate as a low tech predictor of coronary events in women: Prospective cohort stud. BMJ 338:b219, 2009.
Hugueny, S, Clifton, DA, Hravnak, M et al: Understanding vital-sign abnormalities in critical care patients. Crit Care 14(Suppl 1):147, 2010.
Khoshdel, AR, Carney, S, and Gillies, A: The impact of arm position and pulse pressure on the validation of a wrist-cuff blood pressure measurement device in a high risk population. Int J Gen Med 2010(3):119, 2010.
Kressin, NR, Orner, MB, Manze, M et al: Understanding contributors to racial disparities in blood pressure control. Circ Cardiovasc Qual Outcomes 3(2):173, 2010.
Myers, MG, Godwin, M, Dawes, M, et al: Conventional versus automated measurement of blood pressure in primary care patients with systolic hypertension: Randomised parallel design controlled trial. BMJ 342:d286, 2011.
Perloff, D, et al: Human Blood Pressure Determination by Sphygmomanometry. American Heart Association, Dallas, TX, 1993. Retrieved February 26, 2012, from http://circ.ahajournals.org/content/88/5/2460.full.pdf+html.
Takeshi, T, and Saito, Y: Effects of smoking cessation on central blood pressure and arterial stiffness. Vasc Health Risk Manage 7:633, 2011.
US Preventive Services Task Force: Screening for High Blood Pressure: U.S. Preventive Services Task Force Reaffirmation Recommendation Statement. AHRQ Publication No. 08-05105-EF-2, 2007. (First published in Ann Intern Med 147[11]:783, 2007.) Retrieved December 9, 2011, from http://www.uspreventiveservicestaskforce.org/uspstf07/hbp/hbprs.htm.
Wan, Y, Heneghan, R, Stevens, R J, et al: Determining which automatic digital blood pressure device performs adequately: A systematic review. J Hum Hypertens 24(7):431, 2010.
Wedgbury, K, and Valler-Jones, T: Measuring blood pressure using an automated sphygmomanometer. BJN 17(11):714, 2008.
Wills, AK, Lawlor, DA, Matthews, FE, et al: Life course trajectories of systolic blood pressure using longitudinal data from eight UK cohorts. PLoS Med 8(6):e1000440, 2011.
Yönt, GH, Korhan, EA, and Khorshid, L: Comparison of oxygen saturation values and measurement times by pulse oximetry in various parts of the body. Appl Nurs Res 24(4):e39, 2011.
Zhang, GQ, and Zhang, W: Heart rate, lifespan, and mortality risk. Ageing Res Rev 8(1):52, 2009.

A. Assemble equipment.

1. Clean oral glass mercury thermometer
2. Clean tissue to wipe thermometer
3. Watch (or wall clock)

B. Procedure

1. Remove the clean thermometer from storage container. If stored in a disinfectant solution, rinse under cold water, and dry with tissue using a firm rotary motion wiping from the bulb toward the fingers.
2. Hold the thermometer between the thumb and forefinger at the end of the stem (opposite the bulb). Holding the thermometer horizontally at eye level (required to obtain an accurate reading), rotate until the column of mercury is clearly visible. Note the level of the column. The reading should be below 95°F (35°C) before placing the thermometer in the patient's mouth. If the value is higher, "shake down" the thermometer until the mercury is below 95°F (35°C). While holding the thermometer securely, use quick, downward snapping motions of the wrist, which will effectively lower the column.
3. Ask the patient to open his or her mouth, and place the bulb of the thermometer at the posterior base of the tongue to the right or left of the frenulum in the sublingual pocket. Instruct the patient to close the lips (not teeth) around the thermometer to hold it in place.
4. Leave the glass mercury thermometer in place for 3 to 5 minutes.
5. Remove the thermometer.
6. Using a clean tissue, wipe the thermometer away from the fingers (toward the bulb) using a firm rotary motion.
7. Hold the thermometer at eye level, rotate until the mercury is clearly visible, and read the highest point on the scale to which the mercury has risen for recording.
8. Wash the thermometer in tepid soapy water and return to the storage container.
9. Wash hands.

Measuring Axillary Temperature: Glass Mercury Thermometer

A. Assemble equipment.

1. Clean the oral glass mercury thermometer
   Note: Axillary temperatures can also be measured with automated thermometers as well as disposable single-use thermometers.
2. Clean tissue to wipe thermometer
3. A towel to dry axillary region (moisture will conduct heat).
4. Watch (or wall clock)

B. Procedure

1. Expose the axilla and ensure area is dry. If any moisture is present, the area should be gently towel dried with a patting motion (vigorous rubbing will increase temperature of the area).
2. Remove the clean thermometer from storage container. If stored in a disinfectant solution, rinse under cold water, and dry with tissue using a firm rotary motion, wiping from the bulb toward the fingers.
3. Hold the thermometer horizontally at eye level and rotate until the column of mercury is clearly visible; note the level of mercury. If necessary, shake the thermometer until the mercury is below 95°F (35°C).
4. Place the bulb of the thermometer in the center of the axillary region between the trunk and upper arm. The patient's upper extremity should be placed tightly across the chest to keep the thermometer in place (asking the patient to move the hand toward the opposite shoulder is often a useful direction). If the patient is disoriented or very young, the thermometer must be held in place.
5. Leave thermometer in place for 10 minutes (more time is required for the mercury to expand when measuring axillary temperature).
6. Remove the thermometer.
7. Using a clean tissue, wipe the thermometer away from the fingers (toward the bulb) using a firm rotary motion.
8. Hold the thermometer at eye level, rotate until the mercury is clearly visible, and read the highest point on the scale to which the mercury has risen for recording.
9. Wash the thermometer in tepid soapy water and return to the storage container.
10. Wash hands.

Resources for Patients, Families, and Clinicians

American Heart Association (www.heart.org/HEARTORG)

- Provides patient information on multiple health topics including nutrition, physical activity, weight, and stress management and smoking cessation. www.heart.org/HEARTORG/GettingHealthy/GettingHealthy_UCM_001078_SubHomePage.jsp
- Information is provided for specific conditions such as arrhythmia, diabetes, heart attack, high blood pressure, and stroke. www.heart.org/HEARTORG/Conditions/Conditions_UCM_001087_SubHomePage.jsp
- Together with the American Stroke Association (www.strokeassociation.org), offers a large directory of scientific statements and practice guidelines for health professionals. http://my.americanheart.org/professional/StatementsGuidelines/ByTopic/By-Topic_UCM_316895_Article.jsp#.T05ncphi5FJ

American Stroke Association (www.strokeassociation.org)

- Provides a large variety of patient education and support materials (e.g., Stroke Connection Magazine, African Americans and Stroke, Post-Stroke Peer Support, and Life After Stroke). www.strokeassociation.org/STROKEORG/Professionals/PatientEducation-Support/Patient-Education-Support_UCM_310901_Article.jsp#.T05qj5hi5FI
- Sponsors *Target: Stroke*, a campaign to improve stroke outcomes by reducing the time to 60 minutes or less between onset of stroke and initiation of intravenous thrombolysis. Support includes publications, patient education, and clinical tools. www.strokeassociation.org/STROKEORG/Professionals/Target-Stroke_UCM_314495_SubHomePage.jsp
- Makes available a directory of stroke statements and guidelines. http://my.americanheart.org/professional/StatementsGuidelines/ByTopic/TopicsQ-Z/Stroke-Statements-Guidelines_UCM_320600_Article.jsp#.T05vjZhi5FI

National Heart, Lung, and Blood Institute [NHLBI] (U.S. Department of Health and Human Services) (www.nhlbi.nih.gob)

- Sponsors the *National High Blood Pressure Education Program*. The goal of the program is to reduce deaths and disability associated with high blood pressure through education. www.nhlbi.nih.gov/about/nhbpep
- Provides *Clinical Practice Guidelines* for health professionals www.nhlbi.nih.gov/health/indexpro.htm
- Promotes educational campaigns such as *COPD: Learn More Breathe Better* and *The Heart Truth* www.nhlbi.nih.gov/educational/index.htm
- For patients, NHLBI provides *Your Guide to Lowering High Blood Pressure* that includes information on detection, prevention, and treatment of high blood pressure. www.nhlbi.nih.gov/hbp/index.html

Examination of Sensory Function

Kevin K. Chui, PT, DPT, PhD, GCS, OCS
Thomas J. Schmitz, PT, PhD

Chapter 3

LEARNING OBJECTIVES

1. Understand the purpose(s) of performing a sensory examination.
2. Understand the relationship between preliminary mental status screening and tests for sensory function.
3. Describe the classification and function of the receptor mechanisms involved in the perception of sensation.
4. Identify the spinal pathways that mediate sensation.
5. Understand the guidelines for administering an examination of sensory function.
6. Describe the testing protocol for each sensory modality.
7. Using the case study example, apply clinical decision-making skills to application of sensory examination data.

CHAPTER OUTLINE

■ SENSORY INTEGRATION

If all of the sensory stimuli which enter the central nervous system were allowed to bombard the higher centers of the brain, the individual would be rendered utterly ineffective. It is the brain's task to filter, organize, and integrate a mass of sensory information so that it can be used for the development and execution of the brain's functions.[1, p. 25]—A. Jean Ayers, PhD

The human system is continually inundated with sensory information from a variety of environmental inputs as well as from movement, touch, awareness of the body in space, sight, sound, and smell. "In all higher order motor behaviors, the brain must correlate sensory inputs with motor outputs to accurately assess and control the body's interaction with the environment."[2, p.32] **Sensory integration** is the ability of the brain to organize, interpret, and use sensory information. This integration provides an internal representation of the environment that informs and guides motor responses.[2] These sensory representations provide the foundation on which motor programs for purposeful movements are planned, coordinated, and implemented.[3] Ayers defined *sensory integration* as "the neurological process that organizes sensation from one's own body and from the environment and makes it possible to use the body effectively within the environment."[4, p. 11] In an intact system, sensory integration occurs automatically without conscious effort.

Sensory integration is a theory developed by A. Jean Ayers (1920–1989), an occupational therapist whose work focused on examining the manner in which sensory integration develops, identifying patterns of dysfunction in children with learning disorders, and developing intervention strategies to improve processing of sensory information. The theory purports that disordered sensory integration directly affects both motor and cognitive learning and that interventions designed to enhance sensory integration will improve learning.[1] Bundy and Murray[5] suggest the value of the theory lies in its usefulness in (1) explaining behaviors of individuals with impaired sensory integration functions, (2) establishing a plan of care (POC) to address specific impairments, and (3) predicting expected outcomes of the selected interventions.

■ SENSATION AND MOVEMENT

Motor learning and motor performance are inextricably linked to *sensation*. As a motor task is practiced, the individual learns to anticipate and correct or modify movements based on sensory input organized and integrated by the central nervous system (CNS). The CNS uses this information to influence movement by both feedback and feedforward control. *Feedback control* uses sensory information received *during the movement* to monitor and adjust output. *Feedforward control* is a proactive strategy that uses sensory information obtained from experience. Signals are sent in *advance of movement* allowing for anticipatory adjustments in postural control or movement.[3,6] The primary role of sensation in movement is to (1) guide selection of motor responses for effective interaction with the environment and (2) adapt movements and shape motor programs through feedback for corrective action. Sensation also provides the important function of protecting the organism from injury. See Chapter 5, Examination of Motor Function: Motor Control and Motor Learning, for a more detailed discussion of CNS control of motor function.

■ SENSORY INTEGRITY

The term *somatosensation* (somatosensory) refers to sensation received from the skin and musculoskeletal system (as opposed to that from specialized senses such as sight or hearing). Examination of sensory function involves testing *sensory integrity* by determining the patient's ability to interpret and discriminate among incoming sensory information. The sensory examination is based on the premise that within the intact human system, sensory information is taken in from the body and the environment; the CNS then processes and integrates the information for use in planning and organizing behavior. This premise is more aptly termed a *theoretical construct* (a concept that represents an *unobservable* event). We cannot *directly* observe CNS processing,

integration of sensory information, or the motor planning process. However, our current knowledge of CNS function and motor behavior provides evidence that these unobservable events do occur. We *can* observe impairments in motor behavior, but can only *hypothesize* that they truly result from faulty sensory integration mechanisms.[5]

The *Guide to Physical Therapist Practice* defines **sensory integrity** as "the intactness of cortical sensory processing, including proprioception, pallesthesia, stereognosis, and topognosis."[7, p. 90] Sensory integrity is included among the list of 24 categories of tests and measures that may be used by physical therapists during patient examination and is included in all practice patterns (i.e., musculoskeletal, neuromuscular, cardiovascular/pulmonary, and integumentary).

Box 3.1 presents examples of pathologies, impairments, activity limitations, disabilities, risk factors, and health, wellness, and fitness needs associated with changes in sensory integrity.

This chapter focuses primarily on examination of somatosensory integrity of the trunk and extremities as well as screening for cranial nerve integrity; testing approaches for examining *cranial nerve integrity* and *reflex testing* are addressed in Chapter 5, Examination of Motor Function: Motor Control and Motor Learning. As the CNS analyzes and uses all sensory input to identify movement errors and initiate corrective responses, examination of sensory function typically precedes examination of motor function. This sequence assists the physical therapist in differentiating the impact of sensory impairments on motor function.

■ CLINICAL INDICATIONS

Indications for examination of sensory function are based on the history and systems review (including a *sensory screening* described later in this chapter). This includes "information provided by the patient/client, family, significant other, or caregiver; symptoms described by the patient/client; signs observed and documented during the systems review; and information derived from other sources and records."[7, p. 90] These data may indicate the existence of pathology (or risk of pathology) resulting in sensory changes that may impose impairments, activity limitations, participation restrictions, or disability (see Box 3.1).

Sensory dysfunction may be associated with any pathology or injury affecting either the peripheral nervous system (PNS) or CNS, or with a combined involvement of both systems. Deficits may occur at any point within the system including the sensory receptors, peripheral nerves, spinal nerves, spinal cord nuclei and tracts, brainstem, thalamus, and sensory cortex.[8] Examples of conditions that generally demonstrate some level of sensory impairment include pathology, disease, or injury to the peripheral nerves such as trauma (e.g., fracture) that can sever, crush, or damage

---

Box 3.1 Examples of Pathologies, Impairments, Functional Limitations, Disabilities, Risk Factors and Health, Wellness, and Fitness Needs Associated with Changes in Sensory Integrity (*Note:* ICF terminology has been parenthetically added)

I. Pathology/pathophysiology in the following systems *(ICF: Health conditions)*:
- Cardiovascular (e.g., cerebral vascular accident, peripheral vascular disease)
- Endocrine/metabolic (e.g., diabetes, rheumatological disease)
- Integumentary (e.g., burn, frostbite, lymphedema)
- Multiple systems (e.g., AIDS, Guillain-Barré syndrome, trauma)
- Musculoskeletal (e.g., derangement of joint; disorders of bursa, synovia, and tendon)
- Neuromuscular (e.g., cerebral palsy, developmental delay, spinal cord injury)
- Pulmonary (e.g., respiratory failure, ventilatory pump failure)

II. Impairments in the following categories *(ICF: Body structures/functions [impairments])*:
- Circulation (e.g., numb feet)
- Integumentary integrity (e.g., redness under orthotic)
- Muscle performance (e.g., decreased grip strength)
- Orthotic, protective, and supportive devices (e.g., wears ankle-foot orthosis)
- Posture (e.g., forward head)

III. Functional limitations in the ability to perform actions, tasks, or activities in the following categories *(ICF: Activity/activity limitations)*:
- Self-care (e.g., inability to put on trousers while standing because of loss of feeling in foot)
- Home management (e.g., difficulty with sorting change because of numbness)
- Work (job/school/play) (e.g., inability as a day care provider to change child's diaper because of loss of finger sensation, inability to operate cash register because of clumsiness)
- Community/leisure (e.g., inability to drive car because of loss of spatial awareness, inability to play guitar because of hyperesthesia)

IV. Disability, that is, the inability or restricted ability to perform actions, tasks, or activities of required roles within the individual's sociocultural context, in the following categories *(ICF: Participation/participation restriction)*:
- Self-care
- Home management
- Work (job/school/play)
- Community/leisure

V. Risk factors for impaired sensory integrity *(ICF: Personal Factors and Environment)*:
- Lack of safety awareness in all environments
- Risk-prone behaviors (e.g., working without protective gloves)
- Smoking history
- Substance abuse

VI. Health, wellness, and fitness needs *(ICF: Personal Factors)*:
- Fitness, including physical performance (e.g., inadequate balance to compete in dancing competition, limited perception of arms and legs in space during ballroom dancing)
- Health and wellness (e.g., inadequate understanding of role of proprioception in balance)

From American Physical Therapy Association,[7, p. 90] with permission.
ICF = International Classification of Functioning, Disability, and Health.

---

a nerve; metabolic disturbances (diabetes, hypothyroidism, alcoholism); infections (Lyme disease, leprosy, human immunodeficiency virus [HIV]); impingement or compression (arthritis, carpal tunnel syndrome); burns; toxins (lead, mercury, chemotherapy); and nutritional deficits (vitamin B_{12}). Sensory impairments are also associated with injury to nerve roots or spinal cord, cerebral vascular accident (CVA), transient ischemic attack (TIA), tumors, multiple sclerosis (MS), and brain injury or disease. These examples, which are not all-inclusive, indicate the wide spectrum of injuries,

disease, and pathologies that may present with some element of sensory deficit.

Pattern (Distribution) of Sensory Impairment

Examination of sensory function contributes critical information to establishing a physical therapy diagnosis and prognosis, identifying anticipated goals and expected outcomes, and developing a POC. A seminal feature of the examination involves determining the *pattern* (specific boundaries) of sensory involvement. Pattern identification is accomplished using knowledge of skin segment innervation by the dorsal roots and peripheral nerves (Figs. 3.1 and 3.2). The term **dermatome** (or *skin segment*) refers to the skin area supplied by one dorsal root.[9] The graphic illustration of skin segment innervation as presented in Figures 3.1 and 3.2 is referred to as a *dermatome map*. There exist some discrepancies among published dermatome maps based on the methodologies used to identify skin segment innervation. In a clinical commentary, Downs and Laporte[10] discuss the history of dermatome mapping, including the variations in methodologies employed, and the inconsistencies in the dermatome maps used in education and practice. As new

technology allows for more precise identification of nerve distribution, the authors suggest that cutaneous spinal nerve distribution be reevaluated.

Clinical Note: Considerable variation exists in the clinical presentation of sensory impairments. This variability is typically associated with the nervous system involved (CNS vs. PNS), the type of injury, pathology, or disease, as well as the severity, extent, and duration of involvement.

During the review of systems, asking the patient to carefully describe the pattern or distribution of sensory

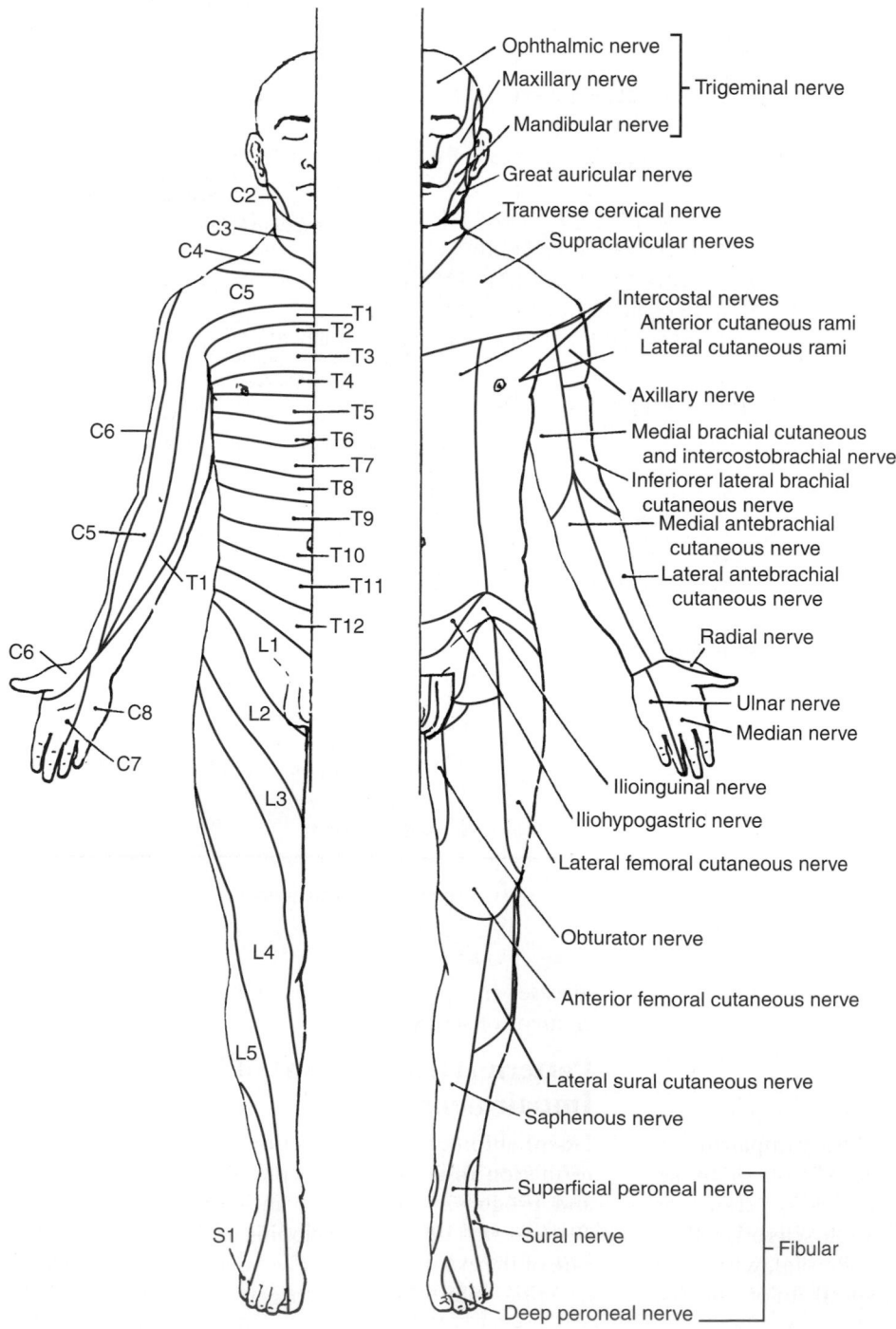

Figure 3.1 Anterior view of skin segment innervation by dorsal roots (*left*) and peripheral nerves (*right*). (*From Gilman and Newman[9, p. 43] with permission.*)

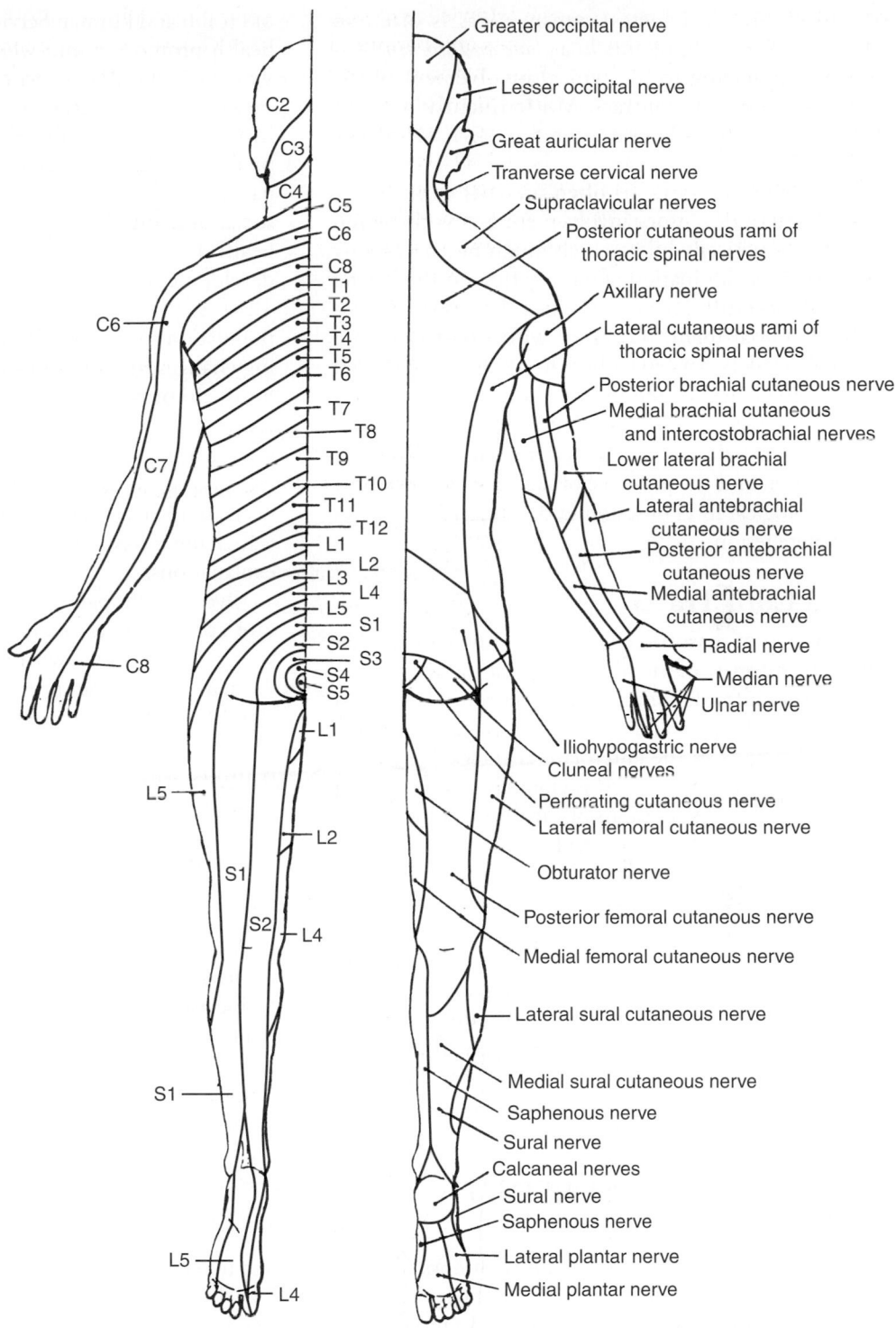

Figure 3.2 Posterior view of skin segment innervation by dorsal roots (*left*) and peripheral nerves (*right*). *(From Gilman and Newman[9, p. 44] with permission.)*

symptoms (e.g., tingling, numbness, diminished, or absent sensation) provides the therapist with preliminary information to help guide the examination and to assist in identifying the dermatome(s) and nerve(s) involved. Peripheral nerve injuries generally present sensory impairments that parallel the distribution of the involved nerve and correspond to its pattern of innervation. For example, if a patient presents with complaints of numbness on the ulnar half of the ring finger, the little finger,

and the ulnar side of the hand, the therapist would be alerted to carefully address ulnar nerve (C8 and T1) integrity during the sensory examination. Complaints of sensory disturbances on the palmar surface of the thumb and the palmar and distal dorsal aspects of the index, middle, and the radial half of the ring finger would be indicative of median nerve (C6–8 and T1) involvement.

Other patterns of sensory loss may be associated with specific pathology. For example, with peripheral neuropathy (e.g., diabetes), sensory loss is often an early symptom and presents in a *glove and stocking* distribution (referring to the typical involvement of the hands and feet). In contrast, MS frequently presents with an unpredictable or scattered pattern of sensory involvement.

Spinal cord injury (SCI) often presents with a more diffuse pattern of sensory involvement below the lesion level that is typically bilateral, although not necessarily symmetrical. Examination of sensory function following SCI provides critical data that reflect the degree of neurological impairment. Together with other tests and measures, sensory data contribute to determining the relative completeness of the injury, the existence of *zones of partial preservation* (areas distal to a complete lesion that retain partial innervation), symmetry or asymmetry of the lesion, and the presence of sacral sensation below the neurological level of lesion (a defining feature of an incomplete lesion).

Spinal Cord Tracts

Examination of sensory function also provides data that reflect the integrity of the spinal cord tracts that carry somatosensory information. For example, contralateral loss or impairment of pain and temperature perception is suggestive of lesions in the anterolateral tracts. Deficits in discriminative sensations such as vibration and two-point discrimination suggest lesions of the dorsal column.

Evidence of both sensory and motor loss is usually indicative of nerve root involvement (recall that the dorsal and ventral roots converge to form the spinal nerves). CNS lesions (e.g., CVA, brain injury) may produce significant sensory impairments characterized by a diffuse pattern of involvement (e.g., head, trunk, and limbs) and can result in significant motor dysfunction (sensory ataxia) and impairment of fine motor control and motor learning, as well as present a significant threat of injury to anesthetic limbs (e.g., an inability to determine the temperature of bath water).

■ AGE-RELATED SENSORY CHANGES

Alterations in sensory function occur with normal aging and should be clearly differentiated from those associated with specific illness, disease, or pathology. In recent years there has been a gradual expansion of interest in and information about the causes and consequences of age-related sensory changes. This has been evident through the large and expanding body of literature devoted to the neuroscience of aging and its impact on function and quality of life of older adults.[11-34] The topics addressed are specific age-related changes in vision, hearing, and the somatosensory system; treatment, prevalence, and risk factor information; as well as the role of public policy and public health in addressing age-related sensory loss. *Healthy People 2020*,[35] published by the U.S. Department of Health and Human Services, presents a comprehensive health promotion and wellness agenda for the second decade of the 21st century. The overarching goals of *Healthy People 2020* are to (1) attain high-quality, longer lives free of preventable disease, disability, injury, and premature death; (2) achieve health equity, eliminate disparities, and improve the health of all groups; (3) create social and physical environments that promote good health for all; and (4) promote quality of life, healthy development, and healthy behaviors across all life stages. The first goal draws national attention to an expanding population of older adults and the impact of age (including changes in sensation such as vision and hearing) on health improvement and health promotion strategies. Decreased acuity of many sensations occurs and is considered a characteristic finding with aging.[36-40] The exact morphology of diminished sensation with age has not been completely established. However, several neurological changes have been identified and suggest potential explanations.

Over the lifespan neurons are replaced at a declining rate and this may account for the decline of average weight of the brain with aging. Although a feature of Alzheimer's disease, normal aging does not produce a significant loss in the number of cortical neurons.[40] Other changes in the brain include degeneration of neurons with presence of replacement gliosis, lipid accumulation in the neurons, loss of myelin, and development of neurofibrils (masses of small, tangled fibrils) and plaques on the cells.[40-42] There is also a decrease in the number of enzymes responsible for synthesis of dopamine, norepinephrine, and to a lesser degree acetylcholine,[43] as well as depletion of the neuronal dendrites in the aging brain.[43,44]

Electrophysiological studies have identified a gradual reduction in conduction velocity of sensory nerves with advancing age,[45-47] and this may reflect degenerative changes in myelin sheaths or loss or reduction in size of sensory axons.[36,41,45,48] Evoked potentials provide a quantitative measure of sensory function and have been found to decrease in amplitude with age.[49] A reduction in the number of Meissner's corpuscles[50] has also been identified. These corpuscles, responsible for touch detection, are limited to hairless areas, and become sparse, take on an irregular distribution, and vary in size and shape with age.[50] Age-related changes in morphology and decreased concentrations of Pacinian corpuscles, responsive to rapid tissue movement (e.g., vibration), have also been reported.[51]

Degenerative changes in myelin have been documented in both the central and peripheral nervous systems.[40,45,52] In a review of the literature on the effects of normal aging on myelin and nerve fibers, Peters[40] suggests that (1) age-associated cognitive decline is more likely due to widespread damage to myelin sheaths of cortical neuron axons than to actual loss of these neurons and (2) the resulting changes in conduction velocity alter the normal timing of neuronal circuits.

In the PNS, a decrease in the distance between the nodes of Ranvier has been associated with advancing age.[53] This finding may be related to a slowing of saltatory conduction identified by some authors.[41,45] Destruction of myelin sheaths has been linked to a reduced expression of primary myelin proteins, axonal atrophy, and to reduced expression and axonal transport of cytoskeletal proteins.[54] As compared to younger subjects, lower sensory nerve conduction velocities have been documented for both the median[55,46] and sural[46] nerves in older subjects.

Although not an exhaustive list, other documented age-related sensory changes include altered postural stability and control,[15,20,24,26,56,57] diminished response to tactile stimuli,[12,55,58,59] reduced vibratory[51,60] and proprioceptive acuity,[13,31,61] decreased cutaneous temperature thresholds[11] and two-point discrimination,[29,62] and altered ability to adapt sensorimotor responses to task demands.[17]

These changes frequently appear in the presence of age-related visual or hearing losses that impair compensatory capabilities. In addition, some medications may further influence the distortion of sensory input. This combination of sensory impairments may pose a variety of activity limitations for the elderly individual such as postural instability, exaggerated body sway, balance problems, wide-based gait, diminished fine motor coordination, tendency to drop items held in the hand, and difficulty in recognizing body positions in space. Box 3.2 Evidence Summary provides an overview of research exploring age-related sensory changes.

Clinical Note: In addition to age-related sensory changes, activity limitations may be exacerbated by muscle weakness associated with a reduction in the number and size of skeletal muscle fibers and overall cross-sectional area of muscle. See discussion in Chapter 5, Examination of Motor Function: Motor Control and Motor Learning.

■ PRELIMINARY CONSIDERATIONS

Accuracy of data from examination of sensory function relies on the patient's ability to respond to application of multiple somatosensory stimuli. Use of several easily administered preliminary tests will provide sufficient data to determine the patient's ability to concentrate on, and respond to, the battery of sensory test items. The two general categories of preliminary tests include the patient's (1) arousal level, attention span, orientation, and cognition;[63] and (2) memory, hearing, and visual acuity. These preliminary tests are typically considered with sensory involvement associated with CNS lesions.

Arousal, Attention, Orientation, and Cognition

A necessary first step is to determine the patient's arousal level for participation in the test protocol. **Arousal** is the physiological readiness of the human system for activity.[7] It is described by using traditionally accepted key terms and definitions to identify the patient's level

| ▸ **Box 3.2 Evidence Summary** Research Exploring Age-Related Changes in Sensory Function |

Reference	Method(s)	Subjects/Design	Results	Conclusions/ Comments
Tochihara et al[11]	Examined age-related differences in cutaneous temperature (Temp) thresholds for warm thermal sensitivity in "thermoneutral" (28°C [82.4°F]) and "cool" (22°C [71.6°F]) environments. Used a thermal stimulator over the cheek, chest, abdomen, upper arm, forearm, hand, thigh, shin, and foot.	Compared 12 young males (22±1 years) and 13 older male adults (67±3 years) in two different environments. There was a significant difference between groups for mean height, subscapular skinfold thickness, and body mass index (BMI).	Cutaneous Temp (warm) thresholds were significantly great for the elder than the younger men on the hand, shin, and foot in both thermoneutral and cool environments. There were no differences observed for the other body parts.	Older adult males were less sensitive to Temp (warmth) than young males in two environments. Differences in Temp sensitivity were nonuniform on the head and trunk (i.e., cheek, chest, abdomen) and significant on the extremities (i.e., hand, shin, foot).
Davila et al[32]	To determine the prevalence of sensory (hearing or visual)	Examined 1997–2004 data from the National Health Interview	The prevalence of hearing impairment (33.4%) was more	The results of this study highlight the growing need for

Continued

Box 3.2 Evidence Summary Research Exploring Age-Related Changes in Sensory Function—cont'd

Reference	Method(s)	Subjects/Design	Results	Conclusions/Comments
	impairment among U.S. workers 65 years and older.	Survey. Of those sampled (N = 5,590), the majority were female, 65–69 years old, white, non-Hispanic, married/living with partner, above the poverty line, had >12 years of education, and had health insurance.	than three times that of visual impairment (10.2%). The highest prevalence of hearing or visual impairment was greatest among farm operators, mechanics, and motor vehicle operators.	workplace accommodations. In addition, there is a need for preventive measures for workers at risk for injury due to their sensory impairments.
Shaffer and Harrison[28]	Reviewed the literature on (1) age-related changes in the proprioceptive and cutaneous systems; (2) the relationship between basic science research and age-related clinical changes; and (3) the relationship between the proprioceptive and cutaneous systems and balance in older adults.	This narrative review included sections on the following: muscle spindle, Golgi tendon organ, proprioception, cutaneous receptors, cutaneous somatosensation, peripheral sensory innervations, and somatosensory integration.	There are age-related declines in various sensory structures and physiology, which accelerates with advancing age. Large myelinated sensory fibers and receptors are preferentially affected with aging. There is evidence that older adults have impaired proprioception, vibration, discriminative touch, and balance. With aging, sensory involvement occurs before motor changes.	This synthesis of the literature provides foundational knowledge about the effects of an aging sensory system on balance. The paper also emphasizes the importance of using reliable and valid methods to examine sensory function. Additional research that examines the relationship between age-related changes in the sensory system and balance is needed.
Laurienti et al[33]	Examined the speed of discrimination responses to the presentation of visual, auditory, or both visual and auditory (multisensory) stimuli. The difference between the visual response time and multisensory response time was examined as an estimate of multisensory gain (i.e., the improvement in performance [reaction time] with additional sensory input).	Compared the speed of discrimination between young (N = 31, 28.1±5.6 years) and older adults (N = 27, 70.9±5.1 years). The researchers also examined performance accuracy, which was used as a covariate when examining multisensory gain.	When using accuracy as a covariate, the older adults demonstrated a significantly greater multisensory gain when compared to the young group.	Older adults demonstrated greater improvements in performance than younger adults with information from multiple sensory modalities. Despite age-related declines in sensory function, the use of information from multiple senses may compensate for impairment in individual sensory functions.

of consciousness. These terms include *alert, lethargic, obtunded, stupor,* and *coma* and represent a continuum of physiological readiness for activity; they are defined as follows:[63]

- *Alert.* The patient is awake and attentive to normal levels of stimulation. Interactions with the therapist are normal and appropriate.
- *Lethargic.* The patient appears drowsy and may fall asleep if not stimulated in some way. Interactions with the therapist may get diverted. Patient may have difficulty in focusing or maintaining attention on a question or task.
- *Obtunded.* The patient is difficult to arouse from a somnolent state and is frequently confused when awake. Repeated stimulation is required to maintain consciousness. Interactions with the therapist may be largely unproductive.
- *Stupor* (semicoma). The patient responds only to strong, generally noxious stimuli and returns to the unconscious state when stimulation is stopped. When aroused, the patient is unable to interact with the therapist.
- *Coma* (deep coma). The patient cannot be aroused by any type of stimulation. Reflex motor responses may or may not be seen.

Reliable information about the integrity of the somatosensory system can be obtained from patients who are alert. Reliability is proportionally reduced in patients with lethargy and nonexistent in patients who are obtunded, stuporous, or comatose.

Attention is selective awareness of the environment or responsiveness to a stimulus or task without being distracted by other stimuli.[6,9,64] Attention can be examined by asking the patient to repeat items on a progressively more challenging list. These repetition tasks can begin with two or three items and gradually progress to longer lists. For example, the patient might be asked to repeat a series of numbers, letters, or words. Another approach to examining attention is to ask the patient to spell words backwards (e.g., book, fork, bottle, garden). The task can be made more challenging by using progressively longer words. Individuals with a high attention span will be able to perform the task. Attention deficits will be apparent when the order of letters is confused.[64]

Orientation refers to the patient's awareness of time, person, and place. In medical record documentation the results of this mental status screening are often abbreviated "oriented × 3," referring to the three parameters of time, person, and place. If a patient is not fully oriented to one or more domains, the notation would read "oriented × 2 (time)" or "oriented × 1 (time, place)." With partial orientation entries, it is customary to include the *domains of disorientation* within parentheses. Box 3.3 presents sample questions for examining orientation.[9,63,64]

Box 3.3 Sample Questions for Examining Orientation

A series of simple questions is posed to the patient. The questions are designed to determine the patient's understanding of recognition of who he or she is, location including the present facility (the name of hospital or clinic), the present time, and the passage of time.

Person

- What is your name?
- Do you have a middle name?
- How old are you?
- When were you born?

Place

- Do you know where you are right now?
- What kind of a place is this?
- Do you know what city and state we are in?
- What city or town do you live in?
- What is your address at home?

Time

- What is today's date?
- What day of the week is it?
- What time is it?
- Is it morning or afternoon?
- What season is it?
- What year is it?
- How long have you been here?

From Nolan[63, p. 26] with permission.

Cognition is defined as the process of knowing and includes both awareness and judgment.[6] Nolan[63] suggests three areas for testing cognition-dependent functions: (1) fund of knowledge, (2) calculation ability, and (3) proverb interpretation. **Fund of knowledge** is defined as the sum total of an individual's learning and experience in life, which will be highly variable and different for each patient. Detailed information about premorbid knowledge base is often not available. However, a number of general categories of information can be used to test this cognitive function. Sample questions might include the following:[63]

- Who became president after Kennedy was shot?
- Who is the current vice president of the United States?
- Which is more—a gallon or a liter?
- In what country is the Great Pyramid?
- What would you add to your food to make it sweeter?
- In what state would you find the city of Boston?
- What are the elements that make up water and salt?
- Can you name a car made by General Motors?
- Who is Charles Dickens?

Calculation ability examines foundational mathematical abilities.[63,64] Two associated terms are **acalculia**

(inability to calculate) and **dyscalculia** (difficulty in accomplishing calculations).[63] This cognitive screening can be administered either verbally or in written format. The patient is asked to mentally perform a series of calculations when provided with mathematical problems. The test should be initiated with simple problems and progress to the more difficult. Adding and subtracting are generally easier than multiplication and division. An alternative approach is to provide written mathematical problems and ask the patient to fill in the answer (e.g., 4 + 4 = ____; 10 + 22 = ____; 46 × 8 = ____; 13 × 7 = ____; 4 × 3 = ____; 6 × 6 = ____; and so forth.).

Proverb interpretation examines the patient's ability to interpret use of words outside of their usual context or meaning. This is a sophisticated cognitive function. During the screening, the patient should be asked to describe the meaning of the proverb. Sample proverbs include the following:[63,64]

- People who live in glass houses shouldn't throw stones.
- A rolling stone gathers no moss.
- A stitch in time saves nine.
- The early bird catches the worm.
- The dog that trots about finds the bone.
- The empty wagon makes the most noise.
- Every cloud has a silver lining.
- Grass doesn't grow on a busy street.

Memory, Hearing, and Visual Acuity

Also related to the ability to respond during sensory testing is the status of the patient's memory and hearing function as well as visual acuity.

Memory

Both long- and short-term memory should be examined. Impairments of short-term memory will be the most disruptive to collecting sensory information owing to patient difficulties in remembering and following directions. *Long-term (remote) memory* can be examined by requesting information on date and place of birth, number of siblings, date of marriage, schools attended, and historical facts. *Short-term memory* can be addressed by verbally providing the patient with a series of words or numbers. For example, a series of words might include "car, book, cup"; use of numbers could include a seven-digit list; a short sentence could also be used to test short-term memory. To ensure understanding of the task, the patient should repeat the sequence immediately. Individuals with normal memory function should be able to recall the list 5 minutes[9] later and at least two of the items from the list after 30 minutes.[63]

Hearing

Observing the patient's response to conversation can provide a gross assessment of hearing. Note should be made of how alterations in voice volume and tone influence patient response.

Visual Acuity

A gross visual examination can be made by use of a standard Snellen chart mounted on the wall or visual acuity cards for use at bedside. If the patient uses corrective lenses, they should be worn during testing and should be clean. Visual acuity is typically recorded at 20 feet (6 m) from the Snellen chart (standard eye chart). This distance (20 feet [6 m]) is then placed over the size of the type the individual is able to read comfortably. For example, on a continuum of visual acuity 20/20 is considered excellent and 20/200 is considered poor acuity.[9]

> **Clinical Note:** Some diagnoses or co-morbidities directly affect vision such as multiple sclerosis, hypertension, and diabetes. Examining the cranial nerves (CNs) will provide additional information about vision. For example, the oculomotor nerve (CN III) is often affected by diabetes (oculomotor nerve palsy).

Peripheral field vision can be examined by sitting directly in front of the patient with outstretched arms. The index fingers should be extended and gradually brought toward the midline of the patient's face. The patient is asked to identify when the therapist's approaching finger is first seen. Differences between right and left visual field should be noted carefully. Depth perception may be grossly checked by holding two pencils or fingers (one behind the other) directly in front of the patient. The patient is asked to touch or grasp the foreground object.

Because tests of sensory integrity require a verbal response to the stimulus, patients with arousal, attention, orientation, cognitive, or short-term memory impairments generally cannot be accurately tested. However, impairments in vision, hearing, or speech will not adversely affect test results if appropriate adaptations are made in providing instructions and indicating responses (e.g., signaling with either one or two fingers during tests for two-point discrimination, pointing to an area of stimulus contact, mimicking joint position sense or awareness of movement with the contralateral extremity, or object identification by selecting from a group of items during tests for stereognosis).

■ CLASSIFICATION OF THE SENSORY SYSTEM

Several different schemes have been proposed for categorizing the sensory system. Among the more common is classification by the type (or location) of *receptors* and the *spinal pathway* mediating information to higher centers.

Sensory Receptors

Sensory receptors (sensory nerve endings) are located at the distal end of an afferent nerve fiber. Once stimulated, they give rise to perception of a specific sensation.

Sensory receptors are highly sensitive to the type of stimulus for which they were designed (termed *receptor specificity*). This specificity of nerve fiber sensitivity to a single modality of sensation is called the *labeled line principle*.[65] This means that individual tactile sensations are perceived when specific types of receptors are stimulated. For example, in response to touch, selective activation of Merkel's discs and Ruffini endings generate the sensation of steady pressure in the cutaneous area above the active receptors.[66]

It should be noted that the term *modality* has a specific meaning within the context of sensation. Modality "defines a general class of stimulus, determined by the type of energy transmitted by the stimulus and the receptors specialized to sense that energy."[66, p. 413] Each type of sensation perceived (e.g., vision, hearing, taste, touch, smell, pain, temperature, proprioception) is referred to as a modality of sensation.

The three divisions of sensory receptors include those that mediate the (1) superficial, (2) deep, and (3) combined (cortical) sensations.[9]

Superficial Sensation

Exteroceptors are responsible for the superficial sensations.[67] They receive stimuli from the external environment via the skin and subcutaneous tissue. Exteroceptors are responsible for the perception of pain, temperature, light touch, and pressure.[9,67]

Deep Sensation

Proprioceptors are responsible for the deep sensations. These receptors receive stimuli from muscles, tendons, ligaments, joints, and fascia,[64] and are responsible for position sense[68] and awareness of joints at rest, movement awareness (kinesthesia), and vibration.

Combined Cortical Sensations

The combination of both the superficial and deep sensory mechanisms makes up the third category of combined sensations. These sensations require information from both exteroceptive and proprioceptive receptors, as well as intact function of cortical sensory association areas. The cortical combined sensations include **stereognosis, two-point discrimination, barognosis, graphesthesia,** tactile localization, recognition of texture, and double simultaneous stimulation.

Spinal Pathways

Sensations also have been classified according to the system by which they are mediated to higher centers. Sensations are mediated by either the *anterolateral spinothalamic system* or the *dorsal column-medial lemniscal system*.[41,67,69]

Anterolateral Spinothalamic

This system initiates self-protective reactions and responds to stimuli that are potentially harmful in nature.

It contains slow-conducting fibers of small diameter, some of which are unmyelinated. The system is concerned with transmission of thermal and nociceptive information, and mediates pain, temperature, crudely localized touch, tickle, itch, and sexual sensations.

Dorsal Column–Medial Lemniscal System

The dorsal column is the system involved with responses to more discriminative sensations. It contains fast-conducting fibers of large diameter with greater myelination. This system mediates the sensations of discriminative touch and pressure sensations, vibration, movement, position sense, and awareness of joints at rest. The two systems are interdependent and integrated so as to function together.

■ TYPES OF SENSORY RECEPTORS

The sensory receptors frequently are divided according to their structural design and the type of stimulus to which they preferentially respond. These divisions include (1) *mechanoreceptors*, which respond to mechanical deformation of the receptor or surrounding area; (2) *thermoreceptors*, which respond to changes in temperature; (3) *nociceptors*, which respond to noxious stimuli and result in the perception of pain; (4) *chemoreceptors*, which respond to chemical substances and are responsible for taste, smell, oxygen levels in arterial blood, carbon dioxide concentration, and osmolality (concentration gradient) of body fluids; and (5) *photic (electromagnetic) receptors*, which respond to light within the visible spectrum.[8,9,67,70]

The perception of pain is not limited to stimuli received from nociceptors, because other types of receptors and nerve fibers contribute to this sensation. High intensities of stimuli to any type of receptor may be perceived as pain (e.g., extreme heat or cold and high-intensity mechanical deformation).

The general classification of sensory receptors is presented in Box 3.4.[64,65,71] Note that this list also includes the receptors responsible for electromagnetic (visual) and chemical stimuli.

Cutaneous Receptors

Cutaneous sensory receptors are located at the terminal portion of the afferent fiber. These include free nerve endings, hair follicle endings, Merkel's discs, Ruffini endings, Krause's end-bulbs, Meissner's corpuscles, and Pacinian corpuscles. The density of these sensory receptors varies for different areas of the body. For example, there are many more tactile receptors in the fingertips than in the back. These areas of higher receptor density correspondingly display a higher cortical representation in somatic sensory area I. Receptor density is a particularly important consideration in interpreting the results of a sensory examination for a given body surface. Figure 3.3 illustrates the cutaneous sensory receptors and their respective locations within the various layers of skin.

Box 3.4   Classification of Sensory Receptors

I. Mechanoreceptors
A. Cutaneous sensory receptors
1. Free nerve endings
2. Hair follicle endings
3. Merkel's discs
4. Ruffini endings
5. Krause's end-bulbs
6. Meissner's corpuscles
7. Pacinian corpuscles

II. Deep Sensory Receptors
A. Muscle receptors
1. Muscle spindles
2. Golgi tendon organs
3. Free nerve endings
4. Pacinian corpuscles
B. Joint receptors
1. Golgi-type endings
2. Free nerve endings
3. Ruffini endings
4. Paciniform endings

III. Thermoreceptors
A. Cold
1. Cold receptors
B. Warmth
1. Warmth receptors

IV. Nociceptors
A. Pain
1. Free nerve endings
2. Extremes of stimuli*

V. Electromagnetic Receptors
A. Vision
1. Rods
2. Cones

VI. Chemoreceptors
A. Taste
1. Receptors of taste buds
B. Smell
1. Receptors of olfactory nerves in olfactory epithelium
C. Arterial oxygen
1. Receptors of aortic and carotid bodies
D. Osmolality
1. Probably neurons of supraoptic nuclei
E. Blood CO_2
1. Receptors in or on surface of medulla and in aortic and carotid bodies
F. Blood glucose, amino acids, fatty acids
1. Receptors in hypothalamus

*Extremes of stimuli to other sensory receptors will be perceived as pain.
Adapted from Waxman,[64] Hall,[65] and Fitzgerald et al.[71]

Free Nerve Endings

These receptors are found throughout the body. Stimulation of free nerve endings result in the perception of pain, temperature, touch, pressure, tickle, and itch sensations.[9,64]

Hair Follicle Endings (Hair End-Organs)

At the base of each hair follicle a free nerve ending is entwined. The combination of the hair follicle and its nerve provides a sensitive receptor. These receptors are sensitive to mechanical movement and touch.[72,73]

Merkel's Discs

These touch receptors are located below the epidermis in hairless smooth (glabrous) skin with a high density in the fingertips. They are sensitive to low-intensity touch, as well as to the velocity of touch, and respond to constant indentation of the skin (pressure). They provide for the ability to perceive continuous contact of objects against the skin and are believed to play an important role in both two-point discrimination and localization of touch.[67,73] Merkel's discs are also believed to contribute to recognition of texture.

Ruffini Endings

Located in the deeper layers of the dermis, these encapsulated endings are involved with the perception of touch and pressure. They are slowly adapting and particularly important in signaling continuous skin deformation such as tension or stretch; they are also found in joint capsules and assist with joint position sense.[65,73]

Krause's End-Bulb

The function of these bulbous encapsulated nerve endings is not clearly understood. They are located in the dermis and conjunctiva of the eye. They are believed to be low-threshold mechanical receptors that may play a contributing role in the perception of touch and pressure.

Meissner's Corpuscles

Located in the dermis, these encapsulated nerve endings contain many branching nerve filaments within the capsule. They are low-threshold, rapidly adapting and in high concentration in the fingertips, lips, and toes, areas that require high levels of discrimination. These receptors play an important role in discriminative touch (e.g., recognition of texture) and movement of objects over skin.[41,65,73]

Pacinian Corpuscles

These receptors are located in the subcutaneous tissue layer of the skin and in deep tissues of the body (including tendons and soft tissues around joints). They are stimulated by rapid movement of tissue and are quickly adapting. They play a significant role in the perception of deep touch and vibration.[73,74]

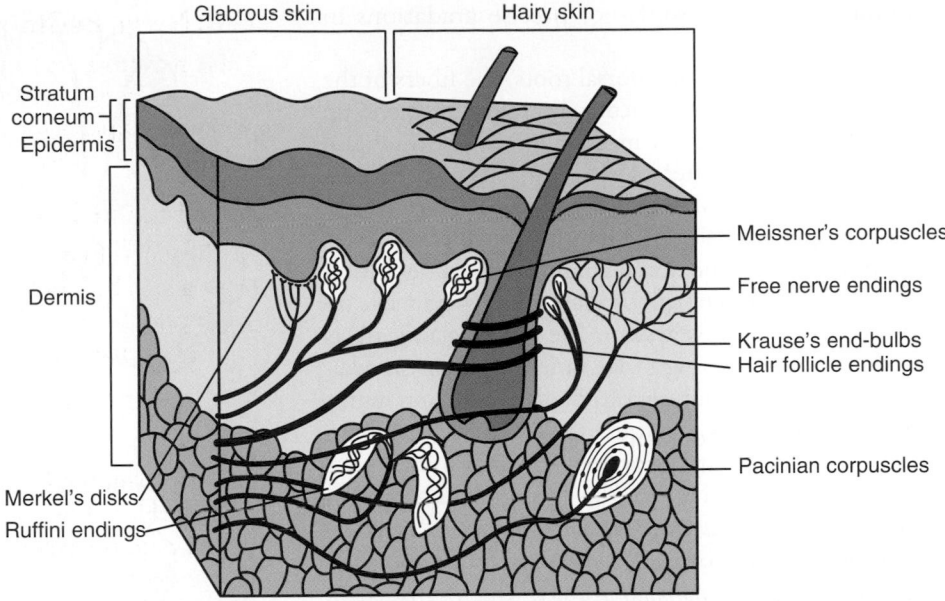

Figure 3.3 The cutaneous sensory receptors and their respective locations within the various layers of skin (epidermis, dermis, and the subcutaneous layer).

Deep Sensory Receptors

The deep sensory receptors are located in muscles, tendons, and joints[64,65,69] and include both muscle and joint receptors. They are concerned primarily with posture, position sense, proprioception, muscle tone, and speed and direction of movement. The deep sensory receptors include the muscle spindle, Golgi tendon organs, free nerve endings, Pacinian corpuscles, and joint receptors.

Muscle Receptors
Muscle Spindles

The muscle spindle fibers (intrafusal fibers) lie in a parallel arrangement to the muscle fibers (extrafusal fibers). They monitor changes in muscle length (Ia and II spindle afferent endings) as well as velocity (Ia ending) of these changes. The muscle spindle plays a vital role in position and movement sense and in motor learning.

Golgi Tendon Organs

These receptors are located in series at both the proximal and distal tendinous insertions of the muscle. The Golgi tendon organs function to monitor tension within the muscle. They also provide a protective mechanism by preventing structural damage to the muscle in situations of extreme tension. This is accomplished by inhibition of the contracting muscle and facilitation of the antagonist.

Free Nerve Endings

These receptors are within the fascia of the muscle. They are believed to respond to pain and pressure.

Pacinian Corpuscles

Located within the fascia of the muscle, these receptors respond to vibratory stimuli and deep pressure.

Joint Receptors
Golgi-Type Endings

These receptors are located in the ligaments, and function to detect the rate of joint movement.

Free Nerve Endings

Found in the joint capsule and ligaments, these receptors are believed to respond to pain and crude awareness of joint motion.

Ruffini Endings

Located in the joint capsule and ligaments, Ruffini endings are responsible for the direction and velocity of joint movement.

Paciniform Endings

These receptors are found in the joint capsule and primarily monitor rapid joint movements.

■ PATHWAYS FOR TRANSMISSION OF SOMATIC SENSORY SIGNALS

Somatic sensory information enters the spinal cord through the dorsal roots. Sensory signals are then carried to higher centers via ascending pathways from one of two systems: the *anterolateral spinothalamic system* or the *dorsal column–medial lemniscal system*.

Anterolateral Spinothalamic Pathway

The spinothalamic tracts are diffuse pathways concerned with nondiscriminative sensations such as pain, temperature, tickle, itch, and sexual sensations. This system is activated primarily by mechanoreceptors, thermoreceptors, and nociceptors, and is composed of afferent fibers that are small diameter and slowly conducting. Sensory signals transmitted by this system do not require discrete localization of signal source or precise gradations in intensity.

After originating in the dorsal roots, the fibers of the spinothalamic pathway immediately cross and ascend up the spinal cord through the medulla, pons, and midbrain to the ventroposterolateral (VPL) nucleus of the thalamus (Fig. 3.4). Axons of the VPL neurons project to the somatosensory cortex via the internal capsule.[41,74]

Compared with the dorsal column–medial lemniscal system, the anterolateral spinothalamic pathways make up a cruder, more primitive system. The spinothalamic tracts are capable of transmitting a wide variety of sensory modalities. However, their diffuse pattern of termination results in only crude abilities to localize the source of a stimulus on the body surface, and poor intensity discrimination.[64]

The three major tracts of the spinothalamic system are the (1) *anterior (ventral) spinothalamic tract,* which carries the sensations of crudely localized touch and pressure; (2) the *lateral spinothalamic tract,* which carries pain and temperature; and (3) the *spinoreticular tract,* which is involved with diffuse pain sensations.[64]

Dorsal Column–Medial Lemniscal Pathway

This system is responsible for the transmission of discriminative sensations received from specialized mechanoreceptors. Sensory modalities that require fine gradations of intensity and precise localization on the body surface are mediated by this system. Sensations transmitted by the dorsal column–medial lemniscal pathway include discriminative touch, stereognosis, tactile pressure, barognosis, *graphesthesia,* recognition of texture, kinesthesia, two-point discrimination, proprioception, and vibration.

This system is composed of large, myelinated, rapidly conducting fibers. After entering the dorsal column the fibers ascend to the medulla and synapse with the dorsal column nuclei (nuclei gracilis and cuneatus). From here they cross to the opposite side and pass up to the thalamus through bilateral pathways called the *medial lemnisci.* Each medial lemniscus terminates in the ventral posterolateral thalamus. From the thalamus, third-order neurons project to the somatic sensory cortex. Projection to sensory association areas in the cortex allows for the perception and interpretation of the combined cortical sensations (Fig. 3.5).[64,65,67,74] Table 3.1 presents a comparison of the most salient features of each ascending pathway.

■ SOMATOSENSORY CORTEX

The most complex processing of sensory information occurs in the somatosensory cortex, which is divided into three main divisions: primary somatosensory cortex (S-I), secondary somatosensory cortex (S-II), and posterior parietal cortex (Fig. 3.6A). The primary somatosensory (S-I) area occupies a lateral strip called the postcentral gyrus (posterior to the central sulcus) and includes four

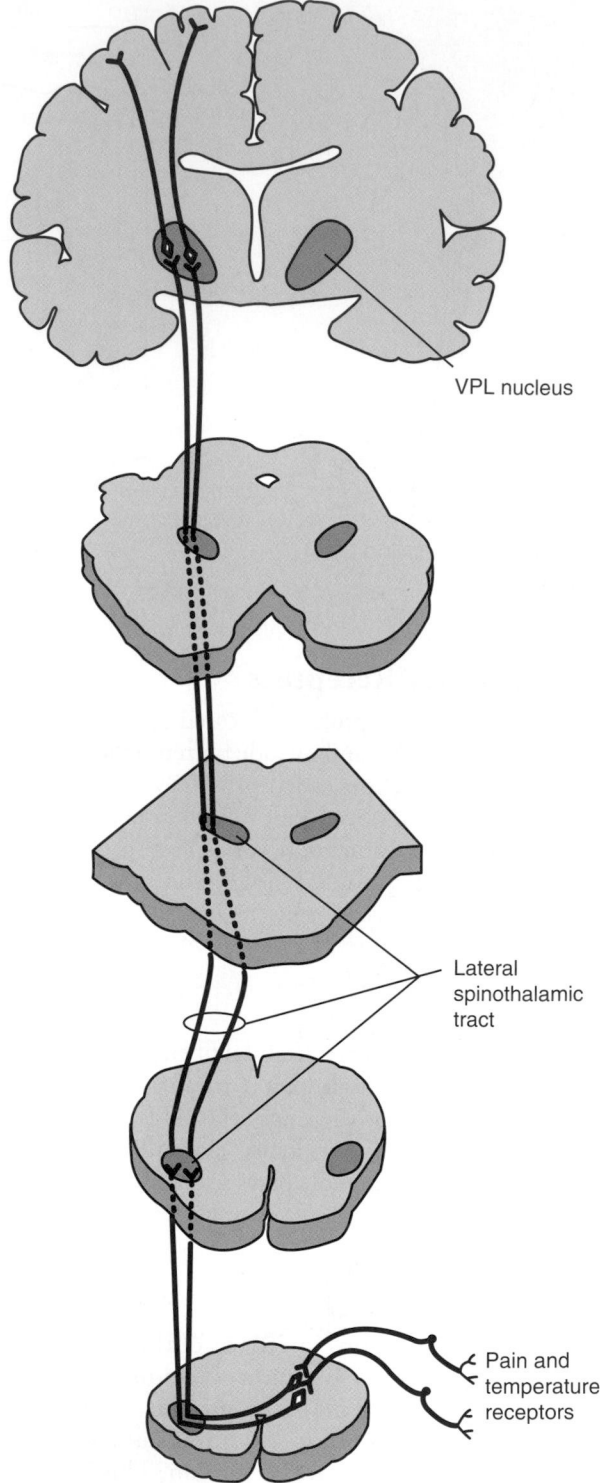

Figure 3.4 Anterolateral spinothalamic tract carrying pain and temperature.

distinct areas: Brodmann's areas 3a, 3b, 1, and 2. S-I neurons identify the location of stimuli as well as discern the size, shape, and texture of objects. At the superior aspect of the lateral sulcus is the secondary somatosensory cortex (S-II), which is innervated by neurons from S-I. S-II projects to the insular cortex that innervates

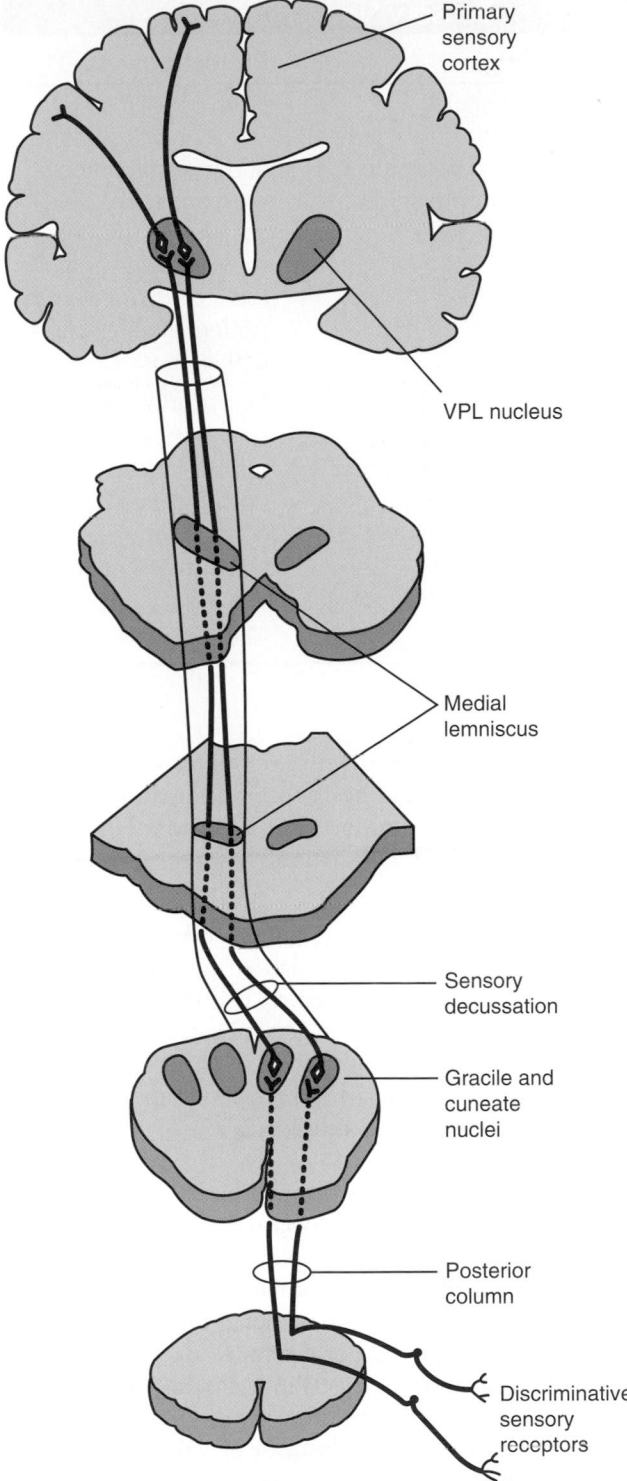

Figure 3.5 Dorsal column–medial lemniscal tract carrying discriminative sensations such as kinesthesia and touch.

and integrate somatosensory information and contribute to motor performance by (1) determining the initial position required before a movement occurs, (2) error detection as movement occurs, and (3) identification of movement outcomes, which helps to shape learning.

Animal models have provided considerable insight into the function of the cortical association areas. Complete removal of area S-I of the somatosensory system produces deficits in position sense and the ability to determine the size, texture, and shape of objects. Temperature and pain perception are diminished but not abolished. Owing to reliance on input from S-I, removal of S-II results in severe impairment of the perception of both shape and texture of objects. Animal models have also shown reduced ability to learn new discriminative tasks, which are based on the shape of an object. Insult to the posterior parietal cortex presents profound impairments in attending to sensory input from the contralateral side of the body.[75]

The sensory homunculus (somatotopic map) represents a cross-sectional view through the postcentral gyrus and identifies the relative size of the cortex devoted to specific body parts (Fig. 3.6B). Note that certain areas of the body are exaggerated such as the hand, face, and mouth owing to greater innervation density of the skin. The relative size of body parts represents both the *density* of sensory input from the body region as well as the *importance* of sensory information from the area as it relates to function.[74,75] For example, the relative size of the foot is reflective of its importance in locomotion; the relative size of the index finger reflects its role in fine motor skills. In contrast, cortical areas for the trunk and back are small, implying a lower receptor density and reduced role in sensory perception related to function.

Using two-point discrimination as an example, Bear et al[74] provide an extraordinary illustration of how our ability to perceive a stimulus varies remarkably across the body:

> Two-point discrimination varies at least twenty-fold across the body. Fingertips have the highest resolution. The dots of Braille are 1 mm high and 2.5 mm apart; up to six dots make a letter. An experienced Braille reader can scan an index finger across a page of raised dots and read about 600 letters per minute, which is roughly as fast as someone reading aloud. Several reasons explain why the fingertip is so much better than, say, the elbow for Braille reading: (1) There is a much higher density of mechanoreceptors in the skin of the fingertip than on other parts of the body; (2) the fingertips are enriched in receptor types that have small receptive fields; (3) there is more brain tissue (and thus more raw computing power) devoted to the sensory information

the temporal lobe, believed important in tactile memory. The posterior parietal lobe is behind S-I and consists of areas 5 and 7. Area 5 integrates tactile input from mechanoreceptors of the skin with proprioceptive input from muscles and joints. Area 7 integrates stereognostic and visual information from visual, tactile, and proprioceptive input.[69,74,75] These processing areas analyze

Table 3.1   Features of Pathways for Transmission of Somatic Sensory Signals

Pathway	Type of Sensation	Afferent Fibers	Origin	Projection
Anterolateral spinothalamic	Nondiscriminative (e.g., pain, temperature); broad spectrum of sensory modalities; crude localization; poor intensity discrimination; poor spatial orientation relative to origin of stimulus	Small-diameter, slowly conducting	Skin: mechanoreceptors, thermoreceptors, nociceptors	From dorsal roots of spinal nerves, synapse at dorsal horns, fibers cross and move up spinal cord, through medulla, pons, and midbrain to the ventroposterolateral nucleus of thalamus
Dorsal column–medial lemniscal	Discriminative (e.g., stereognosis, two-point discrimination); precise localization; fine intensity gradations; high degree of spatial orientation relative to origin of stimulus	Large, rapidly conducting	Skin, joints, tendons: specialized mechanoreceptors	From dorsal roots of spinal nerves, ascend to medulla, synapse with dorsal column nuclei, cross to contralateral side and ascend to thalamus; then project to sensory cortex

of each square millimeter of fingertip than elsewhere; and (4) there may be special neural mechanisms devoted to high-resolution discriminations.[74, p. 392]

■ SCREENING

An important component of physical therapy intervention is to accurately and efficiently meet individual patient needs. Together with information from the history and review of systems, screenings assist the therapist in proficiently identifying the needed tests and measures and setting priorities within the examination process. Screenings consist of a series of brief tests that provide the therapist an "overview" of the system of interest (e.g., musculoskeletal, neuromuscular). Within this context, screenings are conducted to:[7,76]

• Determine the need for further or more detailed examination
• Determine in a timely manner if referral to another health care practitioner is warranted
• Focus the search for the origin of symptoms to a specific location or body part
• Identify system-related impairments that contribute to activity limitations or disability

Clinical Note: The term *screening* is also used in another context. It additionally refers to identification of individuals or groups who are not currently receiving physical therapy services but may be at risk for a health problem.[7] Examples might include identification of risk factors for low back injury, diabetes, obesity, or falls in the elderly. Physical therapy interventions associated with this type

of screening typically involve prevention strategies, fitness advocacy, and health promotion and wellness programs designed to meet the needs of an individual client or target population.

To perform a sensory screening, several easily tested (i.e., requiring little or no specialized equipment) modalities of sensation are selected. It is important to select modalities from each of the general categories of sensations. For example, the therapist might select pain and light touch (superficial), kinesthesia and vibration (deep), and two-point discrimination or stereognosis (combined).

Sensory screening is performed by using the selected modalities to test randomly over somewhat large surface areas. For example, several applications of each stimulus might be distributed over the upper and lower extremities and trunk. The information gathered informs the therapist's decision making. For example, if sensory impairments are identified it may (1) indicate the need for more detailed testing, (2) help narrow the origin of symptoms, or (3) provide insight into the cause of activity limitations.

As mentioned earlier, screening tests for mental status (arousal, attention, orientation, cognition, and memory), vision, and hearing acuity should be performed prior to the sensory examination.

■ PREPARATION FOR ADMINISTERING THE SENSORY EXAMINATION

Before initiating the examination of sensory function, the testing environment should be identified and prepared, needed equipment gathered, and consideration

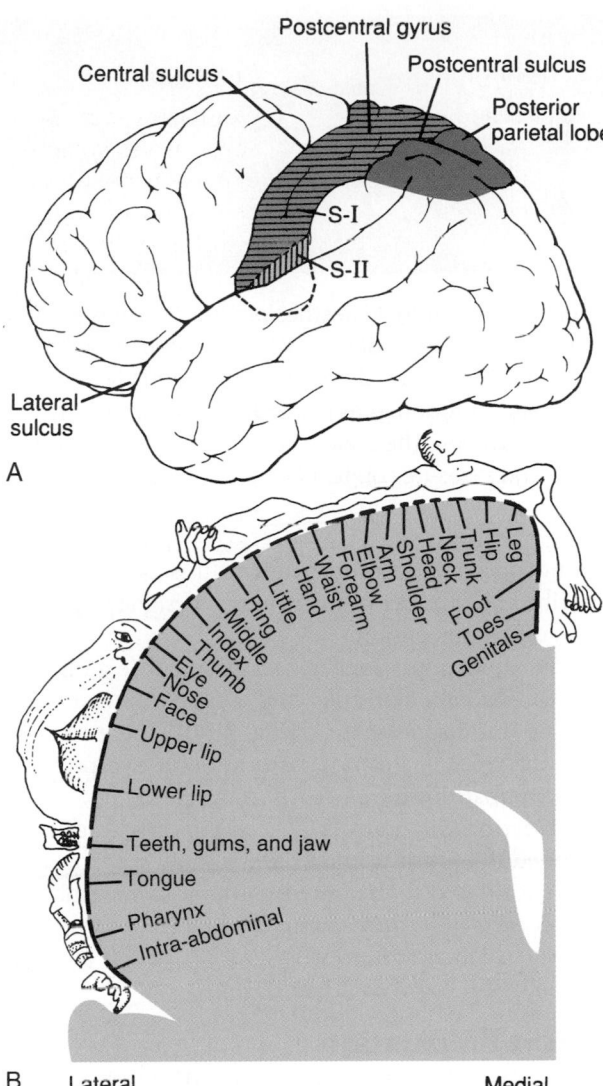

A

B   Lateral   Medial

Figure 3.6 (A) The somatosensory cortex has three main divisions: The primary (S-I) and secondary (S-II) areas, and the posterior parietal lobe. **(B)** The sensory homunculus. Areas of the body used for tactile discrimination (e.g., lips, tongue, and fingers) are represented by large areas of cortical tissue. Areas with reduced cortical representation, such as the trunk, are reflective of body parts with lesser roles in sensory perception. *(From Kandel, ER, and Jessell, TM: Touch. In Kandel, ER, Schwartz, JH and Jessel, TM: Principles of Neural Science, ed 3. Appleton and Lange, Norwalk, CT, 1991 with permission, pp. 368 [A] and 372[B]).*

given to patient preparation (i.e., what information and instruction will be provided).

Testing Environment

The sensory examination should be administered in a quiet, well-lighted area. Depending on the number of body areas to be tested, either a sitting or recumbent position may be used. If full body testing is indicated, both prone and supine positions will be required and use

of a treatment table is recommended to allow examination of each side of the body.

Equipment

To perform a sensory examination the following equipment and materials are used:

1. *Pain.* A large-headed safety pin or a large paper clip that has one segment bent open (providing one *sharp* and one *dull* end). The sharp end of the instrument should not be sharp enough to risk puncturing the skin. If a large-headed safety pin is used, the sharp end may be further blunted by a light sanding. Commercially available single-use protected neurological pins may also be used (Fig. 3.7).
2. *Temperature.* Two standard laboratory test tubes with stoppers.

Clinical Note: The Tip Therm® is an early detection tool for identification of changes in thermal perception designed for monitoring polyneuropathy associated with diabetes (Fig. 3.8). It provides a method for patients to test temperature sensitivity of their feet independently. It provides only a gross estimate of temperature perception; however, its convenience, low cost, and patients' ability to use it are important characteristics. The tool can be used many times, requires no energy, and makes use of the special characteristics of synthetic material and metal. One end is metal and the opposite side is synthetic material. Both materials are essentially at room temperature; however, the metal end takes more heat from the body (metal has a higher

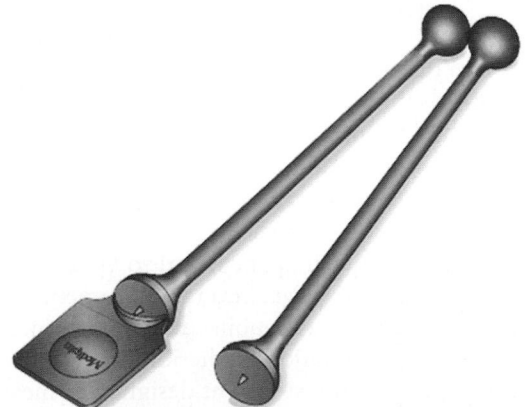

Figure 3.7 Single use protected neurological pin. The image on the *left* shows the pin prior to use with the protective cap intact (although schematically presented to allow visualization of pin location). On the *right*, the protective cap is removed and the pin exposed. On the opposite end of the pin is a smooth rounded surface used to randomly intersperse application of a dull stimulus. After use, the point is destroyed by compressing it against a hard surface and disposed of in a biohazard receptacle. *(Courtesy of US Neurologicals, Kirkland, WA 98033.)*

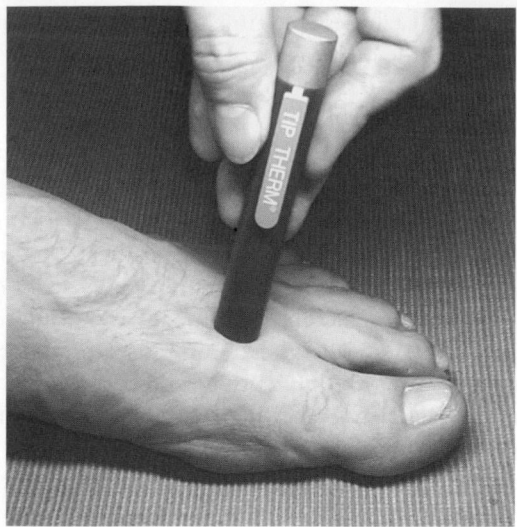

Figure 3.8 The Tip Therm® is a thermal instrument designed for patient monitoring of gross temperature perception of the feet. The instrument is 4 inches (100 mm) long with a .59 inch (15 mm) diameter. *(Courtesy of Tip-Therm® GmbH, Düsseldorf, Germany.)*

conductivity than the synthetic end). As a result, the metal end is perceived as warm and the synthetic end as cooler.

3. *Light touch.* A camel-hair brush, a piece of cotton, or a tissue.
4. *Vibration.* Tuning fork and earphones (if available, to reduce auditory clues). Tuning forks are made of steel or magnesium alloy and grossly resemble a two-pronged fork. When the tines are stuck against a surface (usually the palm of the examiner's hand) the fork resonates at a specific pitch (e.g., 128, 256, or 512 Hz) determined by the length of the two U-shaped prongs (tines).
5. *Stereognosis (object recognition).* A variety of small, commonly used articles such as a comb, fork, paper clip, key, marble, coin, pencil, and so forth.
6. *Two-point discrimination.* Several instruments are available to measure two-point discrimination. A two-point discrimination aesthesiometer (Fig. 3.9) is a small handheld instrument designed to measure the shortest distance that two points of contact on the skin can be distinguished. It consists of a small ruler with one stationary and one moveable (sliding) tip coated with vinyl. The vinyl coverings help to minimize the impact of temperature on perception of contact. Some instruments also have a third tip allowing ease of alternating from two points to a single point of contact during testing. If used on an uneven body surface, care should be taken not to allow the "ruler" portion of the instrument to make contact with the skin. *Note:* The term *aesthesiometer*

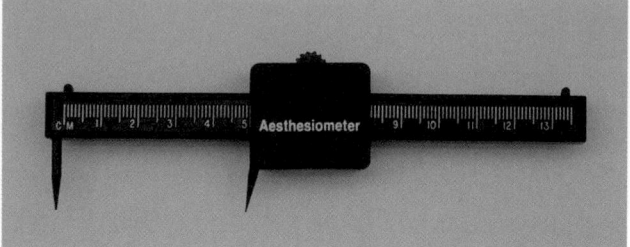

Figure 3.9 A handheld aesthesiometer provides a quantitative measure of two-point discrimination. The two-point threshold is determined by gradually bringing the tips closer together as it is sequentially applied to the patient's skin. The scale is calibrated to the nearest 0.1 cm and measures up to 14 cm.

is not specific to this instrument; it is used to describe any number of instruments designed to examine touch perception.

For finer gradations in measurement (e.g., fingertips), small circular disks can be used to measure two-point discrimination (Fig. 3.10). These instruments typically allow quantification of two-point discrimination from 1 to 25 mm.

Electrocardiogram (ECG) calipers[77] with the tips sanded to blunt the ends[78] and a small ruler have also been used to measure two-point discrimination.

7. *Recognition of texture.* Samples of fabrics of various texture such as cotton, wool, burlap, or silk (approximately 4×4 inches [10×10 cm]).

Patient Preparation

A full explanation of the purpose of the testing should be provided. The patient also should be informed that cooperation is necessary to obtain accurate test results. It is of considerable importance that the patient be requested *not to guess* if uncertain of the correct response.

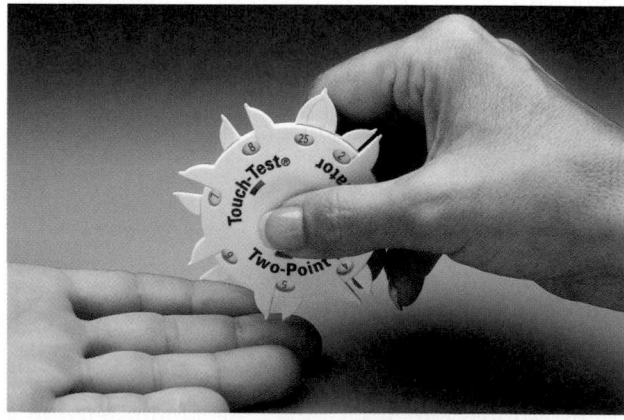

Figure 3.10 This circular two-point discrimination instrument consists of two joined plastic rotating disks with rounded tips placed at standard testing intervals. *(Courtesy of North Coast Medical, Inc., Morgan Hill, CA 95037.)*

During the examination, the patient should be in a comfortable, relaxed position. Preferably, the tests should be performed when the patient is well rested. Considering the high level of concentration required, it is not surprising that fatigue has been noted to affect results of some sensory tests adversely.[77]

Note: A "trial run" or demonstration of each test should be performed just prior to actual administration. This will orient the patient to the sensation being tested, what to anticipate, and what type of response is required. The importance of this initial trial should not be underestimated. If a practice trial is inadequately or not performed, what appears to be a sensory impairment may in reality only be a reflection of the patient's lack of understanding of the testing protocol or how to respond to a stimulus.

Some method of occluding the patient's vision during the testing should be used (vision should not be occluded during the explanation and demonstration). Visual input is prevented because it may allow for compensation of a sensory deficit and thus decrease the accuracy of test results. The traditional methods of occluding vision are by use of a fabric blindfold (such as those worn by travelers to sleep on an airplane), a small folded towel, or by asking the patient to keep the eyes closed. These methods are practical in most instances. However, in situations of CNS dysfunction, a patient may become anxious or disoriented if vision is occluded for a long period of time. In these situations, a small screen or folder may be preferable as a visual barrier. Whatever method is used, it should be removed between the tests while directions and demonstrations are provided.

■ THE SENSORY EXAMINATION

The superficial (exteroceptive) sensations are usually examined first, inasmuch as they consist of more primitive responses, followed by the deep (proprioceptive), and then the combined cortical sensations. If a test indicates impairment of the superficial responses, some impairment of the more discriminative (deep and combined) sensations also will be noted and is a contraindication to further testing (e.g., lack of touch sensation would be a contraindication for testing stereognosis). That is, the primary modality of sensation (touch) must be sufficiently intact to permit meaningful testing of cortical sensory function (ability to identify objects placed in the hand).

For each sensory test, the following data will be generated:

- The modality tested
- The quantity of involvement or body surface areas affected (pattern identification)
- The degree or severity of involvement (e.g., absent, impaired, or delayed responses)
- Localization of the exact boundaries of the sensory impairment

- The patient's subjective feelings about changes in sensation
- The potential impact of sensory loss on function (i.e., activity limitation, disability)

Knowledge of skin segment (dermatome) innervation by the dorsal roots and peripheral nerve innervation (see Figs. 3.1 and 3.2) is required for making sound, accurate diagnostic and prognostic judgments. They serve as critical references during testing as well as provide a framework for documenting results.

Sensory tests are typically performed in a distal to proximal direction. This progression will conserve time, particularly when dealing with localized lesions involving a single extremity, where deficits tend to be more severe distally. It is generally not necessary to test every segment of each dermatome; testing general body areas is sufficient. However, once a deficit area is noted, testing must become more discrete and the exact boundaries of the impairment should be identified. A skin pencil may be useful to mark the boundaries of sensory change directly. This information should be transferred later to a sensory examination form, graphically presented on a dermatome chart, and peripheral nerve involvement identified. Figure 3.11 presents a sample Sensory Examination Form. A single documentation form applicable to the variety of patients seen in different practice settings does not exist. Specialized centers or organizations have developed specific forms to examine sensory function (e.g., the American Spinal Injury Association (ASIA) Standard Neurological Classification of Spinal Cord Injury, described in Chapter 20, Traumatic Spinal Cord Injury). However, the following are common elements of sensory examination forms: (1) a dermatome chart to graphically display findings; (2) a grading scale (e.g., 0—absent; 1—impaired; 2—normal; NT—not testable; and so forth) to score patient perception of individual modalities; and (3) a section for narrative comments.

Most often the dermatome charts are completed using a color code (i.e., each color represents a different sensory modality). The colors used to plot each sensation are then coded by the examiner directly on the form (see Fig. 3.11). In many instances hatch marks of varying density are used to represent gradations in sensory impairment (i.e., the closer together, the greater the sensory impairment). With this method, a completely colored-in area indicates no response to a given sensation. With varied or "spotty" sensory loss it is not uncommon that more than one dermatome chart is required to completely depict all test findings. With use of several dermatome charts, the sensation(s) represented should appear in bold print at the top of each page.

Figure 3.11 provides the foundational elements of documentation typically included for sensory examinations. It should be modified or expanded to meet the needs of a given population or facility. It is also not uncommon for therapists to included sensory testing data within the body of a narrative or progress report.

This form provides a record of the type, severity, and location of sensory impairments. It should be used in conjunction with additional dermatome sheets, if needed, to graphically outline the exact boundaries of the impairment. The designations P and D may be added to the grading key to indicate either a proximal (P) or a distal (D) location of the impairment on a limb or body part. The dermatome chart should be color coded and filled in using varying density hatch marks (higher density for more severe areas of impairment). Indicate the color used for documentation in the box titled Color Code (a different color should be used for each sensation). Separate notation should be made for examination of the face and identification of peripheral nerve involvement. Abnormal responses should be briefly described in the comments section.

ANTERIOR

POSTERIOR

Patient Name: _____

Examiner: _____   Date: _____

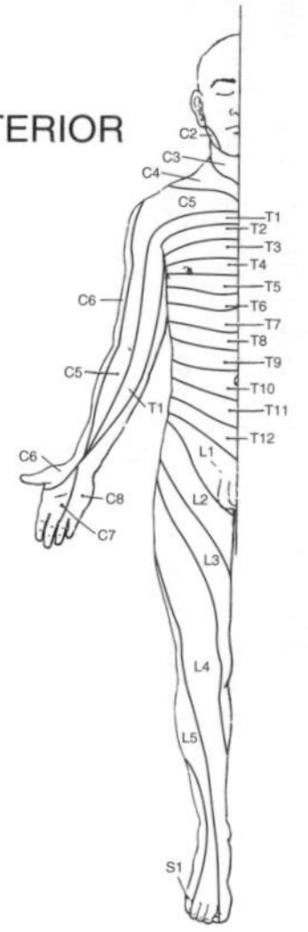

Sensations	Upper Extremity		Lower Extremity		Trunk		Comments
	Right	Left	Right	Left	Right	Left	
Pain							
Temperature							
Touch							
Vibration							
Two-Point Disc							
Kinesthesia							
Proprioception							
Stereognosis							

Note: Areas shaded indicate sensation not typically tested for corresponding body part.

Key to Grading
0 = Absent, no response
1 = Decreased, delayed response
2 = Increased, exaggerated response
3 = Inconsistent response
4 = Intact, normal response
NT = unable to test
P = proximal; D = distal

Color Code

Color	Sensation

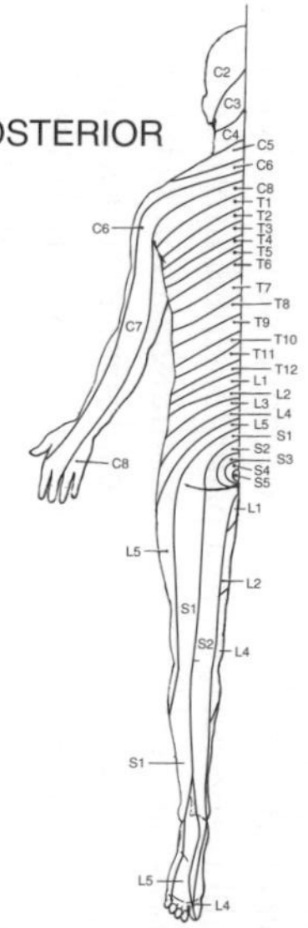

Indicate Peripheral Nerve Involvement:

Figure 3.11 Sample Sensory Examination Form.

During testing, the application of stimuli should be applied in a random, unpredictable manner with variation in timing. This will improve accuracy of the test results by avoiding a consistent pattern of application, which might provide the patient with "clues" to the correct response. During application of stimuli, consideration must be given also to skin condition. Scar tissue or callused areas are generally less sensitive and will demonstrate a diminished response to sensory stimuli. Recall that a trial test is performed to instruct the patient in what to expect and how to respond to application of the specific stimuli; and that patient vision is occluded during testing.

The following sections present the individual sensory tests. The tests are subdivided for superficial, deep, and combined cortical sensations. Table 3.2 presents terminology used to describe common sensory impairments.

Clinical Note: Hands should always be washed prior to and after patient contact. "Hand hygiene is a major component of standard precautions and one of the most effective methods to prevent transmission of pathogens associated with health care."[79, p. 1] The World Health Organization (WHO) recommends hand washing with soap and water for 40 to 60 seconds and hand rubbing using an alcohol-based hand rub for 20 to 30 seconds.[80] See Chapter 2, Examination of Vital Signs (section titled Hand Hygiene) for a more detailed discussion and figures illustrating hand hygiene techniques using soap and water and an alcohol-based hand rub.

Superficial Sensations
Pain Perception

This test is also referred to as *sharp/dull discrimination* and indicates function of protective sensation. To test pain awareness, the sharp and dull ends of a large-headed safety pin, a reshaped paper clip (the segment pulled away from the body of the paper clip provides a sharp end), or a single-use protected neurological pin (see Fig. 3.7) are used. The instrument should be carefully cleaned before administering the test and disposed of immediately afterward (owing to the protective cap on the neurological pin, cleaning is not required). The sharp and dull ends of the instrument are randomly applied perpendicularly to the skin. To avoid summation

Table 3.2	Terminology Describing Common Sensory Impairments
Abarognosis	Inability to recognize weight
Allesthesia	Sensation experienced at a site remote from point of stimulation
Allodynia	Pain produced by a non-noxious stimulus
Analgesia	Complete loss of pain sensitivity
Astereognosis	Inability to recognize the form and shape of objects by touch (synonym: tactile agnosia)
Atopognosia	Inability to localize a sensation
Causalgia	Painful, burning sensations, usually along the distribution of a nerve
Dysesthesia	Touch sensation experienced as pain
Hypalgesia	Decreased sensitivity to pain
Hyperalgesia	Increased sensitivity to pain
Hyperesthesia	Increased sensitivity to sensory stimuli
Hypesthesia	Decreased sensitivity to sensory stimuli
Pallanesthesia	Loss or absence of sensibility to vibration
Paresthesia	Abnormal sensation such as numbness, prickling, or tingling, without apparent cause
Thalamic syndrome	Vascular lesion of the thalamus resulting in sensory disturbances and partial or complete paralysis of one side of the body, associated with severe, boring-type pain; sensory stimuli may produce an exaggerated, prolonged, or painful response
Thermanalgesia	Inability to perceive heat
Thermanesthesia	Inability to perceive sensations of heat and cold
Thermhyperesthesia	Increased sensitivity to temperature
Thermhypesthesia	Decreased temperature sensibility
Thigmanesthesia	Loss of light touch sensibility

of impulses, the stimuli should not be applied too close to each other or in too rapid a succession. To maintain a uniform pressure with each successive application of stimuli, the pin or reshaped paper clip should be held firmly and the fingers allowed to "slide" down the pin or paper clip once in contact with the skin. This will avoid the chance of gradually increasing pressure during application. The instrument used to test pain perception should be sharp enough to deflect the skin, but not puncture it.

Response

The patient is asked to verbally indicate *sharp* or *dull* when a stimulus is felt. All areas of the body may be tested.

Temperature Awareness

This test determines the ability to distinguish between warm and cool stimuli. Two test tubes with stoppers are required for this examination; one should be filled with warm water and the other with crushed ice. Ideal temperatures for cold are between 41°F (5°C) and 50°F (10°C) and for warmth, between 104°F (40°C) and 113°F (45°C). Caution should be exercised to remain within these ranges, because exceeding these temperatures may elicit a pain response and consequently inaccurate test results. The side of the test tube should be placed in contact with the skin (as opposed to only the distal end). This technique provides sufficient surface area contact to determine the temperature. The test tubes are randomly placed in contact with the skin area to be tested. All skin surfaces should be tested.

Response

The patient is asked to reply *hot* or *cold* after each stimulus application.

> **Clinical Note:** The clinical usefulness of thermal testing may be problematic. Nolan[77] points out that the tests are extremely difficult to duplicate on a day-to-day basis owing to rapid changes in temperature once the test tubes are exposed to room air. Although it is a simple test to perform, determining changes over time is not practical unless a method of monitoring the temperature of the test tubes is used.[77]

Touch Awareness

This test determines perception of tactile touch input. A camel-hair brush, piece of cotton (ball or swab), or tissue is used. The area to be tested is lightly touched or stroked. Examination of finer gradations of light touch can be quantified using monofilaments (see later section titled Quantitative Sensory Testing and Specialized Testing Instruments).

Response

The patient is asked to indicate when he or she recognizes that a stimulus has been applied by responding "yes" or "now."

Note: A quantitative score for pain perception, temperature, and light touch awareness can be obtained by dividing the number of *correct responses* by the *number of stimuli* applied (normal response would be 100%).[81] Also, inability to verbally communicate does not necessary preclude obtaining accurate data. For example, having the patient hold up one or two fingers might be used for dichotomous responses (yes/no; hot/cold). Other options might include nodding the head, pointing to index cards containing printed responses; or using hand gestures to indicate recognition of a stimulus.

Pressure Perception

The therapist's fingertip or a double-tipped cotton swab is used to apply a firm pressure on the skin surface. This pressure should be firm enough to indent the skin and to stimulate the deep receptors. This test can also be administered using the thumb and fingers to squeeze the Achilles tendon.[77]

Response

The patient is asked to indicate when an applied stimulus is recognized by responding "yes" or "now."

Deep Sensations

The deep sensations include **kinesthesia**, **proprioception**, and **vibration**. Kinesthesia is the awareness of movement. Proprioception includes position sense and the awareness of joints at rest. Vibration refers to the ability to perceive rapidly oscillating or vibratory stimuli. Although these sensations are closely related, they are examined individually.

Kinesthesia Awareness

This test examines *awareness of movement*. The extremity or joint(s) is moved passively through a relatively small range of motion (ROM). Small increments in ROM are used as joint receptors fire at specific points throughout the range. The therapist should identify the range of movement being examined (e.g., initial, mid-, or terminal range). As discussed, a trial run or demonstration of the procedure should be performed prior to actual testing. This will ensure that the patient and the therapist agree on terms to describe the direction of movements.

Response

The patient is asked to describe verbally the direction (up, down, in, out, and so forth) and range of movement in terms previously discussed with the therapist while the extremity is *in motion*. The patient may also respond by simultaneously duplicating the movement with the contralateral extremity. This second approach, however, is impractical with proximal lower extremity joints, owing to potential stress on the low back. During testing, movement of larger joints is usually discerned more quickly than that of smaller joints. The therapist's grip should remain constant and minimal (fingertip grip over bony prominences), to reduce tactile stimulation.

Proprioceptive Awareness

This test examines *joint position sense* and *the awareness of joints at rest*. The extremity or joint(s) is moved through a ROM and held in a static position. Again, small increments of range are used. The words selected to identify the range of movement examined should be identified to the patient during the practice trial (e.g., initial, mid-, or terminal range). As with kinesthesia, caution should be used with hand placements to avoid excessive tactile stimulation.

Response

While the extremity or joint(s) is held in a static position by the therapist, the patient is asked to describe the position verbally or to duplicate the position of the extremity or joint(s) with the contralateral extremity (position matching). This test may also be performed unilaterally using the same extremity or joint(s); first held in position by the examiner, then returned to resting position, followed by active duplication of position by patient using the same limb.

Clinical Note: Based on a series of position matching studies conducted in the Motor Control Laboratory at the University of Michigan, Goble[82] presents several important factors to assist clinicians in making informed decisions about proprioceptive matching test outcomes:

- For position matching tests, there are different memory influences and different interhemispheric communication requirements between use of the ipsilateral extremity (same arm positioned by examiner is used to actively replicate the joint angle[s]) versus contralateral limb (patient moves opposite extremity from that used by examiner).
- Likely owing to the enhanced role of the right hemisphere in proprioceptive feedback processing, the left arm appears to have an advantage in matching tasks.
- The magnitude of the reference joint angle (larger magnitudes associated with greater error) and how reference positions are established (fewer errors noted when active movement used to establish position versus passive movement by examiner) will influence performance.
- Proprioceptive acuity must be considered within the context of anticipated changes occurring over the lifespan or that are diagnosis specific (e.g., stroke).
- Task workspace (area in which activities of daily living are typically performed) appears to influence joint position matching performance. During position matching experiments, greater performance occurred to the left of body midline with the fewest errors in the far left of the workspace.

Vibration Perception

This test requires a tuning fork that vibrates at 128 Hz.[77] The ability to perceive a vibratory stimulus is tested by placing the base of a vibrating tuning fork on a bony prominence (such as the sternum, elbow, or ankle). The tuning fork base (the "handle" of the fork) is held between the examiner's thumb and index finger without making contact with the tines. The tines are then briskly hit against the open palm of the examiner's opposite hand to initiate the vibration. Care must be taken not to touch the tines, as this will stop the vibration. The base of the fork in then placed over a bony prominence. If vibration sensation is intact, the patient will perceive the vibration. If there is impairment, the patient will be unable to distinguish between a vibrating and non-vibrating tuning fork. Therefore, there should be a random application of vibrating and non-vibrating stimuli.

Auditory clues can pose a challenge in obtaining accurate test results. Typically it is easy to hear the sound of the tines making vigorous contact with the examiner's hand to initiate the vibration. If the sound is not heard, it provides an easy indicator to the patient that the next application will be non-vibrating. To minimize this effect, the vibration can be initiated for *every* stimulus application; however, when a non-vibrating stimulus is desired, brief contact of the therapist's fingers on the tines will stop the vibration prior to placement on the skin. This, though, does not solve the problem of the auditory cues generated during application of a vibrating stimulus. The best solution is use of sound occlusive earphones (the type worn by airport ground workers). Unfortunately, such earphones are seldom available in a clinic setting.

Response

The patient is asked to respond by verbally identifying or otherwise indicating if the stimulus is vibrating or non-vibrating each time the fork makes contact.

Combined Cortical Sensations
Stereognosis Perception

This test determines the ability to recognize the form of objects by touch (stereognosis). A variety of small, easily obtainable, and culturally familiar objects of differing size and shape are required (e.g., keys, coins, combs, safety pins, pencils, and so forth). A single object is placed in the hand, the patient manipulates the object, and then identifies the item verbally. The patient should be allowed to handle several sample test items during the explanation and demonstration of the procedure.

Response

The patient is asked to name the object verbally. For patients with speech impairments, sensory testing shields can be used (Fig. 3.12). Alternatively, the item manipulated can be identified from a group of images presented after each test.

Tactile Localization

This test determines the ability to localize touch sensation on the skin (topognosis). The patient is asked to identify the specific point of application of a touch stimulus (e.g., tip of ring finger, lateral malleus, and so forth) and not simply the perception of being touched. Tactile localization is typically not tested in isolation and frequently examined in combination with similar tests such as pressure perception or touch awareness. Using a cotton swab or fingertip, the therapist touches different skin surfaces. After each application of a stimulus the patient is given time to respond.

Response

The patient is asked to identify the location of the stimuli by pointing to the area or by verbal description. The patient's eyes may be open during the response component of this test. The distance between the application of the stimulus and the site indicated by the patient can be measured and recorded. Accuracy of localization over

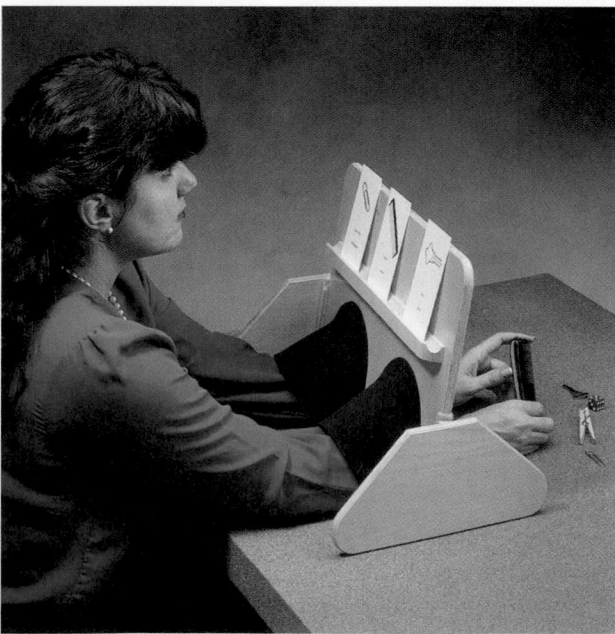

Figure 3.12 A sensory testing shield can be used for examining stereognosis in the presence of speech or language impairments. In this simulation, the subject manipulates the object without the use of visual input. Following manipulation, the subject points to the matching object pictured on the ledge of the testing shield. *(Courtesy of North Coast Medical, Inc., Morgan Hill, CA 95037.)*

various parts of the body may be compared to determine the relative sensitivity of different areas.

Two-Point Discrimination

This test determines the ability to perceive two points applied to the skin simultaneously. It is a measure of the smallest distance between two stimuli (applied simultaneously and with equal pressure) that can still be perceived as two distinct stimuli. Two-point discrimination values vary for different individuals and body parts. As this sensory function is most refined in the distal upper extremities, this is the typical site for testing. It is believed to contribute to precision grip movements and instrumental activities of daily living (IADL).[83]

Two-point discrimination is among the most practical and easily duplicated tests for cutaneous sensation. Some years ago, a series of classic two-point discrimination studies were conducted by Nolan.[84–86] The purpose of his research was to establish normative data on two-point discrimination for young adults. His sample consisted of 43 college students ranging in age from 20 to 24 years. Values from Nolan's studies for the upper and lower extremities as well as the face and trunk are presented in Appendix 3.A. The results from these studies should be used cautiously, inasmuch as they relate to a specific population. They should not be generalized for interpreting data from older or younger patients. Normative data for two-point discrimination have been documented by several authors including van Nes et al,[29] Kaneko et al,[62] and Vriens and van der Glas.[87]

As mentioned earlier, the aesthesiometer (see Fig. 3.9) and the circular two-point discriminator (see Fig. 3.10) are among the most common devices used for measurement. Two reshaped paper clips can also be used; however, this requires the assistance of a second examiner to measure the distance between the two points using a small ruler. During the test procedure the two tips of the instrument are applied to the skin simultaneously with tips spread apart. To increase the validity of the test, it is appropriate to alternate the application of two stimuli with the random application of only a single stimulus (the purpose of the third tip on some aesthesiometers). With each successive application, the two tips are gradually brought closer together until the stimuli are perceived as one. The smallest distance between the stimuli that is still perceived as two distinct points is measured.

Response

The patient is asked to identify the perception of "one" or "two" stimuli.

Double Simultaneous Stimulation

This test determines the ability to perceive simultaneous touch stimuli (double simultaneous stimulation [DSS]). The therapist simultaneously (and with equal pressure) touches: (1) identical locations on opposite sides of the body, (2) proximally and distally on opposite sides of the body, and/or (3) proximal and distal locations on the same side of the body. The term *extinction phenomenon* is used to describe a situation in which only the proximal stimulus is perceived, with "extinction" of the distal.

Response

The patient verbally states when he or she perceives a touch stimulus and the number of stimuli felt.

Several additional tests for the combined (cortical) sensations include graphesthesia (traced finger identification), recognition of texture, and barognosis (recognition of weight). However, these tests are usually not performed if stereognosis and two-point discrimination are found to be intact.

Graphesthesia (Traced Figure Identification)

This test determines the ability to recognize letters, numbers, or designs "written" on the skin. Using a fingertip or the eraser end of a pencil, a series of letters, numbers, or shapes is traced on the palm of the patient's hand. During the practice trial, agreement should be reached about the orientation of the tracings. (For example, the bottom of the traced figures will always be oriented toward the base of the patient's hand [wrist].) Between each separate drawing the palm should be gently wiped with a soft cloth to clearly indicate a change in figures to the patient. This test is also a useful substitute for stereognosis when paralysis prevents grasping an object.

Response

The patient is asked to identify verbally the figures drawn on the skin. For patients with speech or language impairments, the figures can be selected (pointed to) from a series of line drawings.

Recognition of Texture

This test determines the ability to differentiate among various textures. Suitable textures may include cotton, wool, burlap, or silk. The items are placed individually in the patient's hand. The patient is allowed to manipulate the sample texture.

Response

The patient is asked to identify the individual textures as they are placed in the hand. They may be identified by name (e.g., silk, cotton) or by texture (e.g., rough, smooth).

Barognosis (Recognition of Weight)

This test determines the ability to recognize different weights. A set of discrimination weights consisting of small objects of the same size and shape but of graduated weight is used (Fig. 3.13). The therapist may choose to place a series of different weights in the same hand one at a time, place a different weight in each hand

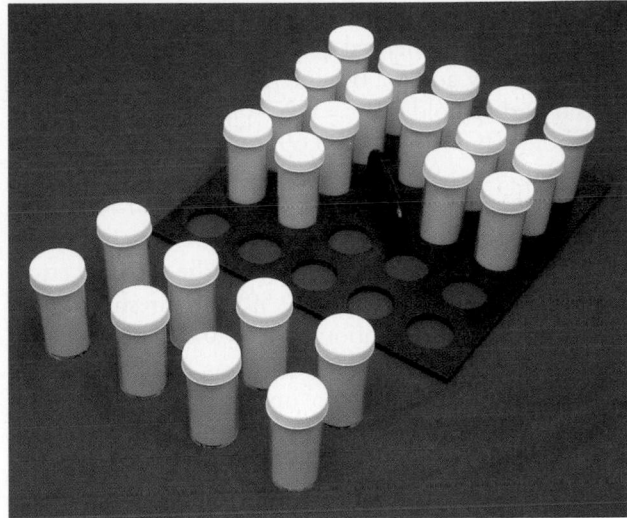

Figure 3.13 Discrimination weights are identical in size, shape, and texture. The only distinguishing feature is their variation in weight. *(Courtesy of Lafayette Instruments, Lafayette, IN 47903.)*

simultaneously, or ask the patient to use a fingertip grip to pick up each weight.

Response

The patient is asked to identify the comparative weight of objects in a series (i.e., to compare the relative weight of the object with the previous one); or when the objects are placed (or picked up) in both hands simultaneously the patient is asked to compare the weight of the two objects. The patient responds by indicating that the object is "heavier" or "lighter."

Clinical Note: Impaired sensation is a contraindication to or precaution for use of some physical agents because the end range of intensity or duration is frequently associated with the patient's subjective report of how the intervention feels (i.e., patient tolerance).

■ RELIABILITY

Reliability is an important parameter of any test or measure. However, few systematic reports addressing the reliability of traditional sensory tests appear in the literature. This is likely due to the inability to accurately quantify test results. In an important early reliability study by Kent[88] the upper limbs of 50 adult patients with hemiplegia were tested for sensory and motor deficits. Three sensory tests were administered and then repeated by the same examiner within 1 to 7 days. Results revealed a high reliability for both stereognosis ($r = 0.97$) and position sense ($r = 0.90$). A lower reliability was reported for two-point discrimination, with correlation coefficients ranging from 0.59 to 0.82, depending on the body area tested.

More recently, Moloney et al[89] examined the interrater reliability of thermal quantitative sensory testing in young healthy adults. The interrater reliability for cold detection threshold (ICC = 0.27–0.55), warm detection threshold (ICC = 0.38–0.69), cold pain threshold (ICC = 0.88–0.94), and heat pain threshold (ICC = 0.52–0.86) ranged from poor to high. Juul-Kritensen et al[90] examined proprioception of the elbow in healthy subjects. The test-retest reliability (of the absolute error) of joint position sense (ICC = 0.59) and threshold to detection of a passive motion (ICC = 0.69) ranged from fair to good, respectively. Khamwong et al[91] examined the vibration sense of two upper extremity sites on healthy male volunteers. The test-retest reliability of vibration sense over the lateral epicondyle (ICC = 0.94) and belly of the carpi radialis brevis muscle (ICC = 0.93) was excellent. Byl et al[92] examined the reliability of a new test of stereognosis on patients with hand problems and controls and reported excellent interrater reliability (ICC = 0.99). Their new test also moderately correlated (r = 0.41–0.53) with other tests of stereognosis and graphesthesia. In a similar study, Rosen[93] examined the properties of a recently introduced test for the assessment of tactile gnosis (stereognosis). Good interrater reliability (kappa = 0.66) was reported using the test for patients with serve upper extremity nerve injuries.

Although limited published data are available related to reliability measures, several approaches can be used to improve this aspect of the tests, including (1) use of consistent guidelines for completing the tests; (2) administration of the tests by trained, skillful examiners; and (3) subsequent retests performed by the same individual. It also should be noted that the patient's understanding of the test procedure and the patient's ability to communicate results further influence the reliability of sensory tests. As developing advances in technology (see discussion below) provide tools for quantitative sensory testing, greater emphasis on reliability will follow. Additional research related to standardization of testing protocols and identification of normative data for various age groups will improve the overall reliability and interpretation of test results.

■ QUANTITATIVE SENSORY TESTING AND SPECIALIZED TESTING INSTRUMENTS

With the expanding availability of specialized testing systems and instruments, quantitative sensory testing (QST) has gained considerable clinical and research interest. This is clearly evident from the expanding body of literature on this topic.[94–104] QST allows quantification of the level of stimuli required for perception of a sensory modality. Although sufficient data are not available to predict the ultimate integration of QST instrumentation into clinical practice, preliminary information suggests its potential usefulness. This section provides a brief overview of selected QST devices and is certainly not all-inclusive. The Internet provides a rich source of information on this developing technology and instrumentation.

TSA-II Thermal Sensory Analyzer + VSA 3000 (Medoc, Ltd., Durham, NC)

This computer-controlled system (Fig. 3.14) is capable of generating and recording a response to repeatable vibratory and thermal stimuli (i.e., warmth, cold, heat- or cold-induced pain). For testing thermal sensation, a "thermode" capable of heating or cooling is placed on the patient's skin (Fig. 3.15). The patient is asked to respond to the stimulus by pushing a response button. A sensory threshold is recorded and a computer comparison to age-matched normative data is generated. The system includes hand and foot (Fig. 3.16) support vibratory stimulators as well as a handheld vibrating device (see Fig 3.14). A variety of report formats can be generated; a sample is presented in Figure 3.17. Several examples of clinical applications include neuropathies (e.g., diabetic, metabolic, cancer), compression injuries, and pharmacological trials.

von Frey Aesthesiometer (Somedic Sales AB, Hörby, Sweden)

Monofilaments are not new to examination of sensory function and are actually considered a classic tool

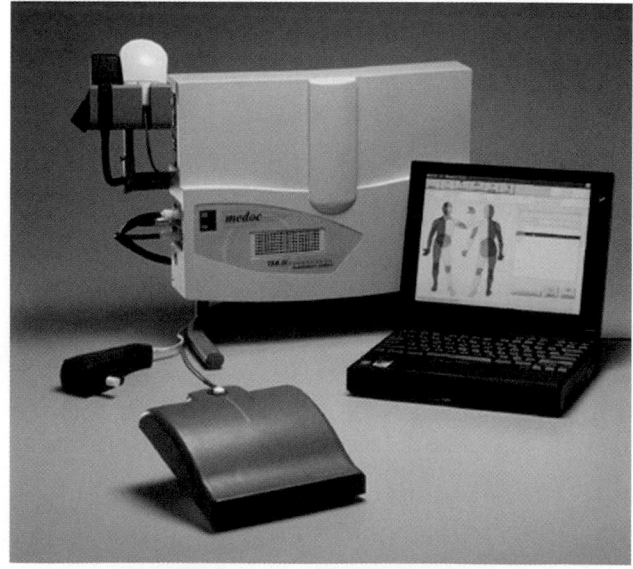

Figure 3.14 TSA-II Thermal Sensory Analyzer + VSA 3000. This system provides quantitative measures of both thermal and vibratory stimuli using a variety of patient interfaces. Note the small handheld vibratory device on the far left. (*Courtesy of Medoc, Ltd., Durham, NC 27707.*)

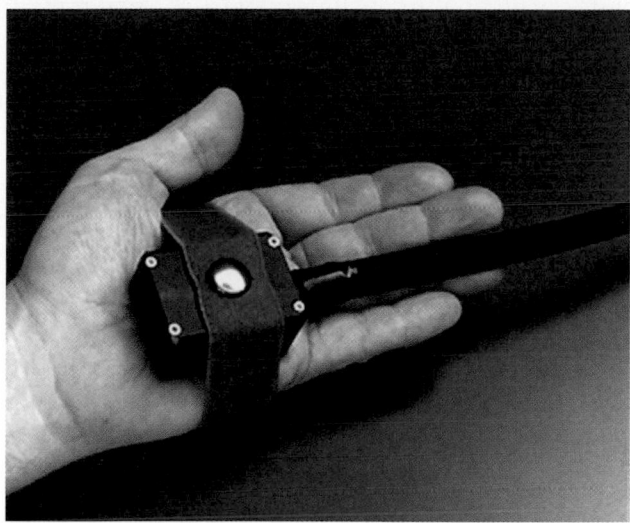

Figure 3.15 Thermode placed in hand for measuring perception of thermal stimuli. *(Courtesy of Medoc, Ltd., Durham, NC 27707.)*

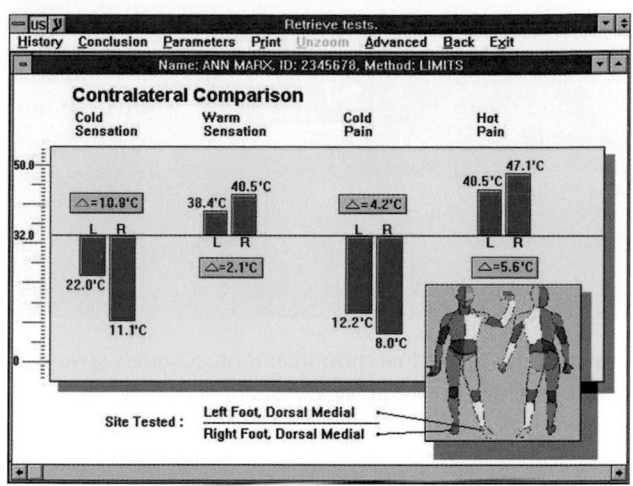

Figure 3.17 Computer-generated data from thermal testing that presents a comparison between the two sides of the body. Note the data for the right foot presents consistently higher threshold values than that of the left. Values are generated for each foot as well as the total difference between the feet. All values are in Celsius. Conversions for the temperature scale on the left border are 32°C = 89.6°F and 50°C = 122°F. *(Courtesy of Medoc, Ltd., Durham, NC 27707.)*

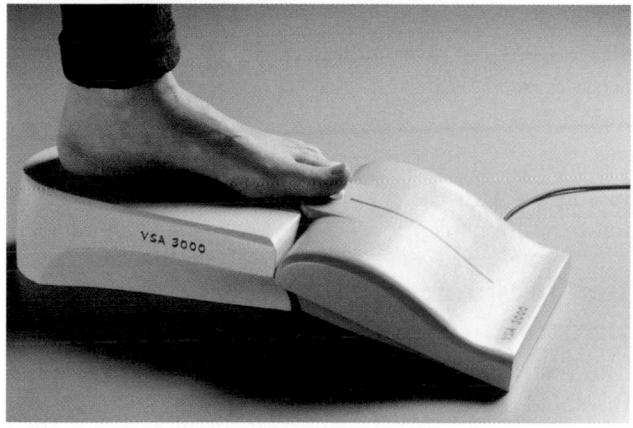

Figure 3.16 Foot support vibratory stimulator. *(Courtesy of Medoc, Ltd., Durham, NC 27707.)*

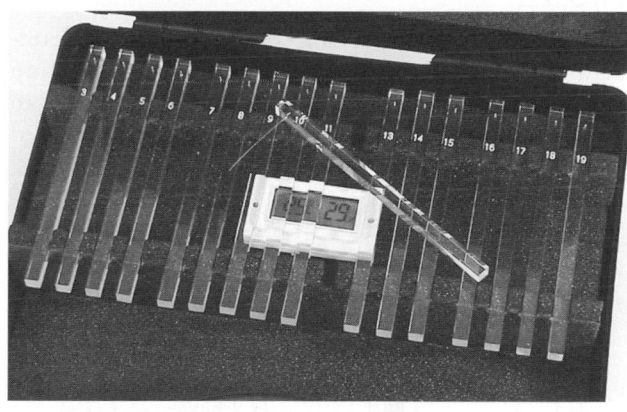

Figure 3.18 von Frey aesthesiometer. This set contains 17 monofilaments mounted on Plexiglas handles. *(Courtesy of Somedic Sales AB, Hörby, Sweden.)*

for measuring touch-evoked potentials (Fig. 3.18). They are designed to detect very small changes in touch threshold. The filaments are available as sets, in various sizes (i.e., thicknesses), with each mounted on a handle. The force required for bending the monofilament increases from 0.026 g for the first handle to 100 g for the last (pressure range of between 5 g/mm² and 178 g/mm²). The filaments are applied individually to the patient's skin until it bends; each filament providing a specific amount of force (thicker filaments are used if the thinner are not perceived). With vision occluded, the patient responds "yes" when a stimulus is felt. The filaments are held perpendicular to the skin and application is usually repeated three times at each testing site.[81] Monofilaments are frequently used in hand rehabilitation clinics; other examples of clinical applications include neuropathies (e.g., diabetic) and peripheral nerve injuries.

Touch-Test Sensory Evaluator (North Coast Medical, Inc., Morgan Hill, CA)

Individual monofilaments are also available in increments ranging from 0.008 to 300 g (Fig. 3.19). These instruments are convenient and can be carried in a pocket. The handle opens to a 90° angle for testing; when folded it protects the monofilament when not in use.

Rydel-Seiffer 64/128 Hz Graduated Tuning Fork (US Neurologicals, Kirkland, WA)

This quantitative tuning fork contains small scaled weights on the distal ends of the two prongs converting

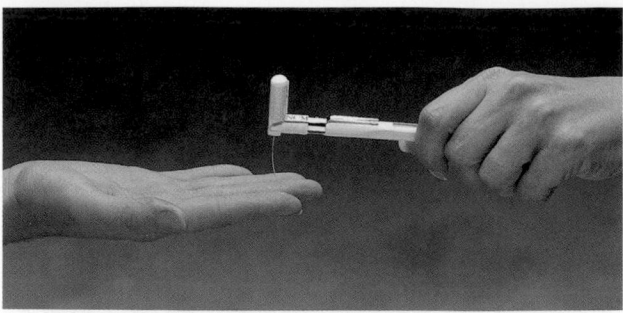

Figure 3.19 Individual monofilament. *(Courtesy of North Coast Medical, Inc., Morgan Hill, CA 95037.)*

it from 128 to 64 Hz (Fig. 3.20). The two triangles move closer together and their intersection moves upward as the intensity of vibration decreases. The intensity where the patient no longer perceives the vibration is recorded as the number adjacent to the intersection of the triangles. This instrument allows more sensitive and specific testing for detecting sensory changes as compared to qualitative tuning forks and has demonstrated high intertester and intratester reliability.[105]

Rolltemp (Somedic Sales AB, Hörby, Sweden)

This instrument is used as a screening tool for determining changes in perception of thermal sensation (Fig. 3.21). The rollers are housed in a storage unit to maintain temperature. The individual rollers are placed

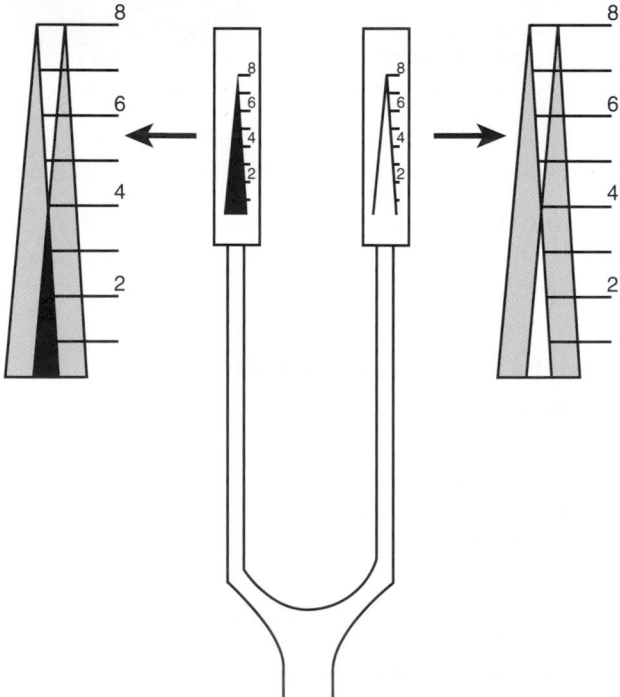

Figure 3.20 Schematic illustration of the Rydel-Seiffer tuning fork. *(Courtesy of US Neurologicals, Kirkland, WA, 98033.)*

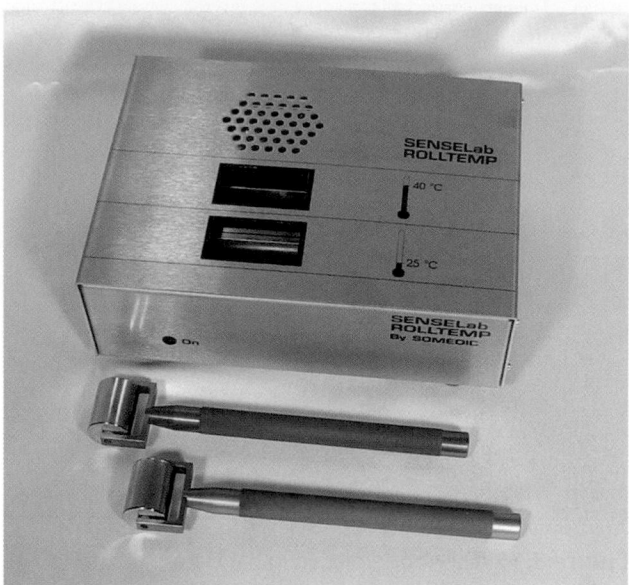

Figure 3.21 The Rolltemp provides a quick screening tool for thermal sensation. The rollers are mounted on handles and stored upright in the two square insertion points on the storage unit. One roller is maintained at 40°C (104°F); the other at 25°C (77°F). *(Courtesy of Somedic Sales AB, Hörby, Sweden.)*

in contact with the skin to provide a gross estimate of temperature perception.

Bio-Thesiometer (Bio-Medical Instrument Co, Newbury, OH)

This instrument is designed to quantitatively measure threshold perception of a vibratory stimulus (Fig. 3.22). The stimulus is applied using a handheld device applied to the skin. Intensity of stimulation can be preset or gradually increased until the threshold is reached (or gradually lowered until no longer felt).

Vibrameter (Somedic Sales AB, Hörby, Sweden)

The Vibrameter also quantitatively measures the perception of vibration (Fig 3.23). Standardized test points have been identified for use with this instrument. The test points (e.g., dorsum of the metacarpal bone of index finger, first metatarsal, and on tibia) allow for ease of comparison and interpretation of results. The sites also represent relatively long neural pathways for transmission to the CNS. Stimulus is applied using the handheld device.

SENSEBox (Somedic Sales AB, Hörby, Sweden)

This instrument measures pain thresholds (**algometer**) and touch evoked potentials (von Frey transducer). It determines the relationship between the intensity of controlled mechanical stimuli and patient response.

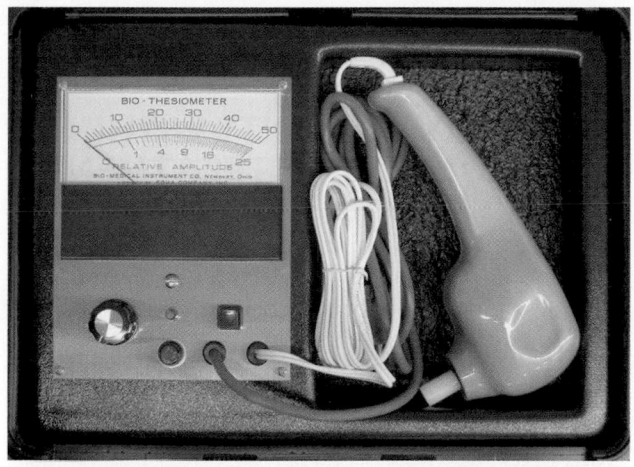

Figure 3.22 Bio-Thesiometer for measuring perception of vibratory stimulus. *(Courtesy of Bio-Medical Instrument Co., Newbury, OH, 44065.)*

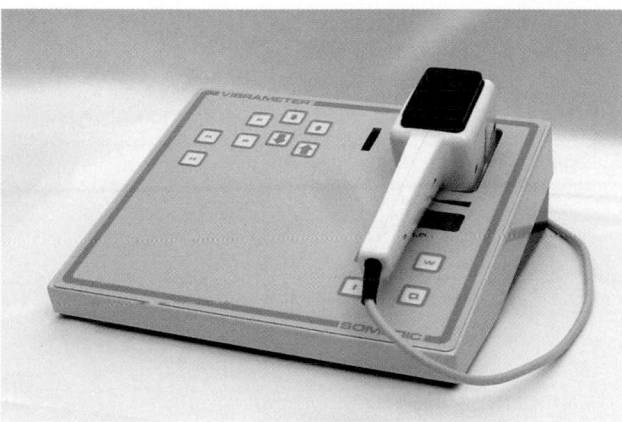

Figure 3.23 Vibrameter for measuring perception of vibratory stimulus *(Courtesy of Somedic Sales AB, Hörby, Sweden.)*

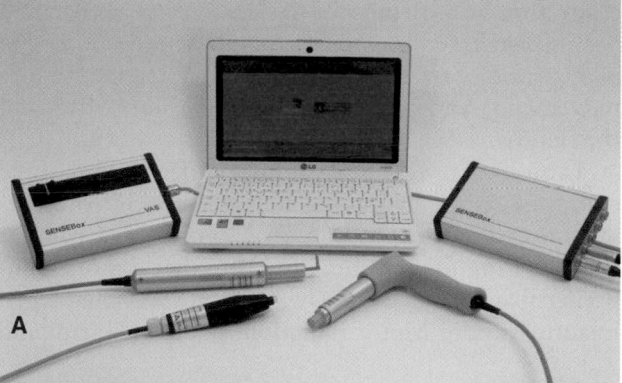

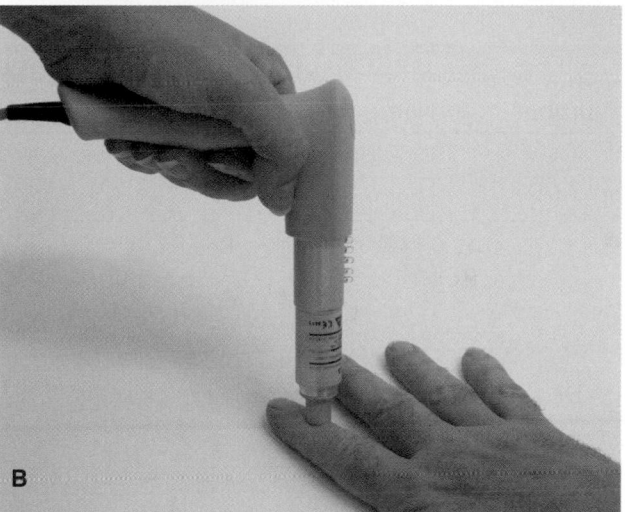

Figure 3.24 (A) SENSEBox. Viewing counterclockwise, to the left of computer is the electronic patient response visual analog scale (VAS), von Frey transducer for touch evoked potentials, pushbutton patient response device, algometer transducer for measuring sensitivity to pain, and data collection unit. **(B)** Algometer transducer for SENSEBox. *(Courtesy of Somedic Sales AB, Hörby, Sweden.)*

Handheld transducers are used to apply the stimuli (Fig. 3.24A and B). Patient responses are recorded using a handheld pushbutton device or a continuous electronic visual analog scale (VAS). During examination, data are automatically stored in a computer database.

MSA (Modular Sensory Analyzer) Thermotest (Somedic Sales AB, Hörby, Sweden)

The MSA Thermotest (Fig. 3.25) measures response to thermal (warm and cold) stimuli. Thermodes of different sizes allow testing of various anatomical locations. A computer interfaces using SenseLab software that sets up and runs the Thermotest, and allows for analysis and storage of data. Temperatures range from 41° to 125.6°F (5° to 52°C).

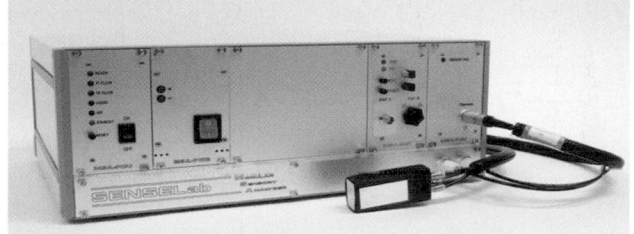

Figure 3.25 MSA Thermotest. In the right foreground is a 1 × 2 inch (25 × 50 mm) standard thermode for application of thermal stimuli.

■ CRANIAL NERVE SCREENING

Screening tests for the cranial nerves provide information about location of dysfunction within the brainstem as well as identification of cranial nerves that require more detailed examination. Data generated may include function of muscles innervated by the cranial nerves; visual, auditory, sensory, and gag reflex integrity; perception of taste; swallowing characteristics; eye movements; and constriction and dilation patterns of the pupils.

Table 3.3 provides a summary of the functional components of the cranial nerves. Box 3.5 presents screening tests for each cranial nerve. Impairments noted during the screening indicate that a more comprehensive examination is warranted. See Chapter 5, Examination of Motor Function: Motor Control and

Motor Learning, for additional information on cranial nerve examination.

■ SENSORY INTEGRITY WITHIN THE CONTEXT OF TREATMENT

Learning a motor behavior is dependent on the patient's ability to take in sensory information from the body and the environment (sensory intake), process it (sensory integration), and use it to plan and organize behavior (output). When patients experience impairment in processing

Table 3.3	Functional Components of the Cranial Nerves		
Number	**Name**	**Components**	**Function**
I	Olfactory	Afferent	Olfaction (smell)
II	Optic	Afferent	Vision
III	Oculomotor	Efferent	
		Somatic	Elevates eyelid
			Turns eye up, down, in
		Visceral	Constricts pupil
			Accommodates lens
IV	Trochlear	Efferent (somatic)	Turns the adducted eye down and causes intorsion (inward rotation) of eye
V	Trigeminal	Mixed	
		Afferent	Sensation from face
			Sensation from cornea
			Sensation from anterior tongue
		Efferent	Muscles of mastication
			Dampens sound (lensor tympani)
VI	Abducens	Efferent (somatic)	Turns eye out
VII	Facial	Mixed	
		Afferent	Taste from anterior tongue
		Efferent (somatic)	Muscles of facial expression
			Dampens sound (stapedius)
		Efferent (visceral)	Tearing (lacrimal gland)
			Salivation (submandibular and sublingual glands)
VIII	Vestibulocochlear	Afferent	Balance (semicircular canals, utricle, saccule)
			Hearing (organ of Corti)
IX	Glossopharyngeal	Mixed	
		Afferent	Taste from posterior tongue
			Sensation from posterior tongue
			Sensation from oropharynx
		Efferent	Salivation (parotid gland)
X	Vagus	Mixed	
		Afferent	Thoracic and abdominal viscera
		Efferent	Muscles of larynx and pharynx
			Decreases heart rate
			Increases GI motility
XI	Spinal accessory	Efferent	Head movements (sternocleidomastoid and trapezius)
XII	Hypoglossal	Efferent	Tongue movements and shape

From Nolan[63,p. 44] with permission. GI, gastrointestinal.

Box 3.5   Screening Tests for Cranial Nerves[9,63]

Cranial nerve I: Examine olfactory acuity using non-noxious odors such as lemon oil, coffee, cloves or tobacco.

Cranial nerve II: Examine visual acuity using a Snellen chart; both central and peripheral vision is tested.

Cranial nerves III, IV, and VI: Determine equality and size of pupils; reaction to light; presence of strabismus (loss of ocular alignment); ability of eyes to follow a moving target without head movement; presence of ptosis of eyelid.

Cranial nerve V: Sensory tests of face (sharp/dull discrimination, light touch); open and close jaw against resistance; jaw jerk reflex.

Cranial nerve VII: Examine any asymmetry of face at rest and during voluntary contraction.

Cranial nerve VIII: Test auditory acuity using a vibrating tuning fork (Weber test) placed on vertex of skull or forehead, patient indicates on which side the tone is louder; rub fingers together at a distance and gradually bring toward patient, note distance when first heard; alter volume of conversation; Rinne test (conductive hearing loss) vibrating tuning fork placed on mastoid process, then near external ear canal, note hearing acuity.

Cranial nerve IX: Examine taste on posterior one-third of tongue; examine gag reflex.

Cranial nerve X: Examine swallowing; observe uvula and soft palate for any asymmetry (tongue depressor).

Cranial nerve XI: Examine strength of the sternocleidomastoid and trapezius muscles.

Cranial nerve XII: With tongue protruded, examine ability to move tongue rapidly from side to side.

---

sensory intake, deficits typically occur in planning and organizing behavior. This produces behaviors that may interfere with successful motor learning and motor function.

The POC designed for a patient with impaired sensation is typically guided by one of two approaches, the *Sensory Integration Approach* and the *Compensatory-Approach*. The selection of a treatment model is based on a complete data set of information from all examinations together with the established prognosis and diagnosis. The treatment approach depicted in Figure 3.26 is based largely on the Sensory Integration Model developed by Ayers.[1,106–110] The basic premise of this approach is that specific treatment techniques can enhance sensory integration (CNS processing) with a resultant change in motor performance.

Using the Sensory Integration Approach, data obtained from the examination of sensory function informs development of a POC to enhance opportunities for *controlled* sensory intake within a framework of meaningful functional skills. During treatment, the patient is provided guided practice in planning and organizing motor behaviors using both *intrinsic* feedback (from the movement itself) and *augmented* feedback (cues planned by the therapist). This approach is designed to improve the ability of the CNS to process and integrate information and promote motor learning. The reader is referred to the work of Ayers[1,106–110] and Bundy and Murray[5] for a detailed presentation of both the theory and practice of the Sensory Integration Model.

The Compensatory Approach is a more traditional intervention that focuses on patient education to accommodate to the limitations imposed by the sensory deficit. The therapist's role is to assist the patient in achieving optimum functional capacity, minimizing activity limitations, protecting anesthetic limbs, and creating appropriate environmental adaptations to enhance safety and function. Guided by this approach, the therapist instructs the patient in practical strategies

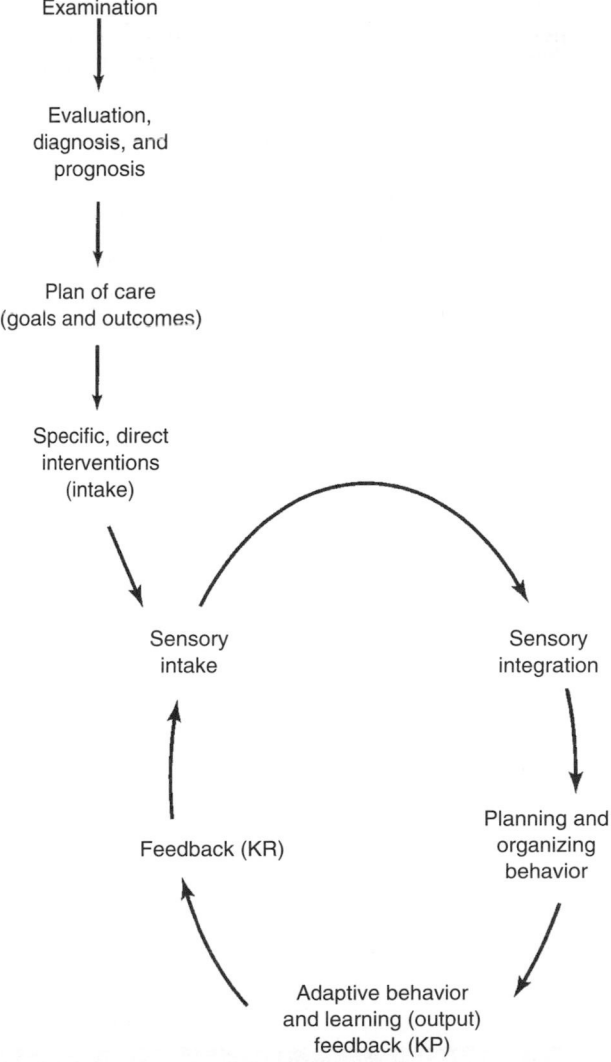

Figure 3.26 Elements of patient management for sensory impairment. KP refers to knowledge of performance (feedback about the quality of movement produced) and KR refers to knowledge of result (feedback about the end result or outcome of the movement). *(Adapted from Bundy and Murray.[5, p. 5])*

such as testing bath water with a thermometer or body part with intact sensation before entering; not going barefoot; regularly checking insensitive skin areas for cuts or bruises (particularly important for patients with diabetes); adaptations ("compensations" for the sensory loss) that can include substituting vision for absent tactile cues when carrying objects; wearing heat-resistant gloves when working in the kitchen; using a rolling cart in kitchen or other work space to transport items from one area to another; and arranging kitchen supplies to eliminate need for access to storage areas directly over the stove.

SUMMARY

Examination of sensory function provides important information about the integrity of the somatosensory system. Findings from the examination assist in making clinical judgments about diagnosis, prognosis, anticipated goals and expected outcomes, and establishing the POC. Periodic reexamination provides critical data on changes in patient status and in determining progress toward goals and outcomes. Individual tests for each sensory modality have been presented. Reliability of these test procedures can be improved by careful adherence to consistent guidelines, administration of tests by trained individuals, and subsequent retests performed by the same examiner. Documentation of test results should address the type(s) of sensation affected, the quantity, and degree of involvement, and localization of the exact boundaries of the sensory deficits. Finally, it should be emphasized that additional research related to sensory testing is warranted. Further development of QST techniques, standardized protocols, reliability measures, and additional normative data will significantly improve the clinical applications of data obtained from the examination of sensory function.

Questions for Review

1. Define a dermatome and describe a precaution with using published dermatome maps.

2. Identify six pathologies or health conditions that would warrant (or indicate the need for) examination of sensory function.

3. Describe the five terms used to document a patient's level of consciousness.

4. Which type of sensory receptor is responsible for position sense and awareness of joints at rest, during movement, and vibration? How would you comprehensively examine this sensory receptor?

5. Which type of muscle receptor senses tension and how does it affect the muscle when under extreme tension?

6. For a suspected localized lesion, in which direction would you conduct your examination of sensory function and why?

7. Describe four purposes of screening the sensory system.

8. Describe how the data from the examination of sensory function is used by the physical therapist.

9. Describe equipment (items) that can be used to assess stereognosis.

10. What type of findings from an examination of sensory function would indicate that a referral is warranted?

11. Explain why impaired sensation is a contraindication to or precaution for use of some physical agents.

12. What information would you provide to the patient prior to administration of sensory tests to obtain informed consent?

13. Which muscles would you test to assess the spinal accessory cranial nerve?

14. Describe the variables you would use to record the results of sensory testing.

CASE STUDY

A 68-year-old woman presents for outpatient physical therapy with an improperly fitted cane. You escort her to the examination room while observing her gait pattern, which is characterized by a slower self-selected walking speed, wide base of support, and increased time spent in double limb support. She has a long-standing history of hypertension (15 years), hypercholesterolemia (10 years), and diabetes (25 years). In addition to reporting several falls in the past 6 months, none of which resulted in injury serious enough to be hospitalized, the patient describes increasing pain in her lower extremities that is deep, sharp, and burning, that is symmetrical, and occasionally wakes her up at night. The patient lives alone in a one-bedroom apartment in a building with an elevator and level entrance to the lobby.

GUIDING QUESTIONS

1. Of all the senses, which one is most often affected by the patient's medical conditions and how would you assess it?

2. Given her history of falls, which sensory systems should you examine? Why? How?

3. How would you examine pain sensation and what findings would you expect given the long-standing history of diabetes? Why is it important to examine pain sensation?

4. How would you quantitatively measure touch awareness (touch-evoked potentials) in this patient?

5. The test findings indicate mild loss of proprioception and vibration in the lower extremities (distal more than proximal). What receptors are responsible for these sensory modalities? Where are the receptors located? Identify the ascending pathway that mediates proprioception and vibration.

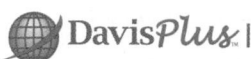 DavisPlus | For additional resources, including answers to the questions for review and case study guiding questions, please visit **http://davisplus.fadavis.com**

References

1. Ayers, JA: Sensory Integration and Learning Disorders. Western Psychological Services, Los Angeles, 1972.
2. Byl, NN: Multisensory control of upper extremity function. Neurology Report (now JNPT) 26(1):32, 2002.
3. Ghez, C, and Krakauer, J: The organization of movement. In Kandel, ER, Schwartz, JH, and Jessell, TM: Principles of Neural Science, ed 4. McGraw-Hill, New York, 2000, p 653.
4. Ayers, AJ: Sensory Integration and Praxis Tests (SIPT Manual). Western Psychological Services, Los Angeles, 1989.
5. Bundy, AC, and Murray, EA: Sensory integration: A. Jean Ayres' theory revisited. In Bundy, AC, Lane, SJ, and Murray, EA: Sensory Integration: Theory and Practice, ed 2. FA Davis, Philadelphia, 2002, p 3.
6. Cooper, C, and Canyock, JD: Evaluation of sensation and intervention for sensory dysfunction. In Pendleton, HM, and Schultz-Krohn, W (eds): Pedretti's Occupational Therapy: Practice Skills for Physical Dysfunction, ed 7. Elsevier/Mosby, St. Louis, 2013, p 575.
7. American Physical Therapy Association (APTA): Guide to Physical Therapist Practice, ed 2. APTA, Alexandria, Virginia, 2001.
8. Greenberg, DA, Aminoff, MJ, and Simon, RP: Clinical Neurology, ed 5. Lange Medical Books/McGraw-Hill, New York, 2002.
9. Gilman, S, and Newman, SW: Manter and Gatz's Essentials of Clinical Neuroanatomy and Neurophysiology, ed 10. FA Davis, Philadelphia, 2003.
10. Downs, MB, and Laporte C: Conflicting dermatome maps: Educational and clinical implications. J Orthop Sports Phys Ther 41(6):427, 2011.
11. Tochihara, Y, et al: Age-related differences in cutaneous warm sensation thresholds of human males in thermoneutral and cool environments. J Therm Biol 36(2):105, 2011.
12. Deshpande, N, et al: Association of lower limb cutaneous sensitivity with gait speed in the elderly: The Health ABC Study. Am J Phys Med Rehabil 87(11):921, 2008.
13. Adamo, DE, Martin, BJ, and Brown, SH: Age-related differences in upper limb proprioceptive acuity. Percept Mot Skills 104 (3 Part 2):1297, 2007.
14. Callisaya, ML, et al: A population-based study of sensorimotor factors affecting gait in older people. Age Ageing 38(3):290, 2009.
15. Dickin, DC, Brown, LA, and Doan, JB: Age-dependent differences in the time course of postural control during sensory perturbations. Aging Clin Exp Res 18(2):94, 2006.

16. Voelcker-Rehage, C, and Godde, B: High frequency sensory stimulation improves tactile but not motor performance in older adults. Motor Control 14(4):460, 2010.
17. Sosnoff, JJ, and Voudrie, SJ: Practice and age-related loss of adaptability in sensorimotor performance. J Mot Behav 41(2): 137, 2009.
18. Saunders, G, and Echt, K: Dual sensory impairment in an aging population. ASHA Leader 16(3):5, 2011.
19. Hondzinski, JM, Li, L, and Welsch, M: Age-related and sensory declines offer insight to whole body control during a goal-directed movement. Motor Control 14(2):176, 2010.
20. Kim, S, Nussbaum, MA, and Madigan, ML: Direct parameterization of postural stability during quiet upright stance: Effects of age and altered sensory conditions. J Biomech 41(2):406, 2008.
21. Cressman, EK, Salomonczyk, D, and Henriques, DY: Visuomotor adaptation and proprioceptive recalibration in older adults. Exp Brain Res 205(4):533, 2010.
22. Strotmeyer, ES, et al: Sensory and motor peripheral nerve function and lower-extremity quadriceps strength: The Health, Aging and Body Composition Study. J Am Geriatr Soc 57(11):2004, 2009.
23. Schumm, LP, et al: Assessment of sensory function in the National Social Life, Health, and Aging Project. J Gerontol B Psychol Sci Soc Sci 64B(Suppl 1):i76, 2009.
24. Illing, S, et al: Sensory system function and postural stability in men aged 30–80 years. Aging Male 13(3):202, 2010.
25. Webber, SC, Porter, MM, and Gardiner, PF: Modeling age-related neuromuscular changes in humans. Appl Physiol Nutr Metab 34(4):732, 2009.
26. Redfern, MS, et al: Perceptual inhibition is associated with sensory integration in standing postural control among older adults. J Gerontol B Psychol Sci Soc Sci 64B(5):569, 2009.
27. Mahoney, JR, et al: Multisensory integration across the senses in young and old adults. Brain Res 2(1426):43, 2011.
28. Shaffer, SW, and Harrison, AL: Aging of the somatosensory system: A translational perspective. Phys Ther 87(2):193, 2007.
29. van Nes, SI, et al: Revising two-point discrimination assessment in normal aging and in patients with polyneuropathies. J Neurol Neurosurg Psychiatry 79(7):832, 2008.
30. Cacchione, PZ: Sensory changes and aging. Insight 35(2):24, 2010.
31. Wright, ML, Adamo, DE, and Brown SH: Age-related declines in the detection of passive wrist movement. Neurosci Lett 500(2): 108, 2011.

32. Davila, EP, et al: Sensory impairment among older US workers. Am J Public Health 99(8):1378, 2009.
33. Laurienti, PJ, et al: Enhanced multisensory integration in older adults. Neurobiol Aging 27(8):1155, 2006.
34. Callisaya, ML, et al: Sensorimotor factors affecting gait variability in older people—a population-based study. J Gerontol A Biol Sci Med Sci 65(4):386, 2010.
35. US Department of Health and Human Services, Office of Disease Prevention and Health Promotion: Healthy People 2020. Washington, DC. Retrieved April 5, 2012, from www.healthy people.gov/2020/default.aspx.
36. Schulte, OJ, Stephens, J, and Joyce, A: Brain function, aging, and dementia. In Umphred, DA (ed): Neurological Rehabilitation, ed 5. Mosby/Elsevier, St. Louis, 2007, p 902.
37. Hooper, CD, and Dal Bello-Haas, V: Sensory function. In Bonder, BR, and Dal Bello-Haas, V: Functional Performance in Older Adults, ed 3. FA Davis, Philadelphia, 2009, p 101.
38. Shumway-Cook, A, and Woollacott, MH: Translating Research into Clinical Practice, ed 4. Wolters Kluwer/Lippincott Williams & Wilkins, Philadelphia, 2012.
39. Elfervig, LS, and Gallman, RL: The aging sensory system. In Stanley, M, Blair, KA, and Beare, PG: Gerontological Nursing: Promoting Successful Aging with Older Adults, ed 3. FA Davis, Philadelphia, 2005, p 121.
40. Peters, A: The effects of normal aging on myelin and nerve fibers: A review. J Neurocytol 31:581, 2002.
41. Ropper, AH, and Samuels, MA: Adams and Victor's Principles of Neurology, ed 9. McGraw-Hill, New York, 2009.
42. Gould, BE, and Dyer, RM: Pathophysiology for the Health Related Professions, ed 4. Saunders/Elsevier, Philadelphia, 2011.
43. Price, DL: Aging of the brain and dementia of the Alzheimer type. In Kandel, ER, Schwartz, JH, and Jessell, TM: Principles of Neural Science, ed 4. McGraw-Hill, New York, 2000, p 1149.
44. Shankar, SK: Biology of aging brain. Indian J Pathol Microbiol 53(4):595, 2010.
45. Lewis, CB, and Bottomley, JM: Geriatric Physical Therapy: A Clinical Approach, ed 3. Pearson Education, Upper Saddle River, NJ, 2008.
46. Bouche, P, et al: Clinical and electrophysiological study of the peripheral nervous system in the elderly. J Neurol 240(5):263, 1993.
47. Taylor, PK: Nonlineal effects of age on nerve conduction in adults. J Neurol Sci 66:223, 1984.
48. Fuller, KS: Introduction to central nervous system disorders. In Goodman, CC, and Fuller, KS: Pathology: Implications for the Physical Therapist. Saunders/Elsevier, St. Louis, 2009, p 1319.
49. Onofri, M, et al: Age-related changes in evoked potentials. Neurophysiol Clin 31(2):83, 2001.
50. Matsuoka, S, et al: Quantitative and qualitative studies of Meissner's corpuscles in human skin, with special reference to alterations caused by aging. J Dermatol 10(3):205, 1983.
51. Stuart M, et al: Effects of aging on vibration detection thresholds at various body regions. BMC Geriatr 3:1, 2003.
52. Bartzokis, G, et al: Lifespan trajectory of myelin integrity and maximum motor speed. Neurobiol Aging 31(9):1554, 2010.
53. Lascelles, RG, and Thomas, PK: Changes due to age in internodal length in the sural nerve of man. J Neurol Neurosurg Psychiatry 29:40, 1966.
54. Verdu, E, et al: Influence of aging on peripheral nerve function and regeneration. J Peripher Nerv Syst 5(4):191, 2000.
55. Dorfman, LJ, and Bosley, TM: Age-related changes in peripheral and central nerve conduction in man. Neurology 29(1):38, 1979.
56. Pedalini, MEB, et al: Sensory organization test in elderly patients with and without vestibular dysfunction. Acta Otolaryngol 129(9):962, 2009.
57. Bohannon, RW: Single limb stance times: A descriptive meta-analysis of data from individuals at least 60 years of age. Top Geriatr Rehabil 22(1):70, 2006.
58. Menz, HB, Morris, ME, and Lord SR: Foot and ankle characteristics associated with impaired balance and functional ability in older people. J Gerontol A Biol Sci Med Sci 60A(12):1546, 2005.
59. Menz, HB, Morris, ME, and Lord, SR: Foot and ankle risk factors for falls in older people: A prospective study. J Gerontol A Biol Sci Med Sci 61A(8):866, 2006.
60. Deshpande, N, et al: Physiological correlates of age-related decline in vibrotactile sensitivity. Neurobiol Aging 29(5):765, 2008.
61. Westlake, KP, and Culham, EG: Influence of testing position and age on measures of ankle proprioception. Adv Physiother 8(1):41, 2006.
62. Kaneko, A, Asai, N, and Kanda, T: The influence of age on pressure perception of static and moving two-point discrimination in normal subjects. J Hand Ther 18(4):421, 2005.
63. Nolan, MF: Introduction to the Neurologic Examination. FA Davis, Philadelphia, 1996.
64. Waxman, SG: Clinical Neuroanatomy, ed 26. New York, Lange Medical Books/McGraw-Hill, 2010.
65. Hall, JE: Guyton and Hall Textbook of Medical Physiology, ed 12. Saunders/Elsevier, Philadelphia, 2011.
66. Gardner, EP, and Martin, JH: Coding of sensory information. In Kandel, ER, Schwartz, JH, and Jessell, TM: Principles of Neural Science, ed 4. McGraw-Hill, New York, 2000, p 411.
67. Kiernan, JA: Barr's The Human Nervous System: An Anatomical Viewpoint, ed 9. Wolters Kluwer/Lippincott Williams & Wilkins, Philadelphia, 2009.
68. Schmidt, RA, and Lee, TD: Motor Control and Learning, ed 5. Human Kinetics, Champaign, IL, 2011.
69. Lundy-Ekman, L: Neuroscience: Fundamentals for Rehabilitation, ed 3. Saunders/Elsevier, Philadelphia, 2007.
70. Gardner, EP, Martin, JH, and Jessel, TM: The bodily senses. In Kandel, ER, Schwartz, JH, and Jessell, TM: Principles of Neural Science, ed 4, McGraw-Hill, New York, 2000, p 430.
71. Fitzgerald, MJT, Gruener, G, and Myui, E: Clinical Neuroanatomy and Neuroscience, ed 5. Elsevier/Saunders, Philadelphia, 2007.
72. O'Connor, A, and McCreesh, K: Function and dysfunction of joint. In Petty, NJ (ed): Principles of Neuromusculoskeletal Treatment and Management: A Guide for Therapists. Churchill Livingstone/Elsevier, New York, 2011, p 3.
73. Siegel, A, and Sapru, HN: Essential Neuroscience. Lippincott Williams & Wilkins, Philadelphia, 2006.
74. Bear, MF, Connors, BW, and Paradiso, MA: Neuroscience: Exploring the Brain, ed 3. Wolters Kluwer/Lippincott Williams & Wilkins, Philadelphia, 2007.
75. Gardner, EP, and Kandel, ER: Touch. In Kandel, ER, Schwartz, JH, and Jessell, TM (eds): Principles of Neural Science, ed 4. McGraw-Hill, New York, 2000, p 451.
76. Boissonnault, WG: Upper quarter screening examination. In Boissonnault, WG (ed): Primary Care for the Physical Therapist: Examination and Triage, ed 2. Elsevier/Saunders, Philadelphia, 2011, p 167.
77. Nolan, MF: Clinical assessment of cutaneous sensory function. Clin Manage Phys Ther 4:26, 1984.
78. Werner, JL, and Omer, GE: Evaluating cutaneous pressure sensation of the hand. Am J Occup Ther 24:347, 1970.
79. World Health Organization (WHO): Standard precautions in health care. WHO, Geneva, Switzerland, 2007. Retrieved April 9, 2012, from www.who.int/csr/resources/publications/EPR_AM2_E7.pdf.
80. World Health Organization (WHO): WHO Guidelines on Hand Hygiene in Health Care. WHO, Geneva, Switzerland, 2009. Retrieved April 9, 2012, from http://whqlibdoc.who.int/publications/2009/9789241597906_eng.pdf.
81. Bentzel, K: Assessing abilities and capacities: Sensation. In Vining Radomski, M, and Trombly Latham, CA (eds): Occupational Therapy for Physical Dysfunction, ed 6. Wolters Kluwer/Lippincott Williams & Wilkins, Philadelphia, 2008, p 212.
82. Goble, DJ: Proprioceptive acuity assessment via joint position matching: From basic science to general practice. Phys Ther 90(8):1176, 2010.
83. Gutman, SA, and Schonfeld, AB: Screening Adult Neurologic Populations: A Step-By-Step Instruction Manual, ed 2. AOTA Press, Bethesda, MD, 2009.
84. Nolan, MF: Limits of two-point discrimination ability in the lower limb in young adult men and women. Phys Ther 63:1424, 1983.
85. Nolan, MF: Quantitative measure of cutaneous sensation: Two-point discrimination values for the face and trunk. Phys Ther 65:181, 1985.
86. Nolan, MF: Two-point discrimination assessment in the upper limb in young adult men and women. Phys Ther 62:965, 1982.
87. Vriens, JP, and van der Glas, HW: Extension of normal values on sensory function for facial areas using clinical tests on touch and two-point discrimination. Int J Oral Maxillofac Surg 38(11):1154, 2009.

88. Kent, BE: Sensory-motor testing: The upper limb of adult patients with hemiplegia. J Am Phys Ther Assoc 45:550, 1965.
89. Moloney, NA, et al: Reliability of thermal quantitative sensory testing of the hand in a cohort of young, healthy adults. Muscle Nerve 44 :547, 2011.
90. Juul-Kristensen, B, et al: Test-retest reliability of joint position and kinesthetic sense in the elbow of healthy subjects. Physiother Theory Pract 24(1):65, 2008.
91. Khamwong, P, et al: Reliability of muscle function and sensory perception measurements of the wrist extensors. Physiother Theory Pract 26(6):408, 2010.
92. Byl, N, Leano, J, and Cheney, LK: The Byl-Cheney-Boczai Sensory Discriminator: Reliability, validity, and responsiveness for testing stereognosis. J Hand Ther 15(4):315, 2002.
93. Rosen, B: Inter-tester reliability of a tactile gnosis test: The STI-test. Hand Ther 8(3):98, 2003.
94. Backonja, MM, et al: Quantitative sensory testing in measurement of neuropathic pain phenomena and other sensory abnormalities. Clin J Pain 25(7): 641, 2009.
95. Blumenstiel, K, et al: Quantitative sensory testing profiles in chronic back pain are distinct from those in fibromyalgia. Clin J Pain 27(8): 682, 2011.
96. Courtney, CA, et al: Interpreting joint pain: Quantitative sensory testing in musculoskeletal management. J Orthop Sports Phys Ther 40(12):818, 2010.
97. Geletka, BJ, O'Hearn, MA, and Courtney, CA: Quantitative sensory testing changes in the successful management of chronic low back pain. J Manual Manipulative Ther 20(1):16, 2012.
98. Gröne, E, et al: Test order of quantitative sensory testing facilitates mechanical hyperalgesia in healthy volunteers. J Pain 13(1):73, 2012.
99. Heldestad, V, et al: Reproducibility and influence of test modality order on thermal perception and thermal pain thresholds in quantitative sensory testing. Clin Neurophysiol 121(11):1878, 2010.
100. Matos, R, et al: Quantitative sensory testing in the trigeminal region: Site and gender differences. J Orofacial Pain 25(2):161, 2011.
101. Said-Yekta, S, et al: Verification of nerve integrity after surgical intervention using quantitative sensory testing. J Oral Maxillofac Surg 70(2):263, 2012.
102. Tamburin, S, et al: Median nerve small- and large-fiber damage in carpal tunnel syndrome: A quantitative sensory testing study. J Pain 12(2): 205, 2011.
103. Walk, D, et al: Quantitative sensory testing and mapping: A review of nonautomated quantitative methods for examination of the patient with neuropathic pain. Clin J Pain 25(7):632, 2009.
104. Yekta, SS, et al: Assessment of trigeminal nerve functions by quantitative sensory testing in patients and healthy volunteers. J Oral Maxillofac Surg 68(10):2437, 2010.
105. Pestronk, A, et al: Sensory exam with a quantitative tuning fork: Rapid, sensitive and predictive of SNAP amplitude. Neurology 62(3):461, 2004.
106. Ayers, JA: Tactile functions: Their relation to hyperactive and perceptual motor behavior. Am J Occup Ther 18:83, 1964.
107. Ayers, JA: Interrelations among perceptual-motor abilities in a group of normal children. Am J Occup Ther 20:288, 1966.
108. Ayers, JA: Improving academic scores through sensory integration. J Learn Disabil 5:338, 1972.
109. Ayers, JA: Cluster analysis of measures of sensory integration. Am J Occup Ther 31:362, 1977.
110. Ayers, JA: Sensory Integration and the Child. Western Psychological Services, Los Angeles, 1979.

Supplemental Readings

Apok, V, et al: Dermatomes and dogma. Pract Neurol 11(2):100, 2011.
Boles, DB, and Givens, SM: Laterality and sex differences in tactile detection and two-point thresholds modified by body surface area and body fat ratio. Somatosens Mot Res 28(3-4):102, 2011.
Collins, S, et al: Reliability of the Semmes Weinstein Monofilaments to measure coetaneous sensibility in the feet of healthy subjects. Disabil Rehabil 32(24):2019, 2010.
Connell, LA, and Tyson, SF: Measures of sensation in neurological conditions: A systematic review. Clin Rehabil 26(1):68, 2012.
Di Pietro, F, and McAuley, JH: (Thermal) Quantitative Sensory Testing—tQST. J Physiother 57(1):58, 2011.
Drago, V, et al: Graphesthesia: A test of graphemic movement representations or tactile imagery? J Int Neuropsychol Soc 16(1):190, 2010.
Feng, Y, Schlosser, FJ, and Sumpio, BE: The Semmes Weinstein monofilament examination is a significant predictor of the risk of foot ulceration and amputation in patients with diabetes mellitus. J Vasc Surg 53(1):220, 2011.
Gahdhi, MS: Progress in vibrotactile threshold evaluation techniques: A review. J Hand Ther 24(3):240, 2011.
Lane, SJ, and Lynn, JZ: Sensory integration research: A look at past, present, and future. Sensory Integration Special Interest Section Quarterly 34(3):1, 2011.
Mørch, CD, et al: Exteroceptive aspects of nociception: Insights from graphesthesia and two-point discrimination. Pain 151(1):45, 2010.
O'Conaire, E, Rushton, A, and Wright, C: The assessment of vibration sense in the musculoskeletal examination: Moving towards a valid and reliable quantitative approach to vibration testing in clinical practice. Man Ther 16(3):296, 2011.
Perkins, BA, et al: Prediction of incident diabetic neuropathy using the monofilament examination: A 4-year prospective study. Diabetes Care 33(7):1549, 2010.
Tamè, L, Farnè, A, and Pavani, F: Spatial coding of touch at the fingers: Insights from double simultaneous stimulation within and between hands. Neurosci Lett 487(1):78, 2011.
Temlett, JA: An assessment of vibration threshold using a biothesiometer compared to a C128-Hz tuningfork. J Clin Neurosci 16(11):1435, 2009.
Yoshioka, T, et al: Perceptual constancy of texture roughness in the tactile system. J Neurosci 31(48):17603, 2011.

Two-point Discrimination Values for Healthy Subjects 20 to 24 Years of Age

Two-Point Discrimination Values for the Upper Extremities of Healthy Subjects 20 to 24 Years of Age ($N = 43$)

Skin Region	X (mm)	s
Upper—lateral arm	42.4	14.0
Lower—lateral arm	37.8	13.1
Mid—medial arm	45.4	15.5
Mid—posterior arm	39.8	12.3
Mid—lateral forearm	35.9	11.6
Mid—medial forearm	31.5	8.9
Mid—posterior forearm	30.7	8.2
Over first dorsal interosseous muscle	21.0	5.6
Palmar surface—distal phalanx, thumb	2.6	0.6
Palmar surface—distal phalanx, long finger	2.6	0.7
Palmar surface—distal phalanx, little finger	2.5	0.7

Two-Point Discrimination Values for the Lower Extremities of Healthy Subjects 20 to 24 Years of Age ($N = 43$)

Skin Region	X (mm)	s
Proximal—anterior thigh	40.1	14.7
Distal—anterior thigh	23.2	9.3
Mid—lateral thigh	42.5	15.9
Mid—medial thigh	38.5	12.4
Mid—posterior thigh	42.2	15.9
Proximal—lateral leg	37.7	13.0
Distal—lateral leg[a]	41.6	13.0
Medial leg	43.6	13.5
Tip of great toe	6.6	1.8
Over 1–2 metatarsal interspace	23.9	6.3
Over 5th metatarsal	22.2	8.6

[a] $n = 41$

Two-Point Discrimination Values for the Face and Trunk of Healthy Subjects 20 to 24 Years of Age ($N = 43$)

Skin Region	X (mm)	s
Over eyebrow	14.9	4.2
Cheek	11.9	3.2
Over lateral mandible	10.4	2.2
Lateral neck	35.2	9.8
Medial to acromion process	51.1	14.0
Lateral to nipple	45.7	12.7[a]
Lateral to umbilicus	36.4	7.3[b]
Over iliac crest	44.9	10.1[c]
Lateral to C7 spine	55.4	20.0[b]
Over inferior angle of scapula	52.2	12.6[b]
Lateral to L3 spine	49.9	12.7[b]

[a]$n = 26$
[b]$n = 42$
[c]$n = 33$
From Nolan,[84–86] with permission of the American Physical Therapy Association.

Chapter 4

Musculoskeletal Examination

D. Joyce White, PT, DSc, MS

The musculoskeletal system includes bones; muscles with their related tendons and synovial sheaths; bursa; and joint structures such as cartilage, menisci, capsules, and ligaments. Acute injuries or chronic conditions that disrupt the anatomy or physiology of musculoskeletal tissues can greatly affect a patient's function by causing direct impairments such as pain, inflammation, swelling, structural deformity, restricted joint movement, joint instability, and muscle weakness. Examples of diagnoses that result in direct impairment of the musculoskeletal system include fracture, rheumatoid arthritis (RA), osteoarthritis (OA), joint dislocation, tendinitis, bursitis, muscle strain/rupture, and ligament sprain/rupture.

Many pathological conditions that initially affect other body systems such as the neurological, cardiovascular, or pulmonary systems can result in secondary or indirect impairment of the musculoskeletal system. This often occurs when patients' activities are restricted by the condition—perhaps as a result of confinement for a period of time to a bed or wheelchair—or the patient moves the upper extremities (UEs) or lower extremities (LEs) in an inefficient or stress-causing pattern. Diagnoses that can cause indirect impairments of the musculoskeletal system include traumatic brain injury (TBI), cerebral vascular accident (CVA), cerebral palsy (CP), spinal and peripheral nerve injury, burns, and myocardial infarction (MI), just to name a few.

Both direct and indirect musculoskeletal impairments can contribute to activity limitations and participation restrictions and disability that affect a patient's ability to perform certain tasks and roles in society. By considering the few examples of diagnoses that cause direct and indirect musculoskeletal impairments provided in the previous paragraph, one can appreciate how often physical therapists and other health professionals encounter clinical problems affecting the musculoskeletal system. Administering specific tests and measures is almost always a major component of an initial patient examination.

This chapter discusses the purposes of, and provides a general framework for, conducting a musculoskeletal examination. The principles and components of a musculoskeletal examination, together with how to organize and integrate the data with those of other body systems, are emphasized. Other resources are available that provide detailed musculoskeletal testing procedures of specific body regions.[1-5]

■ PURPOSES OF THE MUSCULOSKELETAL EXAMINATION

Evaluation of data from the musculoskeletal examination contributes to establishing a diagnosis and prognosis, setting anticipated goals and expected outcomes, and developing and implementing a plan of care (POC). A musculoskeletal examination is also an important component of evaluating treatment outcomes both periodically during the treatment process and at the conclusion of the episode of care. The purposes of performing a musculoskeletal examination include the following:

1. To determine the presence or absence of impairments, activity limitations, and disability involving muscles, bones, and related joint structures.
2. To identify the specific tissues that are causing/contributing to the impairment, activity limitation, or disability.
3. To determine baseline status.
4. To help formulate appropriate anticipated goals, expected outcomes, and plan of care.
5. To evaluate the effectiveness of rehabilitation, medical, or surgical management.
6. To identify risk factors to prevent the development or worsening of impairments, activity limitations, or disabilities.
7. To determine the need for orthotic and adaptive equipment necessary for functional performance of activities of daily living (ADL), occupational, and/or recreational activities.
8. To motivate the patient.

■ EXAMINATION PROCEDURES
Patient History and Interview

Before beginning the physical examination, it is important to gain as much information as possible about the patient's current condition and past medical history. This information will help to direct and focus the physical examination to an area and system of the body. Information on symptoms and functional ability will help to establish a baseline against which treatment effectiveness can be judged. It will also help ensure that the examination and subsequent treatment are conducted safely.

Typically, most of this information is obtained while interviewing the patient. However, utilizing other information sources can be very efficient and provide objectivity and details to supplement interview data. If the patient is hospitalized in an acute care or rehabilitation setting, the medical records, including admission reports, progress notes, medication sheets, surgical summaries, body imaging reports, and laboratory test results, should be available and sought out. Referral summaries from previous medical care settings that review prior treatment approaches and discuss functional status may also be included. Other members of the health care team can be consulted for their input.

Outpatients often arrive with only a general diagnosis from a referring physician, or may be self-referred. In such cases it will be helpful to ask the patient to complete a medical history questionnaire before the examination process. A medical history questionnaire should include space for the patient to note the chief problem and date of onset; diagnostic tests performed for the problem; name and date of all surgeries; all medications currently being taken; past or current treatment for the problem (including those initiated by patient); a checklist of common medical conditions the patient may have experienced; brief family medical history; and patient's age, occupation, and lifestyle questions pertaining to smoking, alcohol use, and exercise. Figure 4.1 provides an example of a medical history questionnaire. The Guide to Physical Therapy Practice also includes a detailed template for a patient self-administered health questionnaire.[6]

A thorough understanding of the patient's medical background is critical for selection and safe application of examination and treatment procedures. For example, a history of an MI would cause the therapist to limit and more closely monitor the patient during muscle performance testing. A history of diabetes mellitus (DM) would cause the therapist to suspect and test for potentially compromised peripheral vascular and peripheral nervous systems, and to possibly avoid the use of heat modalities during treatment.

Patient self-administered health questionnaires have been shown to be generally accurate when conducted in a general medicine[7] and orthopedic outpatient settings.[8] However, even if a patient completes a medical history questionnaire, it is important for the therapist to review and clarify the information with the patient. Sometimes important medical background and medication data are inadvertently forgotten as the patient focuses on current problems. Verbally reviewing the information with the patient may jog the patient's memory.

After reviewing the information gained from medical records, other health care providers, and the patient-completed medical history questionnaire, the therapist is ready to begin the patient interview. Ideally, the patient interview should be conducted in a quiet, well-lit room that offers a measure of privacy. To encourage good communication, the therapist and patient should be at a similar eye level, facing each other, with a comfortable space between them—about 3 feet (91.44 cm) apart is customary in the United States. The patient should have the therapist's undivided attention; telephone calls and other interruptions should be avoided. The therapist may wish to have paper and pen available to record particular dates and information that is easily forgotten, but the interview should flow as an active conversation, not a dictation session. Repeated practice greatly improves the therapist's ability to listen, direct the interview, and establish a positive working relationship with the patient.

Over the course of the interview the therapist gains information about the patient's current complaints including onset, location, type and behavior of symptoms, current medications, previous treatments, secondary medical problems, medical history, and goals for

The purpose of this questionnaire is to assist us in providing you with quality care by obtaining a better understanding of your total health status. This questionnaire is part of your confidential medical record.

NAME: _____ DATE: _____

CHIEF PROBLEM OR COMPLAINT: _____

REFERRING MD: _____ DATE OF NEXT MD VISIT: _____

MEDICATIONS: Please list *all* medications currently being taken, along with the dosage, if known, and frequency.

1. _____   4. _____

2. _____   5. _____

3. _____   6. _____

SURGERY: Please list *all* surgeries and approximate date.

1. _____   DATE: _____

2. _____   DATE: _____

3. _____   DATE: _____

4. _____   DATE: _____

DIAGNOSTIC TESTS: Please check tests for current problem only.

X-rays: _____   CT Scan: _____   MRI: _____   Bone Scan: _____

EMG: _____   Blood Test: _____   Myelogram: _____   Others: _____

OCCUPATION: _____

LIFE STYLE: Non Smoker: _____ Smoke _____/day

No Alcohol: _____ Alcohol _____/day or _____/week

No Exercise: _____ Exercise _____/day or _____/week

FAMILY HISTORY: Mother, Father, siblings: Alive and healthy: _____

If deceased, cause of death: _____

Figure 4.1 An example of a medical history recording form. *(Courtesy of North Andover Physical Therapy Associates, North Andover, MA.)*

DO YOU HAVE, OR HAVE YOU HAD, ANY OF THE FOLLOWING: Please check *all* that apply.

___ High blood pressure
___ Heart problems
___ Heart palpitations, murmur
___ Chest pain

___ Shortness of breath
___ Coughing

___ Difficulty sleeping lying flat
___ Lung problems
___ Asthma
___ Allergies

___ Ulcers
___ Recent weight gain or loss
___ Nausea, vomiting
___ Bowel or bladder changes
___ Loss of appetite

___ Sexual dysfunction
___ Abnormal or painful menstruation
___ Pelvic inflammatory disease
___ Currently pregnant
___ Date of last mammogram:_____

___ Blood in urine
___ Incontinence

___ Seizures
___ Head trauma
___ Paralysis
___ Loss of consciousness
___ Headaches

___ Numbness or tingling
___ Dizziness
___ Balance problems

___ Arthritis

___ Hot or cold intolerance
___ Diabetes
___ Low blood sugar
___ Thyroid problems

___ Tumors ___ Cancer
___ Bleeding or bruising
___ Dialysis
___ Blood transfusion

___ Rashes
___ Scars
___ Changes in hair or nails

___ Wear eye glasses, contacts
___ Changes in vision
___ Blurred or double vision

___ Difficulty swallowing
___ Ear pain
___ Vocal changes
___ Ringing in ears

___ Dentures
___ Major dental work
___ Difficulty eating

___ Varicose veins
___ Muscle cramps
___ Joint or muscle pain

___ Psychiatric or psychological care

___ Fractures (broken bones)
     Where?_____
___ Problem requiring orthopedic shoes
___ Hip or ankle problem
___ Unusual illness as child

Please check if you have ever been in a motor vehicle accident _____

Figure 4.1—cont'd

the physical therapy episode of care. The patient's age and gender should be noted; some conditions are more common in particular age groups and genders. Often, detailed information about a patient's occupation, recreational activities, and social/living situation are required to understand the cause of the impairments, activity limitations, and to develop a relevant POC that focuses on the patient's goals. Open-ended, objective questions that do not promote biased answers should be used. For example, instead of asking "Is your right knee painful?" the therapist should ask, "Where are your symptoms located?" The therapist should carefully guide the interview to keep it focused on pertinent information and conclude in a timely manner. All questions should use conversational language rather than medical terminology so the patient easily understands the questions. The therapist should ask one question at a time and be sure to obtain a response before proceeding to other questions. Follow-up inquiries may be needed to clarify initial answers. It is important for the therapist to keep an open mind during the interview and not rush to conclusions about the patient's symptoms and diagnosis.

The following sequence is suggested as a way of organizing the interview. Similar information on general patient interviewing, that includes slight variations in format, can be found in texts by Talley and O'Connor,[9] Hertling and Kessler,[1] Paris,[10] and Coulehan and Block.[11]

Opening Question

The interview should begin with a general question such as "What brings you to physical therapy today?" or "What seems to be the problem?" If the patient is hospitalized the question may need to be rephrased to avoid having the patient retell the medical history to every health care provider. "I see from your medical chart that you fractured your hip and underwent a surgical repair yesterday. Is that what happened?" The patient should be given the opportunity to present the story. After the patient has concluded his or her statement, it is appropriate to say, "That's good. Now I have an idea of the problem. I have some other questions I need to ask to help me understand your problem better." Depending on the information provided by the patient, some of the following questions may be asked.

Onset of Symptoms

"How did this pain (swelling, limitation, problem, etc.) begin?" The therapist must know if the onset was sudden (e.g., caused by trauma such as a fall, blow, or skiing or motor vehicle accident). Specific information about the patient's body or body segment position at the time of trauma and the mechanism of injury will help to identify the structures involved. If the onset was more gradual or insidious, a systemic condition or chronic biomechanical problem may be more likely. A congenital onset is also a possibility.

Location of the Symptoms

"Where is your pain? Can you point to the location?" A body chart (Fig. 4.2) can be used to help identify and document the specific location of symptoms. The patient (or therapist with the patient's direction) can darken the involved area on the body chart using a pen or pencil.

Often the location of the symptoms coincides with the location of the lesion. This is more likely if the lesion is in superficial and distal tissues. For example, a lesion in a superficial tendon near the ankle will usually cause pain over the tendon site. Lesions in deeper, more proximal tissues can refer pain distally following sclerotome (Fig. 4.3) or dermatome patterns. (Refer to Chapter 3, Examination of Sensory Function.)

Referred pain may be perceived as originating from any or all tissues innervated by the same segmental spinal level in which the lesion is located. For example, pain due to OA of the hip is often felt in the anterior groin and thigh along the sclerotomes or dermatomes for L2 and L3. Considerable individual variation has been noted in dermatome and sclerotome patterns.[12]

"Has the pain changed in location? Spread to other areas? Become more focused?" Pain that is spreading usually indicates a worsening condition, whereas more focused symptoms indicate improvement. Changes in symptoms in relationship to varying body positions, activities, and treatments should be noted.

Quality of the Symptoms

"How severe is the pain? Is the pain sharp? Dull? Throbbing?" A simple yet effective way to document pain severity is to ask the patient to rate his or her pain from 0 (no pain) to 10 (most severe pain imaginable) as illustrated in the numerical pain rating scale presented in Figure 4.4. A visual analog scale (Fig. 4.5) or thermometer pain scale (Fig. 4.6) can also be used if preferred. A checklist of adjectives like that found in the McGill Pain Questionnaire[13] can clarify symptoms further (Fig. 4.7).

The adjectives used to describe pain may have diagnostic implications. Dull, aching pain may indicate muscle or joint lesions. Numbness, tingling, shooting pain, or burning sensations may indicate nervous system involvement. Deep, throbbing pain, or coolness in a body region may indicate vascular problems. Weakness, clumsiness,

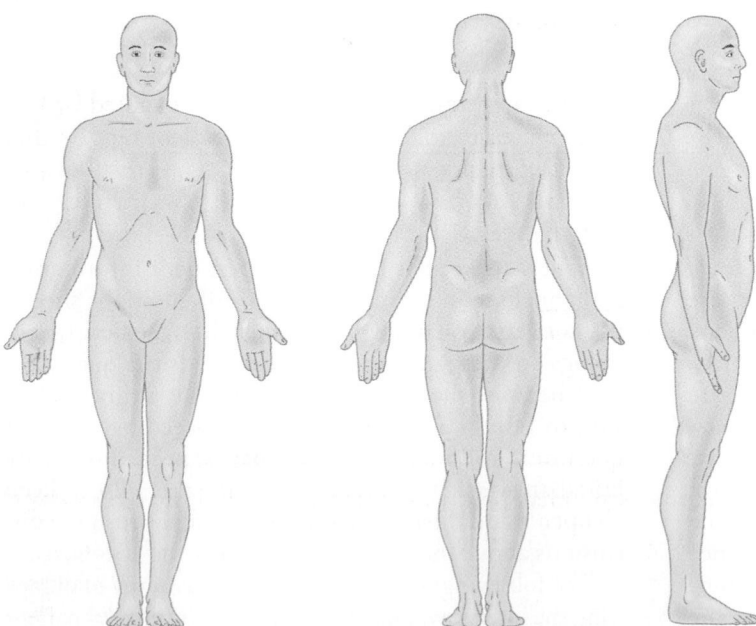

Figure 4.2 This body chart can supplement the patient's verbal description of the location of the pain.

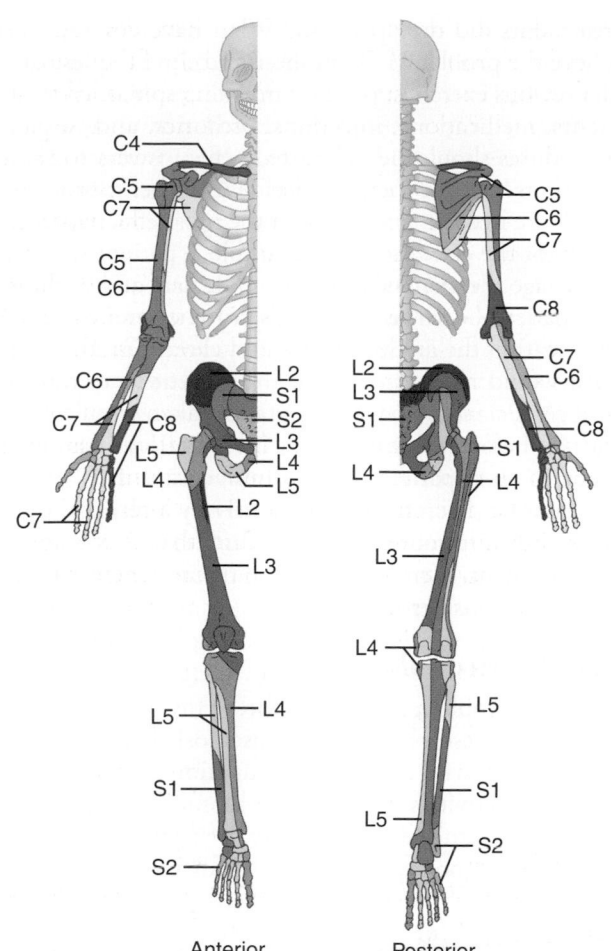

Figure 4.3 Sclerotomes from the anterior and posterior aspects of the body. *(From Hertling and Kessler,[1, p. 52] with permission.)*

On the line provided below please mark where the intensity of your pain is today.

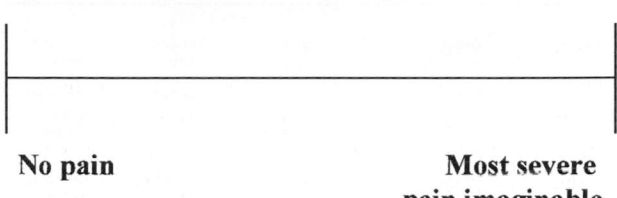

No pain   **Most severe pain imaginable**

Figure 4.5 Visual analog pain rating scale. The line is usually 10 cm in length. The patient's mark is measured from the left (no pain) end of the scale and is recorded in centimeters.

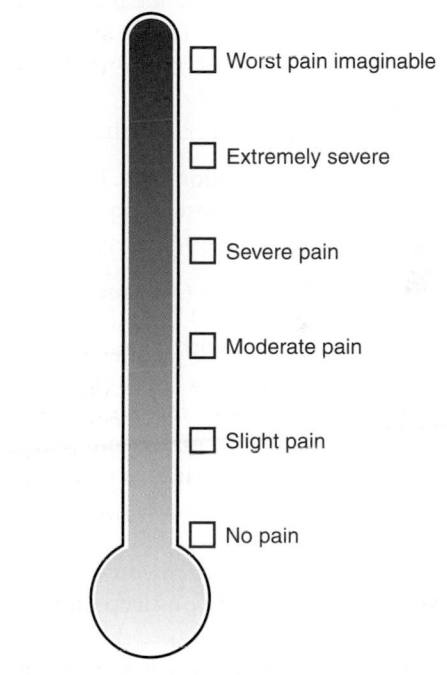

Figure 4.6 Thermometer pain rating scale. *(From Brodie, DJ, et al: Evaluation of low back pain by patient questionnaires and therapist assessment. J Orthop Sport Phys Ther 11:528, 1990, with permission.)*

or incoordination may suggest muscle and possibly peripheral or central nervous system dysfunction.

Behavior of the Symptoms

"What makes your symptoms increase? Decrease?" Symptoms from musculoskeletal conditions typically vary in response to rest, activity, and body positions that either increase or decrease mechanical stress placed on the involved tissue. The behaviors of the symptoms help to establish a diagnosis and determine which treatment techniques are more likely to be effective. For example, pain from overuse syndromes such as tendonitis will decrease with rest, whereas joint stiffness caused by OA often increases following rest. If a patient reports that the sitting position reduces back pain, then the therapist will probably have more success in relieving the pain using back flexion rather than extension exercises.

Figure 4.4 Two types of numerical pain rating scales.

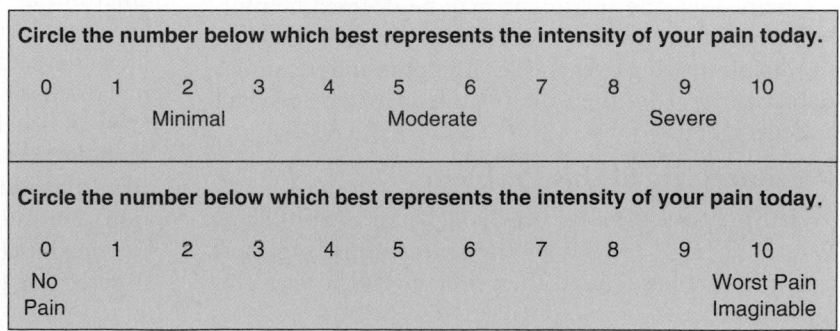

Circle the number below which best represents the intensity of your pain today.										
0	1	2	3	4	5	6	7	8	9	10
		Minimal			Moderate				Severe	

Circle the number below which best represents the intensity of your pain today.										
0	1	2	3	4	5	6	7	8	9	10
No Pain										Worst Pain Imaginable

Look carefully at the twenty groups of words. If any word in any group applies to *your* pain, please circle that word — but do not circle more than *one* word in any one group — so you must choose the *most suitable* word in that group.

In groups that do not apply to your pain, there is no need to circle *any* word — just leave them as they are.

Group 1	Group 2	Group 3	Group 4	Group 5
Flickering	Jumping	Pricking	Sharp	Pinching
Quivering	Flashing	Boring	Gritting	Pressing
Pulsing	Shooting	Drilling	Lacerating	Gnawing
Throbbing		Stabbing		Cramping
Beating		Lancinating		Crushing
Pounding				

Group 6	Group 7	Group 8	Group 9	Group 10
Tugging	Hot	Tingling	Dull	Tender
Pulling	Burning	Itching	Sore	Taut
Wrenching	Scalding	Smarting	Hurting	Rasping
	Searing	Stinging	Aching	Splitting
			Heavy	

Group 11	Group 12	Group 13	Group 14	Group 15
Tiring	Sickening	Fearful	Punishing	Wretched
Exhausting	Suffocating	Frightful	Gruelling	Blinding
		Terrifying	Cruel	
			Vicious	
			Killing	

Group 16	Group 17	Group 18	Group 19	Group 20
Annoying	Spreading	Tight	Cool	Nagging
Troublesome	Radiating	Numb	Cold	Nauseating
Miserable	Penetrating	Drawing	Freezing	Agonizing
Intense	Piercing	Squeezing		Dreadful
Unbearable		Tearing		Torturing

Figure 4.7 The McGill Pain Questionnaire. The first 10 groups of words are somatic (describing what the pain feels like), 11–15 are affective, 16 is evaluative, and 17–20 miscellaneous.[13]

Symptoms that do not vary with a change in activity or body position are rarely due to musculoskeletal lesions, and in fact are a "red flag" for more serious conditions such as space-occupying tumors and pathologies involving internal organs. Often patients will report that "nothing helps the pain." This statement should be fully explored with follow-up questions such as "Is your pain better or worse in the morning when you wake up from sleeping? Does your pain vary if you sleep on your back versus on your stomach?"

Behavior of Symptoms During the Last 48 Hours

It is important to understand the behavior of the symptoms during the past few days, not just at the current moment. Sometimes symptoms suddenly worsen or disappear at the time of the physical examination. A more accurate picture of the situation is told if the time frame spans 48 hours. "Are the symptoms getting better, worse, or staying the same?" The answer to this question will help inform the therapist about the effectiveness of future treatment. If the patient's pain has been steadily worsening over the last 48 hours and treatment stabilizes the pain, then the treatment may be deemed helpful. However, if the patient reports that the pain has been steadily improving over the last 48 hours and treatment stabilizes the pain, then the treatment may be deemed as detrimental.

Previous Care of this Problem

"What previous care has been sought for the problem? Who else (e.g., physician, therapist, athletic trainer, chiropractor) has treated the problem? What tests and treatments did they perform? What have you done to relieve the problem?" From these and similar questions, all previous exercises, physical modalities, manual treatments, medications, injections, orthotics, and surgical procedures should be delineated. The answers to these questions help the therapist decide if further medical referrals are needed, and focus on the most effective treatment for the condition. For example, a patient who fell 3 days ago is experiencing severe ankle pain and swelling. The patient borrowed a friend's crutches and has been self-treating the ankle with ice and elevation. The therapist would recommend that the patient be examined by a physician and have radiographs taken to rule out a fracture before physical therapy intervention. In another scenario, if a patient with adhesive capsulitis of the shoulder has been treated previously by a physical therapist with ultrasound and pendulum exercises without improvement, then other physical therapy interventions should be considered.

Specific Medical History

"Has this problem occurred before? How was it treated? How was it resolved?" Many musculoskeletal problems tend to recur with continued occupational, recreational, and daily activities if underlying biomechanical abnormalities, weaknesses, joint laxity, or tightness persists. Information about previous successful and unsuccessful treatments for similar past problems can help in treatment planning for the current problem.

General Medical History

A brief history should be obtained concerning medical problems and prior surgeries involving other body regions and systems. Conditions involving the cardiac, respiratory, neurological, vascular, metabolic, endocrine, gastrointestinal, genital urinary, visual, and dermatological systems should be noted. Having a patient complete a medical history questionnaire before the examination is an efficient means of obtaining this information, but the information should also be verified during the interview. Therapists also need to be aware of other conditions that mimic signs and symptoms often attributable to the musculoskeletal system. For example, inflammation of the gallbladder (cholecystitis) may result in right shoulder pain. However, shoulder pain related to cholecystitis typically will not increase with shoulder movements or resisted isometric testing of shoulder musculature, as would occur in the presence of musculoskeletal conditions. Patients with cholecystitis would likely have additional symptoms such as upper abdominal discomfort, bloating, belching, nausea, and intolerance of fried foods. Knowledge of systemic human pathology allows the therapist to recognize conditions requiring additional physician evaluation and intervention. Boissonnault[14] and Goodman and Snyder[15] have provided useful information to assist physical therapists in screening for medical conditions.

Medications

The type, frequency, dose, and effect of medications the patient is taking should be noted. The use of analgesic or anti-inflammatory medications may reduce the intensity of symptoms at the time of the examination. Changes in the use of these medications may make it difficult to determine the effects of physical therapy treatment. The secondary effects of some medications may necessitate the modification of examination and treatment techniques. For example, prolonged use of corticosteroids is associated with osteopenia (reduced bone mass) and reduced tensile strength of ligaments. The therapist may need to limit manual force applied through the lever of long bones to prevent fracture or ligament tear. The use of anticoagulants may make the patient susceptible to contusions and **hemarthrosis**. Such patients should be closely monitored for bruising and joint swelling. The amount of force used in exercise and manual therapies may need to be reduced.

Social History and Occupational, Recreational, and Functional Status

Questions in this area might include the following: "What type of work do you do in and outside of the home? How has this problem affected your ability to perform your job? Care for your children? Play golf? Dress? Bathe?" Certain occupational and recreational activities may contribute to the problem or interfere with recovery. Strategies such as joint preservation techniques and use of assistive devices may need to be considered to allow performance of necessary tasks. Medical insurance companies often make treatment reimbursement decisions based on a patient's functional status as related to the medical problem. Figure 4.8 presents sample questions that can be used to quantify the impact of the problem on function. Detailed assessment instruments, such as the Katz Index of Independence in Activities of Daily Living, Outcome and Assessment Information Set (OASIS), and SF-36 have also been developed to quantify a patient's functional status. See Chapter 8, Examination of Function, for additional information on examination of function.

"Do you have to climb stairs to get into your house? To reach the bedroom? Bathroom?" Characteristics of the home environment may determine whether a patient who uses an ambulatory assistive device requires instruction in stair activities before returning home. The condition of floors, size of halls and doorways, placement of furniture, and bathroom facilities will need to be considered for a patient using a wheelchair. A more detailed discussion of examination of the environment including the home, workplace, and community can be found in Chapter 9, Examination of the Environment.

"Do you live alone?" It is helpful to understand the patient's living situation to determine if others are available to assist with exercise programs, ambulation, and transfer activities. Some patients have responsibility for the care of children, elderly parents, or a disabled spouse or sibling. These responsibilities may need to be restructured to allow time for rest and recovery.

"Do you use tobacco products? Alcohol? Recreational drugs?" Cigarette smoking has been associated with decreased bone density, delayed bone healing after fractures, greater spinal disk degeneration, increased low back pain, and increased UE and LE musculoskeletal disorders. Use of alcohol and recreational drugs can lead to risk-taking behaviors resulting in increased incidence of injuries, or difficulty in safely performing functional activities and home exercise programs (HEPs). Therapists may wish to advise a patient to reduce the use of these substances and refer the patient to appropriate social services or self-help organizations for counseling.

Anticipated Goals, Expected Outcomes, and Time Frame of Recovery

Ask the following types of questions, as appropriate: "What do you hope will be the outcome of physical therapy treatment? When do you anticipate returning home? To work? To playing football?" These questions enable the therapist and patient to discuss and determine mutually agreed upon anticipated goals and expected outcomes. The therapist should not presume to know what issues are important to the patient. Answers to these questions help the therapist to determine

Figure 4.8 Questions used to rate a patient's function. The patient circles the percent of activity that he or she is able to perform.

What percentage of your normal <u>work</u> activities are you able to perform?

0% 10% 20% 30% 40% 50% 60% 70% 80% 90% 100%

What percentage of your normal <u>home</u> activities are you able to perform?

0% 10% 20% 30% 40% 50% 60% 70% 80% 90% 100%

What percentage of your normal <u>recreational</u> activities are you able to perform?

0% 10% 20% 30% 40% 50% 60% 70% 80% 90% 100%

whether the patient has realistic expectations or will need further patient education concerning his or her condition and typical recovery. For example, an elderly patient who suffered a fractured hip yesterday and is currently hospitalized may expect to remain in the acute care hospital for 2 weeks until he or she can independently ambulate and be independent in self-care. More realistic goals given current health insurance practices may need to be discussed, such as discharge from the hospital in 3 or 4 days to a rehabilitation or extended care facility for further nursing care, physical and occupational therapy, or discharge home with home health aides, visiting nurses, and home care physical and occupational therapists.

Concluding Question

When the therapist has finished obtaining the above information, one final type of open-ended question needs to be asked: "Is there anything else you wish to tell me?" or "Is there anything else you think I should know concerning your condition that I have not asked about?" Most likely the patient will respond by saying that he or she has no further information to offer and believes you understand the problem clearly. Sometimes, though, a patient may take this opportunity to clarify a previous point or share a concern that is adding stress to his or her life. Without this type of question at the conclusion of the interview, important information that may affect treatment and recovery may be lost.

The information elicited with the questions discussed above may be supplemented with additional questions based on the specific region of the body being examined and suspected etiologies. The physical therapist's knowledge of anatomy, kinesiology, pathokinesiology, physiology, and pathophysiology, as well as the physical presentation and progression of musculoskeletal conditions, provide the appropriate background on which to base and develop patient interview questions.

Mental Status

During the interview, the patient's orientation to person, place, and time as well as general arousal state and cognitive and communication abilities should be noted (see section titled Arousal, Attention, Orientation, and Cognition in Chapter 3, Examination of Sensory Function). If deficits in these areas are present, the examination may need to be modified to gain accurate information. The use of simple words, concise instructions, and task demonstrations may be helpful. Distractions in the environment should be kept to a minimum. Communication difficulties may be overcome through the use of foreign language interpreters, gestures, drawings, and language boards. Changes in medications, upright positioning, and access to natural light via windows and skylights may improve patient arousal and orientation to time. Depending on the type of deficit, the patient may benefit from an evaluation by a neurologist, neuropsychologist, speech-language pathologist, and/or occupational therapist.

Vital Signs

If a patient's medical record or interview suggests a compromised cardiovascular system, then heart rate, blood pressure, and respiratory rate should be determined before beginning other physical examination procedures (see Chapter 2, Examination of Vital Signs). Patients who are getting out of bed for the first time following recent surgery or prolonged bedrest should routinely have vital signs taken to establish baseline values before movement.

Observation/Inspection

Observation begins with the therapist's first contact with the patient, whether at bedside in the case of hospitalized patients, or in the waiting room for outpatients. The patient's general posture and ability to perform functional activities—change bed position, transfer from sitting to standing, ambulate to the examining room—provides information about the severity of symptoms, willingness to move, range of joint motion, and muscle strength. This information, although preliminary, helps to focus and individualize the physical examination. For example, a patient with a shoulder disorder who uses the UE to push off from a chair during transfers, stands with level bilateral shoulder height, and has an alternating arm swing during gait, would be expected to have milder symptoms, tolerate a more extensive examination, and have a greater range of motion (ROM) and muscle function than a patient who stands with an elevated scapula and protectively cradles the UE during transfers and gait. If functional difficulties and gait abnormalities were noted, detailed functional status and gait examinations would be performed later. See Chapter 8, Examination of Function, and Chapter 7, Examination of Gait, for additional information about these examination procedures.

To perform the physical examination and inspect specific areas of the body, the patient must be suitably dressed. Observation of the shoulders, elbows, or spine will require males to remove their shirt and females to wear only a bra or loose hospital gown that can be draped to expose the UE and back. To observe the LEs, patients should undress from the waist down, wearing only undergarments or shorts.

Once the patient is in the privacy of an examining room and appropriately disrobed, the therapist begins a careful inspection of the body region implicated in the interview as well as biomechanically related areas. The LEs and lumbar region, being intricately involved in weight-bearing activities, should be inspected as a functional unit. Likewise, conditions involving the shoulder require the examination of the cervical and thoracic regions, and vice versa. Visual inspection should focus on bone, soft tissue structures, skin, and nails. The therapist should view the body region anteriorly, posteriorly, and laterally. Often palpation, which is discussed in the next section, is combined with observation.

Bone shafts and joints are judged against normative models for symmetry, comparing one side of the body to the other. Contour and alignment should be considered. Common causes of changes in bone contour include acute fractures, callus formation or bone angulation owing to healed fractures, congenital variations, or bone hyperplasia at tendon insertions, and arthritis. Alignment differences can be due to the above conditions as well as muscle and soft tissue tightness, muscle weakness, muscle and ligament laxity, and joint dislocation.

For patients with musculoskeletal involvement, an examination for postural alignment is often indicated. From an *anterior* view both eyes, shoulders (acromion processes), iliac crests, anterior superior iliac spines, greater trochanters of the femur, patellae, and ankle medial malleoli should be horizontally level. Waist angles should be symmetrical. Patellae and feet should face anteriorly. *Laterally* the line of gravity should bisect the external auditory meatus, acromion process, greater trochanter, lie just posterior to the patella and approximately 2 inches (5 centimeters) anterior to the lateral malleolus (Fig. 4.9).[16]

The cervical and lumbar spine should exhibit normal lordotic curves, and the thoracic spine a normal kyphotic curve. From a *posterior* view the ear lobes, shoulders, inferior angles of the scapula, iliac crests, posterior superior iliac spines, greater trochanters, buttock and knee creases, and malleoli should be level. The spine should be straight, with the medial borders of the scapula equidistant from the spine bilaterally. Varus and valgus deformities of the knee and calcaneus should be noted.

The size and contour of soft tissue structures should be inspected and compared bilaterally. An increase in size may indicate soft tissue edema, joint effusion, or muscle hypertrophy. A decrease in size often indicates muscle atrophy. A loss of soft tissue continuity can suggest a muscle rupture. Cysts, rheumatoid nodules, ganglia, and gouty tophi can all change soft tissue contour. *Clubbing,* in which the distal finger and nail become rounded (bulbous), is believed to be caused by chronic hypoxemia and is typically associated with cardiovascular and respiratory diseases or neurovascular abnormalities.[9] Clubbing may also occur in the toes. Skin color and texture provide important clues to pathological conditions. *Cyanosis,* a blue discoloration of the skin and nail bed, indicates a lack of oxygen and excessive carbon dioxide in superficial blood vessels.[9] Inspection of the tongue for cyanosis helps determine if the poor perfusion is due to central or peripheral causes. *Pallor* is noted with a decrease in blood flow or blood hemoglobin—for example, in situations such as peripheral vasoconstriction, shock, internal bleeding, and anemia. *Erythema,* a localized redness, usually indicates increased blood flow and inflammation. Generalized redness can suggest fever, sunburn, or carbon monoxide poisoning. Yellow skin tone may be due to increased carotene intake, or liver disease. Brown, highly pigmented, hairy areas sometimes overlay bony defects such as spina bifida. Open wounds should be measured and diagrammed in patient records. New scars will be red, and older scars will be white in color. Skin tissue thickenings such as *calluses* can indicate chronic overloading and stress. Thin, glossy skin with decreased elasticity and hair loss is often found with peripheral nerve lesions or neurovascular disorders.

Palpation

It is suggested that palpation immediately follow or be integrated with observation and occur before other testing procedures. Other procedures may aggravate the patient's condition, making it more difficult to localize tenderness if palpation is performed later. The information gained from palpation will also help guide decision making about the need for additional test and measurements.

Palpation requires detailed knowledge of anatomy and a systematic approach. All structures on one body surface should be palpated before proceeding to another surface. For example, all structures on the anterior surface of the patient should be palpated before beginning to palpate structures on the posterior surface. The uninvolved side is palpated first to acquaint the patient with the procedure and, in some cases, to serve as a normative model for comparison. The therapist should develop a system of moving from superior to inferior structures, medial to lateral, or superior and then inferior from a

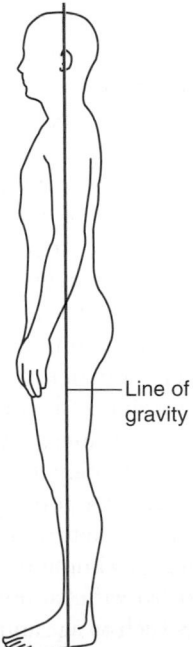

Figure 4.9 The location of the line of gravity from the lateral view. *(From Levangie and Norkin,[16] with permission.)*

Line of gravity

joint line. Which direction the therapist moves is not important, but the palpation process should be consistent and thorough.

Palpation of bone, soft tissue structures, and the skin is performed by varying the therapist's tactile pressure and using various parts of the hands. Light tactile pressure allows palpation of superficial tissues like the skin, whereas more pressure is needed to palpate deeper structures such as bone. Usually the fingertips are used for palpation, but large, deeper structures such as the greater trochanter of the femur or borders of the scapula are easier to locate using the entire surface of the hand. Rolling the skin and soft tissue between the fingertips and thumb helps the therapist judge myofascial mobility. Changes in skin temperature may be easier to detect using the posterior surface of the therapist's hand. When moving from one area to another, the therapist's hand should stay in firm contact with the skin whenever possible to prevent a tickling sensation. The fingers should not "crawl" or "walk" across the skin.

During palpation the therapist seeks feedback from the patient to help localize painful structures. Some lesions in deep or proximal structures will refer symptoms to other body areas, but localized tenderness often helps to implicate particular structures. Localized skin temperature should be noted: cool temperatures suggest reduced circulation, whereas warmth indicates increased circulation and often inflammation. Skin and soft tissue density and extensibility should be considered. Often muscle spasms and adhesions in skin and connective tissue can be found with palpation. The quality (amplitude) of peripheral pulses will provide gross information on arterial blood supply. Bilateral edema in the ankles and legs that forms pits with tactile pressure (termed *pitting edema*) can indicate cardiac failure, liver, or renal conditions. Unilateral pitting edema is typically associated with obstruction of returning circulation.

Anthropometric Characteristics

Abnormalities noted during observation and palpation may be further documented with anthropometric measurements. Using a cloth or flexible plastic tape measure, limb lengths are measured from one bony landmark to another and compared bilaterally. For example, true leg length is commonly measured from the anterior superior iliac spine to the medial malleolus.

Circumferential measurements help substantiate joint effusion, edema, and muscle hypertrophy and atrophy. Typically, these measurements are taken at specified distances (inches or centimeters) above or below a bony landmark so they can be reliably reproduced during subsequent measurements. For example, circumference measurements of the upper arm should be taken at noted distances distal to the acromion process of the scapula or proximal to the olecranon process of the ulna. If measurements are needed

of the hands or feet, volumetric measurements can be taken by submerging the distal extremity in a container of water and noting the volume of water that is displaced.

Range of Motion

Joints and their related structures are examined by performing active and passive joint motions. Joint motion is a necessary component of most functional tasks. Numerous studies have identified the ROM needed in the LE to walk on level surfaces,[17-21] ascend and descend stairs,[21-23] rise from a chair,[24-26] as well as squat, kneel, and sit cross-legged.[27,28] The ROM needed in the UE to eat with a spoon[29,30] and perform many UE activities[31-33] has been examined. Careful examination of joint movement for ROM, end-feel, effect on symptoms, and pattern of restriction help identify and quantify impairments causing activity limitations, and determine which structures need treatment.[34]

Active Range of Motion

The examination of joint motion begins by testing **active range of motion (AROM)**. Active motion is the unassisted voluntary movement of a joint. The patient is asked to move a body part through the osteokinematic motions at the involved and other biomechanically related joints. **Osteokinematics** refers to the gross angular motions of the shafts of bones. These motions are described as occurring in the three cardinal planes of the body: flexion and extension in the sagittal plane, abduction and adduction in the frontal plane, and medial and lateral rotation in the transverse plane. For example, in an examination of the hip the patient would be asked to move the hip into flexion, extension, abduction, adduction, and medial and lateral rotation. Often flexion and extension of the knee, as well as flexion, extension, rotation, and lateral flexion of the lumbar spine, are tested, because knee and spine motions can affect hip function. Some therapists prefer to have the patient move in functional, combined motions rather than straight plane motions. For example, a patient would be asked to reach a hand behind the head to test shoulder abduction and medial rotation simultaneously rather than perform isolated, individual motions.

Active motion is a good musculoskeletal screening procedure to further focus the physical examination. The amount, quality, and pattern of motion, as well as the occurrence of pain and crepitus, should be noted. For purposes of musculoskeletal screening, AROM can be visually estimated to determine if motion is within functional limits (WFL); however, use of a goniometer is required for the more objective and accurate measurements needed to establish a pathological baseline and to evaluate treatment response. Normal ROM varies among individuals and is influenced by factors such as age and gender,[35-44] as well as measurement methods.[45-50] Ideally, to determine if ROM is impaired, the ROM values should be compared with those obtained with the same measurement methods from people of the same age and gender. Studies that provide normative values by age and gender have been summarized by Norkin and White.[34] However, when particular values are not available, the therapist may need to compare ROM values to those of the patient's contralateral extremity or to average adult values from sources such as the *American Academy of Orthopedic Surgeons*[51,52] and the *American Medical Association*.[53] If the patient can complete AROM easily, without presenting pain or other symptoms, then further passive testing of that motion is usually unnecessary.

If, however, the amount of active motion is less than normal the therapist will not be able to isolate the cause without further testing. Capsule, ligament, muscle and soft tissue tightness, joint surface abnormalities, and muscle weakness are all capable of causing limitations in AROM. Pain during AROM may be due to the contracting, stretching, or pinching of contractile tissues such as muscles, tendons, and their attachments to bone, or due to the stretching or pinching of non-contractile tissues such as ligaments, joint capsules, and bursa.[54] Variations in the quality and pattern of active motion can result from central and peripheral nervous system disorders and metabolic conditions, in addition to disorders involving musculoskeletal structures. So, although active motion is an effective screening procedure, positive findings require a variety of additional tests to identify the underlying etiology and thus enable effective treatment.

Passive Range of Motion

Passive motions are movements performed by the therapist without the assistance of the patient. The term **passive range of motion (PROM)** typically refers to the amount of osteokinematic motion available when the patient's joint is moved without the patient's assistance. Normally, PROM is slightly greater than AROM because joints have a small amount of motion at the end of the range that is not under voluntary control. This additional range helps to protect joint structures by allowing the joint to absorb extrinsic forces. Passive ROM is examined not only for amount of motion, but also for the motion's effect on symptoms, the type of tissue resistance felt by the therapist at the end of the motion (end-feel), and pattern of limitation.

Passive range of osteokinematic motions depends on the integrity of joint surfaces and the extensibility of the joint capsule, ligaments, muscles, tendons, and soft tissue. Limitations in PROM may be due to bone or joint abnormalities or tightness of soft tissue structures. Because the therapist provides the muscle force needed to perform PROM, rather than the patient, PROM (unlike AROM) does not depend on the patient's muscle strength and coordination.

Pain during PROM is often due to moving, stretching, or pinching of non-contractile structures. Pain occurring at the end of PROM may be due to stretching contractile structures, as well as non-contractile structures.

Pain during PROM is not due to the active shortening (contracting) of muscle and the resulting pull on tendon and bone attachments. By comparing active and passive motions that cause pain, and noting the location of the pain, the therapist gains important information about which injured tissues are involved.

For example, on examination a patient is found to have limited and painful active knee flexion. This pain and limitation may be due to a lesion in the hamstring muscles (including tendons and bone attachments), the quadriceps muscles (including patella tendon and bone attachments), tibiofemoral and patellofemoral joint surfaces, meniscus, joint capsule, collateral and cruciate ligaments, or various anterior and posterior bursa. If the patient had similar pain and limitation during passive ROM, the quadriceps muscles, tibiofemoral and patellofemoral joint surfaces, meniscus, joint capsule, collateral and cruciate ligaments, or various anterior bursa may be involved. The hamstring muscles would not be implicated as these structures are put on slack and relieved of tension during passive knee flexion. Careful consideration of patient history, observation and palpation findings, and the results of additional tests and measurements such as end-feel determination, capsular versus non-capsular joint limitation patterns, accessory joint motion tests, and ligament stress tests will help to isolate the involved structures. These additional tests are discussed later in this chapter. If, however, passive knee flexion ROM were now normal and pain free as compared to painful during active flexion, a lesion in the hamstring muscles would be likely. The performance of resisted isometric muscle contractions would be used to confirm the presence of a lesion in the hamstring muscles.

In the clinical setting, PROM is usually measured with **universal goniometers** (Fig. 4.10) or less frequently with **inclinometers** (Fig. 4.11A and B), tape measures, and flexible rulers. With the exception of screening examinations, visual estimates are not used because they are less accurate than measurements taken with goniometers.[55,56] Both the beginning and the end of the motion are measured to identify the "range" of movement and are recorded using both the start and end values (e.g., 0°–110°) (Fig. 4.12).

Using the most common notation system, the 0° to 180° system, all motions except rotation begin in anatomical position at 0° and progress toward 180°. For example, a motion that begins at 0° and ends at 135° would be recorded as 0°–135°. A ROM that does not start with 0° or ends prematurely indicates joint **hypomobility**. Joint **hypermobility** at the beginning of the range is noted by the inclusion of a zero (the normal starting position) between the starting and ending measurements. For example, if the elbow joint has 5° of hypermobility in extension and 140° of flexion, it would be recorded as 5°–0°–140°. Hypermobility at the end of the ROM is denoted by an ending value higher than normal. Measurement results are incorporated

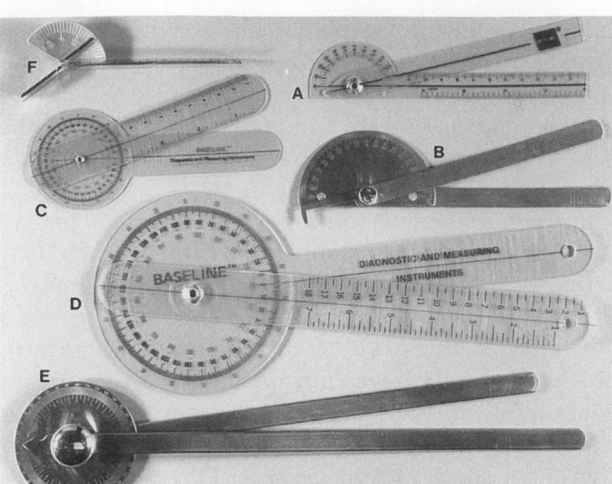

Figure 4.10 A variety of metal and plastic universal goniometers in different sizes and shapes. All universal goniometers have a central "body" with a protractor and fulcrum to center over the patient's joint, as well as two "arms" to align with the patient's body parts. *(From Norkin and White,[34] with permission.)*

into narrative reports or recorded on specialized forms. Specialized ROM recording forms typically have joints and motions listed centrally, with multiple columns on the left and right sides to record the date, examiner's initials, and ROM values of serial measurements (Fig. 4.13). These forms readily allow comparison of serial measurements to assess patient progress. Norkin and White,[34] Clarkson,[57] and Reese and Bandy[58] provide detailed descriptions of goniometric measurement procedures.

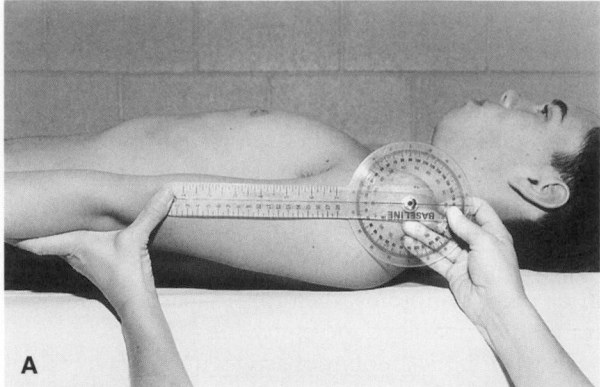

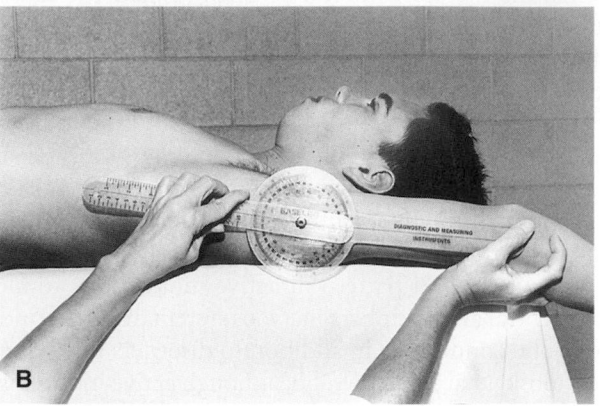

Figure 4.12 Measurement of the beginning (**A**) and end (**B**) of shoulder flexion ROM with a universal goniometer. The universal goniometer is moving from 0° toward 180° during the motion. *(From Norkin and White,[34, p. 63] with permission.)*

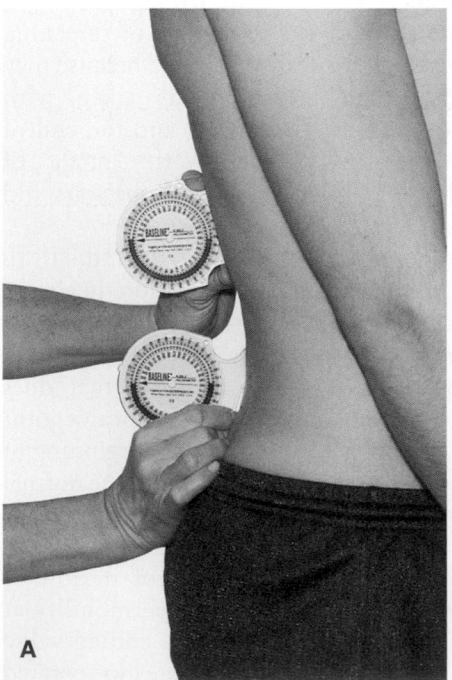

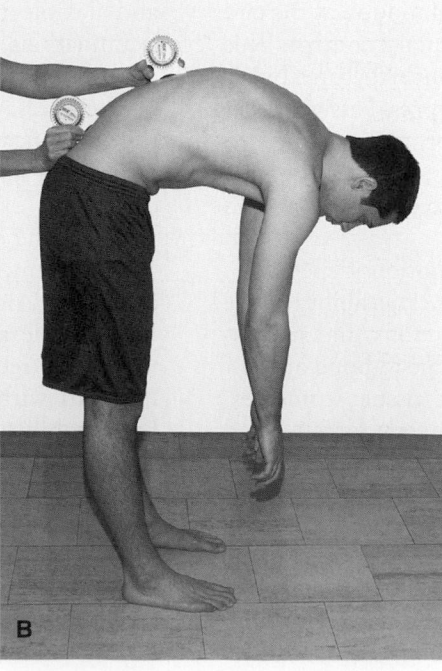

Figure 4.11 An inclinometer, with a bubble to indicate the position of the goniometer relative to gravity, is used to measure the beginning (**A**) and end (**B**) of lumbar flexion ROM. *(From Norkin and White,[34, p. 387] with permission.)*

			Range of Motion—Lower Extremity			
			Patient's Name _____ Date of Birth _____			
Left					Right	
			Date			
			Examiner's Initials			
			Hip			
			Flexion			
			Extension			
			Abduction			
			Medial Rotation			
			Lateral Rotation			
			Knee			
			Flexion			
			Ankle			
			Dorsiflexion			
			Plantarflexion			
			Inversion—Tarsal			
			Eversion—Tarsal			
			Inversion—Subtalar			
			Eversion—Subtalar			
			Inversion—Midtarsal			
			Eversion—Midtarsal			
			Great Toe			
			MTP Flexion			
			MTP Extension			
			MTP Abduction			
			IP Flexion			
			Toe			
			MTP Flexion			
			MTP Extension			
			MTP Abduction			
			PIP Flexion			
			DIP Flexion			
			DIP Extension			
			Comments:			

Figure 4.13 Range of motion recording form for the lower extremity. The multiple columns on either side of the centrally listed joints and motions are used to record the date, examiner's initials, and ROM values from serial measurements. *(From Norkin and White,[34] with permission.)*

ROM measurements taken with a universal goniometer of the extremity joints generally have good to excellent reliability. Reliability does vary depending on the joint and motion being measured. Reliability studies that include ROM measurements of elbow motions with a universal goniometer are presented in Box 4.1 Evidence Summary. ROM measurements of UE joints have been found to be more reliable than measurements of the LE[46,60,66] and spine.[67-69] In an often cited study, Boone et al[60] found the average standard deviation between measurements made on the same subjects by different testers to be 4.2° for UE motions and 5.2° for LE motions. These differences in reliability have been attributed to difficulties in measuring complex as compared to simple hinged joints, in palpating bony landmarks, and in moving heavy body parts.[60,70] The use of standardized positions, stabilization of the body part proximal to the joint being tested, use of bony landmarks to align the goniometer, and repeated testing conducted by the same therapist (rather than multiple therapists) all help to improve the validity and reliability of goniometric measurements.[46,56,71]

End-Feel

The end of each motion at each joint is limited from further movement by particular anatomical structures. The type of structure that limits a joint motion has a characteristic feel, which may be detected by the therapist performing the passive ROM. This feeling, which is experienced by the therapist as resistance, or a barrier to further motion, is called the **end-feel**. Cyriax and Cyriax,[54] Kaltenborn,[72] and Paris[73] have described a variety of normal (physiological) and abnormal (pathological) end-feels. A summary of the types of end-feels has been adapted from the work of these authors. Normal end-feels are generally described as *soft, firm,* or *hard* (Table 4.1). A soft end-feel has a gradual increase in resistance as muscle, skin, and subcutaneous tissues are compressed between body parts.[74] A firm end-feel has a more abrupt increase in resistance as compared to a soft end-feel. Firm end-feels include varying amounts of creep, or give, depending on whether the barrier to the end of the motion is the stretching of muscle, capsule, or ligamentous tissue. The firm end-feel with the most creep would be the rubbery resistance offered by the stretch of muscle tissue, and the least amount of creep would be provided by the stretch of ligamentous tissue. The firm end-feel created by the stretch of a joint capsule usually has a moderate amount of creep. A hard end-feel is abrupt; there is an immediate stop to movement as when bone contacts bone.

End-feels are considered to be abnormal when they occur sooner or later in the ROM than is typical, or if they are not the type of end-feel that is normally found for that joint motion. Abnormal end-feels have been associated with more pain than normal end-feels.[75] Many abnormal, pathological end-feels have been described, but most can be categorized as variations of soft, firm,

and hard end-feels (Table 4.2). An abnormal end-feel that cannot be categorized as soft, firm, or hard, is an *empty end-feel.* This term describes the inability of the therapist to detect any anatomical barrier to the end of the ROM. Rather, the patient through verbal or nonverbal cues indicates that no further motion should occur, usually because of pain.

The ability to determine the type of end-feel is important in helping the therapist identify the limiting structures and choose a focused and effective treatment. Developing this ability takes practice and sensitivity. Passive ROM, particularly toward the end of the motion, must be performed slowly and carefully. Secure stabilization of the bone proximal to the joint being tested is critical in preventing multiple joints and structures from moving and interfering with determination of the end-feel.[76,77]

Capsular Patterns of Restricted Motion

Cyriax and Cyriax[54] initially described characteristic patterns of restricted joint ROM due to diffuse, intra-articular inflammation involving the entire joint capsule. These patterns of restricted motion, which usually involve multiple motions at a joint, are called **capsular patterns**. The restrictions do not involve the loss of a fixed number of degrees, but rather the loss of a proportion of one motion relative to another. Capsular patterns vary from joint to joint. Table 4.3 presents common capsular patterns as described by Cyriax and Cyriax[54] and Kaltenborn.[72] Although therapists have been using capsular patterns in clinical decision making for many years, studies are needed to test the hypotheses regarding the cause of capsular patterns and to determine the capsular pattern for each joint.[78,79]

Hertling and Kessler,[1] expanding on Cyriax's work, have suggested that capsular patterns are due to one of two general situations: (1) joint effusion or synovial inflammation or (2) relative capsular fibrosis. Joint effusion or synovial inflammation results in a capsular pattern of limitation by distending the entire joint capsule, causing the joint to maintain a position that allows the greatest intra-articular volume. Pain triggered by stretching the capsule, and muscle spasms that protect the capsule from further stretch, inhibit movement and cause a capsular pattern of restricted motion. The other general situation that causes capsular patterns is relative capsular fibrosis, seen in the resolution of acute capsular inflammation, chronic low-grade capsular inflammation, and immobilization of a joint. These conditions cause a decrease in the extensibility of the entire capsule owing to an increase in collagen content of the capsule relative to the mucopolysaccharide content, or from internal changes in the collagen tissue.

To plan an effective treatment, the therapist must determine whether the capsular pattern is caused by joint effusion/synovial inflammation or capsular fibrosis. If joint effusion or synovial inflammation is present,

(Text continues on page 142)

Box 4.1 Evidence Summary   Outcome Studies on Reliability of Using Universal Goniometer to Measure Elbow Range of Motion

Reference	Subjects	Design/Intervention/Duration	Results	Comments
Hellebrandt et al,[59] 1949	77 patients	Repeated measures design AROM 1 highly experienced PT tester 8 average experienced PT testers 2 trials by same tester, time between trials not defined	Highly experienced tester had mean difference between trials of 1.0° for flexion and 0.1° for extension. Sig difference between trials for flexion	High intratester reliability. Sig difference not clinically important. No data on elbow motions for average-experienced testers
Boone et al,[60] 1978	12 healthy males 26–54 years	Repeated measures design AROM Standardized method 4 PT testers with 5–20 years of experience 3 trials by each tester in one session 1 weekly session for 4 weeks (4 sessions total)	No sig difference between 3 trials by each tester in one session so session means used in intra- and intertester calculations. Sig difference between testers Intratester $r = 0.94$ SD = 0.2° Intertester $r = 0.88$ SD = 2.6°	High intra- and intertester reliability. Intratester reliability higher than intertester reliability
Rothstein et al,[46] 1983	12 patients had elbow measured	Repeated measures design, blinded PROM; method not standardized. 12 PT testers with 1–4 years experience 3 types of universal goniometer: large metal, large plastic, small plastic 2 trials per goniometer per tester 2 testers evaluated each patient.	Single trial: Intratester reliability $r = .95 – .99$ ICC = .86. – .99 Intertester reliability $r = .89 – .97$ ICC = .85 – .95 Mean of 2 trials: Intertester reliability $r = .94 – .97$ ICC = .89 – .96	High intra- and intertester reliability. Intratester reliability slightly higher than intertester reliability. Minimal improvement in intertester reliability by using mean of 2 trials versus score from single trial (differences in ICC no. 0.12)
Grohmann,[61] 1983	1 healthy adult	Repeated measures design, blinded Elbow held in 2 fixed positions: 1 obtuse and 1 acute angle. 40 PT student testers used over-the-joint and lateral methods to measure each position 1 trial daily for 4 days	No sig difference between methods	No difference in using over-the-joint method or lateral method of measuring elbow position
Walker et al,[43] 1984	4 healthy adults, 60 years	Repeated measures design, blinded. AROM 4 testers Each tester performed 5 trials on each subject in one day.	Intratester reliability $r = 81$	High intratester reliability

Continued

Box 4.1 Evidence Summary   Outcome Studies on Reliability of Using Universal Goniometer to Measure Elbow Range of Motion—cont'd

Reference	Subjects	Design/Intervention/Duration	Results	Comments
Fish and Wingate,[62] 1985	1 healthy adult	Repeated measures design, blinded 46 PT student testers measured with 2 instruments: plastic and steel goniometers 3 conditions: ALIGN = elbow in fixed position with landmarks noted, ASSIGN = elbow in fixed position with no landmarks, PROM = full range of passive flexion	ALIGN plastic SD = $1.8°-2.1°$ ALIGN steel SD = $2.0°-2.6°$ ASSIGN plastic SD = $2.5°-3.0°$ ASSIGN steel SD = $2.5°-3.4°$ PROM plastic SD = $3.4°-3.8°$ PROM steel SD = $3.9°-4.2°$	Variability of scores increased as standardization of measurements decreased
Greene and Wolf,[64] 1989	20 healthy adults (10 males, 10 females) 18–55 years	Repeated measures design. AROM 1 PT tester 2 instruments: universal goniometer and pendulum goniometer 3 trials per instrument in a session 3 sessions within 2 weeks	Universal goniometer within-sessions: Flexion: ICC = .94; SD = 1.2°; 95% CI = 3.0°; Extension: ICC = .95; SD = 1.0°; 95% CI = 1.9°; Both instruments had sig difference between sessions. Low correlation ($r = .11-.21$) and sig difference between instruments within-sessions	High intratester reliability with universal goniometer in one session. 95% of time reliability within 2–3° if taken by same tester in one session. Different instruments should not be used interchangeably.
Goodwin et al,[63] 1992	23 healthy females, 18–31 years	Repeated measures design. AROM 3 experienced testers. 3 instruments: universal goniometer, fluid goniometer, electrogoniometer. Landmarks noted on skin. 3 trials per instrument by each tester in a session. 2 sessions 4 weeks apart.	Universal goniometer intra-tester reliability between sessions: $r = .61-.92$ ICC = $.56-.91$. Difference in means between sessions = 0.9°; Average difference in means between testers = 5.1°; Sig differences and interactions between goniometers, testers, and sessions	Moderate to high intra-tester reliability between 2 sessions 4 weeks apart, depending on tester. Differences between sessions smaller than differences between testers. Different instruments should not be used interchangeably.

Box 4.1 Evidence Summary Outcome Studies on Reliability of Using Universal Goniometer to Measure Elbow Range of Motion—cont'd

Reference	Subjects	Design/Intervention/Duration	Results	Comments
Armstrong et al,[65] 1998	38 patients with history of surgery for upper extremity injury. 19 males, 19 females 14–72 years	Repeated measures design. AROM 5 testers of varying experience. 2 instruments: universal goniometer and electrogoniometer. 2 trials per instrument by each tester on same day	Universal goniometer: Intratester reliability for flexion: ICC = .55 – .98, mean difference between trials = 3.2°; 95% CI = 5.9° Extension: ICC = .45 – .98, mean difference = 3.5°; 95% CI = 6.6° Intertester reliability for flexion: ICC = .58 – .62, mean difference = 6.4°; 95% CI = 9.2°; Extension: ICC = .58 – .87, mean difference = 7.0°; 95% CI = 8.9°	Moderate to high intra-tester reliability. Moderate intertester reliability. 95% of time reliability within 6.7° if taken by same tester, and 9° if taken by different testers.

AROM = active range of motion; CI = confidence interval; ICC = intraclass correlation coefficient; PROM = passive range of motion; PT = physical therapist; r = Pearson's correlation coefficient; sig − significant.

Table 4.1	Normal End-Feels	
End-Feel	**Structure**	**Example**
Soft	Soft tissue approximation	Knee flexion (contact between soft tissue of posterior leg and posterior thigh)
Firm	Muscular stretch	Hip flexion with the knee straight (passive elastic tension of hamstring muscles
	Capsular stretch	Extension of metacarpophalangeal joints of fingers (tension in the anterior capsule)
	Ligamentous stretch	Forearm supination (tension in the palmar radioulnar ligament of the inferior radioulnar joint, interosseous membrane, oblique cord)
Hard	Bone contacting bone	Elbow extension (contact between the olecranon process of the ulna and the olecranon fossa of the humerus)

From Norkin and White,[34] with permission.

Table 4.2	Abnormal End-Feels	
End-Feel		**Examples**
Soft	Occurs sooner or later in the ROM than is usual, or in a joint that normally has a firm or hard end. Feels boggy, with fluid shift.	Soft tissue edema Synovitis
Firm	Occurs sooner or later in the ROM than is usual, or in a joint that normally has a soft or hard end.	Increased muscular tonus Capsular, muscular, ligamentous shortening

Continued

Table 4.2	Abnormal End-Feels—cont'd	
End-Feel		**Examples**
Hard	Occurs sooner or later in the ROM than is usual, or in a joint that normally has a soft or firm end. A grating or bony block is felt.	Chondromalacia Osteoarthritis Loose bodies in joint Myositis ossificans Fracture
Empty	No real end because pain prevents reaching end of ROM. No resistance is felt except for patient's protective muscle splinting or muscle spasm.	Acute joint inflammation Bursitis Abscess Fracture Psychogenic disorder

From Norkin and White,[34] with permission.

Table 4.3	Capsular Patterns of Extremity Joints
Shoulder (glenohumeral joint)	Maximum loss of external rotation Moderate loss of abduction Minimum loss of internal rotation
Elbow complex	Flexion loss is greater than extension loss
Forearm	Full and painless Equally restricted in pronation and supination in presence of elbow restrictions
Wrist	Equal restrictions in flexion and extension
Hand Carpometacarpal joint I Carpometacarpal joints II-V	Abduction and extension restriction Equally restricted in all directions
Upper extremity digits	Flexion loss is greater than extension loss
Hip	Maximum loss of internal rotation, flexion, abduction Minimal loss of extension
Knee (tibiofemoral joint)	Flexion loss is greater than extension loss
Ankle (talocrural joint)	Plantarflexion loss is greater than extension loss
Subtalar joint	Restricted varus motion
Midtarsal joint	Restricted dorsiflexion, plantarflexion, abduction, and medial rotation
Lower extremity digits Metatarsalphalangeal joint I Metatarsalphalangeal joints II-V Interphalangeal joints	Extension loss is greater than flexion Variable, tend toward flexion restriction Tend toward extension restriction

Capsular patterns are from Cyriax and Cyriax[54] and Kaltenborn.[72]

treatment methods typically focus on resolving the acute inflammation with rest, cold modalities, compression, elevation, joint mobilization using grade 1 sustained and grade 1 and 2 oscillations, gentle ROM exercise, and anti-inflammatory medications. Capsular fibrosis, a more chronic condition, can be treated with heat modalities, joint mobilization using grade 3 sustained stretch and grade 3 and 4 oscillations, passive stretching procedures, and more vigorous ROM exercises. Patient history, observation, palpation, and careful determination

of end-feels will help establish the cause of the capsular pattern.

Noncapsular Patterns of Restricted Motion

Restricted passive ROM that is not proportioned similarly to a capsular pattern is called a **noncapsular pattern** of restricted motion.[1,54] Noncapsular patterns usually involve only one or two motions of a joint, in contrast to capsular patterns, which involve all or most motions of a joint. Noncapsular patterns are caused by conditions involving structures other than the entire joint capsule. Internal joint derangement, adhesion of a part of a joint capsule, and extracapsular lesions such as ligament shortness, muscle strain, and muscle shortness are examples of conditions that can result in noncapsular patterns. For example, shortness of the iliopsoas muscle will result in the noncapsular pattern of limited passive hip extension; the passive range of other hip motions will not be affected. This is in contrast to the capsular pattern of the hip caused by diffuse joint effusion or capsular fibrosis, in which there is loss of passive internal rotation, flexion, and abduction.

The sole recognition of a noncapsular pattern is not enough to direct appropriate treatment. Information gained from the patient history, observation, palpation, active and passive ROM, end-feels, resisted isometric muscle tests, joint mobility tests, and special tests must be integrated to determine the most likely cause of the noncapsular pattern. For example, both chronic shortness and acute strain of the iliopsoas muscle may result in a noncapsular pattern of limited passive hip extension. However, those conditions will present differently in terms of patient history, pain during active and passive ROM, end-feel, and resisted isometric muscle tests, and will require different treatment approaches.

Accessory Joint Motions

If passive ROM is found to be limited or painful, an examination of arthrokinematic motions in indicated. **Arthrokinematics** refers to the motion of joint surfaces. These motions, often called **accessory** or **joint play motions**, are used to determine joint mobility and integrity. Accessory joint motions are typically described as slides (or glides), spins, and rolls. A **glide (slide)** is a linear motion of one surface sliding over another (Fig. 4.14). A **roll** is a rotary motion similar to the bottom of a rocking chair rolling over the floor or a tire rolling over a road (Fig. 4.15). A **spin** is a rotary motion around a fixed point or axis (Fig. 4.16).

Accessory motions usually occur in combination with each other and result in angular movement of the bone shaft, or osteokinematic motion. Kaltenborn[72] refers to the combination of translatory glide and the rotary motion of rolling as **roll-gliding**. The combination of a roll and glide allows for increased ROM by postponing the joint compression and separation that would occur at either side of the joint during a pure rolling motion. The direction of the rolling and gliding components of roll-gliding depends on whether a concave or convex joint surface is moving. If a concave joint surface is moving, the gliding component occurs in the same direction as the rolling or angular movement of the shaft of the bone (Fig. 4.17). For example, during flexion of the knee with the femur fixed, the shaft of the tibia rolls posteriorly while the joint surface of the tibia also glides posteriorly. If a convex joint surface is moving, the gliding component occurs in the direction opposite to the rolling or

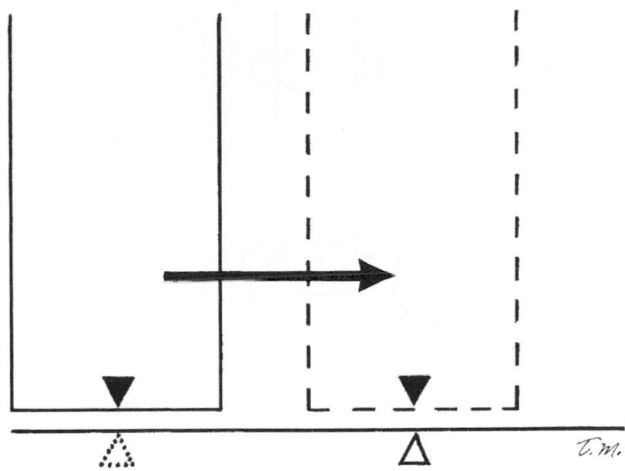

Figure 4.14 A glide (slide) is a type of linear accessory joint motion in which points on a moving joint surface comes in contact with new points on the opposing joint surface. *(From Norkin and White,[34] with permission.)*

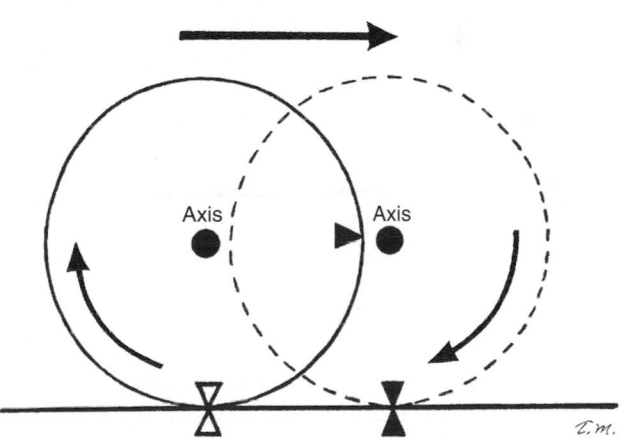

Figure 4.15 During a roll, new points on the moving joint surface come in contact with new points on the opposing surface. The axis of rotation also moves, in this case to the right. *(From Norkin and White,[34] with permission.)*

angular movement of the shaft of the bone. As an example, during abduction of the glenohumeral joint, the shaft and humeral head roll cranially, while the contacting articular surface of the humeral head glides caudally. In the human body, roll-gliding is by far the most frequently occurring arthrokinematic motion, although there are several instances of pure spin motions. An example of a spin joint motion would be supination and pronation of the radius at the humeroradial joint.

Normal arthrokinematic (accessory) motions are necessary for full and symptom-free osteokinematic motions. The careful examination of accessory motions helps to more specifically locate and treat the source of impaired osteokinematic motions. The patient cannot perform accessory motions actively because these

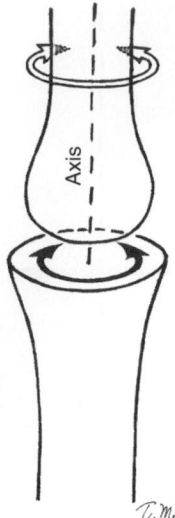

Figure 4.16 A spin is an accessory joint motion in which all the points on the moving surface rotate around a fixed axis. *(From Norkin and White,[34, p. 4] with permission.)*

motions are not under voluntary control. Rather, the therapist tests them passively. The accessory motions most commonly tested are translatory motions: glides that are parallel to the joint surfaces, and *distractions* and *compressions* that are perpendicular to the joint surfaces. Kaltenborn,[72] Kisner and Colby,[80] Edmund,[81] and Hertling and Kessler[1] describe specific testing and treatment techniques that focus on accessory motions—usually under the topic of **joint mobilization**. Careful attention must be given to general patient positioning, specific joint positioning, relaxation of surrounding muscles, stabilization of one joint surface, and mobilization of the other joint surface.

Accessory joint motions are examined for amount of motion, effect on symptoms, and end-feel. The ranges

of accessory motions are very small and cannot be measured with goniometers or standard rulers. Rather, they are typically compared to the same motion on the contralateral side of the patient's body, or compared to the therapist's past experience in testing people of similar age and gender as the patient. Accessory motions are assigned a joint play mobility grade of 0 to 6.[72] These mobility grades have implications for treatment (Table 4.4).[1,81]

The testing accessory motions put stress on specific anatomical structures. A change in symptoms during the performance of an accessory motion helps to implicate particular structures. Distraction stresses the entire joint capsule and numerous ligaments surrounding and supporting the joint. Glides stress a specific part of the joint capsule and particular ligaments, depending on the direction of the glide and joint. Compression applies force to intracapsular structures such as meniscus, bone, cartilage, and projections of the synovial lining of the joint capsule into the joint space. Accessory motions are of such a small magnitude that they do not stress surrounding muscles. Angular changes in joint position that typically occur during osteokinematic ROM movements more effectively change the length of muscle tissue. Normal and abnormal end-feels noted during passive accessory motions are characterized as soft, firm, and hard. Similar to end-feels noted during passive osteokinematic motions, they help determine the limiting structures and guide treatment planning.

Muscle Performance

Muscle performance is the ability of a muscle to do work.[6] **Linear work** is defined as force multiplied by distance, and **rotational work** is defined as torque (force multiplied by perpendicular distance from the axis of rotation) multiplied by arc of movement. Usually during a

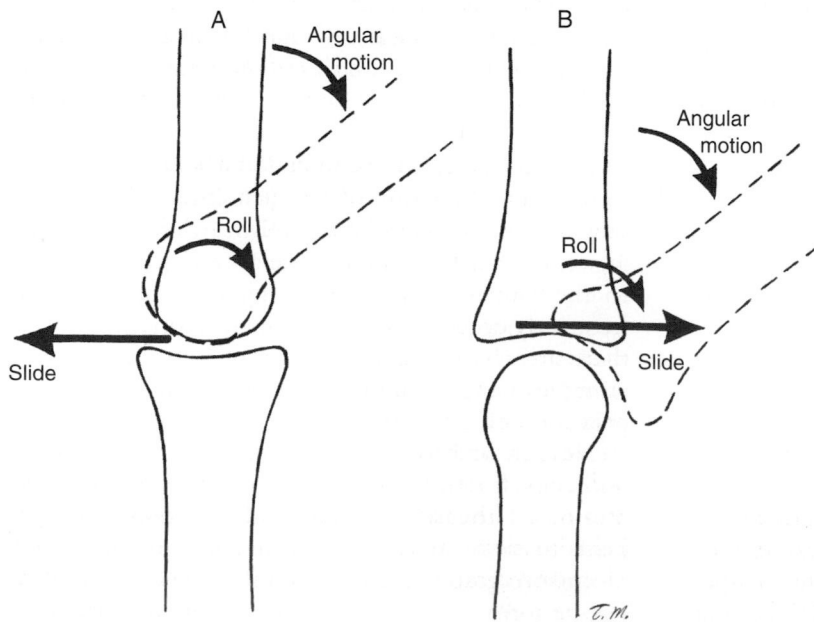

Figure 4.17 Diagrammatic representation of the concave-convex rule. **(A)** If the joint surface of the moving bone is convex, gliding is in the opposite direction of the angular movement of the bone. **(B)** If the joint surface of the moving bone is concave, gliding is in the same direction as the angular movement of the bone. *(From Norkin and White,[34, p. 5] with permission.)*

Table 4.4	Accessory Joint Motion Grades and Implications for Treatment	
Grade	Joint Status	Implications for Treatment
0	Ankylosed	Joint mobilization is not indicated; surgery should be considered.
1	Considerable hypomobility	*Grades 1 and 2*: Joint mobilization to increase the extensibility of joint structures is indicated. Heat modalities before mobilization and ROM exercises after mobilization should be considered.
2	Slight hypomobility	
3	Normal	Joint mobilization is not needed, because findings are normal.
4	Slight hypermobility	*Grades 4 and 5*: Joint mobilization to increase joint extensibility is not indicated. Taping, bracing, strengthening exercises, and education regarding posture and positions to be avoided should be considered.
5	Considerable hypermobility	
6	Unstable	Joint mobilization is not indicated; surgery should be considered.

musculoskeletal examination, a component of muscle performance—muscle strength—is tested. **Muscle strength**, as described in the *Guide to Physical Therapist Practice*,[6] is the force exerted by a muscle or group of muscles to overcome a resistance in one maximal effort. Clinical methods of determining muscle strength include manual muscle testing (MMT), handheld dynamometry, and isokinetic dynamometry. Depending on the patient, other characteristics related to muscle performance may also be tested. *Muscle power* is work produced per unit of time, or the product of strength and speed. **Muscle endurance** is the ability of the muscle to contract repeatedly over time. In addition to these quantitative measures, the patient's qualitative response in terms of changes in pain during resisted isometric testing is important in identifying musculotendinous lesions.

Resisted Isometric Testing

During the performance of active and passive ROM testing, a patient may complain of pain. The patient history, location of pain, and the pattern of painful motions may suggest a lesion in contractile tissues such as muscle or tendons and their insertions into bone, or involvement of inert tissues such as the joint surfaces, joint capsule, or ligaments. Resisted isometric testing can be used to further clarify which type of tissue, contractile or inert, is involved. *Increased pain* during a resisted isometric contraction, caused by shortening of the muscle and pulling on the tendon, helps to confirm the involvement of contractile tissues. Sometimes more pain is felt when the contraction is released and lengthening occurs; this would still be considered a positive finding for a lesion in contractile tissues. The *lack of pain* during resisted isometric testing, pain noted with limited accessory joint motions, a capsular pattern of joint restriction, or particular end-feels during PROM and accessory joint motions help to confirm the involvement of inert tissues. For example, bicipital tendinitis would be painful during

resisted isometric testing of elbow flexion and shoulder flexion. An adhesive capsulitis of the glenohumeral joint would be painless during these same resisted isometric maneuvers.

Resisted isometric testing must be performed carefully to stress particular contractile tissue while avoiding stress to surrounding inert tissue. The therapist should place the patient's joint in a position midway through the ROM, so that minimal tension is put on inert structures. The body part proximal to the joint being tested must be well stabilized by the therapist to minimize extraneous muscle substitutions. The patient is then asked to hold the position while the therapist gradually applies resistance. Joint movement is strictly avoided. Although some compression of articular surfaces will occur during the isometric contraction, this does not usually present a problem in interpreting the results. However, a bursa located deep to the musculotendinous tissue will also be compressed. Although bursae are not considered to be connective tissue, pain will be felt during the isometric contraction if a bursa is inflamed. Fortunately, treatment for bursitis is similar to treatment for musculotendinous strains and inflammation.

In addition to determining the absence or presence of pain during the resisted isometric testing, the therapist should also note the strength of the muscle contraction. If weakness is found, more extensive testing of muscle strength should be performed using MMT or dynamometers. Muscle weakness may be due to many causes, including pathologies involving upper motor neurons, peripheral nerves, neuromuscular junctions, muscles, and tendons. Pain, fatigue, and disuse atrophy can also cause weakness. The pattern of muscle weakness will help to identify the site of the pathology and direct treatment. The patient history and the results of sensory, coordination, motor control, cardiopulmonary, and electromyography (EMG) testing will help clarify findings as well.

Several authors[1,2,54] have suggested using the results of resisted isometric testing to determine the type of pathology. The strength of the muscle contraction (strong or weak) and the presence or absence of pain (painful or painless) are used to implicate possible pathologies (Table 4.5). Franklin et al[82] have suggested that a resisted isometric test finding of "weak and painful" warrants expansion to include not only serious pathologies, but also relatively minor muscle damage and inflammation such as that induced by eccentric isokinetic exercise. Intratester and intertester reliability of resisted isometric testing have been examined to determine types of pathology in the shoulder and knee.[83,84]

Manual Muscle Testing

Manual muscle testing was developed by Wright[85] and Lovett[86] beginning in 1912 as a means of testing and grading muscle strength based on gravity and manually applied resistance. Over the years others have described various MMT methods, but the two methods most frequently used in the United States are those proposed by Daniels and Worthingham[87] and Kendall et al.[88] Both methods, based on the works by Wright and Lovett, use arc of motion, gravity, and manually applied resistance by the therapist to test and determine muscle grades. Generally, the patient is positioned so that the muscle or muscle group being tested has to move or hold against the resistance of gravity. If this is well tolerated, the therapist applies manual resistance gradually to the distal end of the body part in which the muscle inserts, and in a direction opposite to the torque produced by the muscle(s) being tested.

In recent editions, both methods recommend applying manual resistance in the form of a **break test** in which the patient holds a joint position until the therapist gradually overpowers the patient and an eccentric contraction begins to occur. Both methods suggest that the break test occurs at the end of the ROM when testing one-joint muscles, and at mid-range when testing two-joint muscles. In addition, many therapists apply manual resistance while the patient moves through the ROM, in what is called a **make test**, or an **active resistance test**, so that the muscle's ability to contact concentrically against maximal resistance can also be determined. In the case of weaker muscles that cannot hold or move well against gravity, the patient is repositioned and attempts to move the body part through a gravity-minimized (horizontal) plane of motion. During all testing, stabilization of the body part on which the muscle originates and careful avoidance of substitution by other muscle groups are emphasized.

Although there are many similarities, there are some differences between these two popular MMT methods. Kendall et al[88] propose to examine individual muscles insofar as practical, whereas the Daniels and Worthingham method[87] examines muscle groups that perform particular joint motions. Some testing positions are similar but others vary between the two methods, with Daniels and Worthingham providing more instruction and emphasis on gravity-minimized positioning for weaker muscle groups. Daniels and Worthingham recommend that the patient move through the arc of motion when testing both against gravity and with gravity minimized. Kendall et al have the patient move through an arc of motion only when testing with gravity minimized; otherwise the patient is positioned against gravity at the middle or end of the ROM and asked to hold the position.

Both methods use a grading system based on the work of Lovett with categories of Normal, Good, Fair, Poor, Trace, and Zero. However, Kendall et al suggest a 0% to 100% or a 0 to 10 scale; Daniels and Worthingham suggest a 0 to 5 scale (Table 4.6). If numerical scoring is used, it is important to clarify which scale is being used by following the score with a slash indicating the maximal value of the scale. For example, a grade of *Fair* strength should be noted as 3/5 if using a 0 to 5 scale, or 5/10 if using a 0 to 10 scale. Results can be noted in a narrative report or on standardized recording forms (Fig. 4.18).

It is important to note that these numerical scales indicate ordinal data, because the intervals between the numbers do not represent equal units of measure. The MMT grades of *Good* and *Normal* typically encompass a large range of muscle strength, whereas the grades of *Fair, Poor,* and *Trace* include a much narrower range. Sharrard,[89] counting alpha motor neurons in spinal cords of individuals with poliomyelitis at the time of autopsy, found that muscles previously receiving a grade of *Good* had 50% of their innervated motor neurons, whereas muscles graded as *Fair* had only 15% of their motor neurons. Beasley[90] noted that patients with

Table 4.5	Results of Resisted Isometric Testing
Findings	**Possible Pathologies**
Strong and painless	There is no lesion or neurological deficit involving the tested muscle and tendon.
Strong and painful	There is a minor lesion of the tested muscle or tendon.
Weak and painless	There is a disorder of the nervous system, neuromuscular junction, a complete rupture of the tested muscle or tendon, or disuse atrophy.
Weak and painful	There is a serious, painful pathology such as a fracture or neoplasm. Other possibilities include an acute inflammatory process that inhibits muscle contraction, or a partial rupture of the tested muscle or tendon.

Table 4.6 Manual Muscle Testing Grades

Grades	Grade Abbreviations	0–5 Scale	0–10 Scale	Criteria
Normal	N	5	10	Full available ROM, against gravity, strong manual resistance
Good plus	G+	4+	9	Full available ROM, against gravity, nearly strong manual resistance
Good	G	4	8	Full available ROM, against gravity, moderate manual resistance
Good minus	G–	4–	7	Full available ROM, against gravity, nearly moderate manual resistance
Fair plus	F+	3+	6	Full available ROM, against gravity, slight manual resistance
Fair	F	3	5	Full available ROM, against gravity, no resistance
Fair minus	F–	3–	4	At least 50% but not full ROM, against gravity, no resistance
Poor plus	P+	2+	3	Full available ROM, gravity minimized, slight manual resistance
Poor	P	2	2	Full available ROM, gravity minimized, no resistance
Poor minus	P–	2–	1	At least 50% but not full ROM, gravity minimized, no resistance
Trace plus	T+	1+		Minimal observable motion (less than 50% ROM), gravity minimized, no resistance
Trace	T	1	T	No observable motion, palpable muscle contraction, no resistance
Zero	0	0	0	No observable or palpable muscle contraction

poliomyelitis were graded as having *Good, Fair,* and *Poor* knee extension when they had on average only 43%, 9%, and 3% of the knee extension force of normal subjects, respectively. Andres et al,[91] in a study of four muscle groups in patients with amyotrophic lateral sclerosis (ALS), found that the muscles were often graded as *Normal* until up to 50% of strength was lost.

The concurrent validity of MMT with muscle strength measured by handheld dynamometers (described in the following section) and strain gauges have been supported by many research studies. Schwartz et al[92] studied 24 muscle groups in 122 patients with spinal cord injury (SCI) and noted correlation coefficients ranging from .59 to .94 between strength measured with MMT grades and handheld dynamometry. Other investigators have reported similar findings.[91,93,94] However, several researchers have noted a wide range of strength values within a MMT grade and an overlap in strength values between adjacent MMT grades, especially in the grades of *Good* and *Normal.*[92,94-96] Manual muscle testing has been

shown to be less sensitive in detecting strength deficits in stronger muscles than in weaker muscles. Although more costly and time consuming than MMT, handheld dynamometry can be used to improve objectivity and sensitivity as needed. When muscles are strong enough to move against gravity and the dynamometer's lever arm, isokinetic dynamometry may also be used.

Generally, intratester reliability of MMT has been found to be good among trained therapists using established methods, with correlation coefficients ranging from .63 to .98.[96-98] The results of studies on intertester reliability of MMT vary more widely. Several investigators[98-102] report complete agreement in MMT grades between testers who examined the same patient to be the lowest, ranging from 28% to 75%. Using a 0–5 scale, agreement between testers within a half grade (plus or minus) was better, ranging from 50% to 97%. Using a 0–10 scale, agreement between testers within plus or minus one full grade was high, ranging from 89% to 100%. Correlation coefficients for intertester reliability

DOCUMENTATION OF MUSCLE EXAMINATION

LEFT					RIGHT		
3	2	1	Date of Examination Examiner's Name		1	2	3
			NECK				
			Capital extension				
			Cervical extension				
			Combined extension (capital plus cervical)				
			Capital flexion				
			Cervical flexion				
			Combined flexion (capital plus cervical)				
			Combined flexion and rotation (Sternocleidomastoid)				
			Cervical rotation				
			TRUNK				
			Extension—Lumbar				
			Extension—Thoracic				
			Pelvic elevation				
			Flexion				
			Rotation				
			Diaphragm strength				
			Maximal inspiration less full expiration (indirect intercostal test) (inches)				
			Cough (indirect forced expiration) (F, WF, NF, O)				
			UPPER EXTREMITY				
			Scapular abduction and upward rotation				
			Scapular elevation				
			Scapular adduction				
			Scapular adduction and downward rotation				
			Shoulder flexion				
			Shoulder extension				
			Shoulder scaption				
			Shoulder abduction				
			Shoulder horizontal abduction				
			Shoulder horizontal adduction				
			Shoulder external rotation				
			Shoulder internal rotation				
			Elbow flexion				
			Elbow extension				
			Forearm supination				
			Forearm pronation				
			Wrist flexion				
			Wrist extension				
			Finger metacarpophalangeal flexion				
			Finger proximal interphalangeal flexion				
			Finger distal interphalangeal flexion				
			Finger metacarpophalangeal extension				
			Finger abduction				
			Finger adduction				
			Thumb metacarpophalangeal flexion				
			Thumb interphalangeal flexion				

*After Hislop and Montgomery

Figure 4.18 An example of a manual muscle testing recording form. *(From Hislop and Montgomery,*[87] *with permission.)*

ranged from .11 to .94.[92,98,99,103] Training to standardize testing positions, stabilization, and grading criteria resulted in higher agreement and correlation coefficients between testers. Global strength scores that average MMT results from multiple muscle groups also resulted in higher reliability.[98,103]

Grade definitions modified from Kendall et al[88] and Daniels and Worthingham[87] are presented in Table 4.6 with additional criteria as to the amount of motion completed by the patient to delineate the grades of *Fair minus*, *Poor minus*, and *Trace plus*. The grades *Fair plus* through *Normal* depend on the therapist's interpretation of what is minimal, moderate, and maximal resistance. A *Normal* grade is typically equated with the normal strength for that muscle given the patient's age, gender, and body size. It should be noted that there is considerable variability in the amount of resistance that *Normal* muscles can be expected to hold against. For example, large muscles in the LE will normally hold against considerable force and be difficult to overpower during a break test, while small muscles of the hand will normally hold against less force and be easily overpowered during a break test. The application of resistance throughout the arc of motion (**make test** or **active resistance test**) in addition to resistance at only one point in the arc of motion (**break test**) may help in accurately judging a muscle's strength.

Handheld Dynamometry

Handheld dynamometers (HHDs) are portable devices, placed between the therapist's hand and the patient's body, that measure mechanical force at the point of application (Fig. 4.19). Patients are typically asked to push against resistance in a maximal isometric contraction (make test), or hold a position until the resistance overpowers the muscle producing an eccentric

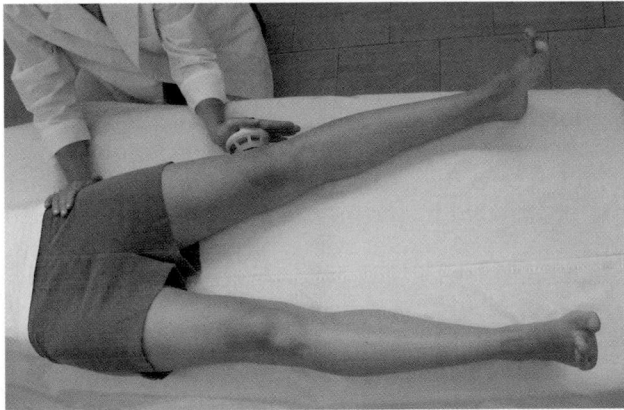

Figure 4.19 Measurement of the strength of the left hip abductors with a handheld dynamometer. The handheld dynamometer measures force at the point of application, which should be converted to torque by multiplying the force by the distance from the joint axis.

contraction (break test). The force measured by the dynamometer will vary depending on the method of applying the resistance (make or break test), the patient's body position in relationship to gravity, joint angle, dynamometer placement on the patient (lever arm), stabilization to prevent muscle substitution, and the therapist's strength.[104-106] Although force values determined with make and break tests are highly correlated, break tests usually result in greater force values than make tests,[107,108] so they should not be used interchangeably.

To reduce the effect of moving a body segment's weight on force measurements, it is recommended that muscle groups be tested in gravity-minimized positions. For example, to test the strength of the hip abductors the patient would be positioned supine so that the muscle action would pull in a horizontal plane relative to the ground (see Fig. 4.19). Soderberg[106] provides detailed information on recommended positions and procedures for HHD. The joint should also be positioned at an easily reproducible angle so that muscle length remains constant. The dynamometer is applied perpendicular to the body segment at an established location on the patient's body. When muscles contract they produce **torque** that creates angular joint motion. The therapist must apply sufficient resistance to oppose the patient's torque to ensure an isometric (make test), or an eccentric contraction (break test). To provide greater resistance than what can be achieved manually, the dynamometer can be attached to a fixed surface[109,110] or an isokinetic dynamometer can be used with the speed set to 0°/sec.

Normative force values for particular muscle groups by age and gender have been reported;[111-115] however, attention must be directed to replicating methods used in the normative studies to ensure appropriate comparisons. Some authors have also included regression equations to take into account body weight and height.[111,112] Most normative studies have reported results in units of force such as pounds, newtons, or kilogram-force. However, these force values will vary depending on the length between the dynamometer's location on the patient's body to the joint axis of motion, or lever arm. A better method of comparison across people would be to use torque.[105,115,116] To determine torque, the measured force is multiplied by the distance between the dynamometer's location and the joint axis. Examples of units of torque are foot-pounds, newton-meters, or kilogram-force (kgf) meters.

For patients with unilateral conditions, it may be helpful to compare results to that of the uninvolved extremity. Andrews et al[112] found no statistically significant difference in force between the dominant and nondominant LEs using a HHD, but did find a difference between the dominant and nondominant UEs. In general, differences were between 0 and 4.5 pounds or between 0% and 11.2% of the average forces generated. Phillips et al[111] found statistically significant differences in force between sides in a variety of upper and LE muscle groups ranging from 0.2% to 8.0%. Sapega[117] has recommended that a difference in muscle force between sides of greater than 20% *probably* indicates abnormality, while a difference of 10% to 20% *possibly* indicates abnormality.

Muscle forces measured with HHD have been compared to forces measured with isokinetic dynamometers to evaluate concurrent validity. Most studies have found good to excellent validity with correlation coefficients ranging from .78 to .98.[118-120] Several investigators have reported that HHD underestimates strength in large muscle groups such as the knee extensors,[121,122] or when forces are greater than 196 to 250 newtons.[118,123]

Depending on the study, HHDs have demonstrated good to excellent intratester reliability, and poor to excellent intertester reliability.[107,122,124-130] Several reviews of such reliability studies are available.[106,131,132] Reliability seems to be better when testing the UEs than when testing the LEs and trunk,[125,127] in particular, the measurements of ankle dorsiflexion and hip abduction.[111,112,122,125] Agre et al[124] found the standard deviation of the repeated measurements expressed as a percentage of the mean force measurements (coefficient of variation of replication) to be 5.1% to 8.3% for the UE muscle groups, and 11.3% to 17.8% for the LE muscle groups. Wang et al[128] reported coefficient of variation of replication ranging from 4.2% to 7.4% for three LE muscle groups. Researchers believe some of the error in using HHDs is due to off-center loading of the dynamometer, difficulties in positioning and stabilization, and limitations in the strength and experience of the examiners.

Isokinetic Dynamometry

Isokinetic dynamometers are stationary, electromechanical devices that control the velocity of a moving body segment by resisting and measuring the patient's effort so that the body segment cannot accelerate beyond the preset angular velocity (Fig. 4.20). For example, the velocity of a Cybex Humac Norm (Computer Sports Medicine, Inc., Stoughton, MA 02071) isokinetic dynamometer can be set from 0° to 500°/sec; the resistance, measured in torque, can be monitored up to 500 ft-lb, or 680 newton-meters.[133] Speeds of 60°, 120°, and 180°/sec are commonly tested in relatively sedentary patients, whereas faster speeds may be warranted in trained individuals. Isokinetic dynamometers can be used to measure the torque produced during isometric (if the velocity is set to 0°/sec), concentric, and eccentric contractions. Isokinetic dynamometers, although expensive and cumbersome, are especially helpful in examining the performance of large, strong muscle groups. In such situations, MMT and HHDs are often insensitive to muscle performance abnormalities.[90,105] Muscle groups acting at the knee, shoulder, back, and to a lesser extent the elbow and ankle are those most frequently tested with isokinetic devices.

Isokinetic dynamometers measure torque and ROM as a function of time. Muscle performance characteristics

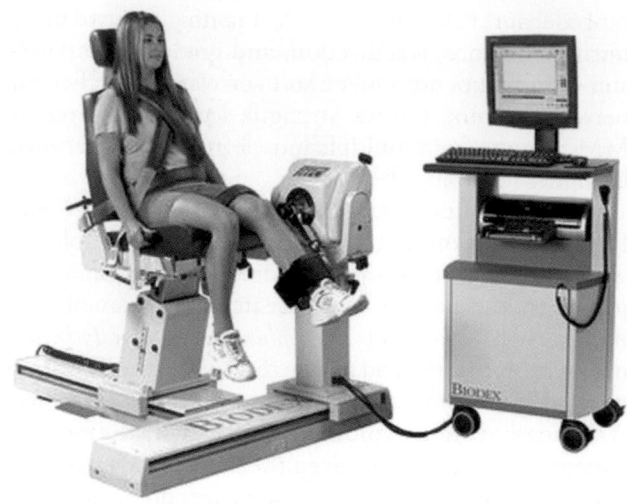

Figure 4.20 An isokinetic dynamometer is being used to measure muscle performance characteristics of the right knee extensors (quadriceps). Peak torque is the most frequently noted characteristic. *(Courtesy of Biodex Medical Systems, Inc., Shirley, NY 11967.)*

most often noted are peak (maximal) torque, and less frequently peak torque/body weight (Nm/kg), and average torque. Work measurements can be derived from the angular displacement and torque values. Power, which is work per unit time, also can be determined. Endurance (muscle fatigue) can be assessed by measuring the time required for peak torque to decrease by 50%.[117] Other approaches to examining endurance include determining: the sum of work performed for 25 repetitions of a motion; and a ratio of the work performed in the last 5 repetitions divided by the work performed in the first 5 repetitions.[134,135]

Peak torque ratios of reciprocal (agonist-antagonist) muscle groups such as the hamstrings/quadriceps and external/internal rotators of the shoulder have been documented. However, careful corrections for the weight of the limb (gravity effects) are necessary to arrive at an accurate relationship.[136-139] If gravity corrections are not utilized, the muscles assisted by gravity will exhibit erroneously high torque values, whereas the muscles that resist gravity will exhibit erroneously low torque values.

It has been suggested that submaximal patient effort can be detected by the increased variability of repeated measures of peak torque, average torque, and slope to peak torque in isometric and concentric contractions.[140-142] However, research in this area has produced conflicting findings and demonstrated large errors in classifying effort into maximal and submaximal categories.[138,143-145] Many factors such as patient pain, fear, or fatigue, and damp settings, preload forces, mechanical artifact, and acceleration and deceleration ramping can affect the variability of torque measurements. The use of isokinetic dynamometer records to form clinical opinions of patient effort is not advised.

To ensure the validity of isokinetic dynamometry measurements, calibration of the equipment is necessary and should be performed each day of testing, at the same speed and damp setting to be used during testing.[138] Proper alignment of joint axis and machine axis, stabilization of proximal body parts, and gravity correction are needed. Several practice trials of the motion to acquaint the patient with the equipment and testing protocol is helpful, and at least one to three maximal test repetitions should be performed before recording measurements.[146,147] It is important to note that torque values will vary with type of muscle contractions (isometric, concentric, eccentric) and changes in velocity settings, joint angle, patient position, test trials, rest intervals, patient feedback, and preload, damp, and ramping machine settings. For example, isometric contractions will result in higher torque values than concentric contractions in the same muscle group, whereas eccentric contractions will result in higher torque values than isometric contractions. Faster velocity settings during concentric contractions will result in lower torque values than slower velocity settings. All of these factors must be kept constant in order to effectively use repeat testing data to judge patient progress. Keating and Matyas,[148] Rothstein et al,[138] Davies et al,[149] and Gaines and Talbot[150] have presented information to improve the validity and reliability of isokinetic testing. Peak torque and work measurements in a variety of healthy and patient populations have shown good to excellent reliability for concentric contractions, and poor to good reliability for eccentric contractions.[146,151-161] Reciprocal (agonist–antagonist) ratios have shown less reliability than peak torque measurements.[161]

Normative data on adults[161-168] and children[169-174] can provide a reference for evaluating and interpreting patient data. However, comparisons with published data are appropriate only when identical procedures and equipment are used, and tested populations are similar. Patient age, gender, weight, height, and athletic participation can affect recorded values. Out of necessity, the involved extremity is often compared to the contralateral extremity. Generally, studies have found no statistically significant difference between dominant and nondominant sides in torque measurements for muscles surrounding the knee joint,[165,169,175-177] elbow,[170,174] and shoulder.[170,178] Alternatively, some studies have found differences due to side dominance for certain motions at the elbow and shoulder especially in highly skilled male athletes.[174,179-182] A difference of at least 10% in torque values between opposing sides of the body has been suggested as an indicator of impairment.[183,184] Others have noted imbalances of more than 10% between sides of the body in healthy populations. Further research is needed to establish the magnitude of difference between opposite limbs that would indicate impairment. At the present time it seems appropriate to use the guidelines provided by Sapega,[117] suggesting that a difference in muscle force between sides of greater than 20% *probably* indicates abnormality, whereas a difference of 10% to 20% *possibly* indicates abnormality.

Special Tests

After completing the patient interview, observation, palpation, and examination of ROM, accessory motions, and muscle performance, the therapist may suspect the nature of the pathology. Special tests, designed to focus on specific conditions in a particular region of the body, may be helpful in confirming the diagnosis. A therapist would ordinarily choose to perform only those tests indicated by previous findings that are relevant to the area of the body being examined. False-positive and false-negative results are possible. However, a positive test finding in conjunction with other aspects of the examination would be highly suggestive of pathology. There are many special tests presented in the work of Hoppenfeld,[3] Magee,[2] Starky et al,[5] and Konin et al.[185]

One category of special tests is used to determine the integrity of ligaments in supporting a joint. The therapist performs these **ligamentous instability tests**, also called *ligament stress tests,* on a relaxed, passive joint. These maneuvers are often similar to tests of accessory or joint play motions. Although these tests focus on ligament integrity, capsular integrity as well as dynamic muscle support may influence the results. If possible, results should be compared with those from the uninvolved, contralateral joint. The amount of laxity is usually graded from I to IV (Table 4.7).[186] Examples of ligamentous instability tests include the *Lachman test,* which examines injury to the anterior cruciate ligament; the *posterior drawer test,* which examines damage to the posterior cruciate ligament of the knee; and the *varus and valgus stress tests,* which examine the integrity of collateral ligaments at the elbow and knee.[2,3]

In addition to ligament instability tests, there are more general tests that examine joint subluxation and dislocation. These tests are often called **apprehension tests** because the patient is placed in a vulnerable joint position while being monitored for apprehension. For example, to test for a history of an anterior subluxation or dislocation of the glenohumeral joint, the shoulder is positioned in 90° of abduction and moved toward external rotation. These provocative tests are considered positive and should be stopped if they begin to elicit patient discomfort.

Table 4.7	Grading of Ligamentous Instability Tests	
Grades	Amount of Movement
I	0–5 mm
II	6–10 mm
III	11–15 mm
IV	>15 mm

The length of muscles that cross and act at one joint can usually be examined in the process of testing PROM. However, some muscles cross and act at two or more joints. Some special tests examine the length of these multi-joint muscles. The *Thomas test*,[34,88] which examines the length of one and two joint hip flexors; the *Ober test*,[34,88] which focuses on the length of the tensor fascia lata; and the *Bunnel-Littler test*,[3] which determines the role of the lumbricles, interossei, extensor digitorum, and joint capsule in limited flexion of the proximal interphalangeal joints of the hand, are examples of special muscle length tests.

Numerous special tests address common conditions affecting the integrity of muscle and tendon structures. These tests typically stretch or contract the inflamed or injured structure, resulting in pain if the tests are positive. For example, the *Finkelstein test*[3] is used to examine inflammation of the tendons of the abductor pollicis longus and extensor pollicis brevis by stretching these structures over the wrist and thumb. The *tennis elbow test*[3] has the patient isometrically contract the extensor carpi radialis muscles against manual resistance. Often the therapist will have previously noted pain, limitation, and possibly weakness during tests for ROM and muscle performance; special tests are used to clarify these earlier findings.

Another category of special tests reproduces the symptoms caused by irritation, compression, or restricted mobility of peripheral nerves. For example, the *Tinnel test* that involves manual tapping over superficial nerve sites is positive for nerve irritation and possible neuroma when pain, numbness, burning, or tingling sensations are elicited. The *Phalen test* for carpal tunnel syndrome places the wrist in full flexion for 60 to 90 seconds to reproduce pain and paresthesia due to compression of the median nerve by the transverse carpal ligament.[2,3] Neurodynamic tests utilize sequential positioning of two or more joints to lengthen and mobilize neural tissue independent from surrounding non-neural structures.[186-188] The ability to complete the sequence of joint positions is compared to the uninvolved side. Once symptoms are provoked, the examiner moves one of the joints out of the nerve lengthening position to determine if the symptoms are relieved and confirm the involvement of neural tissue. However, before conducting neurodynamic testing all joints in the sequence should be tested and cleared for joint and non-neural soft tissue limitations so as not to confound the results.[189] An example of a neurodynamic test is the *slump test* which requires the sequential motions of thoracic, lumbar, and cervical spine flexion, hip flexion, ankle dorsiflexion, and knee extension to assess the mechanosensitivity of the spinal cord, cervical and lumbar nerve roots, and sciatic nerve.[2,80,186] Additional neurodynamic tests have been developed to test the sciatic, femoral, obturator, and peroneal nerves in the LE, and median, radial, and ulnar nerves in the UE.[2,80,186,187,189-192]

In addition to palpating for the quality of arterial blood flow at the brachial, radial, femoral, popliteal, tibial, and dorsalis pedius pulses, special tests can be performed to examine the peripheral circulation of particular body regions. For example, the *Allen test* examines blood flow from the radial and ulnar arteries to the hand.[2,3] *Homan's sign* utilizes ankle dorsiflexion, knee extension, and deep palpation to elicit calf pain, which would be suggestive of deep vein thrombophlebitis; however diagnostic reliability is limited.[2,3]

Additional Tests and Measurements

Depending on findings, other tests and measurements may be indicated. Many of these additional examination procedures are discussed in detail in other chapters of this book. For example, patient complaints of paresthesia or difficulty in muscle performance often indicate neurological involvement that calls for testing of superficial, deep, and proprioceptive sensations (see Chapter 3, Examination of Sensory Function), reflexes and motor tone (see Chapter 5, Examination of Motor Function: Motor Control and Motor Learning), and coordination and balance (see Chapter 6, Examination of Coordination and Balance). Data from these tests together with muscle performance results help to identify conditions affecting peripheral nerves, spinal nerve roots, and the CNS. Therapists must distinguish peripheral nerve versus nerve root patterns of sensory and motor innervation. Manual muscles testing textbooks, such as those by Kendall et al[88] and Hislop and Montgomery,[87] provide extensive information on innervation patterns. Figure 4.21 presents muscle testing recording forms that are helpful in recognizing impaired innervation patterns. Myotomes that are often included as parts of a musculoskeletal examination are shown in Table 4.8, and deep tendon reflexes are presented in Chapter 5, Examination of Motor Function: Motor Control and Motor Learning. Upper motor neuron lesions usually result in hyperreflexia, whereas lower motor neuron lesions involving the spinal nerve root or peripheral nerves usually cause hyporeflexia of deep tendon reflexes.

Impairments in ROM, accessory joint motions, and motor performance may affect activities of daily living (ADL) and occupational and recreational activities. In such cases the examination of gait (see Chapter 7, Examination of Gait), functional abilities (see Chapter 8, Examination of Function), and environmental surroundings (see Chapter 9, Examination of the Environment) is often appropriate. Sometimes findings indicate the need for additional testing by other health professionals such as physician specialists, psychologists, speech-language pathologists, and occupational therapists.

■ EVALUATION OF EXAMINATION FINDINGS

At the conclusion of the musculoskeletal examination, all pertinent historical, subjective, and physical findings are evaluated to establish a physical therapy diagnosis on which treatment is based. A *diagnosis* has been defined

SPINAL NERVE AND MUSCLE CHART
NECK, DIAPHRAGM AND UPPER EXTREMITY

Name _____   Date _____

KEY
- D. = Dorsal Prim. Ramus
- V. = Vent. Prim. Ramus
- P.R. = Plexus Root
- S.T. = Superior Trunk
- P. = Posterior Cord
- L. = Lateral Cord
- M. = Medial Cord

		Muscle	Peripheral Nerves																		Spinal Segment C1–T1
Cervical nerves		HEAD & NECK EXTENSORS	Cervical (D)																		1 2 3 4 5 6 7 8 1
		INFRAHYOID MUSCLES		Cervical (V)																	1 2 3
		RECTUS CAP ANT. & LAT.		Cervical (V)																	1 2
		LONGUS CAPITIS		Cervical (V)																	1 2 3 (4)
		LONGUS COLLI	Cervical (D)																		2 3 4 5 6 (7)
		LEVATOR SCAPULAE		Cervical (V)		Dor. Scap															3 4 5
		SCALENI (A. M. P.)	Cervical (D)																		3 4 5 6 7 8
		STERNOCLEIDOMASTOID		Cervical (V)																	(1) 2 3
		TRAPEZIUS (U. M. L.)		Cervical (V)																	2 3 4
		DIAPHRAGM			Phrenic																	3 4 5
Brachial Plexus — Root		SERRATUS ANTERIOR				Long Thor.															5 6 7 8
		RHOMBOIDS MAJ & MIN					Dor. Scap														4 5
Trunk		SUBCLAVIUS						N. to Subcl.													5 6
		SUPRASPINATUS							Suprascap.												4 5 6
		INFRASPINATUS							Suprascap.												(4) 5 6
P Cord		SUBSCAPULARIS								U. Subscap.	Thoracodor.	L. Subscap.									5 6 7
		LATISSIMUS DORSI									Thoracodor.										6 7 8
		TERES MAJOR										L. Subscap.									5 6 7
M&L		PECTORALIS MAJ (UPPER)											Lat. Pect.								5 6 7
		PECTORALIS MAJ (LOWER)											Lat. Pect.	Med. Pect.							6 7 8 1
		PECTORALIS MINOR												Med. Pect.							(6) 7 8 1
Axil.		TERES MINOR													Axillary						5 6
		DELTOID													Axillary						5 6
Musculo-cutan.		CORACOBRACHIALIS														Musculocu.					6 7
		BICEPS														Musculocu.					5 6
		BRACHIALIS														Musculocu.					5 6
Radial		TRICEPS															Radial				6 7 8 1
		ANCONEUS															Radial				7 8
Lat M		BRACHIALIS (SMALL PART)															Radial				5 6
		BRACHIORADIALIS															Radial				5 6
		EXT CARPI RAD L															Radial				6 7 8
		EXT CARPI RAD B															Radial				6 7 (8)
		SUPINATOR															Radial				5 6 (7)
Post Inter		EXT DIGITORUM															Radial				6 7 8
		EXT DIGITI MINIMI															Radial				6 7 8
		EXT CARPI ULNARIS															Radial				6 7 8
		ABD POLLICIS LONGUS															Radial				6 7 8
		EXT POLLICIS BREVIS															Radial				6 7 8
		EXT POLLICIS LONGUS															Radial				6 7 8
		EXT INDICIS															Radial				6 7 8
Median		PRONATOR TERES																Median			6 7
		FLEX CARPI RADIALIS																Median			6 7 8
		PALMARIS LONGUS																Median			(6) 7 8 1
		FLEX DIGIT SUPERFICIALIS																Median			7 8 1
A Inter		FLEX DIGIT PROF I & II																Median			7 8 1
		FLEX POLLICIS LONGUS																Median			(6) 7 8 1
		PRONATOR QUADRATUS																Median			7 8 1
		ABD POLLICIS BREVIS																Median			6 7 8 1
		OPPONENS POLLICIS																Median			6 7 8 1
		FLEX POLL BREV (SUP. H)																Median			6 7 8 1
		LUMBRICALES I & II																Median			(6) 7 8 1
Ulnar		FLEX CARPI ULNARIS																	Ulnar		7 8 1
		FLEX DIGIT. PROF. III & IV																	Ulnar		7 8 1
		PALMARIS BREVIS																	Ulnar		(7) 8 1
		ABD DIGITI MINIMI																	Ulnar		(7) 8 1
		OPPONENS DIGITI MINIMI																	Ulnar		(7) 8 1
		FLEX DIGITI MINIMI																	Ulnar		(7) 8 1
		PALMAR INTEROSSEI																	Ulnar		8 1
		DORSAL INTEROSSEI																	Ulnar		8 1
		LUMBRICALES III & IV																	Ulnar		(7) 8 1
		ADDUCTOR POLLICIS																	Ulnar		8 1
		FLEX POLL BREV. (DEEP H.)																	Ulnar		8 1

SENSORY

Dermatomes redrawn from Keegan and Garrett Anat Rec 102. 409. 437. 1948
Cutaneous Distribution of peripheral nerves redrawn from *Gray's Anatomy of the Human Body*. 28th ed

Figure 4.21 Manual muscle testing recording forms that aids in determining the site or level of a nerve lesion. *(From Kendall et al,[88] with permission.)*

Table 4.8	Myotomes[2,3]	
Level	**Upper Quarter Myotomes**	
	Action to Be Tested	*Muscle*
C5	Shoulder abduction, shoulder flexion	Deltoid
C5, C6	Elbow flexion	Biceps
	Wrist extension	Extensor carpi radialis longus Extensor carpi radialis brevis
C7	Elbow extension	Triceps
	Wrist flexion	Flexor carpi radialis Flexor carpi ulnaris
C8	Ulnar deviation	Flexor carpi ulnaris Extensor carpi ulnaris
T1	Digit abduction/adduction	Interossei
Level	**Lower Quarter Myotomes**	
	Action to Be Tested	*Muscle*
L2, L3	Hip flexion	Iliopsoas
L2, L3, L4	Knee extension	Quadriceps
L4	Ankle dorsiflexion	Anterior tibialis
L5	Extension of great toe	Extensor hallicus longus
S1	Plantarflexion	Gastrocnemius
	Ankle eversion	Peroneus longus Peroneus brevis

as a label encompassing a cluster of signs and symptoms, syndromes, or categories.[6] The specific tissues causing the impairments should be identified so that treatment can be focused and effective. The therapist must have a thorough understanding of the pathologies commonly affecting the body segment under consideration. The symptoms and clinical manifestations of these pathologies are compared to the current examination findings to establish a diagnosis. Musculoskeletal Practice Patterns listed in the *Guide to Physical Therapist Practice*[6] can assist in categorizing diagnoses into common clusters, and provide information on prognosis, anticipated goals and expected outcomes, POC, and intervention strategies (see Appendix A in Chapter 1, Clinical Decision Making).

Sometimes the evaluation process does not yield a clearly identifiable diagnosis. In such cases, a provisional diagnosis and the alleviation of symptoms and impairments become the basis for treatment. In other instances, the evaluation may indicate the presence of two or more conditions. The therapist should then prioritize and focus initially on the condition causing the most serious impairments, activity limitations, and disability.

The evaluation should clearly determine the baseline for the patient's symptoms, impairments, activity limitations, and participation restrictions. This information becomes the basis of the clinical problem list and guides development of anticipated goals and expected outcomes. The results of future examinations can be compared to this baseline to evaluate the effectiveness of treatment.

In addition to establishing a diagnosis and baseline data, the evaluation of findings should ascertain etiological factors. Unless the underlying causes of the condition are recognized and treated, chronic problems can be expected.[1] The therapist must not only direct attention to the specifically involved tissues, but must also think more broadly of physiological units of function and biomechanics. For example, a patient with a sprain of the medial collateral ligament of the knee may initially respond well to treatment consisting of compression elastic wrapping, ice, elevation, reduced activity, and a protective non–weight-bearing crutch gait. However, if the condition is partially due to abnormal foot pronation, the resumption of normal weight-bearing activities may cause reinjury unless the alignment of the foot and leg is improved with orthotics. Similarly, a patient with supraspinatus tendinitis may react well to rest, modalities applied to the tendon, and gentle glenohumeral ROM exercises, but often also requires eventual strengthening of the rotator cuff, middle and lower trapezius, and serratus anterior muscles, as well as lengthening of the posterior and inferior glenohumeral capsule to restore normal scapulohumeral rhythm and prevent recurrent subacromial impingement of the supraspinatus tendon.

Other information that affects the prognosis and course of treatment should be determined during the evaluation process. The mode and mechanism of onset must be established. Was the onset sudden, gradually acquired, or congenital? Generally, the prognosis is better for a condition caused by a well-defined event than for a congenital condition or one with an insidious, gradual onset. The mode and mechanism of onset also provide clues to help develop strategies for prevention of reoccurring episodes of the injury or condition.

Finally, an analysis of the examination findings should establish the stage of the patient's condition. The stage, whether acute, subacute, or chronic, can indicate how well the patient will tolerate mechanical loads such as those imposed by daily activities or by a therapist during treatment. The **acute stage** is usually defined as occurring up to the first 48 to 72 hours after onset. The **subacute stage** may continue up to 2 weeks to several months after onset. Typically, conditions are considered in the **chronic stage** after 3 to 6 months. Another way of defining the stages, which is probably more relevant to treatment planning, focuses on tissue inflammation and the repair process.[1] Conditions in an *acute inflammation stage* will show signs and symptoms of inflammation associated with hyperemia, increased capillary permeability with protein and plasma leakage, and an influx of granulocytes and other defensive cells. These signs and symptoms include swelling, elevated skin temperature at the lesion site, and pain at rest that worsens with ROM and resisted isometric contractions that even minimally stress the involved tissues. The *chronic inflammation stage* produces signs and symptoms associated with attempts at tissue repair, including an increase in the number of fibrocytes and the presence of granulation tissue; the patient will now have minimal or no swelling and elevated temperature at the lesion site. Pain tends to occur only at the extremes of ROM when the end-feel is reached, or with a moderate to maximal amount of isometric resistance. Tissues in an acute stage will often not tolerate mechanical loading from daily, recreational, occupational, or therapeutic activities. The force, frequency, and duration of treatment procedures must be monitored closely so as not to increase inflammation and worsen the condition. In contrast, tissues in the chronic stage will usually tolerate and require treatment procedures involving more mechanical loading, frequency, and duration to effect positive changes in the tissues. The stage of the condition also adds prognostic information. Typically, an acute condition will show more spontaneous improvement over a shorter period of time than a chronic condition. A chronic condition usually requires a longer period of treatment to promote a smaller improvement in status.

SUMMARY

The musculoskeletal examination provides important information concerning the status of bones, articular cartilage, joint capsules, ligaments, and muscles. The examination process begins with a review of the patient's medical records and a detailed interview. Careful observation, palpation, and ROM, accessory joint motion, and muscle performance tests are typically performed. Depending on the findings, special tests particular to the body region under examination may need to be included. Examination of the peripheral and central nervous systems, gait, functional ability, and the environment is often required. At the conclusion of this process, all findings must be evaluated to determine the diagnosis, baseline status, etiological factors, mode of onset, and stage (acute, subacute, or chronic) of the condition. At this point the prognosis, anticipated goals, expected outcomes, and plan of care can be developed.

Questions for Review

1. What are the purposes of a musculoskeletal examination?

2. What information about the patient's symptoms should be obtained during a patient interview?

3. What are the three types of normal end-feels? What types of tissue contribute to these end-feels?

4. Compare capsular versus noncapsular patterns of restricted motion.

5. Give at least three examples of osteokinematic and arthrokinematic motions. How do arthrokinematic motions combine to produce osteokinematic motion in a typical synovial joint in which the moving joint surface is concave? Convex?

6. Distinguish between muscle performance, strength, endurance, work, and power.

7. Discuss the implications of a finding of *pain* versus *no pain*, and *strong* versus *weak* during the performance of resisted isometric testing.

8. What three factors are important in determining manual muscle testing grades? What would be the criteria for manual muscle testing grades of *Good, Fair,* and *Poor*?

9. What are the advantages and disadvantages of using manual muscle testing, handheld dynamometers, and isokinetic dynamometers to determine muscle strength?

10. What would a positive finding on an apprehension test indicate?

11. What summary information should be determined from evaluation of the musculoskeletal examination findings to develop a clinical problem list, goals, expected outcomes, prognosis, and plan of care?

CASE STUDY 1

A 45-year-old man enters the outpatient physical therapy department with a complaint of right shoulder pain of 1 week's duration. The pain began Monday morning following a weekend of scraping and painting his house. The patient describes his pain as aching and troublesome; his pain is a 6 on a pain scale of 0 to 10. He reports that he is married, and having difficulty in home maintenance activities such as lawn mowing. He is able to perform only 30% of his normal home and recreational activities. The therapist decides to conduct a musculoskeletal examination.

While palpating the shoulder region, increased tenderness and skin temperature in the region of the bicipital groove of the right anterior shoulder is noted. Active ROM of the right shoulder reveals increased pain and some limitations during shoulder flexion, abduction, and extension; all other active motions are pain free and within normal ROM limits. Passive shoulder motions are pain free with normal ROM, except for shoulder extension, which is limited and causes an increase in pain toward the end of motion.

GUIDING QUESTIONS

1. What additional information should be gathered during the interview?

2. What is a capsular pattern of limitation? Does this patient have a capsular pattern of limitation for the glenohumeral joint?

3. The therapist suspects the presence of bicipital tendinitis. Do the findings during testing of active and passive ROM support this diagnosis? Explain.

4. What additional tests should be performed to selectively examine contractile tissue and help to support or repudiate the diagnosis of bicipital tendinitis? Provide a rationale for your selection.

CASE STUDY 2

A 14-year-old girl is referred for outpatient physical therapy 12 weeks after sustaining midshaft fractures of her left tibia and fibula from a bicycle accident. Her long leg cast was removed yesterday. The fracture is well healed. The patient reports her left knee and ankle are stiff and painful when she tries to bend them. She also describes her left leg as weak. At this time she is ambulating with two crutches, weight-bearing as tolerated, with hopes of progressing off the crutches as soon as possible.

GUIDING QUESTIONS

1. On observation, the patient's left thigh and calf appear to be thinner than the right. How can this observation be objectively measured and documented? Why might the patient's left leg be thinner than the right?

2. Passive ROM for left knee flexion is 10° to 70°. The end-feel for left knee flexion is firm. What is an end-feel? What are the three general types of normal end-feels? What tissues could be causing a firm end-feel for knee flexion in this patient?

3. What accessory joint motion should be examined considering the limitation in passive knee flexion ROM? Apply the concave–convex rules for determining the direction of the glide given the shape of the joint surfaces. The accessory joint motion was found to be very hypomobile. What grade should the accessory joint motion be given?

4. In addition to observing, palpating, and testing active ROM, passive ROM, accessory joint motions, and muscle performance, what other testing procedures would be important to include in the examination of this patient?

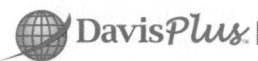 | For additional resources, including answers to the questions for review and case study guiding questions, please visit **http://davisplus.fadavis.com**

References

1. Hertling, D, and Kessler, RM: Management of Common Musculoskeletal Disorders: Physical Therapy Principles and Methods, ed 4. Lippincott, Philadelphia, 2006.
2. Magee, DJ: Orthopedic Physical Assessment, ed 5. WB Saunders, Philadelphia, 2008.
3. Hoppenfeld, S: Physical Examination of the Spine and Extremities. Prentice-Hall, Englewood Cliffs, NJ, 1976.
4. Dutton, M: Orthopaedic Examination, Evaluation, and Intervention. McGraw-Hill, New York, 2004.
5. Starkey, C, Brown, S, and Ryan, J: Evaluation of Orthopedic and Athletic Injuries, ed 3. FA Davis, Philadelphia, 2009.
6. American Physical Therapy Association: Guide to Physical Therapist Practice, ed 2. Phys Ther 81:1, 2001.
7. Pecoraro, RE, et al: Validity and reliability of a self-administered health history questionnaire. Public Health Rep 94:231, 1979.
8. Boissonnault, WG, and Badke, MB: Collecting health history information: The accuracy of a patient self-administered questionnaire in an orthopedic outpatient setting. Phys Ther 85:531–543, 2005.
9. Talley, N, and O'Connor, S: Clinical Examination: A Guide to Physical Diagnosis, ed 4. Williams & Wilkins, Baltimore, 2001.
10. Paris, SV: The Spine. Course notes, Boston, 1976.
11. Coulehan, JL, and Block, ML: The Medical Interview, ed 5. FA Davis, Philadelphia, 2006.
12. Downs, MB, and Laporte, C: Conflicting dermatome maps: Educational and clinical implications. J Orthop Sport Phys Ther 41:427, 2011.
13. Melzack, R: The McGill pain questionnaire: Major properties and scoring methods. Pain 1:277, 1975.
14. Boissonnault, WG: Examination in Physical Therapy Practice: Screening for Medical Disease, ed 2. Churchill Livingstone, New York, 1995.
15. Goodman, CC, and Snyder, TK: Differential Diagnosis in Physical Therapy, ed 4. WB Saunders, Philadelphia, 2007.
16. Levangie, PK, and Norkin, CC: Joint Structure and Function: A Comprehensive Analysis, ed 5. FA Davis, Philadelphia, 2011.
17. Murray, MP: Gait as a total pattern of movement. Am J Phys Med 46:290, 1967.
18. Ostrosky, KM, et al: A comparison of gait characteristics in young and old subjects. Phys Ther 74:637, 1994.
19. Kuster, M, Sakurai, S, and Wook, GA: Kinematic and kinetic comparison of downhill and level walking. Clin Biomech 10:79, 1995.
20. Kerrigan, DC: Gender differences in joint biomechanics during walking: Normative study in young adults. Am J Phys Med Rehabil 77:2, 1998.
21. Rowe, PJ, et al: Knee joint kinematics in gait and other functional activities measured using flexible electrogoniometry: How much knee motion is sufficient for a normal daily life? Gait Posture 12:143–155, 2000.
22. Livingston, LA, et al: Stairclimbing kinematics on stairs of differing dimensions. Arch Phys Med Rehabil 72:398, 1991.
23. Protopapadaki, A, et al: Hip, knee and ankle kinematics and kinetics during stair ascent and descent in healthy young individuals. Clin Biomech 22:203, 2007.
24. Rodosky, MW, Andriacchi, TP, and Andersson, GB: The influence of chair height on lower limb mechanics during rising. J Orthop Res 7:266, 1989.
25. Ikeda, ER, et al: Influence of age on dynamics of rising from a chair. Phys Ther 71:473, 1991.
26. Janssen, GM, Bussmann, HBJ, and Stam, HJ: Determinants of the sit-to-stand movement: A review. Phys Ther 82:866, 2002.
27. Mulholland, SJ, and Wyss, UP: Activities of daily living in non-Western cultures: Range of motion requirements for hip and knee joints. Int J Rehabil Res 24:191–198, 2001.
28. Hemmerich, A, et al: Hip, knee and ankle kinematics of high range of motion activities of daily living. J Orthop Res 24:770, 2006.

29. Safee-Rad, R, et al: Normal functional range of motion of upper limb joints during performance of three feeding activities. Arch Phys Med Rehabil 71:505, 1990.
30. Packer, TL, et al: Examining the elbow during functional activities. Occup Ther J Res 10:323, 1990.
31. Morrey, BF, et al: A biomechanical study of normal functional elbow motion. J Bone Joint Surg Am 63:872, 1981.
32. Ryu, J, et al: Functional ranges of motion of the wrist joint. J Hand Surg 16A:409, 1991.
33. Matsen, FA: et al: Practical Evaluation and Management of the Shoulder. WB Saunders, Philadelphia, 1994.
34. Norkin, CC, and White, DJ: Measurement of Joint Motion: A Guide to Goniometry, ed 4. FA Davis, Philadelphia, 2009.
35. Boone, DC, and Azen, SP: Normal range of motion of joints in male subjects. J Bone Joint Surg Am 61:756, 1979.
36. Bell, RD, and Hoshizaki, TB: Relationship of age and sex with range of motion: Seventeen joint actions in humans. Can J Appl Sci 6:202, 1981.
37. Roach, KE, and Miles, TP: Normal hip and knee active range of motion: The relationship to age. Phys Ther 71:656, 1991.
38. Schwarze, DJ, and Denton, JR: Normal values of neonatal limbs: An evaluation of 1000 neonates. J Res Pediatr Orthop 13:758, 1993.
39. Moll, JMH, and Wright, V: Normal range of spinal mobility. Ann Rheum Dis 30:381, 1971.
40. Chen, J, et al: Meta-analysis of normative cervical motion. Spine 24:1571, 1999.
41. Allander, E, et al: Normal range of joint movement in shoulder, hip, wrist and thumb with special reference to side: A comparison between two populations. Int J Epidemiol 3:253, 1974.
42. Beighton, P, et al: Articular mobility in an African population. Ann Rheum Dis 32:23, 1973.
43. Walker, JM, et al: Active mobility of the extremities in older subjects. Phys Ther 64:919, 1984.
44. Escalante, A, et al: Determinants of hip and knee flexion range: Results from the San Antonio Longitudinal Study of Age. Arthritis Care Res 12:8, 1999.
45. Boon, AJ, and Smith, J: Manual scapular stabilization: Its effect on shoulder rotation range of motion. Arch Phys Med Rehabil 81:978, 2000.
46. Rothstein, JM, et al: Goniometric reliability in a clinical setting: Elbow and knee measurements. Phys Ther 63:1611, 1983.
47. Ekstrand, J, et al: Lower extremity goniometric measurements: A study to determine their reliability. Arch Phys Med Rehabil 63:171, 1982.
48. Sabari, JS, et al: Goniometric assessment of shoulder range of motion: Comparison of testing in supine and sitting positions. Arch Phys Med Rehabil 79:64, 1998.
49. Kebaetse, M, McClure, P, and Pratt, NA: Thoracic position effect on shoulder range of motion, strength, and three-dimensional scapular kinematics. Arch Phys Med Rehabil 80:945, 1999.
50. Simoneau, GG, et al: Influence of hip position and gender on active hip internal and external rotation. J Orthop Sports Phys Ther 28:158, 1998.
51. American Academy of Orthopaedic Surgeons: Joint Motion: A Method of Measuring and Recording. AAOS, Chicago, 1965.
52. Greene, WB, and Heckman, JD (eds): American Academy of Orthopaedic Surgeons: The Clinical Measurement of Joint Motion: AAOS, Chicago, 1994.
53. Cocchiarella, L, and Andersson, GBJ (eds): American Medical Association: Guide to the Evaluation of Permanent Impairment, ed 5. AMA, Milwaukee, 2001.
54. Cyriax, JH, and Cyriax, PJ: Illustrated Manual of Orthopaedic Medicine. Butterworth, London, 1983.
55. Low, JL: The reliability of joint measurement. Physiotherapy 62:227, 1976.
56. Watkins, MA, et al: Reliability of goniometric measurements and visual estimates of knee range of motion obtained in a clinical setting. Phys Ther 71:90, 1991.

57. Clarkson, HM: Musculoskeletal Assessment: Joint Range of Motion and Manual Muscle Strength, ed 2. Lippincott Williams & Wilkins, Philadelphia, 2000.
58. Reese, NB, and Bandy, WD: Joint Range of Motion and Muscle Length Testing. WB Saunders, Philadelphia, 2002.
59. Hellebrandt, FA, Duvall, EN, and Moore, ML: The measurement of joint motion: Part III—Reliability of goniometry. Phys Ther Rev 29:302, 1949.
60. Boone, DC, et al: Reliability of goniometric measurements. Phys Ther 58:1355, 1978.
61. Grohmann, JL: Comparison of two methods of goniometry. Phys Ther 63:922, 1983.
62. Fish, DR, and Wingate, L: Sources of goniometric error at the elbow. Phys Ther 65:1666, 1985.
63. Goodwin, J, et al: Clinical methods of goniometry: A comparison study. Disabil Rehabil 14:10, 1992.
64. Greene, BL, and Wolf, SL: Upper extremity joint movement: Comparison of two measurement devices. Arch Phys Med Rehabil 70:288, 1989.
65. Armstrong, AD, et al: Reliability of range-of-motion measurement in the elbow and forearm. J Shoulder Elbow Surg 7:573, 1998.
66. Pandya, S, et al: Reliability of goniometric measurements in patients with Duchenne muscular dystrophy. Phys Ther 65:1339, 1985.
67. Tucci, SM, et al: Cervical motion assessment: A new, simple and accurate method. Arch Phys Med Rehabil 67:225, 1986.
68. Burdett, RG, Brown, KE, and Fall, MP: Reliability and validity of four instruments for measuring lumbar spine and pelvic positions. Phys Ther 66:677, 1986.
69. Nitschke, JE, et al: Reliability of the American Medical Association Guides' model for measuring spinal range of motion. Spine 24:262, 1999.
70. Gajdosik, RL, and Bohannon, RW: Clinical measurement of range of motion: Review of goniometry emphasizing reliability and validity. Phys Ther 67:1987.
71. Ekstrand, J, et al: Lower extremity goniometric measurements: A study to determine their reliability. Arch Phys Med Rehabil 63:171, 1982.
72. Kaltenborn, FM: Manual Mobilization of the Joints: The Extremities, ed 5. Olaf Norlis Bokhandel, Oslo, 1999.
73. Paris, S: Extremity Dysfunction and Mobilization. Institute Press, Atlanta, 1980.
74. Riddle, DL: Measurement of accessory motion: Critical issues and related concepts. Phys Ther 72:865, 1992.
75. Petersen, CM, and Hayes, KW: Construct validity of Cyriax's selective tension examination: Association of end-feels with pain at the knee and shoulder. J Orthop Sports Phys Ther 30:512, 2000.
76. Chesworth, BM, et al: Movement diagram and end-feel reliability when measuring passive lateral rotation of the shoulder in patients with shoulder pathology. Phys Ther 78:593, 1998.
77. Hayes, KH, and Petersen, CM: Reliability of assessing end-feel and pain and resistance sequence in subjects with painful shoulders and knees. J Orthop Sports Phys Ther 31:432, 2001.
78. Hayes, KW, Petersen, C, and Falconer, J: An examination of Cyriax's passive motion tests with patients having osteoarthritis of the knee. Phys Ther 74:697, 1994.
79. Fritz, JM, et al: An examination of the selective tissue tension scheme, with evidence for the concept of a capsular pattern of the knee. Phys Ther 78:1046, 1998.
80. Kisner, C, and Colby, LA: Therapeutic Exercise: Foundations and Techniques, ed. 5. FA Davis, Philadelphia, 2007.
81. Edmond SL: Manipulations and Mobilization: Extremity and Spinal Techniques, ed 2. Mosby, St. Louis, 2006.
82. Franklin, ME, et al: Assessment of exercise-induced minor muscle lesions: The accuracy of Cyriax's diagnosis by selective tension paradigm. J Orthop Sports Phys Ther 24:122, 1996.
83. Pellecchia, CL, Paolino, J, and Connell, J: Intertester reliability of the Cyriax evaluation in assessing patients with shoulder pain. J Orthop Sports Phys Ther 23:34, 1996.
84. Hayes, KW, and Peterson, CM: Reliability of classifications derived from Cyriax's resisted testing in subjects with painful shoulders and knees. J Orthop Sports Phys Ther 33:235, 2003.
85. Wright W: Muscle training in the treatment of infantile paralysis. Boston Med Surg J 167:567, 1912.
86. Lovett, R: Treatment of Infantile Paralysis. Blakiston's Son & Co., Philadelphia, 1917.
87. Hislop, HJ, and Montgomery, J: Daniels and Worthingham's Muscle Testing: Techniques of Manual Examination, ed 8. WB Saunders, Philadelphia, 2007.
88. Kendall, FP, McCreary, EK, and Provance, PG: Muscles Testing and Function, ed 4. Williams & Wilkins, Baltimore, MD, 1993.
89. Sharrard, WJW: Muscle recovery in poliomyelitis. J Bone Joint Surg Br 37:63, 1955.
90. Beasley, WC: Quantitative muscle testing: Principles and application to research and clinical services. Arch Phys Med Rehabil 42:398, 1961.
91. Andres, PL, et al: A comparison of three measures of disease progression in ALS. J Neurol Sci 139-S:64, 1996.
92. Schwartz, S, et al: Relationship between two measures of upper extremity strength: Manual muscle test compared to hand-held myometry. Arch Phys Med Rehabil 73:1063, 1992.
93. Aitkens, S, et al: Relationship of manual muscle testing to objective strength measurements. Muscle Nerve 12:173, 1989.
94. Bohannon, RW: Measuring knee extensor muscle strength. Am J Phys Med Rehabil 80:13, 2001.
95. Noreau, L, and Vachon, J: Comparison of three methods to assess muscular strength in individuals with spinal cord injury. Spinal Cord 36:716, 1998.
96. Wadsworth, CT, et al: Intrarater reliability of manual muscle testing and hand-held dynametric muscle testing. Phys Ther 67:1342, 1987.
97. Florence, JM, et al: Intrarater reliability of manual muscle test (Medical Research Council scale) grades in Duchenne's muscular dystrophy. Phys Ther 72:115, 1992.
98. Barr, AE, et al: Reliability of testing measures in Duchenne or Becker muscular dystrophy. Arch Phys Med Rehabil 72:315, 1991.
99. Frese, E, et al: Clinical reliability of manual muscle testing: Middle trapezius and gluteus medius muscles. Phys Ther 67:1072, 1987.
100. Silver, M, et al: Further standardization of manual muscle test for clinical study: Applied in chronic renal disease. Phys Ther 50:1456, 1970.
101. Iddings, DM, et al: Muscle testing: Part 2. Reliability in clinical use. Phys Ther Rev 41:249, 1961.
102. Lilienfeld, AM, et al: A study of the reproducibility of muscle testing and certain other aspects of muscle scoring. Phys Ther Rev 34:279, 1954.
103. Escolar, DM, et al: Clinical evaluator reliability for quantitative and manual muscle testing measures of strength in children. Muscle Nerve 24:787, 2001.
104. Smidt, GL, and Rodger, MW: Factors contributing to the regulation and clinical assessment of muscular strength. Phys Ther 62:1283, 1982.
105. Mulroy, SJ, et al: The ability of male and female clinicians to effectively test knee extension strength using manual muscle testing. J Orthop Sport Phys Ther 26:192, 1997.
106. Soderberg, GL: Handheld dynamometry for muscle testing. In Reese, NB (ed): Muscle and Sensory Testing, ed 2. Elsevier Saunders, St. Louis, 2005, p 473.
107. Bohannon, RW: Make tests and break tests of elbow flexor muscle strength. Phys Ther 68:193, 1988.
108. Stratford, PW, and Balsor, BE: A comparison of make and break tests using a hand-held dynamometer and the Kin-Com. J Orthop Sports Phys Ther 19:28, 1994.
109. Ford-Smith, CD, et al: Reliability of stationary dynamometer muscle strength testing in community-dwelling older adults. Arch Phys Med Rehabil 82:1128, 2001.
110. Nadler, SF, et al: Portable dynamometer anchoring station for measuring strength of the hip extensors and abductors. Arch Phys Med Rehabil 81:1072, 2000.
111. Phillips, BA, et al: Muscle force measured using "break" testing with a hand-held myometer in normal subjects aged 20 to 69 years. Arch Phys Med Rehabil 81:653, 2000.
112. Andrews, AW, et al: Normative values for isometric muscle force measurements obtained with hand-held dynamometers. Phys Ther 76:248, 1996.
113. Bohannon, RW: Upper extremity strength and strength relationships among young women. J Orthop Sport Phys Ther 8:128, 1986.
114. Backman, E, et al: Isometric muscle force and anthropometric values in normal children aged between 3.5 and 15 years. Scand J Rehabil Med 21:105, 1989.

115. Van der Ploeg, RJO, et al: Hand-held myometry: Reference values. J Neurol Neurosurg Psychiatry 54:244, 1991.
116. Magnusson, PS: Clinical strength testing. Rehab Management Dec-Jan:38, 1993.
117. Sapega, AA: Muscle performance evaluation in orthopaedic practice. J Bone Joint Surg 72A(10):1562, 1990.
118. Visser, J, et al: Comparison of maximal voluntary isometric contraction and hand-held dynamometry in measuring muscle strength of patients with progressive lower motor neuron syndrome. Neuromuscul Disord 13:744, 2003.
119. Brinkmann, JR: Comparison of a hand-held and fixed dynamometer in measuring strength of patients with neuromuscular disease. J Orthop Sports Phys Ther 19:100, 1994.
120. Bohannon, RW: Hand-held compared with isokinetic dynamometry for measurement of static knee extension torque (parallel reliability of dynamometers). Clin Phys Physiol Meas 11:217, 1990.
121. Reinking, MF, et al: Assessment of quadriceps muscle performance by hand-held, isometric, and isokinetic dynamometry in patients with knee dysfunction. J Orthop Sport Phys Ther 24:154, 1996.
122. Kilmer, DD, et al: Hand-held dynamometry reliability in persons with neuropathic weakness. Arch Phys Med Rehabil 78:1364, 1997.
123. Beck, M, et al: Comparison of maximal voluntary isometric contractions and Drachman's hand-held dynamometry in evaluating patients with amyotrophic lateral sclerosis. Muscle Nerve 22:1265, 1999.
124. Agre, JC, et al: Strength testing with a portable dynamometer: Reliability for upper and lower extremities. Arch Phys Med Rehabil 68:454, 1987.
125. Bohannon, RW, and Andrews, AW: Interrater reliability of hand-held dynamometry. Phys Ther 67:931, 1987.
126. Riddle, DL, et al: Intrasession and intersession reliability of hand-held dynamometer measurements taken on brain-damaged patients. Phys Ther 69:182, 1989.
127. Moreland, J, et al: Interrater reliability of six tests of trunk muscle function and endurance. J Orthop Sport Phys Ther 26:200, 1997.
128. Wang, CY, Olson, SL, and Protas, EJ: Test-retest strength reliability: Hand-held dynamometry in community-dwelling elderly fallers. Arch Phys Med Rehabil 83:811, 2002.
129. Ottenbacher, KJ, et al: The reliability of upper- and lower-extremity strength testing in a community survey of older adults. Arch Phys Med Rehabil 83:1423, 2002.
130. Hayes, K, et al: Reliability of 3 methods for assessing shoulder strength. Shoulder Elbow Surg 11:33, 2002.
131. Bohannon, RW: Intertester reliability of hand-held dynamometry: A concise summary of published research. Percept Mot Skills 88(3 Pt 1):899, 1999.
132. Sloan, C: Review of the reliability and validity of myometry with children. Phys Occup Ther Pediatr 22:79, 2002.
133. Cybex Humac Norm: Computer Sports Medicine, Inc, Stoughton, MA, 02071. Retrieved October 22, 2011, from www.csmisolutions.com.
134. Wilcox, A, et al: Use of a Cybex Norm dynamometer to assess muscle function in patients with thoracic cancer. Biomedical Central Palliative Care 7:3, 2008. Retrieved October 22, 2011, from www.biomedcentral.com/1472-684X/7/3.
135. Cybex Norm testing and rehabilitation system: User's guide. Blue Sky Software Corporation, Ronkonkoma, New York, 1996.
136. Keating, JL, and Matyas, TA: Method-related variations in estimates of gravity correction values using electromechanical dynamometry: A knee extension study. J Orthop Sports Phys Ther 24:142, 1996.
137. Kellis, E, and Baltzopoulos, V: Gravitational moment correction in isokinetic dynamometry using anthropometric data. Med Sci Sports Exerc 28:900, 1996.
138. Rothstein, JM, et al: Clinical uses of isokinetic measurements: Critical issues. Phys Ther 67:1840, 1987.
139. Winter, DA, et al: Errors in the use of isokinetic dynamometers. Eur J Appl Physiol 46:397, 1981.
140. Lin, PC, et al: Detection of submaximal effort in isometric and isokinetic knee extension tests. J Orthop Sports Phys Ther 24:19, 1996.
141. Bohannon, RW: Differentiation of maximal from submaximal static elbow flexor efforts by measurement variability. Am J Phys Med Rehabil 66:213, 1987.
142. Kishino, ND, et al: Quantification of lumbar function. Spine 10:921, 1985.
143. Robinson, ME, et al: Variability of isometric and isotonic leg exercise: Utility for detection of submaximal efforts. J Occup Rehabil 4:163, 1994.
144. Murray, MP, et al: Maximum isometric knee flexor and extensor contractions: Normal patterns of torque versus time. Phys Ther 57:637, 1977.
145. Hazard, RG, et al: Lifting capacity: Indices of subject effort. Spine 17:1065, 1992.
146. Johnson, J, and Siegel, D: Reliability of an isokinetic movement of the knee extensors. Res Q 49:88, 1978.
147. Mawdsley, RH, and Knapik, JJ: Comparison of isokinetic measurements with test repetitions. Phys Ther 62:169, 1982.
148. Keating, JL, and Matyas, TA: The influence of subject and test design on dynamometric measurements of extremity muscles. Phys Ther 76:866, 1996.
149. Davies, GJ, et al: Assessment of strength. In Malone, TR, et al (eds): Orthopedic and Sports Physical Therapy, ed 3. Mosby, St. Louis, 1997, p 225.
150. Gaines, JM, and Talbot, LA: Isokinetic strength testing in research and practice. Biol Res Nurs 1:57, 1999.
151. Molnar, GE, et al: Reliability of quantitative strength measurements in children. Arch Phys Med Rehabil 60:218, 1979.
152. Tredinnick, TJ, and Duncan, PW: Reliability of measurements of concentric and eccentric isokinetic loading. Phys Ther 68:656, 1988.
153. Morris-Chatta, R, et al: Isokinetic testing of ankle strength in older adults: Assessment of inter-rater reliability and stability of strength over six months. Arch Phy Med Rehabil 75:1213, 1994.
154. Emery, CA, Maitland, ME, and Meeuwisse, WH: Test-retest reliability of isokinetic hip adductor and flexor muscle strength. Clin J Sports Med 9:79, 1999.
155. Ayalon, M et al: Reliability of isokinetic strength measurements of the knee in children with cerebral palsy. Dev Med Child Neurol 42:398, 2000.
156. Pohl, PS, et al: Reliability of lower extremity isokinetic strength testing in adults with stroke. Clin Rehabil 14:601, 2000.
157. Hsu, AL, Tang, PF, and Jan, MH: Test-retest reliability of isokinetic muscle strength of the lower extremities in patients with stroke. Arch Phys Med Rehabil 83:1130, 2002.
158. Quittan, M, et al: Isokinetic strength testing in patients with chronic heart failure—a reliability study. Int J Sports Med 22:40, 2001.
159. van Meeteren, J, Roebroek, ME, and Stam, HJ: Test-retest reliability in isokinetic muscle strength measurements of the shoulder. J Rehabil Med 34:91, 2002.
160. Plotnikoff, NA, and MacIntyre, DL: Test-retest reliability of glenohumeral internal and external rotator strength. Clin J Sports Med 12:367, 2002.
161. Kramer, JF, and Ng, LR: Static and dynamic strength of the shoulder rotators in healthy, 45 to 75 year-old men and women. J Orthop Sports Phys Ther 24:11, 1996.
162. Cahalan, TD, et al: Quantitative measurements of hip strength in different age groups. Clin Orthop 246:136, 1989.
163. Murray, MP, et al: Strength of isometric and isokinetic contractions: Knee muscles of men aged 20 to 86. Phys Ther 60:412, 1980.
164. Smith, SS, et al: Quantification of lumbar function. Part I: Isometric and multispeed isokinetic trunk strength measures in sagittal and axial planes in normal subjects. Spine 10:757, 1985.
165. Neder, JA, et al: Reference values for concentric knee isokinetic strength and power in nonathletic men and women from 20 to 80 years old. J Orthop Sports Phys Ther 29:116, 1999.
166. Gajdosik, R, Vander Linden, DW, and Williams, AK: Concentric isokinetic torque characteristics of the calf muscles of active women aged 20 to 84 years. J Orthop Sports Phys Ther 29:181, 1999.
167. Hulens, M, et al: Assessment of isokinetic muscle strength in women who are obese. J Orthop Sports Phys Ther 32:347, 2002
168. Aniansson, A, et al: Muscle function in 75-year-old men and women. A longitudinal study. Scand J Rehabil Med Suppl 9:92, 1983.
169. Holmes, JR, and Alkerink, GJ: Isokinetic strength characteristics of the quadriceps femoris and hamstring muscles in high school students. Phys Ther 64:914, 1984.
170. Weltman, A, et al: Measurement of isokinetic strength in prepubertal males. J Orthop Sports Phys Ther 9:345, 1988.

171. Henderson, RC, et al: Knee flexor-extensor strength in children. J Orthop Sports Phys Ther 18:559, 1993.

172. Ramos, E, et al: Muscle strength and hormonal levels in adolescents: Gender related differences. Int J Sports Med 19:526, 1998.

173. Kellis, S, et al: Prediction of knee extensor and flexor isokinetic strength in young male soccer players. J Orthop Sports Phys Ther 30:693, 2000.

174. Ellenbecker, TS, and Roetert, EP: Isokinetic profile of elbow flexion and extension strength in elite junior tennis players. J Orthop Sports Phys Ther 33:79, 2003.

175. Grace, TG, et al: Isokinetic muscle imbalance and knee-joint injuries. J Bone Joint Surg Am 66:734, 1984.

176. Hageman, PR, et al: Effects of speed and limb dominance on eccentric and concentric isokinetic testing of the knee. J Orthop Sports Phys Ther 10:59, 1988.

177. Lucca, JA, and Kline, KK: Effects of upper and lower limb preference on torque production in the knee flexors and extensors. J Orthop Sports Phys Ther 11:202, 1989.

178. Golebiewska, JA, et al: Isokinetic muscle torque during glenohumeral rotation in dominant and nondominant limbs. Acta Bioeng Biomech 10(2):69, 2008.

179. Aquino Mde, A, et al: Isokinetic assessment of knee flexor/extensor muscular strength in elderly women. Rev Hosp Clin Fac Med Sao Paulo 57:131, 2002.

180. Hinton, RY: Isokinetic evaluation of shoulder rotational strength in high-school baseball pitchers. Am J Sports Med 16:274, 1988.

181. Lertwanich, P, et al: Difference in isokinetic strength of the muscles around dominant and nondominant shoulders. J Med Assoc Thai 89(7):948, 2006.

182. Perrin, DH, et al: Bilateral isokinetic peak torque, torque acceleration energy, power, and work relationships in athletes and nonathletes. J Orthop Sports Phy Ther 9:184, 1987.

183. Mira, AJ, et al: A critical analysis of quadriceps function after femoral shaft fracture in adults. J Bone Joint Surg Am 62:61, 1980.

184. LoPresti, C, et al: Quadriceps insufficiency following repair of the anterior cruciate ligament. J Orthop Sports Phys Ther 9:245, 1988.

185. Konin, JG, et al: Special Tests for Orthopedic Examination, ed 3. Slack, Thorofare, NJ, 2006.

186. Butler, D. Mobilisation of the Nervous System. Churchill Livingstone, Melbourne, 1991.

187. Butler, D: The Sensitive Nervous System. Noigroup Publications, Adelaide, Australia, 2000.

188. Topp, KS, and Boyd, BS: Structure and biomechanics of peripheral nerves: Nerve responses to physical stresses and implications for physical therapist practice. Phys Ther 86:92, 2006.

189. Coppieters, MW, et al: Addition of test components during neurodynamic testing: Effect on range of motion and sensory responses. J Orthop Sports Phys Ther 31(5):226, 2001.

190. Byl, C, et al: Strain in the median and ulnar nerves during upper-extremity positioning. J Hand Surg (Am) 27(A):1032–1040, 2002.

191. Kleinrensink, GJ, et al: Upper limb tension tests as tools in the diagnosis of nerve and plexus lesions. Clin Biomech 15:9–14, 2000.

192. Reisch, R, et al: ULNT2-Median nerve bias: examiner reliability and sensory responses in asymptomatic subjects. J Manual Manipulative Ther 13(1):44–55, 2005.

Examination of Motor Function: Motor Control and Motor Learning

Susan B. O'Sullivan, PT, EdD
Leslie G. Portney, PT, DPT, PhD, FAPTA

Chapter 5

■ OVERVIEW OF MOTOR FUNCTION

Motor control evolves from a complex set of neural, physical, and behavioral processes that govern posture and movement. Some movements have a genetic basis and emerge through processes of normal growth and development. Examples of these include the largely reactive reflex patterns that predominate during much of early life and in some patients with brain damage. Other movements, termed *motor skills*, are learned through interaction and exploration of the environment. Practice and feedback are important variables in defining motor learning and motor skill development. Sensory information about movement is used to guide and shape the development of motor programs. A **motor program** is defined as "an abstract representation that, when initiated, results in the production of a coordinated movement sequence."[1, p. 497] Examples include the complex neural circuitry in the spinal cord known as central pattern generators (CPGs) that control locomotion and gait. Higher-level motor programs can be viewed as abstract rules or code for coordinated actions that are stored (*generalized motor programs [GMPs]*). GMPs contain information about the order of events, the timing of events (temporal structure), the overall force of contractions, and the muscle(s) or limb(s) used in the movements.[1] Sensory feedback from the responding limbs, as well as from the environment, modifies the resulting movements.[1] A **motor plan** (*complex motor program*) is an idea or plan for purposeful movement that is made up of several component motor programs. **Motor memory** (*procedural memory*) involves the recall of motor programs or subroutines and includes information on (1) initial movement conditions; (2) how the movement felt, looked, and sounded (sensory consequences); (3) specific movement parameters (knowledge of performance); and (4) outcome of the movement (knowledge of results).

The cooperative actions of multiple systems allow for accommodation of movement to match the specific demands of the task and the environment. This is defined by *systems theory,* a distributed model of motor control. The central concept is that many systems interact to produce coordinated movement, not just the nervous system. For example, mechanical factors of the musculoskeletal system (body mass, inertia, and gravity) contribute to the overall quality of the movement produced. Cognition (attention, memory, learning, judgment, and decision making) and perception (interpretation of sensation) are also critical. Impairments in any of these interacting systems can significantly alter the quality of the movement produced and the level of function achieved.[2] Another concept is that units of the central nervous system (CNS) are organized around specific task demands (termed *task systems*). The entire CNS may be necessary for complex tasks, whereas only small portions may be needed for simple tasks. Command levels vary depending on the specific task executed. Thus, the highest level of command may not be required in the execution of some simple movements.[2,3] Lateral pathways are involved in voluntary movement of distal musculature and are under direct cortical control (i.e., corticospinal and rubrospinal tracts). Ventromedial pathways are involved in control of posture and locomotion and are under brainstem control (i.e., vestibulospinal tracts, tectospinal tract, and pontine and medullary reticulospinal tracts). The neurons of the ventral horn of the spinal cord are the final common pathway to engage the peripheral muscles for function.

Motor skills are acquired and modified by actions of the CNS through processes of motor learning. **Motor learning** is defined as "a set of internal processes associated with practice or experience leading to relatively permanent changes in the capability for skilled behavior."[1, p. 497] The CNS organizes and integrates vast amounts of sensory information. **Feedback** is response-produced information received during or after the movement and is used to monitor output for corrective actions. **Feedforward**, the sending of signals in advance of movement to ready the sensorimotor systems, allows for anticipatory adjustments in postural activity. Processing of information by the CNS is both serial and parallel, leading to the production of coordinated movement. **Coordination** is the ability to execute smooth, accurate, and controlled motor responses. **Coordinative structures** (synergistic units) are the functionally specific units of muscles that are constrained by the nervous system to act cooperatively to produce relatively stable movement patterns but are scaled to the environment.[1]

Recovery of function is the reacquisition of movement skills lost through injury. The movements recovered may be performed exactly as before. In the patient with neurological damage, it is more often the case that the movements are modified and not performed exactly as before. A determination then needs to be made as to whether the movements are of sufficient quality and efficiency to permit return of function (e.g., the patient with stroke learns to dress using the involved upper extremity [UE]). **Compensation** refers to the adoption of alternative behavioral strategies to complete a task. Movements utilize different muscles and strategies to substitute for the loss function (e.g., the patient with stroke dresses using the less involved UE). The term **neuroplasticity** refers to the ability of the brain to change and repair itself. Neuroplasticity includes "a continuum from short-term changes in the efficiency or strength of synaptic connections to long-term structural changes in the organization and numbers of connections among neurons."[2, p. 84] As learning progresses there is a shift from short-term to long-term memory processes. Memory allows for continued access of this information for repeat performance or modification of existing patterns of movement.

Damage to the CNS interferes with motor function processes. Lesions affecting areas of the CNS can produce specific, recognizable deficits that are consistent among patients (e.g., patients with upper motor neuron syndrome). Individual differences in neural plasticity, recovery, and functional outcomes can be expected. In conditions with widespread damage to the CNS (e.g., traumatic brain injury [TBI]) the resultant problems in motor function are numerous, complex, and difficult to delineate. An accurate picture of the scope of deficits may not be readily apparent on initial examination. A process of reexamination over time will generally yield an understanding of the patient's performance capabilities and deficits. The comprehensive examination focuses on delineation of impairments, activity limitations, and participation restrictions. Those impairments that directly affect motor function and motor learning should be clearly identified. Anticipated goals, expected outcomes, and plan of care (POC) can then be effectively developed.

This chapter will review essential components of examination, factors that may constrain the motor function examination (preliminary examinations), and elements of the motor function examination (with the exception of the examination of coordination and balance, which is discussed in Chapter 6, Examination of Coordination and Balance). Required elements of motor learning and examination are also discussed.

■ COMPONENTS OF THE EXAMINATION

An examination of motor function involves three components: (1) patient history, (2) a review of relevant systems, and (3) specific tests and measures that allow formulation of the diagnosis, prognosis, and POC.[4]

Patient History

During the patient/client history, information is gathered on (1) general demographics; (2) social history; (3) employment/work (job/school/play); (4) living environment; (5) general health status; (6) social/health habits; (7) family history; (8) medical/surgical history; (9) current condition(s)/chief complaint(s); (10) functional status and activity level; (11) medications; and (12) other clinical tests. Information is obtained from the patient and other interested persons (family members, significant others, and caregivers). If the patient is unable to communicate accurate and meaningful information, as is frequently the case with injury to the brain, data must be gathered from other sources (e.g., family members, caregivers). A review of the medical record can be used to verify and triangulate data obtained from personal communications. Often, the medical record of a patient with pronounced deficits in motor function (e.g., the patient with traumatic brain injury [TBI]) is filled with extensive volumes of data that can be unwieldy and difficult to sort through. The therapist can benefit from the application of a framework to identify and classify problems. The International Classification of Functioning, Disability and Health (ICF) model,[5] focusing on impairments, activity limitations, and participation restrictions, provides a useful framework and is discussed fully in Chapter 1, Clinical Decision Making.

Systems Review

A systems review serves the purpose of a screening examination; that is, a brief or limited examination of body systems. The physical therapist can then use this information to identify potential problems that will require more extensive testing. For example, screening examinations for posture and tone may reveal significant impairments. More detailed tests and measures are then required to delineate the exact nature of the problems uncovered. Sometimes screening examinations reveal problems in communication and/or cognition that preclude further testing. For example, a patient with stroke and severe communication and cognitive impairments will be unable to follow directions and cooperate with many individual tests of physical function. The therapist will document this in the medical record as *unable to test at the present time due to severe communication/cognitive deficits.*

Tests and Measures

Specific parameters of dyscontrol should be closely examined using appropriate tests and measures. If the test accurately measures the parameter of performance being examined, it is said to have **validity**. Validity can be established through construct, content, and criterion-based validity (concurrent, predictive, and prescriptive). The **reliability** of an instrument is reflected in the consistency of results obtained by a single examiner over repeat trials (intrarater reliability) or among multiple examiners (interrater reliability). **Sensitivity** refers to the proportion of times that a method of analysis correctly identifies an abnormality as being present (true positive). **Specificity** refers to the proportion of times that a method of analysis correctly identifies an abnormality as being absent (true negative). Therapists should select standardized methods and instruments with established validity and reliability, consistent with the American Physical Therapy Association's goal of evidence-based practice (EBP).

An examination of motor function is a multifaceted process that requires a number of different specific tests and measures. Instruments can be qualitative, utilizing observations of complex aspects of performance. Insights and understanding of patterns of movement or postures are developed from inductive reasoning (formulating generalizations from specific observations). The experienced therapist or expert clinician is far more efficient in reaching decisions about qualitative performance than the novice therapist. Quantitative instruments use objective measurement as a way of examining performance. Documentation constraints imposed by the health care system and third-party payers increasingly emphasize objective instruments as proof of the need for services and the effectiveness of services. However, many aspects of motor function are not easily measured. For example, motor learning is not directly measurable but rather is inferred from measures of performance, retention, generalizability, and adaptability. Thus, these constructs are used to infer changes in the CNS that occur with learning. The therapist must be sensitive to the nature of the variables being examined and identify appropriate measures that provide a meaningful analysis of patient function. It is not likely that any one measure will provide all of the data needed for the examination of motor function.

Reexaminations are performed to determine if goals and outcomes are being met and if the patient is benefiting from the plan of care (POC). Interventions can then be modified or redirected as appropriate. Successful achievement of anticipated goals and expected outcomes is an indication for discharge and referral for follow-up or additional services. Reexamination is also an important quality assurance measure.

■ FACTORS THAT MAY CONSTRAIN THE MOTOR FUNCTION EXAMINATION

Patients who sustain brain damage either through trauma or disease may present with a number of cognitive, perceptual, or communication deficits that can significantly affect how they experience the environment and interact with others. Impairments in sensation and sensory integrity can also profoundly influence a patient's movement responses. It is important to understand how the examination of motor function can be influenced by these factors. Using tests and directions that confuse a patient during an examination or are clearly beyond the capabilities of the patient will only yield inaccurate information about a patient's movement behaviors.

Consciousness and Arousal

Examination of consciousness and arousal is important in determining the degree to which an individual is able to respond. The *ascending reticular activating system* (ARAS) includes core neurons in the brainstem, the locus coeruleus, and raphe nuclei that synapse directly on the thalamus, cortex, and other brain regions. It functions to arouse and awaken the brain and control sleep–wake cycles. High levels of activity are associated with extreme excitement (high arousal), whereas lesions in the brainstem are associated with sleep and coma. The *descending reticular activating system (DRAS)* is composed of the pontine and medullary reticulospinal tracts. The pontine (medial) reticulospinal tract enhances spinal cord antigravity reflexes and extensor tone of lower limbs. The medullary (lateral) reticulospinal tract has the opposite effect, reducing antigravity control.[6]

Five different levels of consciousness have been identified. **Consciousness** refers to a state of arousal accompanied by awareness of one's environment. A conscious patient is awake, alert, and oriented to his or her surroundings. **Lethargy** refers to altered consciousness in which a person's level of arousal is diminished. The lethargic patient appears drowsy but when questioned can open the eyes and respond briefly. The patient easily falls asleep if not continually stimulated and does not fully appreciate the environment. Attempts to communicate

with the patient are difficult owing to deficits in maintaining focus. The therapist should speak in a loud voice while calling the patient's name. Questions should be simple and directed toward the individual (e.g., How are you feeling?). **Obtunded state** refers to diminished arousal and awareness. The obtunded patient is difficult to arouse from sleeping and once aroused, appears confused. Attempts to interact with the patient are generally nonproductive. The patient responds slowly and demonstrates little interest in or awareness of the environment. The therapist should shake the patient gently as if awakening someone from sleep and again use simple questions. **Stupor** refers to a state of altered mental status and responsiveness to one's environment. The patient can be aroused only with vigorous or unpleasant stimuli (e.g., painful stimuli such as flexion of the great toe, sharp pressure or pinch, or rolling a pencil across the nail bed). The patient demonstrates little in the way of voluntary verbal or motor responses. Mass movement responses may be observed in response to painful stimuli or loud noises. The unconscious patient is said to be in a **coma** and cannot be aroused. The eyes remain closed and there are no sleep–wake cycles. The patient does not respond to repeated painful stimuli and may be ventilator dependent. Reflex reactions may or may not be seen, depending on the location of the lesion(s) within the CNS.[7]

Clinically the patient can progress from one level of consciousness to another. For example, with an intracranial bleed, the swelling and mass effect compresses the brain, resulting in decreasing levels of consciousness. The patient progresses from consciousness, to lethargy, to stupor, and finally to coma. If medical interventions are successful, recovery is evidenced by a reverse progression. True coma is generally time limited. Patients emerge into a *minimally conscious (vegetative) state,* characterized by return of irregular sleep–wake cycles and normalization of the so-called vegetative functions—respiration, digestion, and blood pressure control. The patient may be aroused, but remains unaware of his or her environment. There is no purposeful attention or cognitive responsiveness. The term *persistent vegetative state* is used to describe individuals who remain in a vegetative state 1 year or longer after TBI and 3 months or more for anoxic brain injury. This state is caused by severe brain injury.

The *Glasgow Coma Scale (GCS)* is a gold standard instrument used to document level of consciousness in acute brain injury. Three areas of function are examined: eye opening, best motor response, and verbal response. Total GCS scores range from a low of 3 to a high of 15. A total score of 8 or less is indicative of severe brain injury and coma, a score between 9 and 12 is indicative of moderate brain injury, and a score from 13 to 15 is indicative of mild brain injury.[8] The Rancho Los Amigos Scale, or Levels of Cognitive Functioning (LOCF), is widely used in rehabilitation facilities to examine the return of the person with brain injury from coma (Level I, no response) to consciousness (Level VIII, Purposeful–Appropriate). Different levels of behavioral function are described (e.g., confused states, automatic states).[9] See Chapter 19, Traumatic Brain Injury, for a complete discussion of both these instruments.

Examination of the pupillary size and reaction can also reveal important information about the unconscious patient. Pupils that are bilaterally small may be indicative of damage to the sympathetic pathways in the hypothalamus or metabolic encephalopathy. Pinpoint pupils are suggestive of a hemorrhagic pontine lesion or narcotic overdose (e.g., morphine, heroin). Pupils that are fixed in mid-position and slightly dilated are suggestive of midbrain damage, whereas large bilaterally fixed and dilated pupils suggest severe anoxia or drug toxicity (e.g., tricyclic antidepressants). If only one pupil is fixed and dilated, temporal lobe herniation with compression of the oculomotor nerve and midbrain is likely.[7]

Whereas an appropriate level of arousal allows for optimal motor performance, very low or high levels of arousal can cause deterioration in motor performance. This is referred to as the **inverted-U principle** (Yerkes-Dodson law).[10,11] Patients at either end of the arousal continuum (either very high or very low) may not respond at all or may respond in an unpredictable manner. This phenomenon may explain the reactions of patients with brain damage who are labile and lack homeostatic controls for normal function. Under conditions of severe stress, performance can become severely disrupted.

Therapists need to be cognizant of *autonomic nervous system (ANS)* responses. The ANS has two main divisions; the actions of the ANS are typically widespread with multiple systems engaged (Table 5.1) and two main divisions. The *sympathetic nervous system (SNS)* allows actions to be initiated to protect the individual during conditions of stress (*the alarm system*). Motor systems become engaged in carrying out defensive commands, producing *fight or flight responses* (e.g., the aroused patient with TBI may hit or bite). The *parasympathetic nervous system (PNS)* is activated continuously to maintain *homeostasis*. It shuts down when the SNS is activated and works to restore homeostasis afterward.[6]

Critical components for baseline examination include (1) a representative sampling of ANS responses, including heart rate (HR), blood pressure (BP), respiratory rate (RR), pupil dilation, and sweating; (2) a determination of patient reactivity, including the degree and rate of response to stimulation; and (3) a determination of physiological stressors (e.g., environmental factors). Careful monitoring during a motor performance examination assists in defining homeostatic stability. Specific guidelines for the examination of vital functions can be found in Chapter 2, Examination of Vital Signs.

Table 5.1	Effects of Autonomic Nervous System Stimulation	
SNS Stimulation	**PNS Stimulation**
Fight or Flight Response	*Maintains Homeostasis*
Hypervigilance; increased awareness of environment	Decreased awareness of environment
Pupils dilate	Pupils constrict
Heart rate (HR) increases	Heart rate slows
Blood pressure (BP) increases	Blood pressure slows
Respiration increases and quickens	Respiration slows, becomes shallow
Blood flow to muscles increases; blood flow to skin and gastrointestinal track decreases	Blood flow returns to viscera/GI tract
Digestion slows; release of insulin and digestive enzymes slows	Digestion returns
Glucose production and release increases	
Activation of mass muscles	Relaxation of most muscle groups
Sweating increases	Sweating ceases

PNS = parasympathetic nervous system; SNS = sympathetic nervous system.

Autonomic dysregulation is characteristic of certain diseases and conditions and can be seen in patients with TBI, Parkinson's disease, multiple sclerosis (MS), and spinal cord injury (SCI) (particularly injury above T5). Examination of baseline ANS parameters should, therefore, precede other elements of the motor examination in the patient suspected of autonomic instability. Ongoing monitoring is also critical to ensuring that accurate data are collected, as well as to safeguard the patient.

Cognition

A screening examination of cognitive abilities should include orientation, attention, and memory; communication; and executive or higher-order cognition (e.g., calculating abilities, abstract thinking, constructional ability). Abnormalities can occur with neurological disease (e.g., frontal lobe disease, TBI) or psychiatric illness (e.g., panic attacks, depression following stroke). Impaired cognitive function deficits can range from orientation and memory deficits to poor judgment; distractibility; and difficulties in information processing, abstract reasoning, and learning, to name just a few.

Patients with deficits across many or all areas of cognitive function demonstrate diffuse or multifocal pathology (e.g., Alzheimer's disease, chronic brain syndrome). Patients with deficits in only one or a few areas of testing typically demonstrate focal deficits (e.g., stroke).[12] The physical therapist may be one of the first professionals to interact with the patient and should be able to screen for cognitive deficits and initiate appropriate referrals. A referral for a detailed examination by an occupational therapist and/or speech-language pathologist is typically necessary to obtain a complete and accurate picture of these deficits. The reader is referred to Chapter 27, Cognitive and Perceptual Dysfunction, and Chapter 28, Neurogenic Disorders of Speech and Language, for detailed descriptions of examination procedures and deficits.

Orientation

Orientation is the ability to comprehend and to adjust oneself with regard to time, location, and identity of persons. It is examined with respect to (1) *time* (What day/month/season/year is it? What is the time of day?); (2) *place* (Where are you? What city/state are we in? What is the name of this place?); and (3) *person* (What is your name? How old are you? Where were you born? What is the name of your wife/husband?). The therapist records the accuracy of the patient's responses. Findings are documented in the medical record as follows: Patient is alert and oriented × 3 (time, person, place) or × 2 (person, place) depending on the domains correctly identified. An additional domain that can be examined is *circumstance* (What happened to you? What kind of a place is this? Why do people come here?). To answer these last questions correctly, the individual must be able to take in, store, and recall new information. This may be severely disrupted in the patient with TBI. Disorientation is also common in the patient with delirium or advanced dementia.

Attention

Attention is the directing of consciousness to a person, thing, perception, or thought. It is dependent on the capacity of the brain to process information from the environment or from long-term memory. An individual with intact *selective attention* is able to screen and process relevant sensory information about both the task and the environment while screening out irrelevant information. The complexity and familiarity of the task determine the degree of attention required. If new or complex information is presented, concentration and effort are increased. Patients who are inattentive will have difficulty concentrating. Attention deficits are typically seen in individuals with delirium, brain injury, dementia, mental retardation, or performance anxiety.

Selective attention can be examined by asking the patient to attend to a particular task. For example, the therapist asks the patient to repeat a short list of numbers forward or backward (*digit span test*). The therapist documents the number of digits the patients is able to recall. Normally individuals can recall seven forward and five backward numbers. For patients with communication impairments, the therapist can read a list of items while the patient is asked to identify or signal each time a particular item is mentioned. *Sustained attention* (or vigilance) is examined by determining how long the patient is able to maintain attention on a particular task (time on task). *Alternating attention* (attention flexibility) is examined by requesting the patient to alternate back and forth between two different tasks (e.g., add the first two pairs of numbers, then subtract the next two pairs of numbers). Requesting the patient to perform two tasks simultaneously is used to determine *divided attention*. For example, the patient talks while walking (*Walkie–Talkie Test*), or walks while locating an object placed to the side (simulated grocery shopping). Documentation should include the specific component of attention examined, any slowness or hesitation in the response (latency), the duration and frequency of episodes of inattention, the environmental conditions that contribute to or hinder attention abilities, and the amount of required redirection (verbal cueing) to the task.

Memory

Memory is the process of registration, retention, and recall of past experience, knowledge, and ideas. *Declarative (explicit) memory* involves the conscious recollection of facts, past events, experiences, and places. **Motor memory (procedural memory)** involves recall of movements or motor information and storage of motor programs, subroutines, or schema as well as perceptual and cognitive skills. Patients with brain injury and deficits in the medial temporal lobe areas and hippocampus demonstrate profound deficits in explicit memory while they may retain implicit memory, which is more broadly distributed in the CNS motor areas (striatum, cerebellum, premotor cortex).

The length of time required from initial acquisition into memory also distinguishes types of memory. *Immediate memory* (immediate recall) refers to the immediate registration and recall of information after an interval of a few seconds (e.g., repeat after me). *Short-term memory (STM)* (recent memory) refers to the capability to remember current, day-to-day events (e.g., what was eaten for breakfast, date), learn new material, and retrieve material after an interval of minutes, hours, or days. *Long-term memory (LTM)* (remote memory) refers to the recall of facts or events that occurred years before (e.g., birthdays, anniversary, historic facts). It includes items an individual would be expected to know.

A simple test for memory involves presenting the patient with a short list of words of unrelated objects (e.g., pony, coin, pencil) and asking the patient to repeat those words immediately after presentation (immediate recall) and again 5 minutes after presentation (STM).

LTM can be determined by having the patient recall events or persons from his or her past (Where were you born? Where did you go to school? Where do/ did you work?). The patient's fund of general knowledge can also be examined (Who is the president? Who was president during World War II?). The questions selected should represent sensitivity to the cultural and educational background of the patient. It is important to consider that memory may be influenced by attention, motivation, rehearsal, fatigue, and other factors.[11] The *Mini-Mental Status Examination (MMSE)* provides a valid and reliable quick screen of cognitive function.[13]

Patients with **amnesia** experience partial or total, permanent or transient loss of memory. *Anterograde amnesia (post-traumatic amnesia [PTA])* refers to the inability to learn new material acquired after a brain insult. *Retrograde amnesia* refers to the inability to remember previous learning acquired before the occurrence of a brain insult. Patients with *delirium (acute confusional state)* typically demonstrate impairments in immediate memory and STM along with confusion, agitation, disorientation, and usually illusions or hallucinations. Patients with *dementia* demonstrate broad-based memory impairments and learning. Significant memory deficits are also seen in patients with diffuse encephalopathies, bilateral temporal lesions, and Korsakoff's psychosis (thiamine deficiency). Certain drugs can improve memory (e.g., CNS stimulates, cholinergic agents) whereas other drugs can degrade memory (e.g., benzodiazepines, anticholinergic drugs).[7] Patients who demonstrate difficulty in retrieving information will often relate that the information is on the "tip of their tongue" (the *tip of the tongue phenomenon*). Various different strategies can be used to facilitate recall of information (e.g., prompting, rehearsal, and repetition). If attention and memory are impaired, instructions during the examination should be kept simple and brief (one-level commands vs. two- or three-level commands). The therapist should structure or choose an environment in which distractions are reduced (i.e., a closed environment) to ensure maximum performance during the examination. Demonstration and positive feedback can assist the patient to understand what is expected, and can be used to motivate and improve performance. Use of any memory-enhancing strategies during an examination should be carefully documented in the patient's chart. It is also important to remember that diffuse declarative memory deficits can persist while procedural memory for well-learned motor tasks can be retained (e.g., the patient with brain injury remembers how to pedal a bicycle). Documentation should include delineation of declarative versus procedural memory deficits.

Communication

The patient's grasp of information and ability to communicate should be ascertained. The physical therapist should listen carefully to spontaneous speech during the initial examination sessions. The patient's understanding of spoken language can be determined using simple tests. Word comprehension can be determined by varying the difficulty of commands, from one- to two- or three-stage commands (Point to your nose; Point to your right hand and lift your left hand). Repetition and naming can be tested (Repeat after me: Name the parts of a watch). Problems with articulation (*dysarthria*) are evidenced by speech errors, such as difficulties with timing, vocal quality, pitch, volume, and breath control. Problems of *fluency,* word flow without pauses or breaks, should be noted. Speech that flows smoothly but contains errors, neologisms (nonsense words), misuse of words, and circumlocutions (word substitution) is indicative of *fluent aphasia* (i.e., Wernicke's aphasia). The patient typically demonstrates deficits in auditory comprehension with well-articulated speech marked by word substitutions. Speech that is slow and hesitant with limited vocabulary and impaired syntax is indicative of *nonfluent aphasia* (i.e., Broca's aphasia). Articulation is labored and word-finding difficulties are apparent. In some settings, especially the acute hospital setting, the physical therapist may be the first to become aware of communication deficits. Referral to a speech-language pathologist is indicated for comprehensive examination and evaluation (see Chapter 28, Neurogenic Disorders of Speech and Language).

To ensure the validity of the physical therapy examination, it is necessary to identify an appropriate means of communicating with the patient. Consultation with the speech-language pathologist is essential. This may include simplifying instructions, using written instructions, or using alternative forms of communication such as gestures, pantomime, or communication boards. A common error is to assume that the patient understands the task at hand when he or she really has no idea what is expected. To ensure accuracy of testing, frequent checks for comprehension should be performed throughout the examination. For example, the use of message discrepancies (saying one thing and gesturing another) can be used to test the patient's level of understanding.

Executive functions included under this heading include awareness, reasoning, judgment, intuition, and memory. The patient with brain injury may demonstrate an inability to plan, manipulate information, initiate and terminate activities, recognize errors, problem-solve, and think abstractly. The presences of any of these deficits can have a significant impact on learning and performance. Referral to an occupational therapist is indicated for comprehensive examination and evaluation (see Chapter 27, Cognitive and Perceptual Dysfunction). Recognition and understanding of these deficits can improve the validity of the motor function examination and the effectiveness of the rehabilitation POC. Collaboration and consistency of team members can go a long way toward alleviating potential frustrations and inappropriate expectations.

Sensory Integrity and Integration

Sensory information is a critical component of motor function. It provides the necessary feedback for determination of initial position before a movement, error detection during the movement, and movement outcomes necessary to shape further learning. A *closed-loop system* of motor control is defined as "a control system employing feedback, a reference of correctness, computation of error, and subsequent correction in order to maintain a desired state."[1, p. 462] A variety of feedback sources are used to monitor movement including visual, vestibular, proprioceptive, and tactile inputs. The term *somatosensation* (or *somatosensory inputs*) is sometimes used to refer to sensory information received from the skin and musculoskeletal systems. The CNS analyzes all available movement information, determines error, and institutes appropriate corrective actions as necessary. Thus, a thorough sensory examination of each of these systems is an important first step in the examination of motor function. See Chapter 3, Examination of Sensory Function, for a complete discussion of this topic. The primary role of closed-loop systems in motor control appears to be the monitoring of constant states such as posture and balance, and the control of slow movements, or those requiring a high degree of precision or accuracy. Feedback information is also essential during learning of new motor skills. Patients who have deficits in any movement-monitoring sensory system may be able to compensate with other sensory systems. For example, the patient with major proprioceptive losses can use vision as an error-correcting system to maintain a stable posture. When vision is also impaired, however, postural instability becomes readily apparent. Significant sensory losses and inadequate compensatory shifts to other sensory systems may result in severely disordered movement responses. The patient with proprioceptive losses and severe visual disturbances such as diplopia (commonly seen in the patient with multiple sclerosis) may be unable to maintain a stable posture at all. An accurate examination, therefore, requires that the therapist not only look at each individual sensory system but also at the overall sensory interaction and integration and the adequacy of compensatory adjustments. Postural tasks, balance, slow (ramp) movements, tracking tasks, or new motor tasks provide the ideal challenge in which to test feedback control mechanisms and closed-loop processes.

An **open-loop system** of motor control is a "control system with preprogrammed instructions to a set of an effectors; it does not use feedback information and error-detection processes."[1, p. 497] Movements emerge from learned motor **schema** that contain "a rule, concept, or relationship formed on the basis of experience."[1, p. 499] Rapid and skilled movement sequences or well-learned movements can thus be completed without the benefit of sensory feedback. In reality, most movements have elements of both closed- and open-loop control processes (hybrid control system). Absence of sensation degrades movement quality (e.g., the patient with sensory neuropathy and sensory ataxia).

Joint Integrity, Postural Alignment, and Mobility

Joint range of motion (ROM) and soft tissue flexibility are important elements of motor function. Limitations restrict the normal coordinated action of muscles and alter the biomechanical alignment of body segments and posture. Long-standing immobilization results in contracture, a fixed resistance resulting from fibrosis of tissues surrounding a joint, and restricted movement. The resultant compensatory movement patterns are frequently dysfunctional, producing additional stresses and strains on the musculoskeletal system. They are also more energy costly and can significantly limit functional mobility. For example, shortening of the gastrocnemius muscles results in a toe-walking gait pattern; tightness of the hip adductors results in a scissoring gait pattern. Changes in alignment secondary to muscle tightness alter postural control. For example, in standing, anterior pelvic tilting and flexion of the hips and knees are typically the result of hip flexor tightness. Posterior pelvic tilting is associated with kyphosis and forward head in sitting and is typically the result of hamstring tightness. Abnormalities in alignment that alter the center of mass (COM) within the base of support (BOS) place increased demands on the postural control system. For example, the patient with stroke will stand with the weight displaced over the sound leg and away from the affected limb. This patient will be limited in the use of normal postural control strategies. Thus, an examination of the musculoskeletal system is important to complete before an examination of motor function.

■ ELEMENTS OF THE MOTOR FUNCTION EXAMINATION

Tone

Tone is defined as the resistance of muscle to passive elongation or stretch. It represents a state of slight residual contraction in normally innervated, resting muscle, or steady-state contraction. Tone is influenced by a number of factors, including (1) physical inertia, (2) intrinsic mechanical-elastic stiffness of muscle and connective tissues, and (3) spinal reflex muscle contraction (tonic stretch reflexes). It excludes resistance to passive stretch from fixed soft tissue contracture. Because muscles rarely work in isolation, the term *postural tone* is preferred by some clinicians to describe a pattern of muscular tension that exists throughout the body and affects groups of muscles. Tonal abnormalities are categorized as *hypertonia* (increased above normal resting levels), *hypotonia* (decreased below normal resting levels), or *dystonia* (impaired or disordered tonicity).

Hypertonia

Spasticity

Spasticity is a motor disorder characterized by a velocity-dependent increase in muscle tone with increased resistance to stretch; the larger and quicker the stretch, the stronger the resistance of the spastic muscle. During rapid movement, initial high resistance (spastic catch) may be followed by a sudden inhibition or letting go of the limb (relaxation) in response to a stretch stimulus, termed *clasp-knife response*. Chronic spasticity is associated with contracture, abnormal posturing and deformity, functional limitations, and disability.

Spasticity arises from injury to descending motor pathways from the cortex (pyramidal tracts) or brainstem (medial and lateral vestibulospinal tracts, dorsal reticulospinal tract) producing disinhibition of spinal reflexes with hyperactive tonic stretch reflexes or a failure of reciprocal inhibition. The result is hyperexcitability of the alpha motor neuron pool. It occurs as part of **upper motor neuron (UMN) syndrome** (Table 5.2). Increased tonic contraction of muscles is seen at rest, evidenced by abnormal typical resting postures. When movements are attempted, the result is action-induced abnormal movement patterns (stereotyped movement synergies or spastic dystonia). Additional signs include **associated reactions**, defined as involuntary movements resulting from activity occurring in other parts of the body (e.g., sneezing, yawning, squeezing the hand). **Clonus** is characterized by cyclical, spasmodic alternation of muscular contraction and relaxation in response to sustained stretch of a spastic muscle. Clonus

Table 5.2	Positive and Negative Features of Upper Motor Neuron Syndrome
Negative Features	**Positive Features**
Paresis and paralysis	Spasticity
Loss of dexterity	Stereotyped movement synergies; spastic dystonia
Fatigue	Spasms (flexor, extensor/adductor)
	Spastic co-contraction
	Extensor plantar response (Babinski sign)
	Clonus
	Exaggerated deep tendon reflexes (DTR)
	Associated reactions
	Disturbances in movement efficiency and speed; mass movements

is common in the plantarflexors, but may also occur in other areas of the body such as the jaw or wrist. The *Babinski sign* is dorsiflexion of the great toe with fanning of the other toes on stimulation of the lateral sole of the foot.[14-16]

Rigidity

Rigidity is a hypertonic state characterized by constant resistance throughout ROM that is independent of the velocity of movement (*lead-pipe rigidity*). It is associated with lesions of the basal ganglia system (*extrapyramidal syndromes*) and is seen in Parkinson's disease. Rigidity is the result of excessive supraspinal drive (upper motor neuron facilitation) acting on alpha motor neurons; spinal reflex mechanisms are typically normal. Patients demonstrate stiffness, inflexibility, and significant functional limitation. *Cogwheel rigidity* refers to a hypertonic state with superimposed ratchet-like jerkiness and is commonly seen in upper extremity movements (e.g., wrist or elbow flexion and extension) in patients with Parkinson's disease. It may represent the presence of tremor superimposed on rigidity. Tremor, bradykinesia, and loss of postural stability are also associated motor deficits in patients with Parkinson's disease.

Decorticate and Decerebrate Rigidity

Severe brain injury can result in coma with decorticate or decerebrate rigidity. **Decorticate rigidity** refers to sustained contraction and posturing of the upper limbs in flexion and the lower limbs in extension. The elbows, wrists, and fingers are held in flexion with shoulders adducted tightly to the sides while the legs are held in extension, internal rotation, and plantarflexion. **Decerebrate rigidity** (abnormal extensor response) refers to sustained contraction and posturing of the trunk and limbs in a position of full extension. The elbows are extended with shoulders adducted, forearms pronated, and wrist and fingers flexed. The legs are held in stiff extension with plantarflexion. Decorticate rigidity is indicative of a corticospinal tract lesion at the level of diencephalon (above the superior colliculus), whereas decerebrate rigidity indicates a corticospinal lesion in the brainstem between the superior colliculus and vestibular nucleus. *Opisthotonus* is characterized by strong and sustained contraction of the extensor muscles of the neck and trunk, resulting in a rigid, hyperextended posture. Extensor muscles of the proximal limbs may also be involved. These postures are considered exaggerated and severe forms of spasticity.

Dystonia

Dystonia is a prolonged involuntary movement disorder characterized by twisting or writhing repetitive movements and increased muscular tone. *Dystonic posturing* refers to sustained abnormal postures caused by co-contraction of muscles that may last for several minutes, for hours, or permanently. Dystonia results from a CNS lesion commonly in the basal ganglia and can be inherited (primary idiopathic dystonia), associated with neurodegenerative disorders (Wilson's disease, Parkinson's disease on excessive l-dopa therapy), or metabolic disorders (amino acid or lipid disorders). Dystonia can affect only one part of the body (*focal dystonia*) as seen in spasmodic torticollis (wry neck) or isolated writer's cramp. *Segmental dystonia* affects two or more adjacent areas (e.g., torticollis and dystonic posturing of the arm).[17]

Hypotonia

Hypotonia and *flaccidity* are the terms used to define decreased or absent muscular tone. Resistance to passive movement is diminished, stretch reflexes are dampened or absent, and limbs are easily moved (floppy). Hyperextensibility of joints is common. **Lower motor neuron (LMN) syndrome** results from lesions that affect the anterior horn cell and peripheral nerve (e.g., peripheral neuropathy, cauda equina lesion, radiculopathy). It produces symptoms of decreased or absent tone, decreased or absent reflexes, paresis, muscle fasciculations and fibrillations with denervation, and neurogenic atrophy. Mild decreases in tone along with asthenia (weakness) can also be seen in cerebellar lesions. Acute UMN lesions (e.g., hemiplegia, tetraplegia, paraplegia) can produce temporary hypotonia, termed *spinal shock* or *cerebral shock* depending on the location of the lesion. The duration of CNS depression and hypotonia that occurs with shock is highly variable, lasting days or weeks. It is typically followed by the development of spasticity and classic UMN signs.

Examination of Tone

An examination of tone consists of (1) initial observation of resting posture and palpation, (2) passive motion testing, and (3) active motion testing. Variability of tone is common. For example, patients with spasticity can vary in their presentation from morning to afternoon, day to day, or even hour to hour depending on a number of factors, including (1) volitional effort and movement, (2) anxiety and pain, (3) position and interaction of tonic reflexes, (4) medications, (5) general health, (6) ambient temperature, and (7) state of CNS arousal or alertness. In addition, urinary bladder status (full or empty), fever and infection, and metabolic and/or electrolyte imbalance can also influence tone. The therapist should therefore consider the impact of each of these factors in arriving at a determination of tone. Repeat (serial) testing and a consistent approach to examination is necessary to improve the accuracy and reliability of test results.[17]

Initial observation of the patient can reveal abnormal posturing of the limbs or body. Careful inspection should be made regarding the position of the limbs, trunk, and head. With spasticity, posturing in fixed, antigravity positions is common; for example, a spastic upper extremity is typically held fixed against the body with the shoulder adducted, elbow flexed, forearm supinated with wrist/fingers flexed. In the supine position, the lower extremities are typically held in extension, adduction with plantarflexion, and inversion (Table 5.3).[18] Limbs that appear floppy and lifeless (e.g., a lower extremity [LE] rolled out to the side in external rotation) may indicate hypotonicity. *Palpation* of the muscle belly may yield additional information about the resting state of muscle. Consistency, firmness, and turgor should all be examined. Hypotonic muscles will feel soft and flabby, whereas hypertonic muscles will feel taut and harder than normal.

Passive motion testing reveals information about the responsiveness of muscles to stretch. Because these responses should be examined in the absence of voluntary control, the patient is instructed to relax, letting the therapist support and move the limb. During a passive motion test, the therapist should maintain firm and constant manual contact, moving the limb in all motions. When tone is normal, the limb moves easily and the therapist is able to alter direction and speed without feeling abnormal resistance. The limb is responsive and feels light. Hypertonic limbs generally feel stiff and resistant to movement, whereas flaccid limbs feel heavy and

Table 5.3	Typical Patterns of Spasticity in Upper Motor Neuron Syndrome	
Upper Limbs	**Actions**	**Muscles Affected**
Scapula	Retraction, downward rotation	Rhomboids
Shoulder	Adduction and internal rotation, depression	Pectoralis major, latissimus dorsi, teres major, subscapularis
Elbow	Flexion	Biceps, brachialis, brachioradialis
Forearm	Pronation	Pronator teres, Pronator quadratus
Wrist	Flexion, adduction	Flexor carpi radialis
Hand	Finger flexion, clenched fist thumb, adducted in palm	Flexor digitorum profundus/sublimis, adductor pollicis brevis, flexor pollicis brevis

Table 5.3	Typical Patterns of Spasticity in Upper Motor Neuron Syndrome—cont'd	
Lower Limbs	**Actions**	**Muscles Affected**
Pelvis	Retraction (hip hiking)	Quadratus lumborum
Hip	Adduction (scissoring) Internal rotation Extension	Adductor longus/brevis Adductor magnus, gracilis Gluteus maximus
Knee	Extension	Quadriceps
Foot and ankle	Plantarflexion Inversion Equinovarus Toes claw (tarsometatarsal extension, metatarsophalangeal flexion) Toes curl (tarso- and metatarsophalangeal flexion)	Gastrocnemius/soleus Tibialis posterior Long toe flexors Extensor hallucis longus Peroneus longus
Hip and knee (prolonged sitting posture)	Flexion Sacral sitting	Iliopsoas Rectus femoris, pectineus Hamstrings
Trunk	Lateral flexion with concavity Rotation	Rotators Internal/external obliques
Posture forward (prolonged sitting posture)	Excessive forward flexion Forward head	Rectus abdominis, external obliques Psoas minor

The form and intensity of spasticity may vary greatly, depending on the CNS lesion site and extent of damage. The degree of spasticity can fluctuate within each individual (i.e., due to body position, level of excitation, sensory stimulation, and voluntary effort). Spasticity predominates in antigravity muscles (i.e., the flexors of the upper extremity and the extensors of the lower extremity). If left untreated, spasticity can result in movement deficiencies, subsequent contractures, degenerative joint changes, and deformity.

MP: meta

Adapted from Mayer, NH, Esquenazi, A, and Childers, MK: Common patterns of clinical motor dysfunction. Muscle and
Nerve 6:S21, 1997.

unresponsive. Some older adults may find it difficult to relax; their stiffness should not be mistaken for hypertonicity. Varying the speed of movement is an important determinant of spasticity. In a spastic limb, resistance may be near normal when the limb is moved at a slow velocity. Faster movements intensify the resistance to passive motion. It is also important to remember that muscle stiffness with spasticity will offer the greatest resistance during the first stretch and that with each successive stretch resistance can be reduced by as much as 20% to 60%.[15] In the patient with rigidity, resistance is constant and not responsive to increasing the velocity of passive motion.

Clonus, a phasic stretch response, is examined using a quick stretch stimulus that is then maintained. For example, ankle clonus is tested by sudden dorsiflexion of the foot and maintaining the foot in dorsiflexion. The presence of a clasp-knife response should also be noted.

All limbs and body segments are examined, with particular attention given to those identified as problematic in the initial observation. Comparisons should be made between upper and lower limbs and right and left extremities. Asymmetrical tonal abnormalities are always indicative of neurological dysfunction.

A subjective determination of the degree of tone can be made. Therapists need to be familiar with the wide range of normal and abnormal tonal responses to develop an appropriate frame of reference to grade tone. For documentation in the medical record, tone is typically graded on a 0 to 4+ scale:

0   No response (flaccidity)
1+   Decreased response (hypotonia)
2+   Normal response
3+   Exaggerated response (mild to moderate hypertonia)
4+   Sustained response (severe hypertonia)

Modified Ashworth Scale

The *Modified Ashworth Scale (MAS)* is a clinical scale used to assess muscle spasticity that is in commonly used in many rehabilitation facilities and spasticity clinics (Table 5.4). The original Ashworth Scale (AS), a 4-point ordinal scale, was developed as a simple clinical tool to test the efficacy of an antispastic drug in patients with MS.[19] Bohannon and Smith[20] modified the instrument scale by adding an additional 1+ grade to increase the sensitivity of the instrument, making it a 5-point scale. In both versions, the examiner uses passive motion to evaluate resistance to passive motion due to spasticity. The MAS has been shown to have moderate to good intrarater reliability but only poor to moderate interrater reliability.[21-26] Limitations with use of the scale include (1) inability to detect small changes, (2) inability to distinguish between soft tissue viscoelastic and neural changes, and (3) problems with psychometric properties (unequal distances of scores). Agreement on the MAS middle scores (1, 1+, and 2) is the most problematic. Training should be considered to improve interrater reliability between examiners. See Box 5.1 Evidence Summary on the reliability of the Modified Ashworth Scale as a clinical tool for assessing spasticity.

Special Tests

In the lower limbs, spasticity can be examined using the *pendulum test*. The patient is positioned in supine with knees flexed over the end of a table. The examiner passively extends the knee fully against gravity and then allows the leg to drop and swing like a pendulum. A normal and hypotonic limb will swing freely for several oscillations. In patients with quadriceps or hamstring spasticity, the leg is resistant to full extension and when

dropped swings for only a few repetitions. It quickly returns to the initial dependent starting position. The pendulum test can be quantified using an isokinetic dynamometer, an electrogoniometer, or computerized video equipment with high test–retest reliability.[27,28]

Tonic stretch reflexes can be accurately measured using electromyography (EMG). Response to stretch can be documented for various velocities of stretch and spastic co-contraction can be quantified (see EMG section later in this chapter). A *myotonometer* is a handheld computerized electronic device developed by Leonard and co-workers that can be used to measure muscle tone. It provides quantitative measurements of force and displacement of muscle tissue and is able to detect small changes in both extremity and postural tone.[29,30]

Documentation

Documentation of tone abnormalities should include a determination of the specific body segments demonstrating abnormal tone, the type of abnormality present (e.g., spasticity, rigidity), whether the changes are symmetrical or asymmetrical, resting postures and associated signs (e.g., UMN syndrome), and factors that modify (increase or diminish) tone. It is important to remember that measurement of tone in one position does not mean that tone will be the same in other positions or during functional activities. A change in position such as sitting up or standing up can substantially alter the requirements for postural tone. Of great importance is a description of the effects of tone on active movements, posture, and function.

Reflex Integrity

Deep Tendon Reflexes

A **reflex** is an involuntary, predictable, and specific response to a stimulus dependent on an intact reflex arc (sensory receptor, afferent neurons, efferent neurons, and responding muscles or gland). The *deep tendon reflex (DTR)* results from stimulation of the stretch-sensitive IA afferents of the neuromuscular spindle producing muscle contraction via a monosynaptic pathway. DTRs are tested by tapping sharply over the muscle tendon with a standard reflex hammer or with the tips of the therapist's fingers. To ensure adequate response, the muscle is positioned in midrange and the patient is instructed to relax. Stimulation can result in observable movement of the joint (brisk or strong responses). Weak responses may be evident only with palpation (slight or sluggish responses with little or no joint movement). The quality and magnitude of responses should be carefully documented. In the medical record, reflexes are graded on a 0 to 4+ scale:

0   Absent, no response
1+ Slight reflex, present but depressed, low normal
2+ Normal, typical reflex
3+ Brisk reflex, possibly but not necessarily abnormal
4+ Very brisk reflex, abnormal, clonus

Table 5.4	Modified Ashworth Scale for Grading Spasticity
Grade	Description
0	No increase in muscle tone.
1	Slight increase in muscle tone, manifested by a catch and release or by minimal resistance at the end of the ROM when the affected part(s) is moved in flexion or extension.
1+	Slight increase in muscle tone, manifested by a catch, followed by minimal resistance throughout the remainder (less than half) of the ROM.
2	More marked increase in muscle tone through most of the ROM, but affected part(s) easily moved.
3	Considerable increase in muscle tone, passive movement difficult.
4	Affected part(s) rigid in flexion or extension.

From Bohannon and Smith,[20, p. 207] with permission.

Box 5.1 Evidence Summary Reliability of Measurements Obtained With the Modified Ashworth Scale (MAS)

Reference	Subjects	Design/Interventions	Results	Comments
Ghotbi et al (2011)[21]	Tested 23 subjects with LE spasticity and stroke or MS (14 w; 9 m)	Test-retest study of intrarater reliability; MAS scores obtained by one senior PT using standardized test positions; testing 2 days apart; three LE muscles assessed	Kappa (k) value for overall agreement was very good (weighted k = 0.87); mod. for hip adductors, good for knee extension, and very good for PF).	Intrarater reliability with patients with LE spasticity was very good. Reliability for ankle PF was significantly higher than that for hip adductors.
Craven and Morris (2010)[22]	Tested 20 subjects with chronic SCI (C5–T10, ASIA A–D, > 12 mo)	Test-retest study of intrarater and interrater reliability; MAS scores obtained by two blinded raters; ratings taken at same time of day, weekly for 5 weeks, using standardized positions; six LE muscles assessed	Intrarater reliability was substantial to high (0.6 < k < 1.0) for rater A; poor to fair for rater B (k < 0.4); interrater reliability was poor-to-moderate for all muscle groups (k < 0.6).	Intrarater reliability with patients with LE spasticity was very good; showed poor to mod. interrater and modest intersession reliability. Differences existed in abilities of raters. An alternative measure for quantifying spasticity was recommended.
Ansari et al (2008)[23]	Tested 30 subjects with UE and LE muscle spasticity	Test-retest study of intrarater and interrater reliability; MAS scores obtained by two experienced PTs; examined 1 week apart; random order of muscles tested using both UE and LE muscles.	Interrater reliability was mod. (k = 0.514); intrarater reliability also mod. (k = 0.590). Agreement between UE and LE was similar. Agreement on UE distal wrist flexor was significantly higher between rater than proximal shoulder adduction.	Interrater and intrarater reliability was mod. Limbs had no effect on reliability. Researchers question validity of measurements.
Mehrholz et al (2005)[24]	Tested 30 subjects with severe TBI and impaired consciousness	Test-retest study of intrarater and interrater reliability; MAS scores obtained by four experienced PTs; examined over 2 consecutive days; random order of muscles tested using both UE and LE muscles.	Intrarater reliability was mod. to good (k = 0.47–0.62); interrater reliability was poor to mod. (k = 0.16–0.42)	Interrater reliability is limited. Both intrarater and interrater reliability were significantly higher with the Modified Tardieu Scale compared to the MAS. Researchers question the use of MAS as the gold standard for assessing spasticity.
Blackburn et al (2002)[25]	Tested 20 subjects 2 weeks post-stroke; 20 subjects 12 weeks post-stroke	Test-retest study of intrarater and interrater reliability; MAS scores obtained by experienced PTs; testing performed 1 hour apart; testing	Interrater reliability for 2 raters was poor, correlation was .062 (P = .461); intrarater reliability was .567 (P < .001)	Intrarater reliability was mod. for a single examiner; interrater reliability between examiners was poor.

Continued

Box 5.1 Evidence Summary Reliability of Measurements Obtained With the Modified Ashworth Scale (MAS)—cont'd

Reference	Subjects	Design/Interventions	Results	Comments
		repeated 1 week later; three LE muscles tested.		Most agreement at grade of 0; poor agreement on grades of 1, 1+, and 2. Researchers question the use of the MAS
Pandyan et al (1999)[26]	Seven reliability studies identified; four using MAS, two using AS, one using both	Systematic review of the literature of studies on MAS	Intrarater reliability was superior to interrater reliability.	Confusion exists on the characteristics and limitations of MAS and AS. AS scale is an ordinal measure of resistance to PM. MAS is a nominal measure of resistance to PM; ambiguity exists between 1 and 1+ grades. Training should be considered to improve reliability between examiners.
Bohannon and Smith (1987)[20]	Tested 30 subjects (1 MS; 5 TBI; 24 CVA)	Test-retest study of interrater reliability; MAS scores obtained by two senior PTs using standardized test positions; testing several minutes apart; elbow flexor muscles assessed	Interrater agreement was 86.7%, Kendall's tau correlation of .847 (P < .001)	Interrater reliability of a manual test of elbow flexor spasticity was good.

ASIA = American Spinal Injury Association Impairment Scale; AS = Ashworth Scale; k = kappa; LE = lower extremity; m = men; mod. = moderate; MAS = Modified Ashworth Scale; MS = multiple sclerosis; PF = plantarflexors; PM = passive movement; PT = physical therapist; SCI = spinal cord injury; TBI = traumatic brain injury; UE = upper extremity; w = women.

Table 5.5 presents an overview of the examination of DTRs.

If DTRs are difficult to elicit, responses can be enhanced by specific reinforcement maneuvers. In the *Jendrassik maneuver,* the patient hooks together the fingers of the hands and strongly pulls them apart. While this pressure is maintained, LE reflexes are tested. Maneuvers that can be used to reinforce responses in the upper extremities (UEs) include squeezing the knees together, clenching the teeth, or making a fist with the contralateral extremity. The use of any reinforcing maneuvers to elicit responses in patients with hyporeflexia should be carefully documented.

DTRs are increased in UMN syndrome (e.g., stroke) and decreased in LMN syndrome (e.g., peripheral neuropathy, nerve root compression), cerebellar syndrome, and muscle disease. *Reflex spread* (the extension of the response beyond the muscle normally expected to contract) is indicative of UMN syndrome. Because each DTR arises from specific spinal segments, an absent reflex can be used to identify the level of a spinal lesion (e.g., radiculopathy).

Superficial Cutaneous Reflexes

Superficial cutaneous reflexes are elicited with a light stroke applied to the skin. The expected response is brief contraction of muscles innervated by the same spinal segments receiving the afferent inputs from the cutaneous receptors. A stimulus that is strong may produce irradiation of cutaneous signals with activation of protective withdrawal reflexes. Cutaneous reflexes include the plantar reflex, confirming toe signs (Chaddock), and abdominal reflexes. The *plantar reflex* (S1, S2) is tested by applying a stroking stimulus on the sole of the foot along the lateral border and up across the ball of the foot.

Table 5.5	Examination of Deep Tendon Reflexes	
Myostatic Reflexes (Stretch)	**Stimulus**	**Response**
Jaw (CN V)	Patient is sitting, with jaw relaxed and slightly open. Place finger on top of chin; tap downward on top of finger in a direction that causes the jaw to open.	Jaw rebounds and closes
Biceps Musculocutaneous nerve (C5, C6)	Patient is sitting with arm flexed and supported. Place thumb over the biceps tendon in the cubital fossa, stretching it slightly. Tap thumb or directly on tendon.	Slight contraction of elbow flexors
Brachioradialis (supinator) Radial nerve (C5, C6)	Patient is sitting with arm flexed onto the abdomen. Place finger on the radial tuberosity and tap finger with hammer.	Slight contraction of elbow flexors, slight wrist extension or radial deviation
Triceps Radial nerve (C6, C7)	Patient is sitting with arm supported in abduction, elbow flexed. Palpate triceps tendon just above olecranon. Tap directly on tendon.	Slight contraction of elbow extensors
Finger flexors Median nerve (C6–T1)	Hold hand in neutral position. Place finger across palmar surface of distal phalanges of four fingers and tap.	Slight contraction of finger flexors
Hamstrings Tibial branch, sciatic nerve (L5, S1, S2)	Patient is prone with knee semiflexed and supported. Palpate tendon at the knee. Tap on finger or directly on tendon.	Slight contraction of knee flexors
Quadriceps (patellar, knee jerk) Femoral nerve (L2, L3, L4)	Patient is sitting with knee flexed, foot unsupported. Tap tendon of quadriceps muscle between the patella and tibial tuberosity.	Slight contraction of knee extensors
Achilles (ankle jerk) Tibial (S1–S2)	Patient is prone with foot over the end of the plinth or sitting with knee flexed and foot held in slight dorsiflexion. Tap tendon just above its insertion on the calcaneus. Maintaining slight tension on the gastrocnemius-soleus group improves the response.	Slight contraction of plantarflexors

A normal response consists of flexion of the big toe; sometimes the other toes will demonstrate a downgoing (flexion) response, or no response at all. An abnormal response (positive Babinski sign) consists of extension dorsiflexion (upgoing) of the big toe, with fanning of the lateral four toes. It is indicative of a corticospinal (UMN) lesion. The *Chaddock's reflex (or sign)* is elicited by stroking around the lateral ankle and up the lateral dorsal aspect of the foot. It also produces extension dorsiflexion of the big toe and is considered a confirmatory toe sign. The *abdominal reflex* is elicited with brisk, light strokes over the skin of the abdominal muscles. A localized contraction under the stimulus is produced, with a resultant deviation of the umbilicus toward the area stimulated. Each quadrant should be tested in a diagonal direction. Umbilical deviation in a superior/lateral direction indicates integrity of spinal segments T8 to T9. Umbilical deviation in an inferior/lateral direction indicates integrity of spinal segments T10 to T12. Loss of response is abnormal and indicative of pathology (e.g., thoracic spinal cord injury). Asymmetry from side to side is highly significant with respect to neurological disease. Abdominal reflexes may be absent with in patients with obesity or abdominal surgeries. Table 5.6 presents an overview of the examination of superficial cutaneous reflexes.

Primitive and Tonic Reflexes

Primitive and *tonic reflexes* are present during infancy as a stage in normal development and become integrated by the CNS at an early age. Once integrated, these reflexes are not generally recognizable in adults in their pure form. They may continue, however, as adaptive fragments of behavior, underlying normal motor control. Persistent reflexes (sometimes termed *obligatory reflexes*) beyond the expected age of development or appearing in adult patients following brain injury are always indicative of neurological involvement. Patients who exhibit these reflexes typically present with extensive brain damage (e.g., stroke, TBI) and other UMN signs.

Reflexes important to examine in the patient suspected of abnormal reflex activity include flexor withdrawal, traction, grasp, tonic neck, tonic labyrinthine, positive support, and associated reactions. *Flexor withdrawal reflex*

Table 5.6	Examination of Superficial Cutaneous Reflexes	
Superficial Reflexes (Cutaneous)	**Stimulus**	**Response**
Plantar (S1, S2)	With blunt object (key or wooden end of applicator stick), stroke the lateral aspect of the sole, moving from the heel to the ball of the foot, curving medially across the ball of the foot.	Normal response is flexion (plantarflexion) of the great toe, and sometimes the other toes (negative Babinski sign). Abnormal response, termed a **positive Babinski sign**, is extension (dorsiflexion) of the great toe with fanning of the four other toes (indicates UMN lesions).
	Alternate stimuli for plantar (for sensitive feet): • Chaddock: stroke lateral ankle and lateral aspect of foot. • Oppenheim: stroke down tibial crest	Same as for plantar.
Abdominal reflexes	Position patient in supine, relaxed. Make brisk, light stroke over each quadrant of the abdominals from the periphery to the umbilicus.	Localized contraction under the stimulus, causing the umbilicus to move toward the stimulus.
Above umbilicus = T8–T10		Masked by obesity.
Below umbilicus = T10–T12		Can be absent in both UMN and LMN disorders.

is generally the simplest to observe and is judged by appearance of an overt movement response. *Tonic neck reflexes,* on the other hand, bias the musculature and may not be visible through overt movement responses. In fact, movement is rarely produced but rather posture is typically influenced through tonal adjustments. Thus, the term *tuning reflexes* is an appropriate description of their function. Abnormal postures should be examined for their reflex dependence (e.g., the patient with brain injury exhibits excessive extensor tone in supine but not in side lying). To obtain an accurate examination, the therapist must be concerned with several factors. The patient must be positioned appropriately to allow for the expected response. An adequate test stimulus is essential, including both an adequate magnitude and duration of stimulation. Keen observation skills are needed to detect what may be subtle movement changes and abnormal responses. Palpation skills can assist in identifying tonal changes not readily apparent to the eye. Primitive and tonic reflexes are graded using a 0 to 4+ scale:[31,32]

0+   Absent
1+   Tone change: slight, transient with no movement of the extremities
2+   Visible movement of extremities
3+   Exaggerated, full movement of extremities
4+   Obligatory and sustained movement, lasting for more than 30 seconds

Table 5.7 presents an overview of the examination of primitive and tonic reflexes.

Documentation of Reflex Integrity

Documentation of reflex abnormalities should include a determination of (1) specific reflexes tested, (2) the degree of abnormality observed, (3) associated signs (e.g., UMN syndrome), and (4) factors that modify reflexes. Of great importance is a description of the effects of abnormal reflex behavior on active movements, posture, and function.

Cranial Nerve Integrity

There are 12 pairs of cranial nerves (CNs), all distributed to the head and neck with the exception of CN X (vagus), which is distributed to the thorax and abdomen. CNs I, II, and VIII are purely sensory and carry the special senses of smell, vision, hearing, and equilibrium. Cranial nerves III, IV, and VI are purely motor and control pupillary constriction and eye movements. Cranial nerves XI and XII are also purely motor, innervating the sternocleidomastoid, trapezius, and tongue muscles. Cranial nerves V, VII, IX, and X are mixed, containing both motor and sensory fibers. Motor functions include chewing (V), facial expression (VII), swallowing (IX, X), and vocal sounds (X). Sensations are carried from the face and head (V, VII, IX), alimentary tract, heart, vessels, and lungs (IX, X), and tongue, mouth, and palate (VII, IX, X). Parasympathetic secretomotor fibers (ANS) are carried by CN III for control of smooth muscles in the eyeball, VII for control of salivary and lacrimal glands, IX to the parotid salivary

Table 5.7   Examination of Primitive and Tonic Reflexes

Primitive/Spinal Reflexes	Stimulus	Response
Flexor withdrawal	Noxious stimulus (pinprick) to sole of foot. Tested in supine or sitting position.	Toes extend, foot dorsiflexes, entire LE flexes uncontrollably. Onset: 28 weeks of gestation. Integrated: 1–2 months.
Crossed extension	Noxious stimulus to ball of foot of LE fixed in extension; tested in supine position.	Opposite LE flexes, then adducts and extends. Onset: 28 weeks of gestation. Integrated: 1–2 months.
Traction	Grasp forearm and pull up from supine into sitting position.	Grasp and total flexion of the UE. Onset: 28 weeks of gestation. Integrated: 2–5 months.
Moro	Sudden change in position of head in relation to trunk; drop patient backward from sitting position.	Extension, abduction of UEs, hand opening, and crying followed by flexion, adduction of arms across chest. Onset: 28 weeks of gestation. Integrated: 5–6 months.
Startle	Sudden loud or harsh noise.	Sudden extension or abduction of UEs, crying. Onset: birth. Integrated: persists.
Grasp	Maintained pressure to palm of hand (palmar grasp) or to ball of foot under toes (plantar grasp).	Maintained flexion of fingers or toes. Onset: palmar, birth; plantar, 28 weeks of gestation. Integrated: palmer, 4–6 months; plantar, 9 months.

Tonic/Brainstem Reflexes	Stimulus	Response
Asymmetrical tonic neck (ATNR)	Rotation of the head to one side.	Flexion of skull limbs, extension of the jaw limbs, "bow and arrow" or "fencing" posture. Onset: birth. Integrated: 4–6 months.
Symmetrical tonic neck (STNR)	Flexion or extension of the head.	With head flexion: flexion of UEs, extension of LEs; with head extension: extension of UEs, flexion of LEs. Onset: 4–6 months. Integrated: 8–12 months.
Symmetrical tonic labyrinthine (TLR or STLR)	Prone or supine position.	With prone position: increased flexor tone/flexion of all limbs; with supine: increased extensor tone/extension of all limbs. Onset: birth. Integrated: 6 months.
Positive supporting	Contact to the ball of the foot in upright standing position.	Rigid extension (co-contraction) of the LEs. Onset: birth. Integrated: 6 months.
Associated reactions	Resisted voluntary movement in any part of the body.	Involuntary movement in a resting extremity. Onset: birth–3 months. Integrated: 8–9 years.

LE = lower extremity; UE = upper extremity.

gland, and X to the heart, lungs, and most of the digestive system.

An examination of CN function should be performed with suspected lesions of the brain, brainstem, and cervical spine. Deficits in olfactory function (CN I) should be suspected with lesions of the nasal cavity and anterior/inferior cerebrum. Lesions of the optic pathways (optic nerve [CN II], optic chiasma, optic tract, lateral geniculate body, superior colliculus) and visual cortex may produce visual deficits. Midbrain (mesencephalic) lesions may result in deficits of CNs III and IV (oculomotor, trochlear). Pontine lesions may involve several CNs, including V (ophthalmic, maxillary, and mandibular branches) and VI (abducens). Nuclei of CNs VII (facial) and VIII (vestibular and cochlear branches) are located at the junction of the pons and medulla. Lesions affecting the medulla may involve CNs IX (glossopharyngeal), X (vagus), XI (spinal accessory), and XII (hypoglossal). The spinal root of XI is found in the upper five cervical segments. The CNs, their function, clinical tests, and possible abnormal findings are presented in Table 5.8.

Documentation of Cranial Nerve Integrity

Documentation of an examination of CN integrity should include a determination of (1) specific cranial nerves tested, (2) the degree of abnormality observed (specific deficits), and (3) the effects of abnormal cranial nerve integrity on function. The patient's perceptions of loss of function should also be identified.

Muscle Performance
Muscle Atrophy

Atrophy, the loss of muscle bulk (wasting), occurs as a result of the loss of functional mobility (disuse atrophy), LMN disease (neurogenic atrophy), or protein-calorie malnutrition. *Disuse atrophy* is evident after periods of inactivity, developing in weeks or months. It is generally widespread and affects antigravity muscles to a greater extent. Strength can be negatively influenced by disuse atrophy. The lack of resistive load on muscle reduces the overall number of sarcomeres and results in diminished capacity of muscle for developing torque (contractile strength). It also results in reduced passive tension of

Table 5.8	Examination of Cranial Nerve Integrity		
Cranial Nerve	**Function**	**Test**	**Possible Abnormal Findings**
I Olfactory	Smell	Test sense of smell on each side (close off other nostril): use common, nonirritating odors.	Anosmia (inability to detect smells), seen with frontal lobe lesions
II Optic	Vision	Test visual acuity. Central: Snellen eye chart; test each eye separately (covering other eye); test at distance of 20 ft. Test peripheral vision (visual fields) by confrontation.	Blindness, myopia (impaired far vision), presbyopia (impaired near vision) Field defects: homonymous hemianopsia
II, III Optic and oculomotor	Pupillary reflexes	Test pupillary reactions (constriction) by shining light in eye light; if abnormal, test near reaction. Examine pupillary size/shape.	Absence of pupillary constriction Anisocoria (unequal pupils) Horner's syndrome, CN III paralysis
III, IV, VI Oculomotor, trochlear, and abducens	Extraocular movements	Test saccadic (patient is asked to look in each direction) and pursuit eye movements (patient follows moving finger).	Strabismus (eye deviates from normal conjugate position) Impaired eye movements Double vision
III	Medial, superior, and inferior rectus: inferior oblique; turns eye up, down, in. Elevates eyelid.	Observe position of eye. Test eye movements.	Strabismus: eye pulled outward by CN VI Eye cannot look upward, downward, inward movements. May see ptosis, pupillary dilation.
IV	Superior oblique: turns eye down when adducted.	Test eye movements.	Eye cannot look down when eye is adducted.
VI	Lateral rectus: turns eye out.	Observe position of eye. Test eye movements.	Esotropia (eye pulled inward) Eye cannot look out.

Table 5.8	Examination of Cranial Nerve Integrity—cont'd		
Cranial Nerve	**Function**	**Test**	**Possible Abnormal Findings**
V Trigeminal Ophthalmic, maxillary, mandibular divisions	Sensory: face	Test pain, light touch sensations: forehead, cheeks, jaw (eyes closed). Test corneal reflex: touch lightly with wisp of cotton.	Loss of facial sensations, numbness with CN V lesion Trigger area with trigeminal neuralgia Loss of corneal reflex ipsilaterally (blinking in response to corneal touch)
	Sensory: cornea Motor: muscles of mastication	Palpate temporal and masseter muscles. Observe spontaneous movements. Have patient clench teeth, hold against resistance.	Weakness, wasting of muscles When opened, deviation of jaw to ipsilateral side
VII Facial	Facial expression	Test motor function facial muscles. Raise eyebrows, frown. Show teeth, smile. Close eyes tightly. Puff out both cheeks.	Paralysis: Inability to close eye, Drooping corner of mouth, Difficulty with speech articulation Unilateral LMN: Bell's palsy (PNI) Bilateral LMN: Guillain-Barré Unilateral UMN: stroke
	Taste to anterior two thirds of tongue	Apply saline solution and sugar solution using a cotton swab.	Incorrectly identifies solution.
VIII Vestibulocochlear (acoustic)	Vestibular function	Test balance: vestibulospinal function (VSR). Test eye–head coordination: vestibular ocular reflex (VOR).	Vertigo, dysequilibrium Gaze instability with head rotations, nystagmus (constant, involuntary cyclical movement of the eyeball)
	Cochlear function	Test auditory acuity. Test for lateralization (Weber test): place vibrating tuning fork on top of head, mid-position; check if sound heard in one ear, or equally in both.	Deafness, impaired hearing, tinnitus Unilateral conductive loss: sound lateralized to impaired ear Sensorineural loss: sound heard in good ear
		Compare air and bone conduction (Rinne test): place vibrating tuning fork on mastoid bone, then close to ear canal; sound heard longer through air than bone.	Conductive loss: sound heard through bone is equal to or longer than air Sensorineural loss: sound heard longer through air
IX Glossopharyngeal	Sensory to posterior one third of tongue, pharynx, middle ear	Apply saline solution and sugar solution. Not typically tested	Incorrectly identifies solution.
IX, X Glossopharyngeal and vagus	Phonation Swallowing	Listen to voice quality. Examine for difficulty in swallowing glass of water.	Dysphonia: hoarseness denotes vocal cord weakness; nasal quality denotes palatal weakness. Dysphagia
	Palatal, pharynx control	Have patient say "ah"; observe motion of soft palate (elevates) and position of uvula (remains midline).	Paralysis: palate fails to elevate (lesion of CN X); asymmetrical elevation with unilateral paralysis
	Gag reflex	Stimulate back of throat lightly on each side.	Absent reflex: lesion of CN IX; possibly CN X

Continued

Table 5.8	Examination of Cranial Nerve Integrity—cont'd		
Cranial Nerve	**Function**	**Test**	**Possible Abnormal Findings**
XI Spinal accessory	Motor function: Trapezius muscle	Examine bulk, strength. Shrug both shoulders upward against resistance.	LMN: atrophy, fasciculations, ipsilateral weakness Inability to shrug ipsilateral shoulder; shoulder droops
	Sternocleidomastoid	Turn head to each side against resistance.	Inability to turn head to opposite side UMN: weakness of ipsilateral sternocleidomastoid and contralateral trapezius
XII Hypoglossal	Tongue movements	Listen to patient's articulation.	Dysarthria (seen with lesions of CN X or CN XII, also V, VII)
		Examine resting position of tongue.	Atrophy or fasciculations of tongue (LMN, ALS)
		Examine tongue movements: ask patient to protrude tongue, move side-to-side.	Impaired movements, deviation to weak side UMN lesion: tongue deviates away from side of cortical lesion

From O'Sullivan and Siegelman,[18, p. 119] with permission.

muscle with loss of joint stability and increased risk for postural abnormality.[33] *Neurogenic atrophy* accompanies LMN injury (e.g., peripheral nerve injury, spinal root injury) and occurs rapidly, generally within 2 to 3 weeks. Atrophy is also accompanied by other signs of LMN injury (e.g., decreased or absent tone or decreased or absent DTRs, fasciculations, weak or absent voluntary movements). Distribution is limited to a segmental or focal pattern (nerve root).

Examination of Muscle Bulk

During the examination, the therapist should visually inspect the muscle symmetry and shapes, comparing and contrasting their size and contour. Muscles that look flat or concave are indicative of atrophy. Comparisons should be made between and within limbs. Is the atrophy unilateral or bilateral? Are multiple limbs involved? Is the atrophy more proximal, or distal, or both? Limb girth measurements can be used to compare a limb undergoing neurogenic atrophy with the corresponding normal limb. Palpation at rest and during muscle contraction is used to determine muscle tension. Girth measurements or volumetric displacement measures (e.g., hands or feet) can be used to confirm visual inspection findings.

Strength and Power

Muscle performance is "the capacity of a muscle or a group of muscles to generate forces."[4, p. 688] **Muscle strength** is "the muscle force exerted by a muscle or a group of muscles to overcome a resistance under a specific set of circumstances."[4, p. 688] Isotonic contractions involve active shortening of muscles, and eccentric contractions involve active lengthening of muscles. Isometric contractions produce high levels of tension for holding contractions without overt movement. **Muscle power** is "work produced per unit of time or the product of strength and speed."[4, p. 688] Muscle performance depends on a number of interrelated factors, including length–tension characteristics, viscoelasticity, velocity, and metabolic adequacy (fuel storage and delivery). Of equal importance are the integrated actions of the CNS (neuromuscular control factors) acting on motor units, including (1) the number of motor units recruited, (2) the type of motor units recruited, and (3) the discharge rate and continuing modulation of motor units. The CNS controls the recruitment order and timing of muscles. Synergistic movements and postural adjustments are also dependent on the integrity of the peripheral nerves, as well as the muscle fibers.

Patients with impairments in motor control and neurological injury pose unique challenges for the examination of muscle performance. *Weakness* is the inability to generate sufficient levels of force and can vary from *paresis* (partial weakness) to *plegia* (absence of muscle strength). Weakness is seen in patients with UMN syndrome, along with spasticity and hyperactive reflexes. Patients may present with *hemiplegia* (one-sided paralysis), *paraplegia* (LE paralysis), or *tetraplegia* (quadriplegia). Weakness also appears in patients with LMN lesions.

Patients with stroke demonstrate significant changes in muscle performance, including altered recruitment patterns, abnormal times to achieve force, and decreased motor unit firing rates.[34-36] They also demonstrate up to a 50% decrease in motor units of affected extremities within 2 months after insult with greater losses of Type II (fast twitch) fibers.[37,38] Impairments in grip strength impairments are observed, including an exaggeration of grip force, altered times to achieve grip, and difficulty maintaining grip.[39] Muscle performance in patients with stroke is influenced by the presence of other UMN impairments including spasticity, disordered synergistic activity/mass patterns of movements, abnormal muscle co-contraction, and/or profound sensory deficit.[40-42] Strength losses are typically greater in the distal extremity than proximal. Strength losses have also been found on the "supposedly normal" extremities.[43-45] The bilateral effects of an ipsilateral cortical lesion is evidence of the small percentage (estimated 10%) of corticospinal tract fibers that remain uncrossed. Possible other unidentified factors may also exist. This information has prompted use of terms such as "less involved" or "less affected" in place of more traditional terms such as "unaffected," "uninvolved," "sound," "normal," or "good" side. This also casts doubt as to the validity of using the contralateral uninvolved side as a reference for normal muscle strength in patients with hemiplegia.

In patients with peripheral sensorimotor neuropathy (e.g., chronic diabetic neuropathy) or acute motor neuropathy (e.g., Guillain-Barré), strength losses are typically greater in distal segments (i.e., foot and ankle) than proximal with involvement of more proximal segments as the disease progresses. In neuropathy, the progression is slow (months or years) whereas in Guillain-Barré the progression is rapid (days or weeks) and more complete, involving not just the proximal LEs but also the trunk, UEs, and in some cases the lower CN nerves. Patients with primary muscle disease (e.g., myopathies) typically experience proximal weakness whereas patients with myasthenia gravis experience decremental strength losses. Thus, the first contraction of a muscle may start out strong and then each succeeding contraction gets weaker and weaker.

Examination of Muscle Strength and Power

The clinical examination of muscle strength and power utilizes standardized methods and protocols (e.g., manual muscle testing [MMT], handheld dynamometers, instrumented isokinetic systems). See Chapter 4, Musculoskeletal Examination, for a thorough discussion of this topic. Analysis of muscle timing including amplitude, duration, waveform, and frequency can be obtained using EMG (see later section). Activity analysis of functional performance also yields important data about muscle performance.

Strength testing measures (MMT) were originally developed to examine motor function in patients with polio (an LMN disease). There are validity issues when used in the clinical examination of patients with UMN lesions.[46,47] Strength testing using standardized protocols may be inappropriate for some patients with UMN syndrome. Appropriate criteria are therefore critical in determining whether the standards of validity and reliability of MMT are met. First and foremost, the therapist must consider the patient's movement

capabilities. Individual isolated joint movements, mandated by standardized MMT procedures and isokinetic protocols, may not be possible in the presence of UMN lesion where stereotypic abnormal movement patterns (obligatory synergies) are present. The presence of abnormal co-activation, spasticity, and abnormal posturing may preclude the patient's ability to perform isolated joint movements. These barriers to normal movement are termed *active restraint*. The prescribed test positions may also be precluded by the presence of abnormal reflex activity (e.g., supine testing influenced by presence of the tonic labyrinthine reflex). Muscle and soft tissue changes in viscoelasticity (e.g., contracture) offer a form of *passive restraint* and may also preclude the use of standardized testing. In these instances, the decision should be made *not* to use standardized MMT procedures. An estimation of strength can be made from observations of active movements during performance of functional activities. For example, shallow knee bends or sit-to-stand transfers can be used to examine the strength of hip extensors and knee extensors. Standing heel-rises or toe-rises can be used to examine the strength of foot-ankle muscles (dorsiflexors, plantarflexors). Documentation should clearly indicate that UMN involvement precluded use of standardized MMT procedures. Estimates of strength can be made based on observations during active functional movements using the following criteria:

- Muscles with visible movement that are unable to overcome gravity and move throughout the ROM receive a *poor grade*.
- Muscles that are able to move against gravity throughout the range but can take no additional resistance receive a *fair grade*.
- Muscles that can move against gravity throughout the range and against some resistance (moderate resistance) receive a *good grade*.
- Muscles that can move throughout the range and against strong resistance receive a grade of *normal*.

The reader will recognize obvious similarities to the standard MMT grading system. However, in this case muscle performance involves groups of muscles moving during specific functional tasks and not during isolated joint movements with standardized protocols.

If MMT is to be used, therapists should utilize standardized positions whenever possible. If a modified position is required (e.g., the patient lacks full ROM or adequate stabilization), it should be carefully documented. *Substitutions* (muscle actions that compensate for specific muscle weakness) should be identified, eliminated whenever possible, and carefully documented. For example, the patient with SCI typically presents with common muscle substitutions (e.g., wrist extensors are used to close the fingers using tenodesis grasp). Knowledge of common substitutions is very helpful when working with this patient group.

Handheld dynamometers are small portable devices that measure mechanical force; they have been incorporated clinically into MMT procedures. The therapist reads the exact amount of force applied to the muscle during tests for good and normal grades instead of estimating the amount of resistance. High intratester and intertester reliability scores have been reported. Limitations in their use include difficulty in stabilizing both the limb and device, controlling the rate of muscle tension development, and applying sufficient force for a break test. These may be influential factors in reports that indicate the portable dynamometer is less reliable for testing LE muscle groups.[48-51]

The use of an *isokinetic dynamometer* allows the therapist to monitor many important parameters of motor control. It allows examination of a muscle's ability to generate force throughout the range, peak torques, and ability to generate torques at changing velocities. Rate of tension development (time to peak torque) and shape of the torque curve can also be determined. Concentric, isometric, and eccentric contractions and reciprocal agonist/antagonist relationships can be analyzed. This information is especially important for an understanding of functional performance.[52]

Patients with stroke typically demonstrate a variety of deficits when tested with an isokinetic dynamometer, including (1) decreased torque overall in the more affected limb when compared to the less affected limb; (2) decreased torque with increasing movement speeds; (3) decreased limb excursion; (4) extended times to peak torque development and the duration time peak torque is held; and (5) increased time intervals between reciprocal contractions. For example, many patients with stroke are unable to develop tension above 70° to 80° per second. When this value is compared to the speed needed for normal walking (100° per second), reasons for gait difficulties become readily apparent. Normative data, when available, can provide an appropriate reference for evaluating and interpreting patient data.[53,54]

Documentation of Strength and Power

Documentation of strength and power changes should include a determination of the specific muscles and body segments tested and tests used; the type and degree of changes present (e.g., paresis, paralysis); whether the changes are symmetrical or asymmetrical, distal or proximal; presence of associated signs (e.g., UMN or LMN); presence of atrophy; and factors that modify muscle performance. A description of the effects of muscle weakness on active movements, posture, and function should also be included. When examining functional performance, it is important to remember that strength estimates taken in one position do not necessarily generalize to other positions (e.g., ability to move while supporting full body weight in upright standing).

Muscle Endurance

Muscle endurance is "the ability to sustain forces repeatedly or to generate forces over a period of time."[4, p. 688] An examination of muscle endurance is important in determining functional capacity. **Fatigue** is an overwhelming sustained sense of exhaustion and decreased capacity for physical and mental work at the usual level. Fatigue can be the result of excessive activity caused by an accumulation of metabolic waste products (e.g., lactic acid); malnutrition (i.e., deficiency of nutrients); cardiorespiratory disturbances (i.e., inadequate oxygen and nutrients to the tissues); emotional stress; and other factors. Although fatigue is protective and serves a useful function in guarding against overwork and injury, it is a serious problem for some individuals. For example, patients with postpolio syndrome or chronic fatigue syndrome may experience significant restrictions in their functional activities and work as a result of debilitating fatigue. Other groups of individuals who may also experience significant limitations as a result of fatigue include those with MS, amyotrophic lateral sclerosis (ALS), Duchenne muscular dystrophy, and Guillain-Barré syndrome.[55,56] Additional factors that can influence fatigue include health status, environmental context (e.g., stressful environment), and temperature (e.g., heat stress in the patient with MS).

Exhaustion is defined as the limit of endurance, beyond which no further performance is possible. Most patients can report with great accuracy the point at which exhaustion is reached. Of concern with some patients is **overwork weakness (injury)**, defined as "a prolonged decrease in absolute strength and endurance due to excessive activity of partially denervated muscle."[57, p. 22] For example, patients with postpolio syndrome may experience weakness following strenuous activity that is not recovered with ordinary rest. They report having to spend the entire next day or two in bed following an exhaustive exercise session. It is therefore important to document the type, length, and effectiveness of rest attempts. *Delayed onset muscle soreness (DOMS)* is prolonged in patients with overwork weakness, peaking between 1 and 5 days after activity.

Examination of Fatigue

An examination of fatigue begins with the initial interview. The patient is asked to identify those activities that are fatiguing, the frequency and severity of fatigue episodes, and the circumstances surrounding the onset of fatigue. It is important to identify the *fatigue threshold*, defined as "that level of exercise that cannot be sustained indefinitely."[58, p. 691] In most cases, the onset of fatigue is gradual, not abrupt, and dependent on the intensity and duration of the activity attempted. Precipitating activities should be identified within the context of habitual daily activity. The patient is asked to identify any solutions used to overcome debilitating fatigue and how successful they are. Self-assessment questionnaires are particularly useful for the patient with significant fatigue. One example is the *Modified Fatigue Impact Scale (MFIS)*, an instrument initially developed to assess quality-of-life problems related to fatigue in patients with MS. It includes questions on the cognitive and social domains, as well as physical performance (see Chapter 16, Multiple Sclerosis, Appendix 16.B).[59]

The examination then proceeds with specific performance-based testing. As this is likely to be fatiguing to the patient, performance testing should be limited to those key functional activities identified in the earlier interview or questionnaire. The therapist should carefully document the patient's level of fatigue during performance testing, including level of independence, modified independence (device required), or level of assistance required (minimal, moderate, or maximal). The grading criteria for the *Functional Independence Measure (FIM)* provides a useful scoring key, and the functional activities tested (e.g., transfers, locomotion) are basic to independent living.[60] During performance testing, perceived level of fatigue can be documented using the *Borg Scale for Rating of Perceived Exertion*.[61] In order to better determine the level of muscle fatigue, the therapist should ask the patient to identify two separate scores, one for the level of muscular fatigue and one for the level of central fatigue (breathlessness). The therapist is then able to differentiate between peripheral factors and central factors contributing to fatigue.

Examination of muscle fatigue can also include both volitional and electrically elicited fatigue tests using an isokinetic dynamometer. This equipment permits quantification of torque outputs. Patients are asked to perform repetitive, submaximal isokinetic contractions. A drop-off of peak torque by 50% can be used as an index of fatigue.[62] Electrically induced fatigue tests can also be used to examine muscle performance and may provide a more reliable measure in individuals with low motivation or who have a disorder of central drive (e.g., stroke). The muscle is stimulated with groups of electrical pulses (pulse trains) and percentage of decline in force production is measured.[63,64] Timed performance on functional tasks (e.g., timed self-care tasks, time to walk a particular distance, 6-minute walk test) also provides objective and reproducible measures of muscular endurance.

Documentation

Documentation of muscle endurance should include a determination of (1) activities that result in debilitating fatigue, including onset, duration, and recovery; (2) level of assistance or assistive devices required; (3) frequency and effectiveness of rest attempts; (4) compensatory strategies adopted and effectiveness; and (5) impact on quality of life. Results of specific questionnaires and tests are documented. Social and environmental stressors should also be described along with the patient's emotional/psychological responses (e.g., degree of depression or anxiety).

Voluntary Movement Patterns

Synergies are functionally linked muscles that are constrained by the CNS to act cooperatively to produce an intended motor action. They are used to simplify control, reduce or constrain the degrees of freedom, and initiate coordinated patterns of movement. **Degrees of freedom** refers to the number of separate independent dimensions of movement that must be controlled by engaging these cooperative units of muscle action.[1] Synergistic movements are defined by precise spatial and temporal organization that requires a high degree of coordination involving control of speed, distance, direction, rhythm, and levels of muscle tension (see Chapter 6, Examination of Coordination and Balance). In individuals with normal motor control, voluntary movement patterns are functional, task specific, and highly variable, depending on the task purpose and environment. The CNS controls patterns of (1) single limb and multiple limb movements, (2) bilateral (bimanual) symmetrical and asymmetrical movements, (3) reciprocal movements, and (4) patterns of proximal stabilization and postural support. Movements are also appropriately timed with events in the environment (*coincident timing*).

Abnormal Synergistic Patterns

Synergistic organization of movement may be disturbed with pathology of the CNS. Lesions of the corticospinal tracts (e.g., stroke) can produce abnormal **obligatory synergies**, defined as movements that are primitive and highly stereotyped. Voluntary movements are limited with loss of ability to adapt movements to changing demands. Selective movement control (isolated joint movements) is severely disordered or disappears completely. Patients with stroke typically demonstrate obligatory flexion and extension synergies (see Chapter 15, Stroke, Table 15.5). Abnormal synergies are highly predictable and characteristic of middle stages of recovery from stroke.[65-67]

Examination

The examination of abnormal synergies is both qualitative and quantitative. The therapist observes whether voluntary movement can be initiated, whether it can be completed, and how the movement is carried out. If movement is stereotypic and obligatory, what muscle groups are linked together? How strong are the linkages between muscle groups? Are there linkages between upper and lower limbs or one side to another (associated reactions)? Are the movements influenced by other components of UMN syndrome, such as primitive reflexes, spasticity, paresis, or position? For example, does elbow, wrist, and finger flexion always occur when shoulder flexion is initiated? Is head turning used to initiate or reinforce UE flexion (asymmetric tonic neck reflex [ATNR])? Therapists also need to identify when these patterns occur, under what circumstances, and what variations are possible. As CNS recovery progresses, the synergy patterns become less dominant, and reemerge only under conditions of stress or fatigue. Lessening of synergy dominance and emergence of selective movement control are evidence of sequential recovery in patients with stroke.[64-66] The *Fugl-Meyer Post-Stroke Assessment of Physical Performance* provides an objective and quantifiable measure of obligatory synergistic dominance and recovery after stroke[68] (see Chapter 15, Stroke, Appendix 15.A).

Documentation

Documentation of abnormal synergies should include a determination of (1) what abnormal synergies are present; (2) the overall strength of the synergies present; (3) the strongest components in each synergy; (4) the influence of other UMN signs on synergies; (5) what variations in movement from the typical synergies are possible, if any; and (6) the effect of obligatory synergies on function (basic activities of daily living [BADL], functional mobility skills).

Table 5.9 presents a summary of the differential diagnosis summary comparing UMN and LMN syndromes. Table 5.10 presents a summary of the differential diagnosis summary comparing the major types of CNS disorders by location of lesion/motor control disorders.

Activity-based Task Analysis

Examination at the functional level focuses on observation and classification of functional abilities and the identification of activity limitations. Performance-based instruments yield important information about function and levels of independence or dependence (supervision, assistance, assistive devices). Numerous instruments are available with quantitative scoring systems (e.g., the FIM). See Chapter 8, Examination of Function, for a thorough discussion of performance-based measures.

Activity-based task analysis is the process of breaking a specific activity down into its component parts to understand and evaluate the demands of the task and the performance demonstrated. It begins with an understanding of normal movements and normal kinesiology associated with the task. The therapist examines and evaluates the patient's performance and analyzes the differences compared to "typical" or expected performance. Critical skills in this process include accurate observation and recognition of barriers or obstacles to moving in the correct pattern. Interpretations are made about the nature of the motor performance and the possible links between documented impairments and performance difficulties. A determination of how the environment affects performance must also be made. For

Table 5.9	Differential Diagnosis: Comparison of Upper Motor Neuron (UMN) and Lower Motor Neuron (LMN) Syndromes	
	UMN Lesion	**LMN Lesion**
Location of lesion, structures involved	Central nervous system cortex, brainstem, corticospinal tracts, spinal cord	Cranial nerve nuclei/nerves Spinal cord: anterior horn cell, spinal roots Peripheral nerve
Diagnosis/pathology	Stroke, traumatic brain injury, spinal cord injury	Polio, Guillain-Barré Peripheral nerve injury Peripheral neuropathy Radiculopathy
Tone	Increased: hypertonia Velocity dependent	Decreased or absent: hypotonia, flaccidity Not velocity dependent
Reflexes	Increased: hyperreflexia, clonus Exaggerated cutaneous and autonomic reflexes, +Babinski	Decreased or absent: hyporeflexia Cutaneous reflexes decreased or absent
Involuntary movements	Muscle spasms: flexor or extensor	With denervation: fasciculations
Strength	Weakness or paralysis: ipsilateral (stroke) or bilateral (SCI) Corticospinal: contralateral if above decussation in medulla; ipsilateral if below Distribution: never focal	Ipsilateral weakness or paralysis Limited distribution: segmental or focal pattern, root-innervated pattern
Muscle bulk	Disuse atrophy: variable, widespread distribution, especially of antigravity muscles	Neurogenic atrophy: rapid, focal distribution, severe wasting
Voluntary movements	Impaired or absent: dyssynergic patterns, obligatory mass synergies	Weak or absent if nerve interrupted

From O'Sullivan and Siegelman,[18, p. 127] with permission.

Table 5.10	Differential Diagnosis: Comparison of Major Types of Central Nervous System Disorders			
Location of Lesion	**Cerebral Cortex Corticospinal Tracts**	**Basal Ganglia**	**Cerebellum**	**Spinal Cord**
Diagnosis/pathology	Stroke	Parkinson's disease	Tumor, stroke	Trauma, tumor, vascular insult: complete, incomplete SCI
Sensation	Impaired or absent: depends on lesion location; contralateral sensory loss	Not affected	Not affected	Impaired or absent below the level of lesion
Tone	Hypertonia/spasticity velocity-dependent; clasp-knife Initial flaccidity: cerebral shock	Lead-pipe rigidity: increased, uniform resistance Cogwheel rigidity: increased, ratchet-like resistance	Normal or may be decreased	Hypertonia/spasticity below the level of the lesion Initial flaccidity: spinal shock
Reflexes	Hyperreflexia	Normal or may be decreased	Normal or may be decreased	Hyperreflexia
Strength	Contralateral weakness or paralysis: hemiplegia or hemiparesis Disuse weakness in chronic stage	Disuse weakness in chronic stage	Normal or weak: asthenia	Impaired or absent below the level of the lesion: paraplegia or paraparesis; tetraplegia or tetraparesis
Muscle bulk	Normal during acute stage; disuse atrophy in chronic stage	Normal or disuse atrophy	Normal	Disuse atrophy
Involuntary movements	Spasms	Resting tremor	None	Spasms
Voluntary movements	Dyssynergic: abnormal timing, co-activation, fatigability	Bradykinesia: slowness of movement Akinesia: absence of movement	Ataxia: intention tremor dysdiadochokinesia dysmetria dyssynergia nystagmus	Above level of lesion: intact (normal) Below level of lesion: impaired or absent
Postural control	Impaired or absent, depends on lesion location Impaired balance	Impaired: stooped (flexed) Impaired balance	Impaired: truncal ataxia Impaired balance	Impaired below level of lesion Impaired balance
Gait	Impaired: gait deficits due to abnormal weakness, synergies, spasticity, timing deficits	Impaired: shuffling, festinating gait	Impaired: ataxic gait deficits, wide-based, unsteady	Impaired or absent: depends on level of lesion

From O'Sullivan and Siegelman,[18, p. 126] with permission.
SCI = spinal cord injury.

example, the patient who is unable to transfer from bed to wheelchair may lack postural trunk support (stability), adequate LE extensor control (strength), and ability to maintain control while moving from one surface to the other. Or the patient with acute stroke sits up from supine using the less affected UE for support and propulsion. The more affected extremities lag behind, not well integrated into the movement pattern. The final sitting position is asymmetrical with most of the weight borne on the less affected side and the more affected UE held in an abnormally flexed and adducted position. In addition, the patient is highly distractible with poor attention demonstrated in the busy clinic environment. It is important to document these qualitative findings as they provide valuable information necessary for developing an effective POC to improve motor function. The term *activity demands* refers to the requirements imbedded in each step of the activity. The term *environmental demands* (constraints) refers to the physical characteristics of the environment or features required for successful performance of movement (regulatory conditions). Questions posed in Box 5.2 can be used to provide a guide for qualitative task analysis.

Taxonomy of Tasks

Tasks are commonly grouped into functional categories. **Activities of daily living (ADL)** refer to those daily living skills necessary for an adult to manage life. **Basic ADL (BADL)** include grooming skills (oral hygiene, showering or bathing, dressing), toilet hygiene, feeding, and personal device care. **Instrumental ADL (IADL)** include money management, functional communication and socialization, functional and community mobility, and health maintenance.

Functional mobility skills (FMS) refer to those skills involved in:

1. Bed mobility: rolling, bridging, scooting in bed, moving from supine-to-sit and sit-to-supine
2. Sitting: scooting
3. Transfers: moving from sit-to-stand and stand-to-sit, transfers from one surface to another (e.g., bed-to-wheelchair and back, on and off a toilet, to and from a car seat), and moving from floor-to-standing
4. Standing: stepping
5. Walking and stair climbing

Control can also be examined in other postures including prone-on-elbows, quadruped (hands and knees), kneeling, and half-kneeling. It is important to note that there is considerable variability in motor

---

Box 5.2   Functional Task Analysis Worksheet

Task analysis begins with an appreciation of normal movements. An examination and evaluation of the patient's task performance is completed and a comparison of the differences is made. Critical skills include accurate observation, recognition and interpretation of movement deficiencies, determination of how underlying impairments relate to the movement deficiencies observed, and determination of what needs be altered and how. The following questions can be used as a guide for qualitative functional task analysis.

A. What are the normal requirements of the functional task being observed?

1. What is the overall movement sequence (motor plan)?
2. What are the initial conditions required? Starting position and initial alignment?
3. How and where is the movement initiated?
4. How is the movement executed?
5. What are the musculoskeletal components required for successful completion of the task?
6. What are the motor control strategies required for successful completion of the task?
7. What are the requirements for timing, force, and direction of movements?
8. What are the requirements for balance?
9. How is the movement terminated?
10. What are the environmental constraints that must be considered?
11. What are the motor learning factors that must be considered?

B. How successful is the patient's overall movement in terms of outcome?

1. Was the overall movement sequence completed?
2. What components of the patient's movements are normal? Almost normal?
3. What components of the patient's movements are abnormal?
4. What components of the patient's movements are missing? Delayed?
5. If abnormal, are the movements compensatory and functional? Noncompensatory and nonfunctional?
6. What are the underlying impairments that constrain or impair the movements?
7. Do the movement errors increase over time? Is fatigue a constraining factor?
8. Is this a transitional mobility activity? Are the requirements met?
9. Is this a stability level activity? Are the requirements met for static and dynamic control?
10. Is this a skill level activity? Are the requirements met?
11. Are balance requirements met? Is patient safety evident throughout the task?
12. What environmental factors constrained or impaired the movements?
13. Can the patient adapt to changing task and environmental demands?
14. What difficulties do you expect this patient will have with other functional tasks?
15. What difficulties do you expect this patient will have in other environments?
16. How successful were the motor learning strategies?

Adapted from *A Compendium for Teaching Professional Level Neurologic Content*, Neurology Section, American Physical Therapy Association, 2000.

performance of FMS across the life span.[69-73] Changes are influenced by such factors as changing body dimensions, age, health, and level of physical activity. Thus, the activities of rolling over and sitting up may vary considerably between two adults of different size, age, or health.

Tasks can also be grouped according to the actions and type and nature of motor control (neuromotor processes) required during performance of the task. These include (1) transitional mobility, (2) stability (static postural control), (3) dynamic postural control (controlled mobility), and (4) skill. Difficulty varies according to the degree of postural and movement control required. Thus, those tasks with increased degrees of freedom and attentional demands such as standing and walking are more difficult than prone or supine tasks with limited body segments to control.

Transitional mobility is the ability to move from one position to another independently and safely (e.g., rolling, supine-to-sit, sit-to-stand, transfers). Common characteristics of normal mobility include the ability to initiate movement, control movement, and terminate movement while maintaining postural control. Deficits in *mobility* range from failure to initiate or sustain movements to poorly controlled movement to failure to successfully terminate the movement. At the very lowest level, the impaired patient is only able to roll partially over to side lying and exhibits poor ability to sustain movements. At the highest end, the patient is asked to stand up and walk across the room. The impaired patient exhibits difficulty standing up (may require several attempts) but once up is able to walk with only a few abnormal gait characteristics. Key elements the therapist should observe and document include (1) the ability to initiate movements; (2) strategies utilized and overall control of movement; (3) the ability to terminate movement; (4) the level and type of assistance required (manual cues, verbal cues, guided movements); and (5) environmental constraints that influenced performance.

Stability (*static postural control*) is the ability to maintain postural stability and orientation with the center of mass (COM) over the base of support (BOS) and the body at rest. For example, the patient demonstrates stability in sitting or standing if he or she is able to maintain the posture with minimum sway, no loss of balance, and no handhold. Key elements the therapist should observe and document include (1) the BOS; (2) the position and stability of the COM within the BOS; (3) the degree of postural sway; (4) the degree of stabilization from UEs or LEs (e.g., handhold, hooked legs); (5) the number of episodes and direction of loss of balance (LOB) and fall safety risk; (6) the level and type of assistance required (manual cues, verbal cues, guided movements); and (7) environmental constraints that influenced performance.

Dynamic postural control (*dynamic balance,* or *controlled mobility*) is the ability to maintain postural stability (a stable, nonmoving BOS, COM within the BOS) while parts of the body are in motion. Thus, an individual is able to weight shift or rock back and forth or side to side in a posture (e.g., in sitting or standing) without losing control. The adjustment of postural control while performing a secondary task with a limb freed from weight-bearing is also evidence of dynamic postural control (sometimes called *static-dynamic control*). The initial weight shift and redistributed weight-bearing places increased demands for stability on the support segments while the dynamic limb challenges control. For example, a patient with TBI is positioned in quadruped and demonstrates difficulty when asked to lift either an upper or lower limb, or lift the opposite upper and lower limbs together. In sitting, the patient with stroke is unable to reach forward and toward the affected side with the less affected limb without losing balance and falling over. In standing, the patient with cerebellar ataxia is unable to step forward, backward, or out to the side without losing balance. Key elements the therapist should observe and document include (1) the degree of postural stability maintained by the weight-bearing segments; (2) the range and degree of control of the dynamically moving segments; (3) the level and type of assistance required (e.g., verbal cues, manual cues, guided movements); and (4) environmental constraints that influenced performance.

Skill is the ability to consistently perform coordinated movement sequences for the purposes of attaining an action goal. Skilled behaviors allow for purposeful investigation and interaction with the physical and social environment (e.g., manipulation or transport). Skills are learned, and are the direct result of practice and experience with actions organized in advance of movement using a motor plan. Skilled movements are variable and not constrained by one set movement pattern but rather are organized by the action goal and the environment. Thus, a skilled individual is able to adapt movements easily to changes in task demands and the environments in which they occur. For example, control of walking is evident in the clinic as well as in home and community environments. Skills can be performed using consistent or variable movements. Regulatory conditions can vary from a stationary environment to motion in the environment.[74]

Motor skills can be further categorized. Kicking a ball is an example of a *discrete skill*, with a recognizable beginning and end. Walking is a *continuous skill* (no recognizable beginning and end), and playing a piano represents a *serial skill* (a series of discrete actions put together). A movement skill performed in a stable , nonchanging environment is called a **closed motor skill**, and a movement skill performed in a variable, changing environment is called an **open motor skill**.[1] A skilled individual is also able to perform a simultaneous secondary task while moving (**dual task control**). For example, the patient with stroke is able to stand or walk while holding or manipulating an object (e.g., bouncing a ball), talking, or performing a cognitive task (counting backwards by 3's from 100). Table 5.11 provides a summary of categories of motor skills.

During functional task analysis, key elements the therapist should observe and document include (1) the ability to organize and control movements; (2) economy of effort; (3) the success of attaining an action-goal (outcome); (4) ability to easily and successfully adapt a task; (5) ability to easily and successfully adapt to changing environments; and (6) verbal cues and assistance, if any, required. Box 5.2 provides a Functional Task Analysis Worksheet.

Videography

The qualitative analysis of motor skills can be enhanced by the use of videography. Patient responses are recorded, providing a permanent record of motor performance that allows the therapist the opportunity to compare responses over time. Recordings made at 3 or 6 weeks of recovery can be compared easily without reliance on the therapist's memory or written notes. Accuracy of observations can be improved. A therapist who is closely involved in assisting or guarding during performance may not be attentive enough to observe all movement parameters (e.g., when assisting the patient with TBI with severe ataxia). Depending on equipment capabilities, videotapes can be viewed repeatedly at different speeds to determine control during different tasks and at different body segments. For example, a patient's performance in a task such as sitting up from supine can be observed first at regular speeds, then at slow motion speeds. Stop-action or freezing a frame can be used to isolate a problematic point in the movement sequence. This may be helpful, particularly for the inexperienced therapist, in improving both the quality and reliability of observations. Repeat trials on a functional performance test may needlessly tire the patient while yielding a decrease in performance. Sequential recordings over the course of rehabilitation provide visual documentation of patient progress and can be an important motivational and educational tool in therapy for use with the patient and family. Reliability of recordings for intersession comparisons can be improved by the following measures. Placement of equipment should be planned in advance to achieve the best location and should be consistently placed over subsequent sessions. Use of a tripod can improve the stability of the recording. Verbal descriptions of the performance during each trial can be edited directly onto a videotape or documented in a written summary.[75]

■ MOTOR LEARNING

Motor learning is a complex process that requires spatial, temporal, and hierarchical organization within the CNS

Table 5.11	Categories of Motor Skills		
Categories	**Characteristics**	**Examples**	**Impairments**
Transitional mobility	Ability to move from one posture to another; BOS and/or COM is changing	Rolling; supine-to-sit; sit-to-stand; transfers	Failure to initiate or sustain movements through the range; poorly controlled movements
Static postural control (stability, static equilibrium, or static balance)	Ability to maintain postural stability and orientation with the COM over the BOS with the body not in motion; BOS is fixed	Holding in antigravity postures: prone-on-elbows, quadruped, sitting, kneeling, half-kneeling, modified plantigrade, or standing	Failure to maintain a steady posture; excessive postural sway; wide BOS; high guard arm position or handhold; loss of balance (COM exceeds BOS)
Dynamic postural control (controlled mobility, dynamic equilibrium, or dynamic balance)	Ability to maintain postural stability and orientation with the COM over the BOS while parts of the body are in motion; BOS is fixed	Weight shifting; UE reaching in any of the above antigravity postures; LE stepping in modified plantigrade or standing	Failure to maintain or control posture during dynamic trunk or extremity movements; loss of balance
Skill	Ability to consistently perform coordinated UE and LE movement sequences for the purposes of investigation and interaction with the physical and social environment; during locomotion, COM is in motion and BOS is changing	UE skills: Grasp and manipulation LE skills: Bipedal locomotion	Poorly coordinated movements; lack of precision, control, consistency, and economy of effort

BOS = base of support; COM = center of mass; LE = lower extremity; UE = upper extremity.

that allows for acquisition and modification of movement. As mentioned earlier, changes in the CNS are not directly observable, but rather are inferred from improvement in performance as a result of practice or experience. Individual differences in learning are expected and influence both the rate and degree of learning possible. Motor learning abilities among individuals vary across three main foundational categories of abilities: cognitive abilities, perceptual speed ability, and psychomotor ability.[76] Differences occur as a result of both genetics and experience. The therapist should be sensitive to such factors as alertness, anxiety, memory, speed of processing information, speed and accuracy of movements, and uniqueness of the setting. In addition, recovering patients may vary in their learning potential according to the pathology present, the number and type of impairments, recovery potential and general health status, and comorbidities. Although most skills can be learned through practice or experience, the therapist should be sensitive to the patient's underlying capabilities (abilities) that support certain skills. For example, some patients with SCI may not be able to learn to manage curbs using "wheelies" because of the difficulty of the task, their residual abilities, and their general health status.

Stages of Motor Learning

Fitts and Posner[77] described three main stages in learning a motor skill. Their model provides a useful framework for examining and developing strategies to improve motor learning and is used in this chapter as well as in Chapter 10, Strategies to Improve Motor Function. A three-stage process is supported by the work of Anderson,[78,79] whereas Gentile proposed a two-stage process.[80]

In the early **cognitive stage** the learner develops an understanding of task. During practice *cognitive mapping* allows the learner to assess abilities and task demands, identify relevant and important stimuli, and develop an initial movement strategy (motor program) based on explicit memory of prior movement experiences. The learner performs initial practice of the task, retaining some strategies while discarding others in order to develop an initial movement strategy. During successive practice trials, the learner modifies and refines the movements. During this stage there is considerable cognitive activity and each movement requires a high degree of conscious attention and thought. The learner is highly dependent on use of visual feedback. Performance is initially inconsistent with large gains occurring as the patient progresses to the next stage. The basic "What to do" decision is answered.

The second and middle stage is the **associated stage** of motor learning. During this stage, the learner practices and refines the motor patterns, making subtle adjustments. Spatial and temporal organization increases while errors and extraneous movements decrease. Performance becomes more consistent and cognitive activity decreases. The learner is less dependent on visual feedback while use of proprioceptive feedback increases. Thus, the learner begins to learn the "feel" of the movement. This stage can persist for a long time, depending on the learner and the level of practice. The "How to do" decision is answered.

The third and final stage is the **autonomous phase** of motor learning. The learner continues to practice and refine motor patterns. The spatial and temporal components of movement become highly organized. Performance is at a very high level (e.g., skilled athletes). At this stage of learning, movements are largely error free and automatic with only a minimal level of cognitive monitoring and attention. The "How to succeed" decision has been answered.

Patients with brain injury admitted to active rehabilitation often have to relearn basic motor skills using entirely different motor control mechanisms and strategies. Activities and movements that were easily done before now become unfamiliar and challenging. These patients can persist in the cognitive learning stage for some time before they develop the idea of a movement skill. Impairments in motor control can influence performance and learning during the middle or associated stage, which can also be prolonged. Many times patients are discharged from rehabilitation before the skills become refined and learning completed. Many patients fail to reach the third stage of learning evidenced by highly skilled performance.

Measures of Motor Learning
Performance Observations

Traditionally, improvements in performance during practice have been used to assess motor learning. Performance criteria are established and used for comparison to determine the success of learning outcomes. Table 5.12 presents some possible measures of motor performance. For example, an individual recovering from stroke is able to demonstrate functional independence in transfers after a series of training sessions. Improvement in functional scores (e.g., FIM scores) documents changes in the level of assistance needed. Qualitative changes in performance compared to the criterion skill can also be used to document motor learning. Thus, the movement is performed with improved coordination, indicative of changes in spatial and temporal organization. Error scores can be used to document accuracy of movement. Thus, therapists can report the number and type of errors (constant, variable) that occur within a given practice session and across practice sessions. A decrease in the frequency of error provides indirect evidence of improvements in learning. One common measurement problem in skill learning is the *speed–accuracy trade-off*. Typically, initial practice sessions are characterized by slowed performance in order to improve movement accuracy. As learning progresses, performance speed is increased once accuracy demands are satisfied. The therapist needs to document the time it takes to complete the activity along with number of errors. Reduced effort and concentration are indicative of improved performance and should be documented. A high degree

Table 5.12	Measures of Motor Performance	
Category	Examples of Measures	Performance Examples
Outcome Measures	**Movement Time (MT):** The time interval between the initiation of a movement and completion of a movement, in seconds or minutes	10-Meter Walk Test (10-MWT) Time to complete a functional task (e.g., transfer wheelchair to mat) Minnesota Rate of Manipulation Test
	Reaction Time (RT): The time interval between the presentation of a stimulus and the initiation of a response, in seconds or minutes	Time to initiate a functional task after cueing is provided (e.g., supine-to-sit or sit-to-stand transfers)
	Distance: The total distance completed, in meters or feet	6- or 12-Minute Walk Test
	Observational Performance Changes: Observation of deviations of performance with respect to target behaviors	Observational gait analysis: Systematic examination of movement patterns of body segments at each point in the gait cycle
	Changes in Performance Scores using a standardized outcome measure	Changes in scores on the Functional Independence Measure, Barthel Index, Berg Balance Scale, or Purdue Pegboard Test
	Errors in Performance using a criterion task	*Error in program selection*: Patient with stroke incorrectly transfers to the less affected side when asked to transfer to the more affected side *Error in program execution*: Patient with TBI becomes distracted and is unable to complete a transfer
	Constant Error (CE): The average error of a set of scores from a target value; a measure of average bias	Patient exhibits an average distance on a Functional Reach Test of 6 inches on 3 trials; mean for age ([72 years, women] ≥13.8 inches)
	Variable Error (VE): The SD of a set of scores about the subject's own average score; a measure of movement consistency	Patient exhibits an average SD on a Functional Reach Test of 3 inches on 3 trials
	Number of Successful Attempts: During practice of an activity compared to total number of attempts	Patient performs an independent sit-to-stand transfer 4 out of 10 attempts
	Percentage of Successful Attempts	Patient performs an independent sit-to-stand transfer 40% of attempts
	Time on Target, compared to total time of the activity, in sec or min	Patient is able to maintain independent stability in sitting (or standing) for 2 min during a 5 min trial
	Time in Balance	Number of seconds patient is able to maintain BOS within COM while standing on foam
	Trials to Completion: Number of trials required until correct response obtained	10 practice trials required for patient to be independent in wheelchair to mat transfers
Instrumental Response Measures	**Limb displacement, trajectory**	Distance limb(s) traveled to produce response during instrumental motion analysis, kinematic gait analysis
	Velocity	Speed limb(s) moved while performing response during instrumental motion analysis or isokinetic dynamometry
	Acceleration/deceleration	Acceleration/deceleration pattern while moving during instrumental motion analysis or isokinetic dynamometry
	Joint angle	Angle of each joint during movement during instrumental motion analysis, or using electrogoniometry
	Muscle activity/electromyography (EMG) testing: The electrical activity of muscle based on motor unit activity	Patterns and timing of muscle activity at rest and during contraction compared to normative muscle activity values (e.g., amplitude, duration, shape, sound, and frequency); correlated with clinical findings of muscle weakness and performance

Table 5.12	Measures of Motor Performance—cont'd	
Category	Examples of Measures	Performance Examples
	Nerve conduction velocity (NCV) testing: The conduction time (speed) with which a peripheral motor or sensory nerve conducts an impulse.	Direct stimulation to a nerve with recording of the evoked potential at a different point, compared to normative NCV values (e.g., evoked potentials, elapsed time); correlated with clinical findings of muscle weakness and sensory changes

BOS = base of support; COM = center of mass; min = minutes; SD = standard deviation; sec = seconds; TBI = traumatic brain injury.

of cognitive monitoring is necessary in early learning (cognitive stage). In contrast, performance across the associative and autonomous stages of motor learning is characterized by a reducing level of cognitive monitoring and increasing automaticity.[76] As learning progresses, performance is increasingly characterized by persistence and consistency. Thus, the acquired skills are observed for variability within and across practice sessions, which can be expected to decrease.

Performance observations can be misleading in that while they indicate initial learning, they are not considered an accurate reflection of long-term learning or retention. It is possible to practice enough to temporarily improve performance but not retain the learning. Conversely, factors such as fatigue, anxiety, poor motivation, boredom, or drugs can cause performance to deteriorate while learning may still be occurring. For example, the patient with MS who is fatigued or stressed performs very poorly during scheduled treatment but returns after the weekend rested and calm, and is able to perform the task with ease. *Performance plateaus,* defined as a leveling off of performance after a period of steady improvement, characterize normal practice and can be expected to occur. During plateaus, learning may still be going on whereas performance is not changing. Problems can also occur with the measurement instruments selected. Failure to demonstrate improved performance can be the result of *ceiling effects,* defined as a high level of performance in which further improvement cannot be detected owing to limitations in the performance measure. Conversely, *floor effects* are a low level of performance in which further decreases cannot be detected by limitations in the performance measure. They can affect a determination of negative learning.[1]

Retention Tests

More reliable inferences about learning can be made through the use of retention tests and transfer tests. **Retention** refers to the ability of the learner to demonstrate the skill over time and after a period of no practice (**retention interval**). A **retention test** is defined as "a performance test administered after a retention interval for the purposes of assessing learning."[1, p. 499] It provides an important measure of learning. Retention intervals can be of varying lengths. For example, a patient who is seen only once a week in an outpatient clinic is asked to demonstrate a skill practiced the previous week. Performance after the

retention interval is compared to performance on the initial practice session. A *difference score* can be determined and documented, that is, the difference in performance scores from the end of the original acquisition phase and the beginning of the retention phase. Performance may show a slight initial decrease but should return to original performance levels within relatively few practice trials after the retention interval if learning has occurred (termed *warm-up decrement*). It is important not to provide any verbal cueing or knowledge of results (KR) during the retention trial. This same patient may have been given a home exercise program (HEP) that includes daily practice of the desired skill. If, on return to the clinic some weeks later, performance of the desired skill has not been maintained or has deteriorated, the therapist might reasonably conclude that the patient has not been diligent with the HEP and learning has not been retained.

Transfer Tests

Transfer of learning refers to the gain (or loss) in the capability of task performance in one task as a result of practice or experience on some other task. Learning obtained from the criterion task enhances (*positive transfer*) or detracts from (*negative transfer*) learning on other tasks. For example, the patient with stroke practices feeding skills using the less affected UE. Performance on the feeding task using the more affected UE is then evaluated. The therapist should observe and document the effectiveness of the prior practice (e.g., number and frequency of practice trials, time, effort) on performance using the more affected extremity. Transfer of learning is greatest when tasks are similar, that is, have similar stimuli and similar responses.

Adaptability

Adaptation is the ability to modify and adapt how movements are performed in response to changing task and environmental demands. Thus, the individual is able to apply a learned skill to the learning of other similar tasks. Individuals who learn to transfer from wheelchair-to-platform mat can apply that learning to other variations of transfers (e.g., wheelchair-to-car, wheelchair-to-bathtub). The number of practice trials, time, and effort required to perform these new types of transfers should be observed and documented. These parameters are typically reduced from that required to learn the initial skill.

Resistance to Contextual Change

Resistance to contextual change is also an important measure of learning. This is the adaptability required to perform a motor task in altered environmental situations. Thus, an individual who has learned a skill (e.g., walking with a cane) should be able to apply that learning to new and variable environments (e.g., walking at home, walking outdoors, walking downtown on a busy street). The therapist observes and documents how successful the individual is in performing the skill in the new and varying environments. The patient who is able to perform the skill in only one type of environment, for example, the patient with TBI who is only able to function within a tightly controlled, clinic environment (*closed environment*), demonstrates limited and largely nonfunctional skills in other environments. This patient is not likely to return home independent in the community environment (*open environment*), and will likely require placement in an assisted living (structured) setting.

Active Problem Solving

The patient who is able to engage in active introspection and self-evaluation of performance and reach decisions independently about how to improve performance demonstrates an important element of learning. Some physical therapists overemphasize guided movements and errorless practice. Although this may be important for safety reasons, lack of exposure to performance errors may preclude the patient from developing capabilities for self-evaluation. In an era of fiscal responsibility and limitations on the amount of physical therapy sessions allowed, many patients are able to learn only the very basic skills while in active rehabilitation. Much of the necessary learning of functional skills occurs after discharge and during outpatient episodes of care. The therapist cannot possibly structure practice sessions to meet all of the functional challenges the patient may face. The acquisition of independent problem solving/decision making skills ensures that the final goal of rehabilitation— independent function—can be achieved. The therapist needs to promote, observe, and document this very important function.

Learning Styles

Individuals vary in their *learning style,* defined as their characteristic mode of acquiring, processing, and storing knowledge. Learning styles differ according to a number of factors, including personality characteristics, reasoning styles (inductive or deductive), and initiative (active or passive). Some individuals utilize an *analytical/objective* learning style. They process information in a step-by-step order and learn best with factual information and structure. Other individuals are more *intuitive/global* learners. They tend to process information all at once, and learn best when information is personalized and presented within the context of practical, real-life examples. They may have difficulty in ordering steps and comprehending

details. Some individuals rely heavily on visual processing and demonstration to learn a task. Others depend more on auditory processing, talking themselves through a task. Individual characteristics and preferences are best determined by talking with the patient and family, using careful listening and observation skills. The medical record may also provide information concerning relevant premorbid history (e.g., educational level, occupation, interests). A thorough understanding of each of these factors allows the therapist to appropriately structure the learning environment and therapist–patient interactions.

■ ELECTROPHYSIOLOGICAL INTEGRITY OF MUSCLE AND NERVE

In the evaluation of muscle performance and motor control, we are concerned with the integrity of both central and peripheral mechanisms. The assessment of electrophysiological properties of nerve and muscle provides essential information to understand diagnosis of neuromuscular disease or trauma, the location of a lesion within the PNS, and prognosis or rate of healing or decay. Such disorders typically result in weakness or lack of motor coordination in movement, resulting in disruption to feedback and motor control mechanisms. Such disorders may be related to neuropathic or myopathic processes, or diseases affecting the neuromuscular junction.[81] Clinical **electromyography** (EMG) is used to evaluate the scope of a neuromuscular disorder through assessment of muscle activity. **Nerve conduction velocity** (NCV) tests determine the speed with which a peripheral motor or sensory nerve conducts an impulse. Together, data from EMG and NCV tests assist with establishing anticipated goals and expected outcomes for patients with musculoskeletal and neuromuscular disorders. EMG findings are not diagnostic in isolation, however, and must be considered in relation to clinical findings, as well as findings from other physical therapy, medical, and physiological tests and measurements.

Concepts of Electromyography

EMG is the recording of the electrical activity of muscle based on motor unit activity. Motor units are composed of one anterior horn cell, one axon, its neuromuscular junctions, and all the muscle fibers innervated by that axon (Fig. 5.1). The single axon conducts an impulse to all its muscle fibers, causing them to depolarize at relatively the same time. This depolarization produces electrical activity that is manifested as a **motor unit action potential** (MUAP) and recorded and displayed graphically as the EMG signal. The characteristics of the MUAP will change when there is damage to either the nerve or muscle.

Recording the EMG Signal

EMG signals are captured using a needle electrode, which is inserted into the muscle through the skin. The

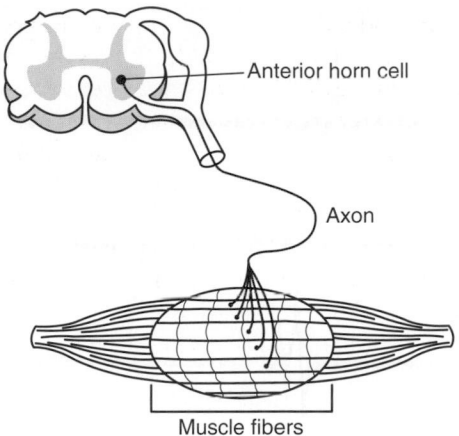

Figure 5.1 The motor unit is composed of one anterior horn cell, one axon, its neuromuscular junction, and all the muscle fibers innervated by that axon.

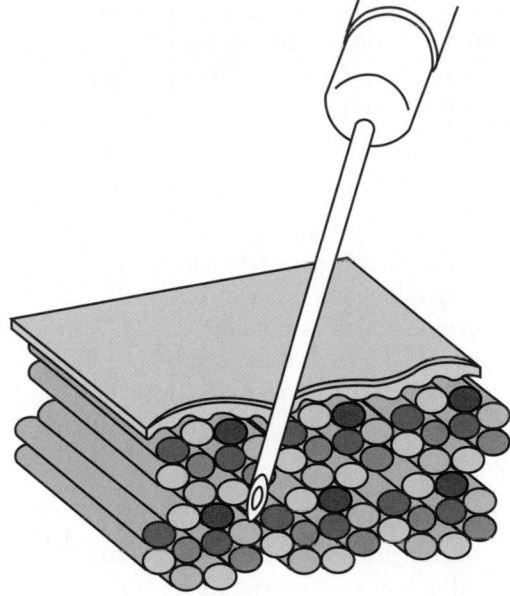

Figure 5.2 Cross-sectional view of muscle belly with needle electrode inserted. Differently shaded fibers represent different motor units.

most common types of needle electrodes are bipolar and monopolar. A *bipolar electrode* is a hypodermic needle, through which a single wire of platinum or silver is threaded. The cannula shaft and wire are insulated from each other, and only their tips are exposed. The wire and the needle cannula act as recording and reference electrodes, and the difference in potential between them is recorded in volts.

A *monopolar needle electrode* is composed of a single fine needle, insulated except at the tip. A second surface electrode placed on the skin near the site of insertion serves as the reference electrode. These electrodes are less painful than concentric electrodes because they are smaller in diameter.

It is important to understand the process by which an MUAP is transmitted to an amplifier in order to understand how such potentials can be interpreted. Because of the dispersion of the fibers in a single motor unit, the muscle fibers from several motor units will be interspersed with one another (Fig. 5.2). Therefore, when one motor unit contracts, the depolarizing fibers are not necessarily close together. Consequently, a needle electrode cannot be situated precisely within one motor unit.

All the fibers of a single motor unit contract almost synchronously, and the electrical potentials arising from them travel through body fluids in all directions, not just in the direction of the inserted needle. Fibrous tissue, fat, and blood vessels act as insulators in this process. Therefore, the actual pattern of the flow of electrical activity is not predictable. The signals that do reach the electrode are transmitted to an amplifier. The activity produced by all the individual fibers contracting at any one time is summated, reaching the electrode almost simultaneously. Electrodes only record potentials they pick up, without differentiating their origin. Therefore, if two motor units contract at the same time, from the same or adjacent muscles, the activity from fibers of both units will be summated and recorded as one large potential.

The size and shape of the MUAP can be affected by several variables. The proximity of the electrodes to the fibers that are firing will affect the amplitude and duration of the recorded potential. Fibers that are further away will contribute less to the recorded potential. The tissue between the electrode and active muscle fibers also acts as a low-pass filter, attenuating the higher-frequency components of the signal. The number and size of the fibers in the motor unit will influence the potential's size. A larger motor unit will produce more activity. Finally, the distance between the fibers will affect the output, because if the fibers are very spread out, less of their total activity is likely to reach the electrodes.

In addition to these variables, many excess signals, or *artifacts*, can be recorded and processed simultaneously with the EMG signal. An artifact is any unwanted electrical activity that arises outside of the tissues being examined. These artifacts can be of sufficient voltage to distort the output signal markedly, such as those coming from other electrical equipment or fluorescent lights. Electromyographers will usually observe the output signal on an oscilloscope or computer screen to monitor artifacts.

An MUAP is actually the summation of electrical potentials from all the fibers of that unit close enough to the electrodes to be recorded. The amplitude (voltage) is affected by the number of fibers involved or by the motor unit territory. The duration and shape are functions of the distance of the fibers from the recording electrodes, the more distant fibers contributing to terminal phases of the potential. Because of these variables, each motor unit will have a distinctive shape (see Fig. 5.3).

The EMG Examination

EMG testing is only part of a complete examination, which will include a thorough understanding of the patient's history and clinical findings. For example, the therapist might also examine muscle strength, pain, reflexes, fatigue, sensory function, and the presence of atrophy, as well as functional abilities. This clinical examination will suggest which muscles and/or nerves should be tested.

Initially, the patient is asked to relax the muscle to be examined during insertion of the needle electrode. Insertion into a contracting muscle is uncomfortable, but bearable. At this time, the electromyographer will observe a spontaneous burst of potentials, called *insertional activity,* which is possibly caused by the needle breaking through muscle fiber membranes. This normally lasts less than 300 milliseconds (msec).[82] Insertional activity can be described as normal, reduced, absent, increased, or prolonged.

Following cessation of insertional activity, a normal relaxed muscle will exhibit *electrical silence,* which is the absence of electrical potentials. Observation of silence in the relaxed state is an important part of the EMG examination. Potentials arising spontaneously during this period are significant abnormal findings.

After observing the muscle at rest, the patient is asked to contract the muscle minimally. This weak voluntary effort should cause individual motor units to fire. These motor unit potentials are examined with respect to amplitude, duration, shape, sound, and frequency (Fig. 5.3). These five parameters are the essential characteristics that distinguish each normal and abnormal potential.

Finally, the patient is asked to increase levels of contraction progressively to a strong effort, allowing determination of recruitment patterns. Gradually increasing the force of contraction will allow the electromyographer to observe the pattern of recruitment in the muscle. With greater effort, increasing numbers of motor units fire at higher frequencies, until the individual potentials are summated and can no longer be recognized, and an *interference pattern* is seen (Fig. 5.4). This is the normal finding with a strong contraction.

The needle electrode will be moved to different areas and depths of each muscle to sample different muscle fibers and motor units. This is necessary because of the small area from which a needle electrode will pick up electrical activity, and because the effects of pathology may vary within a single muscle. Up to 25 different points within a muscle may be examined by moving and reinserting the needle electrode.

In normal muscle, the peak-to-peak amplitude of a single MUAP, recorded with a concentric needle, may range from 100 microvolts (μV) to 5 millivolts (mV). The amplitude is determined primarily by a limited number of fibers located close to the electrode tip. Therefore, motor units must be sampled from different sites in a muscle to determine the amplitude of motor units in that muscle accurately. The normal motor unit has an identifying sound as a clear, distinct thump. The duration of the potential is a measure of time from onset

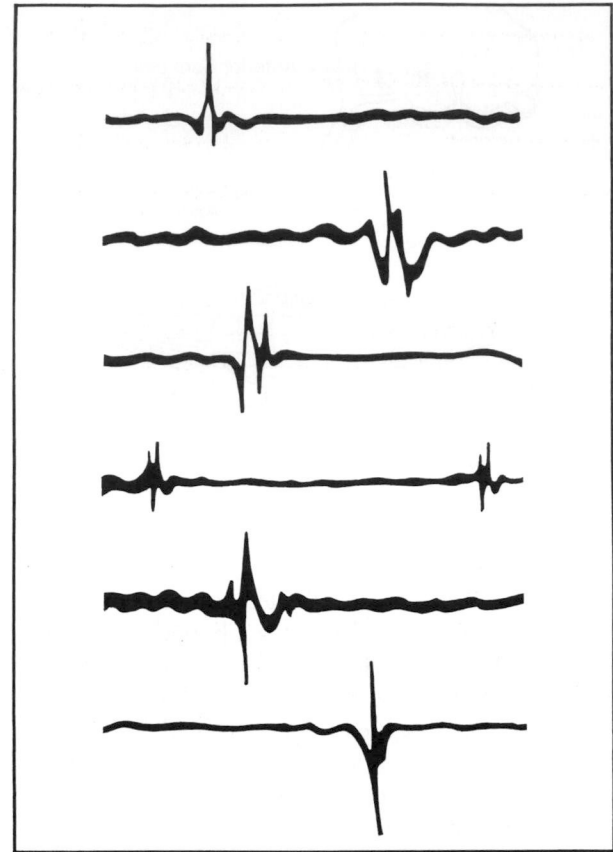

Figure 5.3 Single motor unit potentials as seen on an oscilloscope or computer. Each unit has a distinct shape.

to cessation of the electrical potential, typically from 2 to 14 msec.[84]

The number of phases in a normal motor unit can be from one to four phases. The typical shape of an MUAP is diphasic or triphasic, with a *phase* representing a section of a potential above or below the baseline. It is not abnormal to observe small numbers of *polyphasic potentials,* having five or more phases, in normal muscle. However, when polyphasic potentials represent more than 10% of a muscle's output, it may be an abnormal finding.

Spontaneous Abnormal Potentials

Because a normal muscle at rest exhibits electrical silence, any activity seen during the relaxed state can be considered abnormal. Such activity is termed *spontaneous* because it is not produced by voluntary muscle contraction. Several types of spontaneous potentials have been identified. **Fibrillation potentials** are believed to arise from spontaneous depolarization of a single muscle fiber. They are not visible through the skin. Fibrillation potentials are biphasic spikes, classically indicative of LMN disorders, such as peripheral nerve lesions, anterior horn cell disease, radiculopathies, and polyneuropathies with axonal degeneration (Fig. 5.5). They are also found to a lesser extent in myopathic diseases such as muscular

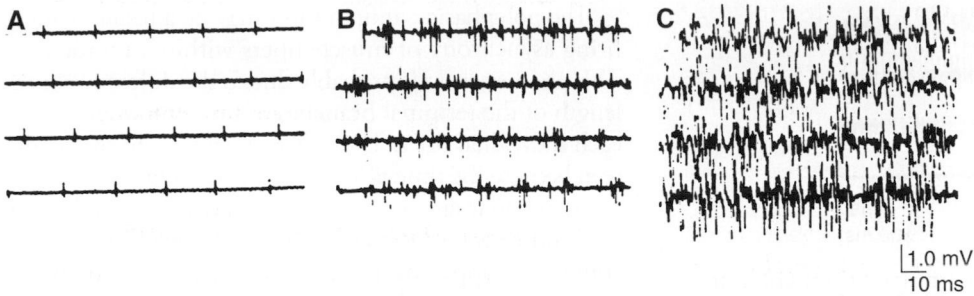

Figure 5.4 Normal recruitment of the triceps brachii in a 44-year-old healthy man. Activity was recorded during minimal contraction **(A)** when single motor unit potentials are visible, during moderate contraction **(B)** when motor units are recruited, and during maximal contraction **(C)** when an interference pattern is visible. *(From Kimura,[83, p. 24] with permission.)*

dystrophy, dermatomyositis, polymyositis, and myasthenia gravis. Their sound is a high-pitched click, which has been likened to rain falling on a roof or wrinkling tissue paper.

Positive sharp waves have been observed in denervated muscle at rest, usually accompanied by fibrillation potentials; however, they are also reported in primary muscle disease, especially muscular dystrophy and polymyositis. The waves are typically biphasic, with a sharp initial positive deflection (below baseline) followed by a slow negative phase (see Fig. 5.5). The negative phase is of much lower amplitude than the positive phase, and of much longer duration, sometimes up to 100 msec. The peak-to-peak amplitude may be variable,

with voltages from 50 μV up to 2 mV. The sound has been described as a dull thud.

Investigators have demonstrated spontaneous potentials in normal muscles of healthy subjects, primarily in muscles of the feet.[85] They have suggested that pathological changes involving axonal loss, segmental demyelination, and collateral sprouting may be associated with aging or mechanical trauma to the feet.

Fasciculations are spontaneous potentials seen with irritation or degeneration of the anterior horn cell, chronic peripheral nerve lesions, nerve root compression, and muscle spasms or cramps. They are believed to represent the involuntary asynchronous. Their sound has been described as a low-pitched thump. Fasciculations are often visible through the skin, seen as a small twitch. They are not by themselves a definitive abnormal finding, however, because they are also seen in normal individuals, particularly in calf muscle, eyes, hands, and feet.[86]

Complex repetitive discharges may be seen with lesions of the anterior horn cell and peripheral nerves, and with myopathies. The discharge is characterized by an extended train of potentials with the same or nearly the same waveform. The feature that distinguishes these discharges from other spontaneous potentials is their regular and repetitive waveform. The frequency usually ranges from 5 to 100 impulses per second. *Myotonic repetitive discharges* that increase and decrease in amplitude in a waxing and waning fashion are found in myotonic disorders such as myotonic dystrophy, as well as other myopathies (Fig. 5.6). The sound is highly characteristic and sounds like a "dive-bomber." High-frequency discharges are probably triggered by movement of the needle electrode within unstable muscle fibers, or by volitional activity.

Polyphasic Potentials

Polyphasic potentials are generally considered abnormal, and are elicited on voluntary contraction, not at rest. By definition, polyphasic potentials are motor unit

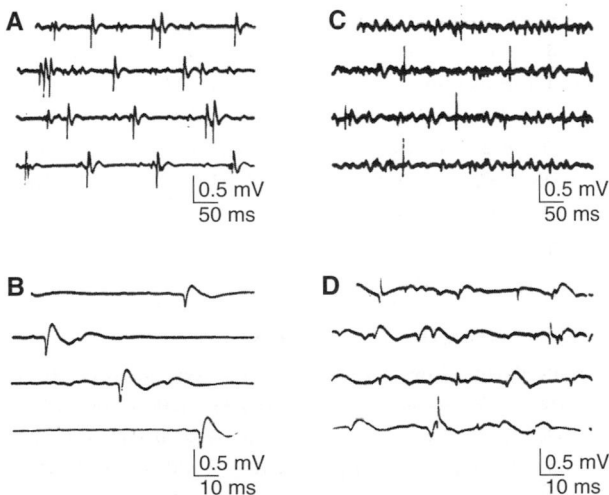

Figure 5.5 Spontaneous activity of the anterior tibialis in a 68-year-old woman with amyotrophic lateral sclerosis. Positive sharp waves **(A, B)** have a consistent configuration with a sharp positive deflection followed by a long-duration, low-amplitude negative deflection **(B)**. Fibrillation potentials **(C, D)** are low-amplitude biphasic spikes. *(From Kimura,[83, p. 256] with permission.)*

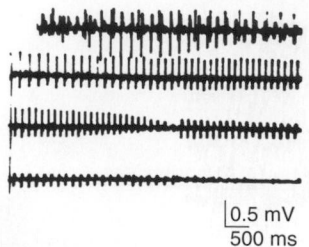

Figure 5.6 Repetitive discharge from the right anterior tibialis of a 39-year-old man with myotonic dystrophy. The waxing and waning quality of these discharges will result in a "dive-bomber" sound. *(From Kimura,[83, p. 254] with permission.)*

potentials with five or more phases (Fig. 5.7). They are typical of myopathies, peripheral nerve involvement, and nerve root compression. In primary muscle disease (myopathies), these potentials are generally of smaller amplitude than normal motor units, are of shorter duration, and have been described by some as myopathic potentials. These multiphasic changes occur because of a decrease in the number of active muscle fibers within the individual motor units due to pathology. Although the entire unit will fire during voluntary contraction, fewer fibers are available in each unit to contribute to the total voltage and the duration of the potential.

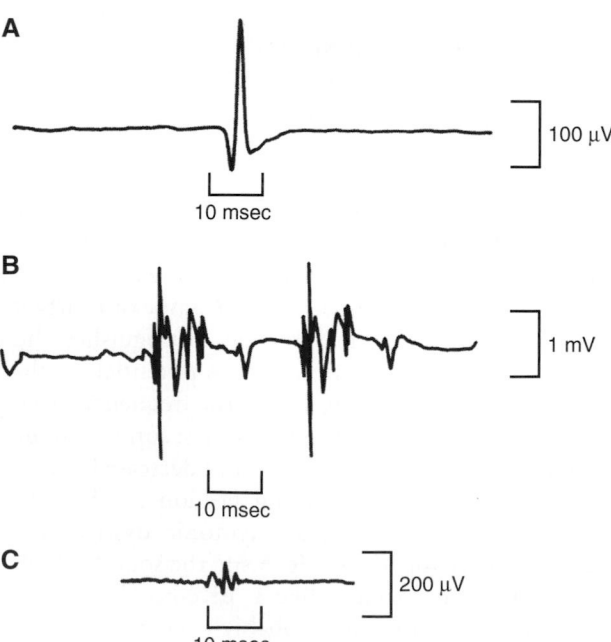

Figure 5.7 Motor unit action potentials. **(A)** Normal potential. **(B)** Long-duration polyphasic potential (shown twice). **(C)** Short-duration, low-amplitude, polyphasic potential. *(From Aminoff, MJ: Electromyography in Clinical Practice, ed 3. Churchill Livingstone (Elsevier), New York, 1997, p. 74, with permission.)*

The polyphasic configuration may be a result of slight firing asynchrony of muscle fibers within a motor unit. This phenomenon is probably due to the difference in the length of the terminal branches of the axon extending to each individual fiber. The effects of this are normally not seen because the time differences are so slight. When some fibers are no longer contracting, or a delay in conduction is found in the terminal branches, these differences become more apparent, resulting in a fragmentation of the motor unit potential.

Polyphasic potentials may also be seen during degeneration and after regeneration of a peripheral nerve. As some muscle fibers become reinnervated, they will generate action potentials with voluntary contraction. However, there are significantly fewer fibers acting than were present in the original unit, and these fibers will clearly reflect asynchronous depolarization. These polyphasic potentials are also much smaller in amplitude and duration than normal units, and they have been termed *nascent motor units*. Although polyphasic potentials are generally considered an abnormal finding, they are a positive finding in patients with regenerating peripheral nerve lesions because they indicate reinnervation.

Some forms of neuropathic involvement, such as chronic peripheral nerve lesions, peripheral neuropathies, and anterior horn cell disease, will result in a change in motor unit territory of an intact motor unit by collateral sprouting of axons to fibers of denervated motor units, forming *"giant" motor units,* which are larger than normal motor unit potentials. In the early stages of this process these sprouts are of small diameter and have slow conduction velocities, resulting in a dispersion in the recorded potential, which increases the amplitude and duration and results in a polyphasic shape. These potentials may be seen in postpolio syndrome.[87-89] If this situation is sufficiently prevalent, the interference pattern may be incomplete. The amplitude of these potentials is greater than 5 mV in small muscles such as the intrinsic muscles of the hands and feet. In other muscles, amplitudes of 3 mV or more could be considered as larger than normal. Duration of these motor units is 4 to 5 msec up to 25 to 30 msec. Other characteristics are similar to normal motor units.

Nerve Conduction Tests

Nerve conduction velocity (NCV) tests involve direct stimulation to initiate an impulse in motor or sensory nerves. The *conduction time* is measured by recording the *evoked potential* either from the muscle innervated by the motor nerve or from the sensory nerve itself. NCV can be tested on any peripheral nerve that is superficial enough to be stimulated through the skin at two different points. The most commonly tested motor nerves are the ulnar, median, fibular (peroneal), tibial, radial, femoral, and sciatic nerves. Commonly tested sensory nerves include the median, ulnar, radial, sural, and superficial fibular nerves. Complete guidelines for performing NCV tests are available in comprehensive references.[82,84,90]

Motor Nerve Conduction Velocity Testing

Because a peripheral nerve trunk houses both sensory and motor fibers, recording potentials directly from a peripheral nerve makes monitoring of purely sensory or motor nerves impossible. Therefore, to isolate the potentials conducted by motor axons of a mixed nerve, the evoked potential is recorded from a distal muscle innervated by the nerve under study. Although the stimulation of the nerve will evoke sensory and motor impulses, only the motor fibers contribute to the contraction of the muscle. For example, to test the ulnar nerve, the test muscle is typically the abductor digiti minimi. Other examples are the following: for the median nerve, the abductor pollicis brevis; for the fibular nerve, the extensor digitorum brevis; and for the tibial nerve, the abductor hallicus or abductor digiti minimi.

Small surface electrodes are usually used to record the evoked potential from the test muscle. The *recording electrode* is placed over the belly of the test muscle and a reference electrode is taped over the tendon of the muscle.

For the purposes of illustration, the test procedure for the motor NCV of the median nerve will be described (Fig. 5.8). The technique is basically the same for all nerves, except for the sites of stimulation and placement of the electrodes. For this example, the recording electrode is taped over the abductor pollicis brevis. The stimulating electrode is placed over the median nerve at the wrist, just proximal to the distal crease on the volar surface.

At the moment the stimulus is produced, the *stimulus artifact* is seen at the left of the oscilloscope screen (Fig. 5.9). A trigger mechanism controls this and it will, therefore, always appear in the same spot on the screen, facilitating consistent measurements. This spike is purely mechanical and does not represent any muscle activity.

The stimulus intensity starts out low and is slowly increased until the evoked potential is clearly observed. When the stimulating electrode is properly placed over the nerve, all muscles innervated distal to that point will contract and the patient will see and feel the hand "jump." The intensity is then increased until the evoked response no longer increases in size. At that time, the intensity is increased further to be sure that the stimulus is *supramaximal.* Because the intensity must be sufficient to reach the threshold of all motor fibers in the nerve, a supramaximal stimulus is required. It is also essential that the stimulator be properly placed over the nerve trunk so that the stimulus reaches all the motor axons.

As in the EMG signal, the potentials seen on the screen represent the electrical activity detected by the recording electrode. The signal will represent the

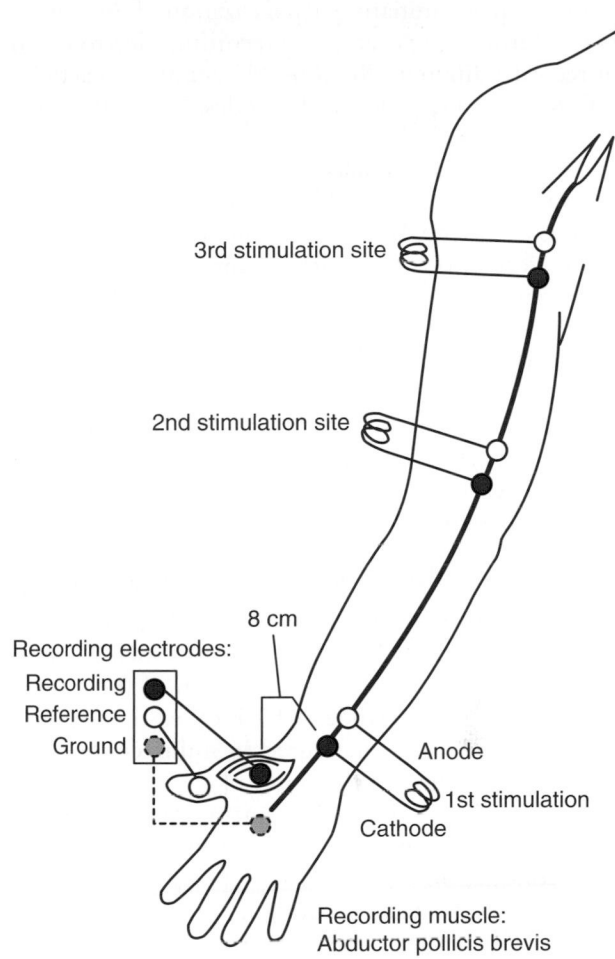

Figure 5.8 Sites of stimulation for motor nerve conduction study of the median nerve. *(From Echternach,[84, p. 34] with permission.)*

difference in electrical potential between the recording and reference electrodes. When the supramaximal stimulus is applied to the median nerve at the wrist, all the axons in the nerve will depolarize and begin conducting an impulse, transmitting the signal across the

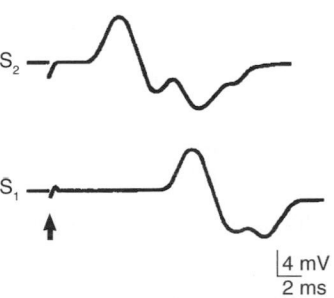

Figure 5.9 Recording of the M wave from a nerve conduction velocity test of the median nerve. The upper trace is from the distal stimulation site, and the lower trace is from the proximal stimulation site. The stimulus artifact appears at the left of both traces. The latencies are measured from the stimulus artifact to the start of the M wave.

motor end plate, initiating depolarization of the muscle fibers. During these events, the recording electrodes do not record a difference in potential because no activity is taking place beneath the electrodes. When the muscle fibers begin to depolarize, the electrical potentials are transmitted to the electrodes, and a deflection is seen on the oscilloscope. This is the evoked potential, which is called the *M wave* (see Fig. 5.9). The M wave is also referred to as the motor action potential (MAP) or compound motor action potential (CMAP). The M wave represents the summated activity of all motor units in the muscle that responded to stimulation of the nerve trunk. The amplitude of this potential is, therefore, a function of the total voltage produced by the contracting motor units. The initial deflection of the M wave is the negative portion of the wave, above the baseline.

Calculation of Motor Nerve Conduction Velocity

The point at which the M wave leaves the baseline indicates the time elapsed from the initial propagation of the nerve impulse to the depolarization of the muscle fibers beneath the electrodes. This is called the response *latency*. The latency is measured in milliseconds from the stimulus artifact to the onset of the M wave. This time alone is not a valid measurement of nerve conduction because it incorporates other events besides pure nerve conduction—namely, transmission across the myoneural junction and generation of the muscle action potential. Therefore, these extraneous factors must be eliminated from the calculation of the motor NCV, so that the measurement reflects only the speed of conduction within the nerve trunk.

To account for these distal variables, the nerve is stimulated at a second, more proximal point. This will produce a response similar to that seen with distal stimulation. The stimulus artifact will appear in the same spot on the screen, but the M wave will originate in a different place because the time for the impulses to reach the muscle would, obviously, be longer. Subtraction of the *distal latency* from the *proximal latency* will determine the conduction time for the nerve trunk segment between the two points of stimulation. *Conduction velocity (CV)* is determined by dividing the distance between the two points of stimulation (measured along the surface) by the difference between the two latencies (velocity = distance/time).

CV = Conduction distance/(Proximal latency − Distal latency)

Conduction velocity is always expressed in meters per second (m/sec), although distance is usually measured in centimeters and latencies in milliseconds. These units must be converted during calculation.

To complete the example of the median nerve, two other sites would be stimulated, where the median nerve crosses the elbow and in the axilla (see Fig. 5.8).

Although motor NCV tests can be performed on these more proximal segments of the nerve trunk, these areas are tested less frequently than the distal-most site.

To compute the motor NCV, the proximal and distal latencies are determined by measuring the time from the stimulus artifact to the initial M wave deflection. The conduction time is calculated by taking the difference between these latencies. *Conduction distance* is then determined by measuring the length of the nerve between the two points of stimulation. For example:

Proximal latency: 7 msec
Distal latency: 2 msec
Conduction distance: 300 mm or 30 cm
CV = 30 cm / (7 msec − 2 msec) = 30 cm/5 msec = 60 m/sec

Interpretation of the motor NCV is made in relation to normal values, which are usually expressed as mean values, standard deviations, and ranges. Many investigators in different laboratories have determined normal values. Even so, average values seem to be fairly consistent. The motor NCV for the UE has a fairly wide range, with values reported from 50 to 70 m/sec. The average normal value is about 60 m/sec. For the LE, the average value is about 50 m/sec. Distal latencies and average normal amplitudes of M waves are also available in such tables, but these must be viewed with caution, because technique, electrode setup, instrumentation, and patient size can affect these values. Age and temperature can also influence NCV measurements, decreasing after age 35 and with lower temperature.[81] The reader is referred to more comprehensive discussions for complete details about techniques for studying various nerves and for tables of normal values.[84,90]

It is important to note that the value calculated as the conduction velocity is actually a reflection of the speed of the fastest axons in the nerve. Although all axons are stimulated at the same point in time, and supposedly fire at the same time, their conduction rates vary with their size. Not all motor units will contract at the same time; some receive their nerve impulse later than others. Therefore, the initial M wave deflection represents the contraction of the motor unit, or units, with the fastest conduction velocity. The curved shape of the M wave is reflective of the progressively slower axons reaching their motor units at a later time.

The M wave can also provide useful information about the integrity of the nerve or muscle. Three parameters should be examined: amplitude, shape, and duration. Any change occurring in these characteristics is called *temporal dispersion*. These parameters reflect the summated voltage over time produced by all the contracting motor units within the test muscle. Therefore, if the muscle is partially denervated, fewer motor units will contract after nerve stimulation. This will cause the M wave amplitude to decrease. Duration may change depending on the conduction velocity of the intact units. Similar changes may also be evident in myopathic conditions, in which all motor units are intact, but fewer fibers are available in each motor unit.

The shape of the M wave can also be variable. Deviation from a smooth curve need not be abnormal, and it is often useful to compare the proximal and distal M waves with each other as well as with the contralateral side if indicated. They should be similar. In abnormal conditions, changes in shape may be the result of a significant slowing of conduction in some axons, repetitive firing, or asynchronous firing of axons after a single stimulus.

Sensory Nerve Conduction Velocity Testing

Sensory neurons demonstrate the same physiological properties as motor neurons, and NCV can be measured in a similar way. However, some differences in technique are necessary to differentiate between sensory and motor axons. Although sensory fibers can be tested using *orthodromic conduction* (physiological direction) or *antidromic conduction* (opposite to normal conduction), antidromic measurements appear to be more common. For the same reason that motor axons are examined by recording over muscle, sensory axons are either stimulated or recorded from digital sensory nerves. This eliminates the activity of the motor axons from the recorded potentials.

The stimulating electrode used for sensory NCV tests is typically provided by ring electrodes placed around the base of the middle of the digit innervated by the nerve. The recording electrodes can be surface or needle electrodes. Surface electrodes are placed over the nerve trunk, where it is superficial to the skin.

Sensory potentials for the median and ulnar nerves can be recorded antidromically by stimulating at the wrist, elbow, and upper arm. Typically the sensory study of these nerves is limited to stimulation at the wrist. Other sensory nerves can be studied in the UEs, which include the superficial radial nerve, the medial and lateral antibrachial cutaneous nerves, and the dorsal branch of the ulnar nerve. In the LEs, the sensory nerves most commonly studied are the sural nerve and the superficial fibular (peroneal) nerves. Other nerves that have been studied include the lateral femoral cutaneous nerve and the saphenous nerve. Normal sensory NCV ranges between 40 and 75 m/sec. Amplitude, measured with surface electrodes, may be 10 to 120 μV, and duration should be short, less than 2 msec. Sensory evoked potentials are usually sharp, not rounded like the M wave. Sensory NCVs are slightly faster than motor NCVs because of the larger diameter of sensory nerves.

H Reflex

The *H reflex* is a useful diagnostic measure for radiculopathy and peripheral neuropathy. Its most common application is in testing the integrity of the sensory and motor monosynaptic pathways of S1 nerve roots, and to a lesser extent at C6 and C7.[91] A submaximal stimulus is applied to the tibial nerve at the popliteal fossa, and a motor response is recorded from the medial portion of the soleus muscle. The action potentials travel along the IA afferent neurons toward the spinal cord, synapsing onto alpha motor neurons within the anterior horn. The consequent activation of the motor neuron leads to an impulse traveling peripherally to the soleus muscle, resulting in a muscle contraction. Because the stimulus causes impulses to travel both distally and proximally within a mixed motor and sensory neuron, the latency of this response is a measure of the integrity of both sensory and motor fibers.

A normal response falls within ± 5.5 msec of this calculated latency. An average response is 29.8 msec (± 2.74 msec).[92] A slowed latency is indicative of abnormal dorsal root function, often from a herniated disc or impingement syndrome. Because of this central involvement, the peripheral motor and sensory NCV would not be affected. This latency may also identify nerve root compression before obvious EMG changes occur.

The F Wave

F waves are a form of NCV test that allows for study of proximal nerve segments that would otherwise be inaccessible to routine nerve conduction studies. F wave abnormalities can be a sensitive indicator of peripheral nerve pathology. The F wave ratio compares the conduction in the proximal half of the total pathway with the distal and may be used to determine the site of conduction slowing—for example, to distinguish a root lesion from a distal generalized neuropathy.[93]

The F wave is elicited by the supramaximal stimulus of a peripheral nerve at a distal site, leading to propagation of impulses in both directions. While the orthodromic impulse travels to the distal muscle, the antidromic response travels to the anterior horn cell, depolarizing the axon hillock, leading to depolarization of dendrites, which in turn depolarizes the axon hillock once again, generating an orthodromic volley back to the muscle. No synapse is involved, so the F wave is not considered a reflex, but only a measure of motor neuron conduction.

The F wave is a useful supplement to nerve conduction and EMG measures, and is most helpful in the diagnosis of conditions where the most proximal portion of the axon is involved, such as Guillain-Barré syndrome, thoracic outlet syndrome, brachial plexus injuries, and radiculopathies with more than one nerve root involved.[84] The latency of the F wave is normally approximately 30 seconds in the upper limb and less than 60 seconds in the lower limb. Only a small percent of motor neurons actually participate in the F response.[94] Because it is an inconsistent response, it must be calculated on the basis of at least 10 successive trials.

Disorders of Peripheral Nerve

Electrophysiological findings usually correlate with clinical signs in patients with neuropathic or myopathic involvement. Lesions of peripheral nerve fall into three categories. **Neurapraxia** is a temporary impairment in nerve conduction typically caused by some form of local compression or blockage, such as in carpal tunnel syndrome. NCV tests can detect evidence of degeneration and slowing of fibers across the site of compression, but may be normal above and below that site. Normal values must be interpreted relative to other disorders such as diabetes or active workers.[95] **Axonotmesis** results from a nerve injury that damages the axon but leaves the neural tube is intact. *Wallerian degeneration*, the dying back of the axons of nerves after insult, occurs distal to the lesion. This may be progressive due to long-standing neurapraxia, or it may occur from a traumatic lesion. NCV will be affected depending on the number of axons involved. Fibrillations and positive sharp waves are typically present 2 to 3 weeks after denervation. **Neurotmesis** is a nerve injury with complete loss of axonal function and disruption of the neural tube. Conduction ceases below the lesion and NCV tests cannot be performed. Spontaneous potentials will appear on EMG at rest. Regeneration may be evident through serial testing, showing appearance of small polyphasic potentials.

Neuropathy is any disease of nerves. *Polyneuropathy* affects multiple nerves and typically results in sensory changes, distal weakness, and hyporeflexia. It can be related to medical conditions, such as diabetes, alcoholism, or renal disease, as well as secondary complications related to cancer and its treatments.[96] These conditions are typically manifested as axonal damage or demyelinization or both. With axonal lesions, EMG recruitment patterns are decreased and spontaneous potentials are typically seen (Fig. 5.10). With demyelinization, NCV measurements are most useful to identify slowing in motor or sensory fibers.

Motor Neuron Disorders

Motor neuron disorders typically involve degeneration of the anterior horn cell, such as in poliomyelitis, or diseases that involve both UMNs and LMNs, such as amyotrophic lateral sclerosis. Spontaneous potentials are classically seen with these disorders, as well as reduced recruitment, allowing single motor unit potentials to be visible even with an interference pattern. Motor NCV can be slowed, depending on the distribution of degeneration. Large polyphasic potentials are often seen later in the course of the disease, due to collateral sprouting and reinnervation.

Myopathies

Myopathy is a primary muscle disease that may be acquired or congenital (e.g., muscular dystrophy, limb girdle myopathy). The motor unit remains intact, but degeneration of muscle fibers is evident. Therefore, motor NCV may be normal, although the M wave amplitude will be reduced. Sensory potentials will also be normal. In early stages, EMG will show prolonged insertion activity, fibrillations and positive sharp waves at rest, and short-duration, low-amplitude polyphasic potentials with voluntary activity, reflecting loss of muscle fibers (Fig. 5.11). Interference patterns will be evident with less than maximal contractions. In advanced stages, no electrical activity may be seen due to fibrosis of muscle tissue.

■ EVALUATION

Evaluation refers to the clinical judgments therapists make based on the data gathered from the examination.[4] Numerous factors influence the judgments therapists make when working with patients with impairments of motor function, including complexity and understanding of the nervous system, clinical findings, psychosocial considerations, and overall physical function and health. Therapists evaluate data in terms of severity of problems (impairments, activity limitations, participation

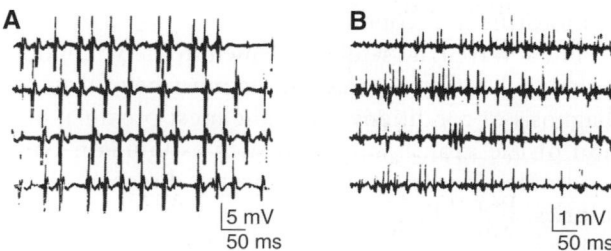

Figure 5.10 Large-amplitude, long-duration motor unit potentials from the first dorsal interosseus **(A)** compared with relatively normal motor unit potentials from orbicularis oculi **(B)** in a patient with polyneuropathy. Note discrete single-unit interference pattern during maximal voluntary contraction. *(From Kimura,[83, p. 267] with permission.)*

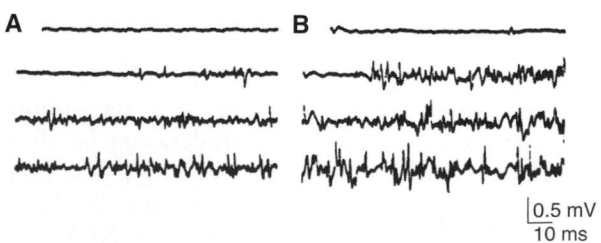

Figure 5.11 Low-amplitude, short-duration motor unit potentials recorded during minimal voluntary contraction from the biceps brachii **(A)** and tibialis anterior **(B)** in a 7-year-old boy with Duchenne's dystrophy. A high number of discharging motor units during minimal contraction reflects early recruitment because of decreased fiber activity. *(From Kimura,[83, p. 268] with permission.)*

restrictions) and level of chronicity. Therapists must also consider the consequences of failure to intervene appropriately when the patient is at risk for additional impairments or prolonged activity limitation. Potential discharge placement and resources also influence evaluation of the data and development of the POC. There is a clear need for the therapist to focus on those problems that directly affect function and can be successfully remediated.

DIAGNOSIS

The *physical therapy diagnosis* is determined from evaluation of examination findings and is based on a cluster of signs, symptoms, or categories. The *Guide to Physical Therapist Practice,*[4] a consensus document developed by expert physical therapy clinicians, identifies diagnostic categories and preferred practice patterns that delineate appropriate interventions (see Chapter 1, Clinical Decision Making, Appendix 1.A). For example, Impaired Motor Function and Sensory Integrity Associated with Acquired Nonprogressive Disorders of the Central Nervous System includes patients with TBI, cerebrovascular accident, or tumor.[4, p. 365] The reader is referred to this document for comparison to and refinement of his or her own practice. Novice therapists can gain understanding and insights into the complex practice issues facing therapists who work with patients with impairments in motor function.

SUMMARY

Examination of motor function is a challenging, multifaceted process, critically related to the therapist's ability to accurately determine and categorize findings. An understanding of normal motor control and motor learning mechanisms is essential to this process. Determining the causative factors responsible for abnormal movement patterns and behaviors must be based on comparison of expected or normal responses (norm-referenced behaviors) with the patient's abnormal ones. This can best be achieved by a systematic and thorough approach to examination. Emphasis should be on the use of valid, reliable, and responsive measurement tools.

Examination of systems yields valuable information about the integrity of individual components (e.g., neuromuscular, musculoskeletal, cognitive). However, it is important to recall that normal motor control and motor learning is achieved through the integrated action of the CNS. The therapist must therefore also focus on integrated function evidenced through an examination at the functional level. Success in rehabilitation is also dependent on our ability to understand the learning abilities of the patient and potential training strategies important for cognitive engagement and practice. Our theoretical understanding of the CNS, motor control, and motor learning processes is both incomplete and imperfect. Therapists must, therefore, be constantly aware of the changing knowledge base in neuroscience and in neurological rehabilitation to incorporate new ideas into their examination and intervention plan.

Questions for Review

1. Differentiate between recovery of function and compensation.

2. Describe the examination of consciousness and arousal. How can the levels of consciousness and arousal influence the motor function examination?

3. Differentiate between selective attention and alternating attention. How should each be examined?

4. Differentiate between spasticity and rigidity. How should each be examined?

5. Describe the examination of a hyperactive patellar deep tendon reflex. What scores are used to document an increased DTR?

6. A patient with stroke exhibits abnormal control of eye muscles and is unable to move the eyes smoothly in all directions. Cranial nerve testing should include what nerves and tests?

7. What are the issues of validity for using manual muscle testing as part of the examination of a patient with UMN syndrome (stroke) who exhibits strong spasticity and strong obligatory synergies?

8. A patient with multiple sclerosis reports fatigue as the number one symptom that impairs functional independence in the home environment. How should this patient's fatigue be examined and documented?

9. Define stability. How should it be examined?

10. Differentiate between the use of performance observations and retention tests in providing evidence of motor learning.

11. What is a fibrillation potential on EMG? What is it indicative of?

12. How is nerve conduction velocity calculated?

CASE STUDY

The patient is a 17-year-old female who is 6 months post–motor vehicle accident (MVA). At the time of admission to the hospital, she was comatose and decerebrate. CT scan revealed intracranial bleeding into the right occipital horn. She received a tracheostomy and a gastrostomy. Two months post-MVA, she was transferred to a *long-term care facility* specializing in TBI.

On initial admission she was able to open her eyes to verbal and tactile stimuli but was unable to visually track. She withdrew her upper and lower extremities in response to stimulation but was not able to move them on command. She was alert but confused, and was unable to carry on a conversation. ROM was within normal limits (WNL) except for right elbow flexion (20° to 100°) and right knee flexion (10° to 110°). She demonstrated increased tone (Modified Ashworth Scale 3) in her left upper extremity (LUE), 4 in her right upper extremity (RUE), and 4 in both lower extremities (BLEs). She exhibited 4+ bilateral ankle clonus. She was unable to sit unsupported. During supported sitting in the wheelchair, her head and trunk control was poor, with persistent posturing to the left side.

She is now 6 months post-MVA and is currently being examined for transfer to active rehabilitation status.

PHYSICAL THERAPY EXAMINATION FINDINGS
Consciousness/Arousal
Fully awake; responds appropriately to varying stimuli.
Oriented to person; some confusion with orientation to place and time.
Can become agitated with minimal stimulation, especially when tired.
Cognition/Behavior
Demonstrates difficulty with concentration and attention.
Able to follow simple instructions (one- or two-level commands) but occasionally forgets what is asked of her.
Reaction time is slowed as the number of choices is increased.
Easily forgets what she is doing.
Sensory Integrity
Aware of sensory input (pinprick, vibration, light touch) to all extremities.
Unable to discern common objects placed in either hand for stereognosis discrimination.
Joint Integrity and Mobility
RLE: plantarflexion contracture (40° to 50°); flexion contractures at the hip (10° to 120°) and knee (10° to 120°).
RUE: flexor contracture at the elbow (10° to 110°).
Full passive ROM in the LUE and LLE.
Tone
Increased bilaterally (R > L).
On Modified Ashworth Scale: RUE and RLE 3; LUE and LLE 2.
Reflex Integrity
Hyperactive, 3+ DTRs RUE, RLE.
3+ bilateral ankle clonus.
Cranial Nerve Integrity
Dysphagia and dysphonia are present.
Muscle Performance
Strength is decreased in the RUE, RLE, and trunk (unable to test with MMT).
She is unable to sustain R knee extension during standing.
Voluntary Movement Patterns
RUE moves in partial range, obligatory mass flexor synergy pattern only.
RLE moves in flexor and extensor synergy patterns with no variation.
LUE and LLE demonstrate full voluntary control with isolated joint movements. Coordination is decreased. Unable to reach directly to an object that is held out to her and demonstrates foot placement problems with the LLE in sitting or in standing.
Demonstrates problems with coordinating limb and trunk movements.

Postural Control and Balance

Demonstrates good head control in all positions.

Sitting: can sit independently for up to 5 minutes. Demonstrates difficulty in maintaining weight equally on both buttocks. Tends to list to the right side while placing weight primarily on her left buttock. Able to reach to the left and forward; demonstrates loss of balance (LOB) with minimal reaching to right.

Standing: able to stand in parallel bars with minimal assistance 1 for up to 2 minutes. Has to be reminded to place weight on RLE. Tends to lose her balance easily if she moves quickly; associated with brief episodes of dizziness and vertigo.

Functional Mobility Skills

Rolling: requires supervision and occasional minimal assistance with rolling to the right; she requires maximal assist when rolling to the left.

Supine-to-sit: able to come to sitting by rolling to the L side and pushing up with her LUE; requires minimal assistance.

Transfers: able to perform stand pivot transfers with minimal assistance of 1.

Gait: does not initiate ambulation on her own. Can ambulate the length of the parallel bars (2 m or 6 ft) with maximal assistance of two persons. Requires posterior splint to stabilize R knee.

Propels wheelchair by using the LUE and both feet for pushing; requires supervision for safety.

Motor Learning

Demonstrates profound deficits in short-term memory; unable to remember new information presented during therapy. Her memory for events and learning that occurred before the MVA is good.

GUIDING QUESTIONS

Based on your evaluation of the data presented in the case history and the physical therapy examination, answer the following questions:

1. How has this patient's level of consciousness/arousal changed from admission to the long-term care facility to the current evaluation? How might this influence the examination of motor function?

2. Develop a physical therapy problem list. Categorize the patient's problems in terms of (a) direct impairments, (b) indirect impairments, and (c) functional limitations.

3. Prioritize the problems in terms of this patient's needs for the POC.

4. Determine the physical therapy diagnosis using the preferred practice patterns identified by the *Guide to Physical Therapist Practice* (Chapter 1, Appendix 1.A).

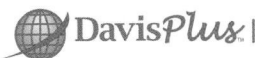 For additional resources, including answers to the questions for review and case study guiding questions, please visit **http://davisplus.fadavis.com**

References

1. Schmidt, R, and Lee, T: Motor Control and Learning, ed 5. Human Kinetics, Champaign, IL, 2011.
2. Shumway-Cook, A, and Woollacott, M: Motor Control: Theory and Practical Applications, ed 4. Lippincott Williams & Williams/Wolters Kluwer, Philadelphia, 2011.
3. Bernstein, N: The Coordination and Regulation of Movements. Pergamon Press, New York, 1967.
4. American Physical Therapy Association. Guide to Physical Therapist Practice, ed 2. American Physical Therapy Association, Alexandria, VA, 2001.
5. World Health Organization (WHO): ICF: Towards a Common Language for Functioning, Disability, and Health. Geneva, Switzerland, 2002. Retrieved March 4, 2011, from www.who.int/classifications/en.
6. Bear, M, Connors, B, and Paradiso, M: Neuroscience: Exploring the Brain, ed 3. Lippincott Williams & Wilkins/Wolters Kluwer, Philadelphia, 2007.
7. Bickley, LS, and Szilagyi, P: Bates' Guide to Physical Examination and History Taking, ed 10. Lippincott Williams & Wilkins/Wolters Kluwer, Philadelphia, 2009.

8. Jennett, B, and Bond, M: Assessment of outcome after severe head injury: A practical scale. Lancet 1:480, 1975.
9. Rancho Los Amigos Hospital: Rehabilitation of the Head Injured Adult. Professional Staff Association, Downey, CA, 1979.
10. Duffy, E: Activation and Behavior. Wiley, New York, 1962.
11. Yerkes, R, and Dodson, J: The relation of strength of stimulus to rapidity of habit-formation. J Comp Neurol Psychol 18(5):459, 1908.
12. Strub, R, and Black, F: The Mental Status Examination in Neurology, ed 4. FA Davis, Philadelphia, 2000.
13. Folstein, M: Mini-mental state: A practical method for grading the cognitive state of patients for the clinician. J Psychiatr Res 12:189, 1975.
14. Shean, G, and McGuire, R: Spastic hypertonia and movement disorders: Pathophysiology, clinical presentation, and quantification. PM & R 1:9, 2009.
15. Gracies, JM. Pathophysiology of spastic paresis. I: Paresis and soft tissue changes. Muscle Nerve 31:535, 2005.
16. Gracies, JM: Pathophysiology of spastic paresis. II: Emergence of muscle overactivity. Muscle Nerve 31:552, 2005.

17. Fuller, G: Neurological Examination Made Easy, ed 4. Churchill Livingstone/Elsevier, New York, 2008.

18. O'Sullivan, S, and Siegelman, R: National Physical Therapy Examination Review and Study Guide. Therapy Ed, Evanston, IL, 2013.

19. Ashworth, B: Preliminary trial of carisoprodol in multiple sclerosis. Practitioner 192:540, 1964.

20. Bohannon, R, and Smith, M: Interrater reliability of a modified Ashworth scale of muscle spasticity. Phys Ther 67:206, 1987.

21. Ghotbi, N, et al: Measurement of lower-limb muscle spasticity: Intrareliability of Modified Ashworth Scale. JRRD 48(1):83, 2011.

22. Craven, BC, and Morris, AR: Modified Ashworth Scale reliability for measurement of lower extremity spasticity among patients with SCI. Spinal Cord 48:207, 2010.

23. Ansari, NN, et al: The interrater and intrarater reliability of the Modified Ashworth Scale in the assessment of muscle spasticity: Limb and muscle group effect. Neuro Rehabil 23:231, 2008.

24. Mehrholz, J, et al: Reliability of the Modified Tardieu Scale and the Modified Ashworth Scale in adult patients with severe brain injury: A comparison study. Clin Rehabil 19:751, 2005.

25. Blackburn, M, et al: Reliability of measurements obtained with the Modified Ashworth Scale in the lower extremities of people with stroke. Phys Ther 82:25, 2002.

26. Pandyan, AD, et al: A review of the properties and limitations of the Ashworth and Modified Ashworth Scales as measures of spasticity. Clin Rehabil 13:373, 1999.

27. Bajd, T, and Vodovnik, L: Pendulum testing of spasticity. J Biomech Eng 6:9, 1984.

28. Bohannon, R: Variability and reliability of the pendulum test for spasticity using a Cybex II Isokinetic Dynamometer. Phys Ther 67:659, 1987.

29. Leonard, C, Stephens, J, and Stroppel, S: Assessing the spastic condition of individuals with upper motoneuron involvement: Validity of the Myotonometer. Arch Phys Med Rehabil 82:1416, 2001.

30. Leonard, C, et al: Myotonometer intra- and inter-rater reliabilities. Arch Phys Med Rehab 2003.

31. Capute, A, et al: Primitive Reflex Profile. University Park Press, Baltimore, 1978.

32. Capute, A, et al: Primitive reflex profile: A pilot study. Phys Ther 58:1061, 1978.

33. Sahrmann, S: Diagnosis and Treatment of Movement Impairment Syndromes. Mosby, St. Louis, 2002.

34. Kokotilo, K, Eng, JJ, and Boyd, L: Reorganization of brain function during force production after stroke. JNPT 33:45, 2009.

35. Gowland, C, et al: Agonist and antagonist activity during voluntary upper-limb movement in patients with stroke. Phys Ther 72:624, 1992.

36. Frascarelli, M, Mastrogregori, L, and Conforti, L: Initial motor unit recruitment in patients with spastic hemiplegia. Electromyogr Clin Neurophysiol 38:267, 1998.

37. Bourbonnais, D, et al: Abnormal spatial patterns of elbow muscle activation in hemiparetic human subjects. Brain 112:85, 1989.

38. Bourbonnais, D, and Vanden Noven, S: Weakness in patients with hemiparesis. Am J Occup Ther 43:313, 1989.

39. Nowak, DA, Hermsdorfer, J, and Topka, H:. Deficits of predictive grip force control during object manipulation in acute stroke. J Neurol 250:850, 2003.

40. Noskin, O, et al: Ipsilateral motor dysfunction from unilateral stroke: Implications for the functional neuroanatomy of hemiparesis. J Neurol Neurosurg Psychiatry 79:401, 2008.

41. Chae, J, et al: Muscle weakness and cocontraction in upper limb hemiparesis: Relationship to motor impairment and physical disability. Neurorehabil Neural Repair 16:241, 2002.

42. Dewald, JP, et al: Abnormal muscle coactivation patterns during isometric torque generation at the elbow and shoulder in hemiplegia. Brain 118:495, 1995.

43. Watkins, M, et al: Isokinetic testing in patients with hemiparesis. Phys Ther 64:184, 1984.

44. Andrews, AW, and Bohannon, RW: Distribution of muscle strength impairments following stroke. Clin Rehabil 14:79, 2000.

45. Marque P, et al: Impairment and recovery of left motor function in patients with right hemiplegia. J Neurol Neurosurg Psychiatry 62:77, 1997.

46. Rothstein, J, et al: Commentary. Is the measurement of muscle strength appropriate in patients with brain lesions? Phys Ther 69:230, 1989.

47. Bohannon, R: Is the measurement of muscle strength appropriate in patients with brain lesions? Phys Ther 69:225, 1989.

48. Andrews, AW: Hand-held dynamometry for measuring muscle strength. J Hum Muscle Perform 1:35, 1991.

49. Riddle, D, et al: Intrasession and intersession reliability of hand-held dynamometer measurements taken on brain-damaged patients. Phys Ther 69:182, 1989.

50. Bohannon, R, and Andrews, A: Interrater reliability of handheld dynamometry. Phys Ther 67:931, 1987.

51. Agre, J, et al: Strength testing with a portable dynamometer: Reliability for upper and lower extremities. Arch Phys Med Rehabil 68:454, 1987.

52. Rothstein, J, et al: Clinical uses of isokinetic measurements. Phys Ther 67:1840, 1987.

53. Pohl, P, et al: Reliability of lower extremity isokinetic strength testing in adults with stroke. Clinical Rehabil 14:601, 2000.

54. Kim, C, et al: Reliability of dynamic muscle performance in hemiparetic upper limb. JNPT 29:1, 2005.

55. Curtis, C, and Weir, J: Overview of exercise responses in healthy and impaired states. Neurology Report 20:13, 1996.

56. American College of Sports Medicine: ACSM's Exercise Management for Persons with Chronic Disease and Disabilities, ed 3. Human Kinetics, Champaign, IL, 2009.

57. Bennett, R, and Knowlton, G: Overwork weakness in partially denervated skeletal muscle. Clin Orthop 12:22, 1958.

58. Bigland-Richie, B, and Woods, J: Changes in muscle contractile properties and neural control during human muscular fatigue. Muscle Nerve 7:691, 1984.

59. Fisk, J, et al: The impact of fatigue on patients with multiple sclerosis. J Can Sci Neurol 21:9, 1994.

60. Guide for the Uniform Data Set for Medical Rehabilitation (including the FIM instrument), Version 5.0 State University of Buffalo, 1996.

61. Borg, G: Borg's Perceived Exertion and Pain Scales. Human Kinetics, Champaign, IL, 1998.

62. Barnes, S: Isokinetic fatigue curves at different contractile velocities. Arch Phys Med Rehabil 62:66, 1981.

63. Binder-Macleod, S, and Synder-Mackler, L: Muscle fatigue: Clinical implications for fatigue assessment and neuromuscular electrical stimulation. Phys Ther 73(12):902, 1993.

64. McDonnell, M, et al: Electrically elicited fatigue test of the quadriceps femoris muscle. Phys Ther 67:941, 1987.

65. Brunnstrom, S: Movement Therapy in Hemiplegia. New York, Harper & Row, 1970.

66. Bobath, B. Abnormal Postural Reflex Activity Caused by Brain Lesions. Heinemann, London, 1965.

67. Twitchell, T: The restoration of motor function following hemiplegia in man. Brain 74:443, 1951.

68. Fugl-Meyer, A: The post-stroke hemiplegic patient. I: A method for evaluation of physical performance. Scand J Rehabil Med 7:13, 1975.

69. VanSant, A: Life span development in functional tasks. Phys Ther 70:788, 1990.

70. Shenkman, M, et al: Whole-body movements during rising to standing from sitting. Phys Ther 70:638, 1990.

71. VanSant, A: Rising from a supine position to erect stance: Description of adult movement and a developmental hypothesis. Phys Ther 68:185, 1988.

72. Green, L, and Williams, K: Differences in developmental movement patterns used by active vs sedentary middle-aged adults coming from a supine position to erect stance. Phys Ther 72:560, 1992.

73. Richter, R, et al: Description of adult rolling movements and hypothesis of developmental sequences. Phys Ther 69:63, 1989.

74. Gentile, A: Skill acquisition: Action, movement and neuromotor processes. In Carr, JH, et al (eds): Movement Science: Foundations for Physical Therapy in Rehabilitation, ed 2. Aspen, Gaithersburg, MD, 2000, p 111.

75. Lewis, A: Documentation of movement patterns used in the performance of functional tasks. Neurol Rep 16:13, 1992.

76. Ackerman, P: Individual differences in skill learning: An integration of psychometric and information processing perspectives. Psychol Bull 102:3, 1988.

77. Fitts, P, and Posner, M: Human Performance. Brooks/Cole, Belmont, CA, 1969.

78. Anderson, JR: Acquisition of cognitive skill. Psychol Rev 89:369, 1982.

79. Anderson, JR: Learning and memory: An Integrated Approach. Wiley, New York, 1995.

80. Gentile, AM: A working model of skill acquisition with application to teaching. Quest 17:3, 1972.

81. Lynch, MC, and Cohen JA: A primer on electrophysiologic studies in myopathy. Rheum Dis Clin North Am 37(2):253–268, vii, 2011.

82. Kimura, J: Electrodiagnosis in Diseases of Nerve and Muscle: Principles and Practice, ed 3. Oxford University Press, New York, 2001.

83. Kimura, J: Electrodiagnosis of Diseases of Nerve and Muscle: Principles and Practice, ed 2. FA Davis, Philadelphia, 1989.

84. Echternach, JL: Introduction to Electromyography and Nerve Conduction Testing, ed 2. Slack, Thorofare, NJ, 2002.

85. Falck, B, Stalberg, E, and Bischoff, C: Influence of recording site within the muscle on motor unit potentials. Muscle Nerve 18:1385, 1995.

86. Van der Heijden, A, Spaans, F, and Reulen, J: Fasciculation potentials in foot and leg muscles of healthy young adults. Electroencephalogr Clin Neurophysiol 93:163, 1994.

87. Rodriquez, AA, et al: Electromyographic and neuromuscular variables in post-polio subjects. Arch Phys Med Rehabil 76:989, 1995.

88. Roeleveld, K, et al: Motor unit size estimation of enlarged motor units with surface electromyography. Muscle Nerve 21:878, 1998.

89. Stalberg, E, and Grimby, G: Dynamic electromyography and muscle biopsy changes in a 4-year follow-up: Study of patients with a history of polio. Muscle Nerve 18:699, 1995.

90. Pease, WS, Lew, HL, and Johnson, EW: Johnson's Practical Electromyography, ed 4. Lippincott Williams & Wilkins, Philadelphia, 2006.

91. Gersh, MR: Electrotherapy in Rehabilitation. FA Davis, Philadelphia, 1992.

92. Misiaszek, JF: The H-reflex as a tool in neurophysiology: Its limitations and uses in understanding nervous system function. Muscle Nerve 28:144, 2003.

93. Mallik, A, and Weir, AI: Nerve conduction studies: Essentials and pitfalls in practice. J Neurol Neurosurg Psychiatry 76(Suppl 2):ii23, 2005.

94. Dumitru, D, Amato, AA, and Zwarts, M: Electrodiagnostic Medicine, ed 2. Hanley & Belfus, Philadelphia, 2001.

95. Werner, RA, and Andary, M: Electrodiagnostic evaluation of carpal tunnel syndrome. Muscle Nerve 44:597, 2011.

96. Custodio, CM: Electrodiagnosis in cancer treatment and rehabilitation. Am J Phys Med Rehabil 90:S38, 2011.

Examination of Coordination and Balance

Chapter 6

Thomas J. Schmitz, PT, PhD
Susan B. O'Sullivan, PT, EdD

LEARNING OBJECTIVES

1. Understand the purposes of performing an examination of coordination and balance.
2. List the types of data generated from the examination.
3. Describe the common coordination and balance impairments associated with lesions of the central nervous system.
4. Explain the primary age-associated changes that affect coordination and balance.
5. Discuss the purpose of screenings within the context of motor function.
6. Provide a rationale for the preliminary patient observation before performing an examination.
7. Identify the motor task requirements and movement capabilities addressed during an examination of coordination and balance.
8. Differentiate between tests used to examine coordination and balance.
9. Using the case study example, apply clinical decision making skills to application of coordination and balance examination data.

■ EXAMINATION OF COORDINATION

Motor control is "the ability of the central nervous system to control or direct the neuromotor system in purposeful movement and postural adjustment by selective allocation of muscle tension across appropriate joint segments."[1, p. 688] Motor control has also been defined "as the ability to regulate or direct the mechanisms essential to movement."[2, p. 3] Components of motor control include normal muscle tone and postural response mechanisms, selective movements, and coordination.[3]

Coordination is the ability to execute smooth, accurate, controlled movement. "Coordinated movement involves multiple joints and muscles that are activated at the appropriate time and with the correct amount of force so that smooth, efficient, and accurate movement occurs. Thus, the essence of coordination is the sequencing, timing, and grading of the activation of multiple muscles groups."[2, p. 121]

The ability to produce these responses is dependent on somatosensory, visual, and vestibular input, as well as a fully intact neuromuscular system from the motor cortex to the spinal cord.[4] Coordinated movements are characterized by appropriate speed, distance, direction, timing, and muscular tension. In addition, they involve appropriate synergistic influences (muscle recruitment), easy reversal between opposing muscle groups (appropriate sequencing of contraction and relaxation), and proximal fixation to allow distal motion or maintenance of a posture.[5] Schmidt and Lee define coordination as the "behavior of two or more degrees of freedom in relation to each other to produce skilled activity."[6, p. 494] Awkward, extraneous, uneven, or inaccurate movements characterize *coordination impairments*.

Two terms often associated with coordination are *dexterity* and *agility*.[1] *Dexterity* refers to skillful use of the fingers during fine motor tasks.[7] *Agility* refers to the ability to rapidly and smoothly initiate, stop, or modify movements while maintaining postural control.

There are several general types of coordination. *Intralimb* coordination refers to movements occurring within a single limb[8-13] (e.g., alternately flexing or extending the elbow; use of one upper extremity to brush the hair; or motor performance of a single lower extremity during a gait cycle). *Interlimb* (bimanual) coordination refers to the integrated performance of two or more limbs working together[14-18] (e.g., alternately flexing one elbow while extending the other; bilateral upper extremity tasks as required during sliding transfers or dressing activities; or between limb movements of the lower extremities and/or upper extremities during walking). *Visual motor* coordination[19-23] refers to the ability to integrate both visual and motor abilities with the environmental context to accomplish a goal (e.g., tracing over a zigzag line, writing a letter, riding a bicycle, or driving an automobile). A subcategory of visual motor coordination with important implications for activities of daily living (ADL) is *eye–hand* coordination[24-30] such as required for using eating utensils, personal hygiene, or reaching for a visual target (e.g., a book from a shelf). Eye–hand coordination is perhaps more aptly termed *eye–hand–head* coordination because movement of the head is typically required for the eyes to fixate on a target or object.

Physical therapists are frequently involved in management of patients with coordination impairments. Data from the examination of coordination inform the therapist about existing impairments. These impairments are often associated with activity limitations that are related to, and indicative of, the type, extent, and location of central nervous system (CNS) pathology. Some CNS lesions present very classic and stereotypical impairments, but others are much less predictable. Examples of medical diagnoses that typically demonstrate coordination impairments include traumatic brain injury, Parkinson's disease, multiple sclerosis, Huntington's disease, cerebral palsy, Sydenham's chorea, cerebellar tumors, vestibular pathology, and some learning disabilities.

The *Guide to Physical Therapist Practice*[1] includes coordination (together with dexterity and agility) as a subcategory of Motor Function (Motor Control and Motor Learning) among the list of 24 categories of tests and measures that may be used by physical therapists during patient examination. In addition, the *Guide to Physical Therapist Practice*[1] includes coordination among the tests and measurements identified for all Musculoskeletal Practice Patterns, Neuromuscular Practice Patterns A–H, and Cardiovascular/Pulmonary Practice Pattern D.

The purposes of performing a coordination examination of motor function are to determine the following:

1. Muscle activity characteristics during voluntary movement
2. Ability of muscles or groups of muscles to work together to perform a task or functional activity
3. Level of skill and efficiency of movement
4. Ability to initiate, control, and terminate movement
5. Timing, sequencing, and accuracy of movement patterns
6. Effects of therapeutic and pharmacological intervention on motor function over time

In addition, data from the coordination examination assist the therapist with establishing the diagnosis of underlying impairments, activity limitations, and participation restrictions (disability); assist with establishing anticipated goals to remediate impairments and formulating expected outcomes that encompass remediation of activity limitations and participation restrictions; and support decision making in establishing a prognosis and determining specific, direct interventions.

■ OVERVIEW OF THE MOTOR SYSTEM

The motor system can be grossly divided into *peripheral* and *central* elements. The peripheral somatic motor system includes muscles, joints, and their sensory and motor innervation.[31] The central elements can be divided into three hierarchical levels to assist understanding their organization as well as delineating the contribution of each neuroanatomical structure. However, this does not imply a strictly top-down control of coordinated movement as each level of the nervous system can influence other levels (above and below) depending on task demands (i.e., flexible hierarchical theory). Bear et al provide a practical description of the three hierarchical levels relative to their functional contributions to motor control as follows: "The highest level, represented by the association areas of the neocortex and basal ganglia of the forebrain, is concerned with *strategy*: the goal of the movement and the movement strategy that best achieve[s] the goal. The middle level, represented by the motor cortex and cerebellum, is concerned with *tactics*: the sequences of muscle contractions, arranged in space and time, required to smoothly and accurately achieve the strategic goal. The lowest level, represented by the brain stem and spinal cord, is concerned with *execution*: activation of the motor neuron and interneuron pools that generate the goal-directed movement and make any necessary adjustments of posture."[31, p. 452]

The motor system can also be viewed as having a *parallel arrangement*. For example, information is conveyed not only from the motor cortex to the spinal cord but also directly from premotor areas as well. Although the cerebellum and basal ganglion are involved in movement, they have no direct output to the spinal cord. Instead, their effect on movement is provided via connections to the motor cortex.[32]

The critical role of sensory input on the motor system cannot be overemphasized. The integration of sensory input provides an internal representation of the environment that informs and guides motor responses.[5] These sensory representations provide the foundation on which motor programs for purposeful movements are planned, coordinated, and implemented.[4] Sensory input to the motor system guides selection and adaptation of motor responses and shapes motor programs for corrective action. For example, the somatosensory system provides the needed information to adjust walking when moving from a smooth surface to an uneven terrain; to maintain standing balance on a moving bus; or to make the required adjustments when throwing a ball from a stable sitting surface (chair) versus an unstable one (therapy ball). To rule out sensory impairments as a contributing factor to coordination impairments, examination of sensory function (see Chapter 3) typically *precedes* the coordination examination.

The Motor Cortex

The principal brain area involved in motor function is the motor cortex, which comprises cortical (Brodmann's) areas 4 and 6 located in a demarcated area of the frontal lobe called the precentral gyrus (Fig. 6.1). However, planning coordinated movement to accomplish a task involves many areas of the neocortex as it requires knowledge of the body's position in space, the location of the intended target, selection of an optimum movement strategy (i.e., which joints, muscles, or body segments will be used), memory storage until time of execution, and specific instructions to implement the movement strategy selected (where to move or what to do).[31,33]

Brodmann's area 4 is designated the *primary motor cortex (PMC)* as it is the most specific cortical motor area containing the largest concentration of corticospinal neurons.[34] This area is electrically excitable and stimuli of low intensity evoke a motor response. It lies anterior to the central sulcus on the precentral gyrus and controls contralateral voluntary movements. Brodmann's area 6 is also electrically excitable but requires stimuli of higher intensities to cause a motor response.[35] It lies just anterior to area 4 and is subdivided into the superiorly placed *supplementary motor area (SMA)* and the inferiorly positioned *premotor area (PMA)*.[35]

The SMA gives rise to axons that directly innervate motor units involved in initiation of movement, simultaneous bilateral grasping movements, sequential tasks, and orientation of the eyes and head. The PMA provides input to the reticulospinal neurons innervating motor units that control trunk and proximal limb movements and contributes to anticipatory postural changes.[31,36] Stimulation of area 4 typically results in uncomplicated movements of a single joint whereas stimulation to the premotor areas (area 6) evokes more intricate coordinated movements involving multiple joints.[33]

The somatotopic organization of the motor cortex is very similar to the sensory cortex. The motor homunculus schematically illustrates the amount of cortical area devoted to motor control of a given body part or region (Fig. 6.2). Beginning on the lateral aspect of the homunculus, the mouth and face areas are represented; moving upward are areas devoted to the hands, trunk, lower extremities, and feet. Note that areas requiring finer gradations of control such as the fingers, hand, and face (including muscles of speech) occupy a disproportionately larger representation (approximately half) in the motor cortex. The SMA and PMA are similarly somatotopically organized.

The motor cortex receives information from three primary sources: the *somatosensory cortex* (peripheral receptive fields), the *cerebellum,* and the *basal ganglia.* Somatosensory input is relayed directly to the primary motor cortex from the thalamus (e.g., cutaneous tactile sensations, joint and muscle receptors). The thalamus also relays information to the motor areas from the cerebellum and the basal ganglia. These connections allow for integration of motor control functions of the motor cortex, cerebellum, and basal ganglia (i.e., to carry out the appropriate course of motor action).[37]

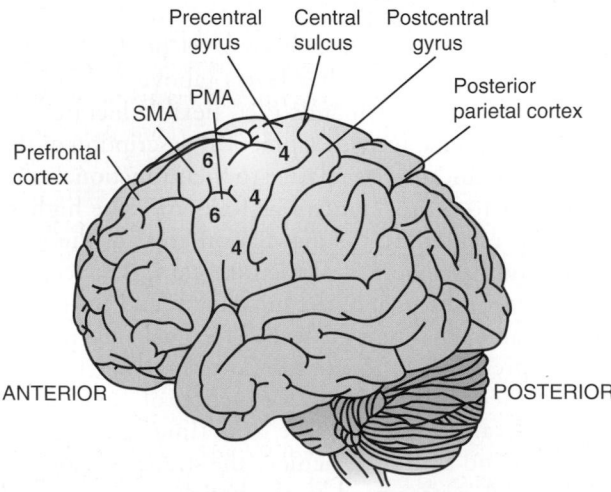

Figure 6.1 Primary areas of the cortex involved in coordinated movement.

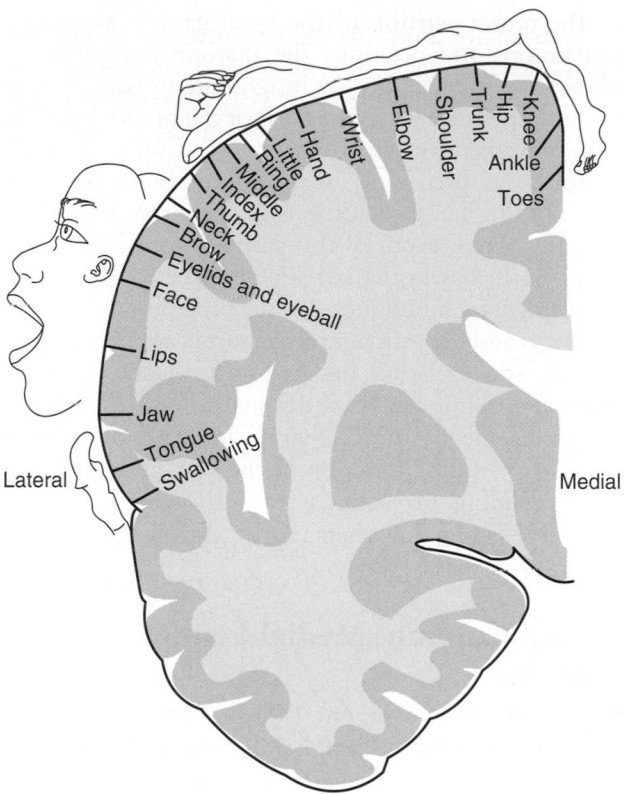

Figure 6.2 The motor homunculus indicates the **somatotopic** organization of the motor cortex. The relative size of body parts reflects the proportion of the motor cortex devoted to controlling that area.

Descending Motor Pathways

The most important descending pathway of the motor system is the corticospinal (pyramidal) tract that transmits signals from the motor cortex directly to the spinal cord. It is among the longest and largest CNS tracts. It originates primarily in areas 4 and 6 and passes through the internal capsule and the brainstem. A majority of fibers then cross to the opposite side in the medulla and descend through the lateral corticospinal tracts of the spinal cord. The fibers that do not cross at the medulla form the ventral corticospinal tracts, but a majority of these eventually cross to the opposite side in the cervical or upper thoracic regions. All fibers of the corticospinal tract terminate on the interneurons of the cord gray matter. The corticospinal tract is concerned with skilled, fine motor control, especially of the distal limbs.[37] The other major descending motor pathways that control neurons innervating muscle include the following:

- Corticobulbar tract: Some fibers project directly to motor cranial nerve (CN) nuclei (e.g., trigeminal, facial, hypoglossal), and others to the reticular formation before reaching cranial nerve nuclei.
- Tectospinal tract: This relatively small tract projects to motor neurons in the cervical cord; fibers influence neurons innervating neck muscles, as well as the

spinal accessory nucleus (CN XI); important in guiding head movements during visual motor tasks.
- Reticulospinal tract (medial and lateral): Projects to the anterior horn of the spinal cord; important influence on muscle tone and reflex activity via influence on muscle spindle activity (increasing or decreasing sensitivity); the pontine (medial) reticulospinal tract facilitates extension of the lower extremities (excitation of extensor motor neurons) augmenting antigravity reflexes of the spinal cord; important influence on posture and gait. The medullary (lateral) reticulospinal tract has the reverse effect (excitation of flexor motor neurons).
- Vestibulospinal tracts (medial and lateral): The lateral vestibulospinal tract descends to all levels of the spinal cord; important contributions to postural control and movements of the head (facilitates axial extensors; inhibits axial flexors). The medial vestibulospinal tract projects primarily to the ipsilateral cervical spinal cord; also involved in coordinated head and eye movements.
- Rubrospinal tract: This tract merges with the corticospinal tract in the cervical region. Its role in human motor control is considered insignificant. It is believed that during primate evolution the role of this tract was completely taken over by the corticospinal tract.

Cerebellum

The primary function of the cerebellum is regulation of movement, postural control, and muscle tone. Although all of the mechanisms of cerebellar function are not clearly understood, lesions have been noted to produce typical patterns of impaired motor function and balance and decreased muscle tone (see Cerebellar Pathology later in this chapter).

Several theories of function of the cerebellum in motor activity have been established. Among the more widely held is that the cerebellum functions as a *comparator* and *error-correcting mechanism*.[33,38] The cerebellum compares the commands for the *intended* movement transmitted from the motor cortex with the *actual* motor performance of the body segment. This occurs by a comparison of information received from the cortex with that obtained from peripheral feedback mechanisms (termed *feedforward control*). The motor cortex and brainstem motor structures provide the commands for the intended motor response (internal feedback).[38] Peripheral feedback during the motor response is provided by muscle spindles, Golgi tendon organs, joint and cutaneous receptors, the vestibular apparatus, and the eyes and ears (external feedback). This feedback provides continual input regarding posture and balance, as well as position, rate, rhythm, and force of slow movements of peripheral body segments. If the input from the feedback systems does not compare appropriately (i.e., movements deviate from the intended command), the cerebellum supplies a corrective influence. This effect is achieved by corrective signals sent to the cortex, which, via motor pathways, modifies or corrects the ongoing movement (e.g., increasing or decreasing the level of activity of specific muscles). The cerebellum also functions to modify cortical commands for subsequent movements.[38,39]

This CNS analysis of movement information, determination of level of accuracy, and provision for error correction is referred to as a **closed-loop system**. Schmidt and Lee define this model as "a control system employing feedback, a reference for correctness, a computation of error, and subsequent correction in order to maintain a desired state."[6, p. 493] It should be noted that not all movements are controlled by this system. Stereotypical movements (e.g., gait activities) and rapid, short-duration movements, which do not allow sufficient time for feedback to occur, are believed to be controlled by an **open-loop system**, defined as "a control system with preprogrammed instructions to a set of effectors; it does not use feedback information and error-detection processes."[6, p. 497] In this system, control originates centrally from a **motor program**, which is a memory or preprogrammed pattern of information for coordinated movement. The motor system then follows the established pattern largely independent of feedback or error-detection mechanisms. Motor programs can be called up in their entirety, modified, or reassembled in a new order. They provide the important function of freeing higher executive levels from attending to all aspects of a motor response.

Basal Ganglia

The basal ganglia are a group of nuclei located at the base of the cerebral cortex. The three main nuclei of the basal ganglia are the *caudate nucleus,* the *putamen,* and the *globus pallidus.* These nuclei have close anatomical and functional connections with two other subcortical nuclei that are also frequently considered as part of the basal ganglia: the *subthalamic nucleus* and the *substantia nigra.*[32,40]

Although the influences of the basal ganglia on movement are not understood as clearly as those of the cerebellum, there is evidence that the basal ganglia play an important role in several complex aspects of movement and postural control. These include the initiation and regulation of gross intentional movements, planning and execution of complex motor responses, facilitation of desired motor responses while selectively inhibiting others, and the ability to accomplish automatic movements and postural adjustments.[37,41,42] In addition, the basal ganglia play an important role in maintaining normal background muscle tone. This is accomplished by the inhibitory effect of the basal ganglia on both the motor cortex and lower brainstem. The basal ganglia also are believed to influence some aspects of both perceptual and cognitive functions.[41]

The motor portion of the basal ganglia assumes a somatotopic organization. The anatomical positioning of the basal ganglia provides insight into its contribution to motor performance. The areas of the brain associated with movement (primary motor cortex, supplementary motor area, premotor area, and the somatosensory cortex) form dense projections to the motor portion of the putamen. Output of this pathway forms the *motor circuit* of the basal ganglia, which is directed back to the supplementary motor area and the premotor area. These two areas and the primary motor cortex are all interconnected, and each has descending projections to the brainstem motor centers and spinal cord. This anatomical arrangement indicates that the influence of the basal ganglia on motor function is indirect and mediated by descending projections from the cortical motor areas.[41-43] Figure 6.3 schematically illustrates the motor circuit of the basal ganglion.

Dorsal Column–Medial Lemniscal Pathway

Regulation of movement is dependent on sensory afferent information. Peripheral somatosensory receptors and pathways provide information about the

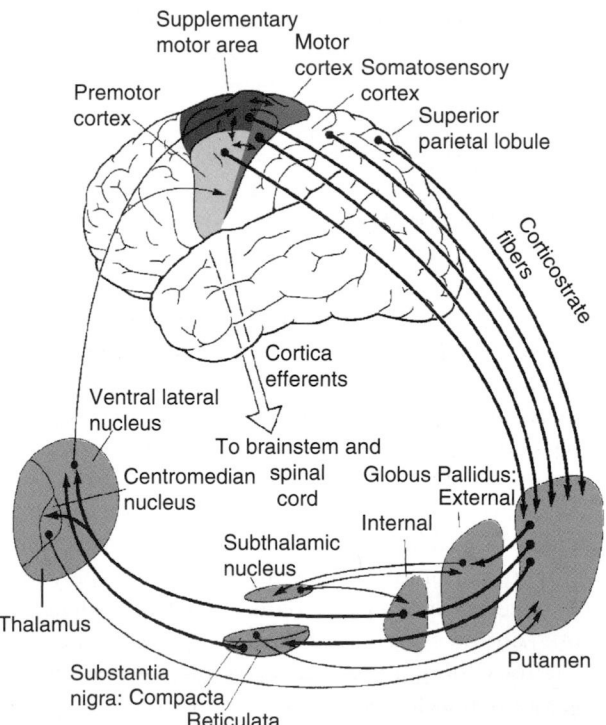

Figure 6.3 The motor circuit of the basal ganglia provides a subcortical feedback loop from the motor and somatosensory areas of the cortex, through portions of the basal ganglia and thalamus, and back to the cortical motor areas (premotor cortex, supplementary motor area, and motor cortex). *(From Ghez and Gordon,[43, p. 548] with permission.)*

status of the environment, the status of the body, and the status of the body in relation to the environment.[6] This information is encoded and conveyed to various parts of the CNS. The data are processed based on peripheral feedback and memory, which leads to selection (or modification) of a movement strategy appropriate to the task demands and environmental conditions.

The dorsal column–medial lemniscal pathway is particularly important to coordinated movement, as it is responsible for the afferent transmission of discriminative sensations. Sensory modalities that require fine gradations of intensity and precise localization on the body surface are mediated by this system. Sensations transmitted by the dorsal column–medial lemniscal pathway include discriminative touch, stereognosis, tactile pressure, barognosis, graphesthesia, recognition of texture, kinesthesia, two-point discrimination, proprioception, and vibration.

This system is composed of large, myelinated, rapidly conducting fibers. After entering the dorsal column the fibers ascend to the medulla and synapse with the dorsal column nuclei (nuclei gracilis and cuneatus). From here they cross to the opposite side and pass up to the thalamus through bilateral pathways called the *medial lemnisci*. Each medial lemniscus terminates in the ventral posterolateral thalamus. From the thalamus, third-order neurons project to the somatic sensory cortex.

■ FEATURES OF COORDINATION IMPAIRMENTS

As the cerebellum, basal ganglia, and dorsal column–medial lemniscal pathway provide input to, and act together with, the cortex in the production of coordinated movement, lesions in any of these areas affect higher-level processing and execution of coordinated motor responses. Although it is incorrect to assign all problems of incoordination to one of these sites, lesions in these areas are responsible for many characteristic motor deficits seen in adult populations. The following sections present an overview of common clinical features associated with lesions in each of these areas.

Cerebellar Pathology

A number of specific motor impairments that affect coordinated movement are associated with cerebellar pathology.[43-47] Many of these impairments either directly or indirectly influence the patient's ability to execute accurate, smooth, controlled movements. The motor deficits identified emphasize the crucial influence of the cerebellum on equilibrium, posture, muscle tone, and initiation and force of movement. **Ataxia** is perhaps the most common term used to describe motor impairments of cerebellar origin. Cerebellar ataxia is a general, comprehensive term used to describe loss of muscle coordination as a result of cerebellar pathology. Ataxia may affect gait, posture, and patterns of movement and is

linked to difficulty initiating movement, as well as errors in the rate, rhythm, and timing of responses.

Perlman[48] provides an adept summary of the motor impairments associated with each of the major anatomic regions of the cerebellum as follows: "The cerebellum has three anatomic divisions that account for the three types of dysfunction commonly seen: (1) the midline (vermis, paleocerebellum), which underlies titubation, truncal ataxia, orthostatic tremor, and gait imbalance; (2) the hemispheres (neocerebellum—right controlling the right side of the body and left controlling the left side), which contribute to limb ataxia (e.g., dysdiadochokinesia, dysmetria, and kinetic tremor), dysarthria, and hypotonia; and (3) the posterior (flocculonodular lobe, archicerebellum), which also influences posture and gait as well as causing eye movement disorders (e.g., nystagmus, vestibulo-ocular reflex disruption)."[48, p. 216]

The following motor impairments are manifestations of cerebellar pathology:

- **Asthenia** is generalized muscle weakness associated with cerebellar lesions.
- **Dysarthria** is a disorder of the motor component of speech articulation. The characteristics of cerebellar dysarthria are referred to as **scanning speech** (often described as having a *one-word-at-a-time* quality). This speech pattern is typically slow, and may be slurred, hesitant, with prolonged syllables and inappropriate pauses. Word use, selection, and grammar remain intact, but the melodic quality of speech is altered.[38,39]
- **Dysdiadochokinesia** is an impaired ability to perform rapid alternating movements. This deficit is observed in movements such as rapid alternation between pronation and supination of the forearm. Movements are irregular, with a rapid loss of range and rhythm especially as speed is increased.[39]
- **Dysmetria** is an inability to judge the distance or range of a movement. It may be manifested by an overestimation (**hypermetria**) or an underestimation (**hypometria**) of the required range needed to reach an object or goal.
- **Dyssynergia (movement decomposition)** describes a movement performed in a sequence of component parts rather than as a single, smooth activity. For example, when asked to touch the index finger to the nose, the patient might first flex the elbow, and then adjust the position of the wrist and fingers, further flex the elbow, and finally flex the shoulder. **Asynergia** is the loss of ability to associate muscles together for complex movements.
- **Gait ataxia** involves ambulatory patterns that typically demonstrate a broad base of support. Upright stance stability is often poor and the arms may be held away from the body to improve balance (high guard position). Stepping patterns are irregular in direction and distance. Initiation of forward progression of a lower extremity may start slowly, and then the extremity may unexpectedly be flung rapidly and

forcefully forward and audibly hit the floor.[49] Gait patterns tend to be generally unsteady (postural instability), irregular, and staggering, with deviations from an intended forward line of progression (veering to one side; swaying or pitching in different directions).

- **Hypotonia** is a decrease in muscle tone. It is believed to be related to the disruption of afferent input from stretch receptors and/or lack of the cerebellum's facilitatory efferent influence on the fusimotor system. A diminished resistance to passive movement will be noted, and muscles may feel abnormally soft and flaccid. Diminished deep tendon reflexes also may be noted.[38] *Note:* After testing the patellar tendon jerk with a reflex hammer in a normal subject, the knee typically returns immediately to the resting state. With cerebellar pathology, the knee may oscillate six to eight times before returning to rest.[38]

- **Nystagmus** is a rhythmic, quick, oscillatory, back-and-forth movement of the eyes. It is typically apparent as the eyes move away from midline to fix on an object in either the medial or lateral field (i.e., extremes of temporal or nasal vision).[50] The patient has difficulty holding the gaze on the object in the peripheral field. An involuntary drift back to midline with immediate return to the object may be observed.[51] Nystagmus causes difficulty with accurate fixation and vision and is believed linked to the cerebellum's influence on synergy and tone of the extraocular muscles.

- **Rebound phenomenon**, originally described by Holmes, is the loss of the check reflex,[49] or check factor, which functions to halt forceful active movements when resistance is eliminated. Normally, when application of resistance to an isometric contraction is suddenly removed, the limb will remain in approximately the same position by action of the opposing muscle(s). For example, in applying resistance to an isometric contraction in the middle range of elbow flexion and then releasing it without warning, the intact subject will "check" or stop the motion quickly through activation of the opposing triceps, as well as feedback regarding joint position and force required to prevent further motion. With cerebellar involvement, the patient is unable to stop the motion, and the limb will move suddenly when resistance is released. The patient may strike himself or herself or other objects when the resistance is removed.

- **Tremor** is an involuntary oscillatory movement resulting from alternate contractions of opposing muscle groups. Different types of tremors are associated with cerebellar lesions. An **intention tremor**, or **kinetic tremor**, occurs during voluntary motion of a limb and tends to increase as the limb nears its intended goal or speed is increased.[38] Intention tremors are diminished or absent at rest. **Postural (static) tremor** may be evident by back-and-forth oscillatory movements of the body while the patient maintains a standing posture. Postural tremors also may be observed as up-and-down oscillatory movements of a limb when it is held against gravity. *Titubation* typically refers to rhythmic oscillations of the head (side-to-side or forward-and-backward movements, or the movements may have a rotary component); however, the term is also less frequently used to refer to axial involvement of the trunk.

In addition to these characteristic clinical features of cerebellar involvement, a greater length of time may also be required to initiate voluntary movements (delayed **reaction time**). Difficulty may also be observed in stopping or changing the force, speed, or direction of movement, prolonging **movement time**.[32] Motor learning will also be affected. Recall that the cerebellum compares the intended movement (internal feedback) with the actual movement (external feedback). For subsequent movements, the cerebellum generates corrective signals to reduce the errors (feedforward control). Lack of this feedforward control is responsible for deficits in motor learning and coordination.

Basal Ganglia Pathology

Patients with lesions of the basal ganglia typically demonstrate several characteristic motor deficits. These include (1) poverty and slowness of movement; (2) involuntary, extraneous movement; and (3) alterations in posture and muscle tone.[36,42] Thus, patients with basal ganglia involvement present on a continuum of motor behavior from severely diminished as seen in advanced Parkinson's disease to excessive extraneous movements apparent with Huntington's disease.[42]

The following motor impairments are manifestations of basal ganglia pathology:[52-59]

- **Akinesia** is an inability to initiate movement and is seen in the late stages of Parkinson's disease. This deficit is associated with assumption and maintenance of fixed postures (freezing episodes). A tremendous amount of mental concentration and effort is required to perform even the simplest motor activity.

- **Athetosis** is characterized by slow, involuntary, writhing, twisting, "wormlike" movements. Frequently, greater involvement in the distal upper extremities is noted;[60] this may include fluctuations between hyperextension of the wrist and fingers and a return to a flexed position, combined with rotary movements of the extremities. Many other areas of the body may be involved, including the neck, face, tongue, and trunk. The phenomena are also referred to as *athetoid movements*. Pure athetosis is relatively uncommon and most often presents in combination with spasticity, tonic spasms, or chorea. Athetosis can be a clinical feature of some forms of cerebral palsy.

- **Bradykinesia** is a decreased amplitude and velocity of voluntary movement. It may be demonstrated in a variety of ways, such as a decreased arm swing; slow, shuffling gait; difficulty initiating or changing direction of movement; lack of facial expression; or difficulty stopping a movement once begun. Bradykinesia is characteristic of Parkinson's disease.

- **Chorea** is characterized by involuntary, rapid, irregular, and jerky movements involving multiple joints. Choreiform movements demonstrate irregular timing, are most apparent in the upper extremities, and cannot be voluntarily inhibited; associated with Huntington's disease.[61]
- **Choreoathetosis** is a term used to describe a movement disorder with features of both chorea and athetosis.
- **Dystonia** (dystonic movements) involves sustained involuntary contractions of agonist and antagonist muscles[42] causing abnormal posturing (*dystonic posture*) or twisting movements. Most common in trunk and extremity musculature but also may affect the neck, face, and vocal cords. Torsion spasms also are considered a form of dystonia, with spasmodic torticollis being the most common.[49]
- **Hemiballismus** involves large-amplitude sudden, violent, flailing motions of the arm and leg of one side of the body. Primary involvement is in the axial and proximal musculature of the limb. Hemiballismus results from a lesion of the contralateral subthalamic nucleus.[32,35]
- **Hyperkinesis** is abnormally increased muscle activity or movement; **hypokinesis** is a decreased motor response especially to a specific stimulus.
- **Rigidity** is an increase in muscle tone causing greater resistance to passive movement. It tends to be more pronounced in the flexor muscles of the trunk and

extremities causing activity limitations in such areas as dressing, transfers, speech, eating, and postural control.[2] Two types of rigidity may be seen: *lead-pipe* and *cogwheel*. **Lead-pipe rigidity** is a uniform, constant resistance felt by the examiner as the extremity is moved through a range of motion (ROM). **Cogwheel rigidity** is considered a combination of the lead-pipe type with tremor. It is characterized by a series of brief relaxations or "catches" as the extremity is passively moved.

- **Tremor** is an involuntary, rhythmic, oscillatory movement observed at rest (**resting tremor**). Resting tremors typically disappear or decrease with purposeful movement, but may increase with emotional stress. Tremors associated with basal ganglia lesions (e.g., Parkinson's disease) are frequently noted in the distal upper extremities in the form of a "pill-rolling" movement, where it looks as if a pill is being rolled between the first two fingers and the thumb. Motion of the wrist, and pronation and supination of the forearm, may be evident. Tremors also may be apparent at other body parts as well, such as the jaw; characteristic of Parkinson's disease. Table 6.1 provides a summary of common coordination impairments associated with pathology of the cerebellum and basal ganglia.

Dorsal Column–Medial Lemniscal Pathology

Coordination impairments associated with dorsal column–medial lemniscal (DCML) lesions are somewhat less characteristic than those produced by either cerebellar

Table 6.1	Common Coordination Impairments Associated with Pathology of the Cerebellum and Basal Ganglia
	Cerebellar Pathology
Asthenia	Generalized muscle weakness
Asynergia	Loss of ability to associate muscles together for complex movements
Delayed reaction time	Increased time required to initiate voluntary movement
Dysarthria	Disorder of the motor component of speech articulation
Dysdiadochokinesia	Impaired ability to perform rapid alternating movements
Dysmetria	Inability to judge the distance or range of a movement
Dyssynergia	Movement performed in a sequence of component parts rather than as a single, smooth activity; decomposition
Gait disorders	Ataxic pattern; broad base of support; postural instability; high-guard position of UEs
Hypotonia	Decrease in muscle tone
Hypermetria	Overestimation of distance or range needed to accomplish a movement
Hypometria	Underestimation of distance or range needed to accomplish a movement
Nystagmus	Rhythmic, quick, oscillatory, back-and-forth movement of the eyes
Rebound phenomenon	Inability to halt forceful movements after resistive stimulus removed; patient unable to stop sudden limb motion

Continued

Table 6.1	Common Coordination Impairments Associated with Pathology of the Cerebellum and Basal Ganglia—cont'd
Cerebellar Pathology	
Tremor	Involuntary oscillatory movement resulting from alternate contractions of opposing muscle groups
• Intention (kinetic)	Oscillatory movement during voluntary motion; increases as the limb nears target; diminished or absent at rest
• Postural (static)	Exaggerated oscillatory movement of the body in standing posture or of a limb held against gravity
Titubation	Rhythmic oscillations of the head; axial involvement of the trunk
Basal Ganglia Pathology	
Akinesia	Inability to initiate movement; associated with fixed postures
Athetosis	Slow, involuntary, writhing, twisting, "wormlike" movements; frequently greater involvement in distal UEs
Bradykinesia	Decreased amplitude and velocity of voluntary movement
Chorea	Involuntary, rapid, irregular, jerky movements involving multiple joints; most apparent in UEs
Choreoathetosis	Movement disorder with features of both chorea and athetosis
Dystonia (dystonic movements)	Sustained involuntary contractions of agonist and antagonist muscles
Hemiballismus	Large-amplitude sudden, violent, flailing motions of the arm and leg of one side of the body
Hyperkinesis	Abnormally increased muscle activity or movement
Hypokinesis	Decreased motor response especially to a specific stimulus
Rigidity	Increase in muscle tone causing greater resistance to passive movement; greater in flexor muscles
• Lead-pipe	Uniform, constant resistance as limb is moved
• Cogwheel	Series of brief relaxations or "catches" as limb is passively moved
Tremor (resting)	Involuntary, rhythmic, oscillatory movement observed at rest

UEs = upper extremities.

or basal ganglia pathology. Lesions of the DCML typically result in coordination and equilibrium impairments related to the patient's lack of joint position sense and awareness of movement, and impaired localized touch sensation. Recall that this ascending pathway carries the peripheral (external) feedback required for feedforward control. It mediates sensations critical to coordinated movement such as proprioception, kinesthesia, and discriminative touch.

Disturbances of gait are a common finding with DCML pathology. The gait pattern is usually wide-based and swaying, with uneven step lengths and excessive lateral displacement. The advancing leg may be lifted too high and then dropped abruptly with an audible impact. Watching the feet during ambulation is typical and is indicative of a proprioceptive loss. Another common deficit seen with DCML pathology is dysmetria. As mentioned, this is an impaired ability to judge the required distance or range of movement and may be noted in both the upper and lower extremities. It is manifested by the inability to place an extremity accurately or to reach a target object. For example, in attempting to lock a wheelchair brake, the patient may inaccurately judge (overestimate or underestimate) the required movement needed to reach the brake handle. Fine motor skills may also be impaired owing to alterations in discriminative tactile and object recognition abilities.

Because vision can assist in guiding movements and maintaining balance, as well as improve accuracy of discriminative tasks, visual feedback can be an effective mechanism to compensate partially for DCML pathology. Thus, coordination and/or balance problems will be exaggerated when vision is occluded or when the patient's eyes are closed. The inability to maintain standing balance with the feet together when the eyes are closed is termed a positive **Romberg sign** and is usually indicative of proprioceptive loss. Visual guidance will also reduce the manifestations of dysmetria and diminished tactile perception. However, some noticeable slowing of movements may be observed as visually guided motions are generally more accurate when speed of movement is reduced.

■ AGE-RELATED CHANGES AFFECTING COORDINATED MOVEMENT

Alterations in the ability to execute smooth, accurate, controlled motor responses occur with aging. The importance of understanding the basis of these changes is reflected in the large and ever expanding body of literature devoted to examining various aspects of motor performance in older adults.[62-78] This section presents an overview of the most salient age-associated changes affecting coordinated movement. For a more comprehensive perspective on the physiological, neurological, and musculoskeletal changes associated with aging, the reader is referred to the work of Guccione, Wong, and Avers[79] and Lewis and Bottomley.[80]

Decreased strength. Diminished strength is a well-documented finding in older adults.[76,78,81,82] *Sarcopenia* refers an age-associated loss of skeletal muscle mass (decreased cross-sectional area) as well as changes in the ability of muscle tissue to regenerate. This loss has a direct impact on strength, endurance, mobility, and the ability to perform smooth controlled motor responses. A combination of factors are believed to contribute to this loss of muscle mass, including nutritional deficiencies, decreased ability to synthesize protein, altered endocrine function, lack of exercise, and the presence of a chronic disease (co-morbidity).[83-85] Other contributing factors to decreased strength include a loss of alpha motor neurons (decreased number of functional motor units), loss or atrophy of fast-twitch fibers (most notably type IIb), reduced number and diameter of muscle fibers,[82] diminished oxidative capacity of exercising muscle, and a subsequent reduction in ability to produce torque.[86] In general, there appears to be a greater loss of strength in antigravity muscles of the back and lower extremities (e.g., latissimus dorsi, hip extensors, quadriceps) as compared to the upper extremity and greater loss in proximal than distal muscles.[80]

Slowed reaction time. Older adults typically move more slowly. This is particularly evident for tasks that require both speed and accuracy; speed will decrease to ensure greater accuracy (speed–accuracy trade-off).[87] In general, the time interval between application of a stimulus and initiation of movement is increased.[6] This finding is also linked to degenerative changes in the motor unit. In addition, *premotor reaction time* (time interval between onset of a stimulus and initiation of a response) and *movement time* (time interval between the initiation of movement and the completion of movement) are lengthened with normal aging. Evidence also suggests that greater cognitive resources are required to accomplish a task, especially those involving fine motor skills and dual-task performance.[88]

Decreased range of motion. Early investigations examining subjects from various age groups have found a reduced ROM in older adults.[89-91] Decreases in ROM with advancing age have been found for wrist flexion and extension and hip and shoulder rotation;[89] small decreases (5° or less) were found in mean active hip and knee motions;[90] and James and Parker[91] found consistent declines in both active and passive ROM for 10 lower extremity joints in a population of 80 healthy adults older than 70 years of age. Increased joint tightness tends to be most evident toward the end of ROM and may affect the overall skill in performing coordinated movements. Decreased ROM has been linked to biological aging of joint surfaces,[91] degenerative changes in collagen fibers, dietary deficiencies, and sedentary lifestyle.[80] Walker et al[92] examined active ROM of 28 joints in two groups of elders (60 to 69 and 75 to 84 years). No significant differences in ROM were found between the two age groups.

Postural changes. A straight line projecting through the ear, acromion, greater trochanter, posterior patella, and lateral malleolus represents the lateral view of normal postural alignment. Common postural changes seen with aging include forward head, rounded shoulders (kyphosis), altered lordotic curve (either flattened or exaggerated), and a slight increase in hip and knee flexion.[80] The base of support may also be widened. Diminished strength and ROM, as well as inactivity and prolonged sitting, may contribute to poor postural alignment. Of particular importance is the potential loss of ability to fully accomplish preparatory postural adjustments before execution of a movement.

Impaired balance (postural control). Decreased balance and increased postural sway (oscillating movements of body over feet during relaxed standing) both occur with advancing age.[93-96] A reduction in postural limits of stability (LOS) and functional reach magnitude has also been documented.[97-99] However, Robinovitch and Cronin[100] found that elderly subjects with impaired LOS lacked awareness of their limitations and as a result tended to plan movements that resulted in a loss of balance.

Changes in skilled motor performance are a predictable aspect of normal aging. However, this information should not negate or undermine the importance of treatment strategies to improve functional performance and quality of life. An important consideration in treatment planning is that the aging neuromuscular system maintains its physiological adaptive response to training stimuli.[101] Physical therapy intervention is highly effective in promoting and sustaining a more successful approach to aging.[102-109] This is an important consideration as the population ages. The 2010 Census indicates that the population age 65 and over is approximately 40.3 million, representing 13% of the total population.[110] It is estimated that by 2030, there will be 71 million older adults accounting for about 20% of the population.[111]

Clinical Note: The identified changes affecting coordinated movement in the older adult may be accentuated further by degenerative joint changes, reduced flexibility, alterations in sensation (see Chapter 3, Examination of Sensory Function), perceptual impairments (see Chapter 27, Cognitive and Perceptual Dysfunction), and diminished vision and hearing acuity. Knowledge of these anticipated age-related changes improves the therapist's ability to establish effective communication to optimize patient performance, as well as assist with interpretation of test results. The potential presence of these changes has important implications for how the therapist communicates with, and provides directions to, the patient during the coordination examination. Sensitive and accurate communication that enhances the therapeutic interaction is central to the role of the physical therapist. This involves conveying information in a language or context that is meaningful and intelligible to the patient and communicates trust, respect, and compassion.

■ SCREENING

Screenings are a series of brief tests that provide the therapist an "overview" of the area of interest (e.g., sensation, ROM, strength). Recall that screenings are used to (1) determine the need for further or more detailed examination; (2) rule out or differentiate specific system involvement; (3) determine if referral to another health care practitioner is warranted; (4) focus the search for the origin of symptoms to a specific location or body part; and (5) identify system-related impairments that contribute to activity limitations or disability.[1,112] In combination with the information from the history and review of systems, screenings assist the therapist in proficiently identifying the needed tests and measures and assist in setting priorities within the examination process.

An important starting point for identification of areas to be screened is consideration of all potential (possible) contributing factors to an observed activity limitation. For example, observation of a coordination impairment imposing activity limitations on dressing abilities would direct the therapist's attention to consider its origin. However, before a detailed systematic examination of all systems, screenings can quickly and efficiently direct the therapist's attention to the following:

- Areas grossly intact that can subsequently be "ruled out" as contributing to the activity limitation; additional examination of these areas is likely not warranted.
- Areas suspected of contributing to the clinical problem (screening findings are abnormal); further examination is indicated.

- Identification of the need for referral to another practitioner (e.g., occupational therapist for management of a perceptual deficit).

For example, ROM, strength, and level of function of the sensory system have direct implications for successful execution of coordinated movements. It may be likely that formal examination of these areas has already been accomplished before a coordination examination. If not, however, screening of these areas is indicated.

Clinical Note: An initial screening of ROM, strength, and sensation before the coordination examination is necessary because impairments in any of these areas may influence the ability to produce smooth, accurate, controlled motor responses. However, it is also important to note that coordination impairments may occur in the presence of normal ROM, strength, and intact sensation.

Examples of Screenings

By virtue of their purpose (i.e., providing quickly and efficiently obtained information), screenings are generally performed with the patient seated on a firm surface. However, to fully screen some areas (e.g., the hip) or if several different screenings are planned in sequence, the supine position may be preferable. If abnormal findings are identified during screening, it is a clear indication that more detailed testing is warranted.

Range of Motion

Generally, ROM screenings involve active movements. The patient is asked to selectively move different joints and body segments actively through their available range. For example, the patient might be asked to flex, abduct, and then extend the shoulder; flex and extend the elbow; flex, extend, or circumduct (flexion–abduction–extension–adduction) the wrist; flex and extend the knee; and plantarflex, dorsiflex, and circumduct the ankle. To minimize time required in providing verbal directions, the therapist may opt to sit directly in front and perform the movements while directing the patient to "mirror" the movements. Alternatively, functional movements can be used that combine motions of several joints. For example, the patient might be asked to individually place each hand on the back or top of the head, to reach as high as possible toward the ceiling with each (or both) upper extremity, to place each hand on the small of the back, or to reach down and touch the ankle.

Using careful observation and knowledge of normative ROM values, the therapist makes a gross determination of whether the ROM is *within normal limits* (WNL); if functional movements are used, the designation is *within functional limits* (WFL). If complete, active, painless ROM is available, additional testing is likely not necessary. If active ROM is incomplete or painful, a more detailed examination is needed to determine the cause and extent of the screening findings.[113]

Strength

Typically the ROM screening will precede the strength screening, so some information about strength will already be gathered. If the patient performed active ROM movements against the resistance of gravity, a logical assumption is that gross strength is at least a fair (3/5) grade (ability to move through the ROM against the resistance of gravity). The screening will then be directed toward further refining this estimate using application of manual resistance. Although standard manual muscle testing positions[114,115] are not used for screening, adherence to foundational principles is indicated. Segments proximal to those being screened should be stabilized; resistance (break test) is applied at the distal end of the segment being tested and at a 90° angle (perpendicular) to the primary axis of movement.

From the sitting position, the patient might be asked to raise the knee toward the ceiling to test hip flexion with application of resistance on the distal femur; to extend the knee to test knee extension strength with resistance on the distal leg; and to bring the hand toward the shoulder to test elbow flexion strength with resistance applied on the distal forearm.

Sensation

To perform a sensory screening, several easily tested (i.e., requiring little or no specialized equipment) modalities of sensation are selected. Modalities from each of the general categories of sensations should be selected. For example, the therapist might select pain and light touch (superficial), kinesthesia and vibration (deep), and two-point discrimination or stereognosis (combined). For modalities such as pain and light touch, the sensory screening is performed by using the selected modalities to screen randomly over somewhat large surface areas. For example, several applications of each stimulus might be distributed over the upper and lower extremities and trunk. For sensations such as kinesthesia or proprioception, screening should include selected joints and movements of both the upper and lower extremities. Abnormal findings indicate the need for a more detailed examination of sensory function.

■ FEATURES OF COORDINATION TESTS

Coordination tests generally can be divided into two main categories: *gross motor movements* and *fine motor movements*. **Gross motor tests** include body posture, balance, and extremity movements involving large muscle groups. Examples of gross motor activities include crawling, kneeling, standing, walking, and running. **Fine motor tests** address movements concerned with utilization of small muscle groups that involve skillful, controlled manipulation of objects. Examples of fine motor activities include finger dexterity tasks such as buttoning a shirt, typing, or handwriting.

Two subdivisions of coordination tests (*nonequilibrium* and *equilibrium*) have traditionally been used for providing structure and organization to administration of the tests. *Nonequilibrium* tests address components of limb movements. *Equilibrium* or *balance* tests consider the ability to maintain the body in equilibrium with gravity both statically (i.e., when stationary) and dynamically (i.e., while moving).[1] However, it should be noted that the "nonequilibrium" division is somewhat of a misnomer in that elements of posture and balance are required during these tests (i.e., maintaining an upright sitting posture).

Coordination tests also address patient capabilities in four basic areas of functional task requirements: transitional mobility, stability (static postural control), dynamic postural control (controlled mobility), and skill. See discussion in Chapter 5, Examination of Motor Function: Motor Control and Motor Learning, and Table 5.11, Categories of Motor Skills.

Movement Capabilities

The nonequilibrium coordination examination focuses on movement capabilities in several main areas:

- *Alternate* or *reciprocal motion,* which is the ability to reverse movement between opposing muscle groups
- *Movement composition,* or synergy, which involves movement control achieved by muscle groups acting together
- *Movement accuracy,* which is the ability to gauge or judge distance and speed of voluntary movement
- *Fixation or limb holding,* which addresses the ability to hold the position of an individual limb or limb segment

The progression of difficulty of coordination tests (increases in challenge to the patient) typically utilizes the following sequence: (1) unilateral tasks; (2) bilateral symmetrical tasks; (3) bilateral asymmetrical tasks; and (4) multilimb tasks (these constitute the highest level of difficulty). Difficulty is also increased by progressively adding increased challenges to balance (i.e., movements performed in sitting progressing to standing).

■ ADMINISTERING THE COORDINATION EXAMINATION

Before initiating the coordination examination, the testing environment should be identified and prepared, needed equipment gathered, and consideration given to patient preparation (i.e., what information and instruction will be provided).

Preparation

Testing Environment

The coordination examination should be administered in a quiet, well-lighted treatment area sufficiently large to accommodate walking activities included in the equilibrium portion of the tests. Ideally, the room should be equipped with two standard chairs and a mat or treatment table. A watch or clock with a second hand should be available for timed components of the examination, as well as a method of occluding vision (an inexpensive blindfold used for sleeping works well).

Patient Preparation

The coordination examination should be administered when the patient is well rested. A full explanation of the purpose of the testing should be provided. Each coordination test is described and demonstrated individually by the therapist before actual testing. Such demonstrations should be attended to carefully, as lack of clarity will negatively affect motor responses. Because testing procedures require mental concentration and some physical activity, fatigue, apprehension, or fear may adversely influence test results.

Preliminary Observation

Observation is an essential skill in clinical decision making. Accurate and careful patient observation provides a rich source of preliminary information before performing a coordination examination. Inasmuch as treatment intervention will be directed, at least in part, toward improving functional performance and activity levels, initial observations should logically focus here. Depending on the practice setting environment, the patient might be observed performing any number of functional activities such as bed mobility, self-care routines (e.g., dressing, combing hair, brushing teeth), transfers, eating, writing, changing position from lying or sitting to standing, maintaining a standing position, and walking. Use of appropriate patient guarding techniques is indicated. While observing the patient, general information can be obtained that will assist in localizing specific areas of impairment. This information will include the following:

- General level of skill in each activity and amount of assistance or assistive devices required
- The occurrence of extraneous limb movements, oscillations; specific extremities involved
- Postural sway or unsteadiness
- Distribution: proximal and/or distal musculature, unilateral or bilateral
- Situations or occurrences that alter (increase or decrease) impairments
- Amount of time required to perform an activity
- Level of safety, fall risk

From this initial observation, the therapist will be guided in selecting the appropriate tests for the general areas of impairment noted. Table 6.2 presents sample tests appropriate for examining nonequilibrium coordination. It should be noted that a single test is often appropriate to examine several different movement capabilities simultaneously to conserve time. The tests presented are intended as samples and are not all-inclusive. Other activities may be developed that are equally effective in examining a particular impairment and may be more appropriate for an individual patient. As noted, performance in any variety of functional skills (e.g., self-care routines, wheelchair skills, transfers, dressing) is also an effective means of examining many aspects of movement capabilities (e.g., alternate or reciprocal motion, movement composition, movement accuracy).

Table 6.3 includes selected impairments and suggested tests appropriate for the clinical problem.

Examination

Guided by information from the preliminary observation of functional activities, tests should be selected (see Table 6.3) to address the required movement capabilities of interest for the individual patient. Generally, nonequilibrium tests are completed first, followed by the equilibrium tests. Attention should be directed to carefully guarding the patient during testing; use of a safety belt may be warranted. During testing, the following questions can be used to help

Table 6.2	Nonequilibrium Coordination Tests*
1. Finger-to-nose	The shoulder is abducted to 90° with the elbow extended. The patient is asked to bring the tip of the index finger to the tip of his or her nose. Alterations may be made in the initial starting position to observe performance from different planes of motion.
2. Finger–to–therapist's finger	The patient and therapist sit opposite each other. The therapist's index finger is held in front of the patient. The patient is asked to touch the tip of his or her index finger to the therapist's index finger. The position of the therapist's finger may be altered during testing to observe ability to change distance, direction, and force of movement.
3. Finger-to-finger	Both shoulders are abducted to 90° with the elbows extended. The patient is asked to bring both hands toward the midline and approximate the index fingers from opposing hands.

Table 6.2	Nonequilibrium Coordination Tests—cont'd
4. Alternate nose-to-finger	The patient alternately touches the tip of his or her nose and the tip of the therapist's finger with the index finger. The position of the therapist's finger may be altered during testing to observe ability to change distance, direction, and force of movement.
5. Finger opposition	The patient touches the tip of the thumb to the tip of each finger in sequence. Speed may be gradually increased.
6. Mass grasp	An alternation is made between opening and closing fist (from finger flexion to full extension). Speed may be gradually increased.
7. Pronation/supination	With elbows flexed to 90° and held close to body, the patient alternately turns the palms up and down. This test also may be performed with shoulders flexed to 90° and elbows extended. Speed may be gradually increased. The ability to reverse movements between opposing muscle groups can be examined at many joints. Examples include active alternation between flexion and extension of the knee, ankle, elbow, or fingers.
8. Rebound test	The patient is positioned with the elbow flexed. The therapist applies sufficient manual resistance to produce an isometric contraction of biceps. Resistance is suddenly released. Normally, the opposing muscle group (triceps) will contract and "check" movement of the limb. Many other muscle groups can be tested for this phenomenon, such as the shoulder abductors or flexors and the elbow extensors.
9. Tapping (hand)	With the elbow flexed and the forearm pronated, the patient is asked to "tap" the hand on the knee.
10. Tapping (foot)	The patient is asked to "tap" the ball of one foot on the floor without raising the knee; heel maintains contact with floor.
11. Pointing and past pointing	The patient and therapist are opposite each other, either sitting or standing. Both patient and therapist bring shoulders to a horizontal position of 90° of flexion with elbows extended. Index fingers are touching or the patient's finger may rest lightly on the therapist's. The patient is asked to fully flex the shoulder (fingers will be pointing toward ceiling) and then return to the horizontal position such that index fingers will again approximate. Both arms should be tested, either separately or simultaneously. A normal response consists of an accurate return to the starting position. In an abnormal response, there is typically a "past pointing," or movement beyond the target. Several variations to this test include movements in other directions such as toward 90° of shoulder abduction or toward 0° of shoulder flexion (finger will point toward floor). After each movement, the patient is asked to return to the initial horizontal starting position.
12. Alternate heel-to-knee; heel-to-toe	From a supine position, the patient is asked to touch the knee and big toe alternately with the heel of the opposite extremity.
13. Toe to examiner's finger	From a supine position, the patient is instructed to touch the great toe to the examiner's finger. The position of finger may be altered during testing to observe ability to change distance, direction, and force of movement.
14. Heel on shin	From a supine position, the heel of one foot is slid up and down the shin of the opposite LE.
15. Drawing a circle	The patient draws an imaginary circle in the air with either UE or LE (a table or the floor also may be used). This also may be done using a figure-eight pattern. This test may be performed in the supine position for the LE.
16. Fixation or position holding	UE: The patient holds arms horizontally in front (sitting or standing). LE: The patient is asked to hold the knee in an extended position (sitting).

*Tests should be performed first with eyes open and then with eyes closed. Abnormal responses include a gradual deviation from the "holding" position and/or a diminished quality of response with vision occluded. Unless otherwise indicated, tests are performed with the patient in a sitting position.

LE = Lower extremity; UE = upper extremity.

Table 6.3	Sample Tests for Selected Coordination Impairments
Impairment	**Sample Test**
Dysdiadochokinesia	Finger-to-nose Alternate nose-to-finger Pronation/supination Knee flexion/extension Walking, alter speed or direction
Dysmetria	Pointing and past pointing Drawing a circle or figure eight Heel on shin Placing feet on floor markers; sitting, standing
Dyssynergia	Finger-to-nose Finger-to-therapist's finger Alternate heel-to-knee Toe-to-examiner's finger
Hypotonia	Passive movement Deep tendon reflexes
Tremor (intention)	Observation during functional activities (tremor will typically increase as target is approached or movement speed increased) Alternate nose-to-finger Finger-to-finger Finger-to-therapist's finger Toe-to-examiner's finger
Tremor (resting)	Observation of patient at rest; limb or jaw movements Observation during functional activities (tremor will diminish significantly or disappear with movement)
Tremor (postural)	Observation of steadiness of normal posture; sitting, standing
Asthenia	Fixation or position holding (upper and lower extremity) Application of manual resistance to determine ability to hold
Rigidity	Passive movement Observation during functional activities Observation of resting posture(s)
Bradykinesia	Walking, observation of arm swing and trunk motions Walking, alter speed and direction Request that a movement or gait activity be stopped abruptly Observation of functional activities: timed tests
Disturbances of posture	Fixation or position holding (upper and lower extremity) Displace balance unexpectedly in sitting or standing (perturbation) Standing, alter base of support (e.g., one foot directly in front of the other; standing on one foot)
Disturbances of gait	Walk along a straight line Walk sideways, backward March in place Alter speed and direction of ambulatory activities Walk in a circle

direct the therapist's observations. The findings should be included in the comment section of the coordination examination form.

- Are movements direct, precise, and easily reversed?
- Do movements occur within a reasonable or normal amount of time?
- Does increased speed of performance affect quality of motor activity?
- Can continuous and appropriate motor adjustments be made if speed and direction are changed?
- Can a position or posture of the body or specific extremity be maintained without swaying, oscillations, or extraneous movements?
- Are placing movements of both upper and lower extremities accurate?
- Does occluding vision alter the quality of motor activity?
- Is there greater involvement proximally or distally?
- Is there greater involvement on one side of body versus the other?
- Does the patient fatigue rapidly?
- Is there a consistency of motor response over time?

Recording Test Results

A generally accepted format for recording results from coordination tests has not been established and approaches to documentation vary considerably among institutions and individual therapists. Owing to the nature of the tests and the wide variation in types and severity of deficits, observational coordination forms are not highly standardized. However, exceptions to this are the upper extremity standardized tests addressing specific components of manual dexterity through the use of functional or work-related tasks. Some of these tests originally were developed to assist with determining if an individual had the needed manual skills required for specific employment tasks. Several examples of these tests are presented later in this chapter under Standardized Instruments: Upper Extremity Coordination.

Several options are available for recording results from a comprehensive examination of coordination. A coordination examination form is useful to provide a composite picture of the areas of impairment noted. These forms are often developed within clinical settings. They may be general (a sample is presented in Table 6.4), or they may be specific to a given group of patients, such as those with brain injuries. In general, these forms lack reliability testing. However, they do provide a systematic method of data collection and documentation. In addition, use of the same form for periodic reexamination facilitates ease of comparison of changes over time. These forms frequently include some type of rating scale in which level of performance is weighted using a scale with descriptors attached. An example of such a scale can be found in Table 6.4.

During testing, postural instability may be evident, particularly in unsupported sitting, and contact guarding may be required. This should be noted in the comments section.

A score from the rating scale would then be assigned to each component of the coordination examination. An advantage of using rating scales is that they provide a mechanism for quantifying patient performance based

---

Table 6.4	Coordination and Balance Examination Form

Patient Name: _____ Examiner: _____ Date: _____

Part I: Nonequilibrium Coordination Tests

Key to Grading	Notations should be made under comments section if:
4 *Normal Performance* 3 *Minimal Impairment:* Able to accomplish activity; slightly less than normal control, speed, and steadiness 2 *Moderate Impairment:* Able to accomplish activity; movements are slow, awkward, and unsteady 1 *Severe Impairment:* Able only to initiate activity without completion; movements are slow with significant unsteadiness, oscillations, and/or extraneous movements 0 *Activity Impossible*	• Lack of visual input renders activity impossible or alters quality of performance • Verbal cuing is required to accomplish activity • Alterations in speed affect quality of performance • Excessive amount of time required to complete activity • Changes in arm position alters sitting balance • Postural instability is evident: unsteadiness, oscillations, extraneous movements • Fatigue alters consistency of response • Performance affects patient safety; requires contact guarding

GRADE: LEFT	COORDINATION TEST	GRADE: RIGHT	COMMENTS
	Finger-to-nose		
	Finger–to–therapist's finger		
	Finger-to-finger		
	Alternate nose-to-finger		
	Finger opposition		
	Mass grasp		
	Pronation/supination		
	Rebound phenomenon		
	Tapping (hand)		
	Tapping (foot)		
	Pointing and past-pointing		
	Alternate heel-to-knee; heel-to-toe		
	Toe–to–examiner's finger		
	Heel-on-shin		
	Drawing a circle (hand)		
	Drawing a circle (foot)		
	Fixation/position holding (UE)		
	Fixation/position holding (LE)		

Continued

Table 6.4 Coordination and Balance Examination Form—cont'd

Part II: Postural Control And Balance Tests

Key to Grading	Notations should be made under comments section if:
4 *Normal:* Able to maintain steady balance without handhold support (static) Accepts maximal challenge and can shift weight easily within full range in all directions (dynamic) 3 *Good:* Able to maintain balance without handhold support, limited postural sway (static) Accepts moderate challenge; able to maintain balance while picking object off floor (dynamic) 2 *Fair:* Able to maintain balance with handhold support; may require occasional minimal assistance (static) Accepts minimal challenge; able to maintain balance while turning head/trunk (dynamic) 1 *Poor:* Requires handhold support and moderate to maximal assistance to maintain position (static) Unable to accept challenge or move without loss of balance (dynamic) 0 *Absent:* Unable to maintain balance	• Lack of visual input renders activity impossible or alters quality of performance • Verbal cuing is required to accomplish activity • Alterations in speed affect quality of performance • Excessive amount of time required to complete activity • Changes in limb position alters standing balance/postural stability • Postural instability is evident: extraneous movements, unsteadiness, or oscillations • Fatigue alters consistency of response • Performance impacts patient safety, fall risk

GRADE	BALANCE TEST	COMMENTS
	Sitting in a normal comfortable position	
	Sitting, weight shifting in all directions	
	Sitting, multidirectional functional reach	
	Sitting, picking an object up off floor	
	Standing in a normal comfortable posture	
	Standing, feet together (narrow base of support)	
	Standing on one foot	
	Standing, with one foot directly in front of the other (tandem position)	
	Standing: eyes open (EO) to eyes closed (EC) (*Romberg Test*)	
	Standing in tandem position: EO to EC (*Sharpened Romberg Test*)	
	Standing, multidirectional functional reach	
	Walking, placing feet on floor markers	
	Walk: sideways	
	Walk: backwards	
	Walk: cross-stepping	
	Walk: in a circle, alternate directions	
	Walk: on heels	
	Walk: on toes	
	March in place	
	Walk with horizontal and vertical head turns	
	Step over or around obstacles	
	Stairclimbing with handrail	
	Stairclimbing without handrail	
	Stairclimbing: one step at a time	
	Stairclimbing: step-over-step	

on subjective ratings. Inherent limitations of using scales include the following: (1) the descriptions may not be reflective of individual patient performance; (2) descriptors may not be defined adequately or detailed appropriately; and (3) without training, individual interpretation decreases reliability of intraexaminer and interexaminer testing. Frequently, coordination forms include a comments section. This component of the form allows for additional narrative descriptions of patient performance. Using a combination of a rating scale and narrative comments or summary will ensure that all coordination impairments are adequately documented.

Measuring the length of time required to complete a motor or functional task provides an important quantitative measure of movement capability. Because accomplishing an activity in a reasonable amount of time is an important criterion of performance, the length of time required to accomplish certain activities is recorded by use of a stopwatch. Using time as a measure of performance has important implications for both function and safety. For example, assume a patient with multiple sclerosis who uses a wheelchair plans to return to school but requires 2.5 hours to complete dressing activities. The time element here would not be considered functional, especially if attempting to make an early morning class. Consider also an ambulatory patient with an ataxic gait unable to cross a street in the allotted time provided by the traffic signal. This time requirement presents a considerable patient safety issue and, as such, would also not be considered functional. Some standardized measurement tools have been developed based on timed activities (e.g., timed Up and Go test [116, 117,]). However, timed performance measures may be incorporated into any variety of motor or functional tasks.

Periodic videotaping of patient performance can be used effectively to document coordination impairments and monitor progress over time. For some patients, such recordings can provide the basis for suggestions about altering movement strategies to improve function and direct attention to safety precautions. Viewed in sequence over time, the visual record can also improve patient motivation to attain further gains. Videotapes have also been used to determine the impact of medications on coordinated movement via preintervention and postintervention administration (e.g., patients with Parkinson's disease).

■ QUANTITATIVE COORDINATION TESTING AND SPECIALIZED TESTING INSTRUMENTS

CATSYS System

The *CATSYS* (Danish Product Development, Ltd., Denmark) is a Windows®-based testing system that allows quantification of several types of coordination

impairments.[118-120] The system interfaces with a computer via a small data logger box (serial cable). The data logger records information from four sensors:

- Tremor Pen™ for documenting tremor intensity and frequency
- Reaction time handheld switch activated by the thumb
- Touch recording plate for measuring pronation/supination and finger tapping
- Force platform for measuring postural sway

Normative data are available and the system allows comparison of interpatient and intrapatient data over time. This system has been used to document movement dysfunction associated with neurodegenerative pathology, as well as pathologies associated with neurotoxic exposure to mercury[121] and magnesium.[122] In response to subthalamic nucleus deep brain stimulation (DBS) for Parkinson's disease, it has been used to quantify features of tremor and finger tapping[123] and to examine the response to DBS in a case study report of essential tremor.[124]

Choice Reaction Time Analyzer

The *Choice Reaction Time Analyzer* (Neuro-Test Inc., Pasadena, CA 91117) is a computerized instrument that allows monitoring of both simple reaction time (SRT) and choice reaction time (CRT). SRT involves only one stimulus and one response (no decisions about the stimuli are required) whereas CRT involves multiple stimuli and requires choosing a response that corresponds to the stimulus. Reaction times are measured from the time a stimulus appears on the screen to the time a response is recorded by pressing one of two small key pads labeled "A" and "S" (pressing a keypad stops the timed measure). For example, in measuring SRT, the patient may be asked to press keypad "A" as quickly as possible each time the color blue appears (note that the color blue here is an arbitrary example, because any number of letters, colors, or objects can serve as the target stimulus; items can also be presented at various angle orientations [sideways, upside-down, and so forth]). For CRT, the subject responds differentially by pressing either the "A" or the "S" key in response to two separate target stimuli. For example, the patient may be instructed to press keypad "A" as quickly as possible each time an inverted number "2" appears and keypad "B" each time the number "2" appears in its normal orientation.

■ STANDARDIZED INSTRUMENTS: UPPER EXTREMITY COORDINATION

Several standardized tests are available to examine arm-hand and eye–hand coordination, as well as fine motor dexterity of the fingers, through use of function-based skills or activities. Many of these tests were originally designed to predict employment success for jobs requiring manipulation of small parts such as might be required for assembly-line work. The vast majority of these tests are scored based both on time required for completion and on quality (accuracy) of results.

Most of these standardized tests include an examiner's manual containing normative data to assist with interpretation of test results. Adherence to the prescribed method of administration is particularly important when using standardized tests. Any deviations from the established protocol will affect the validity and reliability of the measures and consequently make comparisons with published norms invalid. The skill of the examiner is another important consideration. An individual knowledgeable about testing guidelines and interpretation of results should administer the tests. The same individual should perform subsequent retests. These standardized tests are useful in providing objective measures of patient progress over time. The following is a description of several of these tests.

The *Jebsen-Taylor Hand Function Test* (Sammons Preston Rolyan, Bolingbrook, IL 60440) examines hand and finger coordination using seven subtests of functional skills: writing; card turning; picking up small objects; simulated feeding; stacking; picking up large, lightweight objects; and picking up large, heavy objects (Fig. 6.4). The test is easy to construct, administer, and score (commercially available test kits contain all materials together with instructions in a tote bag). Normative data are included relating to age, gender, maximum time, and hand dominance. The test allows examination of hand function in seven common activities of daily living.[125-129]

The *Minnesota Manual Dexterity Test* (Lafayette Instrument Co., Lafayette, IN 47903) was designed to select personnel for semiskilled operations requiring coordinated arm/hand/finger movements, as well as eye–hand coordination such as required for handling small tools or assembly materials that do not require differentiating size or shape (Fig. 6.5). The test includes placing and turning tasks and requires use of a board with wells and round disks. Normative data are available. An expanded variation of this test is the Minnesota Rate of Manipulation Test, which includes five operations: placing, turning, displacing, one-hand turning and placing, and two-hand turning and placing.[129-132]

The *Purdue Pegboard* (Lafayette Instrument Co., Lafayette, IN 47903) Test addresses both gross coordination of the arm/hand/fingers and fine coordination (dexterity) of the fingers by placement of pins, collars, and/or washes on a pegboard (Fig. 6.6). There are several subtests, including right-hand prehension, left-hand prehension, prehension test with both hands, and assembly. The test has been used to select personnel for industrial jobs that require manipulative skills. Normative values are available, and both unilateral and bilateral coordinated movement can be examined.[133,134] This test requires use of a testing board, pins, collars, and washers. The Purdue Pegboard was found to have high test–retest reliability in persons with multiple sclerosis.[135]

The *Crawford Small Parts Dexterity Test* (Harcourt Assessment, San Antonio, TX 78270) uses the manipulation of small tools to examine motor performance. The test uses pins, collars, and screws, as well as a board into which these small objects fit. Use of tweezers is required

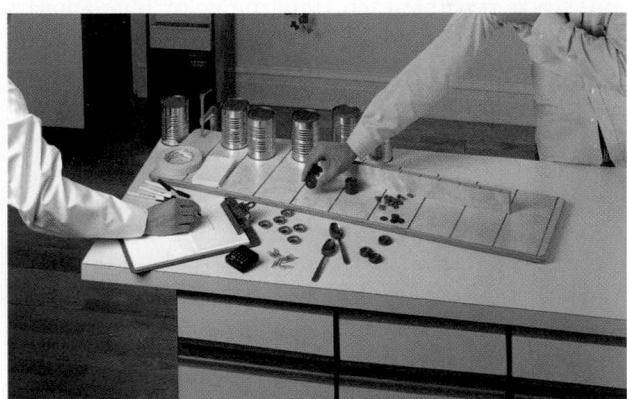

Figure 6.4 The Jebsen-Taylor Hand Function Test includes a subset of seven functional tasks allowing examination of a broad range of skills requiring coordinated movement of the hand and fingers. Common items are used such as spoons, paper clips, cans, and pencils. *(Courtesy of Sammons Preston Rolyan, Bolingbrook, IL 60440-3593.)*

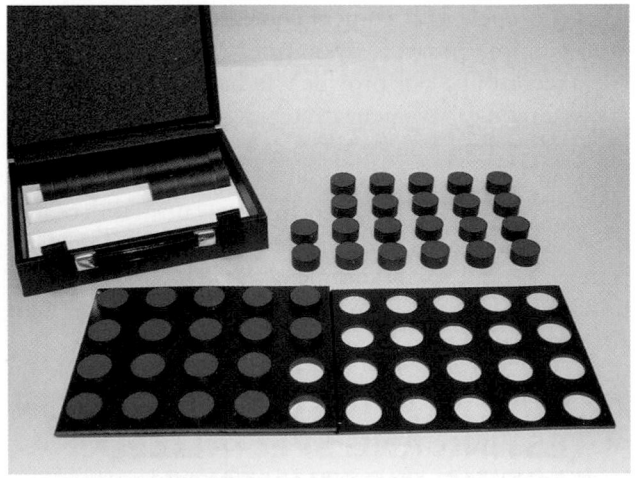

Figure 6.5 Minnesota Manual Dexterity Test consists of two operations: *placing* and *turning*. After a practice trial, scores are based on the time required to complete each of four trials for each operation.

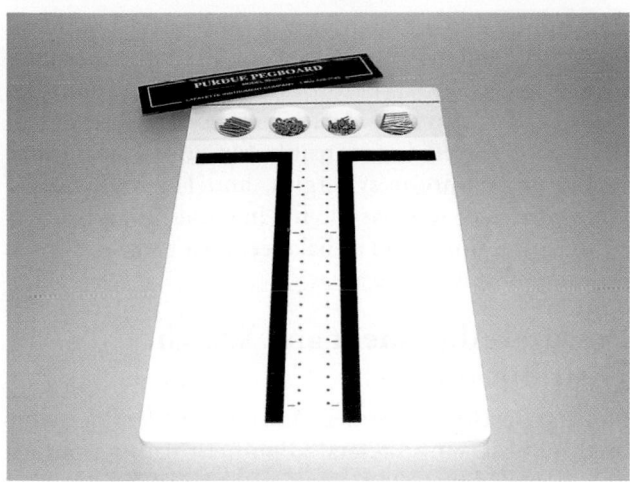

Figure 6.6 The Purdue Pegboard Test includes a pegboard equipped with pins, collars, and washers. Scores are based on the number of assemblies completed within either a 30- or 60-second period.

both to place the pins in holes and to place a collar over the pin. The screws must be placed with the fingers and screwed in with a screwdriver. This test has been used in prevocational testing. Normative data are available. This test is scored by time.[129,136]

The *O'Connor Tweezer Test* (Fig. 6.7, *left*) and the *Finger Dexterity Test* (Fig. 6.7, *right*) examine the ability to rapidly manipulate small objects (Lafayette Instrument Co., Lafayette, IN 47903). The Tweezer Test emphasizes eye–hand and fine motor dexterity by requiring

the subject to use a tweezers to place a single pin in each 1/16th-inch–diameter hole. The Finger Dexterity Test also addresses fine motor dexterity through manual placement of three pins per hole. Both of these tests were originally developed to predict successful employment for assembly-line work requiring rapid manipulation of small parts (e.g., assembling miniature components of watches).

The *Hand Tool Dexterity Test* (Fig. 6.8) utilizes ordinary tools to examine coordinated movement of arm/hand/fingers during a functional task. The test frame consists of a flat board to which two side uprights are attached. The test requires disassembly of the nuts and bolts on one upright using the appropriate tools and reassembling them on the opposite upright. The test is timed and normative data are available.

The *Roeder Manipulative Aptitude Test* (Fig. 6.9) measures arm/hand/finger coordination (including thrusting and twisting) as well as eye–hand coordination. The test materials consist of a high-density plastic board with four wells for washers, rods, caps, and nuts; a T-bar for placement of washer–nut assemblies; and rows of sockets for installing nuts. The test protocol includes four timed operations: dominant hand rod–cap assembly and T-bar washer–nut assembly using both hands, right hand, and left hand. Normative data are available.

Other standardized and commercially distributed tests are available. Selection of standardized instruments should be based on (1) the intended movement capabilities to be examined, such as reciprocal motion, movement composition, reaction time, or accuracy;

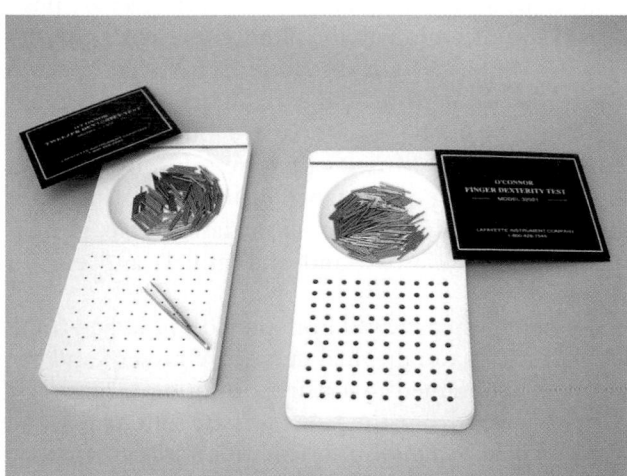

Figure 6.7 The O'Connor Tweezer (*left*) and Finger Dexterity (*right*) Tests examine fine motor coordination. Each board is 11 × 5.5 inches (28 cm × 14 cm) with 100 holes and shallow wells to hold the pins. The black covers slide through grooved channels to keep pins in place during storage.

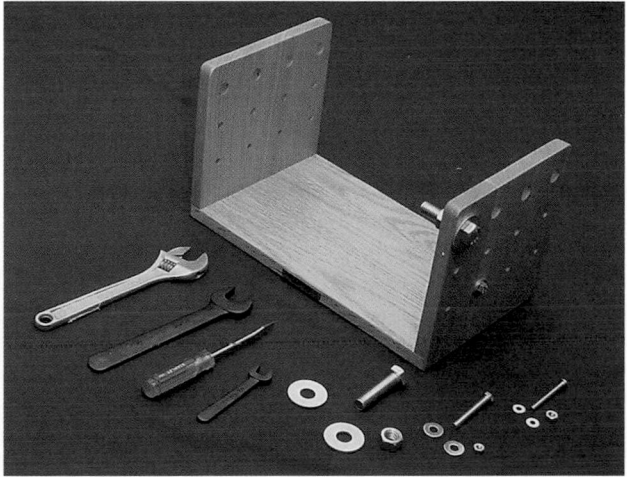

Figure 6.8 The Hand Dexterity Tool Test utilizes ordinary tools for removing and remounting the nuts and bolts. The test is timed from initiation of task (picking up first tool) until the last bolt is secured. *(Courtesy of Lafayette Instrument Co., Lafayette, IN 47903.)*

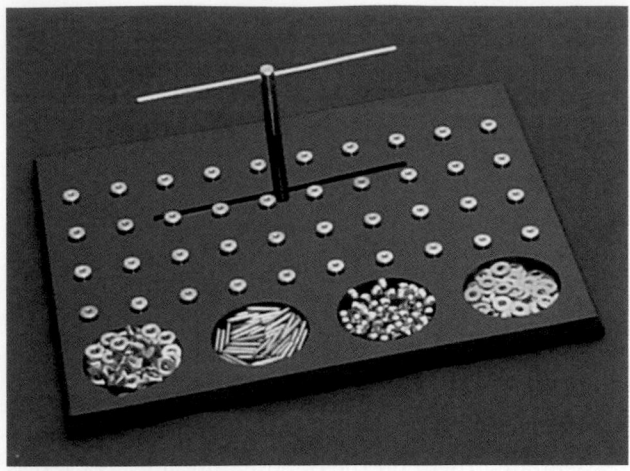

Figure 6.9 The Roeder Manipulative Aptitude Test is scored by counting the number of nuts and washers assembled within the allotted time. *(Courtesy of Lafayette Instrument Co., Lafayette, IN 47903.)*

and (2) the required tasks needed to fully explore coordinated movement for an individual patient (i.e., unilateral tasks, bilateral symmetrical tasks, or bilateral asymmetrical tasks). In addition, careful consideration should be made of criteria used for standardization of the testing instrument and the availability of normative data to assist interpretation of findings.

■ EXAMINATION OF POSTURAL CONTROL AND BALANCE

Postural orientation involves control of the relative positions of body parts by skeletal muscles with respect to each other and gravity. **Balance** is the condition in which all the forces acting on the body are balanced such that the *center of mass (COM)* is within the stability limits, the boundaries of the *base of support (BOS)*. The overall goals of the postural control system, stability and function, are achieved through integrated CNS systems of control. *Reactive postural control* occurs in response to external forces acting on the body (e.g., perturbations) displacing the COM or moving the BOS (e.g., moveable platform, therapy ball). Feedback systems provide the sensory inputs required to initiate corrective responses. *Proactive (anticipatory) postural control* occurs in anticipation of internally generated, destabilizing forces imposed on the body's own movements (e.g., catching a weighted ball). An individual's prior experiences allow the various elements of the postural control system to be pretuned or readied for upcoming movements using feedforward mechanisms. Postural requirements vary depending on the characteristics of the task and the environment. *Adaptive postural control* allows the individual to modify sensory and motor systems in response to changing task and environmental demands.[2] Balance emerges from a complex interaction of (1) sensory/perceptual systems responsible for the detection of body position and motion, (2) motor systems responsible for organization and execution of motor synergies, and (3) higher-level CNS processes responsible for integration and action plans. An examination of balance must therefore focus on each of these three areas.

Postural Alignment and Weight Distribution

Normal postural alignment in standing can be examined by observing skeletal alignment using a plumb or weighted line. More sophisticated analysis can be achieved using motion analysis systems with light-emitting signals, photography, and electromyography. In standing, the COM occurs at a point about two thirds of the body height above the BOS. Static posture in standing is examined by positioning the patient with the feet apart, normal stance width. When viewed from the side (sagittal plane alignment) the plumb line is positioned just in front of the lateral malleolus. The vertical *line of gravity (LOG)* is expected to fall close to most joint axes: slightly anterior to the ankle and knee joints, at or slightly posterior to the hip joint, through midline of the trunk, just anterior to the shoulder joint, and through the external auditory meatus (Fig. 6.10).

Natural spinal curves are present but flattened in upright stance depending on the level of postural tone, lumbar and cervical lordosis, and thoracic or dorsal kyphosis. The pelvis is held in neutral position, with no anterior or posterior tilt. When viewed from the front or back (frontal plane analysis), the feet are positioned equidistant from the plumb line. The examiner looks for equal weight distribution between feet and symmetry of the trunk and extremities. Normal alignment minimizes the need for active muscle contraction during standing. Muscles that are tonically active at low levels during quiet stance include tibialis anterior and gastrocnemius-soleus; tensor fascia latae, gluteus medius, and iliopsoas; and abdominals and erector spinae.[137]

In sitting when viewed from the side, head and trunk are vertical. Natural spinal curves are present and the pelvis is maintained in a neutral position (Fig. 6.11). When viewed from the front or back, the trunk and head are held in a midline orientation with symmetrical weight-bearing on both lower extremities (buttocks, thighs, and feet).[137]

Limits of stability is defined as the maximum distance an individual is able or willing to lean in any direction without loss of balance or changing the BOS. Thus, in standing an individual can shift forward and backward or side-to-side without losing

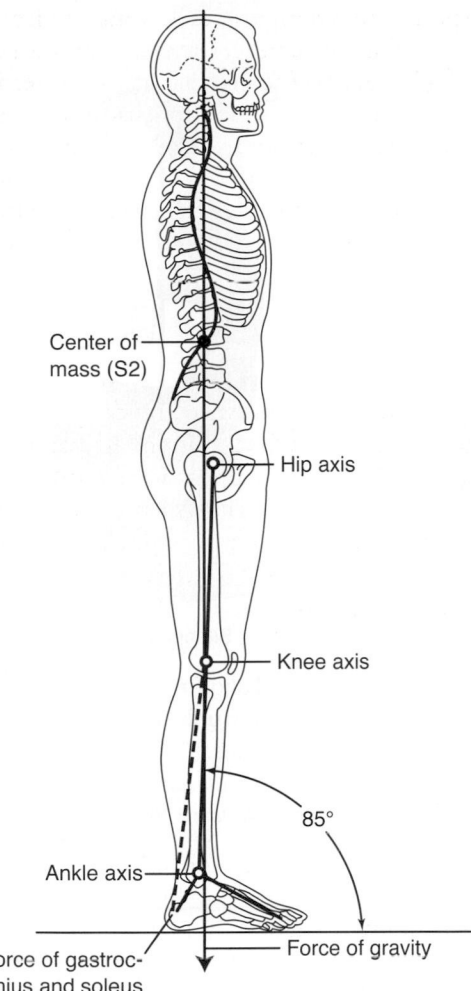

Center of mass (S2)

Hip axis

Knee axis

85°

Ankle axis

Force of gastroc-nemius and soleus

Force of gravity

Figure 6.10 Normal postural alignment in standing-sagittal plane. In optimal alignment, the LOG passes through the identified anatomical structures.

Examination and Documentation

Postural alignment and sway can be examined using visual inspection with the patient standing against a postural grid.[141] More sophisticated instrumentation, posturography, utilizes force plates to measure and quantify ground reaction forces, either center of force (COF) measures or center of pressure (COP) measures. COF is calculated using only vertical forces, and COP is calculated using both vertical and horizontal shear forces. The weight of each foot is determined, forces calculated, and converted into a visual image (Fig. 6.12). Software analysis of data provides an indication of the initial stance position (center of alignment), mean sway path, total sway excursion (LOS), and the zone of stability. These findings are valid and reliable measures of postural control.[142,143]

Using this information, the therapist can objectively determine the patient's postural symmetry, which is a reflection of the amount of weight placed on each foot. Patients with asymmetry may present with the COP positioned away from midline. For example, the patient with stroke typically stands with most of the weight on the less affected limb. Steadiness can be determined by using postural sway measures. A large sway path is evidence of postural unsteadiness. Another example is the patient with ataxia who typically demonstrates hypermetric responses, with excessive sway, uncoordinated movements, and limited postural steadiness. The patient with Parkinson's disease presents with the opposite problem, hypometric responses with diminished sway and excessive stabilization.[144,145] Limits of stability are determined by asking the patient to actively shift weight in any direction as far as possible without losing balance or taking a step. Patients with deficits in motor control typically have reduced LOS (reduced COP excursion). For example, the patient with stroke demonstrates reduced stability limits to the more affected side. The patient with Parkinson's disease typically demonstrates reduced LOS overall with significant anterior stability limits if a stooped posture is evident. LOS and COM alignment are also typically altered in other pathological states (e.g., muscle weakness, skeletal deformity, and tonal abnormalities). Reexamination after training using force platform biofeedback has been used to document recovery of postural control following stroke.[146,147] It has also been used to demonstrate the effectiveness of training using biofeedback force platform training devices.[140,145,148]

Sensorimotor Integration in Postural Control

The sensory systems (vision, somatosensory, and vestibular) provide the CNS with important information about postural control and balance, including information about the results of our own actions and the surrounding environment. The CNS integrates

balance or taking a step. Limits of stability is influenced by a number of factors, including individual characteristics such as height and foot length for anterior/posterior (AP) LOS and distance between the feet and height for medial/lateral (ML) LOS.[138] Both COM position and movement (velocity and displacement) influence LOS.[139] The midpoint of LOS is termed the *COM alignment*. *Steadiness* refers to the ability to maintain a given posture with minimum movement (sway).[140] During standing, an individual normally exhibits small range postural shifts (*postural sway*), cycling intermittently from side-to-side and from heel-to-toe. *Sway envelope* refers to the path of the body's movement during standing. During walking, there are minimal COM movements up and down and side-to-side, resulting in a smooth sinusoidal curve. In sitting, the BOS is larger and COM lower (just above the support base), resulting in greater LOS.

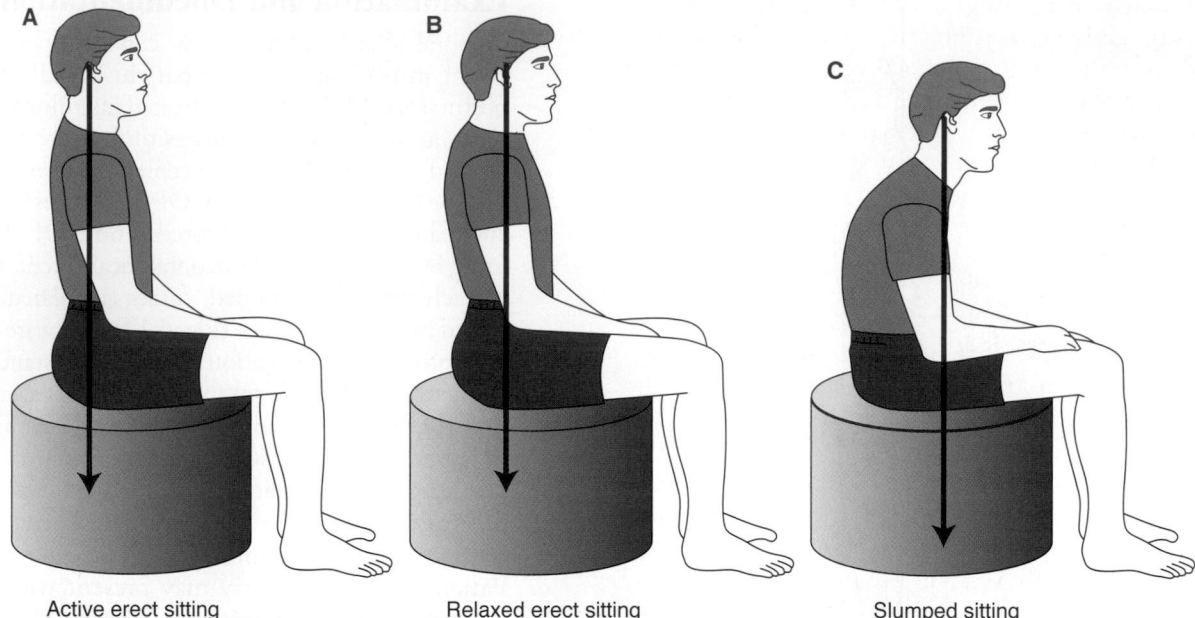

Active erect sitting   Relaxed erect sitting   Slumped sitting

Figure 6.11 Normal sagittal plane postural alignment in sitting: (A) In optimal alignment, the line of gravity passes close to the axes of rotation of the head and neck, and trunk. (B) During relaxed sitting, the line of gravity changes very little, remaining close to those axes. (C) During slumped sitting, the line of gravity is well forward of the spine and hips. *(From O'Sullivan, SB and Schmitz, TJ.* Improving Functional Outcomes in Physical Rehabilitation. *Philadelphia: FA Davis; 2010.)*

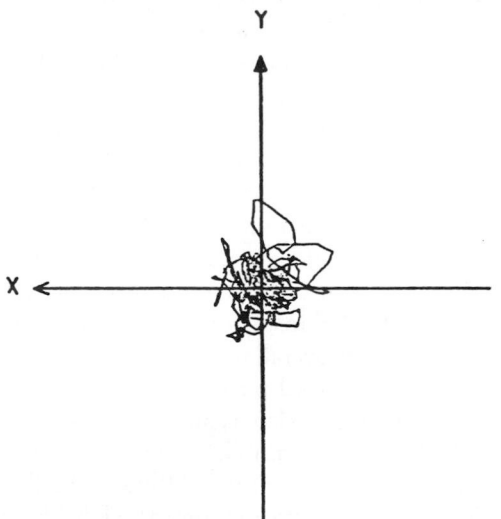

Figure 6.12 Postural sway. Recording of the movement of the center of pressure for 60 seconds in a subject standing on a balance platform. Values: mean amplitude of sway path in inches = .13 × .15; length of path = 32.2; and velocity = .45 in/sec. *(From Smith, L, et al: Brunnstrom's Clinical Kinesiology, ed 5. Philadelphia, FA Davis, 1996, p 406, with permission.)*

these inputs and initiates both goal-directed conscious actions and automatic, unconscious adjustments in posture and movements. Each individual sensory system provides unique and important information and no one system provides all the information needed.

The visual system serves as an important source of information for the ability to perceive movements and detect the relative orientation of body segments and orientation of the body in space. This ability has been termed **visual proprioception**.[149] Two separate functional visual systems have been identified. Various different names have been used: (1) *focal vision* (cognitive or explicit vision) and (2) *ambient vision* (sensorimotor or implicit vision). Focal vision plays a major role in localizing features in the environment and in our conscious reaction to visual events. In contrast, ambient vision utilizes the entire visual field to provide information on the localizing features about the environment and to guide movements using largely nonconscious awareness.[6] Thus, each visual system has a unique functional significance. For example, the patient with brain injury who has a condition called *optic ataxia* can recognize an object using focal vision but cannot use visual information to accurately guide the hand to the object (impaired ambient vision). The opposite occurs in a patient with stroke experiencing *visual agnosia*. The patient cannot recognize common objects, but can use the ambient visual system to reach and grasp an object or navigate an environment. Vision also contributes to righting reactions of the head, trunk, and limbs (optical righting reactions).

Visual acuity (focal vision) can be examined using a Snellen eye chart. A distance acuity poorer than 20/50 will have a significant effect on postural stability.[150]

Whereas focal vision is detected by the central retina only, ambient vision is detected by the entire visual field (central and peripheral vision). Patients with loss of peripheral vision (e.g., a patient with stroke and hemianopsia or a patient with glaucoma) may demonstrate deficits in visual proprioception and functional performance. Peripheral vision can be examined using the *confrontation method*. The patient sits in front of the therapist and is instructed to focus gaze on the therapist's nose. The therapist then slowly brings a target (moving finger or pencil) slowly into the patient's field of view from the right or left side. The patient is instructed to indicate (point or declare) when and where the target is detected. Ambient vision can be examined by instructing the patient to navigate across the busy physical therapy gym. The abilities to navigate safely, to localize features in the environment, and to anticipate changes necessary to avoid obstacles and successfully reach the target area are determined. Patients with stroke who exhibit *topographical disorientation* will have difficulty navigating their environment and understanding the relationship of one place to another.

Somatosensory inputs include the cutaneous and pressure sensations from the body segments in contact with the support surface (e.g., the feet in standing, the buttocks, thighs, and feet in sitting) and muscle and joint proprioception throughout the body. Light touch contact from the hands on a stable surface is also used as a balance aid.[151] This provides information about the relative orientation and movement of the body in relation to the support surface. Cutaneous sensation (touch and pressure) of the feet/ankles and proprioception of the feet/ankles and hips are particularly important in maintaining upright standing balance. Sensory examination of the extremities and trunk is therefore essential (See Chapter 3, Examination of Sensory Function).

The vestibular system is an important source of information for postural control and balance. The semicircular canals (SCCs) detect angular acceleration and deceleration forces acting on the head whereas the otolith organs detect linear acceleration and orientation of the head with reference to gravity. The SCCs are sensitive to fast (phasic) movements of the head, and the otoliths respond to slow head movements and positional change referenced to gravity. The vestibular system functions to stabilize gaze during head movements via the *vestibulo-ocular reflex (VOR)*, and to assist in the regulation of postural tone and postural muscle activation via the vestibulo-spinal reflex (VSR). Tests for vestibular function include positional and movement testing. The patient is observed for symptoms of vestibular dysfunction (e.g., dizziness, vertigo, nystagmus).[152] See Chapter 21, Vestibular Disorders, for a complete discussion of this topic.

During stance, all sensory inputs contribute to the maintenance of posture. Sensory weighting theory specifies that the CNS weights the various sensory inputs depending on the specific sensory environment and task.[153-156] *Quiet stance* is defined as standing with a stable support surface and surroundings. *Perturbed stance* is defined as standing during a brief displacement of the support surface (moving surface) or displacement of the COM over BOS (perturbation). In intact adults during quiet stance, the CNS places greater weight on somatosensory inputs. During an unexpected perturbation, somatosensory inputs are activated quicker and provide much of the early restabilizing control whereas vision and vestibular inputs with slower processing speeds contribute to later components of the postural re-stabilizing response.[157] If somatosensory inputs are impaired (e.g., peripheral neuropathy) or if somatosensory conflict is introduced (e.g., standing on dense foam), vision assumes a greater role. If both somatosensory and visual inputs are impaired or absent, vestibular inputs are critical to maintaining posture and resolving sensory conflict. Central nervous system use of sensory inputs is flexible. Balance responses are task and context dependent and are triggered by CNS weighting based on availability, timing, and accuracy of specific sensory inputs.

Because sensory inputs are redundant, stable balance can be maintained with significant impairment, on unstable surfaces, or in sensory conflict situations. However, if more than one sensory system is deficient, substantial deficiencies in balance control will be evident.[158] For example, the patient with chronic diabetes who has significant diabetic neuropathy (loss of somatosensory inputs from the feet and ankles) and significant diabetic retinopathy (impaired vision) will demonstrate significant postural instability and fall risk. In addition, the cognitive system plays an important role in attending to and interpreting the information for CNS planning of effective postural responses. Attentional demands vary depending on the task (new learning versus familiar response) and the environment (open versus closed or dual-tasking). Patients with impairments in cognition or attention demonstrate increased fall risk, especially for those activities with high stability demands.

Romberg Test

The **Romberg Test** is historically one of the oldest sensory tests for postural control.[159] During the test, the patient is instructed to stand with feet together, eyes open (EO) unaided for 20 to 30 seconds. (If the patient demonstrates significant sway or instability with EO, the test is over.) The patient is then asked to stand with eyes closed (EC). If the test is negative, there is no change or only minimal worsening with EC. If the test is positive, the patient is able to stand with EO but demonstrates a significant increase in sway and/or instability with EC. The *Romberg Quotient* refers to the ratio of body sway during EO and EC conditions and can be used as a measure of stability.[2] During testing, it is important to tell the patient you are prepared to catch him or her in the event of a fall. A positive Romberg test is indicative of a loss of proprioception (*sensory ataxia*) that occurs with posterior column lesions in the spinal cord (e.g., cervical spondylosis, tumor, degenerative spinal cord disease, tabes dorsalis) and peripheral neuropathy. If unsteadiness occurs in standing with EO, it is likely the patient is demonstrating other CNS dysfunction (e.g., cerebellar ataxia or vestibular dysfunction). In the sharpened Romberg test, the feet are placed in tandem (heel–toe position) and the EO to EC conditions imposed.

Sensory Organization Test

The *Sensory Organization Test (SOT)* is based on the work of Nashner[153,154] and determines the effectiveness of the CNS to utilize and integrate different sensory inputs. It examines body sway during quiet standing under six different sensory test conditions (Fig. 6.13). Dynamic posturography equipment is used to provide a moving platform that introduces mechanical perturbations (sliding or tilting movements). A moving visual surround screen is sway referenced and introduces visual conflict. Both the surround and force plate are referenced to the patient by means of hydraulic mechanisms. Test condition 1 provides accurate somatosensory, visual, and vestibular information and is the baseline reference. Each of the other five conditions systematically varies sensory inputs, increasing the level of sensory conflict and postural difficulty (Table 6.5).

Conditions 1 to 3 are all performed with the patient standing on a stable support surface, providing accurate somatosensory inputs. Visual inputs are varied: condition 1 uses EO, and condition 2 uses EC. Condition 3 uses a moving visual surround (screen) referenced to body sway, thus providing inaccurate visual information. Conditions 4 through 6 repeat the visual conditions but with an altered support surface (moving platform) that provides inaccurate somatosensory information. In conditions 5 and 6 maintenance of posture depends on availability and accuracy of vestibular inputs with the reduction of both vision and somatosensory inputs. Thus, patients with vestibular dysfunction will demonstrate maximum instability in conditions 5 and 6. Patients who are visually dependent for postural control will demonstrate instability in conditions 2, 3, 5, and 6. Patients who are surface dependent will demonstrate instability in conditions 4, 5, and 6. Patients who demonstrate sensory selection problems present with abnormal findings in conditions 3 through 6.[2] Each condition is maintained for 30 seconds. If the patient is able to stand for the required 30 seconds, the test is progressed

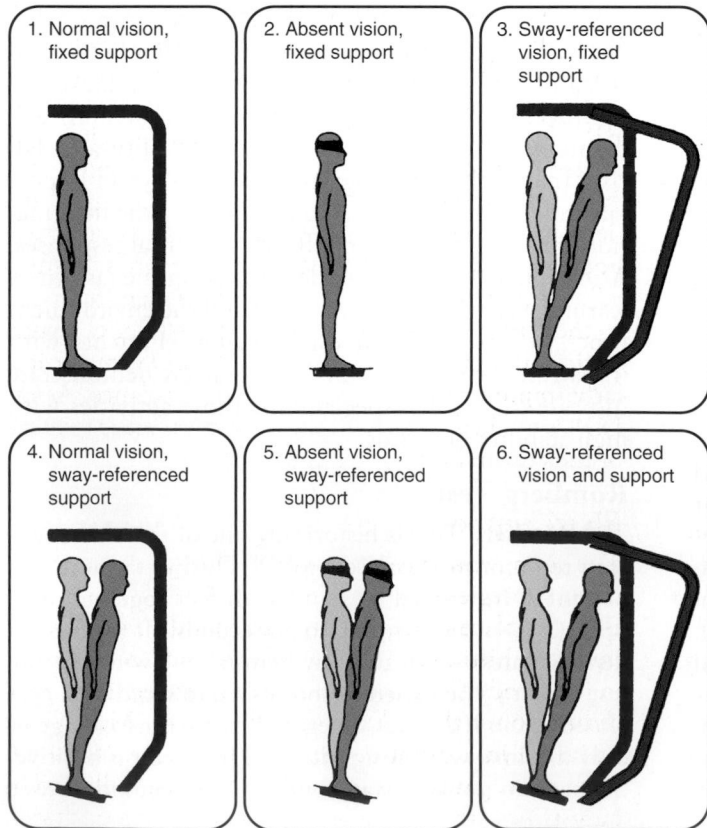

Figure 6.13 The Sensory Organization Test.

Table 6.5	Sensory Organization Test Conditions
Condition	**Sensory Input**
Condition 1 Eyes Open, Stable Surface (EOSS)	All sensory systems unaltered
Condition 2 Eyes Closed, Stable Surface (ECSS)	Vision absent Somatosensory unaltered Vestibular intact
Condition 3 Visual Conflict with Moving Surround, Stable Surface (VCSS)	Vision altered Somatosensory unaltered Vestibular intact
Condition 4 Eyes Open, Moving Surface (EOMS)	Vision unaltered Somatosensory altered Vestibular intact
Condition 5 Eyes Closed, Moving Surface (ECMS)	Vision absent Somatosensory altered Vestibular intact
Condition 6 Visual Conflict with Moving Surround, Moving Platform (VCMS)	Vision altered Somatosensory altered Vestibular intact

to the next sensory condition. If the patient is unsuccessful on the first attempt, a second trial can be given. The SOT is scored by observing changes in the amount and direction of postural sway. A numerical scoring system can be used.

1 Minimal sway
2 Mild sway
3 Moderate sway
4 Loss of balance

Posturography equipment provides a printed bar graph indicating how well the patient performed during each of the six conditions in terms of postural sway. Ratios comparing one condition to another can provide information regarding reliance on one sensory system over another. Additional analyses of motor coordination using electromyography (EMG) can provide information about the relative level of individual muscle activity, as well as overall muscle recruitment patterns.

As in all testing of postural control and balance, patient safety is an important consideration. During posturography the patient typically wears a safety harness to prevent falls. Upper extremity support is not allowed during the test. However, the equipment includes hand rails that can be used as an additional safety net.

Clinical Test for Sensory Interaction in Balance

In the absence of sophisticated and expensive posturography equipment, a modified version can be performed in clinical or home settings. The *Clinical Test for Sensory Interaction in Balance (CTSIB)* is a low-tech version of the SOT developed by Shumway-Cook and Horak.[160] It utilizes medium-density foam to substitute for a moving platform and a modified visual dome (Japanese lantern affixed to the subject's head) to substitute for a moving visual surrounding. Six sensory conditions are tested, similar to the SOT.[161] A simpler to perform modified version of the CTSIB (m-CTSIB) also exists. It utilizes 4 different sensory test conditions (EO and EC on flat surface and on foam). Conditions 3 and 6 are omitted (visual dome conditions). The same posture is adopted in both versions (i.e., feet shoulder-width apart). Three 30-second trials are used. Times in balance and increased sway or loss of balance are recorded. Subjective patient complaints (e.g., nausea, dizziness) and postural strategies used (e.g., ankle or hip strategies, arms widen and elevate) are also documented. The test is stopped if the patient alters the posture (widens or moves feet, opens eyes) or loses balance, requiring manual assistance.[162]

Movement Strategies for Balance

In observational studies of infants and young children and lesioned animals (decerebration experiments), righting and equilibrium reactions comprise the *postural reflex mechanism*. Automatic *righting reactions (RR)* orient the head in space (optical RR, labyrinthine RR, body-on-head RR) and the body in relation to the head and support surface (neck-on-body RR, body-on-body RR). *Equilibrium reactions* include tilting reactions and parachute or protective reactions. In normal adults, however, postural adjustments are far more complex and demonstrate a high degree of adaptability in response to both task and environmental context demands. Postural adjustments vary from the simple stretch reflex responses to the activation of specific movement strategies (synergistic patterns). Muscles closest to the BOS are particularly important to the maintenance of balance. As the LOS is reached with a COM disturbance, the magnitude of the postural response is increased.

Fixed Support Strategies

The term *fixed-support strategies* refers to those movement strategies used to control the COM over a fixed BOS (in-place strategies). In standing, the *ankle strategy* involves shifting the COM forward and back by moving the body (legs and trunk) as a relatively fixed pendulum about the ankle joints (Fig. 6.14). Muscles are activated in a distal-to-proximal sequence. With forward sway, gastrocnemius is activated first, followed by hamstrings, then paraspinal muscles. With backward

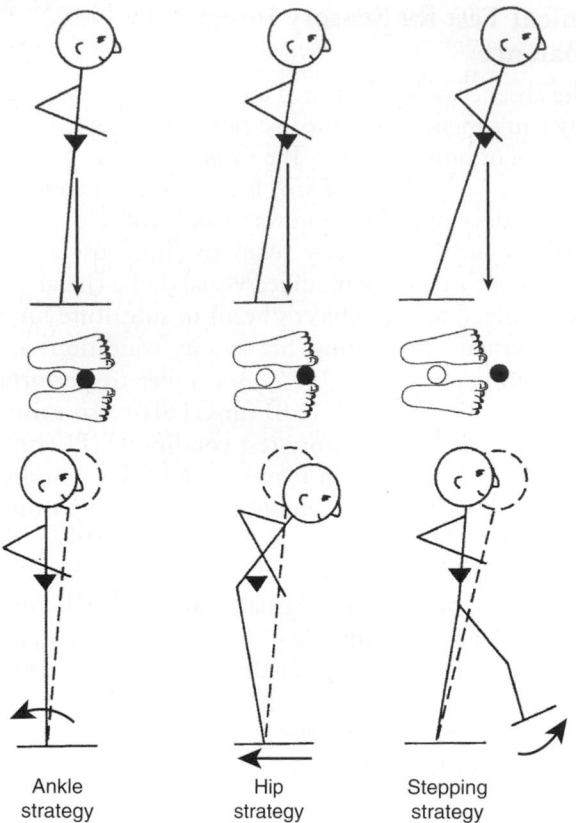

Ankle strategy   Hip strategy   Stepping strategy

Figure 6.14 Strategies for correcting balance perturbations.

sway, the anterior tibialis is activated first, followed by quadriceps, then abdominals. The ankle strategy is a commonly used strategy when sway frequencies are low and disturbances of the COM are small and well within the LOS.

The *hip strategy* involves shifts in the COM by flexing or extending at the hips (see Fig. 6.14). It has a proximal pattern of muscle activation before distal activation. With forward sway abdominals are activated first, followed by quadriceps. With backward sway, paraspinal muscles are activated first, followed by hamstrings. Hip strategies provide primary control for mediolateral stability. Hip muscles (abductors and adductors) are activated to control lateral sway. The hip strategy is typically recruited with faster sway frequencies (greater than 1 Hz) and larger disturbances of the COM or when the support surface is small (less than the size of the feet) or compliant (e.g., standing on foam).[163,164]

Change-in-Support Strategies

Change-in-support strategies are defined as movements of the lower or upper limbs to make a new contact with the support surface.[97] The *stepping strategy* realigns the BOS under the COM by using rapid steps or hops in the direction of the displacing force, for example, forward or backward steps. In instances of lateral destabilization, the individual takes a side step or a cross step to bring

the BOS back under the COM. The stepping strategies are typically recruited in response to fast, large postural perturbations when ankle and hip strategies are not adequate to recover balance (e.g., when the COM exceeds the BOS) (see Fig. 6.14). Change-in-support movements of the upper limbs (reach or grasp) can also assist in stabilizing the COM over the BOS, and serve a protective function in absorbing impact and protecting the head in a fall event. *Reaching movements* assist in extending the BOS and stabilizing posture. These reactions were found to be prevalent in destabilization situations, occurring in 85% of trials. Stepping strategies were also frequent, leading researchers to suggest that change-in-support strategies should not be viewed just as strategies of last resort. They are often initiated well before the COM nears or exceeds the LOS, contrary to the traditional view.[164-166]

Although these movement strategies have been investigated individually as distinct movement patterns, research has also shown that during normal balance combinations of strategies are used.[163] Control of movement strategies should be viewed on a continuum. The CNS quickly moves between patterns depending on the control demands of the activity and environment. Thus, a destabilizing force may yield an initial ankle strategy that progresses quickly to a hip strategy as increased control is warranted to recover balance. When the displacement is large and ankle and hip strategies prove inadequate, a stepping strategy may be necessary to prevent a fall.[167] The CNS uses continuous sensory feedback monitoring to achieve flexibility and adaptability of movement strategies for multidirectional postural control.

In sitting, the BOS is comprised of the thighs and buttocks and the feet if in contact with the support surface. Postural strategies to maintain balance include movement of the trunk about the hips. Backward sway elicits primary responses in hip flexors along with activity of the abdominals and neck flexors. In forward sway, extensor muscles of the hips are activated along with the extensors of the neck and trunk. If the feet are in contact with the floor, tibialis anterior is recruited during forward reaching movements of the arm and the gastrocnemius is recruited to brake forward movements and return the body to erect sitting.[168] Somatosensory inputs from backward rotation of the pelvis may have an important role in triggering the postural strategies in sitting.[169] In frontal plane movements, activity of the hip abductors and adductors along with the quadratus lumborum is important for providing mediolateral stability.

Examination and Documentation of Movement Strategies
Standing Control

An examination of movement strategies should first begin with the musculoskeletal elements (ROM, postural tone, and strength). Weakness and limited ROM in the ankles will influence successful use of an ankle strategy, whereas weakness and limited ROM about the hips will influence the hip strategy. Limitations of neck ROM can be expected in patients with primary vestibular disorders. Available movement strategies in response to AP and ML destabilizations should be determined.

Dynamic posturography provides the ideal way to study motor strategies during standing. The *Movement Coordination Test (MCT)* developed by Nashner and co-workers[164] provides information about postural responses to control the COM when the platform moves, including symmetry of weight-bearing and forces generated, latency of postural responses, amplitude of response in relation to the stimulus size, and strategy utilized (ankle or hip). EMG monitoring can reveal specific muscle activation patterns and latencies. The main disadvantage of this equipment is limited use in the clinic due to expense and lack of portability (e.g., it is typically found in specialized Balance or Vestibular Dysfunction Clinics). Correlation with performance during functional tasks (e.g., walking) is also lacking.

During perturbed stance, the direction of perturbations can be varied (AP and ML). The movement strategies utilized and success of restabilization efforts should be examined and documented. Specific directional instability may be evident. Patients may demonstrate an absence or decreased use of one strategy with increased dependence on another. For example, older adults with somatosensory loss in the feet and ankles typically forgo the ankle strategy and utilize an early hip strategy. The sequencing of movement synergies should be examined and a determination of the pattern of activation made. For example, the ascending pattern of activation (distal-proximal) may be absent in patients with strong spasticity. The therapist is likely to see a proximal-to-distal activation pattern with strong co-activation of spastic muscles in the hips and knees.

Seated Control

Seated postural control and balance should be examined. During quiet sitting, the degree and direction of sway should be determined. During perturbed unsupported sitting, the available movement strategies to prevent destabilization should be examined and documented. Grasp strategies (holding on to the edge of the seat) or lower extremity hooking strategies (the foot and leg hook around the platform mat leg) are common strategies in the presence of significant instability. Seated instability is common in many patients with neurological dysfunction. For example, patients with stroke may demonstrate increased sway, problems activating trunk muscles (e.g., voluntary trunk flexion and extension), limited extent and direction of reaching, and altered postural alignment with greater weight placed on the less affected side.

Documentation

For both standing and seated control, the therapist determines and documents if the movement strategies are (1) present and normal, (2) present but limited or delayed, (3) present but inappropriate for the particular context or situation, (4) abnormal, or (5) absent.[91] The ability to modify postural strategies and adapt movements to changing task conditions should also be documented. For example, the patient can be asked to stand first with normal stance width, then with a narrowed BOS (feet together, in tandem, or single leg stance). Table 6.6 presents an example of a functional balance grade scale with descriptors that can be used to define both static and dynamic control in sitting and standing.

Anticipatory Postural Control

Anticipatory postural control, the ability to activate postural adjustments in advance of destabilizing voluntary movements, should be examined.[2] For example, the therapist asks the patient while standing or sitting to raise both arms overhead or catch a weighted ball. Changes in postural stability control are examined and documented during the performance of the voluntary activity. Impaired anticipatory postural control is found in many individuals with impairments in motor function, including patients with stroke,[170,171] Parkinson's disease,[172] and brain injury.[173]

Dual-Task Control

Dual-task control should be examined. This is the ability to perform a secondary task (motor or cognitive) while

Table 6.6	Functional Balance Grades
4 Normal	Patient able to maintain steady balance without handhold support (static). Patient accepts maximal challenge and can shift weight easily within full range in all directions (dynamic).
3 Good	Patient able to maintain balance without handhold support, limited postural sway (static). Patient accepts moderate challenge; able to maintain balance while picking up object off floor (dynamic).
2 Fair	Patient able to maintain balance with handhold support; may require occasional minimal assistance (static). Patient accepts minimal challenge; able to maintain balance while turning head/trunk (dynamic).
1 Poor	Patient requires handhold support and moderate to maximal assistance to maintain position (static). Patient unable to accept challenge or move without loss of balance (dynamic).
0 Absent	Patient unable to maintain balance

maintaining standing or seated control. For example, while standing the patient is asked to count backward from 100 by 7 (simultaneous verbal-cognitive task) or pour water into a glass (secondary motor task). Patients with Parkinson's disease have been shown to demonstrate significant impairment in dual-task control.[174,175] Patients with traumatic brain injury and stroke have also been shown to demonstrate problems with dual-task control.[176,177]

■ STANDARDIZED INSTRUMENTS: POSTURAL CONTROL AND BALANCE

This section presents selected balance tests (equilibrium coordination tests) in common use today. The reader should analyze each test to determine what aspects of postural control and balance are being examined (e.g., static or dynamic control, proactive or reactive control). The patient's unique impairments and activity limitations will help determine which tests are the most appropriate to use. The patient needs to understand that a variety of functional activities will be used during testing. Some activities will be more difficult than others and will result in instability. The patient should be assured that the therapist will at all times protect the patient from a fall. During testing, all safety precautions should be observed, including close or contact guarding and using a safety gait belt or overhead harness as indicated. Examples of balance test items can be found in Table 6.3.

Standardized instruments for the examination of balance and gait are particularly useful in (1) identifying coordination impairments associated with a skill-level motor task; (2) making decisions about the differences between the patient's performance and the parameters of normal postural control and gait; and (3) providing data to inform decisions about the underlying mechanisms responsible for producing the movement impairments. Standardized tests are available with established reliability, validity, and sensitivity. Scoring is typically based on a scale with specific criterion descriptions for successful performance. Performance observations can also be timed using a stop watch.[178,179]

The Berg Balance Scale

The Berg Balance Scale (BBS) developed by Berg et al[180-183] is an objective measure of static and dynamic balance abilities. The scale consists of 14 functional tasks commonly performed in everyday life. The items range from sitting or standing unsupported, to movement transitions (sit-to-stand, stand-to-sit), variations in standing position (EO/EC), feet together, forward reach, retrieving an object from the floor, turning, standing on one foot, to placing the foot on a stool. Scoring uses a five-point ordinal scale, with scores ranging from 0 to 4. Descriptive criteria are provided for scoring each level: a score of 4 is used to indicate that the patient performs independently and meets time and distance criteria, and a score of 0 is used for unable to perform (see Appendix 6.A). A maximum score of 56 points is possible.

The BBS was developed specifically as a measure of balance function in patients with stroke and has been shown to be a sensitive measure of functional balance in older people in general.[183] Balance scale scores have been shown to be useful in predicting falls in the elderly and evaluating changes in patients undergoing physical therapy.[183-185] Scores of 45 or below are associated with high risk of recurrent or multiple falls with significant increase below a score of 40.[186,187] Studies of community-dwelling older people and those with chronic stroke that looked at individual item analysis revealed that selected BBS items may have greater accuracy than the total BBS in classifying individuals with high fall risk. These items include picking an object up off the floor and stand on one leg,[188,189] as well as turning 360°, placing alternate foot on stool, and tandem stance.[188] Donoghue and Stokes[190] investigated the minimum detectable difference (MDD) of scores on the BBS that would be necessary to indicate significant change in elderly individuals. With baseline BBS scores of 45 to 56, the MDD is 4 points; with scores between 34 and 44, the MDD is 5 points; with scores between 25 and 34, the MDD is 7 points; and with scores of 0 to 24, the MDD is 5 points. Threshold scores have also been reported for older persons at risk for falling[191] and elderly subjects using gait aids.[192]

Performance-Oriented Mobility Assessment

The Performance-Oriented Mobility Assessment (POMA) developed by Tinetti et al[193,194] provides a brief and reliable measure of both static and dynamic balance.[195] Items are organized into two subtests of balance and gait. Balance test items include static sitting balance, sit-to-stand and stand-to-sit, standing balance (static, with sternal nudge, EC), and dynamic standing balance (turning 360°). Gait test items include initiation of gait, path, missed step (trip or loss of balance), turning, and timed walk. Some items are scored on a two-point scale (0 or 1) and some on a three-point (0 to 2) scale (see Appendix 6.B). The original POMA I scale has a total possible score of 28. It was developed for use with the frail elderly, especially nursing home residents with a propensity to fall.[196,197] Patients who score less than 19 are considered at high risk for falls and those who score between 19 and 24 are at moderate risk for falls. A revised form, the POMA Ia, includes five additional items and was designed for use as a predictor of falls among community-dwelling elderly (with a total possible score of 40). The POMA II was developed as an outcome measure in a frailty and injury prevention trial (the Yale Frailty and Injuries: Cooperative Studies of Intervention Techniques [FICSIT] trial) with a total possible score of 54.[198]

Reach Tests

The *Functional Reach Test (FR)* was developed by Duncan et al to provide a quick screen of balance problems in older adults.[199-201] It is the maximal distance one can reach forward beyond arm's length while maintaining a fixed BOS in the standing position. The test uses a level yardstick mounted on the wall and positioned at the height of the patient's acromion. The patient stands sideward next to the wall (without touching), feet normal stance width and weight equally distributed on both feet. The shoulder is flexed to 90° and elbow extended with the hand fisted. An initial measurement is made of the position of the 3rd metacarpal along the yardstick. For forward reach, the patient is instructed to lean as far forward as possible without losing balance or taking a step. A second measurement is taken also using the 3rd metacarpal for reference. This measurement is then subtracted from the initial measurement. See Table 6.7 for normative values of FR.

The *Multidirectional Reach Test (MDFR)* developed by Newton evolved from the earlier FR and measures how far an individual can reach in the forward, backward, and lateral directions.[202,203] For backward reach, the test position is the same as FR with the yardstick position reversed to detect posterior movements. For lateral reach, the patient faces away from the wall and reaches sideways to the right (and then to the left) as far as possible. One practice trial is allowed before the start of three test trials. The therapist records functional reach in inches for all three trials and then average the three trials. The amount of reach is influenced by several factors, including the size and height of the individual, gender, age, and health. The movement strategy used during a reach test should be documented (i.e., ankle or hip strategy, trunk rotation, scapular protraction). See Table 6.8 for normative values of MDRT for older adults. Modified reach can also be reliably measured in sitting.[204,205]

Timed Get Up and Go Test

The *Get Up and Go (GUG) Test* developed by Mathias et al[206] is a quick measure of dynamic balance and mobility. The patient is seated comfortably in a firm chair with arms and back resting against the chair. The patient is then instructed to rise, stand momentarily, and then walk 3 m (10 ft) toward a wall at normal walking speed, turn without touching the wall, return to the chair, turn, and sit down. Tape is used to mark the walking distance and turning point. Performance on the original GUG test is scored using a five-point ordinal scale ranging from 1, Normal (no risk of falls) to 2, Very Slightly Abnormal; 3, Mildly Abnormal (increased risk of falls); 4, Moderately Abnormal; and 5, Severely Abnormal (high risk of falls). If an assistive device is required, the type is recorded. The subjective nature of the grades with very little additional descriptors yielded only limited reliability.

Efforts by Podsiadlo and Richardson[207] to improve the objectivity and reliability resulted in the *Timed Up and Go Test (TUG)*. Timing with a stopwatch begins when the patient is instructed with "go" and ends when the patient returns to the start position seated in the chair. Healthy adults are able to complete the test in less than 10 seconds. Older adults (ages 60 to 80) have also been shown to average scores less than 10 (mean of 8).[207-209] Scores of 11 to 20 seconds are considered within typical for frail elderly or individuals with a disability; scores over 30 seconds are indicative of impaired functional mobility and high fall risk. The TUG has been used to examine functional mobility deficits in patients with stroke[210,211] and Parkinson's disease.[212,213] Minimal detectable changes have been reported for people with Parkinson's disease.[214]

Timed Walking Tests

A timed walking test is an important part of the examination of postural control and balance. The patient

Table 6.7	Functional Reach (FR) Reference Values (NORMS) by Age	
Age	Men (inches)	Women (inches)
20–40	16.7 (± 1.9)	14.6 (± 2.2)
41–69	14.9 (± 2.2)	13.8 (± 2.2)
70–87	13.2 (± 1.6)	10.5 (± 3.5)

From Duncan et al.[199]

Table 6.8	Multidirectional Reach Test (MDRT) Reference Values		
REACH–MDRT	Mean (inches) Standard Deviation Mean Age, 74	Above Average (inches)	Below Average (inches)
Forward	8.9 ± 3.4	>12.2	<5.6
Backward	4.6 ± 3.1	>7.6	<1.6
Right lateral	6.2 ± 3.0	>9.4	<3.8
Left lateral	6.6 ± 2.8	>9.4	<3.8

From Newton.[203]

is asked to walk at his or her *preferred speed* over a set distance clearly marked on the floor (e.g., *10-m Walk Test* [33 ft]). The patient is then asked to walk again at *maximum speed,* as fast as possible. Time is measured using a stopwatch. The results are reported in speed (meters/second or feet/second) or less commonly in total time taken (seconds). Comparisons are made between the two trials. Gait speed has been shown to be a sensitive measure of functional performance.[215] There is a wide range of normal gait speeds reported, ranging from 1.2 to 1.5 m/sec (4 to 5 ft/sec) in healthy young adults. Gait speeds decrease in older adults (0.9 to 1.3 m/sec or 3 to 4.25 ft/sec), in individuals with a disability, and those requiring assistive devices.[216]

Distance tests (e.g., the *3-, 6-,* or *12-Minute Walk Test*) can also be used to document functional mobility.[217-220] The patient is instructed to walk at a comfortable pace. During the test the patient can stop to rest or use an assistive device as needed. The total distance achieved during the preselected timed segment of walking is recorded along with average gait velocity, number of rests, number of deviations from a 15-inch (38 cm) wide gait path, and number of episodes of loss of balance (LOB). Other parameters can also be documented, including BOS, step width, stride length, cadence, trunk and extremity movements, and exertional intolerance (heart rate, chest pain, shortness of breath, Rating of Perceived Exertion [RPE]). See Chapter 7, Examination of Gait, for a more complete description. Gait abnormalities should be carefully documented. Inconsistency and irregularity of stepping and movements, weaving, staggering, widely spaced steps, and arms held out to the sides in high or low guard position are all indicative of decreased postural control and balance.[221]

Dynamic Gait Index

The *Dynamic Gait Index (DGI)* developed by Shumway-Cook et al[187] examines a patient's ability to perform variations in walking on command. Items include changing speed (walk at normal speed and at fast speed), walk with head turns (look right or left, look up or down), walk and pivot turn, step over or around an obstacle, and climb stairs (up and down). A four-point scale (0 to 3) includes specific descriptors of normal control (3), mild impairment (2), moderate impairment (1), and severe impairment (0), with a maximum possible score of 24. The DGI appears to be sensitive in predicting likelihood for falls with older adults (a score below 19 is indicative of increased fall risk). It has also been used with individuals with vestibular dysfunction,[222-225] chronic stroke,[225,226] and multiple sclerosis.[227] Whitney et al[222] found a moderate correlation between the Dynamic Gait Index and the Berg Balance Scale when testing individuals with vestibular and balance dysfunction.

Dual-Task Tests

Stops Walking While Talking

The *Stops Walking While Talking Test (SWWT),* also known as the *Walkie-Talkie Test,* can be used to determine the effects of attentional demands by introducing a secondary task, talking, while walking. The patient walks at a self-selected comfortable speed. The therapist walks alongside the patient and initiates a conversation. Questions are posed that require more than "yes" or "no" answers. The test is positive if the patient stops walking in order to talk. This test lacks sensitivity to the wide range of changes that can occur with dual-tasking.

Sensitivity can be improved by introducing dual tasks during timed walking (Timed Up and Go, 10-m Walk Test). For example, during a 10 m-Walk Test at usual gait speed, a secondary cognitive task (e.g., serial subtraction by 3s from 100) is introduced. Times are compared between usual (single-task walking) and dual-task walking. Performance changes are examined, including hesitations or stops, reduced postural stability, and increased walking variability (steps off path). Cognitive changes (number of errors, mental slowing) are also determined. Examples of other secondary cognitive tasks that can be introduced include reciting the alphabet or alternate letters of the alphabet or walking and remembering (*digit span memory test*).[228] Patients with impaired attention and postural control (particularly automatic control of posture) can be expected to demonstrate difficulty. Dual-task performance impairments have been found in individuals with stroke,[229] traumatic brain injury,[230] multiple sclerosis,[231] Parkinson's disease,[232] and in older adults at risk for falls.[233-236] Dual-task performance impairments have also been found in patients with stroke during sitting balance activities.[237]

Secondary task interference during walking can also be introduced with performance of other motor tasks. For example, the DGI uses walking with head turns on command and obstacle avoidance. Individuals can also be asked to pick up and carry a package, a tray, or a cup of water while walking. It is important to select tasks that are within the capabilities of the individual and appropriate for the functional goals and target environments of the patient. Times are compared for usual walking (single-task performance) and dual-task performance. These forms of complex walking are also likely to result in decreased walking speeds and postural control variations.[228]

Sitting Balance Tests

The *Function in Sitting Test* (FIST) developed by Gorman et al[238] is a 14-item test that examines a person's ability to maintain sitting balance during static sitting (hands in lap) with eyes open and eyes closed, as well as during dynamic challenges to balance. Reactive challenges include nudges (anterior, posterior, and lateral). Anticipatory challenges include moving the head side-to-side, lifting the foot, turning and picking an object up from behind, forward and lateral reach, picking up an object from the floor, and scooting (anterior, posterior, and lateral). The FIST is scored on a 5-point scale with 0 defined as complete assistance and 4 as independent. Descriptors accompany each of the scores and define the amount and type of cueing needed, the degree of upper extremity assistance, or additional physical assistance required. The FIST was developed by a panel of experts and tested on adults with acute stroke (within 3 months of insult). It demonstrates good validity (content, construct, and concurrent) and reliability and provides an objective and easy to administer measure of early sitting in persons with limited functional ability.

Perceived Balance Confidence

During the initial interview, the therapist should ask what activities the patient feels most insecure performing and likely to cause a fall. The therapist should also determine a history of fall events that may have occurred in recent days or months, as well as any injuries received. If possible, the patient can also be asked to self-assess balance abilities using a self-report measure of balance confidence (see scales below). Because each is a measure of perceived confidence, it should not be administered after a performance test that might jeopardize perceptions if difficulties become apparent. Individuals with low self-confidence (self-efficacy) and a history of falls typically demonstrate reduced physical activities and increased fall risk.[239,240]

Activities-Specific Balance Confidence (ABC) Scale

The Activities-Specific Balance Confidence (ABC) Scale developed by Powell and Meyers[241] is a 16-item scale that asks individuals to rate their overall level of self-confidence in performing both household and community activities. Household activities include walking around the house, walking up and down stairs, picking up a slipper off the floor, and several reaching activities (reach at eye level, reach on tiptoes, stand on chair to reach). Community activities include walking to a car, getting in and out of a car, walking on various surfaces (parking lot, ramp) and environments (crowded mall, icy sidewalk), and riding an escalator. The individual is asked to rate his or her confidence on a scale from 100% (complete confidence) to 0% (no confidence).

The Balance Efficacy Scale

The *Balance Efficacy Scale (BES)* developed by Tinetti et al[242] is a self-report measure that examines how confident an individual feels while performing 10 items of ADL and functional mobility. The ADL items on the test include both basic ADL (getting dressed and undressed, taking a bath or shower) and instrumental ADL (cleaning house, preparing simple meals, simple shopping). The functional mobility items include getting in and out of a car, going up and down stairs, walking around the neighborhood, reaching, and hurrying to answer the phone. Individuals are asked to consider how confident they feel in doing each of the activities listed without falling. The individual is asked to rate his or her confidence level on a 0 (not at all) to 10 (completely confident) scale. The highest score is 100 (completely confident on all 10 items) and represents high self-efficacy whereas the bottom score of 0 represents low self-efficacy.

An examination of balance using the International Classification of Functioning, Disability, and Health (ICF) Model is included in Table 6.9. Box 6.1 Evidence Summary provides a review of validity and reliability test results of selected functional balance tests discussed in this chapter.

Table 6.9	Examination of Balance Using the International Classification of Functioning, Disability, and Health (ICF) Model
Components of ICF Model	**Examination of Balance**
Health Condition	• Medical chart review: disorder or disease, medications • Interview, history (fall history)
Body Functions Body Structure Impairments	• Cardiovascular/vitals; orthostatic hypotension • Joint flexibility and range of motion • Muscle strength and endurance • Postural alignment • Posturography: Center of pressure (COP), sway • Coordination, movement strategies (fixed support, change of support) • Sensory integrity: Somatosensory, visual, vestibular • Romberg Test • Sensory Organization Test (SOT) • Clinical Test for Sensory Interaction in Balance (CTSIB) • Cognitive integrity: Memory, attention • Motor function: Adaptive control (changing tasks, changing environment)

Continued

Table 6.9   Examination of Balance Using the International Classification of Functioning, Disability, and Health (ICF) Model—cont'd

Components of ICF Model	Examination of Balance
Activity Limitations	• The Functional Reach Test (FR) • Multidirectional Functional Reach Test (MDFR) • Timed Up and Go (TUG) • Berg Balance Scale (BBS) • Performance-Oriented Mobility Assessment (POMA), Tinetti • 10-m Walk Test (10 MWT) • 6-minute Walk Test • Stops Walking While Talking Test (SWWT) • Function in Sitting Test (FIST) • Functional Independence Measure (FIM): transfers, locomotion
Participation Restrictions	• Self-report activity diary • Activities-specific Balance Confidence Scale (ABC Scale) • Balance Efficacy Scale (BES)

Box 6.1 Evidence Summary   Functional Balance Tests

Instrument	Content	Validity	Reliability	Comments
The Balance Scale (Berg Balance Scale) Berg et al[180] (1989)	Multitask test of 14 balance tasks common in everyday living: 6 static balance items; 8 dynamic balance items Focuses on: • Maintenance of position • Postural adjustment to voluntary movement	Content validity: expert consensus (health professionals and geriatric patients). Concurrent validity: correlation with Tinetti Balance Sub test = .91	Reliability (ICC) Interrater = .98 Intrarater = .99 Individual items ranged from .71 to .99 Internal consistency (Cronbach's alpha) = .96	High degree of agreement of raters Strong internal consistency Simple, easy to administer (15–20 min); comprehensive Requirements: able to stand independently
Equipment needed: chairs with and without arms, stopwatch, ruler, 6-inch step	Items 1–5 = tests of basic balance ability Scoring: 5-point ordinal scale (graded 0–4) with specific task criteria for levels ranging from I > D; some items timed Max score = 56	Barthel Mobility = .67 TUG = .76 Predictive: of falls in the elderly (hospitals, long-term care, community)		Does not include items on gait or reaction to external stimulus/uneven surface Provides baseline, and outcome data; scores of 45 or below are predictive of falls in the elderly
Tinetti Performance-Oriented Mobility Assessment (POMA) Tinetti et al[193] (1986)	Multitask test: Balance subtest: 9 items (4 static; 5 dynamic) Gait subtest: 8 items Focuses on: • Maintenance of position • Postural response to voluntary movement	Content validity: expert consensus Concurrent validity: correlation with Berg = .91 Barthel index = .76 Predictive of falls in the elderly (long-term care)	Reliability (ICC) Interrater = .85 Lacks intrarater reliability testing	High degree of agreement of raters Simple, easy to administer (15 min) Requirements: able to stand and walk independently

Box 6.1 Evidence Summary   Functional Balance Tests—cont'd

Instrument	Content	Validity	Reliability	Comments
Equipment needed: chair, walkway; patient can use usual walking aid	• Postural response to perturbation • Gait mobility Scoring: some items graded can/cannot perform; some 3-point scale with specific task criteria Max score = 28			Some scoring criteria vague; difficult to detect small changes Provides baseline data; predictive of falls in elderly: > 24 low risk 19–24 mod risk 18 > high risk
Timed Up and Go (TUG) Podsiadlo and Richardson[207] (1991)	Single task test: stand-up, walk 3 m (10 ft), turn around, and re-turn to chair Focuses on: functional mobility Scoring: timed test Uses 1 practice/3 trials for average score	Content validity: expert consensus Concurrent validity: Berg = .81 Barthel = ./8	Reliability (ICC) Interrater = .99 Intrarater = .98	High degree of agreement of raters Simple, easy to administer, quick screen (< 3 min) Requirements: able to stand and walk independently Provides baseline and outcome data; Predictive of falls in elderly: < 10 sec = independent 20 – 29 sec = normal for frail elderly or disabled patients > 30 sec = dependent in mobility skills and most ADL
Equipment needed: stopwatch, armchair, measured walkway patient can use AD				
Functional Reach (FR) Duncan et al[199] (1990)	Single task test: Examines forward UE reach with shoulder at 90° flexion, feet still Focuses on: • Postural responses related to voluntary UE movement	Content validity: expert consensus Concurrent validity: Duke mobility = .65 Gait speed = .71	Reliability (ICC) Interrater = .98 Intrarater = .92	High degree of agreement of raters Simple, easy to ad-minister, quick screen (5 min) Requirements: • Able to stand independently • Requires adequate shoulder ROM FR affected by age and height Provides baseline and outcome data Predictive of falls in the elderly
Equipment needed: level yardstick mounted on wall at shoulder height	• Examines Limits of Stability (LOS) Scoring: distance in inches Uses 1 practice/3 trials for average score			
Multidirectional Reach Test (MDRT) Newton[203] (2001)	Single-task test: Examines UE reach with shoulder at 90° flexion, feet still—forward, sideward, and backward			Same as for FR

Continued

Box 6.1 Evidence Summary   Functional Balance Tests—cont'd

Instrument	Content	Validity	Reliability	Comments
Equipment needed: yardstick, wall	Focuses on: • Postural responses related to voluntary UE movements • Examines Limits of Stability (LOS) Scoring: distance in inches Uses 1 practice/3 trials for average score			
Timed Walking Test Murray et al[216] (1966)	Single, continuous test item Compares self-paced, preferred gait speed and fast speed Focuses on • Overall gait speed (distance over time) • Ability to adapt gait speed • Can calculate stride length			Simple, easy to administer, quick screen (3 min) Requirements: independent ambulation, for moderate- to high-functioning adults
Equipment needed: measured walkway and stopwatch	Uses 1 practice/3 trials for average score			Provides screening, baseline and outcome data; results reported as time taken (seconds) or speed (distance/sec) Use of AD is associated with slower gait speeds Age-related norms: • Healthy young adults = 1.2–1.5 m/sec • Older adults = 0.9–1.3 m/sec

AD = Assistive devices; D = dependent; I = independent.

SUMMARY

An examination of coordination and balance provides the physical therapist with important information related to motor performance. Findings provide information about the underlying origin of impairments (although some clinical findings may not be attributable to a single area of CNS involvement). Data from the examination of coordination and balance also assist with establishing anticipated goals and expected outcomes, determining a plan of care, and identifying the effectiveness of treatment interventions.

A variety of coordination and balance tests have been identified. Although the tests have been presented individually for clarity, the therapist selects and chooses individual items to determine a battery of tests appropriate for the specific patient. Because some observational tests are not highly standardized, there is a potential for error and misinterpretation of results. Standardized tests with proven sensitivity and reliability should be selected whenever possible. Sources of potential error can be reduced by the use of well-defined rating scales, administration of tests by skilled examiners, and subsequent retesting performed by the same therapist. Documentation should include the type, severity, and location of the impairments, as well as factors that alter the quality of performance. Emphasis has been placed on the variety of influences that affect movement capabilities. As such, test results must be considered with respect to findings from other examinations such as sensation, ROM, muscle strength, muscle tone, and functional status.

Questions for Review

1. What are the purposes of performing a coordination examination of motor function?

2. What are the believed contributions (function) of the cerebellum to coordinated movement?

3. How is peripheral feedback provided during a motor response?

4. Differentiate between motor impairments associated with cerebellar pathology and basal ganglion pathology. Provide at least five characteristic impairments for each area.

5. What predictable aspects of normal aging may affect coordinated movement?

6. Accurate and careful patient observation is an important source of preliminary information before performing a coordination examination. What type of activities would you select for the observation? What information will the observation provide?

7. Assume you are about to initiate a coordination examination. What screenings would be appropriate?

8. Identify three upper extremity and three lower extremity nonequilibrium coordination tests that could be used to examine a patient with severe ataxia as a result of traumatic brain injury.

9. Differentiate between coordination tests for intention tremor and postural tremor.

10. Differentiate between the Berg Balance Scale and the Performance-Oriented Mobility Test (Tinetti) in terms of aspects of balance tested.

CASE STUDY

The patient is a 62-year-old man with a 5-year history of Parkinson's disease. Since the time of the diagnosis, he reports a progressive decline in functional activity level. With encouragement from his wife and children, he took an early retirement 3 years ago from his career as a commercial airline pilot. He lives with his wife of 38 years in a one-level suburban home. His four adult children all live in neighboring communities.

Initial examination reveals the following:
- Movements are decreased and slowed.
- A uniform, constant resistance is felt as the extremities are moved passively; patient reports an overall feeling of stiffness that is worse during medication "off" times.
- Involuntary, rhythmic, oscillatory movements of the distal upper extremities are observed at rest (pill rolling).
- Patient has difficulty with distal upper extremity (UE) movements required for buttoning shirts, using eating utensils, and writing.
- Patient has difficulty initiating movement transitions, and is unable to stand up from a chair or roll from prone to supine without difficulty.
- Patient stands with a flexed, stooped posture, positioned at the forward limits of the BOS.
- Standing balance is easily displaced with tendency to fall stiffly.
- Patient has difficulty changing direction of movement or stopping while walking.
- Reports regular falls (two to three times per week).

The patient takes Sinemet (a combination of L-dopa/carbidopa). The physical therapy referral is for examination to document baseline function before beginning outpatient rehabilitation.

GUIDING QUESTIONS

1. Describe this patient's motor impairments and activity limitations.

2. Explain the clinical manifestations of bradykinesia.

3. Select the coordination tests you would use to examine the patient's movement capabilities in performing alternating distal UE movements.

4. What are the requirements for documentation?

5. Select the tests appropriate to examine the patient's altered postural control and balance.

6. What functional balance test might yield the best results in terms of this patient's limitations?

DavisPlus | For additional resources, including answers to the questions for review and case study guiding questions, please visit **http://davisplus.fadavis.com**

References

1. American Physical Therapy Association: Guide to Physical Therapist Practice. Phys Ther 81:1, 2001.
2. Shumway-Cook, A, and Woollacott, MH: Motor Control: Translating Research into Clinical Practice, ed 4. Wolters Kluwer/Lippincott Williams & Wilkins, Philadelphia, 2012.
3. Preston, LA: Evaluation of motor control. In Pendleton, HM, and Schultz-Krohn, W (eds): Pedretti's Occupational Therapy: Practice Skills for Physical Dysfunction, ed 7. Mosby/Elsevier, St. Louis, 2013, p 461.
4. Ghez, C, and Krakauer, J: The organization of movement. In Kandel, ER, Schwartz, JH, and Jessell, TM (eds): Principles of Neural Science, ed 4. McGraw-Hill, New York, 2000, p 653.
5. Byl, NN: Multisensory control of upper extremity function. Neurology Report (now JNPT) 26(1):32, 2002.
6. Schmidt, RA, and Lee, TD: Motor Control and Learning: A Behavioral Emphasis, ed 5. Human Kinetics, Champaign, IL, 2011.
7. Wiesendanger, M, and Serrien, DJ: Toward a physiological understanding of human dexterity. News Physiol Sci 16:228, 2001.
8. Crowther, RG, et al: Intralimb coordination variability in peripheral arterial disease. Clin Biomech (Bristol, Avon) 23(3):357, 2008.
9. Daly, JJ, et al: Intra-limb coordination deficit in stroke survivors and response to treatment. Gait Posture 25(3):412, 2007.
10. Farmer, SE, Pearce, G, and Stewart, C: Developing a technique to measure intra-limb coordination in gait: Applicable to children with cerebral palsy. Gait Posture 28(2):217, 2008.
11. Gittoes, MJR, and Wilson, C: Intralimb joint coordination patterns of the lower extremity in maximal velocity phase sprint running. J Appl Biomech 26(2):188, 2010.
12. Lewek, MD, et al: Allowing intralimb kinematic variability during locomotor training poststroke improves kinematic consistency: A subgroup analysis from a randomized clinical trial. Phys Ther 89(8):829, 2009.
13. MacLean, CL, van Emmerik, R, and Hamill, J: Influence of custom foot orthotic intervention on lower extremity intralimb coupling during a 30-minute run. J Appl Biomech 26(4):390, 2010.
14. Bernardin, BJ, and Mason, AH: Bimanual coordination affects motor task switching. Exp Brain Res 215(3-4):257, 2011.
15. Christel, MI, Jeannerod, M, and Weiss, PH: Functional synchronization in repetitive bimanual prehension movements. Exp Brain Res 217(2):261, 2012.
16. Dimitriou, M, Franklin, DW, and Wolpert, DM: Task-dependent coordination of rapid bimanual motor responses. J Neurophysiol 107(3):890, 2012.
17. Hu, X, and Newell, KM: Aging, visual information, and adaptation to task asymmetry in bimanual force coordination. J Appl Physiol 111(6):1671, 2011.
18. Rodriguez, TM, Buchanan, JJ, and Ketcham, CJ: Identifying leading joint strategies in a bimanual coordination task: Does coordination stability depend on leading joint strategy? J Mot Behav 42(1):49, 2010.
19. Brown, T, and Unsworth, C: Evaluating construct validity of the Slosson Visual-Motor Performance Test using the Rasch Measurement Model. Percept Mot Skills 108(2):367, 2009.
20. Parmar, PN, Huang, FC, and Patton JL: Simultaneous coordinate representations are influenced by visual feedback in a motor learning task. Conf Proc IEEE Eng Med Biol Soc (Aug):6762, 2011.
21. Sarpeshkar, V, and Mann, DL: Biomechanics and visual-motor control: How it has, is, and will be used to reveal the secrets of hitting a cricket ball. Sports Biomech 10(4):306, 2011.

22. Coats, RO, and Wann, JP: The reliance on visual feedback control by older adults is highlighted in tasks requiring precise endpoint placement and precision grip. Exp Brain Res 214(1):139, 2011.
23. Wang J, et al: Aging reduces asymmetries in interlimb transfer of visuomotor adaptation. Exp Brain Res 210(2):283, 2011.
24. Bowman, MC, Johansson, RS, and Flanagan, JR: Eye-hand coordination in a sequential target contact task. Exp Brain Res 195(2):273, 2009.
25. Gao, KL, et al: Eye-hand coordination and its relationship with sensori-motor impairments in stroke survivors. J Rehabil Med 42(4):368, 2010.
26. Hsu, HC, et al: Effects of swimming on eye hand coordination and balance in the elderly. J Nutr Health Aging 14(8):692, 2010.
27. Liesker, H, Brenner, E, and Smeets, JB: Combining eye and hand in search is suboptimal. Exp Brain Res 197(4):395, 2009.
28. Ma-Wyatt, A, Stritzke, M, and Trommershäuser, J: Eye-hand coordination while pointing rapidly under risk. Exp Brain Res 203(1):131, 2010.
29. Srinivasan, D, and Martin, BJ: Eye-hand coordination of symmetric bimanual reaching tasks: Temporal aspects. Exp Brain Res 203(2):391, 2010.
30. Rand, MK, and Stelmach GE: Effects of hand termination and accuracy constraint on eye-hand coordination during sequential two-segment movements. Exp Brain Res 207(3-4):197, 2010.
31. Bear, MF, Connors, BW, and Paradiso, MA: Neuroscience: Exploring the Brain, ed 3. Lippincott Williams & Wilkins/Wolters Kluwer, Philadelphia, 2007.
32. Nolte, J: The Human Brain: An Introduction to Its Functional Anatomy, ed 6. Mosby/Elsevier, St. Louis, 2009.
33. Krakauer, J, and Ghez, C: Voluntary movement. In Kandel, ER, Schwartz, JH, and Jessell, TM: Principles of Neural Science, ed 4. McGraw-Hill, New York, 2000, p 756.
34. Mihailoff, GA, and Haines, DE: Motor system II: Corticofugal systems and the control of movement. In Haines, DE (ed): Fundamental Neuroscience for Basic and Clinical Applications, ed 3. Churchill Livingstone/Elsevier, New York, 2005, p 394.
35. Ropper, AH, and Samuels, MA: Adams and Victor's Principles of Neurology, ed 9. McGraw-Hill, New York, 2009.
36. Lundy-Ekman, L: Neuroscience: Fundamentals for Rehabilitation, ed 3. WB Saunders/Elsevier, Philadelphia, 2007.
37. Hall, JE: Guyton and Hall Textbook of Medical Physiology, ed 12. Saunders/Elsevier, Philadelphia, 2011.
38. Ghez, C, and Thach, WT: The cerebellum. In Kandel, ER, Schwartz, JH, and Jessell, TM (eds): Principles of Neural Science, ed 4. McGraw-Hill, New York, 2000, p 832.
39. Melnick, ME: Clients with cerebellar dysfunction. In Umphred, DA (ed): Neurological Rehabilitation, ed 5. Mosby/Elsevier, St. Louis, 2007, p 834.
40. Latash, ML: Neurophysiological Basis of Movement, ed 2. Human Kinetics, Champaign, IL, 2008.
41. Melnick, ME: Metabolic, hereditary, and genetic disorders in adults with basal ganglia movement disorders. In Umphred, DA (ed): Neurological Rehabilitation, ed 5. Mosby/Elsevier, St. Louis, 2007, p 775.
42. DeLong, MR: The basal ganglia. In Kandel, ER, Schwartz, JH, and Jessell, TM (eds): Principles of Neural Science, ed 4. McGraw-Hill, New York, 2000, p 853.
43. Ghez, C, and Gordon, J: Voluntary Movement. In Kandel, ER, Schwartz, JH, and Jessell, TM, et al (eds): Essentials of Neural Science and Behavior. Appleton & Lange, E. Norwalk, CT, 1995, p 529.

44. Marsden, J, and Harris, C: Cerebellar ataxia: Pathophysiology and rehabilitation. Clin Rehabil 25:195, 2011.

45. D'Angelo, E: Neuronal circuit function and dysfunction in the cerebellum: From neurons to integrated control. Funct Neurol 25(3):125, 2010.

46. Haines, DE, and Manto, MU: Clinical symptoms of cerebellar disease and their interpretation. Cerebellum 6(4):360, 2007.

47. Porth, CM: Essentials of Pathophysiology, ed 3. Wolters Kluwer/Lippincott Williams & Wilkins, Philadelphia, 2011.

48. Perlman, SL: Cerebellar ataxia. Curr Treat Options Neurol 2(3):215, 2000.

49. Waxman, SG: Clinical Neuroanatomy, ed 26. Lange Medical Books/McGraw-Hill, New York, 2010.

50. Gutman, SA: Quick Reference Neuroscience for Rehabilitation Professionals: The Essential Neurologic Principles Underlying Rehabilitation Practice, ed 2. Slack, Thorofare, NJ, 2008.

51. Fuller, KS: Introduction to central nervous system disorders. In Goodman, CC, and Fuller, KS (eds): Pathology: Implications for the Physical Therapist, ed 3. Saunders/Elsevier, Philadelphia, 2009, p 1319.

52. Hou, JG, and Lai, EC: Overview of Parkinson's disease: Clinical features, diagnosis, and management. In Trail, M, Protas, EJ, and Lai, EC: Neurorehabilitation in Parkinson's Disease: An Evidence-Based Treatment Model. Slack, Thorofare, NJ, 2008, p 1.

53. Albert, F, et al: Coordination of grasping and walking in Parkinson's disease. Exp Brain Res 202(3):709, 2010.

54. Fuller, KS, and Winkler, PA: Degenerative diseases of the central nervous system. In Goodman, CC, and Fuller, KS (eds): Pathology: Implications for the Physical Therapist, ed 3. Saunders/Elsevier, Philadelphia, 2009, p 1402.

55. Rao, AK, Gordon, AM, and Marder, KS: Coordination of finger-tip forces during precision grip in premanifest Huntington's disease. Mov Disord 26(5):862, 2011.

56. Rao, AK, et al: Spectrum of gait impairments in presymptomatic and symptomatic Huntington's disease. Mov Disord 23(8):1100, 2008.

57. Grimbergen, YA, et al: Falls and gait disturbances in Huntington's disease. Mov Disord 23(7):970, 2008.

58. Quarrell, OWJ: Huntington's Disease, ed 2. Oxford University Press, New York, 2008.

59. Xia, R, and Mao, ZH: Progression of motor symptoms in Parkinson's disease. Neurosci Bull 28(1):39, 2012.

60. Ma, TP: The basal nuclei. In Haines, DE (ed): Fundamental Neuroscience for Basic and Clinical Applications, ed 3. Churchill Livingstone/Elsevier, New York, 2005, p 413.

61. Kiernan, JA: Barr's The Human Nervous System: An Anatomical Viewpoint, ed 9. Lippincott Williams & Wilkins/Wolters Kluwer, Philadelphia, 2009.

62. Bangert, AS, et al: Bimanual coordination and aging: Neurobehavioral implications. Neuropsychologia 48(4):1165, 2010.

63. Cesqui, B, et al: Characterization of age-related modifications of upper limb motor control strategies in a new dynamic environment. J Neuroeng Rehabil 5:31, 2008.

64. Dalton, BH, et al: The age-related slowing of voluntary shortening velocity exacerbates power loss during repeated fast knee extensions. Exp Gerontol 47(1):85, 2012.

65. Diermayr, G, et al: Aging effects on object transport during gait. Gait Posture 34(3):334, 2011.

66. Diermayr, G, McIsaac, TL, and Gordon, AM: Finger force coordination underlying object manipulation in the elderly—A mini-review. Gerontology 57(3):217, 2011.

67. Fling, BW, et al: Differential callosal contributions to bimanual control in young and older adults. J Cogn Neurosci 23(9):2171, 2011.

68. Fujiyama II, et al: Age-related differences in inhibitory processes during interlimb coordination. Brain Res 1262:38, 2009.

69. Hartley, AA, Jonides, J, and Sylvester, CC: Dual-task processing in younger and older adults: Similarities and differences revealed by fMRI. Brain and Cogn 75(3):281, 2011.

70. Hatziteki V, et al: Direction-induced effects of visually guided weight-shifting training on standing balance in the elderly. Gerontology 55(2):145, 2009.

71. Leung, CY, and Chang, CS: Strategies for posture transfer adopted by elders during sit-to-stand and stand-to-sit. Percept Mot Skills 109(3):695, 2009.

72. Noble, JW, and Prentice, SD: Intersegmental coordination while walking up inclined surfaces: Age and ramp angle effects. Exp Brain Res 189(2):249, 2008.

73. Paquette, C, and Fung, J: Old age affects gaze and postural coordination. Gait Posture 33(2):227, 2011.

74. Poonam, K, et al: Sensitivity to change and responsiveness of four balance measures for community-dwelling older adults. Phys Ther 92(3):388, 2012.

75. Poston, B, Enoka, JA, and Enoka, RM: Endpoint accuracy for a small and a large hand muscle in young and old adults during rapid, goal-directed isometric contractions. Exp Brain Res 187(3):373, 2008.

76. Quinn, TJ, et al: Aging and factors related to running economy. J Strength Cond Res 25(11):2971, 2012.

77. Sommervoll, Y, Ettema, G, and Vereijken, B: Effects of age, task, and frequency on variability of finger tapping. Percept Mot Skills 113(2):647, 2011.

78. Stenholm, S, et al: Long-term determinants of muscle strength decline: Prospective evidence from the 22-year mini-Finland follow-up survey. J Am Geriatr Soc 60(1):77, 2012.

79. Guccione, AA, Wong, RA, and Avers, D: Geriatric Physical Therapy, ed 3. Elsevier/Mosby, St. Louis, 2012.

80. Lewis, CB, and Bottomley, JM: Geriatric Rehabilitation: A Clinical Approach, ed 3. Prentice-Hall, Upper Saddle River, NJ, 2008.

81. Puthoff, ML, and Nielsen, DH: Relationships among impairments in lower-extremity strength and power, functional limitations, and disability in older adults. Phys Ther 87(10):1334, 2007.

82. Verdijk, LB, et al: Characteristics of muscle fiber type are predictive of skeletal muscle mass and strength in elderly men. JAGS 58(11):2069, 2010.

83. Fielding, RA, et al: Sarcopenia: An undiagnosed condition in older adults. Current consensus definition: Prevalence, etiology, and consequences. International working group on sarcopenia. J Am Med Dir Assoc 12(4):249, 2011.

84. Jansen, I: The epidemiology of sarcopenia. Clin Geriatr Med (3):355, 2011.

85. Morley, J, et al: Sarcopenia with limited mobility: An international consensus. J Am Med Dir Assoc 12(6):403, 2011.

86. King, GW, et al: Effects of age and localized muscle fatigue on ankle plantar flexor torque development. J Geriatr Phys Ther 35(1):8, 2012.

87. Forstmann, BU, et al: The speed-accuracy tradeoff in the elderly brain: A structural model-based approach. J Neurosci 31(47):17242, 2011.

88. Fraser, SA, Li, KZ, and Penhune, VB: Dual-task performance reveals increased involvement of executive control in fine motor sequencing in healthy aging. J Gerontol B Psychol Sci Soc Sci 65(5):526, 2010.

89. Allander, E, et al: Normal range of joint movements in shoulder, hip, wrist and thumb with special reference to side: A comparison between two populations. Int J Epidemiol 3(3):253, 1974.

90. Roach, KE, and Miles, TP: Normal hip and knee active range of motion: The relationship to age. Phys Ther 71(9):656, 1991.

91. James, B, and Parker, AW: Active and passive mobility of lower limb joints in elderly men and women. Am J Phys Med Rehabil 68(4):162, 1989.

92. Walker, JM, et al: Active mobility of the extremities in older subjects. Phys Ther 64(6):919, 1984.

93. DiFabio, RP, and Emasithi, A: Aging and the mechanisms underlying head and postural control during voluntary motion. Phys Ther 77:458, 1997.

94. Woollacott, MH, and Tang, PF: Balance control during walking in the older adult: Research and its implications. Phys Ther 77:646, 1997.

95. Woollacott, MH: Changes in posture and voluntary control in the elderly: Research findings and rehabilitation. Top Geriatr Rehabil 5:1, 1990.

96. Pyykko, I, et al: Postural control in elderly subjects. Age Ageing 19:215, 1990.

97. King, MB, et al: Functional base of support decreases with age. J Gerontol 49(6):M258, 1994.

98. Duncan, PW, et al: Functional reach: Predictive validity in a sample of elderly male veterans. J Gerontol 47(3):M93, 1992.

99. Weiner, DK, et al: Functional reach: A marker of physical frailty. J Am Geriatr Soc 40(3):203, 1992.

100. Robinovitch, SN, and Cronin, T: Perception of postural limits in elderly nursing home and day care participants. J Gerontol A Biol Sci Med Sci 54(3):B124, 1999.

101. Vandervoort, AA: Aging of the human neuromuscular system. Muscle Nerv 25(1):17, 2002.

102. de Vries, NM, et al: Effects of physical exercise therapy on mobility, physical functioning, physical activity and quality of life in community-dwelling older adults with impaired mobility, physical disability and/or multi-morbidity: A meta-analysis. Ageing Res Rev 11(1):136, 2012.

103. Fahlman, M, et al: Effects of resistance training on functional ability in elderly individuals. Am J Health Promot 25(4):237, 2011.

104. Fahlman, M, et al: Combination training and resistance training as effective interventions to improve functioning in elders. J Aging Phys Act 15(2):195, 2007.

105. Graef, FI, et al: The effects of resistance training performed in water on muscle strength in the elderly. J Strength Cond Res 24(11):3150, 2010.

106. Healey, WE, et al: Physical therapists' health promotion activities for older adults. J Geriatr Phys Ther 35(1):35, 2012.

107. Mangione, KK, Miller, AH, and Naughton, IV: Cochrane review: Improving physical function and performance with progressive resistance strength training in older adults. Phys Ther 90(12):1711, 2010.

108. Van Stralen, MM, et al: The long-term efficacy of two computer-tailored physical activity interventions for older adults: Main effects and mediators. Health Psychol 30(4):442, 2011.

109. VanSwearingen, JM, et al: Physical therapy impact of exercise to improve gait efficiency on activity and participation in older adults with mobility limitations: A randomized controlled trial. Phys Ther 91(12):1740, 2011.

110. US Census Bureau: 2010 Census Shows 65 and Older Population Growing Faster Than Total U.S. Population. US Department of Commerce Economics and Statistics Administration, Washington, DC, 2011. Retrieved March 10, 2012, from http://2010.census.gov/news/releases/operations/cb11-cn192.html.

111. Werner, CA: The Older Population: 2010 (2010 Census Briefs). US Department of Commerce Economics and Statistics Administration, Washington, DC, 2011. Retrieved March 10, 2012, from www.census.gov/prod/cen2010/briefs/c2010br-09.pdf.

112. Janos, SC, and Boissonnault, WG: Upper quarter screening examination. In Boissonnault, WG (ed): Primary Care for the Physical Therapist: Examination and Triage. WB Saunders, Philadelphia, 2005, p 138.

113. Norkin, CC, and White, DJ: Measurement of Joint Motion: A Guide to Goniometry, ed 4. FA Davis, Philadelphia, 2009.

114. Hislop, HJ, and Montgomery, J: Daniels and Worthingham's Muscle Testing, ed 8. Saunders/Elsevier, Philadelphia, 2007.

115. Kendall, FP, et al: Muscles: Testing and Function with Posture and Pain, ed 5. Lippincott Williams & Wilkins, Philadelphia, 2005.

116. Podsiadlo, D, and Richardson, S: The timed "up and go": A test of basic functional mobility for frail elderly persons. J Am Geriatr Soc 39:142, 1991.

117. Hermana, T, Giladia, N, and Hausdorffa, JM: Properties of the 'Timed Up and Go' Test: More than meets the eye. Gerontology 57(3):203, 2011.

118. Aguilar, D, et al: A quantitative assessment of tremor and ataxia in FMR1 premutation carriers using CATSYS. Am J Med Genet A 146A(5):629, 2008.

119. Allen, EG, et al: Detection of early FXTAS motor symptoms using the CATSYS computerised neuromotor test battery. J Med Genet 45(5):290, 2008.

120. Despres, C, Lamoureux, D, and Beuter, A: Standardization of a neuromotor test battery: The CATSYS system. Neurotoxicology 21(5):725, 2000.

121. Netterstrom, B, Guldager, B, and Heeboll, J: Acute mercury intoxication examined with coordination ability and tremor. Neurotoxicol Teratol 18(4):505, 1996.

122. Ellingsen, DG: A neurobehavioral study of current and former welders exposed to manganese. Neurotoxicology 29(1):48, 2008.

123. Papapetropoulos, S, et al: Objective monitoring of tremor and bradykinesia during DBS surgery for Parkinson disease. Neurology 70(15):1244, 2008.

124. Papapetropoulos, S, et al: Objective tremor registration during DBS surgery for essential tremor. Clin Neurol Neurosurg 111(4):376, 2009.

125. Jebson, RH, et al: An objective and standardized test of hand function. Arch Phys Med Rehabil 50:311, 1969.

126. Taylor, N, et al: Evaluation of hand function in children. Arch Phys Med Rehabil 54:129, 1973.

127. Beebe, JA, and Lang, CE: Relationships and responsiveness of six upper extremity function tests during the first six months of recovery after stroke. J Neurol Phys Ther 33(2):96, 2009.

128. Davis Sears, E, and Chung, KC: Validity and responsiveness of the Jebsen-Taylor Hand Function Test. J Hand Surg Am 35(1):30, 2010.

129. Asher, IE: Occupational Therapy Assessment Tools: An Annotated Index, ed 3. American Occupational Therapy Association, Bethesda, MD, 2007.

130. Gloss, DS, and Wardle, MG: Use of the Minnesota Rate of Manipulation Test for disability evaluation. Percept Mot Skills 55(2):527, 1982.

131. Lourenção MIP, et al: Analysis of the results of functional electrical stimulation on hemiplegic patients' upper extremities using the Minnesota manual dexterity test. Int J Rehabil Res 28(1):25, 2005.

132. Surrey, LR, et al: A comparison of performance outcomes between the Minnesota Rate of Manipulation Test and the Minnesota Manual Dexterity Test. Work 20(2):97, 2003.

133. Muller, MD, et al: Test-retest reliability of Purdue Pegboard performance in thermoneutral and cold ambient conditions. Ergonomics 54(11):1081, 2011.

134. Shin, S, Demura, S, and Aoki, H: Effects of prior use of chopsticks on two different types of dexterity tests: Moving Beans Test and Purdue Pegboard. Percept Motor Skills 108(2):392, 2009.

135. Gallus, J, and Mathiowetz, V: Test-retest reliability of the Purdue Pegboard for persons with multiple sclerosis Am J Occup Ther 57(1):108, 2003.

136. Boyle, AM, and Santelli, JC: Assessing psychomotor skills: The role of the Crawford Small Parts Dexterity Test as a screening instrument. J Dent Educ 50(3):176, 1986.

137. Levangie, P, and Norkin, C: Joint Structure and Function: A Comprehensive Analysis, ed 5. FA Davis, Philadelphia, 2011.

138. Nashner, L: Sensory, neuromuscular, and biomechanical contributions to human balance. In Duncan, P (ed): Balance. American Physical Therapy Association, Alexandria, VA, 1990, p 5.

139. Pai, Y, et al: Thresholds for step initiation induced by support-surface translation: A dynamic center-of-mass model provides much better prediction than a static model. J Biomech 33:387, 2000.

140. Nichols, D: Balance retraining after stroke using force platform biofeedback. Phys Ther 77:553, 1997.

141. Horak, F: Clinical measurement of postural control in adults. Phys Ther 67:1881, 1987.

142. Goldie, P, et al: Force platform measures for evaluating postural control: Reliability and validity. Arch Phys Med Rehabil 70:510, 1989.

143. Liston, R, and Brouwer, B: Reliability and validity of measures obtained from stroke patients using the Balance Master. Arch Phys Med Rehabil 77:425, 1996.

144. Horak, F, et al: Postural perturbations: New insights for treatment of balance disorders. Phys Ther 77:517, 1997.

145. Dettman, M, et al: Relationships among walking performance, postural stability, and functional assessments of the hemiplegic patient. Am J Phys Med 66:77, 1987.

146. De Haart, M, et al: Recovery of standing balance in postacute stroke patients: A rehabilitation cohort study. Arch Phys Med Rehabil 85:886, 2004.

147. Geurts, A, et al: A review of standing balance recovery from stroke. Gait Posture 22:267, 2005.

148. Dickstein, R, et al: Foot-ground pressure pattern of standing hemiplegic patients: Major characteristics and patterns of movement. Phys Ther 64:19, 1984.

149. Lee, DN, and Lishman, JR: Visual proprioceptive control of stance. J Hum Mov Stud 1:87, 1975.

150. Brandt, T, et al: Visual acuity, visual field and visual scene characteristics affect postural balance. In Igarash, M, and Black, F (eds): Vestibular and Visual Control on Posture and Locomotor Equilibrium. Karger, Basel, 1985.

151. Jeka, J: Light touch contact as a balance aid. Phys Ther 77:249, 1997.

152. Herdman, S: Vestibular Rehabilitation, ed 3. FA Davis, Philadelphia, 2007.

153. Nashner, L: Adaptive reflexes controlling human posture. Exp Brain Res 26:59, 1976.

154. Nashner, L, and McCollum, G: The organization of human postural movements: A formal basis and experimental synthesis. Behav Brain Sci 9:135, 1985.

155. Kuo, A, et al: Effect of altered sensory conditions on multivariate descriptors of human postural sway. Exp Brain Res 122:15, 1998.

156. Peterka, R: Sensorimotor integration in human postural control. J Neurophysiol 88:1097, 2002.

157. Horak, F, Earhart, G, and Dietz, V: Postural responses to combinations of head and body displacements: Vestibular and somatosensory interactions. Exp Brain Res 141:410, 2001.

158. Horak, F, et al: Postural strategies associated with somatosensory and vestibular loss. Exp Brain Res 82:167, 1990.

159. Romberg, M: Manual of Nervous Diseases of Man. London, Sydenham Society, 1853.

160. Shumway-Cook, A, and Horak, F: Assessing the influence of sensory interaction on balance: Suggestion from the field. Phys Ther 66:1548, 1986.

161. Cohen, H, et al: A study of CTSIB. Phys Ther 73:346, 1993.

162. Whitney, SL, and Wrisley, DM: The influence of footwear on timed balance scores of the modified clinical test of sensory interaction and balance. Arch Phys Med Rehabil 85:439, 2004.

163. Horak, F, and Nashner, L: Central programming of postural movements: Adaptation to altered support-surface configuration. J Neurophysiol 55:1369, 1986.

164. Nashner, L: Fixed patterns of rapid postural responses among leg muscles during stance. Exp Brain Res 30:13, 1977.

165. Maki, B, and McIlron, W: The role of limb movements in maintaining upright stance: The "change-in-support" strategy. Phys Ther 77:488, 1977.

166. Brown, L, Shumway-Cook, A, and Woollacott, M: Attentional demands and postural recovery: The effects of aging. J Gerontol 54A:M165–M171, 1999.

167. Creath, R, et al: A unified view of quiet and perturbed stance: Simultaneous co-existing excitable modes. Neurosci Lett 377:75, 2005.

168. Dean, C, and Shepherd, R: Task-related training improves performance of seated reaching tasks following stroke: A randomized controlled trial. Stroke 28:722, 1997.

169. Forssberg, H, and Hirschfeld, H: Postural adjustments in sitting humans following external perturbations: Muscle activity and kinematics. Exp Brain Res 97:515, 1994.

170. Horak, F, et al: The effects of movement velocity, mass displaced and task certainty on associated postural adjustments made by normal and hemiplegic individuals. J Neurol Neurosurg Psychiatry 47:1020, 1984.

171. Slijper, H, et al: Task-specific modulation of anticipatory postural adjustments in individuals with hemiparesis. Clin Neurophysiol 113:642, 2002.

172. Latash, M, et al: Anticipatory postural adjustments during self-inflicted and predictable perturbations in Parkinson's disease. J Neurol Neurosurg Psychiatry 58:326, 1995.

173. Arce, F, Katz, N, and Sugarman, H: The scaling of postural adjustments during bimanual load-lifting in traumatic brain-injured adults. Hum Move Sci 22:749, 2004.

174. Morris, M, et al: Postural instability in Parkinson's disease: A comparison with and without a concurrent task. Gait Posture 12:205, 2000.

175. Ashburn, A, and Stack, E: Fallers and non-fallers with Parkinson's disease (PD): The influence of a dual task on standing balance. Mov Disord 15(Suppl 3):78, 2000.

176. Brauer, S, et al: Simplest tasks have greatest dual task interference with balance in brain injured adults. Hum Move Sci 23:489, 2004.

177. Hyndman, D, and Ashburn, A: "Stops Walking When Talking" as a predictor of falls in people with stroke living in the community. J Neurol Neurosurg Psychiatry 75:994, 2004.

178. Lee, W, et al: Quantitative and clinical measures of static standing balance in hemiparetic and normal subjects. Phys Ther 68:970, 1988.

179. Bohannon, R, et al: Decrease in timed balance test scores with aging. Phys Ther 64:1967, 1984.

180. Berg, K, et al: Measuring balance in the elderly: Preliminary development of an instrument. Physiother Can 41:304, 1989.

181. Berg, K, et al: A comparison of clinical and laboratory measures of postural balance in an elderly population. Arch Phys Med Rehabil 73:1073, 1992.

182. Berg, K, et al: Measuring balance in the elderly: Validation of an instrument. Can J Public Health 83(Suppl 2):S7, 1992.

183. Berg, K, et al: The Balance Scale: Reliability assessment for elderly residents and patients with an acute stroke. Scand J Rehabil Med 27:27, 1995.

184. Thorbahn, L, and Newton, R: Use of the Berg Balance Test to predict falls in elderly persons. Phys Ther 76:576, 1996.

185. Blum, L, Korner-Bitensky, N: Usefulness of the Berg Balance Scale in stroke rehabilitation: A systematic review. Phys Ther 88:559, 2008.

186. Muir, SW, et al: Use of the Berg Balance Scale for predicting multiple falls in community-dwelling elderly people: A prospective study. Phys Ther 88:449, 2008.

187. Shumway-Cook, A, et al: Predicting the probability of falls in community dwelling older adults. Phys Ther 77:812, 1997.

188. Alzayer, L, Beninato, M, and Portney, L: The accuracy of individual Berg Balance Scale items compared with the total Berg score for classifying people with chronic stroke according to fall history. JNPT 33:136, 2009.

189. Chui, AY, Au-Young, SS, and Lo, SK: A comparison of four functional tests in discriminating fallers from non-fallers in older people. Disabil Regabuk 25:45, 2003.

190. Donoghue, D, and Stokes, E: How much change is true change? The minimum detectable change of the Berg Balance Scale in elderly people. J Rehabil Med 41:343, 2009.

191. Romero, S, et al: Minimum detectable change of the Berg Balance Scale and Dynamic Gait Index in older persons at risk for falling. J Geriatr Phys Ther 34(3):131, 2011.

192. Stevenson, TJ, et al: Threshold Berg Balance Scale scores for gait-aid use in elderly subjects: A secondary analysis. Physiother Can 62(2):133, 2010.

193. Tinetti, M, et al: A fall risk index for elderly patients based on number of chronic disabilities. Am J Med 80:429, 1986.

194. Tinetti, M, and Ginter, S: Identifying mobility dysfunctions in elderly patients: Standard neuromuscular examination or direct assessment? JAMA 259:1190, 1988.

195. Faber, MJ, Bosscher, RJ, and van Wieringen, PC: Clinimetric properties of the Performance-Oriented Mobility Assessment. Phys Ther 86(7):944, 2006.

196. Tinetti, M: Factors associated with serious injury during falls by ambulatory nursing home residents. J Am Geriatr Soc 35:644, 1987.

197. Tinetti, M, et al: Risk factors for falls among elderly persons living in the community. N Engl J Med 319:1701, 1988.

198. Tinetti, M, et al: Yale FISCIT: Risk factor abatement strategy for fall prevention. J Am Geriatr Soc 41:315, 1993.

199. Duncan, P, et al: Functional reach: A new clinical measure of balance. J Gerontol 45:M192, 1990.

200. Duncan, P, et al: Functional reach: Predictive validity in a sample of elderly male veterans. J Gerontol 47:M93, 1992.

201. Weiner, D, et al: Functional reach: A marker of physical frailty. J Am Geriatr Soc 40:203, 1992.

202. Newton, R: Balance screening of an inner city older adult population. Arch Phys Med Rehabil 78:587, 1997.

203. Newton, R: Validity of the multi-directional reach test: A practical measure for limits of stability in older adults. J Gerontol Med Sci 56A:M248, 2001.

204. Lynch, S, Leahy, P, and Barker, S: Reliability of measurements obtained with a modified functional reach test in subjects with spinal cord injury. Phys Ther 78:1128, 1998.

205. Thompson, M, and Medley, A: Forward and lateral sitting functional reach in younger, middle-aged, and older adults. J Geriatr Phys Ther 30(2):43, 2007.

206. Mathias, S, et al: Balance in elderly patients: The "Get Up and Go" test. Arch Phys Med Rehabil 67:387, 1986.

207. Podsiadlo, D, and Richardson, S: The timed "Up and Go": A test of basic mobility for frail elderly persons. J Am Geriatr Soc 39:142, 1991.

208. Isles, R, et al: Normal values of balance tests in women aged 20–80. J Am Geriatr Soc 52:1367, 2004.

209. Pondal, M, and del Ser, T: Normative data and determinants for the timed "Up and Go" test in a population-based sample of elderly individuals without gait disturbances. J Geriatr Phys Ther 31(2):7, 2008.

210. Farla, C, Teixeira-Salmela, L, and Nadeau, S: Effects of the direction of turning on the timed Up and Go test with stroke patients. Top Stroke Rehabil 16:196, 2009.

211. Ng, S, and Hui-Chan, C: The timed Up and Go test: Its reliability and association with lower-limb impairments and locomotor capacities in people with chronic stroke. Arch Phys Med Rehabil 86:1641, 2005.
212. Campbell, C, et al: The effect of attentional demands on the timed Up and Go test in older adults with and without Parkinson's disease. Neurol Rep 3:2, 2003.
213. Dibble, L, and Lange, M: Predicting falls in individuals with Parkinson's disease: a reconsideration of clinical balance measures. JNPT 30:60, 2006.
214. Haug, SL, et al: Minimal detectable change of the timed "up and go" test and the dynamic gait index in people with Parkinson disease. Phys Ther 91(1):114, 2010.
215. Cunha, I, et al: Performance-based gait tests for acute stroke patients. Am J Phys Med Rehabil 81:838, 2002.
216. Murray, M, et al: Comparison of free and fast speed walking patterns of normal men. Am J Phys Med 45:8, 1966.
217. Sadaria, K, and Bohannon, R: The 6-Minute Walk Test: A brief review of literature. Clin Exerc Physiol 3:127, 2001.
218. Harada, N, Chiu, V, and Stewart, A: Mobility-related function in older adults: Assessment with a 6-minute walk test. Arch Phys Med Rehabil 80:837, 1999.
219. Miller, P, et al: Measurement properties of a standardized version of the Two-Minute Walk Test for individuals with neurological dysfunction. Physiother Can 54:241, 2003.
220. Wetzel, JL, et al: Six-Minute Walk Test for persons with mild or moderate disability from multiple sclerosis: Performance and explanatory factors. Physiother Can 63(2):166, 2011.
221. Guralnick, J, et al: Lower-extremity function over the age of 70 years as a predictor of subsequent disability. N Engl J Med 332:556, 1995.
222. Whitney, S, Wrisley, D, and Furman, J: Concurrent validity of the Berg Balance Scale and the Dynamic Gait Index in people with vestibular dysfunction. Physiother Res Int 8:178, 2003.
223. Hall, CD, and Herdman, SJ: Reliability of clinical measures used to assess patient with peripheral vestibular disorders. J Neurol Phys Ther 30:74, 2006.
224. Wrisley, DM, et al: Reliability of the Dynamic Gait Index in people with vestibular disorders. Arch Phys Med Rehabil 84:1528, 2003.
225. Marchetti, GF, et al: Temporal and spatial characteristics of gait during performance of the Dynamic Gait Index in people with and people without balance or vestibular disorders. Phys Ther 88:640, 2008.
226. Jonsdottir, J, and Cattaneo, D: Reliability and validity of the Dynamic Gait Index in persons with chronic stroke. Arch Phys Med Rehabil 88:1410, 2007.

227. McConvey, J, and Bennett, SE: Reliability of the Dynamic Gait Index in individuals with multiple sclerosis. Arch Phys Med Rehabil 86:130, 2005.
228. McCulloch, K: Attention and dual-task conditions: Physical therapy implications for individuals with acquired brain injury. JNPT 31:104–118, 2007.
229. Bowen, A, et al: Dual-task effects of talking while walking on velocity and balance following a stroke. Age Ageing 30:319, 2001.
230. Park, NW, Moscovitch, M, and Robertson, IH: Divided attention impairments after traumatic brain injury. Neuropsychologia 37:1119–1133, 1999.
231. Penner, I, et al: Analysis of impairment related functional architecture in MS patients during performance of different attention tasks. J Neurol 250:461–472, 2003.
232. Rochester, L, et al: Attending to the task: Interference effects of functional tasks on walking in Parkinson's disease and the roles of cognition, depression, fatigue and balance. Arch Phys Med Rehabil 85:1578, 2004.
233. Shumway Cook, A, et al: The effects of two types of cognitive tasks on postural stability in older adults with and without a history of falls. J Gerontol A Biol Sci Med Sci 52:M232–M240, 1997.
234. Shumway-Cook, A, Grauer, S, and Woollacott, M: Predicting the probability for falls in community-dwelling older adults using the timed Up and Go test. Phys Ther 80:896–903, 2000.
235. Hauer, K, et al: Cognitive impairment decreases postural control during dual tasks in geriatric patients with a history of severe falls. J Am Geriatr Soc 51:1638–1644, 2003.
236. Lundin-Olsson, L, Nberg, L, and Gustafson, Y: "Stops walking when talking" as a predictor of falls in elderly people. Lancet 349:617, 1997.
237. Harley, C, et al: Disruption of sitting balance after stroke: Influence of spoken output. J Neurol Neurosurg Psychiatry 77:674, 2006.
238. Gorman, S, et al: Development and validation of the Function in Sitting Test in adults with acute stroke. JNPT 34:150, 2010.
239. Delbaere, K, et al: Fear-related avoidance of activities, falls and physical frailty: A prospective community-based cohort study. Age Ageing 33:368, 2004.
240. Deshpande, N, et al: Activity restriction induced by fear of falling and objective and subjective measures of physical function: A prospective cohort study. J Am Geriatr Soc 56:615, 2008.
241. Powell, L, and Meyers, A: The Activities-specific Balance Confidence (ABC) Scale. J Gerontol Med Sci 50A(1):M28–M34, 1995.
242. Tinetti, M, Richman, D, and Powell, L: Falls efficacy as a measure of fear of falling. J Gerontol 45:P239–P243, 1990.

Supplemental Readings

Arampatzis, A, Peper, A, and Bierbaum, S: Exercise of mechanisms for dynamic stability control increases stability performance in the elderly. J Biomech 44(1):52, 2011.
Beebe, JA, and Lang, CE: Relationships and responsiveness of six upper extremity function tests during the first six months of recovery after stroke. J Neurol Phys Ther 33(2):96, 2009.
Krishnan, V, and Jaric, S: Effects of task complexity on coordination of inter-limb and within-limb forces in static bimanual manipulation. Motor Control 14(4):528, 2010.
Nijland, R, et al: A comparison of two validated tests for upper limb function after stroke: The Wolf Motor Function Test and the Action Research Arm Test. J Rehabil Med 42(7):694, 2010.
Przybyla, A, et al: Motor asymmetry reduction in older adults. Neurosci Lett 489(2):99, 2011.
Sleimen-Malkoun, R, Temprado, JJ, and Berton, E: A dynamic systems approach to bimanual coordination in stroke: Implications for rehabilitation and research. Medicina (Kaunas) 46(6):374, 2010.
Telles, S, Singh, N, and Balkrishna, A: Finger dexterity and visual discrimination following two yoga breathing practices. Int J Yoga 5(1):37, 2012.

Tyson, SF: Measurement error in functional balance and mobility tests for people with stroke: What are the sources of error and what is the best way to minimize error? Neurorehabil Neural Repair 21(1):46, 2007.
Tyson, SF, and Connell, LA: How to measure balance in clinical practice: A systematic review of the psychometrics and clinical utility of measures of balance activity for neurological conditions. Clin Rehabil 23(9):824, 2009.
van de Ven-Stevens, LA: Clinimetric properties of instruments to assess activities in patients with hand injury: A systematic review of the literature. Arch Phys Med Rehabil 90(1):151, 2009.
Velstra, IM, Ballert, CS, and Cieza, A: A systematic literature review of outcome measures for upper extremity function using the International Classification of Functioning, Disability, and Health as reference. PMR 3(9):846, 2011.
Wang, W, et al: Interlimb differences of directional biases for stroke production. Exp Brain Res 216(2):263, 2012.
Wang, YC, et al: Assessing dexterity function: A comparison of two alternatives for the NIH Toolbox. J Hand Ther 24(4):313, 2011.
Yancosek, KE, and Howell, D: A narrative review of dexterity assessments. J Hand Ther 22(3):258, 2009.

Berg Balance Scale

1. Sitting to standing

Instructions: *Please stand up, try not to use your hands for support.*
( ) 4 able to stand without using hands and stabilizes independently
( ) 3 able to stand independently using hands
( ) 2 able to stand using hands after several tries
( ) 1 needs minimal aid to stand or stabilize
( ) 0 needs moderate or maximal assist to stand

2. Standing unsupported

Instructions: *Please stand for 2 minutes without holding.*
( ) 4 able to stand safely 2 minutes
( ) 3 able to stand 2 minutes with supervision
( ) 2 able to stand 30 seconds unsupported
( ) 1 needs several tries to stand unsupported 30 seconds
( ) 0 unable to stand 30 seconds without support

3. Sitting with back unsupported but feet supported on floor or on a stool

Instructions: *Please sit with arms folded for 2 minutes.*
( ) 4 able to sit safely and securely 2 minutes
( ) 3 able to sit 2 minutes with supervision
( ) 2 able to sit 30 seconds
( ) 1 able to sit 10 seconds
( ) 0 unable to sit without support 10 seconds

4. Standing to sit

Instructions: *Please sit down.*
( ) 4 sits safely with minimal use of hands
( ) 3 controls descent by using hands
( ) 2 uses back of legs against chair to control descent
( ) 1 sits independently, but has uncontrolled descent
( ) 0 needs assistance to sit

5. Transfers

Instructions: *Arrange chairs for a pivot transfer. Ask the patient to transfer one way toward a seat without armrests and one way toward a seat with arms. You may use two chairs or a bed/mat and a chair.*
( ) 4 able to transfer safely with minor use of hands
( ) 3 able to transfer safely with definite need of hands

( ) 2 able to transfer with verbal cuing and/or supervision
( ) 1 needs one person to assist
( ) 0 needs two people to assist or supervise to be safe

6. Standing unsupported with eyes closed

Instructions: *Please close your eyes and stand still for 10 seconds.*
( ) 4 able to stand 10 seconds safely
( ) 3 able to stand 10 seconds with supervision
( ) 2 able to stand 3 seconds
( ) 1 unable to keep eyes closed for 3 seconds but stands safely
( ) 0 needs help to keep from falling

7. Standing unsupported with feet together

Instructions: *Place your feet together and stand without holding.*
( ) 4 able to place feet together independently and stand safely 1 minute
( ) 3 able to place feet together independently and stand with supervision for 1 minute
( ) 2 able to place feet together independently but unable to hold for 30 seconds
( ) 1 needs help to assume the position but can stand for 15 seconds, feet together
( ) 0 needs help to assume the position and unable to stand for 15 seconds

8. Reaching forward with outstretched arm while standing

Instructions: *Lift arm to 90°. Stretch out your fingers and reach forward as far as you can. (Clinician places a ruler at the tips of the outstretched fingers—subject should not touch the ruler when reaching.) Distance recorded is from the fingertips with the subject in the most forward position. The subject should use both hands when possible to avoid trunk rotation.*
( ) 4 can reach forward confidently 20–30 cm (10 inches)
( ) 3 can reach forward safely 12 cm (5 inches)
( ) 2 can reach forward safely 5 cm (2 inches)
( ) 1 reaches forward but needs supervision
( ) 0 loses balance when trying, requires external support

9. **Pick up object from the floor from a standing position**

   Instructions: *Pick up the shoe slipper which is placed in front of your feet.*
   ( ) 4 able to pick up the slipper safely and easily
   ( ) 3 able to pick up the slipper but needs supervision
   ( ) 2 unable to pick up the slipper, but reaches 2–5 cm (1–2 inches) from the slipper and keeps balance independently
   ( ) 1 unable to pick up and needs supervision while trying
   ( ) 0 unable to try/needs assistance to keep from losing balance/falling

10. **Turning to look behind over your left and right shoulders while standing**

    Instructions: *Turn and look directly behind you over toward the left shoulder. Repeat to the right. Examiner may pick an object to look at directly behind the subject to encourage a better twist.*
    ( ) 4 looks behind from both sides and weight shifts well
    ( ) 3 looks behind one side only, other side shows less weight shift
    ( ) 2 turns sideways only but maintains balance
    ( ) 1 needs close supervision or verbal cuing
    ( ) 0 needs assistance while turning

11. **Turn 360°**

    Instructions: *Turn completely around in a full circle, pause, then turn a full circle in the other direction.*
    ( ) 4 able to turn 360° safely in 4 seconds or less
    ( ) 3 able to turn 360° safely, one side only, 4 seconds or less
    ( ) 2 able to turn 360° safely, but slowly
    ( ) 1 needs close supervision or verbal cuing
    ( ) 0 needs assistance while turning

12. **Place alternate foot on step or stool while standing unsupported**

    Instructions: *Place each foot alternately on the step stool. Continue until each foot has touched the step stool 4 times.*
    ( ) 4 able to stand independently and safely and complete 8 steps in 20 seconds

( ) 3 able to stand independently and complete 8 steps >20 seconds
( ) 2 able to complete 4 steps without aid with supervision
( ) 1 able to complete >2 steps needs minimal assistance
( ) 0 needs assistance to keep from falling/unable to try

13. **Standing unsupported one foot in front**

    Instructions: *Demonstrate to subject. Place one foot directly in front of the other. If you feel that you cannot place your foot directly in front, try and step far enough ahead that the heel of your forward foot is ahead of the toes of your other foot. To score three points, the length of the step should exceed the length of the other foot and the width of the stance should approximate the subject's normal stance width.*
    ( ) 4 able to place foot tandem independently and hold 30 seconds
    ( ) 3 able to place foot ahead of the other independently and hold 30 seconds
    ( ) 2 able to take a small step independently and hold 30 seconds
    ( ) 1 needs help to step but can hold 15 seconds
    ( ) 0 loses balance while stepping or standing

14. **Standing on one leg**

    Instructions: *Stand on one leg as long as you can without holding*
    ( ) 4 able to lift leg independently and hold >10 seconds
    ( ) 3 able to lift leg independently and hold 5–10 seconds
    ( ) 2 able to lift leg independently and hold >2 seconds
    ( ) 1 tries to lift leg unable to hold 3 seconds but remains standing independently
    ( ) 0 unable to try or needs assistance to prevent fall

_____ **TOTAL SCORE (Maximum 56)**

Performance-Oriented Assessment of Mobility I—POMA I (Tinetti) BALANCE

Instructions: *Subject is seated in hard armless chair. The following maneuvers are tested.*

1. **Sitting balance**

   0 = leans or slides in chair
   1 = leans in chair slightly or slight increased distance from buttocks to back of chair
   2 = steady, safe, upright

2. **Arising**

   0 = unable without help or loses balance
   1 = *able* but uses arm to help *or* requires more than two attempts or excessive forward flexion
   2 = *able* without use of arms in one attempt

3. **Immediate standing balance (first 5 seconds)**

   0 = unsteady marked staggering, moves feet, marked trunk sway or grabs object for support
   1 = steady but uses walker or cane *or* mild staggering but catches self without grabbing object
   2 = steady without walker or cane or other support

4. **Side-by-side standing balance**

   0 = unsteady
   1 = unsteady, but wide stance (medial heels more than 4 inches apart) or uses cane, walker or other support
   2 = narrow stance without support

5. **Pull test (subject at maximum position as above, examiner stands behind and exerts mild pull back at wrist)**

   0 = begins to fall
   1 = staggers, grabs, but catches self
   2 = steady

6. **Turn 360°**

   0 = unsteady (grabs, staggers)
   1 = steady but steps discontinuous
   2 = steady and steps continuous

7. **Able to stand on one leg for 5 seconds (pick one leg)**

   0 = unable or holds onto any object
   1 = some staggering, swaying or moves foot slightly
   2 = able

8. **Tandem stand**

   0 = unable to stand with one foot in front of other or begins to fall
   1 = some staggering, swaying, moves arms, or moves foot slightly
   2 = able to tandem stand 5 seconds

9. **Reaching up—Examiner holds 5-pound weight at height of subject's fully extended reach**

   0 = unable or holds onto any object
   1 = some staggering, swaying or moves foot slightly
   2 = able

10. **Bending over (place 5-pound weight on floor and ask subject to pick it up)**

    0 = unable or is unsteady
    1 = able and is steady

10a. **Time required_____seconds**

11. **Sit down**

    0 = unsafe (misjudged distance; falls into chair)
    1 = uses arms or not a smooth motion
    2 = safe, smooth motion

11a. **Timed rising**

    Time required to rise from chair three times _____ seconds

Total Balance Subtest: 21 points
Timed items: 10, 11

■ GAIT

Instructions: *Subject stands with examiner. Walks down 15 foot walkway (measured). Ask subject to walk down walkway, turn and walk back. Subject should use customary walking aid.*

1. **Initiation of gait (immediately after told to "go")**

   0 = any hesitancy or multiple attempts to start
   1 = no hesitancy

2. **Path (estimated in relation to line on floor or rug). Observe excursion of one foot over middle 10 feet of course.**

   0 = marked deviation
   1 = mild/moderate deviation or uses walking aid
   2 = straight without walking aid

3. **Missed step (trip or loss of balance)**

   0 = yes and inappropriate attempt to recover balance
   1 = yes, but appropriate attempt to recover
   2 = no

4. **Turning (while walking)**

   0 = staggers, unsteady
   1 = discontinuous, but no staggering, or uses walker or cane
   2 = steady, continuous without walking aid

5. **Timed walk performed after 1–7 complete (measure out 15 foot walkway)**

   a) Ask subject to walk at normal pace _____ seconds
   b) Ask subject to walk as "fast as feels safe" _____ seconds

6. **Step over obstacle (to be assessed in a separate walk with a block placed on course)**

   0 = begins to fall or unable
   1 = able but uses walking aid or some staggering but catches self
   2 = able and steady
   Total Gait Subtest: 9 points
   Timed items: 5

   _____ TOTAL SCORE (Maximum = 30 points)

Examination of Gait

Judith M. Burnfield, PT, PhD
Cynthia C. Norkin, PT, EdD

Chapter 7

LEARNING OBJECTIVES

1. Define the terms used to describe normal gait.
2. Explain reliability, validity, sensitivity, and specificity in relation to gait analysis.
3. Describe the variables that are examined in each of the following types of gait analyses: kinematic qualitative analysis, kinematic quantitative analysis, and kinetic analysis.
4. Describe and provide examples of some of the most commonly used types of gait profiles.
5. Compare and contrast the advantages and disadvantages of kinematic qualitative and kinematic quantitative gait analyses.
6. Using the case study example, apply clinical decision making skills in evaluating gait analysis data.

CHAPTER OUTLINE

One of the major purposes of rehabilitation is to help patients achieve the highest level of function given their specific impairments so they can participate optimally in activities of interest. Human ambulation, or gait, is one of the basic components of independent function commonly affected by either disease processes or injury. Consequently, the desired outcome of many physical therapy interventions is to either restore or improve a patient's ambulatory status. *Gait*, defined as the manner in which a person walks (e.g., cadence, step length, stride length, speed, and rhythm) differs from *locomotion*, which refers to an individual's capacity to move from one place to another.[1] Although there are many specific reasons for performing a gait analysis, all of them require some information about the walking capacity of either an individual or a group of people with a particular disability. Because there are multiple approaches to gait analysis, ranging from very simple to extremely complex, the therapist must carefully consider how information obtained from a gait analysis is to be used. General as well as specific clinical indications for conducting a gait analysis may be found in the *Guide to Physical Therapist Practice*, some of which are included below.[1]

■ PURPOSES OF GAIT ANALYSIS

1. To assist with understanding the gait characteristics of a particular disorder. This includes the following:
   - Obtaining accurate descriptions of gait patterns and gait variables typical of different conditions
   - Identifying and describing gait deviations present, or typically present in specific disorders
   - Determining balance, endurance, energy expenditure, and safety
   - Determining the functional ambulation capabilities of the patient in relation to functional ambulation demands of the home, community, and work environments
   - Classifying the severity of disability
   - Predicting a patient's future status
2. To assist with movement diagnosis by:
   - Identifying and describing gait deviations and describing the differences between a patient's performance and the parameters of normal gait
   - Analyzing gait deviations and identifying the mechanisms responsible for producing them
   - Examining balance, endurance, energy expenditure, and safety and determining their impact on gait

3. To inform selection of intervention(s) by guiding the therapist in:
   - Proposing appropriate treatment of impairments that may improve gait performance
   - Determining the need for adaptive, assistive, orthotic, prosthetic, protective, or supportive devices or equipment
4. To evaluate the effectiveness of treatment and guide the therapist in:
   - Determining how interventions such as therapeutic exercise, endurance activities, developmental activities, strengthening or stretching, electrical stimulation, balance training, surgical procedures, and medication will affect gait
   - Determining the effectiveness and fit of devices or equipment selected in providing joint protection and support, correcting deviations and dysfunctions, reducing energy expenditure, and promoting safe locomotive function.

Many examples illustrating these purposes are found in the literature: descriptions of the differences between a patient's performance and the parameters of normal gait,[2-11] identification of the mechanisms causing dysfunction,[12,13] determination of either the need for or the effectiveness of a prosthetic device,[12,14] comparison of the effects of different types of assistive devices,[15,16] determination of either the need for or the effectiveness of an orthotic device,[17-21] determination of the effects of treatment interventions,[22,23] determination of energy expenditure,[14,15,24] and prediction of future status.[25-27]

■ SELECTION OF APPROACH TO GAIT ANALYSIS

The type of gait analysis that is selected depends not only on the purpose of the analysis, but also on the type of equipment available and the experience, knowledge, and skills of the therapist. The equipment necessary for performing a specific type of gait analysis, in turn, depends on the purpose of the analysis, equipment availability, and the amount of time the therapist can expend. Equipment used in a gait analysis may be either as simple as a pencil, paper, and stopwatch,[28] or as complex as an electronic imaging system with force plates embedded in the floor and electromyography electrodes placed on the client.[29-32] To select the appropriate method, the therapist must be aware of the types of analyses available and be able to determine which methods are reliable and valid. Much of the information about gait characteristics of particular disorders, as well as the mechanisms responsible for producing them, has been achieved in clinical research settings using complex instrumentation often not available for general patient use. However, given a firm understanding of the biomechanics of normal gait, including characteristic joint motions and muscle demands, a therapist can use less complex methods to identify variations in movement patterns from normal and problem solve likely causes.

Efficacious treatment approaches can then be employed to address underlying causes.

Regardless of the method, a gait analysis of individual patients should provide accurate, reliable, and valid data that can be used as a basis for describing present status (performance limitations and strengths), planning and implementing interventions, evaluating effectiveness and progress over time, evaluating outcomes, and, in some instances, predicting future status.

Reliability

Reliability, as applied to gait analysis, refers to the level of consistency of either a measuring instrument (e.g., footswitches, force plates, motion analysis systems, electrogoniometers) or a method of analysis (e.g., observational gait analysis checklists, ambulation profiles, and formulas for measuring stride length). To determine if a measuring instrument is reliable, the measurements obtained from successive and repeated use of the instrument must be consistent. For example, if an electrogoniometric measurement of a known angle of 60° consistently measures 60° on every Monday morning for 2 months, the instrument is said to be reliable. However, if the measurement obtained were 60° on the first Monday morning, 30° on the second, and 40° on the third, the instrument would have very low reliability. Two types of reliability may be referred to: relative (association) or absolute (concordance). Relative reliability uses statistical techniques that are correlational;[33] they detect the existence of a relationship between sets of data. The statistical techniques used by absolute reliability can detect the magnitude of differences between measures.

Unlike more tightly controlled scientific conditions, the measures used in gait for determining reliability reflect all of the variability present in the measurement process. This includes trial-to-trial or day-to-day performance variation of the subject, as well as differences in the way the tester carries out the test. To make the best possible determination of the reliability of an instrument, one must rule out factors other than the instrument that could influence the measurement (e.g., that a subject has not injured a knee between successive measurements or that the placement of the instrument has not changed).

To determine whether an analysis method has both relative and absolute reliability, two different forms of reliability need to be determined: *intratester* and *intertester* reliability. The intratester reliability of an analysis method can be determined by examining the consistency of the results obtained when one individual uses a particular method repeatedly. For example, a therapist uses a particular method to examine a student physical therapist's gait. The therapist repeats the examination at 2-week intervals for 8 weeks and obtains the same results each time. In this instance, the method would be considered as having high intratester reliability because the results obtained by the same person are consistent over time. However, this example is strictly hypothetical, as factors other than the therapist's skill, such as fatigue, time of day, and other variables, may affect performance and must be controlled in any analysis.

Intertester reliability is determined by examining the consistency of the data obtained from repeated analyses performed by a number of different persons. If the results obtained by numerous examiners are in agreement both relatively and absolutely, and no significant differences in the results exist among testers, the method has high intertester reliability.

Sensitivity and Specificity

Sensitivity and specificity are important considerations when selecting a method of analysis. **Sensitivity**, as it relates to gait analysis, refers to the proportion of times that a method of analysis correctly identifies a gait abnormality or condition when that abnormality or condition is actually present. **Specificity** refers to the proportion of times that a method of analysis correctly identifies the abnormality as being absent when it truly is absent.[34] Additional information about these parameters will be available as more sophisticated statistical treatment of gait findings becomes common practice.

Validity

Validity refers to the degree that a measurement reflects what it is supposed to measure. There are several types of validity:

- *Construct validity*—determined through logical argumentation based on theoretical research evidence (the ability of an instrument to measure an abstract concept or construct).
- *Content validity*—determined by providing evidence that the measuring instrument contains all relevant elements of a construct and no extraneous elements. In this instance, the test developer might justify the test by demonstrating that all items in the test were correlated with each other.
- *Criterion-based validity*—established by comparisons of either one instrument with another or with data obtained from other forms of testing.
- *Concurrent validity*—the inference is justified by comparisons between the results of a specific test (gait analysis) and another test (functional examination) taken at approximately the same time.
- *Predictive validity*—validity is determined by the capability of the instrument to predict future events, such as falls.

It is difficult to imagine a method of measuring or analyzing gait that is not inherently valid for gait itself. However, gait is not a single construct, but a complex process that mirrors the complexity of human performance. Using a fairly simple approach, one can ask if a particular measure is valid for the specific purpose identified. Examining the tools described below, one may reflect on the purposes of gait analysis identified earlier, and ask if the tool being considered would be valid for that purpose.

By examining the literature, the therapist may determine if the reliability and validity of an instrument or method of analysis has been established. If the instrument or method has not been tested, therapists may wish to incorporate methods such as repeated testing within the context of a research study to confirm reliability.

■ GAIT TERMINOLOGY
The Gait Cycle

The fundamental unit of walking is the *gait cycle,* which has both spatial (distance) and temporal (time) parameters. In normal walking, a gait cycle begins when the heel of the reference extremity contacts the supporting surface and ends when the heel of the same extremity contacts the ground again. In some abnormal gaits, the heel may not be the first part of the foot to contact the ground, so the gait cycle may be considered to begin when some other portion of the reference limb contacts the ground. The cycle ends with the next ipsilateral contact of that portion of the foot with the ground.

The gait cycle is divided into two periods, *stance* and *swing* (Fig. 7.1). In normal gait at a comfortable walking speed, *stance* constitutes approximately 60% of the gait cycle, and is defined as the interval in which the reference foot is in contact with the ground. *Swing* comprises approximately 40% of the gait cycle, and occurs when the reference limb is not in contact with the ground. A single gait cycle includes periods of stance and swing for both the right and left limbs. During gait, body weight is smoothly transferred from one limb to the next during two intervals of double limb stance in the gait cycle when both limbs are in contact with the ground at the same time. *Initial double limb stance* occurs at the beginning of the gait cycle as weight transfers onto the outstretched reference limb from the trailing limb. *Terminal double limb stance* occurs at the end of stance as body weight transfers from the trailing reference limb to the lead limb. Initial double limb stance on the reference limb corresponds with the contralateral limb's terminal double limb stance. *Single limb support,* arising between the two double limb stance periods, is the portion of the gait cycle when only one limb supports body weight. The duration of each of these variables may be measured, for example, *cycle time, stance time* (right and left), *swing time* (right and left), initial *double limb stance time, terminal double limb stance time,* and *single limb support time.*

Two steps, a right step and a left step, form a *stride,* and a stride is equal to a gait cycle. Step and stride may be defined in two dimensions: distance and time. *Step length* is the distance from the point of heel strike of one extremity to the point of heel strike of the opposite extremity, whereas *stride length* is the distance from the point of heel strike of one extremity to the point of heel strike of the same extremity. An alternative portion of the foot that consistently contacts the ground can be used as a reference point if the heel is not the first point of contact, as with some abnormal gait patterns. *Stride*

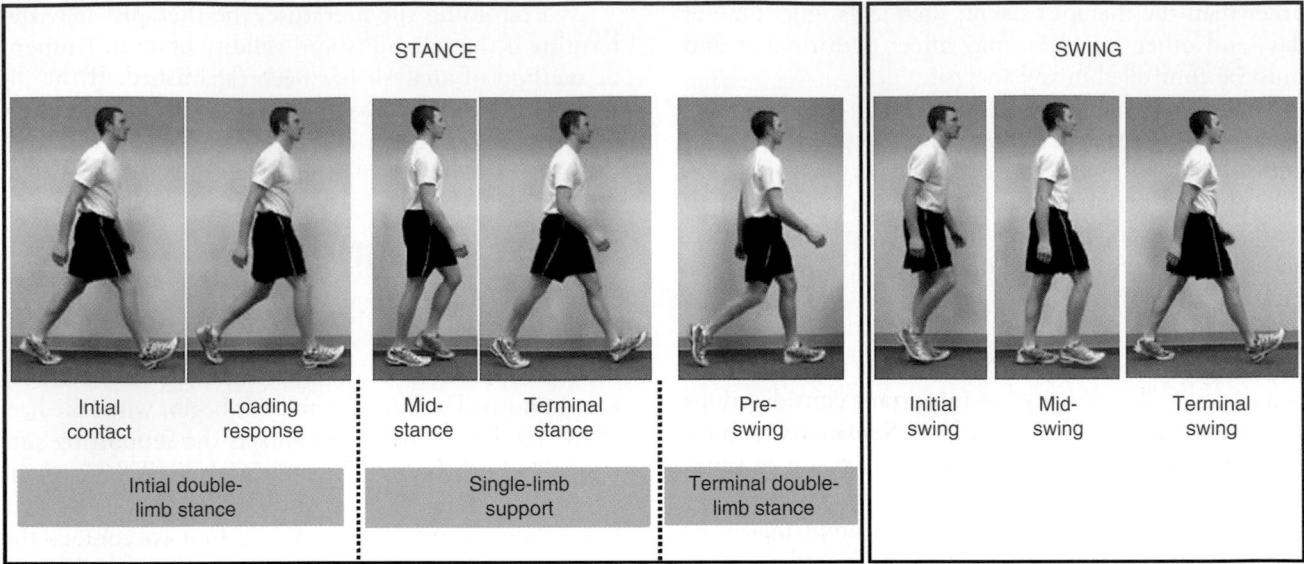

Figure 7.1 The eight phases of the gait cycle. Stance, the period when the reference limb is in contact with the ground, is comprised of the following five phases: initial contact, loading response, mid stance, terminal stance, and pre-swing. Swing, the period when the limb is off the ground, is comprised of the following three phases: initial swing, mid swing, and terminal swing. In addition, there are two periods in gait when both limbs are in contact with the ground: initial double limb stance (initial contact and loading response) and terminal double limb stance (pre-swing). Also, there is one period, single limb support, in which only one limb is in contact with the ground. Single limb support includes the phases of mid stance and terminal stance. Note that the contralateral limb is in swing during the reference limb's single limb support. *(Courtesy of Movement and Neurosciences Center, Institute for Rehabilitation Science and Engineering, Madonna Rehabilitation Hospital, Lincoln, NE 68506.)*

time and *step time* refer to the length of time required to complete a step and a stride, respectively (Fig. 7.2).

Phases of Gait

Early terminology describing the phases of gait included descriptors for both stance (i.e., heel strike, footflat, midstance, heel-off, and toe off) and swing (i.e., acceleration, mid swing, and deceleration). Though useful for describing normal gait, the terminology is sometimes confusing in the presence of pathology. For example, many individuals with pretibial weakness or severe plantarflexion contractures lack a heel first contact at "heel strike." Some individuals with plantarflexor spasticity maintain their heel off the ground throughout stance, not just during heel-off. Others with profound plantarflexor weakness may fail to achieve a period of heel-off and instead lift the full foot from the ground at the end of stance.

To avoid the confusions associated with earlier terminology, Perry and colleagues from Rancho Los Amigos National Rehabilitation Center developed a generic terminology to describe the eight functional phases of gait.[32,35] The first five phases constitute stance: *initial contact, loading response, mid stance, terminal stance,* and *pre-swing*. The latter three comprise swing: *initial swing, mid swing,* and *terminal swing*. The similarities and differences between the two terminologies are presented in Table 7.1.

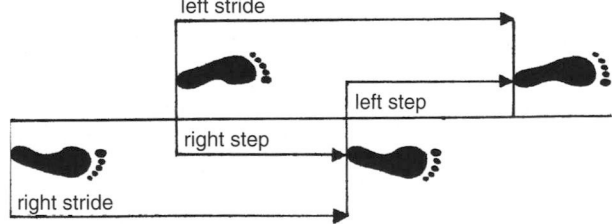

Figure 7.2 A right stride and a left stride. Right stride length is the distance between the point of contact of the right heel (at the lower left corner of the diagram) and the next contact of the right heel. Left stride length is the distance between the point of contact of the left heel (at the top left of the diagram) to the point of contact at the next left heel. Each stride contains two steps, but only both steps in the left stride are labeled. The left stride contains a right step and a left step. The right step length (shown in the middle of the diagram) is the distance between the left heel contact to the point of the right heel contact. Left step length is the distance between the right heel contact and the next left heel contact. Step and stride times refer to the amount of time required to complete a step and to complete stride, respectively.

Table 7.1 Comparison of Gait Terminology

	Rancho Los Amigos[3,32]	Traditional
Stance	*Initial Contact:* Beginning of stance when heel or some other portion of foot contacts ground. Component of initial double limb stance.	*Heel Strike:* Beginning of stance when heel first contacts ground.
	Loading Response: Body weight rapidly loads onto lead limb from trailing limb. Hip remains stable, knee flexes to absorb shock, and forefoot lowers to ground. Immediately follows initial contact and is final component of initial double limb stance. Ends when opposite limb lifts from ground for swing.	*Foot Flat:* Immediately follows heel strike when sole of foot contacts floor.
	Mid Stance: Trunk progresses from behind to in front of ankle over single stable limb. First half of single limb support. Starts when contralateral foot lifts from ground for swing.	*Midstance:* Point at which body passes directly over reference extremity.
	Terminal Stance: Trunk continues forward progression relative to foot. Heel rises from ground and limb achieves trailing limb posture. Second half of single limb support. Ends with contralateral initial contact.	*Heel Off:* Point following mid stance when reference limb's heel leaves ground.
Swing	*Pre-swing:* Body weight rapidly unloads from reference limb and reference limb prepares for swing during this terminal double limb stance period. Starts with contralateral initial contact and ends at ipsilateral limb toe off.	*Toe Off:* Point following heel-off when only the reference limb's toe is contacting ground.
	Initial Swing: Starts when reference foot lifts from ground. Hip, knee, and ankle rapidly flex for clearance and advancement during this initial 1/3 of swing.	*Acceleration:* Beginning portion of swing from reference limb toe off to point when reference limb is directly under the body.
	Mid Swing: Thigh continues advancing, knee begins to extend, and ankle achieves neutral posture during this middle 1/3 of swing.	*Mid swing:* Portion of swing when reference limb passes directly below body. Extends from the end of acceleration to beginning of deceleration.
	Terminal Swing: During this final 1/3 of swing, knee achieves maximal extension and ankle remains at neutral in preparation for heel first initial contact. Ends when foot contacts ground.	*Deceleration:* Portion of swing when reference limb is decelerating in preparation for heel strike.

The first stance phase, *initial contact*, represents the moment in time when the outstretched limb first hits the ground. During the next phase, *loading response*, body weight is rapidly accepted onto the outstretched limb. A small wave of knee flexion helps dissipate the impact forces associated with body weight loading onto the limb. Initial contact and loading response are the two phases that constitute *initial double limb stance,* which is sometimes referred to as *weight acceptance.*[32] Initial double limb stance ends when the foot opposite the reference limb lifts from the ground for swing.

During the next two phases, *mid stance* and *terminal stance,* body weight progresses forward over a single stable limb. By terminal stance, the heel rises from the ground, the leg achieves a "trailing limb" posture, and the trunk advances well in front of the reference foot. Another term for the combined phases of mid stance and terminal stance is *single limb support,* reflective of only one limb being in contact with the ground.[32]

Pre-swing, the last phase of stance, is sometimes referred to as *terminal double limb stance* or *push-off.* During pre-swing, body weight transfers from the trailing limb to the contralateral lead limb, which is experiencing initial contact and loading response. As the proportion of body weight supported by the trailing limb diminishes, residual energy stored in the Achilles tendon during mid and terminal stance rapidly plantarflexes the ankle despite a lack of significant plantarflexor muscle activity.[32,36-38] The knee flexes to 40°, over half of the 60° required for foot clearance during the subsequent phase.

Lifting of the foot from the ground reflects the onset of the first phase of swing, *initial swing.* Rapid flexion of the knee and hip ensue. During *mid swing,* the thigh continues to advance into flexion, achieving a peak of approximately 25° relative to vertical. The knee begins to extend and the tibia achieves a characteristic vertical position by the end of mid swing. The ankle reaches neutral (0° dorsiflexion). During *terminal swing,* further thigh flexion is curtailed; however, the knee continues to extend until it observationally appears neutral. The ankle remains at neutral in preparation for a heel first initial contact.

Characteristic features of normal gait are presented in Tables 7.2 to 7.4. The gait phases, as well as normative values for joint motions, internal moments of force, and

Table 7.2   Ankle and Foot: Normative Sagittal Plane Data and Impact of Weakness[32,35]

Phase	Characteristic Joint Position	Internal Joint Moment	Normative Muscle Activity	Effect(s) of Weakness	Possible Compensation(s)
Initial Contact	Neutral (0° dorsiflexion)	Dorsiflexor moment achieves peak during loading response	Pretibial muscles (tibialis anterior, extensor digitorum longus, extensor hallucis longus) decelerate forefoot lowering and draw tibia forward following initial contact.	Borderline weakness (3+/5) may be accompanied by a foot slap following a heel first initial contact. Profound weakness (2+/5 or less) may result in foot flat or forefoot initial contact if pretibial strength is insufficient for achieving neutral ankle.	With borderline weakness, may slow gait to decrease demands on pretibial muscles during loading response. Alternatively, may contact ground with excess plantarflexion to decrease demands on pretibial muscles.
Loading Response	5° plantarflexion				
Mid Stance	5° dorsiflexion	Plantarflexor moment reaches peak during terminal stance	Plantarflexors (gastrocnemius, soleus, flexor digitorum longus, flexor hallucis longus, tibialis posterior, peroneus longus, and peroneus brevis) progressively increase activity throughout two phases to allow controlled forward progression of tibia. Elastic energy stored in Achilles tendon.	Excess dorsiflexion, uncontrolled tibial advancement, delayed or absent heel-off. However, if vastii are weak (vastus intermedius, vastus lateralis, vastus medialis longus, and oblique), may avoid excess dorsiflexion as it would contribute to excess knee flexion and high demand on weakened vastii.	Shortened step length and slower velocity to reduce demands on calf muscles.
Terminal Stance	10° dorsiflexion				
Pre-Swing	15° plantarflexion		Calf muscles cease in early pre-swing. Stored elastic energy in Achilles tendon contributes to rapid plantarflexion as limb unloads.	Low or no heel-off and lack of rapid plantarflexion.	Use of more proximal muscles to prepare limb for advancement and clearance.
Initial Swing	5° plantarflexion	Low dorsiflexor moment	Pretibial muscles elevate foot to neutral by mid swing and then maintain in that posture.	Excess plantarflexion and foot drag, particularly in mid swing. Poor posture for subsequent initial contact.	Hip hike, excess hip flexion or abduction to assist with limb clearance, or contralateral vault (excessive plantarflexion) to facilitate reference limb clearance.
Mid Swing	Neutral				
Terminal Swing	Neutral				

Table 7.3 Knee: Normative Sagittal Plane Data and Impact of Weakness[32,35]

Phase	Characteristic Joint Position	Internal Joint Moment	Normative Muscle Activity	Effect(s) of Weakness	Possible Compensation(s)
Initial Contact	Appears fully extended	Brief flexor moment	Low-amplitude hamstring activity (semimembranosus, semitendinosus, biceps femoris [long head]) resists knee hyperextension.	Reliance on posterior capsule to stabilize joint and to prevent hyperextension.	*Shading represents column heading information not applicable to the identified phase of gait.*
Loading Response	20° flexion	Extensor moment	Eccentric vastii activity (vastus intermedius, vastus lateralis, vastus medialis longus, and oblique) allows knee flexion for shock absorption but prevents collapse.	Unable to stabilize knee during flexion leading to limb collapse.	Avoid knee flexion (as flexion increases vastii demand) by use of (1) excess plantarflexion; or (2) forward trunk lean to lessen knee extensor moment.
Mid Stance	Appears fully extended	Extensor moment transitions to flexor moment	Vastii activity ceases by middle of mid stance.		
Terminal Stance	Appears fully extended	Flexor moment			
Pre-Swing	40° flexion	Extensor moment	Rectus femoris modulates rate of knee flexion.		
Initial Swing	60° flexion		Biceps femoris [short head], gracilis, and sartorius contribute to knee flexion.	Limited knee flexion for foot clearance.	Compensatory hip hike, excess hip flexion, or abduction to assist clearance.
Mid Swing	25° flexion	Flexor moment	Hamstrings modulate rate of knee extension (and thigh advancement).		
Terminal Swing	Appears fully extended		Hamstrings continue activity and vastii become active in preparation for demands of initial double limb stance.	With profound vastii weakness (less than 2+/5) may see inadequate knee extension in terminal swing.	Past retract of thigh or extension thrust of knee to ensure full knee extension.

Table 7.4   Hip: Normative Sagittal Plane Data and Impact of Weakness[32,35]

Phase	Characteristic Joint Position (thigh relative to vertical)	Internal Joint Moment	Normative Muscle Activity	Effect(s) of Weakness	Possible Compensation(s)
Initial Contact	20° flexion	Extensor moment	Single joint hip extensors and abductors contract vigorously to stabilize pelvis and trunk over femur. Hamstring activity diminishing.	Difficulty stabilizing pelvis and hip joint leading to anterior tilt and increased hip flexion in sagittal plane. If abductors weak, contralateral pelvic drop may occur.	Decrease terminal swing hip flexion to limit demands on weak hip extensors during initial contact and loading response. Posterior trunk lean to reduce extensor moment. For weak abductors, may lean trunk laterally toward stance limb to reduce abductor demands.
Loading Response	20° flexion				
Mid Stance	Neutral	Extensor moment transitions to flexor moment	Residual hamstring activity assists with hip extension at beginning of phase. Low-level abductor activity stabilizes pelvis.	Contralateral pelvic drop.	May lean trunk laterally toward stance limb to reduce abductor demands.
Terminal Stance	20° apparent hyperextension (anatomical hip joint does not allow 20° extension, but hip appears to be extended 20° due to the combined impact of hip extension, backward pelvic rotation, and anterior pelvic tilt on thigh angulation relative to vertical).	Increasing flexor moment	Low amplitude tensor fascia lata activity.	Contralateral pelvic drop.	May lean trunk laterally toward stance limb to reduce abductor demands.
Pre-Swing	10° apparent hyperextension	Flexor moment	Rectus femoris assists with early thigh advancement.		
Initial Swing	15° flexion	Flexor moment	Iliacus, adductor longus, gracilis, and sartorius actively advance thigh.	With profound hip flexor weakness (less than 2/5), may exhibit limited hip flexion, thigh advancement, and foot clearance.	To facilitate limb clearance, may compensate with ipsilateral hip hiking, excess hip abduction, or contralateral limb vaulting (excessive plantarflexion).
Mid Swing	25° flexion	Extensor moment	Increasing hamstring activity at end of phase restrains further thigh advancement.		

Table 7.4	Hip: Normative Sagittal Plane Data and Impact of Weakness[32,35]—cont'd				
Phase	**Characteristic Joint Position (thigh relative to vertical)**	**Internal Joint Moment**	**Normative Muscle Activity**	**Effect(s) of Weakness**	**Possible Compensation(s)**
Terminal Swing	20° flexion	Extensor moment	Hamstrings continue to control thigh posture, while single joint hip extensors and abductors rapidly increase activity in preparation for demands of next phase of gait.	Failure to achieve optimum limb position before initial contact.	Alter speed.

muscle activity, are presented in the first four columns. Familiarity with the normal motion patterns provides the therapist with a basis of comparison to identify deviations from standard. The internal moments (or torques) at each joint reflect the forces generated by muscles' contractile and noncontractile components, as well as ligaments and joint capsules. Internal moments counterbalance the external moments that are created by forces such as gravity and inertia acting on the body segments. In the current chapter, we have elected to describe internal joint moments as this appears to be the more common reference point used in published literature. However, knowledge of the external moments (and thus the internal moments) is helpful for interpreting the characteristic patterns of muscle activation that contribute to stability, forward progression, shock absorption, and limb clearance throughout the gait cycle. For example, during the single limb support period of normal gait, a progressively increasing external dorsiflexion moment occurs as body weight progresses anterior to the ankle joint. Without a counteracting force from the plantarflexors, the ankle would collapse into dorsiflexion. The force generated by the plantarflexors contributes to an internal plantarflexor moment that allows controlled forward progression but prevents tibial collapse. Thus, the internal plantarflexor moment generated by the plantarflexors resists the external dorsiflexion moment created in large part by the force of gravity on the body.

Abnormalities in timing (e.g., activity that is premature or delayed) and amplitude (either too much or too little) can disrupt normal gait patterns. Familiarity with the muscle activity and function associated with normal gait allows therapists to identify potential causes of deviations. In Tables 7.2 to 7.4, the possible effects of muscle weakness and potential compensations are presented in the last two columns. The purpose of the tables is to identify components of normal gait that must be considered when observing gait and to provide an example

of how to proceed with an analysis of the causes of an atypical gait pattern or particular deviation.

■ TYPES OF GAIT ANALYSES

The types of analyses in use today can be classified under two broad categories: **kinematic** and **kinetic**. Kinematic gait analysis is used to describe movement patterns without regard for the forces involved in producing the movement. A kinematic gait analysis consists of a description of movement of the body as a whole and/or body segments in relation to each other during gait. Kinematic gait analysis can be either *qualitative* or *quantitative*. Kinetic gait analysis is used to determine the forces involved in gait. In some instances, both kinematic and kinetic gait variables may be examined in one analysis. In addition to examining kinematic and kinetic variables, physiological variables such as heart rate, oxygen consumption, energy cost, and muscular activation patterns (electromyography) may be considered.

Kinematic Qualitative Gait Analysis

The most common method used in clinical settings is a *qualitative gait analysis*. This method usually requires only a small amount of equipment and a minimal amount of time. The primary variable examined in a qualitative kinematic analysis is *displacement*, which includes a description of patterns of movement, deviations from normal body postures, and joint angles at specific points in the gait cycle.

Observational Gait Analysis

Few clinical settings have the resources (space, money, or time) required to complete an instrumented gait analysis on every patient. As a result, observational gait analysis (OGA) often serves as an essential component of many physical therapy examinations. The results of an OGA are used to identify structural and activity limitations, as well as to plan an intervention and assess the outcomes. While physical therapists seek an easy to administer tool to identify gait abnormalities, guide treatment approaches (e.g., need for orthotic devices), and assess progress,[39] the validity and reliability of existing scales remains less than optimal. This section highlights tools/approaches that clinicians may consider using.

The *Rancho Los Amigos Observational Gait Analysis* system is probably the most common OGA system used by physical therapists.[32,35] The Rancho Los Amigos OGA method involves a systematic examination of the movement patterns of key body segments (foot, ankle, knee, hip, pelvis, and trunk) during each phase of the gait cycle. The system uses a recording form comprising 45 descriptors of common gait deviations such as toe drag, excess plantarflexion and dorsiflexion, excess knee varus or valgus, pelvic hiking, and forward or backward trunk leans (Fig. 7.3). The observing therapist must determine whether or not a deviation is present and note the occurrence and timing of the deviation on the special form.[35]

Considerable training and practice are necessary to develop the observational skills needed for performing any OGA. Therapists who wish to learn the Rancho method can study the *Rancho Los Amigos Observational Gait Analysis Handbook*.[35] Practice gait videos, useful for developing and improving one's observational skills and for learning how to use the recording forms, may be obtained by visiting the Los Amigos Research and Education Institute (LAREI) website (www.larei.org) or by writing to LAREI, Rancho Los Amigos National Rehabilitation Center, 7601 East Imperial Highway, Downey, CA 90242.

Podiatrists have developed their own unique OGA system.[40] A biomechanical gait analysis form for podiatrists, described by Southerland,[40] is presented in Figure 7.4. This form is used in conjunction with a static quantitative analysis that includes measurements of range of motion (ROM) of all joints from the hip to the toes, as well as measurements of limb length. Detailed information is also collected on both the dorsal and plantar surfaces of the feet such as callus formation and corns. The examiner is expected to document abnormalities such as hallux valgus and hammer toes. The dynamic qualitative component of the analysis uses a shorthand system for recording the details of the OGA. The acronym GHORT (*G*ait, *H*omunculus, *O*bserved, *R*elational, and *T*abulator) is used to assist in recording information gathered from the observational analysis (Fig. 7.5). An example of the recording method is shown in Figure 7.6. Following completion of the dynamic portion, the rater's qualitative impressions of the patient's gait are compared with the results of the static analysis to verify the accuracy of the findings and determine the causes of abnormal function. The author states that after the first five analyses, a new rater's results are the same as or similar to those of other raters; however, the author did not reference any reliability and/or validity studies.[40] In general, these observational protocols provide the therapist with a systematic approach to OGA by directing the observer's attention to a specific joint or body segment during a given point in the gait cycle.

The advantages of OGAs are that they require little or no instrumentation, are inexpensive to use, and can yield general descriptions of gait variables. The disadvantages are that the observational method, being dependent on both the therapist's training and observational skills, is subjective and has only low to moderate reliability, and validity has not been demonstrated.[41] Difficulties involved in observing and making accurate judgments about motions occurring simultaneously at numerous body segments, and inadequate training in OGA methods are thought to contribute to the low reliability. Also, therapists differ in their observational skills. A drawback to using the Rancho Los Amigos OGA technique is that reliability and validity of the method have not been published.

Digital Video Recording

If therapists decide to use an OGA method, they should consider using a digital video recorder (DVR) that has the capability of slowing or stopping motion. A visual record is especially important when using the Rancho Los Amigos format because of the time involved in examining a large number of variables at six body parts. Most patients cannot walk continuously for the length of time required to complete a detailed, full-body observational analysis. Furthermore, the observers cannot rate or score a large number of variables while a subject is walking. Digital records of a patient's initial performance that can be replayed in slow motion allow therapists the time needed to make judgments about gait events. Activating the DVR pause feature, a goniometer, aligned with body segments displayed on the video monitor, can be used to assess (validate) joint angles during critical phases. This may also help refine the therapist's observational skills.

Although the use of digital video recordings may provide an opportunity for observers to determine the reliability of their scoring, reliability will probably remain low to moderate unless therapists are knowledgeable about normal gait parameters and variables and are adequately trained to use the measuring instrument. Russell et al[42] found that when observers were trained in the scoring of a Gross Motor Function Measure (GMFM), a significant improvement occurred following training compared with the observers' pretraining scoring of the videotape. Brunnekreef and colleagues[43] identified higher interrater reliability among expert raters of orthopedic gait disorders (intraclass correlation coefficient [ICC] = 0.54) when using a form developed by the experts than the values documented for experienced (ICC = 0.42) and inexperienced (ICC = 0.40) raters using the same form. On the other hand, Eastlack et al[44] found only low to moderate interrater reliability among 54 practicing physical therapists who rated 10 gait variables while observing the

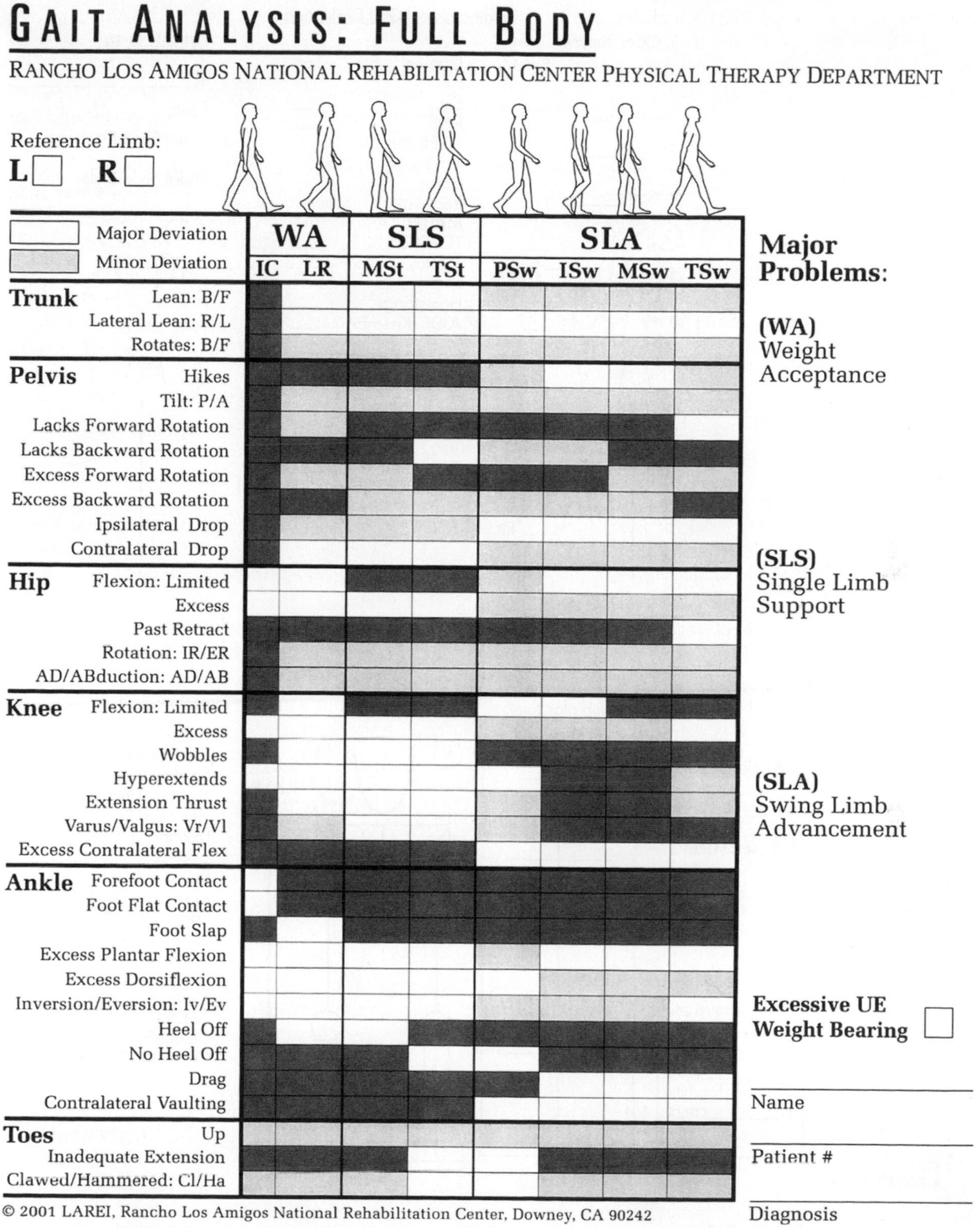

GAIT ANALYSIS: FULL BODY

RANCHO LOS AMIGOS NATIONAL REHABILITATION CENTER PHYSICAL THERAPY DEPARTMENT

Reference Limb:
L ☐ R ☐

		WA		SLS		SLA			
☐ Major Deviation / ▓ Minor Deviation		IC	LR	MSt	TSt	PSw	ISw	MSw	TSw
Trunk	Lean: B/F								
	Lateral Lean: R/L								
	Rotates: B/F								
Pelvis	Hikes								
	Tilt: P/A								
	Lacks Forward Rotation								
	Lacks Backward Rotation								
	Excess Forward Rotation								
	Excess Backward Rotation								
	Ipsilateral Drop								
	Contralateral Drop								
Hip	Flexion: Limited								
	Excess								
	Past Retract								
	Rotation: IR/ER								
	AD/ABduction: AD/AB								
Knee	Flexion: Limited								
	Excess								
	Wobbles								
	Hyperextends								
	Extension Thrust								
	Varus/Valgus: Vr/Vl								
	Excess Contralateral Flex								
Ankle	Forefoot Contact								
	Foot Flat Contact								
	Foot Slap								
	Excess Plantar Flexion								
	Excess Dorsiflexion								
	Inversion/Eversion: Iv/Ev								
	Heel Off								
	No Heel Off								
	Drag								
	Contralateral Vaulting								
Toes	Up								
	Inadequate Extension								
	Clawed/Hammered: Cl/Ha								

Major Problems:

(WA) Weight Acceptance

(SLS) Single Limb Support

(SLA) Swing Limb Advancement

Excessive UE Weight Bearing ☐

Name _____

Patient # _____

Diagnosis _____

© 2001 LAREI, Rancho Los Amigos National Rehabilitation Center, Downey, CA 90242

Figure 7.3 Full Body Gait Analysis Form. *(From Observational Gait Analysis Handbook,[35] with permission.)*

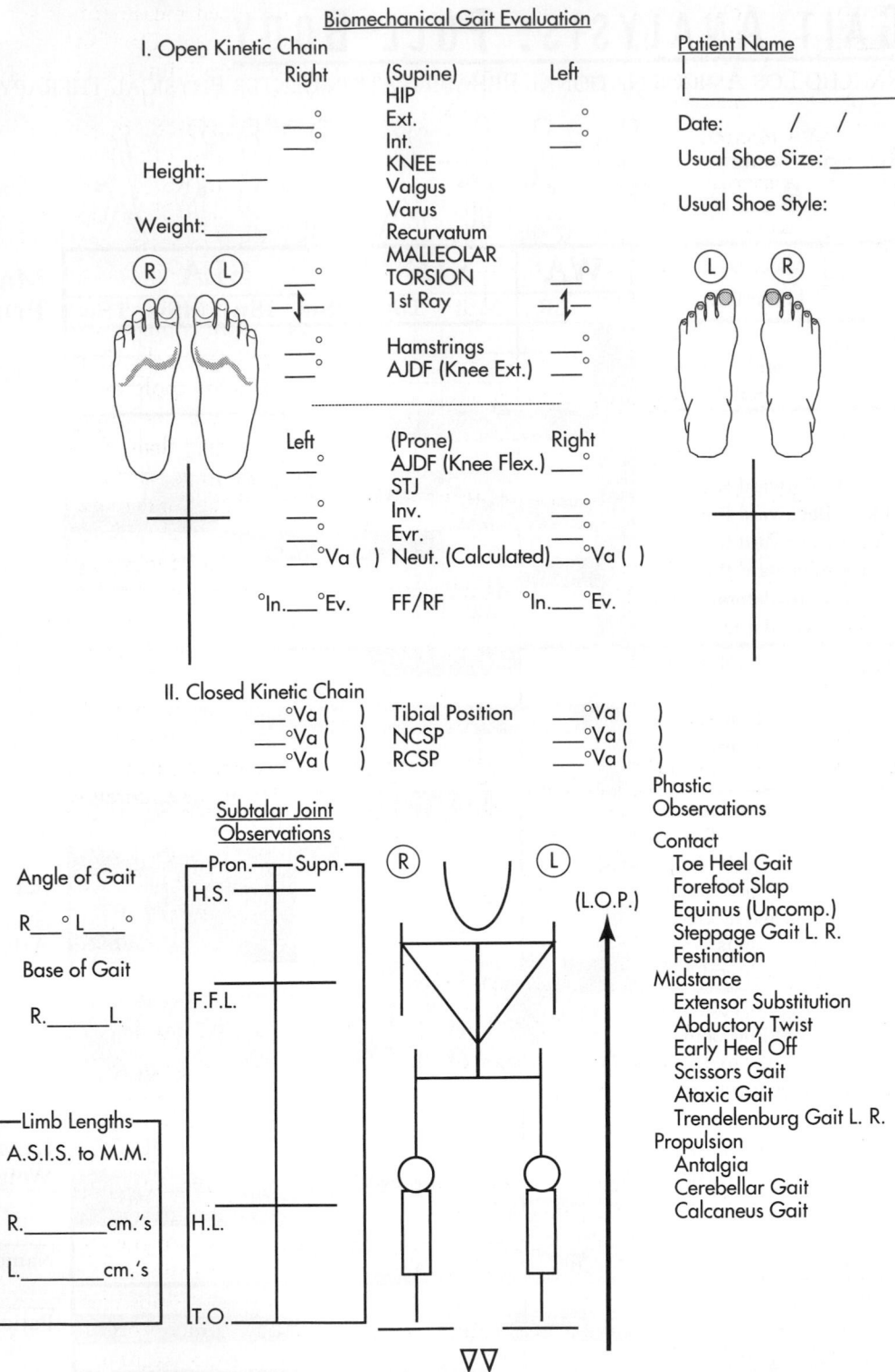

Figure 7.4 Biomechanical Gait Evaluation Form for Observational Gait Analysis. *(From Southerland,[40, p. 155] with permission.)*

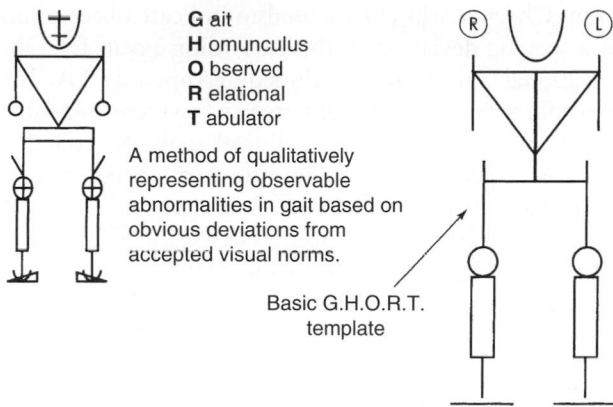

Figure 7.5 GHORT. *(From Southerland,[40, p. 159] with permission.)*

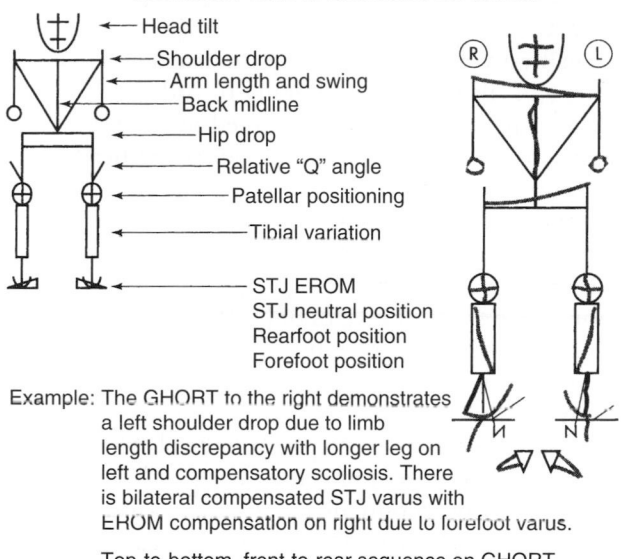

Figure 7.6 Recording points of evaluation on GHORT. *(From Southerland,[40, p. 164] with permission.)*

videotaped gait of three patients. These therapists had reported that they were comfortable performing observational gait analyses. The lack of agreement among raters found in this study, as well as the raters' lack of knowledge of normal gait parameters and terminology, has serious implications for patient treatments based on the results of observational gait analyses.[44] Krebs[45] argues that OGA is impossible to perform in a clinical setting. However, in a study using OGA, physical therapists were able to make accurate and reliable judgments of scored push-off power in the videotaped gait of subjects following stroke. This study suggests that focused analysis on specific gait parameters may be more reliable than general analyses.[46]

Specialized video analysis software may improve interrater reliability of gait measures compared to traditional video viewing methods. Borel et al[47] reported

increased measurement agreement between two raters when using Dartfish®, a program that allows users to measure joint angles, distance, and time variables directly from digital videos. (*Note:* For this chapter, all manufacturer contact information is presented in Appendix 7.C.) Raters used Windows Media Player® and Dartfish® to perform the measurements required to determine Observational Gait Scale scores for 20 videos of children with cerebral palsy (CP). Interrater agreement values increased for select variables (knee position mid stance, foot contact mid stance, timing of heel rise, hindfoot mid stance, and the composite total score) when using the digital goniometer, line drawing, and temporal tools of Dartfish®. One potential negative was that it took longer to complete the analysis using Dartfish® than Windows Media Player (18 versus 10 minutes per video, respectively). Additionally, this study did not determine whether the more consistent values also were valid. If OGA is employed, it should be used in conjunction with quantitative measures. Digital video recordings or videotape can provide a permanent record of the patient's gait. Videography may also be used to examine joint ROM at the hip, knee, and ankle, by taking goniometric measurements directly from the paused screen. Stuberg et al[48] found no significant differences between goniometric measurements calculated from videotaped gait and measurements generated using a digitizer in 10 children with CP and 9 typically developing children. Six blue markers, placed over key anatomical locations of the lower extremity (LE) and shoulder, guided measurements. The use of markers to guide measurements emphasizes the importance of ensuring that joints (or apparent axes of rotation) are clearly visible to facilitate measurements with the eye or a goniometer.

Observational Gait Analysis Process

The purpose of this section is to introduce the process involved in an OGA. The first step in the process involves the identification and accurate description of the patient's gait pattern and any existing deviations. The second step involves a determination of the causes of the deviations. To properly identify and describe a patient's gait, the therapist must have good knowledge of gait terminology and an accurate mental picture of normal gait postures and normal displacements of the body segments during each gait phase, and in each plane of analysis (sagittal, coronal, and transverse). To determine the causes of a patient's gait pattern and specific deviations, the therapist must understand the normal roles and functions of muscles during gait and the normal forces involved.[32,35,49,50] Deviations occur because of an inability to perform the tasks of walking in a normal fashion. For example, a patient with paralysis of the dorsiflexors (which causes a foot drop) cannot attain the normal neutral position of the ankle necessary to complete the task of clearing the floor during swing. Therefore, the patient must find some other method of clearing the floor. The patient could compensate for in-adequate dorsiflexion by increasing the amount of hip and knee flexion, by circumduction of the entire limb, or by hiking the hip. The type of compensation that a particular individual selects depends on the specific disability. Increased hip and knee flexion may be used if the patient has an isolated problem in the ankle and adequate muscle strength and ROM in the extremity. Circumduction or hip hiking may be used if the patient has either a stiff knee or extensor thrust, which prevents use of increased knee flexion to raise the plantarflexed foot above the floor.[6] The therapist must be aware that patients may use a variety of methods to compensate for joint or muscle deficits.

Overview of Common Deviations and Underlying Causes

Tables 7.5 to 7.8 present common gait deviations and possible causes for the deviations. Given that muscle demands vary across phases of gait, the causes of a specific deviation also frequently vary based on the phase. For example, a common cause of excess plantarflexion during swing is weak pretibial muscles. However, this is not a common cause of excess plantarflexion during mid stance and terminal stance, as the pretibial muscles are not normally active during this period. Instead, excess plantarflexion during mid and terminal stance would more likely arise from the influence of plantarflexor spasticity or contractures on joint motion during. Thus, detective work is required to link the observed gait deviations with the specific demands of a phase in order to determine the most likely cause(s). Accurate determination of the impairments leading to the gait deviation is essential for guiding treatment interventions.

Appendix 7.A, Recording Form for Observational Gait Analysis, provides a sample gait analysis recording form. Check marks (√) are used to indicate observation of a specific deviation in the Recording Form for Observational Gait Analysis included in Appendix 7.A. The two columns on the far right are used to record possible causes and findings from the clinical analyses. To guide the OGA process, note that the form presented in Appendix 7.A has been formatted similarly to Tables 7.5 through 7.8. If the reader decides to use the gait analysis recording forms presented in this text, reliability tests should be conducted because these forms are presented only as guides and have not been evaluated.

Guidelines for Performing an OGA

Guidelines for performing an OGA are presented below.

1. Select the area in which the patient will walk and measure the distance that you want the patient to traverse.
2. Position yourself to allow an unobstructed view of the subject. If digitally recording, the cameras should be positioned to view the patient's entire body (LEs as well as the head and trunk) from both the sagittal and coronal perspectives. To avoid errors in estimating the amplitude of joint angles due to angle parallax,[32,48] it is important to perform measurements on paused digital images only when the patient's LEs or body is in the same plane as the image view. Out-of-plane views can lead to distorted angle measurements.
3. Select the joint or body segment to be observed first (e.g., ankle and foot), and mentally review the normative joint positions and muscle activity for the phase of the gait period being observed (e.g., initial contact).

(Text continues on page 268)

Table 7.5	Common Ankle and Foot Deviations[32,35]			
Deviation	Phase(s)	Description	Possible Causes	Analysis
Toes or forefoot contact	Initial contact	Toes or forefoot are first point of contact with ground instead of heel	Leg length discrepancy; plantarflexion contracture or spasticity; profound dorsiflexor weakness; painful heel; excessive knee flexion when combined with any impairment that limits ability to achieve neutral ankle.	Examine range of motion (ROM) and leg lengths and for hip and/or knee flexion contractures and/or ankle plantarflexion contractures. Examine muscle tone and timing of activity in plantarflexors. Examine pretibial strength and for heel pain.
Foot flat contact	Initial contact	Entire foot simultaneously touches ground at initial contact	Plantarflexion contracture; weak dorsiflexors; knee flexion contracture that prevents optimal tibial alignment before initial contact.	Examine ROM at ankle and knee and strength of pretibial muscles.

Table 7.5	Common Ankle and Foot Deviations[32,35]—cont'd			
Deviation	**Phase(s)**	**Description**	**Possible Causes**	**Analysis**
Foot slap	Loading response	Forefoot "slaps" the ground following a heel first initial contact	Weak dorsiflexors or reciprocal inhibition of dorsiflexors.	Examine strength. Evaluate muscle activation timing of pretibial muscles.
Excess plantarflexion	Mid stance and/or terminal stance	Ankle fails to achieve 5° dorsiflexion at mid stance and/or 10° dorsiflexion at terminal stance	Plantarflexion contracture; overactivity or spasticity of the plantarflexors; could be intentional to avoid ankle and knee collapse if plantarflexors and vastii are weak.	Examine ROM and tone for plantarflexion contracture and plantarflexor tone (spasticity); examine strength of calf muscles and vastii. Evaluate if deviation may be intentional due to dual areas of weakness.
Excess dorsiflexion	Mid stance and/or terminal stance	Ankle collapses into more than 5° dorsiflexion at mid stance and/or more than 10° dorsiflexion at terminal stance	Inability of plantarflexors to control tibial advance. Knee flexion or hip flexion contractures.	Examine ROM and plantarflexor strength and for hip and knee flexion contractures.
Early heel rise	Mid stance	Heel comes off ground in mid stance	Spasticity or contracture of plantarflexors.	Examine ROM and tone for plantarflexor spasticity and contractures.
No heel off	Terminal stance and/or pre-swing	Heel fails to elevate from ground appropriately during terminal stance	Weak plantarflexors; weak invertors, which fail to lock midfoot in terminal stance; inadequate toe extension ROM; painful forefoot or toes.	Examine strength of plantarflexors and tibialis posterior; toe extension ROM, particularly the 1st metatarsal phalangeal joint; and for forefoot pain.
Toe clawing	Stance	Toes flex and "grab" floor	Spasticity of toe flexors; excessive activation of toe flexors to compensate for weakness of the gastrocnemius and soleus; plantar grasp reflex that is only partially integrated; positive supporting reflex.	Examine tone of toe flexors, strength of plantarflexors, and presence of primitive reflexes.
Excess inversion or eversion	Stance or swing	Subtalar joint is excessively inverted or everted in contrast to expected position	Excessive inversion: overactivity or contracture of invertors; reduced activity of evertors; primitive extensor pattern. Excessive eversion: overactivity or contracture of evertors; reduced activity or strength of invertors; primitive flexor pattern.	Examine strength and timing of lower extremity movements and tone; and for contractures.
Drag	Swing	Some portion of reference foot contacts ground during swing	Pretibial muscle weakness; plantarflexor spasticity or contractures; inadequate knee or hip flexion.	Examine ROM of ankle, knee, and hip; strength of muscles critical for limb clearance.

Table 7.6	Common Knee Deviations[32,35]			
Deviation	**Phase**	**Description**	**Possible Causes**	**Analysis**
Excess knee flexion	All phases	Knee is in greater flexion than expected for the given phase	Knee flexor spasticity or contracture that exceeds position required for given phase; painful or effused knee; proprioceptive loss at knee; shorter LE on contralateral side. In addition, consider weak calf or hip flexion contracture if it occurs during single limb support.	Examine tone, spasticity, and ROM (contractures); and for pain, effusion, and proprioceptive loss at knee; leg length discrepancy.
Limited knee flexion	Loading response	Knee achieves less than expected 20° flexion	May be intentional to decrease demands on weak quadriceps; secondary to plantarflexor or quadriceps tone, spasticity or contracture; or proprioceptive impairment at knee.	Examine strength, tone, spasticity, of plantarflexors and quadriceps; plantarflexion and knee extension ROM; knee proprioception.
	Pre-swing and initial swing	Knee achieves less than expected flexion for given phase (i.e., 40° and 60° flexion, respectively)	May be secondary to plantarflexor tone, spasticity, or contracture that limits forward tibial progression in terminal stance; quadriceps tone, spasticity; proprioceptive impairment at knee; knee pain or effusion; calf weakness or hip flexion contracture that limits ability to achieve the trailing limb posture in terminal stance (a critical precursor to rapid knee flexion during pre-swing and initial swing). During initial swing, weakness of knee flexors also may contribute.	Examine tone and spasticity of plantarflexors, vastii, and rectus femoris; ROM and knee proprioception. Examine for pain and effusion. Examine plantarflexor strength and for hip flexion contracture. Evaluate if these factors may be inhibiting achievement of optimum limb posture.
Knee hyperextension	Stance	Extension of knee beyond anatomical neutral	Structural abnormality; may develop over time in presence of flaccid/weak quadriceps which is compensated for by excess plantarflexion and/or posterior pull on thigh by gluteus maximus; quadriceps spasticity, accommodation to a fixed plantarflexion deformity, or impaired proprioception can contribute to hyperextension if knee is exposed to deforming forces for extended duration.	Examine strength of vastii; tone, spasticity of plantarflexors and quadriceps; ROM and knee proprioception.
Wobble	Stance	Alternating flexion and extension at knee joint	Consider proprioceptive impairments or alternating spasticity of knee flexors and extensors.	Examine knee for proprioceptive impairments and spasticity.

Table 7.7 Common Hip Deviations[32,35]

Deviation	Phase(s)	Description	Possible Causes	Analysis
Excess flexion	Initial contact and loading response	Hip positioned in greater flexion (thigh relative to vertical) than expected for given phase	Single joint hip extensor weakness (gluteus maximus, adductor magnus) with compensation by hamstrings; severe hip and/or knee flexion contractures; hypertonicity of hip or knee flexors.	Examine single joint hip extensor and hamstring strength; hip and knee flexion range of motion (ROM), tone, and spasticity.
	Mid stance through pre-swing		Hip flexion or knee flexion contractures or spasticity; weak plantarflexors failing to control excess tibial advancement; painful or effused hip.	Examine tone and spasticity of hip and knee flexors; ROM of hip and knee; strength of plantarflexors and hip for joint pain.
	Swing		Compensatory to assist with limb clearance if limb is functionally too long; flexion synergy during swing resulting in too much flexion.	Examine for compensation, determine if ankle and knee of reference limb are achieving correct joint positions. Examine contralateral limb to determine if deviations are occurring on opposite side (e.g., excess stance dorsiflexion) could contribute to clearance problems on reference side.
Limited flexion	Initial contact, loading response, initial swing, mid swing, terminal swing	Hip positioned in less flexion (thigh relative to vertical) than expected for given phase	May be intentional to limit demand on weak hip extensors during loading response; weak hip flexors, or single joint hip extensor; hamstring spasticity or contracture limiting terminal swing advancement before initial contact.	Examine strength of hip flexors and extensors; ROM of hip and for spasticity of hip extensors and hamstrings.
Circumduction	Swing	Lateral circular movement of limb consisting initially of abduction, external rotation, followed by adduction and internal rotation in latter portion of swing	Compensation for weak hip flexors or for inability to shorten leg for limb clearance.	Examine strength of hip flexors, knee flexors, and ankle dorsiflexors; ROM in hip and knee flexion, and ankle dorsiflexion and for abnormal extensor pattern.
Internal rotation	All phases	Internal rotation of femur	Spasticity or contractures of internal rotators; weakness of external rotators; excessive forward rotation of contralateral pelvis.	Examine tone, internal rotation ROM, and strength of external rotators.
External rotation	All phases	External rotation of femur	Spasticity or contractures of external rotators; weakness of internal rotators.	Examine tone, external rotation ROM, and strength of internal rotators.
Abduction	All phases	Abducted position of femur relative to vertical	Contracture of the gluteus medius or iliotibial band; during swing, could be used to assist with foot clearance.	Examine hip abductor range of motion and for any factors that would necessitate compensatory assistance with clearance.
Adduction	All phases	Adducted position of femur relative to vertical	Hip adductor spasticity/contracture. Excess contralateral pelvic drop.	Examine tone of hip flexors and adductors; muscle strength of hip abductors.

Table 7.8   Common Pelvis and Trunk Deviations[32,35]

Deviation	Phase(s)	Description	Possible Causes	Analysis
Backward trunk lean	Stance or swing	Posterior lean of the trunk relative to vertical	Purposeful to reduce demands on weakened stance limb gluteus maximus or to assist with limb advancement when hip flexion capability is limited.	Examine hip extensor and flexor strength.
Forward trunk lean	Primarily stance	Anterior lean of trunk relative to vertical	Compensation for quadriceps weakness. Forward lean reduces knee extensor moment and thus demand on vastii. May also be used to accommodate hip or knee flexion contractures.	Examine quadriceps strength and hip and knee for contractures.
Ipsilateral trunk lean	Most commonly occurs during reference limb stance	Lateral trunk lean toward reference extremity	Most commonly occurs during reference limb stance. Compensation for ipsilateral hip abductor weakness, hip joint pain, iliotibial band tightness, or scoliosis.	Examine ipsilateral gluteus medius strength; hip pain and ipsilateral iliotibial band tightness and for trunk ROM.
Contralateral trunk lean	Most commonly occurs during reference limb swing	Lateral trunk lean toward opposite extremity	May be used to assist with pelvic elevation to ensure foot clearance if reference limb is functionally too long (owing to deviations or leg length discrepancy). Compensation for contralateral hip abductor weakness, hip joint pain, iliotibial band tightness, or scoliosis.	Examine contralateral gluteus medius strength, hip pain and for iliotibial band tightness and for trunk ROM. Examine for factors contributing to swing limb being too long (e.g., limited knee flexion or excess plantarflexion during initial swing or a leg length discrepancy).
Contralateral pelvic drop	Stance	Drop of contralateral iliac crest below ipsilateral iliac crest	Ipsilateral hip abductor weakness, hip adductor spasticity, or hip adduction contracture.	Examine strength, flexibility, and tone of ipsilateral hip abductors and adductors.
Ipsilateral pelvic drop	Swing	Drop of ipsilateral iliac crest below contralateral iliac crest	Contralateral hip abductor weakness, hip adductor spasticity, or hip adduction contracture.	Examine strength, flexibility, and tone of contralateral hip abductors and adductors.
Pelvic hike	Swing	Elevation of ipsilateral iliac crest above contralateral iliac crest	Action of quadratus lumborum to assist with limb clearance when hip flexion, knee flexion, and/or ankle dorsiflexion are inadequate for limb clearance.	Examine strength and ROM at knee, hip, and ankle; examine muscle tone at knee and ankle.

4. Select the plane of observation that will be used first, either the sagittal plane (view from the side) or the coronal plane (view from the front and/or back) and which side of the patient's body (either right or left) will be observed first.

5. Observe the selected body segment at a specific phase (e.g., initial contact) and make a decision about the segment's joint position. Note any deviations from normal.

6. Observe either the same body segment during the next phase or another segment at the same phase (e.g., initial contact) of the gait period. As described in number 5 above, again make a decision about the segment's joint position. Note any deviations from normal.

7. Repeat the process described in number 6 above until you have completed an observation of all segments across all phases of the gait cycle in both the

sagittal and coronal planes. Remember to concentrate on one body segment or joint at a time during one phase of the gait cycle. Do not jump from one segment to another or from one phase to another.

8. Always perform observations on both sides (right and left). Although only one side may be involved pathologically, the other side of the body may be affected.
9. Hypothesize likely causes of gait deviations (e.g., impairments in strength, impairments in ROM, or spasticity).
10. Confirm likely causes of gait deviations based on physical therapy clinical evaluation.
11. Develop and implement a treatment plan to address key underlying causes of gait dysfunction.
12. Periodically use OGA to reassess the patient's gait and determine response to treatment.

OGA in Neuromuscular Disorders

The gait patterns of individuals with neuromuscular deficits are influenced primarily by weakness, abnormalities in muscle tone and synergistic organization, influences of nonintegrated early reflexes, diminished influence of righting and balance reactions, dissociation among body parts, and incoordination. If proximal stability (e.g., co-contraction of the postural muscles of the trunk) is threatened by atypically low, high, or fluctuating muscle tone, controlled mobility is lost. In gait, a loss of control over the sequential timing of muscular activity may result in asymmetrical step and stride lengths. In addition, deviations may occur such as forward or backward trunk leaning, excessive or decreased hip or knee flexion, or altered dorsiflexion or plantarflexion.

In the presence of multiple muscle involvement or neurological deficits that affect balance, coordination, and muscle tone, the deviations observed and the analysis of these deviations will be more complex than indicated in the tables. Examples of gait patterns associated with spasticity and with hypotonus follow.

An individual with spasticity (e.g., an individual with diplegic CP) may have a posteriorly tilted pelvis, forward flexion of the upper trunk, protracted scapulae, and somewhat excessive neck extension. Excessive hip flexion with adduction and internal rotation (scissoring) may be observed during stance and may be accompanied by either excessive knee flexion or hyperextension. During late stance, plantarflexor weakness may allow the ankle to collapse into excess dorsiflexion and the knee into excess flexion. Alternatively, the ankle may be positioned in excess dorsiflexion in late stance as a means of accommodating a knee flexion contracture or hamstring tightness/spasticity.

In other individuals with hypertonia, hyperextension at the knee occurs in stance and may be accompanied by plantarflexion and inversion at the ankle and foot. Electromyographic (EMG) recordings may show prolonged activity in the quadriceps and in the gastrocnemius-soleus muscle group. The hamstring, gluteal, and dorsiflexor muscle groups may be reciprocally inhibited.

In individuals with low muscle tone (hypotonia) in the trunk, core stability (tonic extension and co-contraction of axial muscles) is diminished. The pelvis may be anteriorly tilted so that the upper trunk is slightly extended. The scapulae may be retracted and the head may be forward. During stance, the hip may be flexed and the knee may be hyperextended, accompanied by ankle plantarflexion. The foot may be pronated with the majority of body weight borne on the medial border. Frequently, these individuals show diminished longitudinal trunk rotation and sluggish trunk balance reactions. They tend to rely on protective extension reactions of the limbs to maintain balance. The staggering or stepping reactions of the LEs may be pronounced, stride length and step length may be uneven, and gait may be wide based and unsteady.

Although neurological gait patterns may be complex and an analysis of the causes may be difficult, a detailed OGA can provide valuable data. Generally, to analyze gait patterns in persons who have sustained neurological damage, the following preliminary questions must be asked:

1. What is the influence of abnormal tone (hypertonicity, hypotonicity, fluctuating tone) on joint position and movement?
2. How does the position of the head influence muscle tone, position, and movement?
3. How does weight-bearing influence muscle tone, position, and movement?
4. What is the influence of abnormal (obligatory) synergistic activity on position and movement?
5. What is the impact of weakness (paresis) on position and movement?
6. How do coordination impairments affect position and movement?
7. What is the influence of impaired balance reactions on position and movement?
8. How do contractures alter position and movement?
9. What is the impact of sensory loss (e.g., proprioceptive, visual, vestibular) on position and movement?

Ambulation Profiles and Scales

Profiles and rating scales constitute types of gait analyses that often include both qualitative (observational) and quantitative (spatial and temporal) measures. Profiles and scales are used for a variety of reasons, for example, examination of ambulation skills,[51,52] determination of the patient's need for assistance, identification of a change in a patient's status,[52] screening for identification of the patient's need for physical therapy,[53] and identification of individuals (e.g., older adults) who are at risk for falling.[25,26] Gait analyses of one type or another may be either the sole focus of a profile, or the gait analysis may constitute only a small portion of a broad examination profile that includes balance skills and other functional activities. One particular advantage of some of these profiles is that subordinate gait skills such as standing balance may be examined in individuals who may be unable to walk independently. Since many of these profiles were developed for use with specific populations, comparative data may be available to the therapist.

The following profiles have been selected for review in this chapter because they are in current use and have been examined for reliability and/or validity: the Functional Ambulation Profile;[51] the Emory Functional Ambulation Profile[54] and the Modified Emory Functional Ambulation Profile;[55] the Iowa Level of Assistance Score;[56] the Functional Independence Measure;[57] the Functional Independence Measure plus the Functional Assessment Measure;[58,59] the Community Balance and Mobility Scale;[52,60,61] the Gait Abnormality Rating Scale (GARS)[62] and the Modified GARS;[25] the Dynamic Gait Index;[63-65] the Functional Gait Assessment;[66-70] the High-Level Mobility Assessment Tool;[71-76] the Fast Evaluation of Mobility, Balance, and Fear;[77] and the Figure-of-8 Walk Test.[78]

Functional Ambulation Profile and Modifications

The *Functional Ambulation Profile* (FAP), developed by Arthur J. Nelson, PT, PhD, FAPTA, is designed to examine gait skills on a continuum from standing balance in the parallel bars to independent ambulation.[51] A stopwatch is used to measure the amount of time required either to maintain a position or perform a task. The test consists of three phases. In the first phase, the patient is asked to perform three tasks in the parallel bars: bilateral stance, uninvolved leg stance, and involved leg stance. In the second phase, the patient is asked to transfer weight from one LE to the other as rapidly as possible. In the third phase, the patient is asked to walk 20 ft (6 m) in the parallel bars, with an assistive device, and, if possible, independently. Wolf et al[54] evaluated the tool's reliability and validity in a study of 56 adults (28 with stroke and 28 without). The authors reported high interrater reliability ((0.997) between two examiners who rated subjects' test performance. Construct validity was supported based on the test's ability to distinguish between those with and without a stroke. Concurrent validity was demonstrated by strong correlations with participants' outcomes on the Timed 10-meter Walk Test and the Berg Balance Scale. A more recent version of the FAP developed at Emory University is called the *Emory Functional Ambulation Profile* (EFAP).[54] This profile differs from the original FAP in that five environmental challenges have been added. The individual may negotiate the environmental challenges with or without the use of orthotics or assistive devices.

The *Modified Emory Functional Ambulation Profile*[55] (mEFAP) incorporates manual assistance into the EFAP. Subtasks include 16.4-ft (5-m) walks on a hard floor and on a carpeted floor, rising from a chair and completing a 9.8-ft (3-m) walk and sitting back down, negotiating through a standardized obstacle course and ascending and descending five stairs. Liaw et al[79] evaluated the psychometric properties of the mEFAP in 40 individuals during the early phase of stroke recovery and 20 individuals with chronic strokes. The authors concluded that the mEFAP had good reliability, validity, and responsiveness for assessing walking function in patients with stroke undergoing rehabilitation.

Iowa Level of Assistance Scale

The *Iowa Level of Assistance Scale* (ILAS)[56] examines four functional tasks: getting out of bed, standing from bed, ambulating 15 ft (4.57 m), and walking up and down three steps. The patient's performance on the tasks is rated according to the following seven levels: (1) not tested for safety reasons; (2) activity attempted but not completed; (3) maximum assistance (therapist applies three or more points of contact); (4) moderate assistance (therapist applies two points of contact); (5) minimal assistance (therapist provides one point of contact); (6) standby assistance (no therapist contact but therapist not comfortable leaving patient); and (7) independence (therapist comfortable leaving room). Shields et al[56] examined the reliability, validity, and responsiveness of the ILAS in 86 inpatients recovering from total hip or knee replacements and reported good intratester (k = 0.79 to 0.90) and moderate intertester (k = 0.48 to 0.78) reliability. Scores on the tool correlated highly with Harris Hip Rating Scale scores (r = -.86).

Functional Independence Measure

The *Functional Independence Measure* (FIM) was created as part of a project funded by the National Institute of Handicapped Research (NIHR), designed to develop the Guide for a Uniform Data Set for Medical Rehabilitation.[80] The FIM is an 18-item measure that examines elements of a patient's physical, psychosocial, and social function. The FIM is now proprietary, and is the trademark (FIM™) of the Uniform Data System for Medical Rehabilitation, a division of the University of Buffalo Foundation Activities, Inc. (see Chapter 8, Examination of Function, for further discussion of the FIM). The FIM Locomotion: Walk/Wheelchair Guide is the portion of the document titled *Guide for the Uniform Data Set (Including the FIM™ instrument)* related to gait and includes a seven-point level of assistance rating scale ranging from complete independence to total assistance (Table 7.9). A study designed to evaluate the accuracy of clinical judgments of patient functioning found that bias and poor judgment of a

Table 7.9	The Functional Independence Measure (FIM™) Instrument Seven-Point Scoring System for Locomotion—Version 5.1

LOCOMOTION: WALK/WHEELCHAIR: Includes walking, once in a standing position, or if using a wheelchair, once in a seated position, on a level surface. Performs safely. Indicate the most frequent mode of locomotion (Walk or Wheelchair). If both are used about equally, code: "Both."

NO HELPER

7 Complete Independence—Subject walks a minimum of 150 ft (50 m) without assistive devices. Does not use a wheelchair. Performs safely.

6 Modified Independence—Subject *walks* a minimum of *150* ft (50 m) but uses a brace (orthosis) or prosthesis on leg, special adaptive shoes, cane, crutches, or walkerette; takes more than reasonable time or there are safety considerations. *If not walking,* subject operates manual or motorized wheelchair independently for a minimum of *150* ft (50 m); turns around; maneuvers the chair to a table, bed, toilet; negotiates at least a 3% grade; maneuvers on rugs and over door sills.

5 Exception (Household Ambulation)—Subject walks only short distances (a minimum of *50* ft or 17 m) *independently* with or without a device. Takes more than reasonable time, or there are safety considerations, or operates a manual or motorized wheelchair independently only short distances (a minimum of *50* ft or 17 m).

HELPER

5 Supervision
If walking, subject requires standby supervision, cueing, or coaxing to go a minimum of *150* ft (50 m).
If not walking, requires standby supervision, cueing, or coaxing to go a minimum of *150* ft (50 m) in wheelchair.

4 Minimal Contact Assistance—Subject performs 75% or more of locomotion effort to go a minimum of *150* ft (50 m).

3 Moderate Assistance—Subject performs 50% to 74% of locomotion effort to go a minimum of *150* ft (50 m).

2 Maximal Assistance—Subject performs 25% to 49% of locomotion effort to go a minimum of *50* ft (17 m). Requires assistance of one person only.

1 Total Assistance—Subject performs less than 25% of effort, or requires assistance of two people, or does not walk or wheel a minimum of *50* ft (17 m).

Comment: If the subject requires an assistive device for locomotion (wheelchair, prosthesis, walker, cane, AFO, adapted shoe, and so forth), the Walk/Wheelchair score can never be higher than level 6. The mode of locomotion (Walk or Wheelchair) must be the same on admission and discharge. If the subject changes mode of locomotion from admission to discharge (usually wheelchair to walking), record the admission mode and scores based on the *more frequent mode of locomotion at discharge.*

From The Uniform Data System for Medical Rehabilitation, a division of UB Foundation Activities, Inc. (UDS$_{MR}$^{SM}). Guide for the Uniform Data Set for Medical Rehabilitation (Including the FIM™ Instrument), Version 5.1, Buffalo: UDSMR, 1997, with permission.

patient's functional level played a significant role in 50 rehabilitation professionals' ratings of patient functioning. The authors of the study suggested that blind ratings of the FIM and training in eliminating bias would improve accuracy.[81]

Functional Assessment Measure

The 12-item *Functional Assessment Measure* (FAM) was developed by a multidisciplinary group of clinicians at Santa Clara Valley Medical Center, San Jose, California,[58] to provide a measure of disability that reflected the communication, psychosocial adjustment, and cognitive functions of the populations of individuals who sustained traumatic brain injury (TBI) and stroke. The FAM uses a seven-point rating scale modeled after the FIM to examine the individual's level or degree of independence, amount of assistance required, use of adaptive or assistive devices, and percentage of tasks completed successfully (Table 7.10).[82]

The 12 items of the FAM have been combined with the 18-item FIM to produce the FIM + FAM with the intent of providing more detailed data for TBI[59] and stroke populations. The FIM and FIM + FAM total scales

are psychometrically similar measures of global disability whereas the Barthel Index, FIM, and FIM + FAM motor scales are similar measures of physical disability.[83] However, in a study of 376 patients with stroke in Canadian inpatient rehabilitation units who were concurrently given

Table 7.10	The Functional Assessment Measure (FAM) Items
1. Swallowing	7. Emotional Status
2. Car Transfer	8. Adjustment to Limitations
3. Community Access	9. Employability
4. Reading	10. Orientation
5. Writing	11. Attention
6. Speech Intelligibility	12. Safety Judgment

The 12 items of the FAM are not designed to stand alone but to be added to the 18 items of the FIM to produce the FIM + FAM.

Courtesy of Santa Clara Valley Medical Center (1998). The Functional Assessment Measure. The Center for Outcome Measurement in Brain Injury. Retrieved June 14, 2011, from http://tbims.org/combi/FAM.

the FIM and the FAM, the results of a Rasch analysis showed that in the motor domain, only the FAM community access item was more difficult for subjects to accomplish than the FIM items. In the cognitive domain, the only FAM item that extended the range of the FIM was the one assessing employability. In light of the results, Linn et al[84] concluded that adding the FAM items to the FIM reduced test efficiency and provided only minimal protection against ceiling effects of the FIM.

Community Balance and Mobility Scale

The *Community Balance and Mobility Scale*[52] was developed to evaluate balance and mobility skills in individuals who have experienced mild to moderate TBI. The scale consists of 13 items that include opportunities to assess multitasking (e.g., walking and looking at a target placed to the right or left), sequencing of movements (crouching to pick up an object from the floor and then continuing to walk), and complex motor skills (laterally and rapidly moving sideways by crossing one foot over the other and having to respond to unexpected commands to change direction). Six items are performed on both the right and left side, each of which is rated on a 6-point scale from 0 (poorest performance) through 5 (best performance).[52,60] Although the tool was developed specifically for assessment of individuals who have sustained mild to moderate TBI, it also has been used to measure balance and mobility in community-dwelling individuals following a stroke and in those with varying severity of chronic obstructive pulmonary disease (COPD).[52,60,61]

Gait Abnormality Rating Scale and Modifications

The *Gait Abnormality Rating Scale* (GARS)[62] was designed to distinguish nursing home residents with a recent history of two or more falls from a control group of residents without a recent fall history. The test developers selected 16 features of the gait cycle and a scoring system, in which the features are scored on a 0 to 3 rating scale (0 = normal, 1 = mildly impaired, 2 = moderately impaired, and 3 = severely impaired). Among the 16 features rated, arm-swing amplitude, upper extremity (UE) and LE synchrony, and guardedness best distinguished fallers from other subjects. The distinguishing features could be used to identify residents at risk for falling. Time, space, and resources are often very limited in nursing homes, and the only expenses involved in administering the GARS include purchase of a digital video recorder, recording media, and the therapist's time to film, review, and rate the digital recordings. However, the GARS does not provide information regarding the type of falls (trips, slips, losing balance) sustained by this population.[62] Therefore, it is not helpful in determining the cause of falls.

The *Modified GARS* (GARS-M), which is a seven-item version of the GARS, contains the following

variables: (1) variability, (2) guardedness, (3) staggering, (4) foot contact, (5) hip ROM, (6) shoulder extension, and (7) arm–heel strike synchrony. These variables were selected for inclusion because they were found to be the most reliable in the original GARS. Scoring is the sum of the seven items; the total score represents a rank ordering for risk of falling based on the number of gait abnormalities recognized and the severity of any abnormality identified. A higher score is associated with a more abnormal gait. Similar to the GARS, the GARS-M scores distinguished between older adults with a history of falling and those individuals who had no fall history. The GARS-M has been deemed a good predictor for persons at risk for falls.[25]

Dynamic Gait Index

The *Dynamic Gait Index* (DGI) was designed to examine the ability to adapt gait to changes in task demands. The tool was initially developed for use in community-dwelling older adults with balance and vestibular disorders,[85] but has since been used across a variety of ages and patient populations.[86] The DGI uses a 0 (severe impairment) to 3 (normal) scale to rate performance on eight items, including gait on even surfaces, gait while changing speeds, gait and head turns in a vertical or horizontal direction, stepping over obstacles, and gait with pivot turns and steps. Whitney et al[85] evaluated DGI scores and fall history in adults with vestibular disorders and reported that the odds of falling within the past 6 months were 2.58-fold higher with DGI scores of 19 or lower.[85] The tool has since been used to evaluate dynamic gait and balance in a variety of patient populations, including individuals with Parkinson disease,[87] stroke,[64] and multiple sclerosis.[88]

The *Four-Item Dynamic Gait Index* consists of only half of the original eight DGI items (i.e., gait on level surfaces, changes in gait speed, and horizontal and vertical head turn activities).[65] It is faster to administer and displays adequate capacity to differentiate between individuals with and without balance and vestibular disease.

Functional Gait Assessment

The *Functional Gait Assessment* (FGA) is another modification of the original eight-item DGI. It was developed to address some of the ceiling effect attributes of the DGI when used with individuals with vestibular disorders and to clarify instructions and operational definitions associated with administering the tool.[69] Seven of the eight original DGI tasks were preserved, and three new items were added: gait with a narrow base of support, ambulating backwards, and gait with eyes closed. In a study assessing age-referenced norms for FGA performance in independently living adults between the ages of 40 and 89 years, the tool was found to have excellent interrater reliability (ICC = 0.93).[68] In addition, intrarater reliability and interrater reliability were deemed adequate given seven physical therapists' and three physical therapist students' repeated ratings of six patients with vestibular disorders (total FGA score reliability: intrarater = 0.83; interrater = 0.84).[69] Use of a threshold FGA score of 20/30 or less correctly predicted the unexplained falls experienced by six participants during a 6-month follow-up period in a study of community-dwelling 60- to 90-year-olds.[67] However, the authors recommend use of a threshold score of 22/30 or less as a more conservative criterion for those at risk for falls. The FGA has been used in studies of specific patient populations, including Parkinson disease[66] and stroke.[70]

High-Level Mobility Assessment Tool

The *High-Level Mobility Assessment Tool* (HiMAT) was designed to measure high-level mobility skills required for employment and social roles, as well as leisure and sporting activities for younger adults recovering from a TBI.[73] The tool consists of 13 items, and requires only a stopwatch, a 14-step staircase, inked moleskin markers, a brick-size object, and a tape measure to complete.[71,72] Tasks assessed include walking (forward, backward, on toes, over an obstacle, in a figure 8), running, a run stop, skipping, hopping forward, bounding (affected and non-affected), and going up and down stairs with and without a railing. All items are marked on a five-point scale (0 = unable to perform to 4 = performing item normally) except for two stair items that are rated on a six-point scale (0 to 5). The maximum achievable score is 54. The tool is only appropriate for patients able to ambulate independently for at least 20 meters without an assistive device. Thus, it is most appropriate for higher-functioning patients, such as those in the latter stages of an inpatient rehabilitation program or already living in the community. Interrater reliability and test-retest reliability are high (both ICCs = 0.99).[74] Between-day testing scores demonstrated a small improvement over the 24 hours (1 point), suggestive of improved performance with test familiarity. This highlights the importance of allowing patients an opportunity to practice the test at least once before scoring.

The original 13-item HiMAT has been revised to a shorter, faster to administer version that includes only eight items: walk (forward, backward, toes, obstacle), run, skip, hop, and bound on the nonaffected LE.[76] One key difference between the two versions is that stair items were eliminated. This addresses a challenge clinicians experience when trying to administer the 13-item HiMAT test in environments lacking a 14-step staircase. Because it was the easiest item on the original scale, elimination of stairs is not expected to influence assessment of high-level mobility skills. However, it is possible that the tool may be more susceptible to a floor effect because it is less able to distinguish between abilities of more severely disabled individuals.

Fast Evaluation of Mobility, Balance, and Fear

The *Fast Evaluation of Mobility, Balance, and Fear* (FEMBAF) is another instrument designed to identify risk factors, functional performance, and factors that hinder mobility.[77] It consists of a 22-item risk factor questionnaire and an 18-item performance component, which includes, among other measures, stair ascent and descent, stepping over an obstacle, and one-legged standing. Di Fabio and Seay[77] reported that the FEMBAF served as a valid and reliable measurement of risk factors, functional performance, and factors that hinder mobility in their study of 35 community-dwelling older adults.

Figure-of-8 Walk Test

Many measures of overground walking focus primarily on gait performed along a straight path (e.g., the 5-meter walk test). In contrast, the *Figure-of-8 Walk Test* (F8W)[78] was developed to assess both curved and straight path walking in older adults with walking difficulties. The number of steps, total time, and smoothness of movement are examined as an individual completes a single figure-of-8 walk around two cones spaced 5 ft apart (Fig. 7.7). In a study of performance on the F8W in 51 older community-dwelling adults with walking difficulty, Hess et al[78] reported significant correlations between the time to complete the F8W and overground gait speed, the GARS-M score, select physical function and efficacy measures, step length and width variability, and measures of executive function (i.e., the Trail Making Test B, Trails B). The number of steps required to complete the F8W correlated significantly with gait speed, select physical function and efficacy measures, step width variability, and performance on the Trails B. Movement smoothness correlated significantly only with step width variability.

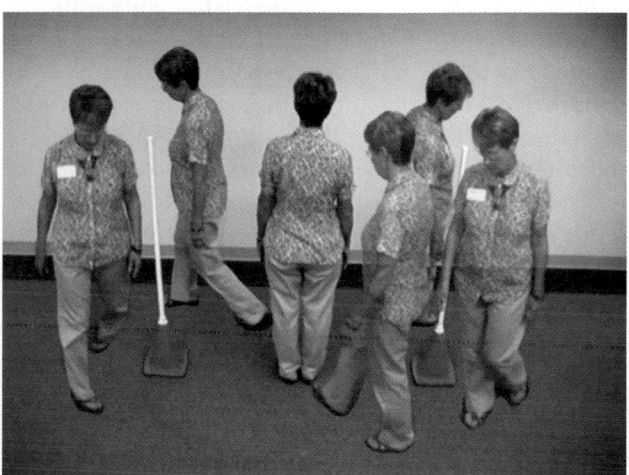

Figure 7.7 Individual performing the Figure-of-8 Walk Test, a tool developed to quantify walking ability in older adults with mobility disorders. Time to complete, number of steps, and smoothness of movement are used to score an individual's walking performance of a single figure-of-8 path around two cones spaced 5 feet apart.

Kinematic Quantitative Gait Analysis

Kinematic quantitative gait analysis is used to obtain information on spatial and temporal gait variables, as well as motion patterns. The data obtained through these analyses are quantifiable and therefore provide the therapist with baseline data that can be used to plan treatment programs and evaluate progress toward goals or goal attainment. The fact that the data are quantifiable is important because third-party payers are demanding that therapists use measurable parameters when examining patient function, establishing treatment strategies, and documenting outcomes. However, data derived from qualitative observations may be necessary to determine degrees of motor impairment and to determine the validity of the quantitative variables measured.

Spatial and temporal measures may be critical factors in determining a patient's independence in ambulation. For example, a patient may need to attain a certain gait speed to cross a local street within the time allotted by a crossing light, or a patient may need to walk a certain distance to shop in the local supermarket. In a study of walking capability of individuals greater than 3-months post-stroke, Perry et al[89] established that walking speed was a valid predictor of community walking status. Speeds of less than 79 ft/min (24 m/min) predicted household walking, and speeds between 79 and 157 ft/min (24 and 48 m/min) predicted limited community walking status. The ability to walk faster than 157 ft/min (48 m/min) predicted unlimited community walking. It is interesting to note that the mean velocity of the community ambulators was only 60% of the 262 ft/min (80 m/min) average velocity of typical, nondisabled adults.[32] This slower velocity is sufficient for many typical activities that individuals recovering from a stroke may need to perform, yet is less than the normal capacity required to cross a wide commercial street within the traffic signal time.[90] In a study by Graham et al[91] of 174 ambulatory adults 65 years of age and older who were admitted to a medical-surgical unit, an even slower walking velocity (69 ft/min [21 m/min]) was identified as a meaningful threshold to differentiate those capable of independent ambulation in a hospital setting from those requiring assistance.

Therapists need to survey the community to determine the distances and time requirements for accessing stores and public buildings before making a judgment about a patient's functional ambulation status. Robinett and Vondran[92] found that target goals on a sample of gait analysis forms were low compared to distance and velocity requirements for crossing the street found in a community survey. Walsh et al[93] reported that individuals 1 year after total knee arthroplasty (TKA) achieved more than 80% of the normal walking speeds of their age- and gender-matched counterparts. However, for 62% of the females and 25% of the males, the normal walking speed attained would not be sufficient to cross a street intersection safely.

Spatial and Temporal Variables

The variables measured in a quantitative gait analysis are listed and described in Table 7.11. Because spatial and temporal variables are affected by a number of factors such as age,[94-98] gender,[99,100] height and weight,[101,102] level of physical activity,[103,104] and level of maturation,[105] attempts have been made to take some of these factors into account. Ratios, such as stride-length divided by functional leg length, may be used to normalize for differences in patients' leg lengths. Step length divided by the subject's height is a method sometimes used to normalize differences among patients' heights. In an attempt to control for both height and weight, body weight is divided by standing height to yield the **body mass index** (BMI). Other ratios are used to assess symmetry, for example, right swing time divided by left swing time and swing time divided by stance time. Sutherland et al[105] listed the ratio of pelvic span to ankle spread as one of the determinants of development of mature gait in children.

Measurement of Spatial and Temporal Variables

The techniques and equipment required for measurement of spatial and temporal variables range from simple to complex. The time requirements also vary, and the therapist must be familiar with different methods of examining these variables in order to select the method most appropriate to each situation. Before selecting a measurement method, the therapist must understand the variable in question and how that variable is related to the patient's gait.

Simple Methods of Measuring Spatial and Temporal Variables

Measurement of spatial variables such as degree of foot angle, width of base of support (BOS), step length, and stride length can be determined simply and inexpensively by recording the patient's footprints during gait. Simple methods of recording footprints include either the application of paints, ink, or chalk to the bottom of the patient's foot or shoe. For example, ink-soaked patches[106] and felt-tipped markers[107] have been attached to the bottom or back of patient's shoes to measure variables such as step length, stride length, step width, and foot angle.

Another way of obtaining step length and stride length data is by placing a grid pattern on the floor.[108] Masking tape is placed on the floor to create a straight-line grid pattern about 1 ft (30 cm) wide and 32 ft (10 m) long. The tape is marked off in 1-in (3-cm) increments for its entire length, and the segments are numbered consecutively so that the patient's heel strikes can be identified. The therapist then calls out the heel strike locations from the numbers on the grid pattern into a tape recorder.

Many variables, such as velocity, stride length, step length, and cadence, may be calculated by using a stop watch to measure the elapsed time required for a

Table 7.11 Gait Variables: Quantitative Gait Analysis

Variable	Description
Speed	A scalar quantity that has magnitude but not direction.
Free speed	A person's normal walking speed.
Slow speed	A speed slower than a person's normal speed.
Fast speed	A rate faster than normal.
Cadence	The number of steps taken per unit of time (e.g., steps/minute).
	Cadence = Number of steps ÷ Time A simple method of measuring cadence is by counting the number of steps taken in a given amount of time. The only equipment necessary is a stopwatch, paper, and pencil. The average cadence of adult women (117 steps/min) is slightly higher than of adult men (111 steps/min).[3]
Velocity Linear velocity Angular velocity Walking velocity	A measure of a body's motion in a given direction. The rate at which a body moves in a straight line. The rate of rotation of a body segment around an axis. The rate of linear forward motion of the body. This is measured in either centimeters per second or meters per minute. To obtain a person's walking velocity, divide the distance traversed by the time required to complete the distance. Walking velocity = Distance ÷ Time Walking velocity may be affected by age, level of maturation, height, gender, type of footwear, and weight. Also, velocity may affect cadence, step, stride length, and foot angle as well as other gait variables. The average self-selected walking velocity of 20 to 85 year old males (86 m/min) is slightly faster than similar aged females (77 m/min).[32]
Acceleration	The rate of change of velocity with respect to time. Acceleration is usually measured in meters per second per second (m/s^2).
Angular acceleration	The rate of change of the angular velocity of a body with respect to time. Angular acceleration is usually measured in radians per second per second (radians/s^2).
Stride time	The amount of time that elapses during one stride; that is, from one foot contact (heel strike if possible) until the next contact of the same foot (heel strike). Both stride times should be measured. Measurement is usually in seconds.
Step time	The amount of time that elapses between consecutive right and left foot contacts (heel strikes). Both right and left step times should be measured. Measurement is in seconds.
Stride length	The linear distance between two successive points of contact of the same foot. It is measured in centimeters or meters. The average stride length for normal adult males is 1.46 meters.[32] The average stride length for adult females is 1.28 meters.[3]
Swing time	The amount of time during the gait cycle that one foot is off the ground. Swing time should be measured separately for right and left extremities. Measurement is in seconds.
Double support time	The amount of time spent in the gait cycle when both lower extremities are in contact with the supporting surface. Measured in seconds.
Cycle time (stride time)	The amount of time required to complete a gait cycle. Measured in seconds.
Step length	The linear distance between two successive points of contact of the right and left lower extremities. Usually a measurement is taken from the point of heel contact at initial contact of one extremity to the point of heel contact of the opposite extremity. If a patient does not have a heel strike on one or both sides, the measurement can be taken from the heads of the first metatarsals. Measured in centimeters or meters.
Width of walking base (step width)	The width of the walking base (base of support) is the linear distance (in the frontal plane) between one foot and the opposite foot. Measured in centimeters or meters.

Continued

Table 7.11 Gait Variables: Quantitative Gait Analysis—cont'd

Variable	Description
Foot angle (degree of toe out or toe in)	The angle of foot placement with respect to the line of progression. Measured in degrees.
Bilateral stance time (for the FAP)	The length of time up to 30 seconds that a person can stand upright in the parallel bars bearing weight on both lower extremities.
Uninvolved stance time (for the FAP)	The length of time up to 30 seconds that an individual can stand in the parallel bars while bearing weight on the uninvolved lower extremity (involved extremity is raised off the supporting surface).
Involved stance time (for the FAP)	The length of time up to 30 seconds that an individual can stand in the parallel bars on the involved lower extremity (uninvolved lower extremity is raised off the supporting surface).
Dynamic weight transfer rate (for the FAP)	The rate at which an individual standing in the parallel bars can transfer weight from one extremity to another. Measured in seconds from the first lift-off to the last lift-off.
Parallel bar ambulation (for the FAP)	Length of time required for an individual to walk the length of the parallel bars as rapidly as possible. Two trials are averaged to obtain this measurement. Measurement is in seconds.

FAP = Functional Ambulation Profile.

patient to walk a known distance and recording the number of right and left steps during that same period (see Table 7.11). If assessing variables across a short distance (e.g., 20 or 30 ft [6 or 10 m]), patients are often positioned a few steps before the "start line" so that they can achieve a steady state for the data collection.[75,106] They are also encouraged to walk a few steps beyond the "finish line." The "rolling start and finish" mitigates the influence of slow velocities at the initiation and termination of a walk on overall values compared to the "standing start and finish."[75]

Todd et al[98] tested 84 normal children (41 girls and 43 boys) ages 13 months to 12 years, and analyzed data from more than 200 other children ages 11 months to 16 years. A two-dimensional gait graph was developed that provides a visual record of a child's walking performance. Although the gait graph is similar in appearance to graphs used for height and weight, it shows norms for gait dimensions of cadence and stride length adjusted by height (Fig. 7.8).

Two relatively simple and standardized methods that have been used to quantify walking speed in the clinical setting are the *6-Minute Walk Test* (6MWT) and the *10-Meter Walk Test* (10MWT). A stopwatch and tape measure are the tools required to complete the tests. A form for recording temporal and spatial gait parameters is presented in Appendix 7.B.

6-Minute Walk Test

In the 6MWT,[109,110] the distance covered walking at a comfortable pace for 6 minutes is determined. Whereas the tool was initially used as a measure of endurance and

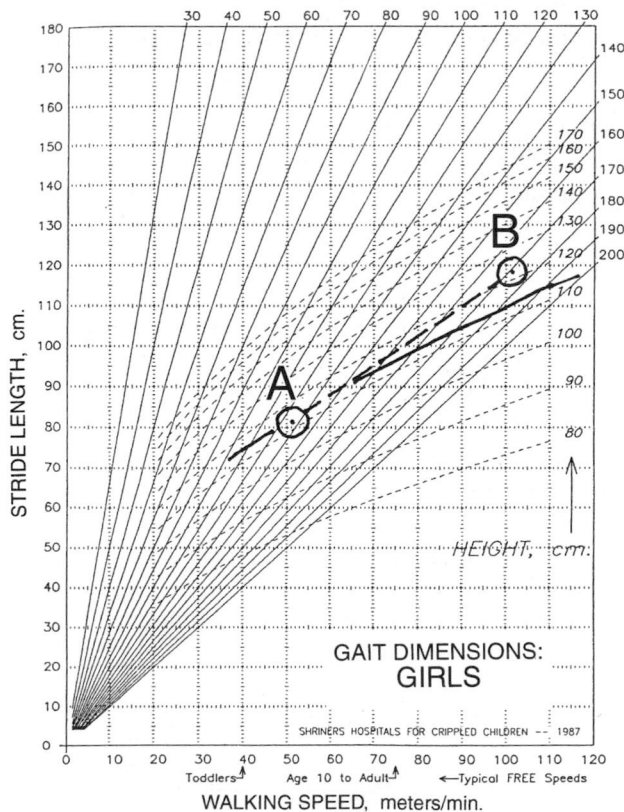

Figure 7.8 The solid line on the gait graph represents normal parameters for height. The dashed line represents data plotted for a normal 6-year-old girl whose height was 45 in (114 cm). A similar chart is available for boys. *(From Todd et al,[98, p. 201] with permission.)*

exercise capacity for individuals with cardiac and pulmonary pathology,[109,110] it has since been used to assess walking endurance in clients with a variety of underlying conditions, including Parkinson's disease,[111] acquired brain injury,[112] and stroke.[113] One protocol for performing the 6MWT includes asking clients to walk as far as they can at their usual pace for 6 minutes while using their customary assistive devices and orthotics.[114] Clients walk in a tight oval path around two chairs spaced 18 meters apart, facilitating calculation of the overall distance traveled. Participants stop and rest as needed, but the stopwatch continues. Standardized encouragement is provided periodically. The final distance walked (in meters) is divided by either 6 to determine average velocity in m/min or by 360 if reporting as m/sec.

This simple test, used in combination with other physical performance and impairment measures (e.g., ROM and muscle strength), can either monitor decline or evaluate improvement associated with treatment interventions. Mossberg[112] found that the 6MWT was a reliable measure of functional ambulation (distance walked) for patients with acquired brain injury. Fulk et al[113] identified that the 6MWT score served as a significant predictor of the average number of steps taken per day by community-dwelling individuals with chronic stroke, accounting for 46% of the variance in community walking activity.

Numerous prediction equations have been developed to estimate the expected 6-minute walk distance based on factors such as height, age, weight, and heart rate; however, these equations have accounted for only 20% to 78% of the variance in 6MWT distances in individuals without known disability.[115-122] Variations in the procedures used across studies, as well as variability in the ages studied, likely contributed to differences in predicted outcomes for the distance walked in 6 minutes. Factors that appear to improve reliability between testing sessions include standardizing the instructions given to the patient, the type and amount of verbal encouragement, and the location of testing (e.g., a long corridor or a circular track).[75,115,123] These factors, as well as other patient characteristics such as age, height, weight, and even ethnicity,[115,119,122] should be considered when comparing a patient's value to normative data.

Alternative tests for individuals with limited endurance include the *2-Minute Walk Test*[124,125] and *3-Minute Walk Test*.[63] A *12-Minute Walk Test* also is available for individuals with greater endurance.[110,124]

Timed Walk Tests (5 m, 10 m, and 30 m)

Timed walked tests measure how long it takes to walk a specified distance and then use these data to calculate an average walking speed. Different distances have been used, including 5 m,[126,127] 10 m,[125,128-130] and 30 m.[130] One common protocol for performing a 10-m timed walk test is to have the client ambulate across a 14-m walkway using his or her traditional assistive and LE orthotic devices.[114] The time (seconds) required to traverse

the middle 10 m of the walkway is recorded with a stopwatch. Two repetitions are completed at the client's preferred comfortable speed and at a fast pace. Speed (m/sec) is calculated by dividing 10 m by the time (in seconds) required to traverse the path. To determine speed in m/min, the previously calculated speed is multiplied by 60. Average cadence and stride length also can be calculated by recording the number of steps required to traverse the 10 m. Physiological responses (e.g., heart rate, blood pressure, respiratory rate) can be monitored immediately before and after the walking trial.

Despite efforts to standardize the test, some variability still is evident in the published literature, including the path taken (i.e., straight line versus a turn), use of assistive devices, speed (self-selected comfortable versus fast), and use of a rolling start and finish (i.e., capacity to take a few steps before and after start and finish lines, respectively) versus a standing start and finish.[75] Thus, when comparing a patient's speed to published normative data, consideration should be given to procedures used.

Low-Cost Instrumentation for Quantifying Spatial and Temporal Variables

Accelerometers During walking, the body generates forces that can be measured using an **accelerometer**. These data can then be used to calculate spatial and temporal gait features such as cadence, step symmetry, step duration, and stride duration. The methods for measuring the acceleration forces vary widely (e.g., strain gauge, piezoresistive, capacitive, and piezoelectric), but in general, many of these devices provide an affordable, noninvasive, easy to apply means for quantifying select gait characteristics over extended periods (days to weeks) in the home and community.[131]

Triaxial accelerometers have been attached to the trunk in order to measure mean acceleration, cadences, and step and stride lengths.[132-136] Accelerometers have also been attached to the head and pelvis to determine acceleration patterns of these anatomical regions while subjects walked on different surfaces.[137] Simultaneous use of multiple accelerometers has enabled successful differentiation of locomotor activities. For example, one system used five accelerometers (one on each foot and thigh, and one on the sternum) to differentiate walking speeds (slow, medium, and fast) and types of activities (e.g., walking, stair negotiation, running, and jumping) with a high level of accuracy (greater than 94%) in 69 participants free of any known impairments of the locomotor system.[138]

The accuracy of accelerometer data can be impacted by a number of factors.[131,138,139] Devices need to be oriented correctly in relation to the manufacturer's specifications, otherwise the acceleration signals may not correspond correctly with the direction of movement, and interpretation will be confounded. Significant adipose tissue, upper extremity (UE) movement to use assistive devices, or excessively loose mounting of the device can introduce movement artifact into the signal, again confounding interpretation. Finally, in patient populations, the acceleration signals may be altered if pathology disrupts normal foot-floor contact patterns or contributes to abnormal alignment of body parts (e.g., the impact of a persistent forward trunk lean on a trunk-mounted accelerometer in an individual with Parkinson's disease).[131]

The Step Watch Activity Monitor 3™ (SAM) is on example of a commercially available accelerometer.[140-144] It records the number of strides taken in 1-minute intervals during daily activities for up to 15 consecutive days. The SAM includes a sensor (custom accelerometer) that measures $0.30 \times 2 \times 0.80$ in ($7.5 \times 50 \times 20$ mm) and weighs approximately 1.3 oz (37 g) (Fig. 7.9). The battery provides up to 4 to 5 years of continual use.[145] The case is contoured to fit just above the lateral malleolus and is attached by an elastic strap. A personal computer is used to set up the SAM for monitoring, and also for downloading data to a computer file. Michael et al[141] used the SAM to evaluate the walking capacity of adults in the chronic phase of stroke recovery and identified significantly reduced step frequency (mean = 2,837 steps/day) compared to sedentary older adults (5,000 to 6,000 steps/day).

Gyroscopes *Gyroscopes* are another type of instrument that may be used for the estimation of spatial and temporal gait parameters. The gyroscope measures the Coriolis acceleration of a vibrating triangular prism. The signal from the prism is proportional to the angular velocity. The instruments are light, portable, and relatively inexpensive. A single uniaxial gyroscope attached on the skin surface of the lower leg can provide data for calculating cadence, determining number of steps, and estimating stride length and walking speed.[146]

Kotiadis et al developed an integrated system that included accelerometers, gyroscopes, and customized

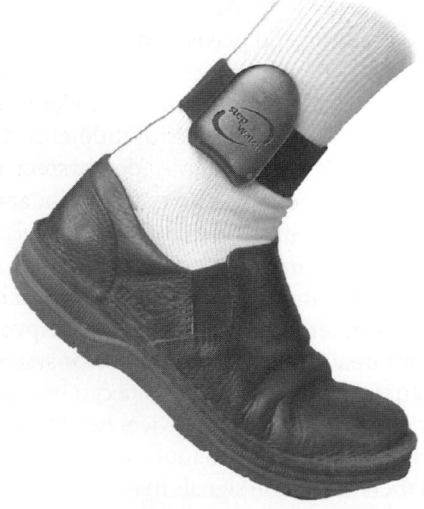

Figure 7.9 The Step Watch Activity Monitor 3® (SAM) is a pager-sized instrument worn at the ankle for long-term monitoring of gait function. *(Courtesy of CYMA Corp., Mountlake Terrace, WA 98043.)*

inertial algorithms to replace the footswitches often used to trigger drop foot stimulators.[147] Testing and refinement was performed for an individual after stroke who used a footswitch-driven drop foot stimulator. The combination of accelerometer and gyroscope data was sufficient for defining gait phases and controlling the drop foot stimulator during walking and stair negotiation activities.

Instrumented Systems for Determining Spatial and Temporal Gait Parameters

Examples of instrumented systems for measuring spatial and temporal variables include two walkways (GaitMat™ II and GAITRite®) and two footswitch systems (Krusen Limb Monitor and the Stride Analyzer). Manufacturer contact information for select equipment is presented in Appendix 7.C.

Walkways Compared to more complex systems that require cameras and footswitches, instrumented walkways provide a reliable, valid, and relatively affordable means for rapidly quantifying spatial and temporal gait parameters.[148-154] These portable devices are used by clinics and research facilities to help classify and quantify the severity of a patient's disability, and to guide and assess the effectiveness of treatment interventions. Two walkways widely available are the GaitMat™ II and the GAITRite®.

The GaitMat™ II is a commercially available walkway with embedded pressure-sensitive switches that open and close in response to contact with the patient's feet. The times of openings and closures of the switches are recorded by a computer that provides information on individual footprints; step and stride length; BOS; and step, swing, stance, single support, and double support times for each extremity. The main advantage of this system is that the patient is unencumbered by equipment attached to either the feet or body.

Barker et al[148] examined the reliability of measurements obtained using the GaitMat™ II and the Vicon motion analysis system and reported excellent reliability for temporal measures (0.99), but only poor reliability for spatial measurements (0.24). However, the difference between measurements acquired by the GaitMat™ II and the Vicon system was only 0.5 in (11.7 mm), suggesting that the level of precision would have little impact on most measurements except for BOS measurements. Bowen et al[155] found that the GaitMat™ II was able to detect decreases in velocity and increases in the percentage of double support in dual-task compared to single-task conditions in 11 patients with stroke.[155] Rosano et al[156] examined gray matter volume in the brains of 220 adults over age 65 and identified a number of significant relationships with measures recorded using the GaitMat™ II. In particular, shorter step lengths and longer double limb support times were associated with decreased volume in the sensorimotor and frontoparietal regions, whereas wider steps related to reduced size of the palladium and inferior parietal lobule.

The GAITRite® is another commercially available walkway system (Fig. 7.10). The 1/8-inch-thick, 2-foot-wide, 16-foot-long portable walkway in this system contains 18,482 sensors embedded between a sheet of vinyl and a layer of rubber. Spatial and temporal parameters can be measured, as well as dynamic pressure mapping of footprints during walking. The pressure parameters measured include peak pressure, pressure time, and sectional integrated pressure over time. The walkway system can be used with or without shoes, orthoses, or walking aids, and the GAITRite software is capable of calculating spatial and temporal parameters and displaying them in graphs and tables.

In general, the GAITRite® provides a valid means for reliably documenting many gait-related temporal and spatial parameters.[150,151,153] Bilney et al[153] reported high correlations between values recorded on the GAITRite® mat and those recorded using the Clinical Stride Analyzer® for walking speed (0.99), stride length (0.99), and cadence (0.99) for 25 healthy adults walking at three speeds (self-selected, slow, and fast). The reliability of repeated measures appears better at self-selected and fast speeds, compared to slower speeds.[153] Decreased consistency across measurements was documented for BOS[151,152] and toe in and toe out variables,[151,152] particularly in older adults.[152] Strong concurrent validity also has been reported for temporal and spatial gait measures recorded in outpatients recovering from strokes, even when the UE was engaged in using an assistive device.[149] Box 7.1 Evidence Summary provides an overview of selected reliability and validity studies performed using the GAITRite® mat.

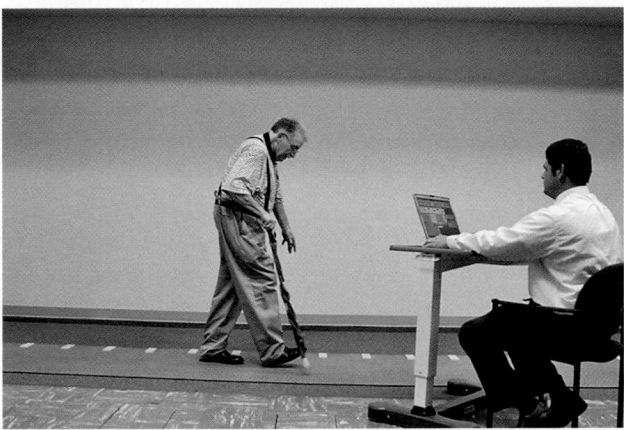

Figure 7.10 Individual with Parkinson's disease walking across the GAITRite® mat while temporal and spatial gait characteristics are recorded including walking velocity, stride length and duration, cadence, and step length and duration. *(Courtesy of Movement and Neurosciences Center, Institute for Rehabilitation Science and Engineering, Madonna Rehabilitation Hospital, Lincoln, NE 68506.)*

Footswitches and Footswitch Systems Footswitches are pressure-sensitive switches placed either on the patient's feet or the inside or outside of the shoes. The switches do not require a walkway, but the patient usually has to carry or wear a data collection device. Footswitches

---

Box 7.1 Evidence Summary   Studies Addressing the Reliability and Validity of Measures of Temporal and Spatial Gait Variables Using the GAITRite® System

Reference	Subjects	Design/Intervention	Results	Comments
Bilney et al[153] (2003)	25 healthy adults (13 males, 12 females; mean age = 40.5 years, range = 21–71 years).	The gait variables measured by the GAITRite® were compared with the same variables obtained with the Clinical Stride Analyzer (speed, cadence, stride length, right (R) and left (L) single leg support time and double support as a percentage of the gait cycle).	Intraclass correlation coefficients (ICCs) for speed (ICCs = 0.99), cadence (ICCs = 0.99), and step length (ICCs = 0.99) showed excellent agreement between the two systems for each speed condition (slow, preferred, and fast). Correlations between the two systems for single leg support time were moderate to high across speeds (ICCs = 0.69 to 0.91) in contrast to the weak correlations documented for double limb support times (ICCs = 0.44 to 0.57).	The authors concluded that the GAITRite® had strong concurrent validity and test-retest reliability for selected spatial and temporal variables in normal adults.

Continued

Box 7.1 Evidence Summary   Studies Addressing the Reliability and Validity of Measures of Temporal and Spatial Gait Variables Using the GAITRite® System—cont'd

Reference	Subjects	Design/Intervention	Results	Comments
McDonough et al[150] (2001)	Single subject: One healthy female with equal leg lengths.	To compare the concurrent validity and reliability of measures recorded with the GAITRite® (cadence, walking speed, R and L step and stride lengths, and R and L step times) to those documented with paper-and-pencil and video-based methods to determine concurrent validity and reliability as the participant walked at various rates and degrees of step symmetry. Additionally, a stride simulator (with predetermined step and stride lengths) was applied to the walkway to simulate 2 steps and 1 stride.	Excellent paper-and-pencil and GAITRite® spatial measure correlations (ICC > 0.95) and video-based and GAITRite® temporal correlations (ICC > 0.93) were reported.	The authors concluded that the GAITRite® was a valid and reliable tool for measuring selected spatial and temporal gait variables.
Menz et al[152] (2004)	Thirty younger adults (12 males, 18 females; mean age = 28.5 years, range 22–40 years) and 31 older adults (13 males, 18 females; mean age = 80.8 years, range = 76–87 years) without known pathology.	Test-retest reliability of temporal and spatial gait parameters was measured using the GAITRite® as subjects walked at a self-selected comfortable speed three times in one session and then repeated the process approximately 2 weeks later. ICCs and coefficients of variation (CV) were calculated.	Reliability of walking speed, cadence, and step length was excellent for younger and older adults (ICCs: 0.82 to 0.92; CVs: 1.4% to 3.5%). Base of support and toe in/out angles also demonstrated high ICCs (0.49 to 0.94); however, CVs were higher in both younger (CVs: 8.3% to 17.7%) and older adults (CVs: 14.3%–33.0%) compared to those calculated for walking speed, cadence, and step length (CVs: 1.4%–3.5% across variables and subject groups).	The authors concluded that the GAITRite® displayed excellent reliability for most temporal and spatial gait parameters in both study groups, but that base of support and toe in/out angles should be interpreted cautiously, particularly in older adults.
Stokic et al[149] (2009)	52 healthy adults (29 males, 23 females; mean age = 47 years, range = 23–87 years) and 20 individuals with chronic stroke (11 males, 9 females; mean age = 58 years, range = 16–90 years).	Gait characteristics (velocity, stride time and length, step length, percent single support, percent total support) were recorded simultaneously by the GAITRite® and an eight-camera motion analysis system as participants performed multiple walks at a self-selected speed.	Mean differences in calculated values between the two methods were ≤ 1.5% of the mean values calculated for each group. For example, healthy adults average gait velocity was 129.1 cm/sec based on GAITRite® calculations compared to 127.7 cm/sec for the motion analysis system. In persons with chronic stroke, the velocity values were 63.9 cm/sec and 63.4 cm/sec, respectively.	The authors concluded that the GAITRite® and motion analysis system provided comparable temporal and spatial measures in healthy adults and those recovering from a stroke.

Box 7.1 Evidence Summary Studies Addressing the Reliability and Validity of Measures of Temporal and Spatial Gait Variables Using the GAITRite® System—cont'd

Reference	Subjects	Design/Intervention	Results	Comments
van Uden and Besser[151] (2004)	Twenty-one adults (12 men, 9 women; mean age = 34 years, range: 19–59 years) without known lower extremity orthopedic disorders or pain that would affect their gait.	Test-retest reliability of GAITRite® temporal and spatial gait measures were recorded at participants' self-selected free and fast speeds on two occasions 1 week apart. Factors evaluated included walking speed, step length, stride length, base of support, step time, stride time, swing time, stance time, single and double support times, and toe in-toe out angle.	At the self-selected walking speed, all measurements had ICCs ≥ 0.92 except base of support (ICC = 0.80). At the fast speed all measurements had ICCs > 0.89 except base of support (ICC = 0.79).	The authors concluded that spatial-temporal gait measurements demonstrated good to excellent test-retest reliability over the 1-week period.
Webster et al[157] (2005)	Five males and five females (mean age = 66.5 years, range = 54–83 years) at least 121 months after unicompartmental knee replacement surgery	Individual step and averaged spatial and temporal variables obtained with the GAITRite® system were compared with the same variables recorded with the Vicon-512 3D motion analysis system.	Walking speed, cadence, step length, and step time variables averaged across one walk using each system revealed an excellent level of agreement between systems (ICCs = 0.92 to 0.99 across variables). No significant systematic differences were found between step length and step time values between the two systems.	The authors concluded that the GAITRite® is a valid tool for measuring both averaged and individual step gait variables. The small number of subjects is one drawback of this study plus the fact that all subjects walked without any problems that were linked to their surgery.

consist of transducers and a semiconductor and are used to signal such events as the heel contacting the ground. One type of footswitch device used to examine both temporal and loading variables is the *Krusen Limb Load Monitor*.[158] This device consists of a pressure-sensitive force plate that can be worn in a patient's shoe. It can be connected to a strip chart recorder to yield a permanent record of temporal and spatial gait variables.[158]

The *Stride Analyzer* is a footswitch system with special insoles containing four pressure-sensitive switches placed under the heel, the heads of the first and fifth metatarsals, and the great toe. The parameters measured by this system include stride length, velocity, cadence, cycle time, single and double limb support time, swing time, and stance time. These measurements are recorded automatically and the information is transmitted to a computer that analyzes

the data. The computer can also provide graphic displays of foot–floor contact patterns. Times are presented in seconds and as a percentage of the gait cycle. The computer analysis also includes a percentage of normal using a built-in database (Appendix 7.D). The advantages of the Stride Analyzer system are that measurements from both feet are available, the system is easy to move from place to place, and normative data comparisons are available because it has been used by a large number of physical therapists with different populations.[13-15,20,53,159-167]

The Stride Analyzer is suitable for use with various age groups as well as for patients with neurological or orthopedic involvement. For example, in a study by Mulroy et al,[18] footswitches were taped to the shoe bottoms of 30 individuals recovering from a stroke to assess the effects of three ankle-foot orthosis (AFO) designs on walking and to determine whether an ankle plantarflexion contracture influenced response to the orthoses. The conditions assessed included walking with usual footwear using three different AFOs, each with unique settings: (1) dorsiflexion assist with a dorsiflexion stop; (2) plantarflexion stop with free dorsiflexion; and (3) a rigid (solid) ankle. The footswitches were used not only to compare stride characteristics across conditions but also to help define gait phases for subsequent analysis of joint kinematics and muscle activation patterns (electromyography [EMG]). Gait parameters were compared across the orthotic conditions and between participants with and without moderate ankle plantarflexion contractures. The authors reported that individuals without a contracture benefitted from AFO designs that allowed stance phase dorsiflexion mobility (e.g., the plantarflexion stop with free dorsiflexion or the dorsiflexion assist with a dorsiflexion stop) as the rigid (solid) ankle inhibited forward progression of the tibia. Those with quadriceps weakness benefitted from an AFO with plantarflexion mobility during loading response (i.e., the dorsiflexion assist with a dorsiflexion stop) as knee flexion motion was diminished compared to the other two AFO conditions.

Powers et al[159] used the Stride Analyzer in an analysis of 22 individuals with transtibial amputations to determine the relationship between isometric muscle force and temporal and spatial gait parameters. Mean walking speed was limited to only 59% of normal, owing to reductions in both cadence (83% normal) and stride length (69% normal). Hip extensor torque of the residual limb served as the only predictor for both free and fast walking speeds. Hip abductor torque of the sound limb was the only predictor of cadence for free and fast walking speeds.

Evaluation of Joint Kinematics (Motion)

Electrogoniometers

Joint displacement can be measured relatively simply by using an electrogoniometer. Early electrogoniometer designs included two rigid links connected by a potentiometer that converted movement into an electrical signal that was proportional to the degree of movement. The rigid links or arms of the electrogoniometer were attached to the proximal and distal limb segments. More recent designs use a flexible shaft and two small end blocks that are affixed to the proximal and distal segments of the joint. The new design allows electrogoniometers to be worn under clothing for extended periods of recording time. Biometrics, Ltd., produces a wide variety of electrogoniometers, including twin-axis designs that simultaneously measure joint motion in multiple planes. Lam et al[168] used these devices to study hip (abduction/adduction) and knee (flexion/extension) during corrective stumbling responses to mechanical perturbations applied to the foot of healthy infants during treadmill stepping. The authors reported that

perturbations to the dorsum of the foot during swing resulted in an increase in flexor EMG activity and an increase in knee flexion during swing. Electrogoniometers provide an affordable means of measuring joint motion during walking.[32]

Video-Based Motion Analysis Systems

Two-dimensional (2D) and three-dimensional (3D) video-based motion analysis systems are available for gait analysis; however, their use is limited due to challenges with providing accurate data. Two-dimensional video-based systems use a single digital video camcorder to track subject motion. Computer software programs then assist with identifying points of reference. Unfortunately, joint angles that are out-of-plane (either because of rotation of the limb or due to the position of the individual relative to the camera) will not be calculated accurately. Three-dimensional video-based motion analysis systems use two or more digital video camcorders to gather 3D coordinate data. Hardware is used to synchronize data recorded from the various cameras, and postprocessing is used to identify points of reference either automatically or manually. Markers can be affixed to the skin to help identify anatomical landmarks. Though portable in nature, the accuracy of 2D and 3D video-based systems is a limitation.

Optical Motion Analysis Systems

Imaging-based systems are the most sophisticated and expensive methods of determining joint displacement and patterns of motion. In computerized motion analysis systems, markers placed on body segments such as the hip, knee, and ankle are tracked by automated systems. Motion analysis systems primarily use either *active* or *passive* markers for tracking motion.[31] *Active markers* are usually light-emitting diodes (LEDs) that flash at given frequencies.[169] Each marker is placed over a prespecified location and its individual frequency is used to identify the marker as it moves across space at each instant in time. To power the LED, the participant is either tethered by cable to a central power source or wears a power pack. Fine cables then extend between each LED and the power unit. LEDs are relatively expensive and the thin cables can break. One challenge to the automated labeling of active markers is that reflections from shiny floor surfaces can confound marker identification, particularly for markers located on the feet. Codamotion, Qualisys, and PheoniX Technologies Incorporated are three manufacturers that produce systems that use active markers.

Passive markers (Fig. 7.11) require an external source of illumination that may be provided by external light sources or a ring of infrared emitting diodes located around the lens of the camera. In the latter case, the diodes on the camera pick up the infrared light reflected

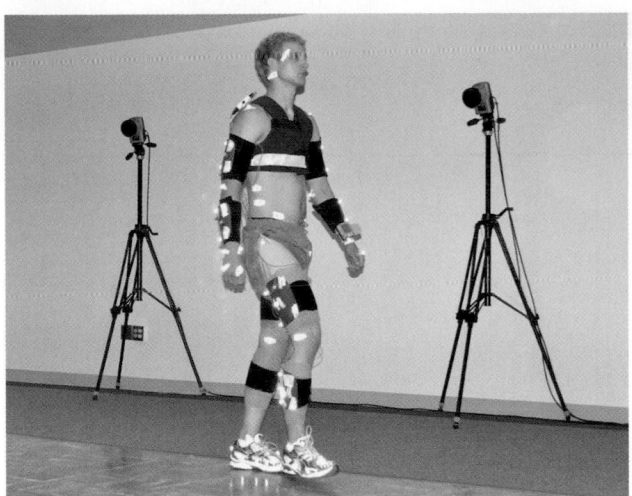

Figure 7.11 Oqus Series-3 cameras Qualisys track motion of passive reflective markers placed over known anatomical landmarks and in clusters on body segments as the subject walks along a 6-meter walkway. Marker data will be used to reconstruct joint motions of the upper extremities, trunk, and lower extremities throughout the gait cycle. *(Courtesy of Movement and Neurosciences Center, Institute for Rehabilitation Science and Engineering, Madonna Rehabilitation Hospital, Lincoln, NE 68506.)*

by the markers that they can "see," which means that a large number of cameras are necessary for obtaining unrestricted views of markers. Qualisys, Vicon, and Motion Analysis are three manufacturers that produce systems that use passive markers.

When the systems were first developed, visualization of passive markers was problematic, but now markers are automatically tracked and a computer performs thousands of computations. However, passive marker systems require many cameras, are expensive, and require training to operate the hardware and software. Figure 7.12 provides an example of a computer-generated display of kinematic data recorded using passive markers (Qualisys Motion Analysis System), as well as signals recorded from EMG sensors. In Figure 7.13, the degrees of motion for the ankle and knee are plotted against time. In Figure 7.14, stick figures are shown with accompanying knee angles.

A number of important problems still exist with the use of both active and passive marker systems. Obstruction of markers by body segments, skin/soft tissue motion, marker vibration, and improper placement of markers in relation to the joint center of motion can introduce potential errors. Determining the location of the hip joint center is particularly problematic. The

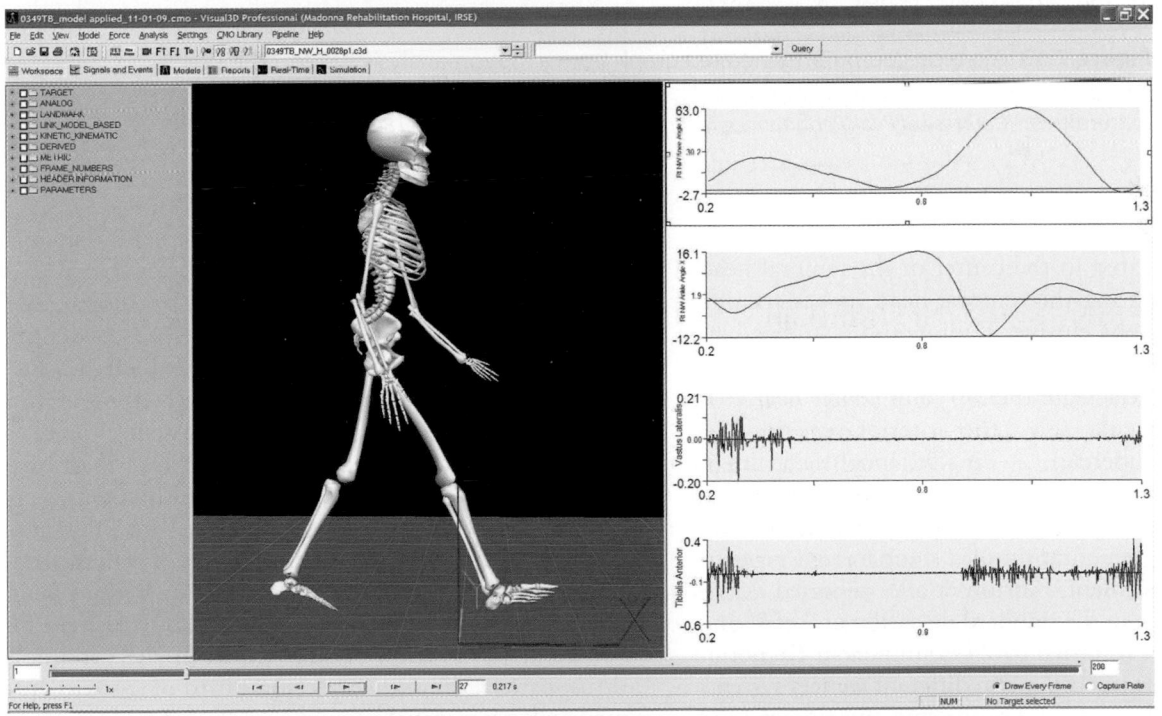

Figure 7.12 Visual 3D computer display of kinematic data recorded using the Qualisys Motion Analysis System and surface electromyographic data recorded using the MA-300 EMG system during overground gait for a 31-year-old male. Reflective markers, applied over known locations, provided the anatomical reference for displayed skeleton and for subsequent analysis of joint motions. To the right of the skeleton, sagittal plane joint motions for the knee and ankle are displayed in the top two rows while surface EMG data for the vastus lateralis and tibialis anterior are displayed in the bottom two rows. *(Courtesy of Dr. Yu Shu, Movement and Neurosciences Center, Institute for Rehabilitation Science and Engineering, Madonna Rehabilitation Hospital, Lincoln, NE 68506.)*

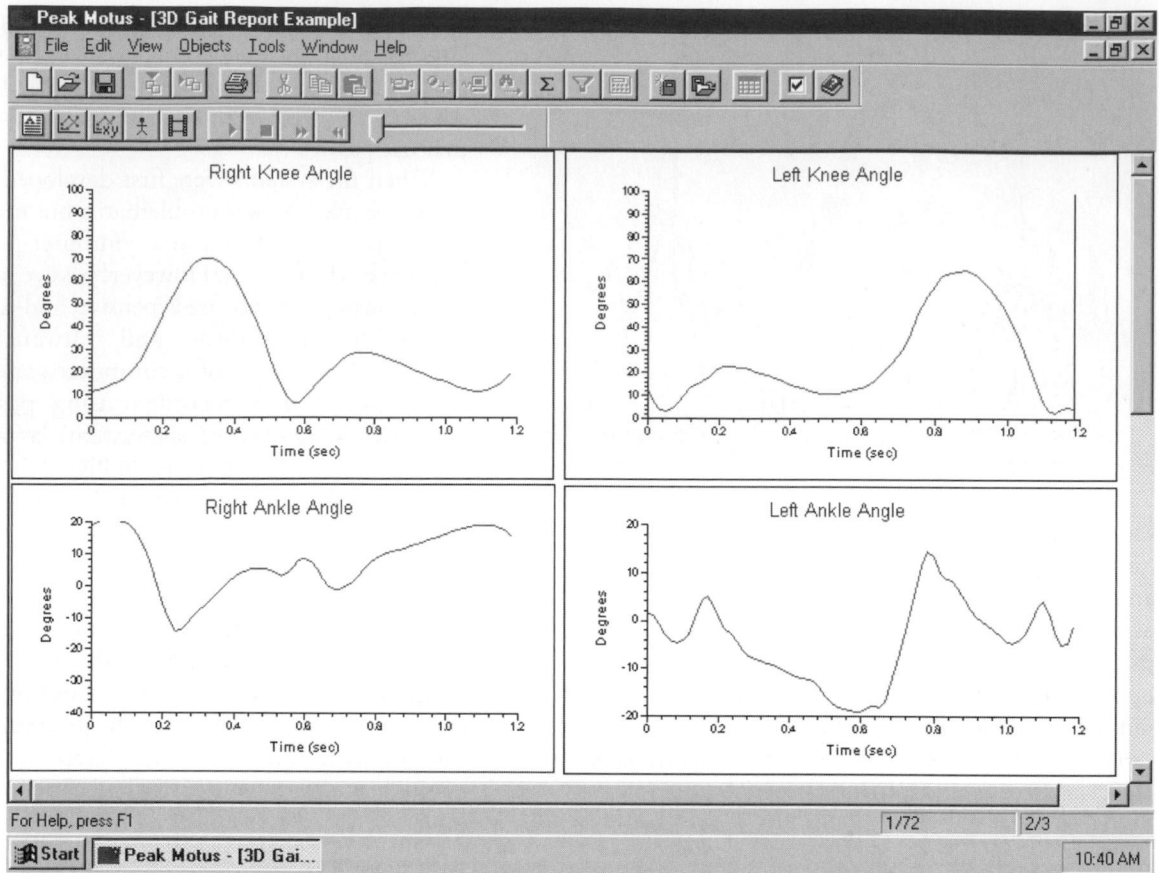

Figure 7.13 A typical computer-generated graph from a motion-analysis system. The graph shows knee and ankle range-of-motion patterns, which are plotted against time for both lower extremities. *(Courtesy of Peak Performance Technologies, Inc., Centennial, CO 80112.)*

ball-and-socket anatomy means that the center of the hip joint is located in the center of the femoral head. Difficulty palpating the femoral head makes accurate marker placement elusive. Radiographic studies have been performed to develop and refine algorithms that can be used to calculate the hip joint center relative to palpable landmarks (e.g., the anterior superior iliac spine, pubic tubercle).[170] Finally, inconsistencies in marker placement have been identified as one of the leading sources of variability in kinematic findings.[171] Following implementation of a standardized protocol for marker placement, Gorton et al[171] reported a 20% average decrease in the standard deviation of 7 of 9 kinematic measures recorded by 24 examiners in 12 motion analysis laboratories using two different camera systems.

As affordable computer processing and storage capabilities rapidly expand, the varying motion analysis products on the market also are evolving. Many video-based systems currently available are able to track markers to within 0.04 in (1 mm) of accuracy, enabling relatively precise tracking of the markers.[172] Most systems have the capacity to integrate with other technology enabling simultaneous acquisition of relevant gait data such as footswitches to identify foot-floor contact patterns and

stride characteristics, EMG systems to examine muscle activation patterns, and force plates to determine ground reaction forces. EMG, when recorded simultaneously with stride characteristics data, can be used to identify the particular portion of the gait cycle in which the muscle activity occurs. An example of how EMG is used in combination with a motion analysis system (Vicon) is presented in Figure 7.15. The figure shows the EMG output and ROM on the graph while the computer-generated figures provide a visual image. The differences in muscle activity among the three types of walking patterns are easily seen in the graphs. The deviations from normal ROM at the knee are also easy to identify. A careful observation of the figures in the extension thrust pattern shows an extension thrust of the knee immediately after initial contact and excessive plantarflexion at the ankle both at heel strike and throughout the gait cycle. Refer to Chapter 5, Examination of Motor Function: Motor Control and Motor Learning, for a more detailed discussion of EMG.

Key differentiating features among motion analysis systems include price, marker system options (e.g., active, passive, or both active and passive), and the capabilities and efficiency of postprocessing software. A number

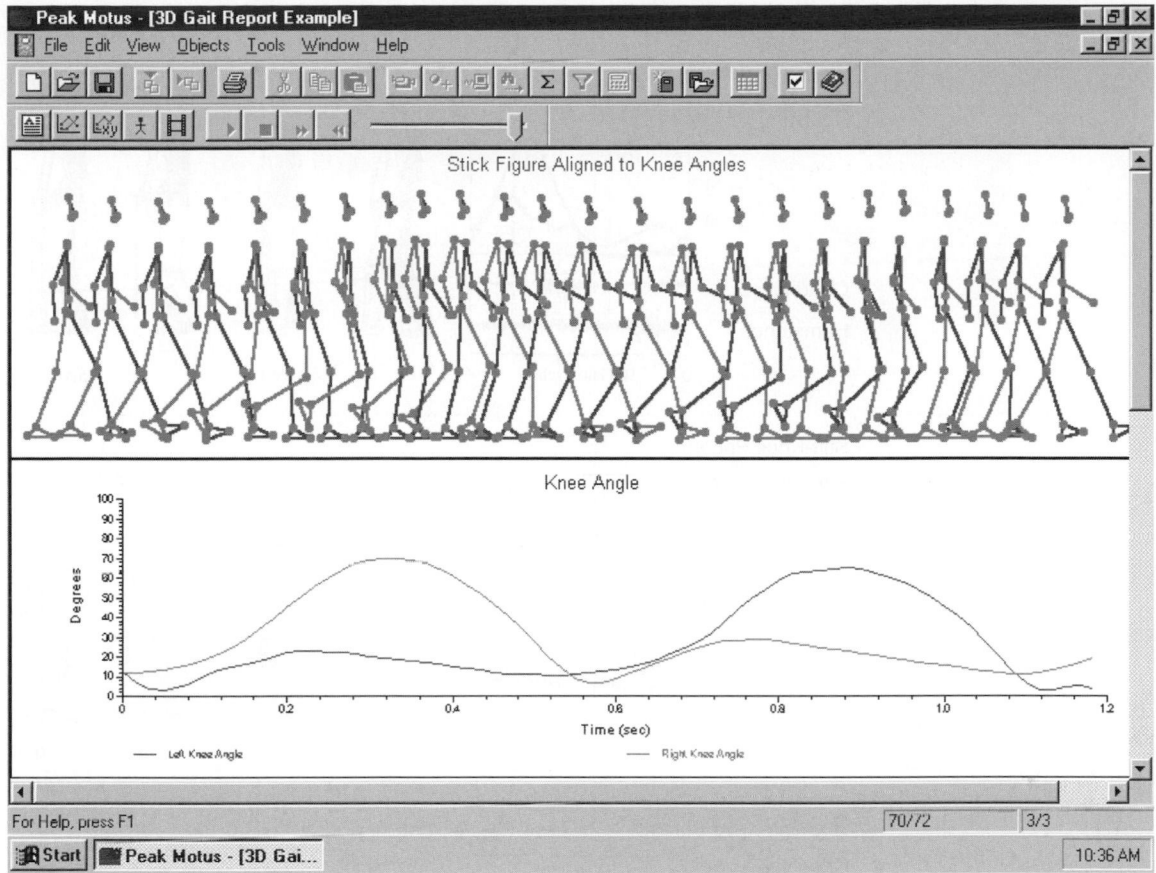

Figure 7.14 Another format for presentation of the data from a motion-analysis system is computer-generated stick figure representations of one complete gait cycle. In this particular case, the pattern of knee motion is graphically presented below the stick figures. *(Courtesy of Peak Performance Technologies, Inc., Centennial, CO 80112.)*

of systems provide manufacturer-generated analysis software that is relatively easy to learn; however, it may be difficult to modify/customize the software to meet the needs of more elaborate studies. Report-generating capabilities differ notably across systems as well, and should be considered depending on the expectations of the laboratory or clinic (e.g., need to produce rapid, easily interpretable reports for inclusion in patient charts versus export of data for statistical analysis for research purposes). Appendix 7.C includes a list of gait analysis software and hardware manufacturers and their contact information. Given the evolving nature of technology, the reader is encouraged to visit the websites provided for the most up-to-date information about the capabilities of different systems.

Electromagnetic Motion Analysis System

One challenge with optical tracking systems is that the motion analysis cameras need to be able to "see" the markers to track their position and subsequently calculate kinematic data. This can be difficult when clients use multiple assistive devices or require substantial physical assistance from one or more therapists to navigate the walkway. An alternative motion analysis technology employs electromagnetic tracking capabilities to determine the 3D coordinates of location and angulation of each sensor. Flock of Birds®, Nest of Birds®, and MotionStar®, all manufactured by Ascension Technology, and FASTRAK® manufactured by Polhemus, are examples of electromagnetic motion analysis technology. MotionStar® allows tracking of up to 120 sensors simultaneously, thus the capacity to perform motion analysis on more than one subject simultaneously. To date, few studies have been published that used electromagnetic motion analysis technology to study gait-related activities.[173,174] The equipment has garnered a following in the virtual reality environments and animation industry.

Kinetic Gait Analysis
Kinetic Variables

Kinetic gait analyses are directed toward determination and analysis of the forces involved in gait, including **ground (floor) reaction forces** (GRFs), joint torques, **center of pressure** (COP), **center of mass** (**COM**), mechanical energy, moments of force, power, support

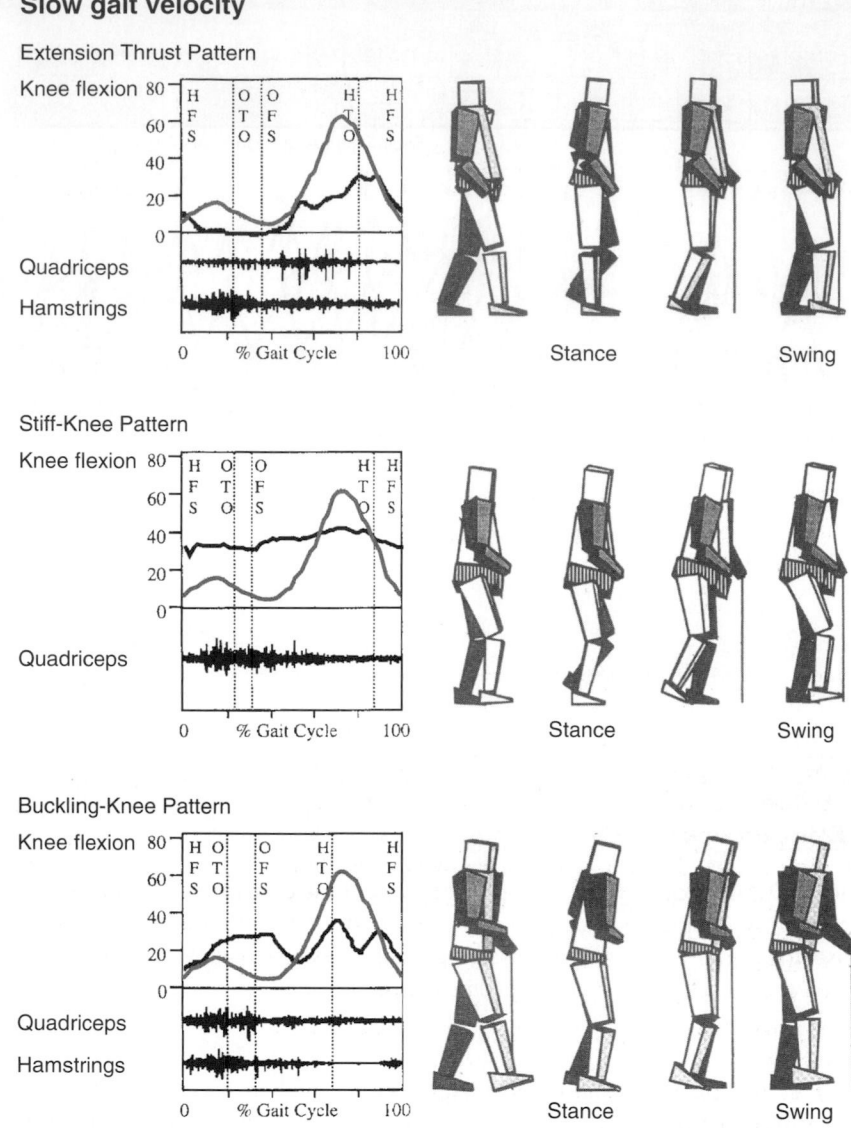

Figure 7.15 Graphs and EMG data for motion of the knee in the sagittal plane for one gait cycle of the three motion patterns. Each patient represents only one of the three motion patterns (extension thrust, stiff knee, and buckling knee) associated with a slow gait velocity. The solid dark red line indicates the motion pattern and the lighter red line represents the normal. HFS, foot strike (initial contact) on the hemiplegic side; OTO, toe off on the contralateral (unaffected) side; OFS, foot strike (initial contact) on the contralateral (unaffected) side; HTO, toe off on the hemiplegic side. *(From De Quervain et al,[6] with permission.)*

moments, work, joint reaction forces, and intrinsic foot pressure (Table 7.12). Although in the past kinetic gait analyses have been used primarily for research purposes, at the present time they are being used clinically as well. Given the risk of foot ulcers arising from high plantar pressures in individuals with diabetic sensory neuropathy, some clinicians are using special pressure mapping insoles to determine if clients may be at risk for developing an ulcer. A patient walks while wearing the special insoles and the pressures are recorded. If high pressures are identified on the bottom of the foot, patients may

be referred to have special orthotics and/or shoes fabricated to help redistribute the pressures.

The instrumentation required to examine kinetic variables is complex and expensive because derivation of kinetics requires knowledge of all of the forces acting on the part of the body analyzed (e.g., the foot or the thigh). The analysis usually starts with the forces being applied to the foot, which is determined by a **force plate** embedded in the floor. These plates contain load transducers that measure the **center of pressure (COP)**, COM, and GRFs during gait. Typically, the force

Table 7.12	Gait Variables: Kinetic Gait Analysis
Ground reaction forces	Vertical, anterior-posterior, and medial-lateral forces created as a result of foot contact with the supporting surface. These forces are equal in magnitude and opposite in direction to the force applied by the foot to the ground. Ground reaction forces are measured with force platforms in newtons (N) or pound force.
Pressure	Pressure = force per unit area. In gait analysis, the parameters that are usually measured include the peak pressure, the pressure-time integral, and the overall pattern of pressure distribution under the foot.
Center of pressure (COP)	The point of application of the resultant force. Movement of the COP as a function of time is used as a measure of stability of a subject who is either standing or walking on a force plate.
Torque (moment of force)	The turning or rotational effect produced by the application of a force. The greater the perpendicular distance from the point of application of a force from the axis of rotation, the greater the turning effect, or torque, produced. Torque is calculated by multiplying the force by the perpendicular distance from the point of application of the force and the axis of rotation. Torque = force × perpendicular distance or moment arm

plates are based on either strain gage or piezoelectric technology.

Calculation of kinetic variables at the ankle requires knowledge of the forces acting on the foot, body mass, and location of the COM (derived from standard anthropometric tables), and knowledge about the acceleration of the COM. Once this knowledge is obtained, equations can be developed to calculate the net forces and net moments occurring at the ankle, at that particular instant in time, in order for the foot to have moved with those particular accelerations. Once forces and moments at the ankle are determined, similar equations can be applied to the adjacent proximal segment (lower leg). One then knows, for each instant in time, whether the dominant internal moment is being caused by the dorsiflexors or the plantarflexors. If the internal moment for each instant in time is multiplied by the net angular velocity between the ankle and the lower leg, the result is knowledge of the net power being produced by the muscles across the ankle. Concentric contractions add power to the limb (power generation), and eccentric contractions reduce power (power absorption). Variations in expected patterns of power generation and absorption are particularly useful in identifying deficiencies and in determining treatment goals. Unfortunately, a detailed explanation of the calculation of COM, COP, and moments and power is beyond the scope of the current chapter. Readers interested in learning more about these concepts are referred to a book written by David Winter included on the supplemental reading list.

The GRF is defined as the net vertical and shear (or horizontal) forces acting between the foot and the supporting surface. The force is three-dimensional and can be resolved into three components: vertical, anterior–posterior, and medial–lateral (Fig. 7.16). Each component varies throughout the gait cycle and is affected by velocity,

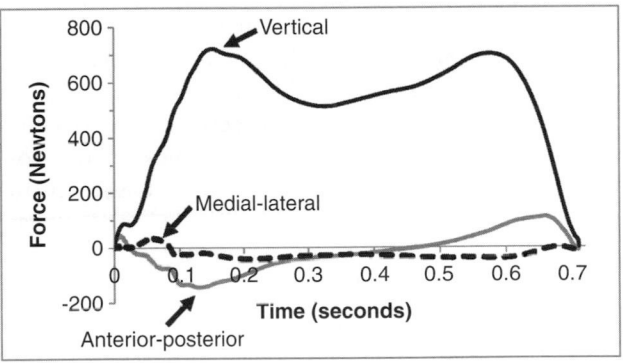

Figure 7.16 Computer-generated graph of the vertical, anterior-posterior and medial-lateral components of the ground-reaction force obtained as an adult walks across an AMTI force plate. *(Courtesy of Movement and Neurosciences Center, Institute for Rehabilitation Science and Engineering, Madonna Rehabilitation Hospital, Lincoln, NE 68506.)*

cadence, and body mass. The averaged wave forms of the vertical and anterior–posterior force components, presented as a percentage of body weight, show consistent patterns across normal subjects for loading rate, peak force, average force, and unloading rate. The vertical force waveform shows a characteristic double hump. The anterior–posterior force has a characteristic negative phase (representing deceleration of the body's mass after the foot hits the ground) followed by a positive phase (reflecting acceleration as body mass moves forward in late stance). In the frontal plane, an initial laterally directed GRF peaks shortly after initial contact. This is most commonly followed by an extended medially directed GRF.

Friction is required while walking and acts in the opposite direction of the desired motion. For example, during loading response, the foot imparts of forward (anterior) shear force onto the floor as body weight loads onto the limb. Friction resists the tendency of the foot to slip forward. An individual's friction needs during walking, sometimes referred to as *utilized* or *required friction,* can be measured as an individual walks across a force plate. It is calculated as the ratio of the individual's shear (resultant of the anterior–posterior and medial–lateral forces) and vertical GRF components. When an individual's walking friction needs exceed the friction available at the foot-floor interface, a slip is likely to occur.[27,175,176] A tribometer is a device used to measure the friction available on different floor surfaces and in the presence of contaminants (e.g., water or oil). Some floor manufacturers will report on the slip resistance of the surfaces they distribute (e.g., different types of tile). Floor surfaces with a higher available friction (as measured by a tribometer) are generally more slip resistant.

Instruments for Measuring Kinetic Variables

Force Plate Technology

Force plate technology, such as that produced by both Kistler Instrument Corp. and Advanced Mechanical Technology, Inc. (AMTI), is capable of measuring the GRF, as well as calculating the COM, **acceleration, velocity, displacement, power,** and **work.** A graphic display is possible showing the waveforms of the GRF. Kistler Instrument Corp. also markets a treadmill called the Gaitway. The treadmill is capable of measuring the GRF and COP during both walking and running. In addition to graphical presentation and statistical functions, the treadmill system can calculate temporal and spatial parameters.

Cook et al[177] used a force plate to investigate the effect of a knee flexion restriction (using a brace) and walking speed on the GRF. The authors concluded that the application of a brace to restrict knee flexion for the purpose of protection after injury, or while surgically repaired structures were healing, may actually increase the stress on both the braced and unbraced limbs.

Hesse et al[178] compared the trajectories of the COP and the COM in 10 healthy individuals and 14 subjects with hemiparesis. They found that the healthy subjects showed no differences in the behavior of the COP, COM, temporal parameters, and step length when initiating gait with either the right or left extremity. In comparison, patients with hemiparesis showed pronounced asymmetric behavior depending on which limb was the starting limb (affected vs. less affected). Whereas patients who initiated gait with the affected limb were similar to healthy subjects, patients who started gait with the less affected limb showed inconsistent movement of the COP and were incapable of producing directional movement of the body's COM. This suggests therapists should be cautious about promoting that type of gait initiation because the affected leg may be too weak to support starting gait with the less affected LE. Rossi et al[7] investigated the COM, COP, and GRF in a study of

gait initiation in patients with transtibial amputations. These authors found that the patients consistently loaded the intact limb more than the prosthetic limb regardless of which limb initiated gait.[7]

Force plates may be used either as part of, or in combination with, motion analysis systems and temporal and spatial analysis systems, as well as in conjunction with EMG and electrogoniometry, for a comprehensive analysis of kinematic and kinetic gait variables. Perry et al[13] incorporated simultaneous recording of GRFs, joint motions, and LE muscle activation patterns to explore an apparent paradox related to the efficiency of toe walking and potential need for therapeutic intervention. Previous researchers identified a lower internal plantarflexor moment during toe walking compared to traditional heel-toe gait and suggested that the plantarflexed foot provided a potential compensatory advantage by reducing the need for plantarflexor strength.[179] However, the earlier researchers had not included measurements of muscle activation (EMG) in their study. The inclusion of EMG into Perry et al's follow-up study,[13] as well as subsequent modeling studies[180,181] of the biomechanical demands of toe walking, highlighted the source of the apparent paradox. Although the internal moments were lower,[13] plantarflexor muscle activation (mean and peak) actually increased because of the biomechanically inefficient position associated with maintaining a plantarflexed foot (less than optimal length–tension of the plantarflexors).[180] The plantarflexed foot also created the need for compensatory adjustments in muscle activation at more proximal joints.[181] This series of studies highlights a potential limitation of using only kinematic and kinetic data to interpret muscle activation patterns; that is, various patterns of muscle co-activation can create the same internal moment. In addition, when a muscle is at an inefficient position on the length–tension curve, it may require greater activation to generate the same internal moment compared to the demands when more optimally aligned.

Plantar Pressure Measurement Systems

Pressure measurement systems may also be used with force plates. Pressure is equal to force divided by area, and is measured by pressure sensors. Therefore, pressure is equal to the force on the sensor divided by the area of the sensor. Plantar pressure measurements are used most commonly in gait analysis to determine the pressure distribution under the foot: foot-to-ground contact, foot-to-shoe contact, and shoe-to-ground contact. Pressure measurements may be used to determine orthotic efficacy, ulceration risk in diabetes, and for regulating weight-bearing following surgery. Many different types of measurement techniques have been developed for measuring contact pressures. Tekscan Inc. has a system called the *F-Scan® Bipedal In-Shoe Plantar Pressure/Force Measurement System* that measures bipedal plantar pressures using paper-thin disposable pressure sensors placed in a patient's shoes. The sensor is ultrathin, flexible, and can be trimmed to fit; it includes 960 sensing locations distributed across the entire plantar surface. An example of the type of information obtained from the F-scan system is presented in Figure 7.17. Reliability of the F-scan system was determined by Randolph et al[182] to be sufficient for the purpose of designing corrective measures to relieve excessive pressures on the foot. Another system produced by Tekscan, Inc., is called *Mat-Scan System*®, which is a pressure-sensing floor mat that allows the clinician to identify barefoot pressures. Mueller et al[183] used the *F-Scan System* to determine how footwear design impacted plantar pressures in 30 individuals with transmetatarsal amputations who were at risk for additional amputations owing to a history of diabetes. Though all footwear designs reduced plantar pressures under the distal portion of the residual foot compared to traditional footwear with a toe-filler, the most effective design included a full-length shoe with a total contact custom-molded Plastazote insert and a rigid rocker bottom sole. This work has important clinical implications given the high incidence of additional amputations in those with diabetes who have already lost a portion of one limb.[184] Armstrong et al[185] found that patients who have high plantar pressures and wounds greater than 3.12 in (8 cm) took significantly longer to heal than other patients.

Novel Electronics' pedar® and emed® pressure mapping systems provide alternative means for examining pressures. The *pedar*® system consists of insoles (in a variety of lengths and widths) that can be placed inside shoes to measure plantar pressures. Each pressure insole consists of a 0.08 in (2 mm) thick array of 99 capacitive pressure sensors used to calculate a variety of measures including peak pressures, mean pressures, contact area, and pressure-time integral. The insoles can also be used to measure barefoot pressures by securing them to the foot with a thin pair of nylon stockings.[186] Burnfield et al[186] used the pedar® system to study plantar pressures patterns in older adults while walking barefoot and with shoes at three predetermined velocities (187, 262, 295 ft/min [57, 80, 97 m/min]). Compared to slower speeds, fast walking was associated with higher peak pressures under the heel, central and medial metatarsals, and toes, whereas walking barefoot was associated with greater peak pressures under the heel and central metatarsals compared to walking with shoes (Fig. 7.18). These findings suggest that when protection of the plantar surface of the heel and forefoot is important (e.g., with diabetic sensory neuropathy), patients should be encouraged to use shoes and avoid walking at fast speeds for prolonged periods. Subsequent work comparing barefoot walking and wearing shoes examined plantar pressures while walking on grass, carpet, and concrete and identified particularly high pressures when walking barefoot on concrete.[187] Burnfield et al focused on understanding how plantar pressures in young and middle-aged adults vary across common forms of cardiovascular exercise, including treadmill walking, treadmill running, elliptical training, stair stepping, and recumbent cycling. The authors concluded that when protection of the forefoot is important (e.g., diabetic foot neuropathies), biking and stair climbing offer optimal pressure reductions; however, in situations where protection of the heels from high pressures and forces is warranted, recumbent biking, stair climbing, and elliptical training provide greater relief.[188]

The emed® pedography platform is a portable device used to record and evaluate pressure distribution under the foot in static and dynamic conditions. Semple et al[189] used the emed® system to examine COP progression as individuals with rheumatoid arthritis (RA) and individuals without known foot pathology walked. Clients with RA displayed reduced loading of painful regions of the foot as evidenced by delaying progression of the COP across the less painful midfoot followed by rapid progression of the COP across the deformed and painful forefoot.

Isokinetic and Isometric Torque Measurement Systems

Simple handheld dynamometers and **isokinetic dynamometer** systems can be used to obtain static and dynamic peak torques before obtaining temporal and spatial measures. Connelly and Vandervoort[104] found that decreases in isometric and dynamic quadriceps strength led to significant decreases in fast-paced and self-selected speed in older women. In a study examining

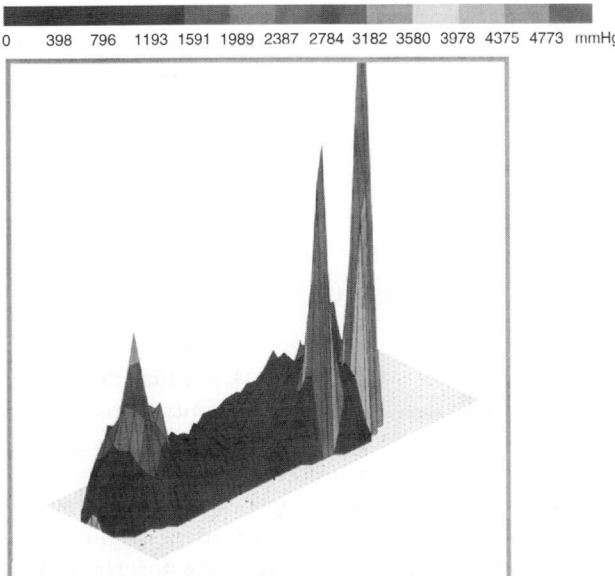

0 398 796 1193 1591 1989 2387 2784 3182 3580 3978 4375 4773 mmHg

Figure 7.17 Magnitude and location of peak pressure during one complete left foot strike. The highest pressures are shown on the heel, first metatarsal head, and great toe. *(Courtesy of Tekscan, Inc., South Boston, MA 02127.)*

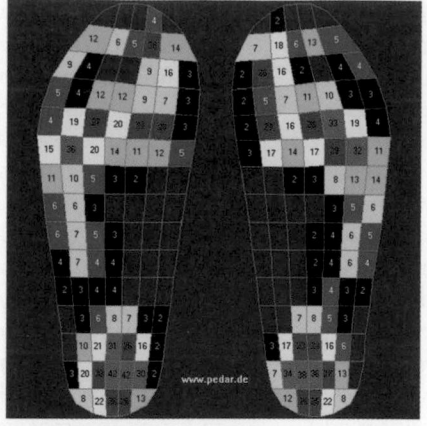
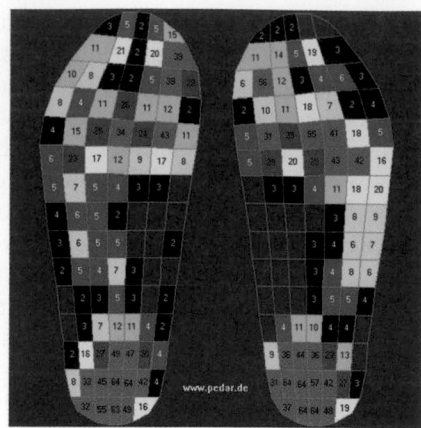

Barefoot, comfortable speed

Barefoot, fast speed

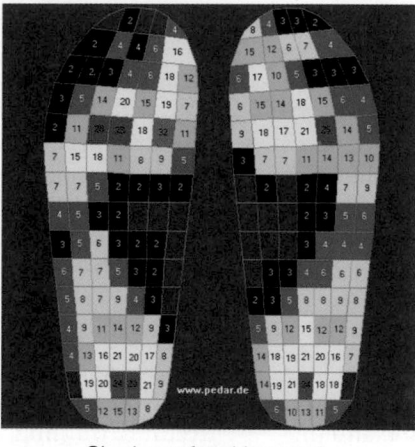
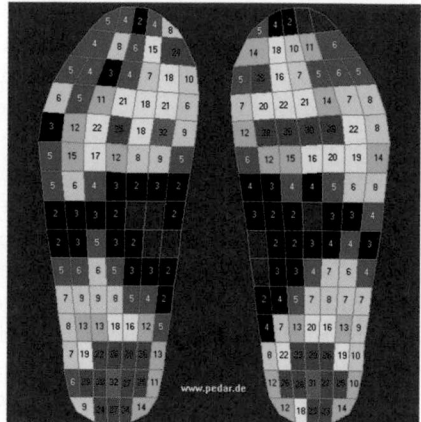

Shod, comfortable speed

Shod, fast speed

Figure 7.18 Pedar (Novel, Inc.) pressure mapping while walking barefoot (top row) and in shoes (bottom row) at self-selected comfortable (left column) and fast (right column) speeds for a 29-year-old male revealed higher pressures under the heel, metatarsal heads, and great toe during barefoot walking at a fast speed compared to the relatively low pressures while walking in shoes at a comfortable speed. Numbers within each square represent the peak pressure (N/cm^2) experienced during the walking trial. *(Courtesy of Adam Taylor, Movement and Neurosciences Center, Institute for Rehabilitation Science and Engineering, Madonna Rehabilitation Hospital, Lincoln, NE 68506.)*

the relationship between sagittal plane LE isokinetic muscle torques and stride characteristics for a group of elderly ambulatory men, maximal isokinetic hip extensor torque was identified as the only significant independent predictor of stride length, cadence, and free walking velocity.[190] These latter findings highlight the importance of maintaining hip extensor strength in older sedentary males.

Software for Processing, Analyzing, and Displaying Kinematic and Kinetic Data

The Visual 3D, innovative software for biomechanical analysis and modeling, is used to process a variety of gait analysis data (e.g., kinematics, EMG, force plates, gyroscopes). It works with nearly all motion capture systems and has an integrated report generator. It allows users to expand beyond manufacturer predetermined marker sets and analysis rules. However, to fully appreciate the versatility and robustness of the Visual 3D

software, it is beneficial to have access to someone with programming skills.

Summary of Kinematic and Kinetic Gait Analysis

Based on the history of gait analysis, one may expect that many gait analysis systems will continue to evolve and more innovative methods of quantifying human gait will be created. However, the most important issues for physical therapists is how reliable and valid the information is and how information can be used to fulfill the four purposes for gait analysis (presented earlier in this chapter under Purposes of Gait Analysis) as described in the *Guide to Physical Therapist Practice*.[1] In brief, these purposes are to assist with understanding the gait characteristics of a particular disorder, to assist with movement diagnosis, to inform selection of intervention(s), and to evaluate the effectiveness of treatment.

The primary advantages of temporal and spatial measures are that they can be determined simply and inexpensively and that they yield objective and reliable baseline data that can be used to formulate anticipated goals and expected outcomes and to evaluate the patient's progress. For example, gait patterns displayed by patients with arthritis often are characterized by a reduced rate and range of knee motion and a slower gait velocity compared to subjects without known pathology. Brinkmann and Perry[191] found that following joint replacement for arthritis, the rate and range of knee motion and gait velocity increased above preoperative levels, but did not reach normal levels.

Usually, increases in measures such as cadence and velocity indicate improvement in a patient's gait. However, comparisons with normal standards are appropriate only if the goal of treatment is to restore a normal gait pattern (e.g., for a patient recovering from a meniscectomy). Comparison with normative standards may not be appropriate for a patient who has had a cerebral vascular accident (CVA). The appropriate norms for examining the gait of a patient with hemiplegia may be either a population of patients with hemiplegia who are of similar age, gender, and involvement, or the patient's pretreatment gait.

Therapists must be cautious when selecting a norm or standard by which to measure patient progress. Significant age, gender, weight, and activity level–related differences have been found in both temporal and spatial measures.[192-194] Himann et al[193] found that an older group (63 to 102 years) of 289 subjects had a significantly slower self-selected walking speed and smaller step length in comparison to a younger group. Age was a significant determinant of walking speed after age 62, but height was a significant determinant before age 62. Step length has been found to be significantly shorter and the double support stance period significantly increased in an elderly sample compared to a database of young adults.[94] Cho et al[195] found a number of gender differences in kinematic and kinetic gait variables. For example, females had shorter stride lengths and narrower step widths, a more anteriorly tilted pelvis, greater hip flexion and internal rotation, greater knee valgus, and smaller ankle joint moment compared to males. Some of these changes were attributed to the anatomically wider female pelvis.[195]

Few disadvantages exist regarding kinematic quantitative gait analysis, except for the possible expense involved in instrumentation, the time required to apply the markers accurately to ensure valid and reliable data, and the fact that a certain amount of uncertainty exists about how to normalize for leg length, height, age, gender, weight, level of maturation, and disability. The interpretation of motion patterns obtained through motion analysis systems usually involves comparisons of an individual's data with a mean curve for normal subjects using one standard deviation (SD) for boundaries. Sutherland et al[196] suggest that motion patterns cannot be fully analyzed without consideration of all points along the curve. They propose the use of prediction regions (multiples of the SD above and below the mean curve of data for each point in the gait cycle). Within a prediction region (Fig. 7.19), if any point along the curve of joint motion falls outside of the

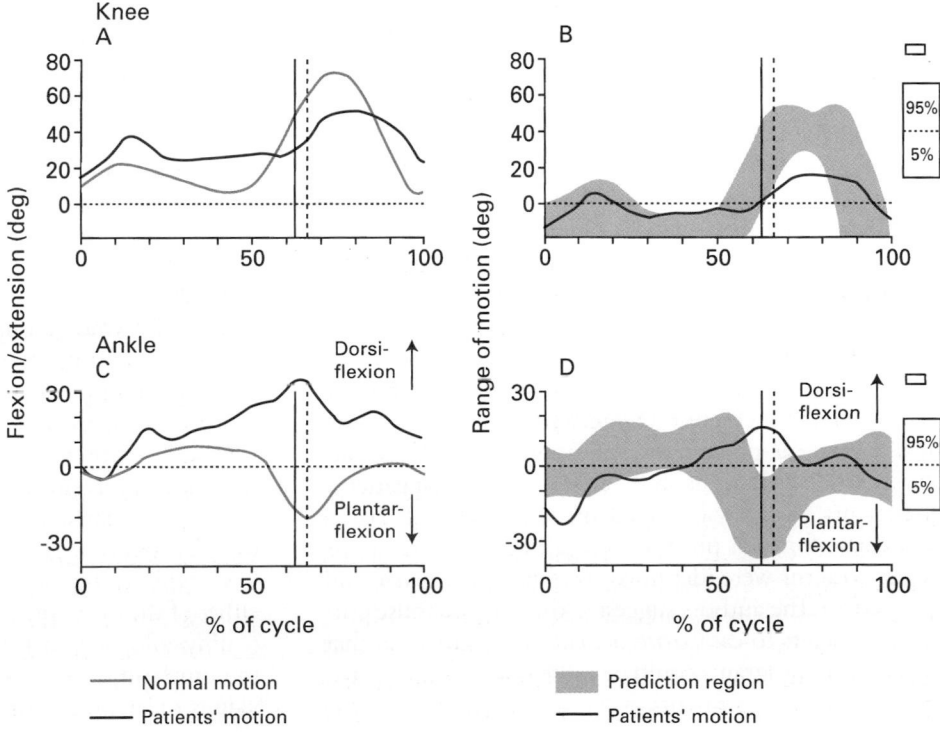

Figure 7.19 Prediction regions. *(Sutherland et al,[196] with permission.)*

defined region, the patient's gait is considered to be abnormal.

Gait Pattern Classification

Identification of gait parameters that deviate widely from a norm is a fairly simple outcome of gait analysis. However, identification of groups or clusters of gait deviations that characterize a known disorder is more complicated and represents one of the very urgent needs in gait analysis. In an attempt to classify gait disorders, a number of statistical techniques are being used for both kinematic and kinetic gait variables. The *bootstrap technique*[197] is used to establish the boundaries (prediction regions) about the mean curve for healthy control subjects in order to establish the limits of normal variability. *Discriminant analysis* is used to recognize gait patterns of healthy people and persons with gait deviations. *Principal components analysis* is useful to reduce the large quantities of data acquired in a gait analysis to a set of features that accurately describe gait patterns. *Cluster analysis* is used to place subjects in homogeneous groups, or clusters, based on specified input parameters.

Normalcy Index

Principal components analysis was used to develop the *Normalcy Index (NI)*, which was able to quantify the amount of deviation in a subject's gait compared to the gait of an average unimpaired person.[198] The *NI* has been found to be sensitive enough to distinguish unimpaired subjects from idiopathic toe walkers and to distinguish between involved and less involved limbs of subjects following stroke. However, the gait pathology of non-independent walkers was not well categorized. The authors suggested that perhaps the inclusion of kinetic variables along with kinematic variables might be helpful.

The principal components method derived the NI by assigning weighted factors inversely proportional to the amount of variation exhibited by each gait measure in the unimpaired population. However, since the data come from a motion analysis system they are subject to sources of error such as soft tissue artifacts and marker misplacement.[198]

Cluster Analysis

Cluster analysis is a commonly used statistical technique in the social sciences, but only relatively recently has been used to create an objective classification system of gait patterns. Cluster analysis has been used to classify gait patterns of patients with stroke based on temporal and spatial parameters for each phase of the gait cycle. Four clusters of gait patterns were identified: *fast, moderate, flexed,* and *extended.*[199] The authors suggested that clinicians use critical parameters to categorize patients with stroke, so that intervention programs could be more specifically targeted to underlying impairments.

Energy Cost Analysis During Gait

Walking at constant speed is a cyclical activity that requires the body to add energy by means of concentric contractions, and absorb energy by means of eccentric contractions. These energy transfers and exchanges are cleverly designed to make walking efficient.[24] Generally, conditions that affect either the motor control of gait and posture or conditions that affect joint and muscle structure and function will increase the energy cost of gait.[14,200-204] The type of footwear,[205] use of assistive devices, and speed of gait affect energy expenditure as well.[206] Energy expenditure is an important consideration in gait analyses, particularly in neurological conditions in which muscular resources may be low. There are three general approaches in determining energy costs: *physiological measurement, mechanical energy analysis,* and *heart rate data.* The selection of a particular approach should be based on the purpose of taking the measure and the relative importance of test characteristics outlined earlier in this chapter under Types of Gait Analyses.

Physiological Energy Cost Measures

Physiological cost measures estimate the heat (energy) produced by a subject at rest and during exercise by indirect calorimetry, based on the assumption that all energy-using reactions of the body depend on oxygen uptake. The most common method of measuring oxygen uptake during walking is open-loop spirometry in which exhaled air is sampled and analyzed for its oxygen content, classically using the Douglas bag method.[24] More recently, stationary or moving metabolic carts or lightweight portable devices perform breath-by-breath oxygen and carbon dioxide analysis. Two parameters of prime interest are *oxygen cost* and *oxygen rate.* One may be interested in the oxygen cost or energy expenditure per unit of distance walked (in mL/kg/m), which relates to the physiological work involved in the task and reflects gait efficiency. Alternatively, the oxygen rate, or energy expenditure per unit of time (in mL/kg/min), reflects the power of walking and is interpreted using knowledge of walking speed.[201,207] Perry et al[14] used a modified Douglas bag assembly to compare the energy expenditure required for an individual with bilateral transfemoral amputations and bilateral transradial (below elbow) amputations to walk at a self-selected speed using different prosthetic devices. When wearing the microprocessor-controlled C-Leg prostheses, the subject walked the farthest and fastest compared to the traditional non–microprocessor-controlled articulating prostheses and stubbies (nonarticulating, short prosthetic limbs). The overall rate of oxygen consumption and oxygen cost was lower while using the C-Legs compared with walking with either of the other prostheses.

Physiological cost analysis methods are most useful in comparing the energy cost of walking with normal values or an individual's maximum capacity, and for determining the effects on energy costs of interventions such as the use of orthoses, prostheses, or assistive devices. Physiological cost analyses reflect overall costs of walking with respect to time or distance, but they cannot discern the possible causes. If insight into the particular movements is needed, mechanical energy analysis can be helpful.

Mechanical Energy Cost Determination

There are two methods of obtaining mechanical energy costs. In the first method, kinematic data alone are required, using estimates of masses of body parts and of locations of the COM of these parts. By employing a spatial motion analysis system with basic equations of motion and anthropometric constants for masses of body parts, the potential energy and translational and rotational kinetic energy levels of each body part can be calculated. The differences between values obtained at each time increment indicate energy cost. Various equations are used to combine the costs across body parts to yield the total body cost. The large head-arms-and-trunk segment shows excellent exchanges between kinetic and potential energy types, providing the body with energy efficiency. When the body is at its highest position (mid stance), it is also moving most slowly, but as the head-arms-and-trunk "roll down the hill" into initial contact of the foot, this potential energy is changed into kinetic energy, and the head-arms-and-trunk picks up speed. In this way, a great deal of energy is saved and the movement is efficient. However, if the person walks very slowly or very quickly, or has a stiff knee and has to lift one side of the body excessively to clear the floor, the energies are no longer complementary in size and/or shape; less energy exchange can take place.[208] These modes of walking are less efficient than normal walking.

The second method of obtaining mechanical energy costs uses a kinetic approach. Briefly stated, the energy changes in a body part between subsequent instants in time are calculated (1) from the product of the forces on each end of the joint and the velocity of the point of application and (2) from the muscle powers, which are the product of each muscle moment and the angular velocity of the body part. In some cases, the muscle is adding energy to the part (generation), and, in other cases, it is absorbing energy. There are a number of different methods of handling the calculations of mechanical energy, exchanges, and transfers, but a sound approach is described by McGibbon et al.[209]

Heart Rate Data

A third general approach to determining the relative energy cost of gait is by measuring the heart rate (HR) during ambulation. Relative energy consumption has been found to be highly correlated with HR and absolute level of energy consumption has been found to be highly correlated with HR and maximum walking speed.

The most accurate way to determine HR is to use a telemetry system that produces beat-by-beat information as well as electrocardiographic activity. Many inexpensive HR monitors are also available and some are designed to download stored information to a computer (see Chapter 2, Examination of Vital Signs). HR responses to ambulation can also be determined by palpation of the radial or carotid arteries, though somewhat more error may be present.

HR measures have been shown to be adequately sensitive for some applications. For example, simple measures of HR and maximum ambulatory velocity allowed accurate prediction ($r = 0.89$) of energy consumption in children with myelomeningocele based on measures recorded from 21 children treadmill walking, 8 children using wheelchairs, and 5 children using both modes.[210] However, Herbert et al[202] found no difference in HR between children with transtibial amputations and those with intact LEs even though energy consumption was 15% higher in the children with amputations. Perhaps because the conditions were more disparate, Waters et al[200] found that in patients with hip arthrodesis, oxygen consumption was 32% greater than normal and that HR was significantly greater than normal.

An energy index based on HR called the *Physiological Cost Index (PCI)* was developed specifically to determine the relative costs of walking per unit of distance walked.[211] Calculated as the difference between the walking HR and the resting HR divided by the average speed, it is expressed in beats per meter. The reliability of PCI has been investigated in individuals without known pathology,[212-214] as well as people with spinal cord[214,215] and brain injuries.[112] The index has been used to quantify improvements following an intervention in individuals with spinal cord injury (SCI),[216,217] RA,[218] and stroke.[219-221] For example, PCI was used as a key outcome measure in a study assessing the effects of a 12-week intervention that combined functional electrical stimulation (FES) with conventional rehabilitation to manage dropfoot in individuals recovering from a stroke.[221] While walking speed increased 38.7% between the initiation and end of the trial, PCI decreased 34.6%, suggesting not only improved function but also efficiency. The relationship between PCI and oxygen consumption has been studied across a variety of populations, including individuals with amputations,[222] individuals with SCIs,[223] and individuals without known disabilities.[212] Some researchers have found oxygen uptake measures to be more repeatable and less variable than PCI.[213,215,224,225] One concern that has been raised is that HR measures may be affected by altered vagal or sympathetic regulation due to brain injury[226-229] or medication.[230]

The *Total Heart Beat Index* provides an alternative approach for determining the relative energy efficiency of walking. It is calculated by dividing the total (cumulative) number of heart beats during exercise by the total distance traveled in a given time period.[214] It has been used to study walking efficiency in individuals with diabetic foot ulcers and amputations,[231] chronic incomplete SCIs,[232] and intellectual and developmental disabilities.[233] Reliable and valid use of the measure with populations with blunted HR responses requires study.

SUMMARY

An overview of select methods for kinematic and kinetic gait analyses has been presented in this chapter. Many of the common variables examined in gait analyses have been defined and described, and examples of studies using gait analyses have been presented. OGA and temporal and spatial variables have been emphasized, because they appear to be the most common types of analyses used in the clinical setting. A brief overview of some of the motion analysis systems has been provided. Readers are encouraged to investigate the capabilities of individual motion analysis systems, and to consult the gait literature for reliability and validity studies regarding these systems. The ability to perform a gait analysis that accurately describes a patient's gait will provide important quantifiable information necessary for optimal treatment planning.

Questions for Review

1. Describe the three different types of gait analyses (kinematic qualitative, kinematic quantitative, and kinetic) and list the variables examined in each type. Identify at least one variable from each type of analysis and describe a technique/technology that could be used to examine the variable.

2. Compare the advantages and disadvantages of a kinematic qualitative gait analysis with the advantages and disadvantages of a kinematic quantitative analysis.

3. Describe how a therapist would determine the concurrent validity of temporal and spatial gait measures recorded using the GAITRite® with values calculated using the Stride Analyzer.

4. A new client is referred to physical therapy with gait dysfunction arising from severe diabetic sensory and motor neuropathy. The patient has a history of recurrent ulcers, bilaterally, under his first metatarsal heads that have impaired his ability to stand/walk at work for prolonged periods of time. He recently received a new pair of custom-molded orthotic shoe inserts and was instructed to use them in his shoes to help reduce plantar pressures. Unfortunately, he is unable to feel whether they are fitting or not, secondary to the sensory neuropathy. What technology could be used to assess the effectiveness of the inserts at reducing plantar pressures? What activities should be assessed and why?

5. A person walks with excessive dorsiflexion, no heel-off, and limited toe extension in terminal stance. Hip and knee analysis reveals excess flexion during stance with absence of the normal "trailing limb" posture characteristic of terminal stance. Identify potential causes for these deviations. What additional tests or measures should be performed?

6. Identify methods that can be used to determine the energy costs that a patient incurs while walking.

7. How could a gait analysis of temporal parameters be used to demonstrate a patient's progress or lack of progress?

CASE STUDY

HISTORY

This 65-year-old woman is 5 days post–right total hip arthroplasty. The surgery was performed following a femoral neck fracture incurred during a fall on the ice in front of her home. She has had daily bedside physical therapy for the past 3 days and now is independent in transfers. However, she needs to be independent in walking before she goes home.

She has a past history of diabetes mellitus (onset age 50), which is controlled with daily insulin injections. She has a recurrent history of foot ulcers and has been hospitalized on two occasions to manage infected foot ulcers. She denies any history of "heart problems." She does not participate in any regular exercise program and spends a great deal of time sitting during her work as a seamstress. She is alert and oriented to time and place and has a pleasant demeanor. She is 5 feet 3 inches tall and weighs 160 pounds.

Goniometric Examination of Passive Range of Motion (Degrees)

Lower Extremities

Joint	Motion	Left	Right
Hip	Flexion	WFL	15–40*
	Extension	WFL	0–10*
	Abduction	WFL	0–20*
	Adduction	WFL	0–10*
	Medial rotation	WFL	Not tested*
	Lateral rotation	WFL	0–20*
Knee	Flexion	WFL	0–120
Ankle	Dorsiflexion	WFL	0–15
	Plantarflexion	WFL	0–45
	Inversion	WFL	0–5
	Eversion	WFL	0–20

WFL = within functional limits.
Upper extremities: All ROM measurements are WFL.
*Painful with movement.

Manual Muscle Test (MMT)

Lower Extremities

Joint	Movement	Left	Right
Hip	Flexion	G	F
	Extension	G	P
	Abduction	G	P
	Adduction	G	F+
	Lateral rotation	G	F+
	Medial rotation	G	F+
Knee	Flexion	G	F+
	Extension	G	F+
Ankle	Dorsiflexion	F	P
	Plantarflexion	F	F
	Inversion	F	F
	Eversion	F+	F
Toes	Flexion	F	F
	Extension	P	P

Upper extremities: All muscle grades are within the G to G– range.

Sensory Examination

	Plantar Aspect Left Foot	Plantar Aspect Right Foot
Sharp/dull	5	5
Light touch	5	5
Temperature	5	5
Proprioceptive sensation	4	4

NUMERIC VALUES REFER TO THE SENSATION SCALE BELOW.

SENSATION SCALE

1. Intact: normal, accurate
2. Decreased: delayed response
3. Exaggerated: increased sensitivity
4. Inaccurate: inappropriate perception of stimuli
5. Absent: no response
6. Inconsistent or ambiguous

INSPECTION

Patient has an ulcer on the medial aspect of the right plantar surface which is 0.7 × 6.0 cm in diameter and 1.5 mm deep.

FUNCTIONAL EXAMINATION

Locomotion
FIM level = 5
Transfers
FIM level = 7
Activities of Daily Living
Eating: FIM = 7
Bathing: FIM = 7
Dressing: FIM = 7

GUIDING QUESTIONS

1. Develop a physical therapy problem list.
2. Complete the sample OGA form for the right lower extremity based on the information presented (see Appendix 7.A). What deviations would you expect to see for the right lower extremity and why? How might gait change if the client is instructed to not bear weight on the right forefoot secondary to the plantar ulcer?
3. Present your recommendations for physical therapy intervention.

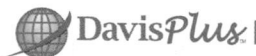 **DavisPlus** | For additional resources, including answers to the questions for review and case study guiding questions, please visit **http://davisplus.fadavis.com**

References

1. American Physical Therapy Association: Guide to Physical Therapist Practice, ed 2. Phys Ther 81:1, 2001.
2. Mueller, MJ, et al: Differences in the gait characteristics of patients with diabetes and peripheral neuropathy compared with age-matched controls. Phys Ther 74:299–313, 1994.
3. Von Schroeder, HP, et al: Gait parameters following stroke: A practical assessment. J Rehabil Res Dev 32:25, 1995.
4. Walker, S, et al: Gait pattern alteration by functional sensory substitution in healthy subjects and in diabetic subjects with peripheral neuropathy. Arch Phys Med Rehabil 78:853, 1997.
5. Hesse, S, et al: Asymmetry of gait initiation in hemiparetic stroke subjects. Arch Phys Med Rehabil 78:719, 1997.
6. De Quervain, IA, et al: Gait pattern in the early recovery period after stroke. J Bone Joint Surg Am 78:1506, 1996.
7. Rossi, SA, et al: Gait initiation of persons with below-knee amputation: The characterization and comparison of force profiles. J Rehabil Res Dev 32:120, 1995.
8. Roth, EJ, et al: Hemiplegic gait. Relationships between walking speed and other temporal parameters. Am J Phys Med Rehabil 76:128, 1997.
9. Al-Zahrani, KS, and Bakheit, AMO: A study of the gait characteristics of patients with chronic osteoarthritis of the knee. Disabil Rehabil 24:275–280, 2002.
10. Kim, C, and Eng, JJ: The relationship of lower-extremity muscle torque to locomotor performance in people with stroke. Phys Ther 83:49–57, 2003.
11. Cook, TM, et al: Effects of restricted knee flexion and walking speed on the vertical ground reaction force during gait. JOSPT 25:236, 1997.
12. Postema, K, et al: Energy storage and release of prosthetic feet. Part 1: Biomechanical analysis related to user benefits. Prosthet Orthot Int 21:17–27, 1997.
13. Perry, J, et al: Toe walking: Muscular demands at the ankle and knee. Arch Phys Med Rehabil 84:7–16, 2003.
14. Perry, J, et al: Energy expenditure and gait characteristics of a person with bilateral amputations walking with the "C-Leg" compared to stubby and conventional articulating prostheses. Arch Phys Med Rehabil 85:1711, 2004.
15. Park, ES, et al: Comparison of anterior and posterior walkers with respect to gait parameters and energy expenditure of children with spastic diplegic cerebral palsy. Yonsei Med J 42:180, 2001.

16. Haubert, LL, et al: A comparison of shoulder joint forces during ambulation with crutches versus a walker in persons with incomplete spinal cord injury. Arch Phys Med Rehabil 87:63–70, 2006.

17. Self, BP, et al: A biomechanical analysis of a medial unloading brace for osteoarthritis in the knee. Arthritis Care Res 13:191, 2000.

18. Mulroy, SJ, et al: Effect of AFO design on walking after stroke: Impact of ankle plantar flexion contracture. Prosthet Orthot Int 34:277–292, 2010.

19. Gok, H, et al: Effects of ankle-foot orthoses on hemiparetic gait. Clin Rehabil 17:137, 2003.

20. Radtka, SA, et al: A comparison of gait with solid, dynamic, and no ankle-foot orthoses in children with spastic cerebral palsy. Phys Ther 77:395–409, 1997.

21. Eng, JJ, and Pierrynowski, MR: The effect of soft foot orthotics on three-dimensional lower-limb kinematics during walking and running. Phys Ther 74:836, 1994.

22. Granata, KP, et al: Joint angular velocity in spastic gait and the influence of muscle-tendon lengthening. J Bone Joint Surg Am 82:174–186, 2000.

23. Damiano, DL, et al: Effects of quadriceps femoris muscle strengthening on crouch gait in children with spastic diplegia. Phys Ther 75:658, 1995.

24. Waters, RL, and Mulroy, SJ: The energy expenditure of normal and pathological gait. Gait Posture 9:207, 1999.

25. Van Swearingen, JM, et al: The modified Gait Abnormality Rating Scale for recognizing the risk of recurrent falls in community-dwelling elderly adults. Phys Ther 76:994–1002, 1996.

26. Shumway-Cook, A, et al: Predicting the probability for falls in community-dwelling older adults. Phys Ther 77:812, 1997.

27. Burnfield, JM, and Powers, CM: Prediction of slips: An evaluation of utilized coefficient of friction and available slip resistance. Ergonomics 49:982–995, 2006.

28. Wall, JC, and Scarbrough, J: Use of a multimemory stopwatch to measure the temporal gait parameters. J Orthop Sports Phys Ther 25:277, 1997.

29. Sutherland, DH: The evolution of clinical gait analysis part III—kinetics and energy assessment. Gait Posture 21:447–461, 2005.

30. Sutherland, DH: The evolution of clinical gait analysis part I: Kinesiological EMG. Gait Posture 14:61–70, 2001.

31. Sutherland, DH: The evolution of clinical gait analysis part II—kinematics. Gait Posture 16:159–179, 2002.

32. Perry, J, and Burnfield, JM: Gait Analysis, Normal and Pathological Function, ed 2. Charles B. Slack, Thorofare, NJ, 2010.

33. Domholdt, E: Physical Therapy Research, ed 4. WB Saunders, Philadelphia, 2010.

34. Strube, MJ, and DeLitto, A: Reliability and measurement theory. In Craik, R, and Oatis, C (eds): Gait Analysis: Theory and Application. Mosby–Yearbook, St. Louis, 1995, p 88.

35. Pathokinesiology Service and Physical Therapy Department: Observational Gait Analysis, ed 4. Los Amigos Research and Education Institute, Inc., Rancho Los Amigos National Rehabilitation Center, Downey, CA, 2001.

36. Ishikawa, M, et al: Muscle-tendon interaction and elastic energy usage in human walking. J Appl Physiol 99:603, 2005.

37. Maganaris, CN, and Paul, JP: Tensile properties of the in vivo human gastrocnemius tendon. J Biomech 35:1639, 2002.

38. Fukunaga, T, et al: In vivo behavior of human muscle tendon during walking. Proc R Soc Lond B 268:229–233, 2001.

39. Toro, B, et al: The status of gait assessment among physiotherapists in the United Kingdom. Arch Phys Med Rehabil 84:1878, 2003.

40. Southerland, CC: Gait evaluation. In Valmassy, RL (ed): Clinical Biomechanics of the Lower Extremities. Mosby–Yearbook, St. Louis, 1996, pp 149–177.

41. Bernhardt, J, et al: Accuracy of observational kinematic assessment of upper-limb movements. Phys Ther 78:259, 1998.

42. Russell, DJ, et al: Training users in the gross motor function measure: Methodological and practical issues. Phys Ther 74:630, 1994.

43. Brunnekreef, JJ, et al: Reliability of videotaped observational gait analysis in patients with orthopedic impairments. BMC Musculoskelet Disord 6:17–26, 2005.

44. Eastlack, ME, et al: Interrater reliability of videotaped observational gait-analysis assessments. Arch Phys Med Rehabil 71:465, 1991.

45. Krebs, DE: Interpretation standards in locomotor studies. In Craik, R, and Oatis, C (eds): Gait Analysis: Theory and Application. Mosby–Yearbook, St. Louis, 1995, pp 334–354.

46. McGinley, JL, et al: Accuracy and reliability of observational gait analysis data: Judgments of push-off in gait after stroke. Phys Ther 83:146, 2003.

47. Borel, S, et al: Video analysis software increases the interrater reliability of video gait assessments in children with cerebral palsy. Gait Posture 33:727, 2011.

48. Stuberg, WA, et al: Comparison of a clinical gait analysis method using videography and temporal-distance measures with 16-mm cinematography. Phys Ther 68:1221, 1988.

49. Levangie, PK, and Norkin, CC: Joint Structure and Function: A Comprehensive Analysis, ed 5. FA Davis, Philadelphia, 2011.

50. Craik, RL, and Otis, CA: Gait assessment in the clinic: Issues and approaches. In Rothstein, JM (ed): Measurement in Physical Therapy. Churchill Livingstone, London, 1985, pp 169–205.

51. Nelson, AJ: Functional Ambulation Profile. Phys Ther 54:1059, 1974.

52. Howe, JA, et al: The Community Balance and Mobility Scale—a balance measure for individuals with traumatic brain injury. Clin Rehabil 20:885, 2006.

53. Harada, N, et al: Screening for balance and mobility impairment in elderly individuals living in residential care facilities. Phys Ther 75:462, 1995.

54. Wolf, SL, et al: Establishing the reliability and validity of measurements of walking time using the Emory Functional Ambulation Profile. Phys Ther 79:1122, 1999.

55. Baer, HR, and Wolf, SL: Modified Emory Functional Ambulation Profile: An outcome measure for the rehabilitation of poststroke gait dysfunction. Stroke 32:973, 2001.

56. Shields, RK, et al: Reliability, validity, and responsiveness of functional tests in patients with total joint replacement. Phys Ther 75:169, 1995.

57. The Guide for Uniform Data System for Medical Rehabilitation (including the FIM™ Instrument) Version 5.1. University of Buffalo Foundation Activities, Inc, Amherst, NY, 1997.

58. Santa Clara Valley Medical Center: Introduction to the Functional Assessment Measure. The Center for Outcome Measurements in Brain Injury (COMBI). Retrieved May 30, 2011, from http://tbims.org/combi/FAM/index.html.

59. Hawley, CA, et al: Use of the functional assessment measure (FIM+FAM) in head injury rehabilitation: A psychometric analysis. J Neurol Neurosurg Psychiatry 67:749, 1999.

60. Butcher, SJ, et al: Reductions in functional balance, coordination, and mobility measures among patients with stable chronic obstructive pulmonary disease. J Cardiopulm Rehabil 24:274–280, 2004.

61. Knorr, S, et al: Validity of the Community Balance and Mobility Scale in community-dwelling persons after stroke. Arch Phys Med Rehabil 91:890, 2010.

62. Woollacott, MH, and Tang, PF: Balance control during walking in the older adult: Research and its implications. Phys Ther 77:646–660, 1997.

63. Shumway-Cook, A, and Woollacott, WJ: Motor Control: Translating Research into Clinical Practice, ed 4. Williams & Wilkins, Baltimore, 2011.

64. Jonsdottir, J, and Cattaneo, D: Reliability and validity of the Dynamic Gait Index in persons with chronic stroke. Arch Phys Med Rehabil 88:1410, 2007.

65. Marchetti, GF, and Whitney, SL: Construction and validation of the 4-Item Dynamic Gait Index. Phys Ther 86:1651, 2006.

66. Leddy, AL, et al: Functional Gait Assessment and Balance Evaluation System Test: Reliability, validity, sensitivity, and specificity for identifying individuals with Parkinson disease who fall. Phys Ther 91:102–113, 2011.

67. Wrisley, DM, and Kumar, NA: Functional gait assessment: Concurrent, discriminative, and predictive validity in community-dwelling older adults. Phys Ther 90:761–773, 2010.

68. Walker, ML, et al: Reference group data for the Functional Gait Assessment. Phys Ther 87:1468, 2007.

69. Wrisley, DM, et al: Reliability, internal consistency, and validity of data obtained with the Functional Gait Assessment. Phys Ther 84:906, 2004.

70. Lin, JH, et al: Psychometric comparisons of 3 functional ambulation measures for patients with stroke. Stroke 41:2021, 2010.

71. Williams, G, et al: The High-level Mobility Assessment Tool (HiMAT) for traumatic brain injury. Part 1: Item generation. Brain Inj 19:925–932, 2005.

72. Williams, GP, et al: The High-level Mobility Assessment Tool (HiMAT) for traumatic brain injury. Part 2: content validity and discriminability. Brain Inj 19:833–843, 2005.

73. Williams, G, et al: The concurrent validity and responsiveness of the High-level Mobility Assessment Tool for measuring the mobility limitations of people with traumatic brain injury. Arch Phys Med Rehabil 87:437–442, 2006.

74. Williams, GP, et al: High-level Mobility Assessment Tool (HiMAT): Interrater reliability, retest reliability, and internal consistency. Phys Ther 86:395–400, 2006.

75. Tyson, S, and Connell, L: The psychometric properties and clinical utility of measures of walking and mobility in neurological conditions: A systematic review. Clin Rehabil 23:1018, 2009.

76. Williams, G, et al: Further development of the High-level Mobility Assessment Tool (HiMAT). Brain Inj 24:1027, 2010.

77. Di Fabio, RP, and Seay, R: Use of the "Fast Evaluation of Mobility, Balance, and Fear" in elderly community dwellers: Validity and reliability. Phys Ther 77:904, 1997.

78. Hess, RJ, et al: Walking skill can be assessed in older adults: Validity of the Figure-of-8 Walk Test. Phys Ther 90:89–99, 2010.

79. Liaw, LJ, et al: Psychometric properties of the modified Emory Functional Ambulation Profile in stroke patients. Clin Rehabil 20:429–437, 2006.

80. Morton, T: Uniform data system for rehab begins: First tool measures dependent level. Progress Report, American Physical Therapy Association, Alexandria, VA, 1986.

81. Wolfson, AM, et al: Clinician judgments of functional outcomes: How bias and perceived accuracy affect rating. Arch Phys Med Rehabil 81:1567, 2000.

82. Gurka, JA, et al: Utility of the Functional Assessment Measure after discharge from inpatient rehabilitation. J Head Trauma Rehabil 14:247, 1999.

83. Hobart, JC, et al: Evidence-based measurement: Which disability scale for neurologic rehabilitation? Neurology 57:639, 2001.

84. Linn, RT, et al: Does the Functional Assessment Measure (FAM) extend the Functional Independence Measure (FIM) instrument? A Rasch analysis of stroke inpatients. J Outcome Meas 3:339, 1999.

85. Whitney, SL, et al: The Dynamic Gait Index relates to self-reported fall history in individuals with vestibular dysfunction. J Vestib Res 10:99–105, 2000.

86. Brown, KE, et al: Physical therapy outcomes for persons with bilateral vestibular loss. Laryngoscope 111:1812, 2001.

87. Huang, SL, et al: Minimal detectable change of the timed "Up and Go" test and the Dynamic Gait Index in people with Parkinson disease. Phys Ther 91:114–121, 2011.

88. Cattaneo, D, et al: Reliability of four scales on balance disorders in persons with multiple sclerosis. Disabil Rehabil 29:1920, 2007.

89. Perry, J, et al: Classification of walking handicap in the stroke population. Stroke 26:982, 1995.

90. Lerner-Frankiel, MB, et al: Functional community ambulation: What are your criteria? Clinical Management in Physical Therapy 6:12–15, 1986.

91. Graham, JE, et al: Walking speed threshold for classifying walking independence in hospitalized older adults. Phys Ther 90:1591, 2010.

92. Robinett, CS, and Vondran, MA: Functional ambulation velocity and distance requirements in rural and urban communities. A clinical report. Phys Ther 68:1371, 1988.

93. Walsh, M, et al: Physical impairments and functional limitations: A comparison of individuals 1 year after total knee arthroplasty with control subjects. Phys Ther 78:248, 1998.

94. Winter, DA, et al: Biomechanical walking pattern changes in the fit and healthy elderly. Phys Ther 70:340, 1990.

95. Blanke, DJ, and Hageman, PA: Comparison of gait of young men and elderly men. Phys Ther 69:144, 1989.

96. Bohannon, RW, et al: Walking speed: Reference values and correlates for older adults. J Orthop Sports Phys Ther 24:86–90, 1996.

97. Ostrosky, KM, et al: A comparison of gait characteristics in young and old subjects. Phys Ther 74:637, 1994.

98. Todd, F, et al: Variations in the gait of normal children. A graph applicable to the documentation of abnormalities. J Bone Joint Surg Am 71:196–204, 1989.

99. Murray, MP, et al: Walking patterns of normal men. J Bone Joint Surg 46A:335–360, 1964.

100. Murray, MP, et al: Walking patterns of normal women. Arch Phys Med Rehabil 51:637–650, 1970.

101. Spyropoulos, P, et al: Biomechanical gait analysis in obese men. Arch Phys Med Rehabil 72:1065, 1991.

102. Hills, AP, and Parker, AW: Gait characteristics of obese children. Arch Phys Med Rehabil 72:403, 1991.

103. McGibbon, CA, and Krebs, DE: Discriminating age and disability effects in locomotion: Neuromuscular adaptations in musculoskeletal pathology. J Appl Physiol 96:149–160, 2004.

104. Connelly, DM, and Vandervoort, AA: Effects of detraining on knee extensor strength and functional mobility in a group of elderly women. J Orthop Sports Phys Ther 26:340–346, 1997.

105. Sutherland, D: The development of mature gait. Gait Posture 6:163, 1997.

106. Holden, MK, et al: Clinical gait assessment in the neurologically impaired: Reliability and meaningfulness. Phys Ther 64:35–40, 1984.

107. van Loo, MA, et al: Inter-rater reliability and concurrent validity of step length and step width measurement after traumatic brain injury. Disabil Rehabil 25:1195, 2003.

108. Robinson, JL, and Smidt, GL: Quantitative gait evaluation in the clinic. Phys Ther 61:351, 1981.

109. Guyatt, GH, et al: The 6-minute walk: A new measure of exercise capacity in patients with chronic heart failure. Can Med Assoc J 132:919, 1985.

110. Butland, RJ, et al: Two-, six-, and 12-minute walking tests in respiratory disease. Br Med J (Clin Res Ed) 284:1607, 1982.

111. Schenkman, M, et al: Reliability of impairment and physical performance measures for persons with Parkinson's disease. Phys Ther 77:19–27, 1997.

112. Mossberg, KA: Reliability of a timed walk test in persons with acquired brain injury. Am J Phys Med Rehabil 82:385, 2003.

113. Fulk, GD, et al: Predicting home and community walking activity in people with stroke. Arch Phys Med Rehabil 91:1582, 2010.

114. Sullivan, KJ, et al: Effects of task-specific locomotor and strength training in adults who were ambulatory after stroke: Results of the STEPS randomized clinical trial. Phys Ther 87:1580–1602, 2007.

115. Jenkins, S, et al: Regression equations to predict 6-minute walk distance in middle-aged and elderly adults. Physiother Theory Pract 25:516, 2009.

116. Geiger, R, et al: Six-minute walk test in children and adolescents. J Pediatr 150:395, 2007.

117. Chetta, A, et al: Reference values for the 6-min walk test in healthy subjects 20–50 years old. Respir Med 100:1573, 2006.

118. Camarri, B, et al: Six minute walk distance in healthy subjects aged 55–75 years. Respir Med 100:658, 2006.

119. Casanova, C, et al: The 6-min walk distance in healthy subjects: Reference standards from seven countries. Eur Respir J 37:150, 2011.

120. Priesnitz, CV, et al: Reference values for the 6-min walk test in healthy children aged 6–12 years. Pediatr Pulmonol 44:1174, 2009.

121. Troosters, T, et al: Six minute walking distance in healthy elderly subjects. Eur Respir J 14:270, 1999.

122. Poh, H, et al: Six-minute walk distance in healthy Singaporean adults cannot be predicted using reference equations derived from Caucasian populations. Respirology 11:211–216, 2006.

123. Bohannon, RW: Six-minute walk test: A meta-analysis of data from apparently healthy elders. Top Geriatr Rehabil 23:155–160, 2007.

124. Kosak, M, and Smith, T: Comparison of the 2-, 6-, and 12-minute walk tests in patients with stroke. J Rehabil Res Dev 42:103, 2005.

125. Rossier, P, and Wade, DT: Validity and reliability comparison of 4 mobility measures in patients presenting with neurologic impairment. Arch Phys Med Rehabil 82:9–13, 2001.

126. English, CK, et al: The sensitivity of three commonly used outcome measures to detect change amongst patients receiving inpatient rehabilitation following stroke. Clin Rehabil 20:52, 2006.

127. Askim, T, et al: Effects of a community-based intensive motor training program combined with early supported discharge after treatment in a comprehensive stroke unit: A randomized, controlled trial. Stroke 41:1697–1703, 2010.

128. Flansbjer, U-B, et al: Reliability of gait performance tests in men and women with hemiparesis after stroke. J Rehabil Med 37: 75–82, 2005.

129. Hollman, JH, et al: Minimum detectable change in gait velocity during acute rehabilitation following hip fracture. J Geriatr Phys Ther 31:53, 2008.

130. Nilsagard, Y, et al: Clinical relevance using timed walk tests and "Timed Up and Go" testing in persons with multiple sclerosis. Physiother Res Int 12:105–114, 2007.

131. Kavanagh, JJ, and Menz, HB: Accelerometry: A technique for quantifying movement patterns during walking. Gait Posture 28:1–15, 2008.

132. Moe-Nilssen, R: Test-retest reliability of trunk accelerometry during standing and walking. Arch Phys Med Rehabil 79:1377, 1998.

133. Moe-Nilssen, R, and Helbostad, JL: Estimation of gait cycle characteristics by trunk accelerometry. J Biomech 37: 121, 2004.

134. Henriksen, M, et al: Test-retest reliability of trunk accelerometric gait analysis. Gait Posture 19:288–297, 2004.

135. Levine, JA, et al: Validation of the Tracmor triaxial accelerometer system for walking. Med Sci Sports Exerc 33:1593, 2001.

136. Hartmann, A, et al: Reproducibility of spatio-temporal gait parameters under different conditions in older adults using a trunk tri-axial accelerometer system. Gait Posture 30:351, 2009.

137. Menz, HB, et al: Acceleration patterns of the head and pelvis when walking on level and irregular surfaces. Gait Posture 18: 35–46, 2003.

138. Zhang, K, et al: Measurement of human daily physical activity. Obes Res 11:33–40, 2003.

139. Foerster, F, et al: Detection of posture and motion by accelerometry: A validation study in ambulatory monitoring. Comput Hum Behav 15:571, 1999.

140. Macko, RF, et al: Microprocessor-based ambulatory activity monitoring in stroke patients. Med Sci Sports Exerc 34:394, 2002.

141. Michael, KM, et al: Reduced ambulatory activity after stroke: The role of balance, gait, and cardiovascular fitness. Arch Phys Med Rehabil 86:1552, 2005.

142. Gebruers, N, et al: Monitoring of physical activity after stroke: A systematic review of accelerometry-based measures. Arch Phys Med Rehabil 91:288–297, 2010.

143. Hartsell, H, et al: Accuracy of a custom-designed activity monitor: Implications for diabetic foot ulcer healing. J Rehabil Res Dev 39:395–400, 2002.

144. Brandes, M, and Rosenbaum, D: Correlations between the step activity monitor and the DynaPort ADL-monitor. Clin Biomech 19:91, 2004.

145. Coleman, KL, et al: Step activity monitor: Long-term, continuous recording of ambulatory function. J Rehab Res Dev 36:8–18, 1999.

146. Aminian, K, et al: Spatio-temporal parameters of gait measured by an ambulatory system using miniature gyroscopes. J Biomech 35:689–699, 2002.

147. Kotiadis, AD, et al: Inertial gait phase detection for control of a drop foot stimulator: Inertial sensing for gait phase detection. Med Eng Phys 32:287–297, 2010.

148. Barker, S, et al: Accuracy, reliability, and validity of a spatiotemporal gait analysis system. Med Eng Phys 28:460, 2006.

149. Stokic, DS, et al: Agreement between temporospatial gait parameters of an electronic walkway and a motion capture system in healthy and chronic stroke populations. Am J Phys Med Rehabil 88:437–444, 2009.

150. McDonough, AL, et al: The validity and reliability of the GAITRite system's measurements: A preliminary evaluation. Arch Phys Med Rehabil 82:419–425, 2001.

151. van Uden, C, and Besser, M: Test-retest reliability of temporal and spatial gait characteristics measured with an instrumented walkway system (GAITRite®). BMC Musculoskelet Disord 5:13, 2004.

152. Menz, HB, et al: Reliability of the GAITRite® walkway system for the quantification of temporo-spatial parameters of gait in young and older people. Gait Posture 20:20–25, 2004.

153. Bilney, B, et al: Concurrent related validity of the GAITRite® walkway system for quantification of the spatial and temporal parameters of gait. Gait Posture 17:68–74, 2003.

154. Titianova, EB, et al: Gait characteristics and functional ambulation profile in patients with chronic unilateral stroke. Am J Phys Med Rehabil 82:778, 2003.

155. Bowen, A, et al: Dual-task effects of talking while walking on velocity and balance following a stroke. Age Ageing 30:319–323, 2001.

156. Rosano, C, et al: Gait measures indicate underlying focal gray matter atrophy in the brain of older adults. J Gerontol A Biol Sci Med Sci 63A:1380, 2008.

157. Webster, KE, et al: Validity of the GAITRite walkway system for the measurement of averaged and individual step parameters of gait. Gait Posture 22:317–321, 2005.

158. Wolf, SL, and Binder-Macleod, SA: Use of the Krusen Limb Load Monitor to quantify temporal and loading measurements of gait. Phys Ther 62:976–984, 1982.

159. Powers, CM, et al: The influence of lower extremity muscle force on gait characteristics in individuals with below-knee amputations secondary to vascular disease. Phys Ther 76:369, 1996.

160. Burnfield, JM, et al: Similarity of joint kinematics and muscle demands between elliptical training and walking: Implications for practice. Phys Ther 90:289–305, 2010.

161. Morris, ME, et al: Changes in gait and fatigue from morning to afternoon in people with multiple sclerosis. J Neurol Neurosurg Psychiatry 72:361, 2002.

162. Powers, CM, et al: The effects of patellar taping on stride characteristics and joint motion in subjects with patellofemoral pain. J Sports Phys Ther 26:286–291, 1997.

163. O'Shea, S, et al: Dual task interference during gait in people with Parkinson disease: Effects of motor versus cognitive secondary tasks. Phys Ther 82:888–897, 2002.

164. Evans, MD, et al: Systematic and random error in repeated measurements of temporal and distance parameters of gait after stroke. Arch Phys Med Rehabil 78:725–729, 1997.

165. Maurer, BT, et al: Quantitative identification of ankle equinus with applications for treatment assessment. Gait Posture 3: 19–28, 1995.

166. Teixeira-Salmela, LF, et al: Effects of muscle strengthening and physical conditioning training on temporal, kinematic and kinetic variables during gait in chronic stroke survivors. J Rehabil Med 33:53–60, 2001.

167. Schwartz, MH, et al: Comprehensive treatment of ambulatory children with cerebral palsy: An outcome assessment. J Pediatr Orthop 24:45–53, 2004.

168. Lam, T, et al: Stumbling corrective responses during treadmill-elicited stepping in human infants. J Physiol 553:319–331, 2003.

169. Woltring, HJ, and Marsolais, EB: Optoelectric (Selspot) gait measurement in two- and three-dimensional space, a preliminary report. Bull Prosthet Res 17:46–52, 1980.

170. Bell, A, et al: A comparison of the accuracy of several hip center location prediction models. J Biomech 23:617, 1990.

171. Gorton, GE, et al: Assessment of the kinematic variability among 12 motion analysis laboratories. Gait Posture 29:398–402, 2009.

172. Richards, JG: The measurement of human motion: A comparison of commercially available systems. Hum Mov Sci 18:589–602, 1999.

173. Cornwall, MW, and McPoil, TG: Motion of the calcaneus, navicular, and first metatarsal during the stance phase of walking. J Am Podiatr Med Assoc 92:67–76, 2002.

174. Fishco, WD, and Cornwall, MW: Gait analysis after talonavicular joint fusion: 2 case reports. J Foot Ankle Surg 43:241, 2004.

175. Burnfield, JM, and Powers, CM: Influence of age and gender of utilized coefficient of friction during walking at different speeds. In Marpet, MI, and Sapienza, MA (eds): Metrology of Pedestrian Locomotion and Slip Resistance, ASTM STP 1424. ASTM International, West Conshohocken, PA, 2003, pp 3–16.

176. Burnfield, JM, et al: Comparison of utilized coefficient of friction during different walking tasks in persons with and without a disability. Gait Posture 22:82–88, 2005.

177. Cook, TM, et al: Effects of restricted knee flexion and walking speed on the vertical ground reaction force during gait. J Orthop Sports Phys Ther 25:236, 1997.

178. Hesse, S, et al: Treadmill training with partial body weight support: Influence of body weight release on the gait of hemiparetic patients. J Neurol Rehabil 11:15–20, 1997.

179. Kerrigan, DC, et al: Compensatory advantages of toe walking. Arch Phys Med Rehabil 81:38–44, 2000.

180. Neptune, RR, et al: The neuromuscular demands of toe walking: A forward dynamics simulation analysis. J Biomech 40:1293, 2007.

181. Sasaki, K, et al: Muscle contributions to body support and propulsion in toe walking. Gait Posture 27:440, 2008.

182. Randolph, AL, et al: Reliability of measurements of pressures applied on the foot during walking by a computerized insole sensor system. Arch Phys Med Rehabil 81:573, 2000.

183. Mueller, MJ, et al: Therapeutic footwear can reduce plantar pressure in patients with diabetes and transmetatarsal amputation. Diabetes Care 20:637, 1997.

184. Mueller, MJ, et al: Incidence of skin breakdown and higher amputation after transmetatarsal amputation: Implications for rehabilitation. Arch Phys Med Rehabil 76:50, 1995.

185. Armstrong, DG, et al: Peak foot pressures influence the healing time of diabetic foot ulcers treated with total contact casts. J Rehabil Res Dev 35:1–5, 1998.

186. Burnfield, JM, et al: The influence of walking speed and footwear on plantar pressures in older adults. Clin Biomech 19:78–84, 2004.

187. Mohamed, OS, et al: Effect of terrain on foot pressure during walking. Foot Ankle Int 26:859–869, 2005.

188. Burnfield, JM, et al: Variations in plantar pressure variables across five cardiovascular exercises. Med Sci Sports Exerc 39:2012, 2007.

189. Semple, R, et al: Regionalised centre of pressure analysis in patients with rheumatoid arthritis. Clin Biomech 22:127, 2007.

190. Burnfield, JM, et al: The influence of lower extremity joint torque on gait characteristics in elderly men. Arch Phys Med Rehabil 81:1153, 2000.

191. Brinkmann, JR, and Perry, J: Rate and range of knee motion during ambulation in healthy and arthritic subjects. Phys Ther 65:1055, 1985.

192. Winter, DA, et al: Biomechanical walking pattern changes in the fit and healthy elderly. Phys Ther 70:340, 1990.

193. Himann, JE, et al: Age-related changes in speed of walking. Med Sci Sports Exerc 20:161, 1988.

194. Hageman, PA, and Blanke, DJ: Comparison of gait of young women and elderly women. Phys Ther 66:1382, 1986.

195. Cho, SH, et al: Gender differences in three dimensional gait analysis data from 98 healthy Korean adults. Clin Biomech 19:145–152, 2004.

196. Sutherland, D, et al: Clinical use of prediction regions for motion analysis. Dev Med Child Neurol 38:773, 1996.

197. Chester, VL, et al: Comparison of two normative paediatric gait databases. Dyn Med 6:8, 2007.

198. Romei, M, et al: Use of the Normalcy Index for the evaluation of gait pathology. Gait Posture 19:85–90, 2004.

199. Mulroy, S, et al: Use of cluster analysis for gait pattern classification of patients in the early and late recovery phases following stroke. Gait Posture 18:114–125, 2003.

200. Waters, RL, et al: Energy expenditure following hip and ankle arthrodesis. J Bone Joint Surg 70:1032, 1988.

201. Marsolais, EB, and Edwards, BG: Energy costs of walking and standing with functional neuromuscular stimulation and long leg braces. Arch Phys Med Rehabil 69:243, 1988.

202. Herbert, LM, et al: A comparison of oxygen consumption during walking between children with and without below-knee amputations. Phys Ther 74:943, 1994.

203. Davies, MJ, and Dalsky, GP: Economy of mobility in older adults. J Orthop Sports Phys Ther 26:69–72, 1997.

204. Torburn, L, et al: Energy expenditure during ambulation in dysvascular and traumatic below-knee amputees: A comparison of five prosthetic feet. J Rehabil Res Dev 32:111, 1995.

205. Ebbeling, CJ, et al: Lower extremity mechanics and energy cost of walking in high-heeled shoes. J Orth Sports Phys Ther 19:190, 1994.

206. Waters, RL, et al: Energy-speed relationship of walking: Standard tables. J Orthop Res 6:215, 1988.

207. Olgiati, R, et al: Increased energy cost of walking in multiple sclerosis: Effect of spasticity, ataxia, and weakness. Arch Phys Med Rehabil 69:846, 1988.

208. Olney, SJ, et al: Mechanical energy of walking of stroke patients. Arch Phys Med Rehabil 67:92, 1986.

209. McGibbon, CA, et al: Mechanical energy analysis identifies compensatory strategies in disabled elders' gait. J Biomech 34:481–490, 2001.

210. Findley, TW, and Agre, JC: Ambulation in the adolescent with spina bifida. II. Oxygen cost of mobility. Arch Phys Med Rehabil 69:855, 1988.

211. MacGregor, J: The objective measurement of physical performance with Long-Term Ambulatory Physiological Surveillance Equipment (LAPSE). Proc 3rd Int Symp on Ambulatory Monitoring, London, 1979, pp 29–39.

212. Graham, RC, et al: The reliability and validity of the Physiological Cost Index in healthy subjects while walking on 2 different tracks. Arch Phys Med Rehabil 86:2041, 2005.

213. Boyd, R, et al: High- or low-technology measurements of energy expenditure in clinical gait analysis? Dev Med Child Neurol 41:676, 1999.

214. Hood, VL, et al: A new method of using heart rate to represent energy expenditure: The Total Heart Beat Index. Arch Phys Med Rehabil 83:1266, 2002.

215. Ijzerman, MJ, et al: Validity and reproducibility of crutch force and heart rate measurements to assess energy expenditure of paraplegic gait. Arch Phys Med Rehabil 80:1017, 1999.

216. Winchester, P, et al: A comparison of paraplegic gait performance using two types of reciprocating gait orthoses. Prosthet Orthot Int 17:101, 1993.

217. Harvey, LA, et al: Energy expenditure during gait using the walkabout and isocentric reciprocal gait orthoses in persons with paraplegia. Arch Phys Med Rehabil 79:945–949, 1998.

218. Steven, MM, et al: The physiological cost of gait (PCG): A new technique for evaluating nonsteroidal anti-inflammatory drugs in rheumatoid arthritis. Br J Rheumatol 22:141, 1983.

219. Olney, SJ, et al: A randomized controlled trial of supervised versus unsupervised exercise programs for ambulatory stroke survivors. Stroke 37:476–481, 2006.

220. Stein, RB, et al: A multicenter trial of a footdrop stimulator controlled by a tilt sensor. Neurorehabil Neural Repair 20:371, 2006.

221. Sabut, SK, et al: Effect of functional electrical stimulation on the effort and walking speed, surface electromyography activity, and metabolic responses in stroke subjects. J Electromyogr Kinesiol 20:1170, 2010.

222. Chin, T, et al: The efficacy of Physiological Cost Index (PCI) measurement of a subject walking with an Intelligent Prosthesis. Prosthet Orthot Int 23:45, 1999.

223. Ijzerman, MJ, et al: Validity and reproducibility of crutch force and heart rate measurements to assess energy expenditure of paraplegic gait. Arch Phys Med Rehabil 80:1017, 1999.

224. Bowen, TR, et al: Variability of energy-consumption measures in children with cerebral palsy. J Pediatr Orthop 18:738, 1998.

225. Danielsson, A, et al: Measurement of energy cost by the Physiological Cost Index in walking after stroke. Arch Phys Med Rehabil 88:1298–1303, 2007.

226. Naver, HK, et al: Reduced heart rate variability after right-sided stroke. Stroke 27:247–251, 1996.

227. Colivicchi, F, et al: Cardiac autonomic derangement and arrhythmias in right-sided stroke with insular involvement. Stroke 35:2094, 2004.

228. Korpelainen, JT, et al: Dynamic behavior of heart rate in ischemic stroke. Stroke 30:1008, 1999.

229. Lakusic, N, et al: Gradual recovery of impaired cardiac autonomic balance within first six months after ischemic cerebral stroke. Acta Neurol Belg 105:39–42, 2005.

230. Gordon, N, et al: Physical activity and exercise recommendations for stroke survivors. An American Heart Association scientific statement from the Council on Clinical Cardiology, Subcommittee on Exercise, Cardiac Rehabilitation, and Prevention; the Council on Cardiovascular Nursing; the Council on Nutrition, Physical Activity, and Metabolism; and the Stroke Council. Circulation 109:2031, 2004.

231. Kanade, R, et al: Walking performance in people with diabetic neuropathy: Benefits and threats. Diabetologia 49:1747, 2006.

232. Kim, MO, et al: The assessment of walking capacity using the Walking Index for Spinal Cord Injury: Self-selected versus maximal levels. Arch Phys Med Rehabil 88:762–767, 2007.

233. Lotan, M, et al: Improving physical fitness of individuals with intellectual and developmental disability through a Virtual Reality Intervention Program. Res Dev Disabil 30:229–339, 2009.

Supplemental Readings

Brach, JS, et al: Diabetes mellitus and gait dysfunction and possible explanatory factors. Phys Ther 88:1365–1374, 2008.

Hergenroeder, AL, et al: Association of body mass index with self-report and performance-based measures of balance and mobility. Phys Ther 91:1223–1234, 2011.

Winter, DA: Biomechanics of Human Movement. John Wiley & Sons, New York, 1979.

Recording Form for Observational Gait Analysis

Patient's name _____ Age ____ Gender ____ Height ____ Weight ____

Diagnosis _____

Footwear _____ Assistive devices _____

Date _____ Therapist _____

DIRECTIONS: Place a check (√) in the space opposite the deviation if the deviation is observed.

Body Segment/ Plane Observed	Deviation	Stance														Swing						Possible Cause(s)	Analysis
		IC		LR		MSt		TSt		PSw		ISw		MSw		TSw							
		R	L	R	L	R	L	R	L	R	L	R	L	R	L	R	L						
Ankle and foot	None																						
Sagittal plane observations	Foot flat																						
	Foot slap																						
	Heel-off																						
	No heel-off																						
	Excessive plantarflexion																						
	Excessive dorsiflexion																						
	Toe drag																						
	Toe clawing																						
	Contralateral vaulting																						
Frontal plane observations	Varus																						
	Valgus																						
	Knee																						
	None																						
Sagittal plane observations	Excessive flexion																						
	Limited flexion																						
	No flexion																						
	Hyperextension																						
	Genu recurvatum																						
	Diminished extension																						

Body Segment/ Plane Observed	Deviation	Stance									Swing						Possible Cause(s)	Analysis
		IC		LR		MSt		TSt		PSw		ISw		MSw		TSw		
		R	L	R	L	R	L	R	L	R	L	R	L	R	L	R	L		
Frontal plane observations	Varus																		
	Valgus																		
Hip	None																		
Sagittal plane observations	Excessive flexion																		
	Limited flexion																		
	No flexion																		
	Diminished extension																		
Frontal plane observations	Abduction																		
	Adduction																		
	External rotation																		
	Internal rotation																		
	Circumduction																		
	Hiking																		
Pelvis	None																		
Sagittal plane observations	Anterior tilt																		
	Posterior tilt																		
	Increased backward rotation																		
	Increased forward rotation																		
	Limited backward rotation																		
	Limited forward rotation																		
	Drops on contralateral side																		
Trunk	None																		
Frontal plane observations	Backward rotation																		
	Lateral lean																		
	Forward rotation																		
	Backward lean																		
	Forward lean																		

Key: IC = initial contact; LR = loading response; MSt = mid stance; TSt = terminal stance; PSw = pre-swing; ISw = initial swing; MSw = mid swing; TSw = terminal swing.

Temporal and Spatial Measures Gait Analysis Form

Patient's name_____ Age_____ Gender _____ Height_____ Weight_____

Diagnosis _____

Ambulatory aids: Yes _____ No _____

Type: Crutch(es) _____ Cane(s):   R _____ Walker: _____

L _____

Other: _____

Instructions: Distance walked, elapsed time and walking velocity can be calculated for a single walking trial or averaged across multiple walking trials if the patient's endurance permits. Therapist should provide an average value (calculated across multiple complete steps/strides) for the stride and step lengths, width of walking base, and foot angles.

Date	
Therapist's initials	
Distance walked (distance from first to last heel strike)	
Elapsed time (time from first to last heel strike)	
Walking velocity (distance walked divided by elapsed time)	
Left stride length (distance between two consecutive left heel strikes)	
Right stride length (distance between two consecutive right heel strikes)	
Left step length (distance between a right heel strike and the next consecutive left heel strike)	
Right step length (distance between a left heel strike and the next consecutive right heel strike)	
Step length difference (difference between right and left step lengths)	
Cadence (total number of steps taken divided by the elapsed time)	
Width of walking base (perpendicular distance between right and left heel strike)	
Left foot angle (angle formed between a line bisecting the left foot and the line of progression)	
Right foot angle (angle formed between a line bisecting the right foot and the line of progression)	
Right stride length to right lower extremity length (right stride length divided by right lower extremity length)	
Left stride length to left lower extremity length (left stride length divided by left lower extremity length)	

Manufacturer Contact Information for Gait Analysis Hardware and Software

7.C

Manufacturer	Address	Gait Analysis Product(s)	Website
Advanced Medical Technology, Inc. (AMTI)	176 Waltham Street Watertown, MA 02472	Force plates and sensors	www.amtiweb.com
Ariel Performance Analysis System	Ariel Dynamics 6 Alicante St. Trabuco Canyon, CA 92679	Gait and motion analysis hardware and software	www.arielnet.com
Ascension Technology Corporation	P.O. Box 527 Burlington, VT 05402	Flock of Birds motion analysis hardware and software	www.ascension-tech.com
B and L Engineering	1901 Carnegie Ave. Suite Q Santa Ana, CA 92705	Stride Analyzer and EMG hardware and software	www.bleng.com
Bioengineering Technology Systems (BTS)	viale Forlanini 40 20024 Garbagnate Milanese MI Italy	Integrated gait systems	www.btsbioengineering.com/
Biometrics Ltd.	PO Box 340 Ladysmith, VA 22501	Electrogoniometers	www.biometricsltd.com/ gonio.htm
Charnwood Dynamics Ltd.	Fowke Street Rothley, Leicestershire LE7 7PJ United Kingdom	Coda motion analysis hardware and software	www.codamotion.com
C-Motion, Inc.	20030 Century Blvd Suite 104A Germantown, MD 20874	Visual 3D software for analyzing biomechanical data	www.c-motion.com/index.php
CYMA Corporation	6405 218th St. S.W. Suite 100 Mountlake Terrace, WA 98043-2180	StepWatch Activity Monitor 3™	www.orthocareinnovations.com/ pages/stepwatch_tradefaq
Dartfish	6505 Shiloh Rd. Suite 110-B Alpharetta, GA 30005	Movement analysis software	www.dartfish.com/en/ index.htm
GaitMat II™	EQ, Inc. P.O. Box 16 Chalfont, PA 18914-0016	Instrumented gait mat	www.gaitmat.com
GAITRite®	CIR Systems, Inc. 60 Garlor Drive Havertown, PA 19083	Instrumented gait mat	www.gaitrite.com

Continued

Manufacturer	Address	Gait Analysis Product(s)	Website
Kistler Instrument Corporation	75 John Glenn Dr. Amherst, NY 14228-2171	GaitWay Treadmill®, force plates, accelerometers	www.kistler.com
Motion Analysis Corporation	3617 Westwind Blvd Santa Rosa, CA 95403	Gait and motion analysis hardware and software	www.motionanalysis.com
Northern Digital Inc.	103 Randall Drive Waterloo, Ontario Canada N2V 1C5	Optotrak and 3D Investigator Motion Capture Systems	www.ndigital.com
Novel Electronics, Inc.	964 Grand Ave. St. Paul, MN 55105	emed®, pedar®, and pliance® pressure mapping hardware and software	www.novel.de
PhoeniX Technologies Inc.	4302 Norfolk St. Burnaby, BC Canada V5G 4J9	Motion analysis hardware and software	www.ptiphoenix.com/index.php
Polhemus	40 Hercules Drive P.O. Box 560 Colchester, VT 05446	Motion analysis hardware and software	www.polhemus.com
Qualisys AB	Packhusgatan 6 S-411 13 Gothenburg, Sweden	Gait and motion analysis hardware and software	www.qualisys.com
Tekscan, Inc.	307 W. First St. South Boston, MA 02127	F-Scan®, MatScan®, and Walkway™ pressure and force mapping hardware and software	www.tekscan.com
Vicon Motion Analysis System	Vicon Colorado 7388 S. Revere Parkway Suite 901 Centennial, CO 80112	Gait and motion analysis hardware and software	www.vicon.com
Windows Media Player®	Microsoft Corporation Redmond, WA 98052	Video player for viewing video recordings of gait	www.windows.microsoft.com
Xsens North America Inc.	2684 Lacy Street Suite 205 Los Angeles, CA 90031	Motion tracking hardware and software	www.xsens.com

Simple Tabulated Output from the Stride Analyzer System

YOUR DEPARTMENT'S NAME
YOUR INSTITUTION'S NAME
STRIDE ANALYZER REPORT—WALKING

NAME:	JOHN SMITH	RUN:	JS01
I.D. NUMBER:	1234	STRIDES:	4
DATE:	05/13/93	DISTANCE (M):	6.00
AGE:	29	TEST CONDITIONS:	
SEX:	M	WALK	
DIAGNOSIS:	Sprained Right Ankle		

STRIDE CHARACTERISTICS	ACTUAL	%NORMAL
VELOCITY (m/min):	60.3	74.0
CADENCE (steps/min):	100.4	92.7
STRIDE LENGTH (m):	1.201	79.8
GAIT CYCLE (sec):	1.20	106.8
SINGLE LIMB SUPPORT	-R-	-L-
(sec):	0.429	0.418
(%NORMAL):	86.4	84.2
(%GC):	35.9	35.0
SWING (%GC):	33.5	34.5
STANCE (%GC):	66.5	65.5
DOUBLE SUPPORT		
INITIAL (%GC):	15.2	15.4
TERMINAL (%GC):	15.4	15.2
TOTAL (%GC):	30.6	30.6

LEFT FOOT (stance = 65.5% GC)

HEEL	–	Normal contact at 0.0% GC (0.0% Stance)
		Delayed cessation at 50.6% GC (77.2% Stance)
5th METATARSAL	–	Premature contact at 3.8% GC (5.7% Stance)
		Delayed cessation at 63.3% GC (96.6% Stance)
1st METATARSAL	–	Normal contact at 22.4% GC (34.2% Stance)
		Delayed cessation at 63.9% GC (97.5% Stance)
TOE	–	Normal contact at 33.7% GC (51.4% Stance)
		Delayed cessation at 65.5% GC (100.0% Stance)

RIGHT FOOT (stance = 66.5% GC)

HEEL	–	Normal contact at 0.0% GC (0.0% Stance)
		Delayed cessation at 50.8% GC (76.4% Stance)
5th METATARSAL	–	Premature contact at 4.0% GC (6.0% Stance)
		Delayed cessation at 64.8% GC (97.5% Stance)
1st METATARSAL	–	Normal contact at 19.6% GC (29.4% Stance)
		Delayed cessation at 63.8% GC (96.0% Stance)
TOE	–	Normal contact at 38.1% GC (57.3% Stance)
		Delayed cessation at 65.2% GC (98.1% Stance)

From Craik and Otis,[50, p. 133] with permission.

Chapter 8

Examination of Function

David A. Scalzitti, PT, PhD, OCS

A clinician needs to consider the purposes of obtaining the measurement in deciding which measure of function to use. For example, is the measure to describe a specific activity limitation or describe an individual's overall level of function? Will the measure be used to assess outcomes of an episode of care, determine the destination at discharge, obtain reimbursement, meet regulatory requirements, or a combination of all of the above? As function may incorporate performance at the level of body systems, the person, and society, or a combination of these, and the clinician should be cognizant of the ability of the measure to capture the appropriate information.

The ultimate objective of any rehabilitation program is to return the individual to a lifestyle that is as close to the premorbid level of function as possible or, alternatively, to maximize the current potential for function and maintain it. For an otherwise healthy person with a fractured arm, this may be a reasonably simple process: improving range of motion, strength, and impairments in body function will reestablish skills in the performance of activities, such as dressing and feeding. However, considering the person with a stroke as an example, the task is much more complex because the problems are much more extensive, complicated, and interwoven. The two cases, however, are broadly similar. In both instances, the therapist begins by describing the problem in functional terms obtained from the history, performing a systems review and detailed examination using selected tests and measures, evaluating the data, establishing a diagnosis and prognosis, implementing interventions to reduce or to eliminate the problems identified, and documenting the progress toward the desired functional outcome.[1]

Every individual values the ability to live independently. The construct of function encompasses all those tasks, activities, and roles that identify a person as an independent adult or as a child progressing toward adult independence. These activities require the integration of both cognitive and affective abilities with motor skills. Functional activity is a patient-referenced concept and is dependent on what the individual self-identifies as essential to support physical and psychological well-being, as well as to create a personal sense of meaningful living. Function is not totally individualistic, however; there are certain categories of activities that are common to everyone. Eating, sleeping, elimination, and hygiene are major components of survival and protection common to all animals. Particular to humans are the evolutionary advancements of bipedal locomotion and complex hand activities, which permit independence in the personal environment. Work and recreation are functional activities in a social context.

This chapter presents a conceptual framework for examining functional status based on the International Classification of Functioning, Disability, and Health (ICF) and introduces the reader to terminology used in the field (see also Chapter 1). It presents an overview of the purposes of the examination of function and the range and rigor of formal test instruments currently available to clinicians and researchers. Considerations in test selection and principles of administration are also presented.

■ A CONCEPTUAL FRAMEWORK

Chronically ill and disabled persons represent a large segment of the population in the United States. In 2008, approximately 37 million Americans (12%) were considered to have a disability (limited in their usual activities due to one or more chronic health conditions).[2] Traditionally, these individuals have been categorized or classified according to their medical diseases or conditions. Medical procedures such as physical examination and laboratory tests are the primary tools to delineate the problems created by disease. Strict focus on a biomedical model, with its emphasis on the characteristics of *disease* (etiology, pathology, and clinical manifestations), may contribute to reducing patients to the *medical labeling* of these individuals; for example, referring to people as amputees, paraplegics, or arthritics rather than as individuals with these conditions. This model virtually ignores the equally important psychological, social, and behavioral dimensions of the **illness**, which accompanies the disease. Illness refers to the personal behaviors that emerge when the reality of having a disease is internalized and experienced by an individual. Factors related to illness often play a key role in determining the success or failure of rehabilitation efforts well beyond the nature of the medical condition that prompted a patient's referral to physical therapy. In helping the individual with a disease, physical therapists come to understand each person's illness as well.

A broad conceptual framework is necessary to fully understand the concept of health and its relationship to function and disability. Terms such as *well-being, health-related quality of life,* and *functional status* are often used interchangeably to describe health status. The most global definition of **health** has been provided by the World Health Organization (WHO), which defined health as "a state of complete physical, mental, and social well-being, and not merely the absence of diseases and infirmity."[3, p. 459] Although such global definitions are useful as philosophical statements, they lack the precision necessary for a clinician or researcher.

In order to describe the components of health and provide a unified and standard language and framework for the description of health and health-related states, the *International Classification of Functioning, Disability, and Health (ICF)* was developed.[4] The ICF was endorsed by the World Health Assembly on May 22, 2001, for international use and complements other classifications of the WHO such as the *International Classification of Diseases,* 10th revision (ICD-10).[5] Whereas the ICD-10 is a classification of diseases, disorders, and other health conditions, the ICF attempts to provide a meaningful description of the components of health and its relationship to a person with the health condition. Since its development the use of the ICF has been endorsed by the physical therapy community, including the World Confederation of Physical Therapy (WCPT) and the American Physical Therapy Association (APTA), and is gradually replacing other frameworks.[6] Table 8.1 presents an overview of some of these other frameworks, including of the ICF's predecessor, the WHO's International Classification of Impairments, Disability and Handicaps (ICIDH)[7] and the Nagi model[8] on which the process of disablement in APTA's *Guide to Physical Therapist Practice*[1] is based.

Function in the ICF is an umbrella term encompassing all **body functions and structures**, **activities**, and **participation**, whereas **disability** is a term that encompasses **impairments** in body functions and structures, **activity limitations**, and **participation restrictions**. Both function and disability are represented in the ICF, in contrast to previous frameworks, to provide for the description of a continuum of the components of health from positive aspects to items an individual is not able to perform or perform in a limited manner or with assistance.

The ICF framework consists of two parts. The first part describes components of function and disability in the context of health, whereas the second part describes contextual factors which may interact with the components of the first part (Fig. 8.1). These components of the ICF do not model a process of disablement, such as in previous frameworks; rather, the ICF provides an approach to classification of function and disability from

Table 8.1	Terminology Used In Historical Disablement Frameworks	
ICIDH[7]	**Nagi[8]**
Disease	**Active pathology**
The intrinsic pathology or disorder	Interruption or interference with normal processes, and efforts of the organism to regain normal state
Impairments	**Impairments**
Any loss or abnormality of psychological, physiological, or anatomical structure or function	Anatomical, physiological, mental, or emotional abnormalities or loss
Disability	**Functional limitations**
Any restriction or lack (resulting from an impairment) of ability to perform an activity in the manner or within the range considered normal for a human being	Limitation in performance at the level of the whole organism or person
Handicaps	**Disability**
A disadvantage for a given individual, resulting from an impairment or disability, that limits or prevents the fulfillment of a role that is normal (depending on age, sex, and social and cultural factors) for that individual	Limitation in performance of socially defined roles and tasks within a sociocultural and physical environment

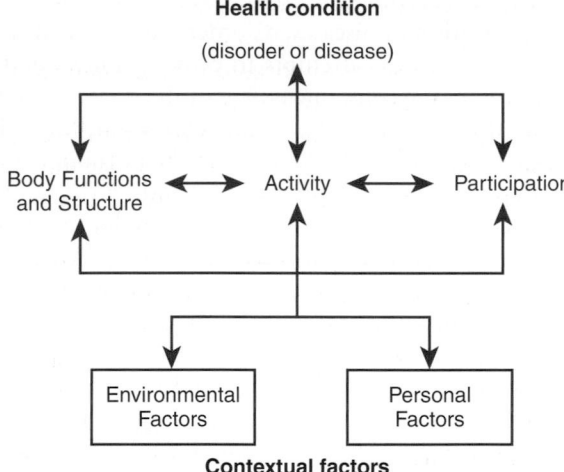

Figure 8.1 Schematic representation of the ICF. *(From World Health Organization: ICF: International Classification of Functioning, Disability, and Health. World Health Organization, Geneva, Switzerland, 2002, p 18, with permission.)*

multiple perspectives. The relationship between components and parts of the ICF does not imply causality. Bidirectional arrows are used in Figure 8.1 to represent a complex relationship. For example, a health condition such as angina may influence aspects of mobility such as gait, whereas at the same time increasing one's mobility by performing a regular walking program may influence the management of the health condition. In addition, a limitation in one component of the framework does not imply limitations in other components.

Body functions are defined by the ICF as the physiological functions of body systems, and body structures are parts of the body such as organs, limbs, and their components. *Impairment* is the term used to refer to

problems in body function or structure. Although two separate sections are used to classify body functions and structures in the ICF, the classifications are designed to be used together. For example, the chapter titled "Neuromuscular and Movement-related Functions" in the body functions classification correlates with the chapter titled "Structures Related to Movement" in the body structures classification. Hence, for a person with rheumatoid arthritis a clinician may use aspects of the body functions classification to describe range of motion of the interphalangeal joints and muscle performance of the hand intrinsic muscles and the body structures classification to describe the integrity of the joints of the hand. The headings for the chapters in the ICF classification of body functions and structures are in Table 8.2.

The ICF defines activity as the execution of a task or action by an individual and participation as involvement in a life situation. The terms used to describe problems in these domains are *activity limitations* and *participation restrictions*. Through the definitions of activity and participation an attempt is made to differentiate what a person can do because of characteristics of the individual and those of society. In the ICF, however, a single list covers both activity and participation. In contrast, a draft of the ICF, the ICIDH-2, used separate lists to distinguish activity from participation.[9] Instead of separate lists, the ICF allows users to operationally differentiate activities and participation. Possibilities suggested in the ICF include (a) designating some domains as activities and others as participation with no overlap, (b) designating some domains as activities and others as participation allowing for overlap, (c) designating all detailed domains as activities and the broad categories as participation, and (d) using all

Table 8.2	ICF Classification of Body Functions and Body Structures
Body Functions	**Body Structures**
Mental functions	Structures of the nervous system
Sensory functions and pain	The eye, ear, and related structures
Voice and speech functions	Structures involved in voice and speech
Functions of the cardiovascular, hematological, immunological, and respiratory systems	Structures of the cardiovascular, immunological, and respiratory systems
Functions of the digestive, metabolic, and endocrine systems	Structures related to the digestive, metabolic, and endocrine systems
Genitourinary and reproductive functions	Structures related to the genitourinary and reproductive systems
Neuromusculoskeletal and movement-related functions	Structures related to movement
Functions of the skin and related structures	Skin and related structures

domains as both activities and participation.[4, pp. 234-237] To date, no standard exists for the distinction of the classification of activity and participation, and physical therapists should be aware of the potential uses of the classification for practice and research.[10]

The headings for the nine chapters in the ICF classification of activities and participation and examples of classification within a chapter are presented in Figure 8.2. The chapters are considered the first-level of classification and can be used to categorize positive and negative aspects of function. The second-level of classification includes categories of different actions, tasks, and activities. Subcategories provide additional detail for the main categories. For example, moving around is a category within the mobility domain of the ICF, and crawling is a subcategory of the moving around category.

The second part of the ICF is labeled "contextual factors," which represent the complete background of an individual's life and are included to represent factors that may interact as facilitators or barriers to the components of function. The contextual factors are considered as either barriers or facilitators to function from the perspective of the individual whose situation is being described. Contextual factors have two components: environmental factors, which are external to the individual and can have positive or negative influence on performance, and personal factors, which are features of the individual such as age, gender, and race that are not part of a health condition or health state. Due to the bidirectional nature of the ICF framework contextual factors may also be modified by the components of part 1. Environmental factors are classified by the ICF; however, a classification of personal factors is notably omitted (Table 8.3).

The ICF, and models such as the Institute of Medicine's enabling-disabling process (Fig. 8.3),[1] emphasize the interaction between the person and the environment as critical to understanding functioning and disability.

Physical therapists can help change discriminatory social attitudes and environmental restrictions such as architectural barriers that stigmatize individuals and restrict participation in all aspects of society. The modification of factors that are barriers and incorporation of factors that are facilitators is as important to functioning as the amelioration of activity limitations.[11]

In addition to providing a framework for the classification of function, the ICF provides a classification scheme for coding, which, although not yet in widespread use by physical therapists, may be particularly intriguing in its delineation of actions, tasks, and activities in an implicit hierarchy of functioning. Within this hierarchy, actions (e.g., rolling, bending, sitting, standing, lifting, and reaching) are constituents of tasks and activities (e.g., bathing, dressing, and grooming). Tests and measures of actions are particularly relevant to physical therapist practice as they capture the complex integration of systems that permits an individual to maintain a posture, transition to other postures, or sustain safe and efficient movement.

Although typical patterns of deficits in body functions and problems in activities may typically exist in certain disease categories, the exact empirical relationship between a particular set of impairments in body functions and structure and activity limitations is not yet known.[12] The cause-and-effect relationship between an impairment and an activity limitation is most often inferred in the clinic from empirical evidence. For example, physical therapists may assume that the reason a patient cannot transfer independently is causally linked to the fact that the individual has lost enough lower extremity range of motion at the hip (e.g., hip flexion contractures) to prevent balancing in a fully upright posture. The return of activity following remediation of the impairment of joint mobility is then considered clinical evidence of a relationship between the impairment and the limitation. For data to be

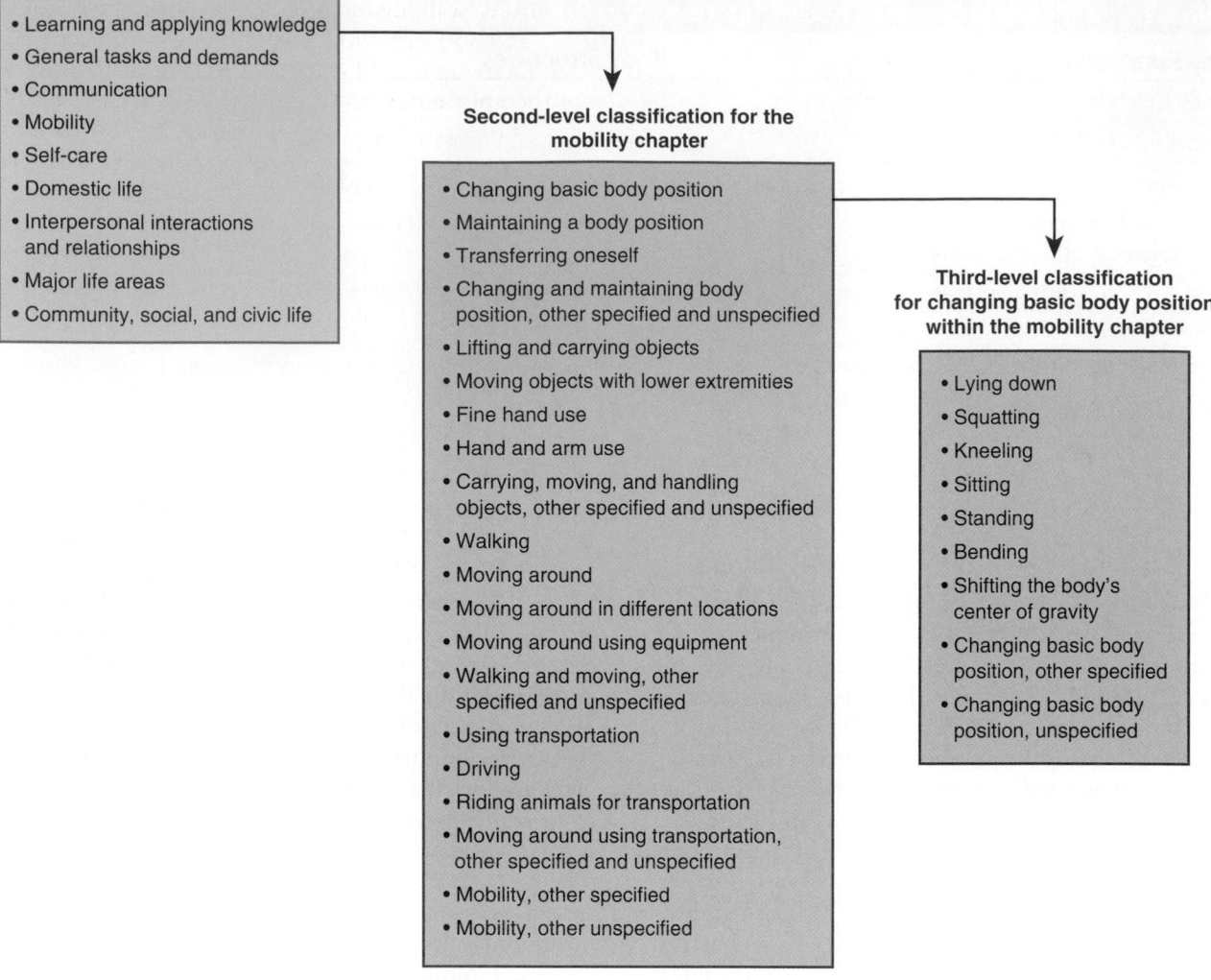

Figure 8.2 ICF Classification of Activities and Participation.

clinically useful, assessment of a patient's function by a physical therapist must include all of the appropriate components.

■ EXAMINATION OF FUNCTION

Purpose of Examination of Function

Analysis of function focuses on the identification of pertinent activities and measurement of an individual's ability to successfully engage in them. In essence, functional testing measures how a person does certain tasks or fulfills certain roles in the various dimensions of living described in the framework of the ICF. Application of selected functional tests and measures yield data that can be used as (1) baseline information for setting function-oriented goals and outcomes of intervention; (2) indicators of a patient's initial abilities and progression toward more complex functional levels; (3) criteria for placement decisions, for example, the need for inpatient rehabilitation, extended care, or community services; (4) manifestations of an individual's level of safety in performing a particular task and the risk of injury

with continued performance; and (5) evidence of the effectiveness of a specific intervention (medical, surgical, or rehabilitative) on function.

General Considerations

Physical therapists possess a unique body of knowledge related to the identification, remediation, and prevention of movement dysfunction. Thus, they have traditionally been involved in the examination of physical function. Other members of the rehabilitation team, including the occupational therapist, nurse, rehabilitation counselor, and recreational therapist, are also typically involved in administering and interpreting functional tests. Some formal instruments were designed to be completed collectively by the team. Other tests are compiled in separate sections by specific health professionals and housed together in the patient's chart. Where teams exist, physical therapists are typically responsible for the testing of aspects of function related to mobility, such as bed mobility, transfers, and locomotion (wheelchair mobility, ambulation, negotiation of stairs and graded

Table 8.3	Environmental Factors in the ICF
First-Level Classification	Examples
Products and technology	Medications, clothes, prosthetics, walking devices, scooters, hearing aids, ramps, assets
Natural environment and human-made changes to environment	Geography, climate, light, air quality
Support and relationships	Immediate family, extended family, friends, persons in positions of authority, personal assistants, domesticated animals, health professionals
Attitudes	Individual attitudes of immediate family members, individual attitudes of health professionals, societal attitudes
Services, systems, and policies	Housing, transportation, legal, associations, health, education, political

elevations, walking for longer distances in the community, and so forth). Instruments to measure activities of daily living (ADL) may be administered by a physical therapist alone or cooperatively with other health professionals. When overlap among team members exists, for example, the performance of toilet transfers, the data may be collected by the physical therapist, an occupational therapist, or a nurse. In these instances, testing should be coordinated to reduce duplication and unnecessary patient stress. In noninstitutional settings or where there is no team, the physical therapist is often responsible for determining all aspects of these instruments.

Testing Perspectives

Function tests can utilize two highly divergent perspectives on what is to be tested or measured by the physical therapist. It is extremely important that the therapist determine in advance whether data are needed to describe the *habitual level* of a patient's ability to do certain tasks and activities, or to identify the patient's *capacity* to perform certain tasks and activities, whether the patient habitually performs up to that level or not, or even performs them at all. These perspectives are incorporated within the ICF by the constructs of performance and capacity and the ICF allows for the separate coding of both constructs.

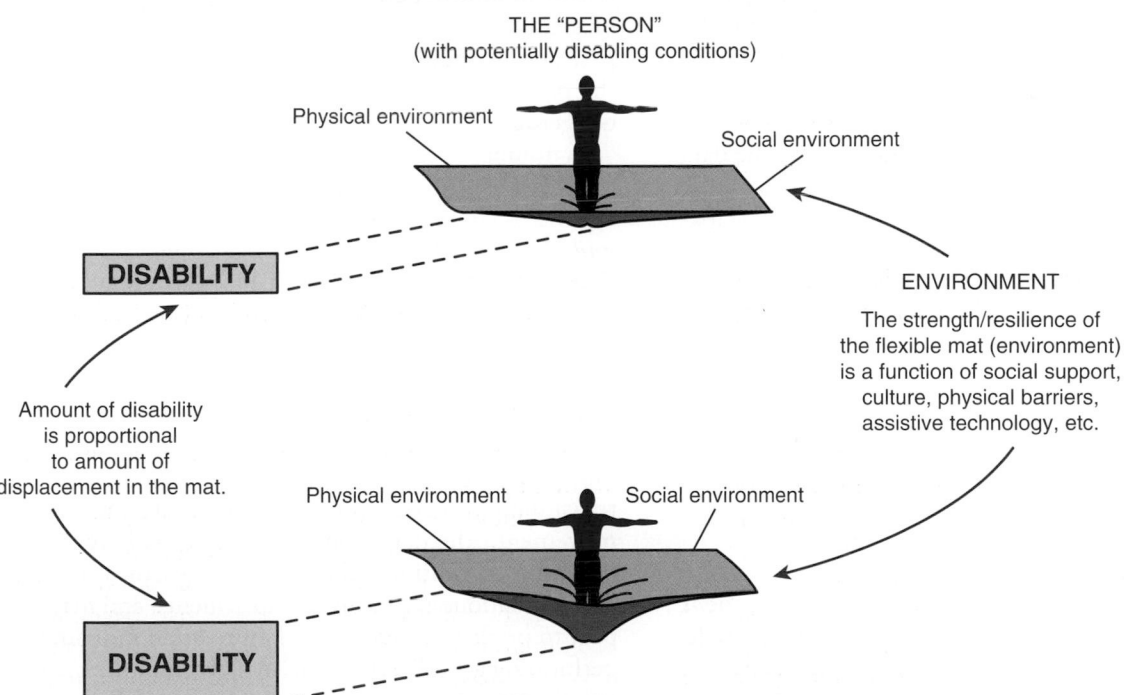

Figure 8.3 The Institute of Medicine model of the enabling-disabling process. Disability is a function of the interaction between the person and the environment. The amount of displacement represents the amount of disability that is experienced by the individual. Displacement is a function of the strength of the physical and social environments that support an individual and the magnitude of the potentially disabling condition. *(From Brandt, EN, Jr, and Pope, AM (eds): Enabling America: Assessing the Role of Rehabilitation Science and Engineering. National Academy Press, Washington, DC, 1997, p 9, with permission.)*

These divergent viewpoints directly affect what types of tests and measures should be chosen and what parameters of measurement are appropriate to yield data useful to making clinical judgments. Most important, physical therapists must consider the differences between capacity for function and habitual function in determining the prognosis for rehabilitation and estimating the likelihood of the success of an intervention. Patients accept a therapist's recommendations regarding the anticipated goals of treatment only if there is the perceived need and motivation to function habitually at the highest level of ability. Understanding the difference between what a person actually does or would be willing to do and what that person potentially could do is an essential component of designing realistic, and achievable, functional goals. For example, even though a person might have the capacity to climb stairs, there may not be any willingness to do so. Ultimately, physical therapists must abide by each patient's own decision regarding which tasks and activities will be incorporated into a daily routine and what is a meaningful level of function, regardless of the therapist's professional opinion.

Irrespective of the particular instrument used, there are several basic considerations to be kept in mind. The setting chosen must be conducive to the type of testing and free of distractions. Instructions should be precise and unambiguous. Testing may be biased by fatigue. If a patient performs best in the morning but tires by afternoon, an accurate determination of functional ability must consider the variation in the patient's performance. Therapists should be aware of patients whose energy fluctuates during the day, and interpret the data accordingly. In general, information related to body functions and body structure, activities, and participation, as well as personal and environmental factors, should be generated during the initial examination (or as soon as feasible) so the information may be considered together to develop a picture of a patient's function. Retesting should occur at regular intervals during treatment to document progress and before discharge from the episode of care.

Types of Instruments
Performance-Based Tests

A performance-based test involves **observing the patient during the performance of an activity**. Generally speaking, the therapist who chooses a performance-based test is searching for an indication of what a patient can do under a specific set of circumstances, which may or may not be similar to the natural environment in which the patient functions. If a performance-based test is chosen with the intention of making inferences about how the patient will perform at home, the conditions and setting should be as similar as possible to the actual environment in which the patient usually performs the tasks

and activities. A performance-based approach may be used either to describe the patient's current level of function or to identify the maximum level of function possible.

During the administration of the test, each task is presented and the patient is asked to perform it. For example, to examine current level of function in wheelchair mobility, a patient would receive this instruction: "Push your wheelchair over to that red chair and stop." To determine the patient's maximum level of function in this activity, the instruction might specify a particular manner of performance: "Push your wheelchair over to that red chair *as quickly as you can* and stop." Understanding the difference between these two commands, even though both are observation-based performance of wheelchair mobility, is essential to sound clinical decision making. Data from the first example identify only what the patient can do under specific circumstances, but does not support the inference that the patient will be able to wheel across a busy intersection in the short time span allotted to a typical pedestrian walkway. The form of the instruction determines whether an inference can be made about the patient's maximal level of function in formulating the goals for intervention and the plan of care.

In either case, a patient is given no additional instructions or assistance unless he or she is unable or unsure of how to perform. Then only as much direction or assistance as is needed is given. Appropriate safety precautions should be taken during the session so that the patient does not attempt tasks that are potentially dangerous.

A number of tests of impairments are sometimes also referred to as functional performance measures, including the *6-Minute Walk Test*,[13] the *Physical Performance and Mobility Examination*,[14] the *Functional Reach Test*,[15,16] the *Get Up and Go Test*,[17] the *Timed Up and Go Test*,[18] and the *Physical Performance Battery*.[19] A performance instrument of this sort typically measures either a complex integration of impairments, the performance of actions, or a combination of both by direct observation. Overall, the tests do provide some insight into the individual's capabilities to maintain a posture, transition to other postures, or sustain safe and efficient movement. The data from such a test, gathered under controlled conditions, characterize a person's performance limitations as a result of impairments, and may purport to predict the success or failure of an individual in performing goal-directed tasks or activities under natural conditions, using a score that summates the combined effects of impairments throughout and across systems on movement dysfunction. Each of these tests can contribute to an understanding of an aspect of a person's function, but they should not be used to represent all aspects of function. Although these tests employ the method of direct observation of performance, they most often do not measure the task or activity as it might be accomplished in the "real" world of the patient, which is also influenced by motivation and habit.

Self-Reports

In contrast to the method of direct observation, useful data on how a person functions may also be gathered by *self-report,* in which the patient is asked directly either by the therapist or a trained interviewer (*interviewer report*) or through the use of a *self-administered report* instrument. The critical issue in the ability of a self-report to capture function correctly and completely lies in providing clearly worded questions without language bias, concise directions on completing the questions, and a format that encourages accurate reporting of answers to all questions. Self-report is a valid method of determining function and may be preferable to performance-based methods in some circumstances.[20] Self-reports should be designed so that questions are asked in a standard format and answers are recorded as specified by the predetermined choices. Long paper-and-pencil tests may be difficult for those with upper extremity disability.

Clinical personnel who will act as interviewers must be trained to administer a questionnaire. Interviewers should practice until they have reached a high degree of agreement with expert examiners of the same cases. Periodic retraining may be necessary if interviewers do not have frequent practice administering the instrument. The interview should be scheduled with the patient in advance and conducted in an environment conducive to complete concentration. Interviews may be conducted by phone or in person, but the mode of administration should be kept consistent if comparisons of the data are to be made. Ad lib prompting by the interviewer or caregivers for answers is discouraged because these intrusions into the patient's self-report tend to bias results. If the patient has had help in filling out a form or responding to questions, this should be noted. Similarly, if the data have been provided by a spouse, family member, or caregiver, this should be documented as well.

The distinction in perspectives on function that was discussed regarding performance-based measures of function also holds for self-reports. It is extremely important to distinguish between questions that indicate a person's habitual performance (e.g., "*Do* you cook your own meals?") and those that identify a person's perceived capacity to perform a task (e.g., "If you had to, *could* you cook your own meals?"). It may also be important to distinguish between an individual's performance of an activity and his or her confidence in performance of an activity. For example, confidence and performance for 21 items are measured in separate scales in APTA's *Outpatient Physical Therapy Improvement in Movement Assessment Log (OPTIMAL).*[21]

The time frame reference of self-reporting is also a relevant consideration. A therapist should decide in advance if the relevant "window" on a person's functional level is the past 24 hours, last week, last month, or the previous year. One can easily imagine how the same person might respond differently regarding the same functional activity depending on frame of reference. Instruments that examine only short-term objectives may not relate well to the long-term objectives of a rehabilitation program.

Instrument Parameters and Formats

Performance-based and self-report instruments grade performance on a number of different criteria in a variety of formats. There is no one parameter or format that is perfect for every type of clinical encounter or research need. It is particularly important that documentation of a patient's progress not be blunted by *floor* or *ceiling* effects. For example, if a therapist wishes to measure changes in function among generally well elderly patients and the most advanced functional activity on an instrument measures "independent ambulation on level surfaces," there would be no room to demonstrate either progression or decline except around ambulation on level surfaces. Similarly, a patient who was severely debilitated might improve in transfers from needing the maximum assistance of two persons to maximum assistance of one. If the instrument only measures change from "maximum assistance" to "moderate assistance," this patient's real improvement will not be recorded.

Descriptive Parameters

Therapists should use descriptive terms that are well defined and unambiguous. Meanings of descriptive terms should be clear to all others using the medical record. Box 8.1 provides a sample set of acceptable terms and definitions. Additional terms used to qualify function include *dependence* and *difficulty*. Most often, the term *independent* refers to the complete absence of a need for human or mechanical assistance to accomplish a task, but some scoring systems consider reliance on devices and aids as a modified form of independence when used without the help of another person. The use of equipment during the performance of a functional task should be explicitly noted; for example, "independent in ambulation with axillary crutches" or "independent in dressing with adapted clothing and a long-handled shoe horn."

Difficulty is a hybrid term that suggests an activity poses an extra burden for the patient, regardless of dependence level. It is unclear whether it is a measure of overall perceptual-motor skill, coordination, endurance, efficiency, or a combination of measures. Difficulty can be measured in two ways. One approach assumes that difficulty is likely to be present and quantifies the degree of difficulty that the individual experiences while performing the activity (e.g., "How much difficulty do you have while doing household chores? None, some, or a

Box 8.1 Functional Examination and Impairment Terminology

Definitions

1. **Independent:** patient is able consistently to perform skill safety with no one present.
2. **Supervision:** patient requires someone within arm's reach as a precaution; low probability of patient having a problem requiring assistance.
3. **Close guarding:** person assisting is positioned as if to assist, with hands raised but not touching patient; full attention on patient; fair probability of patient requiring assistance.
4. **Contact guarding:** therapist is positioned as with close guarding, with hands on patient but not giving any assistance; high probability of patient requiring assistance.
5. **Minimum assistance:** patient is able to complete majority of the activity without assistance.
6. **Moderate assistance:** patient is able to complete part of the activity without assistance.
7. **Maximum assistance:** patient is unable to assist in any part of the activity.

Descriptive Terminology

A. Bed Mobility
  1. Independent—no cuing[a] is given
  2. Supervision
  3. Minimum assistance ⎫
  4. Moderate assistance ⎬ may require cues
  5. Maximum assistance ⎭

B. Transfers, Ambulation
  1. Independent—no cuing is given
  2. Supervision
  3. Close guarding
  4. Contact guarding ⎫
  5. Minimum assistance ⎬ may require cues
  6. Moderate assistance
  7. Maximum assistance ⎭

C. Functional Balance Grades

1. Normal	Patient able to maintain steady balance without support (static). Accepts maximal challenge and can shift weight easily and within full range in all directions (dynamic).	
2. Good	Patient able to maintain balance without support, limited postural sway (static). Accepts moderate challenge; able to maintain balance while picking object off floor (dynamic).	
3. Fair	Patient able to maintain balance with handhold support; may require occasional minimal assistance (static). Accepts minimal challenge; able to maintain balance while turning head/trunk (dynamic).	
4. Poor	Patient requires handhold and moderate to maximal assistance to maintain posture (static). Unable to accept challenge or move without loss of balance (dynamic).	
5. No balance		

[a]Types of cues: verbal, visual, or tactile. In some instances (e.g., a person with a memory deficit, short attention, learning disability, visual loss), a decrease in the number of cues may represent treatment progress, even though the level of dependence remains the same. Interim progress notes can denote these changes by citing frequencies (e.g., 2 out of 3 tries) or an arbitrarily defined rank order scale (e.g., always/occasionally/rarely).

great deal?"). The other approach quantifies the frequency that the difficulty is encountered (e.g., "How often do you have difficulty putting on your shoes? Never, sometimes, very often, or always?").

Often it is helpful to qualify a person's performance by linking observations with nonspecific indicators of impairments such as the energy consumption required to complete the functional task and the degree to which patients must exert themselves to engage in the activity. Simple measurements of a patient's physiological

response to activity generally include heart rate, respiratory rate, and blood pressure, obtained at rest (baseline measurements), during (as possible), or immediately after completion of the most stressful elements of the activity. For example, "heart rate increased to 100 beats per minute with independent ambulation on stairs; no increase in respiratory rate." In addition, the patient's perceived fatigue, perception of exertion, and overt signs of physiological stress, such as shortness of breath, also should be noted. These notations may assist the therapist in a quick identification of some obvious impairments that limit function, which should be followed by more specific tests and measures of impairment.

Additional descriptors frequently used to qualify functional performance further include (1) pain, (2) fluctuations according to the time of day, (3) medication level, and (4) environmental influences. Any factors that modify a patient's function should be carefully noted and considered by the physical therapist evaluating examination data.

Quantitative Parameters

The time it takes to complete a series of activities is often used to enhance a therapist's quantification of function when a given speed of performance is required or an improvement in performance speed is expected. A common example of timed functional skills is found in premedication and postmedication performance of individuals with Parkinson disease who are placed on l-dopa therapy. Examples of activities that may be timed include (1) walking a set distance; (2) writing one's signature; (3) donning an article of clothing; and (4) crossing a street during the time of a "Walk" light. Scores of timed tests should not be taken as absolute, but rather as one dimension of performance. Although the ability to complete a particular activity in a specified period of time does provide one kind of important data on a patient's overall ability, it may not always be correct to conclude that what is being measured as "quicker" can be interpreted as "better." For example, the patient may get dressed quickly (within seconds), but do so with poorly coordinated movements and a haphazard outcome. When the task is slowed down, the movements may become more coordinated, with a more satisfactory functional outcome, even though the time taken to do the task increases. Similarly, certain medical conditions that affect energy expenditure may require that the patient properly pace a functional activity to complete it successfully. Thus, time scores alone do not always yield the complete functional picture. When interpreted in light of other aspects of the patient's clinical presentation, they do provide an added dimension to the evaluation of data collected during a functional examination.

Response Formats

Function can be measured with tests that report data as nominal, ordinal, interval, and ratio measures. The clinician should consider the uses of the measure when deciding which format to use. In cases where the clinical decision is nominal, such as is the patient ready for discharged to home, a nominal measure such as whether the patient can independently ascend 10 stairs may be adequate. When ratio measures are obtained, such as the score on a Berg Balance scale, the clinician may interpret the score as a dichotomous measure related to the decision (e.g., Does the patient have or not have adequate

balance for discharge to home?). In cases where the clinical decision is more complex, such as the amount of assistance a patient needs with activities, nominal measures cannot be used and the measure should reflect the type and amount of information needed for the decision.

Nominal Measures

One of the simplest formats in functional tests uses a **nominal** level of measurement by presenting a **checklist** of various functional tasks on which the patient is simply scored as able to do/not able to do, independent/dependent, completed/incomplete, or the like. The results are not particularly descriptive of the exact nature of an individual's limitations and usually require further examination before interpretation. Nominal measures, however, may be helpful in making dichotomous decisions. For example, knowledge of the ability to perform ADL skills by themselves is important in deciding if a patient can be discharged, or not, to living independently at home.

Ordinal Measures

A few tests use descriptive scales that describe a range of performance or the degree to which a person can perform the task. Most commonly, the scales are **ordinal or rank-order scales** (e.g., "no difficulty," "some difficulty," or "unable to do"; or "always," "sometimes," "rarely," or "never"). Scales may be graded in ascending or descending order. The primary drawback in using such a system to score function is that these grades do not define categories that are separated by equal intervals. For example, it is not possible to tell whether the patient who went from maximal assistance to moderate assistance changed as much as a patient who also went one level between moderate assistance and minimal assistance.

Interval Measures

Summary or **additive measures** grade a specific series of skills, award points for part or full performance, and sum the subscores as a proportion of the total possible points, such as 60/100 or 6/24 and so forth. Although the scales typically may include a score of zero, this value represents a floor effect of the scale and not necessarily the absence of the construct. One example of a summary measure, which is well known to physical therapists, is the Barthel Index.[22]

Some formal, standardized instruments for testing function summarize detailed information about a complex area of function into an overall index score. Use of these instruments facilitates the interpretation of complex data and enables the clinician to perform cross-disease, cross-program, and cross-population comparisons of function. Caution must be exercised in considering only summated scores, however, because potentially important individual differences in functional ability can be masked.[23] A patient who is limited in only a few of the many tasks covered on a functional test will most likely score well, despite what could be substantial limitations in discrete functional activities that are pertinent to the physical therapist's anticipated goals of treatment. Similarly, two patients with the same numeric score might be quite different in their functional deficits, having gained (or lost) their points on different activities. Although these measures yield a "hard number," which is regarded statistically as an interval level of measurement, the degree to which "points" are truly equal intervals or only ordinal should be carefully scrutinized.

Ratio Measures

Visual or linear analog scales attempt to represent measurement quantities in terms of a straight line placed horizontally or vertically on paper (Fig. 8.4). The endpoints of the line are labeled with descriptive or numeric terms to anchor the extremes of the scale and provide a frame of reference for any point in the continuum between them. Some scales will also use descriptors or numeric intervals between the endpoints to assist the individual in grading responses. Commonly a visual analog line of 10 centimeters (100 millimeters) is used. The patient is asked to bisect the line at a point representing self-reported position on the scale. The patient's score is then obtained by measuring from the zero mark to the mark bisecting the scale.

Examples of the use of visual analog scales in rehabilitation settings may be to measure pain, dyspnea, function, or satisfaction with care. Since visual analog scales include a true zero and equal intervals (e.g., mm) they may be analyzed as ratio measures. In contrast, some clinicians may use a numeric rating scale (e.g., rate your function on a scale from 0 to 10) to measure similar impairments. Although providing a numeric rating may be quicker to obtain in clinical settings, scores obtained may not represent interval or ratio data as the reporting of a numeric value may not represent equal intervals. For example, a 4 reported by a patient may not be twice as much function as a 2 reported by another patient. This is due to the nature of interval and ratio scales because a ratio scale allows for the comparison of scores using addition, subtraction, multiplication, or division and an interval scale allows for the comparison of scores using addition or subtraction. These mathematical functions cannot be performed with ordinal or nominal scores.

Knowledge of the level of measurement is important in analyzing data from groups of patients, such as a rehabilitation unit wishing to summarize the functional status of patients admitted during a specified time period. For interval and ratio measures, means and standard deviations may be calculated (assuming the data follow a normal distribution). For ordinal measures, medians and interquartile ranges are appropriate, whereas nominal measures should be reported as modes or frequency counts.

■ INTERPRETING TEST RESULTS

Clearly, the single most important consideration in examining functional status is using the test results correctly to establish and revise the anticipated goals and expected outcomes of intervention and the plan of care. The therapist should carefully delineate the contributing factors that result in the functional deficit. When diminished ability is evident, the therapist must attempt to ascertain the cause of the problem. Some important questions to ask include the following:

1. What are the normal movements necessary to perform the task?
2. Which impairments inhibit performance or completion of the task? For example, do factors such as poor motor planning and execution, decreased strength, decreased range of motion, or altered joint integrity impede function? Does fatigue hamper functional ability?
3. Are the patient's functional deficits the result of impaired communication, perception, vision, hearing, or cognition?

Examples of the kinds of questions a therapist must pose to assess function and integrate findings into a comprehensive treatment program are found using the case vignettes in Table 8.4:

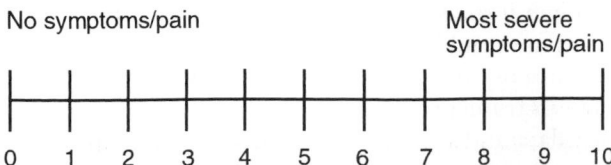

Figure 8.4 A visual analog scale for measuring pain or other symptoms. The patient is instructed to mark the line at the point that corresponds to the degree of pain or severity of symptoms that are experienced.

Table 8.4	Sample Case Vignettes	
Case A		**Case B**
36-year-old male construction worker		72-year-old female homemaker
Dx: traumatic right transtibial amputation; following fracture left femur		Dx: CVA with right hemiplegia with global aphasia
Partial Examination Findings		
Motor Control and Muscle Performance		
Decreased in all extremities following prolonged immobilization		Flaccid paralysis right extremities
Activity Limitations		
Unable to transfer from bed to wheelchair		Unable to transfer from bed to wheelchair

Dx = Diagnosis.

Although the activity limitation in each case is in fact identical, the contributing factors, goals and outcomes, and the interventions would be markedly different. In case A, the patient's inability to transfer can reasonably be attributed to decreased strength. When ameliorated, it is likely that the patient will go on to achieve an outcome of independent ambulation with a prosthesis. The patient in case B has factors that cannot be addressed solely through physical therapy. In addition, it may be difficult to determine whether it is the paralysis or the aphasia that compromises efforts to assess and improve function. Although a similar goal of independence in wheelchair mobility and transfers may be proposed, reexamination throughout the episode of care may demonstrate that functional deficits persist, despite improvement in motor function. In that case, the impairments in comprehension and language function may be the more important factors contributing to functional limitation. Thus, the design of rehabilitation programs is based on the impairments that presumably underlie the functional deficits. If remediation of the impairment does not solve the functional problem, the therapist needs to reexamine the initial clinical impression by looking for other potentially causative factors.

Some functional tasks may need to be analyzed more precisely. Activities can be broken down into subordinate parts, or subroutines. A **subordinate part** is defined as an element of movement without which the task cannot proceed safely or efficiently. For example, bed mobility includes the following subordinate parts: (1) scooting in bed (changing position for comfort or skin care and getting to the edge), (2) rolling onto the side, (3) lowering the legs, (4) sitting up, and (5) balancing at the edge of the bed. A functional loss of independent bed mobility may result from an inability to perform any or all of these subroutines. These are not only checkpoints for examining patients, but they also later represent the anticipated goals of various interventions. The more involved the patient, the slower the learner, or complex the task, the more the functional task may need to be broken down into subordinate parts.

Determining the Quality of Instruments

Within the rehabilitation setting, many tools exist for the measurement of function or its components. For example, the Catalog of Tests and Measures in APTA's *Guide to Physical Therapist Practice* includes close to 500 tests and measures.[24] In deciding which measure to use the instrument's **reliability** and **validity** should be considered. If the reliability and validity of an instrument have not been established, little faith can be put in the results obtained or in the conclusions drawn from the results. A poorly constructed instrument can produce data that are questionable, if not worthless. In light of the fact that the viability of physical therapy as a reimbursable service rests on the demonstration of functional outcomes, the importance of these concepts to

functional testing becomes clear. In accordance with APTA's Standards of Measurement, physical therapists should use only those instruments whose reliability and validity are known.[25] Although no instrument will have perfect reliability or validity, therapists must be able to gauge the certainty of their data and the appropriate scope of inferences drawn from the data.

Reliability

A reliable instrument measures a phenomenon dependably, time after time, accurately, predictably, and without variation. If a functional test is not reliable, the patient's initial baseline status or the true effect of treatment can be concealed. An instrument with acceptable *test–retest reliability* is stable and will not indicate change when none has occurred. Tests performed by the same therapist of the same performance should be highly correlated (*intrarater reliability*). Instruments should also have strong *interrater reliability*, or agreement among multiple observers of the same event. If a particular patient is examined by several therapists in the course of treatment, or reexamined over time to determine long-term change, the reliability of the functional tool must be known.

A flaw in the clinical use of most types of standardized tests and measures is the tendency to disregard interrater reliability. To use functional tests with maximum accuracy, (1) scoring criteria must be defined clearly and must be mutually exclusive; (2) criteria must be strictly applied to each clinical situation; and (3) all therapists in a facility must be retrained periodically in the use of the instrument to ensure similarity.

Values for reliability coefficients have been recommended. For example, Portney and Watkins suggest less than 0.50 as poor reliability, 0.50 to 0.75 as moderate reliability, and greater than 0.75 as good reliability.[26, p. 82] These cutoffs must be based on the precision of the measured variable and how the results of the reliability test will be applied. A clinician should use these values as guidelines, and not as absolutes, in determining the accuracy of the measurement and needs to consider the use of the instrument. If high precision is needed in the instrument for clinical decision making, values of a reliability coefficient higher than the minimal threshold for "good" reliability should be used. In addition to the value of the reliability coefficient, the clinician should consider the variability of the measurement that may be expressed as a standard deviation (SD) or confidence interval (CI).

Validity

Validity is a multifaceted concept and established in many different ways. Questions regarding an instrument's validity attempt to determine (1) whether an instrument designed to measure function truly does just that; (2) what the appropriate applications of the instrument are; and (3) how the data should be interpreted.

First, the valid instrument should, on the face of it, appear to measure what it purports to measure (*face validity*).[25,26] For example, an instrument claiming to measure balance should appear to measure some aspect of balance. Another critical dimension is whether the assessment instrument measures all the important or specified dimensions of function (*content validity*). If there were a **gold standard** (an unimpeachable measure of a phenomenon, such as a laboratory test with normative values), then a new instrument could be tested against the results of this standard (*criterion-related validity*). Such a gold standard does not exist for functional instruments. New functional measurement tools can, however, be compared to existing ones that are accepted measures of the same functional activities. The degree to which the two instruments agree helps to establish *concurrent validity*. Concurrent validity can also be demonstrated by showing that an instrument corresponds appropriately to measures of other phenomena. This method is particularly relevant for self-report instruments. The concurrent validity of some self-report instruments has been determined by comparison with clinician ratings and other clinical findings; for example, a person's level of function as indicated by an instrument correlates directly with clinician's ratings of improvement and inversely with the patient's reports of pain.

Sensitivity and Specificity

In the comparison of a test of function to a gold standard or to another existing instrument one should be concerned with the ability of the measure to make an accurate classification. *Sensitivity* of a test refers to the proportion of individuals with a limitation in function (as identified by the gold standard or existing instrument) who are correctly classified. In other words, sensitivity is an indication of how well a test identifies persons who should have a positive finding on the test. In contrast, *specificity* of a test refers to the proportion of individuals who do not have a limitation in function who are correctly classified. Additional properties of a test are the positive predictive value and the negative predictive value. The *positive predictive value* is the proportion of people who have a positive finding on a test who actually have a limitation in function as classified by the comparison test; the *negative predictive value* is the proportion of people who have a negative finding on a test who do not have a limitation in function.

Both sensitivity and specificity are expressed as values between 0 and 1. Ideally, both sensitivity and specificity should be as close to 1 as possible, but this is very rare in reality. Different tests, however, will be better at identifying those with the condition and others will be better at identifying those without the condition. This will be reflected in the magnitude of their sensitivity and specificity scores. When values of sensitivity or specificity are close to 1, the SpPIn and SnNOut acronyms may help with interpretation.[27] The acronym SpPIn refers to tests that have very high specificity: a positive finding helps to rule in the condition. SnNOut, on the other hand, refers to tests that have very high sensitivity: a negative finding helps to rule out the condition. In general, sensitivity and specificity values greater than 0.95 are considered very high.

Sensitivity and specificity values may be combined to obtain a likelihood ratio (LR) with the following equations. The calculation of likelihood ratios may be helpful in determining how much the test result influences the identification of a patient's condition or identification of a limitation in function. This is especially helpful in cases when sensitivity and specificity are not high enough to apply the SpPIn and SnNOut rules.

Positive LR = (Sensitivity)/(1 − Specificity)
Negative LR = (1 − Sensitivity)/(Specificity)

The larger the value of a positive likelihood ratio, the more helpful the finding of a positive test is in identification of the condition. Likewise, the smaller the value of a negative likelihood ratio (e.g., close to zero), the more helpful the finding of a negative test is in ruling out the condition. In contrast, a positive or negative likelihood ratio close to 1 is not helpful in identifying the condition. Likelihood ratios can be helpful in determination of post-test odds through their application in Bayes' theorem (i.e., the pretest odds (the likelihood ratio = the post-test odds).[27]

There is also the *predictive validity* of a test or measure, which indicates the likelihood of a subsequent phenomenon or event (e.g., return to work) on the basis of a prior phenomenon (e.g., a baseline measure of function). Finally, the degree to which an instrument measures abstract concepts such as physical mobility or social interaction can be established over time (*construct validity*). Construct validation, using a variety of statistical procedures, is a never-ending process as our understanding of the construct is further refined as instruments are developed to measure it.

Meaningful Change

In addition to reliability and validity, a measure of functional status should be sufficiently sensitive to reflect meaningful changes in a patient's status. The change should exceed the **minimal detectable change** (MDC) of the instrument and a **minimal clinical important difference** (MCID). The MDC can be described as the smallest amount of change in a measurement that exceeds the measurement error of the instrument. A physical therapist should be aware of published MDC values for the instruments used to measure function. A sample of MDC and MCID values is presented in Table 8.5. The clinician should keep in mind that MDC values are specific for the patient population in whom the instrument was investigated.

In cases where MDC values may not exist in the literature, values may be calculated if the reliability

Table 8.5	Examples of MDC and MCID Values	
Measure of Function and Population of Interest	**MDC or MCID Value**	**Reference**
6-Minute Walk Test in persons following total hip and knee arthroplasty	61.34 m	Kennedy et al (2005)[28]
6-Minute Walk Test in persons with COPD	37-71 m	Make (2007)[29]
6-Minute Walk Test in older adults	~50 m	Perera et al (2006)[30]
6-Minute Walk Test in persons with Alzheimer disease	33.5 m	Ries et al (2009)[31]
6-Minute Walk Test in persons following stroke	54.1 m	Fulk et al (2008)[32]
Timed Up and Go Test in persons with Alzheimer disease	4.09 sec	Ries et al (2009)[31]
Timed Up and Go Test in persons following total hip and knee arthroplasty	2.49 sec	Kennedy et al (2005)[28]
Gait speed in persons following stroke	0.1 m/sec	Fulk and Echternach (2008)[33]
Gait speed in persons following hip fracture	0.1 m/sec	Palombaro et al (2006)[34]
Berg Balance Scale in persons following stroke	7 points	Liaw et al (2008)[35]
Berg Balance Scale in persons with Parkinson disease	5 points	Steffen and Seney (2008)[36]
FEV_1 in persons with COPD	100 ml	Make (2007)[29]

COPD = chronic obstructive pulmonary disease; FEV_1 = forced expiratory volume in 1 second.

coefficient, such as an intraclass correlation coefficient (ICC), and a measure of its variability is known, such as the SD. The following equations present the relationship between the MDC95 (the amount of change with 95% confidence beyond measurement error) and the standard error of the measurement (SEM). The second equation can be used to determine the SEM if the value of the reliability coefficient and the standard deviation (SD) from one of the groups used to determine reliability is known. Note that because the ICC and the SD are from a specific sample, the calculated SEM and MDC95 are only generalizable to persons with similar conditions.

$$MDC95 = 1.96 \times SEM \times \sqrt{2} \text{ where } SEM = SD \times \sqrt{(1 - ICC)}$$

For example, if a study of persons after total knee arthroplasty reported an ICC of 0.75 for knee flexion with an SD of 5 degrees, the SEM is equal to 2.5 degrees. Using this value in the first equation, the MDC95 is 6.925 degrees. In other words, the measure of knee flexion would need to change more than 7 degrees to have 95% confidence that this change was due to something other than measurement error.

The MCID is the smallest difference in a measured variable that signifies an important rather than a trivial difference in the patient's condition. The value of the MCID should exceed the value of the MDC; in other words, the MCID needs to exceed the measurement error. For example, a 50-meter change in distance on the 6-minute walk test may be beyond measurement error; however, is the ability to walk 50 meters during 6 minutes meaningful to an individual patient's function? A number of different ways have been suggested

to determine values for the MCID.[26, pp. 646-652] No universal method exists. Controversies exist among the strategies to determine MCID based on the perspective of what is meaningful, as well as issues related to measurement.[37,38] The clinician should consult the literature for recommended values of the MCID for measures of function. Additionally, online resources are being developed to help clinicians locate values for a number of tests.[39,40] Similar to the interpretation of the MDC, in consulting published values for the MCID for a measure of function the clinician needs to consider the sample for which the values were established.

Considerations in Selection of Instruments

A large number of instruments have been developed to assess and to classify function. Given the plethora of instruments that currently exist, it is quite reasonable to ask how these instruments compare with one another. It is important to remember that no instrument is perfect for all patients or all situations. No instrument can measure all the items potentially relevant to a particular individual and provide the perfect composite picture. For example, one instrument may provide an extensive measure of ADL, but not deal with psychological or social dimensions of function. Another instrument may investigate social functioning while omitting some ADL tasks. Many items overlap from instrument to instrument. For example, a question on the ability to ambulate is a common item found in most physical function instruments. Although instruments may cover the same kind of activity, the questions posed about the performance of the same activity may be quite different. For example, one instrument may investigate the degree of difficulty and of human assistance required to "dress yourself, including handling of closures, buttons, zippers, snaps." Another may ask, "How much help do you need in getting dressed?" As discussed, differences also may exist in the time frames sampled in the various instruments. Critical questions to ask in selecting an instrument are presented in Box 8.2.

Extrapolating items from a variety of instruments may provide the kind of data desired but should be considered with extreme caution inasmuch as this process changes reliability or validity of the measurements. Factors such as the theoretic orientation of the user, the purpose for using the instrument, and the relevance of particular functional items to certain patient populations all enter into the decision making process. In the final analysis, the choice of instrument may be dictated by practical considerations. For example, self-report instruments, which rely on information from the patient, are limited in use to mentally competent individuals. Time and resources for administration also may influence test selection, or some rehabilitation facilities may adopt the use of a specific instrument for all patients (e.g., the Functional Independence Measure [FIM]). In any case, many suitable instruments are available for assessing functional status, some of which are commonly used by clinicians as well as researchers.

Box 8.2 Critical Questions to Ask in Selecting an Instrument

1. What are the domains or categories that the assessment instrument focuses on?
2. How adequately does the instrument measure the domain or domains being sampled?
3. What areas of physical function are included? Does the instrument measure ADL? Does the instrument measure instrumental activities of daily living (IADL), for example, more advanced skills such as managing personal affairs, cooking, and driving? Mobility skills?
4. What aspect of function is being measured? Is the level of dependence–independence considered? What is the length of time required to complete the functional task? Degree of difficulty? Influence of pain?
5. What is the time frame sampled in the instrument?
6. What is the mode of administration?
7. What type of scoring system is used?
8. Are multiple instruments necessary to provide a more complete picture of functional status?
9. Who completes the instrument—the clinician, the patient (self-report), or family member (proxy)?
10. How long does the instrument take to complete?

■ SINGLE DIMENSION VERSUS MULTIDIMENSIONAL MEASURES OF FUNCTION

Among the factors to consider in selecting a measure of function is whether a single dimension measure or a multidimensional measure should be used. For example, single dimension measures may include a specific construct such as balance, gait, or reaching; whereas multidimensional measures would include a combination of these constructs or have items that represent impairments, activity limitations, and participation restrictions. As an example of a single test, gait speed may be used to represent function. This test may frequently be used in clinical settings because it require a minimal amount of time to perform and little equipment other than a stopwatch and a hallway free of obstructions. For the test, the time for the patient to ambulate a specified distance, such as 10 meters, is recorded and speed is calculated as distance divided by time and frequently reported as meters per second. Although this is a test of a specific mobility item, walking, one might make inferences in regard to a patient's function based on this test. The clinician, however, is responsible to check with the literature to determine if the inferences are supported by evidence, because there are some specific populations where gait speed may be representative of a patient's ability to function. For example, in a study of persons after hip arthroplasty it was demonstrated that gait speed was more representative of the capacity to ambulate than performance because when the patients were tested in real world environments their gait speed was slower than in the clinic. However, in this case the measure of capacity versus performance was highly correlated ($\rho = 0.440$).[41] Recent evidence among older persons also suggests that the measure of gait speed is highly related to overall health.[42] For populations that have not been tested, however, a clinician should be cautious in using gait speed to make inferences regarding function.

Other tests may use multiple items to measure a single dimension, such as the items in the Barthel Index to measure ADL or the 14 items in the Berg Balance Scale to calculate a balance score. A clinician is justified using these instruments to describe the dimension of interest related to the patient's problem. However, unless data exist, they should not be used to make inferences regarding other impairments, activity limitations, or participation restrictions. Other instruments specific to those dimensions should be used as appropriate to the patient's presentation.

Alternatively, a clinician may take an approach to understand a patient's health status in all its domains. Further instrument development has resulted in the emergence of multidimensional health status instruments to measure the spectrum of health status more comprehensively. Used in conjunction with traditional clinical methods of examining signs and symptoms, multidimensional functional status instruments can add an important comprehensive view of a patient's function to the overall health status. In this respect they add a crucial, and previously missing, component in evaluating the health of individuals.

Recently, more comprehensive instruments are being developed to measure multiple dimensions of the ICF to present an overall view of a person's function. Specifically, a number of *ICF Core Sets* are being developed for specific patient conditions, such as stroke,[43] or by settings such as postacute rehabilitation settings.[44] Each core set includes items related to body functions, body structures, activities, participation, and contextual factors important to the specific condition or setting. These core sets are being developed using expert opinion and are being empirically tested to determine if representative items are included.[45,46] These core sets potentially may allow a clinician to focus on the most relevant items from the myriad of specific items in the ICF classification.

The final section of this chapter briefly discusses one single dimension instrument and three multidimensional instruments a physical therapist may use in practice. Many other instruments exist, some of which were mentioned previously in this chapter and some of which are included in other chapters. For a selection of instruments, the reader is referred to the APTA's *Catalog of Tests and Measures*.[24]

For the purposes of illustration, three multidimensional instruments, the *Functional Independence Measure* (FIM), the *Outcome and Assessment Information Set* (OASIS), and the *SF-36* are presented. Choice of a multidimensional instrument carries the same caveats mentioned for instruments a single dimension.[47] No instrument measures all potentially relevant items. In addition, depending on how an item is worded, items that may appear to measure the same aspect of function may be measuring different aspects of performance.[48] Table 8.6 presents a comparison of items covered. In the area of physical function, questions on the ability to ambulate are the only items these instruments have in common. Aspects of physical function not covered in any of these instruments include bed mobility and dexterity. The FIM and the OASIS include more ADL items than either the Sickness Impact Profile (SIP) or the SF-36. The SIP and the SF-36 investigate work performance, whereas the FIM and the OASIS do not. This is not surprising, given that the FIM was originally developed as a tool for the inpatient rehabilitation setting and the OASIS was expressly designed for home health agencies, both generally serving older patients. In contrast, the development of the SIP and SF-36 was focused on younger adult populations in ambulatory care. Anxiety and depression are addressed as areas of psychological function in the SIP, the SF-36, and the OASIS, but not in the FIM. The OASIS does not explore social function, whereas the other three

Table 8.6	Items Covered In Selected Multidimensional Functional Assessment Instruments		
	FIM	SF-36	OASIS
Symptoms	–	+	+
Physical function			
Transfers	+	–	+
Ambulation	+	+	+
ADL			
Bathing	+	+	+
Grooming	+	–	+
Dressing	+	+	+
Feeding	+	–	+
Toileting	+	–	+
IADL			
Indoor home chores	–	+	+
Outdoor home chores/shopping	–	+	+
Community travel/drive car	–	+	+
Work/school	–	+	–
Affective function			
Communication	+	–	+
Cognition	+	–	+
Anxiety	–	+	+
Depression	–	+	+
Social function			
Interaction	+	+	–
Activity/leisure	–	+	–
General health perceptions	–	+	–

instruments do. Finally, only the SF-36 records general health perceptions.

■ SAMPLE INSTRUMENTS TO ASSESS FUNCTION

The Barthel Index

The *Barthel Index* was developed by a physical therapist over 45 years ago.[22] Although not as commonly used today in practice as some other instruments, this instrument is still used to measure function in clinical research, and this assessment tool represents one of the earliest contributions to the functional status literature and identifies physical therapists' long-standing inclusion of functional mobility and ADL measurement within their scope of practice. The Barthel Index specifically measures the degree of assistance required by an individual on 10 items of mobility and self-care ADL (Table 8.7). Levels of measurement are limited to either complete independence or needing assistance. Each performance item

Table 8.7	Items Included in the Barthel Index
Feeding: scores range from independent (able to use utensils and other apparatus) to dependent (needs assistance)	
Bathing: scores range from independent to dependent	
Personal Toilet: scores range from independent (able to wash, comb hair, brush teeth or shave) to dependent (needs assistance)	
Dressing: scores range from independent (able to dress, fasten closures, tie shoes, apply orthosis as needed) to dependent (needs assistance)	
Bowels: scores range from independent (accident-free, able to use suppositories or enemas as needed) to dependent (occasional accidents, needs assistance)	
Bladder: scores range from independent (accident-free, able to use collection device as needed) to dependent (occasional accidents, needs assistance)	
Transfers–Toilet: independent (able to use toilet or bedpan) to dependent (needs assistance)	
Transfers–Chair and Bed: scores range from independent (able to manage wheelchair as needed) to dependent (needs assistance)	
Ambulation: scores range from independent (able to use assistive devices as needed) to dependent (needs assistance)	
Stair Climbing: scores range from independent (able to use assistive devices as needed) to dependent (needs assistance)	

Adapted from Mahoney and Barthel.[22]

is scored on an ordinal scale with a specified number of points assigned to each level or ranking. Variable weightings were established by the developers of the Barthel Index for each item based on clinical judgment or other implicit criteria. An individual who uses human assistance in eating, for example, would receive 5 points; independence in eating would receive a score of 10 points. A single global score, ranging from 0 to 100, is calculated from the sum of all weighted individual item scores, so that 0 equals complete dependence for all 10 activities, and 100 equals complete independence in all 10 activities. The Barthel Index has been used widely to monitor functional changes in individuals receiving inpatient rehabilitation, particularly in predicting the functional outcomes associated with stroke.[49,50] Although its psychometric properties have never been fully examined, the Barthel Index has demonstrated strong interrater reliability (0.95) and test–retest reliability (0.89), as well as high correlations (0.74 to 0.80) with other measures of physical disability.[51]

The Functional Independence Measure

The *Functional Independence Measure (FIM)*[52,53] is an 18-item measure of physical, psychological, and social function that is part of the Uniform Data System for Medical Rehabilitation (UDSMR).[54] The UDSMR collects data from participating rehabilitation facilities and issues summary reports of the records that have been entered into the UDSMR database. The FIM uses the level of assistance an individual needs to grade functional status from total independence to total assistance (Fig. 8.5). A person may be regarded as independent if a device is used, but this is recorded separately from "complete" independence. The instrument lists six self-care activities: feeding, grooming, bathing, upper body dressing, lower body dressing, and toileting. Bowel and bladder control, aspects of which some may consider as impairments rather than function, are categorized separately. Functional mobility is tested through three items on transfers. Under the category of locomotion, walking and using a wheelchair are listed equivalently, whereas stairs are considered separately. The FIM also includes two items on communication and three on social cognition.

The FIM measures what the individual does, not what that person could do under certain circumstances. The interrater reliability of the FIM has been established at an acceptable level of psychometric performance (intraclass correlation coefficients ranging from 0.86 to 0.88).[53] The face and content validity of the FIM, as well as its ability to capture change in a patient's level of function, have also been determined. Any clinical worker can administer the FIM after appropriate training in using the response set for each item.

For persons with stroke, the motor scale of the FIM has been shown to have high concurrent validity with the Barthel Index (ICC ≥ 0.83).[55] Gosman-Hedstrom and Svensson[56] have shown strong construct validity between items on the Barthel and items on the FIM that measure functional limitations. Rasch analysis has been applied to the scale scores of the FIM, which are ordinal measures, in order to create interval scale measurements.[57] In addition, the *WeeFIM*, an 18-item instrument based on the FIM, has been developed for use for children between the ages of 6 months and 18 years.[58]

The Outcome and Assessment Information Set

The *Outcome and Assessment Information Set (OASIS)* was designed to ensure the collection of pertinent data on the adult patient in the home care setting that would allow home health agencies to assess the quality of care by measuring the outcomes of care.[59,60] During the years of its initial development, use of the OASIS by home health agencies had been voluntary. However, as of January 1, 1999, home health agencies were mandated to use the OASIS as a *Condition of Participation in*

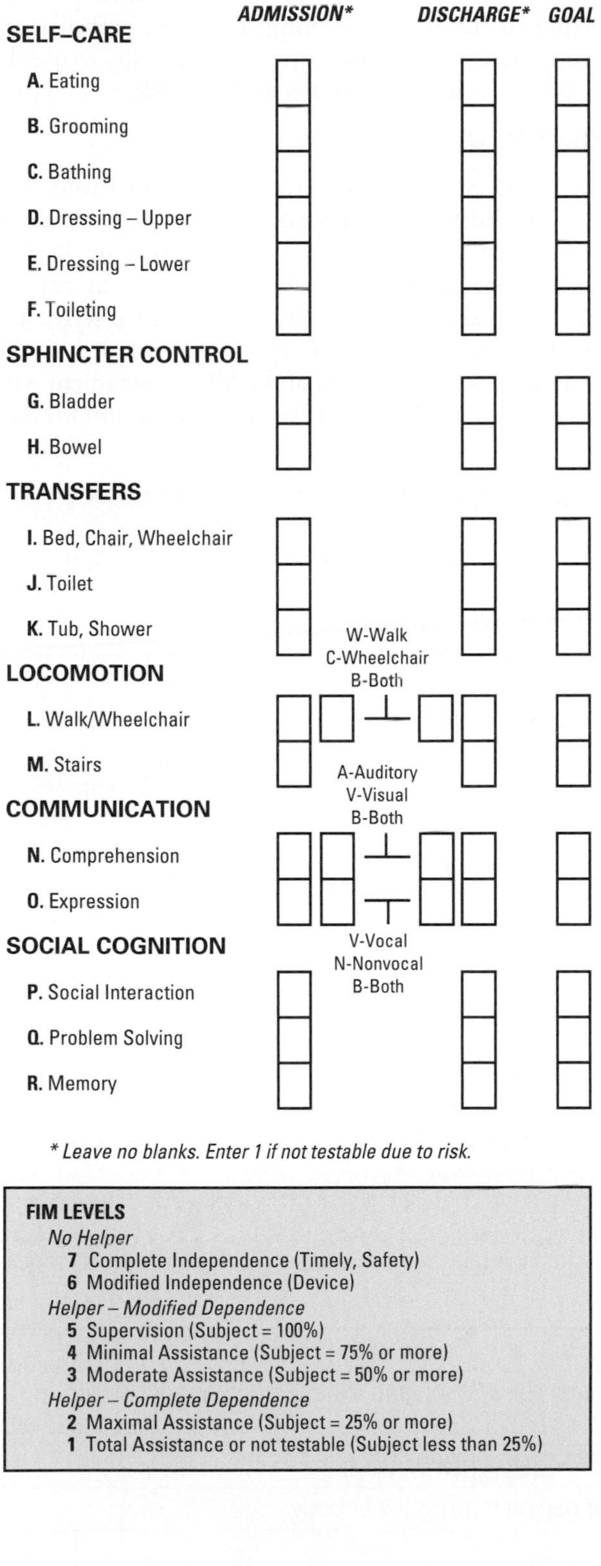

	ADMISSION*	DISCHARGE*	GOAL
SELF–CARE			
A. Eating			
B. Grooming			
C. Bathing			
D. Dressing – Upper			
E. Dressing – Lower			
F. Toileting			
SPHINCTER CONTROL			
G. Bladder			
H. Bowel			
TRANSFERS			
I. Bed, Chair, Wheelchair			
J. Toilet			
K. Tub, Shower			
LOCOMOTION	W-Walk C-Wheelchair B-Both		
L. Walk/Wheelchair			
M. Stairs	A-Auditory V-Visual B-Both		
COMMUNICATION			
N. Comprehension			
O. Expression	V-Vocal N-Nonvocal B-Both		
SOCIAL COGNITION			
P. Social Interaction			
Q. Problem Solving			
R. Memory			

* Leave no blanks. Enter 1 if not testable due to risk.

FIM LEVELS
No Helper
 7 Complete Independence (Timely, Safety)
 6 Modified Independence (Device)
Helper – Modified Dependence
 5 Supervision (Subject = 100%)
 4 Minimal Assistance (Subject = 75% or more)
 3 Moderate Assistance (Subject = 50% or more)
Helper – Complete Dependence
 2 Maximal Assistance (Subject = 25% or more)
 1 Total Assistance or not testable (Subject less than 25%)

Figure 8.5 The Functional Independence Measure (FIM) instrument scores function using a seven-point scale based on percentage(s) of active participation from patient. *(From the Uniform Data System for Medical Rehabilitation, a division of UB Foundation Activities, Inc. [UDS$_{MR}$^{SM}]. Guide for the Uniform Data Set for Medical Rehabilitation [including the FIM™ instrument], Version 5.1. Buffalo, NY 14214: State University of New York at Buffalo; 1997, with permission.)*

the Medicare program by the Health Care Financing Administration. The current version of OASIS, known as OASIS-C, contains core items covering sociodemographic characteristics, environmental factors, social support, health status, and functional status.[61] This version of the instrument was approved in 2009 and represents a substantial change from preceding versions. OASIS is not designed to be a comprehensive examination of a patient or an "add-on" measurement. OASIS items are meant to be integrated into the clinical record to highlight various aspects of a patient's status that identify particular needs for care on admission to the home health service, at follow-up every 60 days, and at discharge. The OASIS was intended to be a discipline-neutral record, administered by any health professional, including physical therapists. Created as part of a research program to develop outcome measures applicable to home health, the OASIS has been field-tested through demonstration projects and refined by a panel of experts. Reliability testing is ongoing.

Ease of administration increases with familiarity with the instrument. Unlike most other instruments, the response sets that accompany each item are specifically matched to the item. Some response sets have only two possible descriptions of behavior, whereas others have as many as nine possible descriptions of behavior. Therefore, the user must be familiar with the possible response set to each item and anticipate that comfort level in using this instrument will increase over a learning curve. The ADL/instrumental ADL (IADL) section is composed of 13 different items (Table 8.8): grooming, dressing the upper body, dressing the lower body, bathing, transferring to the toilet, toileting, transfers, ambulation/locomotion, feeding, meal preparation, ability to use the telephone, prior functioning, and falls risk.

The SF-36

The *SF-36* contains 36 items based on questions used in the RAND Health Insurance Study. These 36 items were culled from the 113 questions used by RAND in the Medical Outcomes Study (MOS) to explore the relationship between physician practice styles and patient outcomes.[62] Thus, it was named the SF-36, because it was a short form of the MOS instrument with only 36 questions. The MOS provided important data

Table 8.8	Outcome and Assessment Information Set (Oasis): ADL/IADL

(M0640) Grooming: Ability to tend to personal hygiene needs (i.e., washing face and hands, hair care, shaving or make up, teeth or denture care, fingernail care).

Prior	Current	
☐	☐	0—Able to groom self-unaided, with or without the use of assistive devices or adapted methods.
☐	☐	1—Grooming utensils must be placed within reach before able to complete grooming activities.
☐	☐	2—Someone must assist the patient to groom self.
☐	☐	3—Patient depends entirely upon someone else for grooming needs.
☐		UK—Unknown

(M0650) Ability to Dress *Upper* Body (with or without dressing aids) including undergarments, pullovers, front-opening shirts and blouses, managing zippers, buttons, and snaps:

Prior	Current	
☐	☐	0—Able to get clothes out of closets and drawers, put them on, and remove them from the upper body without assistance.
☐	☐	1—Able to dress upper body without assistance if clothing is laid out or handed to the patient.
☐	☐	2—Someone must help the patient put on upper body clothing.
☐	☐	3—Patient depends entirely upon another person to dress the upper body.
☐		UK—Unknown

(M0660) Ability to Dress *Lower* Body (with or without dressing aids) including undergarments, slacks, socks or nylons, shoes:

Prior	Current	
☐	☐	0—Able to obtain, put on, and remove clothing and shoes without assistance.
☐	☐	1—Able to dress lower body without assistance if clothing and shoes are laid out or handed to the patient.
☐	☐	2—Someone must help the patient put on undergarments, slacks, socks or nylons, and shoes.
☐	☐	3—Patient depends entirely upon another person to dress lower body.
☐		UK—Unknown

Table 8.8	Outcome and Assessment Information Set (Oasis): ADL/IADL—cont'd

(M0670) Bathing: Ability to wash entire body. ***Excludes*** grooming (washing face and hands only).

Prior	Current	
☐	☐	0—Able to bathe self in *shower or tub* independently.
☐	☐	1—With the use of devices, is able to bathe self in shower or tub independently.
☐	☐	2—Able to bathe in shower or tub with the assistance of another person:
		(a) for intermittent supervision or encouragement or reminders, *OR*
		(b) to get in and out of the shower or tub, *OR*
		(c) for washing difficult to reach areas.
☐	☐	3—Participates in bathing self in shower or tub, *but* requires presence of another person throughout the bath for assistance or supervision.
☐	☐	4—*Unable* to use the shower or tub and is bathed in *bed or bedside chair.*
☐	☐	5—Unable to effectively participate in bathing and is totally bathed by another person.
☐		UK—Unknown

(M0680) Toileting: Ability to get to and from the toilet or bedside commode.

Prior	Current	
☐	☐	0—Able to get to and from the toilet independently with or without a device.
☐	☐	1—When reminded, assisted, or supervised by another person, able to get to and from the toilet.
☐	☐	2—*Unable* to get to and from the toilet but is able to use a bedside commode (with or without assistance).
☐	☐	3—*Unable* to get to and from the toilet or bedside commode but is able to use a bedpan/urinal independently.
☐	☐	4—Is totally dependent in toileting.
☐		UK—Unknown

(M0690) Transferring: Ability to move from bed to chair, on and off toilet or commode, into and out of tub or shower, and ability to turn and position self in bed if patient is bedfast.

Prior	Current	
☐	☐	0—Able to independently transfer.
☐	☐	1—Transfers with minimal human assistance or with use of an assistive device.
☐	☐	2—*Unable* to transfer self but is able to bear weight and pivot during the transfer process.
☐	☐	3—Unable to transfer self and is *unable* to bear weight or pivot when transferred by another person.
☐	☐	4—Bedfast, unable to transfer but is able to turn and position self in bed.
☐	☐	5—Bedfast, unable to transfer and is *unable* to turn and position self.
☐		UK—Unknown

(M0700) Ambulation/Locomotion: Ability to *SAFELY* walk, once in a standing position, or use a wheelchair, once in a seated position, on a variety of surfaces.

Prior	Current	
☐	☐	0—Able to independently walk on even and uneven surfaces and climb stairs with or without railings (i.e., needs no human assistance or assistive device).
☐	☐	1—Requires use of a device (e.g., cane, walker) to walk alone *or* requires human supervision or assistance to negotiate stairs or steps or uneven surfaces.
☐	☐	2—Able to walk only with the supervision or assistance of another person at all times.
☐	☐	3—Chairfast, *unable* to ambulate but is able to wheel self independently.

Continued

Table 8.8		**Outcome and Assessment Information Set (Oasis): ADL/IADL—cont'd**

☐	☐	4—Chairfast, unable to ambulate and is *unable* to wheel self.
☐	☐	5—Bedfast, unable to ambulate or be up in a chair.
☐		UK—Unknown

(M0710) Feeding or Eating: Ability to feed self meals and snacks. **Note: This refers only to the process of** *eating,* *chewing,* **and** *swallowing, not preparing* **the food to be eaten.**

Prior	Current	
☐	☐	0—Able to independently feed self.
☐	☐	1—Able to feed self independently but requires:
		(a) meal setup; *OR*
		(b) intermittent assistance or supervision from another person; *OR*
		(c) a liquid, pureed, or ground meat diet.
☐	☐	2—*Unable* to feed self and must be assisted or supervised throughout the meal/snack.
☐	☐	3—Able to take in nutrients orally *and* receives supplemental nutrients through a nasogastric tube or gastrostomy.
☐	☐	4—*Unable* to take in nutrients orally and is fed nutrients through a nasogastric tube or gastrostomy.
☐	☐	5—Unable to take in nutrients orally or by tube feeding.
☐		UK—Unknown

(M0720) Planning and Preparing Light Meals (e.g., cereal, sandwich) or reheat delivered meals:

Prior	Current	
☐	☐	0—(a) Able to independently plan and prepare all light meals for self or reheat delivered meals; *OR*
		(b) Is physically, cognitively, and mentally able to prepare light meals on a regular basis but has not routinely performed light meal preparation in the past (i.e., prior to this home care admission).
☐	☐	1—*Unable* to prepare light meals on a regular basis due to physical, cognitive, or mental limitations.
☐	☐	2—Unable to prepare any light meals or reheat any delivered meals.
☐		UK—Unknown

(M0730) Transportation: Physical and mental ability to *safely* use a car, taxi, or public transportation (bus, train, subway).

Prior	Current	
☐	☐	0—Able to independently drive a regular or adapted car; *OR* uses a regular or handicap-accessible public bus.
☐	☐	1—Able to ride in a car only when driven by another person; *OR* able to use a bus or handicap van only when assisted or accompanied by another person.
☐	☐	2—*Unable* to ride in a car, taxi, bus, or van, and requires transportation by ambulance.
☐		UK—Unknown

(M0740) Laundry: Ability to do own laundry—to carry laundry to and from washing machine, to use washer and dryer, to wash small items by hand.

Prior	Current	
☐	☐	0—(a) Able to independently take care of all laundry tasks; *OR*
		(b) Physically, cognitively, and mentally able to do laundry and access facilities, *but* has not routinely performed laundry tasks in the past (i.e., prior to this home care admission).
☐	☐	1—Able to do only light laundry, such as minor hand wash or light washer loads. Due to physical, cognitive, or mental limitations, needs assistance with heavy laundry such as carrying large loads of laundry.

Table 8.8		Outcome and Assessment Information Set (Oasis): ADL/IADL—cont'd
☐	☐	2—*Unable* to do any laundry due to physical limitation or needs continual supervision and assistance due to cognitive or mental limitation.
☐		UK—Unknown

(M0750) Housekeeping: Ability to safely and effectively perform light housekeeping and heavier cleaning tasks.

Prior	Current	
☐	☐	0—(a) Able to independently perform all housekeeping tasks; *OR*
		(b) Physically, cognitively, and mentally able to perform *all* housekeeping tasks but has not routinely participated in housekeeping tasks in the past (i.e., prior to this home care admission).
☐	☐	1—Able to perform only *light* housekeeping (e.g., dusting, wiping kitchen counters) tasks independently.
☐	☐	2—Able to perform housekeeping tasks with intermittent assistance or supervision from another person.
☐	☐	3—*Unable* to consistently perform any housekeeping tasks unless assisted by another person throughout the process.
☐	☐	4—Unable to effectively participate in any housekeeping tasks.
☐		UK—Unknown

(M0760) Shopping: Ability to plan for, select, and purchase items in a store and to carry them home or arrange delivery.

Prior	Current	
☐	☐	0—(a) Able to plan for shopping needs and independently perform shopping tasks, including carrying packages; *OR*
		(b) Physically, cognitively, and mentally able to take care of shopping, but has not done shopping in the past (i.e., prior to this home care admission).
☐	☐	1—Able to go shopping, but needs some assistance:
		(a) By self is able to do only light shopping and carry small packages, but needs someone to do occasional major shopping; *OR*
		(b) *Unable* to go shopping alone, but can go with someone to assist.
☐	☐	2—*Unable* to go shopping, but is able to identify items needed, place orders, and arrange home delivery.
☐	☐	3—Needs someone to do all shopping and errands.
☐		UK—Unknown

(M0770) Ability to Use Telephone: Ability to answer the phone, dial numbers, and *effectively* use the telephone to communicate.

Prior	Current	
☐	☐	0—Able to dial numbers and answer calls appropriately and as desired.
☐	☐	1—Able to use a specially adapted telephone (i.e., large numbers on the dial, teletype phone for the deaf) and call essential numbers.
☐	☐	2—Able to answer the telephone and carry on a normal conversation but has difficulty with placing calls.
☐	☐	3—Able to answer the telephone only some of the time or is able to carry on only a limited conversation.
☐	☐	4—*Unable* to answer the telephone at all but can listen if assisted with equipment.
☐	☐	5—Totally unable to use the telephone.
☐	☐	NA—Patient does not have a telephone.
☐		UK—Unknown

From OASIS-B, Center for Health Services and Policy Research, Denver, CO, 1997, with permission.

on the functional status of adults with specific chronic conditions[63] and the well-being of patients experiencing depression compared to subjects with a chronic medical condition.[64] The SF-36 demonstrated high reliability and validity (correlation coefficients ranging from 0.81 to 0.88).[65–68] Normative data for these self-report items have been collected.[69]

All but one of the 36 questions of the SF-36 are used to form eight different scales: physical function, social function, role function, mental health, energy/fatigue, pain, and general health perceptions. The last question considers self-perceived change in health during the past year. Items are scored on nominal (yes/no) or ordinal scales. Each possible response to an item on a scale is assigned a number of points. The total points for all items within a scale are then added and transformed mathematically to yield a percentage score, with 100% representing optimal health. Sample items on physical function and role function are presented in Table 8.9.

The SF-36 has been used in a number of studies that describe the health status and physical functioning of patients with a variety of impairments receiving physical therapy services.[70–75]

A shortened version has been developed that uses a subset of items from the SF-36.[76] This version, known as SF-12, includes items from each of the eight concepts represented in the SF-36 and allows for the calculation of physical and mental subscale scores. An advantage to using fewer questions is that less time is required to complete the survey. This, however, may be at the expense of having a less precise score that may not be as sensitive to change for an individual patient.[77] The development of the SF-36 stands as the premier example, to date, of a complete and published exploration of the psychometric properties of an instrument as an essential part of its development, and a testament to the responsibility of its creators in verifying the quality of the SF-36 as a scientific tool (Box 8.3 Evidence Summary).

Table 8.9	The SF-36: Physical and Role Function		
The following questions are about activities you might do during a typical day. Does *your health* limit you in these activities? If so, how much? (Mark one box on each line.)	Yes, limited a lot	Yes limited a little	No, not limited at all
a. *Vigorous activities*, such as running, lifting heavy objects, participating in strenuous sports	1 ☐	2 ☐	3 ☐
b. *Moderate activities*, such as moving a table, pushing a vacuum cleaner, bowling, or playing golf	1 ☐	2 ☐	3 ☐
c. Lifting or carrying groceries	1 ☐	2 ☐	3 ☐
d. Climbing *several* flights of stairs	1 ☐	2 ☐	3 ☐
e. Climbing *one* flight of stairs	1 ☐	2 ☐	3 ☐
f. Bending, kneeling, or stooping	1 ☐	2 ☐	3 ☐
g. Walking *more than a mile*	1 ☐	2 ☐	3 ☐
h. Walking *several blocks*	1 ☐	2 ☐	3 ☐
i. Walking *one block*	1 ☐	2 ☐	3 ☐
j. Bathing or dressing yourself	1 ☐	2 ☐	3 ☐
During the *past 4 weeks*, have you had any of the following problems with your work or other regular daily activities *as a result of your physical health*? (Mark one box on each line.)		Yes	No
a. Cut down the *amount of time* you spent on work or other activities		1 ☐	2 ☐
b. *Accomplished less* than you would like		1 ☐	2 ☐
c. Were limited in the *kind* of work or other activities		1 ☐	2 ☐
d. Had *difficulty* performing the work or other activities (for example, it took extra effort)		1 ☐	2 ☐

From Ware et al.[69]

Box 8.3 Evidence Summary Reliability and Validity of the SF-36

Study	Study Design	Sample	Setting	Reliability	Validity	Comments
Stewart et al[63] (1989)	Cross-sectional	9,385 persons 18 years and older who had visited a physician	Ambulatory care	Internal consistency of scale scores .67 to .88	Not addressed	Used MOS SF-20
Stewart et al[65] (1988)	Cross-sectional	11,186 English-speaking persons 18 years and older who had visited a physician	Ambulatory care in three large cities	Internal consistency of scale scores .81 to .88	Used internal consistency as a validity measure; also compared good and poor health samples to discriminate; also correlated to sociodemographic factors.	Used MOS SF-20
McHorney et al[68] (1994)	Cross-sectional and longitudinal	3,445 English-speaking persons 18 years and older with chronic medical and psychiatric conditions	Ambulatory care in three large cities	Internal consistency reliability of scale scores .78 to .93	Item discriminant validity from .09–.58 to .20–.62	SF-36
Ware et al[76] (1996)	Longitudinal	$n = 2,333$, including adults with chronic conditions	Participants in the National Survey of Functional Health Status and the Medical Outcomes Study	2-week test–retest. 89 for physical component score and .76 for mental component score, in the general U.S. population	Discriminant validity of SF-12 similar to SF-36 in groups of patients known to differ in physical and mental conditions.	Article on construction of SF-12
Riddle et al[77] (2001)	Longitudinal	101 consecutive patients with low back pain	Three physical therapy clinics in the Richmond, VA area	Not addressed	SF-36 completed before initial examination and at time of discharge. SF-12 items extracted from SF-36. No significant differences were found for the comparison of change scores between the physical component score of the SF-36 and SF-12.	

Continued

Box 8.3 Evidence Summary   Reliability and Validity of the SF-36—cont'd

Study	Study Design	Sample	Setting	Reliability	Validity	Comments
King and Roberts[78] (2002)	Cross-sectional	88 persons with cervical spondylotic myelopathy	Outpatient neurosurgery clinic	Internal consistency reliability (Cronbach's alpha) of scale scores .79 to .92	Construct validity was demonstrated using myelopathy scales constructed by Nurick, Cooper, and Harsh, as well as a Western modification of the scale developed by the Japanese Orthopedic Association.	
Kosinski et al[79] (1999)	Cross-sectional	1,016 persons with osteoarthritis or rheumatoid arthritis	Outpatient or inpatient setting	Internal consistency reliability of baseline scale scores .75 to .91	Not addressed	
Kosinski et al[80] (1999)	Longitudinal	1,016 persons with osteoarthritis or rheumatoid arthritis	Outpatient or inpatient setting	Not addressed	SF-36 administered before treatment and 2 weeks after treatment. Discriminant validity was demonstrated in groups of patients with clinical measures of arthritis severity and across patients who improved with treatment.	
Hagen et al[81] (2003)	Prospective, observational	153 persons recruited within 1 month of a recent stroke. SF-36 administered at 1, 3, and 6 months.	24 general practices in Scotland	Internal consistency of scale scores >.7 at all time points except for Vitality at 1 month = .68 and General Health at 3 months = .66	Construct validity examined with Barthel Index, Canadian Neurological Scale, and Mini-Mental State Examination. Strongest correlations were between Barthel Index and Physical Functioning and Social Functioning subscales.	

Box 8.3 Evidence Summary   Reliability and Validity of the SF-36—cont'd

Study	Study Design	Sample	Setting	Reliability	Validity	Comments
Findler et al[82] (2001)	Cross-sectional	597 participants of whom 326 had a traumatic brain injury (TBI) who were at least 1 year post injury	Residents of New York State	Internal consistency of scale scores for individuals with TBI .79 to .92	Compared with Beck Depression Inventory, TIRR Symptom Checklist, and Health Problems List. Significant correlations were found between the SF-36 scales and the other measures.	
Yip et al[83] (2001)	Cross-sectional	32 persons 60 years of age and older and their proxy respondents	Community-dwelling older adults recruited from senior housing programs, assisted living facilities, and senior centers	Correlations for scale scores of respondents and their proxies .31 to .84	Not addressed	
Andresen et al[84] (1999)	Longitudinal	128 nursing home residents with scores of 17 or more on the Mini-Mental State Examination and at least 3 months residence	Nursing home	1 week test-retest for scales from .55 to .82 (ICC)	Convergent validity of physical health scales with activities of daily living index from −0.37 to −0.43. Mental health scales correlated with Geriatric Depression Scale (−0.63 to −0.71). No SF-36 scales correlated strongly with the Mini-Mental State Examination.	
Hobart et al[85] (2002)	Cross-sectional	126 males and 51 females with stroke at time of admission; mean age 62 years	Three hospitals in Indianapolis	Not addressed	Limited discriminant validity in this sample of persons with stroke due to floor and ceiling effects. Assumptions for generating 5 of the 8 scales and for the 2 summary scores not satisfied.	

SUMMARY

This chapter has presented a conceptual framework for understanding function and for the examination of functional status. The traditional medical model, with its narrow focus on disease and its symptoms, fails to consider the impact of the condition on the person, as well as the broader social, psychological, and behavioral dimensions of illness. All these factors have an impact on an individual's activity and participation. Although individual aspects of function may be assessed, examination of functional status must be viewed as a broad, multidimensional process. Finally, specific aspects of functional examination have been discussed, including purpose, selection of instruments, aspects of test administration, interpretation of test results, and determination of instrument quality.

Questions for Review

1. How does the measurement of function relate to health status?

2. Your rehabilitation facility uses the FIM. How can reliability be ensured so that the results can be used with confidence in both treatment planning and research?

3. What criteria can be used in the selection of a functional instrument?

4. Discuss the uses, advantages, and disadvantages of performance-based instruments, interviewer reports, and self-administered reports.

5. Explain how environment, fatigue, and other related issues affect measurement of function. Suggest ways to control these factors in the clinic.

6. Identify the major types of scoring systems used in functional instruments. What are some common errors in interpretation of testing results?

7. Review Tables 8.4, 8.6, 8.7, and 8.8. Hypothesize a caseload in a particular setting and indicate how and when you could use each of these instruments with the proposed population. Describe the advantages and disadvantages of each. Imagine that you are looking to follow the progress of these same patients to another setting. Which instruments would you choose?

8. Using one of the instruments, develop a set of results and use them to identify treatment goals and outcomes and to formulate a plan of care.

9. For each of the following, identify particular physical tasks relevant to that individual's functional status:
   • A 22-year-old female file clerk
   • A 31-year-old male physical therapist assistant
   • A 39-year-old female homemaker with children
   • A 45-year-old male construction worker
   • A 56-year-old female school teacher
   • A 65-year-old male journalist

10. Discuss the relationship among disease, body structures, body functions, activity, participation, environmental factors, and personal factors.

CASE STUDY

A 78-year-old woman with a diagnosis of osteoarthritis was admitted for a right total hip replacement. The patient reported a long-standing history of discomfort. She described the hip pain as radiating posteriorly to the buttock and low back and exacerbated by weight-bearing and stair climbing. Over the past 12 months she has experienced a very marked increase in pain and stiffness. Radiographic findings demonstrated degenerative changes of both the acetabulum and femoral head consistent with osteoarthritis. The surgical intervention replaced the right femoral head and neck with a metallic prosthesis and the acetabulum was resurfaced with a plastic cup. Past medical history is unremarkable.

SOCIAL HISTORY

The patient is a retired manager of a small accounting firm that she and her husband established. Her husband is deceased. She has three grown children who all live in neighboring communities. Before the functional limitations imposed by the hip pain, the patient had been independent in all ADL and IADL. She also volunteered her accounting services 1 day per week to a local charity that provides meals to homebound individuals. She was a regular participant in family outings, enjoyed going to the theater, concerts, and special museum events, and was an active member of the community historical preservation society. Recently, these activities had to be curtailed owing to the increased hip discomfort. She essentially had no activities outside the home for 3 months before admission and used a walker to minimize weight-bearing and reduce pain. She also required the assistance of a home care aide 4 hours a day two times per week (primarily for shopping, errands, and some household management tasks). She expressed considerable distress at being unable to take a bath and having to rely on the assistance of another person for some basic care activities. She had been using aspirin for its analgesic and anti-inflammatory effects. However, the pain experienced in recent months was not alleviated by the aspirin and other conservative measures. She has been instructed to use local applications of heat, periodic rest intervals, and gentle range-of-motion (ROM) exercises. The patient has extensive medical insurance coverage and is without financial concerns.

POSTSURGICAL RIGHT HIP PRECAUTIONS

No hip flexion beyond 90°.
Avoid crossing one leg or ankle over the other.
Avoid internal rotation of right lower extremity.

REVIEW OF SYSTEMS

Communication, Affect, Cognition, Learning Style: Fully communicative and oriented × 3. Cooperative and motivated. Hearing intact. Wears corrective lens; experiences "night blindness," which she describes as seeing poorly in dim light and her eyes take several seconds longer than normal to adjust from brightness to dimness.

Cardiopulmonary: Heart rate (HR) = 84 beats/minute; blood pressure (BP) = 130/78 mm Hg; respiratory rate (RR) = 16 breaths/minute; no appreciable increases with activity.

Integumentary: Surgical wound healing well; staples removed.

Strength: Upper extremity gross ROM is within normal limits (WNL). Gross strength generally good to normal, except hands. Left hip, knee, and ankle at least good on break test. Partial weight-bearing on right lower extremity.

Joint Integrity and Mobility: Patient reports some sporadic episodes of wrist and finger stiffness on awakening in the morning and after periods of immobility. Crepitus noted in right knee. Heberden's nodes noted at the distal interphalangeal (DIP) and proximal interphalangeal (PIP) joints of the left index finger.

Range of Motion: Right knee and ankle within functional limits; right hip not tested.

Muscle Performance: Grip strength is reduced bilaterally (4–15).

Pain: Patient denies pain in wrist or fingers, or right hip.

Gait, Locomotion, and Balance: The patient is ambulating on level surfaces with supervision using bilateral standard aluminum axillary crutches with partial weight-bearing on the right lower extremity. Stair climbing also requires minimal assistance. It is anticipated that the patient will be independent with ambulation on level surfaces at time of discharge from the hospital.

Functional Status: Impaired bed mobility (modified independence device), sit-to-stand, transfers (minimum assistance).

Home Environment: The patient lives alone in a fifth-floor apartment in a building with an elevator. The living space is a one-bedroom apartment on a single level.

Patient Goals: The patient is extremely motivated to once again be an independent manager of her personal care and household management needs. The prosthetic replacement has successfully relieved much of the pain experienced in the hip before surgery (most of her current discomfort is described as minor and associated with the surgical incision). She would also like to return to her family, volunteer, social, and leisure activities. She is very determined to discontinue the home care assistance as soon as possible.

GUIDING QUESTIONS

1. Based on the findings of the initial examination, discuss the links between the condition, impairments in body structures and body functions, activity limitations, participation restrictions, and contextual factors using the ICF model.

2. Identify the specific ADL and IADL skills that would need to be examined to return this patient to the highest level of function and achieve the patient's goals for rehabilitation. Discuss the appropriateness of the instruments presented in this chapter for measuring her function and documenting the outcomes of patient management.

References

1. American Physical Therapy Association: The Guide to Physical Therapist Practice, ed 2. Phys Ther 81:9, 2001.
2. Adams, PF, Heyman, KM, and Vickerie, JL: Summary health statistics for the U.S. population: National Health Interview Survey, 2008. Vital Health Stat 10(243):1, Dec 2009.
3. World Health Organization (WHO): The First Ten Years of the World Health Organization. World Health Organization, Geneva, 1958.
4. World Health Organization (WHO): International Classification of Functioning, Disability and Health. World Health Organization, Geneva, 2001.
5. World Health Organization (WHO): ICD 10: International Statistical Classification of Diseases and Related Health Problems, Tenth Revision, Volume 1. World Health Organization, Geneva, 1992.
6. Escorpizo, R, et al: Creating an interface between the International Classification of Functioning, Disability and Health and physical therapist practice. Phys Ther 90:1053, 2010.
7. World Health Organization (WHO): International Classification of Impairments, Disabilities, and Handicaps. World Health Organization, Geneva, 1980.
8. Nagi, S: Disability concepts revisited. In Pope, AM, and Tarlov, AR (eds): Disability in America: Toward a National Agenda for Prevention. National Academy Press, Washington, DC, 1991, p 309.
9. ICIDH-2: International Classification of Impairments, Activities and Participation. A Manual of Dimensions of Disablement and Functioning. Beta-1 draft for field trials. World Health Organization, Geneva, 1997.
10. Jette, AM, Haley, SM, and Kooyoomjian, JT: Are the ICF Activity and Participation dimensions distinct? J Rehabil Med 35(3):145, 2003.
11. Brandt, EN, Jr, and Pope, AM (eds): Enabling America: Assessing the Role of Rehabilitation Science and Engineering. National Academy Press, Washington, DC, 1997.
12. Jette, AM, and Keysor, JJ: Disability models: Implications for arthritis exercise and physical activity interventions. Arthrit Rheum 49:114, 2003.
13. Guyatt, GH, et al: The 6-minute walk: A new measure of exercise capacity in patients with chronic heart failure. Can Med Assoc J 132:923, 1985.
14. Winograd, CH, et al: Development of a physical performance and mobility examination. J Am Geriatr Soc 42:743, 1994.
15. Duncan, PW, et al: Functional reach: A new clinical measure of balance. J Gerontol 45:192, 1990.
16. Duncan, PW, et al: Functional reach: Predictive validity in a sample of elderly male veterans. J Gerontol 47:93, 1992.
17. Mathias, S, et al: Balance in elderly patients: The "Get Up and Go" test. Arch Phys Med Rehabil 67:387, 1986.
18. Podsiadlo, D, and Richardson, S: The timed "Up and Go": A test of basic functional mobility for frail elderly persons. J Am Geriatr Soc 39:142, 1991.
19. Guralnik, JM, et al: A short physical performance battery assessing lower extremity function: Association with self-reported disability and prediction of mortality and nursing home admission. J Gerontol 49:85, 1994.
20. Tager, IB, et al: Reliability of physical performance and self-reported functional measures in an older population. J Gerontol 53:295, 1998.
21. Guccione, AA, et al: Development and testing of a self-report instrument to measure actions: Outpatient Physical Therapy Improvement in Movement Assessment Log (OPTIMAL). Phys Ther 85:515, 2005.
22. Mahoney, F, and Barthel, D: Functional evaluation: The Barthel Index. Md Med J 14:61, 1965.
23. Guccione, AA, et al: Defining arthritis and measuring functional status in elders: Methodological issues in the study of disease and disability. Am J Public Health 80:949, 1990.
24. Catalog of tests and measures. Guide to Physical Therapist Practice. Retrieved March 25, 2011, from http://guidetoptpractice.apta.org.
25. Standards for Tests and Measurements in Physical Therapy Practice. Phys Ther 71:589, 1991.
26. Portney, LG, and Watkins, MP: Foundations of Clinical Research: Applications to Practice, ed 3. Prentice-Hall Health, Upper Saddle River, NJ, 2008.
27. Straus, SE, et al: Evidence-Based Medicine: How to Practice and Teach It, ed 4. Churchill Livingstone, Edinburgh, 2011.
28. Kennedy, DM, et al: Assessing stability and change of four performance measures: A longitudinal study evaluating outcome following total hip and knee arthroplasty. BMC Musculoskelet Disord 28(6):3, 2005.
29. Make, B: How can we assess outcomes of clinical trials: The MCID approach. COPD 4(3):191, 2007.
30. Perera, S, et al: Meaningful change and responsiveness in common physical performance measures in older adults. J Am Geriatr Soc 54(5):743–749, 2006.
31. Ries, JD, et al: Test-retest reliability and minimal detectable change scores for the timed "up and go" test, the six-minute walk test, and gait speed in people with Alzheimer disease. Phys Ther 89(6):569–579, 2009.
32. Fulk, GD, et al: Clinometric properties of the six-minute walk test in individuals undergoing rehabilitation poststroke. Physiother Theory Pract 24(3):195–204, 2008.
33. Fulk, GD, and Echternach, JL: Test-retest reliability and minimal detectable change of gait speed in individuals undergoing rehabilitation after stroke. J Neurol Phys Ther 32(1):8–13, 2008.
34. Palombaro, KM, et al: Determining meaningful changes in gait speed after hip fracture. Phys Ther 86(6):809–816, 2006.
35. Liaw, LJ, et al: The relative and absolute reliability of two balance performance measures in chronic stroke patients. Disabil Rehabil 30(9):656–661, 2008.
36. Steffen, T, and Seney, M: Test-retest reliability and minimal detectable change on balance and ambulation tests, the 36-item short-form health survey, and the unified Parkinson disease rating scale in people with parkinsonism. Phys Ther 88(6):733, 2008. Epub March 20, 2008. Erratum in Phys Ther 90(3):462, 2010.
37. MCID—Gatchel, RJ, and Mayer, TG: Testing minimal clinically important difference: Consensus or conundrum? Spine J 10(4):321, 2010.
38. Rennard, SI: Minimal clinically important difference, clinical perspective: An opinion. COPD 2(1):51, 2005.
39. Rehabilitation Measures Database. Retrieved March 25, 2011, from www.rehabmeasures.org/default.aspx.
40. Neurology Section Outcome Measures Recommendations: Stroke. Retrieved March 25, 2011, from www.neuropt.org/go/healthcare-professionals/neurology-section-outcome-measures-recommendations/stroke.
41. Foucher, KC, et al: Differences in preferred walking speeds in a gait laboratory compared with the real world after total hip replacement. Arch Phys Med Rehabil 91(9):1390–1395, 2010.
42. Studenski, S, et al: Gait speed and survival in older adults. JAMA 305(1):50–58, 2011.
43. Geyh, S, et al: ICF Core Sets for stroke. J Rehabil Med 44(Suppl):135–141, 2004.
44. Grill, E, et al: ICF Core Sets for early post-acute rehabilitation facilities. J Rehabil Med 43(2):131–138, 2011.
45. Starrost, K, et al: Interrater reliability of the extended ICF core set for stroke applied by physical therapists. Phys Ther 88(7):841, 2008.
46. Algurén, B, Lundgren-Nilsson, A, and Sunnerhagen, KS: Functioning of stroke survivors—A validation of the ICF core set for stroke in Sweden. Disabil Rehabil 32(7):551, 2010.
47. Guccione, AA, and Jette, AM: Multidimensional assessment of functional limitations in patients with arthritis. Arthrit Care Res 3:44, 1990.
48. Guccione, AA, and Jette, AM: Assessing limitations in physical function in persons with arthritis. Arthr Care Res 1:170, 1988.
49. Granger, CV, et al: The Stroke Rehabilitation Outcome Study—Part I: General Description. Arch Phys Med Rehabil 69:506, 1988.

50. Granger, CV, et al: The Stroke Rehabilitation Outcome Study: Part II. Relative merits of the total Barthel Index score and a four-item subscore in predicting patient outcomes. Arch Phys Med Rehabil 70:100, 1989.
51. Granger, C, et al: Outcome of comprehensive medical rehabilitation: Measurement by Pulses Profile and the Barthel Index. Arch Phys Med Rehabil 60:145, 1979.
52. Granger, CV, et al: Advances in functional assessment for medical rehabilitation. Top Geriatr Rehabil 1:59, 1986.
53. Granger, CV, et al: Functional assessment scales: A study of persons with multiple sclerosis. Arch Phys Med Rehabil 71:870, 1990.
54. Guide for the Uniform Data Set for Medical Rehabilitation (Adult FIM), Version 4.0. Buffalo, Uniform Data System for Medical Rehabilitation, UB Foundation Activities, Inc, 1993.
55. Hsueh, IP, et al: Comparison of the psychometric characteristics of the Functional Independence Measure, 5 item Barthel Index, and 10 item Barthel Index in patients with stroke. J Neurol Neurosurg Psychiatry 73:188, 2002.
56. Gosman-Hedstrom, G, and Svensson, E: Parallel reliability of the Functional Independence Measure and the Barthel ADL Index. Disabil Rehabil 22:702, 2000.
57. Heinemann, AW, et al: Relationships between impairment and physical disability as measured by the Functional Independence Measure. Arch Phys Med Rehabil 74:566, 1993.
58. Ottenbacher, KJ, et al: Measuring developmental and functional status in children with disabilities. Dev Med Child Neurol 41:186, 1999.
59. Krisler, KS, et al: OASIS Basics: Beginning to Use the Outcome and Assessment Information Set. Center for Health Services and Policy Research, Denver, 1997.
60. Shaughnessy, PW, and Crisler, KS: Outcome-based Quality Improvement. A Manual for Home Care Agencies on How to Use Outcomes. National Association for Home Care, Washington, DC, 1995.
61. Deitz, D, et al: OASIS-C: Development, testing, and release. An overview for home healthcare clinicians, administrators, and policy makers. Home Healthc Nurse 28(6):353–362, quiz 363–364, 2010.
62. Tarlov, AR, et al: The Medical Outcomes Study: An application of methods for monitoring the results of medical care. JAMA 262:925, 1989.
63. Stewart, AL, et al: Functional status and well-being of patients with chronic conditions: Results from the Medical Outcomes Study. JAMA 262:907, 1989.
64. Wells, KB, et al: The functioning and well-being of depressed patients: Results from the Medical Outcomes Study. JAMA 262:914, 1989.
65. Stewart, AL, et al: The MOS short general health survey: Reliability and validity in a patient population. Med Care 26:724, 1988.
66. Ware, JE, and Sherbourne, CD: The MOS 36-item short form health survey (SF-36): I. Conceptual framework and item selection. Med Care 30:473, 1992.
67. McHorney, CA, et al: The MOS 36-item short form health survey (SF-36): II. Psychometric and clinical tests of validity in measuring physical and mental health constructs. Med Care 31:247, 1993.
68. McHorney, CA, et al: The MOS 36-item short form health survey (SF-36): III. Tests of data quality, scaling assumptions, and reliability across diverse patient groups. Med Care 32:40, 1994.
69. Ware, JE, et al: SF-36 Health Survey: Manual and Interpretation Guide. Boston, The Health Institute, New England Medical Center, 1993.
70. Mossberg, KA, and McFarland, C: Initial health status of patients at outpatient physical therapy clinics. Phys Ther 75:1043, 1995.
71. Jette, DU, and Downing, J: Health status of individuals entering a cardiac rehabilitation program as measured by the Medical Outcomes Study 36-item short form survey (SF-36). Phys Ther 74:521, 1994.
72. Jette, DU, and Downing, J: The relationship of cardiovascular and psychological impairments to the health status of patients enrolled in cardiac rehabilitation programs. Phys Ther 76:130, 1996.
73. Jette, DU, and Jette, AM: Physical therapy and health outcomes in patients with spinal impairments. Phys Ther 76:930, 1996.
74. Jette, DU, and Jette, AM: Physical therapy and health outcomes in patients with knee impairments. Phys Ther 76:1178, 1996.
75. Jette, DU, et al: The disablement process in patients with pulmonary disease. Phys Ther 77:385, 1997.
76. Ware, J, Kosinski, M, and Keller, SD: A 12-item short-form health survey: Construction of scales and preliminary tests of reliability and validity. Med Care 34:220, 1996.
77. Riddle, DL, Lee, KT, and Stratford, PW: Use of SF-36 and SF-12 health status measures: A quantitative comparison for groups versus individual patients. Med Care 39:867, 2001.
78. King, JT, and Roberts, MS: Validity and reliability of the Short Form-36 in cervical spondylotic myelopathy. Spine 97:180, 2002.
79. Kosinski, M, et al: The SF-36 Health Survey as a generic outcome measure in clinical trials of patients with osteoarthritis and rheumatoid arthritis: Tests of data quality, scaling assumptions and score reliability. Med Care 37:MS10, 1999.
80. Kosinski, M, et al: The SF-36 Health Survey as a generic outcome measure in clinical trials of patients with osteoarthritis and rheumatoid arthritis: Relative validity of scales in relation to clinical measures of arthritis severity. Med Care 37:MS23, 1999.
81. Hagen, S, et al: Psychometric properties of the SF-36 in the early post-stroke phase. J Adv Nurs 44(5):461, 2003.
82. Findler, M, et al: The reliability and validity of the SF-36 Health Survey questionnaire for use with individuals with traumatic brain injury. Brain Inj 15(8):715, 2001.
83. Yip, JY, et al: Comparison of older adult subject and proxy responses on the SF-36 health-related quality of life instrument. Aging Ment Health 5(2):136, 2001.
84. Andresen, EM, et al: Limitations of the SF-36 in a sample of nursing home residents. Age Aging 28:562, 1999.
85. Hobart, JC, et al: Quality of life measurement after stroke: Uses and abuses of SF-36. Stroke 33:1348, 2002.

Supplemental Readings

Dittmar, S, and Bresham, G: Functional Assessment and Outcome Measures for the Rehabilitation Health Professional. Aspen, Gaithersburg, MD, 1997.

Field, MJ, and Jette, AM (eds): The Future of Disability in America. Institute of Medicine Committee on Disability in America. National Academies Press, Washington, DC, 2007.

Finch, E, et al: Physical Rehabilitation Outcome Measures: A Guide to Enhanced Clinical Decision Making, ed 2. Lippincott Williams & Wilkins, Baltimore, 2002.

Hazuda, HP, et al: Development and validation of a performance-based measure of upper extremity functional limitation. Aging Clin Exp Res 17(5):394, 2005.

Jette, AM: Physical disablement concepts for physical therapy research and practice. Phys Ther 74(5):380, 1994.

McDowell, I, and Newell, C: Measuring Health: A Guide to Rating Scales and Questionnaires, ed 2. Oxford University Press, New York, 1996.

Nickel, MK, et al: Changes in instrumental activities of daily living disability after treatment of depressive symptoms in elderly women with chronic musculoskeletal pain: A double-blind, placebo-controlled trial. Aging Clin Exp Res 17(4):293, 2005.

Peel, C, et al: Assessing mobility in older adults: The UAB Study of Aging Life-Space Assessment. Phys Ther 85(10):1008, 2005.

Shaver, JC, and Allan, DE: Care-receiver and caregiver assessments of functioning: Are there gender differences? Can J Aging 24(2):139, 2005.

Vittengl, JR, et al: Comparative validity of seven scoring systems for the instrumental activities of daily living scale in rural elders. Aging Ment Health 10(1):40, 2006.

LEARNING OBJECTIVES

1. Identify the roles and responsibilities of the physical therapist in examination of the physical environment.
2. Understand the importance of environmental accessibility in optimizing patient function.
3. Identify common home, workplace, and community environmental barriers that affect patient function.
4. Identify the tests and measures, tools used for gathering data, and data generated during examination of environmental, home, and work barriers.
5. Describe examination instruments used to measure environmental impact on patient function.
6. Identify strategies to improve patient function through environmental modifications.
7. Describe the scope of adaptive equipment and assistive technology options available for individuals with activity limitations and disability.
8. Recognize the importance of an examination of the environment within the context of a comprehensive plan of care.

CHAPTER OUTLINE

A variety of both built and natural objects comprise the *physical environment* in which an individual functions. Built objects refer to buildings and structures created by humans; natural objects include other humans, as well as geographical objects such as vegetation, mountains, rivers, uneven terrain, and so forth.[1] The environment encompasses a substantial range of components that affect human function and includes the individual's home, neighborhood, community, and method(s) of transportation, in addition to the individual's educational, workplace, entertainment, commercial, and natural settings.[2]

Environmental barriers are defined as physical impediments that prevent individuals from functioning optimally in their surroundings and include safety hazards, access problems, and home or workplace design difficulties.[3] **Accessibility** is the degree to which an environment affords use of its resources with respect to an individual's level of function. **Accessible design** typically refers to structures that meet prescribed standards for accessibility. In the United States, these standards are available from the American National Standards Institute,[4] the Fair Housing Amendments Act of 1988, and the Uniform Federal Accessibility Standards (UFAS). Requirements for public and commercial buildings are regulated by the guidelines of the Americans with Disabilities Act (ADA) Standards for Accessible Design.[5]

■ UNIVERSAL DESIGN

Universal design (UD) refers to "the design of products and environments to be usable by all people, to the greatest extent possible, without the need for adaptation or specialized design."[6, p. 1] This design concept emphasizes social inclusion by creating products and environments that are usable by a wide range of individuals of different ages, stature, sizes, and abilities, and it addresses the changing needs of human beings across the life span. Other terms associated with this design concept include *inclusive design, design-for-all, accessible design, barrier-free design, life span design, aging-in-place design,* and *sustainable* and *transgenerational design.* Joines suggests that "although the individual's capabilities do not change as a result of the design, his/her abilities do. By redefining problems, changing environments, and selecting different products, the quality of life of the individual may be enhanced."[7, p. 155]

Universal design has been identified as an outgrowth of the disability rights movement in the 1960s, although some earlier recognition of the concepts has been identified. Its foundational elements of ensuring equal opportunity and eliminating discrimination based on disability has been embraced in many parts of the world.[8] The design principles not only involve residential or commercial dwellings but also elders and those with disabilities. They provide a human-centered framework for creating spaces, furniture, landscapes, products, and services that can seamlessly accommodate diverse ability levels across generations.[9,10]

Evidence-based design (EBD) supports and informs UD. EBD is defined by the Center for Health Design (CHD) "as the process of basing decisions about the built environment on credible research to achieve the best possible outcomes."[11, p. 2] It emphasizes use of research to influence the design process and evaluate design innovations. Traditionally associated with health care architecture, EBD now supports design decisions for many structures in the built environment, including schools, office spaces, performance centers, restaurants, museums, and prisons.[12]

Although UD is both accessible and free of barriers, it is not the same as bringing existing buildings or structures into compliance with the ADA Standards for Accessible Design[5] or other building codes or laws. Applying such standards to existing structures often results in important but selective accessibility. In contrast, UD is applied from the *inception* of a building design plan versus creating new structures and then approaching the task of eliminating environmental barriers. For example, the need to retrofit a new structure with a ramp would not be needed had the original design plan considered the needs of all users. Ostroff suggests that such thoughtless add-ons "have a stigmatizing quality similar to the 'back of the bus' practices that were once the norm in the United States."[13, p. 1.4]

Incorporated into initial planning, UD elements are essentially "invisible" as compared to adaptations made to existing structures. They apply to all features and spaces of a dwelling. Several examples of UD elements include stepless entrances, wide hallways and doorways, level transitions between rooms (no doorway thresholds), use of nonslip floors, lever door handles, rocker light switches, single-handle sink faucets, and no-step shower access. Reinforced walls capable of supporting handrails or grab bars and large closets aligned from floor-to-floor suitable for housing a residential elevator are examples of UD elements intended to meet the future needs of residents.[4,5,14]

Bjork suggests that UD is empowered by three important characteristics. "First, it expands the focus of design from people with disabilities to a much broader population. Second, UD focuses on striving for new thinking in the development of initiatives and strategies for creating new solutions, instead of focusing on reconstruction and adaptation; an innovative approach. Third, UD strives for full social participation for everybody over a whole life span, through the creation of flexible products and environments with good usability. It is not about one universal solution that fits everybody. It is about solutions that provide flexibility in use and handling."[15, pp. 118-119]

Principles of Universal Design

The Principles of Universal Design (Appendix 9.A) were developed at the Center for Universal Design (CUD) at North Carolina State University by a group of experts that included architects, product designers, engineers, and environmental design researchers. The principles provide guidance for the design of products and environments. They are also intended to educate designers and consumers about characteristics that increase usability for everyone.[16] Key elements of the principles include the following:

- *Equitable Use.* The design is useful and marketable to people with diverse abilities.
- *Flexibility in Use.* The design accommodates a wide range of individual preferences and abilities.
- *Simple and Intuitive.* Use of the design is easy to understand, regardless of the user's experience, knowledge, language skills, or current concentration level.
- *Perceptible Information.* The design communicates necessary information effectively to the user, regardless of ambient conditions or the user's sensory abilities.
- *Tolerance for Error.* The design minimizes hazards and the adverse consequences of accidental or unintended actions.
- *Low Physical Effort.* The design can be used efficiently, comfortably, and with a minimum of fatigue.
- *Size and Space for Approach and Use.* Appropriate size and space is provided for approach, reach, manipulation, and use regardless of the user's body size, posture, or mobility.

Although UD originated in response to the need for environmental access for individuals with activity limitations and disability, many of its design elements proved useful and have been embraced by the general public. Riley[14] provides a fitting example of this development: "Think for a moment of the automatic garage door, which originated out of necessity for a client whose disability prevented him from lifting a heavy door. Now a staple of living for nearly all of us so-called 'able-bodied' people as well as those with disabilities, it is but one of many examples of how Universal Design has raised the bar for home design of all kind."[14, p. XII]

DISABILITY ACCESS SYMBOLS

Reflective of the importance of **environmental accessibility**, an internationally recognized *wheelchair symbol* identifies buildings accessible to individuals with a disability. The Rehabilitation Act of 1973 (Sections 503 and 504) requires that all organizations receiving federal funding provide accessible programs and activities. The Americans with Disabilities Act (1990) expanded accessibility to the private sector to improve employment opportunities, as well as environmental access to retail businesses, cultural events, movie theaters, restaurants, travel, and so forth. Other access symbols identify the availability of assistive listening devices, telephones with interactive text capabilities (TTY), which allow the user to communicate using a keyboard and visual display, volume-controlled telephones, availability of sign language interpretation, and so forth. The Disability Access Symbols are presented in Figure 9.1. These symbols are prominently displayed to identify and make public the availability of accessible services.

PURPOSE OF EXAMINATION

A primary outcome of rehabilitation is for the patient to be fully functional in a former environment and lifestyle. To achieve this outcome, continuity of accessibility must exist within the individual's environmental context. With full accessibility as a goal, examination of the environment must address the patient–environment relationship relative to accessibility, safety, usability, and function. The purposes of an environmental examination are multiple and serve to:

1. Determine the degree of patient safety and level of function in the physical environment.
2. Identify design barriers that may affect usability or compromise performance of customary tasks or activities.
3. Make realistic recommendations regarding environmental accessibility and accommodations to the patient, family/caregivers, employer, government agencies or other potential funding sources, and third-party payers.
4. Determine the need for adaptive equipment or assistive technology to support and promote function.
5. Assist in preparing the patient and family/caregivers for the patient's return to a former environment and to help determine whether further services may be required (e.g., outpatient treatment, home care services, and so forth).

EXAMINATION STRATEGIES

Physical therapists use a variety of tests and measures to examine physical impediments (e.g., safety hazards, access problems, design barriers) affecting the patient–environment relationship. The data generated are used to suggest modifications to the environment, guide recommendations for adaptive equipment and assistive technology, and/or propose alternative approaches to performing a task or activity (e.g., improve safety, conserve energy) to promote optimum function. The *Guide to Physical Therapist Practice*[3] includes examination of environmental, home, and work (job/school/play) barriers among the list of 24 categories of tests and measures that may be used by physical therapists. Table 9.1 presents an overview of examination components, including the types of tests and measures used, tools used for gathering data, and types of data generated.

Depending on the nature of the patient's activity limitation or disability, data collection tools used for examination of the environmental may include (1) interviews, (2) self-reports (checklists, questionnaires) and performance-based measures (observation) of function, (3) measures of environmental impact on function, (4) visual depictions (photographs, videotapes) and dimensions of physical space (structural specifications), (5) viewing the environment from a remote site, and (6) on-site visits.

A combination of two or more of these strategies may be warranted to generate all needed data. The current era of cost containment has placed restrictions on time and travel allocations for on-site visits. In such situations, several data collection alternatives (e.g., interview, self-report, and performance-based measures; and use of photographs and/or diagrams [with dimensions] of the physical space) can be implemented to achieve the goals of the environmental examination.

Telehealth (telecommunication technology) offers considerable potential to view an environment at a remote site using a voice-over-Internet Protocol (voIP) service and software application (e.g., Skype, Linphone) or other videoconferencing protocol. A large and expanding body of literature addresses the extensive application of telehealth in providing health care services,[17-29] including physical therapy.[30-33] In a document titled *Telehealth—Definitions and Guidelines* the Board of Directors of the American Physical Therapy Association (APTA) defines telehealth as "the use of electronic communications to provide and deliver a host of health-related information and health care services, including, but not limited to, physical therapy–related information and services, over large and small distances. Telehealth encompasses a variety of health care and health promotion activities, including, but not limited to, education, advice, reminders, interventions, and monitoring of interventions."[34, p. 1]

Sanford et al[35] reported on an early application of telehealth to examination of the home environment. The authors compared data from an actual on-site home examination with those obtained from remote videoconferencing technology. The data suggested that videoconferencing has the potential for enabling therapists to examine the patient's environment regardless of distance or location. The data from the remote examination identified 51 of the 59 problems (86.4%) documented from the

	Symbol for Accessibility The wheelchair symbol should only be used to indicate access for individuals with limited mobility including wheelchair users. For example, the symbol is used to indicate an accessible entrance, bathroom or that a phone is lowered for wheelchair users. Remember that a ramped entrance is not completely accessible if there are no curb cuts, and an elevator is not accessible if it can only be reached via steps.
	Access (Other Than Print or Braille) for Individuals Who Are Blind or Have Low Vision This symbol may be used to indicate access for people who are blind or have low vision, including: a guided tour, a path to a nature trail or a scent garden in a park; and a tactile tour or a museum exhibition that may be touched.
	Audio Description A service for persons who are blind or have low vision that makes the performing arts, visual arts, television, video, and film more accessible. Description of visual elements is provided by a trained Audio Describer through the Secondary Audio Program (SAP) of televisions and monitors equipped with stereo sound. An adapter for non-stereo TVs is available through the American Foundation for the Blind, (800) 829-0500. For live Audio Description, a trained Audio Describer offers live commentary or narration (via headphones and a small transmitter) consisting of concise, objective descriptions of visual elements (e.g., a theater performance or a visual arts exhibition).
	Telephone Typewriter (TTY) This device is also known as a text telephone (TT), or telecommunications device for the deaf (TDD). TTY indicates a device used with the telephone for communication with and between deaf, hard of hearing, speech impaired and/or hearing persons.
	Volume Control Telephone This symbol indicates the location of telephones that have handsets with amplified sound and/or adjustable volume controls.
	Assistive Listening Systems These systems transmit amplified sound via hearing aids, headsets or other devices. They include infrared, loop and FM systems. Portable systems may be available from the same audiovisual equipment suppliers that service conferences and meetings.
	Sign Language Interpretation The symbol indicates that Sign Language Interpretation is provided for a lecture, tour, film, performance, conference or other program.
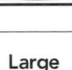	**Accessible Print (18 pt. or Larger)** The symbol for large print is "Large Print" printed in 18 pt. or larger text. In addition to indicating that large print versions of books, pamphlets, museum guides and theater programs are available, you may use the symbol on conference or membership forms to indicate that print materials may be provided in large print. Sans serif or modified serif print with good contrast is important, and special attention should be paid to letter and word spacing.
	The Information Symbol The most valuable commodity of today's society is information; to a person with a disability it is essential. For example, the symbol may be used on signage or on a floor plan to indicate the location of the information or security desk, where there is more specific information or materials concerning access accommodations and services such as "LARGE PRINT" materials, audio cassette recordings of materials, or sign interpreted tours.
	Closed Captioning (CC) This symbol indicates a choice for whether or not to display captions for a television program or videotape. TV sets that have a built-in or a separate decoder are equipped to display dialogue for programs that are captioned when selected by the viewer. The Television Decoder Circuitry Act of 1990 requires TV sets (with screens 13" or larger) to have built-in decoders as of July, 1993. Also, videos that are part of exhibitions may be closed captioned using the symbol with instruction to press a button for captioning.
	Opened Captioning (OC) This symbol indicates that captions, which translate dialogue and other sounds in print, are always displayed on the videotape, movie or television program. Open Captioning is preferred by many including deaf and hard-of-hearing individuals, and people whose second language is English. In addition, it is helpful in teaching children how to read and in keeping sound levels to a minimum in museums and restaurants.
	**Braille Symbol** This symbol indicates that printed material is available in Braille, including exhibition labeling, publications, and signage.

The Disability Access Symbols were produced by the Graphic Artists Guild Foundation with support and technical assistance from the Office for Special Constituencies, National Endowment for the Arts. Special thanks to the National Endowment for the Arts. Graphic design assistance by the Society of Environmental Graphic Design. Consultant: Jacqueline Ann Clipsham, with permission.

Figure 9.1 Disability access symbols.

on-site visit and 54 of the 60 quantitative measures (90%) obtained from the on-site visit.

Interview

Exploration of the environment is typically initiated by interviewing the patient and family/caregivers. If the patient's activity limitations or disability affects only isolated tasks or activities or if accessibility issues involve limited environmental barriers, an interview may be all that is needed to determine the physical impediments and provide suggestions and guidelines for improving performance and resolving access problems. In the presence of more formidable activity limitations or disability, the interview may be the first of several strategies used

Table 9.1	Environmental, Home, and Work (Job/School/Play) Barriers: Types of Tests and Measures Used, Tools Used for Gathering Data, and Types of Data Generated

Environmental, home, and work (job/school/play) barriers are the physical impediments that keep patients/clients from functioning optimally in their surroundings. The physical therapist uses the results of tests and measures to identify any of a variety of possible impediments, including safety hazards (e.g., throw rugs, slippery surfaces), access problems (e.g., narrow doors, thresholds, high steps, absence of power doors and elevators), and home or office design barriers (e.g., excessive distances to negotiate, multistory environments, sinks, bathrooms, counters, placement of controls or switches). The physical therapist also uses the results to suggest modification to the environment (e.g., grab bars in the shower, ramps, raised toilet seats, increased lighting) that will also allow the patient/client to improve functioning in the home, workplace, and other settings.

Tests and Measures	Tools Used for Gathering Data	Data Generated
Tests and measures may include those that characterize or quantify: • Current and potential barriers (e.g., checklists, interviews, observations, questionnaires) • Physical space and environment (e.g., compliance standards, observations, photographic assessments, questionnaires, structural specifications, technology-assisted assessments, videographic assessments)	Tools for gathering data include: • Cameras and photographs • Checklists • Interviews • Observations • Questionnaires • Structural specifications • Technology-assisted analysis systems • Video cameras and videotapes	Data are used in providing documentation and may include: • Descriptions of: —Barriers —Environment • Documentation and description of compliance with regulatory standards • Observations of environment • Quantifications of physical space

From American Physical Therapy Association,[3, p. 68] with permission.

to collect data about the patient's environment. The interview can be used to establish the general characteristics of the environment (number of levels, stairs, railings, and so forth), identify any special problems previously encountered by the patient, alert the therapist to potential safety hazards, and determine the need for further tests and measures to obtain essential information. The interview process also provides the therapist an opportunity to gain knowledge of family/caregiver characteristics, including (1) attitude toward the patient; (2) the extent of their desire to have the patient return to his or her environment; (3) their caregiving goals and capabilities; and (4) attitude toward rehabilitation team members, which may influence receptivity to suggested environmental modifications.

Self-Report and Performance-Based Measures of Function

Self-reports involve asking the patient to provide information about the ability to perform certain tasks and activities in specific environments. Administration can be either in a paper-and-pencil format or by way of an interview conducted by the therapist. An inherent shortcoming of self-report instruments is that an individual may overestimate performance capabilities or underestimate the impact of environmental barriers. Accuracy of reporting can be improved by requesting that the patient (1) focus the performance information on a recent time interval (e.g., *within* the previous week) and (2) distinguish

between actual performance of an activity (e.g., *daily* use of shower for bathing) versus perceived ability in the absence of consistent execution of the task.

Performance-based measures address classification of functional abilities and identification of activity limitations. The therapist administers these measures while observing patient performance of an activity. A variety of instruments are available that include quantitative scoring systems. Examples of instruments used to examine balance, mobility, and fall risk include the *Functional Reach (FR) Test*[36-38] and *Multidirectional Reach Test (MDFR)*,[39,40] the *Get Up and Go (GUG) Test*[41] and *Timed Up and Go (TUG) Test*,[42] the *Performance-Oriented Mobility Assessment (POMA)*,[43-45] timed[46] and distance walking tests,[47-50] and the *Berg Balance Scale (BBS)*.[51-54] The therapist interprets the data by comparison to normative performance. The measures yield important information about the impact of impairments on function and help predict patient performance within his or her natural environment. Self-report and performance-based measures of function are discussed in Chapter 8, Examination of Function.

Measures of Environmental Impact on Function

The environment directly affects the ability to perform tasks and activities that support physical, social, and psychological well-being. Environmental factors can either *constrain* or *promote* patients' abilities to perform customary actions within their social/cultural contexts. A variety of instruments have been developed that address the impact of environmental determinants on function. Examples of these instruments include the following:

- The *Physical Activity Resource Assessment (PARA)*.[55] Based on the close link between aspects of the physical environment and physical activity levels, this instrument was designed to examine and document the available resources that promote activity within a neighborhood or community environment. The PARA is used to examine the type, quantity, accessibility, quality, and features of physical activity resources within a patient's environment. The assessment, together with protocol and definitions, is available online.[56]

- *Home and Community Environment (HACE)* instrument.[57] The HACE is a self-report instrument used to identify features of the patient's home or community that may affect level of function. The environmental domains examined include home and community mobility, basic mobility and communication devices, transportation factors, and attitudes. The instrument and scoring manual are available online.[58]

- *Safety Assessment of Function and the Environment for Rehabilitation (SAFER)* tool.[59-61] A comprehensive functional and environmental examination tool designed for use with the elderly. It includes 15 areas of concern: living situation, mobility, kitchen, eating, household management, fire hazards, dressing, grooming, bathroom, medication, communication, recreation, general items, wandering, and memory aids. Each category is examined within the content of the home environment and the functional capabilities of the patient.

- *Usability in My Home (UIMH)*.[62-65] This self-report instrument examines features of the home environment that either constrain or promote activity performance (see Appendix 9.B). It addresses aspects of both basic activities of daily living (BADL) and instrumental activities of daily living (IADL) and consists of 23 items, 16 of which are scored on a scale of 1 to 7 (1 representing the most negative response, 7 the most positive response). In addition, the instrument includes seven open-ended questions (six for description of specific usability problems and one for expressing additional opinions). Usability is conceptually defined as the extent to which a patient's needs and preferences can be met within the home. The UIMH includes a personal, environmental, and activity component.

- *Housing Enabler*.[62,64] This instrument is administered using a combination of interview and observation and is designed to examine home accessibility. It includes three steps: (1) determination of activity limitations (13 items) and dependence on mobility devices (2 items); (2) examination of environmental barriers (188 items), including indoor and outdoor accessibility, entrances, and communication features; and (3) calculation of an accessibility score (higher scores reflect greater accessibility problems). A content-valid Nordic version of the Housing Enabler has also been developed.[66]

- *Environmental Analysis of Mobility Questionnaire (EAMQ)*.[67,68] The EAMQ is a self-report instrument that examines the impact of the environment on community mobility. It includes 24 characteristics of the environment grouped into 8 dimensions. Each characteristic includes both an encounter question ("How often do you…?") and an avoidance question ("How often do you avoid…?"). A five-item ordinal scale is used to document frequency of encounter and avoidance responses (never, rarely, sometimes, often, always).[68, p. 394] Encounter and avoidance scores are averaged to generate a *summary environmental score* and a *summary avoidance score*.

- *Craig Handicap Assessment and Reporting Technique (CHART)*.[69] This instrument was developed to document an individual's functioning within his or her societal context. It examines level of involvement within six domains of function: physical independence, cognitive independence, mobility, occupation, social integration, and economic self-sufficiency. Each area is scored based on 100 points (600 points maximum) with greater levels of participation receiving higher scores. The CHART Short Form (CHART-SF)[70,71] is a 19-item shortened version of the CHART.

- *Craig Hospital Inventory of Environmental Factors (CHIEF)*.[72,73] This inventory rates frequency and impact of 25 environmental barriers defined as any impediments that prevent functioning within the home and community. In addition to physical and architectural barriers, the instrument includes social, attitudinal, and policy barriers; response items carry numeric values. The CHIEF gathers information about the frequency of encounters with each barrier (daily = 4, weekly = 3, monthly = 2, less than monthly = 1, never = 0) and the magnitude of the problem (big problem = 2 or little problem = 1). Scores are calculated by multiplying the frequency of occurrence by the magnitude of the problem to provide an *impact score*. Higher scores indicate greater impact of environmental barriers. A CHIEF short form (CHIEF-SF) contains 12 items from the original inventory.[74] The CHIEF Manual, containing information about instrument development as well as both the CHIEF and the CHIEF-SF, is available online.[75]

- *ADL-Staircase*.[76-83] Based on the original Katz ADL-Index,[84] the ADL-Staircase (see Appendix 9.C) is an index of four instrumental activities (cleaning, shopping, transportation, and cooking)[80,81] combined with six personal daily life activities (bathing, dressing, going to the toilet, transfer, continence, and feeding).[84] The ability to perform each activity is scored using a three-point scale: *independent, partly dependent,* and *dependent. Partly dependent* means that assistance from another person is required. The ratings can then be dichotomized into *independent* or *dependent,* and arranged into one conditional ordered scale of ADL-steps 0 to 9 or 10 (when continence is included there are 10 steps and when it is excluded there are 9 steps). ADL-step 0 means independent in all activities, and ADL-step 9 (or 10) dependent in all activities. The reliability and validity of the instrument have been established. The 10-step ADL scale has shown good validity and reliability in an elderly population.[82] In a study using three different age groups, findings indicated that the ADL-Staircase is most valid and reliable for age groups between 18–29 and 75–89 years.[79] A version of this instrument has been developed for use in rural areas.[85]

Visual Depictions and Dimensions of Physical Space

The therapist may request that family members or caregivers provide visual depictions (e.g., streaming video using a computer, smart phone, or tablet, photographs, videotapes, diagrams, floor plans) and physical dimensions (structural specifications obtained with a tape measure) of the environment in which the patient is expected to function. If resources for obtaining visuals are limited, an inexpensive disposable camera works well for this purpose.

Suggestions for modifications can be made from the visual representations and measured dimensions of the patient's environment. Such environmental information will allow the therapist to simulate aspects of the patient's surroundings (before discharge) for practicing tasks while directing attention to maximizing safety and function. This will also assist the therapist to determine the need for adaptive equipment.

On-Site Visits

On-site visits require that rehabilitation team members together with the patient travel to the physical location where the patient will be required to function (home, community, and/or work [job/school/play]). A major advantage of the on-site visit is that it allows observation of performance in the actual environment in which the activities must be accomplished. On-site visits are often useful in reducing patient, family, caregiver, and/or employer apprehension concerning the patient's ability to function within the environment. The on-site visit also provides an important opportunity for the therapist to identify safety hazards and make recommendations regarding altering, coping with, or adapting specific environmental barriers. During the visit, patient activity should be interspersed with adequate rest intervals to ensure that fatigue is not an influencing factor.

Whichever examination strategy or combination of strategies are applied, the scope and breadth of the information gathered will be enhanced by involvement of family members and caregivers. Because it is usually not feasible for the therapist to examine all aspects of the patient's total environment, involvement of other individuals can be instrumental in ensuring that the goal of maximum accessibility is met. This is particularly important for determination of general community access. The therapist can direct and guide an investigation of access to community recreational, educational, and commercial facilities, as well as availability of public transportation. The therapist can also provide guidance in the essential role of exploring funding sources for needed environmental modifications (potential funding sources are addressed later in this chapter).

Data from an examination of the environment are used to evaluate the need for specific access, usability, and safety interventions. Corcoran and Gitlin[1] identify five major areas of environmental intervention strategies: (1) *assistive* or *adaptive devices* such as grab bars, reachers, adapted eating utensils (e.g., rocker knife), canes, or walkers; (2) *safety devices* such as lighting, smoke detectors, or sensing devices; (3) *structural alterations,* which include widening doors, installing railings or ramps, or removing a doorway threshold; (4) *modification* or *altered location of environmental objects* such as disabling a stove, placing locks on doors, use of extension levers on door handles, removing throw rugs, or moving furniture; and (5) *task modification* such as use of visual, auditory, or other sensory cueing, work simplification, and energy conservation or joint preservation techniques.

The following sections offer suggestions for examination and modification of the home and workplace environment. The information presented is neither exhaustive nor inclusive of the needs of every patient. The environmental considerations are intended to direct attention to some of the more common access, usability, and safety concerns.

■ EXAMINATION OF THE HOME
Preparation for On-Site Visit

Before an on-site visit to the patient's home, occupational and physical therapy treatment sessions should be scheduled that will include participation from family and caregivers. These visits serve several functions. They provide an opportunity to become familiar with the patient's capabilities and activity limitations. They give the family/caregivers time to learn safe methods (e.g., proper body mechanics, guarding techniques) for assisting with ambulation, transfers, exercise, and functional activities. During these treatment sessions the occupational and physical therapists will have an opportunity to provide instruction in the use of assistive devices, adaptive equipment, and assistive technology. The time spent in education of family and caregivers is often pivotal in facilitating the patient's successful return to the home, community, and/or work (job/school/play) environments.

Clinical Note: Although sometimes restricted by reimbursement issues, when feasible, a day or weekend patient visit to his or her home should be encouraged and arranged before the on-site visit. During such a visit, problems not previously anticipated by the therapist or family and/or caregivers may be uncovered. Emphasis can then be placed on initial development of a plan to solve these problems before the on-site visit and the patient's actual return to the environment.

Preceding the on-site visit, information should be gathered about several important areas that will influence both the preparation for and the types of suggestions made during the visit. This information includes the following:

- Detailed information about present level of function (e.g., communication skills, bed mobility, transfers, gait, and so forth); data should be gathered from all involved disciplines (occupational therapist, physical therapist, speech-language pathologist, and so forth).
- Knowledge of physical assistance or verbal cueing required for activity performance.
- Characteristics and dimensions of adaptive devices and/or assistive technology (e.g., raised toilet seat, long-handled reachers, environmental controls) and ambulatory assistive devices (e.g., canes, crutches, walkers).
- Information about predicted level of optimum function or improvement (expected outcomes).
- Nature of the activity limitations or disability (i.e., static or progressive).
- Insurance coverage, financial resources, and availability of potential funding sources (in terms of capacity to modify environment or obtain needed adaptive and assistive devices or assistive technology).
- Knowledge of the patient's future plans (household management, family care, employment outside the home, school, vocational training, and so forth).
- Knowledge of whether the house or apartment is owned or rented; the type and ownership of the home can affect or preclude the type of modifications the patient may require. However, it should be noted that the Fair Housing Act requires landlords to allow individuals with disabilities to make reasonable access modifications to both personal living space and common space such as entryways.
- Information about the relative permanence of the dwelling; if the patient plans to move in the near future, it will influence the type of modifications recommended (e.g., installing permanent ramps versus removable ones, or paving a gravel driveway).

This information can be obtained from a variety of sources, including the patient, rehabilitation team conferences, patient/family and caregiver conferences or interviews, medical record documentation from all disciplines involved, and social service interviews. Once this information is gathered, decisions can be made concerning what adaptive or assistive devices will be needed and the appropriate team members to accompany the patient on the visit.

Ideally, given their complementary expertise and skills, both the physical and occupational therapist accompany the patient on the home visit. They assume shared responsibility for examining the patient–environment interface. Depending on the specific needs of the patient, family, and/or caregivers, a speech-language pathologist, social worker, or nurse also may be among the rehabilitation team members visiting the home. For purposes of organization and structure, home visits are often divided into two global elements: (1) accessibility of the dwelling's *exterior* and (2) examination of the home's *interior*. An inexpensive disposable camera is useful for providing images of architectural barriers to accompany letters of justification for needed modifications. A tape measure and home examination form are also important tools during the visit. Many rehabilitation departments develop their own home examination forms to meet the particular needs of their patient population. The forms (or checklists) help to organize the visit and are useful in directing attention to all necessary details. An example of a Home Examination Form is provided in Appendix 9.D. This form can be expanded or modified, depending on the specific needs of the individual or patient population. Some caution must be used in interpreting data from home examination forms that have not been standardized or examined for reliability.

On-Site Visit

On arrival at the home for the on-site visit, the patient may need to rest for a short while before beginning the home examination. This is an important consideration, because patients may become very excited or emotional when returning to a cherished home environment after a lengthy absence. This may be true even if a day or weekend visit occurred before the formal home visit.

One method of gathering data about the interior of the home is to begin with the patient in bed as though it were morning. Simulation of all daily tasks and activities, including dressing, grooming, bathroom activities, and preparation of meals, can ensue. The patient should attempt to perform all transfer, exercise, locomotion, self-care, and homemaking activities as independently as possible. This will provide an additional opportunity to teach the family and caregivers how and when to assist the patient.

Exterior Accessibility
Route of Entry

1. If there is more than one entry to the dwelling, the most accessible should be selected (closest to driveway, most level walking surface, fewest stairs, available handrails, and so forth).

2. Ideally, the driveway should be a smooth, level surface with easy access to the home. Walking surfaces to the entrance should be carefully examined. Cracked and uneven surfaces should be repaired or an alternate route selected.

3. The route to entrance should be level, be well lighted, and provide adequate cover from adverse weather conditions. Package shelves near the entrance are useful for freeing hands to unlock and/or open doors.

4. The height, number, and condition of stairs should be noted. Ideally, steps should not be greater than 7 in (180 mm) high with a minimum depth of 11 in (280 mm).[4] *Nosings,* also referred to as "lips," are the 0.5 in (13 mm) curved overhangs on the front edge of stairs. These overhangs are often problematic because they can cause a patient's toe to "catch" and prevent smooth transition to the next step. Nosings should be removed or reduced, if possible. Installing small wood bevels under the overhangs that taper down toward the lower step and provide a smoother contour can minimize nosing (Fig. 9.2A). The steps also should have a nonslip surface to improve traction. This can be accomplished by adding abrasive strips (Fig. 9.2B).

5. Handrails should be installed, if needed. In general, handrail height should measure between a minimum of 34 in (865 mm) and a maximum of 38 in

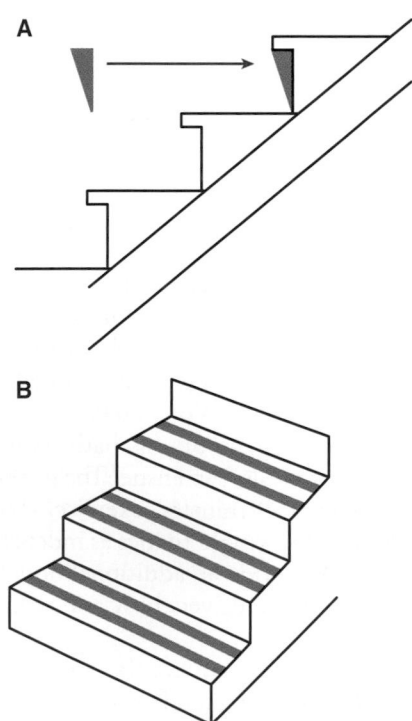

Figure 9.2 (A) Wood bevels placed under nosings minimize the danger of "toe-catching" during transition to the next step. **(B)** Abrasive strips improve traction and depth perception.

(965 mm) high for stairs, ramps, and level walking surfaces (Fig. 9.3). This range in handrail height allows for modifications to accommodate needs of particularly tall or short individuals. At least one handrail should extend a minimum of 12 in (305 mm) beyond the foot and top of the stairs (Fig. 9.4). Outside cross-sectional diameter of circular handrails should be between a minimum of 1.25 in (32 mm) and a maximum of 2 in (51 mm). If mounted adjacent to a wall, clearance between the handrail and wall should be a minimum of 1.50 in (38 mm).[4,5]

6. Installation of a ramp requires adequate space. Large ramps are typically constructed of wood or concrete; smaller ramps can be made from aluminum or fiberglass. The minimum **ramp grade** (incline or slope) for a wheelchair ramp is that for every inch of threshold height there is a corresponding 12 in (305 mm) of ramp length (a running slope of 1:12).[4] Outdoor ramps exposed to inclement weather such as snow or ice formation require a more gradual running slope of approximately 1:20. Ramps should be a minimum of 36 in (915 mm) wide, with a nonslip surface. The overall rise of any ramp should be no greater than 30 in (760 mm). Handrails also should be included on the ramp with a minimum height of 34 in (865 mm) and a maximum height of 38 in (965 mm) and extend 12 in (305 mm) beyond the top and bottom of the ramp (Fig. 9.5).[4,5] Small, commercially available ramps can be used for traversing curbs and small step heights.

7. *Vertical platform lifts* and *stairway lifts* are commercially available and may be a consideration when inadequate space is available for a ramp. Vertical platform lifts (Fig. 9.6) travel approximately 8 ft (243.84 cm) straight up and down. Both open and enclosed models are available. Platform lifts are often installed adjacent to stairs with an upper landing and are available in a variety of dimensions with lengths ranging from 54 to 60 in (137.16 to 152.4 cm) and widths ranging from 34 to 42 in (86.36 to 106.68 cm). The lift brings the wheelchair user from the ground level to the landing level to access the entrance to the home (these lifts can be used indoors as well). Stairway lifts are installed directly onto existing outdoor stairways; however, they are more frequently used indoors. The stairway lifts are mounted on runners that traverse the length of the stairs and slightly beyond. Many models allow the platform to fold up against an adjacent wall to allow free stair access for others entering the home.

Entrance

1. For individuals using a wheelchair, the entrance should have a platform large enough to allow the patient to rest and to prepare for entry. This platform area is particularly important when a ramp is

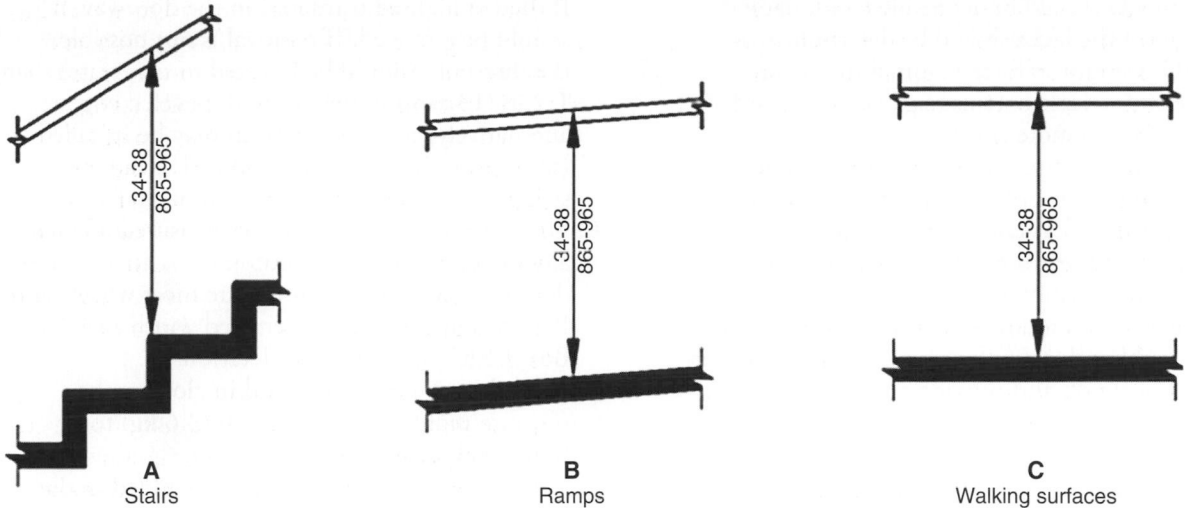

A
Stairs

B
Ramps

C
Walking surfaces

Figure 9.3 Handrail height for (a) stairs, (b) ramps, and (c) level walking surfaces in inches and millimeters. *(From 2010 ADA Standards for Accessible Design.[5, p. 145])*

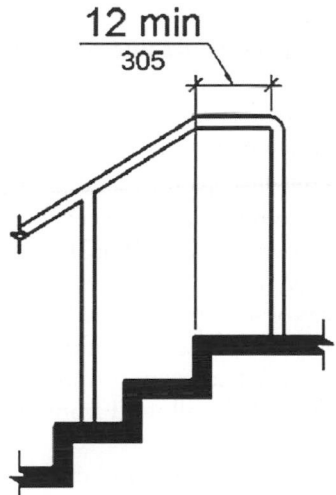

Figure 9.4 Handrail extension at top of stairs. A similar handrail extension of 12 in (305 mm) is placed at bottom of stairs. *(From 2010 ADA Standards for Accessible Design.[5, p. 157])*

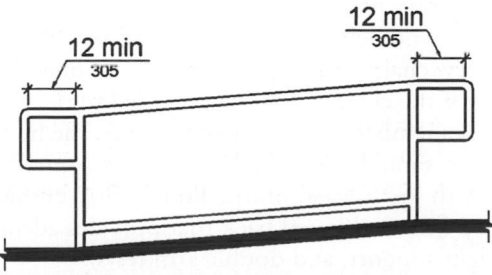

Figure 9.5 Handrail extensions should run a minimum of 12 in (305 mm) beyond the top and bottom edge of ramp. *(From 2010 ADA Standards for Accessible Design.[5, p. 157])*

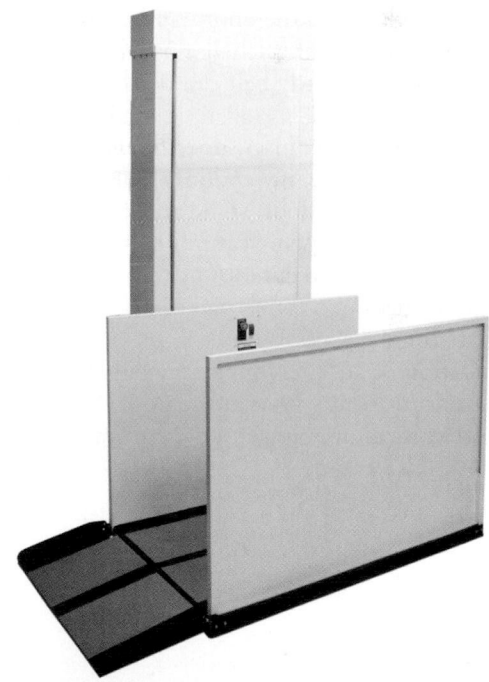

Figure 9.6 Powered residential vertical lift. This lift has a 600-lb weight capacity. The platform measures approximately 36 inches wide and 48 inches deep (91.44 × 121.92 cm). *(Courtesy of AmeriGlide, Inc., Raleigh, NC 27610.)*

in use. It provides for safe transit from the inclined surface to the level surface. If an individual using a wheelchair is required to open a door that swings out, this area should be at least 5 × 5 ft (153 × 153 cm). If the door swings in and away from the patient, a space at least 3 ft (91.5 cm) deep and 5 ft (153 cm) wide is required.

2. The door locks should be accessible to the patient. The height of the locks should be determined, as well as the amount of force required to turn the key. Alternative lock systems (e.g., voice- or card-activated locks, remote control locks, keypad electronic security systems, and push-button padlocks) may be an important consideration for some patients. Particular attention should be directed toward ensuring that the locking mechanism on the door is sufficiently illuminated.

3. The door handle should be turned easily by the patient. Rubber doorknob covers (that stretch over a round doorknob and provide a textured grip) or lever-type handles (Fig. 9.7) are often easier to use for patients with limited grip strength (screw fastened, slip-on levers are also available that convert a round doorknob to lever-type handle). Lever handles do not require the same strength or range of motion (ROM) needed for traditional round doorknobs.[7]

4. The door should open and close in a direction that is functional for the patient. A long canvas "door strap" may be attached to the outside of the door (or around the door handle) to help an individual using a wheelchair close the door when leaving. A long, sturdy belt can be also be used as a door strap.

5. Remote control automatic door openers are available that attach to existing doors that can open, close, and lock the door; some are equipped with customized "stay-open" features to accommodate the time required to enter or exit. A handheld remote control or a touch pad can be used to activate these devices.

6. Installation of an intercom system allows the patient to see and/or hear who is at the door. Some allow remote control opening of a door from any location in the home.

7. If there is a raised threshold in the doorway, it should be removed. If removal is not possible, the threshold should be lowered to no greater than 1/2 in (13 mm) in height, with beveled edges;[4] alternatively, a threshold ramp may be installed (see section titled *Doors*). If needed, weather-stripping the door will help prevent drafts.

8. The doorway width should be measured. Generally, 32 to 34 in (815 to 865 mm) is an acceptable doorway width to accommodate most wheelchairs. Bariatric chairs require increased width. (See Box 9.1 for bariatric considerations.)

9. If the door is weighted to aid in closing, the pressure should not exceed 8 lb (3.6 kg) to be functional for the patient.

10. A kick plate (metal guard) may be added to doors frequently entered by individuals using a wheelchair or ambulatory assistive devices. The kick plate should measure 12 in (305 mm) in height from the bottom of the door.

General Considerations: Interior Accessibility

Furniture Arrangement and Features

1. Sufficient room should be made available for maneuvering a wheelchair or ambulating with an assistive device. An initial step is to move as much furniture as possible against the walls to increase clearance and stability (i.e., prevent sliding of furniture during movement transitions). Further stability can be achieved by placing rubber cups (floor guards) under the legs of sofas and chairs. Items such as coffee tables, footstools, or telephone or electrical wires should not obstruct access to furniture.

2. Clear passage must be allowed from one room to the next.

3. Typically, overstuffed sofas and chairs do not provide the needed support for sit-to-stand movement transitions. Although generally not the case, living room chairs should have double arm rests, a firm seating surface, and an upright back. Sometimes a suitable chair can be found in a different location within the home and moved to the living room. Another option is to modify the current furniture by placing a fitted wooden board under the seat cushion and behind the seat back (if removable). If a new chair is to be purchased, recommended features of the chair should be provided to the patient, family member, and/or caregiver (e.g., the height of the seat should allow the knees to flex approximately 90° with the feet flat on the floor, a firm cushioned seat, a firm cushioned back that provides adequate upright support, and double arm rests).

4. Use of any unstable furniture such as rocking chairs should be discouraged for most patients. Use of leather furniture should also be avoided because the increased friction can hinder movement. Chairs that

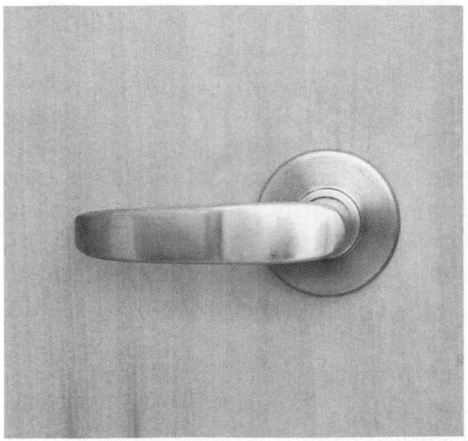

Figure 9.7 Lever-style door handle (a frequent universal design element) is particularly useful for individuals with limited grip strength because they can be activated with other body parts (e.g., fisted hand, forearm, elbow).

Box 9.1   Bariatric Considerations

Obese or morbidly obese individuals present unique environmental needs. Obesity is generally defined using body mass index (BMI) and can be divided into three classes:[1]

Class	BMI
I Obesity (Moderate)	30-34
II Obesity (Severe)	35-39
III Obesity (Very Severe) (morbidly obese)	>40

Patients who are obese often require specialized equipment for being lifted, moved, transferred, or transported. Bariatric equipment is space consuming; this is often exacerbated by older homes designed and built when the statistical averages for adult height and weight were less than today. The following are environmental considerations specific to this population.

- *Patient, Family, and Caregiver Training:* Specific training in the use of bariatric equipment and patient handling is critical. Patients who are obese often require assistance throughout the day for many routine activities (e.g., positional changes, supine-to-sit, sit-to-stand, bathing, toileting, and dressing). These care requirements emphasize the need for highly trained caregivers able to promote safety and injury prevention for both patient and themselves. When possible, the patient should be encouraged to assume the lead in directing those responsible for care.
- *Physical Assistance:* More than one individual may be required to assist the patient. There may be situations where as many as three or four people are needed for patient handling. Third-party payers challenge reimbursement for more than one support person in the home simultaneously (duplication of services). This may require involvement from extended family members and/or require the patient and family to seek creative funding sources to meet this need (see section titled Funding for Environmental Modifications).
- *Bariatric Equipment:* Inherent to its purpose, bariatric equipment is oversized, is designed for increased weight capacity, and is generally heavier and more costly than the nonbariatric equivalent. Bariatric equipment is extensive and includes beds (some with built-in scales), bedside commodes, standard and overhead lifts, reclining chairs, steel-framed chairs, powered lift chairs with a 1,000 lb (453.59 kg) weight capacity, bathroom equipment, adaptive equipment, wheelchairs (widths up to 48 in [121.92 cm]), scooters, and ambulatory assistive devices. Providers of durable medical equipment (DME) typically offer instruction for in-home use. Some provide ongoing support should additional caregivers require training.
- *Risk of Ulceration:* Patients who are obese are at increased risk for developing pressure ulcers secondary to their size and immobility. They may be unable to effectively change positions, creating excess pressure on susceptible areas for long periods. This may require use of a specialized mattress (e.g., low air loss with alternating pressure). Moisture or perspiration may contribute to ulcer formation.
- *Care Environment:* Large beds (e.g., 42 to 54 in [106.68 to 137.16 cm] wide, 80 to 90 in [203.2 to 228.6 cm] long, and up to 1,000 lb [453.59 kg] weight capacity), lifts, and other large bariatric equipment require larger room dimensions. Passage of bariatric equipment generally requires a door width of 60 in (152.4 cm). A large window may need to be temporarily removed to allow passage of oversized items. Ample floor space is also needed for caregivers to interface with the patient in and around the equipment. Five feet of clear floor space is recommended on each side and at the foot of the bed.[2] The floor surface and support structures beneath need to be carefully examined. They must be able to support a patient weight ranging from 500 to 1,000 lb (226.8 to 453.59 kg) together with all needed equipment and supplies. Often space is made available on the first level of a dwelling (versus navigating patient and equipment up a narrow staircase to a small second floor bedroom). This may require conversion of the living room to a patient care area. An environmental control unit is an important consideration.
- *Bathroom:* Space is a primary concern in gaining access to a standard residential bathroom. Sufficient door width is needed to accommodate patient size, an assistive device, and/or the individual(s) guarding the patient. A 60 in (152.4 cm) door width and turning radius is recommended.[2] To place a bariatric commode with armrests over a toilet or allow a two-person assist, ample space of 24 in (60.96 cm) is needed on each side with a 44 in (111.76 cm) front clearance.[2] A bidet may be recommended to assist cleansing. The toilet and sink should be floor mounted with a 1,000 lb (543.59 kg) weight capacity.[2] Longer than typical grab bars with a 1,000 lb (543.59 kg) weight capacity should be installed on reinforced walls. The shower stall should be a minimum of 4 × 6 ft (1.22 × 1.83 m) and include a level entrance, a bariatric shower seat, a shower hand spray, and grab bars with a 1,000 lb (543.59 kg) weight capacity. The use of shower curtains is recommended over solid doors to facilitate caregiver assistance.

Continued

Box 9.1   Bariatric Considerations—cont'd

1. Gabel, L, and Musheno, E: Understanding the Special Needs of the Bariatric Population: Design, Innovation, and Respect, 2010. Retrieved June 6, 2012, from www.ki.com/pdfs/Understanding_Needs_Bariactric_Population.pdf.
2. Facility Guidelines Institute (FGI) with assistance from the U.S. Department of Health and Human Services: Guidelines for Design and Construction of Health Care Facilities, FGI, 2010. Retrieved June 6, 2012, from www.fgiguidelines.org/guidelines2010.php.

provide mechanized elevation of the back of the seat are commercially available but should be used with caution. It may be difficult for a patient to stabilize the feet as the seat is elevating. This causes the feet (and pelvis) to slide forward, resulting in a fall.

Electrical Controls

1. Unrestricted access should be provided to wall switches and electrical outlets. Power strips (surge protectors) can be used to increase the number of outlets, as well as improve access. Outlets may need to be raised and wall switches lowered. For individuals using a wheelchair, use of pull cord extensions may allow control of some high electrical switches.
2. Some patients may benefit from replacement of standard toggle electric switches (e.g., overhead fixtures) with rocker switches that require less fine motor skill to activate (Fig. 9.8). Rocker switches are available with lighted surfaces and with occupancy (motion) sensor devices that automatically turn on or off. Light-switch plates come in a variety of colors and will be easier to see if they contrast with the existing wall color. For example, in rooms with light-colored walls (white, off-white, beige), darker electrical outlet and light-switch plates can be

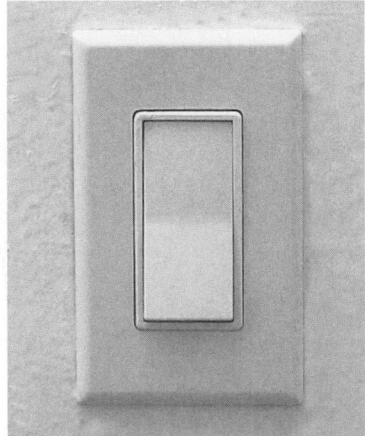

Figure 9.8 Rocker switches do not require fine motor skill and can be activated without using fingers (e.g., fisted hand, lateral aspect of hand, distal forearm). Rocker switches are available with an illuminated surface and with occupancy light sensor that turns on or off upon entering or leaving the room.

selected. A ground fault circuit interrupter (GFCI) should be installed in wet locations such as bathrooms to prevent against electrical shock. A GFCI outlet acts as a monitor for current imbalance between the hot and neutral wires and breaks the circuit if that situation occurs (e.g., faulty appliances, worn cords, or appliance contact with water).

3. For some patients, vision may be enhanced by use of higher wattage bulbs, fluorescent lighting, full-spectrum bulbs, daylight bulbs, or high-intensity halogen lamps. Use of long-life, energy-efficient light bulbs reduces the frequency of required bulb changes.
4. Inexpensive, programmable electrical timers can be used to regularly turn lights on and off throughout the day and night.
5. Inexpensive night-lights with motion sensors can be placed in strategic locations to provide additional illumination.
6. Touch pad dimmer switches can be used to activate lamps with small control knobs. The dimmer module is plugged into a wall outlet and the lamp attached to the module. The lamp can be turned "on" or "off" or level of brightness changed by touching the pad. Voice-activated dimmers are also available.
7. Inexpensive remote control units can be used in any room of the home to control lights or small appliances. The simplest designs of these remote control units send signals through existing wires (receiver modules are plugged into existing outlets and appliances are plugged into the receiver and controlled by a handheld remote); others are wireless and utilize radio signals. Receiver modules can also be wired directly into the electrical system of the dwelling. Remote control units are available with large-print buttons and numbers.

Floors

1. Floors should be nonslip and level. All floor coverings should be glued or tacked to the floor. This will prevent bunching or rippling under wheelchair use. When carpeting is used, a dense, low pile (0.25 to 0.5 in [0.635 to 1.27 cm]), low-level loop generally provides for easiest movement of a wheelchair or ambulatory assistive device. Industrial-style or "indoor/outdoor" carpeting typically meet these requirements. High pile carpeting and carpet padding

increases roll resistance (e.g., wheelchair, rolling walker); firmer carpeting decreases roll resistance. Carpeting with bold patterns of mixed colors may be visually confusing and impair judgment of spatial distances.[86] Padding under carpet is generally not recommended; if used, it should be very firm.[5]

2. Floors should be examined for uneven or unlevel areas. This may be particularly problematic with older wooden floors. Joints in wood flooring should be shallow and no more that 0.25 to 0.5 in (0.635 to 1.27 cm) wide. Deep joints wider than 0.75 in (1.9 cm) will cause wheelchair casters to turn and lodge, blocking movement.[86] Optimally, problem areas should be repaired or replaced. If restoration is not possible, several other solutions might be recommended: (1) establish a path of movement for the patient that eliminates use of the problematic area; (2) place a piece of furniture over the offending area; or (3) place brightly colored tape along the borders of the area to continually remind the patient to avoid this area of potential danger.

3. Scatter rugs should be removed; larger area rugs can be secured with a good-quality carpet tape. Use of nonskid waxes should be encouraged.

4. If flooring is to be replaced, matte finishes should be recommended to reduce glare. Patients with visual impairments will benefit from a contrasting colored border along the perimeter of the room to help mark the boundaries of the space. Wide, colored tape can also be used effectively.

Doors

1. Raised thresholds should be removed to provide a flush, level surface. If structural elements prevent removal, threshold ramps ("transition wedges") can be easily installed (Fig. 9.9).

2. Doorways may need to be widened (if less than 32 in [815 mm] wide) to allow clearance for a wheelchair or assistive device. Doors may have to be removed, reversed (e.g., to open outward for easier exit, especially in the case of an emergency), or replaced with folding doors. Several other options are available to increase door clearance:
   • Installation of pocket doors, which slide into the adjacent wall when not in use; some sliding doors allow installation on the outside of the door frame and wall to minimize structural changes.
   • Removal of the wood strips on the inside of a doorframe will add approximately 0.75 to 1 in (19 to 25.4 mm) of clearance.
   • Use of *offset* hinges (also called *swing-clear* hinges), which swing the open door clear of the frame provide approximately 2 additional inches (51 mm) of space.
   • Removal of the door with installation of a curtain (inexpensive spring-loaded curtain rods and a

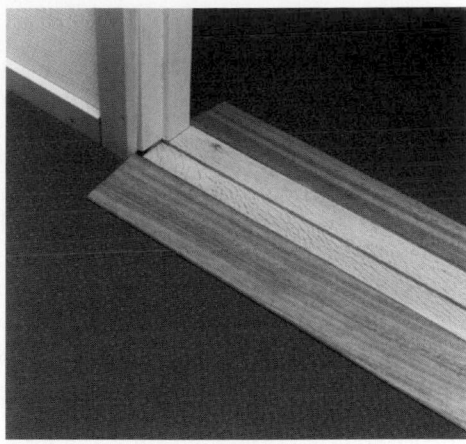

Figure 9.9 Common materials used for threshold ramps are wood (shown) and aluminum with a lacquered nonslip surface. They can be used between rooms, if threshold cannot be removed. *(Courtesy of Guldmann, Inc., Tampa, FL 33634.)*

fabric or plastic shower curtain can be used); if used for a bathroom door, this option is less than optimal because it compromises privacy.

3. As mentioned in regard to exterior doors, handles inside the home should also be examined. Rubber doorknob covers or lever-type handles may be important considerations. Knurled (roughened) surface door handles are used on interiors of buildings and dwellings when frequented by persons with visual impairments. These abrasive, knurled surfaces provide tactile clues that the door leads to a hazardous area and alerts the individual to danger. (Note: Brightly colored roughened areas are also used on flooring to indicate potential danger; for example, the edge of a train or subway platform.)

Windows

1. To reduce glare, window films can be installed; frosted films are effective at diffusing light without appreciably reducing ambient light.

2. Heavy draperies or shades can also be used with the added benefit of absorbing internal background noise to improve hearing and conversation.

3. Remote control systems for closing or opening window coverings either partially or fully are commercially available.

4. Although not frequently seen in older dwellings, casement windows provide several important features for individuals using a wheelchair or for patients with limited upper extremity function. Casement windows open using a crank-style handle and can be locked with a single lever locking mechanism located near the bottom of the window. Automatic openers can be installed on these windows.

Stairs

1. All indoor stairwells should have handrails and should be well lighted. Ideally, handrails should extend a minimum of 12 in (305 mm) past the top and bottom of the stairs for added safety.[4,5] Battery-operated touch switch lamps are a practical supplement where electrical light sources are unavailable. Inexpensive track lighting provides multiple adjustable lamps and requires only a single electrical source. Lighting should be bright with glare and reflection minimized. Motion detection lights that automatically turn on when the patient approaches the stairs (or other area of the home) can also be an important safety consideration.

2. Stairs should be free of clutter. Rather than climbing the stairs to move a single item to the next level, patients sometimes "store" or collect items on the stairs. This creates several safety hazards: (1) initially bending over to pick up the items before stair climbing can alter postural stability; (2) negotiating stairs holding several objects can impair balance and limit use of the handrail; and (3) other household members may not see the item(s), precipitating a fall. As an alternative, a canvas bag or "stair basket" with handles (that can be held in one hand) can be placed near the stairs to collect the items until the patient is ready to move to another floor level.

3. For individuals with decreased visual acuity or age-related visual changes, adhesive, light-reflective *tactile warning strips* provide contrasting textures on the surface of the top and bottom stair(s) to alert them that the end of the stairwell is near. They can also be used on each step to identify its edge. Circular bands of tape also can be placed at the top and bottom of the handrail for the same purpose. Tactile warning strips placed on the floor can also be used to signal a change in level of the walking surface or entrance to another area or room of the dwelling.

4. Many patients with visual impairment will benefit also from bright, contrasting color tape on the border of each stair. Warm colors (reds, oranges, and yellows) are generally easier to see than cool colors (blues, greens, and violets).

5. For patients unable to negotiate stairs who require access to the second floor of a dwelling, a motorized stairlift may be an option (Fig. 9.10). These battery-powered units are available with a variety of options such as swing-away arms for wheelchair transfers, wide adjustable seat width (22.5 to 25.5 in [572 mm to 648 mm]), and wireless call/send controls. Outdoor models are also available, as well as units to accommodate curves or turns in the stairwell. Residential elevators are another, more costly option; they require construction of an enclosed shaft. If the residence has "stacked" closets (same position on different floors), these closet spaces can be combined to form an elevator shaft.

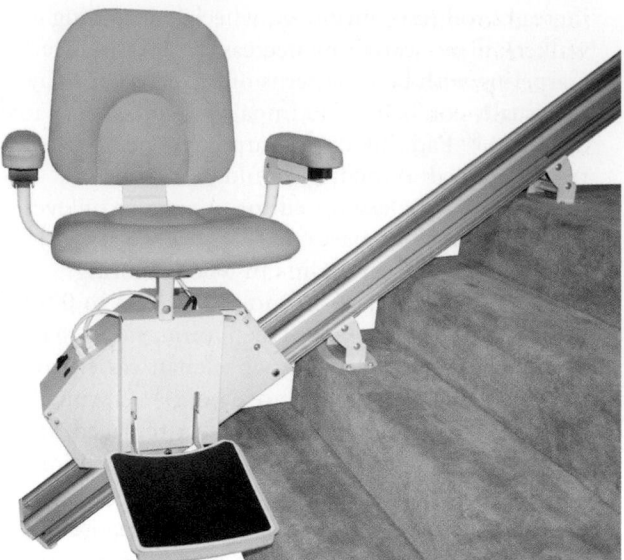

Figure 9.10 Powered stairlift. When not in use, the stairlift folds up against wall. It has a rack-and-pinion drive system that can safely transport up to 350 lb. The seat measures 19 inches (48.26 cm) wide and 14 inches (35.56 cm) deep. *(Courtesy of AmeriGlide, Inc., Raleigh, NC 27610).*

Heating Units

1. All radiators, heating vents, and hot water pipes should be appropriately screened off or insulated with pipe covers to prevent burns, especially for patients who have sensory impairments. Adaptations may be required to allow patient access to heat controls (e.g., remote thermostat control, use of reachers or enlarged, extended, or adapted handles on heat control valves).

2. The heating source should be clear of combustible material and clutter. Use of space heaters should be discouraged.

3. Smoke alarms and carbon monoxide detectors should be in the home and checked regularly by pressing the test button. Some newer models allow testing the unit using a flashlight or remote control.

Specific Considerations: Interior Accessibility

Bedroom Area

1. The bed should be stationary and positioned to provide ample space for transfers. Stability may be improved by placing the bed against a wall or in the corner of the room (except when the patient plans to make the bed). Additional stability may be achieved by placing rubber cups under each leg.

2. The height of the sleeping surface must be optimal for transfers. Furniture risers can be used to raise bed height. Wooden and high-density rubber furniture risers are commercially available in a variety of heights with routed depressions to hold each leg of

the bed (or other furniture such as chairs or tables). The use of an extra-thick mattress or box spring can also provide additional height to the bed. Using reduced-height box springs can lower the bed height.

3. The mattress should be carefully examined. It should provide a firm, comfortable surface. If the mattress is in relatively good condition, a firm bed board inserted between the mattress and box spring may suffice to improve the sleeping surface adequately. If the mattress is badly worn, a new one should be suggested.

4. A bedside nightstand (or small table) should be available; it can be used to hold a lamp, telephone (preferably cordless with a memory dial for frequently used numbers or emergency phone numbers; cellular phones have the added advantage of always remaining with the patient), necessary medications, and call bell if assistance is needed from a caregiver. Brooks et al[87] examined the type of items patients kept in their nightstands and their willingness to consider use of a smart nightstand. Findings indicated that the top surface and upper drawer were used most often. The categories of items most frequently kept on or in nightstands included personal hygiene (e.g., deodorant, eye drops, facial clothes), trash, clothing (e.g., belt, gloves, handkerchief), food accessories (e.g., fork, glass), telephone, book/magazine, water container, lotion, tissue box, and medical items (e.g., alcohol swabs, call button, cold pack). The vast majority of patients were willing to consider use of a smart nightstand. Participant preferences for design features included ability to raise and lower height, contemporary design, well-designed storage space, and voice activation.

5. The closet clothes bar may require lowering to provide wheelchair accessibility. The bar should be lowered to 52 in (132 cm) from the floor. Nonslip hangers are often recommended. Wall hooks also may be a useful addition to the closet area and should be placed between 40 in (101.6 cm) and 56 in (142.2 cm) from the floor. *Wardrobe lifts* can increase closet storage capacity while maintaining accessibility (Fig. 9.11). They consist of a clothes bar attached by hinged supports; using an extended handle, the bar is pulled down and out to access clothing. Electrically powered and hydraulic wardrobe lifts are also commercially available. Shelves also can be installed at various levels in the closet. The highest shelf should not exceed 45 in (115.5 cm). Clothing and grooming articles frequently used by the patient should be placed in the most easily accessible bureau drawer. Freestanding modular closet units are also available in a variety of dimensions. These units typically provide clothes bar, shelves, and drawers that can be adjusted to meet the needs of the user. Figure 9.12 illustrates the basic components and dimensions of an accessible bedroom.

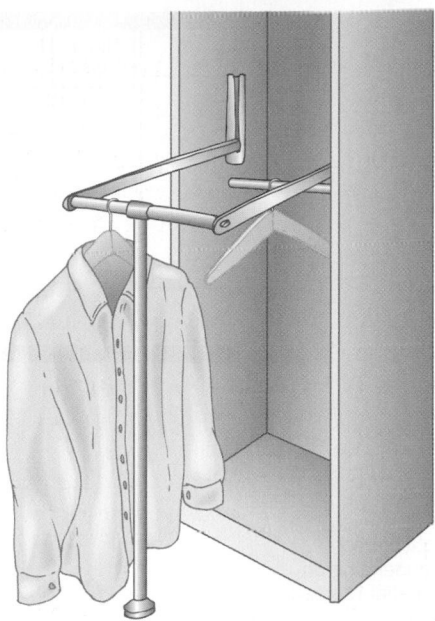

Figure 9.11 Manually operated wardrobe lift. Wardrobe lifts are available in a variety of sizes and some allow placement on either back wall or sidewalls.

Bathroom

1. If the doorframe prohibits passage of a wheelchair, the patient may transfer at the door to a chair with casters attached. As mentioned, several other solutions are available to address the problem of narrow doorframes (see Interior Accessibility: General Considerations, Doors).

2. An elevated toilet seat can be used to facilitate transfers. Some models allow the height to be custom adjusted whereas others provide a fixed height elevation. They are also available with grab bars. Power-lift toilet seats with grab bars are designed to assist the patient to standing (elevation initiated from the posterior aspect of the seat). As with other types of mechanized seat elevators, they should be used with caution, because it may be difficult to stabilize one's feet as the seat is elevating. For new construction, a wall-mounted toilet seat may be recommended that can be placed at the optimum height for the user and provide more floor space for transfer positioning.

3. Grab bars securely fastened to a reinforced wall will assist in both toilet and tub transfers. Grab bars should have a circular cross-section diameter of 1.25 in (32 mm) minimum and 2 in (51 mm) maximum and be knurled. For use in toilet transfers, the bars should be mounted horizontally 33 to 36 in (840 to 915 mm) from floor. The length of the grab bars should be between 42 and 54 in (1,065 and 1,370 mm) on sidewall and between 24 and 36 in (610 and 915 mm) on the back wall (Fig. 9.13). Ideally, two grab bars are secured horizontally to the back wall for use in tub transfers. One is placed

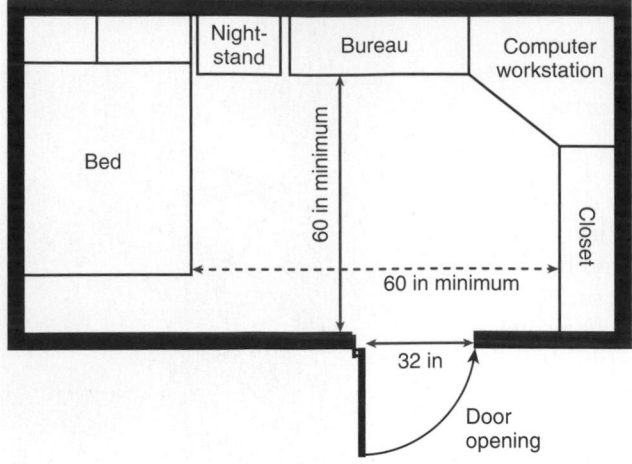

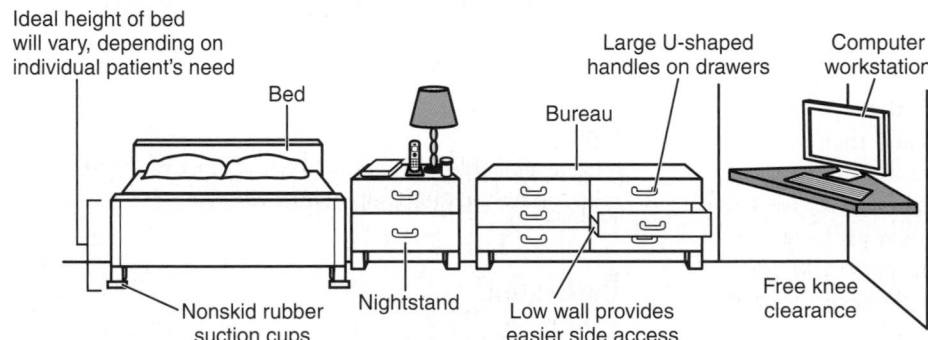

Figure 9.12 Sample dimensions and features of an accessible bedroom.

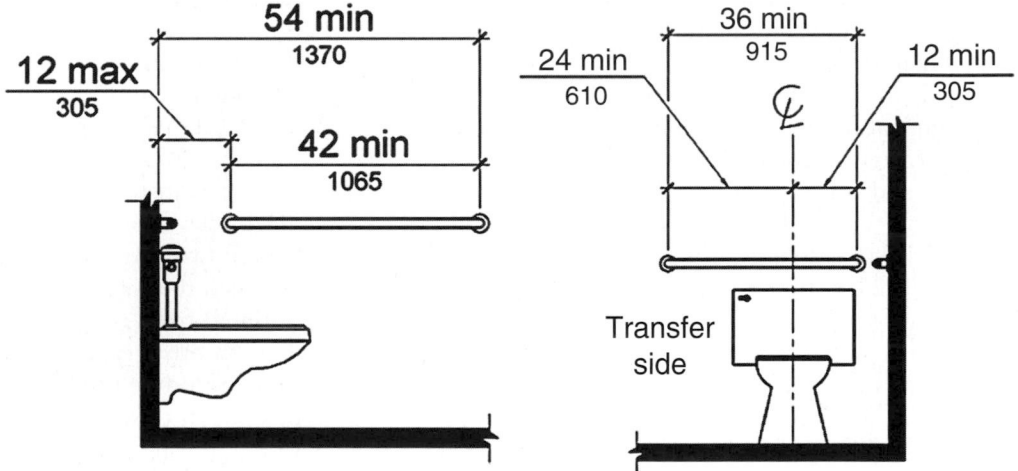

Figure 9.13 Location and dimensions of bathroom grab bars. Values denoted in inches and millimeters. The bars should be mounted horizontally 33 in (840 mm) to 36 in (915 mm) from the floor.[4] *(Left)* The sidewall grab bar is 42–54 in wide placed at a maximum of 12 in (305 mm) from rear wall. If anchored on or near rear wall, it should extend 54 in (1,370 mm) from the wall. *(Right)* The rear wall grab bar is 24–36 in wide (36 in is considered minimum if wall space allows). When 36 in long, 24 in of the bar (from center of toilet) is placed toward the side used for transfers. *(From 2010 ADA Standards for Accessible Design,[5] Left, p 163, Right, p 164.)*

33 to 36 in (840 to 915 mm) from tub floor and the second 9 in (230 mm) above top rim of the bathtub. Grab bars may also be mounted horizontally at the foot-end wall of the bathtub (recommended length is 24 in [610 mm] with placement at the front edge of the bathtub) and at the head-end wall of the bathtub (recommended length is 12 in [305 mm] with placement at the front edge of the bathtub) (Fig. 9.14). Knurled surfaces are typically used on grab bars to improve grasp and prevent slipping.

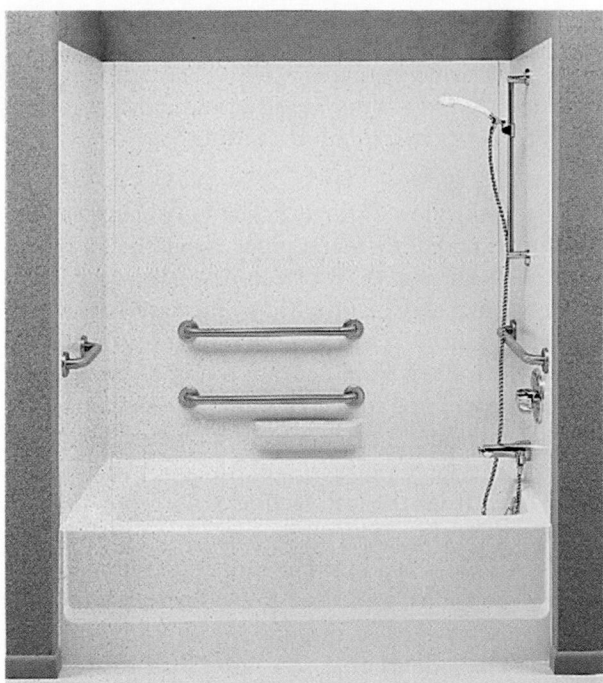

Figure 9.14 Bathtub with grab bars secured to back, foot-end, and head-end walls. The hand-spray faucet attachment facilitates control of water flow direction from a sitting position. *(Courtesy of The Swan Corporation, St. Louis, MO 63101.)*

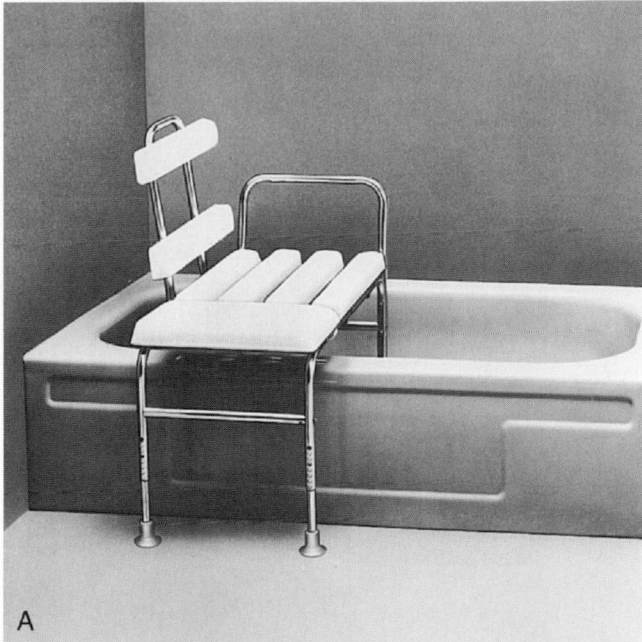

A

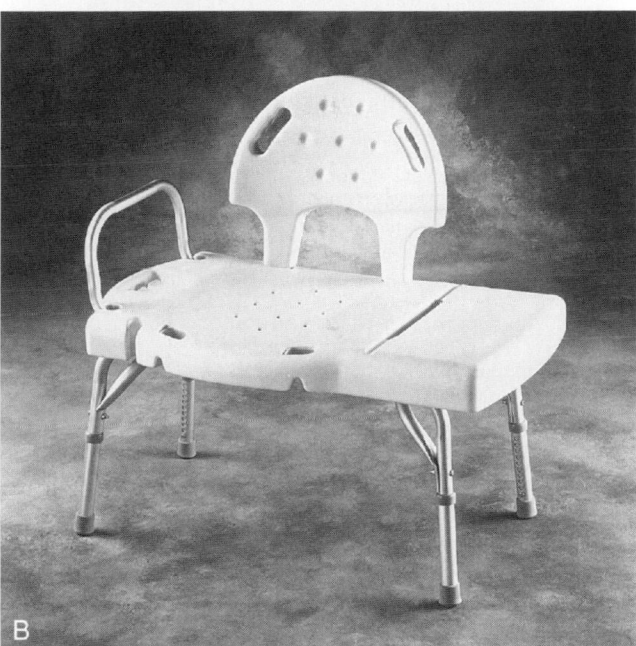

B

Figure 9.15 Two tub transfer bench designs each providing a wide base of support, a secure back rest, and a long seating surface to facilitate transfers. *(Courtesy of Lumex, Inc., Bay Shore, NY 11706.)*

4. A tub transfer bench (tub seat) may be recommended for bathing. Many types of commercially produced benches are available. In selecting a tub transfer bench (tub seat), function and safety are primary considerations. The bench should provide a wide base of support (some are designed with suction feet, and some provide height adjustment), a backrest, and an appropriate seating surface to facilitate transfers in and out of the tub (Fig. 9.15). Tub transfer benches with relatively long seating surfaces are typically positioned with two legs in the tub and two legs on the floor adjacent to the tub. Smaller benches are available that require all four legs to be placed inside the bathtub.

5. A space-saving design combines a toilet and shower seat into one assembled seat (Fig. 9.16). The design has the potential benefit of allowing creation of an accessible toilet and shower area in a relatively small bathroom as well as cost reduction since installation generally requires no wall demolition.

6. In shower stall areas, a collapsible seat may be permanently attached to the wall (Fig. 9.17). When not in use it folds flat against the wall, allowing easy shower access from a standing position as well. Many new extended shower designs incorporate a permanent, built-in seat.

7. Nonskid adhesive strips may be placed on the floor of the tub or shower area.

8. Additional bathroom considerations may include a hand-spray attachment to the bathtub or shower faucet (see Fig. 9.14 and Fig. 9.17), antiscald valves to prevent water temperature from rising above a preset limit (also called *scald-guard valves* or *high temperature stops*), water volume–control mechanisms (to prevent a sudden surge of water with resultant change in temperature), enlarged faucet handles on the tub or sink (single-lever system faucets are optimal owing to their ease of use),

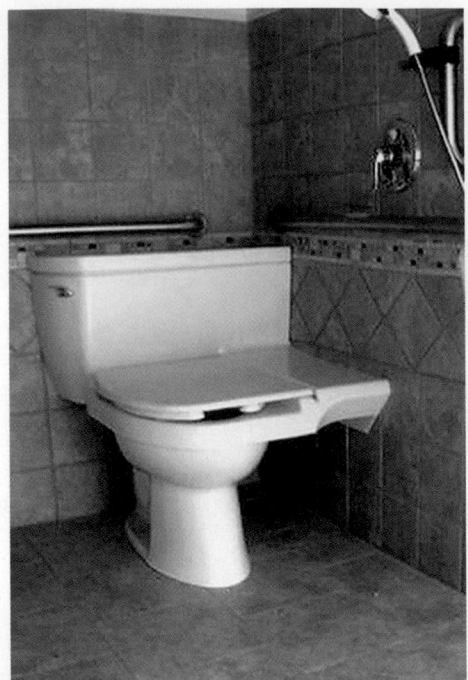

Figure 9.16 Combined toilet and shower seat into a single assembled seat. *(Courtesy of WYNG® Products, The Woodlands, TX 77380).*

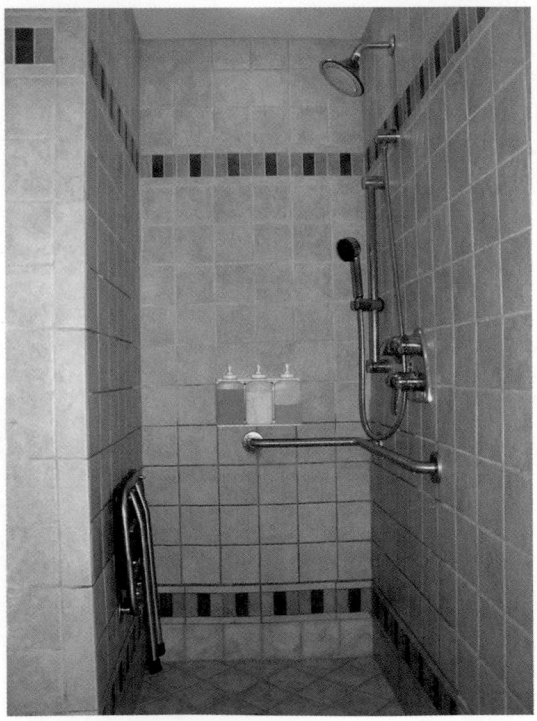

Figure 9.17 Shower stall with collapsible shower seat, grab bars, and hand-spray attachment.

motion-sensor faucets, a spray attachment at the sink (allows washing hair without entering the bathtub or shower), a towel rack and small shelf for toiletry articles, and a call bell within easy reach of the patient.

Clinical Note: To prevent injury in the presence of sensory impairments, patient, family, and caregiver education should include using a thermometer to test water temperature before bathing.

9. Ideally, sinks should provide clear knee space below and any exposed hot water pipes should be insulated to prevent burns (Fig. 9.18). In new construction, shallow sinks may be installed to increase knee clearance with faucets placed on the side for easier access. Storage space lost from beneath the sink can be partially compensated for by an under-the-sink rollout cabinet that can be easily moved for wheelchair access. An enlarged mirror over the sink with the top tilted away from the wall facilitates use from a sitting position (Fig. 9.19). Forward-tilting mirrors are also available with adjustable hinges for alternating placement against and away from the wall. Hinged-wall, gooseneck, or accordion fold-up mirrors (with one side magnified) are also helpful for close work.

Figure 9.20 illustrates the minimum space requirements of a wheelchair-accessible bathroom.

Kitchen

1. The height of countertops (work space) should be appropriate for the individual. When using a wheelchair, the armrests should be able to fit under the working surface. The ideal height of counter surfaces should be no greater than 31 in (794 mm) from the floor with a knee clearance of 27.5 to 30 in (705 to 769 mm). Counter space should provide a depth of at least 24 in (615 mm). All surfaces should be smooth to facilitate sliding of heavy items from one area to another. Slide-out counter spaces are useful in providing an over-the-lap working surface (Fig. 9.21). A section of base cabinetry can be removed to provide a seated countertop workspace. For patients who are ambulatory, stools (preferably with back and footrests) may be placed strategically at the main work area(s). For patients with visual impairments, placing colored tape along the border of the countertop that contrasts sharply with the color of the counter surface will help identify boundaries of the workspace. Under-the-counter cabinets with glide-out height-adjustable shelves improve access to storage areas (Fig. 9.22).

2. Improved function and safety may be provided by a sink equipped with large blade-type handles or a single-lever style faucet, scald-guard valves, or electronic sensors that allow hands-free operation by automatically turning water off and on. A spray-hose fixture allows filling heavy pots without needing to lift them from a sink. Pressure-balanced valves can be used to equalize hot and cold water; other faucets allow pre-programming desired water temperature. Hot water dispensers are helpful for preparing coffee or tea and

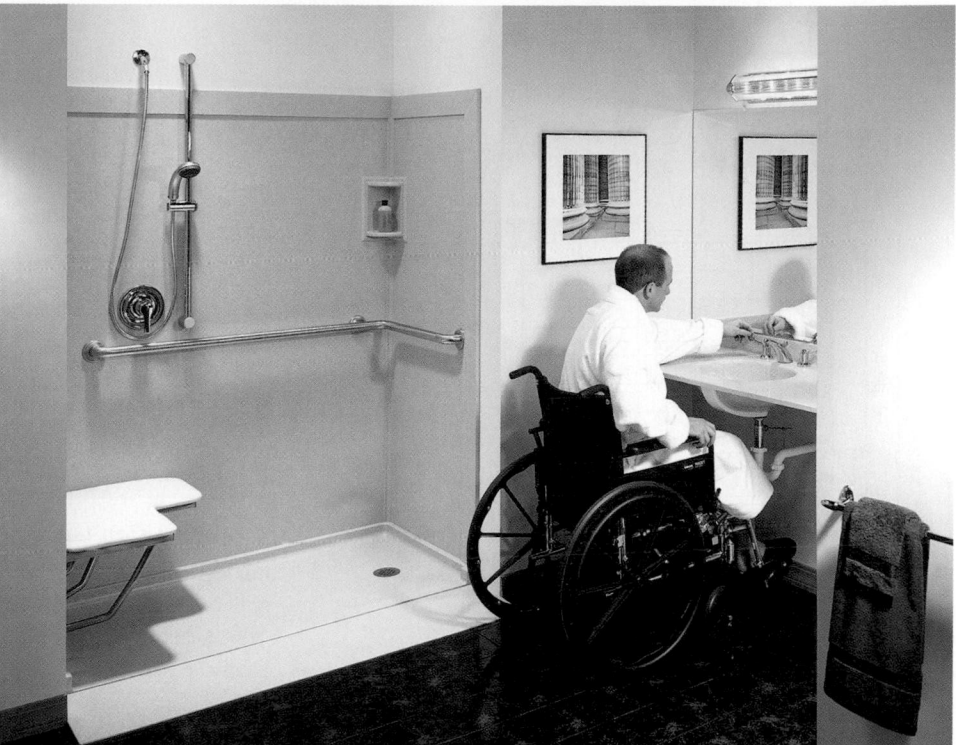

Figure 9.18 Accessible bathroom with knee clearance below sink and insulated piping. The shower entrance includes a small ramp to accommodate a difference in floor surface heights. Note that the shower hand-spray is held by a vertical slide-bar (to change height) allowing for a seated shower. Alternately, the hand-spray can be handheld to direct water flow to specific areas. *(Courtesy of The Swan Corporation, St. Louis, MO 63101.)*

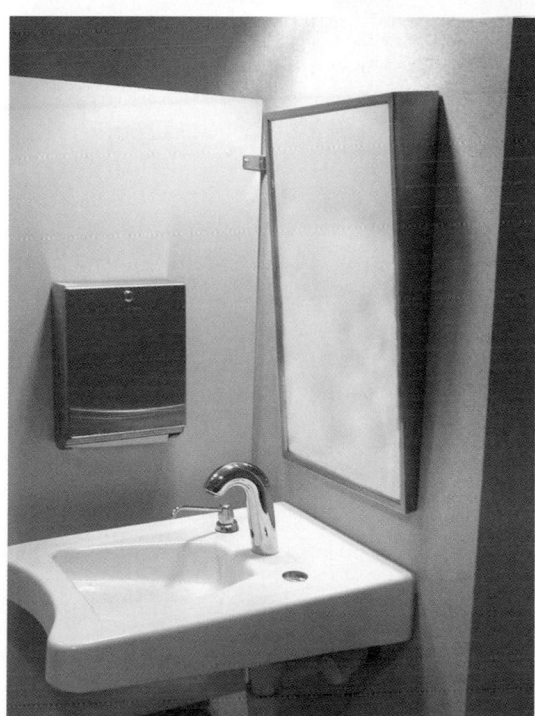

Figure 9.19 Over-sink mirror with top tilted away from wall to allow use from a seated position.

instant soups or cereals, minimizing the need for using the stove. Shallow sinks 5 to 6 in (128 to 153 mm) deep will improve knee clearance below. Providing sink access to an individual using a wheelchair may require removal of under-the-sink cabinets. As in the bathroom, hot water pipes under the kitchen sink should be insulated to prevent burns. Motorized adjustable sinks (Fig. 9.23) are mounted against a wall between two stationary cabinets with free space beneath. By activating the control switch, the sink height can be adjusted for the individual user whether seated in a wheelchair or standing.

3. A small cart with casters may be helpful to improve ease of moving articles from refrigerator to counter or table.

4. The height of tables also should be checked and the tables may have to be raised or lowered.

5. Equipment and food storage areas should be selected with optimum energy conservation in mind. All frequently used articles should be within easy reach, and unnecessary items should be eliminated. Additional storage space may be achieved by installation of open shelving or use of pegboards for pots and pans. If shelving is added, adjustable shelves are preferable and should be placed 16 in (410 mm) above the countertop.[88] Electronically powered storage cabinets are also available that automatically lower for countertop access (Fig. 9.24).

6. Electric stoves are generally preferable to open-flame gas burners. For optimum safety, controls should be located on the front or side border of the stove to eliminate the need for reaching across the burners. Burners that are placed beside each other provide a safer arrangement than those placed one behind the other. A heat-resistant burn-proof counter surface adjacent to the burners

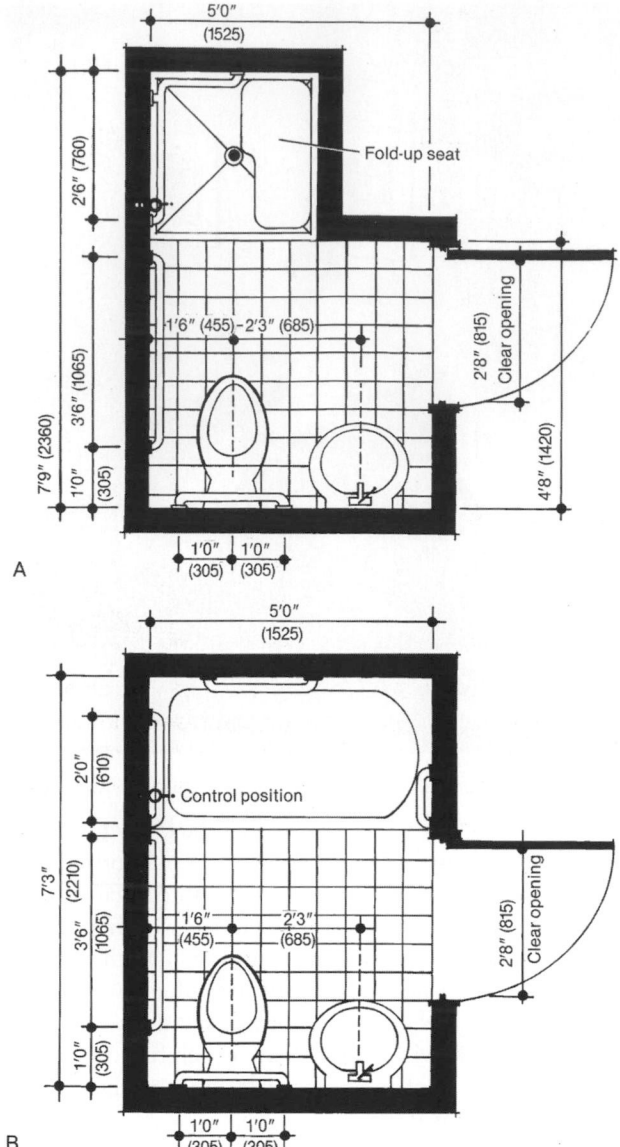

A

B

Figure 9.20 Minimum space requirements of a residential bathroom with **(A)** a shower stall and **(B)** a bathtub. The dotted line indicates lengths of wall that require reinforcement to receive grab bars or supports. *(From Nixon, V: Spinal Cord Injury: A Guide to Functional Outcomes in Physical Therapy Management. Aspen Systems Corporation, Rockville, MD, p 186, with permission.)*

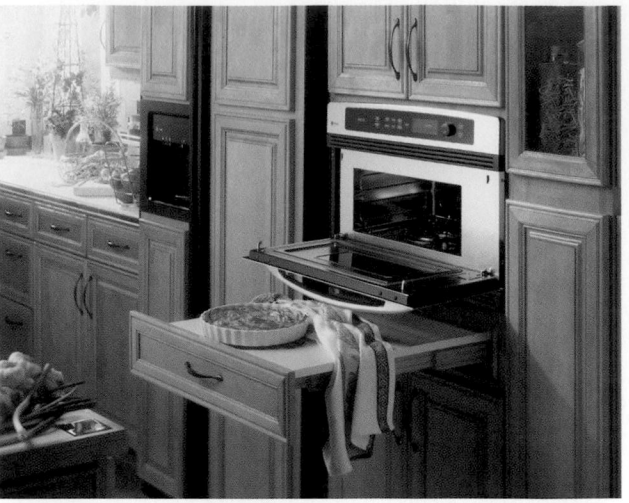

Figure 9.21 Slide-out counter spaces provide over-the-lap working surfaces. Positioned here below a built-in wall oven, the pullout surface allows for ease of transfer of hot dishes. *(Courtesy of General Electric, Appliance Park, Louisville, KY, 40225.)*

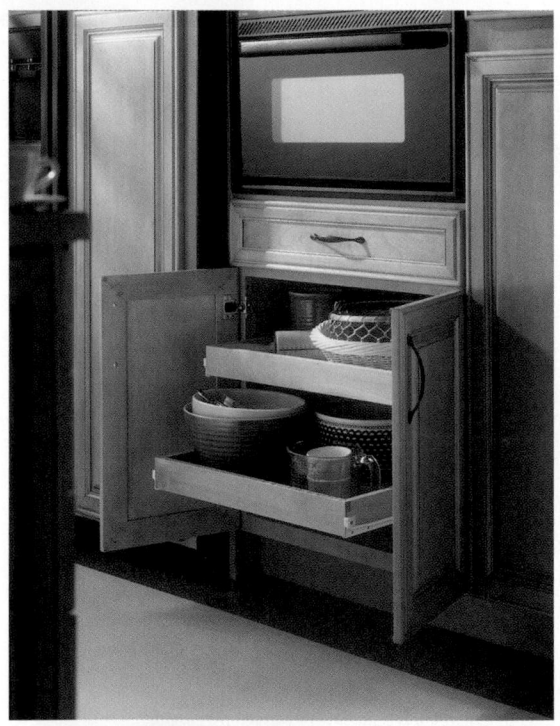

Figure 9.22 Glide-out under-cabinet shelves improve ability to see and access stored items. *(Courtesy of General Electric, Appliance Park, Louisville, KY, 40225.)*

will facilitate movement of hot items once cooking is completed. Smooth, ceramic cooktop surfaces also reduce the amount of lifting required while cooking (Fig. 9.25). If cooktops provide knee clearance beneath, exposed or potential contact surfaces must be insulated. Induction (electromagnetic) stoves are also available that heat food without flames or heating elements.

7. For patients with visual impairments, large-print label-making devices and large-print stencil overlays can be used to enlarge appliance control indicators and dials (e.g., on/off or temperature indicators on thermostats, microwaves, stoves, and ovens). Timers, wall clocks, and telephones with large-print numbers are also available.

8. Wall-mounted ovens (separate from the stove) should be placed 30 to 34 in (76 to 102 cm) from the floor with a side-opening door. These cooking units are generally more easily accessible than a

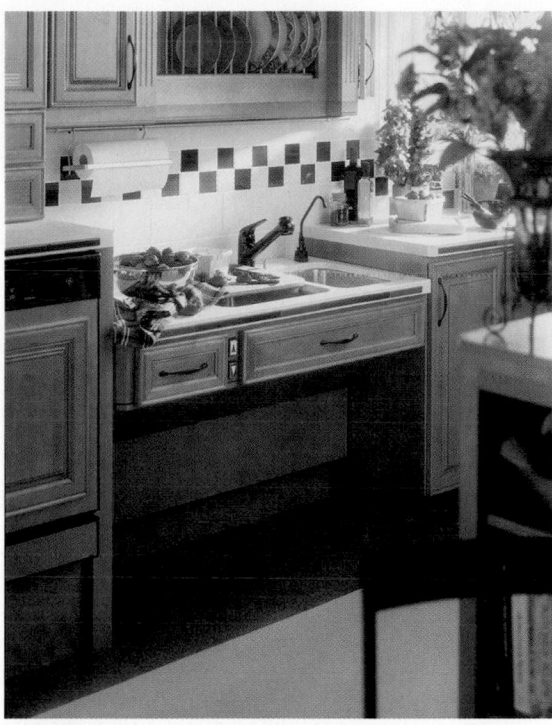

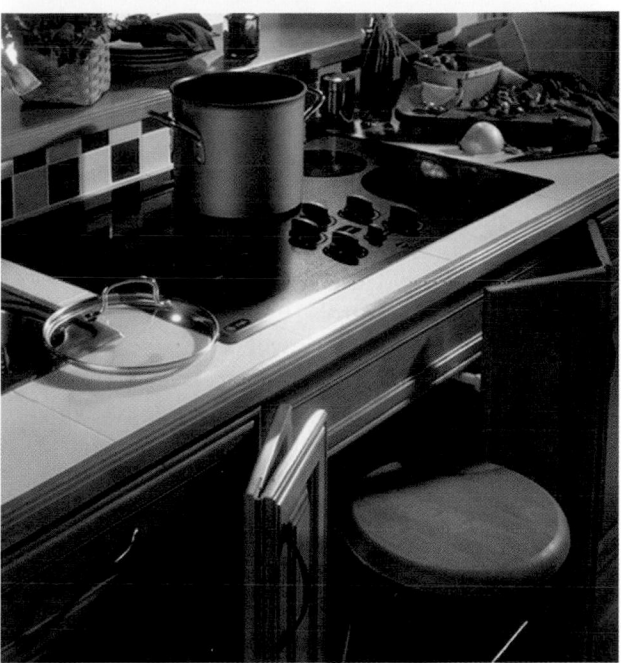

Figure 9.23 A motorized adjustable-height sink can be raised or lowered for comfortable use from either a seated or standing position. Height-adjustment controls are located on the anterior panel of the sink. *(Courtesy of General Electric, Appliance Park, Louisville, KY, 40225.)*

Figure 9.25 Cooktop with front-mounted controls and smooth surface that allows sliding (rather than lifting) from burner to heat-resistant countertop. Knee clearance beneath is accessed by folding doors. *(Courtesy of General Electric, Appliance Park, Louisville, KY, 40225.)*

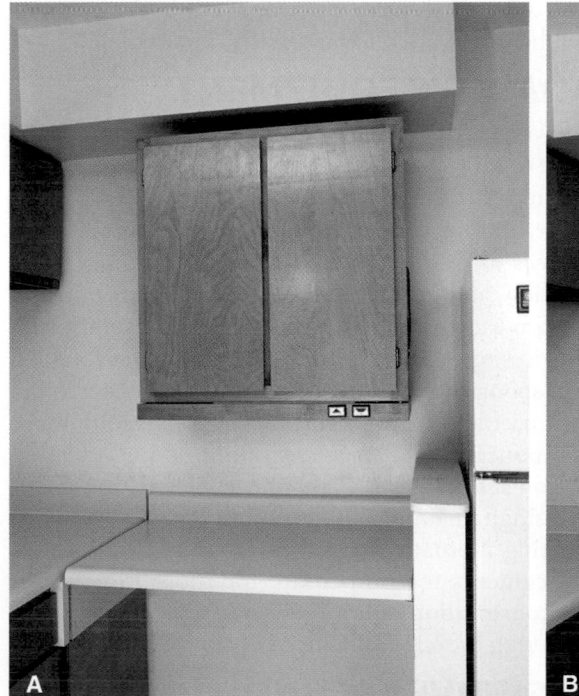

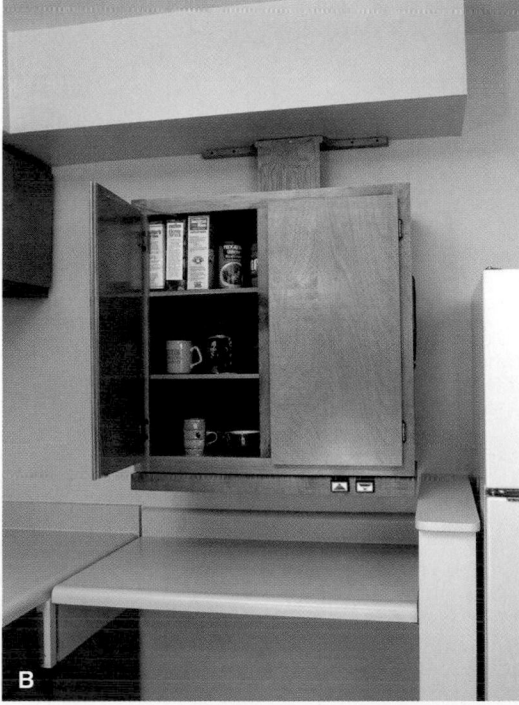

Figure 9.24 Motorized storage cabinets that can be lowered from the resting position to allow countertop access. Height-adjustment controls (*[A]* high and *[B]* low) are located on the right anterior panel of the cabinet. *(Courtesy of AD-AS, Boise, ID 83709.)*

single, low-level combined oven and burner unit. Oven units should be self-cleaning.

9. For many individuals, a countertop microwave oven is essential for food preparation.
10. Dishwashers should be elevated 9 in (228.6 mm) and be front-loading, with pullout shelves and front-mounted controls (Fig. 9.26). Elevated (9 in [228.6 mm]) side-by-side clothes washers and dryers should also be front-loading with front-mounted controls (Fig. 9.27).
11. Access to the refrigerator will be enhanced by use of a side-by-side (refrigerator-freezer) model.
12. A standard or remote control smoke and carbon monoxide detector and one or more, easily accessible, portable fire extinguishers should be available. It is generally recommended that fire extinguishers be mounted in open view near an exit and away from cooking appliances. For patients with hearing impairments, the smoke detector can be attached to a signaling system that activates both an audible and strobe light response to visually warn of danger. These signaling systems also can be used to activate flashing lights in response to a doorbell, knock on the door, telephone ring, or burglar alarm.

Although important for many patients, an examination of the home environment is often essential for older adults with specific areas of the home presenting greater hazards than others. Gitlin et al[89] addressed the types of difficulties older adults experience in their home. Data were collected from 296 participants (mean

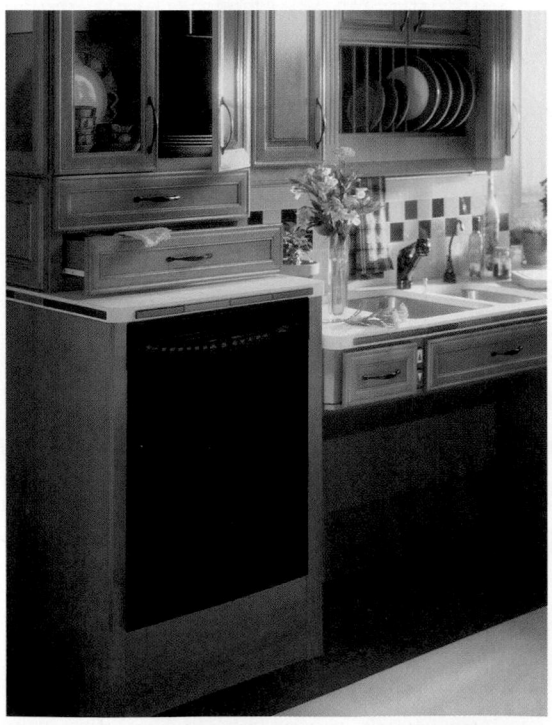

Figure 9.26 Front-loading dishwasher elevated 9 in (228.6 mm) with front-mounted controls. *(Courtesy of General Electric, Appliance Park, Louisville, KY, 40225.)*

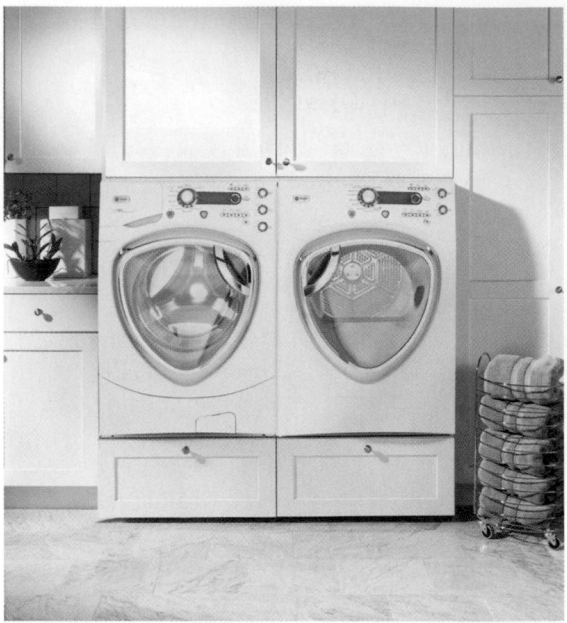

Figure 9.27 Front-loading clothes washer and dryer elevated 9 in (228.6 mm) with front-mounted controls. *(Courtesy of General Electric, Appliance Park, Louisville, KY, 40225.)*

age 73.24 years) using interviews, self-reports, clinical assessment, and direct observation of the home environment. The researchers focused on nine areas of the home: bathroom, kitchen, bedrooms, entry to home, dining/living/family room, outdoor spaces, common rooms, stairs, and the area from street to house. The areas where subjects encountered the greatest environmental difficulties were bathrooms (88%), kitchens (76%), bedrooms (61%), and entryways (58%).

■ ADAPTIVE EQUIPMENT

A large variety of **adaptive equipment** is commercially available to increase independence, speed, skill, and efficiency in performing activities of daily living (ADL). Adaptive equipment is available to assist performance in such areas as bathing, personal care, dressing, meal preparation, and general household tasks (e.g., built-up handles on eating utensils and personal care items, suction devices to stabilize bowls and dishes, long-handled reacher, sponge, duster, dustpan and brush, rocker knife, adapted cutting board). Typically, adaptive equipment is a component of a *compensatory training approach* that focuses on achieving the highest level of function possible by using remaining abilities. This approach involves considering alternative ways to accomplish a task, use of intact segments to compensate for those lost, use of energy conservation and joint preservation techniques, and adapting the environment to optimize performance.

■ ASSISTIVE TECHNOLOGY

In the Technology-Related Assistance for Individuals with Disabilities Act of 1988, assistive technology is defined as "any item, piece of equipment, or product system, whether acquired commercially off the shelf, modified, or customized, that is used to increase, maintain, or improve functional capabilities of individuals with disabilities."[90] Assistive technologies can be simple mechanical or mobility devices but the term usually denotes some type of electronic, computer (e.g., hardware, software, peripherals), tablet application, or microprocessor-based (e.g., prosthetic knee control) device.

Assistive technologies (ATs) enable individuals with disabilities to perform daily activities by compensating for lost or impaired function. They promote greater independence and typically improve quality of life by assisting in such areas as communication, education, environmental accessibility, and work or recreational activities. Three important considerations in determining the need for ATs are (1) the individual's available function, (2) the nature of the tasks or activities that will be performed, and (3) the environmental context in which it will be used.

An enormous variety of ATs are commercially available. Ideally, an interdisciplinary rehabilitation team is responsible for examination, evaluation, and prescription recommendation for specific items. Although influenced by the care setting, participating individuals typically include the patient, family member(s) and/or caregiver(s), physical and occupational therapists, a speech-language pathologist, and an assistive technology professional (see below). Depending on the needs of the patient, other contributors may include a special education teacher, seating specialist, rehabilitation technology supplier, augmentative communication specialist, and social worker or funding specialist. Box 9.2 provides an overview of the general categories of AT.

An assistive technology professional (ATP) or rehabilitation technology specialist is responsible for analyzing the AT needs of the patient. Through the systematic application of technology and engineering principles, this individual addresses the patient's needs in multiple contexts including, but not limited to, education, employment, independent living, transportation, and recreation/leisure activities. The ATP recommends and guides selection of appropriate assistive technology and educates the patient family/caregivers in use of the technology. The ATP or rehabilitation technology specialist may hold a degree in areas such as Assistive Technology Engineering, Assistive Technology and Human Services, Physical or Occupational Therapy, Engineering, Human Factors and Ergonomics, or other related field. In addition, they typically hold a certificate in assistive technology. Many such certification programs have developed across the country. An example of such a certification program is the Rehabilitation Engineering and Assistive Technology Society of North America's (RESNA's) Assistive Technology Professional (ATP) certification program.

Environmental control units (ECUs) are an important example of how ATs can enhance function and improve independence. ECUs are electronic interfaces that allow the user to control a variety of appliances and devices (e.g., telephones, bed controls, various components of an entertainment unit, room temperature and lighting, open and close curtains, open doors). These devices combine operation of all appliances into a central control panel, providing increased independence for individuals with severe disability.

The three main components of an ECU are (1) the input device, (2) the control unit, and (3) the appliance. The *input device* controls the ECU using whatever voluntary movement the individual has available (e.g., joystick, control panel, keypad, keyboard [ECU computer software programs are available], a series of switches, touch pads and screens, light pen, optical pointers, brain implants [e.g., patients with high-level spinal cord injuries] and voice, mouth-stick, and eye control). The *control unit* is the central processor that translates the input signal to an output signal to regulate the target appliance. The *appliance* can be virtually any device that can be controlled electronically.

■ EXAMINATION OF THE WORKPLACE

An investigation of the workplace is an important component of a comprehensive examination of the environment. It is used to explore the *worker–job–environment relationship* and to determine the feasibility of returning to a former job or if reasonable accommodations will provide the needed support to resume work. The tests and measures used by physical therapists to examine the workplace fall into two broad categories: (1) *ergonomics,* which is the application of scientific and engineering principles to the worker–job–environment relationship to improve safety, efficiency, and quality of movement; and (2) *body mechanics,* which is the interaction of muscles and joints in response to forces placed on or generated by the body.[3] Within the context of these two examination categories, Table 9.2 presents the tests and measures used by physical therapists together with the tools for gathering data, and the types of data generated.

Interview

An initial component of the workplace examination is a preliminary *job analysis interview.* The purpose of the interview is to gather information about (1) the functional requirements of the job based on a review of duties and responsibilities and (2) the characteristics of the physical space in which the individual is required to work (job analysis will continue during the on-site visit). Interview questions are developed based on the type of employment (e.g., assembly work, food service tasks, clerical work, motor vehicle operation, manual material handling, factory work, and so forth). During the interview, the patient/client should be encouraged to provide detailed information about responsibilities

---

Box 9.2 Categories of Assistive Technology

Aids for Daily Living

Aids or devices that enhance performance of ADL and level of independence in such activities as eating, meal preparation, dressing, personal hygiene, bathing, or household management. *Examples*: Grab bars, ramps, stairlifts, lowered counters, bathtub seats, adapted doorknobs, eating utensils, personal hygiene items, nonslip surface to stabilize dishes or other objects, and alternative doorbells.

Augmentative Communication

Devices used to enhance personal expressive and receptive communication. *Examples*: Communication enhancement devices (electronic), book holders, communication boards, eye gaze boards, electric page turners, head wands, mouth sticks, light pointers, reading machines, personal voice amplification, signal systems, and telephone adaptations.

Computer Applications

Hardware, software, and devices to enhance computer access. *Examples*: Modified, chording, expanded or alternate keyboards; voice recognition software; alternate workstations (electrically powered height and tilt adjustments); Braille translation software (conversion from print and Braille); Braille printers; access aids (head-control sticks, light pointers, eye gaze input); alternative switches (minimal pressure, voice activated) and cursor (mouse) control; voice synthesizers, large-print software that allows user to alter background and text colors (e.g., electronic books, magazines, and newspapers); magnification screens, touch screens, onscreen keyboard, screen reader; keyguards, forearm supports; text-to-speech software; speech-to-text software; optical character recognition (OCR) system that scans written text to a computer and is read by a speech synthesis/screen review system; and robotic wheelchair mounting to support a laptop computer.

Environmental Control Systems

Electronic systems that enhance ability to control various devices. *Examples*: Electronic control of appliances, lights, doors, and security systems in the home.

Hearing Technology

Devices designed to enhance receptive communication (assistive listening devices). *Examples*: Closed captioning, FM amplification systems (isolate and amplify a sound source), hearing aids, infrared amplification systems, personal amplification systems, TDDs/TTYs, television amplifiers, telephone adaptations, and visual and tactile alerting systems.

Mobility Technology

Devices designed to provide an alternative means for walking or moving within the environment. *Examples*: Manual or powered wheelchairs; powered scooters; vehicle modification (driving adaptations, hand controls, wheelchair lifts); stairlifts; bus lifts; kneeling buses; and ambulatory assistive devices.

Seating and Positioning

Wheelchair (or other seating system) interventions to improve postural alignment, stability, and head control and reduce skin pressure. *Examples*: Custom-fitted wheelchair (reclining back, elevating leg rests), tilt in space wheelchair, custom-molded seating surface, control blocks, pressure-relieving seat cushions, head and neck supports, adductor cushions, abductor pommel, lumbar supports, torso supports, and pelvic and foot positioners.

Vision Technology

Devices designed to enhance interaction with the environment for individuals with visual impairments. *Examples*: Talking devices (clocks, watches, calculators, thermometers, scales, handheld spell checkers, dictionaries, and thesauruses), magnifiers, speech output devices, large-print screens, mini pocket tape recorders, voice-activated daily planners, large-button phone, large-print books, magazines, and newspapers, audio books, and books on disc (can be loaded onto a computer and read to user with a voice synthesizer).

---

and tasks performed while on duty (e.g., duration of performance, weight and distance of items lifted, carried, or pulled, body positions used, and so forth). A sample of suggested job analysis interview questions appropriate for a clerical position is presented in Table 9.3.[91]

Job Analysis

A **job analysis** provides the basis for accommodating individuals with disabilities. It typically includes a job function statement that identifies the overall purpose as well as a description of (1) the essential functions

Table 9.2   Ergonomics and Body Mechanics: Tests and Measures, Tools Used for Gathering Data, and Data Generated

Ergonomics is the relationship among the worker; the work that is done; the actions, tasks, or activities inherent in that work (job/school/play); and the environment in which the work (job/school/play) is performed. Ergonomics uses scientific and engineering principles to improve safety, efficiency, and quality of movement involved in work (job/school/play). Body mechanics are the interrelationships of the muscles and joints as they maintain or adjust posture in response to forces placed on or generated by the body. The physical therapist uses these tests and measures in examining both the worker and the work (job/school/play) environment and in determining the potential for trauma or repetitive stress injuries from inappropriate workplace design. These tests and measures may be conducted after a work injury or as a preventive step. The physical therapist may conduct tests and measures as part of work hardening or work conditioning programs and may use the results of tests and measures to develop such programs.

Tests and Measures	Tools Used for Gathering Data	Data Generated
Tests and measures may include those that characterize or quantify: Ergonomics • Dexterity and coordination during work (job/school/play) (e.g., hand function tests, impairment rating scales, manipulative ability tests) • Functional capacity and performance during work actions, tasks, or activities (e.g., accelerometry, dynamometry, electroneuromyography, endurance tests, force platform tests, goniometry, interviews, observations, photographic assessments, physical capacity tests, postural loading analyses, technology-assisted assessments, videographic assessments, work analyses) • Safety in work environments (e.g., hazard identification checklists, job severity indexes, lifting standards, risk assessment scales, standards for exposure limits)	Tools for gathering data include: • Accelerometers • Cameras and photographs • Checklists for exposure standards, hazards, lifting standards • Dynamometers • Electroneuromyographs • Environmental tests • Force platforms • Functional capacity evaluations • Goniometers • Hand function tests • Indexes • Interviews • Muscle tests • Observations • Physical capacity and endurance tests • Postural loading tests • Questionnaires • Scales • Screenings • Technology-assisted analysis systems • Video cameras and videotapes • Work analyses	Data are used in providing documentation and may include: Ergonomics • Characterizations of efficiency and effectiveness of use of tools, devices, and workstations • Characterizations of environmental hazards, health risks, and safety risks • Descriptions of tools, devices, equipment, and workstations • Descriptions and quantification of: —Abnormal movement patterns associated with work actions, tasks, or activities —Dexterity and coordination —Functional capacity —Repetition and work/rest cycle in work actions, tasks, or activities —Work actions, tasks, or activities • Presence or absence of actual, potential, or repetitive trauma in the work environment
• Specific work conditions or activities (e.g., handling checklists, job simulations, lifting models, preemployment screenings, task analysis checklists, workstation checklists) • Tools, devices, equipment, and workstations related to work actions, tasks, or activities (e.g., observations, tool analysis checklists, vibration assessments)		Body mechanics • Characterizations of abnormal or unsafe body mechanics • Descriptions and quantifications of limitations in self-care, home management, work, community, and leisure actions, tasks, or activities

Continued

Table 9.2	Ergonomics and Body Mechanics: Tests and Measures, Tools Used for Gathering Data, and Data Generated—cont'd	
Tests and Measures	**Tools Used for Gathering Data**	**Data Generated**
Body mechanics • Body mechanics during self-care, home management, work, community, or leisure actions, tasks, or activities (e.g., activities of daily living [ADL] and instrumental activities of daily living [IADL] scales, observations, photographic assessments, technology-assisted assessments, videographic assessments)		

From American Physical Therapy Association,[3, pp. 70–71] with permission.

Table 9.3	Suggested Interview Questions Appropriate for a Clerical Position

Interview questions are used to gather general data about functional requirements of the job and the physical space in which the individual is required to work.

1. Y N   Do you frequently lift more than 35 pounds?
2. Y N   Are you required to lift objects from below knee level or above shoulder level on an occasional or frequent basis?
3. Y N   When you lift, do you reach across other objects or at arms' length in order to accomplish the lift?
4. Y N   Do you frequently reach for objects above shoulder level during the day?
5. Y N   Do you sit for more than 4 hours per day?
6. Y N   Does your job require you to maintain one position or posture for 30 to 60 minutes or longer at one time? If yes, what posture is it?_____
7. Y N   Are repetitive exertions required on a regular basis (e.g., typing)?
8. Y N   Does your job require frequent motions of the fingers, wrists, elbows, or shoulders? (If yes, circle all that apply.)
9. Y N   Do you feel that your desk height is at a comfortable level?
10. Y N   (a) Is your chair comfortable for you?
    Y N   (b) Do you feel that it fits you properly?
    Y N   (c) Do you know how to adjust your chair?
11. Y N   Is there ample space for you to perform your job?
12. Y N   Does your job involve frequent bending, twisting, or jerking movements?

From Hunter,[91, p. 68] with permission.

of a job and relative time spent on each; (2) the physical environment in which the essential functions are performed (e.g., indoors, outdoors, temperature fluctuations, noise levels); (3) the physical requirements (e.g., lifting, push/pull activities, bending, reaching); (4) the skills needed (cognitive processes, language, writing, or computer skills); and (5) the social context of the job (level of supervision, independent, contact with the public).

Job analyses provide a description of the job (not the potential employee). They are typically performed when a job is created to guide hiring of individuals with disabilities. (A sample job analysis form is presented in Appendix 9.E.) The physical therapist may also be called on to analyze a patient/client's current job following the onset of disability to make recommendations for reasonable accommodations.

Functional Capacity Evaluation (FCE)

Typically, the most effective means of examining the patient/client–work environment interface is an on-site visit. However, a variety of standardized functional capacity evaluation (FCE) instruments are commercially available that can be used to gather preliminary data before an on-site visit. The APTA defines FCE as "a comprehensive battery of performance-based tests that are commonly used to determine ability for work, activities of daily living, or leisure activities."[92] Depending on the job task requirements, the FCE may be all that is needed to determine ability to return to a previous job or to assume alternative job placement. The FCE provides a series of objective tests and measures designed to identify both work-related capabilities and activity limitations. Measurement parameters typically include endurance, ROM, flexibility, strength, force generation, posture, coordination, manual dexterity, and consistency of performance.[93-95]

The FCE is used to measure performance in specific components of work-related tasks. The specificity of the job will dictate the functional movements required. FCE instrument capabilities are then selected based on these requirements in order to examine the specific group of skills that comprise the employment tasks (e.g., lifting, stooping, trunk rotation, reaching). An example of an FCE instrument is the *Simulator II* functional testing system (Baltimore Therapeutic Equipment [BTE] Co., Hanover, MD 21076-3105). This computer-integrated system (Fig. 9.28) allows replication of physical task

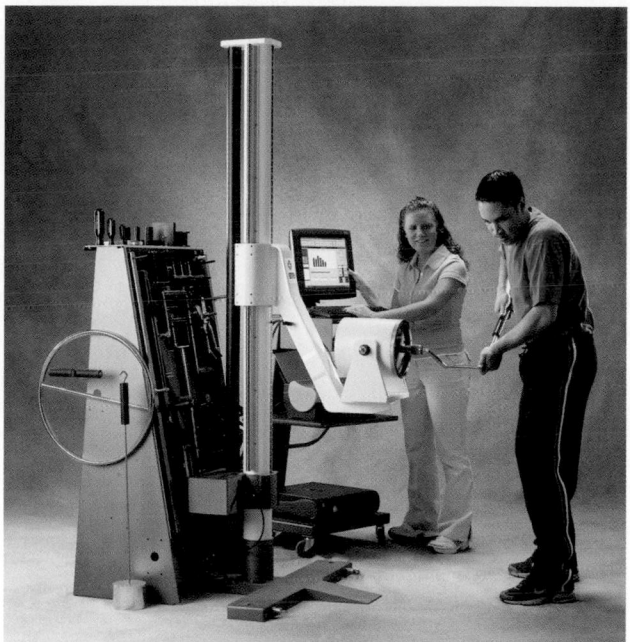

Figure 9.28 Simulator II Functional Capacity Evaluation System. *(Courtesy of BTE Technologies, Inc., Hanover, MD 21076.)*

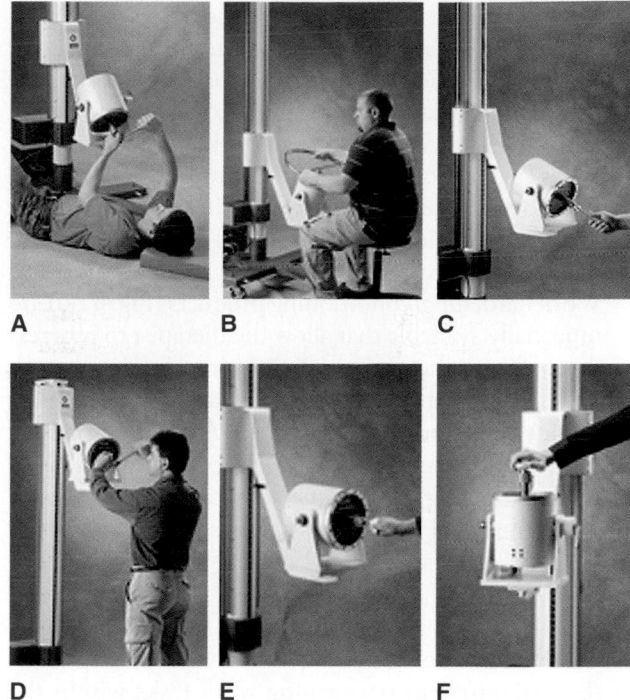

Figure 9.29 Examples of task simulations: (a) auto repair; (b) driving a bus; (c) using a screwdriver; (d) working overhead; (e) turning and (f) opening a jar. *(Courtesy of BTE Technologies, Inc., Hanover, MD 21076.)*

demands required of an individual's work environment using either standardized testing protocols or customized physical tests. A variety of tasks can be simulated, including, but not limited to, lifting, pushing, pulling, carrying capacity, turning a valve, and using a variety of tools (e.g., swinging a hammer, using a paint roller, using a manual saw). Additional examples are provided in Figure 9.29. This system may also be used for strengthening and retraining using task-specific strategies that simulate requirements of the client's real environment. Other examples of physical work capacity instruments include the *Joule Functional Capacity Evaluation System* (Valpar International Corporation, Tucson, AZ 85703-5767), the *Arcon Functional Capacity Evaluation System* (Arcon Vernova, Inc., Saline, MI 48176), the *ErgoMed Work Systems* (ErgoMed USA, San Antonio, TX 78269) and the *Isernhagen Work Systems Functional Capacity Evaluation* (WorkWell Systems, Inc., Aliso, CA 92656).

Software programs allow comparison of FCE data with normative values such as strength and ROM. Data from the FCE assist the physical therapist with the following tasks:

- Predicting the individual's work capacity and ability to safely return to work
- Identifying parameters of the physical environment needed to optimize function and prevent further injury (reasonable accommodations)
- Identifying extent of activity limitations (e.g., compensation process)
- Matching abilities to appropriate job placement
- Projecting potential benefits of a work hardening program

An additional resource is the *Occupational Information Network* (O*NET) available from the U.S. Department of Labor.[96] It provides a database of occupational job requirements (e.g., required skills and knowledge, how and where the work is performed) and worker attributes. The O*NET system includes the O*NET database (files available as free downloads for application development), O*NET OnLine (access to O*NET information), and the O*NET Career Exploration Tools (career investigation and assessment tools).

Work Hardening/Conditioning

Work hardening/conditioning refers to treatment interventions aimed at improving worker capabilities and function. The APTA defines work hardening/conditioning as "a work related, intensive, goal-oriented treatment program specifically designed to restore an individual's systemic, neuromusculoskeletal and cardiopulmonary functions. The objective of the work conditioning program is to restore the injured employee's physical capacity and function for return to work."[92]

Work hardening/conditioning programs typically involve progressive function-based exercise programs established from an analysis of work-related activities with careful attention to ergonomic and body mechanic principles. The anticipated goals and expected outcomes of work hardening programs are based on specific job requirements. Elements of the program may include (1) interventions to improve joint and soft tissue mobility, improve motor function, increase functional skill and coordination at work-related tasks, improve muscle performance (i.e., strength, power, endurance), ROM, flexibility, and cardiovascular/pulmonary status; (2) guided practice and instruction in simulated work activities (replication of physical demands); (3) education (e.g., body mechanics, safety and injury prevention, behavioral education programs); and (4) promotion of self-management strategies.[97-99]

Work hardening/conditioning products (Fig. 9.30) are commercially available that allow the therapist to progressively challenge the patient/client using simulated work activities such as lifting and moving tasks using objects of different shapes and weight (Fig. 9.31A) to and from different heights, assembly tasks (Fig. 9.31B), sorting tasks, shoveling, pushing and pulling activities, use of tabletop and wall-mounted workstations, and so forth.

On-Site Visit

The on-site visit to the workplace typically includes (1) further refinement of the job analysis by observation of the patient/client performing work tasks within the environment in which they must be accomplished and (2) application of ergonomic principles to identify the immediate or predicted risks of musculoskeletal injury for an individual worker. Data from the on-site visit will allow the therapist to establish a *plan for risk reduction* that provides recommendations to eliminate the potential for injury, and a *plan to optimize function* that may include suggestions for fitting the job to the patient/client's anatomical and physiological characteristics in a way that enhances efficiency and performance within the work environment and addresses fear avoidance beliefs.[100,101]

When examining level of function during an on-site visit to the work environment, the principles of energy

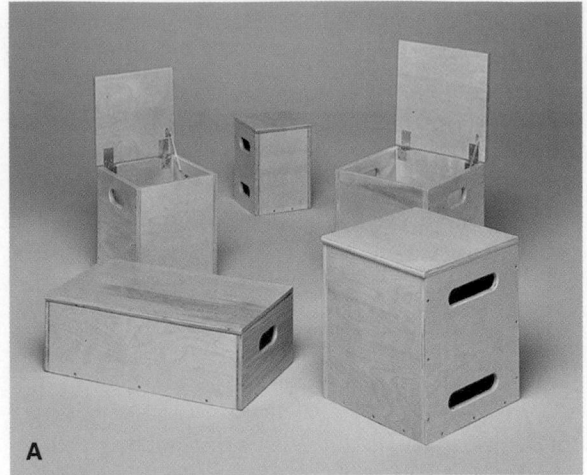

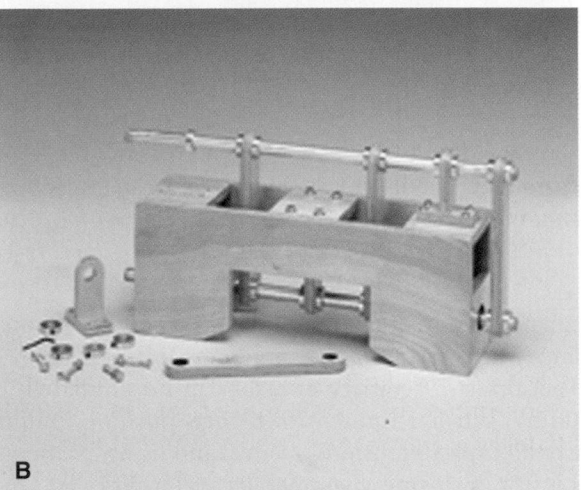

Figure 9.31 (A) Series of boxes of different shapes, sizes, and weights (progressively added) for lifting activities. **(B)** Tabletop unit includes bolts, washers, and nuts used for either manual or tool (e.g., use of a wrench) assembly. *(Courtesy of Bailey Mfg. Co., Lodi, OH 44254.)*

conservation, ergonomics, body mechanics, and anthropometrics are of prime importance in prevention of injury and maximizing the worker's efficiency and comfort. Capabilities should be weighed against the physical demands of the work environment, and the therapist, using knowledge of adaptive equipment and applied biomechanics, may suggest changes appropriate to the situation.

Many of the areas examined, recommendations made, and adaptive strategies employed in the home may be used in the work environment as well. Several considerations specific to the work setting are described below.

External Accessibility

A parking space should be available within a short distance of the building if the patient/client plans to drive to and from work. For wheelchair users, parking spaces should be a minimum of 96 in (2440 mm) wide, with an adjacent access aisle 60 in (1525 mm) wide. The location should be clearly marked as a reserved parking area.

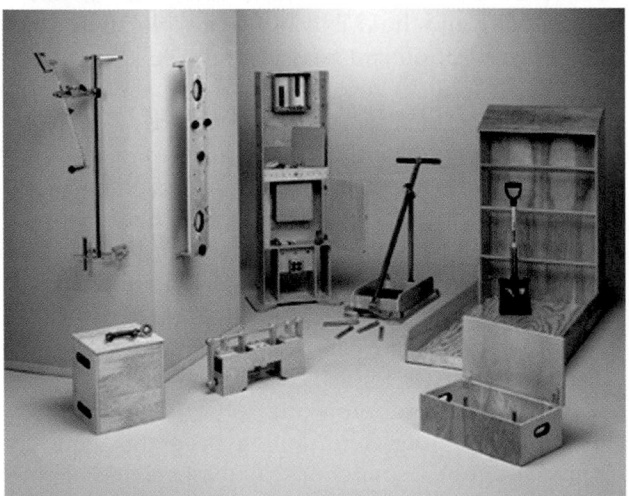

Figure 9.30 Work hardening equipment allows development of progressive therapeutic exercise (conditioning) programs based on simulation of a variety of tasks and assembly activities using sound ergonomic and body mechanic principles. *(Courtesy of Bailey Mfg. Co., Lodi, OH 44254.)*

External accessibility of the building should be addressed using guidelines similar to those presented for home exteriors.

Internal Accessibility

Initially, the component requirements of the work task are identified. The complexity of some tasks or the needed interface with the work environment may render the analysis of such tasks before the on-site visit inappropriate. This will include determination of mobility requirements (movement within and outside the primary work area), as well as determination of demands or skill required in each of the following areas: muscle performance (including strength, power, and endurance [trunk, upper versus lower extremities]), ROM, posture, manual dexterity, eye–hand coordination, vision, hearing, and communication.

The immediate work area should be carefully examined. This includes lighting; temperature; seating surface (if other than a wheelchair); the height and size of the workstation (some patients may benefit from a variable height or tilting work surface); and exposure to noise, vibration, or fumes. Access to supplies, materials, or equipment should be considered with respect to the patient's vertical and horizontal reaching capabilities. Access to public telephones, drinking fountains, and bathrooms should also be addressed.

Owing to the prevalence of computer workstations in many employment settings, therapists may be called on to make recommendations to optimize efficiency and reduce the potential for trauma or repetitive stress injury from poorly designed work areas. A fully adjustable chair is an integral component of an ergonomic workstation.[102] The foundational requirements for workstation chairs are depicted in Figure 9.32. Although individual client parameters may require variations, the general principles for positioning at a computer workstation include screen slightly below eye level, body centered directly in front of monitor and keyboard, forearms level or tilted slightly upward, wrists free while typing, lower back well-supported, thighs horizontal on seating surface, and feet resting flat on the floor (Fig. 9.33).[102]

During examination of workstations for individuals using a wheelchair, functional sitting reach is an important consideration. From an upright wheelchair sitting position, the unobstructed high forward reach is a maximum of 48 in (1,220 mm) from the floor and the low forward reach is a minimum of 15 in (380 mm) from the floor (Fig. 9.34A). When the high forward reach is over a work surface of not greater than 20 in (510 mm), the maximum reach distance is 48 in (1,220 mm) from the floor (Fig. 9.34B). Progressively deeper work surfaces will alter the forward reach accordingly. For example, a work surface depth between 20 and 25 in allows a maximum forward reach of not greater than 44 in (1,120 mm) (Fig. 9.34C). With a floor obstruction of 10 in (255 mm), the high side reach is a maximum of 48 in (1,220 mm) and a low side reach of 15 in (380 mm) minimum

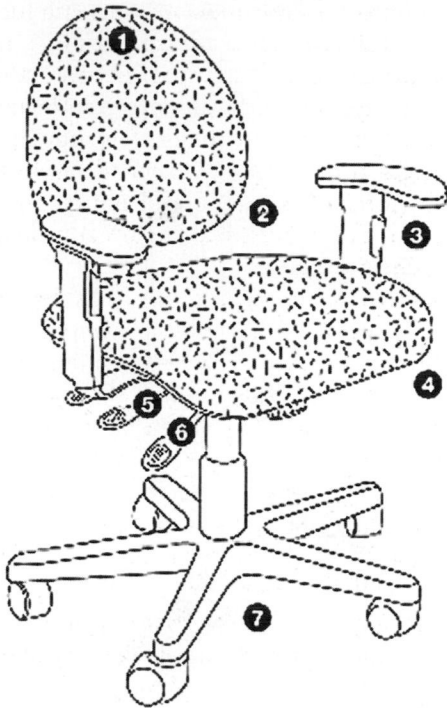

Figure 9.32 Overview of recommended features of workstation chair: (1) breathable, medium-texture upholstery; (2) adjustable lumbar support that moves up/down; (3) adjustable armrests; (4) seat with rounded front border (waterfall design); (5) adjustable seat that moves up and down and tilts forward and backward; (6) a tilt mechanism that tilts forward and backward; and (7) five-caster base with a full 360-degree swivel. *(From Workplace Ergonomics Reference Guide.[102, p. 4])*

(Fig. 9. 34D). With an obstruction of a maximum of 24 in (610 mm), the high side reach is a maximum of 46 in (1,170 mm).[5] For individuals with good trunk control, reaching capacity will be increased.

Detailed resources are available to guide examination of the workplace. These include the *Americans with Disabilities Act (ADA) Regulations and Technical Assistance Materials*,[103] the *ADA Accessibility Guidelines for Buildings and Facilities* (ADAAG),[104] and the *2010 ADA Standard for Accessible Design*.[5] These documents are freely available and include the technical requirements for accessibility to buildings and facilities by individuals with disabilities under the Americans with Disabilities Act of 1990. A comprehensive source of information about the ADA is provided at the U.S. Department of Justice's *ADA Home Page*.[105]

■ COMMUNITY ACCESS

To attain the goal of full accessibility, the viability of community resources, services, and facilities must be investigated. When direct involvement by the therapist is not possible, this may best be accomplished by providing the patient and family/caregivers with guidelines for exploring access to local facilities.

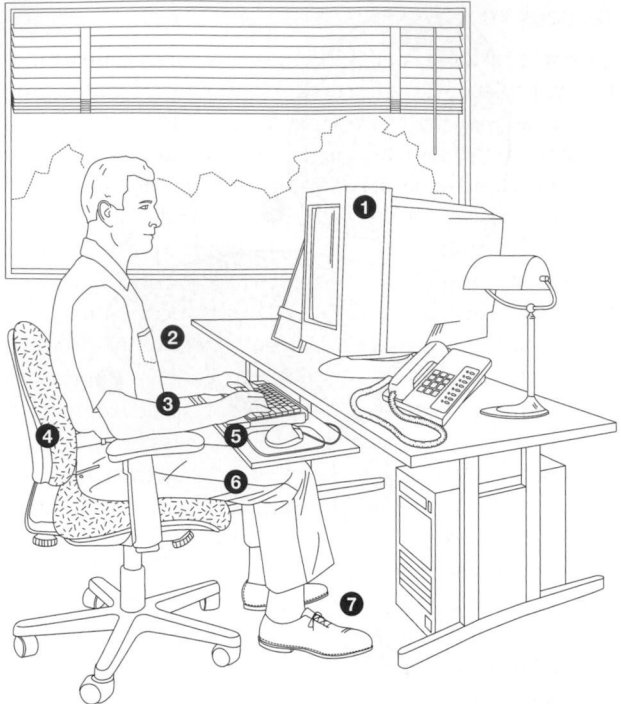

Figure 9.33 Overview of positioning recommendations for computer workstations: (1) monitor screen top slightly below eye level; (2) body centered in from of the monitor and keyboard; (3) forearms level or tilted-up slightly; (4) lower back supported by chair; (5) wrists free while typing; (6) thighs horizontal; and (7) feet resting flat on the floor. *(From Workplace Ergonomics Reference Guide.[102, p. 2])*

groups can provide information on services available to individuals with a disability who reside in the community. Individuals who are returning to school should be encouraged to contact the campus student services office, which addresses the needs of students with disabilities. Information will be offered on housing, special services, and general campus resources.

Transportation

Currently the availability of accessible public transportation varies considerably among geographical areas. As such, careful exploration by the patient, family, and/or caregivers will be needed to determine what resources are obtainable in specific locales. Many communities provide at least part-time service of partially or completely accessible buses. These include the so-called "kneeling buses" equipped with a hydraulic unit that lowers the entrance to curb level for easier boarding (Fig. 9.35). Many buses are now designed with hydraulic lifts to allow direct entry by an individual using a wheelchair (Fig. 9.36).

Not all public transportation systems in the United States allow use by individuals who are nonambulatory or by those with limited ambulatory capacity. However, many urban transit systems are gradually making accommodations for individuals with mobility impairments (e.g., installation of elevators, alternatives to turnstile entrances, identified space for wheelchair riders). In many areas where public transportation is unavailable, door-to-door accessible van transportation is provided to residents with disabilities. Again, availability of such services may be limited in some rural locations.

Some patients will want to master driving an adapted automobile or van. This, of course, will improve opportunities for community travel significantly. Motor vehicle adaptations are selected based on the physical capabilities

Another important consideration is to refer the patient, family, and/or caregivers to community organizations such as the Arthritis Foundation, National Easter Seal Society, Multiple Sclerosis Society, the Mayor's Office, Chamber of Commerce, or the Veterans Administration. These

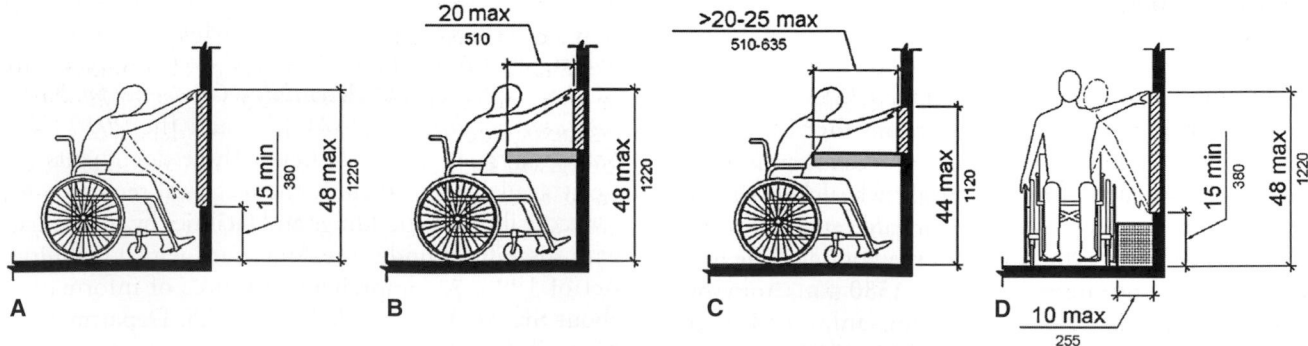

Figure 9.34 (a) Unobstructed high forward reach is a maximum of 48 in (1,220 mm) from the floor and the low forward reach is a minimum of 15 in (380 mm) from the floor. (b) High forward reach over a 20-inch-deep (510-mm-deep) work surface is a maximum of 48 in (1,220 mm) from the floor. (c) A work surface depth of 20 to 25 in (510 to 635 mm) allows a maximum forward reach of not greater than 44 in (1,120 mm) from the floor. (d) For a reach depth of 10 in (255 mm), the high side reach is a maximum of 48 in (1,220 mm). With a floor obstruction of 10 in (225 mm), the high side reach is a maximum of 48 in (1,220 mm) and a low reach of 15 in (380 mm) minimum. Values denoted in inches and millimeters. *(From 2010 ADA Standards for Accessible Design.[5, pp. 114-115])*

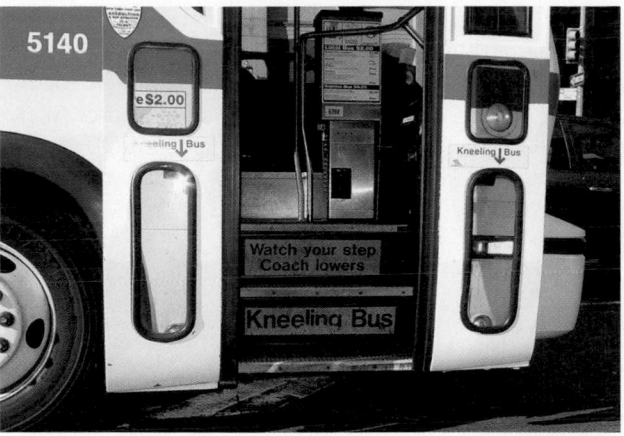

Figure 9.35 A kneeling bus lowers the steps to within 3 to 6 in of the curb. Buses designed to kneel typically display a sign (Kneeling ↓ Bus) either on or next to the door.

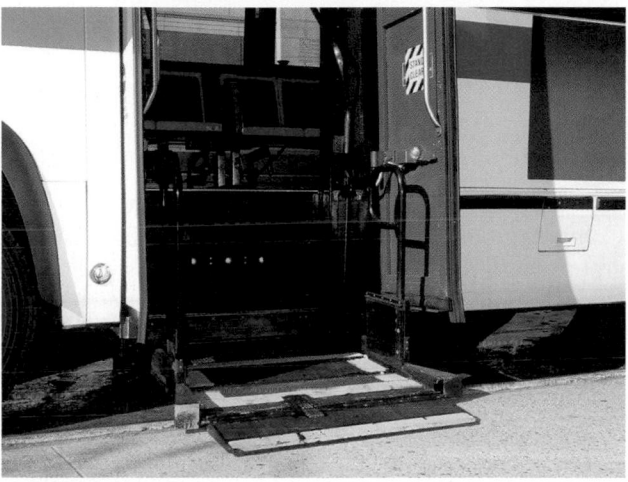

Figure 9.36 Bus lifts are able to accommodate wheelchairs and motorized scooters. The international wheelchair symbol for accessibility is typically displayed on the doors of the bus.

of the individual. Common adaptive equipment includes hand controls to operate the brakes and the accelerator; control panels mounted directly on steering wheel to control windshield wipers, turn indicators, and high/low beams; steering wheel attachments, such as knobs or universal cuffs, for individuals with limited grip strength; lifting units to assist with placement of the wheelchair into the vehicle; and, for patients with tetraplegia or high-level paraplegia, self-contained lifting platforms for entry to a van while remaining seated in a wheelchair. Driver training programs are taught by occupational therapists and offered in most large rehabilitation centers.

For patients whose capacity for long-distance ambulation is limited and/or whose endurance is low, community-going battery-powered scooters (Fig. 9.37) may be a practical alternative for travel within a reasonable proximity of the home.

Access to Community Facilities

Several considerations incorporated into examination of the workplace warrant attention for general community access, as well. Briefly stated, area facilities used by the patient should be explored for the availability of appropriate parking areas; beveled curbs; external and internal structural accessibility of buildings; and availability of accessible public telephones, drinking fountains, bathrooms, and restaurants. Theaters, auditoriums, and lecture halls must be considered with respect to accessible seating areas. Many such public presentation spaces are now designed with an accessible isle leading to open floor space interspersed within a row of standard seats to accommodate a wheelchair. This allows the individual using a wheelchair the option of either sitting next to a person who is ambulatory or someone using a wheelchair. Locations of emergency exits should also be noted for all facilities. In addition to these general considerations, stores and shopping areas should also be inspected for access to merchandise (especially for individuals using a wheelchair), appropriate aisle widths, and adequate space at checkout counters.

Some theater companies offer "touch tours" for individuals who are blind or have impaired vision, allowing them to learn about the visual elements of the production. These multisensory experiences supplement for the lack of detail provided by a live performance and are led by cast, crew, and/or management. They provide an opportunity for participants to touch and handle theatre pieces while tour guides explain the significance of individual pieces.[106]

Another useful source of information on community access is the guidebook offered by many larger cities (often funded by the Mayor's Office or as a community service by local businesses). These guides provide information on accessibility of local cultural, civic, and religious institutions; government offices; theaters; hotels; restaurants; shopping areas; transportation; and social and recreational facilities. These publications usually can be obtained from the city's chamber of commerce, the mayor's office, or the office of tourism. Combined use of such guides and phoning ahead for details of accessibility will facilitate travel both within and outside the local community. Many of these guides are available online (e.g., Accessible NYC!![107] and the Disability Guide for Washington, DC[108]).

■ DOCUMENTATION

Once examination of the environment is complete, a final collaborative report is prepared that includes information from each participating team member. This report consists of information obtained from the home and, if applicable, the workplace or school setting. Information should also be included about the measures taken to explore general community accessibility.

Additional information that should be provided includes (1) a description of the methods used to assist the patient in ambulation or functional activities,

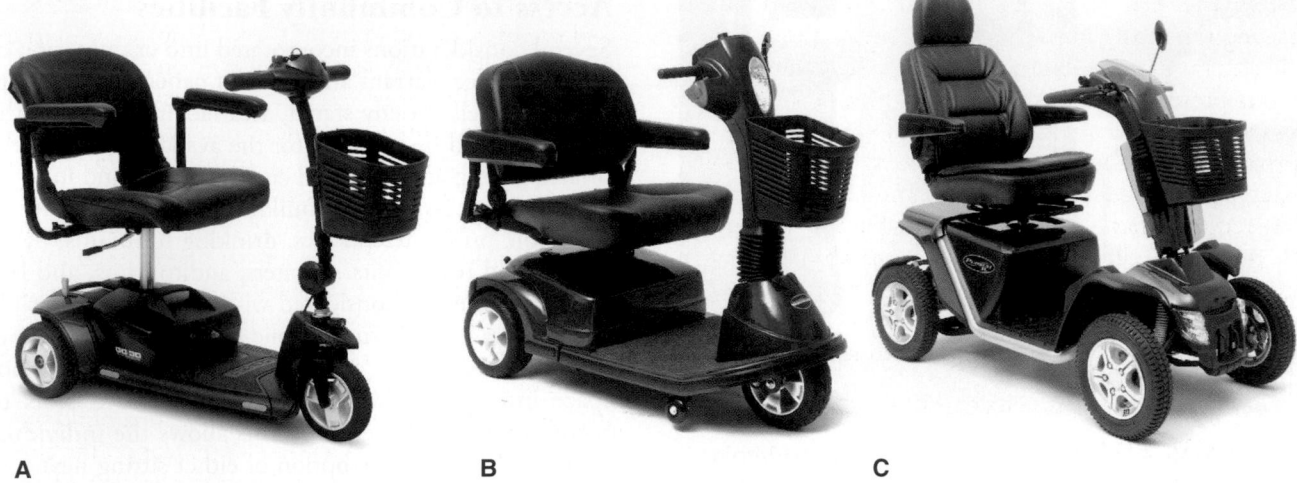

A   **B**   **C**

Figure 9.37 Examples of motorized scooters suitable for outdoor travel. **(A)** This lightweight scooter has a weight capacity of 275 lb (124.74 kg), a maximum speed of 4.25 miles per hour (MPH), and a turning radius of 35.5 in (90.17 cm). **(B)** This model includes a heavy-duty drivetrain with a weight capacity of 500 lb (226.8 kg), a maximum speed of 5.25 MPH, with a turning radius of 50.38 in (127.96 cm). **(C)** This unit features a reclining back with headrest, large pneumatic tires, a weight capacity of 400 lb (181.44 kg), a maximum speed of 8.25 MPH, with a turning radius of 82.5 in (209.55 cm). *(Courtesy of Pride Mobility Products, Exeter, PA, 18643.)*

(2) identification of the type and quantity of adaptive equipment required (including source and cost), (3) AT recommendations, and (4) suggested environmental modifications with precise specifications. If an examination form, survey, or checklist was used during the on-site visit, it should be included with documentation or the data summarized in narrative form.

Documentation related to community access should include verification of the patient's knowledge of available community resources. The sources of this information, as well as whether the therapist was directly or indirectly involved in the community investigation, should be reported.

The completed report is then included as part of the patient's medical record. Copies of the report are typically submitted to the patient's family/caregivers, the physician, third-party payer(s) or other potential funding sources, and any community-based health care or social service agencies that will be providing care.

■ FUNDING FOR ENVIRONMENTAL MODIFICATIONS

The patient and family/caregivers may require assistance in locating appropriate financial resources to achieve environmental accessibility. Typically, the social worker within the patient care facility will provide direction in this area. Information on resource organizations can also be obtained from the National Council on Disabilities. Potential sources of funding include private medical insurance companies, home equity or other types of bank loans, Veterans Administration, the Division of Vocational Rehabilitation (DVR), the Workers' Compensation Commission, and local chapters of national groups (e.g., Kiwanis International, Veterans of Foreign Wars, Masons/Shriners Lodges, and Lions International) or diagnosis-specific organizations (e.g., National Stroke Association, National Multiple Sclerosis Society, National Parkinson Foundation).

An important consideration is that not all patients will have current housing that is amenable to modification (e.g., an individual who previously lived in a third-floor walk-up apartment and now uses a wheelchair). In such instances, the local Housing and Urban Development (HUD) office will be an important resource. This office can provide a listing of accessible housing within the community. Because there are often waiting lists for such dwellings, early application is warranted.

Finally, creative funding for specific items (such as specialized adaptive equipment not covered by other resources) may be available through private organizations or foundations. Considerable time, research, and perseverance may be required in locating a receptive organization. General suggestions the patient, family, and/or caregiver(s) might consider in seeking assistance include contacting local businesses or corporate giving offices, civic or service clubs, churches or synagogues, labor unions, Jaycees, and the Knights of Columbus.

■ LEGISLATION

Much attention has been focused on the importance of environmental accessibility. Through legislation and a variety of private organizations, significant strides have been made in this area. In 1990 the *Americans with*

Disabilities Act was signed into law. This legislation is among the most comprehensive of the civil rights laws enacted for individuals with disabilities. It guarantees civil rights protection and equal opportunity in the areas of government services, employment, public transportation, privately owned transportation available to the public, telephone service, and public accommodations.[109] This law requires that all "public places of accommodation" be made accessible to people with a disability unless it imposes "undue hardship" to the establishment. This law specifies that restaurants, movie theaters, hotels, professional offices, retail stores, and so forth make reasonable accommodations.

With respect to an individual, disability is defined in the ADA as "a physical or mental impairment that substantially limits one or more major life activities of such an individual; a record of such impairment; or being regarded as having such impairment."[109, p. 4] Undue hardship includes excessive direct cost of adapting the environment, limited resources of the establishment, or situations where these changes would fundamentally alter the nature or daily operation of a business. The ADA also provides a federal tax credit incentive for measures taken by businesses to comply with this law.

The *Fair Housing Amendment Act of 1988* prohibits discrimination in housing on the basis of race, color, religion, gender, disability, familial status, and national origin. The Act includes private housing, state and local government housing, and any housing that receives federal financial support. The Act requires that accessible units be included in all new multiple-dwelling buildings with four or more units. It requires landlords to allow individuals with disabilities to make reasonable, access-related modifications to their living space, as well as common areas of the building. However, the landlord is not required to pay for these modifications. To promote adherence, the Fair Housing Amendment Act also provides accessible construction standards for multifamily housing units built for first occupancy after March 1991.

The *Rehabilitation Act of 1973* provided that access must be established in all federally funded buildings and transportation facilities constructed after 1968. The law prohibits discrimination in federal employment, stipulates accessibility within federal buildings, and established the Architectural Transportation Barriers and Compliance Board. Because many federally funded institutions provided low compliance with the 1973 Rehabilitation Act, an amendment was passed in 1978. The Comprehensive Rehabilitation Services Amendments (P.L. 95-602) of 1978 strengthened the enforcement of the original 1973 Rehabilitation Act. The Architectural and Transportation Barriers Compliance Board is the governing body responsible for enforcing this legislation.

The *Architectural Barrier Act of 1968* (P.L. 90-480) provided that certain buildings that were financed by federal funds be designed and constructed "to insure that physically handicapped persons will have ready access to, and use of, such buildings."[110, p. 719] Another important item of legislation related to environmental accessibility is the Public Buildings Act of 1983, which functioned to establish public building policies for the federal government. This Act (section 307) provided several amendments to the Architectural Barrier Act of 1968 to further strengthen and delineate the importance of accessibility. The term *fully accessible* in this Act was defined as "the absence or elimination of physical and communications barriers to the ingress, egress, movement within, and use of a building by handicapped persons and the incorporation of such equipment as is necessary to provide such ingress, egress, movement, and use and, in a building of historic, architectural, or cultural significance, the elimination of such barriers and the incorporation of such equipment in such a manner as to be compatible with the significant architectural features of the building to the maximum extent possible."[111, p. 373]

The *Telecommunications Act of 1996* applies to all telecommunication equipment and services. It stipulates that manufacturers of "telecommunications equipment or customer premises equipment shall ensure that the equipment is designed, developed, and fabricated to be accessible to and usable by individuals with disabilities, if readily achievable."[112, p. s.652-20] The Act also provides a similar accessibility directive to providers of telecommunications services.

Despite the recent gains made in architectural accessibility, barriers continue to exist. Inasmuch as most public transportation systems were built before 1968, accessibility is not required by law. However, the ADA indicates that all concerns that offer public transit along a fixed route must also provide buses that are accessible to individuals with disabilities, including access by wheelchairs. Other areas that continue to be problematic include revolving doors, the design of many supermarkets and shopping areas (barriers imposed by checkout areas and items displayed on high shelves), lack of available parking spaces, multiple levels of stairs at the entrance to some buildings, and the design of some theaters and auditoriums that do not have specifically designated areas for individuals using a wheelchair.

The ADA homepage (www.ada.gov) provides an extensive listing of links to available ADA publications, as well as links to federal resources.

Although increasing numbers of buildings are being designed to provide accessibility, this area warrants further involvement from therapists. Physical therapists can be effective advocates and are equipped to provide a leadership role in compliance with existing and new laws. They have important knowledge and skills to enable them to provide valuable input into the initial planning and/or modification of barrier-free designs. Appendix 9.F provides Web based accessibility resources for clinicians, patients, and families.

SUMMARY ▌

Examination of the environment is an important factor in facilitating the patient's transition to the home, work, and community. The rehabilitation team uses the data to determine the level of patient access, safety, and function within the environment. The information is also used to determine the need for additional treatment interventions, ATs, environmental modifications, outpatient services, and adaptive equipment. In addition, the examination assists in preparing the patient, family, caregivers, and/or work colleagues and employer for the individual's return to a given setting.

This chapter has presented a sample approach to examination of the environment. Common environmental features that typically warrant consideration have been highlighted. Inasmuch as a return to a former environment is often a primary goal of rehabilitation, early consideration of these issues is warranted. Collaboration among team members, the patient, and the patient's family and/or caregivers will ensure an optimum and highly individualized patient–environment interface.

Questions for Review

1. Explain the concept of universal design.

2. What are the purposes for performing an examination of the environment?

3. What data collection tools are used for examination of the environment?

4. Identify an inherent shortcoming of self-report instruments. How can accuracy of reporting be improved?

5. Before an on-site visit to a patient's home, what preliminary information is needed?

6. What specific aspects of the exterior of a patient's home should be examined during an on-site visit? Your response should address the *route of entry* to the home and actual *entrance* to home and include suggestions for potential access problems.

7. During a home visit, you find that a wheelchair user's bathroom door width measures 31 in wide (77.74 cm). The patient owns the 50-year-old home and plans to remain in the dwelling. What options are available to increase the bathroom door width?

8. What is included in a job analysis?

9. What is a functional capacity evaluation (FCE)? How are data from the FCE used (i.e., what decisions are informed by the data)?

10. What is work hardening/conditioning? Describe the elements included in a work hardening/conditioning program.

CASE STUDY

A 78-year-old woman with a diagnosis of osteoarthritis was admitted for a right total hip replacement. The patient reported a long-standing history of discomfort. She described the hip pain as radiating posteriorly to the buttock and low back and was exacerbated by weightbearing and stair climbing. Over the past 12 months she has experienced a very marked increase in pain and stiffness. Radiographic findings demonstrated degenerative changes of both the acetabulum and femoral head consistent with osteoarthritis. The surgical intervention replaced the right femoral head and neck with a metallic prosthesis and the acetabulum was resurfaced with a plastic cup. Past medical history is unremarkable.

SOCIAL HISTORY

The patient is a retired manager of a small accounting firm that she and her husband established. Her husband is deceased. She has three grown children who all live in neighboring communities. Before the activity limitations imposed by the hip pain, the patient had been independent in all BADL and IADL. She also volunteered her accounting services one day per week to a local charity that provides meals to homebound individuals. She was a regular participant in family outings; enjoyed going to the theater, concerts, and special museum events; and was an active member of the community historical preservation society. Recently, these activities had to be curtailed owing to the increased hip discomfort.

She essentially had no activities outside the home for 3 months before admission and used a walker to minimize weight-bearing and reduce pain. She also required the assistance of a home care aide 4 hours a day two times per week (primarily for shopping, errands, and some household management tasks). She expressed considerable distress at being unable to take a bath and having to rely on the assistance of another person for some basic care activities. She had been using aspirin for its analgesic and anti-inflammatory effects. However, the pain experienced in recent months was not alleviated by the aspirin and other conservative measures she has been instructed to use (e.g., local applications of heat, periodic rest intervals, and gentle ROM exercises). The patient has medical insurance coverage and is without financial concerns.

REVIEW OF SYSTEMS

Cognitive function: Intact.

Vision: Wears corrective lens; experiences night blindness, which she describes as seeing poorly in dim light and her eyes take several seconds longer than normal to adjust from brightness to dimness.

Hearing: Intact.

Strength—upper extremities:
- Generally within functional limits; patient reports some sporadic episodes of wrist and finger stiffness on awakening in the morning and after periods of immobility.
- Grip strength is reduced bilaterally (manual muscle testing [MMT] of finger flexors = G–).
- Heberden's nodes noted at the distal interphalangeal (DIP) and proximal interphalangeal (PIP) joints of the left index finger. Patient denies pain in wrist or fingers.

Strength—lower extremities:
- Left: within functional limits.
- Right: within functional limits (hip motions not tested owing to surgical intervention); crepitus noted in right knee.
- Weight-bearing status on right lower extremity: partial weight-bearing

Range of motion: Within functional limits (with the exception of the right hip, which was not tested).

Postsurgical right hip precautions: No hip flexion beyond 90°. Avoid crossing one leg or ankle over the other. Avoid internal rotation of right lower extremity.

Coordination: Within normal limits.

Sensation: Intact.

Gait: The patient is ambulating on level surfaces with supervision using bilateral standard aluminum axillary crutches with partial weight-bearing on the right lower extremity. Stair climbing also requires minimal assistance. It is anticipated the patient will be independent with household ambulation on level surfaces at time of discharge from the hospital.

PATIENT GOALS

The patient is extremely motivated to be independent in her personal care and household management. The prosthetic replacement has successfully relieved much of the pain experienced in the hip before surgery (most of her current discomfort is described as "minor" and associated with the surgical incision). She would also like to return to her family, volunteer, social, and leisure activities. She is very determined to discontinue the home care assistance as soon as possible.

HOME ENVIRONMENT

The patient lives alone in a fifth floor apartment in a building with an elevator. The living space is a one-bedroom apartment on a single level. At your request, one of the patient's children has provided dimensions of doorframes and height of sleeping and seating surfaces together with several photographs of each room of the patient's home. The physical dimensions and photographs indicate the following:
- Bedroom: two small area rugs, a nightstand with an alarm clock, a bureau, an old wooden four-poster bed in the middle of room with a sleeping surface 1.5 ft from the floor, and a ceiling lamp fixture controlled by a switch adjacent to the door.
- Bathroom: an area rug, standard toilet and sink, bathtub does not include a shower, a doorway entrance 30 in wide.
- Kitchen: polished linoleum floors, adequate counter space, and a dining table in the center of the room with standard kitchen chairs.
- Living room: overstuffed upholstered furniture with low seating surfaces, a favorite rocking chair, a large carpet that appears to ripple in several areas, a centered coffee table, a telephone with an extra-long extension wire placed on the coffee table, a remote controlled television, two end tables, and a bookcase.
- Hallway (between rooms): poorly lit with a long, narrow area rug.

GUIDING QUESTIONS

With general knowledge of the patient's living space, what environmental modifications, adaptive equipment, or additional instruction would you suggest or provide to optimize safety and function in each of the following areas of the home?

1. Bedroom
2. Bathroom
3. Kitchen
4. Living room
5. Hallway

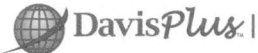 For additional resources, including answers to the questions for review and case study guiding questions, please visit **http://davisplus.fadavis.com**

References

1. Corcoran, M, and Gitlin, L: The role of the physical environment in occupational performance. In Christiansen, CH, and Baum, CM (eds): Occupational Therapy Enabling Function and Well-Being, ed 2. Slack, Thorofare, NJ, 1997, p 336.
2. Lawton, MP, et al: Assessing environments for older people with chronic illness. J Ment Health Aging 3:83, 1997.
3. American Physical Therapy Association (APTA): Guide to Physical Therapist Practice, ed 2. APTA, Alexandria, Virginia, 2003.
4. American National Standards Institute: American National Standard: Accessible and Usable Buildings and Facilities (ICC A117. 1-2009). International Code Council, Inc, Falls Church, VA, 2009.
5. Department of Justice (DOJ): 2010 ADA Standards for Accessible Design. US DOJ, Washington, DC, 20301. Retrieved April 14, 2012, from www.ada.gov/regs2010/2010ADAStandards/2010ADAStandards.pdf.
6. Mace, R: What Is Universal Design? RL Mace Universal Design Institute, Chapel Hill, NC, 2012, p 1. Retrieved April 18, 2012, from www.udinstitute.org/whatisud.php.
7. Joines, S: Enhancing quality of life through universal design. NeuroRehabilitation 25(3):155, 2009.
8. Steinfeld, E, and Maisel, J: Universal Design: Designing Inclusive Environments. John Wiley & Sons, Hoboken, NJ, 2012.
9. Crews, DE, and Zavotka, S: Aging, disability, and frailty: Implications for universal design. J Physiol Anthropol 25:113, 2006.
10. Rossetti, R: A living laboratory. PN 62(8):16, 2008.
11. The Center for Health Design (CHD): An Introduction to Evidence-Based Design: Exploring Healthcare and Design, ed 2. CHD, Concord, CA, 2010.
12. Whitemyer, D: The Future of Evidence-Based Design. Perspective (International Interior Design Association [IIDA]), Spring 2010. Retrieved May 1, 2012, from www.iida.org/resources/category/1/1/1/6/documents/sp10-ebd.pdf.
13. Ostroff, E: Universal design: An evolving paradigm. In Preiser, WFE, and Smith, KH (eds): Universal Design Handbook, ed 2. McGraw-Hill, New York, 2011, p 1.3.
14. Riley, CA: High-Access Home: Design and Decoration for Barrier-Free Living. Rizzoli International Publications, New York, 1999.
15. Bjork, E: Many become losers when the universal design perspective is neglected: Exploring the true cost of ignoring universal design principles. Technol Disabil 21(4):117, 2009.
16. Connell, BR, et al: The Principles of Universal Design. The Center for Universal Design, North Carolina State University College of Design, Raleigh, NC, 1997 (updated 2011). Retrieved May 1, 2012, from www.ncsu.edu/project/design-projects/udi/center-for-universal-design/the-principles-of-universal-design.
17. Ackerman, MJ, et al: Developing next-generation telehealth tools and technologies: Patients, systems, and data perspectives. Telemed J E Health 16(1):93, 2010.
18. Brewer, R, Goble, G, and Guy, P: A peach of a telehealth program: Georgia connects rural communities to better healthcare. Perspect Health Inf Manag 8(Winter):1, 2011.
19. Cosentino, DL: Ten steps to building a successful telehealth program. Caring 28(7):34, 2009.
20. Doarn, CR, Portilla, LM, and Sayre, MH: NIH conference on the future of telehealth: Essential tools and technologies for clinical research and care—a summary. June 25–26, 2009, Bethesda, Maryland. Telemed J E Health 16(1):89, 2010.
21. Doorenbos, AZ, et al: Developing the native people for cancer control telehealth network. Telemed J E Health 17(1):30, 2011.
22. Doorenbos, AZ, et al: Enhancing access to cancer education for rural healthcare providers via telehealth. J Cancer Educ 26(4):682, 2011.
23. Mori, DL, et al: Promoting physical activity in individuals with diabetes: Telehealth approaches. Diabetes Spectr 24(3):127, 2011.
24. Prinz, L, Cramer, M, and Englund, A: Telehealth: A policy analysis for quality, impact on patient outcomes, and political feasibility. Nurs Outlook 56(4):152, 2008.
25. Radhakrishnan, K, and Jacelon, C: Impact of telehealth on patient self-management of heart failure: A review of literature. J Cardiovasc Nurs 27(1):33, 2012.
26. Suter, P, Suter, WN, and Johnston, D: Theory-based telehealth and patient empowerment. Popul Health Manage 14(2):87, 2011.
27. Wade, VA, et al: A systematic review of economic analyses of telehealth services using real time video communication. BMC Health Serv Res 10:233, 2010.
28. Woo, C, et al: What's happening now! Telehealth management of spinal cord injury/disorders. J Spinal Cord Med 34(3):322, 2011.
29. Young, LB, et al: Home telehealth. J Gerontol Nurs 37(11):38, 2011.
30. Huijbregts, MPJ, McEwen, S, and Taylor, D: Exploring the feasibility and efficacy of a telehealth stroke self-management programme: A pilot study. Physiother Can 61(4):210, 2009.
31. Lee, ACW: The VISYTER telerehabilitation system for globalizing physical therapy consultation: Issues and challenges for telehealth implementation (Case Report). J Phys Ther Educ 26(1):90, 2012.
32. Lee, ACW, and Harada, N: Telehealth as a means of health care delivery for physical therapist practice. Phys Ther 92(3):463, 2012.
33. Shaw, DK: Overview of telehealth and its application to cardiopulmonary physical therapy. Cardiopulm Phys Ther J 20(2):13, 2009.
34. American Physical Therapy Association (APTA): Telehealth—Definitions and Guidelines BOD G03-06-09-19 (Retitled: Telehealth; Amended BOD G03-03-07-12; Initial BOD 11-01-28-70) (Guideline). APTA, Alexandria, VA (document updated December 14, 2009). Retrieved May 1, 2012, from www.apta.org/uploadedFiles/APTAorg/About_Us/Policies/BOD/Practice/TelehealthDefinitionsGuidelines.pdf#search=%22Telehealth%20–%20Definitions%20Guidelines%22.
35. Sanford, JA, et al: Using telerehabilitation to identify home modification needs. Assist Technol 16(1):43, 2004.
36. Duncan, P, et al: Functional reach: A new clinical measure of balance. J Gerontol 45:M192, 1990.
37. Duncan, P, et al: Functional reach: Predictive validity in a sample of elderly male veterans. J Gerontol 47:M93, 1992.

38. Weiner, D, et al: Functional reach: A marker of physical frailty. J Am Geriatr Soc 40:203, 1992.

39. Newton, R: Balance screening of an inner city older adult population. Arch Phys Med Rehabil 78:587, 1997.

40. Newton, R: Validity of the multi-directional reach test: A practical measure for limits of stability in older adults. J Gerontol Med Sci 56A:M248, 2001.

41. Mathias, S, Nayak, US, and Isaacs, B: Balance in elderly patients: The "Get Up and Go" test. Arch Phys Med Rehabil 67(6):387, 1986.

42. Podsiadlo, D, and Richardson, S: The timed "Up and Go": A test of basic mobility for frail elderly persons. J Am Geriatr Soc 39:142, 1991.

43. Tinetti, M, et al: A fall risk index for elderly patients based on number of chronic disabilities. Am J Med 80:429, 1986.

44. Tinetti, M, and Ginter, S: Identifying mobility dysfunctions in elderly patients: Standard neuromuscular examination or direct assessment? JAMA 259:1190, 1988.

45. Faber, MJ, Bosscher, RJ, and van Wieringen, PC: Clinimetric properties of the Performance-Oriented Mobility Assessment. Phys Ther 86(7):944, 2006.

46. Cunha, I, et al: Performance-based gait tests for acute stroke patients. Am J Phys Med Rehabil 81:838, 2002.

47. Sadaria, K, and Bohannon, R: The 6-minute walk test: A brief review of literature. Clin Exerc Physiol 3:127, 2001.

48. Harada, N, Chiu, V, and Stewart, A: Mobility-related function in older adults: Assessment with a 6-minute walk test. Arch Phys Med Rehabil 80:837, 1999.

49. Miller, P, et al: Measurement properties of a standardized version of the two-minute walk test for individuals with neurological dysfunction. Physiother Can 54:241, 2003.

50. Wetzel, JL, et al: Six-minute walk test for persons with mild or moderate disability from multiple sclerosis: Performance and explanatory factors. Physiother Can 63(2):166, 2011.

51. Berg, K, et al: Measuring balance in the elderly: Preliminary development of an instrument. Physiother Can 41:304, 1989.

52. Berg, K, et al: A comparison of clinical and laboratory measures of postural balance in an elderly population. Arch Phys Med Rehabil 73:1073, 1992.

53. Berg, K, et al: Measuring balance in the elderly: Validation of an instrument. Can J Public Health 83(Suppl 2):S7, 1992.

54. Berg, K, et al: The Balance Scale: Reliability assessment for elderly residents and patients with an acute stroke. Scand J Rehabil Med 27:27, 1995.

55. Lee, RE, et al: The Physical Activity Resource Assessment (PARA) instrument: Evaluating features, amenities and incivilities of physical activity resources in urban neighborhoods. Int J Behav Nutr Phys Act 2(1):13, 2005.

56. Department of Health and Human Performance: Understanding Neighborhood Determinants of Obesity (UNDO)—Assessment Tools: Physical Activity Resource Assessment (PARA) (Revised 2010), University of Houston, Houston, TX 77204. Retrieved May 3, 2012, from http://grants.hhp.coe.uh.edu/undo/?page_id=21.

57. Keysor, J, Jette, A, and Haley, S: Development of the Home and Community Environment (HACE) instrument. J Rehabil Med 37(1):37, 2005.

58. Home and Community Environment (HACE) Survey: Instrument and Scoring Manual, 2008. Retrieved May 3, 2012, from www.bu.edu/enact/files/2011/05/HACE-Survey-and-Manual-v1_7-30-2008.pdf.

59. Oliver, R, et al: Development of the Safety Assessment of Function and the Environment for Rehabilitation (SAFER) tool. Can J Occup Ther 60(2):78, 1993.

60. Letts, L, et al: The reliability and validity of the Safety Assessment of Function and the Environment for Rehabilitation (SAFER tool). Br J Occup Ther 61(3):127, 1998.

61. Letts, L, and Marshall, L: Evaluating the validity and consistency of the SAFER tool. Phys Occup Ther Geriatr 13(4):49, 1995.

62. Fänge, A, and Iwarsson, S: Changes in accessibility and usability in housing: An exploration of the housing adaptation process. Occup Ther Int 12(1):44, 2005.

63. Fänge, A, and Iwarsson, S: Changes in ADL dependence and aspects of usability following housing adaptation—a longitudinal perspective. Am J Occup Ther 59(3):296, 2005.

64. Fänge, A, and Iwarsson, S: Accessibility and usability in housing: Construct validity and implications for research and practice. Disabil Rehabil 25(23):1316, 2003.

65. Fänge, A, and Iwarsson, S: Physical housing environment: Development of a self-assessment instrument. Can J Occup Ther 66(5):250, 1999.

66. Helle, T, et al: The Nordic Housing Enabler: Inter-rater reliability in cross-Nordic occupational therapy practice. Scand J Occup Ther 17(4):258, 2010.

67. Shumway-Cook, A, et al: Assessing environmentally determined mobility disability: Self-report versus observed community mobility. J Am Geriatr Soc 53(4):700, 2005.

68. Shumway-Cook, A, et al: Environmental components of mobility disability in community-living older persons. J Am Geriatr Soc 51(3):393, 2003.

69. Whiteneck, GG, et al: Quantifying handicap: A new measure of long-term rehabilitation outcomes. Arch Phys Med Rehabil 73(6):519, 1992.

70. Whiteneck, G, et al: Environmental factors and their role in participation and life satisfaction after spinal cord injury. Arch Phys Med Rehabil 85(11):1793, 2004.

71. Gontkovsky, ST, Russum, P, and Stokic, DS: Comparison of the CIQ and CHART Short Form in assessing community integration in individuals with chronic spinal cord injury: A pilot study. NeuroRehabilitation 24(2):185, 2009.

72. Whiteneck, GG, Gerhart, KA, and Cusick, CP: Identifying environmental factors that influence the outcomes of people with traumatic brain injury. J Head Trauma Rehabil 19(3):191, 2004.

73. Whiteneck, GG, et al: Quantifying environmental factors: A measure of physical, attitudinal, service, productivity, and policy barriers. Arch Phys Med Rehabil 85(8):1324, 2004.

74. Ephraim, PL, et al: Environmental barriers experienced by amputees: The Craig Hospital Inventory of Environmental Factors—Short Form. Arch Phys Med Rehabil 87(3):328, 2006.

75. Craig Hospital Inventory of Environmental Factors (Version 3.0). Craig Hospital, Englewood, CO, 2001. Retrieved May 5, 2011, from www.craighospital.org/repository/documents/Research%20Instruments/CHIEF%20Manual.pdf.

76. Iwarsson, S, Horstmann, V, and Sonn, U: Assessment of dependence in daily activities combined with a self-rating of difficulty. J Rehabil Med 41:150, 2009.

77. Norberg, E, Boman, K, and Löfgren, B: Impact of fatigue on everyday life among older people with chronic heart failure. Aust Occup Ther J 57:34, 2010.

78. Jakobsson, U: The ADL-staircase: Further validation. Int J Rehabil Res 31(1):85, 2008.

79. Jakobsson, U, and Karlsson, S: Predicting mortality with the ADL-staircase in frail elderly. Phys Occup Ther Geriatr 29(2):136, 2011.

80. Åsberg, KH, and Sonn, U: The cumulative structure of personal and instrumental ADL in the elderly: A study of elderly people in a health service district. Scand J Rehab Med 21(4):171, 1989.

81. Sonn, U, and Åsberg, KH: Assessment of activities of daily living in the elderly: A study of a population of 76-year-olds in Gothenburg, Sweden. Scand J Rehab Med 23(4):193, 1991.

82. Sonn, U, Grimby, G, and Svanborg, A: Activities of daily living studied longitudinally between 70 and 76 years of age. Disabil Rehabil 18(2):91, 1996.

83. Sonn, U: Longitudinal studies of dependence in daily life activities among elderly persons. Scand J Rehab Med 34:1 (Suppl), 1996.

84. Katz, S, et al: Studies of illness of the aged. The Index of ADL: A standardized measure of biological and psychosocial function. JAMA 185:914, 1963.

85. Iwarsson, S: Environmental influences on the cumulative structure of instrumental ADL: An example in osteoporosis patients in a Swedish rural district. Clin Rehabil 12(3):221, 1998.

86. Schwab, C: A home that makes house calls (part 2). PN 65(2):23, 2011.

87. Brooks, JO, et al: Toward a "smart" nightstand prototype: An examination of nightstand table contents and preferences. HERD 4(2):91, 2011.

88. Building Design Requirements for the Physically Handicapped, Revised Edition. Eastern Paralyzed Veterans Association, New York, undated.

89. Gitlin, LN, et al: Factors associated with home environmental problems among community-living older people. Disabil Rehabil 23(17):777, 2001.

90. Technology-Related Assistance for Individuals with Disabilities Act of 1988 (Public Law 100-407). Retrieved May 27, 2012, from http://codi.buffalo.edu/archives/.legislation/.techact.htm.

91. Hunter, S: Using CQI to improve worker's health. PT Magazine of Physical Therapy 3(11):64, 1995.
92. American Physical Therapy Association (APTA): Glossary of Workers' Compensation Terms. APTA, Alexandria, VA, 22314, 2011. Retrieved May 28, 2012, from www.apta.org/Payment/WorkersCompensation/Glossary.
93. Talmage, JB, Melhorn, JM, and Hyman, MH (eds): AMA Guides to the Evaluation of Work Ability and Return to Work, ed 2. American Medical Association, Chicago, 2011.
94. Genovese, E, and Galper, JS (eds): Guide to the Evaluation of Functional Ability: How to Request, Interpret, and Apply Functional Capacity Evaluations. American Medical Association, Chicago, 2009.
95. Gibson, L, and Strong, J: A conceptual framework of functional capacity evaluation for occupational therapy in work rehabilitation. Austral Occup Ther J 50(2):64, 2003.
96. United States Department of Labor (DOL): O*NET—beyond information—intelligence. DOL, Washington, DC 20210. Retrieved May 28, 2012, from www.doleta.gov/programs/onet.
97. Bethge, M, et al: Work status and health-related quality of life following multimodal work hardening: A cluster randomised trial. J Back Musculoskelet Rehabil 24(3):161, 2011.
98. Cheng, AS, and Hung, L: Randomized controlled trial of workplace-based rehabilitation for work-related rotator cuff disorder. J Occup Rehabil 17(3):487, 2007.
99. Johnson, LS, et al: Work hardening: Outdated fad or effective intervention? Work 16(3):235, 2001.
100. Dennis, L, et al: Screening for elevated levels of fear-avoidance beliefs regarding work or physical activities in people receiving outpatient therapy. Phys Ther 89:770, 2009.
101. Godges, JJ, et al: Effects of education on return-to-work status for people with fear-avoidance beliefs and acute low back pain. Phys Ther 88:231, 2008.
102. United States Department of Defense (DOD): Workplace Ergonomics Reference Guide: A Publication of the Computer/Electronic Accommodations Program, US DOD, Washington, DC 20301. Retrieved May 29, 2012, from http://cap.mil/Documents/CAP_Ergo_Guide.pdf.
103. Department of Justice (DOJ): ADA Regulations and Technical Assistance Materials. US DOJ, Washington, DC 20301. Retrieved May 30, 2012, from www.ada.gov/publicat.htm.
104. ADA Accessibility Guidelines for Buildings and Facilities. Retrieved May 30, 2012, from www.access-board.gov/adaag/html/adaag.htm#toc.
105. Department of Justice (DOJ): ADA Home Page. US DOJ, Washington, DC 20301. Retrieved May 30, 2012, from www.ada.gov.
106. Udo, JP, and Fels, DI: Enhancing the entertainment experience of blind and low-vision theatregoers through touch tours. Disabil Soc (2):231, 2010.
107. Accessible NYC!! Retrieved May 30, 2012, from www.accessiblenyc.org.
108. Disability Guide for Washington, DC. Retrieved May 30, 2012, from www.disabilityguide.org.
109. The Americans with Disabilities Act of 1990 (As Amended): Public Law 101-336. Retrieved June 5, 2012, from www.ada.gov/pubs/adastatute08.htm.
110. Architectural Barriers Act, Public Law 90-480, 1968.
111. Public Buildings Act, 98th Congress, 1st session, 1983.
112. Telecommunications Act of 1996. Retrieved December 18, 2012, from www.gpo.gov/fdsys/pkg/BILLS-104s652enr/pdf/BILLS-104s652enr.pdf.

Supplemental Readings

Bjork, E: Why did it take four times longer to create the universal design solution? A comparative study of two product development projects. Technol Disabil 21:159, 2009.
Choi, SD: Safety and ergonomic considerations for an aging workforce in the US construction industry. Work 33:307, 2009.
Goetz, P, et al: An Introduction to Evidence-Based Design: Exploring Health and Design, ed 2. Center for Health Design, Concord, CA, 2010.
Gossett, A, et al: Beyond access: A case study on the intersection between accessibility, sustainability, and universal design. Disabil Rehabil Assist Technol 4(6):439, 2009.
Kiser, L, and Zasler, N: Residential design for real life rehabilitation. NeuroRehabilitation 25(3):219, 2009.
Levine, D (ed): The NYC Guidebook to Accessibility and Universal Design, ed 2. Center for Inclusive Design and Environmental Access, University at Buffalo, State University of New York, 2003. Retrieved April 14, 2012, from www.nyc.gov/html/ddc/downloads/pdf/udny/udny2.pdf.
Lombardi, AR, and Murray, C: Measuring university faculty attitudes toward disability: Willingness to accommodate and adopt universal design principles. J Vocat Rehabil 34(1):43, 2011.
Pasquina, PF, et al: Using architecture and technology to promote improved quality of life for military service members with traumatic brain injury. Phys Med Rehabil Clin North Am 21(1):207, 2010.
Rodríguez, CIR: Seniors and technology, ergonomic needs and design considerations. Work 41:5576, 2012.
Schraner, I, et al: Using the ICF in economic analyses of assistive technology systems: Methodological implications of a user standpoint. Disabil Rehabil 30(12–13):916, 2008.
Steinfeld, E, and Danford, GS (eds): Enabling Environments: Measuring the Impact of Environment on Disability and Rehabilitation. Kluwer Academic/Plenum Publishing, New York, 1999.
Vavik, T (ed): Inclusive Buildings, Products and Services: Challenges in Universal Design. Tapir Academic Press, Trondheim, Norway, 2009.
York, SL: Residential design and outdoor area accessibility. NeuroRehabilitation 25(3):201, 2009.
Zolna, JS, et al: Review of accommodation strategies in the workplace for persons with mobility and dexterity impairments: Application to criteria for universal design. Technol Disabil 19(4):189, 2007.

The Principles of Universal Design

The Principles of Universal Design

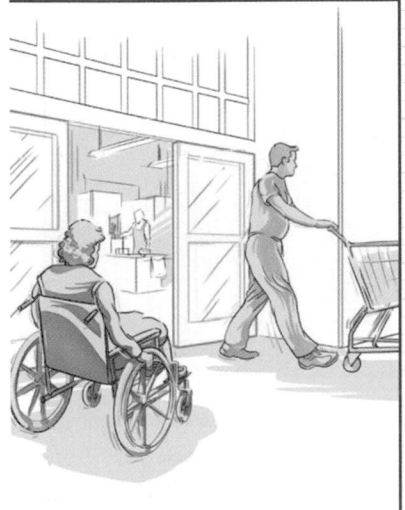

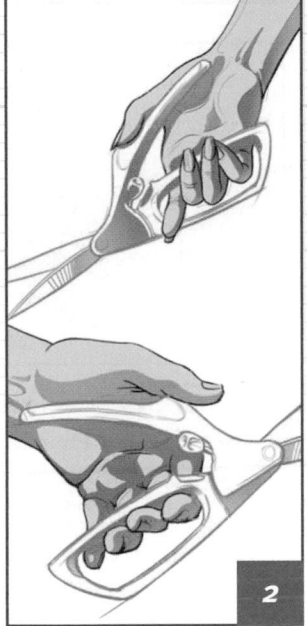

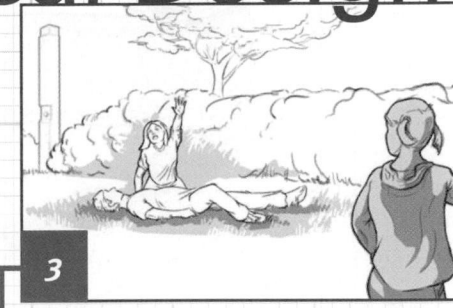

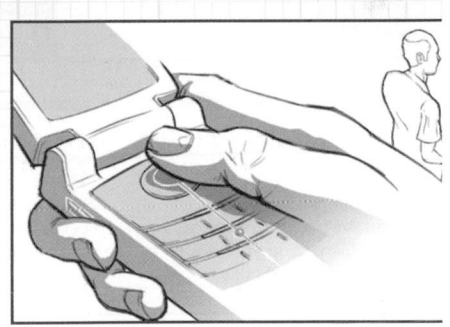

PRINCIPLE

Equitable Use

The design is useful and marketable to people with diverse abilities.

Flexibility in Use

The design accommodates a wide range of individual preferences and abilities.

Simple and Intuitive Use

Use of the design is easy to understand, regardless of the user's experience, knowledge, language skills, or education level.

GUIDELINES

1a. Provide the same means of use for all users: identical whenever possible; equivalent when not.

1b. Avoid segregating or stigmatizing any users.

1c. Provisions for privacy, security, and safety should be equally available to all users.

1d. Make the design appealing to all users.

2a. Provide choice in methods of use.

2b. Accommodate right- or left-handed access and use.

2c. Facilitate the user's accuracy and precision.

2d. Provide adaptability to the user's pace.

3a. Eliminate unnecessary complexity.

3b. Be consistent with user expectations and intuition.

3c. Accommodate a wide range of literacy and language skills.

3d. Arrange information consistent with its importance.

3e. Provide effective prompting and feedback during and after task completion.

EXAMPLES

- Power doors make visiting public spaces easier for all users.
- E-mail makes communication easier for everyone, including people who have trouble communicating via phone.

Large grip scissors accommodates use with either hand and allows alternation between the two in repetitive tasks.

- Public emergency stations utilize recognized emergency colors and a simple design to quickly convey function to passers-by.
- Intuitive ATM interfaces allow use without instruction or training.

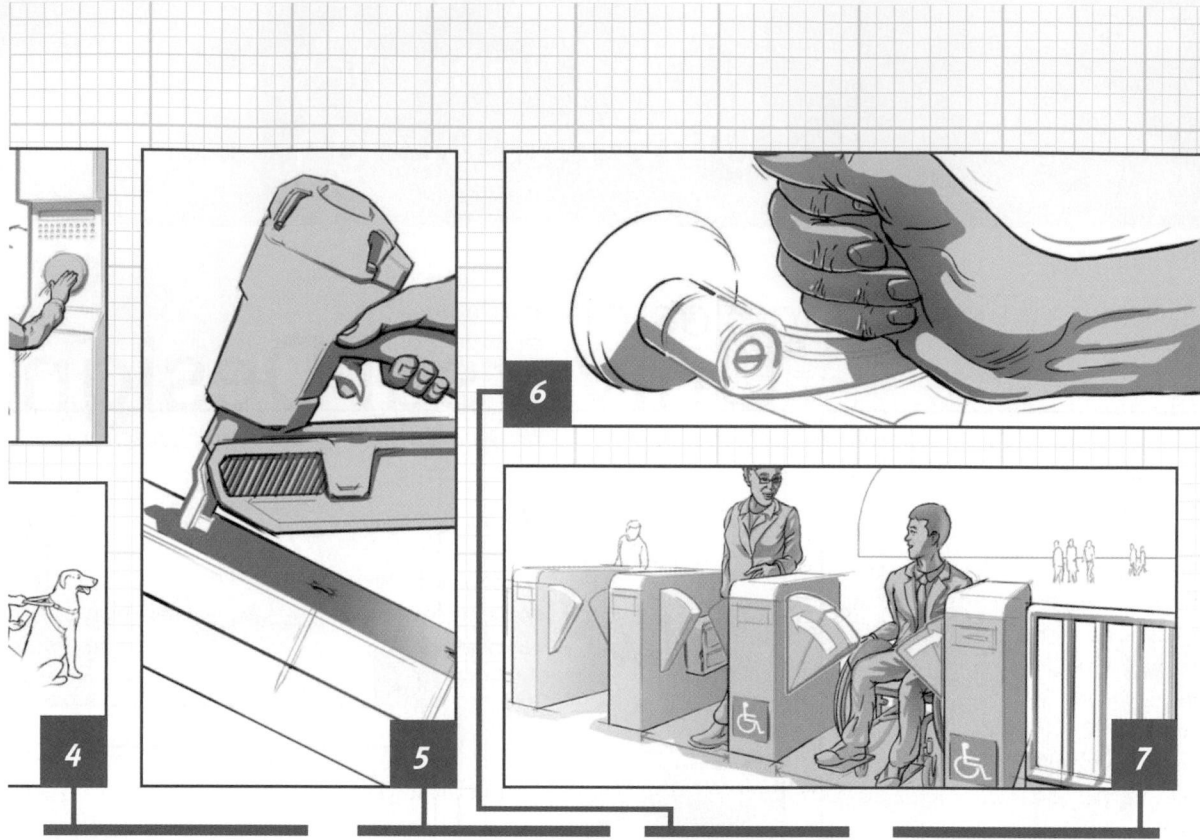

Perceptible Information

The design communicates necessary information effectively to the user, regardless of ambient conditions or the user's sensory abilities.

4a. Use different modes (pictorial, verbal, tactile) for redundant presentation of essential information.

4b. Provide adequate contrast between essential information and its surroundings.

4c. Maximize "legibility" of essential information.

4d. Differentiate elements in ways that can be described (i.e., make it easy to give instructions or directions).

4e. Provide compatibility with a variety of techniques or devices used by people with sensory limitations.

Small bumps on a cell phone keypad tell the user where important keys are without requiring the user to look at the keys.

Tolerance for Error

The design minimizes hazards and the adverse consequences of accidental or unintended actions.

5a. Arrange elements to minimize hazards and errors: most used elements, most accessible; hazardous elements eliminated, isolated, or shielded.

5b. Provide warnings of hazards and errors.

5c. Provide fail safe features.

5d. Discourage unconscious action in tasks that require vigilance.

The "sequential trip" mechanism on a nail gun prevents accidental firing when the tool is not pressed against an object.

Low Physical Effort

The design can be used efficiently and comfortably and with a minimum of fatigue.

6a. Allow user to maintain a neutral body position.

6b. Use reasonable operating forces.

6c. Minimize repetitive actions.

6d. Minimize sustained physical effort.

Door lever does not require grip strength to operate, and can even be operated by a closed fist or elbow.

Size and Space for Approach and Use

Appropriate size and space is provided for approach, reach, manipulation, and use regardless of user's body size, posture, or mobility.

7a. Provide a clear line of sight to important elements for any seated or standing user.

7b. Make reach to all components comfortable for any seated or standing user.

7c. Accommodate variations in hand and grip size.

7d. Provide adequate space for the use of assistive devices or personal assistance.

Wide gates at subway stations accommodate wheelchair users as well as commuters with packages or luggage.

Usability in My Home— A Self-Report Instrument

Directions: The questionnaire consists of two parts, with a number of questions about the design of the *physical housing environment* in which you live. You are asked to answer the questions by assessing how you feel that the design and form of the physical housing environment suits you, your needs, and your wishes.

By physical housing environment is meant here your home, the car park, garage, or parking space that you use if you have a car, your own letterbox, the dustbin/refuse storage place, the storage space, and the shared laundry, if there is one. This includes all the routes along which you move on the site to and from these places. It also includes a balcony, patio, and garden where applicable.

The questions are very general, and the aim is to capture your immediate perception of how the physical housing environment suits you.

For each question there are seven response alternatives in the form of the numbers 1 to 7. The number 1 stands for what is the worst and lowest alternative for you, and 7 stands for the best and highest alternative. The numbers 2 to 6 describe the positions that lie between the best and the worst alternatives. The number 4 is the neutral point on the scale, neither good nor bad. Put a circle round the alternative that agrees best with your perception.

Example: If you are so dissatisfied with your physical housing environment that it could not, in your opinion, be worse for you, then circle the number 1. If you are so satisfied with the design of your physical housing environment that it could not, in your opinion, be better, then circle the number 7. You use the numbers 2 to 7 to describe how close to the best or worst alternative you find the features of your housing environment.

There now follow a number of questions about how well you feel that the design of your physical housing environment suits your needs and wishes. Some questions concern security, social interaction, and so forth, while others concern how the design of the housing environment makes it easy or difficult to do the everyday tasks you wish and need to perform.

Draw a circle round the number that you think agrees best with your own perception.

1. **In relation to how you normally manage your personal hygiene, dressing, visiting the toilet, or how you eat; to what extent is the housing environment suitably designed?** (*If you do not manage any of these at all, cross out the whole question.*)

    1   2   3   4   5   6   7
    Not at all suitable   Very suitable

2. **In relation to how you normally manage your cooking/heating of food or preparation of snacks; to what extent is the housing environment suitably designed?** (*If you do not manage any of these at all, cross out the whole question.*)

    1   2   3   4   5   6   7
    Not at all suitable   Very suitable

3. **In relation to how you normally manage your washing up, cleaning, care of flowers; to what extent is the housing environment suitably designed?** (*If you do not manage any of these at all, cross out the whole question.*)

    1   2   3   4   5   6   7
    Not at all suitable   Very suitable

4. **In relation to how you normally manage your washing, ironing, or repair of clothes; to what extent is the housing environment suitably designed?** (*If you do not manage any of these at all, cross out the whole question.*)

    1   2   3   4   5   6   7
    Not at all suitable   Very suitable

5. **How secure do you feel in your housing environment?**

    1   2   3   4   5   6   7
    Not at all secure   Completely secure

6. **To what extent does the design of the housing environment allow you to be by yourself when you so wish?**

    1   2   3   4   5   6   7
    Not at all   As much as I want to

From Fänge, A: Usability in My Home: Manual and Instrument Form. Division of Occupational Therapy, Lund University, Sweden, 2002. © Agneta Fänge, 2002, with permission.

7. To what extent does the design of the housing environment allow you to socialize with the friends and acquaintances you want to meet?

1   2   3   4   5   6   7
Not at all   As much as I want to

8. To what extent does the design of the housing environment allow you to do hobbies/leisure pursuits and relax?

1   2   3   4   5   6   7
Not at all   As much as I want to

9. If your health should change, to what extent would it be possible for you to make simple changes to your housing environment (e.g., to use a different parking place, to use a different toilet, to rearrange the furniture, to use a different room as a bedroom, and so forth)?

1   2   3   4   5   6   7
Not at all   As much as I need to

There now follow a number of questions about how usable you feel that your housing environment is. First you make an overall assessment (question 10). This is followed by a number of more detailed questions about usability in different parts of the housing environment. State the problems you perceive and make an assessment of how accessible each part of the housing environment is, with regard to the problems you have stated (questions 11 to 22). If you do not feel that there are any special problems, please say so. Do not forget to assess each part of the physical housing environment, even if you have not stated any specific problem.

10. How usable do you feel that your housing environment is in general?

1   2   3   4   5   6   7
Not at all usable   Fully usable

11. What problems do you perceive in the physical environment just outside your home (e.g., paths and pavements, car park/garage/carport, the design of the refuse storage place, the placing of your letterbox, and so forth)?

_____

_____

12. In view of the above problems in question 11, how usable do you feel that the environment outside your home is?

1   2   3   4   5   6   7
Not at all usable   Fully usable

13. What problems do you find in the design of the entrance to your home (e.g. heavy doors, narrow stairs, ramps, cramped lift, poor lighting, and so forth)?

_____

_____

14. In view of the above problems in question 13, how usable do you feel that the entrance to your home is?

1   2   3   4   5   6   7
Not at all usable   Fully usable

15. What problems do you find in the design of the secondary spaces in your home (e.g., store rooms, attic/basement, refuse storage place, laundry [if any], and the routes you have to follow indoors to reach these places)?

_____

_____

16. In view of the above problems in question 15, how usable do you feel that the secondary spaces in your home are?

1   2   3   4   5   6   7
Not at all usable   Fully usable

17. What problems do you have in reading and understanding markings and signs outside the building or at the entrance? (For example, are lift buttons fully visible and easy to use? Are the signs at the waste sorting station clear and easy to understand? Are the markings in staircases easy to see?) (*The questions should only be answered by people living in apartments. If you live in your own house, omit this question and question 18.*)

_____

_____

18. In view of the above problems in question 17, to what extent would you say that the markings and signs outside the building and at the entrance can be read and understood?

1   2   3   4   5   6   7
Not at all   Perfectly easily

19. **What problems do you find in the design of your balcony, patio, or garden?** (*If you do not have any balcony, patio, or garden, please say so. You may then omit question 20.*)

_____

_____

20. **In view of the above problems in question 19, how usable do you feel that the balcony, patio, or garden are?**

    1   2   3   4   5   6   7
    Not at all usable   Fully usable

21. **What problems do you find in the design of the interior of your home?**

_____

_____

22. **In view of the above problems in question 21, how usable do you feel that the interior of your home is?**

    1   2   3   4   5   6   7
    Not at all usable   Fully usable

To conclude, there is a general question that allows you to express your wishes and needs.

23. **If you were able to wish for anything at all concerning your home and your housing environment, what would you wish for?**

_____

_____

_____

_____

_____

_____

_____

Note: In this instrument, the term **personal activities of daily living (P-ADL)** is synonymous with **basic activities of daily living (BADL)**.

■ DEFINITIONS

Cleaning: *performs house cleaning, vacuum cleaning, washing floors*
  Independent: Performs the activity when necessary.
  Partly dependent: Gets assistance in taking the carpets outdoors or assistance very seldom.
  Dependent: Does not perform the activity or gets assistance with some part of the activity regularly.
Shopping: *gets to the store, manages stairs and other obstacles, takes out groceries, pays for them and carries them home*
  Independent: Performs the activity when necessary.
  Partly dependent: Performs the activity but together with another person.
  Dependent: Does not perform the activity or needs assistance with some part of the activity.
Transportation: *gets to the stop for public transportation, gets on and goes by bus, tram, or train*
  Independent: Performs the activity when needed.
  Partly dependent: Performs the activity but together with another person.
  Dependent: Does not perform the activity.
Cooking: *gets to the kitchen, prepares the food, manages the stove*
  Independent: Performs the activity when needed.
  Partly dependent: Does not prepare dinner-food or only heating up prepared food.
  Dependent: Does not perform the activity.
Bathing: *means sponge bath, tub bath, or shower*
  Independent: Receives no assistance (gets in and out of tub by self if tub is usual means of bathing).
  Partly dependent: Receives assistance in bathing only one part of the body (such as back or leg).
  Dependent: Receives assistance in bathing more than one part of the body (or does not bathe self).
Dressing: *means getting all needed clothing from closets and drawers and getting dressed, includes using fasteners, and putting on brace if worn*
  Independent: Gets clothes and gets completely dressed without assistance.
  Partly dependent: Gets clothes and gets dressed without assistance except for help with tying shoes.
  Dependent: Receives assistance in getting clothes or in getting dressed, or stays partly or incompletely dressed.
Toileting: *means going to the "toilet room" for bowel and urine elimination, cleaning self after elimination, and arranging clothes*
  Independent: Goes to the "toilet room," cleans self and arranges clothes without assistance. (May use support object such as cane, walker, or wheelchair, and may manage a night bedpan or commode, emptying it in the morning.)
  Partly dependent: Receives assistance in going to the "toilet room" or in cleaning self or in arranging clothes after elimination, or using the night bedpan or commode.
  Dependent: Does not go to the "toilet room" for elimination.
Transfer: *means moving in and out of bed and in and out of chair*
  Independent: Moves in and out of bed and out of chair without assistance. (May use support object such as cane or walker.)
  Partly dependent: Moves in and out of bed or chair with assistance.
  Dependent: Does not get out of bed.
Continence: *means function of controlling elimination from the bladder and bowel*
  Independent: Controls urination and bowel movement completely by self.
  Partly dependent: Has occasional "accidents."
  Dependent: Supervision helps keep urine or bowel control, or catheter is used, or is incontinent.

Feeding: *means the basic process of getting food from plate or equivalent into the mouth*
    Independent: Feeds self without assistance.
    Partly dependent: Feeds self except for getting assistance in cutting meat or buttering bread.
    Dependent: Receives assistance in feeding or is fed partly or completely through tubes or with intravenous fluids.
    Definitions of personal (P-) and instrumental (I-) ADL according to a cumulative scale of conditional ADL-steps (the ADL Staircase)

■ ADL-STEPS IN I AND P-ADL

Step 0   Independent in all activities
Step 1   Dependent on one activity
Step 2   Dependent on cleaning and one more activity
Step 3   Dependent on cleaning, shopping, and one more activity
Step 4   Dependent on cleaning, shopping, transportation, and one more activity
Step 5   Dependent in all I-ADLs and one P-ADL
Step 6   Dependent in all I-ADLs, bathing, and one more P-ADL
Step 7   Dependent in all I-ADLs, bathing, dressing, and one more P-ADL
Step 8   Dependent in all I-ADLs, bathing, dressing, going to the toilet, and one more P-ADL
Step 9   Dependent in all activities
"Others"   Dependent in two or more activities but not classifiable as above
    If the item continence is included, the definitions of the last two steps will be as follows:
Step 9   Dependent in all I-ADLs, bathing, dressing, going to the toilet, transfer, and one more P-ADL
Step 10   Dependent in all activities

ADL-step 0
ADL-step 1 Cleaning
ADL-step 2 Shopping
ADL-step 3 Transportation
ADL-step 4 Cooking
ADL-step 5 Bathing
ADL-step 6 Dressing
ADL-step 7 Toileting
ADL-step 8 Transfer
ADL-step 9 Continence
ADL-step 10 Feeding

Home Examination Form

Type of Home

(Indicate apartment or single family home)

☐ *Apartment*

Owned _____ Rented _____

Is elevator available? _____

What floor does patient live on? _____

☐ *Single family home*

Two or more floors_____

Does patient live on only one floor, or use all floors of home?_____

Basement. Does patient have or use basement area?

_____

Entrances to Building or Home

Location

Front Back Side (Circle one)

Which entrance is used most frequently or easily?

_____

Can patient get to entrance? _____

Stairs

Does patient manage outside stairs? _____

Width of stairway_____

Number of steps _____ Height of steps _____

Railing present as you go up? R _____ L _____

Both _____

Is ramp available for wheelchair? _____

Door

Can patient unlock, open, close, lock door? (Circle for yes)

If doorsill is present, give height _____ and material _____

Width of doorway _____

Can patient enter _____ leave _____ via door?

Hallway

Width of hallway _____

Are any objects obstructing the way? _____

Approach to Apartment or Living Area

(Omit if not applicable)

Obstructions? _____

_____

Steps

Width of stairway _____

Number of steps _____ Height of steps _____

Railing present as you go up? R _____ L _____

Both _____

Is ramp available? _____

Door

Can patient unlock, open, close, lock door? (Circle one)

Doorsill? Give height _____ material _____

Width of doorway _____

Can patient enter _____ leave _____ via door?

Elevator

Is elevator present? _____ Does it land flush with floor? _____

Width of door opening _____

Height of control buttons _____

Can patient use elevator alone? _____

Inside Home

Note width of hallways and of door entrances.

Note presence of doorsills and height.

Note if patient must climb stairs to reach room.

Can patient move from one part of the house to another?

Hallways _____

Bedroom _____

Bathroom _____

Kitchen _____

Living room _____

Others _____

Can patient move safely?

Loose rugs _____

Electrical cords _____

Faulty floors _____

Highly waxed floors _____

Sharp-edged furniture _____

Note areas of particular danger for patient.

Hot water pipes _____

Radiators _____

Bedroom

Is light switch accessible? _____

Can patient open and close windows? _____

Bed

Height _____ Width _____
Both sides of bed accessible? _____ headboard
    present? _____ footboard? _____
Is bed on wheels? _____ Is it stable? _____
Can patient transfer from wheelchair-to-bed? _____
And bed-to-wheelchair? _____
Is night table within patient's reach from bed _____
Is telephone on it? _____

Clothing

Is patient's clothing located in bedroom? _____
Can patient get clothes from dresser? _____
    Closet? _____ Elsewhere? _____

Bathroom

Does patient use wheelchair _____
    walker _____ in bathroom?
Does wheelchair _____ walker _____ fit into bathroom?
Light switch accessible? _____ Can patient open and
    close window? _____
What material are bathroom walls made of? _____
    If tile, how many inches does tile extend from the
      floor beside the toilet? _____
    How many inches does tile extend from the top of
      the rim of the bathtub? _____
Does patient use toilet? _____
    Can patient transfer independently to and from
      toilet? _____
    Does wheelchair wheel directly to toilet for transfers?
    _____
    What is height of toilet seat from floor? _____
    Are there bars or sturdy supports near toilet? _____
    Is there room for grab bars? _____
Can patient use sink? _____ What is height
    of sink? _____
    Is patient able to reach and turn off faucets? _____
    Is there knee space beneath sink? _____
    Is patient able to reach necessary articles? _____
      Mirror? _____ Electrical outlet? _____

Bathing

Does patient take tub bath? _____ Shower? _____
Sponge bath? _____
If using tub, can patient safely transfer without
    assistance? _____
Bars or sturdy supports present beside tub? _____
Is equipment necessary? (tub seat, hand-spray
    attachment, tub rail, no-skid strips, grab rails,
    other: _____)
Can patient manage faucets and drain plug? _____
Height of tub from floor to rim _____
Is tub built-in _____ or on legs? _____
Width of tub from the inside _____
If uses separate shower stall, can patient transfer
    independently and manage faucets? _____

If patient takes sponge bath, describe method. _____
_____
_____

Living Room Area

Light switch accessible? _____ Can patient open and
    close window? _____
Can furniture be rearranged to allow manipulation of
    wheelchair? _____
Can patient transfer from wheelchair to and from sturdy
    chair? _____
Height of chair _____
Can patient transfer from wheelchair to and from sofa?
    _____
Height of sofa _____
Can ambulatory patient transfer to and from chair or
    sofa? _____
Can patient manage television and radio? _____

Dining Room

Light switch accessible? _____
Is patient able to use table? _____ Height of
    table _____

Kitchen

What is the table height? _____ Can wheelchair
    fit under? _____
Can patient open refrigerator door and take food?
_____
Can patient open freezer door and take food? _____

Sink

Can patient be seated at sink? _____
Can patient reach faucets? _____ Turn
    them on and off? _____
Can patient reach bottom of basin? _____

Shelves and cabinets

Can patient open and close? _____
Can patient reach dishes, pots, eating utensils, and
    food? _____
Comments: _____
_____
_____

Transport

Can patient carry items from one part of kitchen to
    another? _____

Stove

Can patient reach and manipulate controls? _____
Manage oven door? _____
Place food in oven and remove? _____
Manage broiler door? _____
Put food in and remove? _____

Other Appliances

Can patient reach and turn on appliances? _____

Can patient use outlets? _____

Counter space

Is there enough for storage and work area? _____

Diagram (include stove, refrigerator, microwave, sink, table, counters, others if applicable)

Laundry

If patient has no facilities, how will laundry be managed?

_____

_____

Location of facilities in home or apartment and description of facilities present:

Can patient reach laundry area? _____

Can patient use washing machine and dryer? _____

Load and empty? _____

Manage doors and controls? _____

Can patient use sink? _____

What is height of sink? _____

Able to reach and turn on faucets? _____

Knee space beneath sink? _____

Able to reach necessary articles? _____

Is laundry cart available? _____

Can patient hang clothing on line? _____

Ironing board _____

Location: _____

Is it kept open? _____

If not kept open, can patient set up and take down ironing board? _____

Can patient reach outlet? _____

Cleaning

Can patient remove mop, broom, vacuum, pail from storage? _____

Use equipment? (mop, broom, vacuum and so forth)

_____

Emergency

Location of telephone in house: _____

Could patient use fire escape or back door in a hurry if alone? _____

Does patient have numbers for neighbors, police, fire, and physician? _____

Other

Will patient be responsible for child care? _____

If so, give number of children _____ and ages: _____

Will patient do own shopping? _____

Is family member or friend available? _____

Is delivery service available? _____

Does family have automobile? _____

Is family member or friend available to help with lawn care, changing high light bulbs, and so forth?

_____

_____

_____

Purpose and Use

- It qualifies a position, describing the purposes and needs within the respective department.
- It is a comprehensive job description describing both the tasks performed and the physical and cognitive needs of the job.
- It maximizes interview information to determine the candidate's ability to perform the *Essential Functions.*
- It identifies performance evaluation criteria.
- It is required for all job accommodation requests when a health condition necessitates ADA modification/accommodation.
- It must accompany all new positions that need to be advertised and a reclassification request if the position is currently vacant and needs to be advertised.

Help Table

Department: The department where the position is performed.

Position/Job Code Title: Merit classification or professional and scientific classification.

Job Code: University of Iowa Job Code (EX: GB11, PC67).

Incumbent: Name of person currently in position or "vacant."

Position Number: HRIS assigned 8-digit position number (EX: 00000755).

Requisition Number: For advertising, match Requisition Number to Functional Analysis.

Position Summary: Basic purpose of job and rationale for existence.

Function Statements: Action outcome statements, starting with a verb, either essential (primary) or marginal (secondary) to the position, identified by percentage of time performed to add up to 100%.

Essential Function: Functions defined by the frequency with which they are performed, the amount of time it takes to perform them, how the job is affected if not performed by this position, or whether these functions could be assigned to another position.

Marginal Function: Function that needs to be performed only infrequently, with usually minimal consequence to the mission of the job if performed by another person.

Position Context Variables: Needed for the performance of essential functions. Check "YES" even if only one variable applies at this time.

Comments: Add anything not already covered that is needed to perform the essential functions of the job, or to further explain context variables.

Cognitive Processes: Level of training needed to perform the essential functions of the position, split between high school level training and post high school college/technical training. Check "YES" even if only one variable applies at this time.

Bilingual Requirements: Foreign languages used in the performance of the position.

Degree of Push–Pull Activity: Designate all forms of push–pull on the job to add up to a total of 100% for performance of the essential functions.

Physical Requirements: Movements that **CANNOT** be performed concurrently and reflect the essential functions on pages 1 and 2.

Physical Requirements: Movement that **CAN** be performed concurrently to reflect the essential functions of the job.

Vision Clarity: With corrected vision to perform the essential functions.

Equipment, Tools, Electronic Devices and Software: Equipment, tools, electronic devices, and software operated to perform the essential functions.

Physical Surroundings and Hazards: Applicable to all areas where essential functions of a position are performed (e.g., office, job site, lab, hospital, kitchen, and so forth).

Comments: Any that pertain to the physical surroundings or possible hazards involved in the performance of the essential functions of the position.

Vehicle Driven: Only if needed to perform the essential functions (out-of-town work, delivery, and so forth).

Locations: All job sites where essential functions are performed.
Day/Hour Schedule: The work shift or shifts if rotating.
Name and Title of Supervisor: Name of person to whom this incumbent reports.
Person Completing this Form: Incumbent or supervisor (print or type).
Signature of Incumbent: Signature of person currently in position. If "vacant" or "new," leave blank.

THE UNIVERSITY OF IOWA **University Human Resources** Faculty and Staff Disability Services 121 University Services Building, Ste20 Iowa City, Iowa 52242-1911	**ESSENTIAL AND MARGINAL** **JOB FUNCTION ANALYSIS**

Tab field-to-field to enter data (or click with mouse). Press the F1 key at any field to see a description of that field.

Department: _____   Position Title: _____   Job Code: _____
Incumbent: _____   Position #: _____   Requisition #: _____

■ POSITION SUMMARY:

Provide a position summary. If you need more space, please attach a separate sheet. A position summary consists of concise, qualitative statements crystallizing the basic purpose of the job and rationale for its existence.

■ FUNCTION STATEMENTS:

A job function statement should focus on the purpose, the result to be accomplished, and the productivity required rather than the manner in which the function is performed. Begin each statement with a verb. Each statement is to contain one action that produces the desired outcome. Identify whether the functions are essential or marginal (primary or secondary) to the position. Provide the projected percent of time to be devoted to each job function during a typical time period.

Essential (Primary) Functions	%	Marginal (Secondary) Functions	%
1.	0.00	1.	0.00
2.	0.00	2.	0.00
3.	0.00	3.	0.00
4.	0.00	4.	0.00
5.	0.00	5.	0.00
6.	0.00	6.	0.00
7.	0.00	7.	0.00
8.	0.00	8.	0.00
9.	0.00	9.	0.00
10.	0.00	10.	0.00
11.	0.00	11.	0.00
12.	0.00	12.	0.00
13.	0.00	13.	0.00
14.	0.00	14.	0.00
Essential Column Total**	0.00%	Marginal Column Total**	0.00%

**Essential and Marginal Column Totals must total 100%.

■ POSITION CONTEXT VARIABLES:

Indicate the responsibilities and aptitudes required to perform the essential/primary functions for this position.

Yes No Place an "X" in the appropriate box (or click box with mouse to use as toggle).

☐ ☐ Work with frustrating situations: Job objectives are hindered by events beyond the employee's control.
☐ ☐ Advise: Counsel others based on legal, financial, scientific, technical, or other specialized areas; recommend, guide caution.
☐ ☐ Coordinate: Negotiate, monitor and organize activities of others to achieve objectives, but without direct authority.
☐ ☐ Instruct: Teach others, formally or informally.
☐ ☐ Group activities: Participate in activities requiring interpersonal skills and cooperation with others.
☐ ☐ Work under time pressure: Rush or urgent time lines.
☐ ☐ Work on an irregular schedule: Unscheduled overtime, called in to work, unanticipated changes in work pace.
☐ ☐ Work with numerous distractions: Telephone calls, visitors, coworkers.
☐ ☐ Handle multiple assignments, conflicting demands or priorities.
☐ ☐ Concentration: Maintain attention to detail over extended period of time, continually aware of variations in changing situations.
☐ ☐ Reaction or response: Quick reaction/immediate response to emergencies of severe consequences.
☐ ☐ Research and analysis: Fact-finding, interpretation, investigation in preparing reports or evaluations.
☐ ☐ Accountability and consequence of error: Responsible for money, equipment, or personnel. Severe consequences to department, University, or coworkers if work objectives are not met.
☐ ☐ Work independence: Work is performed independently or with minimal on-site supervision.
☐ ☐ Supervise: Recruit, screen, hire, assign and/or review work, train and/or evaluate other employees.
☐ ☐ Confidentiality: Work with confidential information, materials, records.

Comments:

■ COGNITIVE PROCESSES:

Indicate cognitive abilities required to complete the essential functions.

Yes No Type an "X" in the appropriate box (or click box with mouse to use as toggle).

☐ ☐ Inspect products, objects, or materials.
☐ ☐ Analyze information or data.
☐ ☐ Plan sequence of operations or actions.
☐ ☐ Make decisions of moderate to substantial effects, with variety of alternatives and moderate to substantial consequences.
☐ ☐ Use logic to define problems, collect information, establish facts, draw valid conclusions, interpret information, and deal with abstract variables.
☐ ☐ Perform basic counting, addition, and subtraction of numbers.
☐ ☐ Perform calculations using algebra, geometry, and statistics.
Comprehend written communication:
☐ ☐ a. Basic instructions, safety rules, office memoranda at high school graduate level.
☐ ☐ b. Technical or professional materials, financial or legal reports at postsecondary level.
Compose written communication:
☐ ☐ a. Compose letters or memos using standard business English at high school graduate level.
☐ ☐ b. Compose and edit report or technical, professional material at postsecondary level.
Verbal comprehension:
☐ ☐ a. Comprehend simple verbal sentences and instructions at high school graduate level.
☐ ☐ b. Comprehend technical and complex information at postsecondary level.
Verbal communication:
☐ ☐ a. Converse in Standard English at high school graduate level.
☐ ☐ b. Converse using complex technical or professional English at postsecondary level.
Foreign Language Requirements:

Comments:

■ DEGREE OF PUSH/PULL ACTIVITY:

Indicate the percent of time that pushing and pulling activities are performed. The total should equal 100%.

		N/A	<25%	25%–49%	50%–74%	>75%
SEDENTARY	Exert up to 10 lb of force occasionally* and/or a minute amount frequently**	☐	☐	☐	☐	☐
LIGHT	Exert up to 20 lb of force occasionally* and/or up to 10 lb of force frequently**	☐	☐	☐	☐	☐
MEDIUM	Exert 20–50 lb of force occasionally* and/or 10–15 lb of force frequently**	☐	☐	☐	☐	☐
HEAVY	Exert 50–100 lb of force occasionally* and/or 25–50 lb of force frequently**	☐	☐	☐	☐	☐
VERY HEAVY	Exert 100 lb of force occasionally* and/or 50 lb of force frequently**	☐	☐	☐	☐	☐

*Occasionally: activity or conditions exist up to 1/3 of the time
**Frequently: activity or conditions exist from 1/3 to 2/3 of the time

■ PHYSICAL REQUIREMENTS:

Indicate the percent of time the following are performed.

The following activities UNDERLINE CANNOT be performed concurrently, so the total should equal 100%.

		N/A	<25%	25%–49%	50%–74%	>75%
KNEEL	To bend legs at the knee, come to rest on knees	☐	☐	☐	☐	☐
CROUCH	To bend the body down and forward, bending the legs and spine	☐	☐	☐	☐	☐
CRAWL	Move on the hands, knees, and feet					
CLIMB	Ascend/descend ladders, stairs, ramps	☐	☐	☐	☐	☐
SIT	For up to 2 hours at a time	☐	☐	☐	☐	☐
STAND	**For up to 2 hours at a time**	☐	☐	☐	☐	☐
WALK	**Move about on foot**	☐	☐	☐	☐	☐

The following CAN be performed concurrently, so the amounts need not be totaled.

		N/A	<25%	25%–49%	50%–74%	>75%
LIFT	To raise or lower an object >10 lb from one level to another	☐	☐	☐	☐	☐
LIFT	To raise or lower an object >25 lb from one level to another	☐	☐	☐	☐	☐
CARRY	To transport an object	☐	☐	☐	☐	☐
PUSH	To press with steady force, thrust objects forward, downward, outward	☐	☐	☐	☐	☐
PULL	To drag or tug objects	☐	☐	☐	☐	☐
BEND	To bend downward and forward by bending the spine at the waist	☐	☐	☐	☐	☐
BALANCE	Exceeding ordinary body equilibrium	☐	☐	☐	☐	☐
REACH	Extend hands and arms, in any direction	☐	☐	☐	☐	☐
HANDLE	Seize, hold, turn with hands	☐	☐	☐	☐	☐
FINGER	Pinch, type, activity with fingers	☐	☐	☐	☐	☐
REPETITIVE MOTION	Repetitive movements of arms, hands, wrists, and so forth	☐	☐	☐	☐	☐
TALK	Express or exchange ideas verbally	☐	☐	☐	☐	☐
HEAR	Perceiving sound by ear	☐	☐	☐	☐	☐
SEE***	Obtain impressions through the eye	☐	☐	☐	☐	☐

***Check all that apply:
☐ Vision clarity greater than 20 inches
☐ Vision clarity less than 20 inches
☐ Ability to distinguish color

■ EQUIPMENT, TOOLS, ELECTRONIC AND COMMUNICATION DEVICES, AND SOFTWARE:

List the items the employee will use to perform the essential/primary functions.

1.		4.	
2.		5.	
3.		6.	

■ PHYSICAL SURROUNDINGS AND HAZARDS:

Indicate which statements are applicable.

- ☐ Spends approximately 80% or more of time indoors.
- ☐ Spends approximately 80% or more of time outdoors.
- ☐ Activities occur inside or outside in approximately equal amounts.
- ☐ Temperatures may be below 32 degrees for more than 1 hour at a time.
- ☐ Temperatures may be above 100 degrees for more than 1 hour at a time.
- ☐ Noise is sufficient to cause the employee to shout in order to be heard.
- ☐ Exposure to vibrating movements to the extremities or entire body.
- ☐ Risk of bodily injury due to proximity to moving mechanical parts, electrical current, animals, and so forth.
- ☐ Conditions that affect the respiratory system or the skin, for example, fumes, odors, air particles.

■ GENERAL INFORMATION:

Comments: _____

Must a vehicle be driven to perform the essential/primary functions? ☐ YES ☐ NO

Location(s) where work is performed: _____

Day/Hour schedule: _____

Name/phone of Supervisor to whom this position reports: _____

Title of Supervisor: _____

Name of person completing form: _____ Date _____

Signature of incumbent:* _____ Date _____

*Signature of person currently in position. If "vacant" or "new," leave blank.

If you are requesting the establishment of a new Merit position or reclassification of existing Merit position, submit this form to:

Compensation and Classification, 121-11 USB.

All merit requisitions must have an EFMA on file in the hiring department before the requisition will be processed.

It is recommended all P & S requisitions have an EFMA on file in the hiring department at the time of advertising.

Comments: _____

Americans with Disabilities Act of 1990, as amended
www.ada.gov/pubs/adastatute08.htm

Americans with Disabilities Act—Accessibility Guidelines for Buildings and Facilities
www.access-board.gov/adaag/html/adaag.htm#toc

Americans with Disabilities Act—Home Page. U.S. Department of Justice, Washington, DC
www.ada.gov

Americans with Disabilities Act—Regulations and Technical Assistance Materials. U.S. Department of Justice, Washington, DC
www.ada.gov/publicat.htm

Craig Hospital Inventory of Environmental Factors (Version 3.0). Craig Hospital, Englewood, CO
www.craighospital.org/repository/documents/Research%20Instruments/CHIEF%20Manual.pdf

Digest of Federal Resource Laws
www.fws.gov/laws/lawsdigest/adminlaws.htm#ARCHBAR

Glossary of Workers' Compensation Terms. American Physical Therapy Association, Alexandria, VA
www.apta.org/Payment/WorkersCompensation/Glossary

Home and Community Environment (HACE) Survey: Instrument and Scoring Manual
www.bu.edu/enact/files/2011/05/HACE-Survey-and-Manual-v1_7-30-2008.pdf

O*NET—Beyond Information—Intelligence. U.S. Department of Labor, Washington, DC
www.doleta.gov/programs/onet

Technology-Related Assistance for Individuals with Disabilities Act of 1988 (Public Law 100-407)
http://codi.buffalo.edu/archives/.legislation/.techact.htm

Telecommunications Act of 1996
www.gpo.gov/fdsys/pkg/BILLS-104s652enr/pdf/BILLS-104s652enr.pdf

The Principles of Universal Design. The Center for Universal Design, North Carolina State University College of Design, Raleigh, NC
www.ncsu.edu/project/design-projects/udi/center-for-universal-design/the-principles-of-universal-design

2010 ADA Standards for Accessible Design. U.S. Department of Justice, Washington, DC
www.ada.gov/regs2010/2010ADAStandards/2010ADAStandards.pdf

Understanding Neighborhood Determinants of Obesity (UNDO)—Assessment Tools: Physical Activity Resource Assessment (PARA), Department of Health and Human Performance, University of Houston, Houston, TX
http://grants.hhp.coe.uh.edu/undo/?page_id=21

Universal Design Institute, Chapel Hill, NC
www.udinstitute.org/whatisud.php.

Workplace Ergonomics Reference Guide: A Publication of the Computer/Electronic Accommodations Program, U.S. Department of Defense, Washington, DC
http://cap.mil/Documents/CAP_Ergo_Guide.pdf

Intervention Strategies for Rehabilitation

Strategies to Improve Motor Function

Susan B. O'Sullivan, PT, EdD

Chapter 10

LEARNING OBJECTIVES

1. Describe a model for clinical decision making that incorporates components of normal motor control and motor learning.
2. Identify factors critical to motor control and describe intervention strategies designed to optimize the acquisition of motor control.
3. Identify key factors in recovery of function and describe intervention strategies designed to optimize recovery.
4. Identify factors critical to motor learning and describe intervention strategies designed to optimize motor learning.
5. Differentiate among the following: functional task-oriented, augmented, and compensatory interventions.
6. Analyze and interpret patient data, formulate anticipated goals and expected outcomes, and develop a plan of care that presents an integrated approach to treatment when presented with a clinical case study.

CHAPTER OUTLINE

Developing strategies to improve motor function (motor control and motor learning) requires a thorough understanding of the neural processes involved in producing movement and learning and the pathologies that may affect the central nervous system (CNS). In addition, knowledge of recovery and neuroplasticity processes following CNS insult is essential. Treatment based on theories of motor control, motor learning, and recovery allows the therapist to organize thinking and approach clinical decision making in a coherent manner. Patients with disorders of the CNS frequently demonstrate impaired motor function with a wide variety of impairments, activity limitations, and restrictions in the ability to participate in normal roles. Careful examination of cognitive, sensoriperceptual, motor, and learning behaviors, along with the environmental contexts in which they occur, provides an appropriate base for planning (see Chapter 5, Examination of

Motor Function: Motor Control and Motor Learning). Different intervention strategies and techniques have been developed by physical therapists to address disorders of motor function. An optimal plan of care (POC) must address the individual needs of the patient. This includes minimizing or eliminating impairments, reducing activity limitations and physical disabilities, and promoting full participation in life roles to the maximum extent possible. An effective POC also enhances overall quality of life.

■ MOTOR CONTROL
Information Processing

Motor control has been defined as "an area of study dealing with the understanding of the neural, physical, and behavioral aspects of biological (e.g., human) movement."[1, p. 497] Information processing of human motor behavior occurs in stages (Fig. 10.1). In the initial stage, *stimulus identification,* relevant stimuli about current body state, movement, and environment, are selected and identified. This includes somatosensory, visual, and vestibular inputs. Meaning is attached based on past sensorimotor experiences. Perceptual and cognitive processes including memory, attention, motivation, and emotional control all play an integral role in ensuring the ease and accuracy of information processing during this stage. Selection of relevant sensory input is sensitive to the clarity and intensity of the stimuli received. Thus, precise and stronger stimuli result in enhanced attentional mechanisms and information processing. Processing is also influenced by stimulus pattern complexity. Complicated and novel patterns of stimuli prolong stimulus identification. An intrinsic knowledge of movement (e.g., position of limb, length of limb, distance to goal, and so forth) is a critical characteristic of motor behavior.

In the *response selection stage* the plan for movement is developed. A **motor plan** is defined as an idea or plan for purposeful movement and is made up of component motor programs. A general rather than detailed response

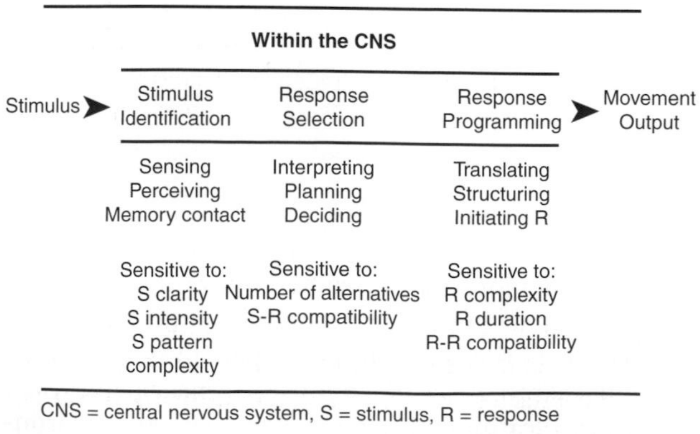

is selected; that is, a prototype of the final movement. Decision making during this stage is sensitive to the number of different movement alternatives possible and the overall compatibility between the stimulus and response. A natural or firmly linked association between stimulus and response enhances the ease of the decision making. For example, in a well-learned movement such as crossing at a streetlight, an individual easily responds to the green light by moving forward. If a crossing guard signals the individual to move forward even though the light is red, the individual is likely to be more hesitant in responding.

The final stage is termed *response programming.* Neural control centers translate and change the idea for movement into muscular actions defined by a motor program. A **motor program** is defined as "an abstract representation that, when initiated, results in the production of a coordinated movement sequence."[1, p. 497] The structuring of motor programs includes attention to specific parameters such as synergistic component parts, force, direction, timing, duration, and extent of movement. Parametric specification is based on the constraints of the individual, the task, and the environment. Information processing during this stage is sensitive to the complexity of the desired movement and duration. Thus, complex and lengthier movement sequences increase the duration of processing during this stage. Programming can also be affected by *response–response compatibility.* This is the compatibility for dual movement tasks that either occur simultaneously (e.g., bouncing a ball while walking) or when choices are required (e.g., one paired movement response must occur before another). During *response execution* (movement output), muscles are selected against an appropriate background of postural control. **Feedforward control** is the sending of signals in advance of movement to ready a part of the system for incoming sensory feedback or for a future motor command.[1] It allows for anticipatory adjustments in postural activity. **Feedback** is response-produced sensory information received during or after the movement and is used to monitor movement output for corrective actions.[1] Although this simplified model gives the appearance that the information flow is linear, actual processing by the CNS is both serial and parallel. Thus, information flows in a specific pathway (serial order) and in multiple pathways (parallel order) in order to process information to more than one center. Many times processing occurs using both serial and parallel order depending on the complexity of the movement.

The association areas of the cortex decide that a movement is called for. The premotor area (PMA) and supplementary motor areas (SMA) (collectively known as Area 6) devise a plan for the movement. The primary motor cortex (Area 4) is located just anterior to the precentral sulcus and issues the motor commands to the descending motor neurons either directly or indirectly

Within the CNS		
Stimulus ▶ Stimulus Identification	Response Selection	Response Programming ▶ Movement Output
Sensing Perceiving Memory contact	Interpreting Planning Deciding	Translating Structuring Initiating R
Sensitive to: S clarity S intensity S pattern complexity	Sensitive to: Number of alternatives S-R compatibility	Sensitive to: R complexity R duration R-R compatibility

CNS = central nervous system, S = stimulus, R = response

Figure 10.1 Model of information-processing stages of movement control.

by way of nuclei and interneurons in the brainstem and spinal cord. A major source of subcortical input arises from the loop from the cortex through the basal ganglia (BG) and back to the cortex, primarily to the SMA via the ventral lateral nucleus (VL) of the dorsal thalamus. This loop functions in assisting in the selection and initiation of voluntary movements. A second motor loop arises from the cortex through the lateral cerebellum and back to the cortex via the VL. This loop also functions in the production of voluntary movement and is concerned with execution of planned, coordinated multijoint movements (i.e., direction, timing, and force). Neurons that give rise to descending pathways are **termed upper motor neurons (UMNs)**. Lateral UMN pathways are involved in the control of voluntary movements through the corticospinal tract. UMN pathways are also involved in indirect control by way of neural subsystems in the brainstem. The reticulospinal tracts and to a lesser extent rubrospinal tracts are the primary alternate route for the mediation of voluntary movement. The tectospinal tract descends from the superior colliculus to the cervical levels and is important for reflex turning of the head. The vestibulospinal tracts are involved in control of postural adjustments and head movements. The ventral horn of the spinal cord gives rise to the peripheral nerve (**lower motor neuron [LMN]**). Activation of muscle fibers is from the motor unit.

Systems Theory

Contemporary theory of motor control has evolved over time, and reflects current understanding and interpretation of nervous system function. The reader is referred to the work of Schmidt and Lee[1] and Shumway-Cook and Woollacott[2] for excellent reviews of this topic. The term **systems theory** is used to describe the process by which various brain and spinal centers work cooperatively to accommodate the demands of intended movements. Both internal factors (joint stiffness, inertia, movement-dependent forces) and external factors (gravity) must be taken into consideration in the planning of movements. Systems theory assumes a shifting locus of neural control, referred to as a *distributed model of control.* Thus, large areas of the CNS may be engaged for complex motor tasks whereas relatively few centers are engaged for more discrete movements. This type of multilevel control allows for the control of a number of separate independent dimensions of movement, termed *degrees of freedom.*[3] The executive level (cortex) can be freed from the responsibility of control of some movements or the demands of having to control many degrees of freedom at one time.[4] For example, the use of central pattern generators (CPGs) in the spinal cord to initiate multijoint and intralimb coordination (coupling) for locomotion is well documented.[5,6] This is in contrast to an older theory of motor control, *hierarchical theory,* in which control was viewed as proceeding only in a descending, top-down direction from higher to lower centers, with the cortex always in control. Multiple descending systems are engaged for control movement and posture. These include corticospinal/corticobulbar, medial (e.g., medial vestibulospinal) and lateral (e.g., reticulospinal, lateral vestibulospinal) descending pathways. Thus, both voluntary (conscious) and involuntary (automatic) pathways regulate posture and movement.

Coordinative Structures

Motor programs allow for movements to occur in the absence of sensation (deafferentation) or in situations in which limitations in speed of processing feedback negate control. Motor programs also free the nervous system from conscious decisions about movement, reducing the problem of multiple degrees of freedom. Preprogrammed instructions to a set of effectors (motor program) run virtually without the influence of peripheral feedback or error detection processes, termed an **open-loop system.**[7] For example, rapid and skilled movements during piano playing occur too rapidly to benefit from feedback and function in an open-loop control system. This is in contrast to a **closed-loop control system**, which employs feedback and a reference for correctness to compute error and initiate subsequent corrections.[1] Feedback and closed-loop processes play a critical role in the learning of new motor skills (response selection) and in the shaping and correction of ongoing movements (response execution). Feedback is also essential for the ongoing maintenance of body posture and balance.[8]

The complexity of human movement negates any simplistic model of movement control. An *intermittent control hypothesis* described by Schmidt and Lee[1] proposes a blending of both open-loop and closed-loop control processes, in which both operate in concert as part of the larger system. Motor programs provide the generalized code for motor events (**schema**) rather than having every specific motor act stored in the brain. Feedback is used to refine and perfect movements.[8] Either may assume a dominant role, depending on the task at hand. Both may operate within a given movement but at different times and with different functions. Generalized motor programs include both invariant characteristics and parameters. *Invariant characteristics* are the unique features of the stored code: relative force, relative timing, and order of components. *Parameters* are the changeable features that ensure flexibility of motor programs and variations in movements from one performance to the next. These include overall force and overall duration of the movement. For example, speeding up or slowing down can change walking performance (changes in speed) while the basic order of stepping cycle and relative timing of the components (invariant characteristics) are maintained.

Muscle **synergies** are used to simplify control, to reduce or constrain the degrees of freedom, and to initiate coordinated patterns of movement. Synergies are functionally linked muscles that are constrained by the CNS to act cooperatively to produce an intended motor action. Control is flexible with the cerebellum acting to generate the appropriate sequence of precise force, timing, and direction. A synergy can act in isolation for discrete movements. More frequently, synergies are combined to produce an appropriate sequence of muscle actions required for a functional task (e.g., the sequence of actions required during a transfer). Synergies are learned through motor skill practice, are flexible, and can be adapted to changes in the task or environment. For example, basic movement strategies (synergies) are well defined for postural control and balance, and include ankle, hip, and stepping strategies.[9-11] The organization and utilization of these strategies varies from quiet to perturbed stance and positions of instability.

■ MOTOR LEARNING

Motor learning has been defined as "a set of internal processes associated with practice or experience leading to relatively permanent changes in the capability for motor skill."[1, p. 497] Learning a motor skill is a complex process that requires spatial, temporal, and hierarchical organization of the CNS. Changes in the CNS are not directly observable but rather are inferred from changes in motor behavior. Improvements in **performance** result from an understanding of the task and practice and are a frequently used measure of learning. For example, with practice an individual is able to develop appropriate sequencing of movement components with improved timing and reduced effort and concentration. A **performance curve** can be used to plot the average performance of a subject or group of subjects across a number of practice trials. Performance, however, is not always an accurate reflection of learning. It is possible to practice enough to temporarily improve performance but not retain the learning. Conversely, factors such as fatigue, anxiety, poor motivation, or medications may cause performance to deteriorate while learning may still occur. Because performance can be affected by a number of factors, it should be viewed as a temporary change in motor behavior observed during practice. **Retention** provides a better measure of learning. Retention, as measured by a **retention test**, refers to the ability of the learner to demonstrate the skill over time and after a period of no practice (**retention interval**).[1] Performance after a retention interval may decrease slightly, but should return to original performance levels within relatively few practice trials. This is referred to as a *warm-up decrement* in performance. For example, riding a bike is a well-learned skill that is generally retained even though an individual may not have ridden for years. The ability to adapt and refine a learned skill to changing task and environmental demands is termed **adaptability**.[2] This is another important measure of motor learning. Individuals who

learn to transfer from wheelchair to platform mat can apply that learning to other types of transfers (e.g., wheelchair to car, wheelchair to tub). The time and effort required to organize and learn these new types of transfers is reduced. Finally, *resistance to contextual change* can be used to measure learning. This is the adaptability required to perform a motor task in altered environmental situations. Thus, an individual who has learned a skill (e.g., walking with a cane on indoor level surfaces) should be able to apply that learning to new and variable situations (e.g., walking outdoors, walking in a busy mall). Motor learning is the direct result of practice and is highly dependent on sensory information and feedback processes. The relative importance of the different types of sensory information varies according to task and to the phase of learning. Individual differences exist in **motor ability**, a relatively stable characteristic or trait that is largely unmodifiable by practice. Abilities underlie and support the development of skills.[1]

Theories of Motor Learning

Adams'[7] theory of motor learning was based on closed-loop control (closed-loop theory). He postulated that sensory feedback from ongoing movement is compared with stored memory of the intended movement (perceptual trace) to provide the CNS with a *reference of correctness* and error detection. Memory traces are then used to produce an appropriate action and to evaluate outcomes. The stronger the perceptual trace developed through practice, the greater the capability of the learner to use closed-loop processes for learning movements. This theory helps to explain learning that occurs during slow, linear-positioning responses. It does not, however, adequately explain learning under conditions of rapid movements (open-loop control processes) or learning that occurs in the absence of sensory feedback (deafferentation studies).

Schema theory, proposed by Schmidt,[8] is an essential concept in motor learning theory. **Schema** is defined as "a rule, concept, or relationship formed on the basis of experience."[1, p. 499] It can be viewed as a generalized motor program (GMP).

Schema allows storage into short-term memory of such things as initial conditions (body position, weight of objects, and so forth), relationships between movement elements, movement outcomes, and sensory consequences of movement. This information is then abstracted into motor memory (**procedural memory**), defined as "the memory for movement or motor information."[1, p. 497] According to schema theory, it consists of two schema, recall and recognition schema. *Recall schema* are used to select and define the relationship among past parameters, past initial conditions, and past movement outcomes produced by these combinations. *Recognition schema* are used to evaluate movement responses and are based on information of the relationships among past initial conditions, past movement outcomes, and the sensory consequences produced by these combinations.[1] Clinically, schema theory supports the concept that "we learn skills by learning rules about the functioning of our bodies—forming relationships between how our muscles are activated, what they actually do, and how these actions feel."[1, p. 448] Practicing a variety of movement tasks and outcomes would improve learning through the development of expanded rules or schema. It also enhances our understanding of how novel and open skills performed in a variable and changing environment are learned.

Stages of Motor Learning

The process of motor learning has been described by Fitts and Posner[12] as occurring in relatively distinct stages, termed *cognitive, associated,* and *autonomous.* These stages provide a useful framework for describing the learning process and for organizing training strategies during rehabilitation. Table 10.1 provides a summary.

Table 10.1 Characteristics of Motor Learning Stages and Training Strategies	
Cognitive Stage Characteristics	**Training Strategies**
The learner develops an understanding of task; **cognitive mapping** assesses abilities, task demands; identifies stimuli, contacts memory; selects response; performs initial approximations of task; structures motor program; modifies initial responses *"What to do"* decision	Highlight purpose of task in functionally relevant terms. Demonstrate ideal performance of task to establish a **reference of correctness.** Have patient verbalize task components and requirements. Point out similarities to other learned tasks. Direct attention to critical task elements. Select appropriate feedback. • Emphasize intact sensory systems, intrinsic feedback systems. • Carefully pair extrinsic feedback with intrinsic feedback. • High dependence on vision: have patient watch movement. • **Knowledge of performance (KP):** focus on errors as they become consistent; do not cue on large number of random errors. • **Knowledge of results (KR):** focus on success of movement outcome. Ask learner to evaluate performance, outcomes; identify problems, solutions. Use reinforcements (praise) for correct performance, continuing motivation. Organize feedback schedule. • Feedback after every trial improves performance during early learning. • Variable feedback (summed, fading, bandwidth designs) increases depth of cognitive processing, improves retention; may decrease performance initially. Organize initial practice. • Stress controlled movement to minimize errors. • Provide adequate rest periods (distributed practice) if task is complex, long, or energy costly or if learner fatigues easily, has short attention, or poor concentration. • Use manual guidance to assist as appropriate. • Break complex tasks down into component parts, teach both parts and integrated whole. • Utilize bilateral transfer as appropriate. • Use blocked (repeated) practice of same task to improve performance. • Use variable practice (serial or random practice order) of related skills to increase depth of cognitive processing and retention; may decrease performance initially. • Use mental practice to improve performance and learning, reduce anxiety. Assess, modify arousal levels as appropriate. • High or low arousal impairs performance and learning. • Avoid stressors, mental fatigue. Structure environment. • Reduce extraneous environmental stimuli, distractors to ensure attention, concentration. • Emphasize closed skills initially gradually progressing to open skills.

Continued

Table 10.1	Characteristics of Motor Learning Stages and Training Strategies—cont'd

Associated Stage Characteristics	Training Strategies
The learner practices movements, refines motor program: spatial and temporal organization; decreases errors, extraneous movements Dependence on visual feedback decreases, increases for use of proprioceptive feedback; cognitive monitoring decreases *"How to do"* decision	Select appropriate feedback. • Continue to provide KP; intervene when errors become consistent. • Emphasize proprioceptive feedback, "feel of movement" to assist in establishing an internal reference of correctness. • Continue to provide KR; stress relevance of functional outcomes. • Assist learner to improve self-evaluation, decision making skills. • Facilitation techniques, guided movements may be counterproductive during this stage of learning. Organize feedback schedule. • Continue to provide feedback for continuing motivation; encourage patient to self-assess achievements. • Avoid excessive augmented feedback. • Focus on use of variable feedback (summed, fading, bandwidth) designs to improve retention. Organize practice. • Encourage consistency of performance. • Focus on variable practice order (serial or random) of related skills to improve retention. Structure environment. • Progress toward open, changing environment. • Prepare the learner for home, community, work environments.

Autonomous Stage Characteristics	Training Strategies
The learner practices movements, continues to refine motor responses, spatial and temporal highly organized, movements are largely error-free, minimal level of cognitive monitoring *"How to succeed"* decision	Assess need for conscious attention, automaticity of movements. Select appropriate feedback. • Learner demonstrates appropriate self-evaluation, decision making skills. • Provide occasional feedback (KP, KR) when errors evident. Organize practice. • Stress consistency of performance in variable environments, variations of tasks (open skills). • High levels of practice (massed practice) are appropriate. Structure environment. • Vary environments to challenge learner. • Ready the learner for home, community, work environments. Focus on competitive aspects of skills as appropriate, e.g., wheelchair sports.

Cognitive Stage

During the initial **cognitive stage** of motor learning, the major task at hand is to develop an overall understanding of the skill, termed the *cognitive map*. This decision making phase of *"what to do"* requires a high level of cognitive processing as the learner performs successive approximations of the task, discarding strategies that are not successful and retaining those that are. The resulting trial-and-error practice initially yields uneven performance with frequent errors. Processing of sensory cues and perceptual–motor organization eventually leads to the selection of a motor strategy that proves reasonably successful. Because the learner progresses from an initially disorganized and often clumsy pattern to more organized movements, improvements in performance can be readily observed during this acquisition phase.

The learner relies heavily on vision to guide early learning and movement. A stable environment free from distractors optimizes learning during this initial stage.

Associative Stage

During the middle or **associative stage** of motor learning, refinement of the motor pattern is achieved through continued practice. Spatial and temporal aspects become organized as the movement develops into a coordinated pattern. As performance improves, there is greater consistency and fewer errors and extraneous movements. The learner is now concentrating on *"how to do"* the movement rather than on what to do. Proprioceptive cues become increasingly important, whereas dependence on visual cues decreases. The learning process takes varying lengths of time depending on a number of factors. The nature of the task, prior experience and motivation of the learner, available feedback, and organization of practice can all influence acquisition of learning.

Autonomous Stage

The final or **autonomous stage** of learning is characterized by motor performance that after considerable practice is largely automatic. There is only a minimal level of attention, with motor programs so refined they can almost "run themselves." The spatial and temporal components of movement are becoming highly organized, and the learner is capable of coordinated motor patterns. The learner is now free to concentrate on other aspects, such as "how to succeed" at a personal goal or competitive sport. Movements are largely error-free with little interference from environmental distractions. Thus the learner can perform equally well in a stable, predictable environment (termed **closed skills**) or in a changing, unpredictable environment (termed **open skills**).

■ CONSTRAINTS ON MOTOR CONTROL AND LEARNING

Patients with neurological lesions may demonstrate impairments in voluntary movements (impaired motor planning or programming) or in the corrective actions (feedback adjustments) needed to initially relearn and coordinate movements. Movements can be uncoordinated with evidence of difficulty initiating or scaling the velocity of movements and controlling force, timing, or direction. Functionally linked synergies may be disorganized or fail to emerge and may show evidence of scaling issues. Reciprocal actions of agonists-antagonists, which normally are fine-tuned, become asynchronous. Disrupted synergistic patterns lead to impairments in body function. Instead of movements that are well matched to the intended movement and the environment, movements become highly stereotyped and limited. Abnormal obligatory or stereotypical synergies may emerge as is seen in the patient recovering from stroke, making it difficult to perform everyday functional tasks. Postural control and balance, a largely automatic function, becomes impaired with evidence of impaired activation of motor strategies, increased conscious control, and difficulty in maintaining balance. Overall, the efficiency and flexibility of motor patterns is significantly reduced.

Additional constraints are imposed by impairments in the musculoskeletal system (e.g., weakness, contracture, postural deformity). Impairments in muscle strength are common in patients with neurological dysfunction. Patients may exhibit complete loss (paralysis or plegia) or partial loss of muscle strength (paresis). Impairments can be localized to one side (hemiplegia), both lower extremities (paraplegia), or all four extremities (tetraplegia). Voluntary movements may become limited or absent with significant loss of the ability to perform common abilities. Fatigue, which can be directly due to a health condition (e.g., MS) or due to secondary factors such as prolonged immobility, often accompanies weakened muscles. Abnormal tone (spasticity or flaccidity) may also limit movement and alter posture. Spasticity and coactivation of agonist-antagonist muscles typically result in fixed, abnormal resting postures, and movements that are characteristically stiff and limited. Hyperactive stretch reflexes and inadequate recruitment of motor neurons present increased challenges for activating and controlling movements. Movements that might be possible at slow speeds become disordered or impossible at faster speeds. Overall, the number, range, and speed of movements are greatly reduced.

Constraints also emerge with impairments in sensory reception or perception, resulting in errors in stimulus identification or response selection. Motor learning is delayed, disorganized, or absent. Response programming may be impaired in the absence of accurate feedback to monitor and correct movement and posture. The central representation of the movement, termed *reference of correctness,* becomes inaccurate as a result of failed or inaccurate feedback. Impairments in cognitive processes (attention, planning, problem solving, emotional stability) may significantly affect learning and motor control. The patient with profound cognitive deficits (e.g., the patient with traumatic brain injury [TBI]) is unable to understand the idea of the movement. This inability to form a *cognitive map* creates severe limitations during the initial stage of learning and is particularly evident with complex or novel movements. Cognitive interference is also readily evident during complex movements such as dual tasking and performing in novel or open environments. Patients with cognitive deficits may also demonstrate a complete lack of awareness of their deficits. Impairments in the cardiovascular system (e.g., limited endurance) can significantly affect movement behavior and the ability to practice. The patient who exhibits profound deficits in motor control and learning can become poorly motivated. Every attempt at movement becomes a frustrating challenge, and activities previously done with ease become labored or impossible. The challenges of learning new motor behaviors can seem insurmountable. In addition to the individual system limitations and impairments discussed above, patients with CNS dysfunction may demonstrate failure of the whole system to function as an integrated whole. The design of a successful intervention needs to be based on careful examination of component parts, as well as the integrated whole.

■ MOTOR SKILLS

Motor development is the evolution of changes in motor behavior occurring as a result of growth, maturation, and experience.[1] Foundational skills are learned in infancy and childhood with the emergence of specific markers of developmental maturation.[13-15] These skills are often referred to as *developmental motor skills* although they are best viewed as *functional motor skills* because they remain a permanent part of movement experience throughout life. Examples include movements such as rolling over and getting up out of bed. Motor skills can be categorized according to specific attributes or characteristics into four main groups:

- **Transitional mobility** refers to skills that allow movement from one posture to another (e.g., supine-to-sit, sit-to-stand).
- **Static postural control,** or *stability,* refers to the ability to maintain a posture with orientation of the center of mass (COM) over the base of support (BOS) and the body held steady (e.g., holding in sitting, kneeling, or standing).
- **Dynamic postural control (controlled mobility)** is the ability to maintain postural stability while parts of the body are in motion. Examples include weight shifting or maintaining a posture with the addition of progressively more challenging movements (e.g., sitting with upper trunk rotation and upper extremity [UE] reaching or standing with lower extremity [LE] stepping).

- **Skill** is the highest level of motor behavior and includes highly coordinated movement patterns such as grasp and manipulation and locomotion.

See Table 10.2 for a description of these categories of motor skills with examples of activities/postures and impairments.

Changes in motor skills are evident throughout the life span. During infancy (birth to 1 year) and childhood (1 to 10 years), changes are rapid and linked to cognitive/perceptual development and experience. During adolescence (11 to 19 years), motor skills become more complex and responsive to increasing cognitive/perceptual development and complex task and environmental demands. In adults, motor skills continue to be refined and are influenced by a number of factors, including age-related changes, overall health and nutrition, activity levels, and emerging pathology.[16-19] In middle adulthood (40 to 59 years), changes associated with aging are moderate in most systems. In older adults (60 years and older), changes are more apparent though there is marked heterogeneity in the aging process. Spirduso et al[19] have identified a continuum of physical function among older adults varying

Table 10.2	Categories of Motor Skills		
Categories	**Characteristics**	**Examples**	**Impairments**
Transitional mobility	Ability to move from one posture to another; BOS and/or COM are changing	Rolling; supine-to-sit; sit-to-stand; transfers	Failure to initiate or sustain movements through the range; poorly controlled movements
Static postural control (stability, static equilibrium, or static balance)	Ability to maintain postural stability and orientation with the COM over the BOS with the body not in motion; BOS is fixed	Holding in antigravity postures: prone-on-elbows, quadruped, sitting, kneeling, half-kneeling, modified plantigrade, or standing	Failure to maintain a steady posture; excessive postural sway; wide BOS; high guard arm position or handhold; loss of balance (COM exceeds BOS)
Dynamic postural control (controlled mobility, dynamic equilibrium, or dynamic balance)	Ability to maintain postural stability and orientation with the COM over the BOS while parts of the body are in motion; BOS is fixed	Weight shifting; UE reaching in any of the above antigravity postures; LE stepping in modified plantigrade or standing	Failure to maintain or control posture during dynamic trunk or extremity movements; loss of balance
Skill	Ability to consistently perform coordinated UE and LE movement sequences for the purposes of investigation and interaction with the physical and social environment; during locomotion, COM is in motion and BOS is changing	UE skills: grasp and manipulation; LE skills: bipedal locomotion	Poorly coordinated movements; lack of precision, control, consistency, and economy of effort

UE = upper extremity; LE=lower extremity; COM = center of mass; BOS = base of support.

from the high ranges of the physically elite and physically fit to a middle range of physically independent to the lower ranges of physically frail, physically dependent and disabled. In the older adult, all stages of information processing are affected.[20] Sensory losses (decline in receptor sensitivity, recognition, and sensory encoding) affect stimulus identification. Response selection and programming are also affected by CNS changes with slowing of reaction time, especially for increasingly complex tasks. An age-related slowing of movement time is well documented.[21] Changes in motor units with a decrease in the overall number and increase in the size of motor units result in impaired coordination, especially for fine motor skills. There is a decreased ability to generate force and an increased tendency to coactivate agonist-antagonist muscles. This coactivation is most likely the result of attempts to modulate movement variability and maintain accuracy.[22] Older adults are also more sensitive to complexity of movement.[23] The principle of *speed–accuracy tradeoff* typically applies as adults age, that is, the accuracy of a movement is decreased as its speed is increased. To accommodate for this change, older adults typically move slower, especially when accuracy is required.[1] Overall movements become less efficient and more variable with age.

Secondary lifestyle factors (nutrition, body weight, exercise) have a significant impact on assisting individuals in maintaining health and in delaying the age of dependency. Decreasing levels of cardiovascular fitness, strength, and endurance and obesity commonly associated with a sedentary lifestyle adversely affect the performance of motor skills. In addition, older adults often experience multiple disease pathologies that affect their ability to move and learn. For example, an older adult may alter the method used to roll over and sit up secondary to an increase in body weight, a decrease in overall strength and fitness, and an emerging pathology such as Parkinson's disease (PD).

■ RECOVERY OF FUNCTION

Recovery of motor performance is defined as the reacquisition of motor patterns that were present before CNS injury. In complete recovery, performance of the reacquired skills is identical in every way to preinjury performance. It is far more likely that the individual with CNS insult will demonstrate recovery using preinjury skills that are modified in some way. Recovery can be further categorized into two main types:

1. **Spontaneous recovery:** the neuronal changes that result from the repair processes occurring within the CNS immediately after the insult, resulting in function being restored in neural tissue initially lost.
2. **Function-induced recovery:** the restoration of the ability to perform a movement in the same or similar manner as it was performed before the injury; occurring in response to changes in activity and the environment (e.g., increased use of involved body segments in behaviorally relevant tasks).

Compensation is defined as the appearance of new motor patterns resulting from the adaptation of remaining motor elements or substitution of alternative motor strategies and body segments. Thus the old movement is performed in a new manner. For example, the patient recovering from severe stroke learns to dress independently using the less affected UE; the patient with a complete T1-level spinal cord injury (SCI) learns to roll using UEs and momentum.[24]

Spontaneous Recovery

Immediately after a brain insult, a cascade of events occurs, producing transient depression of brain activity. Changes at a cellular level occur in the immediate area of damaged brain tissue. Disruption of the blood–brain barrier results in edema, with an accumulation of intracellular fluid and leakage of blood cells, proteins, and other toxic substances that disrupt nerve function. Release of neurotransmitters, glutamate, and calcium activates enzymes associated with neuron death and neuronal degeneration. Free radical damage from toxic particles of oxygen and iron also is associated with cell death. *Denervation supersensitivity,* defined as postsynaptic neuronal hypersensitivity, results in decreased synaptic efficiency. Changes also occur in areas remote from the injured brain. Blood flow changes suggestive of depressed neural activity have been found to exist on both sides of the brain and in both cortical and subcortical structures, areas that are remote from the injured site.[25-27]

Injury-related cortical reorganization is evidenced by a reduction in motor cortex excitability of the involved areas, a decrease in the cortical representation area of paretic muscles, and impairment of motor function. Initial spontaneous recovery that occurs over a relatively short time frame (typically within 3 to 4 weeks) is evidence of return to function of undamaged parts of the brain with the resolution of temporary blocking factors (i.e., shock, edema, decreased blood flow, decreased glucose utilization). This process has been termed *diaschisis.* For example, the patient with cerebral edema following stroke is likely to demonstrate early worsening of clinical signs as edema develops followed by spontaneous improvement within a few weeks as the edema and other factors resolve.[25]

Brain injury was for a long time thought to be permanent with little potential for brain repair. This is now viewed as incorrect and can represent a dangerous *self-fulfilling prophecy* when applied to the individual who suffers from such injuries. **Neuroplasticity** refers to "the ability of the brain to change and repair itself."[25, p. 134] Mechanisms of neuroplasticity include neuroanatomical, neurochemical, and neuroreceptive changes. Anatomical changes include nerve growth (*neural regeneration*) and activation of brain areas previously not active. Trophic molecules (*nerve growth factors*) have been shown to play a key role in growth and repair processes. Nerve cells also change their interactions with each other, with physiological changes occurring at the level of the synapses. *Regenerative synaptogenesis* refers to *sprouting* of the injured axons to innervate (reclaim) previously innervated synapses. *Reactive synaptogenesis (collateral sprouting)* refers to the reclaiming of synaptic sites of the injured axon by dendritic fibers from neighboring axons. Neurotransmitter release and receptor sensitivity are improved *(synaptic plasticity)*. Changes in synaptic strength, known as *long-term potentiation (LTP)*, firm up neuronal connections and serve as a basis for all memory and learning.[26-30]

It is important to remember that the brain is organized with parallel and distributed circuits that provide multiple inputs to many areas with overlapping functions. Different and underutilized areas of the brain (e.g., cortical supplementary and association areas) can take over the functions of damaged tissue, a process known as *cortical remapping*. Another possibility is that the CNS has backup or fail-safe systems *(parallel cortical maps)* that become operational when the primary system breaks down. The unmasking of new, redundant neuron pathways permits cortical map reorganization and maintenance of function. Whole different areas of the brain are also capable of becoming reprogrammed, a process termed *substitution*. An example of substitution is the increased sensitivity of the hands as a sensory information system for the person who becomes blind. In this example, the changes in sensory strategy lead to structural reorganization within the brain. Newer techniques in brain mapping have led to better understanding of these processes. These include (1) positron emission tomography (PET) scanning used to measure regional cerebral blood flow (rCBF), (2) focal transcranial magnetic stimulation (TMS) used to measure responses in motor cortical regions to focal magnetic field stimulation, and (3) functional magnetic resonance imaging (fMRI) used to measure small changes in blood flow during brain activation.[28-31] In summary, recovery is a complex and dynamic process, involving multiple cellular, network, and biochemical processes. It is important to remember that these neuroplastic changes may be *adaptive,* resulting in improved function, or *maladaptive,* resulting in nonfunctional motor behaviors.

Function-Induced Recovery

Function-induced recovery *(use-dependent cortical reorganization)* refers to the ability of the nervous system to modify itself in response to changes in activity and the environment. Repetitive learning behaviors have been shown to prevent degradation and atrophy, enable growth of neurons, strengthen synaptic connections (LTP), alter cortical field representations, and expand topographical areas of motor activity; receptive fields are altered, processing time is improved, and evoked responses demonstrate increased strength and

consistency with improved synchronicity. Improvements in functional outcomes are correlated with observed changes in neural adaptation. These can include improved fine and gross motor coordination, sensory discrimination, postural control and balance, procedural memory, adaptability, and so forth.[32-35] In rehabilitation, constraint-induced movement therapy and locomotor training using partial body weight support (BWS) and a treadmill are examples of targeted interventions to promote function-induced recovery. Changes occur at the level of body function (i.e., the patient moves the limb in a more normal pattern) and at the activity level (the patient reaches or walks with a more normal movement pattern). They differ from conventional or standard care in terms of the high levels of intensity and frequency that are required to improve neural plasticity and function.

There is an accumulating body of research on **constraint-induced movement therapy** (CIMT) in patients following stroke that has demonstrated significant improvements in UE function.[36-45] One important study is the EXCITE Randomized Clinical Trial, a large multisite trial. It consisted of a 2-week CIMT intervention program with training of the more affected UE up to 6 hr/day and use of the mitt on the less affected hand for up to 90% of waking hours. Participants were also encouraged to practice two to three tasks daily at home. Measurements were taken before and after intervention and at 4-, 8- and 12-months' follow-up. Patients in the intervention group showed greater improvement than the control group in all measures of hand function (the Wolf Motor Function Test Performance Time, the Motor Activity Log Amount of Use and Quality of Movement, self-perceived hand difficulty—Stroke Impact Scale).[36,37] Treatment-induced cortical reorganization has also been demonstrated with CIMT.[44,45] Box 10.1 Evidence Summary presents a summary of evidence from selected research in this area. Factors critical to the successful outcomes achieved in these studies include the following:

- A concentrated and repetitive task-specific practice using the more involved UE was utilized (Fig. 10.2). Training was intense, averaging 6 hr/day in CIMT studies. Page et al[41] demonstrated improved function with less intensive, longer duration modified CI therapy (mCIMT). All subjects started with some voluntary movement (wrist and finger extension) in their affected limb.
- Movement was constrained in the less affected UE through the use of a mitt worn up to 90% of waking hours.
- Behavioral techniques were used to enhance adherence and increased use of the affected UE in everyday life. Patients signed a behavioral contract indicating how often and with which activities patients will use their affected limb. Daily administration of the Motor Activity Log (MAL) also increased awareness of using the affected limb, assisting in overcoming

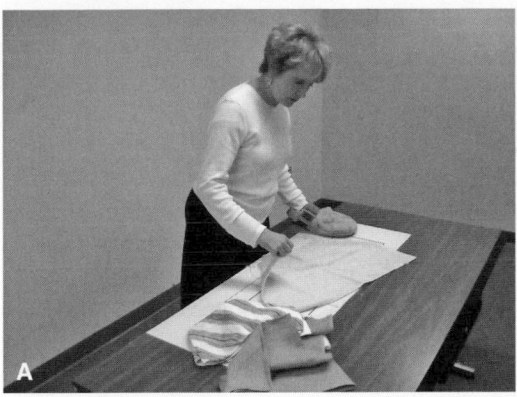 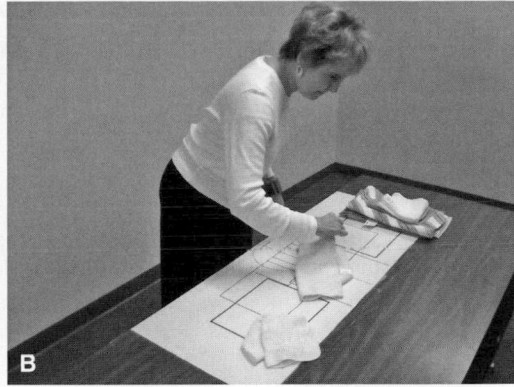

Figure 10.2 Patient is executing a task practice activity involving folding towels and stacking them during **(A)** early and **(B)** later stages of execution. *(From O'Sullivan and Schmitz,[92] with permission.)*

Box 10.1 Evidence Summary   Constraint-Induced Movement Therapy (CIMT)

Reference	Subjects	Design Intervention	Duration	Results	Comments
Wolf et al[36] The EXCITE Randomized Clinical Trial, 2006	106 patients; 3 to 9 months after stroke compared to 116 controls	RCT; prospective, single-blind, RCTs, multisite clinical trial Testing at baseline, after CIMT treatment, and 4-, 8-, and 12-month follow-up	2-week intervention program of CIMT, up to 6 hr/day	CIMT produced statistically significant and clinically relevant improvements in UE motor function that persisted for at least 1 year Improved WMFT performance time; MAL (amount of use and quality of movement); decreased self-perceived hand function difficulty (SIS)	Supports CIMT as an effective treatment for improving UE function post-stroke. This study is important based on its design, sample size, and long-term follow-up.
Sirtori et al[38] Cochrane database, 2009	Systematic review of CIMT and mCIMT; identified 19 studies involving 619 patients; CIMT and mCIMT Intervention included constraint to the normal limb together with exercise of the appropriate quality	Meta-analysis of multiple studies (RCTs, quasi-RCTs) assessing the efficacy of CIMT, mCIMT, or forced use of UE in management of subjects with hemiparesis	Variable	CIMT is associated with a moderate reduction in disability assessed at the end of the treatment period. Disability was measured some months after the end of treatment, there was no evidence of persisting benefit. Majority of studies were underpowered (median number of patients included = 15).	Supports CIMT as an effective treatment for improving UE function post-stroke. Meta-analysis of 19 studies revealed CIMT is a multifaceted intervention. Further RCTs with larger sample sizes and longer follow-up is recommended.

Continued

Box 10.1 Evidence Summary Constraint-Induced Movement Therapy (CIMT)—cont'd

Reference	Subjects	Design Intervention	Duration	Results	Comments
Hakkennes and Keating,[39] 2005	Systematic review of CIMT and mCIMT; identified 14 studies	Meta-analysis of multiple RCTs assessing the efficacy of CIMT compared to control (13 studies) and two CIMT protocols (1 study)	Variable	Significant results in support of CIMT improving UE function when compared to alternative or no treatment	Well-designed and adequately powered trials are required to evaluate the efficacy of different protocols on different stroke populations and to assess the impact on quality of life, cost, and patient/caregiver satisfaction.
Dahl et al,[40] 2008	30 patients with unilateral hand impairment after stroke, inpatient rehabilitation	Single RCT CIMT, restraining mitt used on unaffected hand Testing at baseline, post-treatment, and 6-month follow-up	6 hr/day for 10 consecutive weekdays	CIMT group had shorter performance time and greater functional ability than control group on WMFT. Non-significant trend toward greater hand use (MAL). No differences found on FIM. At 6 months, CIMT group maintained improvement; control group improved more.	Supports CIMT as an effective and feasible method to improve motor function post-stroke in the short term; no long-term effect was found.
Page et al,[41] 2004	17 patients, chronic stroke (> 1 year after stroke)	mCIMT, prospective, multiple-baseline, pre-post, single RCT Intervention: structured PT and OT sessions emphasizing affected UE use in patient-valued functional activities, mitt restraint on less affected hand 5 days/week for 5 hours	30-min sessions, 3×/week for 10 weeks	Improved scores on FMA and ARA for the mCIMT group; amount and quality of UE use as measured by MAL improved only in mCIMT group.	Supports mCIMT as an efficacious method of improving affected UE function and use in patients with chronic stroke. Intense task-specific practice is critical to reacquisition of function; practice schedule intensity is less critical.
Taub et al,[42] 2006	41 patients with chronic stroke (mean = 4.5 years after stroke)	Placebo-controlled trial of CIMT. Two groups: CIMT group: received intensive CIMT training and shaping; placebo group received program of physical fitness, cognitive and relaxation exercises	6 hr/day for 10 consecutive days; CIMT group had restraint of less affected UE for 6 hr/day	CI group showed large and significant improvements in functional use of more affected UE in daily activities (on WMFT, MAL).	Supports efficacy of CIMT for rehabilitating UE motor function in patients with chronic stroke.

Box 10.1 Evidence Summary   Constraint-Induced Movement Therapy (CIMT)—cont'd

Reference	Subjects	Design Intervention	Duration	Results	Comments
		(same length of time; same amount of thera-pist interaction as CIMT group)			
Taub et al,[43] 1993	9 patients, post-stroke with moderate motor deficit (median post-stroke time = 4.1 years) Screening tools for inclusion: Cognitive tests IC: At least 1 year post-stroke; 20° vol-untary wrist extension, 10° finger exten-sion; no cogni-tive or balance problems	Single randomized clinical trial Treatment group: CIMT training of affected UE with restrictive splint/sling worn on nonaffected UE for 90% of waking hours Control group: Received training strategies to focus attention on using affected UE; traditional physi-cal therapy and behavioral shap-ing techniques Pre- and post-treatment testing using WMFT and MAT	7 hr/day, 5 days/week for 2 weeks	Significant and large improvement in motor performance (performance time, quality of move-ment on WMFT) and use of UE (MAT). Gains maintained during 2-year follow-up.	Supports CIMT as an effective treatment for improving UE function post-stroke. Small N; long follow-up period. This is a classic, pioneering study .
Sawaki et al,[44] 2008	30 patients post-stroke in subacute phase (>3 and <9 months)	RCT: Two groups: CIMT treatment group and control group that received usual and custom-ary care and CIMT after study period at 4 months; eval-uated outcomes using TMS at baseline, 2 weeks, and at 4 month follow-up	CIMT given for 10 consecutive weekdays; wore padded mitt for at least 90% of waking hours over 2 weeks	Both CIMT and control group demonstrated improve hand function at 2 weeks. CIMT group showed significantly better grip force after intervention and at follow-up and an increase in size of the TMS motor map area compared to control.	Supports efficacy of CIMT for rehabilitating UE motor function for patients in the suba-cute phase post-stroke. This study is significant in demonstrating enlargement of TMS motor maps and CIMT-dependent plasticity.

ARA = Action Research Arm Test (includes 19 items of UE strength, dexterity, and coordination); BI = Barthel Index (measure of basic ADL and disability); CIMT = constraint-induced movement therapy (intensive, supervised task-specific practice of affected upper extremity [UE] with restriction of nonaffected UE); FMA = Fugl-Meyer Assessment Scale (stroke-specific instrument with UE motor section); mCIMT = modified constraint-induced movement therapy; MAL = Motor Activity Log (structured interview that identifies performance on 30 daily activities); N = number of subjects; NDT = neurodevelopmental treatment; NIHSS = National Institutes of Health Stroke Scale (stroke-specific instrument); OT = occupational therapy; PT = physical therapy; RCT= randomized controlled trial; RAP = Rehabilitation Activities Profile (based on ICIDH, semistructured interview that assesses disabilities and handicaps and consists of 21 items in 5 domains); Rehab = rehabilitation; SIS = Stroke Impact Scale; TMS = transcranial magnetic stimulation; WMFT = Wolf Motor Function Test (a UE functional test that includes 14 timed activities and 2 strength tests).

Table 10.3 Principles of Promoting Function-Induced Recovery	
Focus on active practice of motor skills "Use it or lose it"	Engage the patient in active practice of specific goal-directed activities
Repetition is important	Focus on sufficient repetition to stimulate brain reorganization using high levels of practice both in-therapy and out-of-therapy and a carefully developed home exercise program (HEP)
Intensity is important	Focus on sufficient intensity of training to stimulate brain reorganization, carefully balancing the need for rest with activity
Focus on modifying motor skills "Use it and shape it to the patient's ability"	Continually challenge the patient's movement capability with acquisition of new skills to ensure continued learning; progressively modify skills to achieve functional outcomes
Enhance selection of behaviorally important stimuli	Reinforce behaviorally important stimuli to enhance skill learning; create the best possible environment for learning
Enhance attention and feedback	Actively engage the patient in evaluating goal-achievement and in making accurate adjustments of motor skills based on appropriate use of feedback
Target goal-directed skills	Select skills that are functionally relevant and important to the patient; focus on enhancing patient motivation and commitment; allow for success, select activities that are engaging and fun
Timing is important	Different forms of plasticity occur at different times during training. Very early training may be detrimental in some cases of neural injury (e.g., early intense training in acute after stroke or TBI is associated with exaggeration of cellular injury). Delayed or absent training limits recovery and results in neural degradation and "learned non-use"
Age	Plasticity and adaptive brain changes are strongest in the young; plasticity and brain changes in older adults may be slower and less demonstrable

Adapted from Kleim and Jones.[98]

learned nonuse. Shaping techniques (operant conditioning) and functional training were used to develop challenging intervention tasks. Tasks were selected and tailored to address the specific motor deficits of the patient and shaped to allow for improving movement control and appropriate rest intervals. Feedback, coaching, modeling, and encouragement were provided to set goals, provide motivation, and overcome learned nonuse. Patients were rewarded for improvement and correct movement patterns. Incorrect or poor performance was ignored in an attempt to break the cycle of learned nonuse.

Task-specific locomotor training using partial BWS, a treadmill, and manually assisted trunk and limb movements has also been shown to be effective in promoting function-induced recovery.[46-50] As in CIMT, practice is intense and task-specific. The limbs are loaded to tolerance and active postural control maximized. The treadmill allows control and progression of gait speed and provides rhythmic timing of the stepping movements. Training is progressed by decreasing the amount of loading (BWS) and manual assistance and moving toward overground and community ambulation. See discussion in Chapter 11, Locomotor Training, and Chapter 20, Traumatic Spinal Cord Injury, and the Evidence Summary Boxes in Chapter 15, Stroke, and Chapter 20.

Evidence from animal studies suggests beneficial effects from an enriched environment in promoting brain plasticity and development. Rats raised in enriched environments with opportunities for physical activity and social interaction with other rats demonstrated increased cortical depth, brain weight, dendritic branching, size of synaptic contact areas, and enzyme activity when compared to rats raised in impoverished environments. They also performed significantly better on motor tasks. When brain lesions were induced in rats, exposure to enriched environments and activity before surgical insult had a protective effect with greater sparing of function and improved recovery. Lesioned rats exposed post-surgery to enriched environments also demonstrated improved recovery and performance when compared to those in impoverished surroundings. Finally, socialization influenced outcomes. Rats housed in social groups in enriched environments demonstrated superior recovery over isolated rats.[51-55]

In humans, an unfamiliar and unpredictable hospital or rehabilitation environment may contribute to depression, disorientation, and decline of function. This same environment may be overly structured and protective to the point that it contributes to learned helplessness and disuse. Carr and Shepherd[56] argue that poor recovery after stroke may be partially explained by the impoverished and non-challenging environments that many individuals recovering from stroke are exposed to. Although there are few environmental studies with humans, there is evidence that patients recovering from stroke who were treated on an acute stroke unit demonstrated better recovery and functional outcomes than patients who received a comparable amount of physical therapy while on a general medical unit.[57] This difference could also be due to the better coordination of care and expertise in specialized rehabilitation units. As Carr and Shepherd[58] point out, an important consideration is the amount of "down time" patients typically experience while in rehabilitation. As much as 30% to 40% of the day can be spent in passive pursuits while time in therapy is limited.[59] During non-therapy time, there is often little attention to self-directed practice, thereby further limiting the potential for optimal recovery of function.[60,61] In summary, a rehabilitation POC that focuses on promoting function-induced recovery will emphasize active, task-oriented practice based on the patient's unique needs, an enriched environment, and effective utilization of practice time both in-therapy and out-of-therapy. Principles of promoting function-induced recovery are summarized in Table 10.3.

■ INTERVENTIONS TO IMPROVE MOTOR FUNCTION

Neurorehabilitation interventions have evolved over time for the management of patients with disorders of motor function. Many treatment ideas emerged from empirical knowledge and clinical practice. Theory was applied to explain the success of these interventions and to organize them into a coherent treatment philosophy. Our understanding of motor function and its theoretical base has changed over the years. Emphasis on *evidence-based practice* has resulted in increased validation of therapeutic interventions through research.

The therapist's role is to accurately determine the patient's strengths and limitations and to develop a collaborative POC that includes goals and outcomes that match the patient's unique needs. See Box 10.2 for examples of general goals and outcomes for patients with disorders of motor function. The therapist must also determine an appropriate level of intensity, frequency, and duration of treatment. An important framework for

---

Box 10.2 Examples of General Goals and Outcomes for Patients with Disorders of Motor Function

Impact of pathology/pathophysiology is reduced.

- Risk of recurrence of condition is reduced.
- Risk of secondary impairment is reduced.
- Intensity of care is decreased.

Impact on impairments is reduced.

- Alertness, attention, and memory are improved.
- Joint integrity and mobility are improved
- Sensory awareness and discrimination are improved.
- Motor control is improved.
- Coordination is improved.
- Muscle performance (strength, power, and endurance) is improved.
- Postural control and balance are improved.
- Gait and locomotion are improved.
- Endurance is increased.

Ability to perform physical actions, tasks, or activities is improved.

- Functional independence in activities of daily living (ADL) and instrumental activities of daily living (IADL) is increased.

- Level of supervision for task performance is decreased.
- Tolerance of positions and activities is increased.
- Flexibility for varied tasks and environments is improved.
- Motor learning skills are improved.
- Decision making is improved.
- Safety of patient/client, family, and caregivers is improved.

Disability associated with acute or chronic illness is reduced.

- Ability to assume/resume self-care, home management, work (job/school/play), community, and leisure roles is improved.

Health status is improved.

- Sense of well-being is increased.
- Insight, self-confidence, and self-image are improved.
- Health, wellness, and fitness are improved.
Satisfaction, access, availability, and services are acceptable to patient/client.
Patient/client, family, and caregiver knowledge and awareness of the diagnosis, prognosis, anticipated goals/expected outcomes, and interventions are increased.

Adapted from *Guide to Physical Therapist Practice.*[100]

practice is based on current understanding that movement arises from the interaction of three basic elements: the task, the individual, and the environment (Fig. 10.3).[2] All three components must be considered in developing a successful POC.

Box 10.3 presents a framework of current neurorehabilitation interventions. The interventions are organized from top to bottom starting with *restorative interventions* that are designed to promote and restore optimal functional capacity. These include functional training, defined as activity-based, task-oriented intervention that uses normal patterns to accomplish the task and motor learning strategies. The next level includes impairment-specific and augmented interventions. Augmented interventions include hands-on assistance (guided or assisted movements) and neuromotor development training and are designed to "jumpstart" functional recovery for involved individuals with limited motor function and independent movements. Finally, some individuals will require *compensatory interventions* in the presence of severe impairment, poor prognosis, and multiple co-morbidities. These interventions are designed to promote optimal function using altered movement patterns and strategies using all body segments. A focus on *preventive intervention* is also important. Some activities designed to minimize impairments and disabilities also fall into this category. For example, the patient with stroke who presents with a flaccid and weak shoulder is given

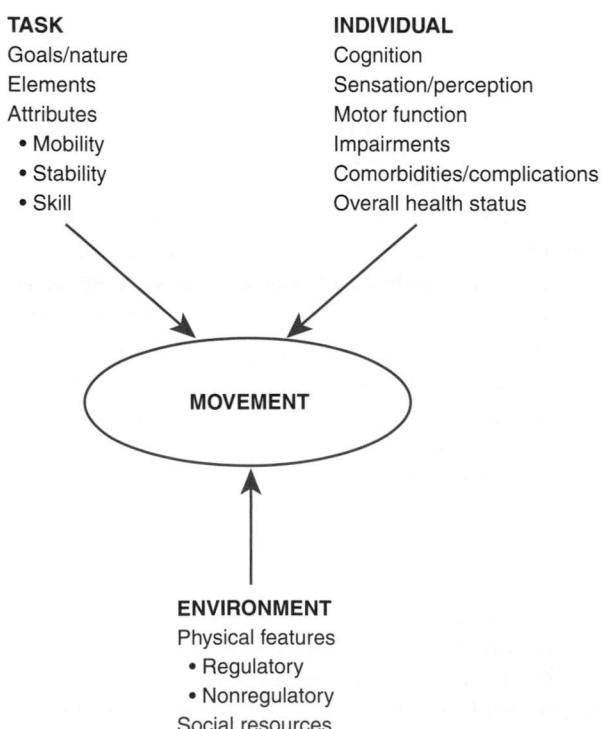

TASK
Goals/nature
Elements
Attributes
 • Mobility
 • Stability
 • Skill

INDIVIDUAL
Cognition
Sensation/perception
Motor function
Impairments
Comorbidities/complications
Overall health status

MOVEMENT

ENVIRONMENT
Physical features
 • Regulatory
 • Nonregulatory
Social resources

Figure 10.3 Movement emerges from interaction between the task, the individual, and the environment.

Box 10.3 Interventions to Improve Motor Function and Functional Independence

Therapeutic Outcome: Improved Motor Function and Functional Independence

Restorative Interventions

Functional Training	Motor Learning Strategies
Task-specific training:	Strategy development
• Functional mobility skills	Feedback
• Activities of daily living	Practice
Environmental context	Transference
Behavioral shaping	Active decision making
Safety awareness training	

Impairment-Specific and Augmented Interventions

Impairment Interventions	Augmented Interventions
Strength, power, endurance	Neurodevelopmental treatment
Flexibility	Neuromuscular facilitation
Postural control and balance	Sensory stimulation
Coordination and agility	Biofeedback
Gait and locomotion	Neuromuscular electrical stimulation
Aerobic capacity/endurance	
Relaxation	

Compensatory Interventions

Substitution training	Assistive/supportive devices

a protective sling to wear during transfer training to reduce the likelihood of shoulder pain and subluxation. Interventions may be used concurrently or in some cases sequentially. For example, the patient with weak hip and knee extensors and limited range of motion (ROM) in hip extension will not be successful in accomplishing sit-to-stand transitions until LE strength is increased and ROM is improved. The following section of the chapter presents an overview of motor learning strategies and therapeutic interventions.

Motor Learning Strategies

Motor learning involves a significant amount of practice and feedback, with a high level of information processing related to control, error detection, and correction. Motor learning can be facilitated through the use of effective training strategies, summarized by stages in Table 10.1.

Strategy Development

The overall goal during the early cognitive stage of learning is to facilitate task understanding and organize early practice. The learner's knowledge of the skill and any existing problems must be ascertained. The therapist should highlight the purpose of the skill in a functionally relevant context. The task should seem important, desirable, and realistic to learn. The therapist should demonstrate the task *(modeling)* exactly as it should be done (i.e., coordinated action with smooth timing and ideal performance speed). This helps the learner develop an internal cognitive map or *reference of correctness.* Attention should be directed to the desired outcome and critical task elements. The therapist should point out similarities to other learned tasks so that schema that are part of other motor programs can be retrieved from memory. Features of the environment critical to performance should also be highlighted.

Highly skilled individuals who have been successfully discharged from rehabilitation can be expert models. Their success in returning to the "real world" will also have a positive effect in motivating patients new to rehabilitation. For example, it is very difficult for a therapist with full use of muscles to accurately demonstrate appropriate transfer skills to an individual with C6 complete tetraplegia. A successful former patient with a similar level injury can accurately demonstrate how the skill should be performed. Modeling has been shown to be effective in producing learning even with unskilled patient models. In this situation, the learner/patient benefits from the cognitive processing and problem solving used while watching the unskilled model attempt to correct errors and arrive at the desired movement.[61] Demonstrations can be live or videotaped. Developing a video library of demonstrations of skilled former patients is a useful strategy to ensure availability of effective models.

Guided movement involves physically assisting the learner through the task to be learned. It can have considerable positive effects during the early period of skill acquisition.[62-64] The therapist's hands can effectively substitute for missing elements, hold a part of the body stable while constraining unwanted movements, reduce errors, and guide the patient toward correct performance. It also allows the learner to preview the tactile and kinesthetic inputs inherent in the task, that is, to learn the *sensations of movement.* The supportive use of hands also allays fears and instills confidence while ensuring safety. Verbal guidance, "talking someone through the task," is also a form of guidance that can be used to improve performance. As discussed previously, improved performance does not represent true learning or retention of a skill. Without *active trial and error, discovery* learning, the changes in performance may be only temporary. The key to success in using guided movements is to limit guidance and intersperse practice with active movements as soon and as much as possible. Overuse of guided movements is likely to result in overdependence on the therapist for assistance, thus becoming a "crutch." The patient who tells you that he or she can only perform the skill if "my therapist" helps or the way "my therapist does it" is demonstrating an overreliance on guided movement. Guidance is most effective for slow postural responses (positioning tasks) and less effective during rapid or ballistic tasks.

During initial practice, the therapist should provide precise feedback, highlighting information critical for movement efficiency. The patient should not be overloaded with excessive feedback or wordy instructions. It is important to reinforce correct performance and intervene when movement errors become consistent or when safety is an issue. The therapist should *not* attempt to correct all the numerous errors that characterize this stage but rather allow for trial-and-error learning. Feedback, particularly visual feedback, is important during the early acquisition phase. The learner should be directed to watch the movements closely. The learner's initial performance trials can also be video recorded for later viewing. Cued or directed viewing of the task improves learning.

During the associated and autonomous phases of learning, the patient continues to refine movement strategies with high levels of practice. Random errors decrease. As consistent errors are identified, feedback may be given and solutions generated. The focus is on refinement of skills and movement consistency in varied environments. This will ensure an overall range of movement patterns that are adaptable and match the changing demands of open environments. The patient's attention should be now focused on proprioceptive feedback, the "feel of the movement." Thus, the patient is directed to attend to the sensations intrinsic to the movement itself and to associate those sensations with the motor actions. Guided movements are counterproductive at this stage because they limit active practice. During late-stage learning, the use of distracters such as ongoing conversation or dual task training (e.g., ball skills during standing and walking) can yield important evidence of a developing level of autonomous control. It is important to remember that many patients undergoing active rehabilitation do not reach this final stage of learning. For example, in patients with TBI, performance may reach consistent levels within structured environments, whereas safe, consistent performance in open, community environments is not possible.

Feedback

The vast body of motor learning literature affirms the critical role of feedback in promoting motor learning. Feedback can be *intrinsic (inherent),* occurring as a natural result of the movement, or *extrinsic (augmented),* incorporating sensory cues provided that are not normally received during the movement. Proprioceptive, visual, vestibular, and cutaneous signals are examples of types of intrinsic feedback; visual, auditory, and tactile cues are forms of extrinsic feedback (e.g., verbal cues, manual cues, biofeedback devices such as the electromyogram [EMG], pressure-sensing devices [force plates, foot pad]). During therapy, both intrinsic and extrinsic feedback can be manipulated to enhance motor learning. The use of augmented feedback serves as an important source of information and helps the learner link associations between the movement parameters and resulting action.[1] *Concurrent feedback* is given during task performance, while *terminal feedback* is given at the end of task performance. Augmented feedback about the nature of the end result produced in relation to the goal is termed **knowledge of results (KR)**. Augmented feedback about the nature or quality of the movement pattern produced is termed **knowledge of performance (KP)**.[1] Although both are important, the relative usefulness of KP and KR can vary according to the skill being learned and the availability of feedback from intrinsic sources.[65-69] For example, tracking tasks are highly dependent on intrinsic visual and kinesthetic feedback (KP) whereas KR has less influence on the accuracy of the movements. In other tasks (e.g., transfers) KR provides the key information about how to shape the overall movements for the next attempt whereas KP may not be as useful. Performance cues (KP) should focus on key task elements that lead to a successful final outcome.

Therapists must consider the cognitive and physical resources of patients and the complexity of the tasks to be learned in determining the type of feedback possible. Clinical decisions about feedback include the following issues:

- What type of feedback should be employed (*mode*)?
- How much feedback should be used (*intensity*)?
- When should feedback be given (*scheduling*)?

Choices about type of feedback involve the selection of which intrinsic sensory systems to highlight, what type of augmented feedback to use, and how to pair extrinsic feedback to intrinsic feedback. The selection of sensory systems depends on specific examination findings of sensory integrity. The sensory systems selected must provide accurate and usable information. If an intrinsic sensory system is impaired and provides distorted or incomplete information (e.g., impaired proprioception with diabetic neuropathy), use of alternate sensory systems (vision) should be emphasized. Supplemental augmented feedback can be used to enhance learning. Decisions are also based on stage of learning. Early in learning, visual feedback is easily brought to conscious attention and therefore is important. Less consciously accessible sensory information such as proprioception should be emphasized during the middle and end stages of learning. Decisions about frequency and scheduling of feedback (when and how much) must be reached. Frequent augmented feedback (e.g., given after every trial) quickly guides the learner

to the improved performance but slows retention and overall learning. Conversely, feedback that is varied (not given after every trial) slows initial performance of the skill while improving performance on a retention test.[70-74] This is most likely due to the increased depth of cognitive processing that accompanies the variable presentation of feedback. In contrast, the therapist who bombards the patient immediately after task completion with excessive augmented verbal feedback may preclude active information processing by the learner.[75,76] The patient's own decision making skills are minimized, while the therapist's verbal skills dominate. Winstein[77] points out that this may well explain why many studies on the effectiveness of therapeutic approaches cite minimal carryover and limited retention of newly acquired motor skills. Finally, the withdrawal of augmented feedback should be gradual and carefully paired with the patient's efforts to correctly utilize intrinsic feedback systems. Table 10.4 summarizes the types and uses of augmented feedback.

Practice

The second major influence on motor learning is practice. *General principles of practice* are (1) increased practice results in increased learning and (2) large and rapid improvements in performance are typically observed initially with smaller improvements noted over time. The therapist's role is to prepare the patient for practice and to ensure that the patient practices the desired movements. Practice of incorrect movement patterns can lead to a *negative learning* situation (interference) in which "faulty habits and postures" must be unlearned before the correct movements can be mastered. The organization of practice will depend on several factors, including the patient's motivation, attention span, concentration, and endurance, and the type of task. Making the task seem important and attainable improves motivation and commitment to practice. Patients who are involved in goal setting and recognize specific practice parameters (task purpose, schedule, limits) demonstrate improved commitment to practice. An additional factor that influences practice is the frequency of allowable therapy sessions, which is often dependent on hospital scheduling and availability of services and payment. Planning for effective use of out-of-therapy practice is important for all patients but especially so for patients with limited access to physical therapy. For outpatients, practice at home is highly dependent on motivation, family support, and suitable environment.

Therapists must consider the cognitive and physical resources of patients and the complexity of the tasks to be learned in determining the type of practice possible. Clinical decisions about practice include the following issues:

- How should practice periods and rest periods be spaced (*distribution of practice*)?

Table 10.4 Types of Augmented Feedback[1]

Concurrent feedback	Feedback is presented during the movement; KP information is provided; e.g., information about joint position; importance of forward weight shift to position the COM over the BOS during sit-to-stand training; or biofeedback; best used to highlight information not readily available from intrinsic feedback and if linked to active problem-solving
Terminal feedback	Feedback is given after the movement
Immediate feedback	Feedback is presented immediately after the movement
Delayed feedback	Feedback given after a brief time delay allows the learner a brief time for introspection and self-assessment; e.g., a 3-second delay Feedback given after long delays is contraindicated, especially if other movements not related to the task occur in between, degrading learning
Summary feedback	Feedback given after a set number of trials; e.g., after every 2nd trial or every 5th or every 20th trial
Faded feedback	Feedback given first after every trial, then less frequently on subsequent blocks of trials; e.g., after every 1st trial progressing to every 3rd trial, then to every 5th trial
Bandwidth-KR feedback	Feedback given only when performance deviates outside the boundaries of correct performance; error range is predetermined (e.g., top and bottom range of errors is determined)
Blocked feedback	One source of feedback is provided; KR is presented about the same segment on consecutive trials; learner processes a limited information about the task; e.g., during gait training, KR is presented about knee segment only on successive trials Blocked KR improves performance of the identified segment but may not improve performance and learning of the whole task (multiple segments); performance deteriorates once KR withdrawn
Variable (random) feedback	Multiple sources of feedback are provided; KR is presented about different segments on successive trials; e.g., during gait training, KR is presented about various different body segments (trunk, hips, knees) on successive trials Random KR is superior in improving both performance and learning of a task; encourages learner to process a wider range of information about the task

- What tasks and task variations should be practiced (*variability of practice*)?
- How should the tasks be sequenced (*practice order*)?
- How should the environment be structured (*closed vs. open*)?
- What tasks should be practiced in a parts-to-whole sequence?

Distribution: Massed Versus Distributed Practice

Massed practice refers to "a sequence of practice and rest times in which the rest time is much less than the practice time."[1, p. 497] Fatigue, decreased performance, and risk of injury are factors that must be considered when using massed practice. *Distributed practice* refers to "a sequence of practice and rest periods in which the practice time is often equal to or less than the time at rest."[1, p. 494] Although learning occurs with both, distributed practice results in the most learning per training time, although the total training time is increased. It is the preferred mode for many patients undergoing active rehabilitation who demonstrate limited performance capabilities and endurance. With adequate rest periods, performance can be improved without the interfering effects of fatigue or increasing safety issues. Distributed practice is of benefit if motivation is low or if the learner has a short attention span, poor concentration, or motor planning deficits (e.g., dyspraxia). Distributed practice should also be considered if the task itself is complex, is long, or has a high energy cost. Massed practice can be considered when motivation and skill levels are high and when the patient has adequate endurance, attention, and concentration. For example, the patient with SCI in the final stages of rehabilitation may spend long practice sessions acquiring the wheelchair skills needed for community access.

Blocked Versus Random Practice

Blocked practice refers to "a practice sequence in which all of the trials on one task are done together, uninterrupted by practice on any of the other tasks."[1, p. 493] *Random practice* refers to "a practice sequence in which the tasks being practiced are ordered randomly across trials."[1, p. 498] Although both allow for motor skill acquisition, random practice has been shown to have superior long-term effects in terms of retention.[78-80] For example, a variety of different transfers (e.g., bed-to-wheelchair, wheelchair-to-toilet, wheelchair-to-bathtub transfer seat) can be practiced all within the same training session. Although skilled performance of individual tasks may be initially delayed, improved retention of transfer skills can be expected. The constant challenge of varying the task demands provides high *contextual interference* and increases the depth of cognitive processing through retrieval practice from memory stores. The acquired skills can then be applied more easily to other task variations or environments. Constant practice will result in superior initial performance because of low contextual interference and is required in certain situations (e.g., the patient with TBI and profound cognitive and behavioral deficits who requires a high degree of structure and consistency for learning; the patient with advanced PD).

Practice Order

Practice order refers to the sequence in which tasks are practiced. *Blocked order* refers to the repeated practice of a task or group of tasks in order (three trials of task 1, three trials of task 2, three trials of task 3: 111222333). *Serial order* refers to a predictable and repeating order (practice of multiple tasks in the following order: 123123123). *Random order* refers to a nonrepeating and nonpredictable order (123321312). Although skill acquisition can be achieved with all three, differences have been found. Blocked order produces improved early acquisition of skills (performance) whereas serial and random order produce better retention and generalizability of skills. This is again due to contextual interference and increased depth of cognitive processing.[81,82] The key element here is the degree to which the learner is actively involved in memory retrieval. For example, a treatment session can be organized to include practice of a number of different tasks (e.g., forward-, backward- and side-stepping and stair climbing). Random ordering of the tasks may initially delay acquisition of the desired stepping movements but over the long term will result in improved retention and generalizability.

Mental Practice

Mental practice is "a practice method in which performance on the task is imagined or visualized without overt physical practice."[1, p. 497] Beneficial effects result from the cognitive rehearsal of task elements. It is theorized that underlying motor programs for movement are activated but with subthreshold motor activity.[1] Brain mapping techniques have also revealed activation of similar brain areas during imagined movements as those activated during actual movement.[83-84] Mental practice has consistently been found to facilitate the acquisition of motor

skills.[85-88] It should be considered for patients who fatigue easily and are unable to sustain physical practice. Mental practice is also effective in alleviating anxiety associated with initial practice by previewing the upcoming movement experience. Mental practice when combined with physical practice has been shown to increase the accuracy and efficiency of movements at significantly faster rates than physical practice alone.[89] When using mental practice, it is important to make sure the patient understands the task and is actively rehearsing the correct movement. Having the patient verbalize aloud the steps being rehearsed can ensure that this occurs. It is generally contraindicated in patients with profound cognitive, communication, and/or perceptual deficits.

Part–Whole Practice

Complex motor skills can be broken down into component parts for practice. The component parts are practiced before practice of the whole task is attempted. For example, during initial wheelchair transfer training the individual steps are practiced in isolation before practicing the whole transfer (e.g., locking the brakes, lifting the foot pedals, moving forward in the chair, standing up, pivoting, and sitting down). It is important to identify the key steps through accurate task analysis and to sequence them in the required order. It is also important to practice the integrated whole in conjunction with the parts practice so that the learner develops the whole idea for the required task (i.e., cognitive mapping). Delaying practice of the integrated whole can interfere with transfer effects and learning.[1] Part–whole practice is most effective with discrete or serial motor tasks that have highly independent parts. Part–whole practice is not as effective for continuous movement tasks (e.g., walking) or for complex tasks with highly integrated parts. Both require a high degree of coordination with spatial and temporal sequencing of elements. For these tasks, practice of the integrated whole will result in superior learning.

Transfer Training

Transfer of learning refers to the gain (or loss) in the capability of task performance as a result of practice or experience on some other task. Learning can be promoted through practice using contralateral extremities, termed *bilateral transfer*. For example, a patient with stroke first practices the desired movement pattern using the less affected extremity. This initial practice enhances formation or recall of the necessary motor program, which can then be applied to the opposite, involved extremity. This method cannot, however, substitute for lack of movement potential of the affected extremities (e.g., a flaccid limb on the hemiplegic side). Transfer effects are optimal with similarity of the tasks (e.g., identical components and actions) and environments.[90] For example, optimal transfer can be expected with practice of a UE flexion pattern first on one side, then with an identical pattern on the other side.

Practice of **lead-up tasks** is commonly used in physical therapy. Lead-ups are tasks or activities presented to prepare learners for a more important or complex task or activity.[1, p. 496] The subtasks are practiced, typically in easier postures with significantly reduced degrees of freedom. Anxiety is also reduced and safety is ensured. Thus initial upright postural control can be practiced with activities in kneeling, half-kneeling, or plantigrade before standing. The patient develops the required trunk and hip extension/abduction stabilization control required for upright stance but without the demands of the full standing position or fear of falling. The more closely the lead-ups (subskills) resemble the final task, the better the transfer. For example, bridging, which involves hip extension to neutral in a supine hook-lying position, can be a lead-up to successful sit-to-stand transitions. Table 10.5 summarizes the types of practice and practice parameters.

Promoting Active Patient Decision Making and Autonomy

Fundamental psychological needs of the patient include autonomy, competence, and social-relatedness.

For effective planning, the therapist needs to have a clear understanding of the patient's values (beliefs and attitudes), self-perceptions, preferences, outcomes expectation, and sense of *self-efficacy* (a belief that the patient can accomplish the task successfully). Focus on the development of decision making skills is critical in ensuring perceived confidence, continued learning, and problem-solving success in the patient's real world environment. The therapist also needs to communicate effectively, develop rapport, and support the patient in collaborative planning. Having the patient actively involved in self-monitoring, analysis, and self-correction of movements encourages self-determined behavior. Trial-and-error learning can only be successful if the patient is challenged to think about the movement, to consider the information feedback received about the movement's performance, and to evaluate the movement outcome.[91] Key questions to promote active decision making and autonomy are presented in Box 10.4.

The therapist should allow adequate time for reflection and confirm the accuracy of the patient's responses. For example, if the patient's efforts do not achieve the

Table 10.5	Types of Practice and Practice Parameters[1]
	Types of Practice
Massed practice	A sequence of practice and rest times in which the rest time is much less than the practice time
Distributed practice	Spaced practice intervals in which the practice time is equal to or less than the rest time
	Practice Sequence
Blocked practice	A practice sequence organized around one task performed repeatedly, uninterrupted by practice of any other task
Random practice	A practice sequence in which a variety of tasks are ordered randomly across trials
	Practice Order
Blocked order	The repeated practice of a task or group of tasks in order; three trials of task 1, three trials of task 2, three trials of task 3 (e.g., 111222333)
Serial order	A predictable and repeating order; practice of multiple tasks in the following order (e.g., 123123123)
Random order	A nonrepeating and nonpredictable order of multiple tasks (e.g., 123321312)
	Practice Strategies
Mental practice	A practice strategy in which performance of the motor task is imagined or visualized without overt physical practice
Part/whole practice	Component parts of a task are practiced before practice of the whole task
Transfer training	The gain (or loss) in the capability of task performance as a result of practice or experience on some other task • Acquisition of motor skills in one training experience enhances acquisition of similar or related skills (*positive learning*) • Acquisition of motor skills in one training experience interferes with acquisition of other skills (*negative learning*)
Practice of lead-up activities	Simpler task versions of the required complex task are practiced

---

Box 10.4   Key Questions to Promote Active Patient Decision Making and Autonomy

- What is the goal of the intended movement?
- Did you accomplish the goal? If no, does the goal need to be modified?
- Did you move as planned? If no, what problems were encountered during the movement?
- What do you need to do to correct the problems in order to achieve movement success?
- For complex movements, what are the component parts or steps of the task? How should the component parts be sequenced?
- What aspects of the environment led to the success (or failure) of reaching the goal of the intended movement?
- What motivates you to keep trying?
- How confident are you in your abilities to move on your own? To be safe in your home environment?

---

expected outcome, the patient can be challenged to consider why. The patient who consistently falls to the right while standing can be challenged with questions such as, "In what direction did you fall?" and "What do you need to do to correct this problem?" The therapist has an important role as a motivational coach ("We can do this together as a team"). This includes emphasizing the patient's capabilities rather than failures and pointing out successes in improving function and obstacles that have been overcome on a regular basis. Beginning and ending the therapy session with a positive and successful movement experience is also a useful strategy to improve self-efficacy.

Functional Training

Functional, task-specific training is based on careful examination of motor function and activity performance (see Chapter 8, Examination of Function). Tasks targeted during early rehabilitation include basic activities of daily living (BADL) (e.g., feeding, dressing, hygiene, and so forth) and functional mobility skills (FMS) (e.g., bed mobility, transfers, locomotion). Later in rehabilitation instrumental activities of daily living (IADL) (e.g., home chores, shopping), community mobility, and work activities are targeted, depending on the patient's level of recovery and discharge placement. Task analysis yields an understanding of task, the essential elements within the task, and the context or environment in which the task occurs (see Chapter 5, Examination of Motor Function: Motor Control and Learning, Box 5.1). The therapist then selects activities and modifies task demands based on this analysis to determine an appropriate POC.

As previously discussed, extensive practice and appropriate feedback are essential in order to reacquire skills

and enhance recovery. Involved segments are targeted for training. For example, training the patient with stroke focuses on use of the more involved extremities during daily tasks whereas use of the less involved extremities is minimized (e.g., CIMT). Initial tasks are selected to ensure patient success and motivation (e.g., grasp and release of a cup for feeding, forward reach for UE dressing). Tasks are modified to permit early practice. For example, training using partial BWS and a motorized treadmill provides a means of early locomotor training for patients with stroke or incomplete spinal cord injury. Tasks are continually modified to increase the level of difficulty, promote adaptation of skills, and promote independence. For example, sit-to-stand training begins with standing up from a raised seat. Progressively lowering the seat height during training increases the difficulty of the task until the patient is able to stand up from a normal seat height. During early training assistive devices may be used to assist function (e.g., for transfer training, gait and locomotion, dressing). The goal is to transition the patient away from using such devices toward independent function as soon as the patient is able. Continued use of and dependence on assistive devices falls under the category of compensatory training (e.g., wheelchair training for the patient with complete paraplegia).

Functional training represents a shift away from some conventional rehabilitation approaches that utilize an extensive hands-on approach to promote recovery and/or substitution. Although initial movements can be assisted in functional training, active movements are the overall goal. The therapist's role is one of training coach, structuring practice and providing appropriate challenge and feedback while encouraging the patient. Task-oriented training effectively counteracts the effects of immobility and the development of indirect impairments such as muscle weakness or loss of flexibility. It also prevents *learned nonuse* of the involved segments while stimulating CNS recovery.

Achieving control in various different functional activities and postures is a primary focus of intervention during rehabilitation. Careful attention to the demands of the postures can effectively address the degrees of freedom problem in controlling body segments and influence the selection of lead-up skills. For example, the prone-on-elbows posture focuses on development of shoulder, upper trunk, and head control while eliminating all demands for movement control in the lower body; because the COM is low and the BOS is wide, the posture is inherently safe. The kneeling posture can be used to improve trunk and hip control without the demands for control of the knee and ankle. As with the prone-on-elbows posture, the low COM and wide BOS reduce the likelihood of falls and injury. See Table 10.6 for a summary of postures and potential treatment benefits. Refer to O'Sullivan and Schmitz's *Improving Functional Outcomes in Physical Rehabilitation*[92] for a more in-depth discussion.

Table 10.6 Functional Postures and Potential Treatment Benefits	
Posture	Treatment Benefits
Prone-on-elbows	• Improve upper trunk, UE, and neck/head control • Weight-bearing through shoulders, elbows flexed • Increase extensor ROM at hip extensors • Improve head/neck and shoulder stabilizers strength • Wide BOS, low COM; inherently safe • Limits degrees of freedom: control of lower trunk and LEs not required
Quadruped	• Improve upper trunk, lower trunk, LE hips, UE (shoulders, elbows), and neck/head control • Weight-bearing through hips and shoulders and extended UEs • Improve hip, shoulder, and elbow stabilizers strength • Decrease extensor tone at knees by prolonged weight-bearing • Decrease flexor tone at elbows, wrists, and hands by prolonged weight-bearing • Increase extensor ROM at elbows, wrists and fingers • Wide BOS, low COM • Limits degrees of freedom: control of LE knees and feet, UE hands not required; allows UEs to share postural loading and support with LEs
Bridging	• Improve lower trunk and LE control • Increase hip stabilizers strength • Weight-bearing through feet and ankles • Lead-up activity for bed mobility, sit-to-stand • Wide BOS, low height of COM • Limits degrees of freedom: control of upper trunk, head/neck, and UE not required
Sitting	• Improve upper trunk, lower trunk, LE, and head/neck control • Weight-bearing in upright, antigravity position; can include weight-bearing through extended UEs • Functional posture, important for reaching and ADL skills • Improve balance reactions • Medium BOS, medium height of COM • Limits degrees of freedom: control of LEs not required
Kneeling and half-kneeling	• Improve head/neck, upper trunk, lower trunk, and LE control • Weight-bearing through hips in upright, antigravity position • Decrease extensor tone at knees by prolonged weight-bearing • Increase hip and trunk stabilizers strength • Improve balance reactions • Weight-bearing through ankle in half-kneeling • Narrow BOS, intermediate height of COM (kneeling) • Wide BOS, intermediate height of COM (half-kneeling) • Limits degrees of freedom: control of LE knees, feet/ankles not required in kneeling
Modified plantigrade	• Improve head/neck, upper trunk, lower trunk, and UE and LE control • Weight-bearing through extended UEs and LEs, upright antigravity position • Improve balance reactions • Functional posture, lead-up for standing, stepping and reaching • Decrease tone in elbow, wrist, and finger flexors by prolonged weight-bearing • Increase extensor ROM at wrists and fingers • Wide BOS, high COM • Requires control of multiple degrees of freedom of head/neck, trunk, UEs and LEs: allows UEs to share postural loading and support with LEs
Standing	• Improve head/neck, upper trunk, lower trunk, and LE control • Weight-bearing through extended LEs, full upright, antigravity position • Improve balance reactions • Functional posture, important for ADL skills; lead-up for gait • Narrow BOS, high COM • Requires maximum control of multiple degrees of freedom of head/neck, trunk, LEs

ADL = activities of daily living; BOS = base of support; COM = center of mass; LE = lower extremity; ROM = range of motion; UE = upper extremity.

Intense task-oriented training may not be appropriate for every patient. Its selection is dependent on the degree of recovery and severity of motor deficits. Research findings suggest that early overemphasis on use-dependent training may actually increase the vulnerability of the brain to additional damage in animals[93,94] and in humans.[95-98] Patients who are not able to participate in task-oriented training include those who lack voluntary control or cognitive function. For example, a patient with TBI who is in the early recovery stages has limited potential to participate with this type of intensive training. Similarly, patients with stroke who experience profound UE paralysis and perceptual deficits would not be candidates for CIMT UE training. One of the consistent exclusion criteria for CIMT has been inability to perform voluntary wrist and finger extension of the more involved hand. Thus, threshold abilities to perform the basic components of the task need to be identified. Careful analysis of underlying impairments with a focus on intervention (e.g., improved strength, ROM) complements task-oriented training. For example, during locomotor training using BWS and a treadmill system, stepping and pelvic motions are guided into an efficient motor pattern. To participate in this type of training, essential prerequisites include basic head stability during upright positioning.

Environmental Context

Altering the environmental context is an important consideration in structuring practice sessions. During early learning many patients benefit from practice in a stable, or predictable, *closed environment*. As learning progresses the environment should be varied and incorporate more variable features consistent with real world, *open environments*. Practicing walking only within the physical therapy clinic might lead to successful performance in that setting (*context-specific learning*) but does little to prepare the patient for ambulation at home or in the community. The therapist should begin to gradually modify the environment as soon as performance becomes consistent. Consideration must be given to practice in a safe environment where the patient can learn without the risk of injury or outright failure. Simulated environments (e.g., Easy Street Environments) are found in many rehabilitation centers. They can serve as an intermediate practice environment before the patient moves to the home or community setting. It is important to remember that some patients (e.g., a patient with TBI and limited cognitive recovery) may never be able to function in anything but a highly structured environment.

Behavioral Shaping

Behavioral shaping refers to the use of techniques designed to systematically progress the level of difficulty of the tasks practiced. The therapist provides immediate and explicit feedback to shape and improve performance.

Attention is directed toward the successful aspects of performance. Thus the therapist serves to direct and motivate the patient toward optimal performance. The tasks chosen should be within the capabilities of the patient. Excessive effort, which can degrade performance and motivation, is avoided. The patient is kept focused on the training activity, fully informed of progress, and continually challenged.[99]

Safety Awareness Training

An important element of functional training is injury prevention or reduction. First and foremost is safety awareness training during self-care activities, postural control and balance activities, and functional mobility. For example, during postural awareness training, the patient learns to define limits of stability (LOS) during weight shifts. During anticipated or reactive perturbations, the patient learns how to react to these destabilizing forces with appropriate adjustments that maintain posture and balance. Identifying fall risk and developing strategies to reduce fall risk are important elements of functional mobility training. Instruction in the use of assistive devices and equipment is also accompanied by safety awareness training. For example, the patient with SCI learns to safely transfer into and out of the tub during bathing and to avoid risk of injury by testing water temperature before emersion. Finally, *secondary prevention* (efforts to decrease the severity of disability and sequelae through early diagnosis and prompt intervention) is an important component of rehabilitation. For example, prevention and management of UE overuse injury is an important component in the rehabilitation of patients with SCI who are wheelchair users.

Box 10.5 presents a summary of task-oriented training strategies to promote function-induced recovery.

Impairment Interventions

Task analysis reveals if the patient is able to perform the functional activity and its basic components. Additional examination and evaluation can reveal if a specific impairment or group of impairments is linked to the functional/task limitation. The therapist then needs to focus on specific interventions to improve performance. For example, a patient with multiple sclerosis (MS) demonstrates inability to stand up or transfer without moderate assistance of one. Lower extremity weakness in hip and knee extension is identified. Strength training of these muscles needs to be a targeted intervention. It is important to remember that resolution of the impairment may still not yield the desired functional performance. It is entirely possible that other impairments, previously masked by an inability to perform the task, were also contributing to the patient's inability to stand up independently (e.g., balance impairments). Without attention to correcting impairments, continued functional training has the potential of delaying recovery and creating a host of faulty movement patterns that

Box 10.5   Functional, Task-Oriented Training Strategies

Emphasize early training.

• To promote use-dependent cortical plasticity and overcome learned nonuse.

Define the goal of task practice.

• Involve the patient in goal setting and decision making, thereby enhancing motivation and promoting active commitment to recovery.

Determine the activities to be practiced.

• Consider the patient's past history, health status, age, interests, and experience.
• Consider the patient's abilities/strengths, level of recovery, learning style, impairments, and activity limitations.
• Determine a set of activities to be practiced for each training goal.
• Select activities that are interesting, stimulating, and important to the patient.
• Choose activities with the greatest potential for patient success and intersperse more difficult tasks with easier tasks.
• Target active movements involving the affected extremities.
• Constrain or limit use of unaffected extremities; set parameters, time limits for use of constraints.
• Prevent or limit compensatory strategies.

Determine the parameters of practice.

• Manage fatigue, determine rest and practice times.
• Model ideal performance; establish a *reference of correctness*.
• Establish requirements for intensity, minimal number of repetitions.
• Establish practice schedule of tasks (blocked or variable); shift to variable practice as soon as possible to enhance retention.
• Determine the practice order of tasks (constant, serial, random); shift to random order as soon as possible to enhance retention.
• Control use of instructions and augmented feedback to promote learning.
• Control use of assisted or guided movements to promote initial learning; ensure that the patient successfully transitions to active movements as soon as possible.

Utilize behavioral shaping techniques.

• Gradually modify the task to increase the challenge and make it progressively more difficult as patient performance improves.
• Provide immediate and explicit feedback; recognize and acknowledge small improvements in task performance.
• Emphasize positive aspects of performance.
• Avoid excessive effort because it degrades performance and dampens motivation.

Promote problem-solving.

• Have the patient evaluate performance, identify obstacles, generate potential solutions, choose a solution, and evaluate outcome.
• Relate successes to overall goals.

Structure the environment.

• Promote initial practice in a supportive environment, free of distractors (closed environment).
• Progress to variable practice in real-world environments (open environments).

Establish parameters for practice outside of therapy.

• Identify specific goals and strategies for unsupervised practice; maximize opportunities.
• Utilize a written behavioral contract, and have the patient agree to targeted behaviors to be carried out during the day.
• Provide home exercise program with adequate training for patient/family/caregivers.
• Have patient document unsupervised practice using an activity log or home exercise diary.

Maintain focus on active learning.

• Minimize hands-on therapy.
• Maximize role as *training coach*.

Monitor recovery closely and document progress.

• Use sensitive, valid, and reliable functional outcome measures.

Be cautious about timetables and predictions, because recovery may take longer than expected.

later may prove difficult to unlearn. For example, early gait training in the parallel bars in which the patient with stroke requires maximal assistance of the therapist to drag the involved and splinted leg forward does very little if anything to promote active locomotor control of that limb. It is also important to remember that impairment-specific interventions must be linked to functional training. The patient needs to practice the functional activity concurrently to resolve or diminish disability. The activity can be modified to ensure patient safety and make it easier. The following section provides an overview of impairment-specific interventions.

Interventions to Improve Strength, Power, and Endurance

Muscle performance is defined as "the capacity of a muscle or group of muscles to generate forces."[100, p. 688] **Muscle strength** is the "muscle force exerted by a muscle or a group of muscles to overcome a resistance under a specific set of circumstances."[100, p. 688] **Muscle power** is "the work produced per unit of time or the product of strength and speed."[100, p. 688] **Muscle endurance** is "the ability to sustain forces repeatedly or to generate forces over a period of time."[100, p. 688] Muscle performance is regulated by a number of factors. Neural factors include motor unit recruitment (number, type), motor neuron firing patterns, and efficiency of cooperative synergistic patterns. Muscle and biomechanical factors include initial muscle length and tension, muscle fiber composition, fuel storage and delivery, speed and type of contraction, and movement arm. Techniques that optimize these factors while addressing the specific demands of the task and environment will yield maximum functional outcomes.

Patients undergoing neurorehabilitation commonly present with disruption of motor neurons from central pathways and reductions in muscle force production, a direct result of a UMN lesion. Weakness or paralysis can affect one side of the body (hemiparesis, hemiplegia), both lower limbs (paraparesis, paraplegia), all four limbs (tetraparesis, tetraplegia), or a single limb or segments of a limb. Patients with hemispheric stroke from an ipsilateral lesion can also demonstrate bilateral weakness with the less involved side showing mild weakness.[101] As recovery progresses, the status of muscle strength and performance may change (e.g., the patient recovering from incomplete SCI regains muscles under voluntary control and functional performance improves). In addition, prolonged periods of disuse and immobility result in diminished neural activity, atrophy, and weakness. Older adults typically demonstrate a preferential loss of type II fibers. It is important to recognize that the patient may have been inactive before the insult or injury, resulting in preexisting deconditioning. Physical size (total body weight) and the demands of the task (e.g., stair climbing vs. walking on level surfaces) also influence the amount of strength required.

Strength Training

The benefits of strength training for patients with disorders of motor function include the following:

- An increase in the production of maximal force due to changes in neural drive (increased motor unit recruitment, increased rate, and synchronization of firing pattern of motor units, improved reaction time).
- Changes in muscle (hypertrophy of muscle fibers, improved metabolic/enzymatic adaptations, increased size and number of myofibrils, muscle fiber type adaptation).
- Increases in connective tissue tensile strength and bone mineral density.
- Improved body composition relative to body mass ratio of fat to lean.
- Improved functional performance and activity levels.
- Improved sense of well-being and self-confidence.

Basic principles of strengthening exercise include overload, specificity, cross training, and reversibility. The loads placed on muscle must be greater than those normally incurred *(overload principle)*. Training effects are specific to the mode of exercise stress imposed on the exercising muscles *(specificity principle)*. Thus, the training effects from an isometric protocol are specific to the exercising muscle and the point in the range that the muscle is holding. Effects do not carry over to improved dynamic performance (concentric or eccentric contractions). Nor will exercise training of the UEs transfer to improved LE performance. *Cross training* refers to a training program that includes a variety of training elements (e.g., isometric, concentric, eccentric, and endurance exercise). Cross training is used to place broadest possible demands on the neuromuscular system and overcome the effects of specificity. *Reversibility principle* refers to the failure to sustain the benefits of strength training if muscles are not regularly used in a maintenance program of resistance or functional exercises. Detraining effects include a reduction in muscle performance, decreased neural recruitment, and muscle fiber atrophy. The effectiveness of strength training is dependent on achieving an adequate training stimulus. Exercise guidelines for strength training are presented in Table 10.7.[102-105]

Patients with impaired motor function may demonstrate deficits in muscle activation. Early training should focus on isometric and eccentric contractions because muscle tension is better maintained than with concentric contractions. With isometric contractions, there is improved peripheral reflex support of contraction as opposed to the spindle unloading that occurs as the muscle moves into the shortened range of a concentric contraction. Eccentric contractions also produce greater muscle force with lower rates of motor unit discharge than concentric contractions. During training, the patient is initially asked to actively hold at midrange where the greatest tension can be generated. The patient is then

Table 10.7 Exercise Guidelines for Strength Training

Determine	Parameters of Exercise
Type of muscle contraction	Isometric, eccentric, concentric exercise
Mode of exercise training	Open chain (isolating one segment): isotonic and isokinetic exercises Closed chain: kinetic chain weight-bearing exercises (e.g., step-ups, modified squats) Circuit training: combination of varied methods Aquatic exercise Synergistic patterns: may be more efficient for improved function (based on specificity principle); e.g., PNF patterns with manual resistance
Type of resistance/equipment	Free weights, pulleys, elastic bands, mechanical resistance machine, isokinetic resistance (dynamometry), manual resistance, body weight, water resistance (aquatics)
Intensity: exercise load that best challenges the patient (based on overload principle)	Use submaximal loads • With weights, load is typically 60%–80% 1-RM with a goal • Very weak individuals can start at 50% 1-RM and fewer than 10 repetitions (reps) Exercise progression: increase reps, number of sets, or load as tolerated; adjust the exercise load on the basis of exercise responses, strength measures, perceived exertion, and fatigue threshold.
Number of repetitions and sets; number of exercises per set	Initial frequency is typically 3 sets of 10–15 reps or as tolerated
Duration	Total time of resistance training: typically 15–30 minutes per session or as tolerated
Frequency	Typically 2-3 days/week, depending on intensity and level of impairment/disease
Warm-up and cool-down periods	Include 5–10 min of warm-ups (calisthenics, stretching, ROM exercises) and 5–10 min of cool-down (muscle relaxation, stretching)
Additional considerations	Movements should be slow and controlled. Progression should occur in small increments. Reduce intensity with sudden onset of fatigue and exhaustion. Reduce intensity with prolonged and severe delayed onset muscle soreness. Regular breathing pattern should be maintained, while avoiding straining/Valsalva. Consider the interactions of exercise and medications. Exercise is contraindicated in some patients (e.g., with severe atrophic polio and recent weakness or ALS with muscle grades less than 3/5).
Outcomes	Relate strength training to functional tasks. Focus the patient on improvements in functional performance in terms that are understandable and meaningful.

ALS = amyotrophic lateral sclerosis; PNF = proprioceptive neuromuscular facilitation; RM = repetition max.

asked to slowly lower the limb (an eccentric contraction) and hold (an isometric contraction). Once control is achieved in both of these types of contractions, concentric contractions can be attempted. For isotonic contractions, prestretching the muscle by starting the contraction in the lengthened range optimizes tension development through increased use of viscoelastic forces *(length–tension relationship)* and peripheral reflex support (e.g., PNF patterns; see later definition and discussion). Weak muscles can be initially lightly resisted to facilitate contraction through *proprioceptive loading* (recruitment) of the muscle spindle. Control of velocity is also important to ensure efficiency of initial movement

attempts. During concentric contractions, total tension decreases as velocity increases. Thus, patients may be able to generate a contraction at slow speeds but not at high speeds. For example, the patient with stroke who demonstrates limited control should be instructed to begin with slow and controlled movements. As movements become more efficient, they can be progressed to faster speeds.

Patients with UMN lesions typically exhibit spasticity. Early neurorehabilitation approaches (e.g., *Bobath*) viewed spasticity as a primary contributor to neuromuscular impairment. Strength training and high resistance were contraindicated because they were viewed as likely to increase spasticity (reflex hyperactivity), co-contraction, and abnormal movement patterns.[105] These views are no longer supported by scientific literature as investigators have shown that it is possible to increase strength without additional detrimental effects on tone and movement control.[106-112]

Open-chain exercises involve an isolated segment of the limb moving in space without simultaneous motions at adjacent joints. Muscle activation occurs predominantly in the prime mover(s) crossing the moving joint. Resistance is applied to the distal moving segment, typically in non–weight-bearing positions. *Closed-chain exercises* involve motions in which the distal part is fixed (foot or hand) while proximal segments are moving (e.g., weight shifting in standing, bilateral short-arc squats). They are performed in weight-bearing postures and involve simultaneous actions of synergistic muscles at multiple joints. The added joint approximation and stimulation of joint and muscle proprioceptors enhances neuromuscular control and joint stabilization (co-contraction). A limitation of closed-chain exercise is the substitution of other agonist muscles for specific muscle weakness. In comparison, open-chain exercises can be used to isolate contraction of a muscle or muscle group. However, the muscles trained and movements used are not well matched to normal functional movements that utilize complex movements and multisegment linkage.[105]

Gains in strength can be obtained through progressive resistive exercises (PRE) using free weights or fixed mechanical resistance machines. A major disadvantage of PRE is that the weight selected is determined by the amount that can be lifted by the muscle at the weakest point of the range. Isokinetic training devices offer the advantage of providing accommodating resistance throughout the range. Muscle performance is therefore not limited to the weakest part of the range. The amount of force generated is recorded, providing an important objective measure of performance. Different isokinetic protocols using concentric and eccentric contractions have been developed. The speed of movement can be predetermined. This is an important consideration for training the patient who demonstrates neuromuscular impairments in timing and velocity control. For example, the patient recovering from stroke may be unable to generate the acceleration and deceleration forces needed during the different phases of gait. This results in delayed sequencing of muscle components and a general slowing of gait. Isokinetic training that focuses on the timing of these various components can improve gait function.

Proprioceptive neuromuscular facilitation (PNF) utilizes manually resisted patterns (PNF patterns) and offers the advantage of functionally based, synergistic movements. Patterns of motion are spiral and diagonal in nature as opposed to straight planes of motion and are linked to normal functional patterns. The therapist can accommodate to the patient's specific level of weakness by providing repetitive graded resistance throughout the range and by providing additional facilitation as needed to improve or maintain performance. Effective verbal commands improve the magnitude of muscle contraction. Stretch is applied in the lengthened range to assist in the initiation of contraction and throughout the range as needed to sustain contraction. Approximation is applied to assist extensor patterns, and traction is applied to assist flexor patterns. Specific PNF techniques (e.g., dynamic reversals, repeated contractions, and so forth) are useful in improving strength. Elastic resistance bands or pulley weights can also be used to provide resistance in synergistic PNF patterns.[113,114]

Strength gains can be achieved through functional training that uses task-related practice. Resistance is provided by gravity and body weight and is applied simultaneously to multiple moving segments. It can be supplemented with manual resistance of the therapist, weights, elastic resistance bands, or resistance of water during pool therapy. Activities are selected that initially focus on specific body segments and progress to involve increasingly larger segments of the body. This serves to increase the level of difficulty and the degrees of freedom that must be controlled during the movement. Benefits of functional training include improved coordination of muscles, improved postural control and balance, and improved muscle extensibility and flexibility. Functional training helps the patient develop control of synergistic muscle groups acting in multiple axes and planes of movements. It also fosters the control of varying types and combinations of muscle contractions (concentric, eccentric, isometric) that are used interchangeably during normal movement. This is a very different focus from the straight planes of motion and isolated movements commonly employed during PRE and isokinetic training. Intrinsic sensory input (somatosensory, vestibular, visual) is maximized during functional training.

Combining strength training protocols with task-specific practice is an important strategy to maximize transfer gains to functional skills. For example, strengthening of weak lower limb extensor muscles can be first achieved using an isokinetic machine that targets both eccentric and concentric contractions of the quadriceps. This training can effectively be combined with repetitive practice of functional activities also demanding similar extensor control (e.g., partial squats, sit-to-stand transfers, and stair climbing). The important consideration here is to match the strength training protocol to the requirements of the functional task in terms of ROM achieved and type, magnitude, and speed of contraction. Use of varied strength training activities and conditions also promotes development of flexibility of performance, an important goal for independence in daily life.

Muscular Endurance and Fatigue

Patients with deficits in motor function may demonstrate poor muscular endurance and fatigue. **Fatigue** is defined as the inability to contract muscle repeatedly over time. Thus, exercise cannot be sustained and exercise tolerance is reduced. The onset of fatigue is variable from patient to patient. Although many different factors may play a role, among the most important are the type and intensity of exercise. With the onset of fatigue, patients will demonstrate a decrement in force production progressing to total *exhaustion* (a ceiling effect). Fatigue can arise from neuromuscular disease affecting three primary sites: (1) the CNS (central fatigue), (2) the peripheral nerves or neuromuscular junction, or (3) the muscle itself. Examples of CNS conditions that can produce debilitating fatigue include MS, Guillain-Barré syndrome (GBS), chronic fatigue syndrome, and post-polio syndrome (PPS). The real danger of exercise training with these patients is the risk of *acute exercise overdose* producing exhaustion and possibly injury. *Overtraining*, defined as chronic overdose of exercise, is associated with both psychological and physiological decompensation, as well as musculoskeletal injury.[104] *Overuse weakness* is manifested as aching on exertion and a prolonged decrease in absolute strength and endurance as a result of excessive activity. This is often seen in patients with PPS. For example, following an exercise session the patient with PPS demonstrates prolonged weakness and fatigue that does not recover with rest. If exercise is exhaustive, the patient may be unable to get out of bed the next day or perform normal activities of daily living (ADL). Even a simple conditioning program should be carefully monitored and progressed slowly to avoid overexertion and injury.

Aerobic Training

The benefits of aerobic training for patients with disorders of motor function include the following:

- Improved cardiovascular and peripheral (muscular) endurance
- Decreased anxiety and depression
- Enhanced physical function
- Enhanced sense of well-being

A cardiovascular training program is determined based on the patient's level of deconditioning and specific symptoms. Aerobic exercises can include ergometry (two-limb or four-limb), recumbent stepper, therapeutic aquatics, and conventional weight-bearing activities such as walking. In general, moderate intensities of exercises are appropriate for most patients undergoing active rehabilitation (e.g., 40% to 70% of maximal oxygen consumption) whereas high intensities are contraindicated. For many patients, a frequency of 3 to 5 days per week with 20- to 30-minute sessions is often recommended (e.g., the patient with stroke or TBI). Alternatively, multiple 10-minute sessions can be used. Most patients will require a discontinuous protocol that carefully balances exercise with rest.[104] Clinical practice guidelines including exercise recommendations are available to assist the therapist in treating patients with chronic disabilities.[115-120] *ACSM's Exercise Management for Persons with Chronic Diseases and Disabilities* is particularly helpful for the rehabilitation therapist as it discusses exercise guidelines for a number of different disabilities (e.g., stroke, TBI, SCI, MS, PD, and so forth).[104]

Effective management of patients with low endurance and fatigue includes the use of energy conservation techniques, activity pacing, lifestyle changes, regular rest periods during the day, and improved sleep through the use of relaxation techniques and medications. An activity log can be used to help the patient identify activities that are particularly exhausting and to document the effectiveness of rest. Unnecessary energy-consuming activities should be discontinued and essential activities restructured and paced to include regular rest periods throughout the day. Patients can monitor their level of general fatigue using the Borg Rating of Perceived Exertion (RPE) scale[121] and should aim to keep their activities at an RPE level of "somewhat hard" (14 or lower using the 6–20 RPE scale). Ergonomic changes (e.g., seating and workstations) should be implemented to reduce energy cost of activities. Finally, stress management should be included in the educational program.[118]

Interventions to Improve Flexibility

Joint ROM and muscle flexibility must be adequate to allow for normal functional excursions of muscle and biomechanical alignment. Prolonged periods of disuse and immobility and motor dysfunction associated with neurological insult can lead to changes in muscle and joint function, postural alignment, and a host of indirect impairments. These include muscle tightness, atrophy, fibrosis, contracture, joint ankylosis, and postural deformity. Older adults demonstrate age-related changes affecting joint flexibility. These include increased viscosity of synovial fluid, stiffening of the joint capsule and ligaments, and calcification of articular cartilage.[122] Proactive intervention following neurological insult (e.g., stroke, TBI, SCI) is an important component of intervention. Patients with chronic and irreversible diseases (e.g., PD, MS, amyotrophic lateral sclerosis [ALS]) also need targeted intervention (tertiary prevention) to limit sequelae and degree of disability. Benefits include maintaining joint flexibility, tissue extensibility, physical ability, and function. Additional benefits include improved circulation and tissue nutrition to the limbs and pain inhibition.

Techniques include ROM exercises, passive stretching, and joint mobilization. The use of a preliminary therapeutic heat modality (e.g., hot pack) increases muscle temperature and elasticity and collagen extensibility. A warm-up period of exercise can also be used. For example, calisthenics or low-resistance cycling will gradually increase tissue temperatures and elasticity, thereby enhancing the safety of stretching. Cold modalities can be used to cool muscles and decrease muscle spasm and physiological splinting.

ROM Exercises

Range of motion is "the arc through which movement occurs at a joint or a series of joints."[100, p. 690] ROM can be *active (AROM)*, performed and controlled entirely by the voluntary muscular efforts of the patient, *active-assisted (AAROM)*, requiring some degree of external assistance for voluntary efforts, or *passive (PROM)*, performed solely by therapist or caregiver. The *Guide to Physical Therapist Practice* classifies the first two as therapeutic exercise whereas PROM is classified as manual therapy.[100] PROM is typically used when active movement is not possible (e.g., due to pain, paralysis, or unresponsiveness). AROM and AAROM have additional benefits of improving circulation, decreasing atrophy, and improving motor function. Progression should be to AROM exercises whenever possible because they are an important component of the home exercise program (HEP). ROM exercises are performed through the patient's full available range. The limb should be well supported with stable positioning of the patient to prevent joint trauma. The movements should be slow and within the patient's tolerance. Excess force and pain are contraindicated. This is especially important when working with the patient at risk for osteoporosis and heterotopic ossifications.

ROM exercises can be administered in anatomical planes of motion or in diagonal patterns of motion (PNF patterns). The latter may be more efficient because ROM can be administered throughout a limb, combining motions at more than one joint. ROM can also be achieved during functional training activities (e.g., shoulder ROM is achieved during weight shifting in quadruped or plantigrade positions). An added benefit may be the patient's lack of attention to joint motion during the activity with less protective splinting.

Passive Stretching

Stretching involves the application of manual or mechanical force to elongate (lengthen) structures that have adaptively shortened and are hypomobile.[100] The term *static stretching* refers to a method of stretching in which the muscle is slowly elongated to tolerance. The end position (greatest tolerated length) is held at least 20 to 30 seconds and the stretch is repeated four to five times, depending on the patient's tolerance. The use of slow, prolonged stretch alters neural activity by minimizing muscle spindle activation and reflex contraction of the muscle being stretched. Maintaining the position at maximal end range results in the firing of the Golgi tendon organs (GTOs) with resulting inhibition of the muscle being stretched through mechanisms of autogenic inhibition. The combined effects result in improved muscle elongation. Passive stretching also affects the muscle directly, resulting in viscoelastic changes

affecting muscle extensibility. Low-load stretching results in less danger of soft tissue tearing, less muscle soreness, and decreased energy requirements.[122-124] Frequency of stretching (number of sessions per day or per week) varies according to underlying cause, the chronicity and severity of contracture, the patient's age and level of tissue integrity and healing, and medical management (e.g., use of corticosteroids).[105] Optimally, stretching is daily and balanced with adequate rest in between to minimize tissue soreness. The results of stretching (i.e., newly gained range) should be combined with active exercise. The adage "use it or lose it" holds true for maintaining the benefits of both ROM and stretching exercises. Patients and/or their families/caregivers should be taught stretching exercises (i.e., self-stretching) as part of the HEP to maintain carryover outside of the clinic setting.

Ballistic stretching, defined as the use of a high-load, short-duration, intermittent stretch, is generally contraindicated for the elderly, the chronically ill, or patients undergoing active rehabilitation with neuromuscular impairments.[125] The high-velocity, high-intensity movements are not easily controlled. In addition, activation of muscle stretch receptors (muscle spindle Ia endings) results in reflex contraction and limits muscle elongation. Also, in chronic contractures, connective tissue is more brittle and tears easily. Thus, it is associated with high rates of microtrauma and injury.[105]

Low-load prolonged stretch (LLPS) (15 to 30 minutes) can be applied using mechanical pulleys and weights or specialized orthotic devices. Prolonged positioning on a tilt table with wedges and straps can be used effectively to improve LE range (e.g., hamstrings, gastroc-soleus muscles).[126,127] Prolonged stretch can also be applied to prevent or reduce contractures using serial casting (discussed later in this chapter).

Facilitated Stretching

Facilitated stretching refers to the use of neuromuscular inhibition techniques to relax (inhibit) and elongate muscles when used in conjunction with stretching. *PNF-facilitated stretching techniques* include *hold-relax (HR)* and *contract-relax (CR)*. The limb is actively moved to the end of PROM (range-limited position). The patient is then instructed to perform a maximal isometric contraction of the restricted, shortened muscles (antagonist pattern). The contraction should be maintained for at least 5 to 8 seconds. This pre-stretch contraction results in muscle inhibition from activation of the GTO (autogenic inhibition). This is followed by voluntary relaxation. In HR, the therapist then passively moves the limb into the new limit of range. In CR, the patient actively moves the limb to the new limit of range in the pattern against resistance. The resisted isotonic contractions of the agonist muscles focuses on all muscles in the pattern with an emphasis on rotators and provides additional reciprocal inhibition effects (i.e., agonist contraction further inhibits the tight muscle via muscle spindle activity). These techniques were originally applied while using PNF patterns though some clinicians have adopted these techniques in patterns using anatomical planes of motion.[113,114] Research has demonstrated the effectiveness and superiority of facilitated stretching techniques over static stretching techniques, particularly when active contractions are used.[128-130] An additional benefit is that patients frequently report less discomfort with the application of facilitated stretching techniques as compared to other stretching methods. Because the inhibitory mechanisms affect primarily muscle and depend on voluntary contraction, these techniques are not effective with very weak or paralyzed muscles or range limitation associated with substantial connective tissue changes (chronic contracture).

Stretching and Positioning for the Patient with Spasticity

The patient with UMN syndrome typically exhibits spasticity (velocity-dependent hypertonia) and hyperactive deep tendon reflexes (DTRs). Functionally the patient demonstrates poor volitional control of movements and limitations in functional skills. The limbs are typically held in fixed, abnormal postures with antigravity muscles primarily affected. For example, the UE typically assumes an abnormal flexor posture whereas the LE assumes an abnormal extensor posture. If left untreated, spasticity can lead to the development of secondary impairments such as contracture, postural asymmetries, and deformity.

Stretching and positioning are important components of management of the patient with spasticity. Patient tolerance needs to be carefully assessed. Precise handling of a spastic limb is important. The therapist should use constant, firm manual contacts positioned over bony or nonspastic areas and avoid direct pressure on spastic muscles. The limb is moved out of the shortened spastic position into the lengthened range using slow, repeated rotations of the limb. The patient's limb can then be positioned and maintained in the newly gained range to provide prolonged stretching. For example, during treatment of the patient with stroke and a spastic UE, the therapist grasps the hand over the thumb and slowly moves the elbow out into full extension with the hand open. The hand is then placed palm down on the mat to the side of the patient in weight-bearing with the elbow extended, hand open, and wrist and fingers extended. Weight shifting forward/backward during sitting can then be used to maintain inhibition and range. Although time to maintain the stretch in order to reduce spasticity is unknown, one group of researchers found 10 minutes to be optimal.[131]

Serial Casts

Serial casts are recommended for patients who have or are at risk for contractures as a result of decreased PROM and/or spasticity. They have been shown to improve ROM, reduce contracture, and prevent deformity.[132-137] The therapist first positions the limb into its fully lengthened end-range. A layer of thin foam and white cotton wrap is applied first, followed by the cast material (e.g., Softcast™, reinforced Softcast, or bivalved fiberglass). Casts are typically changed every 7 to 10 days (serial application) and are used for 1 to 6 weeks. Poor casting techniques include lack of end-range positioning of the limb, loose-fitting cast, or insufficient padding. Faulty technique may result in a lack of improvement or even increased tone, skin breakdown (especially on bony prominences), decreased circulation, and peripheral edema. Highly agitated patients (e.g., the patient with TBI) may potentially injure themselves and demonstrate increased risk of skin breakdown and cast breakage. Patients with cognitive or communication impairments should be monitored closely because they will be unable to indicate pain or discomfort and potential skin breakdown (e.g., the patient with stroke and aphasia). Casting is contraindicated in patients with severe heterotropic ossification; skin surface not intact, such as open wounds, blisters, or abrasions; impaired circulation and marked edema; uncontrolled hypertension; autonomic storming (marked increase in sympathetic nervous system activity); unstable intracranial pressure; pathological inflammatory conditions, such as arthritis or gout; or in individuals at risk for compartment syndrome or nerve impingement. Application to individuals with long-standing contractures (longer than 6 to 12 months) is also contraindicated.[138]

Adjustable orthoses have also been used to provide passive, prolonged stretch with the added benefits of easy removal for hygiene and observation. These devices use a rotating adjustable dial attached to metal rods and a flexible acrylic thermoplastic base.[139] The required adjustments are easier and less time consuming than fabricating an entirely new serial cast. Dynamic orthoses, primarily used on elbow or knee flexion contractures, use a spring-loaded or hydraulic mechanism to provide nearly constant pressure.

ROM for the Patient with Hypotonia

The patient with lower motor neuron (LMN) syndrome typically exhibits hypotonia (low tone) with weak or paralyzed muscles, joint instability, and deformity. Following neurological insult, tone varies relative to recovery stage. For example, the patient with a new or recent stroke or SCI will present with initial flaccidity during the stage of cerebral or spinal shock whereas the same patient later on demonstrates emerging spasticity. In using PROM exercises for the patient with hypotonia, the therapist needs to be cognizant of end-range joint instability and the risk of hyperextension injury. Supportive and protective devices may be necessary to prevent injury to limbs and postural asymmetry during functional training.

Interventions to Improve Postural Control and Balance

Postural control is the ability to control the body's position in space for stability and orientation. **Postural orientation** is the ability to maintain normal alignment relationships between the various body segments and between the body and environment. *Static postural control* (static balance control, stability) is the ability to maintain stability and orientation with the COM over the BOS with the body at rest. *Dynamic postural control* (dynamic balance control, controlled mobility) is the ability to maintain stability and orientation with the COM over the BOS while parts of the body are in motion (see Table 10.2).[2] An intervention program to improve postural control must be based on an accurate evaluation of data obtained during examination of deficits (see Chapter 5, Examination of Motor Function: Motor Control and Motor Learning).

Training activities can be used to improve the following:

- Postural alignment, body mechanics, and static postural control
- Dynamic postural control, including musculoskeletal responses necessary for control of movement and posture
- Adaptation of balance skills for varying task and environmental conditions
- Use of sensory monitoring for postural control
- Safety awareness and compensatory strategies for effective fall prevention

Increased understanding of the range and variability of postural strategies for balance negates any simplistic view of balance based on a developmental perspective of reflex control (i.e., righting and equilibrium reactions). Overall, the organization of postural control strategies must be viewed as flexible, not rigid, involving multiple body segments and postural strategies.[140-142] In that context, patterns will vary according to a number of different factors, including initial conditions, balance requirements and challenges, perturbation characteristics, learning, and intention.[143] The patient needs to practice steady state, anticipatory, and reactive balance control using activities that focus on both static and dynamic postural control. Functional activities selected should be based on an accurate evaluation of the patient's abilities and needs. The activities selected should include those required for ADL, as well as those required for social participation, recreation, and work, if appropriate. Sensory selection and organization should also be a part of a balance training program. Repetition and practice are essential factors in assisting CNS adaptation.

It is important to remember that some balance training activities may cause the patient distress initially. The patient will feel threatened when placed in situations where he or she is in jeopardy of falling. The therapist should ensure patient confidence by providing a clear explanation of the nature of the task, what the challenges to balance are, and the steps the therapist will take to prevent falls in terms that are easy to understand. The patient with instability can wear a gait belt or practice standing activities wearing an overhead safety harness. The therapist needs to stand close enough to the patient to guard safely but not so close as to interfere with the activity. For the very unstable patient, two spotters may be necessary. The environment can be used to assist in keeping the patient from falling. For example, standing exercises can be performed in the parallel bars, between two tables, near a wall or two walls (corner standing), or in a pool with the patient standing in waist-high or chest-high water. Support given early in training should be withdrawn as soon as possible to allow focus on active control.

An understanding of the foundational requirements of upright postures will direct the therapist in improving postural alignment and body mechanics. Sitting is a relatively stable posture with a moderately high COM and a moderate BOS that includes contact of the buttocks, thighs, and feet with the support surface. During normal sitting, weight is equally distributed over both buttocks with the pelvis in neutral position or tilted slightly anterior. The head and trunk are vertical, maintained in midline orientation. The line of gravity passes close to the joint axes of the spine. Muscles of the cervical, thoracic, and lumbar spine are active in maintaining upright postural control and core stability. BOS can be increased by using one or both hands for additional support.

Deficits in sitting can be broadly grouped into those involving alignment, weight-bearing, and extensor muscle weakness. Changes in normal alignment result in corresponding changes in other body segments. For example, a slumped sitting posture (dorsal kyphosis and forward head) is typically the result of sacral sitting with the pelvis tilted posteriorly. The therapist should instruct the patient in the correct sitting posture and demonstrate the position to provide an accurate *reference of correctness*. It is important to focus the patient's attention on key task elements and improve overall sensory awareness of the correct sitting posture and position in space.

Standing is a less stable posture with a high COM and a small BOS that includes contact of the feet with the support surface. During normal quiet standing, there is minimal body sway with ankle muscle activity (dorsiflexors/plantarflexors, invertors/evertors) activated to counteract body sway. Weight is equally distributed over both feet. The line of gravity falls close to most joint axes: slightly anterior to the ankle and knee joints; slightly posterior to the hip joint; posterior to the cervical and lumbar vertebrae; and anterior to the thoracic vertebrae and atlanto-occipital joint. Natural spinal curves are present but somewhat flattened in upright stance depending on the level of postural tone (e.g., lumbar and cervical lordosis, thoracic kyphosis). The pelvis is in neutral position, with no anterior or posterior tilt. Normal alignment minimizes the need for muscle activity during erect stance.

Impairments in standing can also be broadly grouped into those involving alignment, weight-bearing, and specific muscle weakness. Faulty postures such as forward head and kyphosis or lordosis, excessive hip and knee flexion, or pelvic asymmetries can result in decreased postural stability. Inaccurate kinesthetic awareness of true vertical and pain can affect postural position and significantly impair balance. Patients are typically unable to self-correct faulty postures. Physical therapy interventions should focus first on improving specific musculoskeletal impairments (e.g., limited ROM, weakness). For example, active exercises to improve standing can include standing heel-cord stretches, heel-rises, toe-offs, partial wall squats, chair-rises, side-kicks, back-kicks, and marching in place using touch-down support of the hands as needed. These are sometimes referred to as the "kitchen sink exercises." Postural reeducation begins with demonstration of the correct posture. Verbal cues should focus on control of essential postural elements, that is, stable (neutral) pelvis, axial extension (e.g., "stand tall"), and normal alignment (e.g., head erect, shoulders back, weight evenly distributed under both feet). Patients can benefit from tactile cues during initial practice (manual or surface related). For example, patients can stand with the back positioned against a wall or patients with a lateral lean (e.g., patients with pusher syndrome following a stroke) can sit with their side positioned against the seated therapist or a wall. Corner standing or standing between two treatment tables can be effective for patients with significant COM distortion. Mirrors can provide important visual cues regarding vertical position. For example, the patient wears a shirt with a taped vertical line on it and is asked to match it to a taped vertical line on a mirror.[2] The taped lines provide useful visual feedback for achieving vertical. Mirrors are generally contraindicated for the patient with visuospatial perceptual deficits. Application of correct postures to real-life functional situations is important to ensure carryover and lasting change. Instruction in proper body mechanics should include a discussion of the activities of standing up, lifting, reaching, carrying, and arising from the floor.

Interventions to Improve Static Postural Control

Patients who demonstrate impairments in static postural control (stability) are unable to maintain or hold a steady position for a number of reasons, including decreased strength, tonal imbalances (hypotonia, spasticity, dystonia), impaired voluntary control and hypermobility (ataxia, athetosis), sensory hypersensitivity (tactile-avoidance reactions), or increased anxiety or arousal (high sympathetic "fight or flight" state).

Instability is associated with excessive postural sway, wide BOS, low- or high-guard hand position, holding onto an object in the environment (handhold), and loss of balance (falls).

The therapist can select any of a number of weight-bearing (antigravity) postures to develop stability control. Typical training postures include sitting and standing (in modified plantigrade and full standing). Postures are selected on the basis of (1) patient safety and level of control and (2) importance in terms of functional tasks. The therapist varies the level of activities, selecting activities that both allow success and provide an appropriate challenge for the patient.

The therapist should focus on obtaining symmetrical, balanced weight-bearing. Patients may present with specific directional instabilities, such as weight-bearing more on one side than the other. For example, after a stroke the patient typically keeps weight centered toward the less affected side. Practice should focus on redirecting the patient into a centered position by moving toward the more affected side, both in sitting and standing positions. The patient is instructed to "hold steady" while sitting or standing tall and maintaining a visual focus on a forward target. Progression is to holding for longer and longer durations. Techniques that can be used to enhance stabilizing muscle contractions include quick stretch, tapping, resistance, approximation, manual contacts, and verbal cues. For the patient unable to actively stabilize the body, the therapist can begin with resisted isometric contractions of antagonist postural muscle groups (e.g., PNF technique of rhythmic stabilization). For example, the patient with severe instability following TBI who is unable to sit independently may need to begin practice holding a neutral trunk position first in a supported sitting position. The therapist can then progress the patient to active sitting and to postures that demand increasing amounts of upright (antigravity) postural control (standing). If an imbalance exists, the stabilizing activity can be coupled with a strengthening activity for the weak muscles. As the trunk becomes more stable, the patient is expected to assume active control in stabilizing in the posture. For a patient with hyperkinetic disorders (e.g., ataxia, athetosis), the PNF technique of stabilizing reversals is appropriate. Alternating isotonic contractions are used, allowing only very small-range movements. Progression is toward decreasing range (*decrements of range*) until finally the patient is asked to stabilize and hold steady against resistance in the posture.

Additional strategies to improve stability include the use of elastic resistance bands to enhance *proprioceptive loading* and contraction of stabilizing muscles. For example, in the prone-on-elbows position or supported sitting with elbows weight-bearing on a table, a band can be placed around both forearms. The patient is instructed to push out against the band and maintain the forearms apart against the resistance. This selectively loads and facilitates contraction of the shoulder stabilizers (abductors and rotator cuff muscles). In kneeling or standing, elastic resistance bands can be placed around the lower thighs. The patient is instructed to maintain the thighs apart against the resistance of the bands. This selectively loads and facilitates contraction of the hip stabilizers (abductors, extensors), improving stability control at the hips.

As static postural control improves, the therapist can progress the patient to stabilizing on a moveable surface (e.g., sitting on a therapy ball). Gentle bouncing on the therapy ball provides joint approximation through the vertebral joints, facilitating extensors and an upright posture. For patients requiring an additional challenge, sitting control can be practiced on other compliant surfaces (e.g., foam, wobble board, or Dynadisc™) placed on a platform mat. The therapist can also increase task difficulty by reducing the BOS (feet apart to feet together to sitting with single foot support [legs crossed]).

Aquatic therapy can also be used to enhance proprioceptive loading. The water provides a degree of unweighting and resistance to movement. This can be quite effective in reducing hyperkinetic movements and enhancing postural stability. For example, a patient recovering from TBI who demonstrates significant ataxia may be able to sit or stand in the pool with minimal assistance whereas these same activities outside the pool are not possible.

To improve standing control, the patient is directed to practice neuromuscular *fixed-support strategies* that occur at the ankle and hip joints.[142] Feedback is provided to assist the patient in recruiting the correct pattern. To recruit *ankle strategies,* the patient practices small-range, slow-velocity shifts progressing to holding steady. Attention is directed to the action of ankle muscles to maintain the body (COM) over the fixed feet (BOS). Standing on a wobble board (moveable surface) or foam roller with the flat side down progressing to flat side up are effective activities to increase the challenge in recruiting ankle strategies. The patient is also directed to practice tasks that normally recruit *hip strategies.* These are recruited with larger shifts in the COM that approach the LOS and/or faster body sway motions that are characterized by early activation of proximal hip and trunk muscles. Hip flexion and extension responses are generated during anterior–posterior displacements. Lateral hip motions are generated during lateral displacements. Patients can be instructed to move their upper body forward and backward while standing on a foam roller progressing to steady holding. More challenging activities include standing with feet together, tandem standing, and single-limb stance. Tandem standing on a foam roller is an effect way to recruit lateral hip strategies.[97]

Anticipatory postural adjustments should also be practiced, because predictive control must be operational for functional balance. The patient is provided with advance information about the upcoming demands of the task. For example, "I want you to catch this 5-pound weighted ball while maintaining your sitting (or standing) position." The prior knowledge serves as an important source of information in initiating the correct postural pattern. To promote generalizability, practice should occur in a variety of environments. For example, training can progress from a closed or fixed environment (e.g., quiet room) to a more variable environment (e.g., busy physical therapy gym). Training must ultimately be context specific to real-life settings of home or community to ensure functional carryover (e.g., standing at the bathroom sink or kitchen counter).

Interventions to Improve Dynamic Postural Control

Patients who demonstrate impairments in dynamic, anticipatory postural control are unable to control postural stability and orientation while moving segments of the body. A number of impairments may be contributing factors, including tonal imbalances (spasticity, rigidity, hypotonia), ROM restrictions, impaired voluntary control and hypermobility (ataxia, athetosis), impaired reciprocal actions of the antagonists (cerebellar dysfunction), or impaired proximal stabilization. Clinically, the patient demonstrates difficulty weight shifting from side-to-side, forward-backward, or diagonally. Difficulties are also apparent in moving one or more limbs while maintaining a posture (sometimes referred to as *static-dynamic control*). For example, one limb is moving (UE reaching or LE stepping) while the patient maintains the sitting or standing posture. In the quadruped position, the patient lifts one arm or leg or opposite arm and leg. These added movements increase the demand for stabilization control because the overall BOS is reduced and the COM must shift over the remaining support segments before the dynamic limb movement can be successful (e.g., stepping).

The therapist can select any of a number of weight-bearing (antigravity) postures to develop dynamic postural control (see Table 10.7). Postures typically selected include sitting and standing. Practice begins with movements emphasizing smooth directional changes that engage antagonist actions (e.g., weight shifts). *Limits of stability* should be explored. For example, in sitting or standing, the patient is instructed to slowly sway in all directions (forward-backward, side-to-side) as far as possible while still maintaining the position. The outer point at which the COM is still maintained within the BOS is termed the LOS. Loss of balance occurs when the LOS has been exceeded, for example, when the COM extends beyond the BOS. Practice of volitional body sway is important to assist the patient in developing accurate perceptual awareness of stability limits, an important component of an overall CNS internal model of postural control. Because LOS changes with different tasks, a variety of functional activities should be practiced in different environmental settings. As control improves, the movements are gradually expanded through an increasing range (*increments of range*). For the patient who has difficulty initiating or controlling movements, the movements can be facilitated using quick stretch, tapping, light tracking resistance, manual contacts, and dynamic verbal commands. Although active movement is the goal, guided assistance may be required for some patients during initial movement attempts.

Specific task-oriented training incorporates both reaching and stepping activities. Functionally important and motivating activities should be selected. For example, the patient practices reaching for a cup (requiring shoulder stabilization with elbow extension and wrist stabilization) while maintaining a stable sitting position. Or a bilateral UE task (e.g., folding and stacking towels) can be used while maintaining a stable standing position.

PNF extremity patterns can be used to introduce a dynamic challenge to postural stability and promote movement in synergistic patterns. For example, in sitting the patient is asked to move the UEs using a chop/reverse chop pattern in sitting. In addition to the extremity movement, the pattern incorporates diagonal and rotational movement of the trunk along with a weight shift. The patient's full attention is focused on performing the pattern and not on the stabilizing postural components. This ability to redirect cognitive attention is an important measure of developing postural control because intact postural control functions largely on an automatic and unconscious level. Movements can be active or resisted (e.g., PNF techniques of dynamic reversals [slow reversals]).[97]

Therapy ball activities are effective in developing dynamic stability control in sitting. For example, the patient sits on a ball and gently moves the ball side-to-side, forward-backward, or in a combination (pelvic clock motions). Or the patient sits on the ball while performing voluntary movements of the arms or legs (e.g., alternate leg or arm raises). Progression is from unilateral to bilateral and finally to reciprocal limb movements (e.g., Mexican hat dance). Voluntary trunk motions can be practiced while sitting on the ball (e.g., head and trunk rotation with arms held out to the side). Resistance can be introduced by using elastic resistance bands, a weighted ball, or weight cuffs on the ankles or wrists. Difficulty can be increased by adding a second task (*dual task training*) such as catching and throwing a ball, batting a balloon, or kicking a ball. A secondary cognitive task can also be introduced (e.g., spelling forward or backward, remembering a list, counting backward by 3's).[2]

To improve standing control, the patient is directed to practice neuromuscular *stepping strategies*.[142] Stepping strategies can be evoked with perturbations that provide the COM displacement. Stepping movements are accompanied by early activation of hip abductors and ankle co-contraction for medial-lateral stability during static single-limb support.[144] Maki and McIlroy[145] investigated the role of limb movements in maintaining upright stance, specifically compensatory stepping and grasping movements of the upper limbs, which they termed *change-in-support strategies* (as opposed to the fixed-support strategies at the ankle and hip). These investigators found that both stepping and arm movements were common reactions to loss of balance. Moreover, they were initiated well before the COM reached the LOS, contradicting the traditional view that they are strategies of last resort. They also found that stepping may actually be a preferred strategy to using a hip strategy. The direction and magnitude of change-in-support strategies were found to vary according to the magnitude and direction of the perturbation. For example, stepping may occur forward or backward in response to anterior or posterior displacements. Lateral displacements typically resulted in cross-stepping pattern, seen in 87% of lateral stepping responses, as opposed to straight side-stepping. Lateral destabilization with its increased demands for lateral weight transfer is particularly problematic for a large portion of older adults who experience falls. Arm reactions in response to whole-body instability were also found to be prevalent with activation of shoulder muscles occurring in 85% of destabilizing trials.

Training in standing should include practice of a variety of voluntary stepping movements (e.g., marching in place; anterior, posterior, lateral, or crossed side steps). Steps can start out small and gradually increase to mini-lunges or full lunges. Stepping can also be progressed from tandem stepping (e.g., forward tandem to backward tandem steps) to crossed stepping (e.g., stepping forward and across to backward and across). Upper trunk rotation and arm swing can be combined with these cross-stepping movements. Elastic resistance bands positioned around the pelvis can be used to improve the strength of stepping responses.[97] Research evidence demonstrates the effectiveness of training in improving balance control.[146-152]

Interventions to Improve Reactive Balance Control

Patients with deficits in motor function and balance are also typically unable to respond effectively to external perturbations. The therapist can utilize gentle manual pulls or pushes applied to the shoulders or hips, or moving platforms, to provide perturbations. Small perturbations can be used to activate strategies designed to maintain position (e.g., ankle or hip strategies) whereas larger perturbations can be used activate stepping strategies. The therapist should vary inputs so as to not be predicable in terms of the response activated (i.e., direction, type, and speed of response). An elastic band around the hips can also be used to promote stepping strategies. The therapist maintains resistance of band against the hips and then suddenly releases the resistance, requiring the patient to take a step. Patient safety and protection against falls should be maintained during all perturbation training. Research evidence demonstrates the effectiveness of training in improving reactive balance control.[149,152] Tai Chi training has also been shown to improve balance control and stepping strategies.[153-155]

Interventions to Improve Sensory Selection and Utilization for Balance

An important focus of balance training is utilization and integration of appropriate sensory systems. Normally three sources of inputs are utilized to maintain balance: somatosensory inputs (proprioceptive and tactile inputs from the feet and ankles), visual inputs, and vestibular inputs. Careful examination can identify the patient's use of inputs to maintain balance (e.g., *Clinical Test for Sensory Interaction and Balance* [CTSIB]; see Chapter 5, Examination of Motor Function: Motor Control and Motor Learning, for a discussion of this test). Training is directed to using varying sensory conditions to challenge the patient. For example, patients who demonstrate a high degree of dependence on vision can practice balance tasks with absent visual cues (e.g., eyes closed or blindfolded), with reduced visual cues (e.g., low light), or with inaccurate vision (e.g., petroleum-coated lenses on a pair of eyeglasses). Altering the visual inputs allows the patient to shift focus and reliance to other sensory inputs, in this case to intact somatosensory and vestibular inputs. Patients can practice varying somatosensory inputs by standing and walking on different surfaces, from flat surfaces (floor) to compliant surfaces (low to high carpet pile), to dense foam. A patient who is barefoot or wearing thin-soled shoes is better able to attend to sensation from the feet than if wearing thick-soled shoes. Challenges to the vestibular system can be introduced by reducing both visual and somatosensory inputs through sensory conflict situations. For example, the patient practices standing on dense foam with the eyes closed. The patient can also be directed to walk on foam with eyes closed, a condition that requires maximum use of vestibular inputs. Patients should also practice varying environmental influences such as walking outside, progressing from relatively smooth terrain (sidewalks) to uneven terrain to moving surfaces (escalator, elevator). Practice can also include standing or walking in bright or full lighting to reduced lighting. Research evidence demonstrates the effectiveness of altering sensory contexts in improving sensory selection and organization for balance.[156-160]

Patients with significant sensory loss will require assistance in shifting toward the intact systems to monitor and adjust balance using *compensatory training strategies*. For example, the patient with LE proprioceptive losses (e.g., diabetic neuropathy) will need to learn to shift focus to the visual system for functional mobility and balance. The patient with bilateral amputations learns to rely heavily on visual inputs for control in standing and walking. If deficits exist in more than one of the major sensory systems, compensatory shifts are generally inadequate and balance deficits will be pronounced. Thus, the patient with diabetic neuropathy and retinopathy will be at high risk for loss of balance and falls. Compensatory training with an assistive device is indicated. Other patients must be encouraged to ignore distorted information (e.g., impaired proprioception accompanying stroke) in favor of more accurate sensory information (e.g., vision). Patients with low vision should practice balance activities while wearing their eyeglasses. The exception to this is when patients wear bifocal glasses, which should not be worn during balance training. The lower lens (designed for reading) can distort vision when looking down and interfere with depth perception (e.g., stair climbing).

Interventions Using Augmented Feedback

Augmented feedback can be used to during balance training (e.g., biofeedback cane with auditory signals, limb load monitor, posturography). Force-platform devices are used to measure forces and provide *center of pressure (COP) biofeedback* (posturography feedback). COP displacement is associated with movement of the COM or postural sway. Although COP excursion always exceeds COM sway, this relationship is close during ankle motions (ankle strategies) when the body moves like a pendulum over the feet. However, when a hip strategy is used (upper body motion focused at the hips), the COP:COM relationship becomes distorted and does not accurately reflect sway.[161] A computer analyzes the data and provides relevant biofeedback concerning sway path and COP position on a visual monitor. Some units also provide auditory feedback.

Posturography training can be used to shape sway movements to enhance symmetry and steadiness. The patient can be instructed to increase or decrease sway movements or move the COP cursor on the computer screen to achieve a designated range or to match a designated target. It is an effective training mode for patients who demonstrate problems in force generation. For example, the patient with decreased force generation (hypometria) as typically demonstrated by individuals with PD is directed toward achieving larger and faster sway movements during posturography training. The patient with too much force (hypermetria), as typically demonstrated by the individual with cerebellar ataxia, is directed toward decreasing sway movements progressing to holding a stable, centered posture.[162] Research evidence demonstrates the effectiveness of platform training in improving symmetrical weight distribution.[163-166]

It is important to remember that although balance retraining using posturography biofeedback does improve symmetrical standing, it does not automatically transfer to balance skills during functional skills such as gait. Winstein et al[163] found that a reduction in standing balance asymmetry did not result in a concomitant reduction in asymmetrical limb movement patterns associated with hemiparetic locomotion. Given the specificity of training principle, this is not a surprising finding that platform training did not transfer to improved locomotion. Finally, a set of bathroom scales or limb load monitors can provide a low-tech, low-cost form of biofeedback weight information to assist patients in achieving symmetrical weight-bearing.

Strategies to Improve Safety and Reduce Fall Risk

Prevention of falls in the elderly and for the patient with balance deficiency is an important goal of therapy. Patient education and lifestyle counseling can help the patient recognize potentially dangerous situations and reduce the likelihood of falls. For example, high-risk activities likely to result in falls include turning, sit-to-stand transfers, reaching and bending over, and stair climbing. Patients should also be discouraged from clearly hazardous activities such as climbing on step stools, ladders, and chairs, or walking on slippery or icy surfaces. The education plan should stress the harmful effects of a sedentary lifestyle. Patients should be encouraged to maintain an active lifestyle, including a program of regular exercise and walking. Medications should be reviewed and those medications linked to increased risk of falls (e.g., medications that result in postural hypotension) should be addressed. A consultation with the physician for medication review may be indicated.

Compensatory training strategies can be utilized to prevent falls if normal strategies are lacking. The patient should be instructed in how to maintain an adequate BOS at all times. For example, the patient should widen BOS when turning or sitting down. If a force is expected, the patient should be instructed to widen the BOS in the direction of the expected force (e.g., leaning into the wind). If greater stability is needed, instruction should be provided in how to lower the COM (e.g., crouching down to reduce the likelihood of a fall). Greater stability can also be achieved if friction is increased between the body and the support surface. The patient should therefore be instructed to wear shoes with flat rubber soles for better gripping (e.g., athletic shoes). Assistive devices should be used improve balance when necessary. Consideration should always be given to using the least restrictive device while at the same time ensuring safety. Light touch-down support using a vertical or slant cane (used by individuals who are blind) has been shown to improve balance.[167] A fall prevention program must also address environmental factors that contribute to falls. Recommendations for reducing falls in the home environment are presented in Box 10.6.

Box 10.6 Fall Prevention Strategies: Modifying the Home Environment

- Adequate lighting is essential. Both low light and glare can be hazardous, particularly for the elderly. Glare can be reduced with translucent shades or curtains.
- Light switches should be positioned at the entrance to a room and fully accessible. Timers can ensure that lights come on routinely at dusk. Clapper devices can be used to enable the patient to turn on lights from across the room. Night-lights typically used in bathrooms or hallways do not provide enough light to ensure adequate balance.
- Carpets with loose edges should be tacked down. Scatter or throw rugs should be removed.
- Furniture that obstructs walkways should be removed or repositioned.
- Chairs should be of adequate height and firmness to assist in sit-to-stand transfers. Chairs with armrests and elevated seat heights may be required. Motorized chairs that elevate the patient into standing may be hazardous for (1) some patients who are unable to initiate active balance responses in a timely manner during initial standing and (2) those with impaired LE strength unable to maintain firm foot contact with the floor as the chair rises.
- Stairs are the site of many falls. Ensure adequate lighting. Contrast tape using bright, warm colors (red, orange, or yellow) can be used to highlight steps. Handrails are important for safety on stairs and, if not present, may need to be installed.
- Grab bars or rails reduce the incidence of falls in the bathroom. Nonskid mats or strips in the bathtub along with a tub or shower seat can also improve safety. Toilet seats can be elevated to facilitate independent use.

Interventions to Improve Coordination and Agility

Coordination is the ability to execute smooth, accurate, and controlled movements. **Agility** is the ability to perform coordinated movements combined with upright standing balance. **Ataxia** is defined as uncoordinated movement that manifests when voluntary movements are attempted, influencing gait, posture, and patterns of movement. The principal causes of ataxia are cerebellar disease or lesions (e.g., cerebellar atrophy, tumor, MS, TBI, stroke, Friedreich's ataxia, chronic alcoholism). Patients with ataxia typically demonstrate impaired synergistic actions with decomposition of movement (dyssynergia), impaired ability to judge the distance or range of movement (dysmetria), and impaired ability to perform rapid alternating movements (dysdiadochokinesia), along with intention tremor and disturbances of posture and gait. Typical standing postural abnormalities include an exaggerated lumbar lordosis, anterior pelvic tilt, flexion at the hips, hyperextension at the knees, and weight placed more on the heels. Patients with ataxia also typically demonstrate mild decreases in strength (asthenia) and tone (hypotonia) and hypermobility. Postural instability in the patient with ataxia is associated with excessive postural sway, wide BOS, high guard hand position, handhold, and frequent loss of balance (falls). Motor learning is also typically slowed, given the inability of the cerebellum to timely and correctly utilize feedback to modulate movement. The reader is referred to Chapter 6, Examination of Coordination and Balance, for additional information.

Training activities can be used to accomplish the following:

- Improve postural stability and balance
- Improve accuracy of limb movements
- Improve function
- Improve safety awareness and compensatory strategies for effective movement control and fall prevention

Interventions to improve postural stability and balance have been previously discussed. Patients with ataxia generally benefit from the use of light resistance to slow limb and trunk movements, temporarily reducing dysmetria and tremor. This can include use of weight cuffs (ankle, wrist), elastic bands, weighted trunk vest, weighted walkers and canes, and water resistance (pool activities). PNF patterns are an appropriate focus of treatment because of the required synergistic actions of muscles. PNF resistive techniques of rhythmic stabilization, dynamic reversals or dynamic-reversal-hold, and resisted progression are the techniques of choice. The key issue for the therapist is to provide enough resistance to enhance proprioceptive loading and movement without producing debilitating fatigue. During training, movements should be kept slow and controlled; fast movements are considerably more problematic in terms of learning and performance. Complex *gross motor skills* that engage and move large segments of the body (e.g., sit-to-stand, transfers, locomotion) are particularly difficult for patients with ataxia. *Fine motor skills* that engage the small muscles of the hand (e.g., feeding, writing, ADL) are also difficult and can lead to functional dependence (e.g., inability to feed or dress). Augmented feedback in the form of biofeedback, rhythmic auditory stimulation (metronome, music), can be used to help modulate speed and focus attention. Devices that promote reciprocal movements and timing (e.g., cycle ergometer, motorized treadmill with an overhead harness) can also be effective. To enhance motor learning, the patient should practice in a low-stimuli environment. Variable practice should only be attempted as skill development becomes apparent and at a much more gradual rate of progression. A distributed practice schedule is important because patients with ataxia can demonstrate low endurance and increased fatigue. For the patient with significant ataxia and postural instability, hands-on support and guidance may be necessary. Aids for mobility (assistive devices) may be necessary to ensure safety and prevent falls. There is limited research evidence demonstrating the effectiveness of physical therapy in improving ataxia.[168-171]

Interventions to Improve Gait and Locomotion

Most patients with impaired motor function exhibit deficits in gait and locomotion, which is a complex, higher-level motor skill. Substantial rehabilitation efforts are directed toward improving gait and locomotion to restore or improve a patient's functional mobility and independence. Walking is frequently the number one goal of patients who "want to walk" above all other considerations. Ability to ambulate or use a wheelchair independently is often a significant factor in determining discharge placements (e.g., return to home or extended care facility). To establish a realistic POC, the physical therapist must accurately analyze the patient's gait and locomotor ability. Comprehensive gait analysis is discussed in Chapter 7, Examination of Gait. The functional demands of the patient's home, community, or work environment must be considered in planning successful interventions and in predicting a patient's future status. Chapter 11, Locomotor Training, provides a comprehensive discussion of training. Wheelchair training is discussed in Chapter 20, Traumatic Spinal Cord Injury.

Relaxation Training

Patients with impaired motor function typically experience a great deal of stress resulting from loss of motor control, pain, inability to perform functional tasks previously performed with ease, and loss of control in life decisions. Sympathetic nervous system responses (fight or flight) are typically heightened. (See Chapter 5, Examination of Motor Function: Motor Control and Motor Learning, for a discussion of sympathetic and parasympathetic responses.) A goal of therapy is to promote stress reduction and relaxation. A *relaxation response* is associated with engagement of parasympathetic responses along with an increase in alpha brain waves. Positive benefits of relaxation training include the following:

- Muscle relaxation
- Lowered blood pressure
- Reduced ischemic pain
- Enhanced awareness of emotional state and memory
- Increased energy level
- Increased sense of control

Two elements are the important components in producing the relaxation response as described by

Benson:[172] quiet deep breathing and attention on a single focus (thought, word, or object). The patient initially practices while lying down and later can shift to practicing while sitting or standing comfortably. The patient is directed to breathe deeply with the diaphragm moving downward as air is drawn into the lungs. The patient inhales slowly, holds the breath for a few seconds, and then slowly exhales. The patient is also directed to concentrate on a specific focus, while disengaging from all other thoughts and distractions. Relaxation training can be used throughout the day as needed (e.g., 4- to 5-minute sessions) and can be performed individually or in small groups (e.g., before a group exercise class). Use of imagery is another technique that can redirect the patient's focus from the frustrating aspects of performance or pain. With eyes closed, the patient is asked imagine a place or experience that is deeply relaxing (e.g., a sunset at the beach) and to maintain focus on that special experience. The environment should be relaxing and quiet, with softened lights.[173] Jacobson[174] originally described progressive relaxation exercises to promote relaxation. While resting comfortably, the patient is directed to alternately clench and release various different muscle groups, moving progressively throughout the body. This technique may not be the technique of choice for patients who experience high levels of muscle tension or muscle weakness.

Augmented Interventions

Augmented interventions are appropriate for patients who demonstrate insufficient recovery and lack voluntary movement control (e.g., inability to initiate or sustain movement). An intensive hands-on approach (e.g., neurodevelopmental treatment) and neuromuscular/sensory stimulation can be used to "jumpstart" recovery and promote early movement. Biofeedback and electrical stimulation are also important adjuncts. Augmented interventions are contraindicated in patients with sufficient active movement control. The focus of rehabilitation for these patients should be active exercise and task-oriented training (see Tables 10.8 and 10.9).

Key decisions regarding the use of augmented interventions include the following:

- What movements might benefit from augmented intervention?
- What type of stimulation or modality should be used and how much?
- When should the stimulation/modality be withdrawn?
- How can it used to enhance active, task-oriented practice?

Continued use of augmented interventions long after they are needed can result in the patient becoming dependent. For example, a therapist who continually manually assists a patient's movements hears the patient remark to an aide that he or she is not helping correctly.

It has to be done the way "my therapist" does it (i.e., "my therapist" syndrome). This patient is demonstrating an overreliance on the therapist for movement assistance. Augmented interventions can help the patient bridge the gap between absent or severely disordered movements and active movements. Once the patient develops independent voluntary control of movement, these treatment approaches are counterproductive.

Neurodevelopmental Treatment

Neurodevelopmental treatment (NDT) is an approach developed in the late 1940s through 1960s by Dr. Karel Bobath, an English physician, and Berta Bobath, a physiotherapist.[175,176] Their work focused on patients with neurological dysfunction (cerebral palsy and stroke). The essential problems of these patient groups were identified as a release of abnormal tone (spasticity) and abnormal postural reflexes (primitive spinal cord and brainstem reflexes) from higher-center CNS control with resulting loss of the normal postural reflex mechanism (righting, equilibrium, protective extension reactions) and normal movements. The therapist's primary focus in treatment was on specialized handling so that spastic and reflex patterns were inhibited and normal movements promoted. The rationale for this approach (hierarchical theory with top-down control) has been largely refuted by more recent studies on the nervous system.[177,178] Current NDT has realigned itself with newer theories of motor control (systems theory and a distributed model of CNS control). Many different factors are recognized as contributing to loss of motor function in patients with neurological dysfunction, including the full spectrum of sensory and motor deficits (weakness, limited ROM, impaired tone and coordination). Emphasis is on the use of both feedback and feedforward mechanisms to support postural control. Postural control is viewed as the foundation for all skill learning. Normal development in children and normal movement patterns in all patients are stressed. The patient learns to control posture and movement through a sequence of progressively more challenging postures and activities. NDT uses physical *handling techniques* and *key points of control* (e.g., shoulders, pelvis, hands, and feet) directed at supporting body segments and assisting the patient in achieving active control. Sensory stimulation (facilitation and inhibition via primarily proprioceptive and tactile inputs) is used as needed during treatment. Postural alignment and stability are facilitated while excessive tone and abnormal movements are inhibited. For example, in the patient with stroke, abnormal obligatory synergy movements are restricted while out-of-synergy movements are facilitated. Activities are selected that are functionally relevant and varied in terms of difficulty and environmental context. Compensatory training strategies (use of the less involved segments) are avoided. Carryover is promoted through a strong emphasis on patient, family, and caregiver education. NDT is taught today in recognized training courses.[179] Recent literature on the effectiveness of the

Bobath approach to stroke rehabilitation has not revealed any superiority of this approach over other approaches. However, serious methodological shortcomings of the studies reviewed exist, emphasizing the need for further high-quality trials.[180-182]

Neuromuscular Facilitation

The term *neuromuscular facilitation* refers to the facilitation, activation, or inhibition of muscle contraction and motor responses The term *facilitation* refers to the enhanced capacity to initiate a movement response through increased neuronal activity and altered synaptic potential. An applied stimulus may lower the synaptic threshold of the alpha motor neuron but may not be sufficient to produce an observable movement response. *Activation*, on the other hand, refers to the actual production of a movement response and implies reaching a critical threshold level for neuronal firing. *Inhibition* refers to the decreased capacity to initiate a movement response through altered synaptic potential. The synaptic threshold is raised, making it more difficult for the neuron to fire and produce movement. The combination of spinal and supraspinal inputs acting on the alpha motor neuron (final common pathway) will determine whether a muscle response is facilitated, activated, or inhibited. Table 10.8 lists commonly used neuromuscular facilitation techniques.

Table 10.8   Neuromuscular Facilitation Techniques

Stimulus	Response	Comments
Resistance: applied manually, using body position/gravity, or mechanically	Facilitates both intrafusal and extrafusal muscle contraction; hypertrophies extrafusal muscle fibers; enhances kinesthetic awareness (muscle spindle)	With very weak muscles, use light resistance; isometric and eccentric contractions before concentric. Maximal resistance can produce overflow from strong to weak muscles within the same synergistic pattern or to contralateral extremities.
Quick stretch to agonist	Facilitates both intrafusal and extrafusal agonist muscle contraction (*stretch reflex*)	Optimally applied in the lengthened range. A low-threshold response, relatively short-lived; can add resistance to maintain contraction.
Tapping/repeated quick stretch over tendon or muscle belly	Facilitates both intrafusal and extrafusal agonist muscle contraction (*stretch reflex*)	Tapping over muscle belly produces a weaker response than over the tendon. Tapping over a muscle is used to enhance holding in a weight-bearing position.
Prolonged stretch: slow, maintained stretch, applied at maximum available lengthened range	Inhibits or dampens muscle contraction and tone due to peripheral reflex effects (*stretch-protection reflex*)	Positioning; inhibitory splinting, casting; mechanical low-load weights using traction
Joint approximation: compression of joint surfaces, using manual pressure or position/gravity; weighted vest or belt	Facilitates postural extensors and stabilizing responses (co-contraction); enhances joint awareness (joint receptors)	Approximation applied to top of shoulders or pelvis in upright weight-bearing positions facilities postural extensors and stability (e.g., sitting, kneeling, or standing). Used in PNF extensor extremity patterns, pushing actions.
Joint traction: manual distraction of joints; wrist and ankle cuffs	Facilitates joint motion; enhances joint awareness (joint receptors)	Joint mobilization uses slow, sustained traction to improve mobility, relieve muscle spasm, and reduce pain. Used in PNF flexor extremity patterns, pulling actions.

Several general guidelines are important to consider. First, facilitative techniques can be *additive*. For example, several inputs applied simultaneously, such as quick stretch, resistance, and verbal cues, are commonly combined during practice of a PNF pattern. These stimuli collectively can produce the desired motor response, whereas use of a single stimulus may not. This demonstrates the property of *spatial summation* within the CNS. *Repeated stimulation* (e.g., tapping) may also produce the desired motor response owing to *temporal summation* within the CNS, whereas a single stimulus does not. Thus, repeated stretch is used to ensure that the patient with a weak muscle is able to move from the lengthened to the shortened range. Sensory receptors vary in their adaptation over time. Generally, they can be divided into two categories, slow- and fast-adapting receptors. In treatment, fast-adapting, phasic receptors such as touch receptors and phasic Ia muscle spindle endings are generally effective in initiating and shaping dynamic movements, whereas slow-adapting, tonic receptors such as joint receptors, GTOs, and static II muscle spindle endings are effective in monitoring and regulating postural responses. The response to stimulation or inhibition is unique to each patient and dependent on a number of different factors, including level of intactness of the CNS, arousal, and the specific level of activity of the motor neurons in question. For example, a patient who is depressed and hypoactive may require a larger amount of stimulation to achieve the desired response. Stimulation is generally contraindicated for the patient with hyperactivity and high arousal. For this patient, inhibition/relaxation techniques are indicated. The intensity, duration, and frequency of simulation need to be adjusted to meet individual patient needs. Unpredicted responses can result from inappropriate application of techniques. For example, stretch applied to a spastic muscle may increase spasticity and negatively affect voluntary movement. Facilitation techniques are *not* appropriate for patients who demonstrate adequate voluntary control. They should be viewed primarily as a temporary bridge to voluntary movement control.

Sensory Stimulation Techniques

The term *sensory stimulation* refers to the structured presentation of stimuli to (1) improve attention and arousal levels and (2) enhance sensory selection and discrimination. Effects are immediate and specific to the current state of the nervous system. Activity practice using inherent or naturally occurring sensory inputs is necessary for meaningful and lasting functional change to occur. Patients with deficits in sensory function exhibit variable sensory and perceptual impairments. For example, decreased sensitivity may be evident in some older adults and in some patients with neurological conditions such as stroke or TBI. Table 10.9 lists commonly used sensory stimulation techniques.

Several general guidelines are important in using sensory stimulation. Use of appropriate intensities is important to ensure that desired responses are obtained. Excess stimulation can produce unwanted responses, including generalized arousal and sympathetic fight or flight reactions. Sensory receptors adapt over time. Certain body segments such as the face, palms of the hands, and soles of the feet demonstrate both high concentrations of tactile receptors and increased representation in the sensory cortex. These areas are highly responsive to stimulation and are closely linked to both protective and exploratory functions.

Alterations in tactile, proprioceptive, visual, or vestibular systems can affect a patient's ability to move and learn new activities. Deafferentation in animals and in humans is associated with nonuse of a limb, although gross movements are possible under forced situations. Motor learning of new movements is impaired. The therapist should maintain focus on forced training of sensory-deficient limbs even though the patient may have little interest in moving the limb. The movements obtained should not be expected to be normal because significant deficits have been noted in fine motor control in deafferentated limbs.

Sensory stimulation and retraining have been used to improve sensory function in patients with stroke-related impairments.[183-186] Interventions include sensory reeducation, tactile kinesthetic guiding, repetitive sensory practice, and desensitization. The patient is repeatedly exposed to sensory experiences and practices sensory identification tasks (e.g., numbers, letters drawn on the hand or arm), discrimination tasks (e.g., detecting size, weight, and texture of objects placed in the hand), or passive-assisted drawing using a pencil. Intermittent pneumatic compression with an automatic intermittent pattern and electrical stimulation has also been used. The tasks were alternated between the more affected and less affected hands. Outcome measures included testing of sensory modalities (e.g., light touch temperature, two-point discrimination, sustained pressure, stereognosis, kinesthesia, and so forth) and upper limb functional tests (e.g., Motor Assessment Scale, Motor Activity Log, Frenchay Activities Index). In a systematic review of the literature, Doyle et al[185] found insufficient evidence to reach conclusions on the effectiveness of any intervention for sensory impairment of the UE. Limited preliminary evidence was found in support of using mirror therapy for improving detection of light touch, pressure, and temperature pain; thermal stimulation

Table 10.9 Sensory Stimulation Techniques

Stimulus	Response	Comments
Maintained pressure: firm manual pressure to midline back, abdomen; mechanical pressure via cones, pads	Calming effect, generalized inhibition, decreased fight or flight responses; desensitizes skin	Useful with patients with agitation and high arousal (e.g., the patient with TBI). Can be combined with other relaxation techniques (deep breathing, imagery, quiet environment). Also useful for patients with hypersensitivity (e.g., the patient with tactile defensiveness).
Slow, repetitive stroking: applied to midline back	Calming effect, generalized inhibition, decreased fight or flight responses	Performed while patient is prone or in supported sitting (head and arms resting on table top). Can use massage lubricant; stroke on either side of the spine; applied for 3–5 min. May be contraindicated with very hairy surface.
Light touch: brisk, quick stroking	Facilitates muscle; can elicit protection/flexor withdrawal response	Low threshold response, accommodates rapidly. Can be used to initially mobilize patients with low response levels (e.g., the patient with TBI who is minimally responsive).
Neutral warmth: retention of body heat through body wraps (Ace wraps, towel wraps, snug-fitting clothing gloves, socks, tights); air splints; tepid bath	Calming effect, generalized inhibition, decreased fight or flight responses	Useful for patients with high arousal or increased sympathetic activity. Overheating should be avoided, may produce rebound effects.
Prolonged cooling: immersion in cold water; ice wraps, ice massage; cooling suit	Decreases neural and muscle spindle firing. Provides inhibition of muscles and painful muscle spasm. Decreases metabolic rate of tissues	Monitor effects carefully: can produce sympathetic arousal, withdrawal or fight-or-flight responses. *Contraindicated* in patients with sensory deficits, generalized arousal, autonomic instability, and vascular problems.
Slow vestibular stimulation: constant, repetitive rocking; manually assisted in side-lying or sitting; mechanical (rocking chair); therapy ball; hammock	Calming effect, generalized inhibition, decreased fight or flight responses	Useful with patients who are hypertonic, hyperactive, or who demonstrate high arousal or tactile defensiveness (e.g., the patient with TBI who is agitated).
Rapid vestibular stimulation: rapid movements, fast spinning in a chair, mesh net	Heightens postural responses, movements	Useful for patients with hypotonia (e.g., an individual with Down syndrome); patients with sensory integrative dysfunction (e.g., a child with hyperactivity); patients with bradykinesia (e.g., a patient with PD). Can activate sympathetic arousal responses.

for improving rate of recovery of sensation; and intermittent pneumatic compression intervention for improving tactile and kinesthetic sensations.[185] Schabrun and Hillier[186] also found some evidence to suggest that electrical stimulation can improve sensory hand function and dexterity. While some techniques show promise, more quality research is needed. Continued practice with functionally relevant tasks is necessary to maintain the positive effects of any sensory retraining program.

Biofeedback

For patients with severe motor weakness, electromyographic biofeedback (EMG-BFB) can be used to assist the patient in regaining neuromuscular control. With careful electrode placement, it provides an accurate indication of electrical activity associated with muscular effort. It does not, however, provide an accurate indication of force of contraction. Surface electromyography (SEMG) electrodes are commonly used for recording. The signal is amplified and converted in audio and/or visual form, providing useful information about muscular performance to the patient. Patients who exhibit weak (trace, poor, or fair) muscle grades or deficient sensory feedback systems will benefit the most. Biofeedback has been used to increase the contraction of a muscle, train voluntary inhibition of muscle spasm and decrease muscle guarding.[187]

Woodford et al. in a Cochrane Database Systematic Review of the effects of EMG-BFB for motor function recovery following stroke found evidence from a small number of individual studies to suggest that EMG-BFB plus standard physiotherapy produced improvements in motor power, functional recovery and gait quality when compared to standard physiotherapy alone.[188] The researchers concluded that the results are limited because the trials were small, generally poorly designed, and utilized varying outcome measures. Additional research and meta-analysis can be found by reviewing the work of Amagan et all[189], Basmjian[190], Gantz et al[191], Hiraoka[192], Moreland et al[193] and Schleenbaker and Mainous[194], EMG-BFB has also been shown to improve motor function following incomplete SCI.[195] The therapist must carefully structure the use of biofeedback with practice of desired functional movement patterns. External feedback must be gradually reduced in order to foster use of intrinsic feedback mechanisms and active movements as recovery progresses.

Neuromuscular Electrical Stimulation

Neuromuscular electrical stimulation (NMES) is an effective modality to stimulate contraction in very weak muscles and improve motor function. Electrodes are placed directly over the muscle to be stimulated. Contraction is elicited by depolarizing motor neurons, with larger motor units and a greater number of Type II fibers firing first. The motor units will continue to fire until the stimulus stops. NMES can be used to reeducate muscle, improve ROM, decrease edema, and treat disuse atrophy. It is effective in reducing spasticity with stimulation of the weak antagonist. Applications to the tibialis anterior muscle or to the common peroneal nerve have been shown to reduce spasticity in the plantarflexor muscles and improve dorsiflexor function.[196] Electrical stimulation in patients with stroke has been shown to reduce flexor tone and posturing of the hand and improve functional grasp,[197-200] and reduce shoulder subluxation.[201]

Functional electrical stimulation (FES) uses a microprocessor to recruit muscles in a programmed synergistic sequence for the purposes of improving functional movements.[187] Following stroke, FES of the peroneal nerve has been shown to be effective in assisting dorsiflexion (drop foot) and improving walking.[202-205] It has been effectively combined with BWS and a treadmill.[206,207] Patients with incomplete SCI have been stimulated to exercise on bicycle ergometers (FES ergometry) and walk.[208,209]

Compensatory Interventions

Compensatory training strategies allow the patient to perform a task using alternate limbs and/or alternate movement patterns. Thus, the patient is able to perform an old task in a new manner. For example, the patient with hemiplegia dresses using the less-affected UE and increased trunk movement; the patient with paraplegia regains functional rolling, transfers, and wheelchair locomotion using the UEs. *Adaptive compensation* is the result of alternative or new movement patterns. *Substitutive compensation* is the result of using different parts of the body, effectors, to accomplish the task.[210] During training, the patient is made aware of movement deficiencies (cognitive awareness is developed). Changes are then made in the patient's overall approach to functional tasks. Alternate ways to accomplish the task are suggested, simplified, and adopted. The patient practices and relearns the task using the new pattern. The patient then practices the new pattern in the environment in which the function is expected to occur. Energy conservation techniques are incorporated into practice to ensure that the patient can successfully complete all daily tasks. Adaptation of the environment is also used to facilitate relearning of skills, ease of movement, and optimal performance. For example, the patient with unilateral neglect is assisted in dressing by color-coding the shoes (red tape on the left shoe, yellow tape on the right shoe). The wheelchair brake toggle is extended and color-coded to allow easy identification by the patient.

One of the major criticisms of this approach is that the focus on less-involved segments may suppress recovery for certain patients and contribute to *learned nonuse* of impaired segments. For example, the patient with stroke fails to learn to use the more involved extremities. Compensatory training should not become the focus of treatment in patients with potential for recovery. It is important to remember that given appropriate training, motor improvements can continue well into the chronic stages (e.g., patients with stroke). Compensatory training can also lead to development of *splinter skills,* which are skills acquired in a manner inconsistent with skills the individual already possesses. Splinter skills cannot be easily generalized to other task variations or to other environments.

A compensatory training approach may be the only realistic approach possible when recovery is limited or the patient presents with significant impairments and functional limitations with little or no expectation for additional recovery. Examples include the patient with complete SCI or the patient recovering from stroke with severe sensorimotor deficits and extensive co-morbidities (e.g., severe cardiac and respiratory compromise or memory deficits associated with Alzheimer's disease). The patient in the latter example is severely limited in the ability to actively participate in rehabilitation and to relearn motor skills.

Patient/Client-Related Instruction

Patient/client-related instruction is an important component of any rehabilitation plan of care. Components include instruction and training of patients/clients about the following:

- Current condition (pathology/pathophysiology, impairments, activity limitations, and participation restrictions)
- Accommodations to deficits in communication, cognitive, behavioral, or emotional impairments
- Anticipated goals and expected outcomes
- Strategies and preferred interventions to enhance performance and function

- Risk factors for pathology/pathophysiology and prevention of additional impairments, functional limitations, and participation restrictions
- Strategies and preferred interventions to enhance health, wellness, and fitness

Patients with deficits in motor function need to recognize the importance of repetitive practice both in-therapy and out-of-therapy to bring about meaningful recovery. Relevant tools to ensure high levels of practice include a behavioral contract, a caregiver contract, a daily schedule, an activity log or home diary, and a home skill assignment. These tools serve to focus the patient on the POC and ensure full, active participation in reaching successful outcomes. Patient skills in self-evaluation, problem solving, and decision making are promoted to foster independence. This empowerment serves to improve quality of life and prepare the patient for the life-long adjustments needed when living with a disability. If patient independence is not possible because of the complexity of deficits and limitations in recovery, education of family, friends, and caregivers assumes paramount importance.

SUMMARY

This chapter has outlined a conceptual framework for rehabilitation of the patient with deficits in motor function based on an understanding of the normal processes of motor control, motor learning, and recovery. Clinical decision making is based on a thorough examination of the patient's deficits in terms of impairments, activity limitations, and participation restrictions. The unique problems of each patient require that the therapist also recognize a number of interrelated factors, including individual needs and changing status, motivation, goals, concerns, and potential for independent function. The diversity of problems experienced by patients with disordered motor function negates the idea that any one intervention or group of interventions could be successful for all patients. Broad categories of interventions have been presented, with a major emphasis on training functional skills and promoting motor learning. Interventions also need to promote adaptability of skills for function in real-world environments. In selecting interventions, the therapist must consider those that have the greatest chance of success. The choice of interventions must also take into consideration other factors, including ability to deliver care, cost-effectiveness in terms of length of stay and number of allotted physical therapy visits, age of the patient, co-morbidities, social support, and potential discharge placement. Carefully planned and structured education empowers the patient and ensures skills for life-long learning and adjustment.

Questions for Review

1. Differentiate between the terms *motor control* and *motor learning*. How can impairments in motor control be distinguished from those of motor learning?
2. Differentiate between the three stages of motor learning. How do training strategies differ during each stage?
3. Define *neuroplasticity*. What are some of the mechanisms of neuroplasticity (changes in brain function) seen during recovery of function?
4. Discuss feedback strategies designed to improve retention and generalizability. How do they differ from strategies that optimize initial learning and performance?
5. Define *function-induced recovery*. Give an example of an intervention that could be used to promote function-induced recovery for the patient with incomplete paraplegia.

6. Identify three augmented interventions that can be used to calm the patient with traumatic brain injury who is demonstrating high arousal and agitated behavior.

7. Define *compensatory training*. Identify two compensatory training strategies for the patient with left hemiplegia and severe unilateral neglect.

CASE STUDY

HISTORY

The patient is a 36-year-old man who sustained a traumatic brain injury following a motorcycle accident. On admission to a local hospital, the patient was found to have a left frontal laceration with an underlying linear skull fracture. Computed tomography scan revealed edema, a right basal ganglia contusion, and a left frontal contusion. The patient was comatose on admission. His acute hospital course was complicated by increased intracranial pressure and severe spasticity. A gastric tube was inserted.

The patient's neurological status did not substantially improve at the acute hospital. He was transferred to a rehabilitation hospital 4 weeks after injury for intensive rehabilitation. He had a brief readmission to the acute hospital during his sixth week after injury for stabilization of acute hypothermia and hypothyroidism. He was then returned to the rehabilitation facility for continued intensive rehabilitation. His medications consisted of Tegretol (200 mg po qid), multivitamins, and Colace.

PART I: PHYSICAL THERAPY EXAMINATION FINDINGS (INITIAL ADMISSION TO REHAB, 4 WEEKS AFTER INJURY)

Behavior/cognition: He is functioning at Rancho Levels of Cognitive Functioning (RLOCF) Level V Confused-Inappropriate. The patient is able to respond to simple commands fairly consistently. With increased complexity of commands or lack of any external structure, responses are nonpurposeful, random, or fragmented. Highly distractible and lacks ability to focus on a specific task. Memory is severely impaired; often shows inappropriate use of objects. May perform previously learned tasks with structure but is unable to learn new information. Easily frustrated and responds with disinhibited behaviors (name calling and swearing).

Language–communication: Unable to examine.

Social: Married with no children. Wife is a registered nurse and very supportive of her husband.

Vital signs: Heart rate 60 beats per minute; blood pressure 122/70 mm Hg; respiratory rate 14 breaths per minute; O_2 saturation level is 92.

Sensation: Localizes to pinprick with withdrawal.

Passive range of motion:
- Right upper extremity (RUE) is limited in elbow ROM (0° to 70°); left upper extremity (LUE) elbow ROM is 10° to 100°.
- Both lower extremities (BLEs) are within normal limits except for ankle dorsiflexion 0° to 5° on R and 0° to 10° on L.

Motor Function

Tone (Modified Ashworth Scale grades [M-AS]): Severe flexor tone and spasms of the trunk that result in the patient moving in bed from a supine to a left-side-lying, curled-up (fetal) position, M-AS = 4.
- RUE extensor tone, M-AS = 3
- Right lower extremity (RLE) extensor tone, M-AS = 3
- LUE flexor tone, M-AS = 3
- Left lower extremity (LLE) extensor tone, M-AS = 2

Reflexes:
- Frequent asymmetrical tonic neck reflex posturing with head rotated to the right
- Flexor withdrawal reflexes bilaterally in response to pain (delayed on the left with decreased intensity of response)
- Positive support reflex on the left
- Hyperactive deep tendon reflexes throughout
- At times, the lower extremities scissor (extend and adduct), especially when upper body flexor tone increases

Voluntary movements:
- The patient is agitated with restless movements and is frequently diaphoretic.
- Limited head or trunk control, dependent sitting.
- Movement of RUE is spontaneous, purposeful at times, and out-of-synergy.

- Movement of the RLE is spontaneous, nonpurposeful, and out-of-synergy.
- LUE: no active movement.
- LLE movement: demonstrates abnormal obligatory extensor synergy pattern.

Coordination: Unable to assess.

Balance—sitting:

Static: Poor; requires handhold support and moderate assistance; demonstrates sacral sitting with posterior tilt of the pelvis

Dynamic: Poor; unable to accept challenge or move without loss of balance

Balance—standing:

Static: Poor; requires maximal assist of two persons to stand in the parallel bars with splint on LLE

Dynamic: Unable to weight shift or step

- **Gait and locomotion** (wheelchair [w/c]): Unable

Skin: Multiple healed lacerations on the knees and calves and pressure sores bilaterally on the lateral malleoli and calcanei from bivalve positioning splints.

Bladder and bowel: Incontinent of bowel and bladder, and has external catheter in place.

Functional activities: Max assistance in all ADL, FIM level 2.

PART I (QUESTIONS 1–3)

1. Identify and prioritize the problems in motor function presented in this case in terms of impairments and activity limitations based on initial admission data (4 weeks after injury).

2. Identify the goals of physical therapy intervention for this patient at this point in his recovery (initial admission).

3. Identify the motor learning strategies and two treatment interventions appropriate for this patient at this point in his recovery (initial admission).

PART II: REEXAMINATION 12 WEEKS AFTER INJURY

Behavior/cognition: He is functioning at Rancho Levels of Cognitive Functioning (RLOCF) Level VII Automatic-Appropriate. He appears appropriate and oriented within the hospital setting; goes through daily routine automatically, but frequently robot-like. Shows minimal to no confusion and has shallow recall of activities. Shows carryover for new learning but at a decreased rate. With structure is able to initiate social and recreational activities. Judgment remains impaired.

Language–communication: The patient is dysarthric; speech is usually intelligible but difficult to understand and delayed in onset. Auditory comprehension is good.

Vital signs: Within normal limits (WNL).

Skin: Lacerations are healed.

Sensation:

- **Vision and hearing** are WNL.
- **LUE:** Absent sensation.
- **LLE:** Impaired sensation, decreased proprioception.
- **RUE and RLE:** Intact

Range of motion:

- **RUE:** elbow ROM 0° to 90°; LUE: elbow ROM 5° to 110°
- **BLEs:** WNL except for ankle dorsiflexion bilaterally of 0° to 15°

Motor function

Tone (modified Ashworth Scale grades, M-AS):

Trunk: Tone in the trunk is WNL except for occasional flexor spasms

- **RUE and RLE:** Extensor tone, M-AS = 1
- **LUE:** Flexor tone, M-AS = 2
- **LLE:** Extensor tone, M-AS = 1

Reflexes:

- Exhibits strong associated reactions in the LUE and increased flexor posturing with stressful activities.

Voluntary movements:

- **RUE and RLE:** Demonstrates purposeful, full, isolated motions through available ROM against gravity. Strength is grossly F+ in the RUE and RLE.
- **LUE:** Limited voluntary movement; extensor synergy predominates.
- **LLE:** Movement is purposeful; strength is grossly F.
- **Head and trunk:** Movement is functional and strength is grossly F.

Coordination:
Exhibits moderate ataxia in trunk.
Demonstrates moderate impairment in finger-to-nose and toe-tapping test in RUE; LUE not tested.
Balance—sitting:
   Static: Good, able to maintain balance without handhold support, limited postural sway
   Dynamic: Good, able to accept moderate challenge and move without loss of balance
Balance—standing:
   Static: Fair, requires handhold support to stand in the parallel bars, occasional minimal assistance
   Dynamic: Fair, accepts minimal challenge; able to balance while turning head/trunk
Functional Activities:
   • **Bed mobility:** Rolls to right and left with supervision (S)
   • **Supine-to-sit and sit-to-stand:** Moderate assistance × 1, FIM level 3
   • **Transfers:** Moderate assistance × 1 in stand-pivot transfers, FIM level 3
   • **Wheelchair locomotion:** Maneuvers manual wheelchair with close S for safety, FIM level 5
   • **Gait:** Walks in parallel bars 10 ft with moderate assistance × 1, FIM level 3
   • **Dressing and grooming:** Minimal assistance × 1, FIM level 4

PART II (QUESTIONS 4–6)

4. Identify and prioritize this patient's motor function problems in terms of impairments and activity limitations (12 weeks after injury).

5. Identify the goals and outcomes of physical therapy intervention for this patient at this point in his recovery.

6. Identify the motor learning strategies and two treatment interventions appropriate for this patient at this point in his recovery.

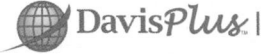 For additional resources, including answers to the questions for review and case study guiding questions, please visit **http://davisplus.fadavis.com**

References

1. Schmidt, R, and Lee, T: Motor Control and Learning: A Behavioral Emphasis, ed 5. Human Kinetics, Champaign, IL, 2011.
2. Shumway-Cook, A, and Woollacott, M: Motor Control Theory and Practical Applications, ed 4. Lippincott Williams & Wilkins, Baltimore, 2012.
3. Bernstein, N: The Coordination and Regulation of Movements. Pergamon Press, Oxford, 1967.
4. Kelso, J: Dynamic Patterns: The Self-Organization of Brain and Behavior. MIT Press, Cambridge, MA, 1995.
5. Calancie, B, et al: Involuntary stepping after chronic spinal cord injury: Evidence for a central rhythm generator for locomotion in man. Brain 117:1143, 1994.
6. Griller S: Neurobiological bases of rhythmic motor acts in vertebrates. Science 228:143, 1989.
7. Adams, J: A closed-loop theory of motor learning. J Motor Behav 3:111, 1971.
8. Schmidt, R: A schema theory of discrete motor skill learning. Psychol Rev 82:225, 1975.
9. Nashner, L: Adapting reflexes controlling human posture. Exp Brain Res 26:59, 1976.
10. Nashner, L: Fixed patterns of rapid postural responses among leg muscles during stance. Exp Brain Res 30:13, 1977.
11. Nashner, L, and Woollacott, M: The organization of rapid postural adjustments of standing humans: An experimental-conceptual model. In Tablott, RE, and Humphrey, DR (eds): Posture and Movement. Raven, New York, 1979, pp 243–257.
12. Fitts, P, and Posner, M: Human Performance. Brooks/Cole, Belmont, CA, 1967.
13. Bayley, N: The development of motor abilities during the first three years. Monogr Soc Res Child Dev 1(1, serial no 1), 1935.
14. Gesell, A: The First Five Years of Life. Harper & Brothers, New York, 1940.
15. McGraw, M: The Neuromuscular Maturation of the Human Infant. Hafner, New York, 1945.
16. VanSant, A: Life span development in functional tasks. Phys Ther 70:788, 1990.
17. Woollacott, M, and Shumway-Cook, A: Changes in posture control across the life span: A systems approach. Phys Ther 70:799, 1990.
18. Woollacott, M, and Shumway-Cook, A (eds): Development of Posture and Gait Across the Life Span. University of South Carolina Press, Columbia, 1989.
19. Spirduso, W, Francis, K, and MacRai, P: Physical Dimensions of Aging. Human Kinetics, Champaign, IL, 2005.
20. Light, K: Information processing for motor performance in aging adults. Phys Ther 70:821, 1990.
21. Salthouse, T, and Somberg, B: Isolating the age deficit in speeded performance. J Gerontol 37:59, 1982.
22. Benjuva, N, Melzer, I, and Kaplanski, J: Aging-induced shifts from a reliance on sensory input to muscle cocontraction during balanced standing. J Gerontol A Biol Sci Med Sci 59A:166, 2004.
23. Light, K, and Spirduso, W: Effects of adult aging on the movement complexity factor of response programming. J Gerontol 45:107, 1990.
24. Levin, M, Kleim, J, and Wolf, S: What do motor "recovery" and "compensation" mean in patients following stroke? Neurorehabil Neural Repair 23:313, 2009.
25. Stein, D, Failowsky, B, and Will, B: Brain Repair. Oxford University Press, New York, 1995.
26. Pascual-Leone, A, et al: The plastic human brain cortex. Annu Rev Neurosci 28:377, 2005.
27. Chen, R, Cohen, LG, and Hallett, M: Nervous system reorganization following injury. Neuroscience 111(4):761, 2002.
28. Kleim, J, et al: Cortical synaptogenesis and motor map reorganization occur during late, but not early, phase of motor skill learning. J Neurosci 24:628, 2004.

29. Luscher, C, et al: Synaptic plasticity and dynamic modulation of the post synaptic membrane. Nat Neurosci 3(6):545, 2000.

30. Nudo, R: Functional and structural plasticity in motor cortex: Implications for stroke recovery. Phys Med Rehabil Clin North Am 14(1, Suppl):s5, 2003.

31. Nudo, R: Adaptive plasticity in motor cortex: Implications for rehabilitation after brain injury. J Rehabil Med 41(Suppl):7, 2003.

32. Fraser, C, et al: Driving plasticity in human adult motor cortex is associated with improved motor function after brain injury. Neuron 34:831, 2002.

33. Kleim, J, Jones, T, and Schallert, T: Motor enrichment and the induction of plasticity before and after brain injury. Neurochem Res 28:1757, 2003.

34. Shepherd, R: Exercise and training to optimize functional motor performance in stroke: Driving neural reorganization. Neural Plast 8:121, 2001.

35. Ploughman, M: A review of brain neuroplasticity and implications for the physiotherapeutic management of stroke. Physiother Can 164(Summer), 2002.

36. Wolf, S, et al: Effect of constraint-induced movement therapy on upper extremity function 3 to 9 months after stroke: The EXCITE randomized trial. JAMA 296:2095, 2006.

37. Wolf, S, et al: The EXCITE trial: Retention of improved upper extremity function among stroke survivors receiving CI movement therapy. Lancet Neurol 7:33, 2008.

38. Sirtori, V, et al: Constraint-induced movement therapy for upper extremities in stroke patients. Cochrane Database of Systematic Reviews. 2009, Issue 4. Art. No.: CD004433. DOI: 10.1002/14651858.CD004433.pub2.

39. Hakkennes, S, and Keating, J: Constraint-induced movement therapy following stroke: A systematic review of randomized controlled trials. Aus J Physiother 51:221, 2005.

40. Dahl, A, et al: Short-and long-term outcome of constraint-induced movement therapy after stroke: A randomized controlled feasibility trial. Clinical Rehab 22:436, 2008.

41. Page, S, et al: Efficacy of modified constraint-induced movement therapy in chronic stroke: A single-blinded randomized controlled trial. Arch Phys Med Rehabil 85:14, 2004.

42. Taub, E, et al: A placebo-controlled trial of constraint-induced movement therapy for upper extremity after stroke. Stroke 37:1045, 2006.

43. Taub, E, et al: Technique to improve chronic motor deficit after stroke. Arch Phys Med Rehabil 74:347, 1993.

44. Sawaki, L, et al: Constraint-induced movement therapy results in increased motor map area in subjects 3 to 9 months after stroke. Neurorehabil Neural Repair 33:505, 2008.

45. Liepert, J: Motor cortex excitability in stroke before and after constraint-induced movement therapy. Cog Behav Neurol 19:41, 2006.

46. Duncan, P, et al: Body-weight-supported treadmill rehabilitation after stroke. N Engl J Med 364:2026, 2011.

47. Moseley, A, et al: Treadmill training and body weight support for walking after stroke. Cochrane Database of Systematic Reviews 2005, Issue 4. Art. No.: CD002840. DOI: 10.1002/14651858.CD002840.pub2.

48. Ada, L: Randomized trial of treadmill walking with body weight support to establish walking in subacute stroke—the MOBILISE Trial. Stroke 41:1247, 2010.

49. Sullivan, K, et al: Effects of task-specific locomotor and strength training in adults who were ambulatory after stroke: Results of the STEPS randomized clinical trial. Phys Ther 87:1580, 2007.

50. Franceschini, M, et al: Walking after stroke: What does treadmill training with body weight support add to overground gait training in patients early after stroke? A single-blind, randomized controlled trial. Stroke 40:3079, 2009.

51. Kolb, B, and Gibb, R: Environmental enrichment and cortical injury: Behavioral and anatomical consequences of frontal cortex lesions. Cerebral Cortex 1:189, 1991.

52. Held, J, Gordon, J, and Gentile, A: Environmental influences on locomotor recovery following cortical lesions in rats. Behav Neurosci 99:678, 1985.

53. Held, J: Environmental enrichment enhances sparing and recovery of function following brain damage. NeuroReport 22:74, 1998.

54. Ohlsson, A, and Johansson, B: Environment influences functional outcome of cerebral infarction in rats. Stroke 26:644, 1995.

55. Johansson, B, and Ohlsson, A: Environment, social interaction and physical activity as determinants of functional outcome after cerebral infarction in the rat. Exp Neurol 139:322, 1996.

56. Carr, J, and Shepherd, R: Stroke Rehabilitation. Butterworth-Heinemann, London, 2003.

57. Mackey, F, et al: Stroke rehabilitation: Are highly structured units more conducive to physical activity than less structured units? Arch Phys Med Rehabil 77:1066, 1996.

58. Carr, J, and Shepherd, R: Neurological Rehabilitation: Optimizing Motor Performance, ed 2. Churchill Livingstone/Elsevier, St Louis, 2010.

59. Tinson, D: How stroke patients spend their days: An observational study of the treatment regime offered to patients in hospital with movement disorders following stroke. Int Disabil Stud 11(1):45, 1989.

60. Esmonde, T, et al: Stroke rehabilitation: Patient activity during non-therapy time. Aust J Physiother 43:43, 1997.

61. Lee, T, and Swanson, L: What is repeated in a repetition? Effects of practice conditions on motor skill acquisition. Phys Ther 71:150, 1991.

62. Winstein, C, Pohl, P, and Lewthwaite, R: Effects of physical guidance and knowledge of results on motor learning: Support for the guidance hypothesis. Res Quart Exer Sport 65:316–323, 1994.

63. Singer, R, and Pease, D: A comparison of discovery learning and guided instructional strategies on motor skill learning, retention, and transfer. Res Q 47:788, 1976.

64. Wulf, G, Shea, C, and Whitacre, C: Physical-guidance benefits in learning a complex motor skill. J Mot Behav 30:367–380, 1998.

65. Salmoni, A, et al: Knowledge of results and motor learning: A review and critical appraisal. Psychol Bull 95:355, 1984.

66. Lee, T, et al: On the role of knowledge of results in motor learning: Exploring the guidance hypothesis. J Mot Behav 22:191, 1990.

67. Bilodeau, E, et al: Some effects of introducing and withdrawing knowledge of results early and late in practice. J Exp Psychol 58:142, 1959.

68. Magill, R: Augmented feedback in motor skill acquisition. In Singer, RN, Hausenblas, HA, and Janell, CM (eds): Handbook of Sport Psychology, ed 2. Wiley, New York, 2001, p 86.

69. Winstein, C, et al: Learning a partial-weight-bearing skill: Effectiveness of two forms of feedback. Phys Ther 76:985, 1996.

70. Bilodeau, E, and Bilodeau, I: Variable frequency knowledge of results and the learning of a simple skill. J Exp Psychol 55:379, 1958.

71. Ho, L, and Shea, J: Effects of relative frequency of knowledge of results on retention of a motor skill. Percept Mot Skills 46:859, 1978.

72. Sherwood, D: Effect of bandwidth knowledge of results on movement consistency. Percept Mot Skills 66:535, 1988.

73. Winstein, C, and Schmidt, R: Reduced frequency of knowledge of results enhances motor skill learning. J Exp Psychol Learn Mem Cogn 16:677, 1990.

74. Lavery, J: Retention of simple motor skills as a function of type of knowledge of results. Can J Psych 16:300, 1962.

75. Boyd, L, and Winstein, C: Explicit information interferes with implicit motor learning of both continuous and discrete movement tasks after stroke. J Neur Phys Ther 30:46–57, 2006.

76. Swinnen, S, et al: Information feedback for skill acquisition: Instantaneous knowledge of results degrades learning. J Exp Psychol Learn Mem Cogn 16:706, 1990.

77. Winstein, C: Knowledge of results and motor learning: Implications for physical therapy. Phys Ther 71:140, 1991.

78. Shea, J, and Morgan, R: Contextual interference effects on the acquisition, retention, and transfer of a motor skill. J Exp Psychol: Hum Learn 5:179, 1979.

79. Wulf, G, and Schmidt, R: Variability in practice facilitation in retention and transfer through schema formation or context effects? J Mot Behav 20:133, 1988.

80. Wulf, G, and Schmidt, R: Variability of practice and implicit motor learning. J Exp Psychol: Learn, Mem, Cogn 23:987, 1997.

81. Lee, T, Wulf, G, and Schmidt, R: Contextual interference in motor learning: Dissociated effects due to the nature of task variations. Q J Exp Psychol 44A:627, 1992.

82. Lee, T, and Magill, R: The locus of contextual interference in motor skill acquisition. J Exp Psychol Learn Mem Cogn 9:730, 1983.

83. Jeannerod, M: Neural simulation of action: A unifying mechanism for motor cognition. Neuroimage 14:103, 2001.

84. Jeannerod, M, and Frak, V: Mental imaging of motor activity in humans. Curr Opin Neurobiol 9:735, 1999.

85. Feltz, D, and Landers, D: The effects of mental practice on motor skill learning and performance: A meta-analysis. J Sports Psychol 5:25, 1983.

86. Braun, S, et al: Using mental practice in stroke rehabilitation: A framework. Clin Rehabil 22:579–591, 2008.

87. Richardson, A: Mental practice: A review and discussion (part 1). Res Q 38:95, 1967.

88. Warner, L, and McNeill, M: Mental imagery and its potential for physical therapy. Phys Ther 68:516, 1988.

89. Maring, J: Effects of mental practice on rate of skill acquisition. Phys Ther 70:165, 1990.

90. Lee, T: Transfer-appropriate processing: A framework for conceptualizing practice effects in motor learning. In Meijer, O, and Roth, K (eds): Complex Movement Behavior: The Motor-Action Controversy. North Holland, Amsterdam, 1988, p 201.

91. Gentile, A: Skill acquisition: Action, movement, and neuromotor processes. In Carr, J, and Shephard, R (eds): Movement Science. Foundations for Physical Therapy in Rehabilitation, ed 2. Aspen, Rockville, MD, 2000, p 147.

92. O'Sullivan, S, and Schmitz, T: Improving Functional Outcomes in Physical Rehabilitation. FA Davis, Philadelphia, 2010.

93. Humm, J, et al: Use-dependent exaggeration of brain damage occurs during an early post-lesion vulnerable period. Brain Res 783:286, 1988.

94. Humm, J, et al: Use-dependent exaggeration of brain injury: Is glutamate involved? Exp Neurol 157:349, 1999.

95. Dromerick, A, et al: Very early constraint-induced movement during stroke rehabilitation. Neurology 73:195, 2009.

96. Griesbach, G, Gomez-Pinilla, F, and Hovda, D: The upregulation of plasticity-related proteins following TBI is disrupted with acute voluntary exercise. Brain Res 1016:154, 2004.

97. Biernaskie, J, Chernenko, G, and Corbett, D: Efficacy of rehabilitative experience declines with time after focal ischemic brain injury. J Neurosci 24:1245, 2004.

98. Kleim, J, and Jones, T: Principles of experience-dependent neural plasticity: Implications for rehabilitation after brain damage. J Speech Lang Hear Res 51:S225, 2008.

99. Morris, D, and Taub, E: Constraint-induced movement therapy. In O'Sullivan, S, and Schmitz, T (eds): Improving Functional Outcomes in Physical Rehabilitation. FA Davis, Philadelphia, 2010, p 232.

100. American Physical Therapy Association: Guide to Physical Therapist Practice. Phys Ther 81:1, 2001.

101. Hermsdorfer, J, et al: Effects of unilateral brain damage on grip selection, coordination, and kinematics of ipsilesional prehension. Exp Brain Res 128:41, 1999.

102. Kisner, C, and Colby, L: Therapeutic Exercise Foundations and Techniques, ed 5. FA Davis, Philadelphia, 2007.

103. American College of Sports Medicine: ACSM's Guidelines for Exercise Testing and Prescription, ed 8. Lippincott Williams & Wilkins, Philadelphia, 2009.

104. American College of Sports Medicine: ACSM's Exercise Management for Persons with Chronic Diseases and Disabilities, ed 3. Lippincott Williams & Wilkins, Philadelphia, 2009.

105. Davies, P: Steps to follow. Springer, New York, 2000.

106. Smith, G, et al: Task-oriented exercise improves hamstring strength and spastic reflexes in chronic stroke patients. Stroke 30:2112, 1999.

107. Riolo, L, and Fisher, K: Is there evidence that strength training could help improve muscle function and other outcomes without reinforcing abnormal movement patterns or increasing reflex activity in a man who has had a stroke? Phys Ther 83:844, 2003.

108. Sharp, S, and Brouwer, B: Isokinetic strength training of the hemiparetic knee: Effects on function and spasticity. Arch Phys Med Rehabil 70:1231, 1997.

109. Teixeira-Salmela, L, et al: Muscle strengthening and physical conditioning to reduce impairment and disability in chronic stroke survivors. Arch Phys Med Rehabil 80:1211, 1999.

110. Miller, G, and Light, K: Strength training in spastic hemiparesis: Should it be avoided? NeuroRehabil 9:17, 1997.

111. Yang, Y, et al: Task-oriented progressive resistance strength training improves muscle strength and functional performance in individuals with stroke. Clin Rehabil 20:860, 2006.

112. Eng, J: Strength training in individuals with stroke. Physiother Can 56:189, 2004.

113. Voss, D, et al: Proprioceptive Neuromuscular Facilitation, ed 3. Harper & Row, Philadelphia, 1985.

114. Adler, S, Beckers, D, and Buck, M: PNF in Practice, ed 3. Springer-Verlag, New York, 2008.

115. Gordon, N, et al: Physical activity and exercise recommendations for stroke survivors: An American Heart Association scientific statement from the Council on Clinical Cardiology, Subcommittee on Exercise, Cardiac Rehabilitation, and Prevention; the Council on Cardiovascular Nursing; the Council on Nutrition, Physical Activity, and Metabolism; and the Stroke Council. Circulation 109:2031–2041, 2004. Retrieved January 20, 2012, from http://circ.ahajournals.org/content/109/16/2031.

116. Teasell, R, et al: Evidence-Based Review of Stroke Rehabilitation Executive Summary, ed 14. Retrieved January 20, 2012, from www.ebrsr.com.

117. Post-Polio Health International: A statement about exercise for survivors of polio. Excerpt from the Handbook on the Late Effects of Poliomyelitis for Physicians and Survivors, 1999. Retrieved January 20, 2012, from www.post-polio.org/ipn/pnn19-2A.html.

118. March of Dimes: Post-polio syndrome: Identifying best practices in diagnosis and care, 2001. Retrieved January 20, 2012, from www.marchofdimes.com/files/PPSreport.pdf.

119. Anderson, P, et al: European Federation of Neurological Societies Task Force on diagnosis and management of amyotrophic lateral sclerosis: Guidelines for diagnosing and clinical care of patients and relatives. Eur J Neurol 12:921, 2005. Retrieved January 20, 2012, from www.ncbi.nlm.nih.gov/pubmed/16324086.

120. Pahwa, R, et al: Practice parameter: Treatment of Parkinson disease with motor fluctuations and dyskinesia (an evidence-based review). Report of the Quality Standards Subcommittee of the American Academy of Neurology. Neurology 66:983, 2006. Retrieved January 20, 2012, from www.neurology.org/content/66/7/983.long.

121. Borg, G: Borg's Perceived Exertion and Pain Scales. Human Kinetics, Champaign, IL, 1998.

122. Taylor, D, et al: Viscoelastic properties of muscle-tendon units. The biomechanical effects of stretching. Am J Sports Med 18:300, 1990.

123. DeDeyne P: Application of passive stretch and its implications for muscle fibers. Phys Ther 81:819, 2001.

124. Anderson, B, and Burke, E: Scientific, medical, and practical aspects of stretching. Clin Sports Med 10:63, 1991.

125. Sady, S, et al: Flexibility training: Ballistic, static or proprioceptive neuromuscular facilitation. Arch Phys Med Rehabil 63:261, 1982.

126. Gracies, J: Pathophysiology of impairment in patients with spasticity and the use of stretch as a treatment for spastic hypertonia. Med Rehabil Clin North Am 12:747, 2001.

127. Bohannon, R. and Larkin, P: Passive ankle Dorsiflexion increases in patients after a regimen of tilt table: Wedge board standing. Phys Ther 65:1676, 1985.

128. Fasen, J, et al: A randomized controlled trial of hamstring stretching: Comparison of four techniques. J Strength Conditioning Research 23(2):660, 2009.

129. Etnyre, B, and Lee, E: Chronic and acute flexibility of men and women using three different stretching techniques. Res Q 59:222, 1988.

130. Osternig, L, et al: Differential response to proprioceptive neuromuscular facilitation (PNF) stretch technique. Med Sci Sports Exerc 22:106, 1990.

131. Hale, L, Fritz, V, and Goodman, M: Prolonged static muscle stretch reduces spasticity—but for how long should it be held? J Physio 51:3, 1995.

132. Booth, B, Doyle, M, and Montgomery, J: Serial casting for the management of spasticity in the head-injured adult. Phys Ther 63:1960, 1983.

133. Moseley, A: The effect of casting combined with stretching on passive ankle dorsiflexion in adults with traumatic head injuries. Phys Ther 77:240, 1997.

134. Singer, B, et al: Evaluation of serial casting to correct equinovarus deformity of the ankle after acquired brain injury in adults. Arch Phys Med Rehabil 84:483, 2003.

135. Jones, C: Case in point. Effect of lower extremity serial casts on hemiparetic gait patterns in adults. Phys Ther Case Rep 2:221, 1999.

136. Singer, B, Singer, K, and Allison, G: Serial plastering to correct equinovarus deformity of the ankle following acquired brain injury in adults: Review and clinical applications. Disabil Rehabil 23:829, 2001.

137. Rothstein, J, et al: The effect of casting combined with stretching on passive ankle dorsiflexion in adults with traumatic head injuries. Phys Ther 77:248, 1997.

138. Cincinnati Children's Hospital Medical Center: Evidence-Based Care Guideline: Serial Casting of the Lower Extremity, January 2009. Retrieved January 22, 2012, from www.guideline.gov/content.aspx.

139. Young, T, and Nicklin, C: Lower Limb Casting in Neurology: Practical Guidelines. Royal Hospital for Neurodisability, London, 2000.

140. Nashner, L: Adapting reflexes controlling the human posture. Exp Brain Res 26:59, 1976.

141. Nashner, L, and Woollacott, M: The organization of rapid postural adjustments of standing humans: An experimental-conceptual model. In Talbott, RE, and Humphrey, DR (eds): Posture and Movement. Raven, New York, 1979, pp 243–257.

142. Nashner, L, Woollacott, M, and Tuma, G: Organization of rapid responses to postural and locomotor-like perturbations of standing man. Exp Brain Res 36:463, 1979.

143. Horak, F, and Nashner, L: Central programming of postural movements: Adaptation to altered support surface configurations. J Neurophysiol 55:1369, 1986.

144. McIlroy, W, and Maki, B: Adaptive changes to compensatory stepping responses. Gait Posture 3:43, 1995.

145. Maki, B, and McIlroy, W: The role of limb movements in maintaining upright stance: The "change-in-support" strategy. Phys Ther 77:488, 1997.

146. Gillespie, L, et al: Interventions for preventing falls in elderly people. Cochrane Database of Systematic Reviews, 2009, Issue 2. Art. No.: CD000340. DOI: 10.1002/14651858.CD000340.pub2.

147. Means, K, Rodell, D, and O'Sullivan, P: Balance, mobility, and falls among community-dwelling elderly persons: Effects of a rehabilitation exercise program. Am J Phys Med Rehabil 84: 238–250, 2005.

148. Marigold, D, et al: Exercise leads to faster postural reflexes, improved balance and mobility, and fewer falls in older persons with chronic stroke. J Am Geriatr Soc 53:416–423, 2005.

149. Shumway-Cook, A, et al: The effect of multidimensional exercises on balance, mobility, and fall risk in community dwelling older adults. Phys Ther 77:46, 1997.

150. Nitz, J, and Choy, N: The efficacy of a specific balance-strategy training programme for preventing falls among older people: A pilot randomized controlled trial. Age Ageing 33:52–58, 2004.

151. Shumway-Cook, A, et al: Effect of balance training on recovery of stability in children with cerebral palsy. Dev Med Child Neurol 45:591, 2003.

152. Lubetzky-Vilnai, L, and Kartin, D: Effect of balance training on balance performance in individuals post stroke: A systematic review. J Neurol Phys Ther 34:127, 2010.

153. Taggart, H: Effects of Tai Chi exercise on balance, functional mobility, and fear of falling among older women. Appl Nurs Res 15:235, 2002.

154. Li, F, et al: Tai Chi and fall reductions in older adults: A randomized controlled trial. J Gerontol A Biol Sci Med Sci 60:187–194, 2005.

155. Gatts, S, and Woollacott, M: Neural mechanisms underlying balance improvement with short term Tai Chi training. Aging Clin Exp Res 18:7–19, 2006.

156. Hu, M, and Woollacott, M: Multisensory training of standing balance in older adults. 1. Postural stability and one-leg stance balance. J Gerontol 49:M52–M61, 1994.

157. Hu, M, and Woollacott, M: Multisensory training of standing balance in older adults. 2. Kinetic and electromyographic postural responses. J Gerontol 49:M62–M71, 1994.

158. Cass, S, Borello-France, D, and Furman, J: Functional outcome of vestibular rehabilitation in patients with abnormal sensory organization testing. Am J Otol 17:581–594, 1996.

159. Bayouk, J, Boucher, J, and Leroux, A: Balance training following stroke: Effects of task-oriented training with and without altered sensory input. Int J Rehabil Res 29:51–59, 2006.

160. Smania, N, et al: Rehabilitation of sensorimotor integration deficits in balance impairment of patients with stroke hemiparesis: A before/after pilot study. Neurol Sci 29:313–319, 2008.

161. Benda, B, et al: Biomechanical relationship between center of gravity and center of pressure during standing. IEEE Trans Rehab Eng 2:3, 1994.

162. Nichols, D: Balance retraining after stroke using force platform biofeedback. Phys Ther 77:553, 1997.

163. Winstein, C, et al: Standing balance training: Effect on balance and locomotion in hemiparetic adults. Arch Phys Med Rehabil 70:755, 1989.

164. Shumway-Cook, A, Anson, D, and Haller, S: Postural sway biofeedback: Its effect on reestablishing stance stability in hemiplegic patients. Arch Phys Med Rehabil 69:395, 1988.

165. Barclay-Goddard, R, et al: Force platform feedback for standing balance training after stroke. Cochrane Database Syst Rev 4:D004129, 2004.

166. van Peppen, R, et al: Effects of visual feedback therapy on postural control in bilateral standing after stroke: A systematic review. J Rehabil Med 38:3–9, 2006.

167. Jeka, J: Light touch contact as a balance aid. Phys Ther 77:476, 1997.

168. Brandt, T, Buchele, W, and Krafczyk, S: Training effects on experimental postural instability: A model for clinical ataxia therapy. In Bles, W, and Brandt, T (eds): Disorders of Posture and Gait. Elsevier, Amsterdam, 1986, pp 353–365.

169. Armutlu, K, Karabudk, R, and Nurlu, G: Physiotherapy approaches in the treatment of ataxic multiple sclerosis; a pilot study. Neurorehab Neural Repair 15:203, 2001.

170. Topka, H, et al: Motor skill learning in patients with cerebellar degeneration. J Neurol Sci 158:164, 1998.

171. Gill-Body, K, et al: Rehabilitation of balance in two patients with cerebellar dysfunction. Phys Ther 77:534, 1977.

172. Benson, H: The Relaxation Response. Avon Books, New York, 1975.

173. Kabot-Zinn, J: Full Catastrophe Living: Using the Wisdom of Your Body to Face Stress, Pain, and Illness. Random House, New York, 1990.

174. Jacobson, E: Progressive Relaxation. University of Chicago Press, Oxford, England, 1929.

175. Bobath, B: The treatment of neuromuscular disorders by improving patterns of coordination. Physiotherapy 55:1, 1969.

176. Bobath, B: Adult Hemiplegia: Evaluation and Treatment, ed 3. Heinemann, London, 1990.

177. Bernstein, N: The Coordination and Regulation of Movement. Pergamon, London, 1967.

178. Kamm, K, Thelen, E, and Jensen, J: A dynamical systems approach to motor development. In Rothstein, J (ed): Movement Science. American Physical Therapy Association, Alexandria, VA, 1991, pp 11–23.

179. Howle, J, et al: Neuro-Developmental Treatment Approach. Neuro-Developmental Treatment Association, Laguna Beach, CA, 2002.

180. Luke, C, Dodd, K, and Brock, K: Outcomes of the Bobath concept on upper limb recovery following stroke. Clin Rehabil 18:888, 2004.

181. Pollock, A, et al: Physiotherapy treatment approaches for stroke. Cochrane Corner. Stroke 39:519, 2008.

182. Kollen, G, et al: The effectiveness of the Bobath concept in stroke rehabilitation. What is the evidence? Stroke 40(4):e89, 2009.

183. Celnik, P, et al: Somatosensory stimulation enhances the effects of training functional hand tasks in patients with chronic stroke. Arch Phys Med Rehabil 88:1369, 2007.

184. Lynch, E, et al: Sensory retraining of the lower limb after acute stroke: A randomized controlled pilot trial. Arch Phys Med Rehabil 88:1101, 2007.

185. Doyle, S, et al: Interventions for sensory impairment in the upper limb after stroke. Cochrane Database of Systematic Reviews, 2010, Issue 6. Art. No.: CD006331. DOI: 10.1002/14651858.CD006331.pub2.

186. Schabrun, SM, and Hillier, S: Evidence for the retraining of sensation after stroke: A systematic review. Clin Rehabil 23:27–39, 2009.

187. Prentice, W: Therapeutic Modalities in Rehabilitation, ed 4. McGraw Hill Medical, New York, 2005.

188. Woodford, Henry J, Price, Christopher IM. EMG biofeedback for the recovery of motor function after stroke. Cochrane Database of Systematic Reviews 2007, Issue 2. Art. No.: CD004585. DOI: 10.1002/14651858.CD004585.pub2.

189. Armagan, O, Tascioglu, F, and Oner, C: Electromyographic biofeedback in the treatment of the hemipletic hand: A placebo-controlled study. Am J Phys Med Rehabil 82:856, 2003.

190. Basmajian, JV, et al. Stroke treatment: comparison of integrated behavioural-physical therapy vs traditional physical therapy programs. Arch Phys Med Rehab 68:267-72, 1987.

191. Gantz, M, et al: Biofeedback therapy in poststroke rehabilitation: A meta-analysis of the randomized controlled trials. Arch Phys Med Rehabil 76:588, 1995.

192. Hiraoka, K: Rehabilitation efforts to improve upper extremity function in post-stroke patients: A meta-analysis. J Phys Ther Sci 13:5, 2001.

193. Moreland, J, Thompson, M, and Fuoco, A: Electromyographic biofeedback to improve lower extremity function after stroke: A meta-analysis. Arch Phys Med Rehabil 79:134, 1998.

194. Schleenbaker, R, and Mainous, A: Electromyographic biofeedback for neuromuscular reeducation in the hemiplegic stroke patient: A meta-analysis. Arch Phys Med Rehabil 74:1301, 1993.

195. Klose, K, Needham, B, and Schmidt, D: An assessment of the contribution of electromyographic biofeedback as a therapy in the physical training of spinal cord injured persons. Arch Phys Med Rehabil 74:453, 1993.

196. Kesar, T, et al: Novel patterns of functional electrical stimulation have an immediate effect on dorsiflexor muscle function during gait for people poststroke. Phys Ther 90:55, 2010.

197. Cauraugh, J, et al: Chronic motor dysfunction after stroke: Recovering wrist and finger extension by electromyography-triggered neuromuscular stimulation. Stroke 31:1360, 2000.

198. Powell, J, et al: Electrical stimulation of wrist extensors in post-stroke hemiplegia. Stroke 30:1384, 1999.

199. Kowalczewski, J, et al: Upper-extremity functional electric stimulation-assisted exercises on a workstation in the sub-acute phase of stroke recovery. Arch Phys Med Rehabil 88:833, 2007.

200. Meilink, A, Hemmen, B, and Ham, S: Impact of EMG-triggered neuromuscular stimulation of the wrist and finger extensors of the paretic hand after stroke: A systematic review of the literature. Clinical Rehabil 22:291, 2008.

201. Wang, R, Chan, R, and Tsai, M: Functional electrical stimulation on chronic and acute hemiplegic shoulder subluxation. Am J Phys Med Rehabil 79:385, 2000.

202. Bogataj, U, Gros, H, and Kljajic, M: The rehabilitation of gait in patients with hemiplegia: A comparison between conventional therapy and multichannel functional electrical stimulation therapy. Phys Ther 75:490, 1995.

203. Yan, T, Hui-Chan, C, and Li, L: Functional electrical stimulation improves motor recovery of the lower extremity and walking ability of subjects with first acute stroke: A randomized placebo-controlled trial. Stroke 36:80, 2005.

204. Embrey, D, et al: Functional electrical stimulation to dorsiflexors and plantar flexors during gait to improve walking in adults with chronic hemiplegia. Arch Phys Med Rehabil 91:687, 2010.

205. Roche, A, Laighin, G, and Coote, S: Surface-applied functional electrical stimulation for orthotic and therapeutic treatment of drop-foot after stroke—a systematic review. Phys Ther Rev 14:63, 2009.

206. Ana, R, et al: Gait training combining partial body-weight support, a treadmill, and functional electrical stimulation on poststroke gait. Phys Ther 87:1144, 2007.

207. Daly, J, and Ruff, R: Feasibility of combining multi-channel functional neuromuscular stimulation with weight-supported treadmill training. J Neurol Sci 255:105, 2004.

208. Triolo, R, and Bogie, K: Lower extremity applications of functional neuromuscular stimulation after spinal cord injury. Top Spinal Cord Inj Rehabil 5:44, 1999.

209. Ferrante, F, et al: Cycling induced by FES improves the muscular strength and motor control of individuals with post-acute stroke. Eur J Phys Rehabil Med 44:159, 2008.

210. Levin, M, Kleim, J, and Wolf, S: What do motor "recovery" and "compensation" mean in patients following stroke? Neurorehabil Neural Repair 23:313, 2009.

Supplemental Readings

Schmidt, R, and Lee, T: Motor Control and Learning: A Behavioral Emphasis, ed 5. Human Kinetics, Champaign, IL, 2011.

Shumway-Cook, A, and Woollacott, M: Motor Control Theory and Practical Applications, ed 4. Lippincott Williams & Wilkins, Philadelphia, 2012.

Locomotor Training

Chapter 11

George D. Fulk, PT, PhD
Thomas J. Schmitz, PT, PhD

LEARNING OBJECTIVES

1. Discuss the major elements of physical therapy intervention for patients with locomotor limitations.
2. Describe the locomotor training principles that guide selection of interventions.
3. Differentiate between advantages and limitations of using parallel bars for locomotor training.
4. Explain the rationale for each component of indoor overground locomotor training.
5. Identify strategies to vary locomotor task demands.
6. Discuss the rationale for locomotor training using body weight support and a treadmill.
7. Compare and contrast locomotor training using body weight support and a treadmill with other locomotor training strategies.
8. Describe strategies for varying task and environmental demands during locomotor training.
9. Describe training activities used for locomotion overground in the community.
10. Using the case study example, apply clinical decision making skills within the context of locomotor training.

CHAPTER OUTLINE

The recovery or improvement of walking ability is a primary goal for people with many different health conditions who seek the services of a physical therapist.[1-3] Initially, approximately two-thirds of people who experience a stroke cannot ambulate or require assistance to walk.[4] Three months later, one-third of those with a stroke still require some level of assistance to walk.[4] Approximately 70% of people with a spinal cord injury (SCI) cannot walk 1 year after their injury.[5] People with Parkinson's disease (PD) often have impaired postural control and limited walking ability.[6] Individuals with low back pain, lower extremity (LE) amputations, multiple sclerosis (MS), and a host of other health conditions all may present with impaired locomotion. The *Guide to Physical Therapist Practice* includes elements of gait and locomotor training (LT) as an intervention category within each of the four preferred practice patterns.[7]

The recovery of walking ability is such an important goal because people who can walk independently are more likely to be able to participate in expected social roles and desired recreational activities, have a higher quality of life, and have improved health status.[2,3,6,8,9]

The major requirements for successful walking include the following:

- Support of body mass by the LEs
- Production of locomotor rhythm

- Dynamic postural control of the moving body
- Propulsion of the body in the intended direction
- Adaptability of the locomotor response to changing environmental and task demands

These requirements should be performed in an energy-efficient manner so as to minimize stress on the individual.

Recent advances in basic science research using animal models of different neurological health conditions provide a strong foundation for physical therapy interventions designed to improve locomotor capability in different patient populations. Research using an SCI cat model has found that spinalized cats trained by suspension in a harness over a treadmill (TM) and provided with manual assistance to step can learn to walk/step on the TM without supraspinal input.[10-12] Studies incorporating an animal model of stroke indicate that skilled, repetitive, task-oriented training can lead to beneficial neural plastic changes that are associated with improved mobility and reaching.[13-17] Exercise in animal models of PD have also demonstrated beneficial effects.[18-20]

Taken together these findings from basic science research provide important insight and guidance for physical therapists. Clinical researchers have used these findings to develop physical therapy interventions designed to improve locomotor ability in a variety of patient populations. Locomotor training using a body weight support (BWS) and a TM system,[21-24] task-oriented circuit training,[24,28-33] TM training and task-specific strengthening exercises[24,30,31] are some of the interventions developed based on translating findings from basic science research to clinical practice. Although the specific interventions strategies vary, they share common principles.[75] These LT principles guide selection of interventions that are:

- Task oriented to the specific task of walking.
- Goal directed and meaningful to the patient.
- Shaped and progressed to maximally challenge the patient's capabilities.
- Performed multiple times (high number of repetitions).

The application of these principles to the specific LT interventions will vary depending on a variety of factors, including patient health condition, prognosis, patient goals, body structure/function impairments, and weight-bearing status. Evaluation of gait analysis data (see Chapter 7, Examination of Gait) can assist the therapist in developing an appropriate, task-oriented, goal-directed plan of care (POC) to address the limitations in walking ability. The LT interventions and principles can be implemented in and progressed through different environments: parallel bars, BWS and TM system, overground with and without a BWS system, and in the community. Interventions that target improved strength, transferring from sitting to/from standing, and standing balance are complementary activities often performed in conjunction with LT because these activities are functionally related to the task of walking.

Box 11.1 provides an overview of complementary interventions to LT and specific LT strategies. It should be noted that the interventions in their entirety are

---

Box 11.1 Overview of Complementary Interventions and Specific Locomotor Training Strategies

I. Interventions Complementary to Locomotor Training

Complementary activities focus on improved:
- Strength
- Sit to/from stand transfers
- Standing balance

II. Locomotor Training

A. Parallel Bars
Instruction and training in:
- Sit-to-stand and reverse with and/or without assistive device
- Static and dynamic standing balance with and/or without assistive device
- Use of appropriate gait pattern with and/or without assistive device while progressing forward and turning (because of limited space, it may not be possible to use an assistive device in standard parallel bars)
- Stepping forward, backward, sideward, and turning

B. Overground Indoors
Instruction and training in:
- Appropriate gait pattern and assistive device use
- Stepping forward, backward, and sideward

Continued

Box 11.1   Overview of Complementary Interventions and Specific Locomotor Training Strategies—cont'd

- Cross-stepping and braiding
- Walking over and around objects (i.e., obstacle course)
- Crossing thresholds and entering/exiting through doorways
- Variations in locomotor task demands (e.g., altering speed, scanning for objects, dual-task activity)
- Stairs
- Falling and transitioning from the floor to standing
- Running

C. Overground Community
Instruction and training in:
- Curb climbing, negotiating ramps, stairs, and sloped surfaces
- Walking over even and uneven terrain
- Walking within imposed timing requirements (e.g., crossing at a stoplight, on/off elevators, escalators)
- Walking for long distances
- Walking at varying speeds, walk using a rhythmic timing device (e.g. metronome)
- Walking while scanning for objects in the environment
- Dual-task training while walking (cognitive and/or motor dual tasks)
- Walking in open environment with distracters
- Entering/exiting transportation vehicles
- Running

D. Body Weight Support/Treadmill
Instruction and training in:
- Stepping on treadmill using body weight support (BWS) with maximally tolerated lower extremity load bearing progressing to no BWS
- Reciprocal stepping pattern with manual assistance at lower extremities and/or trunk with normal or near normal lower extremity and trunk/pelvis kinematics progressing to no manual assistance
- Production of rhythmic stepping pattern with arm swing and minimal to no weight-bearing through the upper extremities
- Progress stepping speeds to normative values based on age
- Walk forward, sideward, and backward
- Strategies to minimize abnormal/compensatory movement patterns
- Strategies to improve aerobic capacity

E. Body Weight Support/Overground
Instruction and training in:
- Walking overground with maximally tolerated lower extremity load bearing progressing to no BWS
- Use of assistive device (if indicated) for walking on level surfaces
- Reciprocal stepping pattern with manual assistance at pelvis with normal or near normal lower extremity and trunk/pelvis kinematics progressing to no manual assistance
- Production of rhythmical, coordinated stepping pattern with arm swing and minimal weight-bearing through the upper extremities
- Strategies to minimize abnormal/compensatory movement patterns
- Strategies to maintain/regain balance when perturbed

F. Assistive Devices (see Appendix 11.A)
Instruction and training in:
- Function and purpose of assistive device
- Sit-to-stand and reverse with assistive device
- Static and dynamic standing balance with assistive device
- Gait pattern
- Use of assistive device and appropriate gait pattern indoor overground and overground in community

likely not indicated for each patient. Depending on individual patient need, multiple interventions may be accomplished concurrently, a more rapid progression may be used, or portions may be completely omitted. While performing LT within the different environments (e.g., parallel bars, indoor, community), principles of motor learning (see Chapter 10, Strategies to Improve Motor Function), strength training, and aerobic conditioning should be incorporated to facilitate learning and maximize walking ability.

■ LOCOMOTOR TRAINING COMPLEMENTARY INTERVENTIONS

The selection of interventions complementary to LT is based on examination findings (e.g., identified impairments and activity limitations) and typically includes strategies to improve the following:

- Strength
- Sit to/from stand transfers
- Standing balance

Strength

A key strategy for improving strength is to combine strength training with task-specific practice. This requires repetitive practice of tasks that are *specific to the outcome* (i.e., locomotion) and *meaningful to the patient* in terms of function. Although muscle-specific strengthening (e.g., progressive resistance, isokinetic equipment) may also be indicated and complementary to LT, using task-specific practice provides optimum transfer of strength gains to functional skills.

Inherent to task-specific strength training is resistance provided by body weight or limb segment weight; this weight may be augmented by the addition of external resistance (e.g., resistive bands, pool activities, cuff weights). Task selection is based on elements of the whole task, including the body segments involved; the required type, speed, and magnitude of contractions; and the degrees of freedom needed for the desired outcome. The goal is progression to whole task training. Activities typically begin with individual joints or body segments with progression to whole body movements.

For example, strengthening of LE extensor muscles is often a complementary activity to LT for some patient groups (e.g., stroke, Parkinson's disease). Task-specific functional activities that focus on extensor control might include partial wall squats, step-ups and step-downs, sit-to-stand transfers, and first bilateral, then single-limb heel rises to strengthen ankle plantarflexors. Another example is strengthening of hip abductors and adductors using side-stepping, cross-stepping, and braiding (manual contact or resistive bands can be used for resistance). Task-specific strengthening is important because it requires interplay of contraction types similar to the demands of walking.

Sit to/From Stand Transfers

Practice to improve transfers focuses initially on sitting with symmetrical weight-bearing, an erect posture on anterior portion of chair with neutral or slight anterior tilt of pelvis, and feet behind knees (allows dorsiflexors to assist forward rotation of legs over feet); emphasis is also placed on coordinated muscle responses and on appropriate timing. The reader is referred to the work of Fulk[25] for a thorough discussion of interventions to improve transfers.

To accomplish a sit-to-stand transfer, the patient must first actively flex the trunk and hips and may use momentum to shift the body mass forward. The patient's arms may be folded across chest, held forward with hands clasped, or hands placed on the chair armrests. (*Note*: Using the hands on a support surface should not be substituted for effective forward translation of body weight.) A higher, firm, seating surface (e.g., high-low treatment table) may be used initially for patients with weakness, and the height gradually reduced. Asking the patient to focus on a visual target can promote upper trunk extension during forward weight shift and enhance postural alignment and vertical orientation. As the patient moves toward the extension phase of the transfer, greater demands are placed on the hip and knee extensors to come to vertical. Tactile and proprioceptive cues can be used to promote contraction of extensor muscles.

To return to the seated position from standing, the motion is similar to that used for sit-to-stand transitions, but executed in reverse order. However, the timing and types of contractions are different. The focus of practice is on eccentric control as the body mass moves downward and backward. Eccentric contractions of the LE extensor muscles control lowering as the hips, knees, and ankles flex.

Initially, transfers may be performed slowly. With repetitive practice, focus can be placed on increasing speed of movement and performance of sit-to-stand and reverse without pausing. Practice should also include a variety of seating surfaces and heights, performance in open environments, and a gradual reduction in verbal cues.

Standing Balance

Adequate standing balance and control are integral components of locomotion. As continuous postural adjustments are needed during locomotion, intervention strategies to improve balance should be selected that impose similar demands. Locomotion requires static postural control (stability) to maintain standing and dynamic postural control (controlled mobility) to control movements within standing (e.g., weight shifting,

LE stepping). Examples of interventions to improve balance follow; balance interventions are also discussed in Chapter 10, Strategies to Improve Motor Function, and in the work of O'Sullivan.[26]

Initial standing activities may require touch-down support of the hands and can be performed in the parallel bars, between two treatment tables, or next to a wall or corner of a room (corner standing). The patient is first directed to stand tall and hold steady in the posture. Techniques such as quick stretch or approximation can be used to enhance postural stabilizing muscle contractions. Enhanced postural awareness can be achieved with limits of stability (LOS) training during weight shifting and in response to anticipated and reactive perturbations. Active exercise to improve standing may include heel-rises, toe-offs, back-kicks and sidekicks, hip and knee flexion, hip flexion with knee extension, partial wall squats, and marching in place. These exercises can also be performed in a pool. Adding ankle cuff weights, altering the base of support (BOS) (feet apart, together, tandem stance), upper extremity (UE) position (e.g., arms overhead, reaching), and support surface (e.g., inflated disc, wobble board) can all impose greater challenge.

Engagement of ankle and hip strategies can be promoted using incremental shifts in center of mass (COM) alignment and postural sway movements. Challenges can be enhanced using a foam cushion (eyes open to closed), split foam rollers (flat side down to flat side up), and wobble boards. Large COM shifts in all directions beyond the LOS will promote stepping strategies. Balance control can be further enhanced using manual perturbations, resistive band around pelvis during stepping (forward, backward, sideward), and using mobile and compliant surfaces with alterations in BOS (feet together, tandem standing, and single-limb stance).

■ LOCOMOTOR TRAINING ENVIRONMENTS

The discussion of locomotion training strategies is divided into the following environments in which LT can be performed: (1) parallel bars, (2) overground indoors, (3) overground community, (4) BWS and TM, (5) BWS overground, and (6) other.

The following section addresses the parallel bar progression. Parallel bars have a time-honored tradition in conventional LT. They provide a reasonably safe and stable environment to become acclimated to upright standing, and they allow early walking practice on a relatively normal indoor floor surface for short distances. They also permit the UEs to assist in maintaining an erect posture and static/dynamic balance control, and to partially or fully unweight an LE. Because a high level of stability is provided by UE support, there is less demand imposed for balance control and the highly coordinated movements required of normal locomotor rhythm. However, prolonged parallel bar training promotes

compensatory practice and learning of skills that often transfer poorly to independent overground walking and use of an assistive device. Owing to the increased weight borne by the UEs, a forward head and flexed trunk posture (limiting hip extension range of motion [ROM] and loading) is imposed and practiced. Locomotor speed, symmetry, and rhythm (timing) are typically diminished and appropriate dynamic balance mechanisms cannot be effectively promoted. In addition, the amount of body weight relief cannot be easily monitored.

In recent years, the availability of partial BWS training devices has diminished the routine use of parallel bars in many facilities. Training using a BWS system can be used in conjunction with a TM or used on overground surfaces and involves the patient donning a harness attached to an overhead frame that supports him or her in an upright vertical posture. Treadmill training using BWS is addressed later in this chapter.

Parallel Bars

Before standing, two important preliminary activities are fitting the patient with a guarding belt and adjusting the parallel bars. The initial adjustment of the parallel bars is an estimate based on the patient's height. Ideally the bars should be adjusted to allow 20 to 30 degrees of elbow flexion and come to about the level of the greater trochanter. Considering individual variations in body proportions and arm length, the elbow measurement is usually most accurate. Once the patient is standing, the height of the bars can be checked. If adjustments are required, the patient should be returned to a sitting position.

Before beginning LT in the parallel bars, wheelchair positioning and use of a guarding belt are important considerations. The patient's wheelchair should be positioned at the end of the parallel bars. The brakes should be locked, the footrests placed in an upright position, and the patient's feet on the floor well under the seating surface (COM over the BOS). The guarding belt should be fastened securely around the patient's waist. Guarding belts provide several critical functions. They increase the therapist's effectiveness in controlling or preventing potential loss of balance; they improve patient safety; they facilitate the therapist's use of proper body mechanics in untoward circumstances; and they are an important consideration regarding issues of liability. The safety implications of the guarding belt should be explained to the patient carefully.

Locomotor training in the parallel bars is initiated with patient instruction and demonstration. First, the entire progression should be presented before breaking it into sequential component parts. This will include instruction and demonstration in how to assume a standing position in the parallel bars, guarding techniques to be used by the therapist, the components of initial standing balance activities, gait pattern to be used, how to turn in the parallel bars, and how to return to a sitting position. Demonstrating these activities by assuming the role of the patient during verbal explanations will facilitate learning. Each component of the parallel bar progression should then be reviewed before the patient's actual performance of the activity. A sequence of activities for use in the parallel bars follows.

Assuming the Standing Position

To prepare for standing, the patient should be instructed to move forward in the chair. The therapist is positioned directly in front of the patient. A method of guarding should be selected that does not interfere with the patient's use of the UEs while moving to standing. Having moved forward in the chair with the supporting foot or feet on the floor well under the seating surface, the patient should be instructed to come to a standing position by leaning or rocking forward and pushing down on the armrests of the wheelchair with verbal cueing from the therapist (*"rock your shoulders forward, continue rocking and on the count of three push down on the armrests, and come to standing, one, two, three"*). The patient should not be allowed to stand by pulling up on the parallel bars because this approach has little functional carryover. As the patient nears an erect posture, the hands should be released from the armrests one at a time and placed on the parallel bars. The patient's COM should be guided over the BOS to promote a stable standing posture.

Standing Activities

During initial parallel bar activities, the therapist typically stands inside the bars facing the patient or outside the bars on the patient's weaker side. In guarding the patient from inside the bars, one hand should grasp the guarding belt anteriorly, and the opposite hand should be in front of, but not touching, the patient's shoulder. (*Note:* An underhand grip is always used when grasping a guarding belt.) From outside the bars one hand should grasp the belt posteriorly with the opposite hand in front of, but not touching, the patient's shoulder. This method of guarding provides effective hand placement for an immediate response should the patient lose his or her balance. It also eliminates the patient's feeling of being "held back" or "pushed forward," which may occur with manual contacts at the shoulders. The following initial activities in the parallel bars can be modified relative to the patient's weight-bearing status and specific requirements (e.g., use of a prosthesis or orthosis). The therapist maintains guarding techniques during these activities.

1. Standing, holding, acclimation to upright position; feet in symmetrical stance position, equal weight on both LEs; hands supported on parallel bars.
2. Limits of stability training (weight shifts with feet in stance position; alteration in hand placement on parallel bars).
   a. Lateral weight shift from side-to-side without altering the BOS; hand placement on the parallel bars is not altered.
   b. Anterior–posterior weight shifting forward and backward without altering the BOS; hand placement on the parallel bars is not altered.
   c. Anterior–posterior hand placement and weight shift; patient lifts and moves hands forward on bars and shifts weight anteriorly; alternated with posterior hand placement, and weight is shifted backward.
   d. Single-hand support; patient balances with support from only one hand on the parallel bars; hands are alternated. A progression of this activity involves gradual changes in position of the freed hand and UE. For example, move the freed hand several inches above the bar and gradually progress to alternate positions such as shoulder flexion, abduction, crossing the midline, and so forth. A progression can be made to balancing with both hands freed from the bars.
3. Stepping forward and backward. Patient steps forward with one LE, anterior weight shift, and then returns foot to starting position (normal BOS); alternated with stepping backward with one LE, posterior weight shift, with return of foot to starting position.
4. Side-stepping and cross-stepping. Patient turns 90° from a forward-facing position and places both hands on one parallel bar; weight is then shifted over support limb and dynamic limb abducts and side-steps. Progression made to cross-stepping; weight shifted over support limb and dynamic limb moves up and over the stance limb.
5. Forward progression. Ambulation in the parallel bars using selected gait pattern and appropriate weight-bearing (e.g., partial, full).

Clinical Note: The patient should be instructed to push down rather than to pull on the parallel bars while ambulating, inasmuch as this is the motion that eventually will be required with an assistive device. This will be easier if the patient is instructed to use a loose or open grip on the bars rather than a tight grip; the loose or open grip facilitates correct use of the parallel bars and, ultimately, the assistive device.

6. Turning. Once the desired distance in the parallel bars has been reached, the patient should be instructed to turn toward the stronger side. For example, with a non–weight-bearing left LE, the turn should be toward the right. The patient should be instructed to turn by stepping in a small circle and not to pivot on a single extremity. This technique will carry over to ambulation outside the bars, when pivoting will always be discouraged because of the potential loss of balance by movement on a small BOS. Guarding can be accomplished two ways. The therapist can remain in front of the

patient, maintain the same hand positions, and turn with the patient. This will keep the therapist positioned in front of the patient. A second method is not to turn with the patient but, rather, to guard from behind on the return trip. In this method hand placements will change during the turn. Hand placement is changed gradually by first placing both hands on the guarding belt as the patient initiates the turn. One hand then remains on the posterior aspect of the belt and the freed hand is placed anterior to, but not touching, the shoulder on the patient's weaker side for the return trip toward the chair. Although both techniques are acceptable, the latter is probably more practical, considering the limited space available in the parallel bars.

7. Return to seated position. When reaching the chair the patient should again turn as described above. Once completely turned, patients are typically instructed to continue backing up until they feel the seat of the chair on the back of their legs (this will require substitution with visual or auditory clues for patients with impaired sensation). At this point the patient releases the stronger hand from the parallel bar and reaches back for the wheelchair armrest. Once this hand has securely grasped the armrest, the patient should be instructed to bend forward slightly, release the opposite hand from the parallel bar, and place it on the other armrest. Keeping the head and trunk forward, the patient gently returns to a seated position.

Clinical Note: Owing to limited space, use of the parallel bars may not be possible with an assistive device. However, when adjustable-width bars are available, they provide added security for preliminary use of the assistive device. An alternative approach would be to begin use of the device outside and next to standard parallel bars or oval-shaped bars.

Overground Indoors

Activities for the indoor overground progression typically include walking forward and backward, resisted progression, side-stepping and cross-stepping, and stair climbing. Manual contacts can be used to guide and assist control of pelvic movement if necessary. Verbal cueing can be used to promote normal timing and locomotor rhythm. Upper extremity support may initially be required (e.g., hands resting lightly on therapist's shoulders; or therapist may be positioned in front of patient with elbows flexed and forearms supinated and patient uses therapist's hands for touch-down support as needed). Manual contacts, verbal cueing, and UE support are progressively decreased and then eliminated.

1. Walking forward and backward. This activity can begin with standing; stepping in place with emphasis on diagonal weight shifts forward and backward onto stance limb; and pelvic rotation in combination with advancing the swing limb.

2. Resistance with forward and backward walking is applied using a resistive band around the pelvis and held from behind as the patient moves forward or held in front facing the patient as he or she moves backward. In standing, wooden dowels held horizontally by both the patient and therapist can be used to promote reciprocal UE movements and trunk rotation moving both forward and backward.

3. Side-stepping and cross-stepping. Side-stepping involves abduction of the leading dynamic limb with foot placement followed by movement of the remaining limb to a parallel position with the first (symmetrical stance). Emphasis should be placed on keeping the pelvis level. Cross-stepping involves side-stepping and then crossing the remaining limb up and over the other limb.

4. Braiding. This activity involves a cross-step and side-step progression with one limb advancing alternately anteriorly and posteriorly across the other while the second limb side-steps. It incorporates lower trunk rotation, as well as crossing the midline. This is a challenging activity and may require support from the therapist standing in front of the patient (forearms supinated, patient's hands lightly touching therapist's hands) or by use of a modified plantigrade position with UEs lightly supported on the treatment table.

5. Step-ups. To practice stepping up, a portable step can be placed directly in front of the patient. The patient weight shifts laterally toward the support limb and places the dynamic limb on the step. The limb is then returned to the original stance position. Verbal cues and manual guidance are provided as needed. The height of the step can be varied to increase or decrease the difficulty of the activity. For example, a 4-in (10-cm) step can be used initially with a gradual progression to a standard 7-in (17.5-cm) step. A progression is made to a step-over-step pattern on stairs. Early activities may require support from a railing. An erect trunk posture should be maintained and "pulling" on the railing should be avoided.

Indoor overground practice activities should also include strategies to vary locomotor task demands such as the following:

• Walking with head turns on verbal command such as *look right, look left, look up,* or *look down.*
• Increasing speed and rhythm of gait by using pacing cues to vary speed such as *walk slow* and *walk fast.*
• Use of a metronome or personal listening device (e.g., marching music) to increase speed and improve rhythm.
• Progress to longer distances with decreased number of rest intervals to improve walking endurance.

- Practice dual-task walking (e.g., walk and talk; walk and catch/throw a ball; tapping a balloon back and forth; bouncing a ball; carrying a tray that holds a glass of water, walk and perform a cognitive task).
- Practice walking on varied indoor surfaces such as tile, wood flooring, and carpeting.
- Practice walking through doorways including opening and closing door.
- Progress from a closed to an open environment.

Box 11.2 presents an overview of strategies for varying locomotor task demands. It provides suggested practice activities for enhancing specific (missing) components of gait that can be incorporated into the indoor overground progression.[27]

Circuit Training

These (see Box 11.2) and other activities can be incorporated into a task-oriented circuit-training program. Circuit training generally consists of different stations at which patients participate in different specific, task-oriented activities designed to improve walking ability.[24,28-33] For example, there may be six to eight stations at which patients participate in the activity for 5 to 10 minutes. Specific training stations may have activities such as standing and reaching, standing on different surfaces, walking through an obstacle course, transitioning from supine to sitting to standing, walking and carrying objects, walking and picking up objects from the floor, stepping up and down, walking at varying speeds and over varying

---

Box 11.2 Strategies for Varying Locomotor Task Demands

Upright Postural Alignment

- Practice walking upright; assist patient in vertical trunk posture using manual and verbal cues (*"Look up and stand tall"*)
- Trekking poles or body weight support harness can be used to promote upright alignment and reduce upper extremity support, forward head, and flexed trunk position (common with use of an assistive device such as a walker)
- Progress upper extremity support provided by assistive device to light touch-down support, then to use of a trekking pole or wall for support as needed, and finally to no support

Foot Placement/Toe Clearance

- Practice heel-toe initial contact; tactile cues can be provided to dorsal foot by tapping over pretibial muscles
- Practice high step marching in place and then high step walking accompanied by marching music
- Practice walking with even steps using foot prints attached to floor
- Practice increasing step length and/or step width using floor grids
- Practice walking with altered base of support; progressing from wide base (8–12 inches apart [20.32-30.48 cm]) to narrow base (2 inches [5 cm] apart) to tandem (heel-to-toe)
- Practice step-to walking (i.e., taking a long step with one limb; then bring opposite limb even with the first on next step)
- Practice walking on a 3-inch (7.6 cm) line taped to floor; half-foam roller; low balance beam

Single- and Double-Limb Support

- Practice controlled lateral and diagonal weight shifts
- Combine diagonal weight shifts with pelvic rotation movements and stepping forward and backward

Forward Progression and Push-off

- Practice push-ups (toe rises) in stance; progress to toe-walking
- Practice heel-rises in stance; progress to heel-walking
- Practice forceful push-off on cue during walking
- Practice alternating between heel-walking and toe-walking (i.e., walk a certain number of steps on heels, then same number on toes)

Walking Against Resistance

- Practice walking against manual resistance using resisted progression
- Walking against resistance from resistive band around pelvis
- Pool walking (ideal initial supportive environment for patients with ataxia)

Trunk Counterrotation and Arm Swing

- Practice walking with exaggerated arm swings
- Practice walking with wooden dowels; therapist is behind and holds one end of dowels; patient is in front and holds other end of dowels

Continued

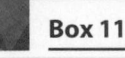

Box 11.2   Strategies for Varying Locomotor Task Demands—cont'd

Walking Sideward

- Practice walking using lateral side-steps; resisted progression (manual and elastic resistive bands)
- Practice walking using cross-steps
- Practice walking using braiding

Walking Backward

- Walking backward (retro-walking)
- Practice appropriate knee flexion in combination with hip extension

Step-Ups/Step-Downs

- Practice stepping-up and stepping-down; vary step height progressing from low (4 in [4 cm]) to high (8 in [20 cm])
- Practice lateral step-ups
- Practice forward step-ups
- Practice stepping onto and off varied surfaces (e.g., foam pad, half foam roller, inflatable disc, BOSU® Balance Trainer)

Stopping, Starting, and Turning on Cue

- Practice abrupt stops and starts on verbal cue
- Practice turns on verbal cue, progressing from a quarter turn to half turn to full turn; progress from wide base turns with progression to narrow base
- Practice figure-8 turns

Visual Input

- Practice walking alternating between eyes open and eyes closed; three steps with eyes open and then three steps with eyes closed

Head Movements

- Practice walking alternating head movements; alternate between taking three steps with head to right and then three steps with head to left
- Practice walking with head movements on verbal cue (*"look right, look left, look down, look up"*)

Practice Timed Walking, Increasing Speed and Locomotor Rhythm

- Begin walking at comfortable speed, gradually increase velocity
- Use pacing cues to vary speed, (e.g., *"walk slow, walk fast"*)
- Use metronome or brisk marching music to increase speed, improve locomotor rhythm
- Practice imposing short bursts of fast walking (on verbal cue) with walking at a comfortable speed

Improve Duration of Walking

- Progress to longer distances with decreased number of rest intervals

Practice Dual-Task Walking

- Walk and talk
- Walk and count by threes
- Walk and bounce or toss a ball, carry a tray

Improving Compensatory Responses to Unexpected Perturbations

- Change speed of treadmill or stop and start treadmill while patient is walking on it
- Practice resisted forward progression using an elastic resistive band with unexpected release of resistance
- Practice walking while recovering from small external perturbations given manually

Adapted from Schmitz,[27, pp. 206-207] with permission.

surfaces, and standing and kicking a ball. As patients' performance improves, the specific tasks are progressed by increasing the complexity and difficulty. For example, to progress a patient in an obstacle course the patient can be required to do it more quickly, carry an object while walking through it, or step over higher objects. A dual cognitive task can be added to the activity to increase the difficulty as well. Progressive resistive strength training targeting key muscles can also be incorporated.[31] Box 11.3 Evidence Summary presents research examining the effectiveness of circuit training for improving locomotor ability.[24,28-32]

Box 11.3 Evidence Summary   Selected Studies of Circuit Class Training for Patients with Stroke

Reference	Subjects	Methods/Procedure	Results	Comments
Fritz et al[24] (2011)	A case series of four participants with chronic neurological diagnoses	Each participant completed 10 sessions of Intense Mobility Training (IMT): 3 hr/day with 1 hour each of body weight supported locomotor training, balance training, and coordination/ strength training. Emphasis was on task-specific training that was massed in schedule.	Despite the wide range of diagnoses, all tolerated the IMT well and each showed improvement in at least one measure for each target area of gait, balance, and mobility.	Study informs us about general feasibility only; a randomized trial of IMT with a more homogenous population is needed.
van de Port et al[28] (2012)	250 subjects with stroke recruited from multiple outpatient centers; randomly allocated to circuit training or usual physical therapy	12 weeks of graded task-oriented circuit training (2×/wk for 90 min) intended to improve walking competency (n = 126) versus 12 weeks of usual outpatient physical therapy (n = 124).	Small but significantly higher scores in comfortable walking speed, distance, and modified stairs test for circuit training group at 12 weeks; no differences in primary outcome (mobility index of Stroke Impact Scale [SIS]) or secondary measures (except gait speed) at 24-week follow-up.	Circuit training appears safe and effective as usual therapy; differences in gait speed and distance were not clinically meaningful; insufficient detail of "usual therapy" to effectively compare groups on intervention content and dose.
Rose et al[29] (2011)	180 clients with stroke (average 10 days post-stroke) participating in a traditional, acute care rehabilitation program	Study compared standard physical therapy (SPT) 1.5 hr/day, 5 days/wk of 1:1 therapy for mobility, gait, balance, and UE function to circuit training physical therapy (CTPT) 1.5 hr/day, 5 days/wk; 60 min/session devoted to circuit training of four task-specific stations. CTPT consisted of four levels of circuit training based on client's stroke severity.	The CTPT group had significantly higher intensity of task repetition than the SPT group. Significantly greater changes in gait speed for CTPT versus SPT. No other significant differences for measures of LE function, balance, or overall mobility. No group differences noted on follow-up (90 days post-stroke).	Nonblinded, nonrandomized controlled trial. The primary finding of this feasibility study is that individuals only 10 days post-stroke tolerated an intervention mode that provided intense, whole-body task practice focused on repetition and progression.

Box 11.3 Evidence Summary   Selected Studies of Circuit Class Training for Patients with Stroke—cont'd

Reference	Subjects	Methods/Procedure	Results	Comments
Combs et al[30] (2010)	A case series of 12 participants with chronic stroke	4-hour sessions daily for 2 weeks included progressive resistance training, locomotor training (BWS with TM and overground), task-specific skills training, education, and home exercise program.	Most clients showed improvement from baseline to follow-up and retention for the activity-based outcome measures (balance, walking ability, UE function) but the effect sizes were all small. Self-perceived improvements on participation-based measures (SIS and Canadian Occupational Performance Measure) were significant and had large effect sizes at follow-up and were maintained.	This protocol is a good representation of how a patient-centered, task-specific, and whole-body program for persons with stroke can be both standardized and feasible, as well as effective.
Wing et al[31] (2008)	Retrospective review of 35 adults with chronic stroke receiving comprehensive, outpatient therapy	Clients received intensive, whole-body rehabilitation 3–6 hr/day, 4 days/wk for a minimum of 2 weeks. Sessions included BWS with TM, overground gait training, progressive resistance training, balance and transfers training, and task-specific UE training.	Clients demonstrated improved walking speed and UE function; small improvements in balance were also noted.	Another good example of how a whole-body rehabilitation program can be applied to this population. No correlations were found between injury chronicity or amount of therapy and outcomes measured.
English and Hillier[32] (2010)	Systematic literature review through 2009; randomized or quasi-randomized studies of adults with stroke were reviewed	Six trials including 292 participants were selected for final analysis.	Positive findings from four studies favored circuit training compared to control intervention for walking capacity and speed. Two studies showed superiority of circuit training for measures of balance and hospital length of stay.	The authors conclude that circuit training classes are effective for improving mobility and reducing rehabilitation length of stay for persons with moderate stroke.

Evidence Summary Box prepared by Coby D. Nirider, PT, DPT, Director of Therapy Services, Touchstone Neurorecovery Center, Conroe, TX 77308.
BWS = body weight support; LE = lower extremity; SIS = stroke impact scale; TM = treadmill; UE = upper extremity.

Body Weight Support/Treadmill

Locomotor training using a BWS and TM system involves suspending a patient over a TM and using the BWS system to partially unweight the patient. The ability to partially unweight the patient allows patients with LE or trunk weakness to stand and take steps in a more symmetrical, natural manner without the need for excessive UE weight-bearing or compensatory movement patterns. Using this system also allows physical therapists and other rehabilitation professionals to manually assist the patient while stepping on the TM (see Fig. 20.37 in Chapter 20, Traumatic Spinal Cord Injury).

Locomotor training using a BWS and treadmill system was first used in patients with SCI. The rationale for its use is supported by animal studies of cats with thoracic spinal cord lesions that regained hind limb stepping patterns when supported by a harness over a moving treadmill.[10-12] These findings suggest that the spinal cord is capable of reciprocal locomotor patterns produced by central pattern generators (CPGs) at the spinal cord level in the absence of supraspinal input. Central pattern generators are also influenced by sensory input, allowing motor output modification based on environmental demands.

Behrman et al[21] and Behrman and Harkema[34] have proposed the following guiding principles for LT:

- Maximally load the LEs for weight-bearing, while minimizing weight-bearing on the UEs (e.g., the BWS system sustains sufficient body weight so that the patient can stand and step with minimal or no UE support).
- Provide sensory cues that are consistent with normal walking (e.g., manual facilitation to the extensors and flexors during stance and swing, respectively).
- Promote trunk, limb, and pelvic kinematics associated with normal walking.
- Promote balance and upright control consistent with normal walking.
- Maximize the recovery and use of normal movement patterns and minimize compensatory movement patterns.

The overarching principle is to *train like you walk*. A key element of LT using BWS and a TM is facilitation of automatic walking movements within the context of intensive, task-specific training (whole-task practice). With body weight supported, the TM speed provides a rhythmic input. Manually guided movements are used to enhance the rhythmicity of the gait pattern. The BWS and TM system provides an environment in which these LT strategies can be accomplished.

Sensory input such as appropriately timed manually assisted limb movements can promote function-induced recovery.[28,31] Within a task-specific and safe patient environment, LT using BWS and a TM allows the therapist access to trunk, pelvis, and LEs to manually assist, guide, or adjust locomotor rhythm, limb placement, weight shifts, and stepping symmetry. Movements are coordinated to simulate normal gait; upright posture and balance are maintained, and speed of walking is controlled. Kosak and Reding[35] emphasize the role of sensory input during LT using BWS and a TM by stating, "Stride and cadence vary with treadmill speed, indicating local sensory feedback to a lumbosacral gait pattern-generator. The intensity and timing of sensory feedback from pressure receptors in the sole of the foot and joint proprioceptors from the ankle, knee, and hip are thought to provide facilitory and inhibitory effects on flexor-extensor motor neuron pools in the spinal cord at appropriate time during the gait cycle."[35, p. 14]

Some of the advantages of LT using BWS and a TM include the following:[34]

- Interlimb and intralimb timing can be practiced before limbs are capable of fully supporting body weight.
- Gait training can be initiated earlier within an episode of care.
- Specific elements of the gait cycle (e.g., midstance limb loading; swing phase unweighting and stepping) can be promoted within a dynamic task-specific strategy.
- Limb loading can be varied based on ability to support weight.
- Owing to forced stepping movements, "learned nonuse" may be prevented by focusing attention on both involved and uninvolved limbs.
- Opportunity to practice walking is provided without undue fear of falling.
- Dynamic balance can be enhanced by decreasing BWS and increasing TM speed.
- Compensatory strategies (e.g., UE support) to compensate for LE impairment are reduced.
- Constant speed of the TM provides rhythmic input that may reinforce a coordinated reciprocal gait pattern.
- Hip extension is facilitated.

Locomotor training using a BWS and TM system can be progressed by increasing TM speed, decreasing the amount of BWS and manual guidance, and increasing the time of stepping on the TM. For example, training may be initiated at very low speeds (e.g., 0.3 m/sec) with limited LE weight-bearing (30% to 40% of BWS), constant manual guidance at both LEs and the trunk/pelvis, and a stepping session of only 1 to 3 minutes. With continued training and patient improvement, this can be progressed to normal, age-appropriate walking speeds of 1.2 to 1.4 m/sec (4 to 4.5 ft/sec), full weight-bearing through the LEs, no manual guidance for stepping, and a stepping session of 30 minutes without rest.

Locomotor training using a BWS and TM system has also been successfully combined with robotic interventions; a robotic device instead of a physical therapist moves the LEs.[36-39] Although the effectiveness of LT using a BWS and TM system has been examined in a variety of patient populations, including those with spinal cord injury[39-43] (see Evidence Summary Box 20.8), stroke[35,44,45] (see Evidence Summary Box 15.9), Parkinson's disease,[46-48] and multiple sclerosis,[49,50] it is not clear that it is more effective than other intervention approaches and what specific patients it is best suited for.

Overground Community

Locomotor training overground in the community is integral to returning the patient to a former environment and lifestyle. Overground community training activities must be specifically examined to determine their appropriateness for an individual patient.

1. Curbs. A useful lead-up activity to curb climbing is provided by training using a series of interlocking portable steps arranged in increments of height. For additional security they can be placed next to a treatment table, wall, or other support surface. A progression can be made from a 3- or 4-in (7.62- or 10.16-cm) increment to a 7-in (17.78-cm) curb height.

2. Ramps and slopes. Ramps and other sloping surfaces can be negotiated in several ways. If the incline is very gradual, it may be sufficient simply to instruct the patient to use smaller steps. For steeper inclines the patient should be instructed to use smaller steps and to traverse the ramp (use a diagonal, zigzag pattern) for both ascending and descending. Practice should include inclines of varying height. Walking up an inclined surface is associated with decreased speed, cadence, and step length.

3. Terrain variations. Community walking presents a variety of terrains that require adaptation of locomotor skills. Practice should include uneven surfaces such as sidewalks, grassy surfaces, parking lots, and so forth.

4. Timing requirements. Several community settings impose precise time restrictions (coincident timing) on movement. Walking should be practiced within these time constraints and can include crossing at a stoplight, stepping on and off a moving walkway or escalator, walking onto an elevator, and walking through a revolving door.

5. Open environment. Walking should be practiced in a variable open community environment such as a shopping mall, community center, grocery store, or other patient-specific location. Because learning is task and environment specific, walking should be practiced in all environments normally used by the patient.

Additional overground community practice activities include the following:

- Exit and entrance through outside doors and thresholds (both residential and commercial structures)
- Outdoor stair climbing (e.g., cement stairs)
- Entering and exiting public or private transportation
- Variations in visual conditions (e.g., full to reduced lighting)
- Scanning the environment

Nordic Walking

Nordic walking (trekking poles) has gained considerable presence in overground LT programs with varied patient populations.[51-58] It is also used in health promotion and fitness programs.[55,59] The International Nordic Walking Federation (INWA) defines Nordic walking as "a form of physical activity, where to regular natural walking there has been added the active use of a pair of specially designed Nordic Walking poles. However, the characteristics of natural, biomechanically correct walking and appropriate posture are maintained in all aspects."[60]

Nordic walking engages muscles of the UE and trunk and is effective in improving gait and aerobic conditioning.[60] Ample evidence supports the use of Nordic walking in overground LT. It has been shown to be a safe and effective training method for patients with chronic obstructive pulmonary disease (COPD)[51] and coronary artery disease.[57] Improvements in postural stability, stride length, gait pattern, and gait variability were found in patients with Parkinson's disease.[52] Nordic walking has also been found to be an effective intervention for low back pain,[53] fibromyalgia,[55,56] intermittent claudication,[58] and overweight individuals with type 2 diabetes.[54]

General goals of Nordic walking include the following:[60,61]

- Increase cardiorespiratory endurance
- Promote correct upright alignment and posture
- Improve balance, agility, and coordination
- Improve gait characteristics and walking speed
- Promote active engagement of multiple muscle groups
- Increase ROM and strength

Nordic walking may progress from overground indoors to overground in the community (see previous section). Other organizations promoting Nordic walking include the American Nordic Walking Association (http://anwa.us/html/index.php) and the International Nordic Fitness Sports Organization (www.nordicfitness.net/).

Body Weight Support/Overground

The task-oriented approach to LT using a BWS system can also be performed overground. Some systems are equipped with casters (Fig 11.1). Moving the BWS system away from the treadmill creates a mobile, safe, and efficient environment for continuing the controlled reduction in BWS to overground surfaces. Although a BWS system can be used overground, very few studies have examined its effectiveness in improving walking ability.[62]

During initial overground training, verbal cueing and manual guidance are provided as needed. Gait speeds may be slower on overground surfaces as compared to over the TM with elimination of the rhythmic steady-state input provided by the TM. Ambulatory assistive devices such as a cane or a walker can be incorporated into overground training (see Appendix 11.A, Ambulatory Assistive Devices: Types, Gait Patterns, and Locomotor Training). The BWS device is manually moved to keep pace with the patient's forward progression. For use without an assistive device, the patient can move and steer the unit with the UEs (Fig. 11.2) before progressing to an assistive device or hands-free reciprocal arm movements.

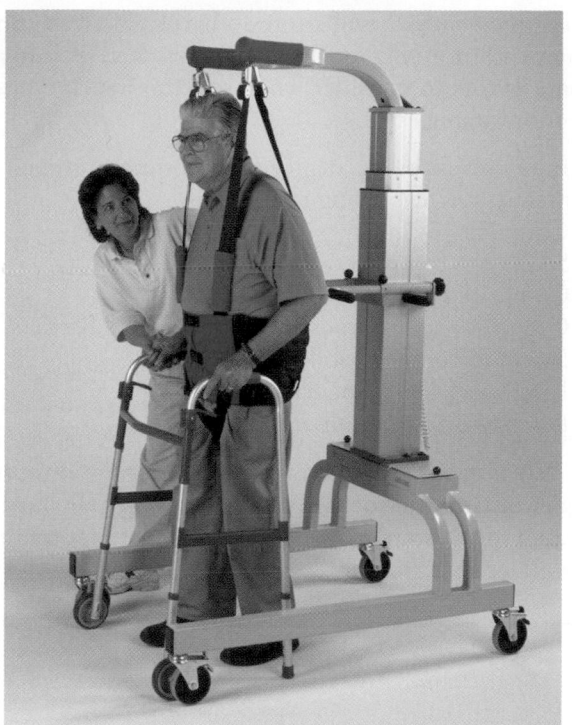

Figure 11.1 Body weight support overground locomotor training using a walker. *(Courtesy of Mobility Research, Tempe, AZ 85281.)*

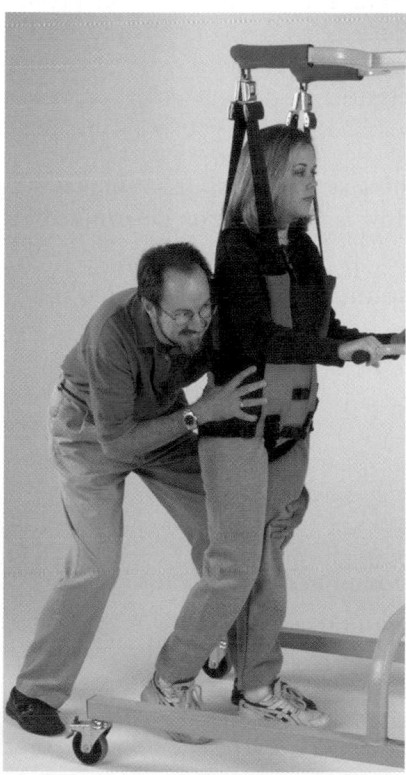

Figure 11.2 Body weight support overground locomotor training without an assistive device. Hand placements allow the patient to move and steer the unit during forward progression. *(Courtesy of Mobility Research, Tempe, AZ 85281.)*

■ EMERGING INTERVENTION STRATEGIES

Other intervention strategies that can be used to improve locomotor capability include virtual reality–based interventions[63-66] and mental practice with motor imagery.[67-69] Virtual reality–based locomotor interventions are typically paired with a TM or robotic device to move the LEs (Fig. 11.3). A computer-generated virtual environment provides a stimulating, task-oriented environment that engages the patient. Visual, proprioceptive, and auditory feedback through interaction in the virtual environment can be used to enhance motor learning.

Motor imagery is the imagining of a motor task without actually performing it, and mental practice is the repetitive imagining of the motor task with the goal of improving physical performance.[69] Similar areas of the brain are activated when people imagine walking and actually walk. The medial primary sensorimotor cortices and the supplementary motor area (SMA) are activated during actual and imagined walking.[69] Optimally, mental practice of gait-related movement should be paired with physical practice.

■ CLINICAL DECISION MAKING

As discussed above, a variety of different intervention strategies can be used to improve locomotor capability. Although these different rehabilitation interventions have been shown to be effective, research has not shown one particular strategy to be superior to another, what the most effective dosage is, or when in the recovery

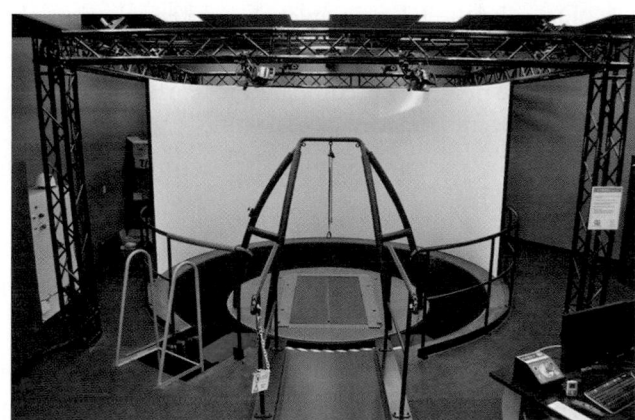

Figure 11.3 CAREN (Computer Assisted Rehabilitation Environment) Extended System is comprised of a treadmill mounted on a motion base (tilting platform), a 12-camera real-time motion capture system, 120- to 180-degree cylindrical screen projection system, and a surround sound system. Standing on the treadmill and safeguarded by a harness, the curved screen engages the patient in the activity of a virtual environment. The system is used for balance as well as all gait applications. *(Courtesy of Motek Medical, Keienbergweg 77 1101 GE Amsterdam, The Netherlands.)*

process a particular intervention strategy should be employed.[32,70-73] This challenges intervention selection when developing a specific POC.

A variety of factors should be considered when deciding on what intervention to select. Current theories of motor control and motor learning advocate for a task-oriented, repetitive approach to interventions.[74] Two basic treatment strategies are a *compensatory* and a *restorative* (recovery) approach. The compensatory approach seeks to improve functional skills by compensating for the lost ability. A simple example of this is the use of an assistive device such as a cane to provide postural support while walking. A restorative approach seeks to restore the "normal" movement while walking. Locomotor training using a BWS and TM system can be viewed as a restorative approach as the guiding principles emphasize normal movement strategies and minimizing compensatory movement patterns. In many cases interventions will require a balance between both compensatory and restorative approaches. Below are some factors to consider when selecting specific intervention strategies:

- Injury severity (i.e., degree of sensorimotor impairments, weight-bearing restrictions)
- Chronicity of injury
- Secondary complications
- Co-morbid health conditions
- Cognitive, communication, or behavioral barriers
- Motor learning capability
- Psychosocial and financial support
- Discharge destination

When determining dosage of the intervention, principles of neuroplasticity[75] (see Chapter 19, Traumatic Brain Injury), strength training, and endurance training should be incorporated.[76]

SUMMARY

Recovery of independent locomotion is an extremely important goal for many patients seen in rehabilitation settings. It is a functional skill that directly affects performance of expected roles within the patient's social, cultural, and physical environment. A framework of LT strategies has been presented that can be modified to meet the needs of an individual patient. Through a process of careful examination and communication with the patient, family, and/or caregivers, specific training strategies can be identified and implemented.

Questions for Review

1. Describe the LT principles that guide selection of interventions.
2. As a complementary activity to LT, what is the benefit of approaching strength training using task-specific practice (as compared to muscle-specific strengthening)? How is task selection determined for task-specific practice?
3. Describe the approach for instructing and guiding a patient to assume a standing position in the parallel bars.
4. What activities are typically included in overground indoor LT?
5. Describe strategies for varying task demands for overground indoor LT.
6. Describe the guiding principles for LT using BWS and a TM.
7. What advantages does LT using BWS and a TM provide?
8. Identify the parameters used for progressing LT using a BWS and TM system.
9. Describe practice activities required for locomotion training overground in the community.
10. At times, LT requires a balance between both compensatory and restorative approaches. What factors are considered when selecting specific intervention strategies?

CASE STUDY

HISTORY

Patient is a 74-year-old male, right-handed, admitted for acute care with progressive right-sided weakness over several hours before admission.

Admission computed tomography (CT) scan was unremarkable; carotid Dopplers were unremarkable without significant stenosis or plaque. Electrocardiogram (ECG) was within normal limits. Chest x-ray showed no active disease. Complete blood count (CBC) was within normal limits.

PHYSICAL EXAMINATION

- Blood pressure (BP): 130/76
- Heart rate (HR): 80
- Respirations (regular): 20
- Temperature: 97.9
- Head, ears, eyes, nose, and throat (HEENT) examination unremarkable
- Chest clear to percussion and auscultation
- Neck supple without carotid bruits
- Abdominal examination: obese without tenderness or organomegaly
- Peripheral pulses intact
- Extremities without deformities

INITIAL NEUROLOGICAL EXAMINATION

Patient is alert and cooperative with mild dysarthria. Speech is fully intelligible. He is able to follow complex commands. There is no neglect or apraxia. Visual fields are full to confrontation. Extraocular movements are full without nystagmus. Pupils are equal and reactive. There is a mild right central facial droop. Sensation is intact over the face. His palate and tongue are midline. Motor examination revealed a spastic right hemiparesis, with right UE (RUE) 3+/5 deltoid, trace triceps, 2+/5 biceps, and 2+/5 finger flexors; on the right LE (RLE) 2/5 iliopsoas, 3/5 quadriceps, 4-/5 gastrocnemius. There is no voluntary dorsiflexion of the foot. Deep tendon reflexes are slightly hyperactive on the right with a right + Babinski. The left side is strong in all muscle groups. Sensation is intact to all modalities.

DIAGNOSIS

Lacunar left cerebrovascular accident (L CVA)

PAST MEDICAL HISTORY

- 7-year history of non–insulin-dependent diabetes
- Patient is obese: 5 ft 7 in tall and weighs 225 lb (102 kg)
- No history of hypertension, heart disease, or prior strokes
- Status post–radical perineal prostatectomy

MEDICATIONS

Aspirin q.d.
Tolinase 250 mg q.d.
Sliding scale insulin for b.i.d. cap sticks

SOCIAL HISTORY

Patient is married, lives with his wife in a two-story home. Patient has been sleeping on the first floor. There are two steps into the house. He is a retired Merchant Marine.

COGNITION

- Alert, follows simple commands, attention is within functional limits (WFL)
- Oriented to place, time, person, situation
- Memory: demonstrates occasional difficulty with immediate/short-term memory; long-term memory WNL
- Safety: demonstrates use of safety precautions during functional situations
- Problem-solving: demonstrates minimal impairment
- Executive function: occasional difficulty with planning, decision making
- Insight: expresses awareness of current limitations with minimal cues

COMMUNICATION

- Auditory comprehension: WNL
- Reading comprehension: WNL
- Written expression: Right (R) hand dominant, legible with left (L)
- Verbal expression: WNL
- Motor speech: Mild dysarthria

SENSORY
- Hearing: WNL
- Visual: WNL
- Somatosensory: trunk and all extremities: WNL

RANGE OF MOTION
- Left upper extremity (LUE) and left lower extremity (LLE): passive range of motion (PROM): WFL
- Right upper extremity (RUE): PROM: WFL; no contractures at wrist or fingers
- Right lower extremity (RLE): PROM: WFL
- Right shoulder subluxation: 1/2 inch (1 finger width)

TONE
- LUE and LLE: WFL
- RUE: Decreased at shoulder; minimal increase: elbow flexors, pronators, wrist and finger flexors, modified Ashworth Scale (mAS) = 1
- RLE: decreased at hip and knee, minimal increase: ankle plantarflexors (PF) (mAS=2)

STRENGTH/ACTIVE ROM
- LUE and LLE: WFL
- RUE: exhibits minimal active control of shoulder flexion, abduction, external rotation with elbow flexion against gravity (flexion synergy pattern)
- RLE: exhibits flexion and extension synergy patterns, can move limb against gravity

BALANCE
Sitting:
- Good (G) static: able to maintain position without handhold support, minimal sway
- Fair (F) dynamic: able to accept only minimal challenge

Standing:
- Poor plus (P+) static: requires handhold support and moderate assistance
- Poor (P) dynamic: unable to accept challenge or move without loss of balance

POSTURAL CHANGES
- Kyphosis
- Forward head position

GAIT
- Able to ambulate 10 feet in parallel bars with moderate assistance
- Gait deviations: unsteady, requires verbal cues for sequencing; decreased foot clearance on right slides RLE forward or hip hikes on right to advance RLE; will benefit from an ankle-foot orthosis (AFO)

PERCEPTUAL
- Spatial awareness: WNL

SKIN
- Dry
- Intact

PSYCHOLOGICAL FUNCTIONING
- Affect: appropriate, no symptoms of depression, emotional distress
- Adjustment to medical condition: good
- Motivation for rehabilitation: good

FUNCTIONAL: FUNCTIONAL INDEPENDENCE MEASURE (FIM) ADMISSION SCORES
- Eating = 6
- Grooming = 4
- Bathing = 4
- Dressing: upper body = 4; dressing lower body = 4
- Toileting = 5

- Bladder management = 5
- Bowel management = 5
- Transfers: bed, chair, wheelchair = 3
- Transfers: toilet = 2
- Transfers: tub-shower = 2
- Locomotion: walk = 1; wheelchair = 5
- Locomotion: stairs =1
- Comprehension = 7
- Expression = 5
- Social interaction = 7
- Problem solving = 7
- Memory = 5

BED MOBILITY

- Patient requires minimal assist to roll onto the sound side and push up into sitting

PATIENT GOALS

- "I want to walk as before"

GUIDING QUESTIONS

1. Identify/categorize this patient's problems affecting locomotion in terms of direct impairments, indirect impairments, and activity limitation.

2. Identify an anticipated goal (within 2 weeks) and expected outcome for LT.

3. Identify three interventions complementary to LT.

4. Identify three LT environments that could be used to improve walking and indicate a training progression.

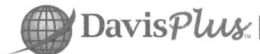 **DavisPlus** | For additional resources, including answers to the questions for review and case study guiding questions, please visit **http://davisplus.fadavis.com**

References

1. Bohannon, RA, Andrews, AW, and Smith, MB: Rehabilitation goals of patients with hemiplegia. Int J Rehabil Res 11(2):181, 1988.
2. Lord, SE, et al: Community ambulation after stroke: How important and obtainable is it and what measures appear predictive? Arch Phys Med Rehabil 85(2):234, 2004.
3. Bain, NB, et al: Factors associated with health-related quality of life in chronic spinal cord injury. Am J Phys Med Rehabil 86(5):387, 2007.
4. Jorgensen, HS, et al: Recovery of walking function in stroke patients: The Copenhagen Stroke Study. Arch Phys Med Rehabil 76(1):27, 1995.
5. National Spinal Cord Injury Statistical Center (NSCIS): The 2010 Annual Report for the Spinal Cord Injury Model Systems. NSCIS, Birmingham, AL. Retrieved July 30, 2012, from https://www.nscisc.uab.edu/PublicDocuments/reports/pdf/2010%20NSCISC%20Annual%20Statistical%20Report%20-%20Complete%20Public%20Version.pdf.
6. Duncan, RP, and Earhart, GM: Measuring participation in individuals with Parkinson disease: Relationships with disease severity, quality of life, and mobility. Disabil Rehabil 33(15-16):1440–1446, 2011.
7. American Physical Therapy Association (APTA): Guide to Physical Therapist Practice, ed 2. APTA, Alexandria, VA, 2003.
8. Schmid, A, et al: Improvements in speed-based gait classifications are meaningful. Stroke 38(7):2096, 2007.
9. Kierkegaard, M, et al: The relationship between walking, manual dexterity, cognition and activity/participation in persons with multiple sclerosis. Mult Scler 18(5):639–646, 2012.
10. Barbeau, H, and Rossignol, S: Recovery of locomotion after chronic spinalization in the adult cat. Brain Res 412(1):84, 1987.
11. Lovely, RG, et al: Effects of training on the recovery of full-weight-bearing stepping in the adult spinal cat. Exp Neurol 92(2):421–435, 1986.
12. Edgerton, VR, et al: Use-dependent plasticity in spinal stepping and standing. Adv Neurol 72:233, 1997.
13. Adkins, DL, et al: Motor training induces experience-specific patterns of plasticity across motor cortex and spinal cord. J Appl Physiol 101(6):1776, 2006.
14. Nudo, RJ: Functional and structural plasticity in motor cortex: Implications for stroke recovery. Phys Med Rehabil Clin North Am 14(1 Suppl):S57, 2003.
15. Nudo, RJ: Plasticity. NeuroRx 3(4):420, 2006.
16. Nudo, RJ: Neural bases of recovery after brain injury. J Commun Disord 44(5):515, 2011.
17. Rossini, PM, et al: Neuroimaging experimental studies on brain plasticity in recovery from stroke. Eura Medicophys 43(2):241–254, 2007.
18. Al-Jarrah, M, et al: Endurance exercise training promotes angiogenesis in the brain of chronic/progressive mouse model of Parkinson's disease. Neurorehabilitation 26(4):369, 2010.
19. Petzinger, GM, et al: Enhancing neuroplasticity in the basal ganglia: The role of exercise in Parkinson's disease. Mov Disord 25(Suppl 1):S141, 2010.
20. Vergara-Aragon, P, Gonzalez, CL, and Whishaw, IQ: A novel skilled-reaching impairment in paw supination on the "good" side

of the hemi-Parkinson rat improved with rehabilitation. J Neurosci 23(2):579, 2003.

21. Behrman, AL, et al: Locomotor training progression and outcomes after incomplete spinal cord injury. Phys Ther 85(12):1356, 2005.

22. Dobkin, B, et al: Weight-supported treadmill vs over-ground training for walking after acute incomplete SCI. Neurology 66(4):484, 2006.

23. Duncan, PW, et al: Body-weight-supported treadmill rehabilitation after stroke. N Engl J Med 364(21):2026, 2011.

24. Fritz, S, et al: Feasibility of intensive mobility training to improve gait, balance, and mobility in persons with chronic neurological conditions: A case series. J Neurol Phys Ther 35(3):141, 2011.

25. Fulk, GD: Interventions to improve transfers and wheelchair skills. In O'Sullivan, SB, and Schmitz, TJ: Improving Functional Outcomes in Physical Rehabilitation. FA Davis, Philadelphia, 2010, p 138.

26. O'Sullivan, SB: Interventions to improve standing control and standing balance skills. In O'Sullivan, SB, and Schmitz, TJ: Improving Functional Outcomes in Physical Rehabilitation. FA Davis, Philadelphia, 2010, p 163.

27. Schmitz, TJ: Interventions to improve locomotor skills. In O'Sullivan, SB, and Schmitz, TJ: Improving Functional Outcomes in Physical Rehabilitation. FA Davis, Philadelphia, 2010, p 194.

28. van de Port, IG, et al: Effects of circuit training as alternative to usual physiotherapy after stroke: Randomised controlled trial. BMJ 344:e2672, 2012.

29. Rose, D, et al: Feasibility and effectiveness of circuit training in acute stroke rehabilitation. Neurorehabil Neural Repair 25(2):140, 2011.

30. Combs, SA, et al: Effects of an intensive, task-specific rehabilitation program for individuals with chronic stroke: A case series. Disabil Rehabil 32(8):669, 2010.

31. Wing, K, Lynskey, JV, and Bosch, PR: Whole-body intensive rehabilitation is feasible and effective in chronic stroke survivors: A retrospective data analysis. Topics Stroke Rehabil 15(3):247, 2008.

32. English, C, and Hillier, SL: Circuit class therapy for improving mobility after stroke. Cochrane Database Syst Rev (7):CD007513, 2010.

33. Wevers, L, et al: Effects of task-oriented circuit class training on walking competency after stroke: A systematic review. Stroke 40(7):2450, 2009.

34. Behrman, AL, and Harkema, SJ: Locomotor training after human spinal cord injury: A series of case studies. Phys Ther 80(7):688, 2000.

35. Kosak, MC, and Reding, MJ: Comparison of partial body weight–supported treadmill gait training versus aggressive bracing assisted walking post stroke. Neurorehabil Neural Repair 14(1):13, 2000.

36. Hidler, J, et al: Multicenter randomized clinical trial evaluating the effectiveness of the Lokomat in subacute stroke. Neurorehabil Neural Repair 23(1):5, 2009.

37. Wu, M, et al: A cable-driven locomotor training system for restoration of gait in human SCI. Gait Posture 33(2):256, 2011.

38. Wu, M, et al: A novel cable-driven robotic training improves locomotor function in individuals post-stroke. Conf Proc IEEE Eng Med Biol Soc (8539–8542), 2011.

39. Field-Fote, EC, and Roach, KE: Influence of a locomotor training approach on walking speed and distance in people with chronic spinal cord injury: A randomized clinical trial. Phys Ther 91(1):48, 2011.

40. Dobkin, B, et al: Weight-supported treadmill vs over-ground training for walking after acute incomplete SCI. Neurology 66(4):484, 2006.

41. Jayaraman, A, et al: Locomotor training and muscle function after incomplete spinal cord injury: Case series. J Spinal Cord Med 31(2):185, 2008.

42. Harkema, SJ, et al: Balance and ambulation improvements in individuals with chronic incomplete spinal cord injury using locomotor training–based rehabilitation. Arch Phys Med Rehabil, July 20, 2011 [Epub ahead of print].

43. Behrman, AL, et al: Locomotor training restores walking in a non-ambulatory child with chronic, severe, incomplete cervical spinal cord injury. Phys Ther 88(5):580–590, 2008.

44. Plummer, P, et al: Effects of stroke severity and training duration on locomotor recovery after stroke: A pilot study. Neurorehabil Neural Repair 21(2):137, 2007.

45. Duncan, PW, et al: Body-weight-supported treadmill rehabilitation after stroke. N Engl J Med 364(21):2026, 2011.

46. Fisher, BE, et al: The effect of exercise training in improving motor performance and corticomotor excitability in people with early Parkinson's disease. Arch Phys Med Rehabil 89(7):1221, 2008.

47. Toole, T, et al: The effects of loading and unloading treadmill walking on balance, gait, fall risk, and daily function in parkinsonism. Neurorehabilitation 20(4):307, 2005.

48. Miyai, I, et al: Treadmill training with body weight support: Its effect on Parkinson's disease. Arch Phys Med Rehabil 81(7):849, 2000.

49. Giesser, B, et al: Locomotor training using body weight support on a treadmill improves mobility in persons with multiple sclerosis: A pilot study. Mult Scler 13(2):224, 2007.

50. Fulk, GD: Locomotor training and virtual reality-based balance training for an individual with multiple sclerosis: A case report. J Neurol Phys Ther 29(1):34, 2005.

51. Breyer, M, et al: Nordic walking improves daily physical activities in COPD: A randomised controlled trial. Respir Res 2010 (doi:10.1186/1465-9921-11-112). Retrieved June 16, 2012, from www.ncbi.nlm.nih.gov/pmc/articles/PMC2933683/pdf/1465-9921-11-112.pdf.

52. Reuter, S, et al: Effects of a flexibility and relaxation programme, walking, and Nordic walking on Parkinson's disease. J Aging Res 2011 (doi: 10.4061/2011/232473). Retrieved June 16, 2012, from www.ncbi.nlm.nih.gov/pmc/articles/PMC3095265/pdf/JAR2011-232473.pdf.

53. Hartvigsen, J, et al: Supervised and non-supervised Nordic walking in the treatment of chronic low back pain: A single blind randomized clinical trial. BMC Musculoskelet Disord 2010 (doi: 10.1186/1471-2474-11-30). Retrieved June 16, 2012, from www.ncbi.nlm.nih.gov/pmc/articles/PMC2831827/pdf/1471-2474-11-30.pdf.

54. Fritz, T, et al: Effects of Nordic walking on health-related quality of life in overweight individuals with type 2 diabetes mellitus, impaired or normal glucose tolerance. Diabet Med 28(11):1362, 2011 (doi:10.1111/j.1464-5491.2011.03348.x). Retrieved June 16, 2012, from www.ncbi.nlm.nih.gov/pmc/articles/PMC3229676/pdf/dme0028-1362.pdf.

55. Kim, DJ: Nordic walking in fibromyalgia: A means of promoting fitness that is easy for busy clinicians to recommend. Arthritis Res Ther 13(1):103, 2011 (doi:10.1186/ar3225). Retrieved June 16, 2012, from www.ncbi.nlm.nih.gov/pmc/articles/PMC3157638/?tool=pmcentrez.

56. Mannerkorpi, K, et al: Does moderate-to-high intensity Nordic walking improve functional capacity and pain in fibromyalgia? A prospective randomized controlled trial. Arthritis Res Ther 12(5):R189, 2010 (doi: 10.1186/ar3159). Retrieved June 16, 2012, from www.ncbi.nlm.nih.gov/pmc/articles/PMC2991024/pdf/ar3159.pdf.

57. Walter, PR, et al: Acute responses to using walking poles in patients with coronary artery disease. J Cardiopulm Rehabil 16(4):245, 1996.

58. Oakley, C, et al: Nordic poles immediately improve walking distance in patients with intermittent claudication. Eur J Endovasc Surg 36(6):689, 2008.

59. Rutlin, T: Activating older adults with "Nordic" pole walking and exercise programs. Journal on Active Aging 10(5):66, 2011.

60. International Nordic Walking Federation (INWA): Definition of Nordic Walking, 2010. Retrieved June 18, 2012, from http://inwa-nordicwalking.com/.

61. Nottingham, S, and Jurasin, A: Nordic Walking for Total Fitness. Human Kinetics, Champaign, IL, 2010.

62. Fulk, G: Locomotor training with body weight support after stroke: The effects of different training parameters. J Neurol Phys Ther 28:20, 2004.

63. Laver, K, et al: Cochrane review: Virtual reality for stroke rehabilitation. Eur J Phys Rehabil Med 48:1, 2012.

64. Mirelman, A, Bonato, P, and Deutsch, JE: Effects of training with a robot–virtual reality system compared with a robot alone on the gait of individuals after stroke. Stroke 40(1):169, 2009.

65. Mirelman, A, et al: Virtual reality for gait training: Can it induce motor learning to enhance complex walking and reduce fall risk in patients with Parkinson's disease? J Gerontol A Biol Sci Med Sci 66(2):234, 2011.

66. Mirelman, A, et al: Effects of virtual reality training on gait biomechanics of individuals post-stroke. Gait Posture 31(4):433–437, 2010.

67. Deutsch, JE, Maidan, I, and Dickstein, R: Patient-centered integrated motor imagery delivered in the home with telerehabilitation to improve walking after stroke. Phys Ther 92(8): 1065, 2012.

68. Verma, R, et al: Task-oriented circuit class training program with motor imagery for gait rehabilitation in poststroke patients: A randomized controlled trial. Topics Stroke Rehabil 18 (Suppl 1): 620, 2011.

69. Malouin, F, and Richards, CL: Mental practice for relearning locomotor skills. Phys Ther 90(2):240, 2010.

70. Mehrholz, J, et al: Treadmill training for patients with Parkinson's disease. Cochrane Database of Syst Rev (1): CD007830, 2010.

71. Laver, K, et al: Cochrane review: Virtual reality for stroke rehabilitation. Eur J Phys Rehabil Med 48(3): 523, 2012.

72. Mehrholz, J, Kugler, J, and Pohl, M: Locomotor training for walking after spinal cord injury. Cochrane Database Syst Rev (2):CD006676, 2008.

73. States, RA, Salem, Y, and Pappas, E: Overground gait training for individuals with chronic stroke: A Cochrane systematic review. J Neurol Phys Ther 33(4):179–186, 2009.

74. Shumway-Cook, A, and Woollacott, MH: Motor Control: Translating Research Into Clinical Practice, ed 4. Lippincott Williams & Wilkins, Philadelphia, 2012.

75. Kleim, JA, and Jones, TA: Principles of experience-dependent neural plasticity: Implications for rehabilitation after brain damage. J Speech Lang Hear Res 51(1):S225, 2008.

76. Durstine, JL, et al (eds): ACSM's Exercise Management for Persons With Chronic Diseases and Disabilities, ed 3. American College of Sports Medicine, Champaign, IL, 2009.

Supplemental Readings

Darter, BJ, and Wilken, JM: Gait training with virtual reality–based real-time feedback: Improving gait performance following transfemoral amputation. Phys Ther 91(9):1385, 2011.

Espay, AJ, et al: At-home training with closed-loop augmented-reality cueing device for improving gait in patients with Parkinson disease. J Rehabil Res Dev 47(6):573, 2010.

Galvez, JA, et al: Trainer variability during step training after spinal cord injury: Implications for robotic gait-training device design. J Rehabil Res Dev 48(2):147, 2011.

Geroin, C, et al: Combined transcranial direct current stimulation and robot-assisted gait training in patients with chronic stroke: A preliminary comparison. Clin Rehabil 25(6):537, 2011.

Hidler, J, et al: ZeroG: Overground gait and balance training system. J Rehabil Res Dev 48(4):287, 2011.

Kang, HK, et al: Effects of treadmill training with optic flow on balance and gait in individuals following stroke: Randomized controlled trials. Clin Rehabil 26(3):246, 2012.

Liu, HH, et al: Assessment of canes used by older adults in senior living communities. Arch Gerontol Geriatr 52(3):299, 2011.

Moe, RH, Fernandes, L, and Osterås, N: Daily use of a cane for two months reduced pain and improved function in patients with knee osteoarthritis. J Physiother 58(2):128, 2012.

Mulroy, SJ, et al: Gait parameters associated with responsiveness to treadmill training with body-weight support after stroke: An exploratory study. Phys Ther 90(2):209, 2010.

Perez, C, and Feung, J: An instrumented cane devised for gait rehabilitation and research. J Phys Ther Educ 25 (1):36, 2011.

Tefertiller, C, et al: Efficacy of rehabilitation robotics for walking training in neurological disorders: A review. J Rehabil Res Dev 48(4):387, 2011.

Wirz, M, et al: Effectiveness of automated locomotor training in patients with acute incomplete spinal cord injury: A randomized controlled multicenter trial. BMC Neurol 11:60, 2011.

■ TYPES AND GAIT PATTERNS

There are three major categories of ambulatory assistive devices: *canes, crutches,* and *walkers.* Each has several modifications to the basic design, many of which were developed to meet the needs of a specific patient problem or diagnostic group. Assistive devices are prescribed for a variety of reasons, including problems of balance, pain, fatigue, weakness, joint instability, excessive skeletal loading, and cosmesis. Another primary function of assistive devices is to eliminate weight-bearing fully or partially from a lower extremity (LE). This unloading occurs by transmission of force from the upper extremities (UEs) to the floor by downward pressure on the assistive device. Prescribing an appropriate assistive device requires knowledge of the patient's weight-bearing status. Common clinical descriptors used to identify weight-bearing status are presented in Box 11A.1. Considerations specific to the bariatric population are presented in Box 11A.2.

Canes

Most canes used in clinical practice are constructed of lightweight aluminum. Evidence supports the effectiveness of canes to improve balance[1,2,3] and improve postural stability.[1,4,5,6] Although canes reduce biomechanical load on LE joints,[2,7] they are not intended for use with a restricted weight-bearing status (such as non–weight-bearing [NWB] or partial weight-bearing [PWB]). Patients are typically instructed to hold a cane in the hand *opposite the affected extremity.* This positioning of the cane most closely approximates a normal reciprocal gait pattern with the opposite arm and leg moving together. It also widens the BOS with less lateral shifting of the center of mass (COM) than when the cane is held on the ipsilateral side.

Several investigations have confirmed that contralateral positioning of the cane reduces hip abductor activity on the side opposite the cane.[4,8,9,10] During normal gait, the hip abductors of the stance extremity contract to counteract the gravitational moment at the pelvis on the contralateral side during swing. This prevents tilting of the pelvis on the contralateral side but results in compressive forces acting at the stance hip. Use of a cane in the UE opposite the affected hip will reduce these forces. The floor (ground) reaction force created by the downward pressure of body weight on the cane counterbalances the gravitational movement at the affected hip.[3] Thus, the need for tension in the abductor muscles is reduced, with a subsequent decrease in joint compressive forces.

Several components of floor reaction forces that create joint compression at the hip can be reduced by use of a cane. In an early study by Ely and Smidt,[11] contralateral use of a cane was found to decrease the vertical and posterior components of the floor reaction force produced by the affected foot. They noted that the reductions in vertical floor reaction peaks were probably due to a shifting of body weight toward the cane, which was a contributing factor in reducing contact force at the affected hip. In a study of patients with total hip arthroplasty (THA), Neumann[8] found that contralateral use of a cane reduced average hip abductor electromyography (EMG) activity to 31% below that generated when not using a cane. Cane use contralateral to a THA, with the addition of carrying an ipsilateral load, decreased hip abductor activity by 40% compared to walking without carrying a load or using a cane.[10]

Research supports use of a cane as an effective method for reducing forces acting at the hip.[4,8,9,10] This reduction is particularly important for activities such as stair climbing, when the forces generated at the hip are significantly

---

Box 11A.1 Clinical Descriptors of Weight-Bearing Status

- *Full weight-bearing* (FWB): There are no restrictions on weight-bearing; 100% of body weight can be borne on the LE.
- *Non–weight-bearing* (NWB): No weight is borne on the involved limb; foot/toes make no contact with floor/ground surface.
- *Partial weight-bearing* (PWB): Only a portion of weight can be borne on the extremity; sometimes expressed as a percentage of body weight (e.g., 20% or 50%).
- *Toe-touch weight-bearing* (TTWB) or *touch-down weight-bearing* (TDWB): Only the toes of the affected extremity contact the floor to improve balance (not to support body weight).
- *Weight-bearing as tolerated* (WBAT): Weight-bearing is limited by patient tolerance of weight borne on extremity.

Box 11A.2   Bariatric Ambulatory Assistive Devices

As with all patients, safety and function are paramount concerns in selection of assistive devices (canes, crutches, and walkers) for patients who are morbidly obese. Important considerations include the following:

- Selecting devices with the appropriate *weight capacity*. Manufacturers of bariatric equipment typically include the maximum weight designation for each product. Standard devices have a weight capacity of 250 to 350 pounds; bariatric equipment carry weight capacities in the range of 400 to 1,000 pounds.
- Identification of the needed dimensions (height and width) of the equipment; this requires knowledge of the anthropometric characteristics (measurements and proportions) of the patient's body.
- Large patients often walk with a wide-based gait owing to lower extremity limb girth and the need to increase the base of support to carry body weight and maintain balance. If a disproportionate amount of weight falls anterior (e.g., abdominal region), upright postures will be further challenged by the need to counteract the anterior effects of gravity.[a]

Following are general characteristics and features of commercially available walkers, crutches, and canes designed for the bariatric population. The information presents a range of available options and is not representative of any individual assistive device. As new products are continually introduced to the market, consultation with a durable medical equipment (DME) supplier will help ensure prescription of the optimal device for an individual patient.

   Note: For labeling or identifying bariatric equipment in patient care settings, the term *expanded capability* (EC) is recommended over less desirable terms such as *oversized, extra- large,* or *heavy duty*.[b]

Walkers

- Bariatric walkers typically include deeper and wider frames.
- May accommodate user heights from 5 feet 3 inches to 6 feet 10 inches.
- Overall walker height adjustments range from 31 to 41.25 inches.
- Available widths: 23.5 to 30 inches.
- May include double anterior cross bracing to increase stability.
- Weight capacity range: 500 to 700 pounds (without seat); 400 to 500 pounds (with seat).
- Walker weight: 7 to 12 pounds (without seat); 19 to 26 pounds (with seat).
- Seat dimensions: height, 22 inches; width, 17.5 to 18 inches; depth, 13 to 14 inches.
- Some models are constructed using a reinforced steel frame; for rolling walkers, large casters are typically used.

Axillary Crutches

- Bariatric axillary crutches are generally constructed of heavy-duty steel.
- May accommodate user heights from 5 feet 2 inches to 7 feet 4 inches (youth sizes available).
- Overall crutch height adjustments range from 44 to 60 inches.
- Weight capacity range: 550 to 1000 pounds.
- Crutch tips: 2-inch diameter.
- Crutch weight: 4 pounds, 6 ounces to 5 pounds each.

Forearm Crutches

- Bariatric forearm crutches are generally constructed of heavy-duty steel.
- May accommodate user heights from 5 feet to 6 feet 7 inches (youth sizes available).
- Crutch height adjustments (handle to floor) range from 28 to 42 inches and forearm piece adjustments (handle to center of cuff) range from 8 to 9.5 inches; as with standard forearm crutches, the leg and forearm sections adjust independently.
- Weight capacity range: 500 to 700 pounds.
- Crutch tips: 2-inch diameter.
- Crutch weight: 2 pounds 6 ounces to 5 pounds 7 ounces.

Canes

- Bariatric canes are generally constructed of stainless steel or heavy-duty steel tubing; most incorporate an offset handle and a reinforcing cuff tightened by a rotation sleeve.
- May accommodate user heights from 4 feet 10 inches to 6 feet 4 inches.
- Overall height adjustments range from approximately 25 to 46 inches.
- Weight capacity range: 500 to 700 pounds.
- Cane weight: 1.8 to 2 pounds.

Continued

Box 11A.2   Bariatric Ambulatory Assistive Devices—cont'd

Quadruped Canes

- Bariatric quadruped canes are generally constructed of steel and often incorporate a double-plated base; most incorporate an offset handle and a reinforcing cuff tightened by a rotation sleeve.
- May accommodate user heights from 4 feet 11 inches to 6 feet 5 inches.
- Overall height adjustments range from approximately 29 to 39 inches.
- Weight capacity range: 500 to 700 pounds.
- Weight: 4 to 5 pounds.
- Footprint size: small base, 6 × 8 inches; large base, 8 × 12 inches.

[a] Trimble, T: Outsize patients—a big nursing challenge. ENW, 2008. Retrieved July 13, 2012, from http://enw.org/Obese.htm.
[b] Patient Safety Center of Inquiry (Tampa, FL): Patient Care Ergonomics Resource Guide, Safe Patient Handling and Movement. Veterans Health Administration and Department of Defense, Washington, DC, 2005. Retrieved July 13, 2012, from www.visn8.va.gov/visn8/patientsafetycenter/resguide/ErgoGuidePtTwo.pdf.

increased. Contralateral cane use has also been found to reduce knee pain in patients with osteoarthritis (OA).[7,12] Clearly, use of a cane has important implications for hip and knee involvement such as joint replacements or degenerative joint disease. Box 11A.3 Evidence Summary presents studies addressing the impact and function of canes.[1,4,7,12,13,14]

Maguire et al[4] found that contralateral cane use reduced gluteus medius activity by 21.86% and tensor fascia lata activity by 19.14% in patients with subacute stroke. This finding has important implications for patients with stroke, who often use canes, because strategies to improve postural control and balance reactions may be adversely affected by reduced hip abductor activity.

In addition to altering the forces on the affected extremity, canes are selected on the basis of their ability to improve gait by providing increased dynamic stability and improving balance. This is achieved by the increased

base of support (BOS) provided by the additional point(s) of floor contact. The level of stability provided by canes is on a continuum. Broad-based (four-point) canes provide the greatest stability and standard (single-point) canes provide the least. The following section presents several of the more common types of canes in clinical use and identifies their advantages and disadvantages.

Types of Canes
Standard Cane

This assistive device also is referred to as a single-point or straight cane (Fig. 11A.1A). It is made of wood or acrylic and has a half-circle ("crook") or T-shaped handle.

- *Advantages.* This cane is inexpensive and fits easily on stairs or other surfaces where space is limited.
- *Disadvantages.* The standard cane is not adjustable and must be cut to fit the patient. With a half-circle

Box 11A.3 Evidence Summary   Canes

Reference	Subjects	Design Intervention	Duration	Results	Comments
Jones et al[7] (2012)	64 patients with knee OA; 89% female (F) and 11% male (M) randomly assigned to either experimental group (EG) or control group (CG); groups homogeneous for demographic and clinical characteristics	Single-blind parallel group RCT; EG used a single-point cane; CG did not use cane; outcome measures (OMs): pain (VAS), function (Lequesne knee questionnaire and WOMAC); general health (SF-36); and energy expenditure (6MWT/ATS)	Two months; OMs performed at baseline, again at 30 and 60 days	Compared to CG, EG showed significant improvement in pain (ES 0.18), function (ES 0.13), two SF-36 items (physical functioning [ES 0.07] and bodily pain [ES 0.08]) and energy expenditure (ES 0.21)	For patients with OA, a cane can be effective in decreasing pain, improving function, and improving quality of life. Patients should be advised that an initial adaptation period to the cane is required before gains in function, reduction in pain, and diminished energy expenditure are achieved.

Box 11A.3 Evidence Summary   Canes—cont'd

Reference	Subjects	Design Intervention	Duration	Results	Comments
Maguire et al[4] (2010)	13 patients with hemiplegia following first unilateral stroke; 5 F and 8 M; mean age: 64 (SD = 14) years; mean time since stroke: 9.2 weeks (range 5–16 weeks; SD = 3.8)	Randomized within-subject experimental design; subjects walked at self-selected pace under three conditions: (1) with cane; (2) with TheraTogs* (elastic orthosis providing vertical support to increase stability); and (3) with taping for GM and TFL; OMs: Peak EMG from baseline and temporal/spatial gait characteristics	Baseline data and testing of three conditions occurred in single experimental session	Use of cane reduced GM activity by 21.86%; TheraTogs increased it by 16.47%; tape increased it by 5.8% Use of cane reduced TFL activity by 19.14%; TheraTogs reduced it by 1.10%; tape reduced it by 3% Gait speed (m/sec): baseline = 0.44; cane = 0.45; tape = 0.48; TheraTogs = 0.49	Following stroke, cane use reduced hemiplegic hip abductor activity; hip abductor taping and TheraTogs increased hemiplegic hip abductor activity and gait speed; cane use may not be optimal during early stroke rehabilitation; TheraTogs and taping may be more beneficial in promoting muscle activity and balance reactions; examination of long-term effects warranted
Bohannon[1] (2011)	11 consecutive qualifying patients obtained from review of author's patient records who were not habitual cane users; 7 F and 4 M; mean age: 79.1 (SD = 12.0)	Descriptive study to determine if use of a single-point cane increases unipedal (single limb) balance time during static standing OM: time in single limb balance (30-sec cutoff)	Bilateral single limb balance times measured using a stopwatch under two conditions: (1) with a cane; and (2) without a cane	Balance times were significantly higher with the cane for both the left (t = (4.99; p <.001) and right (t = (7.82; p <.001) stance times as compared to without the cane	Confirms use of canes for increasing single limb balance time; for patients reluctant to use a cane, study presents a simple method using readily available equipment (stopwatch) to reinforce the increased stability provided by a cane
Beauchamp et al[13] (2009)	14 male inpatients with stroke; based on a gait-symmetry calculation patients divided into 2 groups: symmetrical (n = 5) and asymmetrical (n = 9)	Within-subject experimental design; subjects walked on a pressure-sensitive walkway under three conditions: (1) no cane; (2) single-point cane; and (3) quadruped (quad) cane OMs: spatial and temporal measure of gait using GAITRite† system	Testing of three conditions occurred in single experimental session	Standard cane significantly improved symmetry in asymmetrical subjects (p = 0.028); use of a quad cane did not improve symmetry (p = 0.36); for symmetrical subjects, there was no effect on symmetry with either standard (p = 0.88) or quad (p = 0.32) canes	A standard cane is effective in improving temporal gait symmetry in asymmetrical patients; further research is warranted into the impact of canes on early stroke rehabilitation and the long-term effects of ambulatory assistive devices on gait symmetry

Continued

Box 11A.3 Evidence Summary Canes—cont'd

Reference	Subjects	Design Intervention	Duration	Results	Comments
Nolen et al[14] (2010)	19 physical therapy student volunteers (12 M and 7 F) who recently completed instruction in use of all types of canes; age range from 22 to 30 years	Subjects walked on a pressure-sensitive walkway under four conditions: (1) no cane; (2) standard single-tip cane (STC); (3) tripod cane (TPC); and (4) small-base quad cane (SQC) OMs: spatial and gait parameters using GAITRite† system	Testing of four conditions occurred in single experimental session conducted 3 days after an initial information meeting with subjects	In sequential order of no cane, STC, TPC, and SQC there was a significant difference of decreased velocity, cadence, and increased stance and swing time ($p < 0.001$); no significant difference for step and stride lengths ($p > 0.050$); compared to STC and TPC, the SQC caused slower velocity and cadence with increased stance time (all $p < 0.008$)	An SQC appears most stable but least efficient; an STC is most efficient but least stable; a TPC is most appropriate when considering both efficiency of walking and cane stability; small sample size not representative of individuals typically requiring ambulatory assistance
Jones et al[12] (2012)	64 symptomatic patients with diagnosis of knee OA and pain scores of 3–7 on VAS; 89% F and 11% M; mean age 61.7 years; subjects had not used a cane within the past 3 months	Observational, cross-sectional study; OM: energy expenditure using the Cosmed K4b2‡ portable telemetric gas analysis system during 6MWT/ATS under two conditions: (1) with a standard cane and (2) without a cane	Tests performed on two separate days within a 7-day period; each condition tested twice: Day 1: two tests under one condition Day 2: two tests under the other condition	Subjects walked farther on tests without cane ($p < 0.001$); compared to walking with cane, cane use increased oxygen expenditure (VO_2) by approximately (approx) 50% and O_2 cost by approx 80% ($p < 0.001$); pain decreased by approx 20% with cane compared to without ($p < 0.001$)	Energy expenditure must be viewed with caution because it is typically higher during acclimation period to a cane (concentration on use of cane may alter normal automaticity of walking) Prolonged follow-up studies needed to determine impact of daily cane use on energy expenditure and if adaptation occurs

EMG = electromyography; ES = effect size; GM = gluteus medius; OA = osteoarthritis; OM = outcome measure; RCT = randomized controlled trial; 6MWT/ATS = 6-Minute Walk Test in compliance with the American Thoracic Society guidelines; SD = standard deviation; TFL = tensor fascia lata; VAS = visual analog scale (pain); WOMAC = Western Ontario and McMaster Universities (WOMAC) questionnaire.

*TheraTogs, Inc., Telluride, CO 81435.
†CIR Systems Inc., Clifton, NJ 07012.
‡Cosmed USA Inc., Concord, CA 94520.

handle, the point of support (shaft of cane) is anterior to the hand, not directly beneath it. The T-shaped handle shifts the point of support only slightly closer to hand.

Standard Adjustable Aluminum Cane

This assistive device (Fig. 11A.1B) has the same basic design as the standard cane. It is made of aluminum and has a half-circle handle with a molded plastic covering. The telescoping design of this cane enables the height to be adjusted using a push-button mechanism. Variations in available height range differ slightly with manufacturers. However, they are generally adjustable within the range of approximately 27 to 38.5 in (68 to 98 cm). (*Note:* Most adjustable aluminum assistive devices [e.g., canes, crutches, walkers] use a push-button mechanism to alter height; many include a reinforcing cuff tightened by a thumbscrew or rotation sleeve.)

- *Advantages.* This cane is quickly adjustable, facilitating ease of determining appropriate height. It is lightweight and fits easily on stairs.
- *Disadvantages.* The point of support is anterior to the hand, not directly beneath it. This cane is more costly than a standard wooden cane.

Adjustable Aluminum Offset Cane

The proximal component of the shaft of this cane is offset anteriorly, creating a straight *offset* handle. It is made of aluminum with a plastic or rubber molded grip-shaped handle (Fig. 11A.1C). Using a push-button mechanism, the telescoping design allows the height to be adjusted from approximately 27 to 38.5 in (68 to 98 cm).

- *Advantages.* The design of this cane allows pressure to be borne over the center of the cane for greater stability. This cane also is quickly adjusted, is light-weight, and fits easily on stairs.
- *Disadvantages.* This cane is more costly than standard or adjustable aluminum canes.

Note: For standard and offset canes, the diameter of both the distal rubber tips and shaft of the cane is generally at least 1 in (2.54 cm).

Quadruped (Quad) Cane

This assistive device is constructed of aluminum and is available in a variety of designs depending on the manu-facturer. Both large-based quad canes (LBQCs) and small-based quad canes (SBQCs) are commercially avail-able (Figs. 11A.2 and 11A.3). The characteristic feature of these canes is that they provide a broad base with four points of floor contact. Each point (leg) is covered with a rubber tip. The legs closest to the patient's body are gen-erally shorter and may be angled to allow foot clearance. On many designs the proximal portion of the cane is offset anteriorly. The hand piece is usually one of a variety

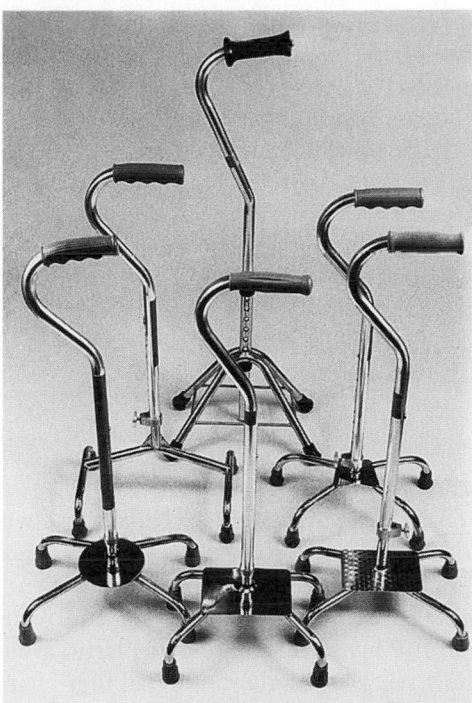

Figure 11A.2 Shown here are a variety of large-based quadruped canes.

of contoured plastic grips. A telescoping design allows for height adjustments. Quad canes are generally adjustable from approximately 28 to 38 in (71 to 91 cm).

- *Advantages.* This cane provides a broad-based sup-port. Bases are available in several different sizes. This cane is also easily adjustable.

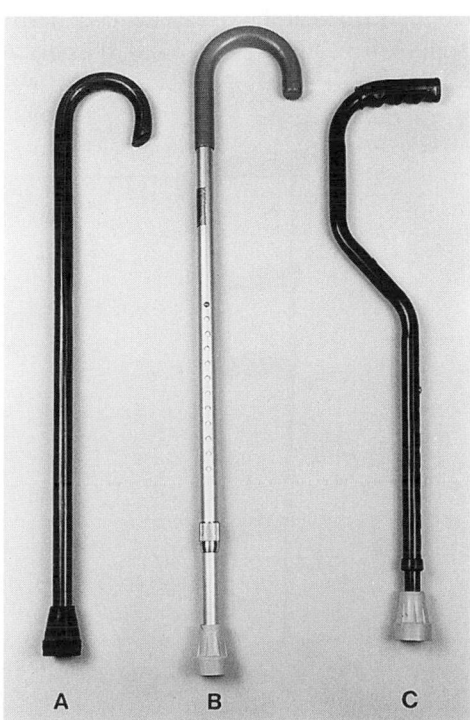

Figure 11A.1 Shown here are (**A**) standard wooden cane, (**B**) standard adjustable aluminum cane, and (**C**) adjustable offset cane.

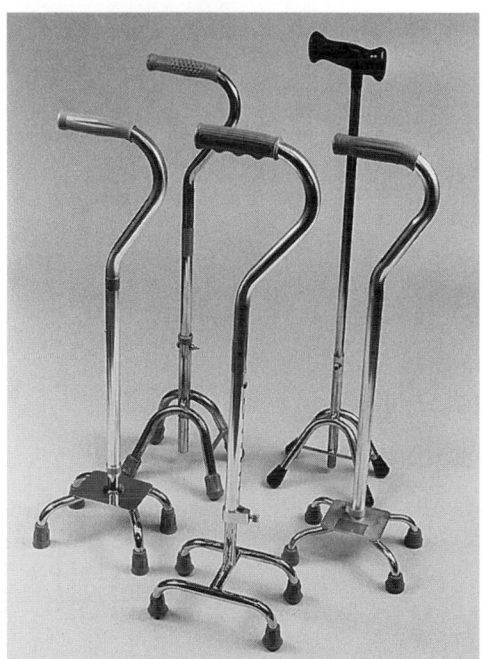

Figure 11A.3 A variety of small-based quadruped canes.

- *Disadvantages.* Depending on the specific design of the cane, the pressure exerted by the patient's hand may not be centered over the cane and may result in patient complaints of instability. As a result of the broad BOS, some quad canes may not be practical for use on stairs. Another disadvantage of broad-based canes is that they warrant use of a slower gait pattern. If a faster forward progression is used, the cane often "rocks" from rear legs to front legs, which decreases effectiveness of the cane. Patients should be instructed to place all four legs of the cane on the floor simultaneously to obtain maximum stability.

Hemi Cane

The hemi cane also is constructed of aluminum (Fig. 11A.4). It provides a very broad base with four points of floor contact. Each point (leg) is covered with a rubber tip. The legs farther from the patient's body are angled to maintain floor contact and to improve stability. The handgrip is molded plastic around the uppermost segment of aluminum tubing. Hemi canes fold flat and are adjustable in height from approximately 29 to 37 in (73 to 94 cm).

- *Advantages.* Hemi canes provide very broad-based support and are more stable than a quad cane. These canes also fold flat for travel or storage.
- *Disadvantages.* As with the quad canes, the specific design of a hemi cane or handgrip placement may not allow pressure to be centered over the cane. Hemi canes cannot be used on most stairs. They require use of a slow forward progression and are generally more costly than quad canes.

Rolling Cane

Constructed of aluminum and aluminum tubing (Fig. 11A.5), this cane provides a wide, wheeled base allowing uninterrupted forward progression. It includes a contoured handgrip, height adjustment from 28 to 37 in (71 to 94 cm), and a pressure-sensitive brake built into the handle engaged using pressure from the base of the hand.

- *Advantages.* The wheeled base allows weight to be continuously applied as the need to lift and place the cane forward is eliminated. This also provides for a faster forward progression. The second and third handles placed between the uprights can assist in rising to standing (brake engaged).
- *Disadvantages.* This cane is more costly than standard quadruped canes and requires sufficient UE and grip strength to engage the braking mechanism. This cane is not suitable for patients displaying a propulsive gait pattern (e.g., Parkinson's disease).

Laser Cane

This cane incorporates a bright red laser line projected across the floor designed to assist with overcoming freezing episodes while walking (Fig 11A.6). A walker with a laser is also available (Fig 11A.7). Donovan et al[15] examined 26 patients with Parkinson's disease using either a laser cane or walker (selection based on type of device habitually used). The Freezing of Gait Questionnaire (FOG-Q)[16,17] was used as an outcome measure (lower scores suggest improved function). Subjects were instructed not to look at the visual cue (laser beam) unless experiencing a freezing of gait (FOG) episode, at which

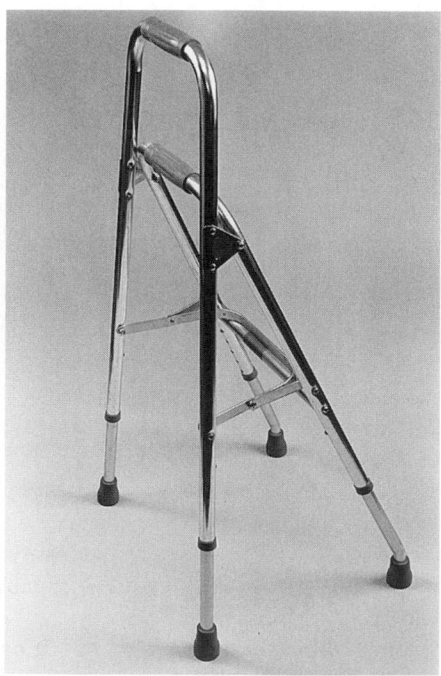

Figure 11A.4 Hemi cane.

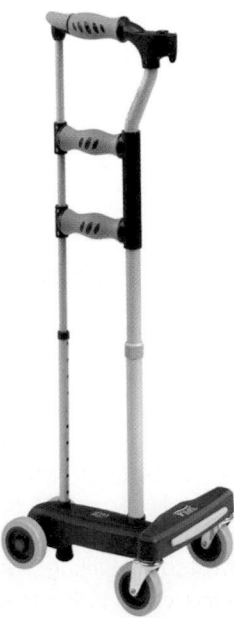

Figure 11A.5 Rolling cane. *(Courtesy of Full Life Products, LLC, Moorestown, NJ 08057.)*

time they were instructed to "step over" the light. Findings indicated a small but significant mean reduction in FOG-Q scores of 1.25 (±0.48; p = 0.0152). The mean reduction in fall frequency was 39.5% (±9.3%; p = 0.002). No significant changes in gait speed were noted. Although additional research is warranted, these initial findings suggest that assistive devices incorporating a laser beam may hold potential for addressing FOG episodes common in patients with Parkinson's disease.

Handgrips

A general consideration relevant to all canes is the nature of the handgrip. A variety of styles and sizes are available. The type of handgrip should be judged and selected primarily on the basis of patient comfort and on the grip's ability to provide adequate surface area to allow effective transfer of weight from the UE to the floor. The more common types of handgrips are (1) the *crook* handle, (2) the straight *offset* handle, and (3) the *T-shaped* handle, which conforms to the patient's hand. It is useful to have several handgrip styles available for examination and trial with individual patients.

Measuring Canes

In measuring cane height, the cane (or center of a broad-based cane) is placed approximately 6 in (15.24 cm) from the lateral border of the toes. Two landmarks typically are used during measurement: the *greater trochanter* and the *angle at the elbow*. The top of the cane should come to approximately the level of the greater trochanter, and the elbow should be flexed to about 20 to 30 degrees. Because of individual variations in body proportion and limb lengths, the degree of flexion at the elbow is generally considered the more important indicator of correct cane height.

The 20 to 30 degrees of elbow flexion serves two important functions. It allows the arm to shorten or to lengthen during different phases of gait, and it provides a shock-absorption mechanism. Finally, as with all assistive devices, the height of the cane should be considered with regard to patient comfort and the cane's effectiveness in accomplishing its intended purpose.

Gait Pattern for Use of Canes

As discussed, the cane should be held in the UE opposite the affected limb. For ambulation overground on level surfaces, the cane and the involved (or more involved) extremity are advanced simultaneously (Fig. 11A.8). The cane should remain relatively close to the body and should not be placed ahead of the toe of the involved extremity. These are important considerations, because placing the cane too far forward or to the side will cause lateral and/or forward bending, with a resultant decrease in dynamic stability.

When bilateral involvement exists, a decision must be made as to which side of the body the cane will be held. This question is most effectively resolved by using a

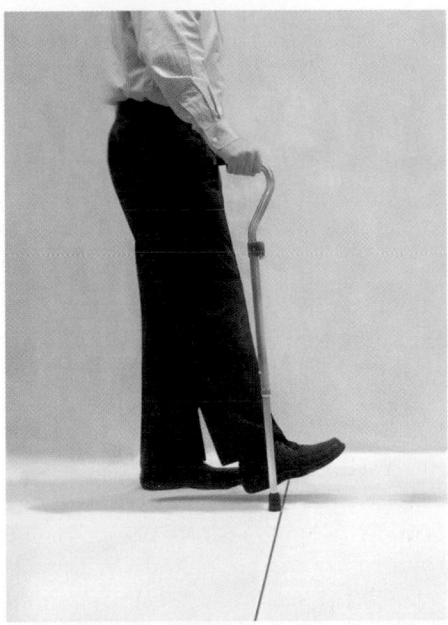

Figure 11A.6 The Laser Cane projects a bright red laser beam across the floor in front of the patient. During a freezing of gait episode, the beam provides a visual cue for the patient to step over. *(Courtesy of In-Step Mobility Products Corp, Skokie, IL 60076.)*

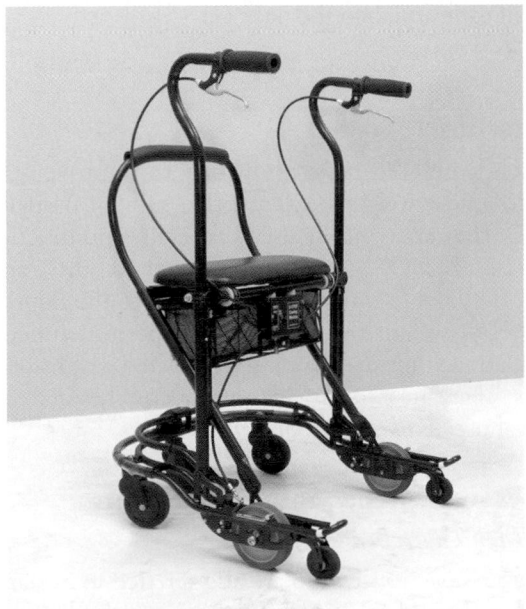

Figure 11A.7 The U-Step II walking stabilizer includes both visual (laser) and auditory (beat pattern for gait speed) cues. U-shaped base surrounds the individual for increased stability. It also includes a seat, a small projection over posterior casters to assist moving onto a curb, and a control to set rolling resistance. *(Courtesy of In-Step Mobility Products Corp, Skokie, IL 60076.)*

(4) Cycle is repeated.

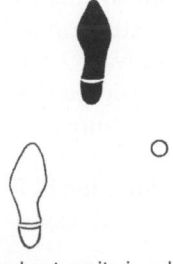

(3) The uninvolved extremity is advanced.

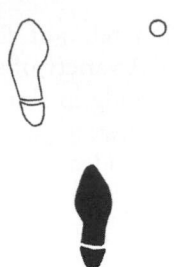

(2) The cane and involved extremity are moved forward simultaneously.

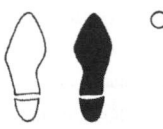

(1) Starting position. In this example, the left lower extremity is the involved limb.

Figure 11A.8 Gait pattern for use of cane.

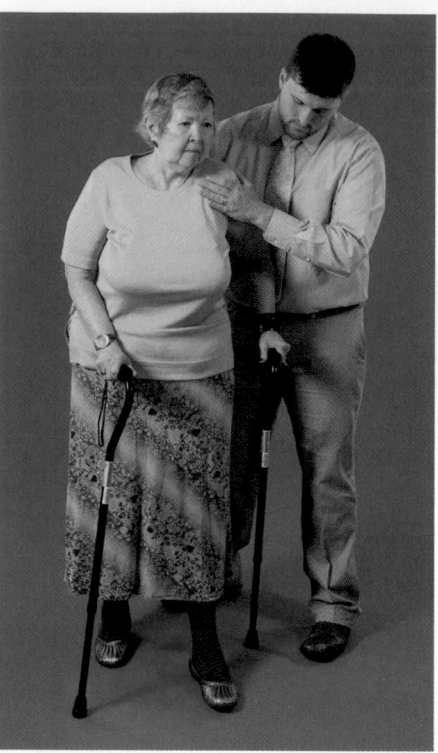

Figure 11A.9 The client is ambulating using bilateral off-set canes with a four-point gait. One cane is advanced and then the opposite LE is advanced. For example, the right cane is moved forward, then the left LE, followed by the left cane and then the right LE.

problem-solving strategy with input from both the patient and therapist. Questions to be considered include the following:

- On which side is the cane most comfortable?
- Is one placement superior in terms of improving balance and/or ambulatory endurance?
- If gait deviations exist, is one position more effective in improving the overall gait pattern?
- Is safety influenced by cane placement (e.g., during transfers, stair climbing, or overground in community)?
- Is there a difference in grip strength between hands?
- Are two canes needed for stability?

Consideration of these questions will generally provide sufficient information to determine the most effective cane placement and use when bilateral involvement exists.

For some patients, optimal function is achieved using canes bilaterally (Fig 11A.9). In these situations, a two- or four-point gait pattern is used. For example, with a four-point pattern, the contralateral cane is moved forward and then the ipsilateral LE steps forward. Using a two-point pattern, the contralateral cane and ipsilateral LE are moved forward simultaneously. These gait patterns are described in the following section on crutches.

Crutches

Crutches are used most frequently to improve balance and to relieve weight-bearing either fully or partially on an LE. They are typically used bilaterally and function to increase the BOS, to improve lateral stability, and to allow the UEs to transfer body weight to the floor. This transfer of weight through the UEs permits functional ambulation while maintaining a restricted weight-bearing status. There are two basic designs of crutches in frequent clinical use: *axillary* and *forearm* crutches.

Types of Crutches and Attachments
Axillary Crutches

These assistive devices also are also referred to as standard crutches (Fig. 11A.10, *left*). They are made of lightweight wood or aluminum. Their design includes an axillary bar, a hand piece, and double uprights joined distally by a single leg covered with a rubber suction tip (which should have a diameter of 1.5 to 3 in [1.5 to 3 cm]). The single leg allows for height variations. Height adjustments for wooden crutches are accomplished by altering the placement of screws and wing bolts in predrilled holes. The design of most aluminum crutches incorporates a push-button pin mechanism for height adjustments similar to those found on aluminum canes. Some aluminum crutches also have

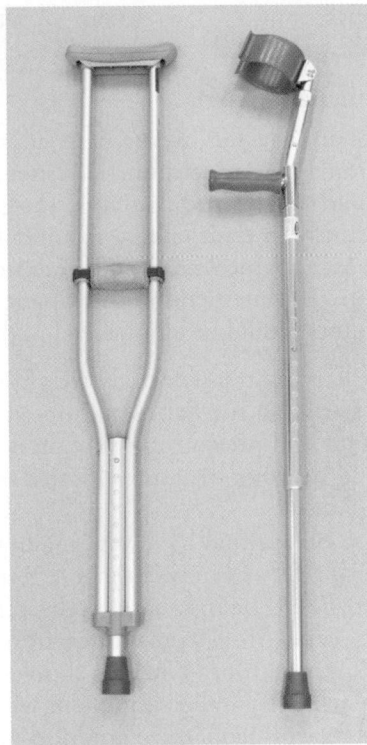

Figure 11A.10 Axillary crutch (*left*) and forearm crutch (*right*).

patient height markers adjacent to the notches to assist in adjustment. The height of the handgrips for wooden and some aluminum crutches is adjusted by placement of screws and wing bolts in predrilled holes. The handgrip height on some aluminum crutches is adjusted using a push-button mechanism with a reinforcing clip-lock (Fig. 11A.11). Both the overall height of the crutch and the height of the

handgrip typically adjust in 1-in (2.54-cm) increments. Axillary crutches are generally adjustable in adult sizes from approximately 48 to 60 in (122 to 153 cm), with children's and extra-long sizes available.

- *Advantages.* Axillary crutches improve balance and lateral stability and provide for functional ambulation with restricted weight-bearing. They are easily adjusted, inexpensive when made of wood, and can be used for stair climbing.
- *Disadvantages.* Because of the tripod stance required to use crutches and the resultant large BOS, crutches are awkward in small areas. For the same reason, the safety of the user may be compromised when ambulating in crowded areas. Another disadvantage is the tendency of some patients to lean on the axillary bar. This causes pressure at the radial groove (spiral groove) of the humerus, creating a situation of potential damage to the radial nerve, as well as to adjacent vascular structures in the axilla.

Platform Attachments

These attachments (Fig. 11A.12) are also referred to as *forearm rests* or *troughs*. Although they are described here, they also are used with walkers. Their function is to allow transfer of body weight through the forearm to the assistive device. A platform attachment is used when weight-bearing is contraindicated through the wrist and hand (e.g., arthritis, Colles' fracture). The forearm piece is usually padded, has a dowel or handgrip, and has hook-and-loop straps to maintain the position of the forearm.

Forearm Crutches

These assistive devices are also known as *Lofstrand* and *Canadian* crutches (Fig. 11A.10, *right*). They are

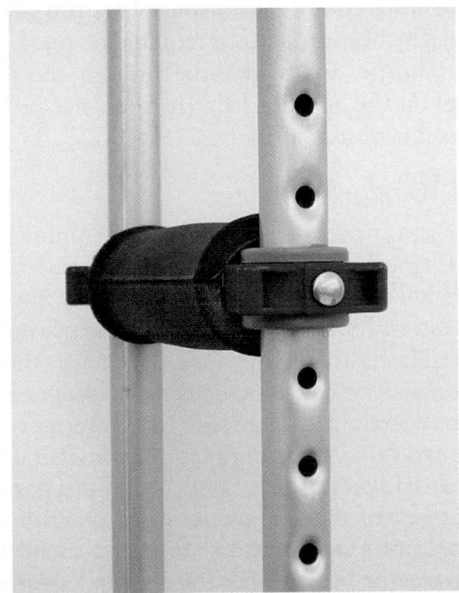

Figure 11A.11 Push-button handgrip adjustment with reinforcing clip-lock.

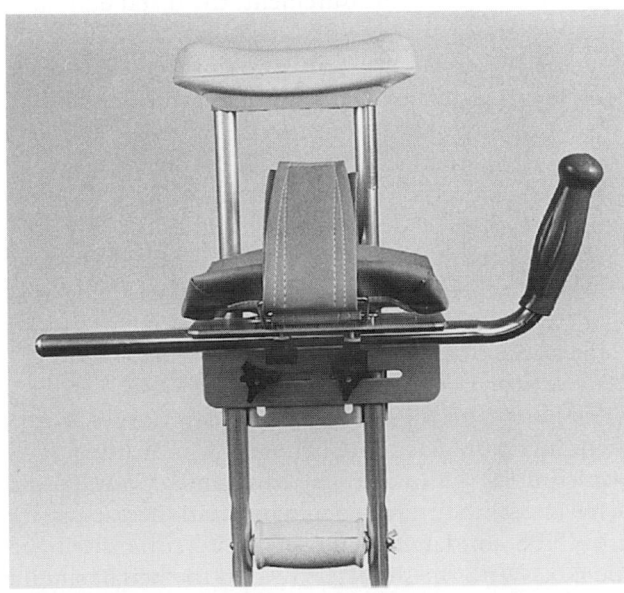

Figure 11A.12 Platform attachment to axillary crutch. These attachments can also be used on walkers.

constructed of aluminum. Their design includes a single upright, a forearm cuff, and a handgrip. This crutch adjusts both proximally to alter position of the forearm cuff and distally to alter the height of the crutch. Adjustments are made using a push-button mechanism. The available heights of forearm crutches are indicated from handgrip to floor and are generally adjustable in adult sizes from 29 to 35 in (74 to 89 cm), with children's and extra-long sizes available. The distal end of the crutch is covered with a rubber suction tip. The forearm cuffs are available with either a medial or anterior opening. The cuffs are made of metal and can be obtained with a plastic coating.

- *Advantages.* The forearm cuff allows use of hands without the crutches becoming disengaged. They are easily adjusted and allow functional stair climbing activities. Many patients feel they are more cosmetic and they fit more easily into an automobile owing to the overall decreased height. They are also the most functional type of crutch for stair climbing activities for individuals wearing bilateral knee-ankle-foot orthoses (KAFOs).
- *Disadvantages.* Forearm crutches provide less lateral support owing to the absence of an axillary bar. The cuffs may be difficult to remove.

Measuring Crutches
Axillary Crutches

Several methods are available for measuring axillary crutches. The most common use a standing or a supine position. Measurement from standing is most accurate and is the preferred approach.

- *Standing.* From a supported standing position, crutches should be measured from a point approximately 2 in (5.08 cm) below the axilla. The width of two fingers is often used to approximate this distance. During measurement, the distal end of the crutch should be resting at a point 2 in (5.08 cm) lateral and 6 in (15.24 cm) anterior to the foot. A general estimate of crutch height can be obtained before standing by subtracting 16 in (40.64 cm) from the patient's height. With the shoulders relaxed, the hand piece should be adjusted to provide 20 to 30 degrees of elbow flexion.
- *Supine.* From this position the measurement is taken from the anterior axillary fold to a surface point (mat or treatment table) 6 to 8 in (5.08 to 7.5 cm) from the lateral border of the heel.

Forearm Crutches

Standing is the position of choice for measuring forearm crutches. From a supported standing position, the distal end of the crutch should be positioned at a point 2 in (5.08 cm) lateral and 6 in (15.24 cm) anterior to the foot. With the shoulders relaxed the height should then be adjusted to provide 20 to 30 degrees of elbow flexion. The forearm cuff is adjusted separately. Cuff placement should be on the proximal third of the forearm, approximately 1 to 1.5 in (2.5 to 3.8 cm) below the elbow.

Crutch Gait Patterns

Gait patterns are selected on the basis of the patient's balance, coordination, muscle function (strength, power, endurance), and weight-bearing status. The gait patterns differ significantly in their energy requirements, BOS, and the speed with which they can be executed.

Before initiating instruction in gait patterns, several important points should be emphasized to the patient:

- During axillary crutch use, body weight should always be borne on the hands and not on the axillary bar. This will prevent pressure on both the vascular and nervous structures located in the axillary region.
- Balance will be optimal by always maintaining a wide (tripod) BOS. Even when in a resting stance, the patient should be instructed to keep the crutches at least 4 in (10 cm) to the front and to the side of each foot. The foot should not be allowed to achieve parallel alignment with the crutches. This will jeopardize anterior–posterior stability by decreasing the BOS.
- When using standard crutches, the axillary bars should be held close to the chest wall to provide improved lateral stability.
- The patient should also be cautioned about the importance of holding the head up and maintaining good postural alignment during ambulation.
- Stepping in a small circle rather than pivoting should be used when turning.

Three-Point

In this type of gait three points of support contact the floor (two crutch points and a single LE). It is used when a non–weight-bearing status is required on one LE. Body weight is borne on the hands through the crutches instead of on the affected LE. The sequence of this gait pattern is illustrated in Figure 11A.13.

Partial Weight-Bearing

This gait is a modification of the three-point pattern. During forward progression of the involved extremity, weight is borne partially on both crutches and on the affected extremity (Fig. 11A.14). During instruction in the partial weight-bearing gait, emphasis should be placed on use of a normal heel–toe progression on the affected extremity. Patients may interpret "partial weight-bearing" as meaning that only the toes or ball of the foot should contact the floor. Use of this positioning over a period of days or weeks will lead to heel cord tightness. Limb load monitors are often a useful adjunct to partial weight-bearing gait training and are described in the section, Adjunct Training Devices. These devices provide auditory feedback to the patient regarding the amount of weight borne on an extremity.

(5) Cycle is repeated.

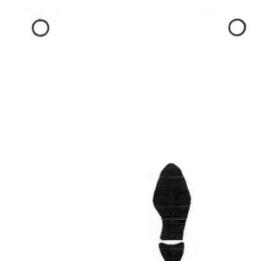

(4) Both crutches are advanced.

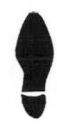

(3) Weight is shifted through the upper extremities onto the crutches, and the uninvolved limb advances beyond the crutches. If this presents difficulty, the unaffected limb may initially be brought to the crutches and later progress beyond.

(2) Weight is shifted onto the uninvolved right lower extremity, and the crutches are advanced.

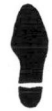

(1) Starting position. In this example, the left lower extremity is non-weightbearing.

Figure 11A.13 Three-point gait pattern.

Four-Point

This pattern provides a slow, stable gait as three points of floor contact are maintained. Weight is borne on both LEs and typically is used with bilateral involvement due to poor balance, incoordination, or muscle weakness. In this gait pattern one crutch is advanced and then the opposite LE is advanced. For example, the left crutch is moved forward, then the right LE, followed by the right crutch and then the left LE (Fig. 11A.15).

Two-Point

This gait pattern is similar to the four-point gait. However, it is less stable because only two points of floor contact are maintained. Thus, use of this gait requires

(4) Cycle is repeated.

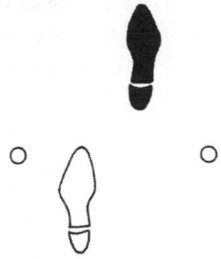

(3) Weight is shifted into the crutches and partially to the affected extremity, and the unaffected limb advances.

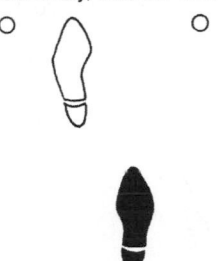

(2) Weight is shifted onto the uninvolved limb. The crutches and the affected extremity are advanced simultaneously as shown or can be broken into two components:
(a) advance crutches, (b) advance affected extremity.

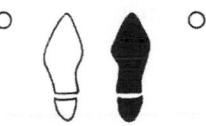

(1) Starting position. In this example, the left lower extremity is partial-weightbearing.

Figure 11A.14 Partial weight-bearing gait; modification of the three-point gait pattern.

better balance. The two-point pattern more closely simulates normal gait, inasmuch as the opposite LE and UE move together (Fig. 11A.16).

Two additional, less commonly used crutch gaits are the *swing-to* and *swing-through* patterns. These gaits are often used when there is bilateral LE involvement, such as in spinal cord injury (SCI). The swing-to gait involves forward movement of both crutches simultaneously, weight is shifted onto the hands, and the LEs "swing to" the crutches. In the swing-through gait, the crutches are moved forward together, weight is shifted onto the hands, and the LEs are swung beyond the crutches.

Walkers

Walkers are used to improve balance and relieve weight-bearing either fully or partially on an LE. Of the three categories of ambulatory assistive devices, walkers afford the greatest stability. They provide a wide BOS, improve anterior and lateral stability, and allow the UEs to transfer body weight to the floor.

Walkers are typically made of aluminum with molded vinyl handgrips and rubber tips. They are adjustable in adult sizes from approximately 32 to 37 in (81 to

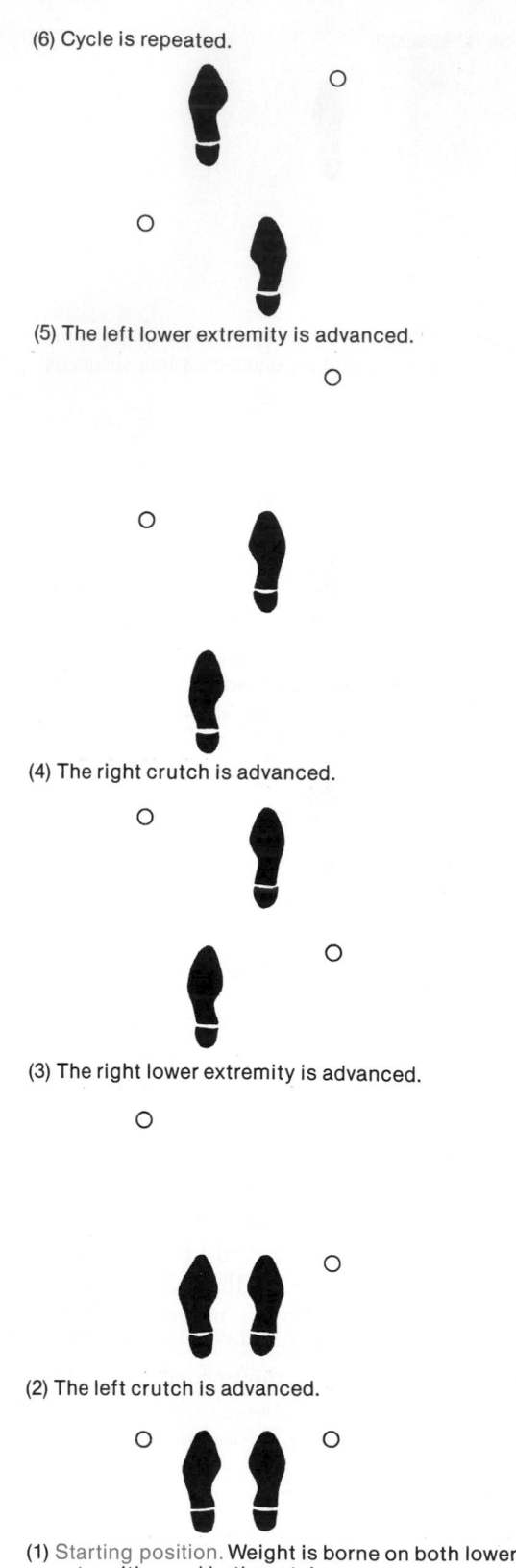

(6) Cycle is repeated.

(5) The left lower extremity is advanced.

(4) The right crutch is advanced.

(3) The right lower extremity is advanced.

(2) The left crutch is advanced.

(1) Starting position. **Weight is borne on both lower extremities and both crutches.**

Figure 11A.15 Four-point gait pattern.

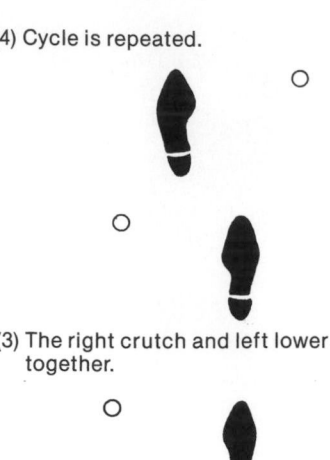

(4) Cycle is repeated.

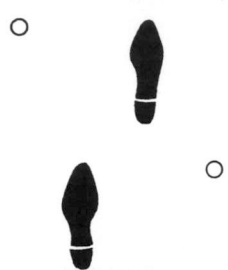

(3) The right crutch and left lower extremity are advanced together.

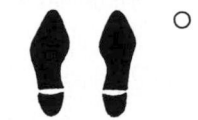

(2) The left crutch and right lower extremity are advanced together.

(1) Starting position. **Weight is borne on both lower extremities and both crutches.**

Figure 11A.16 Two-point gait pattern.

92 cm), with children's, youth, and tall sizes available. Several design variations and modifications to the standard design are available and are described below.

Types of Walkers and Features
Glides

Glides are small, plastic attachments placed on the posterior legs of walkers typically in combination with wheels on the front legs (Fig. 11A.17A). They promote a smooth forward progression without having to lift and place the walker with each step. They are typically made of high-density plastic in an inverted-mushroom shape. Other common glide designs include a 1-in (2.54 cm) diameter "disk" with a central stem that slides into the tubular leg and is tightened into place with a screwdriver, and a fitted cap that is placed directly onto the walker leg (in the same manner the rubber tip is attached). Another style of glide incorporates a tennis ball within a fixed housing (Fig. 11A.18).

Folding Mechanism

Folding walkers are particularly useful for patients who travel. These walkers can be easily collapsed to fit in an automobile or other storage space (see Fig. 11A.17B).

Handgrips (Handles)

Enlarged and molded handgrips are available, and may be useful for some patients with arthritis. Some walkers

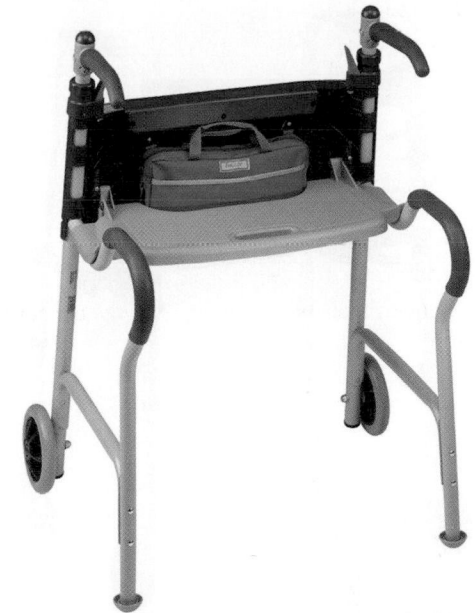

A

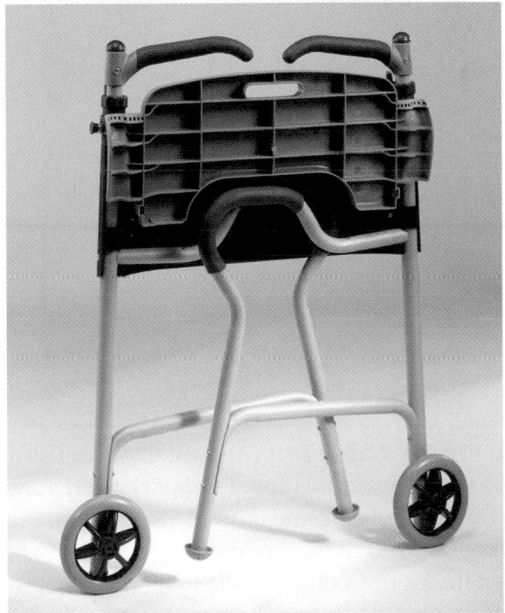

B

Figure 11A.17 Walker in **(A)** open and **(B)** folded position. The features on this walker include plastic posterior glides, a built-in seat with a molded back bar to support the user during rest intervals (the seat flips up for folding), large front wheels (6 in) to improve ease of use on multiple terrains, a second set of handles set at approximately the seat level to assist sit-to-stand transitions in the absence of chair armrests or for movement on and off a toilet, and a removable walker pouch for storing personal items. Handle height adjusts using a collar and pin mechanism that eliminates having to turn the walker over to change the height. *(Courtesy of Full Life Products, LLC, Moorestown, NJ 08057.)*

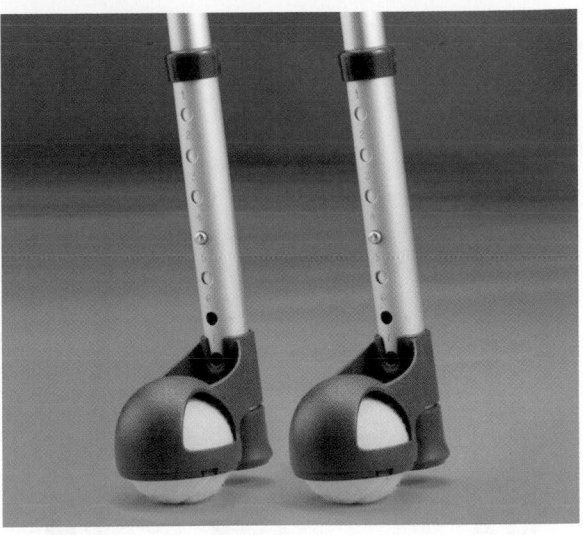

Figure 11A.18 The design of these walker glides incorporates a tennis ball within a fixed housing, a spring-loaded brake for intermittent braking during walking, and brake lock-out clips used to deactivate the braking feature for uninterrupted forward motion. The tennis ball can be manually rotated to unworn areas or completely removed to "snap in" a replacement. *(Courtesy of Invacare Corp, Elyria, OH 44036.)*

offer a second set of handles to assist with sit-to-stand transitions (see Fig 11A.17A).

Platform Attachments

This adaptation is used when weight-bearing is contraindicated through the wrist and hand (described in crutch section; see Figure 11A.12).

Wheel Attachments

This adaptation to walkers (often called *rolling* walkers) includes the addition of wheels (either to the two front wheels only or to all four wheels). The addition of wheels frequently allows functional ambulation for patients who are unable to lift and to move a conventional walker (e.g., frail elderly). *Swivel wheels* turn freely in a complete circle (Fig. 11A.19). *Fixed wheels* rotate around a central axis (Fig. 11A.20A). Wheels are generally available in 3-, 5-, and 6-in (7.62-, 12.7-, 15.24-cm) diameters. Eight-inch-diameter (20.32 cm) wheels are also available and can be used to add height for tall users.

Braking Mechanism

A braking system is an essential feature of walkers designed with wheels. Walkers with four wheels frequently include handbrakes that lock the rear wheels (see Fig. 11A.19). *Spring-loaded locks* can be placed on the rear walker wheels (Fig. 11A.20A). These locks engage when weight is placed on the posterior walker legs through the handgrips. Posterior pressure brakes are effective when wheels are placed only on the front walker legs.

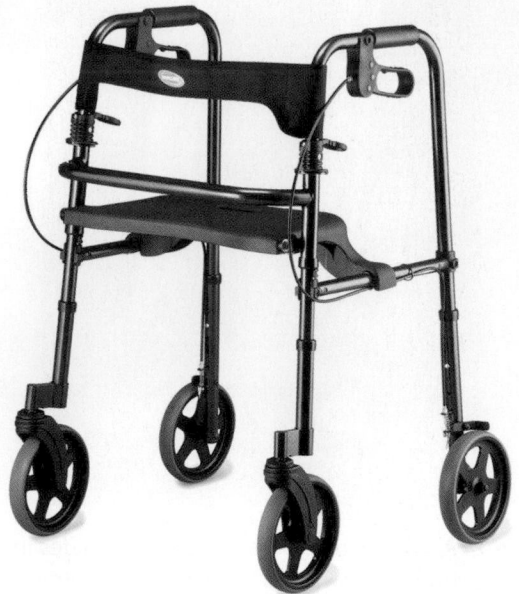

Figure 11A.19 The front wheels of this walker swivel freely in all directions. The back wheels rotate around a single axis. Handbrakes allow locking the rear wheels. A seat surface accommodates rest intervals. *(Courtesy of Invacare Corp, Elyria, OH 44036.)*

Tripod Rolling Walkers

Three-wheel walkers incorporate a tripod design (Fig 11A.21); some manufacturers refer to these as *rollators*. A major advantage of this device is ease of maneuverability and turning. Height adjustments are made at the handles; the unit folds for storage and travel.

Storage Attachments

The ability to transport items is an important consideration for many patients and is often essential for those needing frequent access to medications, a cordless or cellular phone, or remote control device. A variety of sizes and styles of attachable baskets and pouches are available (Fig. 11A.22). These storage attachments should be used judiciously and only for essential items. Overuse of the attachment creates an excessive anterior load that may pose a safety hazard and/or alter the patient's gait or ability to effectively use the walker.

Seating Surface

A variety of walker seat designs are available that fold out of the way when not in use. The structural design of many walkers also includes a contoured back support (see Figs 11A.19 and Fig 11A.20A). Seats are an important consideration for individuals with limited endurance (e.g., postpolio syndrome), as well as for community ambulators who require periodic rest intervals. Walker seats should be carefully examined for stability and safety with respect to individual patient needs. Patient practice in use of the walker seat should be provided.

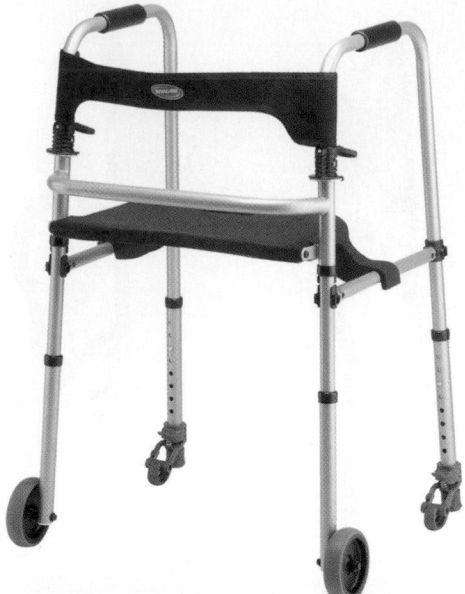

A

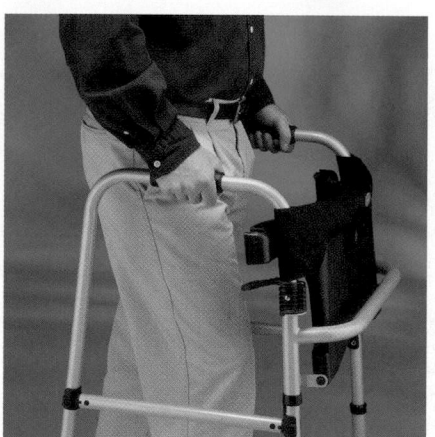

B

Figure 11A.20 Walker seat **(A)** positioned for use and **(B)** flipped up for ambulation. The 5-inch fixed front wheels of this walker rotate around a single axis. Features of this walker include rear spring-loaded brakes, a flexible backrest for sitting, a dual-paddle folding mechanism, and adjustable seat-to-floor height. *(Courtesy of Invacare Corp, Elyria, OH 44036.)*

Reciprocal Walkers

These walkers are designed to allow unilateral forward progression of one side of the walker (Fig. 11A.23). A disadvantage of this design is that some inherent stability of the walker is lost. However, they are useful for patients incapable of lifting the walker with both hands and moving it forward (in situations in which a rolling walker might be contraindicated).

- *Advantages.* Conventional walkers provide four points of floor contact with a wide BOS. They provide a high level of stability. They also provide a sense of security for patients fearful of ambulation. They are relatively lightweight and easily adjusted.
- *Disadvantages.* Walkers tend to be cumbersome, are awkward in confined areas, and are difficult to

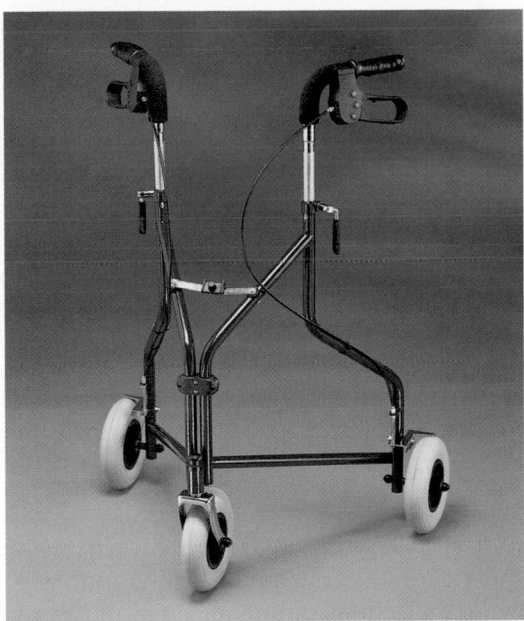

Figure 11A.21 Three-wheel walker with handbrakes and polyurethane tires to improve performance on a variety of terrains. *(Courtesy of Invacare Corp, Elyria, OH 44036.)*

maneuver through doorways and into cars. They eliminate normal arm swing and generally cannot be used safely on stairs.

Measuring Walkers

The height of a walker is measured in the same way as that of a cane. The handgrip or handle of the walker should come to approximately the greater trochanter and allow for 20 to 30 degrees of elbow flexion.

Gait Patterns: Conventional Walkers

Before initiating instruction in gait patterns using a conventional walker (four points of floor contact without wheel attachments), several points related to use of the walker should be emphasized with the patient:

- The walker should be picked up and placed down on all four legs simultaneously to achieve maximum stability. Rocking from the back to front legs should be avoided because it decreases the effectiveness and safety of using the assistive device.
- The patient should be encouraged to hold the head up and to maintain good postural alignment; forward flexion of the trunk, neck, and head should be avoided.
- The patient should be cautioned not to step too close to the front crossbar. This will decrease the overall BOS and may result in a fall.

Three types of weight-bearing gait patterns can be accomplished with conventional walkers: full weight-bearing (FWB), partial weight-bearing (PWB), and non–weight-bearing (NWB) gait (rolling devices are generally not recommended for patients with altered

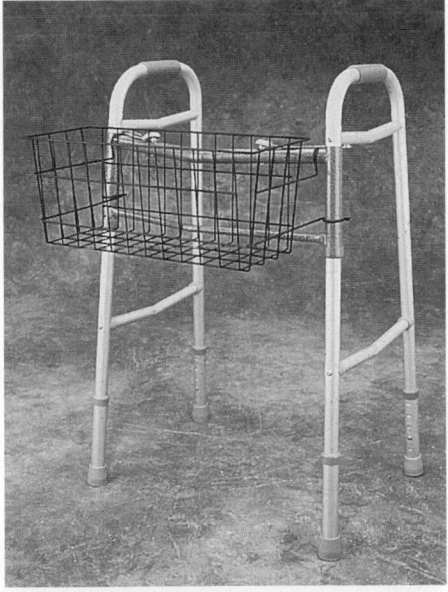

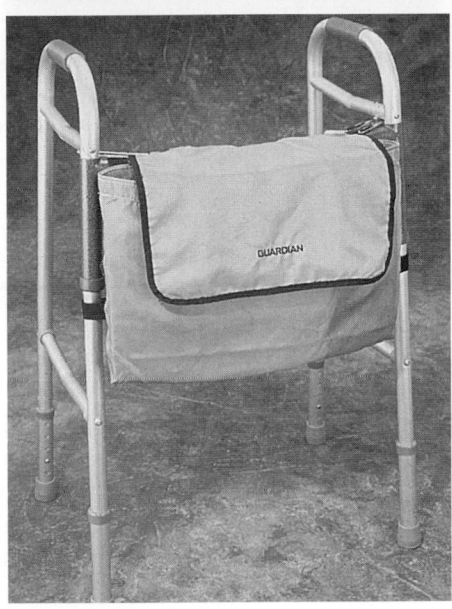

Figure 11A.22 Walker basket *(top)* and walker pouch *(bottom). (Courtesy of Sunrise Medical, Longmont, CO 80503.)*

weight-bearing status). The sequence for each pattern with a walker follows.

Full Weight-Bearing

- The walker is picked up and moved forward about an arm's length.
- The first LE is moved forward.
- The second LE is moved forward past the first.
- The cycle is repeated.

Partial Weight-Bearing

- The walker is picked up and moved forward about an arm's length.
- The involved PWB limb is moved forward, and body weight is transferred partially onto this limb and partially through the UEs to the walker.

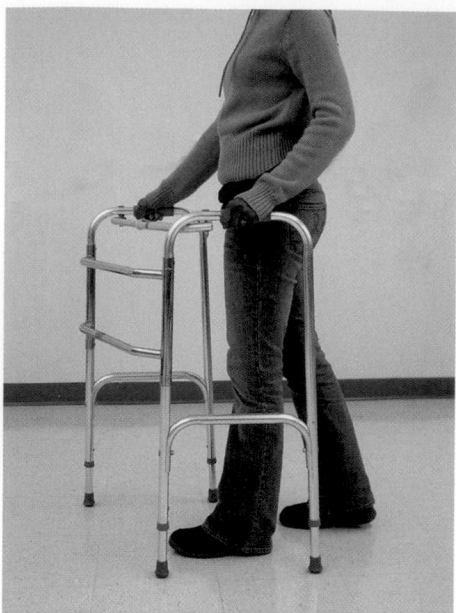

Figure 11A.23 Reciprocal walkers allow unilateral movement of one side of the walker while the opposite side remains stationary.

- The uninvolved LE is moved forward past the involved limb.
- The cycle is repeated.

Non–Weight-Bearing

- The walker is picked up and moved forward about an arm's length.
- Weight is then transferred through the UEs to the walker. The involved NWB limb is held anterior to the patient's body but does not make contact with the floor.
- The uninvolved limb is moved forward.
- The cycle is repeated.

Note: Rolling walkers generally allow use of a reciprocal gait pattern because the walker can be rolled forward while walking. As the need to lift the walker forward following each step is eliminated, a smoother forward progression can be achieved.

■ LOCOMOTOR TRAINING USING ASSISTIVE DEVICES

Overground Indoors

Several important preparatory activities should precede locomotor training (LT) on level surfaces with the assistive device. These activities may be completed in the parallel bars for added security. However, if the width of the bars is not adjustable, the BOS of the assistive device may make movement within the bars difficult and unsafe. An alternative is to move the patient outside but next to the parallel bars (or oval bar)

or near a treatment table or wall. These preparatory activities include the following:

1. **Instruction in assuming the standing and seated positions with use of the assistive device. These techniques are outlined in Box 11A.4 for each category of assistive device.**

2. **Standing balance activities with the assistive device (similar to those using the parallel bars, described earlier).**

3. **Instruction in use of assistive device (with selected gait pattern) for forward progression and turning.**

As mentioned, demonstrating these activities by assuming the role of the patient during verbal explanations is an effective teaching approach. Following the demonstration, manual contacts, verbal cueing, and explanations can be used again to guide performance of the activity. Following these preliminary instructions gait training using the assistive device can be begun overground on level surfaces. The following guarding technique (Fig. 11A.24) should be used:

1. **The therapist stands posterior and lateral to the patient's weaker side.**

2. **A wide BOS should be maintained with the therapist's leading LE following the assistive device. The therapist's opposite LE should be externally rotated and follow the patient's weaker LE.**

3. **One of the therapist's hands is placed posteriorly on the guarding belt and the other anterior to, but *not touching*, the patient's shoulder on the weaker side.**

Should the patient's balance be lost during training, the hand guarding at the shoulder should make contact. Frequently, the support provided by the therapist's hands at the shoulder and on the guarding belt would be enough to allow the patient to regain balance. If the balance loss is severe, the therapist should move in toward the patient so that the therapist's body and guarding hands can be used to provide stabilization. The patient should be allowed to regain balance while "leaning" against the therapist. If balance is not recovered and it is apparent the patient must be moved to the floor, further attempts should not be made to hold the patient up because this is likely to result in injury to the patient and/or the therapist. In this situation, the therapist should continue to brace the patient against his or her body to break the fall and to protect the head and move with the patient to a sitting position on the floor. It is also important to talk to the patient (*"Help me lower you to the floor"*) so

Box 11A.4   Assuming Standing and Seated Positions With Assistive Devices

I. Cane

A. *Coming to standing*
• Patient moves forward in chair.
• Cane is positioned on uninvolved side (broad-based cane) or leaned against armrest (standard cane).
• Patient leans forward and pushes down with both hands on armrests, comes to a standing position, and then grasps cane. With use of a standard cane, the cane may be grasped loosely with fingers before standing and the base of the hand used for pushing down on armrests.

B. *Return to sitting*
• As the patient approaches the chair, the patient turns in a small circle toward the uninvolved side.
• The patient backs up until the chair can be felt against the patient's legs.
• The patient then reaches for the armrest with the free hand, releases the cane (broad-based), and reaches for the opposite armrest. A standard cane is leaned against the chair as the patient grasps the armrest.

II. Crutches

A. *Coming to standing*
• The patient moves forward in the chair.
• Crutches are placed together in a vertical position on the affected side.
• One hand is placed on the hand pieces of the crutches; one on the armrest of the chair.
• The patient leans forward and pushes to a standing position.
• Once balance is gained, one crutch is cautiously placed under the axilla on the unaffected side.
• The second crutch is then carefully placed under the axilla on the affected side.
• A tripod stance is assumed.

B. *Return to sitting*
• As the patient approaches the chair, the patient turns in a small circle toward the uninvolved side.
• The patient backs up until the chair can be felt against the patient's legs.
• Both crutches are placed in a vertical position (out from under axilla) on the *affected* side.
• One hand is placed on the hand pieces of the crutches; one on the armrest of the chair.
• The patient lowers to the chair in a controlled manner.

III. Walker

A. *Coming to standing*
• The patient moves forward in the chair.
• The walker is positioned directly in front of the chair.
• The patient leans forward and pushes down on armrests to come to standing.
• Once in a standing position, the patient reaches for the walker, one hand at a time.

B. *Return to sitting*
• As the patient approaches the chair, the patient turns in a small circle toward the stronger side.
• The patient backs up until the chair can be felt against the patient's legs.
• The patient then reaches for one armrest at a time.
• The patient lowers to the chair in a controlled manner.

---

that the patient does not continue to struggle to regain balance.

Overground indoor activities on level surfaces should include instruction and practice in passage through doorways, elevators, and over thresholds. When using crutches, doorways are most easily approached from a diagonal. A hand must be freed to open the door and one crutch must be placed in a position to hold it open. The patient then gradually proceeds through the doorway, using the crutch to open the door wider if necessary.

Because many patients using a walker or cane may have balance problems, careful examination will determine the safest methods for passage through doorways. A patient using a conventional walker with sufficient balance may be able to use a technique similar to that described above.

Stair Climbing

Several general guidelines should be relayed to the patient during instruction in stair climbing. First, if a railing is available it should always be used. This is true even if it requires placing an assistive device in the hand in which it is not normally used. For stair climbing with axillary crutches using a railing, both crutches are placed together under one arm. Second, the patient should be cautioned that the stronger LE always leads going up the stairs, and the weaker or involved limb always leads coming down (*"up with the good and down with the bad"*).

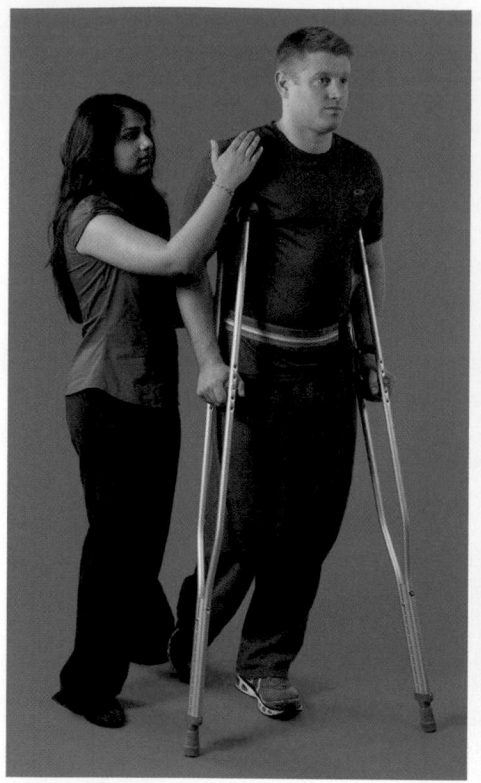 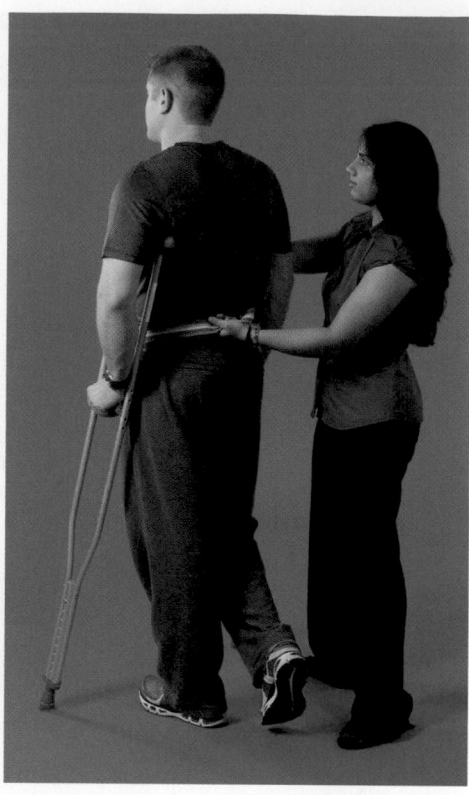

Figure 11A.24 Anterior (*left*) and posterior (*right*) views of guarding technique for level surfaces, demonstrated with use of crutches. The same positioning is used with canes and walkers.

Stair climbing techniques are presented in Box 11A.5. The therapist should use the following guarding technique during stair climbing.

Ascending Stairs (Fig. 11A.25)

1. **The therapist is positioned posterior and lateral on the affected side behind the patient.**

2. **A wide BOS should be maintained with each foot on a different stair.**

3. **A step should be taken only when the patient is not moving.**

4. **One hand is placed posteriorly on the guarding belt and one is anterior to, but not touching, the shoulder on the weaker side.**

Descending Stairs (Fig. 11A.26)

1. **The therapist is positioned anterior and lateral on the affected side in front of the patient.**

2. **A wide BOS should be maintained with each foot on a different stair.**

3. **A step should be taken only when the patient is not moving.**

4. **One hand is placed anteriorly on the guarding belt and one is anterior to, but not touching, the shoulder on the weaker side.**

Should the patient's balance be lost during stair climbing, the following procedure should be followed. First, contact should be made with the hand guarding at the shoulder. Next, the therapist should move toward the patient to help brace the patient (the patient should never be pulled toward the therapist on stairs) or leaned toward the wall of the stairwell (if available). Finally, if needed, the therapist can move with the patient to sit the patient down on the stairs. Remember to inform the patient of your intentions ("*I'm going to sit you down*").

Locomotor training using assistive devices should also include outdoor training and practice with curb climbing, negotiating ramps, and sloped surfaces; even and uneven terrains; walking with imposed time requirements (e.g., crossing street at a stoplight); walking for long distances, dual-task training while walking, walking at various speeds, and negotiating open community environments with distractors, as well as outside doors and thresholds; and transportation vehicles.

Adjunct Training Devices
Limb Load Monitors

A limb load monitor is a form of biofeedback used clinically as an adjunct intervention during gait training. The limb load monitor incorporates a strain gauge attached to the sole or heel of the shoe. When a force or pressure is applied, the strain gauge is deformed and an auditory signal provides feedback to the wearer. As pressure increases, the signal becomes louder or more rapid. This feedback provides information about the

Box 11A.5 Stair-Climbing Techniques*

I. Cane

A. *Ascending*

1. The unaffected lower extremity leads up.
2. The cane and affected lower extremity follow.

B. *Descending*

1. The affected lower extremity and cane lead down.
2. The unaffected lower extremity follows.

II. Crutches: Three-Point Gait (non–weight-bearing gait)

A. *Ascending*

1. The patient is positioned close to the foot of the stairs. The involved lower extremity is held back to prevent "catching" on the lip of the stairs.
2. The patient pushes down firmly on both hand pieces of the crutches and leads up with the unaffected lower extremity.
3. The crutches are brought up to the stair that the unaffected lower extremity is now on.

B. *Descending*

1. The patient stands close to the edge of the stair so that the toes of the unaffected lower extremity protrude slightly over the top. The involved lower extremity is held forward over the lower stair.
2. Both crutches are moved down *together* to the *front* half of the next step.
3. The patient pushes down firmly on both hand pieces and lowers the unaffected lower extremity to the step that the crutches are now on.

III. Crutches: Partial Weight-Bearing Gait

A. *Ascending*

1. The patient is positioned close to the foot of the stairs.
2. The patient pushes down on both hand pieces of the crutches and distributes weight partially on the crutches and partially on the affected lower extremity while the unaffected lower extremity leads up.
3. The involved lower extremity and crutches are then brought up together.

B. *Descending*

1. The patient stands close to the edge of the stair so that the toes protrude slightly over top of the stair.
2. Both crutches are moved down *together* to the *front* half of the next step. The affected lower extremity is then lowered (depending on patient skill, these may be combined). *Note:* When crutches are not in floor contact, greater weight must be shifted to the uninvolved lower extremity to maintain a partial weight-bearing status.
3. The uninvolved lower extremity is lowered to the step the crutches are now on.

IV. Crutches: Two- and Four-Point Gait

A. *Ascending*

1. The patient is positioned close to the foot of the stairs.
2. The right lower extremity is moved up and then the left lower extremity.
3. The right crutch is moved up and then the left crutch is moved up (patients with adequate balance may find it easier to move the crutches up together).

B. *Descending*

1. The patient stands close to the edge of the stair.
2. Both crutches are moved down together. Alternatively, the right crutch is moved down and then the left. This pattern must be used with caution as crutch placement on two different steps can introduce excessive and unwanted trunk rotation.
3. The right lower extremity is moved down and then the left.

*The sequences presented here describe stair-climbing techniques without the use of a railing. When a secure railing is available, the patient should be instructed to use it always.

amount of weight-bearing on a limb. Limb load monitors can also be used to reinforce the correctness or timing of a movement. For example, an audible noise or buzzer sounding when the heel makes contact with the floor can provide immediate feedback on foot placement. Similar devices can also be attached to a cane (often referred to as a ***biofeedback cane***). The principle of operation is the same and incorporates a strain gauge. Auditory signals provide the patient with information on placement, as well as pressure applied to the cane.

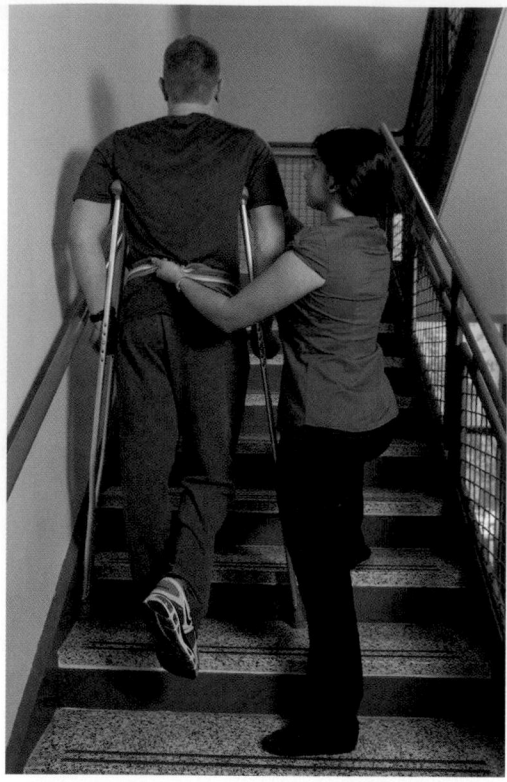

Figure 11A.25 Guarding technique for ascending stairs.

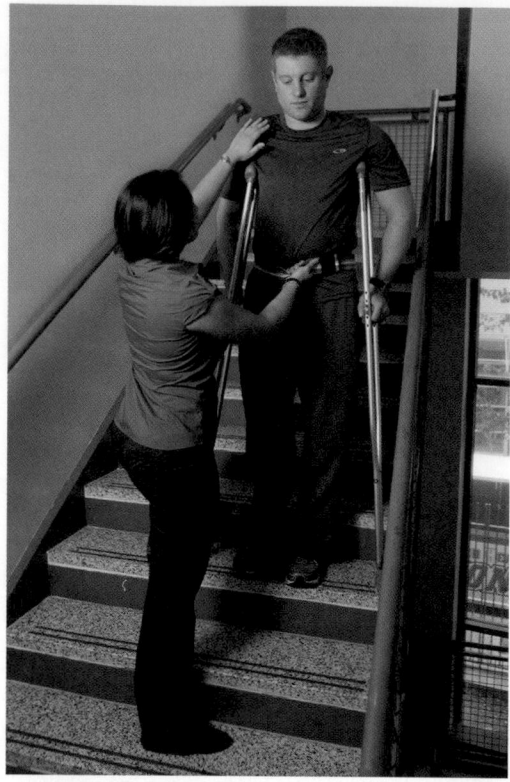

Figure 11A.26 Guarding technique for descending stairs.

References

1. Bohannon, RW: Use of a standard cane increases unipedal stance time during static testing. Percept Mot Skills 112(3): 726, 2011.
2. Hsue, B, and Su, F: The effect of cane use method on center of mass displacement during stair ascent. Gait Posture 32(4):530, 2010.
3. Milczarek, JJ, et al: Standard and four-footed canes: Their effect on the standing balance of patients with hemiparesis. Arch Phys Med Rehabil 74(3):281, 1993.
4. Maguire, C, et al: Hip abductor control in walking following stroke—the immediate effect of canes, taping and TheraTogs on gait. Clin Rehabil 24(1):37, 2010.
5. Laufer, Y: Effects of one-point and four-point canes on balance and weight distribution in patients with hemiparesis. Clin Rehabil 16(2):141, 2002.
6. Laufer, Y: The effect of walking aids on balance and weight bearing patterns of patients with hemiparesis in various stance positions. Phys Ther 83(2):112, 2003.
7. Jones, A, et al: Impact of cane use on pain, function, general health and energy expenditure during gait in patients with knee osteoarthritis: A randomised controlled trial. Ann Rheum Dis 71(2):172, 2012.
8. Neumann, DA: Hip abductor muscle activity as subjects with hip prostheses walk with different methods of using a cane. Phys Ther 78(5):490, 1998.
9. Buurke, JH, et al: The effect of walking aids on muscle activation patterns during walking in stroke patients. Gait Posture 22:164, 2005.
10. Neumann, DA: An electromyographic study of the hip abductor muscles as subjects with a hip prosthesis walked with different methods of using a cane and carrying a load. Phys Ther 79(12):1163, 1999.
11. Ely, DD, and Smidt, GL: Effect of cane on variables of gait for patients with hip disorders. Phys Ther 57(5):507, 1977.
12. Jones, A, et al: Evaluation of immediate impact of cane use on energy expenditure during gait in patients with knee osteoarthritis. Gait Posture 35(3):435, 2012.
13. Beauchamp, MK, et al: Immediate effects of cane use on gait symmetry in individuals with subacute stroke. Physiother Can 61(3):154, 2009.
14. Nolen, J, et al: Comparison of gait characteristics with a single-tip cane, tripod cane, and quad cane. Phys Occup Ther Geriatr 28(4):387, 2010.
15. Donovan, S, et al: Laserlight cues for gait freezing in Parkinson's disease: An open-label study. Parkinsonism Relat Disord 17(4):240, 2011.
16. Giladi, N, et al: Validation of the freezing of gait questionnaire in patients with Parkinson's disease. Mov Disord 24(5):655, 2009.
17. Giladi, N, et al: Construction of freezing of gait questionnaire for patients with parkinsonism. Parkinsonism Relat Disord 6(3):165, 2000.

Chronic Pulmonary Dysfunction

Julie Ann Starr, PT, DPT, CCS

Chapter 12

LEARNING OBJECTIVES

1. Define the disease processes (including definition, etiology, pathophysiology, clinical presentation, and clinical course) of chronic obstructive pulmonary disease, asthma, cystic fibrosis, and restrictive lung disease.

2. Describe examination procedures (including patient interview, vital signs, observation, inspection, palpation, auscultation, and laboratory tests) for a patient with pulmonary disease.

3. Identify the anticipated goals and expected outcomes of pulmonary rehabilitation.

4. Describe the rehabilitative management of a patient with chronic pulmonary dysfunction.

5. Value the therapist's role in the management of a patient with chronic pulmonary dysfunction.

6. Analyze and interpret patient data, formulate realistic goals and outcomes, and develop a plan of care when presented with a clinical case study.

Pulmonary rehabilitation is a multidisciplinary comprehensive program of care for patients with chronic respiratory disease that is designed to reduce symptoms, optimize physical functioning and social participation, and reduce health care costs.[1] A diversity of health professionals is essential to meet the medical, physical, social, and psychological needs of the patient with pulmonary disease. The team may include a nurse, physician, physical therapist, occupational therapist, nutritionist, pharmacist, respiratory care practitioner, exercise physiologist, psychologist, and, most important, the patient and the patient's family and caregivers.

Years ago, patients with chronic pulmonary disease were given a standard prescription for rest and avoidance of exercise.[2] The stress imposed by exercise was considered deleterious to people with pulmonary disorders. A pivotal study by Pierce et al[3] provided the impetus to change direction in the treatment of pulmonary dysfunction. Exercise training effects of decreased heart rate (HR), respiratory rate, minute ventilation, oxygen consumption, and carbon dioxide production at submaximal exercise levels were documented in their subjects with chronic obstructive pulmonary disease (COPD). Increased maximal aerobic capacity was also documented.[3] Reconditioning of patients with pulmonary disease was found to be possible.

COPD, asthma, and cystic fibrosis are the most common chronic obstructive lung diseases for which pulmonary rehabilitation is rendered. Patients with a restrictive lung disease, such as idiopathic pulmonary fibrosis, have also demonstrated improvement in functional abilities following pulmonary rehabilitation.[4] It is clear that pulmonary rehabilitation is of value for all patients in whom respiratory symptoms have resulted in a decreased functional capacity or a decreased quality of life.[1]

In this chapter, the most common chronic pulmonary diseases that present to pulmonary rehabilitation programs will be discussed, as well as the physical therapy examination and treatment of patients with chronic pulmonary disease. A brief review of ventilation and respiration is warranted for a better understanding of the disease pathologies and for understanding the rationale of the physical therapy procedures.

■ RESPIRATORY PHYSIOLOGY

Air is inspired through the nose or mouth, through all of the conducting airways until it reaches the distal respiratory unit, which contains the respiratory bronchiole, alveolar ducts, alveolar sacs, and alveoli (Fig. 12.1). The movement of air through the conducting airways is termed **ventilation.** At full inspiration, the lungs contain their maximum amount of air. This volume of air is called **total lung capacity (TLC),** which can be divided into four separate volumes of air: (1) tidal volume, (2) inspiratory reserve volume, (3) expiratory reserve volume, and (4) residual volume. Combinations of two or more of these lung volumes are termed *capacities.* Figure 12.2 illustrates the relationship of lung volumes and capacities.

The amount of air inspired or expired during normal resting ventilation is termed **tidal volume (TV or V_t).** As this tidal volume of air enters the respiratory system, it travels through the conducting airways to reach the respiratory units. Tidal volume is about 500 mL/breath for a young, healthy, white male. The amount of inspired air that actually reaches the distal respiratory unit and takes part in gas exchange is about 350 mL of that 500 mL total of the tidal breath. The remaining 150 mL of the inhaled tidal breath remains in the conducting airways and does not take part in gas exchange. When

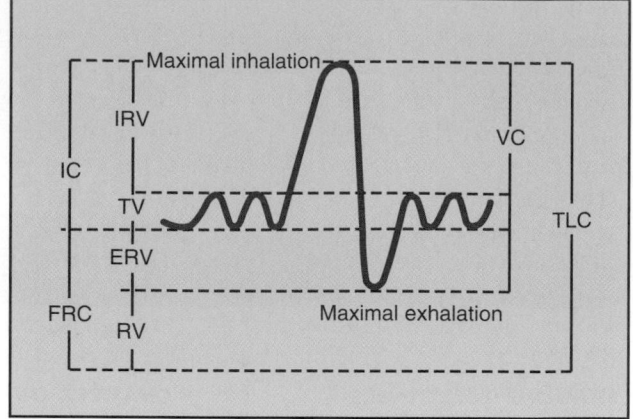

Figure 12.2 Lung volumes and capacities. ERV = expiratory reserve volume; FRC = functional residual capacity; IC = inspiratory capacity; IRV = inspiratory reserve volume; RV = residual volume; TLC = total lung capacity; TV = tidal volume; VC = vital capacity.

only a tidal breath occupies the lungs, there is "room" for additional air that can be further inhaled. This inspiratory volume in excess of that used in tidal breathing is the **inspiratory reserve volume (IRV).** Aptly named, it is the volume of air that can be inspired when needed, but is usually kept in reserve. There is a quantity of air that can potentially be exhaled beyond the end of a tidal exhalation. Although it is usually kept in reserve, the volume of air that can be exhaled in excess of tidal breathing is called the **expiratory reserve volume (ERV).** The lungs are never completely emptied of air even after maximally exhaling the expiratory reserve volume. The volume of air remaining within the lungs when ERV has been exhaled is called the **residual volume (RV).**

The sum of two or more volumes is referred to as a *capacity.* Tidal volume plus the inspiratory reserve volume is known as the **inspiratory capacity (IC).** This refers to the volume of air that can be inspired beginning from a tidal exhalation. The combination of residual volume and expiratory reserve volume is the **functional residual capacity (FRC).** Functional residual capacity is the volume of air that remains in the lungs at the end of a tidal exhalation. The sum of inspiratory reserve volume, tidal volume, and expiratory reserve volume is called the **vital capacity (VC).** It is all of the possible volume of air within the lungs that is under volitional control. The common method of measuring VC is to achieve maximal inspiration, then forcibly exhale as hard and fast as possible into a measuring device until ERV has been exhausted. Because this is a forced expiratory maneuver, it is termed the *forced vital capacity (FVC).* As stated earlier, all volumes together equal total lung capacity:

$$TV + IRV + ERV + RV = TLC.$$

Flow rates measure the volume of air moved in a period of time. Expiratory flow rates, therefore, are

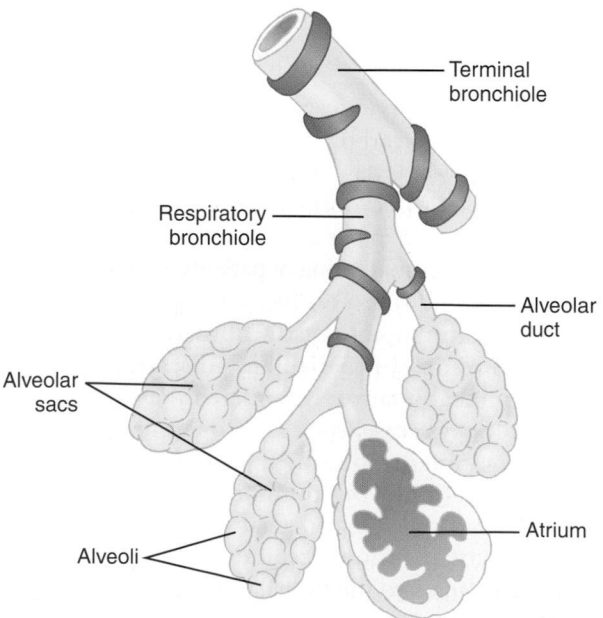

Figure 12.1 Anatomy of the distal conducting airway, the terminal bronchiole and the respiratory unit, the respiratory bronchiole, alveolar ducts, alveolar sacs, and alveoli.

measurements of exhaled gas volume divided by the amount of time required for the volume to be exhaled. Flow rates reflect the ease with which the lungs can be ventilated, the state of the airways, and the elasticity of the lung parenchyma (tissue). An important airflow measurement is the volume of air that can be forcefully exhaled during the first second of a forced vital capacity maneuver. This is called the *forced expiratory volume in 1 second (FEV₁)*. This flow rate is thought to reflect the status of the airways of the lungs. In healthy individuals, FEV_1 is 70% or more of the total FVC (FEV_1/FVC > 70%).[5] *Peak expiratory flow rate (PEF)* is the greatest flow rate generated during a maximal forced expiratory maneuver. Individuals with lung disease often measure PEF on a daily basis with a handheld peak flow meter to track their pulmonary status. Daily peak flow rates are compared to the patient's own "best" test value.[6] A drop in a patient's peak flow rate indicates airway narrowing and may indicate the need for a physician visit and/or change in medication regimen.

Inspiratory mechanics can be helpful in understanding a patient's pulmonary disease. *Maximum inspiratory pressure* (PI_{max}) reflects the greatest static inspiratory effort that can be generated from residual volume. It is measured as a pressure in millimeters of mercury or cubic centimeters of water and reflects the strength of the muscles of inspiration. *Maximal sustained inspiratory pressure* (SIP_{max}) is a test of inspiratory muscle endurance. The patient is initially challenged with –6 cm H_2O pressure resistance. Gradually the resistance is increased –2 cm H_2O every 2 minutes until the patient can no longer achieve adequate ventilatory flow levels.[7] The maximal pressure is defined as the highest level that the patient could tolerate during the testing procedure.

Lung volumes, capacities, flow rates, and mechanics depend on the size and configuration of the thorax. Therefore, height, gender, and race influence static and dynamic lung measurements. Any alteration in the properties of the lungs or chest wall due to the aging process or a disease process will also change the lung volumes, capacities, flow rates, and/or mechanics.

Respiration is a term used to describe the gas exchange within the body. This should not be confused with *ventilation,* which describes only the movement of air. External respiration is the exchange of gas that occurs at the alveolar capillary membrane between atmospheric air and the pulmonary capillaries. Internal respiration takes place at the tissue capillary level between the tissues and the surrounding capillaries. The following discussion traces the course of gas exchange, specifically that of oxygen and carbon dioxide, during both external and internal respiration (Fig. 12.3).

For external respiration to take place, there must first be an inhalation of air from the environment, through the conducting airways, and into the respiratory bronchioles and alveoli. Oxygen diffuses through the walls of the respiratory unit, through the interstitial space, and through the pulmonary capillary wall. Most of the oxygen (98.5%) then travels through the blood plasma into red blood cells where it occupies one of the gas-carrying sites of hemoglobin. A small portion of dissolved oxygen (1.5%) is carried in the plasma.

The now oxygenated blood in the pulmonary capillaries travels to the left side of the heart via the pulmonary veins. From there it is pumped into the aorta, and then through a network of connecting arteries, arterioles, and capillaries, until its destination, the tissue, is reached. Internal respiration begins when the arterial blood reaches the tissue level. Oxygen diffuses from the gas-carrying sites of hemoglobin, out of the red blood cell, out of the capillary, through the cell membranes, and into the mitochondria of the working cells.

Carbon dioxide (CO_2), which is produced at the tissue level as a by-product of metabolism, diffuses out of the working cells into the capillaries. Carbon dioxide is transported in the blood through the venous system into the right side of the heart. Once the carbon dioxide–ladened blood makes its way through the right atrium, the right ventricle, the pulmonary artery, and the pulmonary capillaries, it diffuses out through the capillary membrane, through the interstitial space, and into the alveoli, where it is finally exhaled into the atmosphere.

When the cycle of external and internal respiration has occurred, oxygen has been extracted from the environment and provided to the body tissues. Meanwhile, carbon dioxide has been removed from the body tissues and released into the external environment. Of course, this system is dependent on an intact cardiovascular system to pump the blood through the lungs and through the heart, deliver it to the working cells, and then return it back to the lungs, all in a timely fashion.

CHRONIC LUNG DISEASES
Chronic Obstructive Pulmonary Disease

Chronic obstructive pulmonary disease (COPD) is the most common chronic pulmonary disorder. It is the fourth-leading cause of morbidity and mortality in the United States.[5]

The Global Initiative for Chronic Obstructive Lung Disease (GOLD) is an ongoing collaborative work of the National Heart, Lung, and Blood Institute (NHLBI) and the World Health Organization (WHO). Initially begun in 2001, GOLD set out to increase worldwide awareness of COPD, to advocate for its prevention as well as to decrease morbidity and mortality from the disease. According to GOLD, COPD is defined as a preventable and treatable disease. The pulmonary component of COPD is characterized by airflow limitation that is not fully reversible. The airflow limitation is usually progressive and associated with an abnormal inflammatory response of the lung to noxious particles or gases. Additional significant extra pulmonary effects, such as a decrease in body mass index (BMI) and exercise

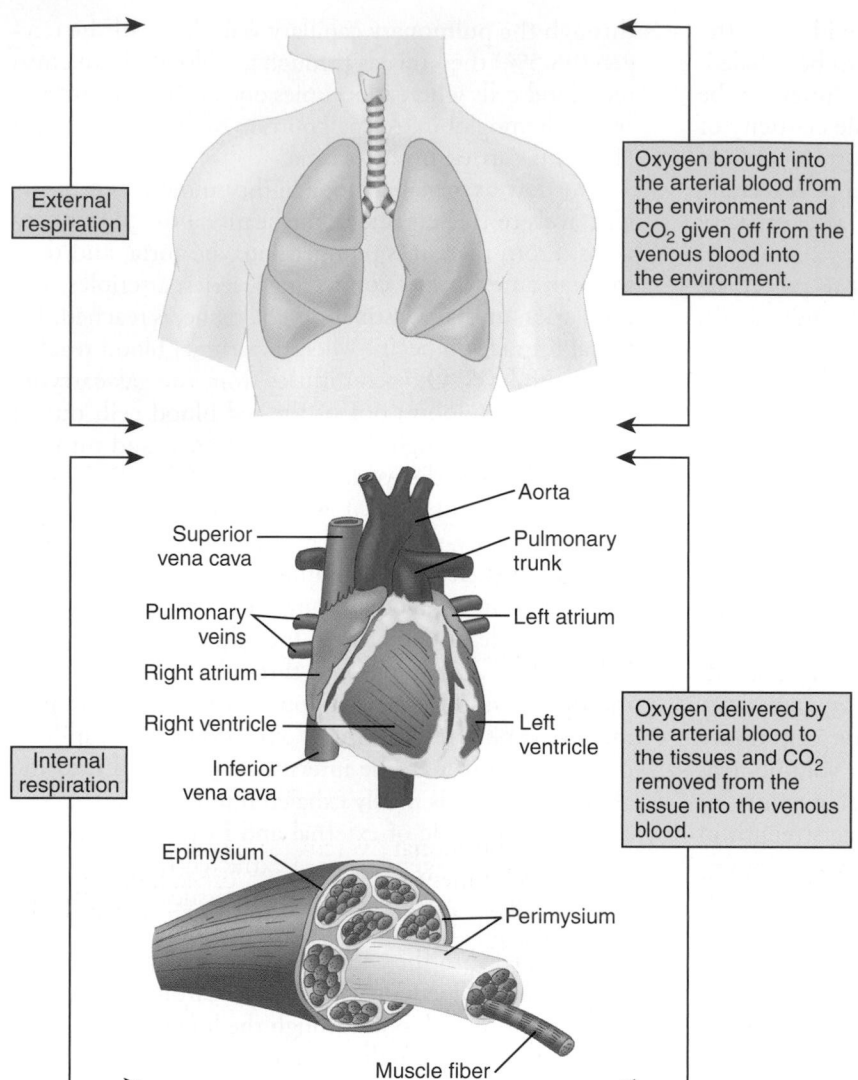

External respiration

Oxygen brought into the arterial blood from the environment and CO_2 given off from the venous blood into the environment.

Aorta

Superior vena cava

Pulmonary trunk

Pulmonary veins

Left atrium

Right atrium

Right ventricle

Left ventricle

Inferior vena cava

Internal respiration

Oxygen delivered by the arterial blood to the tissues and CO_2 removed from the tissue into the venous blood.

Epimysium

Perimysium

Muscle fiber

Figure 12.3 The process of external and internal respiration.

tolerance, contribute to the severity of COPD in individual patients.[5] Classification of disease severity is based on both clinical symptoms and measurements of airflow limitation. Table 12.1 shows the GOLD COPD classification of disease severity based on a patient's altered FEV_1 and presenting symptoms.

Risk Factors

Risk factors for the development of COPD include both environmental factors and host factors. Cigarette smoking is the major environmental causal agent in the development of COPD.[5] Smoking history is quantified in units of *pack/years,* the number of packs per day times the number of years smoked. Other environmental factors that contribute to the development of COPD include occupational exposures (e.g., organic and inorganic dusts), indoor pollutants (e.g., secondhand smoke), and outdoor pollutants (e.g., urban pollution).[5]

Host factors that would make a person more susceptible to the development of COPD include hyperreactivity of the airways, overall lung growth (the amount of lung tissue developed during childhood, which is

dependent on the person's nutritional status, health status, height, exposure to pollutants, and so forth), and genetics. One genetic cause of COPD is an alpha-1 antitrypsin deficiency.[8] It is perplexing that not all smokers go on to develop clinically significant COPD. The COPDGene® Study is investigating the potential for a genetic influence that would help explain the development of COPD in only a portion of smokers while others, who may exhibit similar airway inflammation from cigarette smoke, do not develop the disease.[9] At this point, it would appear that the development of COPD results from a combination of both host and environmental factors.

Pathophysiology

COPD is a combination of chronic airway inflammation and remodeling (reorganization of tissue during healing) that results in airway narrowing, parenchymal destruction, and pulmonary vascular thickening. Chronic inflammation, characterized by an increase in neutrophils, macrophages, and T lymphocytes, damages the endothelial lining of the airways. Airway inflammation is made

Table 12.1 The Global Initiative for Chronic Obstructive Lung Disease (GOLD) Classification System for Severity of Chronic Obstructive Pulmonary Disease

Stage	Characteristics
I: Mild COPD	• $FEV_1/FVC < 70\%$ • $FEV_1 \geq 80\%$ predicted • With or without symptoms of cough and sputum production
II: Moderate COPD	• $FEV_1/FVC < 70\%$ • $50\% \leq FEV_1 < 80\%$ predicted • Shortness of breath with exertion • With or without symptoms of cough and sputum production
III: Severe COPD	• $FEV_1/FVC < 70\%$ • $30\% \leq FEV_1 < 50\%$ predicted • Greater shortness of breath with exercise, decreased exercise capacity, fatigue and repeated exacerbations of their disease
IV: Very Severe COPD	• $FEV_1/FVC < 70\%$ • $FEV_1 < 30\%$ predicted or $FEV_1 < 50\%$ predicted plus chronic respiratory failure

Classification based on postbronchodilator FEV_1.

FEV_1 = forced expiratory volume in 1 second; FVC = forced vital capacity; respiratory failure = arterial partial pressure of oxygen (PaO_2) < 8.0 kPa (60 mm Hg) with or without arterial partial pressure of CO_2 ($PaCO_2$) > 6.7 kPa (50 mm Hg) while breathing air at sea level.

Adapted with permission, NHLBI/WHO Global Initiative for Chronic Obstructive Lung Disease (GOLD) workshop summary, Update 2009, page 1.[5]

worse by an imbalance of proteases/antiproteases and oxidants/antioxidants in patients with COPD.[5] Airway damage results in airway repair, leading to airway remodeling. These airway changes appear to be most pronounced in the smaller peripheral airways (bronchioles).[5] The glands and goblet cells within the bronchial walls hypertrophy producing excessive secretions, which either partially or completely obstruct the airways. Decreases in ciliary function and alterations in physiochemical characteristics of bronchial secretions impair airway clearance and contribute to airway obstruction. Damaged and inflamed mucosa shows an increased sensitivity of irritant receptors within the bronchial walls, which in turn cause bronchial hyperreactivity.

During normal inspiration, the lungs and the airways are pulled open, increasing the diameter of the airway lumen. During normal exhalation, as the thorax returns to its resting position, the airways decrease in size. In COPD, during inspiration, the airways are pulled open wide by thoracic expansion, allowing air to enter. During exhalation, the airways, already narrowed by inflammation, remodeling, and excessive secretions, are prematurely closed, trapping air in the distal airways and airspaces. This air trapping causes **hyperinflation**, which is defined as an abnormal increase in the amount of air within the lung tissue at the end of a tidal exhalation (increased FRC).

The most common parenchymal changes found in COPD are dilation and destruction of the airspaces, which is thought to be due to an imbalance of proteases and antiproteases in the lung.[5] This change results in loss of the normal elastic recoil properties of the lung

tissue. The pulmonary vasculature is also altered early in the development of COPD. Endothelial changes result in thickening of the vessel walls. In advanced stages of the disease, there is destruction of the pulmonary capillary bed.[5]

Ventilation in the alveoli and **perfusion** in the capillary membrane are no longer matched. This results in **hypoxemia**, a condition in which a decreased amount of oxygen is carried by the arterial blood to the tissues. As the disease progresses and more areas of the lungs become involved, hypoxemia will worsen and **hypercapnea**, a condition in which there is an increased amount of carbon dioxide within the arterial blood, will develop. Increased pulmonary vascular resistance secondary to capillary wall damage and reflex vasoconstriction in the presence of hypoxemia results in right ventricular hypertrophy, termed **cor pulmonale**. **Polycythemia**, an increase in the amount of circulating red blood cells, is another complication of advanced COPD.

Clinical Presentation

Patients with COPD will usually present with a history of cigarette smoking and symptoms of chronic cough, expectoration, and exertional dyspnea. The intensity of each symptom varies from patient to patient. Cough and expectoration appear slowly and insidiously. Dyspnea is first evidenced during exertion. As the disease progresses, symptoms worsen. Dyspnea occurs at progressively lower activity levels. Severely involved patients may feel dyspneic even at rest. On physical examination, the thorax appears enlarged owing to loss of lung elastic recoil and hyperinflation. The anterior-posterior diameter of the chest increases and a dorsal kyphosis results. These anatomical changes give the patient a barrel-chest appearance (Fig. 12.4).

As the resting position of the thorax is now held in a more inspiratory mode, the available range of thoracic motion is limited, that is, decreased thoracic **excursion**. There are morphologic changes to the ventilatory muscles due to a greater demand, both in frequency and in power needed for this altered thorax. The muscles of ventilation hypertrophy as a result. Figure 12.5 shows many of the accessory muscles of ventilation that may be recruited for breathing. In severe disease, these muscles are recruited even at rest to aid in the work of breathing. The length–tension relationship of muscles of ventilation is altered as the thorax increases in size with chronic hyperinflation. There are changes in the alignment of fibers, especially the fibers of the diaphragm, with hyperinflation. The diaphragm becomes flatter, or less domed. In severe disease, the diaphragm fiber alignment may become more horizontal than vertical, resulting in an inward motion of the lower ribs during a diaphragm muscle contraction of inhalation (Fig. 12.6).

Breath sounds and heart sounds may be distant and difficult to hear. Partially obstructed bronchi and bronchioles may result in an expiratory **wheeze,** a musical, whistling sound. **Crackles,** an intermittent bubbling or popping sound, may also be present from secretions in the airways. Hypertrophy of accessory muscles of ventilation, pursed-lip breathing, **cyanosis**, and digital **clubbing** may all be present in the advanced stages of COPD. (See Examination in section titled Physical Therapy Management for clarification of terms.)

Significant and progressive airway limitation is reflected in altered pulmonary function tests. Lung volumes and capacities, especially RV and FRC, are increased from the normal value due to air trapping. Figure 12.7 shows the changes in lung volumes and capacities that occur in obstructive pulmonary disease.

Expiratory flow rates, especially FEV_1, are decreased. The ratio of FEV_1 to FVC is also decreased (less than 70%).[5] These changes in pulmonary function do not show a major reversibility in response to pharmacological agents.

Arterial blood gas analyses may reflect hypoxemia (decreased oxygen in the arterial blood) in the early stages of COPD. Hypercapnea (increased carbon dioxide in the arterial blood) appears as the disease progresses. With disease progression, chest radiographs show several characteristic findings. These include depressed and flattened hemidiaphragms; alteration in pulmonary vascular markings; hyperinflation of the thorax, evidenced by an increased anterior-posterior diameter of the chest; and an increase in the size of the retrosternal airspace, hyperlucency reflecting a decreased tissue density, elongation of the heart, and right ventricular hypertrophy.

The inflammatory reaction in the airways of patients with COPD can also affect other organ systems.[10] COPD is, therefore, not only a pulmonary disorder, but also has extrapulmonary (i.e., systemic) effects, including changes to skeletal muscle mass and function, cardiovascular disease, osteoporosis, and depression.[11]

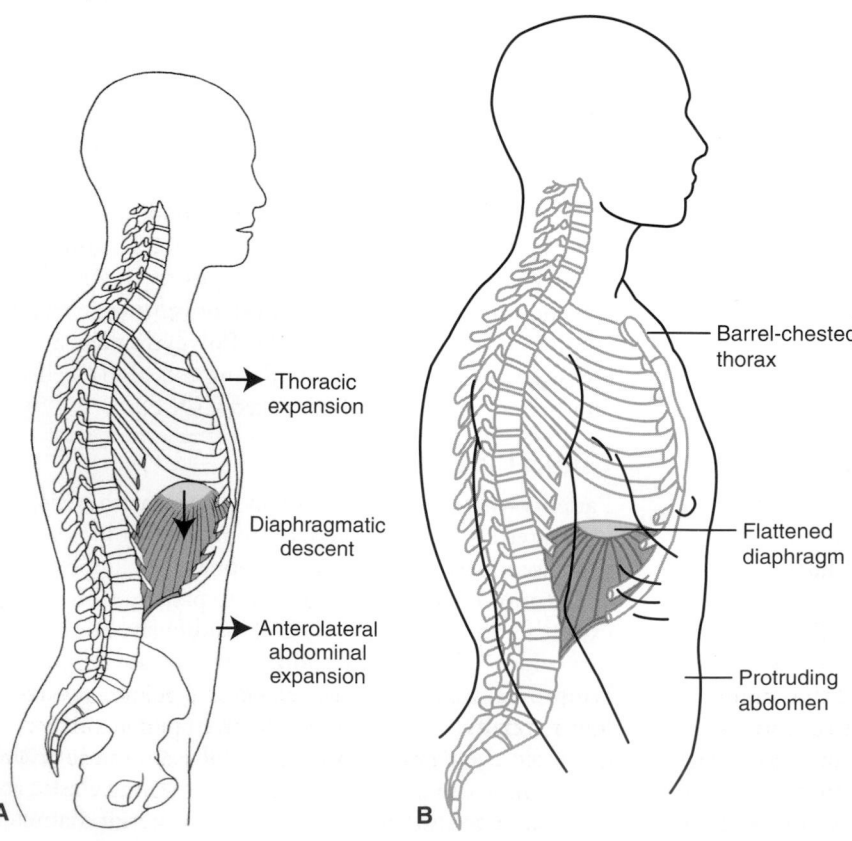

Figure 12.4 (A) Normal thoracic configuration. **(B)** Changes in the configuration of the thorax with chronic obstructive pulmonary disease.
(A, From Levangie, P, and Norkin, C. Joint Structure and Function, ed 5, 2011, p 202, with permission. (B, Adapted from Levangie, P, and Norkin, C. Joint Structure and Function, ed 5, 2011, p 209, with permission.)

Thoracic expansion

Diaphragmatic descent

Anterolateral abdominal expansion

Barrel-chested thorax

Flattened diaphragm

Protruding abdomen

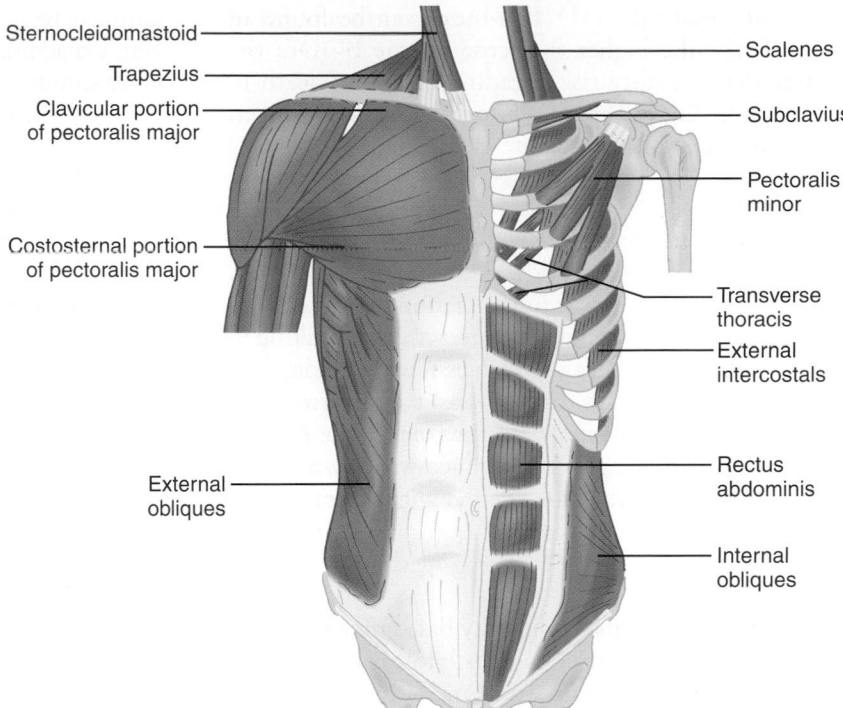

Figure 12.5 Accessory muscles of ventilation are those used during times of increased ventilatory demand. The right side of the figure shows some of the anterior superficial muscles of the thorax that can be accessory muscles of ventilation, and the left side shows the deeper accessory muscles of ventilation.

Course and Prognosis

The clinical course of COPD has an insidious onset with a disease progression that can progress over many years. Early identification of those individuals at risk for the development of COPD has been elusive. Although smoking is the most prevalent risk factor for the development of disease, not all smokers develop clinically significant lung disease. Therefore, a smoking history in and of itself is not predictive for the development of COPD. Prognostic indicators for mortality include advanced age, need for supplemental oxygen, exercise capacity, and disease distribution within the thorax.[12] The *BODE* index has been developed as a prognostic indicator for mortality risk in patients COPD. The index uses four domains to calculate mortality risk: body mass index (B), pulmonary obstruction (O), dyspnea (D), and

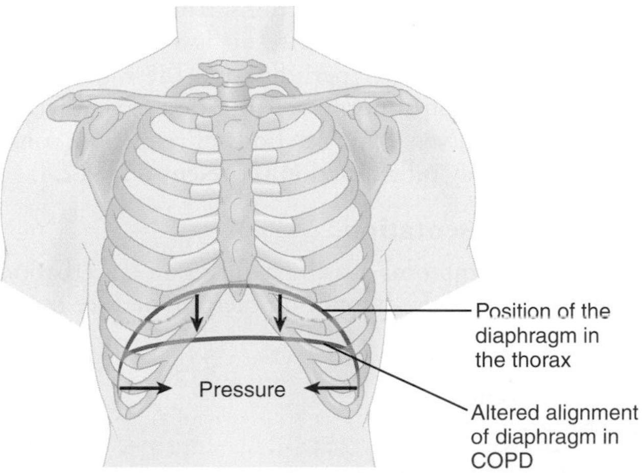

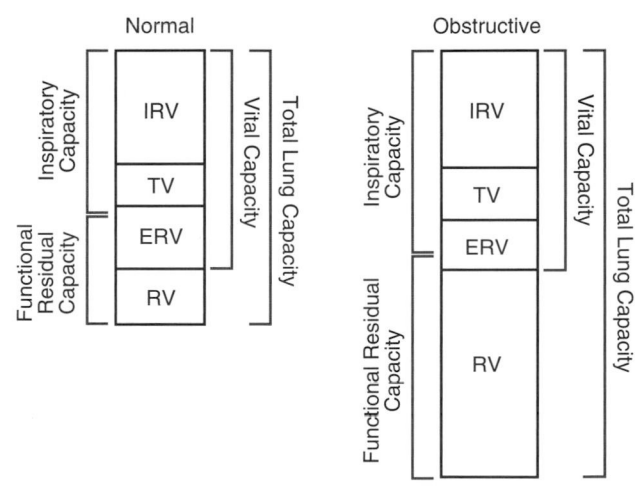

ERV: Expiratory reserve volume
IRV: Inspiratory reserve volume
RV: Residual volume
TV: Tidal volume

Figure 12.7 Lung volumes of a healthy pulmonary system compared with the lung volumes found in obstructive disease. *(Adapted from Rothstein, J, Roy, S, and Wolf, S: The Rehabilitation Specialist's Handbook, ed 3. FA Davis, Philadelphia, 2005, p 428, with permission.)*

Figure 12.6 Alteration in alignment of fibers of the diaphragm due to hyperinflation. Note that the configuration of fibers is more horizontal than vertical and the normal dome shape is minimized. *(Adapted from Levangie, P, and Norkin, C. Joint Structure and Function, ed 5, 2011, p 202, with permission.)*

exercise capacity (E).[13,14] This index can be found in Table 12.2. The higher the score on the BODE, the greater the mortality risk. Leading causes of death in patients with COPD are respiratory failure, lung cancer, and cardiovascular disease.[15]

Asthma

Asthma is a common chronic pulmonary disease, affecting 300 million people worldwide.[16] The disease is characterized by chronic airway inflammation associated with airway hyperresponsiveness (hyperreactivity) resulting in **bronchospasm**. Wheezing, breathlessness, and coughing with sputum production that is at least partially reversible in nature are characteristic symptoms of asthma. Asthma exacerbations may improve spontaneously or with medical intervention and are interspersed with symptom-free intervals.

Diagnosis

The diagnosis of asthma is clinically based on a history of episodic wheezing, shortness of breath (SOB), tightness in the chest, and/or coughing, which may be worse at night in the absence of any other obvious cause. The FEV_1 during exacerbations will be less than 80% of the predicted value. With the use of a rescue drug (used to quickly relieve acute symptoms, e.g., inhaled short-acting beta-2 agonist), an improvement of at least 12% (or 200 mL) in FEV_1

Table 12.2	The Prognosis of COPD Using the BODE Index[13]			
Variable	Points on BODE Index			
	0	1	2	3
FEV_1 (% predicted)	≥65	50-64	36-49	≤35
6-Minute Walk Test (meters)	≥350	250-349	150-249	≤149
MMRC dyspnea scale	0-1	2	3	4
Body mass index	>21	≤21		

BODE = (B) body-mass index; (O) obstruction of airflow severity; (D) dyspnea; and (E) exercise capacity. FEV_1 = forced expiratory volume in 1 second; MMRC dyspnea scale = Modified Medical Research Council dyspnea scale.

Reprinted with permission, Celli, B, et al: N Engl J Med 350(10):1007, 2004.[13]

indicates reversibility of the airway limitation consistent with a diagnosis of asthma.[16,17] An improvement of PEF of 60 L/min (or greater than 20%) following the use of a beta-2 agonist would also suggest the diagnosis of asthma.[16]

Etiology

The etiology of asthma is not completely understood. Historically, two types of asthma have been described. Allergic (or extrinsic) asthma has an immunologic (immunoglobulin E [IgE]–mediated) response to certain environmental triggers (dust mites, pollen, mold, animal dander). The resulting eosinophilic inflammatory response (an increased number of eosinophils found in the airway mucosa) produces the common symptoms and pathophysiological findings of asthma. **Atopy**, or allergic sensitivity, is the strongest factor for the development of allergic asthma. Nonallergic (or intrinsic) asthma is a less common form of asthma. There are no clinical findings of atopy in nonallergic asthma; however, an inflammatory response does result from exposure to an irritant such as smoke, fumes, infections, or cold air. Literature in asthma has begun to consider that the two types of asthma are not all that different: one has a known and widespread allergic response (extrinsic) whereas the other has a more local inflammatory response (intrinsic).[18] The Global Initiative for Asthma (GINA) does not differentiate allergic from nonallergic asthma in its guide to management and prevention.[16] Viral infections have been suggested to play a role in both the development and exacerbation of asthma.[19] Symptoms of asthma may begin at any age.

Pathophysiology

The major physiological manifestation of asthma is narrowing of the airways in response to a trigger. The airway narrowing occurs as a result of eosinophilic inflammation of the bronchial mucosa, bronchospasm, and increased bronchial secretions. The narrowed airways increase the resistance to airflow and cause air trapping, leading to hyperinflation. These narrowed airways provide an abnormal distribution of ventilation to the alveoli. Even during periods of remission, some degree of airway inflammation is present (Fig. 12.8).

Clinical Presentation

The clinical symptoms of asthma during an exacerbation may include cough, dyspnea on exertion or at rest, and

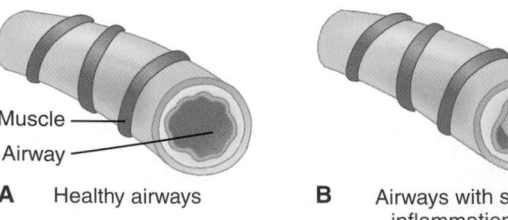

A   Healthy airways

B   Airways with some inflammation in stable asthma

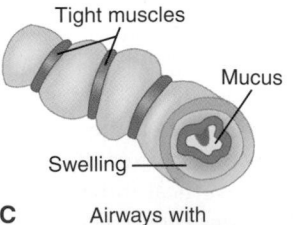

C   Airways with bronchoconstriction, inflammation and secretions in an exacerbation of asthma

Figure 12.8 (A) Airways of a healthy pulmonary system; **(B)** airways showing chronic inflammation of asthma; and **(C)** airways during an asthma exacerbation.

wheezing. The chest is usually held in an expanded position, indicating that hyperinflation of the lungs has occurred. Accessory muscles of ventilation may be used for breathing, even at rest. Intercostal, supraclavicular, and substernal **retractions** (visible inward motion of the soft tissue) may be present on inspiration. While expiratory wheezing is characteristic of asthma, crackles may also be present. With severe airway obstruction, breath sounds may be markedly decreased owing to poor air movement and wheezing may be present not only during exhalation, but may also become present on inspiration.

Chest radiographs taken during an asthmatic exacerbation usually demonstrate hyperinflation, as evidenced by an increase in the anterior-posterior diameter of the chest and hyperlucency of the lung fields. Less commonly, chest radiographs may reveal areas of infiltrate or **atelectasis** from the bronchial obstruction. Chest radiographs may be read as normal between asthmatic exacerbations.

The most consistent change during an exacerbation of asthma is decreased expiratory flow rates, both PEF and FEV_1. RV and FRC are increased because of air trapping at the expense of VC and IRV, which are reduced. The reversibility of these pulmonary function test abnormalities is characteristic of asthma. During remission, the patient with asthma may have normal or near-normal pulmonary function tests.

The most common arterial blood gas finding during an asthmatic exacerbation is mild to moderate hypoxemia. Usually some degree of **hypocapnea** is present secondary to an increased minute ventilation. With severe attacks, hypoxemia will be more pronounced and hypercapnea may occur, indicating that the patient is likely experiencing fatigue and respiratory failure may follow.

Clinical Course

By the time adulthood is reached, many children with asthma no longer have symptoms of the disease.[19-21] When the onset of asthma symptoms begins later in life, the clinical course is usually more progressive, showing changes in pulmonary function tests even during periods of remission. Airway remodeling in response to the chronic airway inflammation is thought to be responsible for the progressive nature of the disease.

Cystic Fibrosis

Cystic fibrosis (CF) is a chronic disease that affects the excretory glands of the body. Secretions made by these glands are thicker, more viscous than usual, and can affect a number of systems of the body: pulmonary, pancreatic, hepatic, sinus, and reproductive. Dysfunction of the pulmonary system is the most common cause of morbidity and mortality in patients with CF. Thickened pulmonary secretions narrow or obstruct airways leading to hyperinflation, infection, and tissue destruction. Other presentations may occur due to the effect of this disease on other organ systems such as failure to thrive, diabetes, sinusitis, biliary disorders, and infertility.

Etiology

CF is a genetic disease transmitted by an autosomal recessive trait (Fig. 12.9). The incidence of disease in children is approximately 1 in 3,700 live births in the United States.[22] Caucasians make up the majority of all cases of CF in the United States. CF is less common in the Hispanic population (white and black) and is rare in the African American and native American populations.[22] The CF gene (cystic fibrosis transmembrane conductance regulator [CFTR]) has been identified on the long arm of chromosome 7. The CFTR functions to transport electrolytes and water in and out of the epithelial cells of many organs in the body, including lungs, pancreas, and digestive and reproductive tracts. Defective transport of sodium, potassium, and water leaves the mucus made by excretory glands thickened and difficult to move, and can often obstruct the lumen of its excretory gland. Over 1,400 mutations of this gene have been described thus far.[23]

Pathophysiology

The chronic pulmonary component of CF is related to the abnormally viscous mucus secreted in the tracheobronchial tree. The altered secretions, resulting in airway

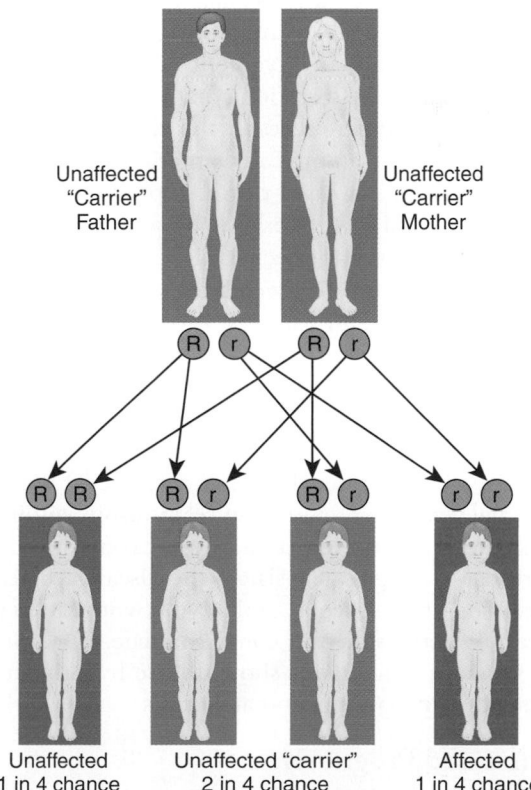

Unaffected "Carrier" Father

Unaffected "Carrier" Mother

R r   R r

R R   R r   R r   r r

Unaffected
1 in 4 chance

Unaffected "carrier"
2 in 4 chance

Affected
1 in 4 chance

Figure 12.9 Autosomal recessive trait (Mendelian) requires that both parents be carriers of the disease or have the disease in order for their child to have the disease.

obstruction and hyperinflation, impair the function of the mucociliary transport system. Exaggerated and sustained neutrophilic airway inflammation in response to infection is also a feature of this disease.[24] Partial or complete obstruction of the airways reduces ventilation to the alveolar units. Ventilation and perfusion within the lungs are not matched. Fibrotic changes are ultimately found in the lung parenchyma.

Diagnosis

The diagnosis of CF may be suspected in patients who present with a positive family history of the disease, in patients with recurrent respiratory infections from *Staphylococcus aureus* and/or *Pseudomonas aeruginosa,* or with a diagnosis of malnutrition and/or failure to thrive. A chloride concentration of greater than or equal to 60 mEq/L found in the sweat of children is a positive test for the diagnosis of CF. Genotyping for the most common CFTR mutations can also be done, but is usually reserved for patients with borderline sweat chloride test results.

Clinical Presentation

The clinical presentation of CF can be related to any number of involved systems. Failure to thrive due to gastrointestinal dysfunction, diabetes due to pancreatic dysfunction, or frequent respiratory infections and chronic cough from pulmonary dysfunction are all possible presentations of the disease. The severity of the disease, while quite variable, has been linked to the classification of the CFTR mutation.[25]

With pulmonary involvement, a patient presents with thick bronchial secretions that may be difficult to clear. With advancing disease, the chest wall will become barreled with an increased anterior-posterior (AP) diameter and an increased dorsal kyphosis due to loss of elastic recoil of the underlying lungs and hyperinflation. There is a resultant decrease in thoracic excursion. Breath sounds may be decreased with adventitious sounds of crackles and wheezes. Hypertrophy of accessory muscles of ventilation, pursed-lip breathing, cyanosis, and digital clubbing may all be present.

Pulmonary function studies show obstructive impairments including decreased FEV_1, decreased PEF, decreased FVC, increased RV, and increased FRC. The abnormal ventilation–perfusion relationship within the lungs results in hypoxemia and hypercapnea, as shown by arterial blood gas analysis. As the disease progresses, destruction of the alveolar capillary network causes pulmonary hypertension and cor pulmonale. In advanced disease, chest radiographs show diffuse hyperinflation, increased lung marking, and atelectasis.

Course and Prognosis

Seventy percent of new cases of CF are diagnosed when the child is less than 1 year of age, likely due to mandatory infant testing for CF within the United States. Life expectancy continues to increase owing to advances in early diagnosis and improved medical management. Although some patients unfortunately die in early childhood, 45% of all patients diagnosed with CF are currently older than 18 years of age.[23] The predicted mean survival age of patients with CF was 37.4 years in 2008, a remarkable improvement from a mean survival age of 16 years in 1970.[22] Respiratory failure is the most frequent cause of death in patients with CF. Therefore, treatment of the pulmonary dysfunction including removal of the abnormally thick secretions and prompt treatment of pulmonary infections is key to the management of CF. Gastrointestinal dysfunction from CF can be aided by proper diet, vitamin supplements, and replacement of pancreatic enzymes. Habitual exercise has been linked to higher aerobic capacity, increased quality of life, and improved survival.[26] Nutritional status is also a powerful predictor of prognosis.[27]

Restrictive Lung Disease

Restrictive lung diseases are a group of diseases with differing etiologies that result in difficulty expanding the lungs and a reduction in lung volumes. This restriction can arise from (1) diseases of the alveolar parenchyma and/or the pleura; (2) changes in the chest wall; or (3) an alteration in the neuromuscular apparatus of the thorax. For the purpose of this discussion, those diseases most likely to be encountered in a rehabilitation setting—restrictive diseases of the lung parenchyma and pleura—will be presented.

Etiology

This group of disorders has a variety of causes. Numerous agents, such as radiation therapy, inorganic dust, inhalation of noxious gases, oxygen toxicity, and asbestos exposure, can cause damage to the pulmonary parenchyma and pleura and result in restrictive pulmonary disease. The most common restrictive lung disease is idiopathic pulmonary fibrosis (IPF). The etiology of IPF is not known; however, there is an immunological reaction in some cases.

Pathophysiology

The particular changes occurring within the lung parenchyma and pleura depend on the etiological factors of restrictive disease. Parenchymal changes often begin with chronic inflammation and a thickening of the alveoli and interstitium. As the disease progresses, distal airspaces become fibrosed, making them more resistant to expansion (i.e., less distensible). Consequently, lung volumes are reduced. A reduced pulmonary vascular bed eventually leads to hypoxemia and cor pulmonale. Asbestosis (asbestos-induced pulmonary fibrosis) is a type of restrictive lung disease that shows both parenchymal and pleural fibrosis.

Clinical Presentation

Dyspnea with activity and a nonproductive cough are the classic symptoms of parenchymal restrictive lung diseases. Signs of restrictive lung disease include rapid, shallow breathing; limited chest expansion; inspiratory crackles, especially over the lower lung fields; digital clubbing; and cyanosis.[28]

The plain chest radiograph reveals fine interstitial markings in a **reticular**, or netlike, pattern. Reduction in overall lung volume and radiographic evidence of pleural involvement, when present, can also be seen on plain chest radiographs, although their diagnostic and prognostic abilities are limited. High-resolution computed tomography (HRCT) is a radiologic test for the diagnosis of IPF that typically shows basilar subpleural changes in a reticular pattern along with traction bronchiectasis (misshapen airways due to a pulling by fibrotic tissue on the airway wall) and **honeycombing**.[28,29]

Pulmonary function tests reveal a reduction in VC, FRC, RV, and TLC. Expiratory flow rates may be somewhat normal. The ratio between FVC and FEV_1 may be normal or even increased. Figure 12.10 shows the changes in lung volumes and capacities that occur in restrictive pulmonary parenchymal disease.

Arterial blood gas studies show varying degrees of hypoxemia and hypocapnea. Exercise may significantly lower oxygenation, even for patients with normal oxygenation at rest.

Course and Prognosis

Restrictive pulmonary disease may have a slow onset but is chronic and relentlessly progressive. Survival depends on the type of restrictive disease, the etiological factor, and the treatment. For patients with IPF mean time from onset of symptoms to death is approximately 80 months. From onset of diagnosis to death is about 35 months.[30] Predictors of mortality include age, gender, smoking history, amount of dyspnea, pulmonary function tests, level of oxygenation, and distance walked on a 6-minute walk test.[29,30]

■ MEDICAL MANAGEMENT

Medical management of chronic pulmonary disease includes smoking cessation, pharmacological agents, and the use of supplemental oxygen. The following discussion provides an overview of these medical interventions.

Smoking Cessation

Smoking is the major causal agent in the development of COPD, as well as a contributing cause to many other disease processes. Smoking cessation is the most important intervention for improving the outcomes of patients with COPD.[31] The addictive properties of smoking and the withdrawal symptoms of smoking cessation make it difficult for smokers to quit. A majority of smokers who try to quit do so on their own. Unfortunately, 94% of those individuals are not successful on their first attempt.[32] Smokers report an average of six to nine attempts at smoking cessation before they are successful.[32] Using a structured smoking cessation program can increase the success of a person attempting to quit smoking.

There are two general types of smoking cessation programs: behavioral therapy and pharmacological therapy. *Behavioral therapy* includes education on the benefits of being a nonsmoker, counseling, and support through the arduous process of withdrawing from smoking. Acupuncture and hypnosis are considered part of a behavioral therapy approach because the purpose is to change smoking behavior. *Pharmacological therapy* includes the use of nicotine replacement therapy and nonnicotine replacement medications such as bupropion (Zyban) and varenicline (Chantix) to assist in the cessation of smoking. Nicotine replacement therapy, using nicotine gum, lozenges, patches, sprays, or inhalers, decreases the withdrawal symptoms linked to nicotine, such as craving for tobacco products, anger, irritability, anxiety, depression, and concentration problems.[33] Bupropion and varenicline counter the withdrawal symptoms of smoking cessation and increase the likelihood of quitting without the use of systemic nicotine.

Smoking cessation without any support has a success rate of approximately 6%. A 2008 meta-analysis regarding smoking cessation found that the use of behavioral therapy had a 14.6% success rate; pharmacological therapy alone had a 21.7% success rate, and a combination of both behavioral and pharmacological therapy had a 27.6% success rate.[34] Recommendations for smoking cessation need to be tailored to the individual patient, because access to counseling may be difficult to obtain and adverse reactions to some medications may be encountered. The regional offices of the American Lung

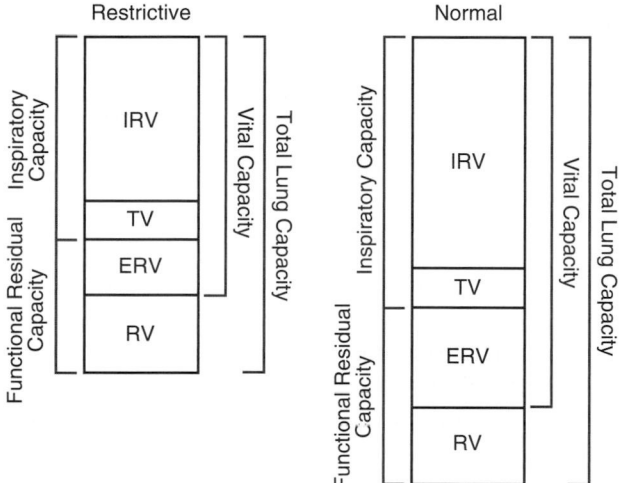

ERV: Expiratory reserve volume
IRV: Inspiratory reserve volume
RV: Residual volume
TV: Tidal volume

Figure 12.10 Lung volumes of a healthy pulmonary system compared with the lung volumes found in restrictive disease. *(Adapted from Rothstein, J, Roy, S, and Wolf, S: The Rehabilitation Specialist's Handbook. FA Davis, Philadelphia, 2005, p 428, with permission.)*

Association and the American Cancer Society are good resources for local smoking cessation programs.

Pharmacological Management

Pharmacological agents provide relief from the symptoms of chronic lung disease and improvement in the health and functional status of individuals with lung disease. Each pulmonary diagnosis and the severity of that disease will require a tailored plan of care. It is not unusual for patients to be on a combination of drugs for the management of their pulmonary disease. These drugs can affect exercise performance, HR, and blood pressure (BP), both at rest and with exercise. This discussion will provide information on both maintenance drugs and rescue drugs used in the care of patients with pulmonary disease. Table 12.3 provides foundational information on the pharmacological management of lung disease. Table 12.4 presents the recommended treatments according to the severity of COPD as described by the GOLD standards.[5] Table 12.5 includes recommendations from GINA for pharmacological control of asthma symptoms.[16]

Table 12.3	Drugs Commonly Used in the Medical Management of Patients with Chronic Pulmonary Disease			
Category	Drug	Trade Name	Action	Adverse Reactions
Maintenance (taken on a regular basis)	Anticholinergic	Atrovent	Bronchodilation	Throat irritation Drying of tracheal secretions Tachycardia Palpitations
	Long-acting beta-2 agonist	Serevent	Bronchodilation	Tachycardia Palpitations GI distress Nervousness Tremor Headache Dizziness
	Steroids	Flovent Prednisone	Reduces inflammatory response	Increases BP Sodium retention (edema) Muscle wasting Osteoporosis GI irritation Atherosclerosis Hypercholesterolemia Increased susceptibility to infection
	Cromolyn sodium	Intal	Prevents inflammatory response	Throat irritation Cough Bronchospasm
	Leukotriene receptor antagonist	Singulair	Blocks allergic reaction (blocking leukotrienes)	GI distress Sore throat Upper respiratory tract infection Dizziness Headache Nasal congestion
	Methylxanthine	Aminophylline Theophylline	Bronchodilation	Seizures Cardiac arrhythmias GI distress Tremor Headache

Table 12.3	Drugs Commonly Used in the Medical Management of Patients with Chronic Pulmonary Disease—cont'd			
Category	**Drug**	**Trade Name**	**Action**	**Adverse Reactions**
Rescue (used to relieve acute symptoms)	Short-acting beta-2 agonist	Albuterol Ventolin	Bronchodilation	Tachycardia Palpitations GI distress Nervousness Tremor Headache Dizziness

BP = blood pressure; GI = gastrointestinal.

Table 12.4	Suggested Pharmacological Management Based on the Global Initiative for Chronic Obstructive Lung Disease (GOLD) Classification of Lung Severity[5]			
	I: Mild	**II: Moderate**	**III: Severe**	**IV: Very Severe**
Characteristics	• $FEV_1/FVC < 70\%$ • $FEV_1 \geq 80\%$	• $FEV_1/FVC < 70\%$ • $50\% \leq FEV_1 < 80\%$	• $FEV_1/FVC < 70\%$ • $30\% \leq FEV_1 < 50\%$	• $FEV_1/FVC < 70\%$ • $FEV_1 < 30\%$ or $FEV_1 < 50\%$
	Reduction of risk factor(s), influenza vaccination *Add* short-acting bronchodilator when needed			
		Add regular treatment with one or more long-acting bronchodilators *Add* rehabilitation		
			Add inhaled glucocorticosteroids if repeated exacerbations	
				Add long-term oxygen if chronic respiratory failure *Consider* surgical treatments

FEV = forced expiratory volume; FVC = forced vital capacity.

Table 12.5	Suggested Pharmacological Management of Patients with Asthma According to the Global Initiative for Asthma (GINA)			
Step 1	**Step 2**	**Step 3**	**Step 4**	**Step 5**
Asthma education Environmental controls Rapid-acting beta-2 agonist, as needed				
	Select one	Select one	Add one or more	Add one or both
	Low-dose inhaled steroid	Low-dose inhaled steroid plus long-acting beta-2 agonist	Medium- to high-dose steroid plus long-acting beta-2 agonist	Oral steroids (lowest dose)
	Or leukotriene modifier	Medium- to high-dose inhaled steroid	Leukotriene modifier	Anti-IgE treatment
		Low-dose inhaled steroid plus leukotriene modifier	Sustained-release theophylline	
		Low-dose inhaled steroid plus sustained-release theophylline		

Step 1 is intended for everyone with a diagnosis of asthma to promote gaining and maintaining control of symptoms. If Step 1 is insufficient in controlling symptoms, the patient moves to the next step(s). *Shaded cells* are the preferred pharmacological options. Adapted from Global Strategy for Asthma Management and Prevention, Update 2008, p 14 (reference 16), with permission.

Maintenance Drugs

Maintenance drugs are used to reduce or minimize pulmonary symptoms throughout the day. These drugs are taken on a regular schedule to keep respiratory symptoms at bay. Steroids, anticholinergics, long-acting beta-2 agonists, cromolyn sodium, and leukotriene antagonists are commonly prescribed maintenance drugs for patients with chronic pulmonary disease. Theophylline, though an effective drug for the treatment of chronic pulmonary diseases, is less frequently prescribed because safer medications are available. Routes of administration of maintenance drugs are usually inhalation or ingestion. When inhalation is effective, it is the advisable route of administration because it limits systemic side effects of the drug.

Inhaled or systemic anti-inflammatories, such as steroids, are the mainstay of medical management of the chronic inflammation of asthma.[35] Inhaled anticholinergics are commonly prescribed for patients with COPD. The action of an anticholinergic is to block the smooth muscle constriction brought on by the parasympathetic nervous system, thus encouraging bronchodilation. Inhaled long-acting beta-2 agonists are used to mimic the sympathetic nervous system encouraging bronchodilation in patients with bronchoconstriction as a chronic symptom of their pulmonary disease. Inhaled cromolyn sodium is used to prevent the inflammatory response within the respiratory system by stabilizing the mast cell within the alveolar units. Used before an exposure of a known trigger for bronchoconstriction, cromolyn sodium can prevent airway narrowing before it can begin. It is therefore helpful in patients with predictable bronchoconstriction, such as exercise-induced bronchospasm. Leukotriene antagonists are systemic drugs that reduce airway inflammation and relax airway smooth muscle. Again, all of these maintenance drugs are used for the long-term management of chronic lung disease. Among the determinants for use and dosage of maintenance drugs are the severity of disease, the patient's symptoms, and response to the medication.

Rescue Drugs

Rescue drugs are used for immediate relief of *breakthrough* symptoms of bronchoconstriction (symptoms that "break through" and become apparent despite careful management). Inhaled short-acting beta-2 agonists are used for this purpose. Patients are advised to use their prescribed inhaled short-acting beta-2 agonist on an as-needed basis, rather than on a regular schedule. If a patient reports an increased frequency in the use of a rescue drug, it is indicative of a flaw in the maintenance drug regimen or a change in the patient's pulmonary status. Short-acting beta-2 agonists can be used before the onset of activity to decrease pulmonary symptoms in cases where exercise is the trigger for bronchospasm.[36]

Although the mechanism of action of each bronchodilator is different, there may be an increase in resting HR and BP with their use. Employing the **heart rate reserve method** (Karvonen's formula) when prescribing exercise intensity acknowledges the elevated resting HR and an appropriate target HR can be calculated. (See Physical Therapy Management section, Exercise Prescription, for further information.) Other common side effects of bronchodilators include nervousness, tremor, anxiety, and nausea. The side effects of systemic steroids, including osteoporosis, myopathies, and muscle wasting, may require modifications to an exercise program.

Antibiotics

Pulmonary infections are frequent in patients with chronic pulmonary diseases. They can be devastating to the patient and cause major setbacks in pulmonary rehabilitation efforts. The early signs of an infection are often noted by changes in the patient's baseline status (i.e., a change in exercise ability, peak flow rates, dyspnea, color or amount of sputum, or an increase in the use of rescue inhalers). Antibiotics are used to interfere with the growth and/or proliferation of bacteria. The action of these drugs is either bacteriostatic or bactericidal. There are many categories of antibiotics (e.g., penicillins, cephalosporins, tetracyclines) that are effective on different infecting organisms. It is important to identify the infecting organism in order to prescribe the appropriate antibiotic. Prophylactic use of antibiotics has not been demonstrated to prevent infections, and the Alliance for the Prudent Use of Antibiotics (APUA) encourages the use of antibiotics for only diagnosed bacterial infections to reduce antibiotic-resistant strains of bacteria.[37]

Supplemental Oxygen

The use of supplemental oxygen has been shown to prolong the survival of patients with COPD whose resting arterial partial pressure of oxygen (P_aO_2) is lower than 60 mm Hg.[38,39] An absolute indication for use of long-term oxygen therapy is a P_aO_2 of 55 mm Hg or less, which correlates with an S_aO_2 of 88% or less.[40] If a patient is limited in the ability to exercise due to dyspnea, supplemental oxygen may be warranted.[38,41] The amount of oxygen used should be titrated individually to maintain an S_aO_2 of at least 90%, if possible.[42] Various supplemental oxygen delivery methods are available; continuous flow, pulsed flow, and reservoir are among the most common.

Surgical Management

There are few surgical options for the patient with pulmonary disease. Lung volume reduction surgery (LVRS) is a surgical technique that removes nonfunctional, overdistended lung tissue, in order to restore more normal biomechanics to the thorax. LVRS may be indicated in patients with heterogeneous areas of relatively nonfunctional emphysema alongside of functional lung tissue. The surgical procedure removes approximately 20%

to 35% of the most diseased lung tissue, relieving the more normal lung tissue of its burden. This surgical procedure reduces RV and FRC (i.e., decreases hyperinflation), allowing for a more normal resting position of the diaphragm, an increased diaphragmatic excursion, and a more normal chest wall motion.[5] Research has shown postoperative results of increased exercise capacity, lung function, quality of life, and gas exchange in patients with moderate *upper lobe* lung disease.[5,43] Patients with severe lung disease distributed to other areas of the lung do not appear to benefit equally from this intervention. Rather, they show only slight improvement in functional abilities and quality of life scores with a high mortality rate.[5,43-46] Many centers that perform LVRS advocate a preoperative pulmonary rehabilitation program. Participants in these preoperative programs demonstrated shorter hospital stays and fewer days on mechanical ventilation.[47]

Lung transplantation for end-stage pulmonary disease has an overall survival rate of 83% at 1 year and approximately 54% at 5 years.[48] The goals of lung transplantation are to restore normal lung function, restore normal exercise capacity, and prolong life.[49] People awaiting a lung transplant include patients with COPD, CF, idiopathic pulmonary fibrosis, and pulmonary hypertension. The number of patients awaiting lung transplantation continues to grow, far exceeding the number of organs available for transplantation, making transplantation a reality for only a small number of individuals.[48]

■ PHYSICAL THERAPY MANAGEMENT

Chronic pulmonary disease and its associated dysfunction have a slow yet progressive course. The person with pulmonary dysfunction often avoids activities that result in the uncomfortable sensation of dyspnea. A slow but steady decrease in these patients' functional activities follows, resulting in progressive aerobic deconditioning. It is not uncommon for someone with pulmonary disease to have lost many functional abilities before ever seeking medical help. The intended outcome of pulmonary rehabilitation is to interrupt this downward spiraling of physical ability, improve exercise performance, decrease the symptom of dyspnea, and improve quality of life.[50-52]

Goals and Outcomes

The *Guide for Physical Therapist Practice* provides a general framework for physical therapy intervention for patients with impaired ventilation, respiration, and aerobic capacity and endurance associated with ventilatory pump dysfunction (Practice Pattern 6F).[53] The development of specific anticipated goals and expected outcomes for the individual patient with pulmonary dysfunction can be based on the general goals presented in Box 12.1.

Examination

The examination of a patient's pulmonary status has several purposes: (1) to evaluate the appropriateness of

---

> **Box 12.1**   Examples of General Goals and Outcomes for Patients with Chronic Pulmonary Dysfunction
>
> - Patient/client, family, and caregiver understanding of disease process, expectations, goals, and outcomes is enhanced.
> - Cardiovascular endurance is increased.
> - Strength, power, and endurance of peripheral muscles are increased.
> - Performance of physical tasks, both basic activities of daily living and instrumental activities of daily living, is improved.
> - Strength, power, and endurance of ventilatory muscles are increased.
> - Independence in airway clearance is improved.
> - Overall work of breathing is decreased.
> - Patient/client decision making ability regarding the use of health care resources is improved.
> - Patient/client self-management of symptoms and self-management of pulmonary disease are enhanced.

the patient's participation in a pulmonary rehabilitation program; (2) to determine the therapeutic interventions most appropriate for the participant's plan of care (POC); (3) to monitor the participant's physiological response to exercise; and (4) to appropriately progress the participant's POC over time.

Patient History

A patient interview should begin with the chief complaint and the patient's perception of why pulmonary rehabilitation is being sought. Commonly, the chief complaint is often SOB and/or loss of function. A medical history contains pertinent pulmonary symptoms specific to that patient: cough, sputum production, wheezing, and SOB. Occupational, social, medication, and family histories should also be obtained and documented.

Tests and Measures
Vital Signs

HR, BP, oxygen saturation (S_aO_2), respiratory rate, temperature, and presence of pain (usually associated with SOB) should be examined and documented (see Chapter 2, Examination of Vital Signs). An individual's height should be measured, because there is a direct relationship between height and lung volumes. Weight should be measured on a standard scale and each subsequent measurement should be performed on the same scale.

Observation, Inspection, and Palpation

By observing the neck and shoulders of a patient with pulmonary disease, the use of accessory muscles of ventilation can be observed (see Fig. 12.5). A normal configuration of the thorax reveals a ratio of AP to lateral diameter of 2:1. Destruction of the lung parenchyma results in an increase in the AP diameter and a reduction of this ratio (up to 1:1) (see Fig. 12.4). During inhalation and exhalation, both sides of the thorax should move symmetrically; asymmetries should be noted and documented.

Cyanosis is a bluish discoloration of the skin that can be observed periorally, periorbitally, and in nail beds; it indicates acute tissue hypoxia. An indicator of more chronic tissue hypoxia is digital clubbing of the fingers and toes. In digital clubbing, there is an increase in the angle created by the distal phalanx and the point where the nail exits from the digit. The tip of the distal phalanx becomes bulbous (Fig. 12.11).

Auscultation of the Lungs

Auscultation involves listening over the chest wall as air enters and exits the lungs. To perform auscultation of the lungs, a stethoscope is placed firmly on the patient's thorax anteriorly, laterally, and posteriorly (Fig. 12.12). The patient is asked to inspire fully through an open mouth, then to exhale quietly. Inhalation and the beginning of exhalation normally produce a soft rustling sound. The end of exhalation is normally silent. This characteristic of a normal breath sound is termed **vesicular**. When a louder, more hollow, and echoing sound occupies a larger portion of the ventilatory cycle, the breath sounds are referred to as **bronchial**. When the breath sounds are very quiet and barely audible, they are termed **decreased**. These three terms—*vesicular, bronchial,* and *decreased*—allow the listener to describe the intensity of the breath sound.[54]

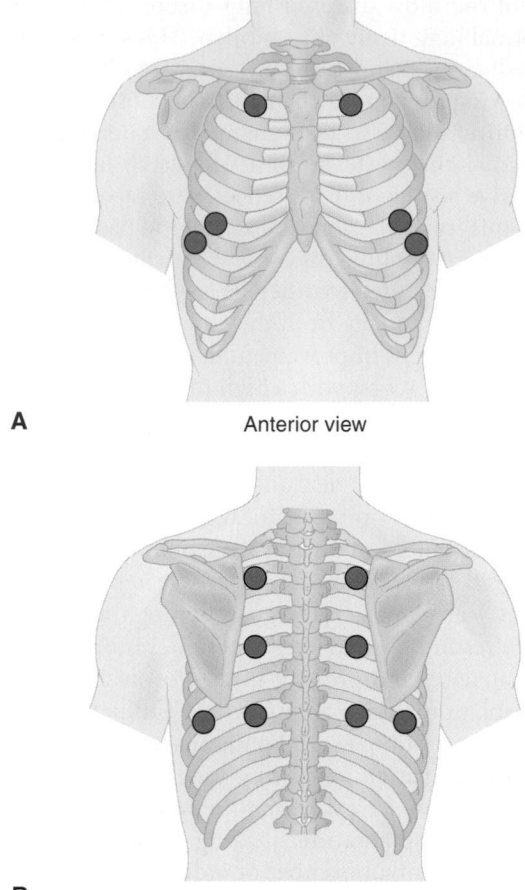

A   Anterior view

B   Posterior view

Figure 12.12 Auscultation of the lungs. A global assessment of lung sounds requires that the therapist listen through a stethoscope, which is placed anteriorly, posteriorly, and laterally on the upper, middle, and lower thorax.

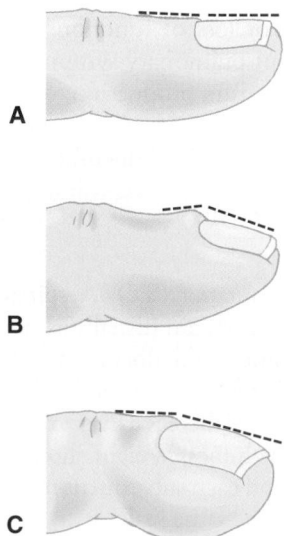

Figure 12.11 Digital clubbing is a sign of chronic tissue hypoxia. **(a)** Normal. **(b)** Early clubbing with increased angle present between nail and proximal skin. **(c)** Advanced clubbing; tip of distal phalanx becomes bulbous.

In addition to the description of the intensity of the breath sound, there may be additional sounds and vibrations heard during auscultation. These are called **adventitious** breath sounds. These sounds are superimposed on the already-described intensity of the breath sound. According to the American College of Chest Physicians and the American Thoracic Society, there are two types of adventitious sounds: crackles and wheezes.[55] Crackles, historically termed *rales* and *rhonchi,* sound like the rustling of cellophane and have a multitude of potential causes (tissue fibrosis, secretions in the airways, and so forth) while wheezes have been described as high-pitched, coarse, whistling sounds. A decrease in the size of the lumen of the airway will create a wheezing sound, much as stretching the neck of an inflated balloon narrows the passageway through which air must escape and produces a whistling sound.

Measurement of Dyspnea and Quality of Life

Quantifying dyspnea at the beginning and the end of a rehabilitation program and during periods of exacerbation can be accomplished using the *Baseline Dyspnea*

Index (BDI) (Table 12.6).[56,57] Quality-of-life (QOL) measures specific to chronic pulmonary dysfunction such as the *Chronic Respiratory Questionnaire* or the *St. George's Respiratory Questionnaire* may be helpful in determining the patient's baseline health-related quality of life. The Chronic Respiratory Questionnaire has a subscore for rating dyspnea and the St. George's Respiratory Questionnaire has a subscore for symptoms. Both of these QOL measure as well as the BDI may be helpful in demonstrating improvement made with physical therapy intervention.[58,59]

Measurement of Function

Examining a patient's functional abilities at baseline using the 6-Minute Walk Test (6-MWT) or the 10-Meter Shuttle Walk Test (10-MSWT) should be used as an outcome measure to document physical improvements following physical therapy intervention.

Table 12.6 Baseline Dyspnea Index	
Functional Impairment	**Magnitude of Effort**
_____ Grade 4: *No Impairment.* Able to carry out usual activities and occupation without shortness of breath.	_____ Grade 4: *Extraordinary.* Becomes short of breath only with the greatest imaginable effort. No shortness of breath with ordinary effort.
_____ Grade 3: *Slight Impairment.* Distinct impairment in at least one activity but no activities completely abandoned. Reduction in activity at work *or* in usual activities that seems slight or not clearly caused by shortness of breath.	_____ Grade 3: *Major.* Becomes short of breath with effort distinctly submaximal. Tasks performed without pause unless the task requires extraordinary effort that may be performed with pauses.
_____ Grade 2: *Moderate Impairment.* Patient has changed jobs *and/or* has abandoned at least one usual activity due to shortness of breath.	_____ Grade 2: *Moderate.* Becomes short of breath with moderate effort. Tasks performed with occasional pauses and require more time to complete than the average person.
_____ Grade 1: *Severe Impairment.* Patient unable to work *or* has given up most or all customary activities due to shortness of breath.	_____ Grade 1: *Light.* Becomes short of breath with little effort. Tasks performed with little effort or more difficult tasks with frequent pauses and requiring 50%–100% longer to complete than the average person might require.
_____ Grade 0: *Very Severe Impairment.* Unable to work *and* has given up most or all customary activities due to shortness of breath.	_____ Grade 0: *No Effort.* Becomes short of breath at rest, while sitting, or lying down.
_____ W: *Amount Uncertain.* Patient is impaired owing to shortness of breath, but amount cannot be specified. Details are not sufficient to allow impairment to be categorized.	_____ W: *Amount Uncertain.* Patient has limited exertional capacity due to shortness of breath, but amount cannot be specified. Details are not sufficient to allow impairment to be categorized.
_____ X: *Unknown.* Information unavailable regarding impairment.	_____ X: *Unknown.* Information unavailable regarding limitation of effort.
_____ Y: *Impaired for Reasons Other than Shortness of Breath.* For example, musculoskeletal problem or chest pain.	_____ Y: *Impaired for Reasons Other than Shortness of Breath.* For example, musculoskeletal problem or chest pain.
Magnitude of Task	
_____ Grade 4: *Extraordinary.* Becomes short of breath only with extraordinary activity, such as carrying very heavy loads on the level, lighter loads uphill, or running. No shortness of breath with ordinary tasks.	

Continued

Table 12.6 Baseline Dyspnea Index—cont'd	
Functional Impairment	**Magnitude of Effort**
_____ Grade 3: *Major.* Becomes short of breath only with such major activities as walking up a steep hill, climbing more than three flights of stairs, or carrying a moderate load on the level.	
_____ Grade 2: *Moderate.* Becomes short of breath with moderate or average tasks, such as walking up a gradual hill, climbing less than three flights of stairs, or carrying a light load on the level.	
_____ Grade 1: *Light.* Becomes short of breath with light activities, such as walking on the level, washing, standing, or shopping.	
_____ Grade 0: *No Task.* Becomes short of breath at rest, while sitting, or lying down.	
_____ W: *Amount Uncertain.* Patient has limited exertional capacity due to shortness of breath, but amount cannot be specified. Details are not sufficient to allow impairment to be categorized.	
_____ X: *Unknown.* Information unavailable regarding limitation of magnitude of task.	
_____ Y: *Impaired for Reasons Other than Shortness of Breath.* For example, musculoskeletal problem or chest pain.	

From Mahler et al,[56] p 399. Reprinted with permission of the American College of Chest Physicians.

Measurement of Strength

Patients with pulmonary disease may show peripheral and ventilatory muscle weakness due to deconditioning, malnutrition, steroid use, and systemic effects of the disease process.[10,11,60] Muscle weakness can contribute to exercise limitations and an inability to perform activities of daily living (ADL). Therefore, measurement of muscle strength (e.g., manual muscle tests) and inspiratory pressures (e.g., PI_{max}) should be performed to determine the need for strength training during rehabilitation.

Laboratory Tests

Various laboratory studies may be performed to examine patients with pulmonary disease. These include radiology, pulmonary function tests (PFTs) including flow rates, **exercise tolerance tests** (ETTs), functional performance measures, arterial blood gas (ABG) analysis, S_aO_2 measurements, and electrocardiograms (ECGs).

Exercise Testing in Patients with Pulmonary Disease

A determination of functional capacity is part of the examination of a patient with pulmonary disease. An ETT can provide the objective information to (1) document a patient's symptomatology and physical impairment;

(2) prescribe safe exercise; (3) document changes in oxygenation during exercise and determine the need for supplemental oxygen; and (4) identify any changes in pulmonary function during exercise performance. If the ETT is repeated following physical therapy intervention, it can provide important outcome data.

A number of testing methods are available to determine the maximal oxygen consumption and functional abilities of patients with pulmonary disease. An ETT protocol, usually utilizing a treadmill or cycle ergometer, gradually increases exercise intensity to stress the patient with pulmonary dysfunction to the point of limitation. Vital signs are monitored throughout the test. The ECG, continuously displayed during exercise, records the exercise HR and electrical activity of the cardiac conduction system. BP measurements recorded at 1- to 3-minute intervals during exercise and during recovery from the test provide information on the hemodynamic status of the patient. ABGs measured during exercise provide the best method for determining arterial oxygenation and the adequacy of alveolar ventilation, though the invasive nature of this test limits its use. Arterial S_aO_2 monitoring provides less information, but the noninvasive nature of the test makes its use more widespread. Oxygen consumption, VO_2, is a helpful measure that can be collected during an ETT, but requires equipment not always found in an exercise testing laboratory. A number of ETT protocols are outlined in Table 12.7.[61-66] (Refer to the section on exercise testing in Chapter 13, Heart Disease, for more information on exercise protocols.) The symptom-limited ETT requires the patient to continue the exercise protocol until symptoms dictate cessation of exercise. Criteria for stopping a pulmonary exercise test are presented in Box 12.2.

The 10-MSWT is a functional performance measure that uses a recorded audio signal to dictate incrementally increasing walking speeds on a level 10-meter course. Two destination points are placed 10 meters apart. The person is asked to reach each destination point by the time the increasingly frequent audio signal sounds. The results of the 10-MSWT have a positive correlation with $VO_{2\,max}$ (maximal oxygen consumption).[67,68]

The 6-MWT is also a functional performance measure that asks a patient to walk as far as possible in 6 minutes. The patient is allowed to stop and rest during the administration of the test as total distance walked is the recorded result of the test. The 6-MWT has been shown to be a good predictor of functional abilities.[69,70] Both the 10-MSWT and the 6-MWT are easy to administer, and the ready availability of the required equipment makes them useful outcome measurements to demonstrate changes in a patient's abilities following physical therapy intervention.

Exercise test data provide information that can be used to determine disability, predict mortality, assess the ability to perform ADL, quantify health-related quality of life, determine the need for oxygen therapy, demonstrate the effectiveness of medication changes, and prescribe exercise.[13,68-72] PFTs performed before and after an exercise test document the effects of exercise on lung function. A reduction of greater than or equal to 10% in FEV_1 is an indication that exercise provoked airway

---

Box 12.2 Graded Exercise Test Termination Criteria

1. Maximal shortness of breath
2. A fall in P_aO_2 of greater than 20 mm Hg or a P_aO_2 less than 55 mm Hg
3. A rise in P_aCO_2 of greater than 10 mm Hg or greater than 65 mm Hg
4. Cardiac ischemia or arrhythmias
5. Symptoms of fatigue
6. Increase in diastolic blood pressure readings of 20 mm Hg, systolic hypertension greater than 250 mm Hg, decrease in blood pressure with increasing workloads
7. Leg pain
8. Total fatigue
9. Signs of insufficient cardiac output
10. Reaching a ventilatory maximum

From Brannon, F, et al: Cardiopulmonary Rehabilitation: Basic Theory and Application. FA Davis, Philadelphia, 1998, p 300, with permission.

---

hyperresponsiveness.[73] Finally, a prescription for exercise that will safely promote improved cardiopulmonary fitness can be developed based on the ETT.

Exercise Prescription

Exercise prescription incorporates four variables that together allow the therapist to develop a patient-specific exercise formula designed to produce an increase in functional capacity. These variables are *mode*, *intensity*, *duration*, and *frequency*.

Mode

Any type of sustained **aerobic exercise** can be used for pulmonary rehabilitation. Lower extremity (LE) activities, including walking, jogging, and cycling, are often used

---

Table 12.7	Exercise Testing Protocols Used for the Patient with Pulmonary Disease	
Test	**Author(s)**	**Protocol**
Cycle tests	Jones[62]	Begin at 100 kpm, increase 100 kpm every minute
	Berman and Sutton[63]	Begin at 100 kpm, increase 100 kpm every minute, or 50 kpm if FEV_1 is <1 L/sec
Treadmill tests	Bruce et al[64]	Begin at 1.7 mph, 10% treadmill grade; increase both speed and grade every 3 minutes
	Naughton et al[65]	Begin at 1.2 mph 0% grade; increase speed and 3% grade every 2 minutes
	Balke and Ware[66]	Begin at constant speed of 3.3 mph, increase grade 3.5% every minutes
10-Meter Shuttle Test	Revill et al[67]	Walking between two markers, 10 m apart, at increasing walking velocities, which are synchronized to an auditory signal or metronome
Walk Test (6- or 12-minute)	American Thoracic Society[69]	Ambulate (walk) as far as possible in the allotted time

to improve exercise tolerance because these modes of exercise more easily translate into functional abilities. Upper extremity (UE) aerobic exercise (e.g., arm ergometry, free weights) can also be included. The combination of UE and LE training in a rehabilitation program results in improved functional status compared to either exercise alone.[74] Many programs utilize a circuit approach (combining a variety of resistive and aerobic exercises) to train different muscle groups and maintain the participant's interest.

Intensity

Three parameters can be used to prescribe exercise intensity: oxygen consumption, HR, and rating of perceived exertion (RPE) or rating of perceived dyspnea (RPD). Below is a discussion of each means of prescribing exercise intensity.

Exercise Intensity as a Percent of VO$_{2max}$

An ETT may report functional capacity in terms of maximal VO$_2$. Exercise intensity can be prescribed using a moderate intensity, 40% to 60% of the maximum VO$_2$ achieved on an ETT, or moderate to vigorous intensity, greater than 60% of the maximum VO$_2$ achieved on an ETT.[75] Patients with mild to moderate pulmonary disease may be able to exercise for a period of time at these intensities in order to produce a training effect. However, patients with severe pulmonary disease may not tolerate long periods of activity at high intensities (greater than 60% of their maximum). Lowering the exercise intensity may not be the answer for patients with severe pulmonary disease as using a lower exercise intensity has resulted in a lesser to no training effect.[76,77] Rather, exercise will be tolerated and a training effect achieved when short bursts of activity using a high percentage of a participant's peak workload are interspersed with low-intensity exercise or rest periods.[75-84] Current research on interval training versus continuous exercise training is presented in Box 12.3 Evidence Summary. There is a dose relationship between exercise intensity and training outcomes, meaning the higher the exercise intensity, the greater the training.[50]

Exercise Intensity as a Percent of Heart Rate Reserve

While using a percentage of VO$_2$ may be the most accurate method of prescribing exercise from a graded exercise test, it does not give the clinician a means to monitor exercise intensity during actual performance of

---

Box 12.3 Evidence Summary Exercise Training Intensity: Interval versus Continuous Exercise

Reference	Subjects	Design/ Intervention	Duration	Results	Comments
Beauchamp et al[80] (2010)	8 randomized clinical trials using 388 patients	Systematic review		No difference was found between interval training and continuous training in their effect on exercise capacity or health-related QOL measures in patients with COPD.	
Nasis et al[81] (2009)	42 patients with COPD (FEV$_1$ 42% predicted)	Randomized clinical trial (RCT) of 2 treatment groups: 1. Interval training group using 126% of peak workload from cycle ergometer test 2. Continuous training group using 76% of peak workload from cycle ergometer test	Both groups: 3 sessions per week for 10 weeks. Interval training group used 30 sec of training with 30 sec of rest for 45 min on cycle ergometer. Continuous session was 30 min on cycle ergometer.	BODE index scores (by reducing dyspnea scores and increasing the 6-MWT distance) were significantly improved in both groups. There was no significant difference between the groups on these measures.	If interval training is as good as continuous exercise in lowering the BODE index, which is a prognostic indicator, then both training strategies would be beneficial to patients with COPD.

Box 12.3 Evidence Summary   Exercise Training Intensity: Interval versus Continuous Exercise—cont'd

Reference	Subjects	Design/ Intervention	Duration	Results	Comments
Arnardottir et al[82] (2007)	60 patients with COPD (FEV_1 of 32%–35% predicted)	RCT of 2 treatment groups: 1. Interval training group using alternating 80% and 30%–40% of peak workload from cycle ergometer test 2. Continuous training group using 65% of peak workload from cycle ergometer test	Both groups: 2 sessions of 39 min of exercise twice weekly for 16 weeks. Interval training group alternated between 3 min of high-intensity training with 3 min of low-intensity training for 39 minutes. Continuous training group performed 39 min of continuous exercise on cycle ergometer.	Peak work and VO_2 peak were significantly increased in each group. Functional capacity, dyspnea ratings, and health-related QOL measures were significantly improved in each group. There was no difference in the improvement between groups.	If interval training is as effective as continuous exercise, then interval training is beneficial for those patients who cannot sustain long periods of activity.
Varga et al[83] (2007)	71 patients with COPD (FEV_1 of 55% of predicted)	Pre-test, post-test clinical trial of 3 treatment groups. 1. Interval training group using alternating 90% and 50% of peak workload using cycle ergometer 2. Continuous training group using 80% of peak workload using cycle ergometer 3. Self-paced group used the maximum load tolerated using either a cycle ergometer, level walking, or stair climbing	All groups: 45 min per session, 3 times per week for 8 weeks. Interval training group: 2 min of high-intensity training alternating with 1 min of low-intensity training for 30 min with 7.5 min warm-up and 7.5 min cool-down. Continuous training group: 45 min on cycle ergometer. Self-paced group: exercised starting with 30 min and increasing for 45 min duration by the study's end.	All three interventions were equally effective in improving the scores on an activity questionnaire. The supervised groups (interval and continuous) groups had a significantly higher peak work rate compared to the self-paced group. Peak VO_2 and lactic acidosis thresholds were improved in all groups without statistical significance between groups.	Participants were assigned to the self-paced group if they lived too far from the research center. Remaining patients were then randomized into the interval training group or the continuous training group. Therefore, this is not a true randomized clinical trial.

Continued

Box 12.3 Evidence Summary Exercise Training Intensity: Interval versus Continuous Exercise—cont'd

Reference	Subjects	Design/ Intervention	Duration	Results	Comments
Puhan et al[84] (2006)	87 patients with COPD, FEV_1 of 34% of predicted	RCT of 2 treatment groups: 1. Interval training group using alternating 50% and 10% of peak workload using steep ramped cycle ergometer 2. Continuous training group using 70% of peak workload using incremental cycle ergometer	Both groups participated in 12 to 15 sessions of exercise lasting 20 min each over 3 weeks of an in-patient pulmonary rehabilitation program. Interval training: alternating between 20 sec of high-intensity and 40 sec of low-intensity training for 20 minutes. Continuous training: 20 min of continuous cycling.	Both groups showed a greater than minimally important change in the CRQ scores. Both groups showed statistically significant increases in the 6-MWT (42 m improvement in the interval exercise group after training and 37 m improvement in the continuous exercise group after training).	Changes in the 6-MWT, although statistically significant, did not approach the clinically significant difference of 54 m. Patients assigned to the interval training group had better adherence than those in the continuous training group. Therefore, it might be worth considering using interval training to improve exercise adherence.

BODE = prognostic tool that incorporates (B) body-mass index; (O) obstruction of airflow severity; (D) dyspnea; and (E) exercise capacity. COPD = chronic obstructive pulmonary disease; CRQ = Chronic Respiratory Questionnaire; FEV_1 = forced expiratory volume in 1 second; 6-MWT = 6-Minute Walk Test; QOL = quality of life; VO_2 = volume of oxygen consumed.

the exercise. There is a relationship between increasing workloads, increasing VO_2, and increasing HR, making exercising HR a practical choice for measuring and monitoring exercise intensity.[85] The **target heart rate range (THRR)** defines a wide, safe, and effective range of exercise intensity that can be performed during the treatment session. The **target heart rate (THR)** for a specific patient defines a more narrow HR (within the prescribed THRR) that will be most appropriate to ensure aerobic training and patient adherence.

A common method to determine a patient's THRR and the THR is using the heart rate reserve (HRR) method or Karvonen's formula.[75] The HRR is the difference between the resting HR (HR_{rest}) in the seated position and the maximal HR (HR_{max}) achieved on an ETT. To calculate the THRR, percentages (40% and 85%) of the HRR are added to the resting HR. Karvonen's formula for determining the upper and lower limits of the THRR is:

$$\text{Lower limit of THRR} = [(HR_{max} - HR_{rest}) \times 0.40] + HR_{rest}$$

$$\text{Upper limit of THRR} = [(HR_{max} - HR_{rest}) \times 0.85] + HR_{rest}$$

For example, a person achieves a maximal HR of 165 beats per minute (beats/min) on an ETT. The person's resting HR was 85 beats/min. The HRR is calculated to be 165 (85 = 80 beats/min; 40% of 80 beats/min (32) + resting HR (85) = 117 beats/min; 85% of 80 beats/min (68) + resting HR (85) = 153 beats/min. Thus, for this person, a THRR of 117 to 153 beats/min has been calculated from the exercise test data.

Determination of the appropriate THR is based on a complete patient's history as well as data from all tests and measurements. Patients with mild to moderate pulmonary disease may not have a pulmonary limitation to their ability to perform exercise; therefore, a maximal cardiovascular exercise test is likely to have been performed. If the patient has no other concomitant diseases, has no musculoskeletal or neurological constraints, and is committed to exercise, the higher end of the THRR could be used. For example, if the THRR was determined to be 117 to 153, the THR for this person could be at the high end or 141 to 153. If, on the other hand, the patient had other co-morbidities, such as musculoskeletal, neurological, or renal issues, and has no exercise experience, then the middle (129 to 141) or even lower (117 to 129) end of the THRR might be used.

Patients with severe pulmonary impairment will likely approach their ventilatory maximum before their cardiovascular maximum is reached; that is, their peak exercise HR may be lower than their cardiovascular HR maximum owing to pulmonary constraints. For these patients, exercise intensities that approach their maximum ventilatory symptoms can be used. This may translate into the upper end of the THRR as calculated by Karvonen's formula or even higher.[61,79] According to the *Guidelines for Pulmonary Rehabilitation* from the American College of Chest Physicians (ACCP) and the American Association of Cardiovascular and Pulmonary Rehabilitation (AACVPR), an exercise intensity that uses a high percentage of the patient's peak exercise capacity is well tolerated and physiological training effects have been documented.[79] However, they caution that lower intensity exercise may be associated with better adherence.[79] It should be emphasized that exercise intensity, when prescribed by HR, should have an upper and a lower HR limit, not a single number.

Exercise Intensity by Rating of Perceived Exertion or Rating of Perceived Dyspnea

With severe pulmonary disease, dyspnea is often reported as the limiting factor in the patient's ability to perform exercise. Using HR to prescribe exercise, as described in the previous section, does not always directly address the cause of physical limitation in patients with low ventilatory reserve. Borg's RPE is often used as a means of prescribing exercise intensity for patients with cardiovascular and pulmonary diseases.[75,86] Using the RPE scale allows the patient to self-regulate exercise intensity based on his or her perception of exertion (Table 12.8). RPE has been correlated with VO_2, making it a useful means of prescribing and monitoring exercise intensity. Perceived exertion ratings of 3, 4, and 5 were correlated with 60%, 72%, and 78% of VO_{2max}, respectively.[80] A variation of the RPE scale uses *rating of perceived dyspnea* (RPD) as a gauge for exercise intensity[87,88] (Table 12.9). Perceived dyspnea ratings between 3 (moderate SOB) and 6 (between severe and very severe SOB) define the range within which patients with pulmonary dysfunction generally exercise. A rating of up to 3 corresponds approximately to 50% of VO_{2max}. A rating of about 6 (between 4 and 8) corresponds to approximately 80% of VO_{2max}[89] (see also Chapter 13, Heart Disease, for additional information).

Clinicians often prefer to prescribe exercise by utilizing a combination of parameters (e.g., THR and RPE and RPD).

Duration

Exercising within prescribed exercise intensity for at least 20 to 30 minutes is recommended.[75] The duration of the training session varies according to patient tolerance, with some participants not being able to

---

Table 12.8	Rating of Perceived Exertion: The Borg CR10 Scale	
The Borg CR10 Scale®		
0	Nothing at all	"No P"
0.3		
0.5	Extremely weak	Just noticeable
1	Very weak	
1.5		
2	Weak	Light
2.5		
3	Moderate	
4		
5	Strong	Heavy
6		
7	Very strong	
8		
9		
10	Extremely strong	"Max P"
11		
12	Absolute maximum	Highest possible

Note: For correct usage of the scale, the exact design and instructions given in Borg's folders must be followed. The scale with correct instructions can be obtained from Borg Perception (see the Borg Perception website at www.borgperception.se). Also see Borg, G. Borg's Perceived Exertion and Pain Scales. Human Kinetics, Champaign, IL, 1998. Reprinted with permission.

Table 12.9	Rating of Perceived Shortness of Breath
Scale	Perceived Shortness of Breath
0	Nothing at all
0.5	Very, very slight (just noticeable)
1	Very slight
2	Slight
3	Moderate
4	Somewhat severe
5	Severe
6	
7	Very severe
8	
9	Very, very severe (almost maximal)
10	Maximal

maintain continuous exercise for 20 to 30 minutes. Frequent rest periods can be interspersed with exercise to accomplish a total of 20 to 30 minutes of discontinuous exercise.

Frequency

The frequency of exercise refers to the number of sessions performed on a weekly basis during the exercise-training period. The frequency of exercise is often dependent on the intensity that can be achieved and the duration that can be maintained. If 20 to 30 minutes of continuous aerobic exercise can be accomplished within the THR, then three to five evenly spaced workouts per week are recommended. More frequent exercise sessions are recommended for patients with lower functional abilities. One to two daily sessions are advisable for patients with very low functional work capacities.

Pulmonary Rehabilitation

Aerobic Training

The aerobic exercise training portion of a pulmonary rehabilitation session includes the following components: check-in, warm-up, aerobic exercise, and cooldown. The check-in period is a time to obtain baseline data, including resting HR, respiratory rate, BP, oxygen saturation, auscultation of the lungs, and weight. It is also the time to discuss medication schedules, any problems the patient may have encountered since last visit, and any changes that need to be addressed by a member of the pulmonary rehabilitation team, such as a change in flow rates, cough, or sputum production. If the patient were found to have a significant decrease in FEV_1 on the ETT, a maintenance drug would typically be prescribed to reduce or minimize pulmonary symptoms. PFTs with a handheld device may be performed pre and post exercise to assess the impact of the maintenance medication. The potential need for use of a beta-2 adrenergic inhaler before exercise should be determined. If a patient is found to have a significant decrease in oxygenation with exercise, supplemental oxygen should be readied before initiation of physical activity.

The warm-up component is a time to slowly increase the HR and BP to ready the cardiovascular system for aerobic exercise. For those patients with mild to moderate lung disease who had a cardiovascular end point to their exercise test, the warm-up is usually accomplished by performing the same mode of exercise that will be used in the aerobic portion of the program but at a lower intensity, with an emphasis on controlled breathing. For example, cycling with no resistance could be used as a warm-up activity for a biking program. The warm-up for patients performing continuous exercise lasts between 5 and 10 minutes. For patients with severe lung disease who are prescribed short bursts of high-intensity exercise, there is little opportunity for a warm-up. In these situations, the program should be designed so that each exercise bout of the circuit gradually builds on the previous exercise to ramp up activity.

The aerobic portion of the exercise session consists of a mode or modes of aerobic activity at the appropriate intensity to maintain the THR of the exercise prescription for the advised duration. This portion of the program lasts for at least 20 minutes of either continuous or discontinuous activity. Participant monitoring can be accomplished using RPE and RPD scales, and measures of HR, respiratory rate, and S_aO_2 (oximetry).

The aerobic training period should be followed immediately by a cool-down period consisting of a slow decline in exercise intensity as the patient nears completion of the circuit. This may consist of 5 to 10 minutes of low-level aerobic activities that slowly return the cardiovascular system to near pre-exercise levels or ramping down of the intensity of short bouts of exercise. Again, there is an emphasis on controlled breathing.

Finally, stretching exercises are performed to maintain joint and muscle integrity and to help prevent injury. Stretching exercises should be performed during exhalation to prevent a **Valsalva** maneuver, which would worsen a participant's pulmonary capabilities. Patients often use accessory muscles of ventilation during the exercise program; therefore, the muscles of the neck and UEs should be incorporated into the stretching program.

General Strength Training

Extremity Training

While cardiopulmonary endurance training through aerobic exercise is the mainstay of pulmonary rehabilitation, generalized strength training has been found to counter the systemic effects of COPD that result in peripheral and ventilatory muscle weakness. Strength of both UEs and LEs has been shown to increase with appropriate training. Strength training can use similar modes of exercise as the endurance training with a change to higher resistance and lower repetitions (i.e., increase the grade of treadmill, increase resistance on stationary cycle or arm ergometer), or weight training of the targeted muscle groups can be prescribed. Participants should be encouraged to refrain from using the Valsalva maneuver during training because this may impair ventilatory exchange and affect exercise performance.

Ventilatory muscle training

Patients with COPD may have weak inspiratory muscles that translate into breathlessness and exercise limitations.[79] Ventilatory muscle training devices provide resistance to the inspiratory phase, the expiratory phase, or both phases of ventilation in order to increase the strength and endurance of the muscles of ventilation. Figure 12.13 shows one type of ventilatory muscle training device (Philips Healthcare, Andover, MA). Many research studies have demonstrated the ability to increase ventilatory muscle strength and endurance using these loading devices, especially in the presence of known

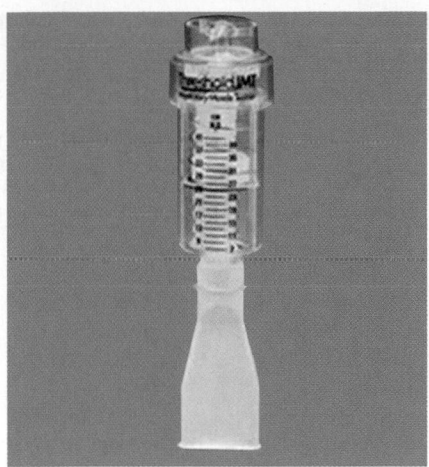

Figure 12.13 A type of ventilatory muscle training device. This is a Threshold® inspiratory muscle trainer for use in improving strength and endurance of the muscles of inspiration. *(Photo courtesy of Phillips Respironics, Murrysville, PA.)*

respiratory muscle weakness.[90-94] Ventilatory muscle trainers have also been studied for their ability to alter the perception of dyspnea. A number of researchers have demonstrated a decrease in the severity of dyspnea with ventilatory muscle training during the performance of ADL and during exercise.[92,95,97,98] Current research on the benefits of ventilatory muscle training can be found in Box 12.4 Evidence Summary.

Whether training the muscles of ventilation alone translates directly into a clinically significant functional improvement is still not clear. Statistically significant changes in 6-MWT and 10-MSWT data have been demonstrated with ventilatory muscle training.[92,93,95,98] However, these changes do not always translate into a clinically significant improvement. For example, a change of greater than 54 meters needs to be realized on a 6-MWT in order to be clinically significant.[69] Although Hill et al[98] found a statistically significant increase in distance on the 6-MWT in those patients in the ventilatory muscle treatment group, the increase

Box 12.4 Evidence Summary   Ventilatory Muscle Training

Reference	Subjects	Design/Intervention	Duration	Results	Comments
Scherer et al[91] (2000)	30 patients with COPD, FEV_1 50%–52% predicted, <15% improvement in FFV_1 with bronchodilation	RCT using two groups: 1. Treatment: respiratory muscle endurance training using a ventilatory muscle training device 2. Control: use of incentive spirometry	Both groups trained twice daily, 15 min per session, 5 days per week for 8 weeks. Treatment group: training apparatus was set at frequency of 60% MV and tidal volume of 50%–60% VC.	Significant increase in respiratory muscle endurance post training. Significant increases in PE_{max}, 6-MWT, VO_2 peak and physical components of SF12 after training. No difference between groups in PI_{max} or mental component of the SF12 after training. No difference between groups in dyspnea index or treadmill endurance after training.	Training apparatus was not a threshold or resistance trainer, but a device that used a fixed tidal volume (TV) and frequency rather than resistance to provide the endurance training.
Riera et al[92] (2001)	20 patients with severe COPD FEV_1 <50%	Randomized control trial using 2 groups: 1. Treatment: IMT at 60% of SIP_{max} 2. Control: zero resistance applied through flowmeter	Treatment and control groups: 15 min of training on device, 2×/day, 6 days/wk for 6 months. Both groups used flowmeter, with different	Significant increase in SIP_{max} and PI_{max} after training. Significant increase in SWT distance after training. Significant decrease in dyspnea after training.	Home-based program training was at 60% of sustained inspiratory pressure, that is, approximately 30% of PI_{max}. Device controlled

Continued

Box 12.4 Evidence Summary   Ventilatory Muscle Training—cont'd

Reference	Subjects	Design/ Intervention	Duration	Results	Comments
		resistances (see design).		Significant improvement in CRQ scores (QOL). No significant change in $VO_{2\,max}$, VE_{max}, or W_{max} was found in either group after training. No significant change in rate of perceived exertion was found in either group after training.	inhalation and exhalation time via visual feedback.
Weiner et al[93] (2003)	32 patients with COPD, FEV_1 < 50% predicted	Randomized control trial using 3 treatment groups + 1 control group: 1. SIMT group: high-load IMT and low-load EMT 2. SEMT group: high-load EMT and low-load IMT 3. SEMT and SIMT group: high-load IMT and EMT 4. Control group: low-load IMT and EMT	1 hr/day (30 min of IMT and 30 min of EMT), 6 days/wk for 3 months. High load was ramped up to 60% of max by the end of first month. Low load was 7 cm H_2O pressure.	Groups that trained inspiratory muscles showed a significant increase in PI_{max}. Groups that trained expiratory muscles showed a significant increase in PE_{max}. Significant increase in 6-MWT in treatment groups. Significant change in dyspnea scores in only the SIMT and SEMT + SIMT group. Significant change in perception of dyspnea in only the SIMT and SEMT + SIMT group.	Small sample size of only 8 participants per group. Increases in 6-MWT were statistically significant but the SEMT and the SEMT + SIMT did not reach clinical significance for improvement in that test (>54 m).
Beckerman et al[95] (2005)	42 patients with COPD, FEV_1 < 50% predicted	Randomized control trial using 2 groups: 1. Treatment: began IMT with 15% of PI_{max} load, increasing to 60% by 4 weeks, and increased to maintain 60% of new weekly PI_{max}	Both groups trained for 15 min, 2 times/day, 6 days a week for 12 months. Training for the first month was onsite in the rehabilitation center, the next 11 months was at home with daily phone calls and	6-MWT—significant increase in the treatment group beginning at 3 months with small gains following during next 9 months. No change in the control group. Inspiratory muscle strength: statistically significant in-	Daily contact for 1 year by a health care professional is unreasonable; therefore the ability to replicate this study is questioned. 11 out of 42 participants did not complete the program (6 were deaths).

Box 12.4 Evidence Summary Ventilatory Muscle Training—cont'd

Reference	Subjects	Design/ Intervention	Duration	Results	Comments
		2. Control: trained with S-IMT at a low load known to not improve inspiratory muscle strength	weekly home visits. Assessments were at 3, 6, 9, and 12 months.	crease in PI_{max} in the treatment group (not in the control group) starting at 3 months and continuing throughout the course of study. Dyspnea: treatment group showed a significant decrease in dyspnea beginning at 6 months compared to the control group. HRQOL as measured by SGRQ improved significantly over the control group beginning at 6 months.	There was a decrease in hospital length of stays among the treatment group; the number of exacerbations requiring hospitalization was similar between groups.
Weiner and Weiner[96] (2006)	28 patients with COPD (FEV$_1$ of 36%–39% predicted) and documented inspiratory muscle weakness	Randomized control trial using 2 groups: 1. Treatment: began IMT with 15% of PI_{max} load, increasing to 60% by 4 weeks, and increased to maintain 60% of new weekly PI_{max} 2. Control: IMT at a steady load of 7 cm H_2O	Training was 6 days per week, 1 hr/day for 8 weeks for each group.	Statistically significant increase in the PI_{max} in the training group (46.1 to 58.7 cm H_2O), no change in the control group.	The increase in PI_{max} was also correlated to an increase in peak inspiratory flow rates. These higher flow rates would improve the drug deposition to the lungs when using a dry powder inhaler.
Magadle et al[97] (2007)	34 patients with COPD (FEV$_1$ 45%–46% predicted) currently enrolled in a 12-week pulmonary rehabilitation program of GER	Randomized control trial using 2 groups of IMT or S-IMT in addition to continued GER for another 6 months: 1. Treatment group began IMT training with 15% of PI_{max} load increasing to 60%	Pulmonary rehabilitation program was 1.5 hr/day, 3 times per week for the first 12 weeks. Second 6 months included 1 hr/day, 3 days/ week of GER for both groups. IMT was performed daily, 6×/wk for the next 8 weeks.	Following the first 12 weeks of GER, there was significant increase in 6-MWT for all participants. There was no significant improvement in perceived dyspnea or SGRQ scores. After the addition of IMT and S-IMT to GER, there was	The addition of the IMT caused changes in QOL measures and dyspnea ratings that were not found in pulmonary rehabilitation programs of GER alone. As patient's chief complaint is often dyspnea or loss of

Continued

Box 12.4 Evidence Summary   Ventilatory Muscle Training—cont'd

Reference	Subjects	Design/Intervention	Duration	Results	Comments
		by 4 weeks, and increased to maintain 60% of new weekly PI_{max} 2. Control group used S-IMT, the same device as the treatment group but set at a fixed, sufficiently low load that would not provide a training effect	It is difficult to distinguish between how the treatment and control groups were handled.	no further improvement in the 6-MWT in either group. The treatment group showed a significant increase in PI_{max}, and significant improvement in perceived dyspnea and in the SGRQ when compared to the control group.	function, this article is compelling in its recommendation to add IMT to an already existing pulmonary rehabilitation program.
Hill et al[98] (2006)	35 subjects with COPD (FEV_1 of 37.4% predicted)	Randomized control trial using 2 groups: 1. Treatment (H-IMT) used the maximum load tolerable for 2 min followed by 1 min rest, repeated 7 times 2. Control: S-IMT used a constant load of 10% of baseline PI_{max} throughout training	Sessions were 21 min, 3×/wk for 8 weeks for both groups.	Inspiratory muscle strength significantly increased by 29% in the H-IMT, whereas the S-IMT group increased by 8%. Inspiratory muscle endurance increased by 56% in the H-IMT group whereas the S-IMT group remained unchanged. 6-MWT increased by 27 m in the H-IMT group, with no change in the S-IMT group. QOL measures in the dyspnea and mastery domains increased in both groups. The H-IMT group also showed improvements in the domains of fatigue and emotional functioning.	Although the results show an increase of 27 m in the 6-MWT, an increase of 54 m is necessary in order to be clinically significant. Therefore, although there is a significant change in the 6-MWT, this will not necessarily relate to clinical improvement.

6-MWT = 6-Minute Walk Test; CRQ = Chronic Respiratory Questionnaire; EMT = expiratory muscle training; GER = general exercise reconditioning; GXT = Graded Exercise Test; H-IMT = high-intensity inspiratory muscle training; HRQOL = health-related quality of life; IMT = inspiratory muscle training; MIP = maximal inspiratory pressure; MVV = maximal voluntary ventilation; PE_{max} = maximal expiratory pressure; PI_{max} = maximal inspiratory pressure; QOL = quality of life; SEMT = specific expiratory muscle training; SF12 = Short Form 12; SGRQ = St. George's Respiratory Questionnaire; S-IMT = sham inspiratory muscle training; SIMT = specific inspiratory muscle training; SIP_{max} = maximal sustained inspiratory pressure; SWT: 10-Meter Shuttle Walk Test; VE_{max} = maximum minute ventilation; $VO_{2\ max}$ = maximal oxygen uptake; W_{max} = maximum workload.

was less than 54 meters, meaning that the increase may not be of clinical value. Following a meta-analysis, Lotters et al[90] indicate that the ability to affect functional improvement by the use of ventilatory muscle training is yet to be determined. In patients with severe pulmonary disease and documented ventilatory muscle weakness, training improved their ventilatory muscle strength and endurance and decreased dyspnea.[79,94] However, in patients with mild to moderate pulmonary disease, training did not significantly improve ventilatory muscle function. The use of a specific ventilatory muscle training device should be made individually, based on the type of disease, the severity of disease, the presence of inspiratory muscle weakness, and the motivation of the participant.[79]

Exercise Progression

A patient's age, functional ability, symptoms, and severity of disease should be considered before any change in the exercise prescription. Exercise progression is appropriate when the individual perceives the exercise session to be easier (lower RPE or target dyspnea) or when the same exercise workload is performed with a lower HR, that is, as the individual physiologically adapts to exercise.

Exercise progression should first be directed toward increasing the number of continuous minutes of exercise and decreasing the amount of time spent in low-intensity exercise or rest periods. When 20 minutes of continuous activity can be accomplished, an increase in exercise duration or intensity can be proposed. Frequency should be adjusted as necessary, based on duration and intensity.

Program Duration

Improved exercise tolerance can occur in multiple settings: an inpatient rehabilitation hospital program, an outpatient pulmonary rehabilitation program, or a home-based program.[1] Because of the limited length of stay for many inpatient rehabilitation hospital admissions, most increases in functional capacity occur in an outpatient or home pulmonary rehabilitation program. Generally, conditioning exercises are conducted up to three times per week over a course of 6 to 12 weeks.[79] At the end of the rehabilitation program, QOL measurements and dyspnea measurements should be readministered to assess the benefits of pulmonary rehabilitation for each participant. A follow-up 6-MWT or a 10-MSWT should be repeated at the end of the program to assess the change in aerobic conditioning of each participant. Exercise abilities gained in a pulmonary rehabilitation program have been found to gradually decline over 12 to 18 months following completion of the program. Pulmonary rehabilitation programs that last longer than 12 weeks have shown greater sustained benefits than shorter programs.[79]

An unfortunate reality is that patients with pulmonary dysfunction often have decreased exercise ability following an exacerbation of their disease. It is currently not clear that repeated bouts of pulmonary rehabilitation are beneficial to patients with pulmonary disease.[99] Continued support in the form of self-help groups and community exercise groups is essential to maintaining the new level of physical activity obtained with pulmonary rehabilitation.[1]

Home Exercise Programs

A home exercise program (HEP) begins while the participant is enrolled in a pulmonary rehabilitation program. When deemed appropriate (based on exercise response and laboratory data), the participant can be assigned home exercise activities. The patient uses an exercise log to record parameters such as exercise HRs, RPEs, exercise workloads, and any questions that may arise about the HEP (Fig. 12.14). At regular intervals, the therapist analyzes the data and adjusts the HEP as necessary. Progression to an independent HEP is an important rehabilitation goal to promote a participant's lifelong commitment to exercise.

Multispecialty Team

Although aerobic exercise training is integral to pulmonary rehabilitation, patients require additional services and information to optimize their exercise capability and to improve quality of life. The following sections address other elements of a pulmonary rehabilitation program: patient education, secretion removal techniques, and **activity pacing**. Smoking cessation should also be considered as a component of pulmonary rehabilitation. (See the section on smoking cessation in the medical management section of this chapter.)

Patient Education

The concept of self-management is promoted in the individual and group educational sessions of a pulmonary rehabilitation program.[79] Participants are given individual, one-on-one time to identify their own needs and address issues that are particular to themselves. Benefits from group discussions include support from peers regarding the patient's feelings or needs, learning from others' experiences and questions, and the socialization only a group can provide. Key components of a patient's education program are presented in Box 12.5.

Education makes it possible for patients to assume the responsibility for their own wellness. A patient will carry out the required activities to produce the desired outcome only if the patient knows what to do, knows how to do it, and also wants to do it. This theory of self-efficacy for the patient with pulmonary disease begins with a daily routine that includes self-assessment, adherence to a medication schedule, performance of airway clearance techniques, ADL with pacing, and an appropriate HEP.

Self-assessment is used to recognize the first sign of an exacerbation of the disease: increased dyspnea, decreased

Activity Log

Week of: _____

Aerobic exercise

	Monday	Tuesday	Wednesday	Thursday	Friday	Saturday	Sunday
Mode							
Average HR							
Average RPE							
Average dyspnea							
Start time							
End time							
Comments:							

Strengthening exercise:

	Monday	Tuesday	Wednesday	Thursday	Friday	Saturday	Sunday
Type							
Weight							
# of reps							
Comments:							

Figure 12.14 An exercise log that can be used to follow a patient's ability to exercise both during and independent of the pulmonary rehabilitation program.

Box 12.5   Education Topics

- Anatomy and Physiology of Respiratory Disease
- Airway Clearance Techniques
- Nutritional Guidelines
- Energy-Saving Techniques
- Stress Management and Relaxation
- Benefits of Being Smoke Free
- Impact of Environmental Factors on COPD
- Pharmacology/Use of MDIs
- Oxygen Delivery Systems
- Psychosocial Aspects of COPD
- Diagnostic Techniques
- Management of COPD
- Community Resources
- Exercise: Effects, Contraindications, Adherence

COPD = chronic obstructive pulmonary disease; MDIs = metered-dose inhalers.

exercise tolerance; change in pulmonary flow rates, sputum color or consistency; pedal edema; or any other significant change from baseline. An exacerbation protocol is individually devised that includes a set of standard instructions consistent with the participant's disease and abilities. These instructions may include the use of airway clearance techniques, pacing techniques, or a change in the exercise prescription, as well as contact with the primary care physician for a review of symptoms and pharmacological management.

Managing lung disease can be taught through educational programs that address the needs of individuals with pulmonary disorders. Compared to general education alone, education as part of an individualized comprehensive pulmonary rehabilitation program produced significantly improved exercise abilities, decreased dyspnea, and greater self-efficacy.[100] Once the patient has progressed through pulmonary rehabilitation, access to new information and continued support is possible through community support groups (e.g., the *Better Breathing Club*, sponsored by the American Lung Association).

Secretion Removal Techniques

Secretion retention can interfere with ventilation and the diffusion of oxygen and carbon dioxide in some patients with pulmonary disease. Patients with secretion retention may improve their exercise performance if proper secretion removal techniques have been performed before the physical activity. The preferred practice pattern from the *Guide to Physical Therapist Practice* for these individuals would be 6C-1: Impaired ventilation, respiration, and aerobic capacity associated with airway clearance dysfunction.[53] An individualized program of secretion removal techniques directed to the areas of involvement can optimize ventilation and therefore gas exchange capabilities. Secretion removal techniques include dependent programs that rely on a caregiver (postural drainage, percussion, and shaking) or independent programs, such as the active cycle of breathing technique (ACBT); positive expiratory pressure (PEP), such as the TheraPEP® PEP Therapy System (Smiths Medical, Dublin, OH); airway oscillation devices, such as the Flutter® (Cardinal Health, Dublin, OH) or the Acapella® (Smiths Medical, Dublin, OH); or high-frequency chest compression (HFCC) devices such as The Vest® System (Hill-Rom, St. Paul, MN).

Manual Secretion Removal Techniques

Postural Drainage

Positioning a patient so that the bronchus of the involved lung segment is perpendicular to the ground is the basis for **postural drainage**. Using gravity, these positions assist the mucociliary transport system in removing excessive secretions from the tracheobronchial tree. Standard postural drainage positions are presented in Fig. 12.15. Although these postural drainage positions are optimal for gravity drainage of specific lung segments, such positioning may not be realistic for some patients. Modification of these standard positions may prevent any untoward effects yet still enhance secretion removal. Box 12.6 lists precautions that should be considered before instituting postural drainage with patients with signs and symptoms of increased daily pulmonary secretions. These are not absolute contraindications, but relative precautions. The list is not meant to be inclusive; however, it does provide a range of considerations that should be addressed before instituting postural drainage.

Percussion

Percussion is a force rhythmically applied with the therapist's cupped hands to the patient's chest wall. The percussion technique is applied to a specific area on the thorax that corresponds to an underlying involved lung segment. The technique is typically administered for 3 to 5 minutes over each involved lung segment. Percussion

is thought to release the pulmonary secretions from the wall of the airways and into the lumen of the airway. By coupling percussion with the appropriate postural drainage position for a specific lung segment, the probability of secretion removal is enhanced. Because percussion is a force directed to the thorax, there are conditions that would necessitate caution with this technique, such as a fractured rib, a flail chest, osteoporosis, elevated coagulation studies, or a decreased platelet count. These examples are by no means inclusive, but they provide some patient presentations that might require modification (a gentler force applied to the thorax) or elimination of the percussion technique.

Shaking

Following a deep inhalation, a bouncing maneuver is applied with the therapist's open hands to the rib cage throughout the expiratory phase of breathing. This **shaking** is applied to a specific area on the thorax that corresponds to the underlying involved lung segment. Five to seven deep breaths with shaking on exhalation are appropriate to hasten the removal of secretions via the mucociliary transport system. Shaking is commonly used following percussion in the appropriate postural drainage position. Because this technique consists of a force applied to the thorax, the same circulatory and musculoskeletal considerations are needed as in the application of percussion.

Airway Clearance

Once the secretions have been mobilized with postural drainage, percussion, and shaking, the task of removing the secretions from the airways is undertaken using an airway clearance technique. Coughing is the most common and easiest means of clearing the airway. However, it should be noted that high intrathoracic pressures, such as those generated during coughing, could force the closing of small airways in some patients with obstructive pulmonary diseases. By trapping air behind the closed airway, the forced expulsion of air during a cough becomes ineffective in clearing secretions. Huffing is an alternative method of airway clearance that is useful for patients with obstructive pulmonary disease. A huff uses many of the same steps of coughing, without creating the high intrathoracic pressures. The patient is asked to take a deep breath and then rapidly contract the abdominal muscles while forcefully saying "HA HA HA." This allows a forced expiration through a stabilized open airway and makes secretion removal more effective.[101]

Active Cycle of Breathing Techniques

ACBT is an independent breathing exercise program the patient can perform to clear secretions from the airways that includes (1) a breathing control phase; (2) thoracic expansion exercises; and (3) a forced expiratory technique. ACBT begins with a few minutes of the breathing

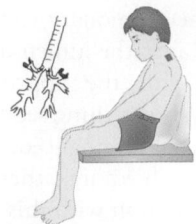

UPPER LOBES Apical Segments

Bed or drainage table flat.

Patient leans back on pillow at 30° angle against therapist.

Therapist claps with markedly cupped hand over area between clavicle and top of scapula on each side.

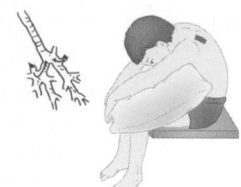

UPPER LOBES Posterior Segments

Bed or drainage table flat.

Patient leans over folded pillow at 30° angle.

Therapist stands behind and claps over upper back on both sides.

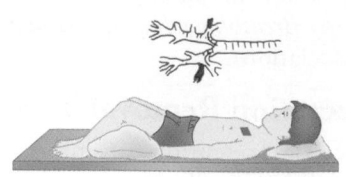

UPPER LOBES Anterior Segments

Bed or drainage table flat.

Patient lies on back with pillow under knees.

Therapist claps between clavicle and nipple on each side.

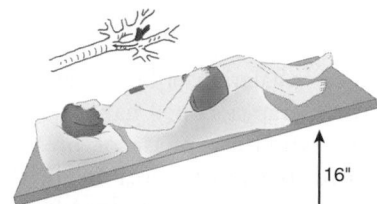

16"

RIGHT MIDDLE LOBE

Foot of table or bed elevated 16 inches.

Patient lies head down on left side and rotates 1/4 turn backward. Pillow may be placed behind from shoulder to hip. Knees should be flexed.

Therapist claps over right nipple area. In females with breast development or tenderness use cupped hand with heel of hand under armpit and fingers extending forward beneath the breast.

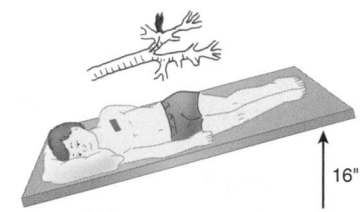

16"

LEFT UPPER LOBE Singular Segments

Foot of table or bed elevated 16 inches.

Patient lies head down on right side and rotates 1/4 turn backward. Pillow may be placed behind from shoulder to hip. Knees should be flexed.

Therapist claps with moderately cupped hand over left nipple area. In females with breast development or tenderness use cupped hand with heel of hand under armpit and fingers extending forward beneath the breast.

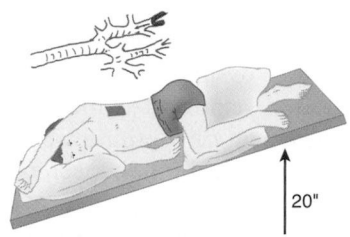

20"

LOWER LOBES Anterior Basal Segments

Foot of table or bed elevated 20 inches.

Patient lies on side, head down, pillow under knees.

Therapist claps with slightly cupped hand over lower ribs. (Position shown is for drainage of left anterior basal segment. To drain the right anterior basal segment, patient should be on the left side in same posture).

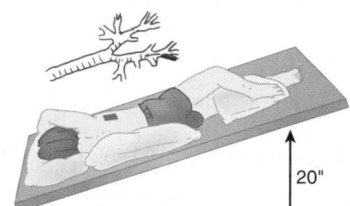

20"

LOWER LOBES Lateral Basal Segments

Foot of table or bed elevated 20 inches.

Patient lies on abdomen, head down, then rotates 1/4 turn upward. Upper leg is flexed over pillow for support.

Therapist claps over uppermost portion of lower ribs. (Position shown is for drainage of right lateral basal segment. To drain the left lateral basal segment, patient should lie on the right side in the same posture).

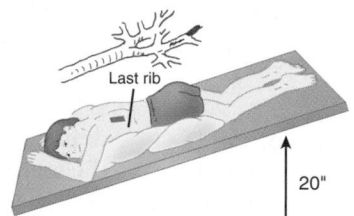

Last rib

20"

LOWER LOBES Posterior Basal Segments

Foot of table or bed elevated 20 inches.

Patient lies on abdomen, head down, with pillow under hips.

Therapist claps over lower ribs close to spine on each side.

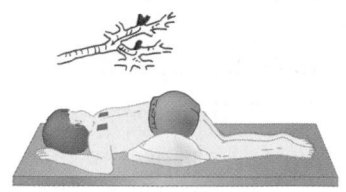

LOWER LOBES Superior Segments

Bed of table flat.

Patient lies on abdomen with two pillows under hips.

Therapist claps over middle of back at tip of scapula on either side of spine.

Figure 12.15 Positions used for postural drainage. *(From Rothstein, J, Roy, S, and Wolf, S: The Rehabilitation Specialist's Handbook, ed 3. FA Davis, Philadelphia, 2005, p 444, with permission.)*

control phase, defined as relaxed, diaphragmatic, tidal volume breathing. Three to four thoracic expansion exercises, defined as deep inhalations with a 3-second hold followed by a passive exhalation, are performed next. A return to the breathing control phase follows. Depending on the patient's needs, this breathing control phase can last for seconds to minutes. If the patient feels that there are secretions ready to be moved upward, then the forced expiratory technique completes the cycle. If secretions are not ready to be moved, the patient returns to thoracic expansion exercises followed by another period of breathing control for rest and for the patient to assess the status of secretions is their airways. The forced expiratory technique, defined as one or two huffs from tidal volume down to low lung volumes, is used to move secretions higher into the larger airways. The forced expiratory technique is followed by a rest period of breathing control. Using ACBT, secretions are "milked" from smaller to larger airways. Once the secretions have moved into the larger airways, huffs from mid or high lung volumes remove the secretions from the airways. This independent technique has been demonstrated to

Precautions for Postural Drainage

Precautions for the use of the supine, head lower than feet (Trendelenburg) position:

- Circulatory: Congestive heart failure, hypertension
- Pulmonary: Pulmonary edema, shortness of breath made worse with lowered head position
- Abdominal: Obesity, abdominal distention, hiatal hernia, nausea, recent food consumption, or any patient-specific precautions

Precautions for the use of the side-lying position:

- Vascular: Axillofemoral bypass graft
- Musculoskeletal: Arthritis, recent rib fracture, shoulder bursitis, tendonitis, or any patient-specific precautions

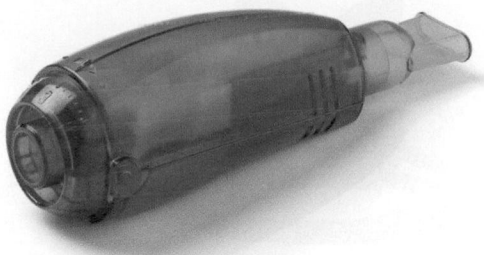

Figure 12.17 The Acapella® device used for an independent program of secretion removal. *(Courtesy of Smith Medical, Dublin OH, 43017.)*

be as effective as postural drainage, percussion, and shaking.[102] Figure 12.16 emphasizes that the patient begins at breathing control and always returns to breathing control for rest and the patient's own assessment of his or her status before moving to either thoracic expansion with breath hold or the forced expiratory technique.

Oral Airway Oscillation Devices

Airway oscillation devices, such as the Flutter® or the Acapella® (Fig. 12.17), alter the exhaled airflow throughout the airways. The patient inhales a normal size breath. During active exhalation through the device, the exhaled air causes an intermittent backward air pressure that jars the airways. The usual procedure is to exhale 10 or so breaths through the device, followed by two large exhaled volumes through the device and finally a huff or

cough to clear mobilized secretions. This routine is repeated until secretions are cleared from the lungs. An airway oscillation device has been shown to help in the removal of secretions from airways.[103,104]

Positive Expiratory Pressure

PEP devices include a valve to regulate expiratory resistance (Fig. 12.18). Inhalation of a normal size breath through the mask or mouthpiece is unresisted. Active exhalation is against a positive expiratory pressure, measuring 10 to 20 cm H_2O. A treatment session lasts approximately 10 to 20 minutes with frequent pauses to remove the mask so that the patient can huff to clear secretions. The session is completed when all secretions have been cleared from the airways. PEP has been shown to be as effective as postural drainage, percussion, and shaking.[105,106]

High-Frequency Chest Compression Devices

HFCC devices use an inflatable vest with air channels that is worn over the patient's thorax (Fig. 12.19). The vest is attached to an air compressor that rapidly delivers small air volumes in and out of the vest. The inflation of the vest causes compression to the chest wall and the deflation allows the chest wall to recoil back to its resting position. The patient assumes a comfortable seated position for treatments lasting between 20 and 30 minutes. Secretions may be huffed clear any time throughout the

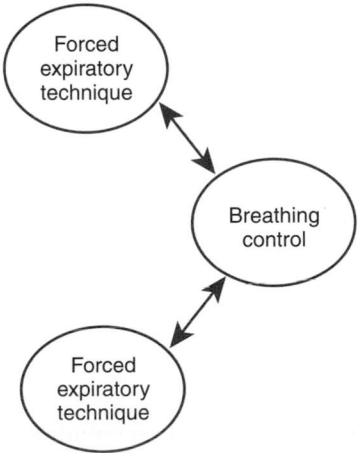

Figure 12.16 Active cycle of breathing begins with breathing control. All choices are made from the breathing control phase. After each choice is made, thoracic expansion or forced expiratory technique, the patient returns to breathing control to rest and make the next choice.

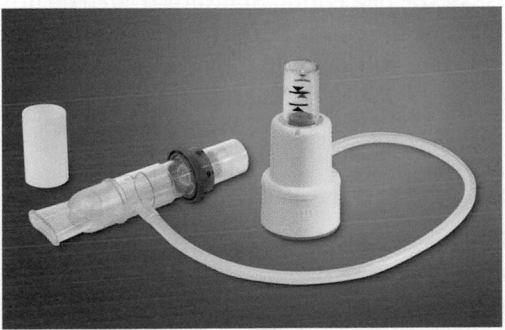

Figure 12.18 The PEP system for an independent program of secretion removal. *(Courtesy of Smith Medical, Dublin OH, 43017.)*

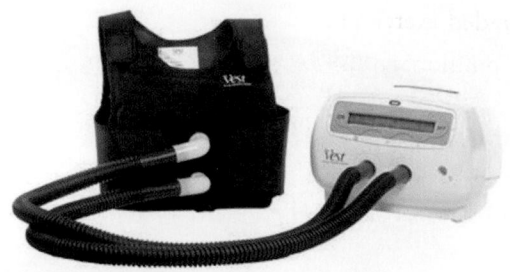

Figure 12.19 The high-frequency chest wall compression device (the vest) can be used for an independent program of secretion removal. *(Courtesy of Hill-Rom, St. Paul, MN 55126.)*

treatment. High-frequency chest wall compression has been shown to be as effective as other secretion removal techniques.[107]

Breathing Exercises

Pursed-lip breathing involves an unresisted inspiration followed by an active oral exhalation through a narrowed (or pursed) mouth opening. When pursed-lip breathing is used by patients with COPD, it may delay or prevent airway collapse, allowing for better gas exchange.[108,109] Most patients demonstrate this strategy during periods of dyspnea and rarely need to be taught the technique.

Although diaphragmatic breathing has been taught to patients with chronic pulmonary dysfunction for years, there is little evidence to support its use to improve pulmonary mechanics.[109] Some patients require the use of accessory muscles with exercise, with exacerbation of their disease, or with periods of dyspnea. Strengthening accessory muscles of ventilation may be a more effective treatment program than encouraging the use of an ineffective diaphragm with little ability to generate muscle force and/or limited muscle excursion. In patients with very flat diaphragms, focusing on diaphragmatic breathing may even be detrimental.

Activity Pacing

Activity pacing refers to the performance of any activity within the limits or boundaries of that patient's breathing capacity. For example, an activity that usually causes dyspnea needs to be broken down into component parts such that each component can be performed at a rate that does not exceed breathing abilities. By breaking activities down into component parts and interspersing rest periods between each component, the total activity can be completed without dyspnea or undo fatigue. For example, patients often find that climbing stairs causes a great deal of dyspnea and discomfort. Rather than climbing the entire flight of stairs (usually done too fast and with a breath hold), the patient might be instructed as follows: *"Take a deep breath. Now, on exhalation, walk up one (or two or three) stair(s). Now recover. Take in another good breath and walk up the next one (or two or three) stair(s) and recover. Repeat this technique until the flight of stairs is completed."* The patient is able to reach the top of the stairs without becoming dyspneic and without undue fatigue. Pacing can and should be part of every activity that would otherwise cause dyspnea. Pacing should be used when performing ADL, ambulation, stair climbing, and other daily tasks. Pacing is not a technique to be used during the aerobic portion of a pulmonary rehabilitation program. During exercise, some shortness of breath is expected to occur.

SUMMARY

Pulmonary rehabilitation programs are a well-established treatment for patients with chronic pulmonary disease. Components of these programs typically include exercise training, strength training, education, secretion removal instruction, and psychosocial support. Outcomes of pulmonary rehabilitation may include increased aerobic capacity, increased skeletal muscle strength, reduced dyspnea both during exercise and ADL, and an increase in the perception of health-related quality of life. Gains made in pulmonary rehabilitation programs can make the difference between a lifestyle of dependence and one of independence. Physical therapists have the important role of evaluating patients, determining their potential, and, through exercise prescription and exercise programs, ensuring that rehabilitation goals and outcomes are realized.

Questions for Review

1. How does the clinical presentation of obstructive lung disease differ from the clinical presentation of restrictive lung disease?

2. Explain how altered airway structure leads to airflow limitation.

3. (a) What would be the expected breath sounds of a patient with COPD (describe intensity and adventitious sounds)? (b) What would be the expected breath sounds of a patient with asthma during an exacerbation (describe intensity and adventitious sounds)?

4. Identify the tests and measures required to determine the extent of pulmonary disease.

5. What are the pulmonary end points to a symptom-limited graded exercise test?

6. How does exercise prescription differ for a patient with mild pulmonary disease as compared to the patient with severe pulmonary disease?

7. (a) How do you know when to progress a patient's exercise program? (b) What is the nature of that progression? (c) Do you need a new ETT to progress a patient's exercise workload?

8. How would you respond to a patient's comment that it would take longer to climb stairs with pacing than without?

9. Design a secretion removal treatment plan for a patient with CF that can be carried out independently before coming to pulmonary rehabilitation.

10. What evidence is presented in the current literature regarding the benefits of pulmonary rehabilitation?

CASE STUDY: PATIENT WITH COPD

A 67-year-old white female was admitted to the hospital with a diagnosis of acute bacterial pneumonia. She was treated with mechanical ventilation for 5 days, steroids, antibiotics, and bronchodilators. After the acute care hospital stay of 7 days, the patient was transferred to an inpatient rehabilitation facility for 7 days. She is now referred to outpatient pulmonary rehabilitation.

PAST MEDICAL HISTORY
COPD, pneumonia four times over the past 2 years, s/p lumpectomy of right breast 8 years ago, smoking history of 45 pack/years; quit on day of admission to hospital for acute bacterial pneumonia.

MEDICATIONS
2 L/min of pulsed oxygen, Atrovent (maintenance, anticholinergic) 4 puffs qid, albuterol (rescue, beta-2 adrenergic) 2 puffs PRN, prednisone (maintenance, anti-inflammatory) 5 mg/day.

OCCUPATION
Secretary, works 32 hours/week. Presently on medical leave.

SOCIAL AND ENVIRONMENTAL
Lives with husband in own home. Three steps to enter home, 12 stairs within the home.

OBJECTIVE FINDINGS
Interview
Mental status: awake, alert, talks in three- to four-word sentences. Adequate historian. Chief complaint: shortness of breath limiting function. Patient is able to walk 150 ft before needing to rest to catch her breath. No complaints of increased secretions. Baseline dyspnea index: functional impairment, grade 1; magnitude of task, grade 1; magnitude of effort, grade 1 (see Table 12.6). Patient reports an RPE of 6 (the Borg 0–10 Scale) with one flight of stairs. Patient is dependent in shopping, house cleaning, and laundry. St. George's Respiratory Questionnaire was administered with a score of 54. Patient's desired functional outcome is to be oxygen free and able to care for grandchildren without shortness of breath.

Vital Signs
HR 72, BP 96/74, S_aO_2 at rest 86% on room air, 98% on 2 L/min pulsed O_2 on 1 pulse/breath, respiratory rate 32, temperature 98.5°F.

Observation, Inspection, Palpation
Thin, frail-looking female wearing nasal cannula; kyphosis noted. Patient uses posture of forward sitting with arms supported on chair arms to enhance ventilatory accessory muscle use. Increased AP diameter of thorax, accessory muscle use at rest; labored, symmetrical breathing pattern with pursed-lip breathing. No venous distention, no edema, no cyanosis, minimal clubbing evident.

Auscultation
Decreased breath sounds throughout both lung fields, especially at bases. End expiratory wheezes at left lateral base.

Strength
Bilateral LE manual muscle testing: hip flexion 3+/5, knee extension 3+/5, plantarflexion 3+/5, dorsiflexion, 4/5. Bilateral shoulder elevation, abduction, elbow flexion, wrist flexion and extension, 3+/5. Patient unable to lie prone or supine for further testing secondary to orthopnea. Alternative positions were used to assess the strength of other muscles: all other muscle groups able to move against gravity and able to accept moderate resistance. Maximal inspiratory effort (PI_{max}) 52 mm Hg; SIP_{max} 26 mm Hg.

Exercise Test Data

Patient performed a 7-minute, staged (3 min/stage) treadmill exercise test using a modified protocol. Treadmill speed was held constant at 2 mph, grade increased from 0% (stage 1) to 2% (stage 2) to 3% (stage 3). ECG was within normal limits. HR_{rest} was 84 beats/min, HR_{peak} 121 beats/min. On 2 L pulsed O_2, S_aO_2 resting 98%, 93% at max exercise, 90% during the first minute of cool-down, returned to baseline within 4 minutes of recovery. Rate of perceived exertion at peak exercise was 7 (1–10 scale). Rate of perceived dyspnea at peak exercise was a 9. Exercise was terminated due to patient complaint of shortness of breath. Single-breath TV measurement just before ending test was .99 liters with a respiratory rate of 36 breaths/min. There was no change in pulmonary function tests after exercise. 6-Minute Walk Test: 200 m on 2 liters pulsed O_2.

Laboratory Test Data (after bronchodilator)

Pulmonary Function Test	Results
FEV_1	1.107 L/sec (45% of predicted)
FVC	1.78 L (64% of predicted)
FEV_1/FVC	62%
MIP	36 mm Hg (60% of predicted)

GUIDING QUESTIONS

1. In what stage of GOLD does this patient present?

2. Did the pulmonary system or cardiovascular system stop her exercise test?

3. Identify this patient's impairments, functional limitations, and disability restrictions. Identify general anticipated treatment goals and expected outcomes for a 3-month (12-week) pulmonary rehabilitation program. Identify outcome measures that will be used to assess the effectiveness of a pulmonary rehabilitation program.

4. Formulate a physical therapy plan of care for week 1. Patient will be seen 3 times/week for this first week of therapy. Briefly describe exercise progression for the first month of the program.

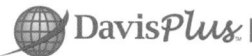 For additional resources, including answers to the questions for review and case study guiding questions, please visit **http://davisplus.fadavis.com**

For this chapter, see also:
Web Based Resources for Clinicians, Families, and Patients with Chronic Pulmonary Dysfunction in Appendix A p. 1445.

 The reader is referred to video **Case Study 1 Critical Care Patient with COPD and Acute Respiratory Distress Syndrome** for additional review and study. The full written case study including all tables, figures, charts, and 3 video segments (examination, intervention, and outcome) appears online at Davis*Plus*. The case study poses questions for the reader's consideration with suggested answers to the case study questions, also posted online at Davis*Plus*.

References

1. Nici, L, et al: Pulmonary rehabilitation. American Thoracic Society/European Respiratory Society Statement on Pulmonary Rehabilitation. Am J Respir Crit Care Med 173:1390, 2006.
2. Hughes, R, and Davison, R: Limitation of exercise reconditioning in COLD. Chest 83:241,1983.
3. Pierce, A, et al: Responses to exercise training in patients with emphysema. Arch Intern Med 114:28, 1964.
4. Foster, S, and Thomas, H: Pulmonary rehabilitation in lung disease other than chronic obstructive pulmonary disease. Am Rev Respir Dis 141:601, 1990.
5. Global Strategy for the Diagnosis, Management and Prevention of COPD, Global Initiative for Chronic Obstructive Lung Disease (GOLD), 2010. Retrieved August 26, 2011, from www.goldcopd.org.
6. Nunn, AJ, and Gregg, I: New regression equations for predicting peak expiratory flow in adults. Br Med J 298:1068, 1989.
7. Martyn, JB, et al: Measurement of inspiratory muscle performance with incremental threshold loading. Am Rev Respir Dis 135:919, 1987.
8. Laurell, CB, and Eriksson, S: The electrophoretic alpha-1 globulin pattern of serum in alpha-1 antitrypsin deficiency. Scand J Clin Lab Invest 15:132, 1963.
9. Study protocol, June 19, 2009: Genetic epidemiology of chronic obstructive pulmonary disease (COPDGene®). Retrieved January, 10, 2011, from www.copdgene.org.
10. Gan, W, et al: Association between chronic obstructive pulmonary disease and systemic inflammation: A systematic review and a meta-analysis. Thorax 59:574, 2004.
11. Angusti, A: Systemic effects of chronic obstructive pulmonary disease. What we know and what we don't know (but should). Proc Am Thorac Soc 4:522, 2007.
12. Martinez, F, et al: Predictors of mortality in patients with emphysema and severe airflow obstruction. Am J Respir Crit Care Med 173:1326, 2006.
13. Celli, B, et al: The body-mass index, airflow obstruction, dyspnea, and exercise capacity index in chronic obstructive pulmonary disease. N Engl J Med 350:1005, 2004.

14. Doherty, D, et al: Chronic obstructive pulmonary disease: Consensus recommendations for early diagnosis and treatment. J Fam Pract Suppl S1, Nov 2006. Retrieved August 26, 2011, from www.jfponline.com/Non_cme.asp.

15. Fletcher, C, and Peto, R: The natural history of chronic airflow obstruction. Br Med J 1:1645, 1977.

16. Global Strategy for Asthma Management and Prevention, Global Initiative for Asthma (GINA) 2010. Retrieved August 26, 2011, from www.ginasthma.org.

17. National Heart, Lung, and Blood Institute: National asthma education and prevention program. Expert Panel Report 3: Guidelines for the diagnosis and management of asthma. US Department of Health and Human Services, National Institutes of Health, NIH publication 08-5846, 2007. Retrieved August 26, 2011, from www.nhlbi.nih.gov/guidelines/asthma/asthgdln.pdf.

18. Humbert, M, et al: The immunopathology of extrinsic (atopic) and intrinsic (non-atopic) asthma: More similarities than differences. Immunol Today 20:528, 1999.

19. Sigurs, N, et al: Severe respiratory syncytial virus bronchiolitis in infancy and asthma and allergy at age 13. Am J Respir Crit Care Med 171: 137, 2005.

20. Weinberger, M: Clinical patterns and natural history of asthma. J Pediatr 142:515, 2003.

21. Panhuysen, CI, et al: Adult patients may outgrow their asthma. Am J Respir Crit Care Med 155:1267, 1997.

22. American Lung Association: Cystic fibrosis. In Lung Disease Data: 2008. American Lung Association, New York, 2008, p 55. Retrieved August 26, 2011, from www.lungusa.org/assets/documents/publications/lung-disease-data/LDD_2008.pdf.

23. Cystic Fibrosis Foundation Patient Registry 2002. Annual Report, Bethesda, MD, 2002. Retrieved January 10, 2011, from www.cff.org/aboutCF/FAQs.

24. Ratjen, F, and Doring, G: Cystic fibrosis. Lancet 361:681, 2003.

25. McKone, F.F, et al: Effect of genotype on phenotype and mortality in cystic fibrosis: A retrospective cohort study. Lancet 361:1671, 2003.

26. William, C, et al: Exercise training in children and adolescents with cystic fibrosis: Theory into practice. Int J Pediatr 2010. Retrieved April 14, 2011, from www.hindawi.com/journals/ijped/2010/670640/cta.

27. Elbom, J, and Bell, S: Nutrition and survival in cystic fibrosis. Thorax 51:971, 1996.

28. Collard, H, and King, T: Demystifying idiopathic interstitial pneumonia. Arch Intern Med 163:17, 2003.

29. Caminati, A, and Harari, S: IPF: New insight in diagnosis and prognosis. Respir Med 104:S2, 2010.

30. King, T: Idiopathic interstitial pneumonias: Progress in classification, diagnosis, pathogenesis and management. Trans Am Clin Climatolo Assoc 115:43–78, 2004.

31. Pauwels, R, and Rabe, K: Burden and clinical features of chronic obstructive pulmonary disease (COPD). Lancet 364:791, 2004.

32. Johnson, TS: A brief review of pharmacotherapeutic treatment options in smoking cessation: Bupropion versus varenicline. J Am Acad Nurse Pract 10:557, 2010.

33. Stead, L, et al: Nicotine replacement therapy for smoking cessation. Cochrane Database Syst Rev CD000146, 2008. Retrieved December 26, 2011, from www.thecochranelibrary.com.

34. AHCPR Supported Guide and Guidelines: Treating tobacco use and dependence. Agency for Health Care Policy and Research, Rockville, MD, 2008. Retrieved April 26, 2011, from www.ncbi.hlm.nih.gov/books/NBK12193.

35. DeKorte, C: Current and emerging therapies for the management of chronic inflammation in asthma. Am J Health-Syst Ph 60:1949, 2003.

36. Belman, M, et al: Inhaled bronchodilators reduce dynamic hyperinflation during exercise in patients with chronic obstructive pulmonary disease. Am J Respir Crit Care Med 153:967, 1996.

37. Alliance for the Prudent Use of Antibiotics. Retrieved April 28, 2011, from www.tufts.edu/med/apua/Patients/patient.html.

38. Tarpy, S, and Celli, B: Long-term oxygen therapy. N Engl J Med 333:710, 1995.

39. Nocturnal Oxygen Therapy Trial Group: Continuous or nocturnal oxygen therapy in hypoxemic chronic obstructive lung disease: A clinical trial. Ann Intern Med 93(3):391, 1980.

40. Man, SF, et al: Contemporary management of chronic obstructive pulmonary disease: Clinical applications. JAMA 290:2313, 2003.

41. Garrod, R, et al: Supplemental oxygen during pulmonary rehabilitation in patients with COPD with exercise hypoxaemia. Thorax 55:539, 2000.

42. British Thoracic Society Standards of Care Subcommittee on Pulmonary Rehabilitation: Pulmonary rehabilitation. Thorax 56: 8278, 2001.

43. Naunheim, K: Long-term follow-up of patients receiving lung-volume-reduction surgery versus medical therapy for severe emphysema by the National Emphysema Treatment Trial research group. Ann Thorac Surg 82:431, 2006.

44. Washko, G, et al: The effect of lung volume reduction surgery on chronic obstructive pulmonary disease exacerbations. Am J Respir Crit Care Med 177:164, 2008.

45. Fishman, A, et al: National Emphysema Treatment Trial research group: Patients at high risk of death after lung volume reduction surgery. N Engl J Med 345:1075, 2001.

46. National Emphysema Treatment Trial Research Group: A randomized trial comparing lung-volume-reduction surgery with medical therapy for severe emphysema. N Engl J Med 348:2059, 2003.

47. Szekely, L, et al: Preoperative predictors of operative morbidity and mortality in COPD patients undergoing bilateral lung volume reduction surgery. Chest 111(3):550, 1997.

48. Patient Survival by Year of Transplant at 3 Months, 1 Year, 3 Years, 5 Years and 10 Years. United States Department of Health and Human Services. Retrieved April 26, 2011, from www.ustransplant.org.

49. Kesten, S: Pulmonary rehabilitation and surgery for end stage lung disease. Clin Chest Med 18:173, 1997.

50. Cassaburi, R, et al: Reductions in exercise lactic acidosis and ventilation as a result of exercise training in patients with obstructive lung disease. Am Rev Respir Dis 143:9, 1991.

51. Lacasse, Y, et al: Pulmonary rehabilitation for chronic obstructive pulmonary disease. Cochrane Database of Systemic Reviews 2006, Issue 4. Art. No: CD003793. Retrieved December 26, 2011, from www.thecochranelibrary.com.

52. Morgan, M, et al: Pulmonary rehabilitation. British Thoracic Society Standards of Care Subcommittee on Pulmonary Rehabilitation. Thorax 56:827, 2001.

53. American Physical Therapy Association: Guide to Physical Therapist Practice, ed 2. Phys Ther 81:1, 2001.

54. Murphy, R: Auscultation of the lung: Past lessons, future possibilities. Thorax 36:99, 1981.

55. American College of Chest Physicians and American Thoracic Society: ACCP-ATS joint committee on pulmonary nomenclature: Pulmonary terms and symbols: A report of the ACCP-ATS Joint Committee on Pulmonary Nomenclature. Chest 67:583, 1975.

56. Mahler, D, et al: The impact of dyspnea and physiologic function in general health status in patients with chronic obstructive pulmonary disease. Chest 102:395, 1992.

57. Mahler, D: Dyspnea: Diagnosis and management. Clin Chest Med 8:215, 1987.

58. Guyatt, G, et al: A measure of quality of life for clinical trials in chronic lung disease. Thorax 42:73, 1987.

59. Brazier, J, et al: Validating the SF-36 health survey questionnaire: New outcome measure for primary care. BMJ 305:160, 1992.

60. Casaburi R: Skeletal muscle function in COPD. Chest 117:267S, 2000.

61. American Thoracic Society/American College of Chest Physicians: ATS/ACCP statement on cardiopulmonary exercise testing. Am J Respir Crit Care Med 167:211, 2003.

62. Jones, N: Exercise testing in pulmonary evaluation: Rationale, methods and the normal respiratory response to exercise. N Engl J Med 293:541, 1975.

63. Berman, L, and Sutton, J: Exercise for the pulmonary patient. J Cardiopulmonary Rehabil 6:55, 1986.

64. Bruce, R, et al: Maximal oxygen intake and nomographic assessment of functional aerobic impairment in cardiovascular disease. Am Heart J 85:546, 1973.

65. Naughton, J, et al: Modified work capacity studies in individuals with and without coronary artery disease. J Sports Med 4:208, 1964.

66. Balke, B, and Ware, R: An experimental study of physical fitness of Air Force personnel. US Armed Forces Med J 10:675, 1959.

67. Revill, S, et al: The endurance shuttle walk: A new field test for the assessment of endurance capacity in chronic obstructive pulmonary disease. Thorax 54:213, 1999.

68. Singh, S, et al: Comparison of oxygen uptake during a conventional treadmill test and the shuttle walk test in chronic airflow limitation. Eur Respir J 7:2016, 1994.

69. American Thoracic Society: Guidelines for the 6-Minute Walk Test. Am J Respir Crit Care Med 166:111, 2002.

70. Solway, S, et al: A qualitative systematic overview of the measurement properties of functional walk tests used in the cardiorespiratory domain. Chest 119:256, 2001.

71. Revill, S, et al: The endurance shuttle walk test: An alternative to the six minute walk test for the assessment of ambulatory oxygen. Chronic Respir Dis 7:239, 2010.

72. Bradley, J, and O'Neill, B: Short-term ambulatory oxygen for chronic obstructive pulmonary disease. Cochrane Database of Systematic Reviews 2005, Issue 4. Art. No.: CD004356. Retrieved December 26, 2011, from www.thecochranelibrary.com.

73. Rundell, K, and Slee, J: Exercise and other indirect challenges to demonstrate asthma and exercise-induced bronchoconstriction in athletes. J Allergy Clin Immunol 122:238, 2008.

74. Lake, F, et al: Upper limb and lower limb exercise training in patients with chronic airflow obstruction. Chest 97:1077, 1990.

75. American College of Sports Medicine: Guidelines for Exercise Testing and Prescription, ed 8. Lea & Febiger, Philadelphia, 2009.

76. Dattal, D, and ZuWallack, R: High versus low intensity exercise training in pulmonary rehabilitation: Is more better? Chronic Respir Dis 1:143, 2004.

77. Normandin, E, et al: An evaluation of two approaches to exercise conditioning in pulmonary rehabilitation. Chest 121:1085, 2002.

78. Punzal, P, et al: Maximum intensity exercise training in patients with chronic obstructive pulmonary disease. Chest 100:618, 1991.

79. Ries, A, et al: Pulmonary rehabilitation joint ACCP/AACVPR evidence-based clinical practice guidelines. Chest 131:4S, 2007.

80. Beauchamp, M, et al: Interval versus continuous training in individuals with chronic obstructive pulmonary disease—a systematic review. Thorax 65:157, 2010.

81. Nasis, I, et al: Effects of interval-load versus constant-load training on the BODE index in COPD patients. Respir Med 103:1392, 2009.

82. Arnardottir, R, et al: Interval training compared with continuous training in patients with COPD. Respir Med 101:1196, 2007.

83. Varga, J, et al: Supervised high intensity continuous and interval training vs. self-paced training in COPD. Respir Med 101:2297, 2007.

84. Puhan, M, et al: Interval versus continuous high-intensity exercise in chronic obstructive pulmonary disease. Ann Intern Med 145:816, 2006.

85. da Cunha, FA, et al: Methodological and practical application issues in exercise prescription using heart rate reserve and oxygen uptake reserve methods. J Sci Med Sport 14:46, 2011.

86. Borg, G: Psychophysical basis of perceived exertion. Med Sci Sports Exerc 14:377, 1982.

87. Mahler, D: Hit the dyspnea target. J Cardiopulm Rehabil 23:226, 2003.

88. Mejia, R, et al: Target dyspnea ratings predict expected oxygen consumption as well as target heart rate values. Am J Respir Crit Care Med 159:1485, 1999.

89. Horowitz, MB, et al: Dyspnea ratings for prescribing exercise intensity in patients with COPD. Chest 109: 1169, 1996.

90. Lotters, F, et al: Effects of controlled inspiratory muscle training in patients with COPD: A meta-analysis. Eur Respir J 20:570, 2002.

91. Scherer, TA, et al: Respiratory muscle endurance training in chronic obstructive pulmonary disease: Impact on exercise capacity, dyspnea, and quality of life. Am J Respir Crit Care Med 162:1709, 2000.

92. Riera, HS, et al: Inspiratory muscle training in patients with COPD: Effect on dyspnea, exercise performance and quality of life. Chest 120:748, 2001.

93. Weiner, P, et al : Comparison of specific expiratory, inspiratory, and combined muscle training programs in COPD. Chest 124:1357, 2003.

94. Wild, M, et al: The outcome of inspiratory muscle training in COPD patients depends on stage of the disease. Chest 120S:181S, 2001.

95. Beckerman, M, et al: The effects of 1 year of specific inspiratory muscle training in patients with COPD. Chest 128:3177, 2005.

96. Weiner, P, and Weiner, M: Inspiratory muscle training may increase peak inspiratory flow in chronic obstructive pulmonary disease. Respiration 73:151, 2006.

97. Magadle, R, et al: Inspiratory muscle training in pulmonary rehabilitation program in COPD patients. Respir Med 101:1500, 2007.

98. Hill, K, et al: High-intensity inspiratory muscle training in COPD. Eur Respir J 27:1119, 2006.

99. Figlio, K, et al: Is it really useful to repeat outpatient pulmonary rehabilitation programs in patients with chronic airway obstruction? A 2 year controlled study. Chest 119:1696–1704, 2001.

100. Ries, A, et al: Effects of pulmonary rehabilitation of physiologic and psychosocial outcomes in patients with chronic obstructive pulmonary disease. Ann Intern Med 122:823, 1995.

101. Hietpas, B, et al: Huff coughing and airway patency. Resp Care 24:710, 1979.

102. Wilson, G, et al: A comparison of traditional chest physiotherapy with the active cycle of breathing in patients with chronic suppurative lung disease. Eur Respir J 8(suppl 19): 171S, 1995.

103. Konstan, M, et al: Efficacy of the flutter device for airway mucus clearance in patients with cystic fibrosis. J Pediatr 124:689, 1994.

104. Gondor, M, et al: Comparison of flutter device and chest physical therapy in the treatment of cystic fibrosis during pulmonary exacerbation. Pediatr Pulmonol 28:255, 1999.

105. Van Asperen, P, et al: Comparison of a positive expiratory pressure (PEP) mask with postural drainage in patients with cystic fibrosis. Aust Paediatr J 23:283, 1987.

106. Steen, H, et al: Evaluation of the PEP mask in cystic fibrosis. Acta Paediatr Scand 80(1):51, 1991.

107. Braggion, C, et al: Short term effects of three chest physiotherapy regimens in patients hospitalized for pulmonary exacerbations of CF: A cross-over randomized study. Pediatr Pulmonol 19:16, 1995.

108. Morgan, M, and Britton, J: Chronic obstructive pulmonary disease: Non-pharmacological management of COPD. Thorax 58:453, 2003.

109. Dechman, G, and Wilson, C: Evidence underlying breathing retraining in people with stable chronic obstructive pulmonary disease. Phys Ther 84:1189, 2004.

Supplemental Readings

American College of Sports Medicine: Guidelines for Exercise Testing and Prescription, ed 8. Lea & Febiger, Philadelphia, 2009.

Global strategy for asthma management and prevention. Update 2008. Retrieved December 26, 2011, from www.ginasthma.com.

Global strategy for the diagnosis, management, and prevention of chronic obstructive pulmonary disease. NHLBI/WHO global initiative for chronic obstructive lung disease (GOLD) workshop summary. 2009. Retrieved December 26, 2011, from www.goldcopd.org.

Goodman, C, Boissonnault, W, and Fuller, K: Pathology: Implications for the Physical Therapist, ed 3. WB Saunders, Philadelphia, 2009.

Pulmonary rehabilitation joint ACCP/AACVPR evidence-based clinical practice guidelines. Chest 131:4S–42S, 2007.

Heart Disease

Konrad J. Dias, PT, DPT, CCS

Chapter 13

■ INTRODUCTION AND EPIDEMIOLOGY OF HEART DISEASE

Cardiovascular disease (CVD) is a term referring to the pathological process of atherosclerosis affecting the entire arterial circulation. **Coronary artery disease (CAD)**, also called **coronary heart disease (CHD)**, refers to the pathological process of atherosclerosis, specifically affecting the coronary arteries. CAD includes the diagnoses of angina pectoris, **myocardial infarction (MI)**, silent myocardial ischemia, and sudden cardiac death.

The pathophysiological conditions that underlie CVD are atherosclerosis, altered myocardial muscle mechanics, valvular dysfunction, **arrhythmias**, and **hypertension (HTN)**. **Atherosclerosis** is a disease in which lipid-laden plaque (lesions) is formed within the intimal layer of the blood vessel wall of moderate and large size arteries; over time the plaque may extend into the lumen causing a decreased lumenal diameter. Atherosclerosis is also a primary contributor to cerebrovascular disease (cerebrovascular accident [CVA]) and peripheral vascular disease (PVD).

Alteration in myocardial muscle mechanics involving the systolic and/or diastolic properties of the myocardium

523

results in an impairment of left ventricular (LV) function. **Heart failure** is a clinical diagnosis caused by impaired LV functioning and is referred to as **congestive heart failure** (CHF) when it is accompanied by signs and symptoms of edema (i.e., congestion). There are many causes of heart failure, including myocardial scarring and remodeling as a result of an MI, cardiomyopathy (involving an enlarged, thickened, and/or hardened heart muscle) from various causes, or impaired valvular function, especially within the mitral and aortic valves.

Arrhythmias are caused by a disturbance in the electrical activity of the heart, resulting in impaired electrical impulse formation or conduction. Arrhythmias may present as benign or malignant (i.e., life threatening). Examples of malignant arrhythmias are sustained ventricular tachycardia (V-tach) and ventricular fibrillation (V-fib). An example of a common benign arrhythmia in the elderly is atrial fibrillation (A-fib) with a controlled ventricular response involving a ventricular rate between 60 and 100 beats per minute (bpm).

HTN is the most prevalent CVD in the United States and one of the most powerful contributors to cardiovascular morbidity and mortality. HTN occurs when the systolic blood pressure is consistently greater than 140 mm Hg or the DBP is equal to or greater than 90 mm Hg.

CVD remains the leading cause of death and disability in the United States. According to the American Heart Association's Heart Disease and Stroke Statistics 2011 Update, an estimated 82,600,000 American adults (more than 1 in 3) have one or more types of CVD.[1] Currently, HTN occurs in 76,400,000 individuals, CHD affects 16,300,000, and heart failure is seen in 5,700,000 patients.[1] The average annual rates of first cardiovascular events rise from 3 per 1,000 men at age 35 to 44 years to 74 per 1,000 at age 85 to 94. For women, comparable rates occur 10 years later in life with a narrowing gap with advancing age.[1] On average, 2,200 Americans die of CVD each day with an average of 1 death every 39 seconds.[2] In every year since 1900 except 1918, CVD accounted for more deaths than any other major cause in the United States.[3]

It is also important to note that the United States is in the midst of a demographic shift with a remarkable increase in the diversity of the American population. By 2050, there will be a decrease in the white non-Hispanic population to 52.5% from 75.7% in 1990.[4] The Hispanic population will increase to 22.5%, a change in African Americans to 15.7%, and Asian and Pacific Islanders will account for 10.3% of the population.[4] These statistics will have a major impact on the epidemiology, pathophysiology, and treatment of CVD in the forthcoming years. Thus, within the United States and worldwide, we are faced with major challenges as CVD dominates as a major cause of death and disease. This chapter provides a review of normal anatomy and physiology of the cardiovascular system and its relevance to physical therapist practice followed by a discussion of various pathologies and pertinent physical therapy implications.

■ CARDIAC ANATOMY AND PHYSIOLOGY

Surface Anatomy

The heart lies within the left thoracic cavity. The base of the heart is located superiorly, approximately between the second and third rib; the apex is located inferiorly, approximately at the level of the fifth rib (Fig. 13.1). In this position, the heart is rotated in the sagittal plane so that the right ventricle (RV) is positioned anterior to the left ventricle (LV) and tipped anteriorly, bringing the apex closer to the chest wall. In the posterior–anterior view of a chest x-ray, the RV occupies a significant portion of the frontal plane. The right atrium (RA) is generally located in the area of the second intercostal spaces and the *angle of Louis*. When one palpates the sternum, the angle of Louis is the "bump" that demarcates the manubrium from the body of the sternum. The second

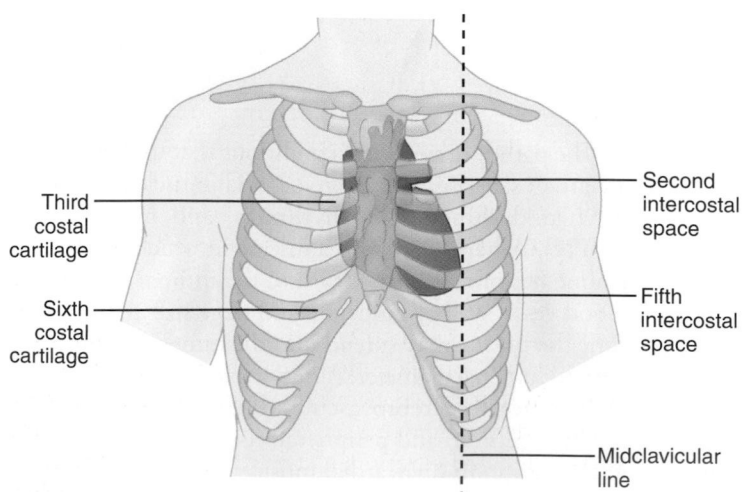

Figure 13.1 Surface anatomy of the heart.

Third costal cartilage

Sixth costal cartilage

Second intercostal space

Fifth intercostal space

Midclavicular line

intercostal spaces are lateral and slightly below the angle of Louis. The second intercostal spaces are an important auscultatory landmark; the right space is known as the *aortic area*, the left as the *pulmonic area*. The apex of the normal heart is in the fifth intercostal space at the midclavicular line. In a healthy heart, this area, known as the *point of maximal impulse (PMI)*, is where the contraction of the LV is most pronounced.

Heart Tissue

The heart wall is made up of three tissue layers (Fig. 13.2). The outermost layer of the heart is a double-walled sac termed the *pericardium.* The two layers of the pericardium include an outer tough fibrous layer of dense irregular connective tissue termed the *parietal pericardium* and an inner thin *visceral pericardium.*[5] Between these two layers is a closed space filled with pericardial fluid, which serves as a lubricant allowing the two surfaces to slide past one another. Clinically, patients may develop an infection with resultant inflammation of the pericardium termed *pericarditis.* The clinical signs that accompany this pathology and used to differentially diagnose pericarditis include a *pericardial friction rub* (an audible grating sound suggesting irritation of the pericardium) that can be auscultated with each heartbeat accompanied by constant chest pain.[6] In some patients excessive fluid accumulation within the closed pericardial space may lead to a secondary condition known as *cardiac tamponade.* Tamponade involves compression of the heart caused by fluid buildup in the space between the myocardium and pericardium. In this state, patients will demonstrate compromised cardiac function and contractility due to the excess fluid within the closed space pushing against the heart.[7,8]

The muscular middle layer of the heart is termed the *myocardium.* It is the layer that facilitates the pumping action of the heart to move blood to the entire body. Alterations in the muscular wall of the heart are termed **cardiomyopathies.** There are three common classifications of cardiomyopathies: *dilated, hypertrophic,* and *restrictive.*[9] Dilated cardiomyopathy is evidenced by ventricular dilation and altered cardiac muscle contractile function. CAD is the prime cause of *dilated cardiomyopathy,* causing mitochondrial dysfunction and resultant myocardial damage. Myocarditis (inflammation of the heart muscle) and alcohol abuse are additional causes of dilated cardiomyopathy. *Hypertrophic cardiomyopathy* presents as diastolic dysfunction with an increased ventricular mass. Chronic HTN and aortic stenosis are examples of hypertrophic cardiomyopathy. *Restrictive cardiomyopathy* also presents as diastolic dysfunction owing to the presence of excessively rigid ventricular walls, resulting in a decrease in compliance. The connective tissue changes of the heart associated with diabetes are an example of a restrictive cardiomyopathy. Damage to myocardial cells from cardiomyopathies and various other etiologies lead to cardiac muscle dysfunction and resultant heart failure, which will be comprehensively discussed later in this chapter.

The innermost layer of the heart is termed the *endocardium.* The tissue of the endocardium forms the inner lining of the chambers of the heart and is continuous with the tissue of the valves and the endothelium of the blood vessel. Because the endocardium and valves share similar tissue, patients with infections of the endocardium are at risk for developing valvular dysfunction. Endocardial infections can spread into valvular tissue developing vegetations (a mixture of bacteria and blood clots) on the valve.[9] In patients with newly developed vegetations, bronchopulmonary hygiene procedures including percussions and vibrations are contraindicated because they may dislodge, move as emboli, and cause an embolic stroke.[9]

Coronary Arteries

The coronary arteries originate in the sinus of Valsalva located in the wall of the aorta near the aortic valve.[5] The right coronary originates from the area near the right aortic leaflet, the left coronary from the area near the left aortic leaflet. When the aortic valve is open during systole, the origins of the coronary arteries are located behind the aortic leaflets within the wall; when the aortic valve is closed during diastole, the openings of the coronaries are clearly exposed, allowing them to be easily perfused.[5] The coronary arteries therefore receive the majority of their blood flow during diastole, unlike the other arteries of the body that are perfused during systole. The left coronary artery begins as the left main (LM) and then branches into the left anterior descending (LAD) and the circumflex (CX) (Fig. 13.3). The LAD may have further divisions, known as diagonal branches,

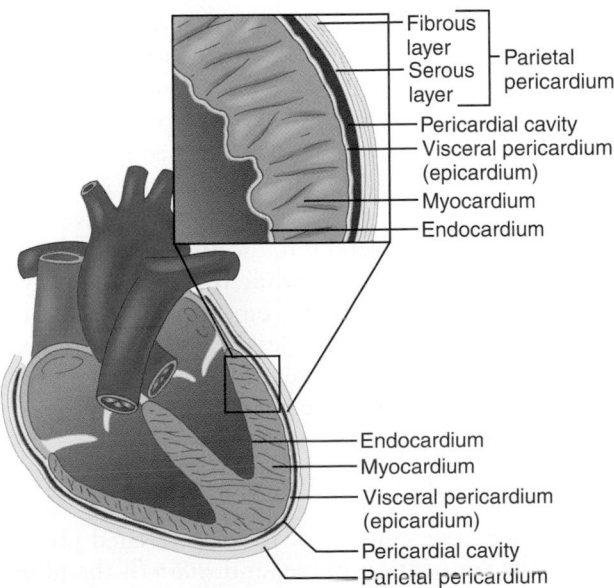

Fibrous layer
Serous layer — Parietal pericardium
Pericardial cavity
Visceral pericardium (epicardium)
Myocardium
Endocardium

Endocardium
Myocardium
Visceral pericardium (epicardium)
Pericardial cavity
Parietal pericardium

Figure 13.2 Layers of the heart.

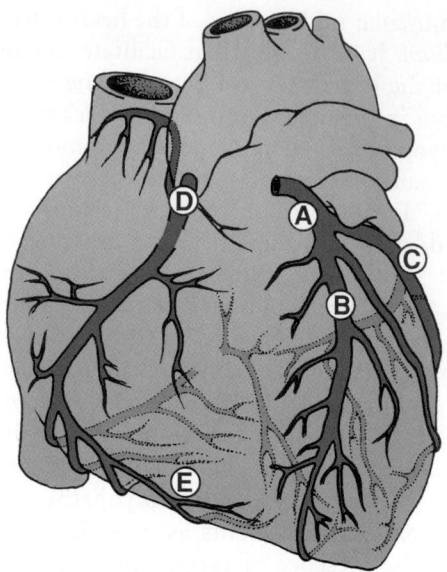

Figure 13.3 Coronary circulation. **(A)** left main (LM); **(B)** left anterior descending (LAD); **(C)** left circumflex (CX); **(D)** right coronary (RCA); **(E)** posterior descending (PDA). The branches of the LAD are known as diagonals; the branches of the CX are known as marginals.

that come off of the primary LAD. The LAD and its diagonal branches primarily supply the anterior and apical surfaces of the LV, as well as portions of the interventricular septum. The circumflex may also have branches, known as marginal branches. The circumflex and its marginal branches supply the lateral and part of the inferior surfaces of the LV and portions of the left atrium (LA). The right coronary artery (RCA) supplies the RA, most of the RV, part of the inferior wall of the LV, portions of the interventricular septum, and the conduction system. The posterior descending artery (PDA) is most commonly a branch of the RCA and perfuses the posterior heart. If the RCA does not perfuse the posterior heart, the CX will supply this area. When the PDA comes from the RCA, the anatomy is referred to as being right dominant; if the PDA comes from the circumflex, the anatomy is referred to as being left dominant. For physical therapists, there is no clinical importance to whether the anatomy of the myocardium is either left or right dominant.

The inner diameter (i.e., the opening) of the arteries through which the blood flows is the *lumen*. The size of the lumen is critical for adequate blood flow. A significant narrowing of the lumen, such as that which occurs with a fixed atherosclerotic lesion of CAD, will decrease the available blood supply to the myocardium. Lumen size may also be altered by the smooth muscle within the walls of the arteries, because smooth muscle regulates vasomotor tone of the coronary arteries. Vasodilation will increase lumen diameter as a result of relaxation of smooth muscle, and vasoconstriction will decrease lumenal diameter as a result of smooth muscle contraction. The responsiveness

of arterial smooth muscle is also influenced by the integrity of the endothelium, the lining of the coronary artery that is in direct contact with the lumen. The endothelium has a number of normal functions and "plays the central role in controlling the biology of the vessel wall."[10, p. 1,265] Some of these important functions are anti-inflammatory actions, antithrombotic activity, and its influence on vasodilation. Endothelial cells release *endothelial-derived relaxing factor (EDRF)*, which facilitates vascular smooth muscle relaxation. Nitric oxide (NO) is the most prevalent EDRF. An injury to endothelium can result in impaired NO release and a decrease in vasodilation.[11] NO release is influenced by many factors, including acetylcholine, norepinephrine, serotonin, adenosine diphosphate, bradykinin, and histamine.[11]

The etiology of the clinical condition known as coronary spasm, in which smooth muscle contraction within the walls of the artery results in narrowing of the coronary artery, is not clearly understood. Coronary spasm occurs in arteries that have endothelial injury (e.g., atherosclerosis), as well as in those arteries that appear to be normal but exhibit hyperreactivity to a variety of vasoconstrictor stimuli, such as serotonin and ergonovine, and loss of EDRF.[12]

Heart Valves

Four heart valves ensure one-way blood flow through the heart. Two atrioventricular valves are located between the atria and ventricle. The atrioventricular valve, positioned between the RA and RV, is termed the *tricuspid valve*; the left atrioventricular valve is the *mitral valve* (also known as the bicuspid valve), located between the left atrium and ventricle. The *semilunar valves* lie between the ventricles and arteries and are named based on their corresponding vessels (i.e., *pulmonic valve* on the right in association with the pulmonary artery, and aortic valve on the left relating to the aorta).

Flaps of tissue called *leaflets or cusps* guard the heart valve openings. The right atrioventricular valve has three cusps and is therefore termed *tricuspid,* whereas the left atrioventricular valve has only two cusps and hence is termed *bicuspid.* These leaflets are attached to the papillary muscles of the myocardium by chordae tendineae. The primary function of the atrioventricular valves is to prevent backflow of blood into the atria during ventricular contraction or systole, while the semilunar valves prevent backflow of blood from the aorta and pulmonary artery into the ventricles during diastole. Opening and closing of each valve depends on pressure gradient changes within the heart created during each cardiac cycle.

Cardiac Cycle

The cardiac cycle consists of two interrelated phases: *systole*, the contraction phase, and *diastole*, the filling phase. During diastole, the ventricles fill with blood from the atria via open atrioventricular valves. The atrioventricular valves lie between the atria and the ventricles and include the tricuspid valve on the right and mitral valve on the left. The first two-thirds of ventricular filling is passive; during the last one-third the atria contract and push the blood into the ventricles. This contraction is known as the *atrial kick*. After the atrial kick, diastole ends and the atrioventricular valves close. Systole begins with both the atrioventricular and semilunar valves closed. An initial *isovolumetric contraction,* similar to an isometric contraction of striated muscle, increases the pressure within the ventricles, and the semilunar valve opens. The LV then undergoes a concentric contraction, causing a volume to be ejected, termed the *stroke volume* (SV). After the SV is ejected, the aortic valve closes and systole is complete. The cardiac cycle is defined by the presence of normal heart sounds, S_1 and S_2. Heart sounds are associated with valvular closings; S_1 is associated with atrioventricular valve closure, and S_2 is associated with semilunar valve closure. Systole occurs between S_1 and S_2, and diastole occurs between S_2 and S_1 (Fig. 13.4).

Blood Flow and Hemodynamic Values

Blood enters the heart via the superior and inferior vena cava into the RA. Blood moves forward from the RA through the tricuspid valve to the RV, and through the pulmonic valve to the pulmonary artery (PA) and pulmonary capillaries. The capillaries perfuse the alveoli, and the alveolar capillary membrane is the site of gas exchange. Newly oxygenated blood within the pulmonary veins (PVs) travels to the left atrium (LA) and passes through the mitral valve into the LV. Blood within the LV travels down to the apex, where it is squeezed in a wringing motion during systole and moved from the apex to the LV outflow tract and finally out through the aortic valve to the aorta.

Blood volume in any chamber or vessel generates a pressure. The normal pressure recordings for the cardiovascular system are presented in Table 13.1. Owing to the relationship between blood volumes and pressures, a direct measure of blood volumes within the heart is accomplished by invasive monitoring of the intravascular

Table 13.1 Hemodynamic Variables	
Right-Sided Heart Catheterization	**Normal Ranges**
Central venous pressure (CVP)	0–8 mm Hg
Right atrial (mean)	0–8 mm Hg
Pulmonary artery (PA)	Systolic 20–25 mm Hg Diastolic 6–12 mm Hg Mean 9–19 mm Hg
Pulmonary capillary wedge pressure (PCWP)	6–12 mm Hg
Left-Sided Heart Catheterization	**Normal Ranges**
Left ventricular end-diastolic pressure	5–12 mm Hg
Left ventricular peak systolic pressure	90–140 mm Hg
Systemic arterial pressure	Systolic 110–120 mm Hg Diastolic 70–80 mm Hg Mean 82–102 mm Hg
Cardiac output (CO)	4–5 L/min
Cardiac index (CO ÷ body surface area)	2.5–3.5 L/min
Stroke volume	55–100 mL/beat
Systemic vascular resistance	800–1200 dynes/sec/cm⁻⁵

Adapted from Braunwald, E, Zipes, D, and Libby, R (eds): Heart Disease: A Textbook of Cardiovascular Medicine, ed 6. Saunders, Philadelphia 1997, p 188; and Parrillo, JE: Current Therapy in Critical Care Medicine. BC Decker Inc., 1987, p 36.

or chamber pressures. In a *right-sided heart catheterization,* an invasive catheter known as a Swan-Ganz catheter or PA catheter, with pressure-sensitive recording ability, is inserted into the internal jugular or subclavian vein and progressed antegrade through the right side of the heart. Common measurements taken with a right-sided heart catheterization are RA pressure, PA pressure, and *pulmonary capillary wedge pressure (PCWP)*. The PCWP is an indirect measure of the *left ventricular end-diastolic pressure (LVEDP)*, one of the most sensitive measures of LV function. An advantage of right-sided heart catheterization is the ability to monitor filling pressures not only on the right side, but also left-side heart pressures, by estimation, without the need for the more difficult and risky LV catheterization. Invasive monitoring through left-sided heart catheterization is accomplished by placing a catheter into the femoral or radial artery and advancing it retrograde to the flow of blood through the aorta, across the aortic valve, and into the LV where LVEDP can be directly monitored. The LV catheter lies within a high-pressure system (the left side of the heart and the

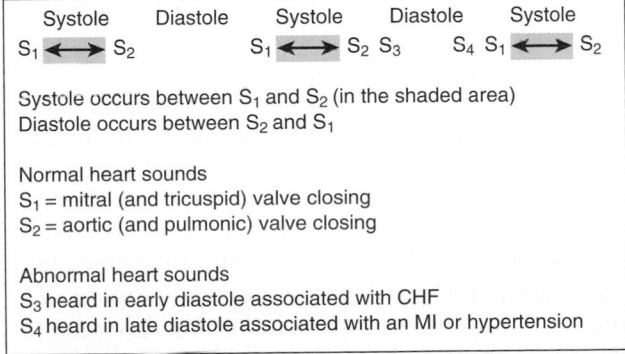

Figure 13.4 Heart sounds of the cardiac cycle.

aorta), and therefore can stay in place for only a short period of time (e.g., 1 hour) because of the difficulties associated with cannulation (catheter insertion) of a high-pressure system. In contrast, the right-sided heart catheter, which lies within a relatively low-pressure system (the right side of the heart), provides continuous monitoring of pressures and can be kept in place for several days.

Neurohormonal Influences on the Cardiovascular System

The autonomic nervous system (ANS) influences the heart and blood vessels through direct neural and indirect neurohormonal mechanisms. The heart has dual direct innervation from the sympathetic and parasympathetic nervous systems.[13] The sympathetic receptors of the heart are primarily beta-adrenergic receptors[14] and are located on the sinus node and within the myocardium. Stimulation of the receptors by the neurotransmitter norepinephrine (noradrenaline) increases the overall activity of the heart by increasing the heart rate (HR) (*chronotropy*) and force of contraction (*inotropy*), and also results in coronary artery dilation.[13] Sympathetic stimulation of the alpha-adrenergic receptors on peripheral blood vessels causes vasoconstriction and an increase in *peripheral vascular resistance (PVR)*.

The sympathetic nervous system may also stimulate the adrenal cortex to secrete the catecholamine epinephrine. This blood-borne hormone has sympathetic effects that at times may even be more long lasting and potent than direct sympathetic activation. Epinephrine is released as part of the normal exercise response, especially when exercise is continued beyond a few minutes. The increase in HR and contractility noted with exercise is in part due to this hormonal influence. Many cardiovascular drugs either enhance or suppress sympathetic functioning. Those that mimic the action of the sympathetic nervous system are known as *sympathomimetics;* those that suppress sympathetic functioning are known as *sympatholytics.* Frequently used sympathomimetics are dopamine, epinephrine, and atropine, which are commonly used in critical care settings. Dopamine and epinephrine increase cardiac output (CO), and atropine increases HR in the presence of critical *bradycardia.* Frequently used sympatholytics are the category of drugs known as beta-blockers (beta-adrenergic antagonists) that suppress beta-adrenergic activity. They are commonly used as part of an anti-ischemic drug regimen and for the medical management of HTN.

The normal parasympathetic influence via the vagus nerve has a primary impact on the resting heart, influencing resting HR substantially more than the sympathetic nervous system. Parasympathetic stimulation results in a depression of HR, decreased force of atrial contraction, and decreased speed of conduction through the atrioventricular (AV) node. Vagal fiber innervation to ventricular myocardium is relatively small; therefore the effect on LV function is minimal.[14] During exercise, the effects of the sympathetic nervous system and catecholamine release significantly override any effect from the parasympathetic system. The impact of direct parasympathetic influence on peripheral blood vessels is limited to a vasodilatory effect on the bowel, bladder, and genitals.[14]

The catecholamine role in myocardial functioning during exercise is especially crucial for the patient who has lost direct sympathetic activation to the heart. For a patient who has undergone a heart transplant, the heart is essentially denervated; the sympathetic and parasympathetic fibers to the heart are excised. Sympathetic influence on the denervated heart is therefore solely dependent on catecholamine stimulation of the beta-adrenergic myocardial receptors to increase HR and contractility. Clinically, the patient with a denervated heart following transplantation will present with elevated resting HRs to achieve normal cardiac output, delayed elevation in HRs with exercise due to circulating catecholamines, decreased maximum HR responses, and slower decreases in HR values during the recovery phase of exercise.[15]

Cardiac Output

The goal of the heart is to provide adequate CO to generate aerobic energy to meet the metabolic demands of the body. Because the energy demands of the body are constantly changing, the heart's CO must also be able to adapt to the changing systemic energy demands, as well as to its own myocardial oxygen needs. CO is defined as the amount of blood that leaves the ventricles per minute, expressed in L/min. Normal CO at rest is approximately 4 to 6 L/min. It is influenced by HR (expressed as beats per minute [bpm]) and stroke volume (expressed as milliliters per minute [mL/min]).

Stroke volume (SV) is the volume of blood ejected with each myocardial contraction and is influenced by three factors: (1) *preload,* the amount of blood in the ventricle at the end of diastole (also known as *left ventricular-end diastolic volume [LVEDV]*); (2) *contractility,* the ability of the ventricle to contract; and (3) *afterload,* the force the LV must generate during systole to overcome aortic pressure and open the aortic valve.[8] Afterload may also be described as the "load . . . against which the LV contracts during left ventricular ejection."[16]

Throughout the cardiac cycle, diastole and systole place different demands on the ventricles. During diastole, the ventricles must be compliant, able to stretch to accommodate the blood entering the ventricles (preload). During systole, the ventricles must be able to contract adequately to eject the SV. The principle of Starling's length–tension relationship is applicable to the myocardium and the relationship between the properties of diastole and systole. During diastole as muscle length increases (e.g., the ventricular chamber size increases) the ability of the myocardium to develop force is increased, up to a point. Beyond a certain length, however, force development is impaired owing to the inadequate alignment of the actin and myosin filaments (Fig. 13.5).

In general, SV will increase with an increase in preload or contractility and will decrease with an increase in afterload. Normally about 55% to 75% of the preload is ejected as the SV. The *ejection fraction* (EF) demonstrates this relationship between SV and LVEDV such that EF = SV ÷ LVEDV. This value represents the ratio of the volume of blood ejected by the LV per contraction relative to the volume of blood received by the LV following diastole. Normal EF is approximately 55% to 75% (67% ± 8%) and is widely used clinically as an index of contractility.[17]

Clinically, especially in critical care settings, the concept of **cardiac index (CI)** is often preferred to CO. CI expresses the CO in relationship to the body surface area (BSA) expressed in meters such that CI = CO/BSA. Normal CO range at rest is 4 to 5 L/min; normal CI range is 2.5 to 3.5 L/min/m². CI provides a more complete determination of the adequacy of an individual's CO than CO alone. For example, in comparing a 6-ft tall individual and a 5-ft tall individual each with a CO of 3 L/min, the 5-ft tall person will have a higher CI and therefore better tissue perfusion because there is less BSA requiring the 3 L of CO. Determination of BSA and CI is often done using nomograms (two-dimensional diagrams) based on the Geigy scientific tables.[18]

Electrical Conduction of the Heart

It is important to note that mechanical contraction of the ventricles only occurs with appropriate electrical conduction through the heart. Effective contraction depends on an intact electrical conduction system that results in depolarization of the myocardium and timely repolarization. In *normal sinus rhythm (NSR)* the impulse begins in the sinus node and travels through the atria, the A–V node, bundle of His, Purkinje fibers, septum, and ventricles.

Electrical conduction can be viewed via the electrocardiogram (ECG) complex (Fig. 13.6). Each component of the complex reflects a certain phase of conduction pathway.[19]

- The P wave depicts sinus node and atrial depolarization.
- The PR segment demonstrates conduction through AV node.
- The QRS complex denotes electrical flow through the ventricles causing ventricular depolarization.
- The ST segment describes the initiation of ventricular repolarization.
- The T wave illustrates the completion of ventricular repolarization.

Each ECG complex represents one cardiac cycle or one heartbeat. In a series of ECG complexes representing sinus rhythm, each QRS complex should be preceded by a P wave and the QRS complexes should be equally spaced apart, indicating a regular rhythm. ECG interpretation enables the clinician to differentially diagnose the cause of reduced CO that may occur from a true mechanical problem versus that occurring from an electrical problem disrupting mechanical activity of the heart.

Myocardial Oxygen Supply and Demand

Myocardial oxygen supply and myocardial oxygen demand must be in balance. *Myocardial oxygen supply* depends on the delivery of oxygenated blood through the coronary arteries, the oxygen-carrying capacity of arterial blood, and the ability of the myocardial cells to extract oxygen from the arterial blood. *Myocardial oxygen demand* (MVO_2), the energy cost to the myocardium, is dependent on many factors. Clinically, MVO_2 is calculated as the product of HR and systolic blood pressure (SBP), known as the *rate pressure product (RPP)* or double product.[9] Any activity that increases HR and/or BP will increase MVO_2. Therefore, any increase in systemic oxygen demand (e.g., exercise) will increase the energy cost of the heart and increase MVO_2.

The myocardium is routinely very efficient at extracting oxygen from its blood supply. Therefore, during times of increased energy demand, very little increase in extraction can occur. The primary mechanism for increasing myocardial oxygen supply during times of increased demand is by increased *coronary blood flow*

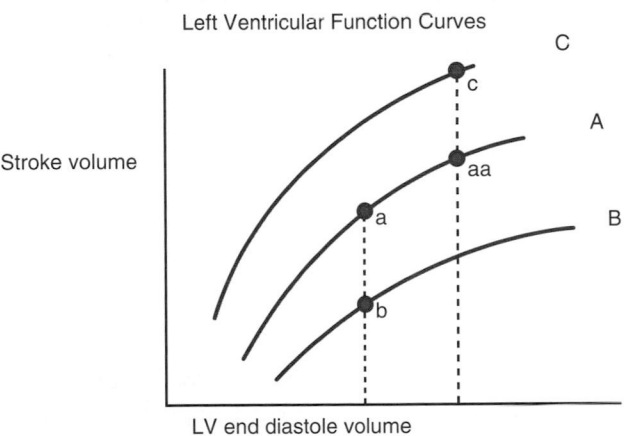

Figure 13.5 Left ventricular (LV) function curves. **(A)** With normal LV function, as the left ventricular volume increases, stroke volume will also increase. **(B)** With LV function impairment, the curve will shift to the right, and for any given length, stroke volume is decreased compared to normal (point *b* has a deceased SV compared to point *a*). **(C)** When normal LV function experiences an increase in sympathetic activity, the curve will shift to the left and SV will increase (note that point *c* is greater than point *aa*).

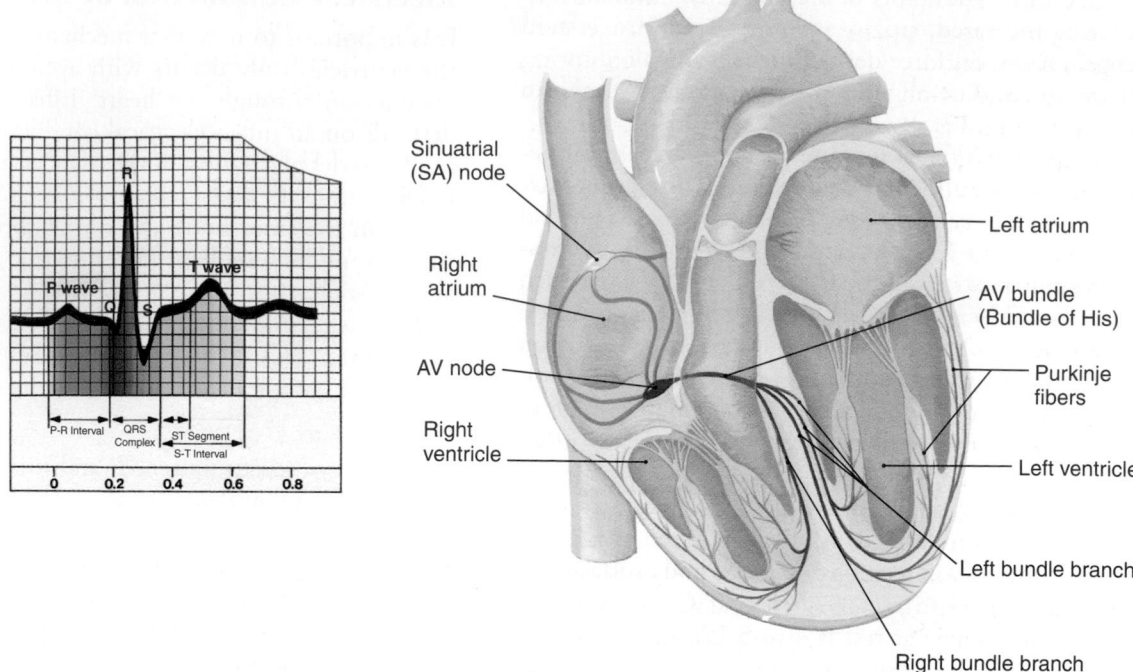

Figure 13.6 Schematic representation of the heart and normal cardiac electrical activity. The ECG is the body surface manifestation of the depolarization and repolarization waves of the heart. The P wave is generated by atrial depolarization, the QRS by ventricular muscle depolarization, and the T wave by ventricular repolarization. The PR interval is a measure of conduction time from atrium to ventricle, and the QRS duration indicates the time required for all of the ventricular cells to be activated. The QT interval reflects the duration of the ventricular action potential. *(Adapted from Taber's Cyclopedic Medical Dictionary, ed 21. FA Davis, Philadelphia, PA, 2005, p 1,022, with permission.)*

(CBF).[11] In general, there is a linear relationship between CBF and MVO$_2$. During exercise, CBF may increase five times above resting level in response to the increased demand. Unlike skeletal muscle, which has the capability of both aerobic and anaerobic metabolism, the heart muscle (myocardium) is essentially dependent on aerobic metabolism and has very limited anaerobic capacity.

Laboratory Values

When managing patients with heart disease, certain laboratory values are particularly important. Table 13.2 provides reference values for various laboratory tests. The hemoglobin and hematocrit levels depict the oxygen-carrying capacity within the system. Each gram of hemoglobin carries approximately 1.34 mL of oxygen within arterial blood. A normal hemoglobin level is approximately 12 to 14 g/100 mL of blood in adult males and 14 to 16 g/100 mL of blood in adult women. For example, for a hemoglobin level of 15 g/100 mL of blood, the oxygen-carrying capacity is approximately 20 mL O$_2$/100 mL of blood (15 × 1.34 = 20). Now, if we consider a patient with a hemoglobin level reduced to 7.5 g/100 mL of blood, the oxygen-carrying capacity is reduced by half and is approximately 10 mL of O$_2$/100 mL of blood. With reduced oxygen-carrying capacity, the heart must work harder to compensate for low oxygen levels to provide sufficient oxygen to the

Table 13.2	Laboratory Tests and Reference Values
Test	**Reference Value**
Sodium	135–145 mEq/L
Potassium	3.5–5.0 mEq/L
Chloride	95–105 mEq/L
Calcium	9–11 mg/dL
BUN	10–20
Creatinine	0.5–1.2 mg/dL
Glucose	70–110 mg/dL
Carbon dioxide	20–29 mEq/L
Magnesium	1.5–2.5 mEq/L
Hgb (g/dL)	Adult female: 12–16 Adult male: 13–18
HCT (%)	Adult female: 36–46 Adult male: 37–49

peripheral tissue. During heart failure, increased workload placed on a failing heart will exacerbate the failure. A general rule of thumb is to use caution and lower the intensity when exercising patients with hemoglobin levels less than 8 g/100 mL of blood.

Electrolyte levels are also important to consider before treating patients with heart disease. Appropriate levels of potassium, calcium, and magnesium allow for normal electrical conduction through the heart. *Hypokalemia,* low potassium (usually less than 3.5 mEq/L), produces arrhythmias with flattened T waves and depressed ST segments, as well as bilateral lower extremity muscle cramping. *Hypocalcemia* (low blood serum calcium levels) and *hypomagnesemia* (low magnesium in blood) have the potential of increasing ventricular ectopy within the heart. In addition, calcium enhances contractile function of muscle cells. Patients with hypocalcemia have reduced cardiac contractility whereas those with hypocalcaemia present with erratic heart beats.

Renal function tests are done to determine kidney function and examine *blood urea nitrogen* (BUN) and *creatinine* levels. These levels are especially important to review in patients with heart failure and patients prescribed with diuretics. Finally, a large number of patients with heart disease also have diabetes and therefore it is important to review blood glucose levels before exercise.

■ CARDIOVASCULAR RESPONSES TO AEROBIC EXERCISE

Normal Responses

An increase in oxygen uptake occurs with an increase in external workload. There is a direct, almost linear relationship between HR and external workload (Fig. 13.7). Therefore, if the physical therapy intervention requires an increase in systemic oxygen consumption expressed as either an increase in MET levels, kcal, L/O$_2$, or ml of O$_2$ per kg of body weight per minute, then HR should also increase. Although some cardiac medications, particularly the beta-blockers, which suppress the sympathetic nervous system's effect on the heart, will limit the actual amount of increase, HR should rise nonetheless. Failure of the HR to increase with increasing workloads (chronotropic incompetence) should be immediately evaluated. Other physiological parameters should be quickly examined, such as BP, respiratory rate, skin color, and temperature, as well as the patient's level of cognition and perceived exertion. An adverse response in any of these parameters is an indication of the patient's inability to hemodynamically respond to the given amount of work.

Blood pressure (BP) should be taken before and immediately after exercise with the patient in the same position (i.e., supine, sitting, standing) and from the same arm each time. Ideally, BP should be taken during exercise to determine the actual hemodynamic response to the increased workload. However, depending on the type of exercise modality, this may be technically difficult. In these cases HR and BP must be taken immediately after exercise. As with HR, a linear increase in systolic pressure is expected with increasing levels of work (see Fig. 13.7). Hellerstein et al[20] reported that for each 10% increment of maximal HR, systolic BP

increased 12 to 15 mm Hg. Naughton and Haider[21] interpreted an increase in systolic BP in excess of 12 mm Hg/MET as a hypertensive exercise response and an increase below 5 mm Hg as a hypotensive exercise response. Diastolic pressure exhibits limited changes with exercise; it may not change, or may either increase or decrease by 10 mm Hg.

In addition, as systemic oxygen requirements increase, the depth and rate of respirations will normally increase from rest. Therefore, tidal volume depicting the depth of respiration and respiration rate indicating the number of breaths per minute will change to meet the metabolic needs of the tissue.

Abnormal Responses

Signs and symptoms of exercise intolerance are presented in Box 13.1. If a patient experiences any of these symptoms, the activity should be stopped and the patient stabilized. It is also important to inform patients that some responses may be delayed for as long as several hours after exercise (e.g. prolonged fatigue, insomnia, sudden weight gain due to fluid retention). Observation of the patient throughout the physical therapy intervention provides a mechanism for ongoing examination. The therapist must be alert to subtle changes in the patient's facial expression, skin color, tone of voice, or thought processing because these may indicate activity intolerance and may require immediate patient examination and modification of the intervention. In addition to the patient's subjective complaint of fatigue or discomfort, there are other responses that warrant termination of an exercise session.[15] These abnormal responses are included in Box 13.1.

■ CARDIAC PATHOLOGIES AND PHYSICAL THERAPY IMPLICATIONS

The pathophysiological conditions that underlie heart disease are HTN, atherosclerosis within the coronary arteries, altered myocardial muscle mechanics, valvular dysfunction, and arrhythmias. The clinical presentations of CVD are diverse and depend on the source of the impairment: perfusion of coronary arteries, contractility of LV myocardium, or alteration of electrical activity. Common signs and symptoms associated with heart disease are chest pressure, dyspnea, fatigue, syncope, and palpitations. However, although these clinical manifestations are strongly associated with heart disease, they are not exclusive for heart disease. Therefore, taking a thorough patient history and performing an appropriate examination and evaluation are crucial to establishing the physical therapy diagnosis, anticipated goals, expected outcomes, and plan of care (POC).

An important consideration is that there is no direct objective measurement of activity limitations based solely on the cardiac diagnosis and pathology. Individuals with seemingly similar cardiac pathology may experience different activity limitations. Activity limitations

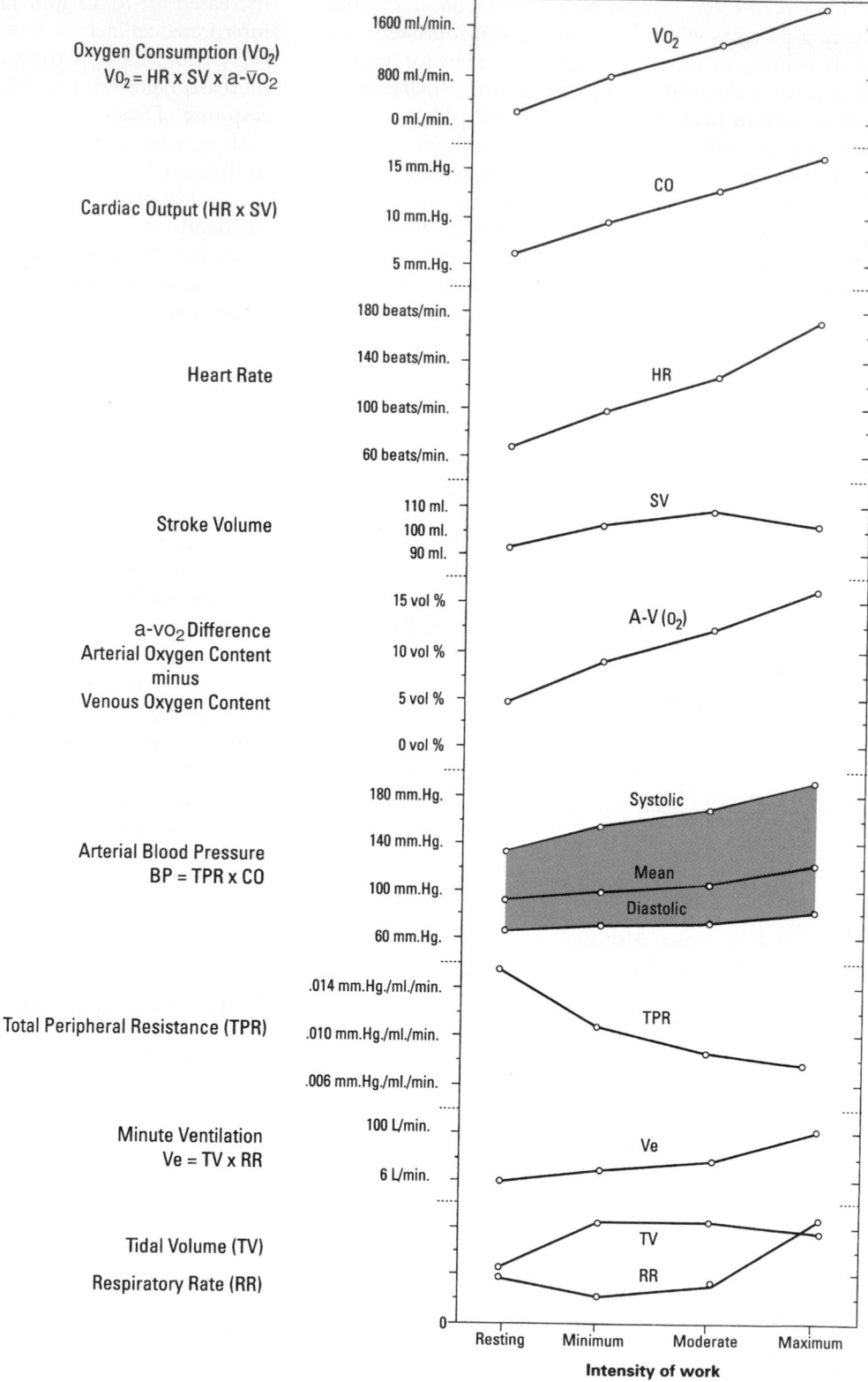

Figure 13.7 Cardiopulmonary response to acute aerobic exercise. *(Adapted from Berne, RM, and Levy, MN: Cardiovascular Physiology, ed 5. CV Mosby, St. Louis, 1986, p 237; Zadai, CC: Clinics in Physical Therapy, Pulmonary Management in Physical Therapy. Churchill Livingstone, New York, 1992, p 27; and McArdle, WD, et al: Essentials of Exercise Physiology. Lea & Febiger, Philadelphia, 1994, p 230.)*

Box 13.1 Indications of Exercise Intolerance That Warrant Modification or Termination of an Exercise Session

Signs and Symptoms

- Moderately severe or increasing angina
- Marked dyspnea
- Dizziness, light-headedness, or ataxia
- Cyanosis or pallor
- Excessive fatigue
- Leg cramps or claudication

Other Abnormal Responses

- Failure of the systolic pressure to rise as exercise continues
- A hypertensive BP response, including a systolic pressure of greater than 200 mm Hg and/or a diastolic pressure greater than 110 mm Hg
- A progressive fall in systolic pressure of 10–15 mm Hg
- A significant change in cardiac rhythm detected either by palpation or by ECG monitoring (e.g., arrhythmias, ST-T wave changes).

Adapted from ACSM's Guidelines for Exercise Testing and Prescription, ed 8. Lippincott Williams & Wilkins, Philadelphia, 2010.

experienced by the patient with CAD or heart failure may vary widely and are influenced by many factors other than the amount of intact, perfused myocardium or LV function. In response to cardiac impairments, neurohormonal and cardiovascular compensatory mechanisms are activated that allow cardiac functioning to continue for a period of time before the patient becomes symptomatic or there is a significant change in function. Activity limitations are therefore influenced by the amount of compensation as well as the pharmacological management. The following section will delineate the major pathologies affecting heart function, medical management of these conditions, and pertinent implications for physical therapist practice.

Hypertension

HTN is "the most prevalent cardiovascular disease in the United States and one of the most powerful contributors to cardiovascular morbidity and mortality."[22] It is estimated that 76 million Americans have HTN.[1] In addition, the prevalence of HTN in blacks in the United States is highest in the world with prevalence increasing from 35.8% to 41.4% from 1994 to 2002.[23]

HTN is defined as a persistent elevation of the systolic arterial blood pressure above 140 mm Hg or diastolic blood pressure above 90 mm Hg. In some patients, the blood pressure is not consistently elevated and fluctuates between hypertensive and normal values. This is termed *labile HTN* and is diagnosed following the evaluation of

elevated blood pressure values over a prolonged period of time.

The Joint National Committee (JNC VII) that evaluates and makes recommendations for HTN management defines the following stages of HTN: prehypertension, stage 1, stage 2, and stage 3 (Table 13.3).[24] Hypertensive individuals may have elevations in both systolic and diastolic values; however, in the elderly, isolated systolic hypertension (ISH) is commonly noted with elevations in the systolic blood pressure above 140 mm Hg with diastolic blood pressures in the normal range.[24]

Broadly, HTN may be divided into two major categories: *primary (or essential) HTN* and *secondary (or nonessential) HTN*. *Primary or essential HTN* is diagnosed when there is no known cause for the elevation in BP values and exists in approximately 90% to 95% of all patients with HTN. Genetic factors, environmental influences (including dietary sodium intake), stress, obesity, alcohol consumption, and other risk factors (including age, lack of exercise, and glucose intolerance) have implications on the occurrence of essential HTN. Regardless of the underlying cause, HTN results secondary to failure of control mechanisms responsible for lowering BP. *Secondary or nonessential HTN* occurs in approximately 5% to 10% of the hypertensive population and is caused by an identifiable medical problem such as renal, endocrine, vascular, or neurological complications.

Uncontrolled elevated BP levels produce a variety of additional complications, including heart failure, renal failure, dissecting aneurysms, PVD, retinopathy, and stroke. These negative consequences are directly related to the level of BP. Prior research indicates that higher systolic blood pressure at any given level of diastolic blood pressure increases morbidity in both genders.[25]

Medical Management of Hypertension

Pharmacological intervention is the most common form of medical management of HTN. Six classes of medications currently exist: beta-adrenergic blockers,

Table 13.3 Stages of Hypertension as Defined by JNC VII [24]

Hypertension is defined by either systolic or diastolic elevation. A BP of 110/90 is Stage 1 diastolic hypertension; a BP of 160/60 is Stage 3 systolic hypertension.

Stages of Hypertension	Systolic Blood Pressure (mm Hg)	Diastolic Blood Pressure (mm Hg)
Prehypertension	120–130	80–89
Stage 1	130–140	90–100
Stage 2	140–160	100–110
Stage 3	>160	>110

Normal: 119/79 or below.

alpha-adrenergic blockers, angiotensin-converting enzyme (ACE) inhibitors, diuretics, vasodilators, and calcium channel blockers.[9] In addition to pharmacology, it is important for clinicians to recommend lifestyle modifications, including weight reduction, sodium restriction, moderation of alcohol intake, and regular aerobic exercise, for patients diagnosed with HTN. The benefits of these lifestyle changes include lowering the dosage of medications and reduced occurrence of adverse side effects.

Implications for the Therapist

HTN is generally asymptomatic until complications develop in various organs throughout the body. It has therefore been called the "silent killer." When HTN affects heart function, the individual develops hypertensive heart disease and presents with exertional dyspnea, fatigue, impaired exercise tolerance, tachycardia, chest discomfort, and possible signs of heart failure. The *Guide to Physical Therapist Practice* indicates that BP monitoring is crucial for all adults over age 35 and in younger patients who are obese or have a history of glucose intolerance, diabetes, or renal dysfunction.[26] In addition, clinical monitoring of BP values must be done both at rest and during exercise. According to the American College of Sports Medicine, if resting BP is elevated (above 200 mm Hg systolic or above 100 mm Hg diastolic), physician clearance must be obtained before exercising the patient.[15] Also, if SBP rises to more than 250 mm Hg or if DBP exceeds 115 mm Hg, exercise must be terminated.[15]

Acute Coronary Syndrome

Acute coronary syndrome (ACS) is the new terminology for ischemic heart disease or CAD. It involves a spectrum of entities ranging from the least involved condition on the spectrum (unstable angina) to the worst involved condition (sudden cardiac death). Additional entities on the spectrum include non-Q myocardial infarction (NQMI) or non–ST-elevation myocardial infarction (NSTEMI) and Q myocardial infarction (QMI), also referred to as ST-segment elevation myocardial infarction (STEMI). The hallmark sign for any patient presenting with any condition on the spectrum is ischemic chest pain because of a dyssynchrony between the myocardial oxygen supply and demand.

The primary impairment in acute coronary syndrome is an imbalance of myocardial oxygen supply to meet the myocardial oxygen demand (MVO_2). The decrease in supply results from a narrowing of the lumen of the coronary artery, usually due to a fixed atherosclerotic lesion. Atherosclerosis is a disease in which lipid-laden plaque (lesions) is formed within the intimal layer of the blood vessel wall of moderate and large size arteries; over time the plaque may extend into the lumen causing a decreased lumenal diameter. The lesion results from an initial endothelial injury that causes changes within the intima of the blood vessel and progresses to lumenal narrowing. The cause of the initial injury is not well understood, but risk factors have been identified that are associated with an increased risk for the formation of an atherosclerotic lesion. The earliest identified risk factors by epidemiological studies such as the classic *Framingham Heart Study* included smoking, high cholesterol, HTN, diabetes, emotional stress, and family history.[27-29] Obesity, sedentary lifestyle, and elevated blood homocysteine and fibrinogen levels have also been identified as possible contributors.[30]

Clinical Manifestations

Occlusions may occur in coronary arteries and not produce symptoms. In general, symptoms of CAD are not experienced until the lumen is at least 70% occluded. There are, therefore, many patients who are unaware of their subacute occlusions. It is imperative that an individual's risk factors are known and interventions and monitoring adjusted accordingly.

The clinical conditions resulting from atherosclerosis of the coronary arteries are due to inadequate myocardial oxygen supply to meet the MVO_2. The three common clinical presentations of ACS are angina, injury, and infarction.

Angina

Angina, or cardiac-related chest pain, is due to ischemia. Ischemia is characterized by reduced blood flow to the myocardium. Ischemia is a temporary condition due to the imbalance between the myocardial oxygen supply and demand. On restoring the balance between oxygen supply and demand, ischemia will be reversed and the angina will disappear.

There are three major types of angina: unstable, stable, and variant angina. *Unstable angina,* sometimes referred to as preinfarction angina or crescendo angina, typically occurs at rest without any obvious precipitating factors or with minimal exertion. It is chest pain that increases in severity, frequency, and duration and is refractory to treatment. Unstable angina usually warrants immediate medical intervention, because the patient is at impending risk for further complications such as an MI or a lethal arrhythmia (V-tach or V-fib).

The term *stable angina* is used when angina occurs during exercise or activity. Chest pain is experienced at a certain intensity of exercise when the myocardial oxygen demand exceeds the blood supply to the myocardium and is alleviated by decreasing the MVO_2. As mentioned earlier, the MVO_2 is calculated as the product of HR and SBP, known as the rate pressure product (RPP). When patients experience episodes of stable angina, exercise must be terminated and HR and BP need to be taken to determine the RPP (RPP = HR × SBP). In addition to terminating exercise and resting, MVO_2 can also be reduced through the use of nitroglycerin (NTG). In stable angina, the patient often describes the sensation as an intensity less than 5/10, which improves to 0/10 when the oxygen supply is able to balance the demand. It is important to remember that any report of angina requires intervention; the clinician cannot ignore the symptoms even when the patient describes the sensation as light (1 to 2/10).

The third type of angina is *variant* or *Prinzmetal angina* and is caused by a vasospasm of coronary arteries in the absence of occlusive disease. Patients with this type of angina respond to NTG for short-term management of their chest pain. However, the preferred long-term pharmacological choice is a calcium channel blocker to reduce the influx of calcium into the smooth muscle cells of the coronary arteries and reduce vasospasm.

Injury and Infarction

Injury represents the presence of a new acute MI.[31] The term *injury* is used because the myocardial tissue is being acutely injured during a sudden heart attack. Acute injury to the myocardial tissue then progresses to irreversible, dead infarcted tissue. The tissue, once dead, is irreversible and dead forever. Thus the term *injury* illustrates the presence of a new MI, whereas the term *infarction* depicts an old heart attack with dead tissue that cannot be reversed.

Individual myocardial cells may differ in their tolerance for ischemia; however, irreversible changes start to appear 20 minutes to 2 hours from the onset of myocardial ischemia.[32] The actual process of injury and infarction evolves over a period of hours. Angina commonly precedes an MI, but the intensity of the symptoms is dramatically increased. Patients frequently describe their discomfort as 10 out of 10 on a pain scale during an acute MI. Infarction is irreversible. Whereas ischemia is due to a partial blockage of the coronary artery, an infarction results from complete occlusion of the vessel. This occlusion commonly results from a rupture of a vulnerable plaque with resultant formation of a thrombus. The type of plaque, more so than the size, will influence the risk of rupture. Lipid-rich and soft plaques are more vulnerable to rupture than collagen-rich and hard plaques. Angiographically large plaque lesions are not necessarily more susceptible to rupture than smaller lesions. Because atherosclerosis begins within the walls of the artery, many vulnerable plaques are invisible via angiogram or appear smaller than their actual size. Although not as common as plaque rupture, coronary occlusion can occur as a result of coronary spasm, coronary emboli, congenital anomalies, and a wide variety of inflammatory diseases.[33] The actual cause of plaque rupture is not clearly understood; however, as a result of the rupture, a thrombus is formed. There may be several mechanisms for thrombosis formation, such as mechanical obstruction of the lumen, release of tissue thromboplastin and the initiation of the clotting cascade, and

platelet plug formation from the contact of platelets and exposed collagen.[34] Only lesions that occlude the lumen by 70% or more can cause ischemia, but smaller lesions can and do cause MIs. It is important to remember that the size of the initial lesions does not determine whether or not an MI can occur; a small plaque lesion of 30% as well as a larger lesion of 80% may rupture and subsequently form a thrombus that occludes the remainder of the lumen. The majority of MIs occur as a result of initial plaque lesions that occlude less than 60% of the lumen and are not hemodynamically significant to cause ischemia.[35] The effects on the ventricle as a result of the infarction often extend beyond the acute infarction period; these long-term effects occur primarily in ventricles that have sustained a moderate to large MI. As the ventricle heals, a process of *remodeling* occurs as a result of the presence of the infarcted tissue and subsequent dilation. Over time, this reengineering process produces an alteration in ventricular size, shape, and function. Thus, the resultant ventricle often operates at an increased myocardial energy cost due to its inefficient muscle mechanics. Often pictured as three concentric circles (although not absolutely histologically correct), the area of infarction would be at the center of the circle surrounded first by an area of injury and then an outside area of ischemia (Fig. 13.8).

Although most MIs heal initially without incident, complications may occur. The major complications following an MI are recurrence of ischemia, LV failure, and ventricular arrhythmias. Therefore, when a patient is said to have had a *complicated MI*, it is indicative that ischemia, LV failure, or significant ventricular arrhythmias have developed in the acute post-MI period. Ischemia after MI is particularly important because it indicates that there may be vulnerable myocardium with a reduced oxygen supply that may go on to infarct

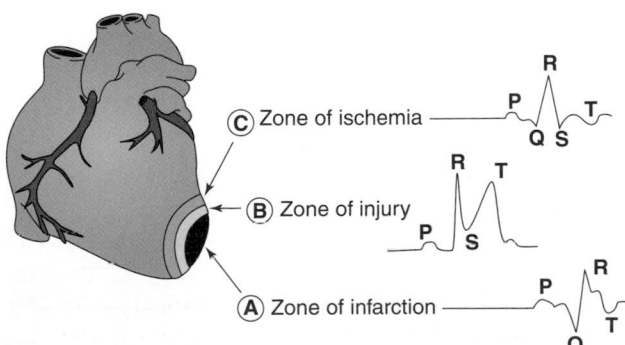

Figure 13.8 ECG following an MI. **(A)** *Zone of infarction*: when infarction occurs through the full thickness of the myocardium (transmural) an abnormal Q wave usually appears. **(B)** *Zone of injury*: ST elevation occurs in the area of injury. **(C)** *Zone of ischemia*: ST depression and/or T-wave inversion occurs in an area of decreased perfusion (ischemia).

and thereby potentially enlarge the MI. The ultimate complication would be **cardiogenic shock** with inadequate CO and insufficient arterial BP to perfuse the major organs as a result of severe LV failure. This may necessitate extraordinary medical interventions such as the *intra-aortic balloon pump (IABP)*. The IABP facilitates CO, decreases MVO_2, and increases coronary artery perfusion. The IABP is a balloon catheter placed within the aorta that inflates during diastole, thereby increasing coronary artery perfusion, and deflates during systole, thereby decreasing afterload. The IABP may be used in other conditions besides post-MI cardiogenic instability, for example, patients with hemodynamic decompensation who are awaiting heart transplantation, patients with unstable angina and malignant arrhythmias (such as V-tach or V-fib), or post–cardiac surgical patients with severe hemodynamic instability.[16]

Evaluation of Acute Coronary Syndrome (the Evaluation Triad)

In addition to the history taking and review of systems, the evaluation of patients with ACS places emphasis on three major components: evaluating patient complaints, ECG changes, and cardiac enzyme levels (Fig. 13.9). Below is a review of each component.

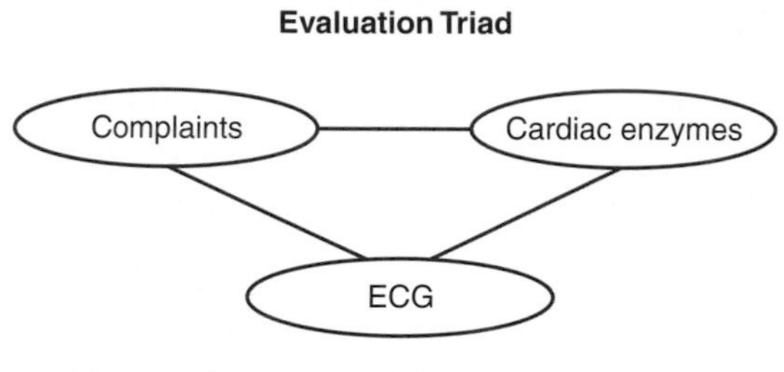

Evaluation Triad

Complaints — Cardiac enzymes

ECG

Figure 13.9 Evaluation triad for patients with acute coronary syndrome.

Patient Complaints

Chest pain from ischemic origin is diffuse and retrosternal. The patient usually reports an intense pressure like "an elephant sitting on the chest." It may radiate to anywhere in the upper extremities and thorax, most specifically to the left arm and left jaw. Figure 13.10 delineates common areas for referred patterns of chest pain. The hallmark approach to differentially diagnosing ischemic chest pain from nonischemic chest pain is to observe for accompanying signs and symptoms of compromised cardiac output. These signs include dizziness, lightheadedness, weakness, diaphoresis (sweating), fatigue, and weakness. Thus, cardiac chest pain during ischemia or an infraction will be accompanied by signs of compromised CO, but chest pain from other etiologies, including pulmonary chest pain, pleural pain, or musculoskeletal pain will not.

ECG Changes

MIs are identified by 12-lead ECG findings. The ECG (also referred to as EKG) is used to examine HR, rhythm, conduction delays, and coronary perfusion. Two of the most common types of ECG are the single-lead and the 12-lead ECG (Fig. 13.11). In the single-lead ECG, only one area of the heart (e.g., anterior, lateral, or inferior) may be viewed at a time. This area may be changed, however, by altering the location of the electrodes. In the 12-lead ECG, 12 areas may be viewed.

The single-lead ECG is sensitive to rate and rhythm changes and is commonly used for monitoring patients during ambulation and activity. Continuous monitoring is accomplished either via telemetry (radio transmission), allowing the patient freedom to move around when wearing this portable device, or by hardwire, where the patient is attached to the monitor by a cable approximately 15 ft long, therefore limiting mobility. A variation of the single-lead ECG is the 3-lead ECG,

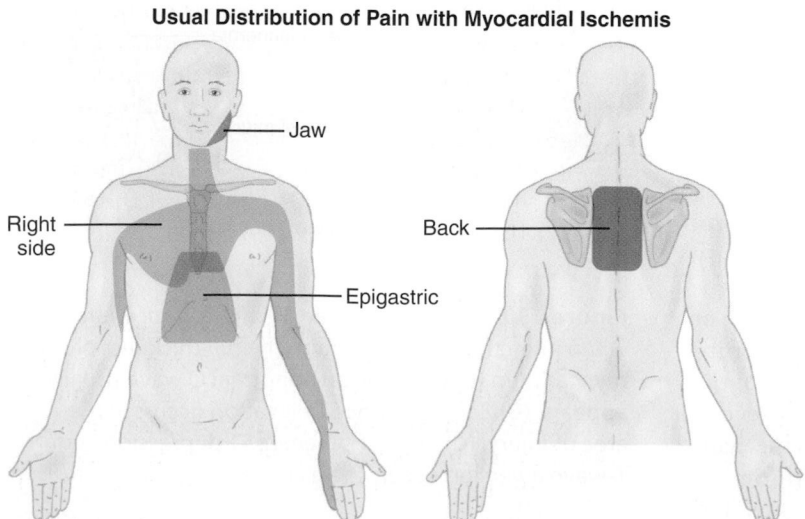

Usual Distribution of Pain with Myocardial Ischemis

Jaw

Right side

Back

Epigastric

Figure 13.10 Referral pattern for chest pain.

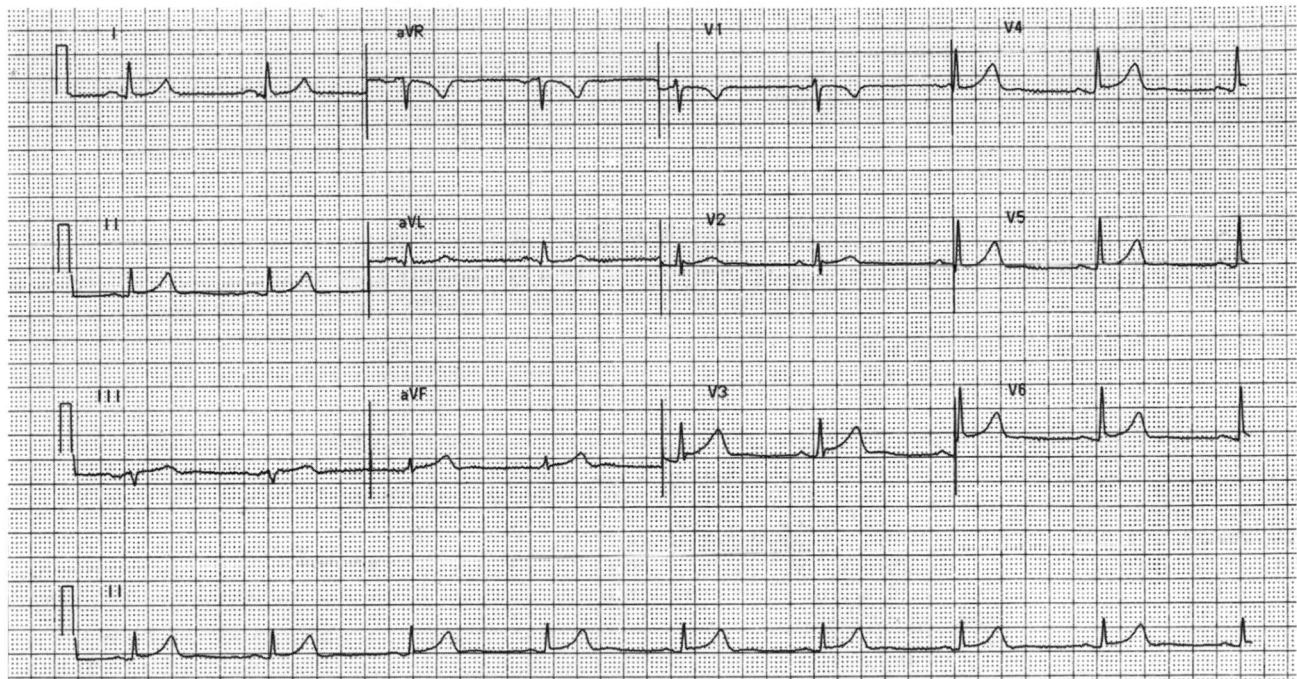

Figure 13.11 Normal 12-lead ECG from 50-year-old woman; slight ST elevation is insignificant. Twelve leads are presented; at the bottom of the page is a rhythm strip from lead II. Heart rate from the rhythm strip is approximately 52 (there are 5.8 large boxes between complex 3 and 4; therefore 300/5.8 = 52).

which is usually hardwire and is used for monitoring in an inpatient setting. It can be worn continuously throughout an entire treatment session or throughout the entire hospitalization. Unlike the single-lead or 3-lead system, the 12-lead ECG does not provide continuous monitoring, except during an **exercise tolerance test (ETT)**. Two common uses for the 12-lead ECG are the resting ECG taken with the patient quietly supine and the ETT. Twelve-lead ECGs are invaluable in identifying perfusion impairments in the coronary arteries and in assisting with arrhythmia detection. During the ETT, the ECG is continuously monitored to determine the presence of ischemia or arrhythmias with each increase in workload. The 12-lead ECG is sensitive to changes in perfusion as well as rate, rhythm, and conduction. Each coronary artery is represented by a cluster of leads that, although not absolutely correlated with each individual's anatomy, gives a general schema for myocardial perfusion.

During the examination of a 12-lead ECG, the ST segment is clinically useful in identifying the presence of impaired coronary perfusion, either ischemia or injury. The *J point,* the point where the S wave turns into the ST segment, is the point of reference for interpreting the ST segment. If ischemia is present, the ST segment will be depressed (one or two small boxes) at two small boxes beyond the J point, and the T wave may also be inverted (flipped). Ischemic changes will be present only while the ischemia is present; when the ischemia has resolved,

the ECG will return to normal. Conversely, a large acute MI, with subsequent injury to the myocardial tissue, will produce ST-segment elevations on the 12-lead ECG. Large ST elevation myocardial infarction (STEMI) will produce pathological Q waves hours to days following the acute process. Therefore a QMI represents a large MI (formerly known as a *transmural MI* because it was believed to involve the full thickness of the ventricular wall). Conversely, an acute MI may be relatively smaller and not cause acute injury to the myocardial tissue. In this case, ST segments are not seen on the ECG and the MI is termed an NSTEMI or an NQMI. An NQMI was formerly known as a *nontransmural* or *subendocardial MI* because it usually involved the endocardium. An MI that initially presents as an STEMI may be an indication for emergent thrombolytic therapy or revascularization.[16]

Anatomical classifications for MIs are based on the surfaces of the LV and not the anatomical heart. An anterior MI involves the anterior surface of the LV, an inferior MI involves the inferior surface of the LV (the diaphragmatic region), a lateral MI involves the lateral surface of the LV (also may be referred to the free wall of the LV for the lateral wall is not adjacent to another structure), a septal MI involves the septum, and a posterior MI involves the LV posterior wall. MIs to different aspects of the ventricle result from compromised levels of blood flow within specific vessels. The RCA supplies blood to the inferior and posterior aspects of the LV and therefore is responsible for producing an inferior- or posterior-wall MI. The anterior and septal aspects of the LV are perfused by the LAD and therefore LAD occlusions are likely to produce anterior or septal MIs. The CX artery supplies blood to the lateral wall of the LV and thereby produces a lateral infarction when it is occluded. The involvement of specific vessels can be determined by a 12-lead ECG. RCA involvement is most likely depicted on leads II, III, and aVF (augmented unipolar limb lead). LAD pathology will be illustrated in chest leads V1, V2, V3, and V4, whereas CX pathology will most likely be demonstrated in leads I, aVL, V5, and V6 (Fig. 13.12).

Enzyme Levels

Blood work also helps determine the presence of an MI. Creatine kinase MB subunit (CK-MB), an isoenzyme, is released into blood and elevates with intracellular myocardial damage. Creatine kinase (CK) is found in many tissues besides the myocardium, especially striated muscle, brain, and liver. Injury to these areas will elevate total CK.

To differentiate the type of tissue injured, use of CK-MB will isolate the source to the myocardium. Troponin levels should not be elevated in the setting of striated muscle trauma. Other markers that may be used to diagnose an acute MI are the proteins troponin I, troponin T, and myoglobin. Total CK-MB, troponin I, and troponin T have a high sensitivity for the diagnosis of an MI.[10,11] CK-MB and myoglobin may be the most sensitive biomarkers for patients presenting for emergent medical intervention within 6 to 10 hours of the onset of an MI.[10] For patients presenting after 10 hours, troponin biomarkers are preferred over CK-MB because of their increased sensitivity.[11] Table 13.4 provides a summary of enzyme levels that are elevated with a myocardial infarction.

Medical Management of Acute Coronary Syndrome

Once the diagnosis of an MI has been reached (i.e., the patient is "ruled in" for an MI), the goal of medical management is to keep the patient hemodynamically stable and optimize the wound healing of the myocardium. Revascularization procedures and pharmacological interventions are addressed in the following sections.

Revascularization Procedures

Percutaneous Transluminal Coronary Angioplasty

Percutaneous transluminal coronary angioplasty (PTCA) uses a balloon and collapsed stents (stainless steel "cage-like" tube with multiple slots) on the tip of a catheter inserted into the radial or femoral artery and advanced retrograde along the aorta to the openings of the coronary arteries. The catheter is inserted into the coronary artery until the site of the lesion is reached. The balloon is then inflated and the stent expands, compressing the plaque against the interior artery walls, thereby increasing the lumenal area. The balloon is deflated and removed and the stent holds the lumen open. The stent is commonly coated with a drug (e.g., paclitaxel [Abraxane]). Drug-coated stents (collectively referred to as *drug-eluting stents*) are used to prevent endothelial cell proliferation, which may occur in response to endothelial

I Lateral Circ	aVR	V1 Septal LAD	V4 Anterior LAD
II Inferior RCA	aVL Lateral Circ	V2 Septal LAD	V5 Lateral Circ
III Inferior RCA	aVF Inferior RCA	V3 Anterior LAD	V6 Lateral Circ

Figure 13.12 Anatomic pathology and ECG interpretation. Leads I, aVL, V5, and V6 depict problems in the lateral aspect of the left ventricle due to occlusion of blood flow within the circumflex artery. Leads II, III, and aVF depict problems in the inferior aspect of the left ventricle due to occlusion of blood flow within the right coronary artery. Leads V1 to V4 depict problems in the anterior aspect of the left ventricle due to occlusion of blood flow within the left anterior descending artery.

Table 13.4   Cardiac Enzymes Associated with Myocardial Injury and Infarction

Enzyme	Normal Level	Minor Cardiac Dysfunction	Major Cardiac Dysfunction	Peak Levels
Creatine kinase - myocardial band CK-MB	0%–3%	5%	10%	14–36 hours
Lactic dehydrogenase LDH	100–225 mU/mL or 127 IU	300–750 mU/mL	≥1000 mU/mL	
Troponin	0–0.2 µg/mL	5 µg/mL	≥10 µg/mL	24–36 hours
Myoglobin	<100 ng/mL	200 ng/mL	≥500 ng/mL	

trauma and the presence of a foreign object placed within the coronary artery and result in restenosis (recurrence of stenosis).

Clinical Implications for the Therapist

The surgical and catheterization reports identify which vessels were revascularized and which vessels have less than 70% lesions and were therefore not revascularized. Because a vessel is not currently a candidate for revascularization does not guarantee that it will not be problematic at a later date, either by rupturing or continuing to demonstrate progressive atherosclerosis. It would be short sighted to assume that a patient who has had a revascularization procedure cannot become ischemic.

There are at present no strict guidelines for when a patient may resume aerobic training following an angioplasty. Conventional wisdom, however, favors waiting approximately 2 weeks to allow the inflammatory process resulting from the intervention an appropriate time to subside. The new exercise prescription should be based on the results of the post-angioplasty ETT, not the pre-angioplasty ETT, which was more than likely positive. Patients may continue to ambulate at a low intensity and comfortable pace during the first 1 to 2 weeks following the PTCA, but should avoid the moderate to higher intensities associated with aerobic training.

Coronary Artery Bypass Graft

Coronary artery bypass graft (CABG) uses a donor vessel to bypass the lesion (narrowed lumen) and establish an alternate improved blood supply. The donor vessel may be the radial artery of the nondominant upper extremity (UE), the saphenous vein, or the internal mammary artery. The patient's harvested saphenous vein or radial artery must be completely detached from both its proximal and distal insertions; the graph is sutured proximally into the aorta and distally into the involved artery beyond the occlusion. When the internal mammary artery is used, it maintains its native proximal attachment while the distal segment is reattached below (bypass) the area of occlusion. Bypass surgery techniques are constantly evolving; traditionally, the full sternum was cut and retracted, but newer minimally invasive techniques termed *minimally invasive direct coronary artery bypass* (MIDCAB) have emerged that involve less sternal cutting, and some techniques involve no sternal cutting at all, but access the heart via the intercostal space.

Most CABG procedures involve placing the patient on an artificial heart–lung machine (bypass pump), which maintains the oxygenation and circulation of the blood while the heart is stopped during the surgical procedure. As a result of the bypass pump, patients may have additional fluid weight gain following surgery, may feel fatigued, and some patients may have transient A-fib and cognitive changes. Newer techniques have facilitated the use of *off-pump procedures* to limit the time on the bypass pump. Thus the surgeon operates on a beating heart for the entire or part of the procedure to limit time on the heart–lung machine and reduce the negative sequelae that result from excessive pump time.

Clinical Implications for the Therapist

For patients who have had bypass surgery (e.g., CABG), recovery is somewhat slower than that for PTCA owing to the complexity of the surgical procedure and the incisional healing. Prolonged time in the crucifix position during surgery may predispose individuals to developing an ulnar nerve palsy after surgery. Examination of sensation and manual muscle testing is indicated to rule out the potential for brachial plexus injuries.

The number and location of incisions depend on the surgeon's technique (i.e., either a full sternal cut, partial sternal cut, or intercostal approach). The donor graph site may require additional incisions: a leg incision if saphenous vein is used, a nondominant arm incision if radial artery is used, or no additional incision if grafted with the internal mammary artery. Physical therapy intervention will address any soft tissue impairments associated with the incision to maintain appropriate tissue extensibility and range of motion (ROM), with awareness that patients often indicate soreness and/or discomfort around the donor site. If a sternal wound is present, appropriate posture, scapula retraction, and functional shoulder movements should be encouraged. Proprioceptive neuromuscular facilitation (PNF) UE diagonal patterns often work well, as do the traditional cardinal plane ROM exercises. Patients should be reminded that only a few repetitions at a time throughout the day are better tolerated than more intensive repetitions 1 to 2 times per day; the latter regimen often results in incisional soreness. Some surgeons choose to limit UE ROM exercises during the 4 to 6 weeks following surgery while the sternum is healing; however, it is unclear as to the rationale for the limitation.

Sternal precautions are commonly applied to reduce dehiscence of the incision. Cited risk factors for dehiscence include diabetes, pendulous breasts, obesity, and COPD.[36] Interestingly, there is no direct evidence that links the use of arm movements or activity to an increased risk of sternal complications after surgery.[36] Prior research has indicated that patients with chronic sternal instability demonstrate greatest sternal separation when pushing up from a chair with sit-to-stand transfers and least sternal separation when elevating both arm overhead.[37] In addition, in normal health individuals, the greatest amount of sternal skin movement was seen with sit-to-stand and supine–to–long sitting transfers and the least movement was noted when raising a unilateral weighted UE (less than 8 lb) above shoulder height.[38] Patients with chronic sternal instability tend to experience pain that is greater when raising a unilateral loaded UE compared to raising bilateral loaded UEs.[39]

Sternal precautions vary greatly by physician, institution, and type of surgery performed. Instructions may include limiting lifting of objects between 5 and 10 pounds for up to 8 weeks after surgery. It is important to develop a professional collegial relationship with the surgical team to discuss surgical techniques and mobility concerns to ensure the best outcome for the patient.

To avoid sternal discomfort, all patients will benefit from splinting the incision with a hand or pillow when laughing, coughing, or sneezing. Patients will also appreciate information regarding energy conservation and rest periods. Even though the heart function is perhaps the best it has been in quite some time, the effects of major surgery on energy level and mobility must be emphasized. The impact of fatigue on the patient's sense of well-being may be profound, and it is important that patients understand the need for rest as well as ambulation. Early ambulation and mobility beginning the first day after surgery will assist in the patient's physical and emotional recovery.

During the initial weeks following cardiac surgery, the early in-hospital limitations following cardiac surgery have perhaps more to do with the surgical procedure and altered mobility and less to do with the heart itself, which is theoretically healthier than it was before surgery. Postoperative fatigue may be due to a combination of factors, including anesthesia, blood loss, initial weight gain due to cardiopulmonary bypass machine, common arrhythmias such as A-fib, and the energy cost of healing. As with the post-MI recovery period, when the patient returns home following surgery it is a good idea to break the day into many subunits including rest, leisure activity, and perhaps visiting with friends by phone or in person. Developing a schedule but keeping it flexible helps the patient exert some control over the day and energy level.

The patient is encouraged to gradually increase walking, with a goal of 30 minutes of ambulation 1 to 2 times per day at 4 to 6 weeks after surgery. If the patient is walking in the neighborhood, suggest that the initial walks be back and forth in front of the house rather than around the block. In this way, if the patient overestimates his or her energy level, the close proximity of home will provide a welcomed rest and prevent overexertion. Many patients ambitiously begin their walk only to find themselves suddenly fatigued and further from home than they would like. Continuing exercises for posture, UE and trunk mobility, and sternal protection are also important components of the home exercise program (HEP).

Once a patient's incisions have healed (approximately 6 weeks) and his or her blood counts including hematocrit and hemoglobin are in acceptable ranges, cardiac rehabilitation may begin. The patient may have a maximal ETT and begin aerobic and strength training.

Pharmacological Management

Cardiovascular pharmacological agents are critical in the medical management of patients with CAD. There are a variety of drugs designed to reestablish the balance of myocardial supply and demand, with new drugs being added all the time. The major anti-ischemic categories

are beta-blockers, calcium channel blockers, and nitrates. *Beta-blockers* decrease beta-sympathetic activity on the heart, resulting in a decrease in HR and contractility and therefore energy demand. *Calcium channel blockers* reduce BP and therefore decrease the work of the heart. Calcium channel blockers are also somewhat unique in preventing coronary smooth muscle spasm and thereby may increase myocardial blood supply. *Nitrates,* one of the oldest categories of drugs, are potent vasodilators that decrease preload and afterload, and therefore decrease myocardial work, as well as dilate coronary arteries. *Afterload reducers,* particularly those that affect the renin–angiotensin–aldosterone system such as *angiotensin-converting enzyme (ACE) inhibitors* and *angiotensin receptor blockers (ARBs),* are frequently used to normalize BP and reduce workload on the heart. The effect of some of the more widely used cardiac drugs on HR, BP, and ECG findings are presented in Table 13.5.

Heart Failure

Heart failure is a syndrome characterized by impaired cardiac pump function, resulting in inadequate systemic perfusion and an inability to meet the body's metabolic demands. Being a syndrome, patients in heart failure present with an array of signs and symptoms. This section presents the epidemiology, causes and types of heart failure, pathophysiological and clinical presentation of heart failure, and medical management and evaluation for this patient population. A discussion of physical therapy interventions for managing patients with heart failure will be delineated later in this chapter.

Epidemiology of Heart Failure

With the marked improvement in anti-ischemic medications, increased knowledge and management of CAD risk factors, availability of sophisticated monitoring, and revascularization techniques, more patients are living longer with coronary disease than similar patients 20 or 30 years ago. New technology and medications continually improve the understanding and management of CAD; however, an undesired effect of long-term CAD may be the increased prevalence of heart failure, also known as **congestive heart failure (CHF)**. Technology and other advances in medicine are reducing mortality with a concomitant increase in morbidity. Therefore, patients with heart failure are less likely to die and more likely to live longer with the worldwide prevalence and incidence of heart failure approaching epidemic proportions. In the United States, heart failure affects 5.7 million individuals with approximately 670,000 incident cases of heart failure diagnosed annually.[40] Estimates of the prevalence of heart failure in the general European population are similar to the Unites States and range from 0.4% to 2%.[41] In North America and Europe the lifetime risk of developing heart failure in both sexes at age 40 is approximately 1 in 5. In addition, 6% to 10% of people older than 65 have heart failure, indicating an exponential rise in the prevalence of

Table 13.5   Effects of Medications on Heart Rate, Blood Pressure, ECG, and Exercise Capacity

Medications	Heart Rate	Blood Pressure	ECG	Exercise Capacity
I. Beta-blockers (including carvedilol and labetalol)	↓* (R and E)	↓ (R and E)	↓ HR* (R) ↓ ischemia† (E)	↑ in patients with angina; ↓ or ↔ in patients without angina
II. Nitrates	↑ (R) ↑ or ↔ (E)	↓ (R) ↓ or ↔ (E)	↑ HR (R) ↑ or ↔ HR (E) ↓ ischemia† (E)	↑ in patients with angina; ↔ in patients without angina; or ↔ in patients with congestive heart failure (CHF)
III. Calcium channel blockers Amlodipine Isradipine Nicardipine Nifedipine Nimodipine	↓ or ↔ (R and E)	↓ (R and E)	↑ or ↔ HR (R and E) ↓ ischemia (E)	↑ in patients with angina; ↔ in patients without angina
Diltiazem Verapamil	↓ (R and E)		↓ HR (R and E) ↓ ischemia† (E)	
IV. Digitalis	↓ in patients w/atrial fibrillation and possibly CHF Not significantly altered in patients w/sinus rhythm	↔ (R and E)	May produce non-specific ST-T wave changes (R) May produce ST segment depression (E)	Improved only in patients with atrial fibrillation or in patients with CHF
V. Diuretics	↔ (R and E)	↔ or ↓ (R and E)	↔ or PVCs (R) May cause PVCs and "false-positive" test results if hypokalemia occurs May cause PVCs if hypomagnesemia occurs (E)	↔ except possibly in patients with CHF
VI. Vasodilators, ACE inhibitors and angiotensin II blockers	↑ or ↔ (R and E) ↔ (R and E)	↓ (R and E) ↓ (R and E)	↑ or ↔ HR (R and E) ↔ (R and E)	↔ except ↑ or ↔ in patients with CHF ↔ except ↑ or ↔ in patients with CHF
Alpha-adrenergic blockers	↔ (R and E)	↓ (R and E)	↔ (R and E)	↔
Antiadrenergic agents without selective blockade	↓ or ↔ (R and E)	↓ (R and E)	↓ or ↔ HR (R and E)	↔
VII. Nicotine	↑ or ↔ (R and E)	↑ (R and E)	↑ or ↔ HR May provoke ischemia, arrhythmias (R and E)	↔ except ↓ or ↔ in patients with angina

Adapted from American College of Sports Medicine: Guidelines for Exercise Testing and Prescription, ed 8. Lippincott, Williams & Wilkins, Baltimore, 2010, pp 286, 287, and 289, with permission.

Key: ↑ = increase; ↔ = no effect; ↓ = decrease; E = exercise; R = rest.

*Beta-blockers with intrinsic sympathomimetic action (ISA) lower resting HR only slightly.

†May prevent or delay myocardial ischemia.

heart failure with increasing age.[42] In looking at gender differences, although the relative incidence of heart failure is lower in women compared to men, women constitute half of all cases with heart failure because of their longer life expectancy.[43] Heart failure has surpassed MI as the leading cause of cardiac deaths in the United States and is the most frequent cardiac diagnosis for hospital admissions and readmissions.

Causes of Heart Failure

The most common cause of heart failure is cardiac muscle dysfunction. *Cardiac muscle dysfunction* is a general term describing altered systolic and/or diastolic activity of the myocardium that usually develops as a result of an underlying abnormality within the cardiac structure or function.[9] Several reasons exist for the development of cardiac muscle dysfunction. Box 13.2 presents potential precursors and risk factors for the development of cardiac muscle dysfunction.

Types of Heart Failure

Heart failure may be categorized based on a structural perspective and a functional perspective. From a structural perspective, heart failure is described as being *left-sided heart failure* or *right-sided heart failure*.[44] Left-sided heart failure occurs with LV insult. Pathology of the LV reduces the CO leading to a backup of fluid into the LA and lungs. The increased fluid in the lungs produces the two hallmark pulmonary signs of left-sided heart failure: shortness of breath (SOB) and cough. Primary right-sided heart failure occurs from direct insult to the RV caused by conditions that increase PA pressure. Increased pressure within the PA subsequently increases the afterload, thereby placing greater demands on the RV and causing it to go into failure. With RV failure, blood is not effectively ejected from the RV and backs up into the RA and venous vasculature, producing two hallmark peripheral signs: jugular venous distention and peripheral edema. Often, left-sided heart failure may be severe as seen in patients experiencing a heart failure exacerbation. With severe LV pathology, fluid from the LV backs up into the lungs, increasing PA pressure and causing fluid to back up into the right side of the heart and the systemic venous vasculature. This is termed biventricular failure. Therefore, patients with biventricular failure will present with both pulmonary and systemic signs of heart failure. Table 13.6 provides hemodynamic pressures noted with left, right, and biventricular failure.

Box 13.2   Causes of Cardiac Muscle Dysfunction

Precursors	Description
Hypertension	Increased peripheral arterial pressure contributes to increased afterload and pathological hypertrophy of the left ventricle.
Coronary artery disease	Acute injury to myocardial tissue damages ventricular contractility causing systolic dysfunction. Scar formation seen in infracted tissue alters relaxation and may lead to diastolic dysfunction.
Cardiac dysrhythmias	Normal electrical conduction through the heart allows for normal mechanical contraction of the ventricles. Altered electrical conduction alters the mechanical activity of the ventricles exacerbating heart failure.
Valve abnormalities	Cardiac valve pathology (stenosis or regurgitation) causes structural changes to the chamber behind the valve resulting in cardiac muscle dysfunction and failure.
Pericardial pathology	Pericarditis (fluid in the pericardial space) with resultant cardiac tamponade compresses the ventricles leading to cardiac muscle dysfunction and heart failure.
Cardiomyopathies	Damage to the myocardial cells from various pathological processes alters the systolic and/or diastolic function of the ventricles.

Table 13.6   Example of Hemodynamic Pressures Associated with Heart Failure

An increase in PAP and/or PCWP is associated with LV failure; an increase in CVP is associated with RV failure; and an increase in CVP, PAP, and PCWP is associated with biventricular failure.

Pressure (Norms)	LV Failure	RV Failure	Biventricular Failure
CVP (0–8 mm Hg)	6 mm Hg	12 mm Hg	12 mm Hg
PAP (9–19) mm Hg	22 mm Hg	16 mm Hg	22 mm Hg
PCWP (6–12) mm Hg	18 mm Hg	10 mm Hg	18 mm Hg

CVP = central venous pressure; LV = left ventricle; PAP = pulmonary artery pressure; PCWP = pulmonary capillary wedge pressure; RV = right ventricle;

From a functional perspective, heart failure is described as systolic or diastolic dysfunction.[44,45] *Systolic dysfunction* is characterized by compromised contractile function of the ventricles causing reductions in the SV, CO, and EF. Patients with systolic dysfunction will usually present with compromised ejection fractions (EFs) less than 40%. *Diastolic dysfunction* is characterized by compromised diastolic function of the ventricles. With this condition, the ventricles cannot relax and fill appropriately during the relaxation (diastolic) phase of the cardiac cycle. The impaired ability to fill the ventricles with blood reduces the volume of blood ejected with each contraction (the SV) and the overall volume of blood ejected per minute (the CO). EF is unaltered and remains normal between 55% and 75%. No reduction in the ratio is noted because there is no change in the contractile ability of the ventricles. However, there is a low volume of blood being ejected with each contraction as less blood entered into the ventricle before the contraction phase.

Pathophysiology of Heart Failure

Heart failure involves a complex series of events involving pathophysiological and compensatory factors in response to cardiac muscle dysfunction.[46-51] When the myocardium is dysfunctional, compensatory mechanisms are activated with the goal of maintaining adequate cardiac output. Neurohormonal mechanisms including activation of the sympathetic nervous system are triggered to increase HR and maintain CO at rest. Thus patients experiencing an acute bout of heart failure are very likely to be tachycardic at rest.

When patients are in heart failure and the ventricle is ejecting low blood volumes, blood begins to accumulate within the ventricles, causing congestion. This congestion increases the LVEDV and contributes to an elevation in LV pressure. The increased pressure is transmitted retrograde toward the LA and the pulmonary veins. This increase in hydrostatic pressure in the pulmonary veins causes fluid to move from the veins into the interstitial space of the lung, resulting in **pulmonary edema**.[45]

It is also important to consider kidney function for patients with heart failure. Low blood volume pumped out of the heart causes less blood to perfuse the kidney and is likely to put the kidney in failure. Patients experiencing an acute heart failure exacerbation often go into renal failure. It is therefore crucial for therapists to monitor BUN and plasma creatinine levels. An increase in urea production, elevated BUN and creatinine levels, and decreased urine output indicate renal dysfunction.[45]

From a musculoskeletal standpoint, patients with heart failure often present with skeletal muscle wasting, myopathies, and osteoporosis. These negative sequelae are associated with inactivity and prolonged bedrest. Several studies have investigated the effects of CHF on skeletal muscle abnormalities and found reductions in the size and number of Type I and Type II muscle fibers.[52-54] It is therefore imperative that the physical therapy POC place emphasis on interventions to improve overall endurance and functional mobility in this patient population.

Clinical Manifestations of Heart Failure

The clinical presentation of the patient with CHF depends not only on the amount of LV failure, but also on the status of compensatory mechanisms and the impact of drug therapy. Over time, the energy cost of the compensatory mechanisms proves to be too much for the impaired myocardium. The patient then begins to present with signs and symptoms of CHF, and now moves from being asymptomatic to symptomatic. Although the terminology may be somewhat confusing, it is important to note that when a patient is referred to as being in *compensated heart failure,* the patient's congestive symptoms can be relieved by medical intervention. A patient who is *noncompensated* is showing signs and symptoms of congestion and requires medical and pharmacological readjustment.

Common signs and symptoms of CHF include fatigue, dyspnea, edema (pulmonary and peripheral), fluid weight gain, presence of an S_3 heart sound, and renal dysfunction. Pulmonary edema may be evident by chest x-ray and auscultation of adventitious sounds. Peripheral edema may be evident in gravity-dependent LEs by the presence of indentations in the skin when pressure is applied, that is, **pitting edema**. Pitting edema associated with CHF is usually bilateral and may extend from the foot to the pretibial area.[55,56] Documentation should include a numerical grade based on the duration of indentation after fingertip pressure. See Chapter 14, Vascular, Lymphatic, and Integumentary Disorders, for pitting edema grading scale. Weight gain and peripheral edema are among the signs of systemic volume overload.

On auscultation of the heart and lungs characteristic sounds are heard with CHF. The usual abnormal heart sound associated with CHF is the presence of an S_3 heart sound. This is a low-frequency heart sound heard in early diastole and occurs due to poor ventricular compliance and subsequent turbulence of blood within the ventricle.[7] Heart murmurs (extra heart sounds), especially those of mitral regurgitation, may also be present owing to the effect of the enlarged LV pulling on the mitral valve. Lung auscultation for patients with heart failure reveals the presence of crackles or rales. These are crackling/bubbling sounds suggesting fluid in the lung. The sounds are usually heard during inspiration and represent the movement of fluid in the alveoli and subsequent opening of the alveoli that were previously closed because of the excess fluid.[44]

Dyspnea is one of the most common symptoms experienced with left-sided CHF. The SOB is associated with pulmonary edema. When fluid accumulates in the lungs, gas exchange is altered at the alveolar capillary interface. Gas exchange (respiration) will occur at the alveolar capillary interface only when ventilation within the alveoli is matched with perfusion within the pulmonary capillary

(V/Q matching). Excessive amounts of fluid within the pulmonary parenchyma cause a ventilation/perfusion mismatch, thereby reducing the amount of oxygen delivered to blood and causing dyspnea.

Two other symptoms reported by patients in CHF are paroxysmal nocturnal dyspnea and orthopnea. **Paroxysmal nocturnal dyspnea (PND)** is characterized by sudden episodes of SOB occurring in the night. **Orthopnea** is increased SOB in the recumbent position. The severity of orthopnea is often crudely documented by observing the number of pillows a patient needs to keep the upper body in an upright or semirecumbent position. Therefore, a patient with three- or four-pillow orthopnea suggests a greater severity of heart failure when compared to a patient with one-pillow orthopnea. Physiologically, as patients assume a recumbent position from an upright position, with their legs elevated to the same horizontal level as their trunk, fluid moves back to the heart causing an increase in preload. A failing heart cannot keep up with the additional preload and excess fluid returning to the heart and therefore causes a backup into the lungs producing increased symptoms of SOB.

Increased arterial resistance is also seen in patients with CHF and results in an increase in afterload and therefore in MVO_2. The increased resistance may result from a combination of factors, including (1) increased sympathetic adrenergic stimulation; (2) decreased vasodilation of vascular smooth muscle as a result of a decrease in the availability of the endothelium-derived relaxant factor, nitric oxide; (3) an increase in the endothelial-derived smooth muscle vasoconstrictor, endothelin-1; (4) an increase in vascular stiffness as a result of salt and water retention; and (5) the presence of the powerful peripheral vasoconstrictors angiotensin II and vasopressin.[57]

One of the common complaints of patients with CHF is early onset of muscle fatigue. The cause of the muscle fatigue may be multifactorial, including a decrease in peripheral blood flow, changes within the peripheral vascular beds, peripheral vasoconstriction, atrophy of muscle fibers, and increased utilization of anaerobic metabolism for energy production.[58,59] The contribution of intracellular mechanisms to muscle fatigue has been studied. Examples of these intracellular mechanisms include an alteration in the control of calcium release and reuptake[60] and myocyte apoptosis.[61] In addition to peripheral muscle functioning in patients with heart failure, exercise studies have also investigated various other factors, including oxygen uptake kinetics, neurohormonal parameters, and endothelial function, that may influence the exercise response.[62-64] Although there are many potential reasons for the fatigue associated with CHF (especially Class III and IV), a recently identified contributor is obstructive sleep apnea. Sleep apnea may be treated in this patient population with the use of continuous positive airway pressure worn while sleeping.[65,66]

Patients with heart failure will present with decreased exercise tolerance owing to a culmination of the pathophysiological and compensatory events associated with heart failure. It is difficult for patients to exercise when they have gained weight, have SOB, and have a rapid HR. There are a variety of methods to measure exercise tolerance in patients with heart failure. Physicians utilize the New York Heart Association (NYHA) and Functional Classification Scale (Table 13.7). Classification is based on the development of symptoms and the amount of energy required to provoke them. Patients in Class I have mild heart failure and relatively better exercise

Table 13.7	Functional Classifications of Patients with Diseases of the Heart	
Functional	Continuous–Intermittent Permissible Workloads	Maximum
Class I	4.0–6.0 cal/min Patients with cardiac disease but without resulting limitations of physical activity. Ordinary physical activity does not cause undue fatigue, palpitation, dyspnea, or anginal pain.	6.5 METs
Class II	3.0–4.0 cal/min Patients with cardiac disease resulting in slight limitation of physical activity. They are comfortable at rest. Ordinary physical activity results in fatigue, palpitation, dyspnea, or anginal pain.	4.5 METs
Class III	2.0–3.0 cal/min Patients with cardiac disease resulting in marked limitation of physical activity. They are comfortable at rest. Less than ordinary physical activity causes fatigue, palpitation, dyspnea, or anginal pain.	3.0 METs
Class IV	1.0–2.0 cal/min Patients with cardiac disease resulting in inability to carry on any physical activity without discomfort. Symptoms of cardiac insufficiency or of the anginal syndrome may be present even at rest. If any physical activity is undertaken, discomfort is increased.	1.5 METs

Four-level classification system based on functional limitations.
Reprinted by permission of the American Heart Association, New York.

tolerance compared to patients in Class IV with severe CHF and poor exercise tolerance.

Medical Examination and Evaluation of Heart Failure

Medical interventions include a variety of tests to identify the etiology and evaluate the severity of heart failure. Following an examination of signs and symptoms of heart failure in a given patient, several key tests are typically performed. These include a chest x-ray, laboratory tests, echocardiography, and nuclear imaging studies.

Radiological Findings in CHF

Three hallmark characteristics of the chest x-ray help confirm the diagnosis of CHF[9] (Fig. 13.13):

1. An enlarged cardiac silhouette: The enlargement of the heart in patients with CHF occurs secondary to congestion of fluid in the lungs and possible pathological hypertrophy of the ventricles.
2. Opacities (white areas) in the lung field with interstitial and parenchymal edema. This occurs when excessive fluid collects in the lung when LV end-diastolic pressures exceed 25 mm Hg.[44]
3. Blunting of the costophrenic angle. The lower ribs meeting the diaphragm creates this sharp image observed on the chest x-ray. In patients with CHF, fluid settles to the lower, dependent aspect of the lung, producing an opaque appearance, and blunts the costophrenic angle.

Laboratory Findings in CHF

Natriuretic peptides including atrial natriuretic peptide (ANP) and B-type or brain natriuretic peptide (BNP) are released from atrial and ventricular myocytes in response to volume overload within the respective chambers.[67] ANP and BNP are cardiac neurohormones that target the kidney when released to increase diuresis and decrease the overall volume of fluid within the vasculature and chambers of the heart.[44] Circulating levels of

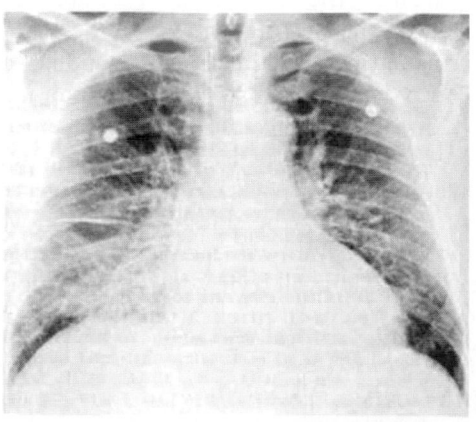

Figure 13.13 Radiographic examination to confirm CHF.

BNP are elevated in plasma in patients with heart failure. There is no level of BNP that perfectly separates patients with and without heart failure. Normal levels of BNP are less than 100 pg/mL. Values above 500 are generally considered to be positive for heart failure. The BNP level provides an indication of the extent of heart failure where higher BNP levels without renal failure indicate worsening failure of the ventricles. Therefore a patient with a BNP of 1,000 pg/mL has more significant heart failure than a patient with a BNP of 500 pg/mL. BNP has been found to be a statistically significant ($p < 0.05$) prognostic indicator of heart failure,[68-69] and studies have discovered moderate to strong (from $r = -0.38$ to -0.64) correlations between BNP and peak oxygen uptake (VO_{2max}).[68,69]

Echocardiogram and Nuclear Imaging

With ultrasound technology, the echocardiogram is used to examine wall motion integrity, valvular status, wall thickness, chamber size, and LV function. The EF may also be calculated using the data obtained from the echocardiogram. An echocardiogram may accompany a stress test and is known as a *stress echo*. The purpose of a stress echo is to compare LV function and wall motion between rest and exercise when an increased VO_2 results in an increased MVO_2. A positive stress echo indicates a worsening of LV function as activity increases; a negative stress echo indicates that the LV has adequately adapted to the increase in energy demand. Nuclear imaging (e.g., thallium sestamibi) compares coronary perfusion between rest and exercise. If there is no decrease in perfusion with increasing workloads, the test is negative; if there is a decrease, the test is considered positive.

Pharmacological Management of CHF

With the advent of new medications such as combined alpha- and beta-blockers, ACE inhibitors, and vasodilators, the symptoms of volume overload are more effectively managed.[70,71] The principles of drug management with CHF are twofold: (1) to increase the contractility or pumping ability of the heart to relieve congestion and (2) to decrease the workload on the heart by reducing either the total volume of fluid in the system (the preload) or the vascular resistance (the afterload). Drugs that increase contractility are known as *positive inotropes;* the common oral drug in this category is digoxin. Diuretics decrease preload, thereby decreasing LVEDV. Patients are often on a sliding scale dosage of diuretics depending on the amount of fluid weight gain; they are instructed to weigh themselves daily and adjust diuretics accordingly. Afterload reducers, particularly those that block the effects of the renin–angiotensin system (e.g., ACE inhibitors or ARBs), are often a critical component of drug management in this population. By blocking salt and water retention through aldosterone suppression, preload is decreased; by blocking vasoconstriction through angiotensin II suppression, afterload is reduced.

The increase in sympathetic activity that accompanies heart failure causes an increase in MVO_2 (from beta-receptor stimulation), peripheral vasoconstriction, and resultant reduction in peripheral blood flow (from alpha-receptor stimulation). Drugs that combine both beta-receptor blockade and alpha-receptor blockade minimize these affects. Beta-blockade will result in a decrease in MVO_2 and alpha-blockade will result in decreased after-load due to suppression of peripheral vasoconstriction.

Mechanical and Surgical Support

For the symptomatic patient in NYHA Class III/IV, there are dramatic surgical options that may improve function, such as heart transplant, left ventricular assist devices (LVADs), myoplasty, and biventricular pacing. It is beyond the scope of this chapter to discuss in detail the complexity of each of these procedures. Heart transplantation involves replacing the patient's heart with a donor heart. The donor heart will be denervated; therefore, it will not have any direct sympathetic or parasympathetic connection and will be dependent on the intrinsic pacemaker of the SA node and hormonal stimulation to increase HR. The patient with a heart transplant requires careful pharmacological management. Immune-suppressing drugs are used to prevent the body from rejecting the organ, as well as for careful control of infection.

The LVAD is a temporary pump inserted into the patient to perform the work of the LV or to augment the function of the failing heart. The patient is connected to an external energy source but also has the option of wearing a battery pack that allows freedom of movement for hours, in which the patient can go shopping, go to the movies, and so forth. It is important for the therapist to consider the effects of a 6-lb mass (created by the external energy source) resting below the diaphragm that is likely to alter ventilator performance. Finally, gentle progression of exercise intensity must be utilized. Therapists must be vigilant to check for flow limitations (10 to 12 L/min) or changes in cardiovascular function that may occur secondary to use of a mechanically driven pump.

Myoplasty is a surgical procedure in which an enlarged LV undergoes a size reduction by removing dilated, scarred myocardium that is ineffective in contributing to contractility.

A new class of pacemaker, the biventricular pacer, includes an intraventricular conduction delay (e.g., left bundle branch block on the ECG) for patients with severe CHF. This pacer coordinates the contraction of the right and left ventricles and in doing so provides a more effective LV contraction and increased CO.[73]

Valvular Heart Disease

Broadly, three major disorders encompass valvular dysfunction of one or more of the four heart valves.[74] These are stenosis, prolapse, and regurgitation.

1. *Stenosis* involves narrowing of a heart valve limiting the flow of blood through the valve. As the pathological condition progresses, the chamber behind the valve pathologically hypertrophies to pump against the obstruction.
2. *Prolapse* involves enlarged valve cusps that become floppy and bulge backward. When the cusps and support mechanisms of the valve are destroyed, the valve droops down. As the disease progresses, prolapse may progress to regurgitation.[75]
3. *Regurgitation* refers to the forward and backward movement of blood resulting from incomplete valve closure. During certain phases of the cardiac cycle valves must close appropriately to prevent blood from flowing in a retrograde fashion. In a regurgitant valve, the valve does not close properly leading to regurgitation of blood into the chamber behind the pathological valve.

Valve replacements are often used for treating valvular disease. Patients with stenosis or regurgitation of the aortic or mitral valves are prime candidates for valve replacement surgeries. A median sternotomy is the route to access the heart. Two major types of valves are used for valve replacement procedures: (1) mechanical valves and (2) biological valves derived from cadavers, porcine tissue, or bovine tissue.[74,76] Mechanical valves are preferred in patients younger than 65 because of their durability and long life. However, the major disadvantage is that they tend to be thrombogenic. Patients who receive a mechanical valve must be on lifelong anticoagulation therapy. For this reason, patients who have a history of a prior bleed, wish to become pregnant, or have poor medication adherence may not be candidates for a mechanical valve. For these patients, biological valves may be more appropriate. The postoperative care for patients with a valve replacement is similar to that for patients who have had a CABG. In addition, neurological monitoring must be continuous postoperatively owing to the potential for an embolic stroke that may occur during or after the procedure.

Electrical Conduction Abnormalities

Arrhythmias are any alteration in the electric conduction of the heart from the normal beat. They are caused by a disturbance in the electrical activity of the heart, resulting in impaired electrical impulse formation or conduction.[76] Arrhythmias may present as benign or malignant (i.e., life threatening). Examples of malignant arrhythmias are sustained ventricular tachycardia (V-tach) and ventricular fibrillation (V-fib). An example of a common benign arrhythmia in the elderly population would be atrial fibrillation (A-fib) with a controlled ventricular response. This section will review a few conduction abnormalities and relevant implications for the physical therapist.

Ectopic Beats

A beat that originates from a site other than the sinus node is known as an *ectopic beat*. The common ectopic beats are atrial *(premature atrial contractions [PACs])* and ventricular *(premature ventricular contractions [PVCs])*. PVCs may occur either by themselves or in groups such as couplets (two PVCs) or triplets (three PVCs), or alternating with sinus beats such as bigeminy (every other beat a PVC) or trigeminy (every third beat a PVC).[77,78]

A PAC is an ectopic beat that originates in the atria and may present as an irregular rhythm (Fig. 13.14B). It may be difficult to distinguish a PAC from a premature junctional contraction (PJC), an ectopic beat that originates within the area around the A-V node. Usually, PACs or PJCs will not compromise CO, and physical therapy intervention may be appropriate if accompanied by adequate hemodynamic responses.

The presence of ectopic beats results in an irregular rhythm. Usually, ectopic beats are transient, and their severity depends on their impact on CO. It is certainly common to have a few PVCs even in a normal heart. Many people may have ectopic beats during times of stress or with stimulants such as nicotine and caffeine. Even though this may be a common response in a normal heart, it is important to educate patients with myocardial impairments who may have ectopic beats or irregular rhythms to avoid these aggravators. An increase in ectopy is undesired. It is unwise for any patient with cardiac disease to engage in exercise following recent cigarette smoking. Although the specific time frame that a patient may be at risk for increased ectopy is not clearly known, a good rule of thumb may be abstinence of smoking for at last 2 hours either before or after exercise. Patient education on wellness strategies and smoking cessation is always useful for any patient identified as a smoker.

Supraventricular Ectopy

Supraventricular ectopy involves the rapid firing of an ectopic focus that originates in any location above the ventricles (atrial or junctional area). Examples of supraventricular ectopy include (1) paroxysmal atrial tachycardia and (2) supraventricular tachycardia. A sudden run of PACs occurring at a fast rate (100 to 200 bpm) is known as *paroxysmal atrial tachycardia (PAT)*. A run of either PACs or PJCs at a rate of 150 to 250 bpm is known as supraventricular tachycardia (SV-tach) (Fig. 13.14C). Patients with SV-tach usually respond to a carotid massage where stimulation of the baroreceptors within the carotid bodies of the carotid artery produce a parasympathetic response. Other treatment interventions to reduce heart rate for patients with SV-tach include coughing and breath-holding techniques achieved through the Valsalva maneuver.

Ventricular Ectopy

PVCs are ectopic beats that originate in the ventricle and may present as irregular rhythms. Two hallmark characteristics identify PVCs on the ECG: (1) A P wave is absent as the impulse originates in the ventricle and (2) a wide and bizarre QRS complex signifying abnormal electrical conduction through the ventricle (Fig. 13.14D). Single PVCs will not compromise CO if less than 7 per minute. Therefore, physical activity may be appropriate if accompanied by an adequate hemodynamic response. If the PVCs increase with activity, the activity should be stopped and the patient examined for possible signs of compromised cardiac output. PVCs may come from the same irritable site and are termed *unifocal PVCs*. If they originate from different ectopic sites within the ventricle they are known as *multifocal PVCs* (Fig. 13.15A). Multifocal PVCs suggest a more irritable ventricle and are therefore more serious than unifocal PVCs. It is appropriate for the therapist to have the patient medically evaluated before beginning or continuing an activity. Finally, a rare type of PVC known as an *R-on-T PVC* occurs when PVC fires *very prematurely*, on the T wave of the preceding cardiac cycle (Fig. 13.15B). These patients must be monitored closely because they are at an increased risk for developing a life-threatening dysrhythmia such as ventricular tachycardia.[77]

In ventricular bigeminy (Fig. 13.14E), every other beat is a PVC; in trigeminy, every third beat is a PVC (Fig. 13.14F).[77] These rhythms occur transiently or episodically, and many patients have frequent bursts of these rhythms. If ectopy increases with activity, the activity should be immediately stopped. When two PVCs occur together, it is known as a couplet (Fig. 13.14G); when three PVCs occur together, it is known as a triplet. Couplets and triplets are important in that they suggest a high level of ventricular irritability. Altered LV function and ischemia are two of the more common causes for ventricular ectopy; therefore, medical management is directed toward improved LV function and perfusion whenever possible, as well as arrhythmia control. Physical therapy intervention is conservative at best and depends on the hemodynamic stability of the patient.

Ventricular Tachycardia

A run of four or more PVCs in a row is known as V-tach (Fig. 13.14H). V-tach may be either sustained or nonsustained. *Sustained V-tach,* by definition, occurs at an HR of at least 100 bpm and lasts for at least 30 seconds.[79] The patient may or may not have a palpable pulse and, if present, the pulse will be weak. Because of the severe decrease in CO and rapid hemodynamic deterioration associated with this rhythm, the presence of sustained V-tach is considered an emergency situation. Medical intervention must be initiated as soon as possible. No physical therapy intervention is appropriate, except assisting the patient in stabilization, initiating cardiopulmonary resuscitation (CPR) when indicated, and activating the advanced cardiac life support (ACLS) system. V-tach may deteriorate quickly into V-fib.

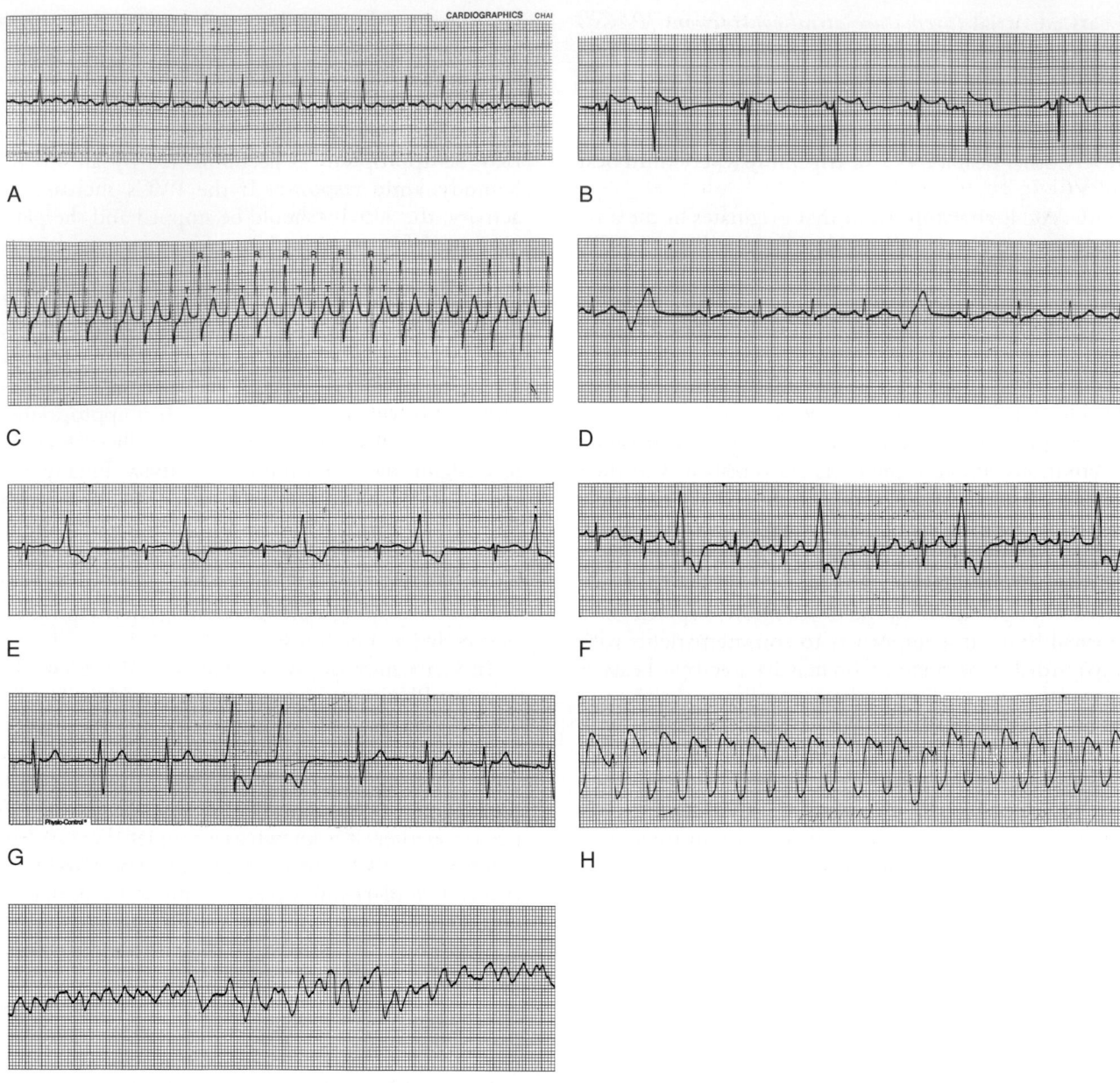

Figure 13.14 Examples of ectopy and arrhythmias. **(A)** Atrial fibrillation. **(B)** Atrial premature beat, also known as premature atrial contraction (PAC) (note third complex). **(C)** Supraventricular tachycardia (SVT). **(D)** Premature ventricular contraction (PVC) (note third complex). **(E)** Bigeminy (note second, fourth, and sixth complexes are PVCs). **(F)** Trigeminy (note second, fifth, and eighth complexes are PVCs). **(G)** Couplets (note fourth and fifth complexes are PVCs). **(H)** Ventricular tachycardia (V-tach). **(I)** Ventricular fibrillation (V-fib) (V-tach deteriorates into V-fib). *(From Brown, K, and Jacobson, S: Mastering Dysrhythmias: A Problem-Solving Guide. FA Davis, Philadelphia, 1988, p 30, with permission.)*

Nonsustained V-tach occurs either in groups of three to five PVCs known as *salvos,* or a run of six or more PVCs lasting for up to 30 seconds.[79] Nonsustained V-tach is considered a high-risk indicator for potentially lethal arrhythmias. Because the rhythm is nonsustained, the decrease in CO may not be sufficient to cause symptoms. However, until the etiology of the arrhythmia is identified and the rhythm

controlled, physical therapy intervention is generally inappropriate.

Ventricular Fibrillation

V-fib is characterized by quivering of the ventricles resulting from inadequate electrical stimulation. The ECG demonstrates a sustained run of different-looking PVCs coming from different ectopic foci (Fig. 13.14I). When the ventricles do not contract but rather quiver, there is ineffective CO. The patient will arrest and expire if this rhythm is not altered immediately. The treatment of choice is activation of ACLS, including electrical defibrillation and medication. Patients who survive fibrillation through defibrillation become candidates for an indwelling defibrillator placement known as an *automatic implantable cardiac defibrillator* (AICD).

Automatic Implantable Cardiac Defibrillator

The AICD is implanted in patients who have life-threatening ventricular arrhythmias (V-tach, V-fib). The AICD is programmed to deliver an electrical shock if it detects an HR higher than its programmed HR limit. Therefore, it is important for the physical therapist to know this limit and avoid an exercise intensity that may inadvertently activate the device.[80] In addition to knowing the HR settings for the patient with an AICD, there are other considerations. ST-segment changes on the ECG may be common and are not specific for ischemia; therefore, other diagnostic studies must be done. In addition, UE aerobic or strengthening exercises should be avoided initially after placement of the pacer to avoid inadvertently dislodging the device or the lead wires.[80] Checking with the physician when these exercises may be included is prudent. There may be a danger for patients with AICDs or pacemakers from electromagnetic signals such as anti-theft devices, either causing the AICD to discharge or causing pacers to slow down or speed up. It may be no problem for patients to walk through these devices but lingering within a few feet could be dangerous.[81]

Atrial Fibrillation

A-fib is characterized by quivering of the atria due to inadequate electrical stimulation. A varied number of non–sinus originating P waves (known as fibrillatory waves) exist for each QRS complex (Fig. 13.14A). The ventricular rhythm is said to be "irregularly irregular" because there is no regularity to the irregularity of the ventricular rhythm. It is important to note that effective contraction of the atria accounts for approximately 15% to 20% of CO—the *atrial kick*.[9,74] In patients with abnormal electrical conduction causing a quivering of the atria (A-fib), the mechanical contractile ability of the atria is reduced, resulting in a low atrial kick and compromised CO.[9,74]

Patients may exhibit A-fib continuously as their baseline rhythm or go in and out this rhythm at rest or with activity. Physical therapy intervention may be appropriate for patients in A-fib who have a good ventricular rate at rest, with appropriate hemodynamic and HR increase with exercise. In patients with A-fib and rapid ventricular rates (greater than 100 bpm) at rest, exercise intensity must be lowered and hemodynamic responses monitored carefully. This is because a rapid ventricular rate in addition to the loss of atrial

kick further compromises the CO and results in altered hemodynamic responses. A good rule of thumb is to avoid physical activity and seek medical consultation if the patient's resting HR is greater than 115 bpm, if the patient appears uncomfortable, or if there is an inadequate hemodynamic response. Because this rhythm is irregular, it is important to monitor the HR for a full minute rather than 15 to 30 seconds to obtain an accurate pulse rate.

Conduction Delays and Blocks

Changes in the length of the PR interval, the width of the QRS complex, and the length of the QT interval are some of the ECG measurements indicative of conduction abnormalities.

Conduction delays through the A-V node are classified as first-, second-, or third-degree heart blocks. *First-degree heart block* occurs when the conduction time through the A-V node is prolonged; therefore, the ECG will have an increased length of the PR interval (Fig. 13.15C). There are two categories of *second-degree heart block*: Mobitz type I and Mobitz type II; each is hallmarked by the presence of dropped beats. Mobitz I, also known as *Wenckebach*, presents with a gradual increase in PR interval length in the preceding beats and then an eventual dropped beat (Fig. 13.15D); Mobitz II has normal PR intervals in all the beats preceding the dropped beat (Fig. 13.15E). In *third-degree heart block*, a mismatch of atrial and ventricular conduction exists, so there is no consistency between the atrial contraction and the ventricular contraction (i.e., no relationship between P waves and QRS complex on the ECG) (Fig. 13.15F). Patients in first-degree block have no limitations to exercise. Whether or not exercise is permitted with second- and third-degree blocks depends on the etiology and subsequent hemodynamic responses. Medical clearance is warranted before beginning any exercise.

Conduction delays through the bundle of His are known as either right bundle branch block (RBBB) or left bundle branch block (LBBB). Bundle branch blocks are not true arrhythmias because there is no change in the actual rhythm, just in the timing of conduction through the bundle of His. The heart is still depolarized from the same pacemaker; only the route of activation is changed. Bundle branch blocks present on the ECG as a distortion of the QRS complex with an increased duration (i.e., widening) (Fig. 13.15G). The presence of an LBBB on the ECG is usually permanent and indicates a pathological condition. RBBB may occur from a variety of reasons; it may be a permanent change due to underlying disease, or it may be benign. RBBB can also occur transiently. LBBB usually indicates the presence of more significant disease than RBBB.

The presence of a new bundle branch block should be medically evaluated before beginning or progressing an exercise program. Following medical clearance, there

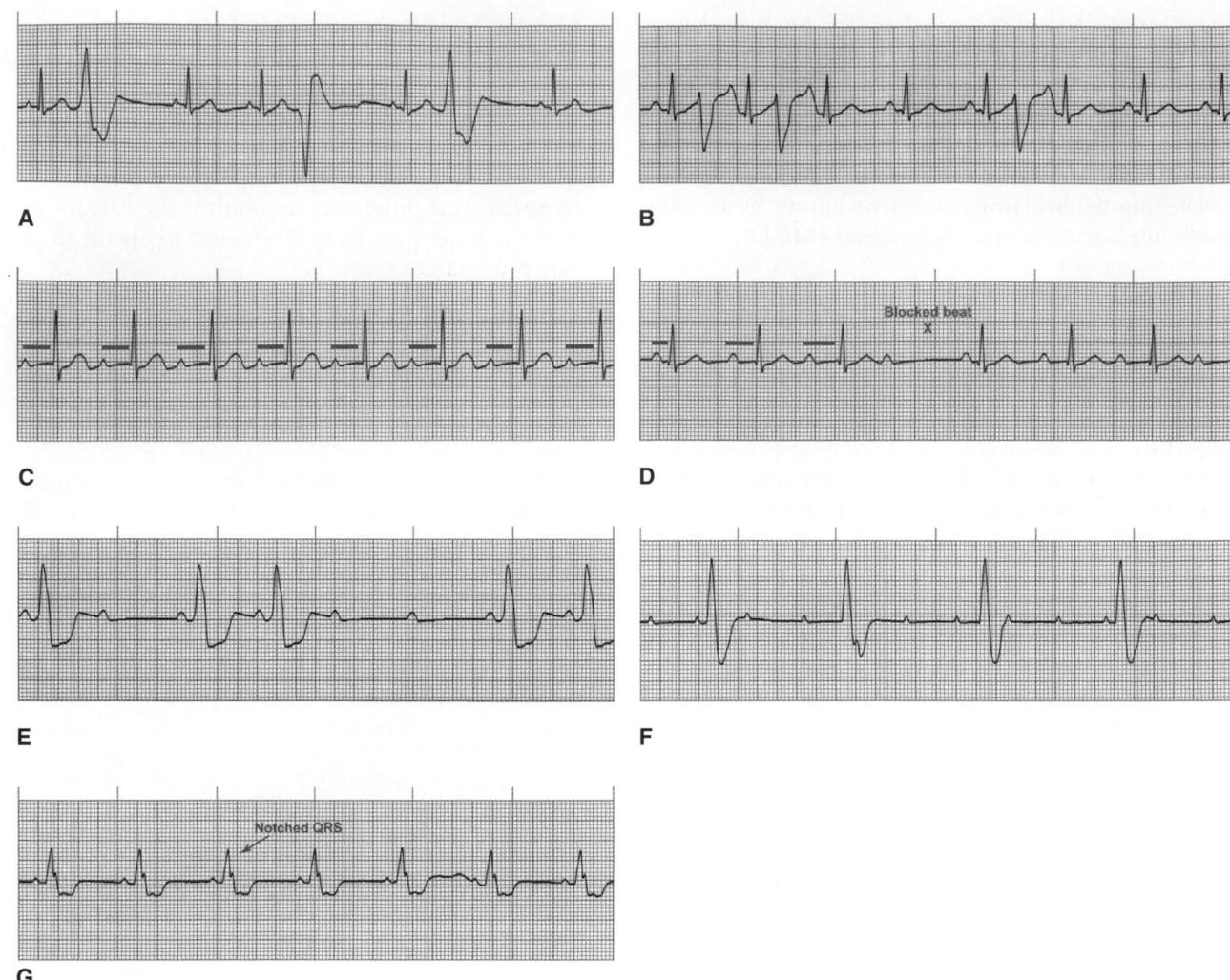

Figure 13.15 (A) Multifocal or multiform PVCs; **(B)** R-on-T PVC; **(C)** first-degree AV block; **(D)** Wenckebach rhythm; **(E)** second-degree type II; **(F)** third-degree AV block; **(G)** bundle branch block. *(From Jones, S: ECG Success: Exercises in ECG Interpretation. FA Davis, Philadelphia, 2008.)*

is usually no contraindication to exercise in either the RBBB or LBBB population. Because of the alteration of the QRS complex and as a result the ST segment, the sensitivity of the ECG in detecting ischemia via ST depression is lost in the patient with LBBB.

Pacemakers

The use of pacemakers has increased considerably, with the most common indications for placement of a permanent pacemaker being (1) an HR that is too slow (symptomatic bradycardia); (2) an HR that fails to increase appropriately with exercise (chronotropic incompetence); or (3) an electric pathway that it blocked resulting in atrioventricular delays or bundle branch blocks.[82]

A pacemaker is a device that is placed subdermally near the heart and consists of an implantable pulse generator and lead wires that connect the pacemaker to the myocardium. The pulse generator contains a long-life battery and circuitry for timing, sensing, and output functions. The life of the battery usually dictates the life of the pacemaker and varies depending on the type of battery and the extent to which the pacemaker is being used. In some cases, the patient is dependent on the pacemaker for every cardiac contraction and is likely to utilize the life of the battery in a shorter period of time.[83] The average pacemaker battery life is between 5 and 10 years. Replacement of pacemaker batteries is done after serial assessments have confirmed a reduction in battery life. Battery life may be consumed more rapidly when the patient is more reliant on the pacemaker for maintaining an appropriate HR.

Patients are reliant on pacemakers at different levels. Some patients have normal electric conduction at most times and do not need to be reliant on the pacemaker at all times. Other patients have altered electrical conduction through the heart and may be very reliant on the pacemaker to keep them alive. Therefore, it is important for therapists to determine how reliant the patient may be on his or her pacemaker. When pacemakers trigger a pace due to altered electrical conduction through the heart, the ECG reveals a pacer spike. Thus, if the patient has a pacemaker and no pacer spikes are evident on the ECG, the therapist can infer that the heart is conducting normally, and the pacemaker is there for emergency needs only. Conversely, if the ECG demonstrates a pacer spike in every cardiac cycle, the therapist must understand that this patient is 100% reliant on the pacemaker and thus ensure that the pacemaker is adequately rate responsive during activity.

The basic functions of the pacemaker lead wires are to provide the pacemaker with information on intrinsic myocardial activity and pace the myocardium when intrinsic activity fails. There are four primary functions of pacemakers: (1) the ability to sense intrinsic cardiac function, (2) the ability to stimulate cardiac depolarization in response to failed intrinsic activity, (3) the ability to respond to increased metabolic demand by providing rate-responsive pacing, and (4) the ability provide diagnostic information stored within the pacemaker.[84]

Pacemakers have rate and rhythm sensitivity as well as the ability to override certain arrhythmias. Pacemakers may also be combined with AICD capabilities. Pacemakers are coded by either a three- or five-category system according to which chamber (atria or ventricle) is sensed, what chamber is paced (atria or ventricle), and whether the electrical stimulus will trigger a response or be inhibited[85] (Table 13.8). Because pacemakers may fail to work properly, ECG monitoring is helpful to determine if the pacer is working properly.

As stated previously, patients with Class III CHF and LBBB may be candidates for a specialized pacemaker known as a biventricular pacemaker, the purpose of which is to synchronize LV contractility to provide a more effective CO. The biventricular pacer does not influence HR or heart rhythm.[86]

Heart Transplant

Patients who have undergone a heart transplant may present with the following: (1) calf cramps (occurring in approximately 15% of patients) owing to the immunosuppressive drug cyclosporine; (2) decreased LE strength; (3) obesity owing to long-term corticosteroid use; (4) increased risk of fracture owing to osteoporosis associated with long-term, high-dose corticosteroids; and (5) an increased probability of developing atherosclerosis in the coronary arteries of the donor heart after the first postsurgical year.[87] Because the heart is denervated, HR alone provides a limited measure of exercise intensity. Therefore, BP and perceived exertion should be included in the routine data collection.

■ CARDIOVASCULAR EXAMINATION

Owing to the increasing incidence and prevalence of heart disease on our society, many patients referred to physical therapy will have cardiovascular dysfunction or may be at risk for developing CVD. The history taking, review of systems, and data from specific tests and measures will guide and inform development of the physical therapy diagnosis, anticipated goals and expected outcomes, prognosis, and POC. This section addresses tests and measures specific to the cardiovascular system.

Medical Record Review

The medical record of a patient with a history of cardiovascular impairments may at times be overwhelming. The patient interview is typically helpful if clarification of the medical record is needed. Depending on the type of setting (inpatient, outpatient, acute rehabilitation, home care), the specific contents of the medical record may vary. Important items to note within the medical record include the following:

1. Medical problems, past medical history, physician's examination
2. Medications, including type, dosage, and schedule

Table 13.8	Pacemaker Classification System		
Chamber Paced	Chamber Sensed	Response	Rate Responsive Pacing
O = none	O = none	O = none	R = rate responsive
A = atria	A = atria	I = inhibit	
V = ventricle	V = ventricle	T = trigger	
D = dual chamber	D = dual chamber	D = capacity to both inhibit and trigger	

Pacemakers are commonly identified by a three-letter code as displayed in the first three columns. Pacemakers may also have the capacity to respond to physiological stimuli to increase rate (column 4) and to override atrial tachycardia. A fifth column, for antitachycardic function, is rarely used due to the increased sophistication of the newer implantable defibrillators/pacemakers, which renders this function unnecessary. Example: VVI pacer will provide an electrical impulse to the ventricle if it senses that there is no ventricular activity within an appropriate time frame. If there is intrinsic ventricular electrical activity, the pacemaker will be inhibited.

3. Laboratory tests
  - Blood tests for specific cardiac enzymes that may indicate an MI has occurred, such as a positive CK-MB or troponin level
  - Electrolytes, including potassium, and magnesium and calcium if ventricular arrhythmias are present
  - Complete blood count (CBC), which may indicate the presence of anemia via the hemoglobin and hematocrit values
  - Status of the kidney (BUN and creatinine) and liver function (liver function tests)
  - Presence of CAD risk factors, such as elevated lipid values (e.g., total cholesterol, low-density lipoproteins [LDLs], triglyceride), and elevated blood sugars (glucose)
  - Arterial blood gases (ABGs)

4. Results of any diagnostic studies or interventions: chest x-ray, ECGs, ETT, cardiac catheterization, surgical reports, hemodynamic monitors (e.g., pressure readings from central line and/or arterial line)

5. Nursing and other health care provider notes

The medical record contains information regarding what has happened to the patient, as well as the status of the patient within the last 24 hours or since the last health care provider intervention. Flow charts, which record vital signs, temperature, oxygenation requirements, and volume status over time, provide up-to-date patient data, especially when working with the more medically challenged patient.

Patient Interview

The formal patient interview should follow the medical record review. A determination of overall cognition (e.g., orientation, memory, learning needs, comprehension) should be made. Information regarding the patient's lifestyle, previous level of functioning, recreational interests, work requirements, and goals is important in establishing the intervention. Data should also be obtained about the patient's response to health and illness, coping status, support systems, and knowledge of heart disease. It is important to note that not all the information from the interview needs to be obtained on the first session. During subsequent sessions, the patient may begin to feel better and less anxious and may therefore be able to communicate more easily. Patient education can often be woven into the interview process, either subtly or overtly. The patient should describe, in his or her own words, the quality and location of the symptom for which medical attention is being sought. It is common for physical therapists to ask a patient about pain; for patients with cardiac disease, one should be cautious about assuming that the patient's symptom is pain. Many patients will not use pain as their qualifier, but instead describe their symptoms as pressure, heaviness, SOB (dyspnea), aching, heartburn, or general malaise,

to identify a few. Knowing the symptom presentation for each individual will make patient education and activity progression easier. It is also important to identify any consistent precipitating factors and alleviators, as well as duration and frequency of symptoms.

The interview also helps to establish rapport and trust between therapist and patient, creating an environment for mutual goal setting. This in turn facilitates patient adherence to the rehabilitation program. Patients who are recovering from an MI or from surgery need to have an understanding of time frames for healing and convalescence. Education for family members and significant others is also crucial for patient adherence and understanding.

Physical Examination

The physical therapist carefully monitors vital signs (see Chapter 2, Examination of Vital Signs) at rest and with activity, auscultates the heart and lungs, and performs a general observation of the patient's appearance. An overview of the pertinent components is presented.

Heart Rate and Rhythm

In taking an initial HR, either by palpation or auscultation, it is important to count for a full minute. When examining the patient's response to an activity and no arrhythmia is present, an immediate postexercise HR can be taken for 10 to 15 seconds. Always note if the rhythm is regular or irregular and report it as such. Unless there is ECG monitoring, it is impossible to identify a specific rhythm by palpation or auscultation alone. Note that there is a normal respiratory variation in HR; inspiration results in an increase in HR, exhalation in a slowing down of HR.

HR can also be determined from an ECG strip. The ECG graph paper consists of a series of small boxes (represented by light black lines) and large boxes (represented by heavy black lines). Each large box is made up of five small boxes. The horizontal axis represents time; when the ECG paper is moving at the usual speed of 25 mm/sec, five large boxes constitutes one second. Knowing that time is on the x-axis, there are many ways to calculate HR from the ECG graph paper. An easy way to calculate a minute rate is to count the number of complexes in 6 seconds (i.e., 30 large boxes) and multiply by 10. Often the ECG paper will have 3-second intervals premarked. An alternative approach is to identify an R wave from one ECG complex that is close to or on a heavy black line (i.e., a large box), and then assign each of the following heavy black lines (large boxes) a number in the following order: 300, 150, 100, 75, 60, 50, 40. The heavy line closest to the next R wave will provide an approximation of HR (Fig. 13.16). Finally, dividing 300 by the number of large boxes between two R waves will also indicate the HR. If the rate is regular, any of the preceding strategies will work. If the rate is irregular,

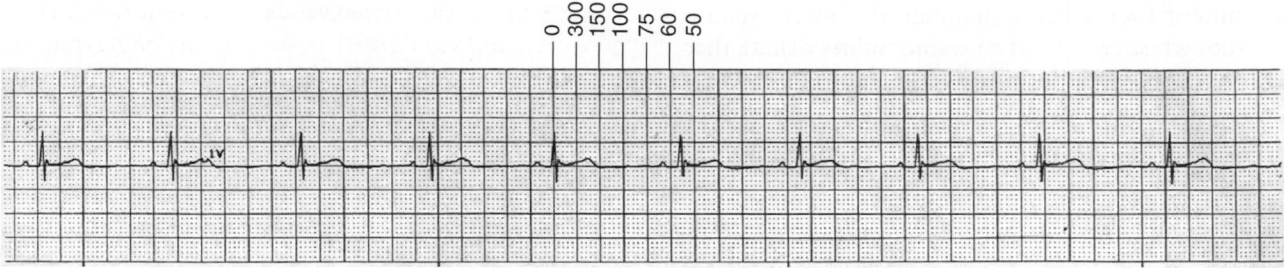

Figure 13.16 Calculation of a heart rate from a rhythm strip. Begin with the fifth complex (which falls on a large black line) and count each large black line to the right of this complex in the order of 300, 150, 100, 75, 60, 50. The sixth complex falls between two large lines (i.e., 50 and 60). There are five small lines between each large line. Between 50 and 60 there are 10 beats, therefore each small line in this case would be two beats. The heart rate would be 60 – 4 = 56. An alternate method would be to count the number of complexes in a 6-second strip and multiply by 10.

however, the complexes will need to be counted over a long time frame, and a minimum of a 6-second strip should be used.

Respiratory Rate, Rhythm, and Dyspnea

As with the heart, both rate and rhythm of respirations should be noted, as well as the breathing pattern and use of accessory muscles. Patients with cardiac impairments frequently complain of dyspnea. Patients with LV dysfunction from CAD, CHF, cardiomyopathies, valvular dysfunction, hypertensive heart disease, pericarditis with tamponade, and arrhythmias may all present with dyspnea. Sometimes, dyspnea begins with activity and is termed *dyspnea on exertion (DOE)* and progresses to occurring at rest. It is important to document and understand the amount and types of activity that provoke DOE. Dyspnea associated with a cardiovascular etiology is usually accompanied by signs and symptoms of compromised CO, including lightheadedness, dizziness, fatigue/weakness, and hypotension; symptoms may worsen in the supine position (orthopnea).[88] Some patients may experience dyspnea as their anginal equivalent; that is, they do not have the typical chest discomfort often associated with ischemia but instead experience SOB. For these patients, treatment should be immediate and follow the guidelines for ischemia. A commonly used tool to objectively identify subjective feelings of dyspnea is the Dyspnea Scale (Box 13.3).

Angina

The classical presentation of angina is substernal chest pressure accompanied by the *Levine sign* (the patient clenching his or her fist over the sternum). The Levine sign has a high diagnostic accuracy for ischemia.[89] For some patients, angina does not present in the classic way but rather may present as a pain or heaviness in the shoulder, jaw, arm, elbow, or upper back between scapulae. Angina may radiate from the chest to the arm or up to the throat, or it may present as indigestion or even SOB. The patient is often asked to rank his or her discomfort on the Angina Scale (Box 13.4).

Blood Pressure

Arterial BP is a product of CO and total peripheral resistance (TPR) where BP = CO × TPR. An increase in either of these factors will increase BP, and a decrease in either may decrease BP. Clinically, therefore, aerobic exercise of increasing intensity increases CO and concomitantly increases BP. Conversely, a drop in BP during aerobic exercise indicates a drop in CO, or signifies the inability of the heart to meet the metabolic needs of the peripheral tissue.[90] This drop in BP is usually accompanied by signs of compromised CO, including fatigue, weakness, tiredness, dizziness, and so forth, that occur during the activity. Therefore, BP values of a patient with heart disease who demonstrates signs of compromised CO during ambulation should be closely monitored to

Box 13.3 Dyspnea Scale
0 = No dyspnea
1 = Mild, noticeable
2 = Mild, some difficulty
3 = Moderate difficulty, but can continue
4 = Severe difficulty, cannot continue

Box 13.4 Angina Scale
0 = No angina
1 = Light, barely noticeable
2 = Moderate, bothersome
3 = Severe, very uncomfortable: preinfarction pain
4 = Most pain ever experienced: infarction pain

determine if CO is being maintained. Lower exercise BP values when compared to resting values denote that CO is not being met during exercise.

Accurate measurement of BP is a vital process within the examination process. Using inappropriate cuff sizes when measuring BP is the most frequent error in BP measurement.[91] Proper cuffs must have a bladder length of 80% and a width of 40% of arm circumference. In addition, maintaining the arm at the level of the heart promotes accurate measurement of BP to negate the effects of hydrostatic pressure. For every 2.5 cm above or below the level of the heart, BP readings can change by 1 to 2 mm Hg. An arm maintained above the level of the heart lowers BP readings and if placed at a level below the heart falsely increases BP measurements.[91] For more information on measurement of BP, see Chapter 2, Examination of Vital Signs.

Observation and Inspection

The patient's skin color should be inspected. **Cyanosis**, a bluish color of the skin, nail beds, and possibly lips and tongue, may be present when arterial oxygen saturation is 85% or less.[74] **Pallor**, the absence of a pink, rosy color, may indicate a decrease in CO. **Diaphoresis** (excess sweating, cool clammy skin) should also be noted because it may indicate excessive effort or inadequate cardiovascular response. Cold fingertips may be due to compensatory vasoconstriction in response to a decreased CO or from the suppressed beta-sympathetic response of some beta-blockers.

The extremities are inspected for the presence of edema; patients with LV failure may have an increase in peripheral edema owing to the increase in hydrostatic intravascular pressure associated with increased pressure from the LV transmitted retrograde through the heart to the venous system. Bilateral peripheral edema may be a result of CHF. Edema of one leg, however, is usually associated with local factors within the same leg such as varicose veins, lymphedema, or thrombophlebitis.[90] The patient with chronic CHF who has a weight gain owing to sodium and water retention may notice edema of the ankles and lower legs during the day (due to an increase in hydrostatic pressure) that diminishes during the night.

Heart Auscultation

Invaluable information as to the status of the heart is obtained from **auscultation** (listening) of the heart and lungs. Normal heart sounds are identified as S_1 (lub), which occurs at the time of the closure of the mitral (and tricuspid) valve and marks the beginning of systole and S_2 (dub), which occurs at the time of aortic (and pulmonic) valve closure and marks the end of systole. Figure 13.17 depicts locations on the chest for appropriate auscultation of each valve. The aortic valve is best auscultated at the second intercostal space, right sternal border. The pulmonic valve is heard at the second intercostal space, left sternal border. The tricuspid valve

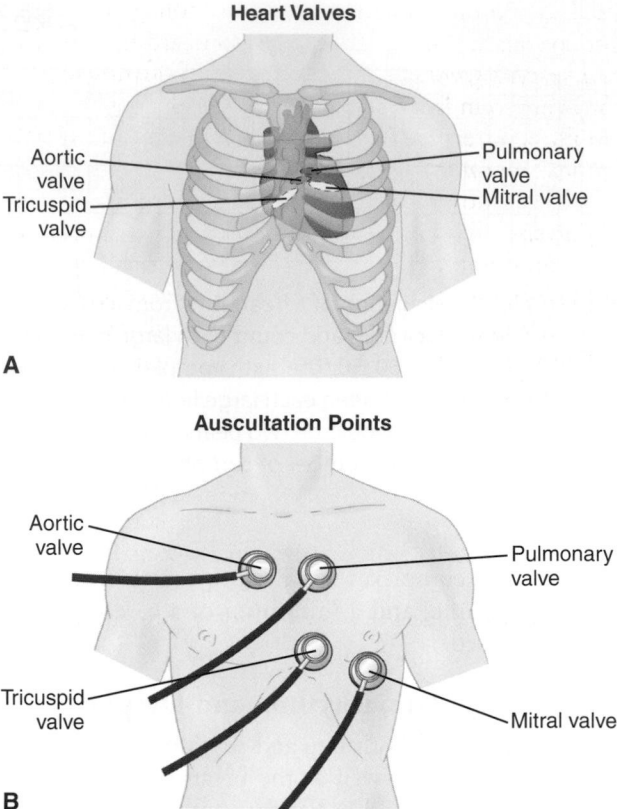

Figure 13.17 Anterior view of the chest wall of a man showing skeletal structures, heart, location of the heart-valves, and auscultation points.

is auscultated at the fourth intercostal space, left sternal border, and the mitral valve is best heard at the fifth intercostal space, along the midclavicular line.

Murmurs are abnormal heart sounds commonly the result of valvular disorders due to the changes in blood flow around and through the altered valve. A *systolic murmur* will present as audible turbulence between S_1 and S_2, and a *diastolic murmur* as turbulence between S_2 and S_1. A *stenotic* valve has impaired opening, and a regurgitant valve has impaired closing. A valve may be both stenotic and regurgitant.

Other abnormal sounds are S_3 and S_4. S_3, also known as a *ventricular gallop,* occurs after S_2 and is clinically associated with LV failure. S_4, also known as an *atrial gallop,* occurs before S_1 and is clinically associated with an MI or chronic HTN.

Another type of auscultatory finding is the *pericardial friction rub.* These friction sounds are high pitched with a leathery and scratchy quality, although they may vary in intensity from hour-to-hour or day-to-day, or may even transiently disappear.[92] The pericardial rub has been described as similar to the squeaking sound of rubbed leather.[93] This rub results from an inflammation of the pericardial sac, either with or without excessive fluid. Pericardial disease may result from many causes such as trauma, infections, tumors, collagen diseases, anticoagulants, and MI. Post-MI pericarditis is known as *Dressler's syndrome*.[94] An example of documentation for heart sounds would be *Cor: RRR Ø m, g, r,* which would be interpreted as *Heart: regular rate and rhythm without murmurs, gallops, or rubs.*

Auscultation of the heart borders is also done to examine size. The location of the apex and point of maximal impulse (PMI) is noted. The PMI is usually present at the fifth intercostal space along the midclavicular line. If the LV has increased in size, as frequently occurs with patients in LV failure, the PMI will be displaced laterally toward the axilla.

Lung Auscultation

Auscultating the lungs is an important component of the cardiac physical examination. Normal lung tissue produces vesicular (soft, low-pitched) sounds in the peripheral aspect of the lungs and bronchial breath (loud, high-pitched) sounds centrally along the manubrium of the sternum.[7] Vesicular sounds are longer and louder with inspiration, whereas bronchial breath sounds are longer and louder with expiration. Figure 13.18 demonstrates appropriate sites for the auscultation of lung fields.

Patients with LV failure often have the adventitious sounds of *crackles*. Crackles may also appear as a result of atelectasis; in that case, deep breathing with an inspiratory hold and coughing may correct this impairment. A patient with decreased breath sounds or consolidations may have a decrease in the oxygen content of his or her blood; a decrease in oxygenation may result in an increase in myocardial work and aggravate a preexisting cardiac impairment.

Jugular Venous Distention

Patients with CHF with backup of fluid into the venous vasculature should be examined for the presence of jugular venous distention. To examine for this sign, the patient is placed at a 45-degree semirecumbent position.[74] The

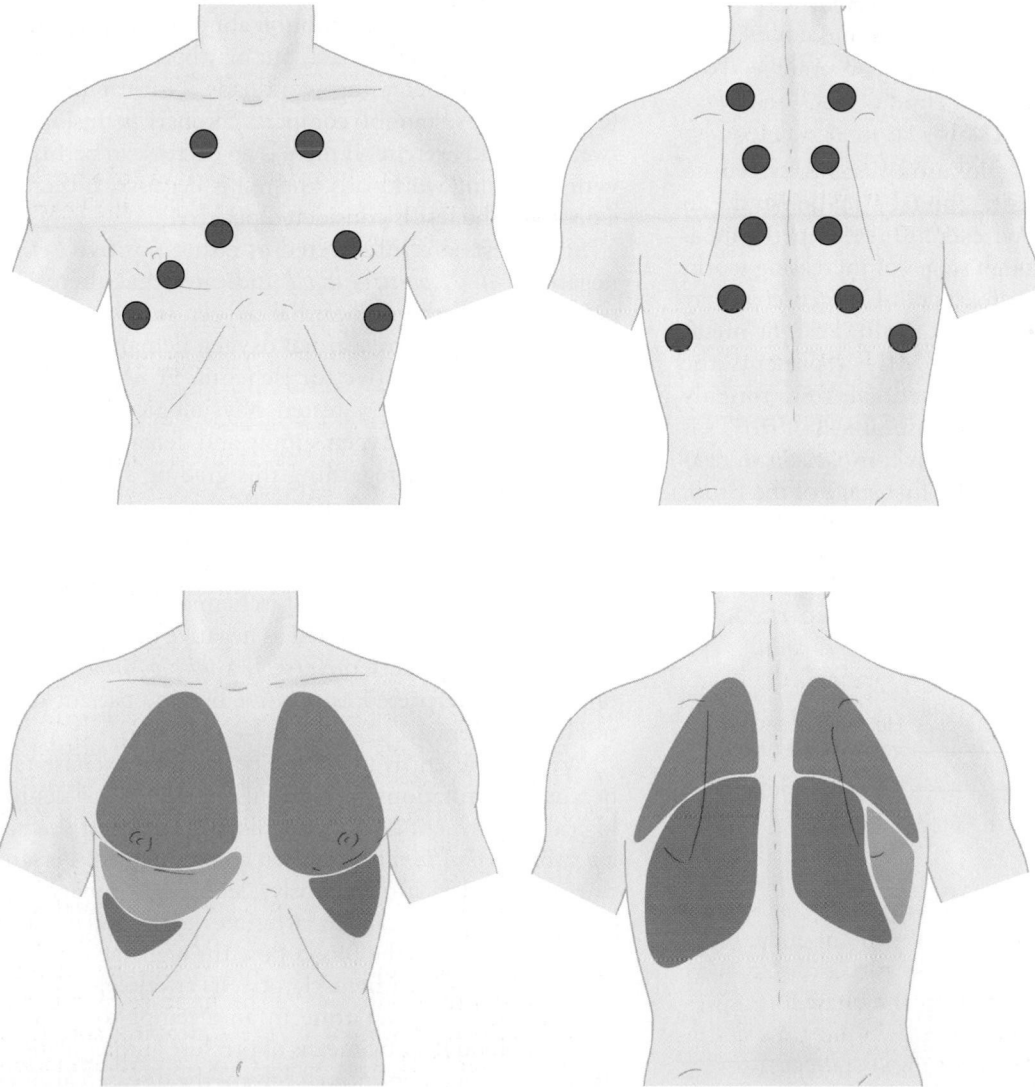

Figure 13.18 Auscultation of lungs.

patient's head is turned away from the side to be evaluated and the clinician observes for a distention or pulsations of the jugular vein 3 to 5 cm above the sternum.[44] The highest point of visible pulsation is determined and the vertical distance between this level and the level of the sternal angle of Louis is recorded (Fig. 13.19).

Pitting Edema

In patients with congestive heart failure, low SV causes a reduced blood volume perfused to the periphery. This stimulates the pressoreceptors as they sense a decrease in volume. These pressoreceptors subsequently relay a message to the kidney to retain fluid. This retention of fluid increases the hydrostatic pressure within the peripheral vasculature, thereby pushing fluid into the interstitial space resulting in peripheral edema and weight gain. Edema can be assessed through girth measurements or by using the pitting edema scale. See Chapter 14, Vascular, Lymphatic, and Integumentary Disorders, for the pitting edema grading scale. The severity of peripheral edema is categorized into four stages based on the time taken for the skin to rebound to its original contour after pitting. It is also important to note that edema can accumulate in the abdominal area (ascites) or sacral areas of the body.

Exercise Tolerance Tests

To examine the ability of the cardiovascular system to accommodate to increasing metabolic demand, an ETT, stress test, or graded exercise test is performed. The patient exercises through stages of increasing workloads, expressed in units of oxygen. Oxygen cost may be expressed in L/min, mL O_2/kg/min, kcal, or **metabolic equivalents (METs)**; the MET represents the basic systemic oxygen requirement at rest, roughly 3.5 mL O_2/kg/min. The clinical usefulness of METs is that an activity can be expressed in comparison to resting energy cost. For example, the first stage of the Bruce protocol requires roughly 5 METs of energy (i.e., it requires five times the energy expended at rest). The

most common modalities used in exercise testing of patients with cardiac impairments are the treadmill, bicycle, and arm ergometer (Fig. 13.20). In the earlier years of exercise testing for examination of CAD, the step test was routinely used; however, it has for the most part been replaced by the other modalities. The step test is useful for fitness screening in the relatively healthy population and in exercise training for both the cardiac and noncardiac populations.

Knowledge of systemic energy requirements is important in prescribing exercise and activity guidelines, as well as in exercise testing for patients with cardiac impairments. Many charts are available that express systemic energy requirements using a variety of oxygen equivalents (Table 13.9).

The two major goals of exercise testing are to detect the presence of ischemia and to determine the functional aerobic capacity of the individual. The patient is monitored with a 12-lead ECG throughout the test and recovery; information regarding perfusion, rhythm, or conduction changes is therefore immediately available. In addition to the ECG, other diagnostic tools may be used, most commonly the echocardiogram and nuclear imaging. The stress echo examines wall motion abnormalities that may or may not be present at rest, but may become more pronounced with increasing workloads. Nuclear imaging (e.g., thallium sestamibi) compares coronary perfusion between rest and exercise. If there is no decrease in perfusion with increasing workloads, the test is negative; if there is a decrease, the test is considered positive.

Stress tests are interpreted as either positive (+) or negative (−). A *positive ETT* indicates that there is a point at which the myocardial oxygen supply is inadequate to meet the myocardial oxygen demand, and the test is therefore positive for ischemia. A *negative ETT* indicates that at every tested physiological workload there is a balanced oxygen supply and demand. Patients are often confused regarding this grading system. It is helpful to reassure them that in this case, a negative test is in fact good. Stress tests are not unlike other diagnostic tools; however, they are not 100% specific and sensitive in identifying the presence of ischemia. A *false-negative ETT* is one that is interpreted as negative but the patient in fact has ischemia. Conversely, a *false-positive ETT* is one that is interpreted as positive but the patient does not have ischemia.

When a patient is unable to perform an exercise test because of limitations such as musculoskeletal or neurological impairments, a pharmacological stress test such as a *persantine thallium* test is often recommended. Persantine, when given intravenously, decreases coronary vascular resistance by causing arterioles to vasodilate, and therefore increases the blood flow through the capillary beds. If an artery is atherosclerotic, its arteriole may have gradually dilated over time in an attempt to increase capillary blood flow by means of pressure autoregulation. Therefore, when persantine is given, the diseased arteries may have a limitation in the amount of further arteriolar

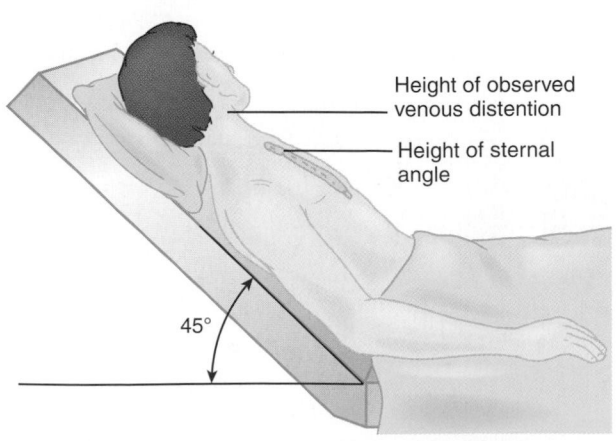

Height of observed venous distention

Height of sternal angle

45°

Figure 13.19 Examination of jugular venous distention.

Figure 13.20 Estimated oxygen requirements for step, bicycle, and treadmill. The standard Bruce protocol begins at 1.7 mph and 10 percent grade (roughly 5 METs). Oxygen requirements increase with progressive increases in workload for all modalities. (*Adapted from Fletcher et al,[112] p. 156.*)

Treadmill Protocols (Figure 13.20)

Column legend / notes:
- **Bicycle Ergometer:** 1 watt = 6 kpds. KPDS shown for 70 kg body weight.
- **Step Test:** Nagle, Balke, Naughton — 2 min stages, 30 steps/min; step height increased 4 cm q 2 min. Height given in cm.
- **Bruce:** 3-min stages.
- **Cornell:** 2-min stages.
- **Balke-Ware:** % grade at 3.3 mph, 1-min stages (grades 26 → 1).
- **ACIP:** 2-min stages, first 2 stages 1 min.
- **mACIP:** 2-min stages, first 2 stages 1 min.
- **Naughton:** 2-min stages.
- **Ware:** 2-min stages.
- **Clinical Status:** Healthy (dependent on age, activity) → sedentary healthy → Limited → Symptomatic.

Functional Class	O2 Cost ml/kg/min	METS	Step Test Height (cm)	Bicycle KPDS	Bruce MPH/%GR	Cornell MPH/%GR	ACIP MPH/%GR	mACIP MPH/%GR	Naughton %GR @3 mph	Naughton %GR @3.4 mph	Naughton %GR @2 mph	Ware MPH/%GR
Normal and I	56.0	16			5.5 / 20							
	52.5	15			5.0 / 18	5.0 / 18						
	49.0	14							32.5	26		
	45.5	13			4.2 / 16	4.6 / 17	3.4 / 24	3.4 / 24	30	24		
	42.0	12	40	1500		4.2 / 16	3.1 / 24	3.1 / 24	27.5	22		
	38.5	11	36	1350					25	20		
	35.0	10	32	1200	3.4 / 14	3.8 / 15	3 / 21	2.7 / 24	22.5	18		
	31.5	9	28	1050			3 / 17.5	2.3 / 24	20	16		
	28.0	8	24	900			3 / 14	2 / 24	17.5	14		
	24.5	7	20	750	2.5 / 12	3.0 / 13	3 / 10.5	2 / 18.9	15	12	17.5	
	21.0	6	16	600		2.5 / 12	3.0 / 7.0	2 / 13.5	12.5	10	14	
II	17.5	5	12	450	1.7 / 10	2.1 / 11	3.0 / 3.0	2 / 7	10	8	10.5	3.4 / 14.0
III	14.0	4	8	300		1.7 / 10	2.5 / 2.0	2 / 3.5	7.5	6	7	3.0 / 15.0
	10.5	3	4	150	1.7 / 5	1.7 / 5	2.0 / 0	2 / 0	5	4	3.5	3.0 / 12.5
IV	7.0	2			1.7 / 0	1.7 / 0			2.5	2	0	3.0 / 10.0
	3.5	1							0			3.0 / 7.5

Additional (lowest) Ware stages: 3.0 / 10.5 · 2.0 / 7.0 · 2.0 / 3.5 · 1.5 / 0 · 1.0 / 0

Balke-Ware grades (% grade at 3.3 mph, 1-min stages): 26, 25, 24, 23, 22, 21, 20, 19, 18, 17, 16, 15, 14, 13, 12, 11, 10, 9, 8, 7, 6, 5, 4, 3, 2, 1

Table 13.9   Metabolic Equivalent (MET) Chart

Intensity (70-kg Person)	Endurance Promoting	Occupational	Recreational
1½–2 METs 4–7 mL/kg/min 2–2½ kcal/min	Too low in energy level	Desk work, driving auto, electric calculating machine operation, light housework, polishing furniture, washing clothes	Standing, strolling (1 mph), flying, motorcycling, playing cards, sewing, knitting
2–3 METs 7–11 mL/kg/min 2½–4 kcal/min	Too low in energy level unless capacity is very low	Auto repair, radio and television repair, janitorial work, bartending, riding lawn mower, light wood-working	Level walking (2 mph), level bicycling (5 mph), billiards, bowling, skeet shooting, shuffleboard, powerboat driving, golfing with power cart, canoeing, horseback riding at a walk
3–4 METs 11–14 mL/kg/min 4–5 kcal/min	Yes, if continuous and if target heart rate is reached	Brick laying, plastering, wheelbarrow (100-lb load), machine assembly, welding (moderate load), cleaning windows, mopping floors, vacuuming, pushing light power mower	Walking (3 mph), bicycling (6 mph), horseshoe pitching, volleyball (6-person, noncompetitive), golfing (pulling bag cart), archery, sailing (handling small boat), fly fishing (standing in waders), horseback riding (trotting), badminton (social doubles)
4–5 METs 14–18 mL/kg/min	Recreational activities promote endurance; occupational activities must be continuous, lasting longer than 2 min	Painting, masonry, paperhanging, light carpentry, scrubbing floors, raking leaves, hoeing	Walking (3½ mph), bicycling (8 mph), table tennis, golfing (carrying clubs), dancing (foxtrot), badminton (singles), tennis (doubles), many calisthenics, ballet
5–6 METs 18–21 mL/kg/min	Yes	Digging garden, shoveling light earth	Walking (4 mph), bicycling (10 mph), canoeing (4 mph), horseback riding (posting to trotting), stream fishing (walking in light current in waders), ice or roller skating (9 mph)
6–7 METs 21–25 mL/kg/min 7–8 kcal/min	Yes	Shoveling 10 times/min (4½ kg or 10 lb), splitting wood, snow shoveling, hand lawn mowing	Walking (5 mph), bicycling (11 mph), competitive badminton, tennis (singles), folk and square dancing, light downhill skiing, ski touring (2½ mph), water skiing, swimming (20 yards/min)
7–8 METs 25–28 mL/kg/min 8–10 kcal/min	Yes	Digging ditches, carrying 36 kg or 80 lb, sawing hardwood	Jogging (5 mph), bicycling (12 mph), horseback riding (gallop), vigorous downhill skiing, basketball, mountain climbing, ice hockey, canoeing (5 mph), touch football, paddleball
8–9 METs 28–32 mL/kg/min 10–11 kcal/min	Yes	Shoveling 10 times/min (5½ kg or 14 lb)	Running (5½ mph), bicycling (13 mph), ski touring (4 mph), squash (social), handball (social), fencing, basketball (vigorous), swimming (30 yards/min), rope skipping
10+ METs 32+ mL/kg/min 11+ kcal/min	Yes	Shoveling 10 times/min (7½ kg or 16 lb)	Running (6 mph = 10 METs, 7 mph = 11½ METs, 8 mph = 13½ METs, 9 mph = 15 METs, 10 mph = 17 METs), ski touring (5+ mph), handball (competitive), squash (competitive), swimming (greater than 40 yards/min)

From Fox, SM, et al: Physical activity and cardiovascular health: 3. The exercise prescription: Frequency and type of activity.
Mod Con Cardiovasc Dis 41:26, 1972, with permission.

dilation that can occur. In comparison to the nondiseased arteries, there will be a relative decrease in blood flow through the capillary beds of the diseased arteries. Imaging studies will thus detect a relative decrease in blood flow to the area of the myocardium that is perfused by the diseased artery compared to that perfused by a nondiseased artery. Adenosine, which is a coronary and peripheral vasodilator (as well as an antiarrhythmic), has similar effects as persantine and may be used instead.[95]

Assessment of Aerobic Capacity and Endurance

The best indicator of an individual's aerobic capacity is through examination of the peak oxygen uptake or VO_2 maximum and anaerobic threshold. However, to obtain these numbers, sophisticated and expensive equipment such as a metabolic cart is required. Most physical therapists do not have access to this equipment to determine these numbers. Therefore, the physical therapist can continually monitor the patient's responses during exercise to better understand the individual's tolerance and level of endurance. HR, BP, pulse oximetry, and respiratory rate and rhythm at every given level of intensity will provide clinicians with a good picture of the patient's aerobic capacity and endurance.

Another useful test to determine an individual's functional status, exercise tolerance and oxygen consumption is the *6-Minute Walk Test (6-MWT)*. Patients are asked to walk as far as they can in 6 minutes, taking as many rests as needed during this time.[96-98] The 6-MWT, although considered submaximal, closely approximates the maximal exercise of persons with CHF and can be correlated to peak oxygen consumption.[98,99] In addition to prediction of the peak oxygen uptake, a distance of 300 m is an important indicator of short-term and long-term survival in patients with CHF. Coats[100] found that patients unable to ambulate greater than 300 m during the 6-MWT had poorer short-term survival, and Bittner et al[101] reported that patients who were unable to ambulate distances over 300 m had poorer long-term survival.

■ PHYSICAL THERAPY INTERVENTION FOR PATIENTS WITH HEART DISEASE

Intervention for Patients with Coronary Artery Disease

According to the APTA *Guide to Physical Therapist Practice,* the preferred practice pattern for management of patients with CVD is Pattern 6-D. The development of specific anticipated goals and expected outcomes for the individual with CAD is based on the general goals of physical therapy intervention presented in Box 13.5.

Physical therapists treat not only patients who have a primary diagnosis of heart disease, but also, and perhaps more commonly, patients with multiple medical diagnoses, only one of which is cardiac. Physical therapy

---

Box 13.5 Coronary Artery Disease— Anticipated Goals and Expected Outcomes

- Aerobic capacity is increased.
- Ability to perform physical tasks related to self-care, home management, community and work integration or reintegration, and leisure activities is increased.
- Physiological response to increased oxygen demand is improved.
- Strength, power, and endurance are increased.
- Symptoms associated with increased oxygen demand are decreased.
- Ability to recognize a recurrence is increased, and intervention is sought in a timely manner.
- Risk of recurrence is reduced.
- Behaviors that foster healthy habits, wellness, and prevention are acquired.
- Decision making is enhanced regarding health of patient and the use of health care resources by patient/client, family, significant others, and caregivers.

---

intervention during the traditional acute cardiac rehabilitation phase involves following the patient while recovering from his or her cardiac event, such as an MI, providing hemodynamic monitoring of progressive activity, discharge guidelines, education, and information regarding outpatient referral. It may include outpatient management as well, ideally in a multidisciplinary setting including nursing and nutrition. Patients with cardiac histories commonly have physical therapy needs at other points throughout their lives. For example, the patient with a previous MI might require ambulation training as a result of a fractured hip, an outpatient knee rehabilitation program following a skiing injury, tennis elbow intervention, prosthetic ambulation training, or intervention following a CVA. If the physical therapist understands the pathophysiology of the cardiac condition and the energy demands being placed on the patient, the therapist will be able to adjust the POC accordingly.

It is important to remember that a patient with known CAD may not have symptomatic ischemia, either because the lesions are not of significant size to interfere with blood flow, or the anti-ischemic medications are able to keep the patient's physiological response to activity below his or her ischemic threshold. Following a noncomplicated MI, ischemia should not occur in the area perfused by the involved artery because infarcted tissue cannot become ischemic. However, if there is disease in other arteries, ischemia can occur in any noninfarcted tissue that has a compromised blood supply. A physical therapist working with patients with significant CAD must be aware that their basic cardiac impairment is an imbalance of myocardial oxygen supply and demand, and any increase in systemic oxygen consumption will increase myocardial oxygen consumption. A past medical history of CAD does not mean that the disease occurred in the past and is no longer present; once a person has been diagnosed with CAD, he or she has the potential for atherosclerosis progression at any later point in time. Although the precipitating factors for plaque rupture are not clearly understood, the plaque with increased levels of oxidized LDLs is thought to be unstable with a greater potential for rupture.[102] It is important to note that plaque rupture may occur with lesions of any size, not just those that are greater than 70%.[102] Therefore, it is prudent for the physical therapist to know the status of all the coronary arteries, not just those that were revascularized or have a greater than 70% lesion.

The degree of a patient's risk for increased morbidity and mortality is based on a number of factors. The *American Association of Cardiovascular and Pulmonary Rehabilitation (AACVPR)* and the *American College of Physicians* provide a framework for stratifying patients with cardiac impairments (Table 13.10).

Table 13.10	**Risk Stratification Criteria for Cardiac Patients by the American College of Physicians (ACP) and American Association of Cardiovascular and Pulmonary Rehabilitation (AACVPR)**
ACP	**AACVPR**
Low Risk	
Uncomplicated MI or CABG	Uncomplicated MI, CABG, angioplasty, or atherectomy
Functional capacity ≥8 METs 3 weeks after clinical event	Functional capacity ≥6 METs 3 or more weeks after clinical event
No ischemia, left ventricular dysfunction, or complex arrhythmias	No resting or exercise-induced myocardial ischemia manifested as angina and/or ST-segment displacement No resting or exercise-induced complex arrhythmias
Asymptomatic at rest with exercise capacity adequate for most vocational and recreational activities	No significant left ventricular dysfunction (EF ≥ 50%)
Intermediate (Moderate) Risk	
Functional capacity <8 METs 3 weeks after clinical event	Functional capacity <5–6 METs 3 or more weeks after clinical event
Shock or CHF during recent MI (<6 months) (EF 31%–49%) Inability to self-monitor heart rate	Mild to moderately depressed left ventricular function
Failure to comply with exercise prescription	Failure to comply with exercise prescription
Exercise-induced ST-segment depression <2 mm	Exercise-induced ST-segment depression of 1–2 mm or reversible ischemic defects (echocardiography or nuclear radiography)
High Risk	
Severely depressed LV function (EF <30%)	Severely depressed LV function (EF ≤30%)
Resting complex ventricular arrhythmias (low grade IV or V)	Complex ventricular arrythmias at rest or appearing or increasing with exercise
PVCs appearing or increasing with exercise	
Exertional hypotension (≥15 mm Hg decrease in systolic pressure during exercise)	Decrease in systolic blood pressure of >15 mm Hg during exercise or failure to rise consistent with exercise workloads
Recent MI (<6 months) complicated by serious ventricular arrhythmias	MI complicated by CHF, cardiogenic shock, and/or complex-ventricular arrhythmias
Exercise-induced ST-segment depression >2 mm	Patients with severe CAD and marked (>2 mm) exercise-induced ST-segment depression
Survivor of cardiac arrest	Survivor of cardiac arrest

From American College Sports Medicine: Guidelines for Exercise Testing, ed 5. Williams & Wilkins, Baltimore, 1995, pp 20, 21, with permission.
CABG = coronary artery bypass graft; CHF = congestive heart failure; EF = ejection fraction; LV = left ventricular; MET = metabolic equivalent; PVC = premature ventricular contraction.

Exercise Prescription

The *Clinical Practice Guidelines for Cardiac Rehabilitation* were established after extensive and critical review of published scientific literature.[103] These guidelines support the beneficial effect of exercise training on exercise tolerance for patients with heart disease. The most consistent benefit appeared to occur with exercise training at least three times per week for 12 or more weeks' duration. The duration of aerobic exercise training sessions varied from 20 to 40 minutes at an intensity approximating 70% to 85% of the baseline maximal exercise test HR. Exercise prescriptions are based on frequency, intensity, time (duration), and type (mode), the FITT equation. Activity should be gradually progressive in a logical stepwise fashion of increasing energy costs (i.e., METs, kilocalories) with appropriate HR and BP monitoring.

Although exercise is highly recommended for the patient with heart disease, there are conditions in which exercise is unwise. The AACVPR established guidelines for evaluating a patient's appropriateness for exercise participation. Contraindications for exercise training include unstable angina, symptomatic and uncompensated heart failure, uncontrolled arrhythmias, moderate to severe aortic stenosis, uncontrolled diabetes, resting blood pressure values in excess of 200/110, and uncontrolled resting tachycardia.[104]

The patient should be evaluated once these conditions have been corrected and, when appropriate, begin (or resume) the exercise program. Recognizing that cardiac disease is a dynamic process, and that the patient who was stable and able to participate in physical therapy last week may not be stable this week, is a critical concept. The importance of a patient-specific examination and evaluation before each session will allow the physical therapist to critically plan the appropriate intervention.

Exercise Intensity

Intensity may be prescribed by either HR or by subjective report, a *rating of perceived exertion (RPE)*. Subjective ratings of intensity of exertion have been used to quantify effort during exercise. The original *Rating of Perceived Exertion Scale (The Borg RPE Scale)*, developed by Borg, has been used extensively (Table 13.11). It consists of numbers ranging from 6 to 20, which patients use to rate their perceptions of how hard they are working. Descriptive words accompany the numbers, such as hard or very hard. Commonly, patients are asked to limit their exertion to between fairly light and somewhat hard. Borg also developed a category-ratio scale of 0 to 10. Both local symptoms, such as muscle aches, cramps, pain, or fatigue, and central symptoms, such as feelings of fatigue or breathlessness, contribute to the overall feelings of work performance. High correlation of RPE ratings with HR and aerobic power has been found in normal individuals and in patients with cardiac disease.

Table 13.11	Rating of Perceived Exertion: The Borg RPE Scale*
6	No exertion at all
7	
8	Extremely light
9	Very light
10	
11	Light
12	
13	Somewhat hard
14	
15	Hard (heavy)
16	
17	Very hard
18	
19	Extremely hard
20	Maximal exertion

*Copyright Gunnar Borg. Reproduced with permission.
For correct usage of the scale(s) the exact design and instructions given in Borg's folders must be followed. See Borg, G: Borg's Perceived Exertion and Pain Scales. Human Kinetics, Champaign, IL, 1998, or www.borgproducts.com.

A common aerobic exercise prescription based on HR is 70% to 85% of HR_{max}. However, the more deconditioned patient may be aerobically trained at as low as 50% to 60% of HR_{max}. Any patient who has documented CAD should have a medically supervised ETT before beginning an aerobic exercise program. Without an ETT, it is impossible to assume what the maximum HR would be for a patient with cardiac disease. The ECG monitoring during the ETT is useful in the detection of exercise-induced ischemia. If no ETT data are available, it is unwise to prescribe an exercise based on HRs. Cautious progression of activity is warranted, along with use of RPE and knowledge of adverse signs and symptoms for exercise intolerance. An easy tool for self-monitoring is for the patient to be able to talk without becoming breathless while exercising. This is termed the *Talk Test* and provides a fair indication that the patient is appropriately exercising below his or her anaerobic threshold, which usually occurs at approximately 55% to 70% of the maximal oxygen uptake.

Exercise Frequency

Exercise is commonly prescribed three to five times per week. The patient should not experience increased fatigue as a result of exercise. If fatigue does occur, the frequency and/or intensity of exercise should be decreased. Patients who choose to exercise daily must watch for signs and symptoms of fatigue and overexertion, recognizing that fatigue may not just occur during the activity, but be delayed until later in the day or the next day.

Exercise Duration (Time)

The goal of 30 to 40 minutes of aerobic exercise with an additional 5 to 10 minutes of warm-up and an adequate cool-down is appropriate. If this amount of activity is uncomfortable for the patient, whatever amount he or she can do comfortably without adverse symptoms is appropriate. Patients who are deconditioned may require interval work, brief rests every 5 minutes during their early training. Adequate warm-up is crucial for all patients but especially for patients with CAD. By gradually increasing the MVO_2 and allowing the coronary arteries time to vasodilate, a balanced myocardial supply and demand may be possible with subsequent activity.

Mode of Exercise (Type)

The variety of exercise equipment has expanded in the last 20 years. The good news is that the patient has the opportunity to experience a variety of equipment including treadmills, stair climbers, bicycles, rowers, crosscountry ski simulators, reclining bicycles, steppers, arm ergometers, and others. Patients frequently ask which is the best equipment; the one that they enjoy and the one that they will use is by far the best for them.

If a patient becomes symptomatic with angina during a physical therapy intervention, the immediate goal is to decrease MVO_2; the activity should be immediately stopped. The patient should sit or, if possible, lie down on a bed or plinth. The physical therapist should take the patient's HR and BP and calculate the rate pressure product (RPP = HR (SBP) as soon as possible to determine the MVO_2 at which the patient became ischemic, termed the *ischemic threshold*. If the patient is in an inpatient facility, help may be sought immediately to ensure that facility guidelines are quickly initiated. Such guidelines may include supplemental oxygen, a 12-lead ECG, administration of NTG, and other anti-ischemic medications. If the patient is in an outpatient setting and has his or her own NTG (which the patient should be carrying at all times), the patient should take it and follow the prescribed guidelines. NTG usually produces a tingling or burning sensation if it is effective. Failure of the NTG to produce these sensations may indicate that the NTG is outdated. Patients are generally instructed to take one NTG pill sublingually (under the tongue), although some patients use an NTG spray. They can then wait 5 minutes and repeat administration if the symptoms are not completely gone. A third NTG may also be taken after waiting another 5 minutes. Patients are frequently told that if the symptoms have not resolved completely after three doses of NTG they should come to the emergency department for further management. If the patient is in an outpatient setting without his or her own NTG and has symptoms that do not resolve after a few minutes of rest, the facility guidelines

to activate advanced care for the patient should begin quickly. If the patient's symptoms escalate, even after the first NTG, emergency care needs to be initiated immediately. If the patient is climbing stairs, the patient should stop, take a few easy deep breaths, and then descend when the symptoms have abated and walk slowly to the first available support. However, if the patient's symptoms are quickly accelerating despite stopping the activity and taking deep breaths, the patient should be assisted to a position of comfort and further medical assistance sought immediately. It is important that therapists maintain a calm demeanor, reassuring the patient that the situation can be handled efficiently and easily.

Cardiac Rehabilitation: Myocardial Infarction

Although it is common today to take cardiac rehabilitation for granted, it was not so long ago that treatment for patients with MI included weeks of prolonged bedrest. In the pivotal 1952 study by Levine and Lown,[105] chair rest and low-level activity was found to be more beneficial than the traditional 8 weeks of bedrest. Today, the patient with a noncomplicated MI may be hospitalized for as few as 3 to 5 days.

Cardiac rehabilitation (cardiac rehab) is multidisciplinary and may include the physician, nurse, physical and occupational therapists, exercise physiologist, nutritionist, and social service caseworker. Cardiac rehab begins in the hospital and extends indefinitely into the maintenance phase. The inpatient component is referred to as *Phase I*. Outpatient phases include *Phase II*, the exercise-training period, and *Phase III*, the maintenance period. Phase II is usually described as occurring immediately after discharge, requiring intensive monitoring and supervision including ECG monitoring and intensive risk factor interventions.[106] Aerobic and strength training may begin based on the results of the ETT, which is usually done at approximately 4 weeks. In Phase III, the patient has stabilized and requires ECG monitoring only if signs and symptoms necessitate; endurance training and risk factor modification continue. Ideally, Phase II is initiated within 2 weeks of hospital discharge. It is important to note that these phases are not absolutes and the timelines and activities of these phases may vary according to managed care models, contracts with reimbursement plans, and treatment protocol designs. Owing to insurance coverage, some patients do not enter into a formal cardiac rehab program until after their symptom-limited maximum ETT at 4 to 6 weeks post-MI.

Inpatient/Phase 1

The length of hospital stay for a patient with an MI has changed dramatically in the last decade and is commonly 3 to 5 days for an *uncomplicated MI* (no post-MI angina, malignant arrhythmias, or heart failure), compared to at least three to four times that duration in the early 1980s.

Inpatient cardiac rehab uses a team approach based on activity progression, patient education, and hemodynamic and ECG monitoring, together with medical and pharmacological management. The role of the physical therapist is to monitor activity tolerance, prepare for discharge, educate the patient to recognize adverse symptoms with activity, support risk factor modification techniques, provide emotional support, and collaborate with other team members.

Vital sign monitoring occurs before and after and, if possible, during activity. The intensity of the activity is considered to be low level, and perceived exertion for the patient should be comparable to the "fairly light range" of the Borg RPE Scale (see Table 13.11). For an increase of 1 to 2 METs, an HR increase of 10 to 20 bpm is appropriate, if beta-blockers or other HR suppressers are not used; however, the absence of beta blockade in Phase I is uncommon. If a beta-blocker is used, there is no standardization as to the degree of HR suppression; subjective ratings of perceived exertion and objective observation of patient effort become increasingly important. A patient on beta-blockers who has an HR increase of 20 bpm during low-level inpatient activity would be considered inadequately medicated, unless the activity level was considerably higher than appropriate. A decrease in HR or BP during activity for any patient, regardless of medications, should be evaluated for the presence of an arrhythmia. Following the physical therapy intervention, the patient's tolerance of activity and hemodynamic stability should be documented.

There are a variety of inpatient cardiac rehab programs, frequently progressive based on levels of increasing energy costs (e.g., MET levels). Each facility will establish its own levels and criteria for activity progression and education; an example of an inpatient program is shown in Table 13.12. Following are some general comments and recommendations about the various levels. It is important to note that activity progression occurs along a continuum and is not done in a rigid format. Although a patient must demonstrate the ability to sit at the bedside with appropriate hemodynamic response before ambulating in the hallway, the patient's individual response and medical history will dictate how quickly he or she is able to progress. A patient may progress through more than one level within any treatment session.

Level 1. The patient is in the intensive care unit (ICU) and is stable; generally physical therapy intervention does not begin until after the first 24 hours from admission or until the patient has been stable for 24 hours. Physical therapy intervention should begin after the blood work has indicated the MI is completed. CK and troponin (both I and T) levels are monitored. For both CK and troponin levels, reliable diagnostic sensitivity (greater than 90%) is reached within 12 to 16 hours of the onset of symptoms.[106] CK peak levels occur between 14 and 36 hours, with a return to normal level after 48 to 72 hours; troponin peaks at 24 to 36 hours, with a return to normal levels within 10 to 12 days.[107] Commonly, three sets of CK levels collected 8 hours apart are collected. Because CK is released very quickly into the bloodstream with cellular damage, it is typical for the first and second CK levels to show a progressive increase and the third set to be less than the second (i.e., the CK peak has occurred, and the values are now trending downward). Because CK may be released with cellular damage to areas other than to the myocardium, specific myocardial isoenzymes known as CK-MB are monitored. Appropriate activity for the patient in the ICU during the first 24 hours is to move comfortably within the bed, perform ankle pumps, perform deep-breathing exercises, use the commode (if hemodynamically stable), and perform limited personal care.

Level 2. Once the patient has been hemodynamically stable for 24 hours he or she may progress out of bed (OOB). The therapist should also be alert to signs of orthostatic hypotension when the patient changes position from supine to sitting on the side of the bed. The patient's feet should be supported on a stool to assist venous return if they are not able to touch the floor. The patient walks to a bedside chair. The patient sits in an upright chair for up to 30 minutes a few times a day. There is a real temptation for many health care providers to have the patient "do" something while seated, such as washing, eating, or visiting with family. It is probably wise to just let the patient sit for the first time, without being encumbered with other tasks. The therapist is thus better able to evaluate the patient's response to being upright. If the patient has had a large MI or requires a slow progression to upright posture, the use of a reclining chair is a way to gradually assume the upright position. The patient performs LE exercises such as ankle pumps, knee extensions, or marching in place. Vital signs are monitored for hemodynamic stability and appropriate activity response. Ensuring sufficient healing time, pacing activities, and creating a healthful environment are components of a comprehensive patient education program.

Level 3. Patients are instructed to gradually increase their ambulation. One approach is to educate patients to judge their ambulation in terms of time instead of distance. Time is a more reproducible measurement, whereas distance may be difficult to judge (e.g., "I want you to walk for 2 minutes" vs. "I want you to walk 200 ft"). It also allows for an easier transition to the HEP, which is commonly based on length of time. For documentation purposes, it is most effective to document the distance covered in the time period whenever possible (e.g., "Patient ambulated 500 ft in 6 minutes with an RPE of 10/20"). Information regarding CAD risk factors allows patients to begin to take responsibility for their choices about activity and lifestyle. However, for some patients this may be too early in their recovery, and they are unable to focus on what is being said. Giving patients written information is a good way to provide education and yet give patients the choice when to read it. Use of the Borg RPE Scale assists the patient in monitoring of activity intensity.

Levels 4 through 6. Patients gradually increase the frequency and time of their walks at a comfortable and leisurely pace. The goal is to progress walks from 2 minutes, to 5 minutes, to 10 minutes with appropriate hemodynamic response. Stairs may be climbed foot over foot with a planned rest halfway or so, or one foot at a time, depending on the status of the patient. Patients are often hesitant to move, especially in stretching their arms overhead; therefore performing a variety of trunk, arm, and standing leg exercises for a few repetitions each often allays the fear and helps the patient feel more comfortable moving.

Patients need to be made aware of the fatigue that often accompanies seemingly innocuous activities (e.g., showering) and plan their rests accordingly. Visitors are often a hidden energy cost; patients are often very excited and reassured to have visitors, but the fatigue that follows is sometimes very disconcerting. Helping the patient understand the concept of energy and the cost of not just physical but emotional and mental activities is invaluable. Comparing energy costs to money may help the patient to pace activity. Patients are told that they have a dollar's worth of energy and everything they do is going to cost them some part of that dollar; however, they can never spend more than 50 or 60 cents at one time. Every time they rest, it is like going to the ATM for a quick refill. In this way, patients become knowledgeable about the expendability of energy and yet are given the responsibility to spend (and save) as they choose.

Documentation

There are many ways to document physical therapy examination and intervention. In this patient population, appropriate documentation would include the following:

1. Objective activity data, including time period and distance ambulated, type of sitting and standing exercises, and stair climbing (number of steps); number and duration of rests.
2. Patient's vital sign response to each activity, including a statement that addresses patient performance with respect to vital signs (e.g., "Patient ambulated 6 minutes covering 500 ft and climbed 10 steps foot over foot using handrail with adaptive VS

response without signs or symptoms of hemodynamic compromise").
3. Education provided and response of patient, family, and caregivers.

Home Exercise Program

Two of the more important concepts for a patient to understand at the time of discharge are symptom recognition and appropriate activity guidelines. It is crucial that the patient recognizes cardiac symptoms and understands the action to take if they occur.

Physical therapists establish activity guidelines during the first 4 to 6 weeks after MI while the myocardium is healing. During this healing phase, physical activity involves a gradual increase in ambulation time, with a goal of 20 to 30 minutes of ambulation one to two times per day at 4 to 6 weeks after MI. Patients are encouraged to walk comfortably, dress appropriately, and to try to exercise in ambient temperature at indoor malls if weather is not appropriate (i.e., below 40°F including wind chill factor, over 80°F, or excessive humidity and poor air quality). Some patients are very sensitive to environmental factors and should exercise only in ambient conditions or indoors. For some patients, home exercise equipment is affordable and may be a reasonable alternative to outdoor exercise. For safety reasons, the patient should be monitored on similar equipment before independently beginning to exercise at home. This is not the time for a patient to try a new type of exercise modality but to stay with what is familiar. Walking appears to be the exercise of choice owing to its ease and familiarity.

The patient's days will be a combination of rest and low-level activity including ambulation and LE and UE mobility. The patient should be encouraged to try to change positions or activity every 1 to 2 hours. For example, it is generally not a good idea for the patient to be up all morning and then rest all afternoon. It is invaluable to have patients verbally outline what their days will include once they are discharged. This affords an opportunity to better understand the interests of the patient and make specific suggestions, as well as provide an opportunity to determine the patient's understanding of activity guidelines and energy conservation techniques.

Outpatient Phase II

Patients commonly undergo a symptom-limited maximal stress test (ETT) at 4 to 6 weeks after MI. Based on the results of the tests, either positive (+) for ischemia or negative (−) for ischemia, an exercise prescription is prescribed. For a (−) ETT, a common exercise prescription would be 70% to 85% of the peak achieved on the test (i.e., HR_{max}); however, an equally effective alternative would be 65% to 80% of HR_{max}. Understanding that a negative test does not mean the patient is disease free and that vulnerable plaques may exist, a conservative prescription may be a wiser choice.

Table 13.12   Inpatient Cardiac Rehabilitation Program

CCU–Essentially Bedrest

Level 1
1–1.5 METs
- Evaluation and patient education
- Arms supported for meals and activities of daily living (ADL)
- Bed exercises and dangle with feet supported (if CK levels have peaked and patient has no complications)

Education
- Introduction to inpatient cardiac rehab and role of physical therapy
  - Education
  - Monitored progression of activity
  - Home exercise/activity guidelines/outpatient cardiac rehab

Sitting—Limited Room Ambulation

Level 2
1.5–2 METs
- Sitting 15–30 min, 2–4 times/day
- Leg exercises
- Commode privileges
- Reclining upright chair
- Limited ADL
- Electric razor
- Limited supervised room ambulation for small uncomplicated MI

Education
- Identification of CAD risk factors
- Concept of "healing interval" and need to pace activities

Room—Limited Hall Ambulation

Level 3
2–2.5 METs
- Room or hall ambulation up to 5 min as tolerated 3–4 times/day
- Standing leg exercises optional*
- Sit on side of bed or in bathroom to wash (per discretion nurse/physical therapist [PT])
- Manual shave
- Bathroom privileges
- Independent or assisted ambulation in room or hall as advised by PT

Education
- Size of infarct and how it relates to the need for gradual resumption of activities
- Impact of exercise on reducing the patient's risk factors
- Teach use of Borg's Scale for Rating of Perceived Exertion and appropriate parameters with activity

Progressive Hall Ambulation

Level 4
2.5–3 METs
- Hall ambulation 5–7 min as tolerated 3–4 times/day
- Standing trunk exercises optional*
- Independent or assisted ambulation in hall as advised by PT

Education
- Teach pulse taking and appropriate parameters with activity
- Reinforce benefits of outpatient cardiac rehabilitation

Progressive Hall Ambulation

Level 5
3–4 METs
- Hall ambulation 8–10 min as tolerated
- Arm exercises optional*
- Standing shower
- Independent hall ambulation as advised by PT

Education
- Written home exercise/activity guidelines reviewed
- Patient given written information on outpatient cardiac rehab

Stair Climbing

Level 6
4–5 METs
- Progressive hall ambulation as tolerated
- Full flight of stairs (or as required at home) up and down one step at a time†

Education
- Answer patient's questions
- Check for understanding of activity guidelines

Patient Outcome—No Evidence of Hemodynamic Compromise with Activity Progression (All Levels)

No systolic drop in BP >10 mm Hg or increase >30 mm Hg
No HR increase >12 if beta blocked, or no HR increase >20 if not beta blocked
No complaints of dizziness, lightheadedness, or angina
Perceived exertion <13/20

Hemodynamic Monitoring

Level 1
- HR and BP before and after supine bed exercises
- Orthostatic signs supine and dangling at bedside

Level 2
- Orthostatic signs (supine, sit, and stand) before exercises and transfer
- HR and BP after leg exercises/transfer to chair
- HR and BP after return to bed

Levels 3–6
- HR and BP in sitting and standing prior to activity
- HR and BP immediately following activity
- HR and BP 5 min after activity

From Rehabilitation Services Department, Newton Wellesley Hospital, Newton, MA, with permission.
*Optional exercises are at the discretion of the PT and may be used to establish the patient's CV response in the room, prior to moving on to more challenging hallway ambulation; or in those patients who require general strengthening exercises.
†Stair climbing activities should take place after the ETT if the scheduling of the ETT permits. Otherwise patients may, at the discretion and supervision of the PT, climb stairs on the day prior to the ETT.

If a patient has had a *positive ETT*, the exercise prescription becomes relatively simple: during aerobic training, it is important to keep MVO_2 below the patient's ischemic MVO_2. Remember that a clinical measure of MVO_2 is the product of HR and SBP, known as the rate pressure product ($RPP = HR \times SBP$). The importance of considering the ischemic threshold is the recognition that BP will vary during use of different pieces of exercise equipment owing in part to the differences in muscle recruitment. If there is a difference in BP for a given HR, then there will be a difference in the MVO_2 to the patient. For example, if a patient has an HR of 100 bpm and a BP of 140/80 mm Hg while exercising on the treadmill, and an HR of 100 bpm and a BP of 160/80 mm Hg while exercising on the stationary bicycle, the bicycle is costing the myocardium more energy than the treadmill, even though HR is the same. Depending on the patient's ischemic threshold, it is possible that angina may occur on the bicycle but not on the treadmill. A good safety tip is to not exceed 90% of the ischemic RPP. The remainder of the exercise prescription may follow the common guidelines for aerobic training in regard to frequency, intensity, and duration for patients with cardiac involvement.

Strength Training

The inclusion of strength training in a cardiac rehab program is a relatively recent addition to the traditional cardiac rehabilitation program. Initial concern was that resistance work would inordinately increase MVO_2 and ventricular arrhythmias and therefore be detrimental.[108] A publication by Beniamini et al[109] gives excellent insight into this area. The AACVPR's thorough review of the literature on this topic concluded that "resistance exercise has been shown to be a safe and effective method for improving strength and cardiovascular endurance, modifying risk factors and enhancing self efficacy in low-risk cardiac patients."[106] Resistance training may begin with the use of elastic bands and light hand weights (1 to 3 lb) and progress to a load that allows 12 to 15 repetitions comfortably.[110] *AACVPR guidelines* further state that resistance training should not begin until the patient has been in a cardiac rehab program for at least 3 weeks and is at least 5 weeks post-MI or 8 weeks post-CABG.[110] Some guidelines for resistance training include the following: (1) exercising large muscle groups before small; (2) stressing exhalation with exertion; (3) avoiding a sustained, tight grip; (4) focusing on RPE 11 to 13; (5) using slow, controlled movements; and (6) stopping exercise with any warning of concerning or uncomfortable signs or symptoms.[110] The American Heart Association (AHA), American College of Sports Medicine (ACSM), and AACVPR all advocate the importance of muscular fitness for the patient with cardiac impairment and support the inclusion of resistance training into the patient's exercise program.[106,110-112]

Intervention for Patients with Congestive Heart Failure

The APTA *Guide to Physical Therapist Practice* includes management of patients with CHF under the category of Impaired Aerobic Capacity and Endurance Associated with Cardiovascular Pump Dysfunction or Failure, Pattern 6-D.[26] The development of specific anticipated goals and expected outcomes for the patient with CHF is based on the general goals of physical therapy intervention presented in Box 13.6.

Exercise Prescription

Exercise programs for patients with CHF are relatively recent. Patients whose cardiac status was once thought to be too fragile to participate in organized exercise are now not only participating, but exercise is recommended as an integral component of their medical management.[113-116] Studies have shown that patients with heart failure can exercise safely, and regular exercise may improve functional status, quality of life, and exercise capacity, and decrease symptoms.[117-123]

The safety and importance of strength training and peripheral adaptations have also been studied.[124,125] Using a multidisciplinary approach that includes a thorough physical examination before each exercise session with a review of symptoms and medications, low-level exercise may begin if the patient is hemodynamically stable. CHF is a multisystem disease that affects not just the heart but peripheral muscle and arteries as well. Studies have demonstrated muscle fiber atrophy of skeletal and respiratory muscle, as well as an alteration in arterial vasodilation capacity. Exercise has been shown to limit some of these adverse changes; therefore, an exercise program should consider not only systemic conditioning, but also peripheral endurance training, low-level resistance training, and respiratory muscle training.[126-128] Exercise training can be initiated when

---

Box 13.6 Congestive Heart Failure—Anticipated Goals and Expected Outcomes

- Physiological response to increased oxygen demand is improved.
- Self-management of symptoms is improved.
- Ability to perform physical tasks is increased.
- Behaviors that foster healthy habits, wellness, and prevention are acquired.
- Disability associated with acute or chronic illness is reduced.
- Risk of secondary impairments is reduced.
- Awareness and use of community resources is improved.
- Performance of and independence in ADL is increased.

ADL = activities of daily living.

the patient is in compensated CHF. Box 13.7 provides the relative criteria for initiation and relative criteria for modification and termination of exercise in patients with heart failure.

Aerobic Exercise

There is no paucity of research indicating that aerobic exercise is beneficial for patients with CHF. Exercise prescription must keep intensity low and gradually increase duration as the patient tolerates. In general, aerobic exercise training may include low-impact exercise with gradual progression of intensity, frequency, and duration. Intensity should be monitored through the use of the dyspnea or perceived exertion scales and should be kept to a rating of fairly light. HR cannot be relied on for evaluating intensity due to the effects of various medications, including beta-blockers. It is also important to note that in the normal heart, an increase in HR is accompanied by an increase in inotropy. In the failing heart, an increase in HR may actually result in a decrease in force; this is known as the *negative treppe effect.*[129]

Monitoring BP response is crucial to determine if CO is being maintained during aerobic exercise. A drop in BP during aerobic exercise signifies the inability of the heart to maintain CO during exercise. For these patients, therapists may chose to reduce the aerobic component and focus more on strength training to achieve peripheral adaptations as opposed to central adaptations. By strength training the peripheral muscles, therapists can increase the number of mitochondria and utilization of blood and oxygen at the level of the muscle, thereby enabling the muscle to make more energy to sustain activity without putting excessive stress on the heart.

Two important studies depict the benefits of exercise training in patients with heart failure. A meta-analysis conducted by van Tol et al[130] in 2006 investigated 35 original randomized crossover trials of patients with systolic heart failure.[130] The average exercise within these studies included aerobic exercise 3 times/week for 60 minutes/session for 12 weeks. The investigators found an increase in 6-minute walk distance with an effect size of 46.2 m, within 15 studies including 599 patients. In 31 studies with approximately 1,240 patients, maximum oxygen uptake was found to increase after exercise with an effect size of 2.06 mL/kg/min. The researchers also found improvements in the resting diastolic BP, resting CO, and resting HR values following exercise. Finally, patients were able to demonstrate an increase in the LVEF and tolerate greater intensity following the 12 weeks of exercise. A systematic review published by Smart and Marwick[131] investigated 81 studies involving 2,387 exercising subjects with 1,197 patients enrolled in controlled studies and included 60,000 patient hours of exercise training. Mean number of subjects was 30 ± 25; mean age was 59 ± 7 years, and mean EF was $27\% \pm 7\%$. The investigators reported that studies utilizing aerobic exercise training ($n = 40$) demonstrated $VO_{2\,max}$ increase of 16.5%. In addition, studies utilizing strength training alone ($n = 3$) demonstrated $VO_{2\,max}$ increase of 9.3%, and studies that combined aerobic and strength programs ($n = 30$) demonstrated $VO_{2\,max}$ increase of 15%. Clinically, this could mean that an individual with a $VO_{2\,max}$ of 15 mL/kg/min could increase to 17.4 mL/kg/min, which is an approximately .68 MET increase and could lead to sustained walking on a level surface. Box 13.8 Evidence Summary presents related research investigating the effects of exercise in patients with heart failure.[132-141]

Strength Training

Strength training is a crucial component of the exercise plan for patients with heart failure to help improve peripheral muscle strength and endurance. Inclusion of light resistance work has been shown to be safe in this population.[142] Modalities for resistance training may include elastic bands for mild UE and LE resistance work or light weights. A review by Braith and Beck[143] provides clinicians with the benefits of resistance training in helping to improve skeletal muscle morphology and provides clinical guidelines for prescription of resistance exercise. Box 13.9 delineates recommendations for resistance exercise in patients with heart failure.

Ventilatory Muscle Training

Breathing exercises[144,145] and inspiratory muscle training[146,147] have been shown to be beneficial in patients with heart failure. Diaphragmatic breathing may help reduce excessive accessory muscle use and reduce the work of breathing. Pursed-lip breathing has been shown to

---

Box 13.7 Criteria for Modification or Termination of Exercise in Patients with Heart Failure

- Marked dyspnea or fatigue
- RR > 40 breaths/min
- Development of S_3 heart sound
- Increase in pulmonary crackles
- Decrease in HR or BP of > 10 bpm or mm Hg respectively during steady state or progressive exercise
- Increase in the CVP by 10 mm of Hg
- Diaphoresis, pallor, or confusion

Criteria for Initiation of Exercise

- Compensated CHF
- Able to speak comfortably without signs of dyspnea with RR < 30 breaths/min
- Less than moderate fatigue
- CI > 2.0 L/min
- CVP < 10 mm Hg
- Crackles in less than one half of the lungs
- Resting heart rate < 120 bpm

Box 13.8 Evidence Summary   Studies Investigating the Effects of Exercise on Patients with Congestive Heart Failure

First Author (Reference)	Design	Controls (n)	Exercise	Training Time, Frequency, Duration	Intensity and of Training	Change in Oxygen Consumption
Adamopoulos[132]	Crossover	20	24	30 min, 5 sessions/wk, 12 wk	60%–80% maximum heart rate; aerobic	15%
Barlow[133]	Longitudinal		23	60 min, 3 sessions/wk, 16 wk	50% of 1 repetition max; 90% anaerobic threshold; aerobic + strength	3%
Delagardelle[134]	Longitudinal		20	40 min, 3 sessions/wk, 12 wk	50%–75% max oxygen consumption; 60% of 1 repetition max	0% strength; 8% aerobic
Harris[135]	Longitudinal		24	30 min, 5 sessions/wk, 6 wk	70% maximum heart rate; aerobic	4%
Kemppainen[136]	Controlled nonrandomized	7	9	45 min, 3 sessions/wk, 20 wk	70% max oxygen consumption; aerobic + strength	27%
Stolen[137]	Controlled nonrandomized	11	9	45 min, 3 sessions/wk, 20 wk	50%–70% max oxygen consumption; aerobic + strength	27%
Malfatto[138]	Controlled nonrandomized	15	30	60 min, 5 sessions/wk, 12 wk	40%–50% max oxygen consumption; aerobic	18%
Radzewitz[139]	Longitudinal	88		25 min, 3 sessions/wk, 4 wk	60%–80% max oxygen consumption; aerobic + strength	11%
Santoro[140]	Longitudinal	6		90 min, 3 sessions/wk, 16 wk	50%–60% max oxygen consumption; 50% of 1 repetition max; aerobic + strength	18%
Vibarel[141]	Longitudinal		10	46 min, 3 sessions/wk, 8 wk	70%–80% max oxygen consumption; aerobic	22%

promote the positive end-expiratory pressure not only in patients with COPD but also in patients with CHF.[144] Pursed-lip breathing is also beneficial in helping slow down the respiratory rate in patients with heart failure.[145]

Patients with heart failure are known to have poor ventilatory muscle strength.[148] Strength of the ventilator muscles can be enhanced through use of a device known as a threshold inspiratory muscle trainer. Improvements in the maximal inspiratory pressure are achieved by having the patient breathe with this device, which resists

inspiration, thereby strengthening the inspiratory muscles. A general protocol is to use the threshold inspiratory muscle trainer at 20% of the maximal inspiratory pressure, to be used 3 times per day for 5 to 15 minutes at each session.[9]

Activity Pacing and Energy Conservation Techniques

Patients with heart failure require activity pacing and energy conservation techniques to decrease the workload

Box 13.9 Resistance Training Recommendations for Patients with CHF

	NYHA Class I	NYHA Class II–III
Frequency	2–3 days/wk	1–2 days/wk
Duration	15–30 min	12–15 min
Intensity	50%–60%, 1 RM*	40%–50%, 1 RM*
Sets	2–3	1–2
Reps	6–15	4–10

*1 RM = 1 repetition maximum.

on the heart. A few techniques that may be beneficial for patients include the following:

- Recommending frequent rest intervals before they get tired.
- Participate in activities that require greater energy costs at times of the day when they have the most energy.
- Plan ahead to decide activities that possibly may be avoided and delegated to others.
- Alternate easy and difficult tasks with rest intervals.
- Adjust the environment to make tasks easier and sit when feasible while doing strenuous activity.

■ EDUCATION FOR PATIENTS WITH HEART DISEASE

For patients with heart disease, patient and family education develops along a continuum, depending on the patient's baseline status and readiness to attend to the information. The physical therapist, along with other members of the health care team, must determine the patient's and family's ability to understand and adhere to the information. Appropriate discharge or ongoing outpatient topics to be addressed include the following.

1. *Activity Guidelines.* Patients (and family) need to be able to understand specific activity guidelines, which include planned exercise sessions as well as leisure time and rests.

2. *Self-Monitoring.* Patients may monitor the intensity of their activity in a variety of ways; two of the more common ways are palpating a pulse and RPE. Because many older patients have decreased sensitivity in their palpation skills, the use of RPE may be easier and more reliable. Those patients who are able to take a pulse or choose to invest in an HR monitor may prefer to use those methods. Self-monitoring not only involves HR or RPE, but awareness of other symptoms or signs that may suggest exercise intolerance, such as lightheadedness, mental confusion, dyspnea, and inability to carry on a brief conversation while performing an activity. Patients with CHF commonly use the dyspnea scale and the Borg RPE Scale.

3. *Symptom Recognition and Response.* Being able to recognize their specific cardiac symptoms and to know how to respond is a key component in patient education. Patients should have written information regarding the action they should take when symptoms occur, for example, when to call their physician or go to the hospital. Angina is the most common symptom associated with coronary heart disease, whereas weight gain (2 lb over 1 to 2 days), dyspnea, LE edema, and increased pillows for sleep are common signs and symptoms for CHF.

4. *Nutrition.* Patients commonly meet with a nutritionist to discuss their usual dietary habits and to make recommendations when needed for a more heart-healthy diet. Most commonly, patients with heart disease are instructed to reduce fat intake; patients with CHF are instructed to monitor salt and fluid intake.

5. *Medications.* Patients receive written information regarding the desired action of their medications, potential side effects, dosage, and timing of medications. Patients should also know which nonprescription drugs such as cold, sinus, allergy, or anti-inflammatory medications they should avoid because of possible interactions with prescription drugs. Patients should also be encouraged to disclose all herbal remedies and supplements that they may be taking.

6. *Lifestyle Issues.* Many factors influence whether a patient will return to work after a cardiac event. Many patients with CAD return to work if they were employed before their event; patients with CHF are, in general, an older population when compared to patients with CAD and therefore may have already retired.

   Resumption of sexual activity may be an uncomfortable discussion for some patients. There may be many issues of concern for the patient (e.g., fear, anxiety, performance concerns, lack of libido). Patients and their partners are encouraged to verbalize their concerns to each other and to seek appropriate information from their health care team. Some medications (e.g., beta-blockers) may blunt the sexual response, and it is important that patients communicate this with their physician. Often, another medication or category of medication may be better tolerated. When patients feel ready for sex, their energy level throughout the day is satisfying for them, and they are able to walk outdoors and climb stairs comfortably, they are probably ready for sexual activity. It may be helpful for patients to remember that sexual activity is not unlike other physical activity with respect to energy cost, and therefore planning, pacing, and warm-up are powerful contributors for a more comfortable outcome. In some cases, the physician may recommend taking prophylactic NTG before sexual activity.

7. See Box 13.10 *Suggested Topics for Patient, Family, and Caregiver Education and Counseling* from the U.S.

Box 13.10 Suggested Topics for Patient, Family, and Caregiver Education and Counseling

General Counseling

- Explanation of heart failure and the reason for symptoms
- Cause or probable cause of heart failure
- Expected symptoms
- Symptoms of worsening heart failure
- What to do if symptoms worsen
- Self-monitoring with daily weights
- Explanation of treatment/care plan
- Clarification of patient's responsibilities
- Importance of cessation of tobacco use
- Role of family members or other caregivers in the treatment/care plan
- Availability and value of qualified local support group
- Importance of obtaining vaccinations against influenza and pneumococcal disease

Prognosis

- Life expectancy
- Advance directives
- Advice for family members in the event of sudden death

Activity Recommendations

- Recreation, leisure, and work activity
- Exercise
- Sex, sexual difficulties, and coping strategies

Dietary Recommendations

- Sodium restriction
- Avoidance of excessive fluid intake
- Fluid restriction (if required)
- Alcohol restriction

Medications

- Effects of medications on quality of life and survival
- Dosing
- Likely side effects and what to do if they occur
- Coping mechanisms for complicated medical regimens
- Availability of lower-cost medications or financial assistance

Importance of Compliance with the Treatment Care Plan

From Clinical Practice Guidelines, Number 11, Heart Failure: Evaluation and Care of Patients with Left-Ventricular Systolic Dysfunction, AHCPR Publication No. 94-0612, p 42, with permission.

Department of Health and Human Services Clinical Practice Guidelines for Patients with CHF.[149]

■ PSYCHOLOGICAL/SOCIAL ISSUES

Cardiac disease may not only create new emotional issues but also enhance some that might have existed before the cardiac event. Reassure patients that many of these issues are normal sequelae of their event. Encourage them to seek guidance and counseling in whatever arena they feel appropriate (e.g., health care, counseling, religion).

Many studies have addressed the relationship of emotional depression following CABG.[150-152] Although depression is reported to exist, there is difficulty in objectively measuring the direct impact of CABG on subsequent depression. Some of the difficulty arises in the use of depression scales (Beck or CES-D), grading criteria, the presurgical emotional status, and gender. Burg et al[150,151] reported two studies in 2003 in which 89 men were followed preoperatively and up to 2 years following surgery. They found that presurgical depression was an independent predictor of postoperative prolonged surgical pain and failure to return to previous activity. In a study by Blumenthal et al,[152] 817 patients were studied preoperatively, up to a mean of 5.2 years postoperatively. They reported that patients with moderate to severe depression at baseline (preoperatively) that persisted postoperatively had an increased death rate compared to the nondepressed patients.[152] Ai et al[153] reported that the presence of preoperative co-morbidities strongly influenced whether depression existed. McKhann et al,[154] in their study of 124 patients, concluded that the majority of patients depressed after surgery were in fact depressed before surgery. Pirraglia et al[155] reported on 237 patients and noted that 43% were classified as depressed preoperatively and only 23% postoperatively. Factors that influenced postsurgical scores were length of ICU stay and the amount of reported social support.[155] The decrease in postoperative depression compared to preoperatively was supported by Lindquist et al[156] in 2003; they studied more than 650 men and women and found less anxiety and depression following surgery than preoperatively. Of interest, they also noted that women's report of quality of life (QOL) was lower than men's up to 1 year following surgery. Westin et al[157] also reported a gender difference in CABG outcomes in regard to depression and QOL measures. In their study of more than 300 patients, women scored lower on the QOL and higher on depression scale than men at 1 month and 1 year following CABG, compared to men.[157] Phillips et al[158] reported women to be at greater risk for both cognitive difficulties and anxiety than men at 1-year postoperative CABG than men. The physical therapist, therefore, needs to be aware that depression may exist following surgery and, as a member of the health care team, assist in directing appropriate care and support for the patient.

PRIMARY PREVENTION OF CORONARY ARTERY DISEASE

Patients who do not have documented CAD but who have identifiable risk factors should be encouraged to adopt lifestyle behaviors that can modify their risk factors. Health education and primary prevention programs through individualized education and exercise guidelines attempt to modify an individual's risk factors and thereby prevent CAD.

Patients are instructed in appropriate dietary guidelines, including low fat, adequate fiber, minerals and vitamins, and decreased salt, particularly if the patient has high BP. Besides lowering total dietary fat, patients are instructed to decrease their percentage of saturated fats and avoid trans fatty acids. Elevated levels of the amino acid homocysteine appear to increase the risk of arterial endothelial disease. Folic acid, a B vitamin, lowers homocysteine levels. If weight loss is needed, patients are encouraged to see a nutritionist to design a sensible eating plan. Patients are encouraged to gradually increase their endurance activity, such as walking toward a goal of 30 to 40 minutes (not including warm-up and cool-down) four times a week. The *American College of Sports Medicine* and the *American Heart Association* recommend that anyone over age 40 with two or more risk factors should have an ETT before beginning an aerobic or strengthening exercise program. The purpose of the ETT is to identify the presence of any latent ischemia.

If no ischemia is present, a typical aerobic exercise prescription might be as follows:

- Intensity: 70% to 85% of HR_{max} as the aerobic training zone
- Duration: 30 to 40 minutes in the aerobic training zone; appropriate warm-up of 5 to 10 minutes, and cool-down
- Frequency: three to four times per week

Maximum HR may be estimated by subtracting the person's age from 220; this, however, is not an exact science for any individual and cannot be accurate if the person is on any cardiac medications, such as beta-blockers, that may decrease the maximum HR. Supplemental resistance work is also encouraged at moderate intensities, with initial monitoring of HR and BP.

Modification of the other CAD risk factors is also key to the success of any primary prevention intervention. Patients are encouraged to identify risk factors and to seek resources to assist in modifying them. There are many community-based smoking cessation programs or medically supervised programs that a patient might explore. Stress management programs are also varied and can be adapted to the individual's needs. Proper and consistent use of any medications that might be used in controlling risk factors, such as antihypertensives, antihypercholesterolemias, blood glucose–lowering agents (hypoglycemics), and antianxiety agents or antidepressants, is crucial to the success of any program.

HTN, as the most prevalent CVD in the United States, is one of the most powerful contributors to cardiovascular morbidity and mortality. The Joint National Committee on Prevention, Detection, Evaluation, and Treatment of High Blood Pressure recommends a multifactorial approach and suggests that lifestyle modifications, including weight reduction, physical activity, and moderation of dietary sodium, are recommended as either definitive or adjunctive therapy for HTN.[24]

SUMMARY

Physical activity is important for all individuals and is especially beneficial for those individuals already diagnosed with CAD and CHF. Individuals with heart disease should understand that a consistent exercise program is part of the management for their disease and is as necessary as their medications. Having heart disease means that the person needs to understand the parameters in which he or she may safely participate in activity either recreationally or as a prescribed exercise. The role of the physical therapist is to provide a safe exercise prescription for all patients.

During the time of illness, the effects of decreased activity can be devastating. A paradox exists, however, in that the less activity that is done, the less activity can be done as a result of a decreased work capacity. Therefore, the relative energy cost of all activity increases, and the heart actually works harder for any given task. Not encouraging the patient to resume activity when he or she is medically stable is a disservice. As physical therapists, our role is clear: to understand the pathophysiology of the disease process, to accurately examine the patient, and to establish a safe POC. The ultimate goal is to improve the patient's physiological response to activity and, in doing so, decrease the work of the cardiovascular system.

Questions for Review

1. Discuss key differences between an NSTEMI and an STEMI.

2. Discuss three different types of angina. How would you instruct your patient in symptom recognition? Delineate the physical therapy management if a patient has angina during a treatment session.

3. Discuss sternal precautions that you would instruct your patient to use following a median sternotomy procedure.

4. Discuss differences between compensated and uncompensated CHF.

5. Discuss the physical therapy implications when managing patients with pacemakers.

6. Discuss appropriate goals, education, and treatment interventions for patients with acute coronary syndrome in Phase I cardiac rehabilitation.

7. Discuss appropriate goals and treatment guidelines for patients with CHF.

8. Delineate the adaptation that may be noted following an aerobic training exercise program in patients with heart failure.

CASE STUDY

A 58-year-old man presents to the local emergency department (ER) with chief complaint of SOB and difficulty sleeping last night; patient had to sit up all night to make symptoms even a little better. Patient came to the ER because he was unable to get ready for work owing to increased SOB. Patient reports that he has felt SOB off and on for a couple of months, usually associated with physical activity; symptoms, however, usually resolved with rest. Today's episode was the first related to sleeping.

PAST MEDICAL HISTORY
- Coronary artery disease: anterior MI 4 years ago
- Hypercholesterolemia
- Peripheral vascular disease

MEDICATIONS
- Digoxin, captopril, furosemide (Lasix), diltiazem, simvastatin (Zocor)

FAMILY/SOCIAL
- Patient works full-time as an engineer; travels 3 to 4 days per month.
- Married, lives with his wife in a two-story home on a 2-acre lot; three college-aged children.
- Patient is an avid golfer; enjoys gardening and landscaping.

PHYSICAL EXAMINATION
- Heart sounds: S_1, S_2 normal; S_3 present, no S_4; 2/6 systolic murmur
- Lung sounds: crackles 1/3 way
- Rhythm/rate: irregular, 140 bpm
- Blood pressure: 100/60 mm Hg
- Respiratory rate: 26 breaths/min
- SaO_2:90%
- Jugular venous distention: 5 cm
- Echocardiogram: akinetic apex, akinetic distal septum and anterior wall; dilated atria and LV
- Chest x-ray: unavailable

LABORATORY DATA
- Enzyme pending; CBC WNL except BUN and creatinine slightly elevated.
- BNP: 900 pg/mL.
- Patient remained in the hospital for 2 days while medications were adjusted. During this time patient underwent further testing, including an ETT.

RESULTS OF ETT
- Bruce protocol: 4 minutes; estimated VO_2 max; 20 mL O_2/kg/min (approximately 6 METs); max VS: 130 bpm HR; 120/60 mm Hg BP
- ECG: (–) negative for ischemia, chest pain
- Reason for stopping: absolute exhaustion

- Examination immediately post-ETT: (+) S_3
- Physical and occupational therapy were requested to assist with exercise guidelines and discharge planning

PATIENT'S GOALS

- Return to work.
- Resume hiking.
- Begin to prepare his garden for spring planting within the next 5 weeks.

PHYSICAL THERAPY INTERVENTION

- Exercise tolerance via low-level exercises sitting and standing, as well as 5-minute walk.

Vital Signs

- Sitting (rest): HR 90 bpm; BP 110/60 mm Hg
- Sitting exercises: HR 108 bpm; BP 110/60 mm Hg
- Standing (rest): HR 110 bpm; BP 108/60 mm Hg
- Standing exercise: HR 116 bpm: BP 110/60 mm Hg
- 5-minute walk: 1000 ft; HR 120 bpm; BP 116/60 mm Hg

HOME INSTRUCTIONS

- Meetings planned with patient and his family to discuss discharge guidelines over the next 4 to 8 weeks.

FOLLOW-UP

- Patient returns to his primary care provider 3 months after discharge. Echocardiogram is unchanged with EF 30%. Patient states that he has been following discharge guidelines.

Vital Signs

- HR 100 bpm; BP 116/70 mm Hg (resting).
- Patient states that he feels great and just wants to get on with his life.

GUIDING QUESTIONS

1. What is a reasonable presenting diagnosis? Identify each piece of information (and how you interpreted it) that you used to make this diagnosis.

2. Explain the pathophysiology of the patient's presenting symptoms. Discuss the significance of his HR and heart rhythm in relation to his symptoms.

3. If the patient's symptoms and signs worsened, and he was admitted to the coronary care unit (CCU),

   a. What do you think his Swan-Ganz reading could reasonably look like?

   b. What would you expect these signs/symptoms would be that would bring the patient to the CCU?

   c. What might be a reasonable cause of his signs/symptoms worsening?

   d. What other drugs/interventions might be given in the CCU?

4. What rhythm do you think the patient is in and why? What do you think might be a reason that he is in this rhythm?

5. What do you think the chest x-ray would look like and why?

6. What is your interpretation of the patient's vital sign response to PT intervention? What is your plan for your next session?

7. What exercise prescription would you recommend for the patient at home (modality, intensity, duration, frequency)?

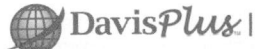 DavisPlus | For additional resources, including answers to the questions for review and case study guiding questions, please visit **http://davisplus.fadavis.com**

For this chapter, see also:
Web-Based Resources for Clinicians, Families, and Patients with Heart Disease in Appendix A p. 1446.

References

1. Roger, VL, et al: Executive summary: Heart disease and stroke statistics—2011 update: A report from the American Heart Association. Circulation 123:e18–e209, 2011.
2. Xu, J, et al: Deaths: Final data for 2007. Natl Vital Stat Rep 58: 1–135, 2010.
3. National Center for Health Statistics. Health Data Interactive. Retrieved August 20, 2011, from www.cdc.gov/nchs/hdi.htm.
4. Barnett, E, et al: Men and Heart Disease: An Atlas of Racial and Ethnic Disparities in Mortality, ed 1. Office of Social Environment and Health Research, Morgantown, WV, 2001.
5. Gray, H, Williams, PL, and Bannister, LH: Gray's Anatomy: The Anatomical Basis of Medicine and Surgery, ed 38. Churchill Livingstone, New York, 1995.
6. Frownfelter, D, and Dean, E: Cardiovascular and Pulmonary Physical Therapy: Evidence and Practice, ed 4. Mosby–Elsevier, St. Louis, 2006.
7. DeTurk, W, and Cahalin, L: Cardiovascular and Pulmonary Physical Therapy: An Evidence-Based Approach, ed 2. McGraw-Hill, New York, 2010.
8. Guyton, AC, and Hall, JE: Textbook of Medical Physiology, ed 11. Elsevier, Philadelphia, 2006.
9. Hillegass, E: Essentials of Cardiopulmonary Physical Therapy, ed 3. Elsevier, St. Louis, 2011.
10. Fuster, V, Walsh, R, and Harrington, R: Hurst's the Heart, ed 13. McGraw-Hill, New York, 2011.
11. Bonow, R, et al: Braunwald's Heart Disease: A Textbook of Cardiovascular Medicine, ed 9. Elsevier, Philadelphia, 2012.
12. Hungerford, J, and Little, C: Developmental biology of the vascular smooth muscle cell: Building a multilayered vessel wall. J Vasc Res 36:1, 1999.
13. Berne, RM, and Levy, MN: Cardiovascular Physiology, ed 9. Elsevier, St. Louis, 2007.
14. Fox, S: Human Physiology, ed 11. McGraw-Hill, Boston, 2009.
15. ACSM's Guidelines for Exercise Testing and Prescription, ed 8. Lippincott Williams & Wilkins, Philadelphia, 2010.
16. Braunwald, E, et al: Heart Disease: A Textbook of Cardiovascular Medicine, ed 8. Elsevier, Philadelphia, 2008.
17. Ganong, WF: Review of Medical Physiology, ed 21. McGraw-Hill, New York, 2003.
18. Lentner, C (ed): Geigy Scientific Tables, ed 8. Ciba Geigy, Basel, Switzerland, 1981.
19. Phillips, RE, and Feeney, MK: The Cardiac Rhythms, ed 3. WB Saunders, Philadelphia, 1990, p 44.
20. Hellerstein, HK, et al: Principles of exercise prescription. In Naughton, JP (ed): Exercise Testing and Exercise Training in Coronary Heart Disease. Academic, New York, 1973, p 147.
21. Naughton, J, and Haider, R: Methods of exercise testing. In Naughton, JP, and Hellerstein, HK (eds): Exercise Testing and Exercise Training in Coronary Heart Disease. Academic, New York, 1973, p 80.
22. Fryar, CD, et al: Hypertension, high serum total cholesterol, and diabetes: Racial and ethnic prevalence differences in U.S. adults, 1999–2006. NCHS Data Brief, pp 1–8, 2010.
23. Hertz, RP, et al: Racial disparities in hypertension prevalence, awareness and management. Arch Intern Med 165:2098–2104, 2005.
24. Chobanian, AV, et al: US Department of Health and Human Services: The Seventh Report of the Joint National Committee on Prevention, Detection, Evaluation, and Treatment of High Blood Pressure. NIH Publication No. 03-5233. National Institutes of Health, National Heart, Lung, and Blood Institute, 2003.
25. Kannel, WB, et al: Epidemiological assessment of the role of blood pressure in stroke. JAMA 276:1269, 1996.
26. American Physical Therapy Association: Guide to Physical Therapist Practice, ed 2. Phys Ther 81(1):471, 2001.
27. Kannel, WB, et al: Factors of risk in the development of coronary heart disease—six-year follow-up experience. The Framingham Study. Ann Intern Med 55:33, 1961.
28. Kannel, WB, Castelli, WP, and Gordon, T: Cholesterol in the prediction of atherosclerotic disease. New perspectives based on the Framingham study. Ann Intern Med 90(1):85, 1979.
29. Wilson, PW: Established risk factors and coronary artery disease, the Framingham Study. Am J Hypertens 7(7 pt 2):7S, 1994.
30. Grundy, SM, et al: Assessment of cardiovascular risk by use of multiple-risk-factor assessment equations: A statement for health care professionals from the American Heart Association and the American College of Cardiology. Circulation 100(13):1481, 1999.
31. Berry, C, Tardif, JC, and Bourassa, MG: Coronary heart disease in patients with diabetes. I. Recent advances in prevention and noninvasive management. J Am Coll Cardiol 49:631–642, 2007.
32. Moore, K, and Dalley, A: Clinically Oriented Anatomy, ed 5. Lippincott Williams & Wilkins, Baltimore, 2006.
33. Huether, S, and McCance, K: Understanding Pathophysiology, ed 3. Elsevier, St. Louis, 2004.
34. Pandey, S: A review on pathology of myocardial ischemia and various types of novel biomarkers. Int J Pharm Sci Rev Res 2:1, 2010.
35. Ross, R: Atherosclerosis—an inflammatory disease. N Engl J Med 340:115–126, 1999.
36. Cahalin, LP, LaPier, TK, and Shaw, DK: Sternal precautions: Is it time for change? Precautions versus restrictions—a review of the literature and recommendations for revision. Cardiopulm Phys Ther J 22(1):5–13, 2011.
37. El-Ansary, D, Waddington, G, and Adams, R: Measurement of non-physiological movement in sternal instability by ultrasound. Ann Thorac Surg 83:1513–1517, 2007.
38. Irion, G, et al: Effects of upper extremity movement on sternal skin stress. Acute Care Perspectives 15:3–6, 2006.
39. El-Ansary, D, Waddington, G, and Adams, R: Relationship between pain and upper limb movement in patients with chronic sternal instability following cardiac surgery. Physiother Theory Pract 23(5):273–280, 2007.
40. Bahrami, H, et al: Differences in the incidence of congestive heart failure by ethnicity: The multi-ethnic study of atherosclerosis. Arch Intern Med 168:2138–2145, 2008.
41. Swedberg, K, et al: Guidelines for the diagnosis and treatment of chronic heart failure: Executive summary (update 2005): The Task Force for the Diagnosis and Treatment of Chronic Heart Failure of the European Society of Cardiology. Eur Heart J 26:1115, 2005.
42. Lev, D, et al: Long term trends in the incidence of and survival with heart failure. N Engl J Med 347:1397, 2002.
43. Loehr, LR, et al: Heart failure incidence and survival (from the Atherosclerosis Risk in Communities study). Am J Cardiol 101: 1016–1022, 2008.
44. Chatterjee, K, and Massie, B: Systolic and diastolic heart failure: Differences and similarities. J Cardiac Fail 13:569–576, 2007.
45. Parish, TR, Kosma, M, and Welsh, M: Exercise training for the patient with heart failure: Is your patient ready? J Cardiopulm Phys Ther 18(3):12, 2007.
46. Watchie, J: Cardiovascular and Pulmonary Physical Therapy— A Clinical Manual, ed 2. Saunders Elsevier, St. Louis, 2010.
47. Goodman, CC, Boissenault, WG, and Fuller, KS: Pathology: Implications for the Physical Therapist, ed 3. Elsevier, St. Louis, 2009.
48. Cahalin, LP: Heart failure. Phys Ther 76:516–533, 1996.
49. Cahalin, LP: Physiotherapy for the disablement of heart failure— part II. Physiother Singapore 3:31–38, 2000.
50. Mitchell, SH, et al: Oxygen cost of exercise is increased in heart failure after accounting for recovery costs. Chest 124:572–579, 2003.
51. Piña, et al: Exercise and heart failure: A statement from the American Heart Association Committee on Exercise, Rehabilitation, and Prevention. Circulation 107:1210–1225, 2003.
52. Warburton, DER, and Mathur, S. Skeletal muscle training in people with chronic heart failure or chronic obstructive pulmonary disease. Physiother Can 56(3):143–157, 2004.
53. Lipkin, DP, et al: Abnormalities of skeletal muscle in patients with chronic heart failure. Int J Cardiol 18(2):187, 1988.
54. Poole-Wilson, PA, Buller, NP, and Lipkin, DP: Regional blood flow, muscle strength and skeletal muscle histology in severe congestive heart failure. Am J Cardiol 62(8):49E–52E, 1988.
55. Bickley, L: Peripheral vascular system. In Bickley, L (ed): Bates' Guide to Physical Examination and History Taking, ed 8. Lippincott, Philadelphia, 2003.
56. Jarvis, C: Physical Examination and Health Assessment, ed 3. WB Saunders, Philadelphia, 2004.

57. Schlant, RC, and Sonnenblick, EH: Pathophysiology of heart failure. In Alexander, RW, Schlant, RC, and Fuster, V (eds): Hurst's the Heart, ed 9. McGraw-Hill, New York, 1998.

58. Atsumi, H, et al: Cardiac sympathetic nervous disintegrity is related to exercise intolerance in patients with chronic heart failure. Nucl Med Commun 19:451, 1998.

59. Linjiing, X, et al: Effect of heart failure on muscle capillary geometry: Implications for O_2 exchange. Med Sci Sports Exerc 30:1230, 1998.

60. Lunde, PK, et al: Skeletal muscle fatigue in normal subjects and heart failure patients: Is there a common mechanism? Acta Physiol Scand 162:215, 1998.

61. Vescovo, G, et al: Apoptosis in the skeletal muscle of patients with heart failure: Investigation of clinical and biochemical changes. Heart 84(4):431, 2000.

62. Rocca, HPBL, et al: Oxygen uptake kinetics during low level exercise in patients with heart failure: Relation to neurohormones, peak oxygen consumption, and clinical findings. Heart 81:121, 1999.

63. Bank, AJ: Effects of short-term forearm exercise training on resistance vessel endothelial function in normal subjects and patients with heart failure. J Card Fail 4:193, 1998.

64. Genth-Zotz, S, et al: Changes of neurohumoral parameters and endothelin-1 in response to exercise in patients with mild to moderate congestive heart failure. Int J Cardiol 30:137, 1998.

65. Yan, AT, Bradley, TD, and Liu, PP: The role of continuous positive airway pressure in the treatment of congestive heart failure. Chest 120(5):167, 2001.

66. Mansfield, DR, et al: Controlled trial of continuous positive airway pressure in obstructive sleep apnea and heart failure. Am J Respir Crit Care Med 169(3):361, 2004.

67. Januzzi, JL, Jr: Natriuretic peptide testing: A window into the diagnosis and prognosis of heart failure. Cleve Clin J Med 73(2):149–152, 155–157, 2006.

68. Norman, JF, et al: Relationship of resting B-type natriuretic peptide level to total cardiac work and total physical work capacity in heart failure patients. J Cardiopulm Rehabil Prev 29:310–313, 2009.

69. Felker, MG, et al: N-terminal pro-brain natriuretic peptide and exercise capacity in chronic heart failure: Data from the Heart Failure and a Controlled Trial Investigating Outcomes of Exercise Training (HF-ACTION) study. Am Heart J 158(4):S37–S44, 2009.

70. Avezum, A, et al: Beta-blocker therapy for congestive heart failure: A systemic overview and critical appraisal of the published trials. Can J Cardiol 14:1045, 1998.

71. Cleland, JG, et al: Beta-blockers for chronic heart failure: From prejudice to enlightenment. J Cardiovasc Pharmacol 32:S36, 1998.

72. Ciccone, CD: Current trends in cardiovascular pharmacology. (Special series: Cardiopulmonary Physical Therapy.) APTA 1:1–22, 1996.

73. Salukhe, TV, Dimopoulos, K, and Francis, D: Cardiac resynchronization may reduce all-cause mortality: Meta analysis of preliminary COMPANION data with CONTAK-CD, InSync ICD, MIRACLE and MUSTIC. Int J Cardiol 93(2-3):101, 2004.

74. Paz, JC, and West, MP: Acute Care Handbook for Physical Therapists, ed 3. Butterworth & Heinemann, Boston, 2009.

75. Plowman, SA, and Smith, DL: Exercise Physiology for Health, Fitness and Performance, ed 3. Lippincott Williams & Wilkins, 2011.

76. Watchie, J: Cardiovascular and Pulmonary Physical Therapy, ed 2. Saunders Elsevier, St. Louis, 2010.

77. Dubin, D: Rapid Interpretation of EKG's, ed 6. Cover Publishing, Tampa, FL, 1996.

78. Jones, SA: ECG Success: Exercises in ECG interpretation. FA Davis, Philadelphia, 2008.

79. Brugada, P, et al: A new approach to the differential diagnosis of a regular tachycardia with a wide QRS complex. Circulation 83(5):1649, 1991.

80. ACC/AHA/NASPE 2002 guideline update for implantation of cardiac pacemakers and antiarrhythmia devices: Summary article. Circulation 106:2145–2161, 2002.

81. Mallela, VS, et al: Trends in cardiac pacemaker batteries. Ind Pacing Electrophysiol J 4(4):201–212, 2004.

82. Martinez, C, et al: Pacemakers and defibrillators: Recent and ongoing studies that impact the elderly. Am J Geriatr Cardiol 15(2):82–87, 2006.

83. West, M, Johnson, T, and Roberts, SO: Pacemakers and implantable cardioverter defibrillators. In American College of Sports Medicine: ACSM's Exercise Management for Persons with Chronic Diseases and Disabilities. Human Kinetics, Champaign, IL, 1997, p 37.

84. Harvard Heart Letter: Hazards for patients with cardiac pacemakers and defibrillators. Harvard Heart Lett 19:6, 1999.

85. Mitrani, RD, et al: Cardiac pacemakers. In Fuster, V, Alexander, RW, and O'Rourke, RA (eds): Hurst's The Heart, ed 10. McGraw-Hill, New York, 2001.

86. Dias, KJ, Collins, SM, and Cahalin, LP: Physical therapy implications in managing patients with pacemakers and defibrillators. Cardiopulm Phys Ther J 17(2), 2006.

87. Keteyian, SJ, and Brawner, C: Cardiac transplantation. In American College of Sports Medicine: ACSM's Exercise Management for Persons with Chronic Diseases and Disabilities. Human Kinetics, Champaign, IL, 1997, p 54.

88. Cahalin, LP: Physiotherapy for the disablement of heart failure—part II. Physiother Singapore 3:31–38, 2000.

89. Edmondstone, WM: Cardiac chest pain: Does body language help the diagnosis? BMJ 311(7021):1660, 1995.

90. Goodman, CC, Boissenault, WG, and Fuller, KS: Pathology: Implications for the Physical Therapist, ed 3. WB Saunders, 2009.

91. Frese, E, Fick, A, and Sadowski, S: Blood pressure measurement guidelines for physical therapists. Cardiopulm Phys Ther J 22(2):5–12, 2011.

92. Tingle, LE, Molina, D, and Calvert, CW: Acute pericarditis. Am Fam Physician 76(10):1509, 2007.

93. Collin, V: Contribution to diseases of the heart and pericardium: I. Historical Introduction. Bull N Y Med Coll 18:1, 1955.

94. Bendjelid, K, and Pugin, J: Is Dressler syndrome dead? Chest 126(5):1680, 2004.

95. McGuinness, ME, and Talbert, RL: Cardiovascular testing. In Dipiro, J (ed): Pharmacotherapy: A Pathophysiologic Approach. McGraw-Hill, New York, 2002.

96. Pollentier, B, et al: Examination of the Six Minute Walk Test to determine functional capacity in people with chronic heart failure: A systematic review. Cardiopulm Phys Ther J 21(1):13–20, 2010.

97. Schaufelberger, SM, and Swedberg, K: Is Six-Minute Walk Test of value in congestive heart failure? Am Heart J 136:371, 1998.

98. Cahalin, L: The Six-Minute Walk Test predicts peak oxygen uptake and survival in patients with advanced heart failure. Chest 110:325, 1996.

99. Faggiano, P, et al: Assessment of oxygen uptake during Six Minute Walk Test in patients with heart failure. Chest 111(4):1146, 1997.

100. Coats, AJ: Heart failure: What causes symptoms of heart failure? Heart 86(5):578, 2001.

101. Bittner, V, et al: Prediction of mortality and morbidity with a 60-minute walk test in patients with left ventricular dysfunction. JAMA 270(14):1702, 1993.

102. Maehara, A, et al: Morphologic and angiographic features of coronary plaque rupture detected by intravascular ultrasound. J Am Coll Cardiol 40(5):904, 2002.

103. US Department of Health and Human Services: Effects of Cardiac Rehabilitation Exercise Training. Clinical Practice Guidelines, Cardiac Rehabilitation, AHCPR No. 17, publication No. 96-0672, October 1995.

104. Cardiopulmonary exercise testing in the clinical evaluation of patients with heart and lung disease. Circulation 123:668–680, 2011.

105. Levine, SA, and Lown, B: Armchair treatment of acute coronary thrombosis. JAMA 1948:1356, 1952.

106. ACCF/AHA/AMA-PCPI 2011 performance measures for adults with coronary artery disease and hypertension: A report of the American College of Cardiology Foundation/American Heart Association Task Force on Performance Measures and the American Medical Association–Physician Consortium for Performance Improvement. J Am Coll Cardiol 58:316–336, 2011.

107. American Association of Cardiovascular and Pulmonary Rehabilitation: Patient education, psychological issues and outcomes. In Guidelines for Cardiac Rehabilitation Programs, AACVPR ed 2. Human Kinetics, Champaign, IL, 1995.

108. McCartney, N: Role of resistance training in heart disease. Med Sci Sports Exerc S396, 1998.

109. Beniamini, Y, et al: Effects of high intensity strength training on quality of life parameters in cardiac rehabilitation patients. Am J Cardiol 841, 1997.

110. American Association of Cardiovascular and Pulmonary Rehabilitation: Graded exercise testing, exercise prescription, and resistance training. In Guidelines for Cardiac Rehabilitation Programs, AACVPR, ed 4. Human Kinetics, Champaign, IL, 2004.

111. American College of Sports Medicine: General principles of exercise prescription. In ACSM's Guidelines for Exercise Testing and Prescription, ed 6. Lippincott Williams & Wilkins, Philadelphia, 2000.

112. Fletcher, GF, et al: Exercise standards for testing and training: A statement for healthcare professionals from the American Heart Association. Circulation 104(14):1694, 2001.

113. Rossi, P: Physical training in patients with congestive heart failure. Chest 101(5 Suppl):350S, 1992.

114. Afzal, A, et al: Exercise training in heart failure. Prog Cardiovasc Dis 41:175, 1998.

115. Piepoli, MF, et al: Exercise training meta-analysis of trials in patients with chronic heart failure (exTraMATCH). Br Med J 328(7433):189, 2004.

116. Kokkinos, PF, et al: Chronic heart failure and exercise. Am Heart J 140(1):21, 2000.

117. Wielenga, RP: Safety and effects of physical training in chronic heart failure: Results of the chronic heart failure and graded exercise study (CHANGE). Eur Heart J 20:872, 1999.

118. Dubach, D, et al: Hemodynamic response to training in CHF. JACC 29(7):1591, 1997.

119. Piepoli, M: Experience from controlled trials of physical training in chronic heart failure. Eur Heart J 19:466, 1998.

120. Coats, A, et al: Controlled trial of physical training in chronic heart failure: Exercise performance, hemodynamics, ventilation and autonomic function. Circulation 85:2119, 1992.

121. Giannuzzi, P, et al: Attenuation of unfavorable remodeling by exercise training in postinfarction patients with left ventricular dysfunction: Results of the Exercise in Left Ventricular Dysfunction (ELVD) trial. Circulation 96:790, 1997.

122. Willenheimer, R, et al: Exercise training in heart failure improves quality of life and exercise capacity. Eur Heart J 774, 1998.

123. Kelvie, RS, et al: Effects of exercise training in patients with heart failure: The Exercise Rehabilitation Trial (EXERT). Am Heart J 144:23, 2002.

124. Hambrecht, R, et al: Effects of exercise training on left ventricular function and peripheral resistance in patients with chronic heart failure: A randomized trial. JAMA 283(23):3095, 2000.

125. Tyni-Lenne, R, et al: Improved quality of life in chronic heart failure patients following local endurance training with leg muscles. J Card Fail 2:111, 1996.

126. Johnson, PH, et al: A randomized controlled trial of inspiratory muscle training in stable chronic heart failure. Eur Heart J 19:1249, 1998.

127. Balady, GJ: Exercise training in the treatment of heart failure: What is achieved and how? Ann Med 30(Suppl 1):61, 1998.

128. Cahalin, LP: Heart failure. Phys Ther 76:516, 1996.

129. Schlant, RC, and Sonnenblick, EH: Pathophysiology of heart failure. In Alexander, RW, Schlant, RC, and Fuster, V (eds): Hurst's The Heart, ed 9. McGraw-Hill, New York, 1998.

130. van Tol, BAF, et al: Effects of exercise training on cardiac performance, exercise capacity and quality of life in patients with heart failure: A meta-analysis. Eur J Heart Failure 8(8):841–850, 2006.

131. Smart, N, and Marwick, TH: Exercise training for patients with heart failure: A systematic review of factors that improve mortality and morbidity. Am J Med 116(10):693–706, 2004.

132. Adamopoulos, S, et al: Physical training modulates proinflammatory cytokines and the soluble Fas/soluble Fas ligand system in patients with chronic heart failure. J Am Coll Cardiol 39:653–663, 2002.

133. Barlow, CW, et al: Effect of physical training on exercise-induced hyperkalemia in chronic heart failure. Relation with ventilation and catecholamines. Circulation 89:1144–1152, 1994.

134. Delagardelle, C, et al: Strength/endurance training versus endurance training in congestive heart failure. Med Sci Sports Exerc 34:1868–1872, 2002.

135. Harris, S, et al: A randomized study of home-based electrical stimulation of the legs and conventional bicycle exercise training for patients with chronic heart failure. Eur Heart J 24:871–878, 2003.

136. Kemppainen, J, et al: Insulin signalling and resistance in patients with chronic heart failure. J Physiol 550:305–315, 2003.

137. Stolen, KQ, et al: Exercise training improves biventricular oxidative metabolism and left ventricular efficiency in patients with dilated cardiomyopathy. J Am Coll Cardiol 41:460–467, 2003.

138. Malfatto, G, et al: Recovery of cardiac autonomic responsiveness with low-intensity physical training in patients with chronic heart failure. Eur J Heart Fail 4:159–166, 2002.

139. Radzewitz, A, et al: Exercise and muscle strength training and their effect on quality of life in patients with chronic heart failure. Eur J Heart Fail 4:627–634, 2002.

140. Santoro, C, et al: Exercise training alters skeletal muscle mitochondrial morphometry in heart failure patients. J Cardiovasc Risk 9:377–381, 2002.

141. Vibarel, N, et al: Effect of aerobic exercise training on inspiratory muscle performance and dyspnoea in patients with chronic heart failure. Eur J Heart Fail 4:745–751, 2002.

142. McKelvie, RS, et al: Comparison of hemodynamic responses to cycling and resistance exercises in congestive heart failure secondary to ischemic cardiomyopathy. Am J Cardiol 76:977, 1995.

143. Braith, R, and Beck, D: Resistance exercise: Training adaptations and developing a safe exercise prescription. Heart Failure Rev 13(1):69–79, 2008.

144. Mancini, DM, et al: The sensation of dyspnea during exercise is not determined by the work of breathing in patients with heart failure. J Am Coll Cardiol 28(2):391, 1996.

145. Bernardi, L, et al: Effect of breathing rate on oxygen saturation and exercise performance in chronic heart failure. Lancet 351(9112):1308, 1998.

146. Winkelmann, ER, et al: Addition of inspiratory muscle training to aerobic exercise training improves cardiorespiratory responses in patients with heart failure and inspiratory muscle weakness. Am Heart J 158(5):768e1; 2009.

147. Manacini, DM, et al: Benefits of selective respiratory muscle training on exercise capacity in patients with chronic heart failure. Circulation 91(2):320, 1995.

148. McParland, C, et al: Inspiratory muscle weakness and dyspnea in congestive heart failure. Am Rev Respir Dis 146(2):467, 1992.

149. US Department of Health and Human Services: Clinical Practice Guideline, Number 11, Heart Failure: Management of Patients with Left Ventricular Systolic Dysfunction. AHCPR Publication No. 94-0613, 1994.

150. Burg, MM, et al: Presurgical depression predicts medical morbidity 6 months after coronary artery bypass graft surgery. Psychosom Med 65(1):111, 2003.

151. Burg, MM, et al: Depressive symptoms and mortality two years after coronary artery bypass graft surgery (CABG) in men. Psychosom Med 65(4):508, 2003.

152. Blumenthal, JA, et al: Depression as a risk factor for mortality after coronary artery bypass surgery. Lancet 362(9384):604, 2003.

153. Ai, AL, et al: Psychological recovery from coronary artery bypass graft surgery: The use of complementary therapies. J Altern Complement Med 3(4):343, 1997.

154. McKhann, GM, et al: Depression and cognitive decline after coronary artery bypass grafting. Lancet 349(9061):1282, 1997.

155. Pirraglia, PA, et al: Depressive symptomatology in coronary artery bypass graft surgery patients. Int J Geriatr Psychiatry 14(8):668, 1999.

156. Lindquist, R, et al: Comparison of health-related quality-of-life outcomes of men and women after coronary artery bypass surgery through 1 year: Findings from the POST CABG Biobehavioral Study. Am Heart J 146(6):935, 2003.

157. Westin, L, et al: Differences in quality of life in men and women with ischemic heart disease: A prospective controlled study. Scand Cardiovasc J 33(3):160, 1999.

158. Phillips, BB, et al: Female gender is associated with impaired quality of life 1 year after coronary artery bypass surgery. Psychosom Med 65(6):944, 2003.

Vascular, Lymphatic, and Integumentary Disorders

Deborah Graffis Kelly, PT, DPT, MSEd **Chapter 14**

LEARNING OBJECTIVES

1. Understand basic concepts about the anatomy, physiology, and pathophysiology of the vascular, lymphatic, and integumentary systems.
2. Describe wound physiology as it relates to normal and abnormal wound healing.
3. Recognize the characteristics and risk factors of common disorders of the vascular, lymphatic, and integumentary systems.
4. Identify the components of a comprehensive examination of a patient with a disorder related to the vascular, lymphatic, and/or integumentary systems.
5. Analyze and integrate wound examination data to complete the physical therapy evaluation.
6. Interpret the rationale for skin and wound care treatment with particular attention to moist wound healing, arterial wound hydration, venous wound compression, lymphedema treatment, and foot care for the patient with diabetes.
7. Design an appropriate plan of care for an individual with a vascular, lymphatic, and/or integumentary disorder.
8. Using the case study example, apply clinical decision making skills to design a plan for advanced wound care.

CHAPTER OUTLINE

Patients and clients with disorders of the vascular, lymphatic, and integumentary systems have complex and often interrelated health problems to be understood before healing can occur. In recent years options for intervention have expanded significantly, providing the physical therapist with challenging and rewarding clinical treatments for clients. This chapter provides foundational material on which to build sound clinical decisions. Though interrelated, the systems discussed have unique characteristics and functions. This chapter facilitates understanding of the separate systems and then illustrates how the systems are intricately and essentially related. The elements of examination and the intervention strategies for all of the disorders are combined to ensure that the overlapping signs, symptoms, impairments, and activity limitations will be addressed and considered in the plan of care (POC). In this text, information about thermal injuries is complementary and supplemental to the information in this chapter (see Chapter 24, Burns).

■ ANATOMY AND PHYSIOLOGY OF THE VASCULAR, LYMPHATIC, AND INTEGUMENTARY SYSTEMS

In the microscopic world of circulation, blood and lymph vessels permeate most tissues, carrying oxygen and nutrients while removing carbon dioxide and wastes. Not all vessels involved are the "large tubes" so often associated with the circulatory system. Capillaries are woven throughout most of the tissues of the body, around muscle fibers, through connective tissues, and below the basement membrane of the epithelium.[1] Since arteries and veins are too large and too thick to allow diffusion between the bloodstream and surrounding tissues, a delicate network of blood and lymph capillaries controls all chemical and gaseous exchange between blood, interstitial fluid, and lymph.[1] In the normal system, homeostatic mechanisms adjust blood flow across the capillary walls to meet the needs of peripheral tissues. Every year, new information is uncovered that further elucidates the complexities of the circulatory system and how it interacts with the other systems of the body. It is important to have a clear understanding of the delicate vessels that carry blood to the peripheral tissues and the normal processes that occur there to gain insight into the disorders discussed later in the chapter.

Vascular
Arterial

Arteries carry rich, oxygenated blood away from the heart, branching off into sections with smaller diameters called **arterioles**, leading ultimately to capillaries. Arteries have three-layered walls that give them strength and elasticity. The walls of arteries are generally thicker than those of veins because they have to bear strong blood flow pressures generated by the heart. Arteries are strong and durable, able to keep their cylindrical shape when stretched. The movement of blood through arteries is dependent on heart function. Arteries have the ability to change in diameter when the volume of blood passing through them changes. They can also change in diameter when the sympathetic division of the autonomic nervous system (ANS) is triggered, either contracting (*vasoconstriction*) or relaxing (*vasodilation*). Because they have contractile abilities, arteries do not need valves to effect blood flow. These terms and concepts will be important when the chapter discussion turns to topics such as peripheral vascular disease, capillary blood flow, and wound healing.

Venous

Veins return oxygen-depleted blood from tissues and organs to the heart. At the beginning of the venous system, superficial blood capillaries empty into **venules** that carry blood toward medium-sized veins (about the size of muscular arteries). Superficial veins run above the fascia of the muscles. Deep veins run below the fascia. Perforating veins run between the superficial and the deep, penetrating the fascia to connect the superficial and deep vessels. Veins also have three-layered walls but they do not need to be as muscular or elastic as arteries because the blood pressure in veins is lower than in

arteries. Venous walls are so thin that they do not hold their shape well under stress, collapsing or tearing when stretched. As blood moves through the outermost regions of the body (the peripheral vascular system) from the arteries to the veins, blood pressures decrease. The blood pressure in the medium-sized veins is so low that it cannot oppose the force of gravity without structural assistance.[1] In the limbs, medium-sized veins contain *valves* that project from the inner walls of the veins, pointing in the direction of blood flow. Under normal conditions, the valves allow blood to flow in one direction, preventing backflow of blood. When the valves are working normally, any movement that compresses or pulls on a vein will help to push blood toward the heart. Skeletal muscle contraction will squeeze venous blood toward the heart. The act of walking helps to empty veins and move blood out of the lower extremities (LEs). When the walls of veins weaken, or are enlarged, the valves cannot function properly and blood pools in the veins. Eventually the veins become distended, leading to **varicose veins**. If a valve or valves do not close properly, this leads to a condition known as **venous reflux**. These terms and concepts will be important when the chapter discussion leads to topics such as chronic venous disease and LE swelling.

Lymphatic

Although parallel, and working in concert with the venous system, the lymphatic system is separate and unique. Because of its many roles and diffuse locations throughout the body, anatomists place discussion of the lymphatic system with the immune system, the circulatory system, and the integumentary system. The two primary functions of the lymphatic system are to protect the body from infection and disease via the immune response and to facilitate movement of fluid back and forth between the bloodstream and the interstitium, removing excess fluid, blood waste, and protein molecules in the process of fluid exchange. *Lymphatics* are located in all portions of the body except the central nervous system (CNS) and cornea.[2] The lymphatic system includes lymph vessels (superficial, intermediate, and deep, also referred to as lymphatics); lymph fluid; and lymph tissues and organs (lymph nodes, tonsils, spleen, thymus, and the thoracic duct).

Lymph fluid is first absorbed at the capillary level, then channeled through small vessels called *precollectors*, and finally picked up by the larger, valved vessels called *collectors*. The collectors have contractile properties, smooth muscle, and valves. Lymphatics are even thinner and more likely to collapse under pressure than veins.[2-4] Lymph moves throughout the body by a number of mechanisms. Superficially, the process of diffusion and filtration moves lymph fluid. Below the dermis, intrinsic contractions drive lymph propulsion in the deeper collectors. The force to generate a lymph vessel contraction does not come from the heart but from *lymphangions,* small pump-like segments within the larger lymph vessels. Classic literature reports information about lymph flow.[4-8] Newer literature indicates that scientists continue to explore the intricate world of the lymphatics.[9,10] The human body is wonderfully equipped to provide a variety of stimuli that have an impact on lymphangion contraction:

- Parasympathetic, sympathetic, and sensory *nerve stimulation*
- *Contraction of muscles* adjacent to a vessel
- *Pulsation of arteries* adjacent to a lymph vessel (even pre-capillary arterioles have pulsation)
- Abdominal and thoracic cavity pressure changes that occur during *breathing*
- *Volume changes* within each lymphangion (internal receptors respond to tension and trigger a contraction)
- *Mild mechanical stimulation* of dermal tissue increases the frequency of lymphangion contractions

Excess lymph fluid is transported through the thoracic duct and emptied into the venous angles at the left and right jugular vein trunks. Under normal conditions, lymph flow is not adversely affected by gravity. Under abnormal conditions, the lymphatic system may exhibit excess lymph pooling related to gravity, especially in the LEs.

Integumentary

Also referred to as an organ, the integumentary system is the most often seen and touched by a physical therapist of all the body systems. The integumentary system has a functional relationship to many other body systems. The health of this system is dependent on the normal functions of the arterial, venous, and lymphatic capillaries (dermal circulation). A thorough review of the functions of the skin illustrates the importance of even a small area of damage to this organ. The discussion on skin anatomy, with diagrams, in this textbook will supplement the overview here (see Chapter 24, Burns). The *epidermis* is avascular and water-resistant. It provides protection from infection, abrasion, and chemicals and assists with heat regulation, retention, and dissipation. Melanocytes, present in this layer, determine skin color and provide protection from ultraviolet radiation. The epidermis regenerates rapidly, allowing individuals to heal quickly when conditions are normal. The *dermis* is 20 to 30 times thicker than epidermis. It contains blood vessels and lymphatics, nerves and nerve endings, and sensory neurons that all supply the epidermis. The dermis also contains hair follicles, sweat glands and sebaceous glands, and nails. All of these project through the epidermis to the surface of the skin. These appendages are a deep source of epithelial cells, needed to resurface a wound during healing. The contents of the dermis are surrounded and supported by collagen, elastin, and ground substance that provide structure, strength, flexibility, and elasticity. The *hypodermis* (also referred to as

the *subcutaneous* layer) is not part of the integument but is important in stabilizing skin over skeletal muscles and organs. It consists of loose connective tissue and fat cells and provides insulation and protection to underlying structures. The hypodermis plays an important role in the prevention of **pressure ulcers**, especially over the ischial tuberosities and greater trochanters.

When there is an injury to the integument, some or all of the components of the integument are impaired, resulting in many possible sequelae such as decreased lubrication, loss of elasticity, increased scar formation, loss of **tensile strength**, decreased ability to resist infection, and an increase or decrease in sensitivity.

■ WOUND PHYSIOLOGY
Normal Wound Healing

In the human body, an elegant sequence of events takes place to ensure that when injury occurs, wounds will heal. Within the **endogenous** fluids of the body, every cell and chemical mediator is programmed and ready to act when needed. When conditions are normal, the body is equipped to heal itself.

Phases of Healing

The classic model of overlapping phases of wound healing describes a process that is continuous, its phases not entirely distinct. The model is used in this chapter to draw attention to the normal process and to provide guidelines for what can be expected in normal healing. The number of days to complete each phase will vary based on factors such as age, size of wound, co-morbidities, continued trauma, nutrition, blood flow, medications, stress, and infection. The process of repair is the same for all wounds but the sequence will be much quicker in more shallow wounds with less tissue loss. In all stages of healing, wounded tissues are striving to achieve homeostasis. Italicized words below stress important concepts.

Inflammation (Phase I)

- The *normal* immune system reaction to injury.
- The *central activity* in wound healing.
- Temporary repair initiated by coagulation (clotting factors, platelets) and *short-term decreased* blood flow.
- **Necrosis** occurs after cells have been injured or destroyed.
- The spread of pathogens is slowed: debris and bacteria are attacked by a host of cells. If the wound is acute, some periwound edema, **erythema**, and drainage can be expected.[11] If fluid accumulates at the injury site it is called **pus**.
- Oxygen is delivered via *increased* blood flow to keep the phagocytic cells alive and functioning.
- Permanent repair is facilitated by creating a clean wound, *setting the stage* for the next phase of healing; signals are generated that re-epithelialization can begin.

- Time frame: day of injury to approximately day 10.
- *Rate* of inflammatory process is affected by the size of the wound, blood supply, available nutrients, and the extrinsic environment.
- If this phase is interrupted or delayed, *chronic inflammation can result,* lasting from months to years (see section titled Abnormal Wound Healing and the Chronic Wound).

Proliferation (Phase II)

- *New tissue* fills in the wound as **fibroblasts** secrete collagen.
- Skin integrity is restored by re-epithelialization and/or contraction (see discussion below).
- **Angiogenesis** occurs: new blood vessel growth from endothelial cells, fragile capillary buds grow into the wound bed; new reddish, slightly bumpy tissue is called granulation tissue.
- Epithelial cells differentiate into type I collagen. *Collagen synthesis* occurs but the resulting new scar tissue is fragile and must be protected; trauma during this phase may return the wound to the inflammatory process.
- Time frame: day 3 of injury to approximately day 20.
- *Rate* of proliferation is affected by the size of the wound, blood supply, available nutrients, and the extrinsic environment.
- If this phase is interrupted or delayed, the result may be a chronic wound.

Maturation/remodeling (Phase III)

- Maturation or remodeling of new tissue begins while granulation tissue is forming during the prior (proliferative) phase.
- Epithelial cells continue to differentiate into Type I collagen.
- New skin has *tensile strength* that is 15% of normal. Scar tissue is rebuilding but at best reaches 80% of original tensile strength.
- Underlying granulation tissue is replaced by *less vascular* tissue.
- In deep wounds, dermal appendages are rarely repaired (hair follicles, sebaceous and sweat glands, nerves) but instead are replaced by *fibrous tissue.*
- Over time the scar tissue matures, changing from red to pink to white and from raised and rigid to flat and flexible.
- Time frame: approximately day 9 of injury up to 2 years.
- *Rate* of *maturation/remodeling* is affected by the size of the wound, blood supply, available nutrients, and the extrinsic environment.

The Role of Oxygen in Wound Healing

Oxygen reaches the wound bed through blood flow to the area. The need for oxygen to sustain life is apparent, not only at the systemic level, but also at the cellular level of human physiology. Most cells in the wound environment have an enzyme that converts oxygen to a form that allows the cell to support wound healing.[12] Wound contraction, collagen deposition, angiogenesis, and granulation are examples of wound healing steps supported by oxygen. Wound tissue oxygenation is a sensitive indicator for the risk of post-operative infection.[13] A decrease in oxygen availability in a wound results in increased likelihood of infection. Wound perfusion may be limited for a variety of reasons. The presence of edema and necrotic tissue makes it more difficult for oxygen to reach the wound. Since compression can reduce edema and débridement can reduce the presence of necrotic tissue, these procedural interventions are important components of most wound care. Unless contraindicated owing to arterial disease, compression and débridement will decrease the obstruction to wound oxygenation. Peripheral vasoconstriction can also limit wound perfusion. Problems with vasoconstriction cannot always be improved readily. Interventions that will increase wound perfusion and are appropriate for all individuals include keeping the wound area warm, avoiding smoking, hydrating the individual, and controlling pain and anxiety. Clinical studies have shown that keeping patients warm and giving them supplemental oxygen decreases the rate of infection and shortens hospital stay.[14] Improvement of oxygen levels in wound tissue alone may trigger wound healing. Adequate oxygen levels will also enhance the effectiveness of growth factors and a host of other cells that require oxygenation to maintain their function. The delivery of exogenous oxygen will be discussed later in the chapter under the section on Intervention. The nutritional status of the individual, as discussed below, will also have an impact on oxygenation since hemoglobin, iron, vitamin B_{12}, and folic acid are needed to enable red blood cells to carry oxygen to healing tissues.

The Role of Moisture in Wound Healing

In the past, the goal of wound care was to create and maintain a dry wound, packed with dry dressings, dried by heat lamps, and exposed to the air. Modern wound management is based on the concept of creating and maintaining a *moist wound environment* to facilitate wound healing. More than 50 years ago, research confirmed that a dry wound creates an environment that is hostile to wound healing. A dry wound allows the formation of wound scab and **eschar**, which inhibit migration of epithelial cells, provide food for pathogens, and affect blood flow to the wound bed. A dry wound also allows cooling of the wound surface; without a protective barrier, the surface temperature of the wound is decreased and healing is slowed. Adhesion of gauze or other dry dressings to the wound bed causes trauma to the wound bed and pain to the individual upon removal. Bacteria enter a dry wound more readily because of the lack of a protective barrier. As the wound dries, the rich endogenous fluids that are lost contain the elements necessary for timely wound healing.

Wound management experts agree that adequate wound hydration is the most important external factor responsible for optimal wound healing.[15-18] Wounds are typically covered with an occlusive or semi-occlusive dressing. This type of dressing is also called a moisture-retentive dressing because the dressing retains fluids on the wound bed. There are many types and styles of dressings that will facilitate a moist environment (see the section on Dressings for further discussion). Maintaining a moist wound with an occlusive dressing should hold an appropriate amount of endogenous fluids on the wound, preserving the cells needed for healing and keeping them in contact with the wound bed. Some chronic wound fluid may contain substances that can delay healing so a balance must be maintained between moisture and exudate removal.[19] Moisture softens wound scab and eschar; under the right conditions, the body's own enzymes will dissolve the eschar in a process called **autolytic débridement**. Occlusive dressings maintain appropriate wound surface temperature to prevent delays in healing and protect the wound surface from trauma and from bacteria and other contaminants. Wound cleansing is facilitated during autolytic débridement and further breakdown of skin in the periwound area is prevented.

Basic principles of moist wound healing include covering the wound with a barrier (occlusive dressing) that preserves adequate wound hydration; limiting fluid loss from the wound surface while the dressing is in place; allowing gaseous exchange; maintaining periwound integrity; controlling heavy **exudate**; and removing the dressing when exudate begins to leak out from edges of dressing.

It has long been believed that occlusive dressings should not be applied over infected wounds because trapped bacteria could fulminate. Studies are now producing evidence that the opposite may be true.[20-22] Because in acute wounds, and some chronic wounds, endogenous fluids have bacteria-fighting chemical elements, evidence of colonized bacteria in the wound does not automatically preclude the use of occlusive dressings. Specially selected dressings such as hydrocolloids are a good choice in this situation.

With the use of a systemic antibiotic and a close watch for signs of change in the patient's symptoms, clinicians may be able to utilize occlusive or moisture-retentive dressings over some types of wounds that are infected. The use of this dressing technique may broaden if the evidence continues to build in strength. Meanwhile, there is ongoing investigation into the contents of chronic wound exudate and its power to break down growth factors and prolong the inflammatory phase of wound healing. Information on this level will guide the use of occlusive dressings in the chronic wound healing environment.[23]

Despite half a century of research to support the concepts of moist wound healing, there are still practitioners who ignore the evidence and utilize outdated methods of wound management. Clinicians must strive to educate patients, families, and all members of the wound care team about appropriate wound care concepts.

The Role of Nutrition in Wound Healing

It is well established that nutritional status can have a significant impact on wound healing. Adequate protein intake is required for collagen synthesis, as well as the formation of new blood vessels and muscle tissue. Literature abounds with information about important nutritional issues such as the role of specific nutrients in wound healing, how poor nutritional status can delay wound healing, the use of special pharmacological interventions, and appropriate routes for nutritional support (enteral versus parenteral).[24-32]

The nutritional status of special populations such as children with special healthcare needs must be addressed by interdisciplinary interaction. Pediatric patients in long-term care, recovering from surgery, or with wounds, burns, or trauma are at risk for pressure ulcers.[33] As with adults, adequate protein intake is essential for healing to occur on time. Another patient population of concern is the elderly, whose tissues are fragile and whose immune systems are easily compromised. Nutrition plays a role in the prevention and management of pressure ulcers in this population as well.[34]

Nutrients that must be present for a wound to heal include iron, vitamin B_{12} and folic acid (essential so that red blood cells can deliver oxygen to tissues), vitamin C and zinc (essential for tissue repair), vitamin A (essential to stimulate collagen cross-linking), and arginine (enhances healing and immune function).[35,36] High protein intake provides the amino acids required to build new tissue. Protein and calorie needs will vary depending on the size of the wound and the medical condition of the patient. What are yet to be established are guidelines about energy levels, or nutrient needs required to heal a wound. In response to the available information and the need for more research, nutrition and metabolic support of acutely and chronically ill patients is emerging as an important branch of medicine.

As a part of the wound care team, a physical therapist will make contributions to the plans for nutritional support of the patient. Clinicians will collect data through chart review, observation, history taking, and the use of dietary examination methods.[37] Because exercise, hydration, and improved appetite often are interrelated, a physical therapist should pay close attention to a patient's activity level, strength, conditioning, and any mobility issues while encouraging fluid and nutrient intake.

Wound Characteristics

The characteristics of wounds may be defined as dry, wet, or granulating. Wounds can also be defined by their etiology, such as diabetic, vascular, or traumatic. Wound characteristics describe the physical appearance of the wound but often provide the clues to the etiology, phase of healing, and likelihood of closure. Wound characteristics can provide valuable information needed to make sound clinical judgments about treatment. For example, the location of the wound may prompt the clinician to select a particular dressing, change patient positioning, or prescribe orthotic footwear. When wound characteristics are described in documentation, they can indicate progress (or failure to progress) toward closure and healing. Wound characteristics should be identified during the initial examination and then monitored at least weekly during the wound healing phase. Depending on the etiology and chronicity of the wound, some characteristics may not be evident on initial examination but could appear at a later date as complications of the wound healing process. The following are characteristics that should be tracked and documented throughout the phases of wound healing:

- *Location*: where on the body
- *Size*: depth, width, and length
- *Shape*: irregular versus distinct
- *Edges*: condition and shape of wound edges, evidence of premature healing
- *Tunneling, undermining, sinus tracts*: presence and depth
- *Base*: characteristics of the wound base compared to sides and edges
  - Necrosis, eschar, **slough**: amount, color, texture, adherence to wound bed
  - Exudate: amount, color, odor
  - **Granulation tissue**: presence or absence, amount, location
  - Epithelialization: presence or absence, premature or on schedule
  - Exposed structures: color and condition of bone, tendon, ligament
- *Periwound area*: edema, induration, **maceration**
- *Pain*: although not a visible characteristic, it is measurable and significant to the intervention
- *Quantity of bacteria*: amount present in a wound. This is referred to as the **bio-burden**.

The quantitative biopsy is the gold standard for obtaining a wound culture but it is not used universally owing to cost, lack of laboratory facilities, and potential pain for the patient.[12] A swab culture is often used as an alternative but it is limited to detecting surface contamination, not tissue infection. Some literature supports swab culture, when used appropriately, as an adjunct in the management of chronic wounds.[38] Clinical intuition is also important in determining if infection is probable.

The examination will include data about the characteristics that have been gathered using methods such as observation, palpation, measurement, photography, and tracing. A clinician who is new to the wound care team should remember that these are skills that take practice.

Wound Closure

Primary Intention

Healing by primary intention occurs when a surgeon closes a wound by bringing the edges together. Approximating the edges can occur through the use of sutures, staples, glue, skin grafts, or skin flaps. For more information on skin grafting see Chapter 24, Burns. Wounds closed by primary intention still pass through the phases of wound healing but on a smaller scale. The major mechanism for healing wounds by primary intention is connective tissue deposition. A wound closed by primary intention that later opens up again owing to maceration or infection has opened by the process of *dehiscence* (Fig. 14.1). Following dehiscence, a wound is almost always allowed to close by secondary intention.

Secondary Intention

Healing by secondary intention occurs when a wound is left to heal on its own. The mechanisms of healing by secondary intention are contraction, re-epithelialization, or a combination of both. Deeper wounds heal by replacing injured tissue with scar tissue as collagen fills the wound bed.

During the process of contraction, existing tissue migrates, pulling the wound edges toward the center of the wound. This process forms no new tissue. New tissue may be forming in the wound simultaneously but not via contraction. Contraction occurs when growth factors trigger myofibroblasts to pull the wound edges inward. Growth factors and myofibroblasts can be influenced positively or negatively by physiological factors such as

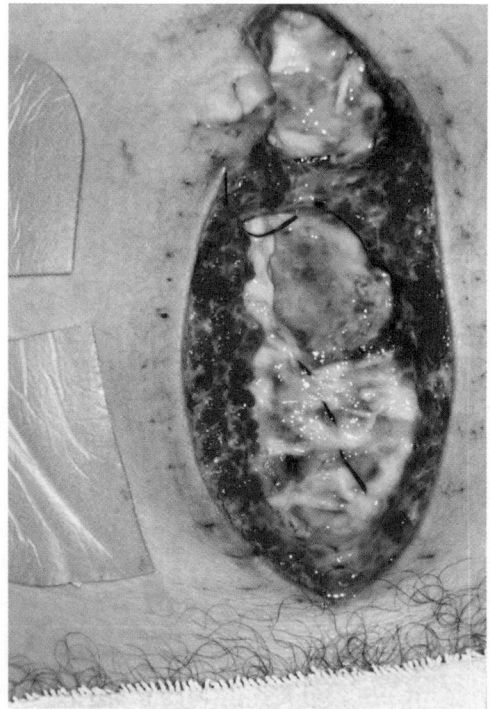

Figure 14.1 Wound dehiscence following appendectomy.

the amount of oxygen and nutrients available, and by mechanical factors such as external compression and the shape of the wound. Even though contraction is a normal occurrence in certain types of wound healing, if it is too rapid, it can cause disfiguring scars and impaired tissue function. Since there is centripetal movement of the entire thickness of the surrounding skin, tissue elongation may not keep up with the pace of contraction, causing significant functional and cosmetic deformity. Clinicians should intervene by applying special types of pressure to the tissues to slow the deforming forces of contraction (scar management discussed later in chapter).

Epithelialization is another response used by the body to close a wound. As noted in the phases of normal wound healing, chemical mediators send signals for re-epithelialization to begin in Phase I (the inflammatory phase). Actual repair begins in Phase II when new tissue is formed to cover the wound. Growth factors stimulate specialized epithelial cells, *keratinocytes,* to begin to migrate from the edges of the wound toward the center. In partial-thickness wounds in which the dermal appendages have not been destroyed, the cells will also migrate from the hair follicles, sebaceous glands, and sweat glands. In smaller, shallower wounds this process may be triggered to begin as early as 12 hours after wounding. In larger wounds, it may be 10 days or longer before the cells begin to migrate. In a chronic wound there are many reasons why this process is not triggered or is interrupted. (See discussion under Abnormal Wound Healing and the Chronic Wound.) When the wound is covered with new skin, re-epithelialization stops by contact inhibition.

When epithelial cells meet at the center of the wound, migration ends and cells will stop dividing. This is referred to as *contact inhibition.* At the time of contact inhibition and/or full re-epithelialization, wound *closure* has occurred. Wound *healing,* however, may continue for several years. A significant amount of intervention is still required to support the wound successfully from "closed" to "healed" status. Factors affecting the rate and type of closure by secondary intention include the following:

- *Wound shape*: linear wounds (surgical) contract most rapidly; circular wounds (pressure ulcers) contract most slowly.[39]
- *Wound depth*: all things equal, the shallower the wound, the quicker the closure.[40-43]
  - *Superficial* (loss of the epidermis): closes by re-epithelialization.
  - *Partial-thickness* (loss of the epidermis and dermis): closes primarily by re-epithelialization with minimal contraction.
  - *Full-thickness* (loss of all layers of the epidermis, dermis, and deeper structures): closes by contraction and scar formation; however, epithelial cells

will migrate from the wound edges to assist in wound closure if the environment is homeostatic.
- *Wound location*: areas with least pressure, most perfusion (face) will close more rapidly than areas with most pressure, least perfusion (sacrum, heel).
- *Wound etiology*: least traumatic (surgery) will close more rapidly than most traumatic (pressure ulcer, burn).

As deeper wounds heal, the wound is filled with tissue but the repair process does not replace lost muscle, fat, or dermis with those same types of tissue. The wound is filled with scar tissue made up primarily of collagen. Because the original tissue is not replaced with more of the same, a wound that is closed, and finally healed, does not return to its prewounded state. This concept is particularly important to understanding the position on reverse staging of pressure ulcers as described in the section on Tests and Measurements. It is also important to understand this concept when planning protection, positioning, patient education, footwear, and exercise programs for individuals with all types of wounds whether they are acute, closed, healed, or chronic wounds.

Tertiary Intention
Also called *delayed primary*, this type of closure occurs when a wound is allowed to heal by secondary intention and then is closed by primary intention as the final treatment. The delay in primary closure is usually owing to the presence of infection.

Abnormal Wound Healing and the Chronic Wound
When the sequence of events that leads to normal wound healing does not occur, a chronic wound results. The characteristics and causes of chronic wounds vary owing to the diverse nature of individuals with wounds, their medical histories, and the etiologies of the wounds. Even if the chronic wound moves through the classic phases of wound healing, it does so in an abnormal manner. Vital actions and reactions necessary for wound healing are interrupted, stunted, or absent in the chronic wound.

Although the characteristics of abnormal wound healing may be varied, concepts can be used to illustrate the failure of a wound to pass through phases of wound healing in a timely manner. The following discussion focuses on the results of interruption to the classic phases of wound healing:
- Inflammation (Phase I): if there is inadequate blood flow and oxygen supply to support cellular life and activity, cells may not initiate the repair sequence. Debris and bacteria build up, and pathogens spread more rapidly. Bio-burden is measured as greater than 10^5 organisms/g of tissue, the classic definition of infection.

- Clinical signs: increase in amount of drainage, change in color or odor, lingering swelling, eschar/necrosis from ischemic conditions, periwound maceration, chronic inflammation, **tunneling**, **undermining**, and infection may develop if the host's immune system is unable to resist the impact of the bacterial load.
- Proliferation (Phase II): if collagen synthesis is delayed in this phase, skin integrity will be poor. If angiogenesis is delayed, there will not be enough myofibroblasts to initiate wound contraction. The need for oxygen and nutrients will be very high and without them, available cells will be unable to reproduce rapidly, resulting in delayed epithelialization.
  - Clinical signs: keratinocytes do not migrate because the wound bed is not moist, healthy, clean, and granulating. Epithelial cells may attempt to migrate from the wound edges but without a wound bed that is ready, they will build up at the wound edge and may migrate over the edge, forming a lip that curls under. Granulation tissue is either absent, pale, or delayed; new tissue is weak and breaks down or bleeds easily; tunneling, eschar, and periwound maceration may be evident. Necrosis, if it has not been removed, will delay angiogenesis. Changes in drainage color, amount, odor, or lingering swelling may signal a return to the inflammation stage.
- Maturation/Remodeling (Phase III): if the synthesis and lysis of collagen is out of balance, weakened tissue will break down too easily or hypertrophic scarring will build up too rapidly.
  - Clinical signs: newly formed skin breaks down with little provocation, and scar tissue builds up within the outline of the original wound (hypertrophic) or beyond the margins of the original wound (keloid).

Infection in Wound Healing

Wound infection is a significant problem for any individual. Bio-burden has a greater impact on wound healing than most underlying medical conditions.[11,44] Infection may turn life threatening if the patient is elderly or critically ill. Regardless of the condition of the individual, wound infection is detrimental to wound closure and healing time. True infection is identified if the presence of bacteria or microorganisms is greater than 10^5 per gram of tissue determined by a quantitative culture. This determination can only be made with a biopsy. Surface swabs that are cultured may or may not be conclusive for actual infection since there are many types of bacteria that exist on the skin all the time.

- Effects of infection
  - Inefficient cellular activity, decreased collagen metabolism, chemical mediators absent or dilute, cells absent or confused by lack of instructions from chemical mediators and presence of other cells; when the bio-burden is greater than 10^5 organisms/g of tissue, epithelialization may not occur[38]
  - Decreased oxygen in the wound bed; insufficient oxygen to support the regeneration of tissue and to assist in the prevention of infection
  - Increased rate of cell necrosis
  - Overall decline of body systems contributes to strain on the specialized cells
  - Risk of wound sepsis, **osteomyelitis**, **gangrene**
- Signs of potential infection
  - Change in wound drainage (amount, color, odor)
  - Swelling
  - Periwound redness or warmth (less obvious with darker skin)
  - Increase in pain or tenderness
  - Change in the quality of granulation tissue or failure to produce good quality tissue (may be pale, soft, easily broken down)
  - No measurable wound contraction within 2 to 4 weeks
  - Tissue culture/punch biopsy results of greater than 10^5 organisms/g of tissue
  - Fever, nausea, fatigue, loss of appetite

Clinicians should use a structured approach to identify clinical infection. Careful identification of infection may help to avoid the risk of overuse of antibiotics.[45] The punch biopsy is the gold standard for confirming infection, but a physical therapist should watch for the early signs of infection: *warmth, redness, swelling, fever, malaise,* and *loss of appetite.*

Factors Contributing to Abnormal Wound Healing

The factors or triggers that may contribute to abnormal wound healing are varied but can be placed into broad categories for better understanding. Most abnormal wound healing will be influenced by factors from all the categories. Treatment intervention that addresses factors from one category and not the others will be incomplete.

Intrinsic Factors

Intrinsic or internal factors are conditions within the body that may contribute to abnormal healing. These factors relate primarily to the wound and periwound areas, and include hypoxemia owing to inadequate blood flow, oxygen supply and aging skin. As the integument ages, there is a decrease in moisture content leading to an increase in brittle quality and a delay in the renewal time affecting the stratum corneum. **Rete pegs**, undulations between contact layers of the epidermis and dermis, become less functional with increased risk of shearing.

Changes in the dermis include a decrease in elasticity, collagen, and mast cell production, along with a decrease in the vascularity and number of pain receptors. Available fat in the subcutaneous layer begins to resorb after age 70, leading to a decrease in protection against pressure and shearing. Finally, underlying disease will affect acute and chronic wound healing. The more common conditions known to affect healing are diabetes, cancer, circulatory insufficiencies, human immunodeficiency virus infection, and connective tissue diseases.

Extrinsic Factors

Extrinsic or environmental factors are those influences that come from outside the body. The medical professionals caring for a person with a wound may be able to moderate the impact of extrinsic factors on the wound environment. Factors include the effects of radiation therapy or chemotherapy; incontinence; medication, smoking, recreational drugs, and alcohol (all slow or eliminate cellular reactions needed for healing); dehydration and malnutrition (both slow the delivery of oxygen to wound tissues); bio-burden/infection (healing is slowed by pathogens, necrotic tissue, granulomas); and stress (negative effects of stress can lead to impaired healing).[42,46-51]

Iatrogenic Factors

Iatrogenic refers to any injury or illness that occurs as the result of medical care. Theoretically, these factors are under the control of the medical professionals who care for the patient and are therefore preventable. Factors include, but are not limited to, the following: poor wound management, frequent disruption of the wound through inappropriate cleansing, use of inappropriate dressings and dressing techniques, cytotoxic topical agents that lead to inefficient cellular activity, and lack of moisture resulting in delayed or absent migration of keratinocytes. Frequent dressing changes will slow wound healing by reducing wound temperature. It can take more than 30 minutes for a wound to return to normal temperature after a dressing change. Infection can be an iatrogenic factor when caused by cross-contamination, improper use of gloves and other protective devices, inadequate use of sterile and clean technique, lack of proper hand washing, lack of adherence to **standard precautions**, and inadequate clean or sterile technique. Other iatrogenic factors that contribute to abnormal wound healing include shear injuries (skin tears) that occur during transfers and repositioning and **ischemia** from unrelieved pressure owing to inadequate turning schedules or absent or inadequate *pressure-redistributing devices (PRDs)*.

Complications of Chronicity

A chronic wound creates a complex and serious health problem for an individual (Fig. 14.2). Chronic wounds may lead to complications including any or all of the following: impairments of body function and structures, restrictions in activities and participation, need for assisted living or home care, decreased quality-of-life

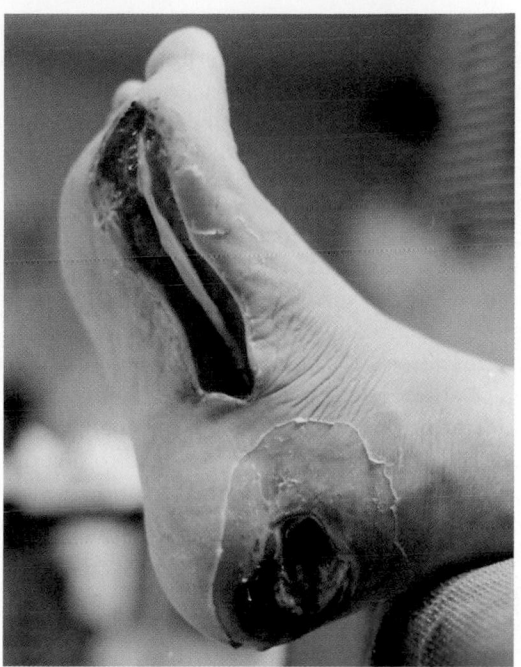

Figure 14.2 Chronic wound as a result of diabetic neuropathy.

perceptions, depression, infection, malnutrition and weight loss, protein depletion, tissue **fibrosis**, loss of limb, and death. Every year over 5 million Americans are treated for chronic wounds at a cost of billions of dollars, making this type of wound one of the most costly challenges in health care.[52] A chronic wound fails to heal because of an underlying pathology and will not heal until the cause is corrected or improved. The clinician must determine the factors contributing to abnormal wound healing and then develop an appropriate POC to overcome or address the obstacles.

■ VASCULAR, LYMPHATIC, AND INTEGUMENTARY DISORDERS

Arterial Insufficiency and Ulceration

Arterial insufficiency refers to a lack of adequate blood flow to a region or regions of the body. Many different disorders may arise from arterial insufficiency and can be classified by a variety of descriptors. For the purposes of this chapter, references will be to arterial insufficiency owing to organic disruption of blood flow to the extremities or to **peripheral vascular disease (PVD)**. PVD is a general term used to describe any disorder that interferes with arterial or venous blood flow of the extremities. PVD caused by arterial insufficiency may be related to smoking, cardiac disease, diabetes, hypertension, renal disease, and elevated cholesterol and triglycerides. Obesity and a sedentary lifestyle are related contributors in the cycle of disease and vessel obstruction. When several of these factors are combined, as they often can be, the possibility for health problems is almost 100%. The damage caused by these factors is reflected in structural changes in the walls of the arteries, causing abnormal blood flow. The following is a brief overview of disorders that occur with abnormal arterial blood flow:

- **Arteriosclerosis:** thickening, hardening, and loss of elasticity of arterial walls.
- **Atherosclerosis:** the most common form of arteriosclerosis, associated with damage to the endothelial lining of the vessels and the formation of lipid deposits, eventually leading to plaque formation.
- **Arteriosclerosis obliterans:** a peripheral manifestation of atherosclerosis characterized by **intermittent claudication**, rest pain, and trophic changes. This is the arterial disease most likely to lead to **ulceration**.[53] Known risk factors for development of the disease are smoking, diabetes mellitus, hypertension, hyperlipidemia, and hyperhomocysteinemia.
- **Thromboangiitis obliterans** (Buerger's disease): inflammation leads to arterial occlusion and tissue ischemia, especially in young men who smoke.
- **Raynaud's disease:** a vasomotor disease of small arteries and arterioles that is most often characterized by pallor and cyanosis of the fingers. In some cases both the hands and feet may be affected. The cause of Raynaud's is unknown but attacks are usually triggered by cold or emotional upset.
- Ulceration: a peripheral sign of a long-standing disease process; by definition, arterial ulcers are associated with arterial insufficiency.

Between 10% and 25% of LE ulcers are caused by arterial disease.[54] The incidence of arterial disease and LE ulceration is significantly lower than that for venous disease and ulceration; however, arterial wounds more frequently lead to loss of limb and death. These important facts signal the significance of taking a thorough history, performing a systems review, and adequate skin inspection during the initial visit with any individual who might have arterial disease.

Clinical Presentation

- Wounds will most frequently be located on the LEs: lateral malleoli, dorsum of feet, toes.
- When wounds are present on an ischemic limb, atherosclerotic occlusion of the peripheral vasculature is almost always present.
- The majority of patients with arterial insufficiency also have diabetes.
- Trophic changes are present and include abnormal nail growth, decreased leg and foot hair, and dry skin.
- Skin is cool on palpation.
- Wounds are painful and patient may also describe pain in the legs and/or feet (see discussion below about intermittent claudication).
- Wound base is usually necrotic and pale, lacking granulation tissue.
- Skin around the wound may be black, mummified (dry gangrene).

- Other signs of arterial insufficiency will be evident: decreased pulses, **pallor** on leg elevation, and **rubor** when dependent.

History

Painful cramping or aching of the LEs during walking is the most common complaint of patients with chronic arterial occlusion of the LEs. The pain is caused by **intermittent claudication** that occurs when exercising muscles are not receiving the blood perfusion needed for normal function. Patients should be examined for other signs of arterial insufficiency if intermittent claudication is occurring. Rest pain that develops at night, awakens the patient, or requires analgesics for relief is considered more severe than claudication. The individual with vascular dysfunction may also be diabetic. Diabetes will contribute to slower healing times and difficulty fighting infection. A wound in a distal, ischemic area is not likely to heal unless the vascular supply is enhanced or restored. Individuals with arterial disease and diabetes are more likely to have hypertension, and may have previous bypass grafts or amputations of the toes, pain on ambulation or rest, pain with elevation, cold hands and feet, and color changes of fingers and toes. Owing to the long latency period between injury to the arterial circulation and clinical appearance of disorders, healthcare providers, families, caregivers, and patients must join forces with education, prevention, and vigilance.

Tests and Measurements

One of the most important tests for individuals with arterial disease is the **Ankle-Brachial Index (ABI)**. The ABI is a test designed to examine the vascular system. Results provide useful information about the potential loss of perfusion in the LEs. Refer to Arterial Perfusion in the section on Tests and Measurements under Examination and Evaluation.

Intervention

If ulceration is present, intervention should enhance chemical and gaseous homeostasis in the wound bed, facilitate superficial blood flow to target tissues, and educate patients about the importance of facilitating blood flow to the extremities. Treatment will include appropriate wound care as well as important adjuncts to wound care. Results of the ABI will guide the therapist and referring practitioner in the appropriate use of compression. In a diagnosis of mixed arterial and venous disease the condition that is more severe should be treated first. If the arterial condition is worse, compression may be inappropriate even when edema is present. A nonhealing wound on an ischemic limb can lead to gangrene, amputation, further amputation, and/or loss of life (Fig. 14.3). In the most severe cases, conditions are inhospitable to wound closure. In this case necrotic tissue should not be débrided, since the dead tissue will not be replaced with new tissue. Conditions for closing and healing the wound are poor. Skin grafts

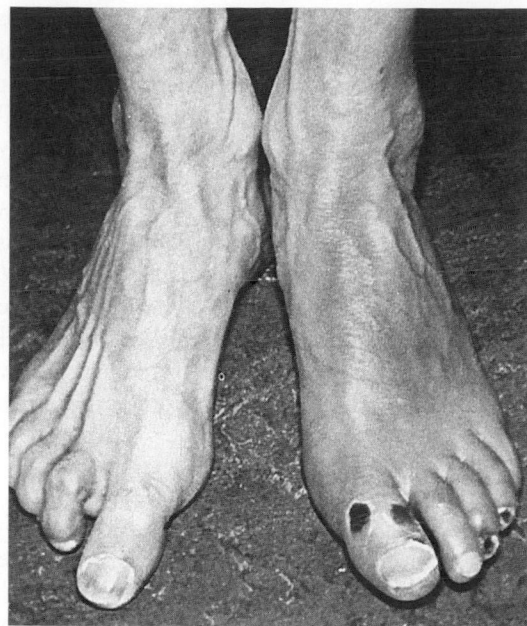

Figure 14.3 Clinical presentation of arterial insufficiency.

do not adhere to the virtually lifeless wound bed. Antibiotics cannot reach the wound systemically and topical agents are too superficial to stop infection. At this point, vascular surgery may be an option for some individuals. A bypass graft is used to restore arterial circulation to the ischemic tissue. For others, living with a chronic nonhealing wound or coming to terms with amputation are the only options. Most experts agree that the single most important intervention in PVD is prevention of smoking. The second most important intervention is exercise for weight control. Exercise will also improve collateral circulation, lipid profiles, and management of hypertension. A physical therapist plays a crucial role in wound care for arterial wounds and should address patient education and exercise in the intervention plan.

Venous Insufficiency and Ulceration

Venous insufficiency refers to inadequate drainage of venous blood from a body part, usually resulting in edema and/or skin abnormalities and ulcerations. **Chronic venous insufficiency (CVI)** refers to venous insufficiency that persists over a long period of time. The majority of individuals with PVD are diagnosed with CVI. CVI is the most common cause of leg ulcers.[55] In current literature, venous insufficiency is synonymous with venous hypertension, defining the beginning of a chain of pathophysiological events that often end in ulceration. Some authors still use the term *venous stasis ulcer* although it has been shown that blood stasis (blood pooling) is not the cause of these wounds.[56] Although it is clear that ulcerations are the result of inadequate venous circulation, the mechanism by which this happens is not clear. Research is currently focused on how skin breakdown is affected by

dysfunction of circulating white blood cells (WBCs), endothelial cell dysfunction, **fibrin** deposition, edema, and lymphatic congestion.[57,58]

The incidence of venous ulceration is much higher than that of arterial ulceration (Fig. 14.4). In fact, 80% of all leg ulcers are caused by venous disease.[54] The higher incidence is not clearly understood even though years of clinical and laboratory research have been devoted to understanding venous disease. The path from CVI to ulceration can take many turns. Aging, lack of exercise, obesity, pregnancy, long hours of standing or sitting, and heredity will predispose an individual to venous hypertension and subsequent CVI. Predictors for ulceration include the factors just listed, as well as history of deep vein thrombosis (DVT), number of pregnancies for women, family history of ulceration, and history of vigorous activity in the presence of other risk factors.[59]

Clinical Presentation

- Swelling of unilateral or bilateral LEs relieved in the early stages by elevation
- Complaints of itching, fatigue, aching, heaviness in involved limb(s)
- Skin changes including **hemosiderin staining** and **lipodermatosclerosis**
- *Fibrosis* of the dermis
- Increase in skin temperature of lower legs
- Wounds:
  - Most frequently located on the LEs: proximal to the medial malleolus although can occur anywhere (arterial wounds may also occur at this location).
  - Not significantly painful; usually complaints of minor dull leg pain are relieved with elevation.
  - Granulation tissue is usually present in the wound bed.
  - Tissue is *wet* from a typically large amount of draining *exudate*.
- Signs and symptoms of **lymphedema** may be present (it is common to see the impact of chronic inflammation and fluid overload as triggers for the onset of lymphedema).

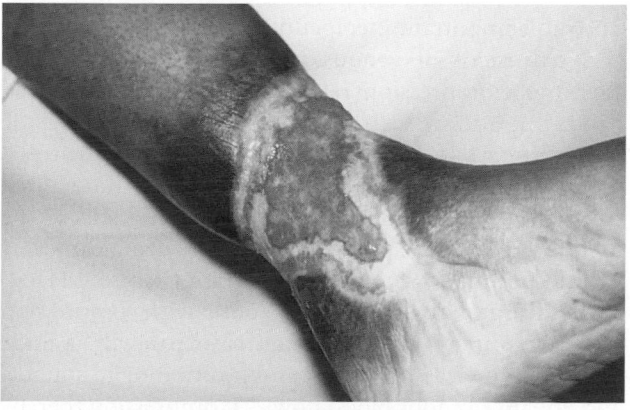

Figure 14.4 Venous insufficiency with leg ulcer.

History

Because the incidence of CVI increases with age, clinicians should be suspicious of the disease in older patients. The slow development of venous disease and ulceration usually implies a history of lingering swelling, slow healing, repeated infection, and frequent recurrence of skin breakdown. Once ulceration occurs, venous wounds can exist for years. This progression of symptoms frequently leads to a mechanical overload of the lymphatic system and subsequent development of lymphedema. If the individual is older than age 50, it is likely there are co-morbidities such as diabetes, hypertension, congestive heart failure (CHF), or history of DVT. Owing to the long latency period between injury to the venous circulation and clinical manifestations, health care providers, patients, families, and caregivers must join forces using the tools of education, prevention, and vigilance.

Tests and Measurements

One of the first tasks during the examination process is to address the possibility of an arterial component to the venous pathology. If there is arterial insufficiency, healing will be impaired and compression may be contraindicated.[54,60] Results from the ABI will give preliminary information, but more sophisticated laboratory tests may be indicated to confirm or rule out arterial disease in the individual who also has venous insufficiency. With the exception of mixed arterial and venous disease, the vascular examination results for venous insufficiency will show strong distal pulses and a normal ABI. On palpation, the skin temperature of the lower leg may be elevated. This sign can imply a worsening or impending complication of CVI.[61] The use of instrumentation to measure skin temperature can be invaluable during the examination. Existing edema may decrease with elevation unless it occurs in the advanced stages of disease or in combination with lymphedema. With venous disease, pitting edema may occur in the periwound area, the foot and ankle, or anywhere on the body. Advanced edema and lymphedema are generally unaffected by elevation and require compression as part of treatment.

Intervention

The most important therapeutic measure for prevention and treatment of venous leg ulcers is **compression therapy**. Compression refers primarily to specialized bandaging and specialized garments but can also include intermittent pneumatic compression. All of these treatment interventions will be discussed later in the chapter. Even though edema is a natural characteristic of the first phase of wound healing, excessive edema can delay wound healing by slowing perfusion of tissues and facilitating the growth of bacteria.[15] Along with compression and appropriate wound care, treatment will include exercise to increase mobility, and positioning to support and enhance venous blood flow.[55] Compression therapy

is essential for timely healing if arterial disease has been ruled out. As mentioned earlier, in a diagnosis of mixed arterial and venous disease, the more severe pathology is treated first. Significant arterial disease will most likely preclude the use of compression. For the individual with a diagnosis of venous disease or mixed (mild) arterial/venous disease, a combination of therapeutic measures will accelerate results.[62] These include compression bandaging and garments, gait training, *manual lymphatic drainage (MLD)*, and exercise, including range of motion (ROM). A wound care plan should not include whirlpool owing to the risks of dependent positioning, cross-contamination, cytotoxic additives, and unnecessary costs.

Lymphedema

Lymphedema is a chronic disorder characterized by an abnormal accumulation of lymph fluid in the tissues of one or more body regions.[2,63] The accumulation of fluid can be caused by a number of events but is most often owing to a mechanical insufficiency of the lymphatic system. This means that some components of the lymphatic system are not functioning sufficiently to manage the lymph fluid present in the body region. Lymphedema can be classified as primary or secondary lymphedema. **Primary lymphedema** (Fig. 14.5) is caused by a condition that is congenital or hereditary. With primary lymphedema, lymph node or lymph vessel formation is abnormal. The most common abnormality is *hypoplasia*, a condition in which there are fewer lymphatic vessels and they are smaller than normal. One of the more common forms of primary lymphedema appears in **Milroy's disease**. **Secondary lymphedema** (Fig. 14.6) is caused by injury to one or more components of the lymphatic system: some portion of the lymphatic system has been blocked, dissected, fibrosed, or otherwise damaged or altered.

Secondary lymphedema is more prevalent than primary. In developed countries, the most common cause

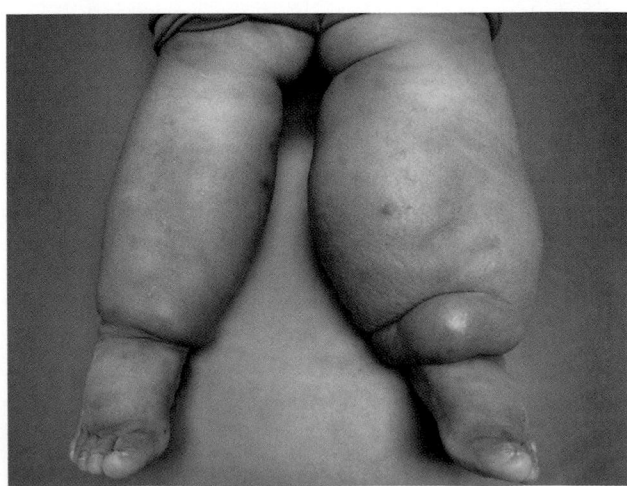

Figure 14.5 Primary lymphedema of bilateral LEs with one extremity more involved than the other.

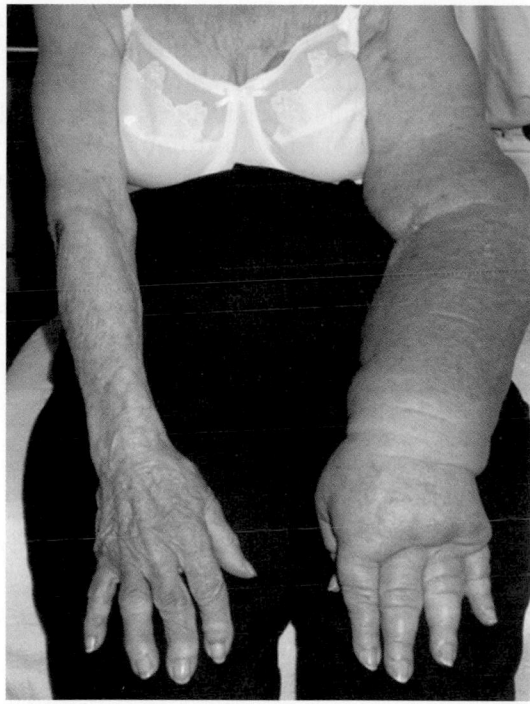

Figure 14.6 Secondary lymphedema of unilateral UE.

of secondary lymphedema is surgery and/or radiation therapy as part of breast cancer treatment. The rise in incidence of other types of cancer and the subsequent treatments for those cancers has led to an increase in reports of lymphedema following treatment for cancer of the prostate, bladder, uterus, ovaries, and skin. Cancer is not the only causative factor for lymphedema. It is common for an individual with CVI to develop lymphedema, triggered by long-standing fluid overload in the LEs.[64] Secondary lymphedema can also be triggered by the complications of paralysis, disuse in chronic regional pain syndrome, or trauma to regional lymph nodes following liposuction, pelvic fracture, hernia repair, and other surgical interventions where lymph nodes or lymph vessels are located.[65-67] Lymphedema is a common disease and health care providers can expect an increase in the number of patients rather than a decrease in this condition over the next decade.[68] The collection of data on the incidence of non–cancer-related secondary lymphedema is limited by the lack of specific education related to lymphedema among health care professionals and by a lack of clinical suspicion when examining individuals with a history of swelling. In the tropical and subtropical regions of the world, secondary lymphedema is most often caused by *filariasis*. In filariasis, nematode worm larvae live a full life cycle in the lymphatic vessels, causing inflammation and blocked lymphatic vessels.

Clinical Presentation

- Swelling distal to or adjacent to the area where lymph system function has been impaired
- Swelling usually not relieved by elevation

- Pitting edema in the early stages of disease, nonpitting edema in later stages, as fibrotic changes occur
- Feelings of fatigue, heaviness, pressure, or tightness in the affected region
- Numbness and tingling
- Discomfort varying from mild to intense
- Fibrotic changes of the dermis
- Dermal abnormalities such as **cysts, fistulas, lymphorrhea, papillomas, hyperkeratosis**
- Increased susceptibility to infection, at first local to the affected region but often becoming systemic
- Loss of mobility and ROM
- Impaired wound healing

History

A patient history consistent with lymphatic system damage or deformity will be pivotal in the diagnosis of lymphedema. A patient's history might include cancer, cancer treatment, radiation therapy, lymph node disruption, CVI, trauma, surgery, or (in primary lymphedema) onset of swelling at birth or puberty. There may be a long latency period between injury to the lymphatics and clinical manifestations; thus, health care providers and patients must adhere to prevention guidelines and be suspicious of any signs and symptoms that might suggest lymphedema. The condition can develop within a few weeks of the initial insult to the system or as long as 30 years later.

Tests and Measurements

The diagnosis of lymphedema can be made without the use of special tests for most individuals. A patient history consistent with lymph system damage or deformity, a systems review, differential diagnosis, inspection, and palpation of the integument and girth measurements are adequate for accurate diagnosis in most cases. Unique findings might include the **Stemmer's sign**, skin texture changes, skin folds, fibrosis, increase in girth, **papules**, lymph leakage, and **elephantiasis**. *Severity* is determined by a collection of data including presence of fibrotic tissue changes (brawny or woody [hardened], and/or lobular [rounded projection]); number of episodes of cellulitis; condition of the superficial integument of the lymphedematous limb (papules, leakage, fungus, venous wounds); circumference or volume differences between involved and uninvolved limbs; and quality-of-life issues (sleep, mobility, activities of daily living [ADL], relationships). A noninvasive test called **lymphscintigraphy** is a special test using radioactive tracer and a gamma camera to provide images of the lymphatic system. This test is useful for differential diagnosis and to characterize the severity of lymphedema.[68-70]

Intervention

A physical therapist should be cautious about the application of pressure to an edematous or lymphedematous body part. Although compression is an essential intervention, pressures that are too high will occlude superficial lymph capillaries and prevent the initial step of fluid absorption needed to control edema and lymphedema.[4]

Current intervention for the patient/client with lymphedema requires attention to detail and a level of expertise not often provided in entry-level professional educational programs. Practitioners are best served by gaining additional education to better prepare them to treat these patients. The current recommended course of care is a two-phase program of **complete decongestive therapy**(CDT).[71-74] Phase I (intensive) includes skin care, MLD, lymphedema bandaging, exercise, and compression garment at the *end* of Phase I. Phase II (self-management) includes skin care, compression garment during the day, exercise, lymphedema bandaging at night, and MLD as needed. A good source of information on training programs or other information on CDT, trained therapists, and patient education related to lymphedema is the National Lymphedema Network (NLN). The NLN can be reached at www.lymphnet.org.

As with many progressive, chronic disorders, the effectiveness of treatment is significantly improved by early intervention. Accurate and early diagnosis occurs when health care professionals are sensitized to the signs and symptoms and carefully evaluate the examination data. In the POC, the number and frequency of treatments should not be determined by lymphedema staging or by circumferential differences between limbs (the severity of the condition is not determined by these data alone). Some individuals with lymphedema may present with more involved signs and symptoms than the measurements imply.

Pressure Ulcers

A *pressure ulcer* is a wound caused by unrelieved pressure to the dermis and underlying vascular structures, usually between bone and support surfaces. When pressure is not relieved in time, the damage is of such magnitude that the tissues cannot repair and recover on their own. As deeper vessels are occluded, decreased blood flow leads to cell death, tissue necrosis, and finally a visible wound. The superficial dermis can tolerate *ischemia* for 2 to 8 hours before breakdown occurs. Deeper muscle, connective, and fat tissues tolerate pressures for 2 hours or less. Thus, there may be significant damage to underlying tissues while the epidermis and dermis remain intact. The clinical implications of this phenomenon are discussed below and in the section on Tests and Measurements. Readers can gain greater understanding about depth of damage to the integument by referring to Chapter 24, Burns, to view cross sections of skin, illustrating which components of the skin are lost at descending levels of damage.

Pressure ulcers occur most frequently among individuals who are immobilized for long periods of time.

Although pressure ulcers can occur at any age during prolonged periods of immobility, they are more likely to occur on individuals who are hospitalized, elderly, incontinent, and/or underweight and among individuals of all ages following spinal cord injury (SCI).[45,75-77] Up to 25% of hospital-acquired pressure ulcers may originate during surgery.[78] According to Reed et al,[79] the presence of low albumin levels, confusion, and a *Do Not Resuscitate (DNR)* order are also pressure ulcer risk factors.[79] Pressure ulcers increase the risk of death for elderly individuals whether at home or in a hospital or long-term care setting.[80] In developed countries, the incidence of chronic wounds, including pressure ulcers, is increasing as the population ages.

Clinical Presentation

The severity of pressure ulceration can be estimated by observing clinical signs. A progression from least tissue damage to most severe damage is presented here.[81] More details on the challenges of identifying pressure ulcer depth will be covered later in the chapter.

- The first clinical sign of pressure ulceration is **blanchable** *erythema* along with increased skin temperature. If pressure is relieved, tissues may recover in 24 hours. If pressure is unrelieved, nonblanchable erythema occurs.
- Progression to a superficial abrasion, blister, or shallow crater indicates involvement of the dermis.
- When full-thickness skin loss is apparent, the ulcer appears as a deep crater. Bleeding is minimal, and tissues are **indurated** and warm. Eschar formation marks full-thickness skin loss. Tunneling or undermining is often present (the official staging classification for pressure ulcers will be covered later in this chapter).
- The majority of all pressure ulcers develop over six primary bony areas (Fig. 14.7): sacrum (Fig. 14.8), coccyx, greater trochanter, ischial tuberosity, calcaneus (heel), and lateral malleolus.

History

If an individual has a history of a period of immobility followed by the discovery of a warm, red, spot over a bony prominence, a pressure ulcer can usually be confirmed. If the spot is unnaturally soft to the touch, sometimes referred to as "boggy," this is enough evidence to suspect that damage is deeper than the epidermis.

Tests and Measurements

During examination, along with general wound characteristics, pressure ulcers are classified by grading or staging systems that describe the degree of tissue damage observed. It can also be important to use a tool to measure an individual's risk of developing a pressure ulcer before a pressure ulcer exists. Refer to the section

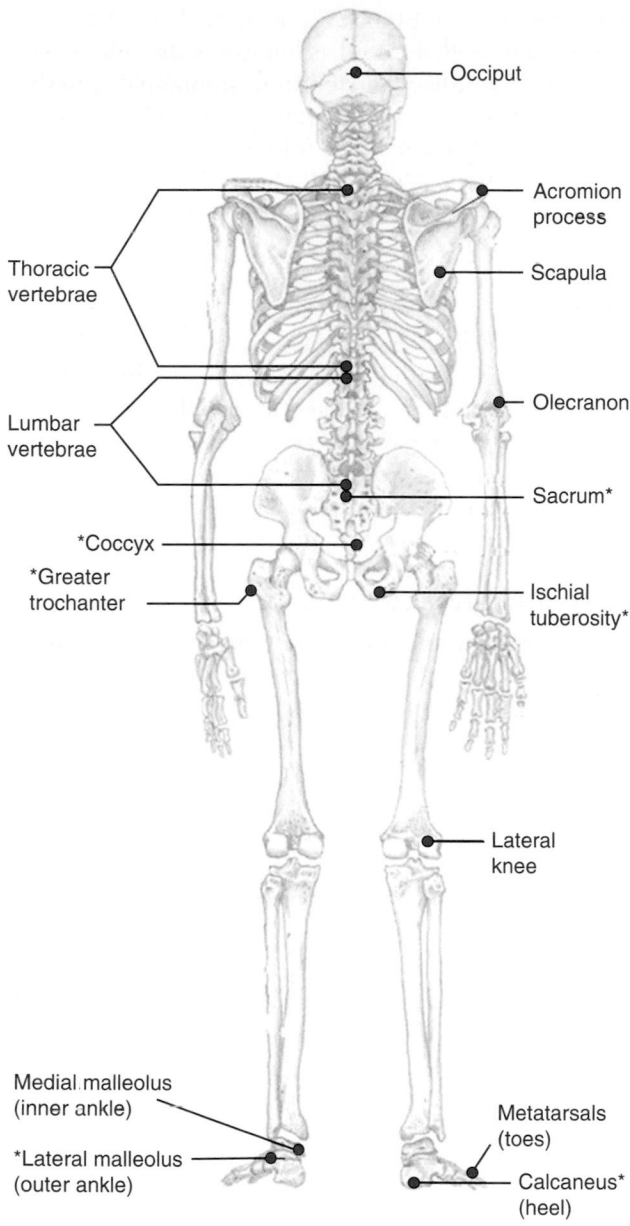

Occiput

Acromion process

Scapula

Thoracic vertebrae

Olecranon

Lumbar vertebrae

Sacrum*

*Coccyx

*Greater trochanter

Ischial tuberosity*

Lateral knee

Medial malleolus (inner ankle)

Metatarsals (toes)

*Lateral malleolus (outer ankle)

Calcaneus* (heel)

* Most common sites of pressure ulcers

Figure 14.7 Pressure points of bony prominences.

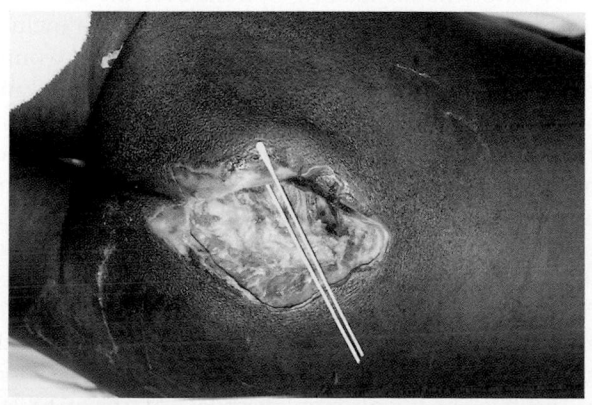

Figure 14.8 Sacral pressure ulcer. *(From Kloth, LC, and McCulloch, JM, Plate 31, with permission.)*

in this chapter on Integumentary Integrity for more information on risk assessment for pressure ulcers.

Intervention

A physical therapist treats integumentary disorders that involve the epidermis, dermis, hypodermis, or below into exposed bone, tendon, muscle, and organs. For healing to occur, intervention for disorders of the integument must facilitate local and regional homeostasis of the vascular and lymphatic systems. In addition to appropriate wound care, it is imperative that the underlying cause of pressure be addressed. Wounds will not close and remain healed unless the reduction of pressure and prevention of future breakdown are top priorities in the intervention plan. Pressure management is accomplished with the use of pressure-redistributing devices (PRDs), *pressure mapping* to determine pressure loads, *positioning/turning schedules,* and *education* of the patient, family, and caregivers. Other factors that contribute to ulceration or risk of ulceration should be considered and/or addressed. These factors include shear, friction, mobility, sensation, moisture, nutrition, age, and underlying medical condition. With appropriate wound care, control of pressure, and attention to risk factors, a wound should progress through the phases of wound healing, showing signs of improvement in a matter of weeks.[41,82,83]

Neuropathy

Neuropathy can be defined as any disease of nerves and can include peripheral nerves, cranial nerves, and/or autonomic nerves. Neuropathy exists in many disease processes; however, the most common disease process seen with neuropathy is diabetes. For most chronic diseases, including diabetes, the effects of neuropathy are peripheral. Most physical therapists treat patients with peripheral neuropathies caused by diabetes more often than any other cause. The etiology of diabetic neuropathy is not well understood but thought to be related to high levels of glucose in the blood over a long period of time. *Diabetic neuropathy* is a generic term for any diabetes mellitus–related disorder of the peripheral or autonomic nervous systems or the cranial nerves. The majority of symptoms from diabetic neuropathy will be located in the LE with foot insensitivity and subsequent ulceration being the most common (Fig. 14.9).

It is estimated that 15% of individuals with diabetes will develop a foot ulcer sometime in their life, making them almost 40 times more likely to undergo amputation because of a nonhealing wound than the nondiabetic population.[54,84] To complicate matters, many individuals with diabetes have coexisting arterial disease because the conditions are not mutually exclusive. Although the incidence is lower than for venous and arterial wounds in general, the underlying diabetic condition creates a difficult environment in which to close a wound. The incidence of neuropathic LE wounds is likely to grow as the population ages and the incidence

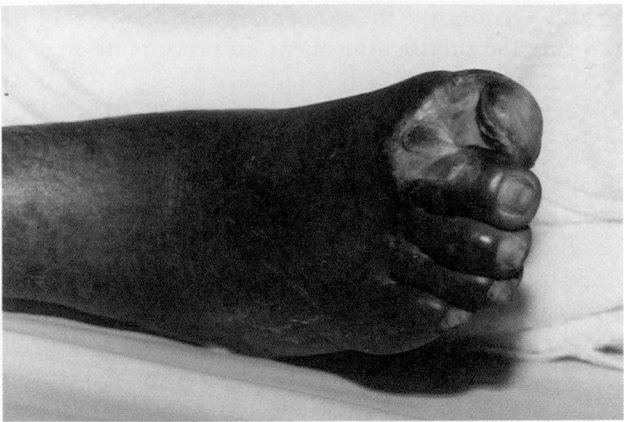

Figure 14.9 Chronic wound as a result of diabetic neuropathy.

of diabetes continues to escalate. According to the U.S. Department of Health and Human Services (HHS), someone in America is diagnosed with diabetes every 25 seconds.[85] Almost half of all adults now are at risk for the disease.[86] Based on information from the Centers for Disease Control and Prevention (CDC), diabetes affects more than 25.8 million people of all ages in the United States. This figure represents 8.3% of the population. About 60% to 70% of people with diabetes have mild to severe forms of neuropathy and more than 60% of the nontraumatic lower-limb amputations that are performed in the United States occur among people with diabetes.[87] A foot ulcer, many of which could have been prevented by appropriate team management, preceded at least half of the amputations. If current trends prevail, the impact of diabetic neuropathy on future wound care needs will continue to expand.

Clinical Presentation

- Ulceration is usually located on the weight-bearing surfaces of the foot
- Usually anesthetic, round, over bony prominences but can be located anywhere
- Sensory neuropathy, if present:
  - Patient unable to sense pain and pressure
  - Risk of skin breakdown without patient awareness
  - Mechanical, repetitive stresses are most common causative factors of wounds
- Motor neuropathy, if present:
  - Loss of intrinsic muscles
  - Hammer-toe, claw-toe deformities adding to risk of breakdown owing to poor weight distribution and rubbing from shoes
  - Foot drop
- Autonomic neuropathy, if present:
  - Decreased or absent sweat and oil production leading to dry, inelastic skin
  - Increased susceptibility to skin breakdown and injury
  - Propensity for heavy callus formation

- Dysvascular symptoms, if present:
  - Usually arterial disorders but can be complicated by reduced cardiac function from autonomic causes
  - Ischemia
  - Impaired healing time (also present owing to diabetes)
  - Impaired transport of oxygen, antibiotics, and nutrients needed for healing

History

A history of diabetes is sufficient to warrant investigation of diabetic neuropathy. If the individual has had diabetes for a number of years or has had trouble regulating insulin levels even for a few years, the presence of diabetic neuropathy is very likely. When ulceration is visible, the history will include specific details about the wound in addition to information about other symptoms.

Tests and Measurements

During the examination, every patient with diabetes should be checked, using monofilaments, for the presence of **protective sensation** in the LEs. This should be part of a systems review for patients with diabetes even when diabetes is not the primary diagnosis. Data on skin temperature of the LEs should also be recorded during the examination. Information about blood glucose levels should be obtained as part of the examination and must be considered for safe development of the POC.

Intervention

Physical therapists are in an ideal position to provide education and comprehensive foot care intervention for the diabetic population. According to the National Diabetes Fact Sheet, comprehensive foot care programs can reduce amputation rates by 45% to 85%.[87] In addition to appropriate wound care and maintenance of acceptable blood glucose levels, intervention must include some method of decreasing weight-bearing stresses. Options for off-loading include crutches or walker, changes in gait patterns, walking casts or splints, and specialized footwear. It would not be unusual to utilize all of the off-loading options over the course of treatment for foot ulceration. Intervention must include a comprehensive program including elements of wound care, foot care, education, PRDs, orthotics, exercise, and modalities. Every effort should be made by clinicians and patients alike to improve or retain skin integrity of the foot. Refer to Appendix 14.A for patient education information on foot care. In addition to other medical complications of diabetes, altered circulation to the foot can complicate symptoms from diabetic neuropathy. Intervention should address the worst problem first but with lower expectations for healing when vascular disorders coexist with neuropathy.

The five most common disorders of the vascular, lymphatic, and integumentary systems have been discussed. Disorders caused by surgery, trauma, malignancy, hematologic disease, connective tissue disease, and thermal injury *will* affect the systems discussed in this chapter. Owing to space restrictions, however, they will not be discussed at this time. Interested readers should seek one of the texts mentioned in the reference list to supplement information presented here.[1,2,42,56,63] Examination and treatment of other disorders would utilize the same tests and measurements and treatment interventions discussed in this chapter based on the patient's unique characteristics.

■ EXAMINATION AND EVALUATION

Examination

History

A thorough history will include seeking information on systems beyond the local affected area. As noted in Chapter 1, Clinical Decision Making, physical therapy examinations for all disorders begin with gathering data from the patient, family, and other involved individuals. For the disorders discussed in this chapter, information needed from the history will be similar. Many of the disorders discussed in this chapter have a slow or insidious onset, making history taking challenging but important. See Chapter 1 to review the type of data that may be generated from taking a thorough history.

Systems Review

It might be tempting to skip a systems review before using other tests and measurements in the examination process to save time. This step, however, is of utmost importance as physical therapists move toward greater autonomy. Results may alert the physical therapist to problems that may require referral to another practitioner. A systems review is particularly important here because the disorders discussed in this chapter are the result of dysfunction in other systems of the body. For example, diabetes may lead to wounds of the feet, breast cancer surgery may lead to lymphedema, heart disease may lead to arterial wounds of the legs, and paralysis may lead to pressure ulcers. A comprehensive approach to observing and examining the patient will set the stage for the investigation and data collection that follow.

Tests and Measurements

Owing to the close relationship among disorders of the vascular, lymphatic, and integumentary systems, the importance of differential diagnosis, and the likelihood of a patient or client presenting with more than one disorder, a physical therapist will make use of a wide variety of available tests and measurements during the examination. The tests and measurements discussed in this chapter are described in the order in which they are presented in the *Guide to Physical Therapist Practice*.[88] A review of the test and measurement categories themselves should serve as a reminder of the responsibility of the examining therapist to document thoroughly. For purposes of space, only the most essential categories have been addressed. An annotated version of selected tests and measurements has been included to assist the reader in greater understanding of the tests and the conditions under examination.

Aerobic Capacity/Endurance

Aerobic capacity during functional activities is important to measure since activity will be encouraged as part of long-term management of the disorders in this chapter. In addition to information obtained during the systems review, the gathering of additional data will depend on the individual patient. This might include the use of angina, claudication and dyspnea scales, pulmonary function tests, and electrocardiogram (ECG). A determination of heart rhythm sounds, as well as breath and voice sounds, may also be required.

Anthropometric Characteristics

Height and Weight Data on height and weight are necessary to address and track normal weight values, especially for the patient with a disorder that results in abnormal fluid retention such as diabetes, edema, lymphedema, venous disease, or underlying cardiopulmonary disease.

Volumetric Measurement Volumetrics are performed utilizing special containers that hold water, and a graduated cylinder for water collection (Fig. 14.10). This method is accurate for measuring changes in body dimensions with the most common measurements taken for the hand, full arm, foot, or full lower leg; however, it is time consuming, awkward to administer, and may be inappropriate when open wounds are present owing to cross-contamination risks.

Girth Measurement Girth is recorded using a tape measure to determine circumferential body dimensions (Fig. 14.11). Ideally, a tape measure specially designed to measure girth should be used. Although bony landmarks are sometimes used as reference points in taking girth measurements, the standard among experts who

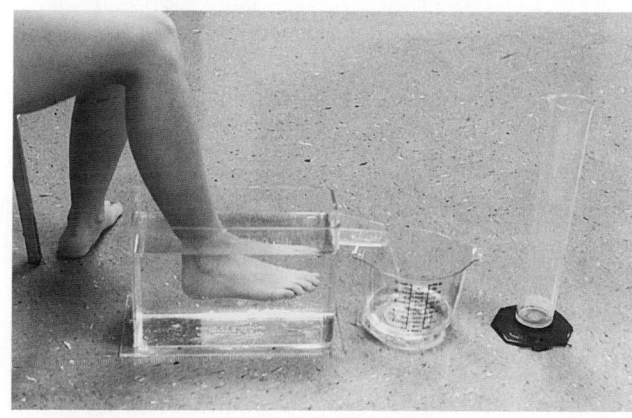

Figure 14.10 Volumetric examination for edema.

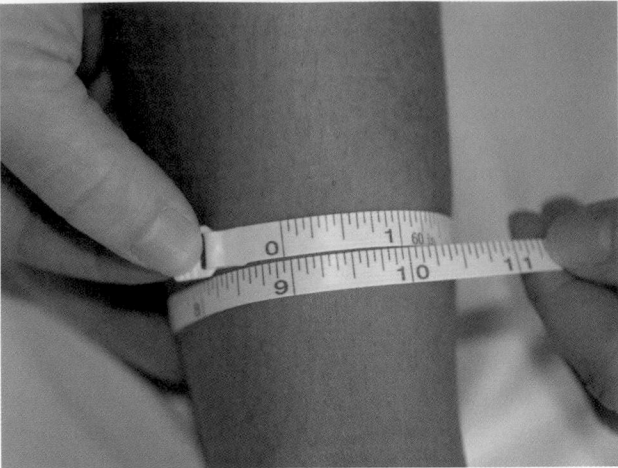

Figure 14.11 Tape measure examination for girth measurement.

treat edema is to use consistent centimeter intervals instead. For example, in measuring the LE, circumferential measurements are taken every centimeter, starting from the floor or weight-bearing surface to the groin. Clinicians choose intervals of 4, 6, or 10 cm. The smaller the interval, the better the representation of body dimensions. Special measuring boards (Fig. 14.12) can be obtained for measuring the LE, or a well-placed clipboard can be used to establish the beginning measurement. A physical therapist should remember that girth measurements by themselves should not be used to determine severity, frequency of visits, or duration of the episode of care. Advanced fibrotic changes can occur to the dermis and underlying connective tissue without a significant increase in the girth of a limb.[2,66]

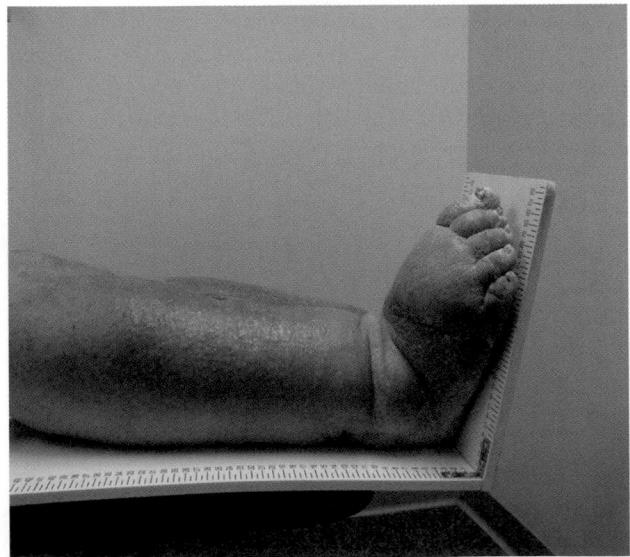

Figure 14.12 Use of footboard with ruler to establish consistent intervals for measuring lower extremity circumferences.

Additional Tools

Data on anthropometric measurements may be collected using *tonometry* or *bioelectrical impedance*. Although not a standardized procedure, soft-tissue tonometry uses a device that measures tissue tension at the surface of the skin. Less pliable skin creates a higher tension reading, suggesting the presence of fluid and/or tissue fibrosis. Data from tonometry can be useful for subclinical evidence of edema, lymphedema, and fibrotic changes before they are visible or palpable. Bioelectrical impedance analysis provides accurate measurements to help predict the onset of lymphedema, often many months before a clinical diagnosis is possible. The technique involves passing a very small amount of alternating current (AC) through the limb to be tested and measuring the impedance to its flow at various frequencies. This technique is more sensitive than limb volume measurements in detecting changes in the extracellular fluid volume. In studies thus far the false-negative rate has been zero.[89-92]

Staging or Grading of Lymphedema

In an effort to categorize levels of severity, some professionals use staging or grading systems for edema and lymphedema in addition to one or more of the measurement techniques above.[2] Grading or staging of edema and lymphedema is not universally used by health professionals and should be accompanied by objective information in the examination results. One of the more frequently used systems is the *International Society of Lymphology Staging System* as described in Foldi et al[63] and the American Cancer Society:[93]

- Preclinical: patient begins to feel "heaviness" in limb, fibrotic changes and fluid accumulation occur before visible swelling or pitting; even with minimal edema, many patients report a feeling of fullness in the extremity.
- Stage I, reversible lymphedema: accumulation of protein-rich fluid, elevation reduces swelling; pits on pressure.
- Stage II, spontaneously irreversible lymphedema: proteins stimulate fibroblast formation, connective and scar tissues proliferate; minimal pitting even with moderate swelling.
- Stage III, lymphostatic elephantiasis: hardening of dermal tissues, papillomas of the skin, appearance of skin is elephant-like.

Palpation/Pitting Scale

Palpation of soft tissues must be a regular part of vascular, lymphatic, and integumentary examinations. There is no universal pitting scale currently used by healthcare professionals. Some scales are based on how deep an indentation is left after applying fingertip pressure. Other scales are based on how severe the examiner believes the pitting to be. The following scale, most commonly used by physical therapists and physicians, gives a numerical grade to the pitting based on how long it remains after fingertip pressure is applied:

1+: Indentation is barely detectable.
2+: Slight indentation visible when skin is depressed, returns to normal in 15 seconds.
3+: Deeper indentation occurs when pressed and returns to normal within 30 seconds.
4+: Indentation lasts for more than 30 seconds.

If using a pitting scale during an examination, it is wise to document an explanation of the grades or scoring system used. Pedal edema may be attributed to chronic wounds, inflammation, infection, cellulitis, diabetes, liver disease, renal disease, CVI, lymphedema, phlebolymphedema, CHF, or trauma.

Arousal, Attention, and Cognition

After evaluating screening results during the history and systems review, the physical therapist will decide whether there is a clinical indication for tests and measurements in this category. It is important for the therapist to understand the patient's level of motivation, orientation, attention, and ability to process instructions. Many of the disorders in this chapter, such as diabetic neuropathy, chronic venous insufficiency and lymphedema, require life-long adherence to the self-care component of the treatment in order to retain the gains made during intervention. Most of this information can be obtained through interviews and observations. Additional tools would include cognitive and behavior scales, safety checklists, and learning profiles.

Assistive and Adaptive Devices

It is very likely that patients with vascular, lymphatic, or integumentary disorders will need assistive devices during the intervention and self-care phases of management. Observation, gait analysis, and manual muscle testing are often used to guide this determination.

Circulation

Collecting data about the movement of blood and lymph through the arterial, venous, and lymphatic systems is interrelated with the tests and measurements for integumentary integrity. Tests and measurements for skin changes that may occur with impairment of the circulation are discussed under the section on Integumentary Integrity. The presence or risk of pathology of the circulatory systems can be detected in many cases by skilled observation and palpation (e.g., temperature and pulses).

Temperature

To further examine circulation, skin temperature can be assessed by palpation. Objective data should also be collected and quantified using a **radiometer** or a **thermistor**, because superficial skin temperature changes are often indicative of pathology (Fig. 14.13). A decrease in skin temperature can indicate poor arterial perfusion. An increase can indicate infection or active disease processes such as cellulitis or a **Charcot joint**. An increase in temperature can also indicate a worsening or impending complication of CVI.[61]

Arterial Perfusion

The therapist collects data to determine whether adequate blood flow is reaching distal tissues. If blood flow is adequate, the oxygen supply will be adequate. Some noninvasive tests and measurements are designed to determine *blood flow* and *skin perfusion,* whereas others address *oxygen levels* in the tissues. Pulses should be palpated initially to provide information about possible vascular system involvement. The examination should include palpation of the following arteries: brachial and radial, femoral, popliteal, dorsalis pedis, and posterior tibialis. The following scale, commonly used by physical therapists and physicians, gives a numerical grade to the pulse quality:

0 = *No pulse*
1+ = *Weak* pulse, difficult to palpate
2+ = Palpable but not normal, *diminished*
3+ = *Normal,* easy to palpate
4+ = *Bounding,* very strong, may imply the possibility of an aneurysm or other pathological condition

Auscultation by stethoscope of major pulse points may identify a **bruit**. If turbulent blood flow is heard, the patient may have partial blockage of the artery. Barriers to effective pulse taking include scar tissue, edema, fibrosis, and tissue induration.

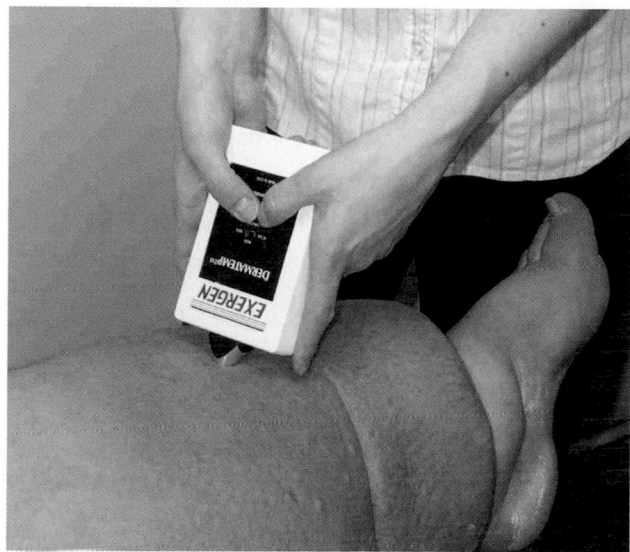

Figure 14.13 Skin temperature examination using a skin thermometer.

Doppler ultrasound is considered an essential component of the vascular examination.[53,56,94,95] The examiner uses a handheld probe to direct a sound wave into the vessel to be tested. The sound wave is reflected by red blood cells moving in the vessel. The sound wave signal is changed into audible sound that is transmitted from a small, handheld unit. The ABI is the most frequently performed test using Doppler ultrasound. A blood pressure cuff is inflated to occlude blood flow temporarily and is then deflated as the examiner listens for the return of flow. Blood flow is observed on the upper extremity (UE) at the brachial artery and on the LE at the posterior tibial and the dorsalis pedis arteries (Fig. 14.14). The ABI is a ratio of the LE pressure divided by the UE pressure. Table 14.1 presents the ranges of ABI values and potential vascular indications. Obtaining an ABI will provide useful information about the arterial system since the ABI is an indicator of loss of perfusion in the LE. Results will guide the therapist in decisions about the use of compression and débridement, and will help predict the likelihood of wound closure. When the examiner cannot occlude blood flow with the blood pressure cuff, calculations may show a falsely elevated ABI. Arteriosclerosis or calcified vessels (from diabetes) can make it difficult for the cuff to compress enough to get an accurate ABI. The target arteries would be documented as *noncompressible vessels*. Test options when the vessels are noncompressible include taking toe pressures with a special cuff, proceeding with transcutaneous oxygen testing (see below), or recommending referral for a vascular laboratory workup.

Trophic Changes

Trophic changes occur in the skin of the LEs when circulation is impaired by poor arterial blood flow. Observation is the most accurate way to note changes. Trophic changes include dry, shiny skin (pale in Caucasians), decreased or absent leg hair, and thick toenails. It should be noted that these signs are also a predictable part of aging but not to the same degree as can be seen with trophic changes. The presence of changes indicates the need for other tests of circulation.

Pain

When related to circulation, a thorough pain history may be all that is necessary to suggest the possibility of arterial disease. Reports of pain indicate the need for further tests and measurements of the vascular system. Pain as the result of intermittent claudication (IC) is described earlier in this chapter. Rest pain that develops at night, awakens the patient, or requires analgesics for relief is considered more severe than IC. Pain can be measured for severity on a Visual Analog Scale (VAS). The degree of impairment from IC is often measured in terms of how far an individual can walk before experiencing acute leg pain or fatigue. IC can be classified objectively with a rating scale to indicate severity based on distance walked before onset of pain. The *Walking Impairment Questionnaire (WIQ)* is a disease-specific questionnaire commonly used to examine claudication. It does not, however, measure the impact of claudication on quality of life (QOL).[96] The most extensively researched disease-specific QOL questionnaire for IC is the *Claudication Scale (CLAU-S)*.[96-98]

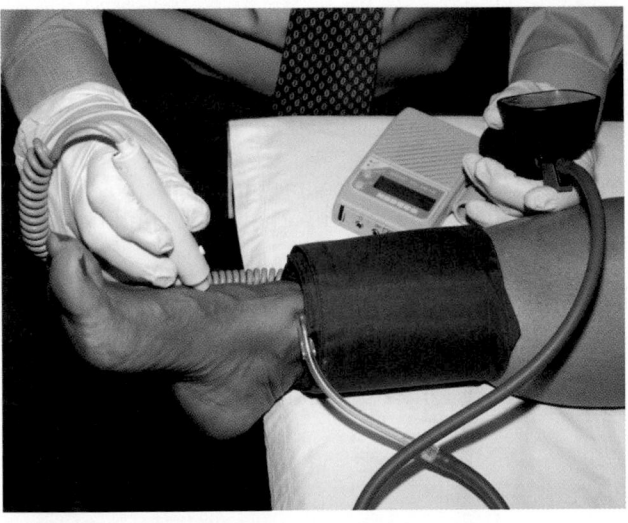

Figure 14.14 ABI test performed using Doppler ultrasound probe. *(From McCulloch and Kloth: Wound Healing: Evidence-Based Management, ed 4. FA Davis, Philadelphia, Figure 7-3, with permission.)*

Special Tests

There are many other noninvasive and invasive tests used to detect, examine, diagnose, or confirm arterial disease and dysfunction. Appendix 14.B presents a brief description of special tests for arterial and venous function including *rubor of dependency, air plethysmography (APG), transcutaneous oxygen (TcPO$_2$)* measurement, and *skin perfusion pressure (SPP)* measurement. Although some of the tests are useful for predicting healing of ulcers and amputation wounds, they may not be readily reimbursed when performed by a physical therapist.

Table 14.1	Ankle-Brachial Indices with Corresponding Indications
ABI Ranges	**Possible Indication**
>1.2	Falsely elevated, arterial disease, diabetes
1.19–0.95	Normal
0.94–0.75	Mild arterial disease, + intermittent claudication
0.74–0.50	Moderate arterial disease, + rest pain
<0.50	Severe arterial disease

The APG, TcPO$_2$, and SPP are used primarily for research purposes because they are time consuming to perform.

Venous Patency

Venous disease and dysfunction can be detected with a wide range of tests and measurements. The amount of time available for examination, as well as reimbursement issues, may influence decisions about which tests to use. Refer to Appendix 14.B for a brief description of *Venous Filling Time, Percussion Test,* and the *Trendelenburg Test.* Owing to inconsistencies in interpretation and administration, the *Homans' Test,* or Homans' sign (pain in the calf when the foot is passively dorsiflexed), should not be relied on to detect a DVT. A physician should be contacted and a Doppler study used if an individual exhibits two of the following signs: change in skin temperature, change in skin color (darker), pain in the calf (experienced by approximately half of patients), or swelling.

Lymph Vessel Integrity

Patient history and clinical findings are used most often to make a diagnosis of lymphedema. Most invasive tests have lost popularity because of the risk of triggering the onset of lymphedema or an exacerbation of existing lymphedema owing to the irritation caused by dye and/or needle puncture. When invasive tests are indicated, the most common test procedure is *lymphoscintigraphy.* This test, using dye and a special camera and computer, can visualize many lymphatic system functions.[2,99]

Gait, Locomotion, and Balance

The importance of movement to improve blood and lymphatic flow, and to facilitate the overall return to function for most individuals, will validate the use of tests and measurements to document patient abilities in this area. During the initial examination, gathering data through observation, gait analysis, and postural control tests is usually adequate. The examination results may indicate the need for additional tests such as inventories, or batteries of tests to further document safety (fall risk) or equipment needs. Individuals who are morbidly obese have unique challenges with gait that should be addressed during the examination.

Integumentary Integrity

Collection of data about skin and subcutaneous tissues is interrelated with the tests and measurements for circulation and cutaneous sensation.

Observation and Palpation

Characteristics of the skin are noted almost entirely by observation and palpation. A comparison between involved and normal integument is made with careful attention to color, moisture, texture, firmness, temperature, elasticity, symmetry, and shape. In the presence of a wound, the wound tissue, the periwound area, and the wound exudate should all be observed and data recorded regarding the observations. The location of a wound, presence of edema, and presence of lymphedema can be documented using a *body diagram.*

Trophic Changes

Because they are an important part of many disorders involving the integument, trophic changes are mentioned again under this section. Individuals who are making a quick reference specifically to integumentary integrity in this chapter are reminded to refer to all sections related to trophic changes. As in the section on circulation, observation is an important approach to noting changes.

Fibrosis

The best way to detect fibrotic changes of the skin is through palpation of the affected tissue. The superficial skin and underlying tissue will feel thickened, firm, and unyielding or immobile. Testing for the presence or absence of the *Stemmer's sign* is an objective measurement that can be added to the examination for lymphedema. When the dorsal skin folds of the toes or fingers are resistant to lifting or cannot be lifted at all, the Stemmer's sign is said to be "present." The clinician must be cautious, however, because a negative or "absent" skin fold test does not rule out lymphedema.

Coloration

Skin color will vary based on the underlying disease. Observation is the best way to note comparisons between normal tissues and those under examination. The most abnormal color changes include red, purple, and brown. Color changes may indicate a chronic condition such as hemosiderin staining or an acute situation such as redness associated with DVT. If color changes are intermittent they may signal a disease such as **Raynaud's.**

Temperature

The temperature of the skin is most often examined by palpation but data can be objectively collected and quantified using a radiometer or a thermistor (see Fig. 14.13). Maintenance of normal skin temperatures is essential for good wound healing. Abnormal skin temperatures can signal problems related to the dermis or other structures. A decrease in superficial skin temperature may indicate poor arterial perfusion. An increase may indicate infection or active disease processes.

Wounds
Size and Depth

A number of tools and scales are available for gathering data about wounds, edema, lymphedema, and other aspects of integumentary integrity. Wounds not classified with staging or grading can be described based on the depth of tissue damage. The descriptions used for depth of burn injury, *superficial, partial,* and *full thickness,* can also be used to describe depth in other types of wounds. Objective measures included in documentation are vital for communication about the patient. A calibrated grid, photographs, tracings, graphs, and specifically designed forms are most commonly used to document wound size and depth.

Drainage

Drainage is measured by observation and is often described in terms of color and thickness. Examination of wound drainage may be very important because it may indicate a normal response to trauma (few days) or a prolonged response to necrotic tissue, a foreign substance in the wound, or infection. The most common language for describing wound drainage is described in Table 14.2.

Staging

Pressure ulcers are typically classified using a *staging* or *grading* system that gives information about the severity of the wound based on depth of tissue destruction. Both the National Pressure Ulcer Advisory Panel (NPUAP) and the Agency for Health Care Research and Quality (AHRQ) support the use of the universal classification system described in Table 14.3.[100,101]

Despite some standardization and acceptance by some government agencies, staging of pressure ulcers is controversial among wound management experts because it is often misused. The misuse most often occurs because the staging system describes only the depth of tissue destruction and not other characteristics of the wound that need to be considered. Treatment plans should not be based solely on the staging system. Staging can be challenging because tissue damage may be deeper than what appears on the surface, wounds cannot be staged when necrotic tissue is present, and darker skin does not always show the reddened alterations indicating Stage I. The NPUAP has redefined the definition of a pressure ulcer and the stages of pressure ulcers to address the challenges of staging. The staging descriptions are intended for use with pressure ulcers and not to describe the severity of other wound types.

Wound Healing Tools

A variety of tools can be utilized to document wound status and wound healing. Since there is no single wound characteristic that can be used alone to monitor healing or predict outcomes, it is best to use a tool that includes multiple characteristics as measures of wound healing. The three tools with the most well-established reliability and validity are the *Sussman Wound Healing Tool (SWHT)*,[43] the *Pressure Ulcer Scale for Healing (PUSH)*,[43,102] and the *Pressure Sore Status Tool (PSST)*.[43] The *Wagner Ulcer Grade Classification* system is a tool designed for examination of the diabetic foot when neuropathy and ischemia are present.[103]

Risk Factor Assessment

Although all individuals may be subjected to the same intensities of pressure for similar amounts of time, they all will not develop pressure ulcers. As a result, factors related to individual risk, susceptibility, or tolerance capacity should be determined. A physical therapist will find that data from a risk assessment can be helpful in planning cost-effective intervention strategies. As discussed earlier in the chapter, there are many factors that put individuals at risk for developing pressure ulcers, such as poor peripheral circulation, diabetes, nutritional status, mobility, and continence issues, to name a few. To objectify and standardize risk assessment, a number of reliable tools have been validated by research:

- *Norton Risk Assessment Scale*: original risk assessment instrument scores individuals on physical condition, mental condition, activity, mobility, and incontinence.[104]
- *Gosnell Scale–Pressure Sore Risk Assessment*: refinement of Norton's scale includes changes to the following scoring categories: nutrition, mental condition, activity, mobility, continence, skin appearance, medication, diet, and fluid balance.[105]
- *Braden Scale for Predicting Pressure Sore Risk*: the six scoring categories of this instrument include sensory perception, moisture, activity, mobility, nutrition, and friction/shear.[106]

Table 14.2 Descriptions of Drainage by Color and Thickness		
Drainage Type	Color	Thickness
Transudate	Clear	Thin, watery
Serosanguineous	Clear or tinge of red/brown	Thin, watery
Exudate	Creamy, yellowish	Moderate to very thick, expected with autolytic debridement
Pus	Yellow, brown	Moderate to very thick
Infected pus	Hues of yellow, blue, green	Thick, usually indicates infection (but may be normal as white blood cells macrophage necrotic cells and turn them into slough); drainage can be foul and yet the wound may not be infected

Table 14.3 Pressure Ulcer Staging Criteria Revised by NPUAP

Pressure Ulcer Stage	Definition
Suspected Deep Tissue Injury Further description	Purple or maroon localized area of discolored intact skin or blood-filled blister due to damage of underlying soft tissue from pressure and/or shear. The area may be preceded by tissue that is painful, firm, mushy, boggy, warmer, or cooler as compared to adjacent tissue.
	Deep tissue injury may be difficult to detect in individuals with dark skin tones. Evolution may include a thin blister over a dark wound bed. The wound may further evolve and become covered by thin eschar. Evolution may be rapid, exposing additional layers of tissue even with optimal treatment.
Stage I Further description	Intact skin with nonblanchable redness of a localized area usually over a bony prominence. Darkly pigmented skin may not have visible blanching; its color may differ from the surrounding area.
	The area may be painful, firm, soft, warmer, or cooler as compared to adjacent tissue. Stage I may be difficult to detect in individuals with dark skin tones. May indicate "at risk" persons (a heralding sign of risk).
Stage II Further description	Partial-thickness skin loss of dermis presenting as a shallow open ulcer with a red pink wound bed, without slough. May also present as an intact or open/ruptured serum-filled blister.
	Presents as a shiny or dry shallow ulcer without slough or bruising. (Bruising indicates suspected deep tissue injury.) This stage should not be used to describe skin tears, tape burns, perineal dermatitis, maceration, or excoriation.
Stage III Further description	Full-thickness tissue loss. Subcutaneous fat may be visible but bone, tendon, and muscle are not exposed. Slough may be present but does not obscure the depth of tissue loss. May include undermining and tunneling.
	The depth of a Stage III pressure ulcer varies by anatomical location. The bridge of the nose, ear, occiput, and malleoli do not have subcutaneous tissue and Stage III ulcers can be shallow. In contrast, areas of significant adiposity can develop extremely deep Stage III pressure ulcers. Bone/tendon is not visible or directly palpable.
Stage IV Further description	Full-thickness tissue loss with exposed bone, tendon, or muscle. Slough or eschar may be present on some parts of the wound bed. Often include undermining and tunneling.
	The depth of a Stage IV pressure ulcer varies by anatomical location. The bridge of the nose, ear, occiput, and malleoli do not have subcutaneous tissue and these ulcers can be shallow. Stage IV ulcers can extend into muscle and/or supporting structures (e.g., fascia, tendon, or joint capsule) making osteomyelitis possible. Exposed bone/tendon is visible or directly palpable.
Unstageable Further description	Full-thickness tissue loss in which the base of the ulcer is covered by slough (yellow, tan, gray, green, or brown) and/or eschar (tan, brown, or black) in the wound.
	Until enough slough and/or eschar is removed to expose the base of the wound, the true depth, and therefore stage, cannot be determined. Stable (dry, adherent, intact without erythema or fluctuance) eschar on the heels serves as "the body's natural (biological) cover" and should not be removed.

Staging should not be used in reverse order (also called back-staging or down-staging). The staging system is not a measure of healing. A Stage IV ulcer is always a Stage IV. If it is healed, it would be referred to as a healed Stage IV, not a Stage 0.
Used with permission of the National Pressure Ulcer Advisory Panel 2/2011. The permission granted through this process cannot be transferred to others or used for other purposes than expressed above and approved by the NPUAP.
© NPUAP. For more information, contact www.npuap.org.

Muscle Performance

Muscle strength screening during the systems review and specific manual muscle testing during the examination should be included for the individual with a disorder of the vascular, lymphatic, or integumentary system. Functional muscle strength identified during an examination of functional mobility skills and ADL is also important. Lack of strength and immobility go hand in hand, often leading to problems such as pressure ulcers, CVI, increased LE edema and lymphedema, varicosities, and poor control of diabetic sequelae.

Orthotic, Protective, and Supportive Devices

There are many situations in which an individual with disorders from this chapter would need to be assessed for an orthotic, protective, or supportive device. Those individuals already using a device may need a modification. For the individual with impaired sensation of the feet, *extra-depth* shoes may be indicated. Existing shoes should be checked periodically for fit and wear. A referral to another professional for protective footwear may be needed. Supportive devices may allow an individual to increase his or her activity level, offsetting the risks of a sedentary lifestyle. Compression garments and bandaging, considered *supportive devices,* must be checked periodically for fit and function to ensure that they retain their effectiveness. Garments and bandages will be essential intervention choices for most individuals with edema and lymphedema. In the later stages, a patient's need for devices may provide a way to quantify the remediation of impairments or activity limitations imposed by the symptoms of the disorder.

Pain

The presence or absence of pain, its location and intensity, its effect on sleep, and other QOL factors should be measured (see Chapter 25, Chronic Pain). Pain scales, drawings, and maps are effective for documentation. Owing to the high incidence of co-morbidity in patients with disorders of the vascular, lymphatic, and integumentary systems, the measurement of pain may also assist in making a differential diagnosis.

Posture

Indications for examination of posture include pain, heavy or large limbs, scar tissue, poor body image (e.g., following cancer treatment), obesity, and decreased sensation. Data can be obtained with the combined use of a posture grid, tape measure, observation, and palpation. A physical therapist will begin a posture assessment initially by observation the moment the client enters the room, and will continue to assess and observe posture formally and informally during the examination and intervention.

Range of Motion

The need for adequate ROM and the impact of decreased ROM cannot be underestimated. Following ROM screening during the systems review, specific ROM measurements are often indicated, especially with persons for whom movement is an essential part of symptom management. Examples are numerous but include ankle ROM for the person with CVI, shoulder ROM following breast cancer surgery, or knee ROM in the individual with lymphedema of the LE. A universal goniometer and a tape measure are required to obtain objective ROM data.

Self-Care and Home Management

Activity limitations and disability are common with disorders of the vascular, lymphatic, and integumentary systems. Examination, education, and training that allow the patient to safely perform self-care and home management activities are of great importance in planning and implementing the self-management phase. Descriptions and quantifications are needed for documentation and goal setting. Examination tools should include functional measures of both basic activities of daily living (BADL) and instrumental activities of daily living (IADL), as well as fall risk scales (see Chapter 8, Examination of Function).

Sensation

Information from the history and systems review may indicate the need for a detailed examination of sensory function. Therapists should not rely on history alone as an indication for sensory testing, however, because many individuals are unaware of their deficits until tested. Sensory tests are particularly important when symptoms are long-standing, or include complaints of numbness, tingling, or burning. Patients who should routinely be tested are those who may receive LE compression treatments, and all individuals who have a diagnosis of peripheral neuropathy, diabetes, and/or arterial disease. In addition to observation and palpation, initial tests should include testing for protective sensation using filaments such as the *Semmes-Weinstein monofilaments.* The filaments are supplied in varying sizes and are each mounted on a handle. The filament is applied to the skin until it bends. The patient is asked to report, with eyes closed, whether the filament is touching the body part. Each monofilament supplies a specific amount of force when it is placed on the test area and gently bent. The monofilaments are available in a large set but most testing can be accomplished using a few filaments. An individual has *normal sensation* when the 4.17 monofilament (1 g of force) can be felt. An individual has *protective sensation* intact when the 5.07 filament (10 g of force) can be felt (Fig. 14.15). With loss of protective sensation, the individual cannot sense trauma to the foot, often leading to foot ulceration. For the individual who has lost protective sensation, the use of special protective footwear is indicated. Lack of sensation, especially protective sensation, can be a characteristic of long-standing diabetes. Decreased sensation

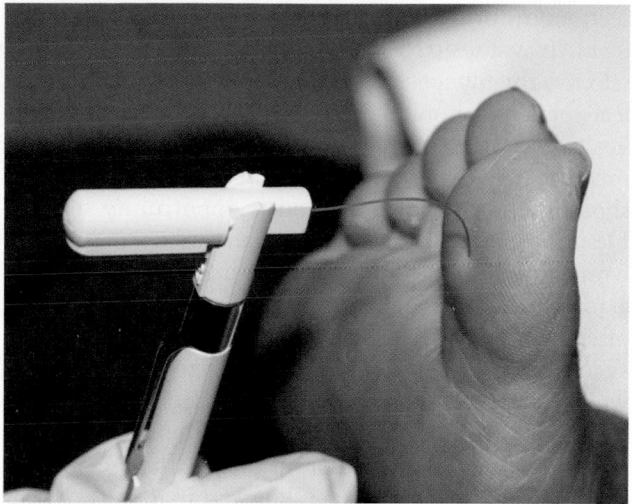

Figure 14.15 Semmes-Weinstein monofilament used to assess presence of protective sensation. Bowing of the filament indicates that appropriate pressure has been applied. *(From McCulloch and Kloth: Wound Healing: Evidence-Based Management, ed 4. FA Davis, Philadelphia, Figure 7-6, with permission.)*

may signal a disorder such as **scleroderma**. To test for sharp/dull sensation, vibratory sensation, pressure, and other sensations, tools for gathering data include a pressure scale, tuning fork, and/or aesthesiometer. Additional information can be obtained in this textbook (see Chapter 3, Examination of Sensory Function).

Ventilation and Respiration

Tests and measures should be used to determine if the patient has adequate ventilation and respiration to meet normal oxygen demands. The presence of pathology might be indicated from a predictable source such as breath sounds or the color of nail beds. A less predictable sign, such as swelling around the ankles, could also indicate pathology. Initial data may be gathered by examining arterial blood gases, observing the work of breathing, or utilizing a spirometer. Additional appropriate tests include the airway clearance test and use of a pulse oximeter (see Chapter 12, Chronic Pulmonary Dysfunction).

Evaluation

Diagnosis, Prognosis, and Plan of Care

Once the examination is complete, the physical therapist evaluates the data and determines the diagnosis and prognosis. The physical therapist needs to consider a number of factors including clinical findings, overall physical function and health status, social support, multisystem involvement and co-morbid conditions, and chronicity, severity, and stability of the condition. This information is outlined in the *Guide to Physical Therapist Practice*[88] and presented in this textbook (see Chapter 1, Clinical Decision Making). The next step is the design and

implementation of the POC, including procedural interventions.

■ INTERVENTION

Physical therapist intervention for disorders of the vascular, lymphatic, and/or integumentary systems should include a variety of techniques to address the problems identified during the examination. It is common for patients with disorders in these systems to present with multiple factors contributing to the primary diagnosis. The intervention plan should reflect a holistic view of the patient. For example, an individual with signs and symptoms of venous disease may also present with poor ankle ROM, an LE wound, and lymphedema. The wound must be cleansed and dressed but the limb should also receive compression for optimum healing. Ankle ROM must be improved because ambulation will enhance calf pump function. Another example of the need to view patients holistically would be an individual with signs and symptoms of arterial disease who also presents with decreased LE strength, diabetes, and peripheral neuropathy. Exercise is important for this person, but it must be carefully coordinated to address arterial health, diabetes management, and skin protection.

A natural component of viewing patients holistically is to be able to identify the need for interdisciplinary care. This concept may be more important for individuals with disorders of the vascular, lymphatic, or integumentary systems for the very reasons listed in the previous paragraph: these populations present with complicated, multisystem problems that are often best addressed using a team approach. Integrated care facilitates an exchange of information among all the health professionals that are involved in the care of the patient. This model of care might be delivered by a team of individuals who work together every day or it might be coordinated by a physical therapist who pulls together certain professionals for a particular patient's needs.

Coordination, Communication, and Documentation

In keeping with practice standards, the physical therapist coordinates intervention efforts to ensure the patient receives the highest quality of care. Critical to this goal is open communication among the health care team, patient, family, and caregivers. The team will most likely include a physician, nurse, physical therapist, occupational therapist, dietitian, and social worker. Referrals to other health care professionals (e.g., podiatrist) who can support the patient can also be made. Meticulous documentation will have a significant impact on issues such as continuity of care, receiving adequate number of visits for procedures, and a stronger working relationship with referring practitioners. Photographs, special forms for data collection, and body graphs are very effective tools to enhance communication and documentation. Appendix 14.C provides an example of an examination form that might be used to document data collected for a patient with a disorder of the vascular, lymphatic, or integumentary system.

Patient/Client-Related Instruction

Disorders of the vascular, lymphatic, and integumentary systems represent major health events for patients and their families and require life-long management strategies. Patients and families often react with anger, despair, or at least confusion when learning about a condition that may be permanent. The value of patient and family education cannot be underestimated. Patient education will be the key to preparing individuals to manage their symptoms, prevent recurrence, and remain vigilant about their condition. Information should be provided that is appropriate to the patient/family/caregiver's educational level with provisions for follow-up and repetition. Motivational strategies are important to ensure adherence to self-management. For many chronic disorders, high-quality patient education has been shown to result in positive changes in health behaviors, QOL perceptions, and adherence to home programs. Instruction for the patient should include resources, education materials, and a home program.

- Resources
  - Community services and support groups related to the patient's diagnosis
  - Counseling services, as needed, especially for assistance with QOL issues
  - Internet sites (Appendix 14.D lists Web-based resources for clinicians, families, and patients with vascular, lymphatic, and integumentary disorders)
  - Family member participation in care
- Education materials
  - Instructional materials, multimedia tools
  - Self-management strategies
  - Available resources include *Wound Care* by Sussman[107] and *Living Well with Lymphedema* by Ehrlich, Vinje-Harrewijn, and McMahon[108]
- Home program
  - Skin and/or wound care; prevention practices; scar management
  - Compression garment or bandage wear and care
  - Exercise
  - Edema control
  - Pressure-redistributing devices
  - Foot care for patients with diabetes (see Appendix 14.A for a foot care guide)

Outpatient or home therapy may be required for some patients. Follow-up visits at regularly scheduled intervals may be the best way to facilitate adherence to the home program and to prevent recurrence or exacerbation of symptoms.

Procedural Interventions

This section has been organized in the order in which a physical therapist would provide patient care. Within each section, information has been organized from most invasive/least selective (nonspecific) to least invasive/most selective (highly specific). In developing the POC, a physical therapist should select interventions that are least invasive/most selective, always trying to create an environment that is conducive to healing. The ultimate goal should be to optimize the body's opportunity to heal. Despite tremendous gains in the management of vascular, lymphatic, and integumentary disorders, there are still an alarming number of practitioners using outdated and often harmful methods to treat these disorders. Overused agents such as povidone-iodine, wet-to-dry dressings, whirlpool, and compression pumps have been replaced for at least a decade with more advanced, biocompatible, and cost-effective methods of treatment. The use of inappropriate agents can delay healing and may cause harm. Supporting literature abounds for the clinician seeking evidence-based practice. Elements of skin and wound care that are often overlooked or underestimated for their impact include PRDs, positioning, exercise, patient education, compression, and orthotics.

The therapist treating a patient with a wound should strive to establish an ideal wound environment. The choices made about intervention should be guided by the goal of achieving this ideal environment, described as moist, free from necrotic tissue, free from exudate, warm, protected from trauma, and protected from infection. Physical therapists may manage wound care in a primary care role, or in consultation with a physician and/or other providers. Interventions involving pharmaceuticals will always require physician consultation for a prescription. "Although practice may change based on new evidence, the search for healing in the most humane way and fastest time possible persists as the goal."[109, p. S1]

Cleansing

Wound cleansing is differentiated from wound débridement, which follows in the next section. The wound cleansing method should be selected based on its ability to support or return a wound bed to homeostasis. Chemical and mechanical trauma should be minimized even in the presence of infection. A decision to cleanse should be made carefully, because many wounds do not need to be cleansed at every dressing change. Often the negative effects to the wound from cleansing outweigh the positives. Not only is there a potential loss of endogenous fluids from the wound surface but also there is significant slowing of cellular activity for up to 3 hours after wound cleansing.[110]

Whirlpool

Since whirlpool can be classified as a means of cleansing and mechanical débridement, it is discussed in both categories of intervention. Despite at least a decade of investigation, with little evidence to support its use, whirlpool is still used for both nonselective mechanical débridement and for wound cleansing. However, many clinicians involved in wound care have decreased their use of whirlpool significantly in response to the evolution of wound care and subsequent publication of the Agency for Health Care Research and Quality (AHRQ) guidelines. Standards have changed with the increased knowledge of the microenvironment in the wound bed and a greater understanding of the chemical mediators necessary for homeostasis.

The historical rationale for use of whirlpool was based on its use in deodorization, skin and wound cleansing, mechanical nonselective débridement, wound decontamination and infection control, and softening adherent necrotic tissue in preparation for débridement. There is little evidence to support whirlpool as the *optimal* method for achieving these. If using whirlpool for an infected wound, the AHRQ recommends that whirlpool be discontinued when the ulcer is clean. First issued in 1994, the guidelines are considered to still be current.[101] The guidelines include more than 300 references, bibliographic sources, and updates that can be easily obtained.[111]

Evidence-based rationale for a decrease in the use of whirlpool is based on a number of factors. There is risk of contamination from waterborne pathogens and from patient cross-contamination. The dependent position can initiate or increase venous congestion and extremity edema. With whirlpool there is loss of endogenous fluids from the wound bed and heat loss affecting core body temperature and the local wound area. Even mild changes in core body temperature (hypothermia) have negative effects on the cells that are important to wound healing. In addition, mechanical disruption of granulation tissue, epithelial cells, and new skin grafts occurs, primarily from the use of water agitation. Immersion in a whirlpool saturates wound tissue and surrounding skin, creating the potential for maceration, skin breakdown, and temporary inactivation of normal skin defenses. Thus, there is the potential to prolong inflammation and delay wound healing. Whirlpool can also increase heart and respiratory rates. Finally, the use of whirlpool is labor intensive and costly in terms of use of water, utilities, linen, and staff.[3,112-116]

Based on current standards of care and guidance from the literature, it may be possible to justify the use of whirlpool in some situations. Wounds that need intensive cleansing that cannot be accomplished with other methods might benefit from whirlpool. Minimal agitation of water is recommended with only small body areas treated for short amounts of time (5 to 10 minutes) to limit the negative effects of temperature and pressure changes. Unless infection is confirmed with tissue culture, cytotoxic agents in the water should be avoided (e.g., povidone-iodine, chlorine). Wounds that need softening of loosely adherent tissue before sharp, enzymatic, or autolytic débridement might benefit from whirlpool when other tissue-softening methods are not appropriate. (**Note:** there is little to no reimbursement for the use of whirlpool to soften tissue before débridement.) Wounds that would benefit from stimulation of peripheral circulation might benefit from whirlpool. Neutral warmth or normothermia (normal body temperature, 98.6°F [37°C]) is recommended.

Pulsatile Lavage with Suction

Pulsatile lavage with suction (*PLWS,* also referred to as *forceful irrigation*) is a method of wound irrigation combined with suction (Fig. 14.16).[117] Pulsed irrigation and simultaneous suction removes the irrigation fluid, wound exudate, and loose debris. In use for over 20 years, this wound cleansing and débridement method has several advantages over whirlpool cleansing. PLWS uses less water, less staff support, and less treatment time and requires less cleanup time. PLWS can be performed bedside and in the home. (**Note:** family or visitors are not allowed in the room during the procedure owing to aerosolization of microorganisms.)[118] This type of cleansing collects wound exudate and debris efficiently and delivers topical antibiotics, antiseptics, and antibacterial solutions efficiently. PLWS speeds healing by rapid removal of contaminants and treats tunneling wounds and undermining wounds using special cannula tips. Risk of periwound maceration and cross-contamination is eliminated with use of disposable equipment.

Although the advantages are clear, there are disadvantages to using PLWS. These include risk of overuse, especially with clean, granulating wounds, and risk of trauma to newly formed tissue from plastic tips, pulsed irrigant, and/or suction. Treatment may be painful to the patient. PLWS use should be limited to experienced therapists who are well versed in anatomy, especially when irrigating tracts, areas of undermining, or exposed bone, tendon, blood vessels, cavity linings, grafts, or flaps. All staff involved in treatment must wear disposable personal protective equipment (PPE).

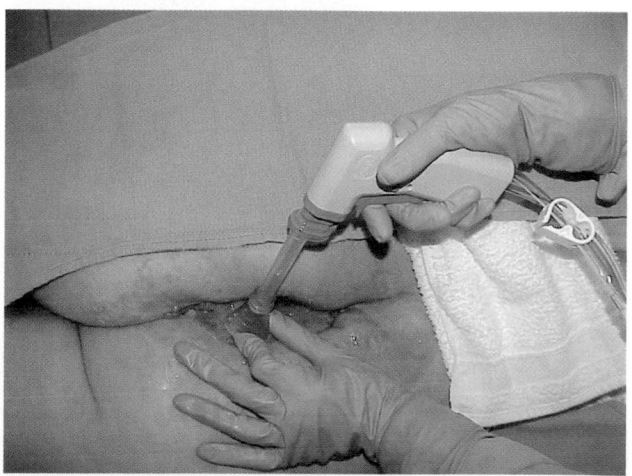

Figure 14.16 Physical therapist's fingers mold PLWS shield to sacral wound surface. *(From Kloth, LC, and McCulloch, JM, p 221, with permission.)*

Compared to other irrigation options, disposable, single-use equipment contributes to landfill burden. There is considerable cost when labor, PPE, and equipment are calculated.

Nonforceful Irrigation

As soon as possible, wound cleansing should be accomplished with minimal pressure or force on the wound bed by nonforceful irrigation. This can be accomplished by pouring a solution over a wound, or using a bulb syringe or other device designed to deliver an irrigant to the wound (Fig. 14.17). There are several products that package saline specifically for wound cleansing: Blairex® Wound Wash Saline, manufactured by Blairex Laboratories, Inc., Columbus, IN 47202; and Saljet®, single-dose sterile saline manufactured by Winchester Laboratories, LLC, St. Charles, IL 60174. Several manufacturers produce a spray container that delivers saline or a surfactant at very gentle pressures (Fig. 14.18). Infected wounds can also be effectively cleaned with nonforceful irrigation. Wounds with necrotic tissue or debris, however, may respond best to a few sessions of a more forceful type of cleansing. For wounds that are clean, with new tissue growth, cleansing should be done only to remove excess endogenous fluids or residue left by dressing products.

Commercial Skin and Wound Cleansers

There are many skin and wound cleansers designed as topical solutions and marketed to treat acute and chronic wounds. For many years solutions have been used indiscriminately without consideration or measurement of the potential side effects on the new cells trying to proliferate in the wound bed. These topical cleansers may have some antimicrobial effects but most have significant

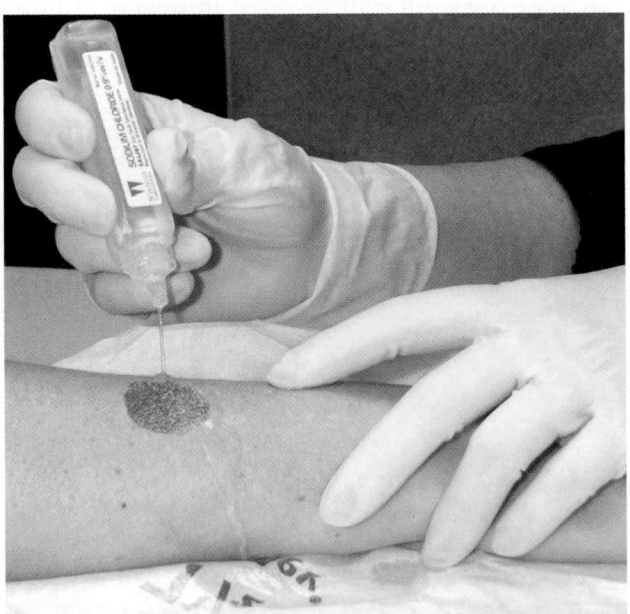

Figure 14.17 Wound cleansing with nonforceful irrigation.

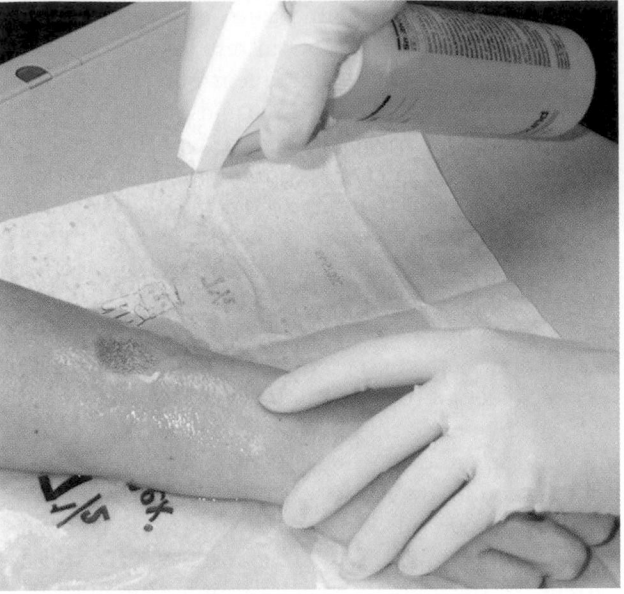

Figure 14.18 Wound cleansing with a spray cleanser.

antimitotic (inhibiting mitosis) effects as well.[119] This means that cleansers may adversely affect important cells such as fibroblasts and epidermal keratinocytes during tissue repair. The cells most affected are the all-important cells that fill and cover a wound. Information on the toxicity of the most common cleansers has been created to assist health care providers in selecting or rejecting the use of cleansers.[119] It is no surprise that acetic acid is extremely cytotoxic to the cells in a wound but of greater concern is the fact that ordinary bath soaps, even moisturizing body washes, are very cytotoxic. A physical therapist utilizing commercial cleansers or ordinary soap must consider the rationale behind the use of each topical agent applied to the wound and weigh the cost to the wound: some contribute to wound healing whereas others contribute to aspects other than wound healing.

Débridement

Débridement is defined as the removal of foreign material and dead or damaged tissue. Removal of devitalized or infected tissue is an important intervention to prevent or control bacterial growth, encourage normal cellular activity in the wound bed, and enhance the rate of tissue repair. *Nonselective débridement* removes all tissue both necrotic and living. Methods in this category may be quick but are often painful and frequently cause damage to nearby healthy tissue. *Selective débridement* removes necrotic tissue in a controlled method. Selective methods are more comfortable and gentle to the wound bed but may remove tissue more slowly.

The importance of physical therapist proficiency in sharp débridement is reflected in the Physical Therapist Licensure Examination Content Outline (the content outline can be accessed at www.fsbpt.org/download/CandidateHandbook20110114.pdf), the Commission on

Accreditation in Physical Therapy Education (CAPTE) evaluative criteria (the Accreditation Handbook can be accessed at www.capteonline.org/Accreditation Handbook) and the *Guide to Physical Therapist Practice*.[88] In response, most professional-level programs include instruction in sharp débridement within the curriculum. In the majority of states, débridement is included in the scope of practice for physical therapists. Physical therapists should consult their state's practice act to ensure that débridement is within their scope of practice in that state before providing this intervention.

When choosing a method of débridement, clinicians must consider not only the wound status but also the physiological, emotional, and financial status of the patient. Modern wound management experts avoid débridement techniques that cause the wound to bleed owing to the highly damaging effects to the wound tissues.

Nonselective Débridement

Wet-to-Dry Dressings   A wet-to-dry (WTD) dressing consists of wet gauze applied to the wound bed and allowed to dry on the wound. Removal of the dry dressing débrides the wound, pulling away any cellular material that has adhered to the gauze. This method of débridement removes necrotic tissue, as well as rich endogenous fluids, fibrin, and other cells critical to wound healing. It is also frequently uncomfortable for the patient, often causing bleeding and trauma to the wound bed. There is literature to describe the use of WTD dressings for débridement, but the efficacy of the procedure has not been demonstrated.[120,121] Wound management experts have agreed for over two decades with a multidisciplinary panel: "One of the most routinely and inappropriately used forms of non-selective mechanical débridement is the wet-to-dry dressing."[122, p. 28] Once believed to be less costly than other dressing options, it has been shown that WTD gauze dressings are actually more costly than advanced dressings. Evidence for the many negative aspects of WTD dressings is summarized in Box 14.1 Evidence Summary.

Since WTD dressings can be classified as a tool for mechanical débridement and/or a primary wound dressing, the procedure has been discussed here and in the section on dressings.

Surgical Débridement   Surgical débridement provides rapid results when treating life-threatening necrosis, large wounds, tunneling wounds, and necrotic or infected bone. Wide excision, removing viable and nonviable tissue, is usually done in the operating room with anesthesia. Laser débridement, another form of surgical débridement, may be appropriate when an individual is not a candidate for operating room procedures. Surgical débridement is not within the scope of practice of a physical therapist.

Pulsatile Lavage with Suction   PLWS will provide nonselective débridement while cleansing a wound. Refer to the detailed discussion of PLWS in the previous section on Cleansing.

Box 14.1 Evidence Summary   Outcome Studies Using Wet-to-Dry (WTD) Dressings as Part of Wound Care

Reference	Subjects	Design/ Intervention	Duration	Results	Comments
Ovington[123] (2001)	N/A	Prospective cohort study	N/A	WTD dressings have been standard procedure for wound care although research indicates gauze dressings are not optimal for the patient, the clinician, or the healthcare system.	Gauze dressings do not support optimal healing and are more labor intensive than advanced dressings. This article provides clinicians with the rationale and evidence to collaborate with physicians in choosing cost-effective products to achieve positive patient outcomes.
Shinohara et al[124] (2008)	134 patients with surgical incisions	RCT	7 days postoperative (post-op)	Occlusive hydrocolloid dressings were less expensive to use than gauze dressings. Rate of post-op wound infection was no different between the two.	Post-op dressings still commonly consist of gauze. Evidence continues to show that gauze dressings are not cost-effective. Concerns about infection under occlusive dressings appear to be unfounded.

Continued

Box 14.1 Evidence Summary Outcome Studies Using Wet-to-Dry (WTD) Dressings as Part of Wound Care—cont'd

Reference	Subjects	Design/ Intervention	Duration	Results	Comments
Singh et al[125] (2004)	N/A	Meta-analysis	N/A	72% more chronic wounds healed completely with an occlusive dressing than with conventional gauze dressing.	The results are clinically and statistically significant.
Vermeulen et al[126] (2004)	N/A	Systematic review: All RCTs evaluating the effectiveness of dressings and topical agents for surgical wounds healing by secondary intention.	N/A	The use of gauze dressings is associated with an increase in pain, number of dressing changes, and cost, with a decrease in patient satisfaction.	The authors conclude that the use of gauze for the local treatment of surgical wounds healing by secondary intention should be considered carefully. In this category of dressings for surgical wounds healing by secondary intention, most studies are underpowered with little replication. There is a need for further research to validate empirical and anecdotal reports from the field.
Cowan and Stechmiller[121] (2009)	202 subjects with open wounds healing by secondary intention	Descriptive study. A retrospective chart review was performed.	N/A	WTD dressings accounted for 42% of wound care orders. 69% of wounds treated with WTD were surgical. Mechanical débridement was not clinically indicated in more than 78% of wounds treated with WTD dressings.	WTD dressings were inappropriately ordered in 78% of the cases in this review. These findings suggest that WTD dressings are prescribed inappropriately in situations where there is little evidence to support their use.
Bergstrom et al[127] (2005)	882 residents of long-term care facilities, age 18 and older with at least one PrU	Retrospective cohort study with convenience sampling	12 weeks	Multiple regression models, one for each PrU stage grouping were completed. The area of PrUs was reduced more with moist than with dry dressings for all stages.	The treatment factor most significantly associated with healing in this study was the use of moist dressings, which was a stronger factor in healing than dry dressings or no dressings.

Box 14.1 Evidence Summary   Outcome Studies Using Wet-to-Dry (WTD) Dressings as Part of Wound Care—cont'd

Reference	Subjects	Design/ Intervention	Duration	Results	Comments
Jones and Fennie[128] (2007)	114 adults in 3 areas of the country, in hospitals, clinics, nursing homes, and home care; 50 years or older with at least one Stage II to IV PrU	Multisite, retrospective chart review using a structured data abstraction form and protocol	N/A	Bivariate analysis showed there were several variables that were significantly associated with healing. Logistic regression models identified the most significant predictors of healing. Among the list was the use of moisture management dressings. Gauze dressings were associated with nonhealing after 6 months of treatment.	Evidence does exist to support the use of dressings that maintain a moist environment at the wound/dressing interface.
Lawrence[129] (1994) and Lawrence et al[130] (1992)	Simulated infected wounds in the first study and 7 subjects with burn wounds in the second study, 14 dressing changes IC: colonized burn wounds	Cohort design	Two dressing changes per wound	Removing dry or damp gauze from a wound released significant numbers of organisms into the air. Significantly fewer organisms were released when removing an occlusive dressing. Significant numbers of bacteria were still in the air as long as 30 minutes after removal of gauze dressings.	Although these studies are older, they are classic and have not been repeated in the literature. Wounds are often undressed in open areas, sometimes with other patients nearby. Some health care practitioners do not wear masks when undressing a wound. There is an appreciable cross-contamination hazard from removing dry or damp gauze dressings without protection to all individuals in the room.
Kohr[131] (2001)	1 subject IC: wound that had failed to heal	Case study: moist wound environment applied to wound that had failed to heal with WTD dressing for 21 days	10 days	Switch from WTD to moist-wound-healing (MWH) dressing: 10 days to significant wound healing.	The temperature in the wound was optimized, autolytic débridement promoted. Cost comparison issues between WTD and MWH also well illustrated in the article.

Continued

Box 14.1 Evidence Summary Outcome Studies Using Wet-to-Dry (WTD) Dressings as Part of Wound Care—cont'd

Reference	Subjects	Design/ Intervention	Duration	Results	Comments
Payne et al[132] (2009)	36 patients with Stage II pressure ulcers at 5 centers in the United States	Prospective RCT; participants were randomized to treatment with a foam dressing or a saline-soaked gauze dressing	4 weeks	Total cost over the study period was lower by $466 per patient in the foam group. Cost spent on dressings per day, cost per ulcer healed, and costs per ulcer-free day were all lower in the foam group over the saline gauze group.	Patients in the foam group had less frequent dressing changes. On the evidence of this study, foam dressings are a more cost-effective treatment than saline-soaked gauze in this group of patients with Stage II pressure ulcers.
Capasso and Munro[133] (2003)	50 adult patients with wounds, IC: 25 WTD dressings, 25 amorphous hydrogel dressings	Nonexperimental, retrospective chart review	4 biweekly data collection points	The overall cost of wound care was significantly higher for patients in the normal saline group, with a higher number and cost of home nursing visits.	Demonstrating the value and cost-effectiveness of hydrogel dressings should enhance therapeutic decision making and guide treatment decisions.

IC = inclusion criteria; MWH = moist-wound-healing; N/A = not applicable; PrU = pressure ulcer; RCT = randomized clinical trial; RCTs = randomized clinical trials; WTD = wet-to-dry.

Whirlpool Whirlpool can be used for mechanical débridement through its feature of water agitation. It can also be used to soften necrotic tissue in preparation for sharp, enzymatic, or autolytic débridement. There are, however, often better methods of preparing tissue for débridement than whirlpool. See discussion in the previous section on Cleansing.

Selective Débridement

Sharp *Sharp débridement* is defined as the removal of dead or necrotic tissue or foreign material from and around a wound using sterile instruments such as a scalpel, scissors, and/or forceps (Fig. 14.19). Considered the *gold standard* of methods for removal of necrotic tissue, sharp débridement is a minor, tissue-sparing procedure that is performed bedside or in a procedure room. In the vast majority of U. S. states, it is within the scope of practice for a physical therapist to perform sharp débridement. It is incumbent on the therapist to be aware of his or her state practice act regarding regulations. The American Physical Therapy Association (APTA) position statement indicates that sharp débridement should be performed exclusively

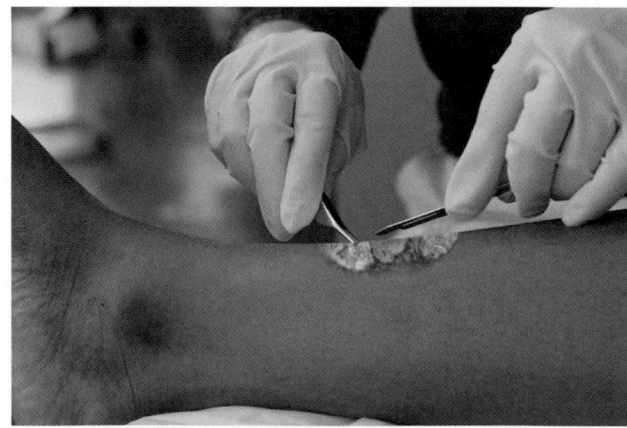

Figure 14.19 Use of scalpel and forceps for sharp débridement.

by physical therapists, not other personnel. For a full copy of this statement, go to www.apta.org/uploadedFiles/APTAorg/About_Us/Policies/HOD/Practice/ProceduralInterventions.pdf. Additional information can be found in the *Guide to Physical*

Therapist Practice.[88] To maintain current standards, a physical therapist should not débride except in the presence of necrotic tissue.

Even though sharp débridement is effective for all types of necrotic tissue, there are situations where this form of débridement is not appropriate. It is contraindicated for vascular wounds with limited blood flow where eschar may be serving as a cap or cover for a chronic open wound. Without adequate perfusion in this scenario, there is little hope of wound closure. Sharp débridement is not appropriate for wounds with tunneling (when the wound bed cannot be seen) or areas affected by dry gangrene. Patients with low platelet counts, on anticoagulants, or with other conditions that inhibit clotting are not suitable candidates. It is also contraindicated for pressure ulcers on the heels covered with dry eschar. (*Note:* Some experts maintain that in this scenario, eschar provides protection as long as there is no infection present; others maintain that eschar must be removed because it inhibits epithelial cell growth.)

Chemical or Enzymatic   Enzymatic **débridement** is a type of selective débridement that includes the application of a topical agent containing enzymes that act by dissolving necrotic tissue. There are several types and brands of enzymatic agents, each designed to affect a certain type of necrotic tissue. Advantages for this type of treatment are that débridement is selective, patient discomfort is minimal, and application procedures are simple. Disadvantages include the potential development of dermatitis of the intact periwound skin, frequent dressing changes disrupting the wound bed, and the need to crosshatch existing eschar with a scalpel so that the enzyme can penetrate the wound. Enzymatic débridement agents do not have an impact on pathogen levels in the wound bed and should not be considered antimicrobial. Some enzymatic débridement preparations contain the protein papain. Topical drug products containing papain were taken off the market in the United States in November 2008 because they have not been approved by the Food and Drug Administration (FDA); for more information on this issue go to www.fda.gov/papain. When utilizing other types of enzymatic agents still on the market, a referral for treatment and a prescription for the enzymatic agent are currently required in most regions of North America.

Biosurgery   Biosurgery as a form of selective débridement is also referred to as *maggot débridement therapy (MDT)*, or maggot or larval therapy (Fig 14.20). Although it has been in use in the Western world for over 150 years, its popularity declined with the advent of antibiotics. Biosurgery is now generating new interest owing to the rise of multidrug-resistant bacteria such as **methicillin-resistant *Staphylococcus aureus* (MRSA)**. Sterile, newly hatched larvae are placed on chronic wounds and held in place with dressings or a *biobag* for 2 to 5 days before removal. Biosurgery has been shown to remove devitalized tissue, decrease the risk of infection, and improve wound

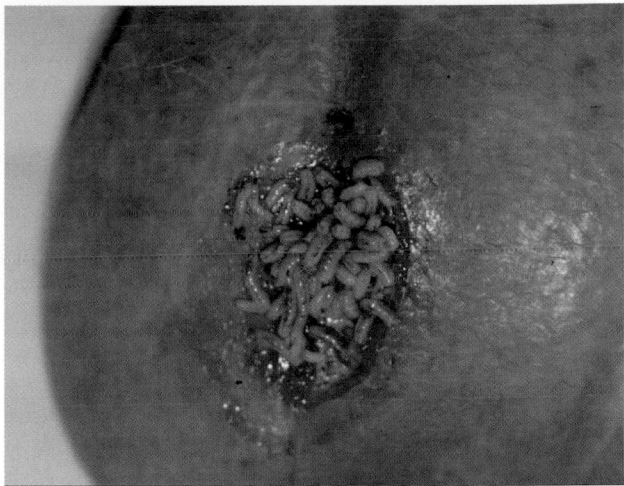

Figure 14.20 Maggot therapy for a cavity wound. *(Courtesy of the Biosurgical Research Unit, Surgical Materials Testing Laboratory, Bridgend, UK.)*

healing without side effects in a wide variety of wound types. Biosurgery is recommended for osteomyelitis and deep wound infections that remain unresponsive to more conventional antibiotic and surgical therapy. Although moist wound healing is compatible with biosurgery, a very wet wound environment has an adverse effect on larval survival. Certain types of moisture-retentive wound dressings are more compatible with larval survival than others.[134-141]

Medical-Grade Honey

The use of medical-grade honey as a wound dressing has been shown to enhance débridement and healing. Honey dressings are available in hydrocolloid, alginate, and liquid categories. They have been shown to facilitate **autolytic débridement**, decrease or eliminate wound odor, prevent biofilm (thin layer of bacteria) formation, and soften necrotic tissue.[142-145]

Autolytic

Autolytic débridement uses the endogenous enzymes on the wound bed to digest devitalized tissue and promote granulation tissue formation. In practice, the body's natural fluids are held in contact with the wound base with a moisture-retentive dressing for 3 to 7 days. By increasing the moisture content of slough and necrotic tissue with enzyme-rich body fluids, autolytic activity is facilitated. Although this method is the least invasive/most selective, as well as inexpensive, painless, and biocompatible, each patient is examined to determine if this type of débridement is best for the existing wound. The type of moisture-retentive dressing selected to promote autolytic débridement will be based on the health of the periwound tissues and the level of fungal or bacterial loads. The presence of infection does not rule out the use of occlusive dressings, as described earlier in the discussion on moist wound healing.

Topical Agents

Current standards for chronic wound care have decreased the use of topical agents even in the presence of infection. In the literature these agents may be referred to as *antiseptics, disinfectants,* and/or *antimicrobials.* Other topical agent categories include *antibiotics* and *analgesics.* Guidelines reveal that almost all human-made products are cytotoxic to WBCs even when diluted.[101] Many agents once thought to be safe are now known to be unsafe to healing tissue, causing adverse reactions at any concentration. Many agents once thought to be effective as antibacterial or decontaminating agents are now known to be ineffective. When striving for wound bed homeostasis, preserving cellular life in endogenous fluids is almost always more desirable than destroying it with additives. Many physicians and wound management experts use the following adage to guide in the decision making process: "It is desirable never to put anything in the wound that cannot be tolerated comfortably in the conjunctival sac."[15, p. 179] In plain terms, "If you can't put it in your eyes don't put it in the wound." Even under Direct Access, in most states physical therapists are not permitted to prescribe medications, even over-the-counter products, for wound care. If, during the examination or intervention, a physical therapist determines that a topical agent may be indicated, the patient's physician should be contacted and the findings discussed. Consideration of topical agents should always include the risks and benefits of the topical agent in relation to potential cytotoxicity, biocompatibility, safety, and efficacy.

Antiseptics

Povidone-Iodine Povidone-iodine (PVI) is a combination of iodine plus a polymer that provides bactericidal effects. One commonly known product name is Betadine (Purdue Products LP, Stamford, CT 06901). Used indiscriminately for many years on acute and chronic wounds, it is now recommended mainly for wounds infected with *Staphylococcus aureus.* The AHRQ guidelines published in 1994 state: "Do not clean ulcer wounds with skin cleansers or antiseptic agents (e.g., povidone-iodine, iodophor, sodium hypochlorite solution [Dakin's solution], hydrogen peroxide, acetic acid)."[101, p. 15] Although the guidelines address pressure ulcers, the wound-healing evidence is applicable to all wound treatments. This evidence implies that the use of PVI, as well as other antiseptics, is inconsistent with practice standards. In rare instances when such agents are recommended by a physician and are indeed appropriate, clinicians should document sound reasoning behind the use of these products because they will be held accountable to these published and respected guidelines. An example of a situation such as this would be when other, less cytotoxic treatments have failed to reduce the bacterial load in an infected wound. The literature does not provide adequate clinical or legal reasons to use PVI for managing wounds.[146] In addition, the FDA has not approved the use of PVI solution or PVI surgical scrub solution for wounds. PVI has been shown to reduce bacterial counts in infected wounds, and currently there is no antimicrobial resistance to PVI.[147] Its use is contraindicated for the noninfected wound.[101]

Sodium Hypochlorite Solutions: Dakin's Solution (Bleach and Boric Acid), Sodium Hypochlorite (Household Bleach) Sodium hypochlorite is cytotoxic even at very dilute concentrations. It damages fibroblasts and endothelial cells and causes cellular damage to granulation tissue. It is irritating to the skin and can initiate severe reactions in some individuals. It is used in the management of wounds with purulent exudate. Treatment should be discontinued when the wound is clean. Its use is contraindicated for the noninfected wound.[101]

Acetic Acid Solution Acetic acid is traditionally used to inhibit bacterial infections; however, the solution has been found to be more damaging to fibroblasts than to bacteria. A common form of acetic acid is found in vinegar. It is corrosive and cytotoxic at any dilution. Most recently, it has been used to manage contamination by *Pseudomonas aeruginosa.* Its use is contraindicated for the noninfected wound.[101]

Oxidizing Agents: Hydrogen Peroxide Solution When this solution comes in contact with tissue, there is a release of oxygen and temporary antimicrobial activity. Its bubbling action is used for nonselective débridement to loosen small debris. It is cytotoxic unless diluted to a very weak concentration. Its use is contraindicated in wounds that are noninfected, tunneling, or granulating.[101]

Antibacterials

This section includes a sample of commonly used topical antimicrobials, antibiotics, and antibacterials. Each of these topical agents is effective against a variety of bacteria and is selected by the physician based on the species cultured for an individual patient. All share a risk of similar side effects such as burning, itching, contact dermatitis, and/or allergic sensitivity. There is little evidence in the literature to show levels of cytotoxicity in these topical agents. Examples include the following:

- Bacitracin/Baciguent: associated with allergic reactions.
- Neosporin/neomycin sulfate: causes greatest incidence of allergic reactions.
- Silvadene/silver sulfadiazine: primarily for thermal injuries, silver is selectively toxic to bacteria but may inactivate topical proteolytic enzymes.[148]
- Furacin/nitrofurazone: cytotoxic in animal studies.[149]
- Sulfamylon/mafenide acetate: diffuses easily through eschar, primarily for thermal injuries.
- Bactroban/mupirocin ointment: currently effective against all species of staphylococcus.
- Gentamicin/Geramycin: currently effective against all species of staphylococcus and streptococcus.

Owing to the paucity of information on cytotoxicity, the risk of side effects, and the growing incidence of antibiotic-resistant bacteria, use of these products for chronic wounds should be considered carefully and is usually contraindicated for the noninfected wound.

Creams and Ointments (Over-the-Counter) Some antibacterial ointments and creams such as Bacitracin and Neosporin can be purchased without a prescription. These are minimally bacteriostatic owing to their dilution. Once they lose their antibacterial strength, the ointments may trap bacteria and encourage bacterial growth from surface contamination. If ointments or creams are used, the wound should be cleansed regularly to remove potential contamination; however, frequent cleansing may disrupt the healing process. These preparations can be used to provide moisture to a dry wound, but they may create a greasy wound bed, making early epithelial cell migration difficult. A more biocompatible ointment that will provide moisture to a healing wound is Aquaphor® (Beiersdorf Inc., Wilton, CT 06897).

Analgesics

The use of topical anesthetics to control wound pain is controversial in the literature. Conflicting reports and the lack of substantial research have led to concerns about the impact of anesthetics on the wound bed. This issue is further complicated by the broad profile of patients with wounds, their etiologies, and co-morbidities. The more common agents used topically are lidocaine and EMLA (eutectic mixture of local anesthetics) cream, which is a mixture of lidocaine and prilocaine (AstraZeneca, Wilmington, DE 19850). Amitriptyline, a tricyclic antidepressant, has local anesthetic properties and has shown promise as an option for treating wound pain.[150] While topical anesthetics may be under scrutiny for their effects, vasoconstriction in particular, there is a need for more investigation since pain is a major issue for most patients with wounds.

Growth Factors

Endogenous growth factors normally abound in the fluids of a wound. In most chronic wounds the normal timetable for healing has been delayed or stopped. Growth factors that are decreased or absent can be added topically to the wound bed. Increasing strength of evidence supports the practice of adding growth factors to a wound to facilitate healing. The application of exogenous growth factors in conjunction with good wound care increases wound healing outcomes and can convert a chronic wound into a healed wound.[19,151-156] Growth factors can be isolated from an individual's own tissue, added to a liquid formula in a laboratory, and then applied to the wound. An example of an autologous growth factor product with a name familiar to many clinicians is AutoloGel™ System (Cytomedix Inc., Gaithersburg, MD 20877).[157] Recombinant DNA technology has resulted in other products such as becaplermin gel, trade name Regranex® Gel (Ortho-McNeil-Janssen Pharmaceuticals, Inc., Titusville, NJ 08560). Reimbursement for application of growth factors varies and should be checked before use. For example, becaplermin gel is FDA approved for the treatment of LE diabetic neuropathic ulcers that extend into the subcutaneous tissue or beyond but currently not approved for the treatment of pressure, venous, or other nondiabetic-related wounds.

Topical Agents and Acute Wounds

The use of antiseptics and antibiotics to reduce bacterial levels in acute, traumatic wounds follows a different rationale from that of chronic wounds. For wounds resulting from trauma or thermal injury, the risk for contamination is high. It is accepted practice to use cytotoxic products such as povidone-iodine or Silvadene® (silver sulfadiazine) in the *early* management of acute traumatic wounds. The goal is to discontinue use of cytotoxic agents as soon as the wounds are clean and able to produce and support endogenous fluids.

Mechanical Modalities

Procedures for use of modalities vary based on unique patient characteristics and individual patient response. A useful place to begin is with protocols recommended in comprehensive wound management texts such as *Wound Healing: Evidence-Based Management* by McCulloch and Kloth[158] and *Wound Care: A Collaborative Practice Manual for Health Professionals* by Sussman and Bates-Jensen.[159] Owing to the ever-changing rules of reimbursement, it is prudent to check current reimbursement and documentation guidelines when billing for these services. The decision to use mechanical modalities rests in the hands of the physical therapist unless physician authorization is required in order to receive reimbursement. The reimbursement requirement may vary from state to state and sometimes between payers in the same state. In some cases, individual physicians may develop their own protocols that require physical therapists to contact them before changing a POC.

Ultrasound

Therapeutic ultrasound (US) application for wound management differs from its use as a modality to treat pain. Ultrasound stimulates cell activity, accelerating processes such as inflammation. Once thought to target only the sluggish wound in the inflammatory stage, evidence now demonstrates that the effects can be seen throughout all wound-healing phases. Basic science evidence and clinical research have established that skin repair and wound contraction can be accelerated, collagen secretion can be stimulated, and elastin properties can be affected to strengthen scar tissue. Standard procedure for the treatment is to cover the wound with a sheet of hydrogel or an application of amorphous hydrogel. US is then delivered with a handheld applicator (Fig. 14.21). Another option for treatment is to apply US transmission

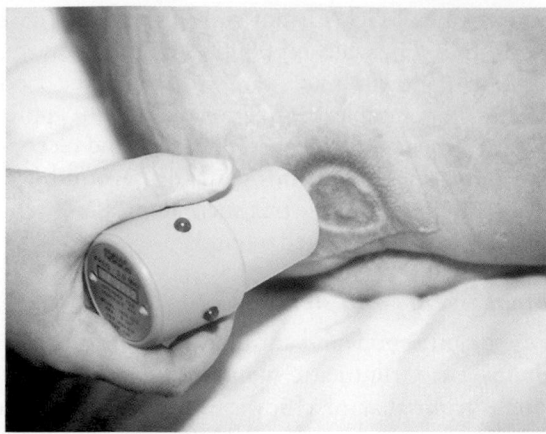

Figure 14.21 Application of ultrasound to wound and peri-wound tissues with hydrogel sheet coupling. *(From Kloth, LC, and McCulloch, JM, Plate 15, with permission.)*

gel to the periwound area and treat from this region in addition to or instead of the wound bed.[160-164] Another option for delivery of US is to use a system that provides noncontact, nonthermal, low-frequency ultrasound (Fig. 14.22). A mist of sterile saline is propelled toward the wound and the ultrasound is transferred from the device to the patient without contact or pain. Studies have provided evidence that this type of US treatment reduces bacterial quantity in a wound and promotes healing, especially in wounds that have been slow to heal.[84,165-169]

Electrical Stimulation

The use of electrical stimulation (ES) to treat chronic and, more recently, acute wounds is well documented. Electrical stimulation is recommended to eliminate bacterial load, promote granulation, decrease inflammation, reduce edema, reduce wound-related pain, and augment blood flow. Human skin, wounds, and the cells that facilitate wound healing all have measurable electrical currents. Electrical stimulation affects various types of cells and their activities by supporting, altering, or providing electrical currents to accelerate wound healing. A clear understanding of medical electricity will assist the clinician in applying an appropriate ES treatment. The available literature is diverse and instructive.[170-177] There are a variety of options for treatment setup depending on the goals of treatment, the type of wound, and the condition of the patient. Standard equipment for the direct method of application will include an ES unit, treatment and nontreatment electrodes, and a substance such as saline-soaked gauze or a hydrogel dressing applied to the wound bed or cavity to enhance electrical conductivity under the treatment electrode (Fig. 14.23). For the indirect method, gel electrodes straddle the wound and interface with the periwound skin. Clinical decisions related to voltage, electrode placement, dosage, and other variables must be made on a case-by-case basis. Information about treatment protocols, strength of evidence, and guidelines for treatment can be found in detailed wound care texts.[178,179]

Thermal and Nonthermal Diathermy

Pulsed shortwave diathermy (PSWD), continuous shortwave diathermy (CSWD), and nonthermal pulsed radiofrequency stimulation (PRFS) have been used successfully to treat chronic open wounds, facilitating progress from one phase of wound healing to the next. These diathermy treatments utilize radio waves to provide thermal and nonthermal effects, respectively. All models transmit radiation from an applicator head to the target tissues. PSWD heats superficial and deep tissues. CSWD heats deep muscle and joint tissues. PRFS is nonthermal and can influence tissue at the cellular

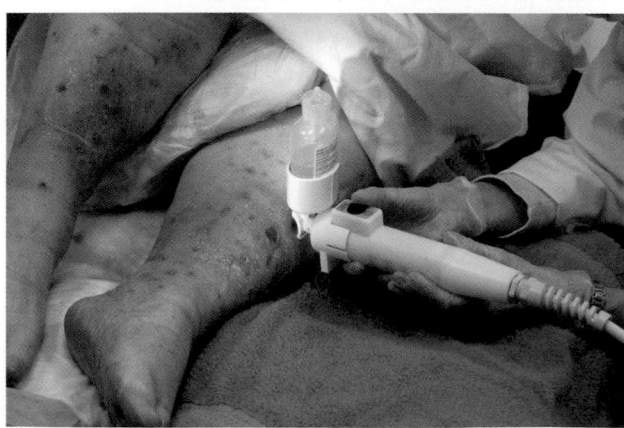

Figure 14.22 Application of noncontact, nonthermal, low-frequency ultrasound treatment to leg wounds. *(Courtesy of Celleration®, Eden Prairie, MN 55344.)*

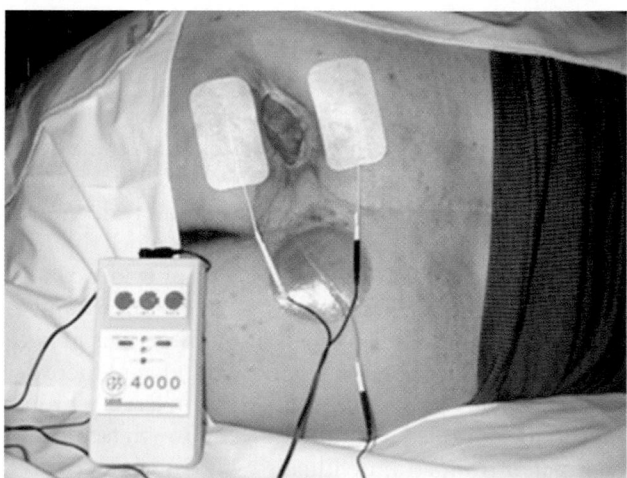

Figure 14.23 Conductively coupled bipolar treatment electrodes of opposite polarity positioned on opposite sides of a wound. *(From McCulloch and Kloth: Wound Healing: Evidence-Based Management, ed 4. FA Davis, Philadelphia, Figure 26-28, with permission.)*

level. Individuals with arterial insufficiency are not good candidates for PSWD or CSWD because their tissues are not able to dissipate heat well enough to avoid burns. Wound sites treated with diathermy have demonstrated increased fibroblast proliferation, collagen formation, tissue perfusion, and metabolic rate. Although the number of clinical studies is smaller than that of other modalities, the evidence is mounting for the role diathermy plays in wound healing. Physical therapists are using diathermy more often since the publication of a number of studies regarding the nonthermal effects of pulsed diathermy and the production of smaller, more portable, user-friendly diathermy units.[180-182] Equipment needed for treatment includes a diathermy unit/electronic console and one or two applicator heads. Treatment is usually delivered without touching the skin. Wounds should be carefully prepared before treatment according to guidelines provided by the distributor. With newer units such as the Provant® Therapy System (Regenesis® Biomedical Inc., Scottsdale, AZ 85257), the pad can be placed over wound dressings, compression garments, and casts. Because the effects of heat may continue after the treatment, patients should be observed carefully and protocol guidelines should be followed closely (Fig. 14.24).

Ultraviolet Radiation

Ultraviolet (UV) radiation energy is a form of radiation between x-ray and visible light on the electromagnetic spectrum.[183] UV wavelengths have been divided into wavelengths and bands. The three bands most useful for their effects on human skin are UVA, UVB, and UVC. UV has cutaneous and bactericidal effects that include increased blood flow, enhanced granulation tissue formation, destruction of bacteria, stimulation of vitamin D production, and thickening of the stratum corneum. The varied physiological effects make this treatment appropriate for a variety of skin diseases, as well as acute and chronic wounds.[160] The effects of UV radiation on antibiotic-resistant bacteria make it a potentially effective tool in wound care; however, there are only a few up-to-date, well-controlled clinical studies emerging at this time.[184,185] Early supporting literature is now quite dated, leaving room for new clinical studies to provide evidence of the efficacy of the intervention. UVC in particular has been found to be effective in the treatment of *methicillin-resistant Staphylococcus aureus* (MRSA), *vancomycin-resistant Enterococcus* (VRE), and, more recently, some strains of *Pseudomonas aeruginosa*.[186,187] The treatment is typically delivered to a clean wound with dressings removed, using a UVB or UVC lamp. Treatment distance, dosage, frequency, and subsequent clinical outcomes will vary based on the goals of the treatment and the status of the wound. Due to manufacturing challenges in North America, portable, handheld UV units to treat wounds are not readily available at this time. Physical therapists planning to utilize UV for wound care might partner with a wound care team, a resourceful vendor, and the latest evidence to devise a treatment plan.

Hyperbaric Oxygen Therapy

Hyperbaric oxygen therapy (HBOT) delivers 100% oxygen to an individual resting inside a sealed chamber. The oxygen is delivered at a pressure greater than the atmosphere. This *systemic* treatment increases the amount of oxygen available for cell metabolism, improving oxygen delivery to hypoxic tissue. Systemic HBOT is, however, associated with risks related to oxygen toxicity. The literature demonstrates positive responses to this treatment when used as an adjunct to other forms of wound care but few controlled, randomized trials have been completed.[160,188-191] Chambers to deliver *topical* oxygen have been available for at least a decade. These smaller chambers enclose a limb or a segment of the body instead of requiring coverage of the entire body.

Following physician referral, a physical therapist may assist or coordinate a systemic or topical treatment. Often, a trained technician will manage the equipment controls and the delivery chamber. Wound care may occur before or after the HBOT or the topical HBOT depending on the preferences of the physician and the protocol of the facility. Discussion among investigators comparing the effects of systemic versus topical oxygen is ongoing. In some studies, topical oxygen is also referred to as *topical hyperbaric oxygen (THBO)* and O_2 *therapy*.[13,192,193] Instead of the full-body chamber used for HBOT, THBO is portable and is delivered in a localized limb chamber.[13,192] THBO has been combined with electrical stimulation and also with cold laser for the treatment of pressure ulcers and neuropathic foot wounds.[193,194] Topical O_2 therapy has enhanced the effects of growth factors in investigations within the last few years.[12] Renewed interest by investigators has led to more refined protocols and improved strength of

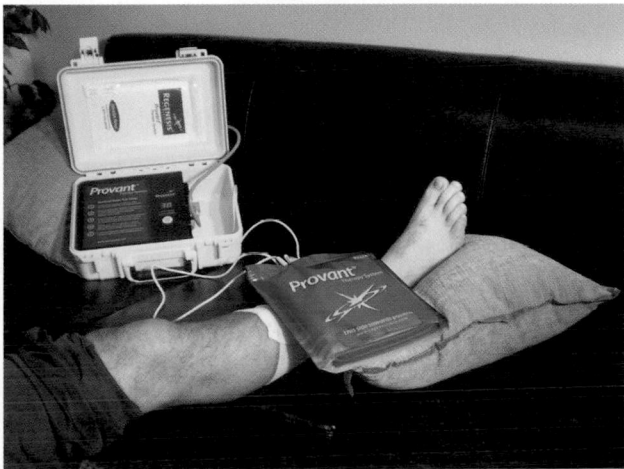

Figure 14.24 Leg wound covered with Provant® treatment pad. *(Courtesy of Regenesis® Biomedical Inc., Scottsdale, AZ 85257.)*

evidence in the field. If investigations continue to provide positive results, the use of topical O_2 in wound care could result in more cost-effective and efficient care, fewer risks, and applicability to a wider population as compared to systemic O_2.

Negative Pressure Wound Therapy

Negative pressure wound therapy (NPWT) is used as an adjunct to wound healing to facilitate wound closure in acute surgical wounds, as well as with more challenging, slow-to-heal wounds. The procedure is known by several terms but the most well known is *vacuum-assisted closure* or *VAC®* (Kinetic Concepts, Inc., San Antonio, TX 78265). An open cell foam dressing is placed in the wound and a suction tube is connected from the foam to a portable pump. An airtight seal is created over the foam and the suction tube with a clear, occlusive film (Fig. 14.25). A controlled amount of negative (subatmospheric) pressure is applied through the foam to the entire wound bed. Typically, for the first few days (48 hours) the negative pressure is applied continuously via the portable pump system. After a significant amount of excess wound fluid has been withdrawn, the pump is programmed to apply pressure intermittently. The foam dressing is changed every 12 hours (infected wounds) to 48 hours or longer (clean wounds). The strength of evidence is mounting as basic research explores the effects of this treatment. NPWT has been shown to enhance granulation tissue formation, promote wound edge approximation, remove edema from wounds, and improve oxygen levels in the wound.[195-201] Studies have also shown that with the use of NPWT, the healing time for selected wounds decreased in comparison to standard wound care.[202,203] One claim that is still under investigation is the ability of the VAC to remove bacteria from the wound bed. Although a physician must order this type of therapy, many are unaware of this intervention and would be responsive to an appropriate recommendation by the therapist. In different environments, physical therapists, nurses, or other clinical staff may perform administration of the technique.

Cold Laser Therapy

Cold laser is also referred to in the literature as low-level cold laser, low-level infrared laser, or monochromatic infrared photo energy (MIRE). Low-energy laser treatment uses light in the infrared spectrum. This therapy has been promoted for augmenting wound healing[204] and reversing the symptoms of peripheral neuropathy in individuals with diabetes.[205,206] It is thought that the effects of laser increase circulation and reduce pain by increasing the release of nitric oxide into the microcirculation. Although supportive, peer-reviewed literature is modest at this point, published studies citing success with this treatment are mounting while debates continue.[207-210] Despite the term *cold laser*, light in the infrared spectrum can also be used to deliver heat as a treatment modality. Owing to the perceived lack of adequate evidence, some third-party payers do not cover cold laser treatment except when used as a heat modality. This may soon change as the strength of evidence increases for its use to treat peripheral neuropathy. The most well-known product on the market is called Anodyne® Therapy System (Anodyne® Therapy, LLC, Tampa, FL 33626). Figure 14.26 depicts use of a special foot pad to deliver infrared photo energy.

Dressings

The type of wound dressings selected for a wound may have a profound effect on healing time. There are hundreds of choices for the discerning clinician.

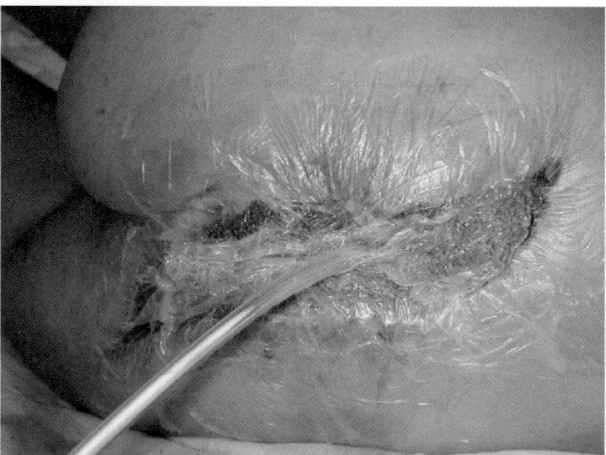

Figure 14.25 A Stage IV sacral pressure ulcer with reticulated foam dressing, tubing, and polyurethane sheet covering the entire wound to maintain the vacuum during treatment with vacuum-assisted closure. *(From Kloth, LC, and McCulloch, JM, Plate 14, with permission.)*

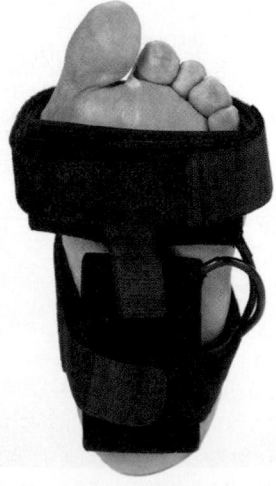

Figure 14.26 Application of infrared photo energy to the foot using an Anodyne® Therapy foot pad. *(Courtesy of Anodyne Therapy, LLC, Tampa, FL 33626.)*

Information on indications, contraindications, and expected outcomes can be obtained from individual vendors listed in Appendix 14.E, as well as from texts devoted entirely to wound care.[158,159] Physical therapists who are monitoring a wound on a regular basis and are knowledgeable about dressing alternatives are often the most appropriate clinicians to make the decision about dressing selections. This chapter includes introductory information necessary to make clinical decisions about dressings: the characteristics of the dressing categories and the effects of the dressings on the wound bed. Refer to Appendix 14.F for a listing of dressings categorized by treatment goal (purpose) or type of wound (indication).

Choosing or recommending appropriate dressings should be directed by the characteristics of the wound and periwound tissues, not by what is available in the supply closet. A product that preserves wound hydration and limits fluid loss is usually ideal. In addition to following the principles of moist wound healing in most dressing selections, the following list identifies wound characteristics and the corresponding action that a dressing should perform:

- Infection: absent or present; prevent or treat
- Necrosis: remove or not; autolytic or mechanical
- Drainage: dry (no drainage), adequate (moist) or excessive (too wet); restore, retain, or remove
- Granulation tissue: present or absent; protect, facilitate formation
- Epithelialization: present or absent; facilitate formation
- Periwound area: intact, at risk or macerated; protect or absorb
- Incontinence: present or absent; protect or absorb
- Cavities and tunneling: present or absent; fill and protect
- Friction: present, some risk, significant risk; cushion, protect, or prevent
- Odor: minimal or needs reduction; ignore or add odor-reducing dressings

The dressing that is applied directly to the wound is referred to as the *primary* dressing. The dressing that is applied over the primary dressing is referred to as the *secondary* dressing. Some advanced dressings serve as the primary and secondary, including adhesive and absorptive qualities in the same dressing.

Gauze/Fiber

Gauze dressings (Fig. 14.27) are considered by many wound management experts to be outside the description of modern wound dressings.[120] Used and misused for decades, there are more reasons not to use gauze than there are indications for use. As a primary dressing, gauze leaves contaminating fibers in the wound, contributes to desiccation, is permeable to bacteria, can be adherent to the wound, releases excessive amounts of bacteria into the air on removal, causes a loss of normothermia, and

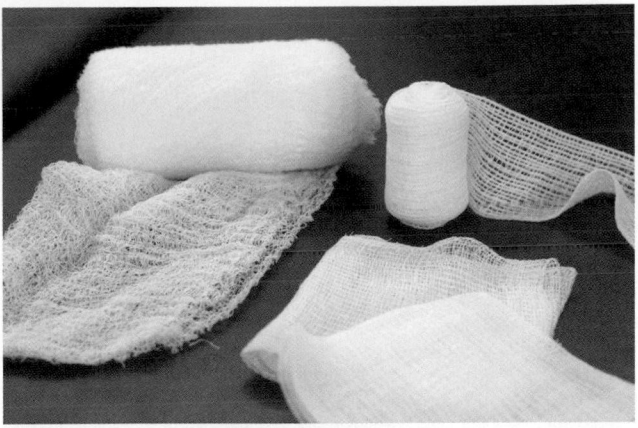

Figure 14.27 Samples of gauze dressings.

is painful on removal if it adheres to the wound surface. Once thought to be cost-effective, it has been shown in more than one study to be more costly than other dressing choices (see Box 14.1 Evidence Summary). Gauze ribbon can be used to maintain an opening for drainage in a tunneling wound. It can also be used successfully to gently support a cavity wound but should not be used to aggressively pack any shape of wound. It was once thought that cavity wounds should be packed very full but it has since been established that granulation tissue and epithelial cells do not flourish with aggressive gauze packing. The additional pressure from a tightly packed wound will impede the flow of oxygen and nutrients to the granulating wound bed. Gauze can be an effective secondary dressing, especially if the dressings will be changed frequently or if exudate is heavy. Gauze 4 × 4s and a roll of gauze are typically used to create a WTD dressing. WTD dressings were previously discussed under the section on débridement because of their nonselective removal of tissue during dressing changes. Because WTD dressings can be classified as a tool for mechanical débridement or as a primary wound dressing, they are discussed in both categories. Refer to that section of the chapter for more details.

Impregnated Gauze

Designed to be less adherent, this category includes products made of tightly meshed synthetic fibers or woven products such as cellulose acetate. Fiber materials are impregnated with a petroleum emulsion such as Vaseline®, intended to prevent the gauze from sticking to the wound surface. Used as a primary dressing this choice is minimally absorptive, provides minimal protection, does not enhance a moist environment, and may create a greasy wound bed. One of its more appropriate uses is as a primary dressing over new sutures to prevent them from catching or sticking in a gauze secondary dressing.

Transparent Films

Films are made of a transparent membrane with an acrylic adhesive layer (Fig. 14.28). Transparent films do not allow

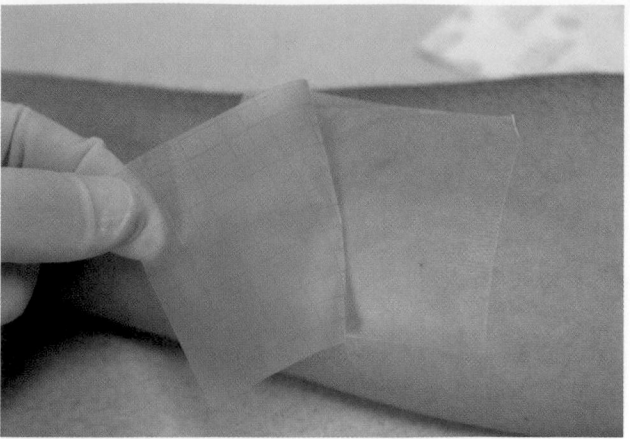

Figure 14.28 Application of a film dressing.

bacteria or moisture into the wound. They facilitate a moist wound environment, trapping endogenous fluids in the wound bed to assist with autolytic débridement, wound bed homeostasis, and *angiogenesis*. Films assist in protecting skin from the effects of shearing, friction, and the contaminating effects of incontinence. Removal of a film dressing must be done with great caution because this can cause skin tears, especially with fragile or aging skin. Currently, few films have absorptive qualities and cannot be used on highly exuding wounds.

Foam

Foams are highly absorbent pads, sheets, or ropes of polyurethane available in many sizes with many features (Fig. 14.29). They are available with or without adhesive backing so that they can be used as a primary and/or a secondary dressing. Foam dressings are highly absorptive but also help to create an occlusive environment for moist wound healing. They should not be used alone on a dry wound but could serve as a secondary dressing if the primary dressing was a gel product.

Hydrogels

Hydrogels are categorized as *amorphous,* referring to a liquid-like gel, or as *sheets,* consisting of a thin, flexible sheet of polymer containing at least 90% water (Fig. 14.30). Both types are used to increase moisture in a dry wound bed, soften necrotic tissue, and support autolytic débridement. Both have some absorptive qualities and will swell slightly until they are saturated. The amorphous gel (Fig. 14.31) must be contained in the wound with a secondary dressing. The flexible sheets usually require a secondary dressing but are available through some vendors with tape attached to the borders. Patient response is usually very positive to the soothing sensation of the hydrogel application.

Hydrocolloids

Considered the most occlusive of the moisture-retentive dressings, hydrocolloids are also available in less occlusive or semipermeable styles as well. As with foams, these dressings come in a variety of styles and shapes including pastes, granules, powder, and sheets. They typically consist of an absorbent colloidal material combined with a film

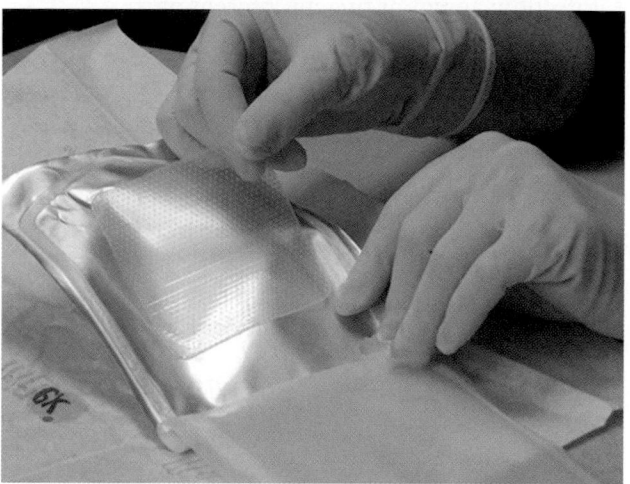

Figure 14.30 Sample of a hydrogel sheet dressing.

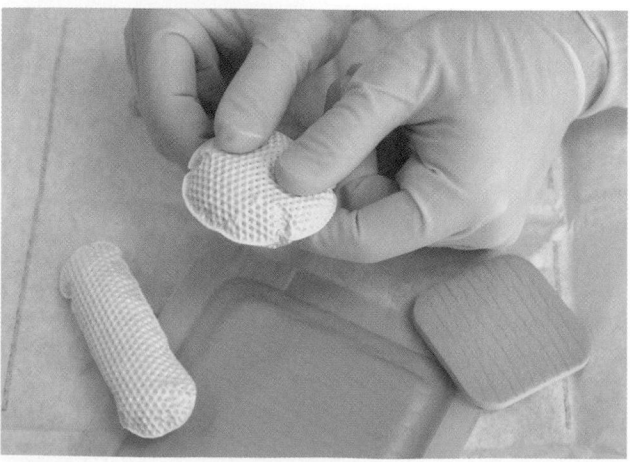

Figure 14.29 Samples of foam dressings.

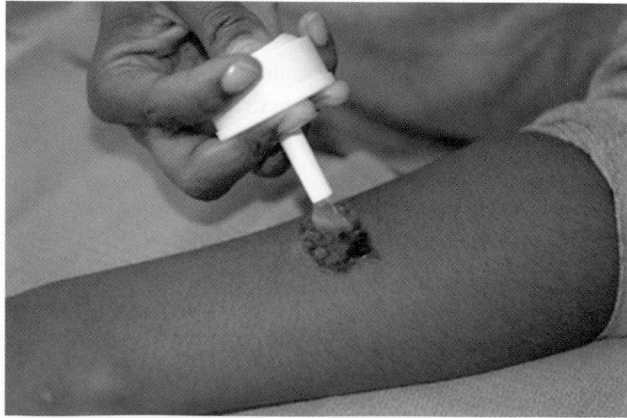

Figure 14.31 Application of an amorphous gel dressing.

or foam backing (Fig. 14.32). Hydrocolloid dressings work best on mild to moderate exudating wounds. When wound exudate combines with the colloidal polymer, a soft, gelatinous, often yellow, and malodorous mass is formed. Patients, families, caregivers, and other health care providers must be informed about this harmless reaction so that infection is not assumed. Hydrocolloids have been used successfully as occlusive dressings over infected wounds without fulmination of existing bacteria. They are also the dressing of choice to cover and protect larvae during maggot débridement therapy.

Alginates

This dressing category is also known as *calcium alginate* because the dressings are manufactured using the calcium salts of alginic acid derived from marine algae and kelp (seaweed). The raw material is woven and then converted into flat sheets, ropes, or ribbon shapes (Fig. 14.33). Alginates absorb 20 to 30 times their own weight, are gentle to apply and remove, and are biocompatible with the wound bed. A chemical reaction between the dressing and wound exudate creates a gel substance that helps to maintain a moist wound environment while absorbing excess exudate. Because they are permeable, alginates do not provide a barrier against bacteria. This characteristic makes them an effective choice when an infected wound cannot be covered with an occlusive dressing. Most alginates currently require a secondary dressing to hold them in place. Several manufacturers are combining alginates with other products, such as hydrocolloids, to maximize their effectiveness. There is growing interest in the use of silver in advanced dressings to combine the antimicrobial action of silver with the absorptive qualities of alginates. Long-term effects remain unclear. There is a need for more clinical trials and longer follow-up times to look at the long-term effects on healing.[211] An example of this type of dressing is SILVER*CEL*® (Johnson & Johnson Wound Management, ETHICON, Inc., Somerville, NJ 08876).

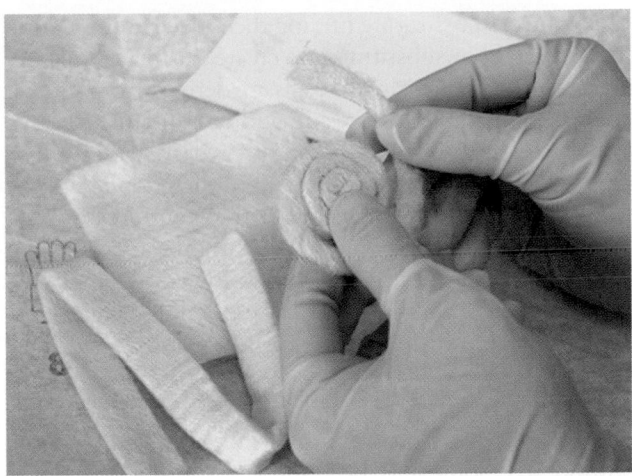

Figure 14.33 Samples of alginate dressings.

Hydrofibers

Hydrofiber or hydroactive dressings are designed to have a selective absorptive capacity. They have the combined positive characteristics of alginate, foam, and gel dressings. When in contact with the wound, the synthetic fibers absorb exudate and align themselves perpendicular to the wound surface. This vertical wicking process keeps debris and wound fluid contained within the dressing.[212] There is considerably less pain on removal of a hydrofiber dressing because the fibers do not stick to the wound or dry out.[212,213] The dressing properties allow growth factors and other peptides to survive on the wound bed. Aquacel® is a spun Hydrofiber® dressing that readily absorbs moisture (Fig. 14.34). Aquacel® Ag adds ionic silver to the absorbent dressing (ConvaTec, Skillman, NJ 08558).

Skin Substitutes

Considered by some to be topical applications and by others to be dressings, human skin equivalents and

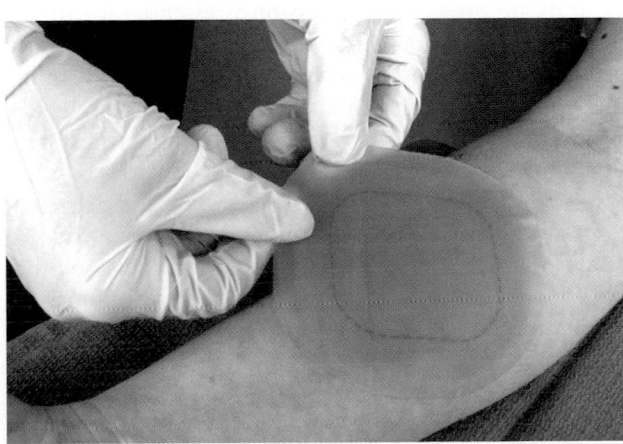

Figure 14.32 Sample of a hydrocolloid dressing.

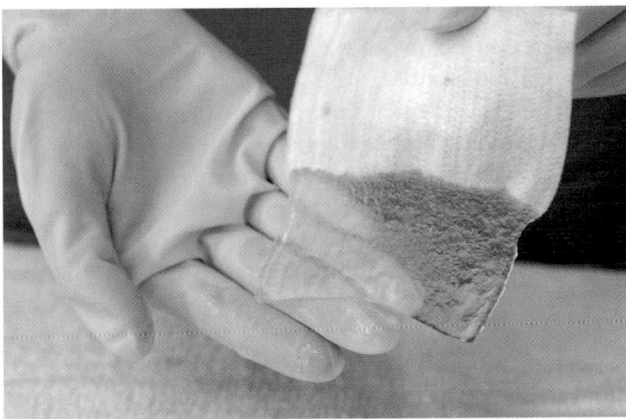

Figure 14.34 Sample of AQUACEL®, a Hydrofiber® dressing simulating the change in consistency from dry to gel as wound drainage is absorbed.

bioengineered tissues are finding their place in the wound care arena. Skin substitutes are created using a variety of techniques and substances. Cells are derived from sources such as neonatal male foreskin and porcine (pig) dermal collagen. The products are produced in laboratories, shipped either frozen or cooled, and then applied to the patient's wound by a member of the wound care team. Although a physician would prescribe the use of a skin substitute, other health care professionals can apply the product to the wound based on individual facility protocol. Skin substitutes consist of living skin applications that resemble skin structure and function and may include epidermal and dermal layers. They are useful as temporary coverage, providing skin protection for the wound bed. Some have been shown to stimulate endogenous cell activity. Most are marketed to use on wounds that have not responded to conventional therapy such as chronic diabetic foot ulcers, venous leg ulcers, and deep burn wounds.[214] Examples to look for when investigating skin substitutes are Apligraf (Novartis, East Hanover, NJ 07936), Dermagraft and Transcyte (Advanced Biohealing, LaJolla, CA 92037), and Biobrane (UDL Laboratories, Rockford, IL 61103).

Innovative Dressings

New products are entering the market yearly as research and development continue to grow and expand in the area of wound care. Too many to mention all, categories include options such as polysaccharide dressings, absorptive fillers, hydrophilic fiber, composite dressings, collagen, and biological products. Hyalofill-F (ConvaTec, Skillman, NJ 08558) is a hyaluronic acid derivative dressing that is applied directly to the wound. Hyaluronic acid is important for its role in cell proliferation. It is useful in helping a chronic wound to move through the stages of healing. First used on neuropathic foot ulcers, it has been used successfully in clinical trials for venous leg ulcers.[215,216]

Manual Lymphatic Drainage

MLD is a specialized manual therapy technique that affects primarily superficial lymphatic circulation. It is considered to be one of the five elements of an effective treatment intervention for lymphedema and many types of edema. This manual therapy provides a gentle stretch to the skin that enhances lymph capillary activity. MLD will increase the frequency of lymphangion contractions; improve lymph transport capacity; redirect lymph flow toward collateral vessels, anastomoses, and uninvolved lymph regions; and mobilize excess lymph fluid that has overwhelmed a body segment or region.[74,217,218] The techniques of MLD are gentle and specific, requiring specialized education to be performed accurately (Fig. 14.35). To obtain contact information for training facilities that provide specialized education in MLD as a part of CDT, refer to the special section in Appendix 14.D for contact information. The benefits of this treatment are not limited to the population with lymphedema. MLD is used

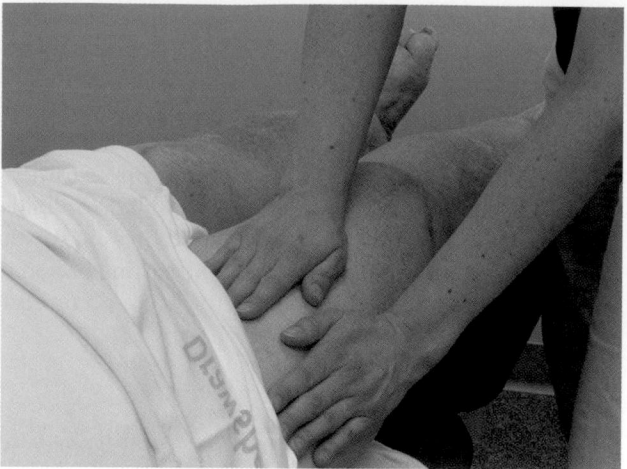

Figure 14.35 Manual lymphatic drainage on the LE.

successfully for edema from CVI, sports injury, neurological injury, and post-operative swelling, but there is a need for more well-designed randomized controlled trials to provide high-ranking evidence.[219,220] The use of MLD is contraindicated for treating cardiac-, pulmonary-, or renal-related edema because the amount of fluid that will be mobilized may overwhelm one or all of those systems when disease is present.[221]

Compression Therapy

Controlling edema or lymphedema is critical to all stages of healing. Edema not only inhibits wound healing by affecting perfusion of tissues, but also inactivates the ability of the skin to manage bacteria.[222] Unless there are red flags, compression should be part of every treatment for individuals with lymphedema, edema, and CVI. Compression therapy should be introduced as soon as clinical signs of swelling or fibrosis appear. A physical therapist may find indications for compression therapy during the examination or later, during the intervention. In most situations the therapist will decide what type and/or style of compression should be applied. Physician authorization, however, may be necessary for reimbursement. When leg wounds are present, compression is essential for timely wound healing. For the individual with mixed arterial and venous disease, an ABI test is indicated to provide information about the safety of using compression on the LE. A greater understanding of how the lymphatic system functions has created a paradigm shift in the way intervention for all types of swelling is planned and delivered. Aggressive compression techniques were once used to "milk" the fluid out of a limb. It is now understood that deep pressure and mechanical "milking" techniques are counterproductive and harmful to the superficial capillary network that filters lymph and interstitial fluids.[4]

Elevation

Elevation is used as a means of controlling some types of swelling and is often a precursor to compression therapy. Mild, acute swelling of the extremities may be relieved temporarily with elevation. Active ROM exercises (e.g., ankle pumps) can be added to elevation to facilitate blood flow in the extremities. Patients should be educated about how to elevate safely, paying attention to positioning so that optimal venous and lymphatic circulation is facilitated. Elevation should be viewed as a temporary or complementary measure while other means of controlling swelling are employed.

Unna's Boot

Compression for the LE with a venous wound can be applied using zinc paste–impregnated gauze or Unna's boot (Fig. 14.36). Examples of conveniently packaged products are Medicopaste (Graham-Field Inc., Bay Shore, NY 11706), Unna-FLEX (ConvaTec, Skillman, NJ 08558), and Gelo-Cast (BSN-JOBST, Charlotte, NC 28209). There is little information in the literature to support the topical application of zinc for wound healing. The success of this treatment application is most likely owing to the compression. It is an inexpensive means of covering a wound, providing compression and supporting the calf pump to empty venous blood from the LE. Unna's boot is not appropriate for arterial or mixed arterial/venous ulcers. Although the treatment is used frequently, there are other methods for combining compression with wound care to treat venous wounds.[223]

Four-Layer Bandage System

Four-layer bandage systems have been associated with leg ulcer closure. The system includes a wound covering with modest absorptive qualities and several layers of compression. The bandage system has been shown to be comfortable and cost-effective.[224] An example of a well-known system is Profore™ (Fig. 14.37) (Smith & Nephew, Inc., Largo, FL 33773). For the appropriate

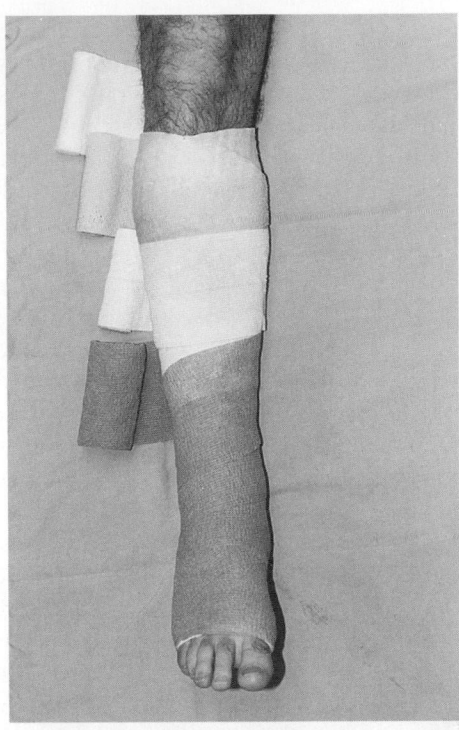

Figure 14.37 Profore™ is a four-layer bandage system consisting of a cotton, crepe, and two compression layers *(top to bottom)*.

patient, a four-layer bandage system can be left in place for up to a week.

Long-Stretch and Short-Stretch Bandages

Both long-stretch and short-stretch bandages are used to control edema and to supply therapeutic levels of compression to support the venous and lymphatic systems. Long-stretch bandages such as Ace (3M, St. Paul, MN 55144) bandages provide a *high resting pressure,* which means that they continue to constrict when the wearer is resting. Owing to their extensibility or stretchiness, they do not provide significant *working pressure,* the ability to resist muscle contraction during activity. Long-stretch bandages are readily available and require minimal training to apply. Short-stretch bandages such as Comprilan (Smith & Nephew, Auckland 1140, NZ) and Rosidal (Lohmann & Rauscher, Topeka, KS 66619) provide *low resting pressure* and *high working pressure* (Fig. 14.38). They are less extensible or stretchy, providing a more rigid shell when applied to a limb. This feature makes short-stretch bandages more appropriate for treating edema and lymphedema. Higher working pressures increase the efficiency of the muscle pump during activity whereas lower resting pressures make the bandages more tolerable to wear. Short-stretch bandages require special training to apply. The amount of working and resting pressure delivered to a limb that is bandaged will depend on several important factors: the number of layers of bandage, the age and condition of the bandages,

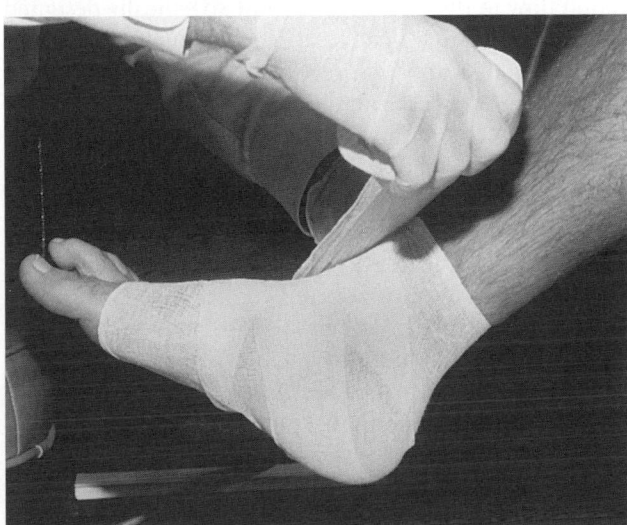

Figure 14.36 Unna's boot application.

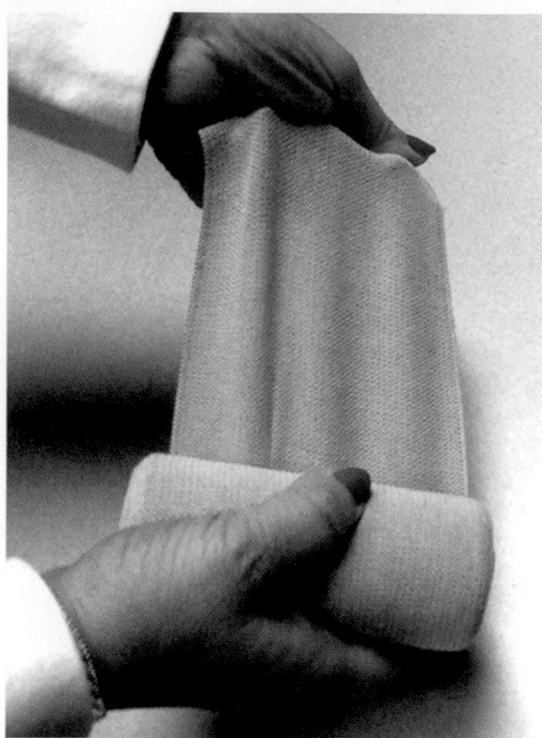

Figure 14.38 Sample of short-stretch bandage.

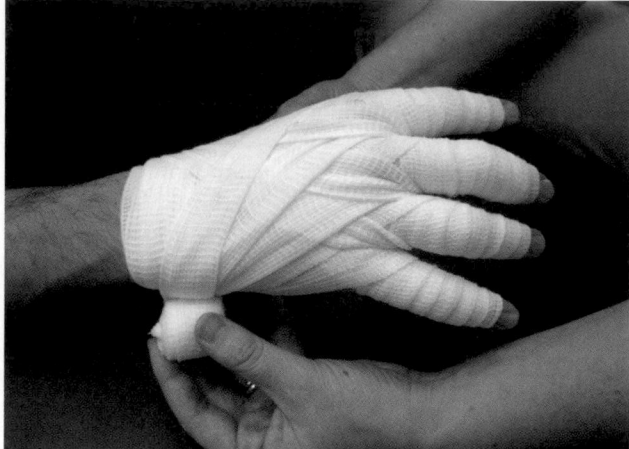

Figure 14.39 Application of lymphedema bandaging to fingers and hand.

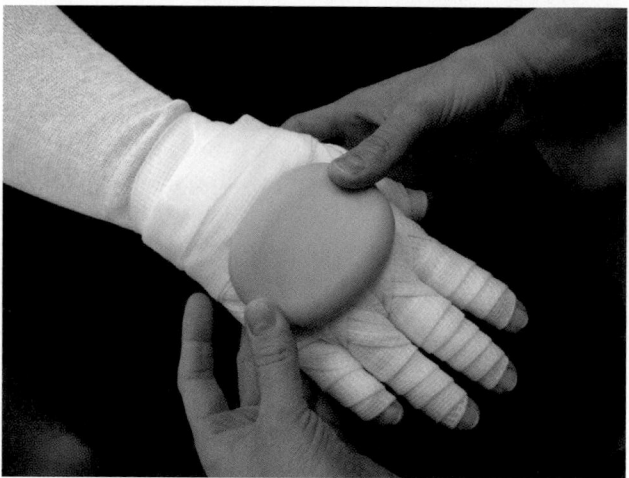

Figure 14.40 Use of foam padding to enhance the effects of lymphedema bandaging.

the tension on the bandage when it is applied, and the skill of the clinician.[225]

Lymphedema Bandaging

This highly specialized form of bandaging utilizes multiple layers of unique padding materials and short-stretch bandages to create a supportive structure for edematous and lymphedematous body segments. Lymphedema bandaging provides support for tissues that have lost elasticity; facilitates a mild increase in tissue pressure, assisting lymph vessels to empty; prevents refilling of the interstitium between MLD treatments; improves the efficiency of the muscle pump during activity; and provides localized pressure where indicated to soften fibrotic tissue.

Bandaging protocols include techniques for applying compression to the head and neck, fingers, and hands (Figs. 14.39 and 14.40), UE (Fig. 14.41), and LE (Fig. 14.42). The chest, abdomen, genital area, and back can also receive specialized support from compression products.[225]

As with MLD, the benefits of this treatment are not limited to the population with lymphedema. When compression is indicated, standard or modified lymphedema bandaging can be beneficial to the population with edema (e.g., post-operative, CVI, venous ulcers, orthopedic injury).[226-231] To obtain contact information for training facilities that provide specialized education in bandaging as a part of CDT refer to Appendix 14.D.

Compression Garments

Many patient/client populations use compression garments (Fig. 14.43). Originally designed to assist venous blood flow in the LEs, they are now specifically designed to manage burn and surgical scars, provide support to venous circulation, and prevent reaccumulation of fluid in the lymphedematous limb. There are a variety of garment styles and fabrics, custom and off-the-shelf, to meet the unique needs of different populations. Varying amounts of pressure are woven into the fabric during manufacturing. The amounts of pressure are conveyed as millimeters of mercury (mm Hg). Low pressure would start at 12 to 25 mm Hg and higher pressures go up to 30 to 40 mm Hg. When appropriately selected and fitted by a trained professional and worn correctly by a prepared patient, the garments serve an essential role in managing chronic, life-long conditions such as CVI and lymphedema.[225,231]

Garments should not be used as a treatment to remove excess fluids from an extremity. If applied to an extremity that has not been adequately evacuated, the garments will be uncomfortable and may worsen the

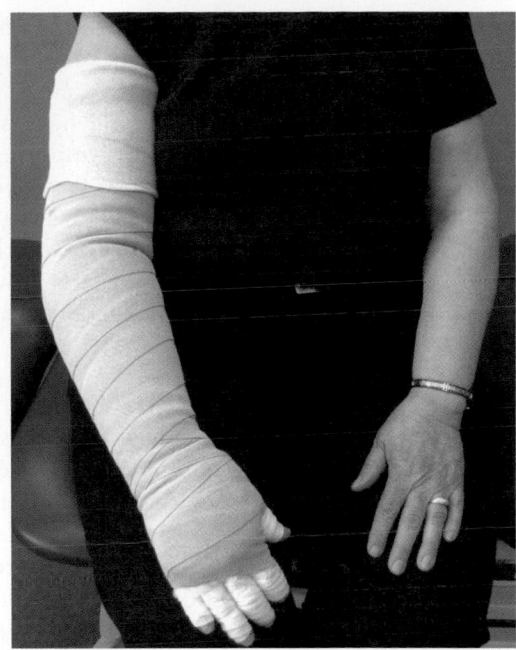

Figure 14.41 Lymphedema bandaging of the UE.

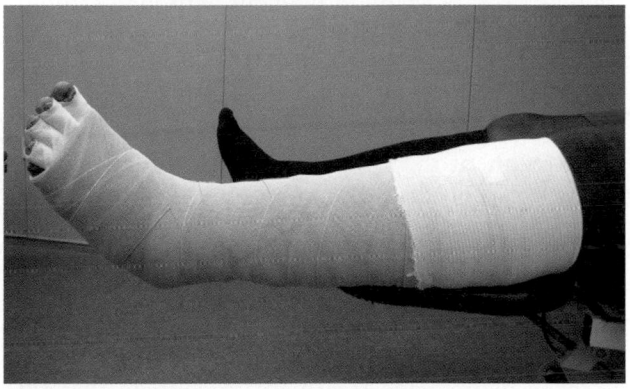

Figure 14.42 Lymphedema bandaging of the foot, ankle, and calf.

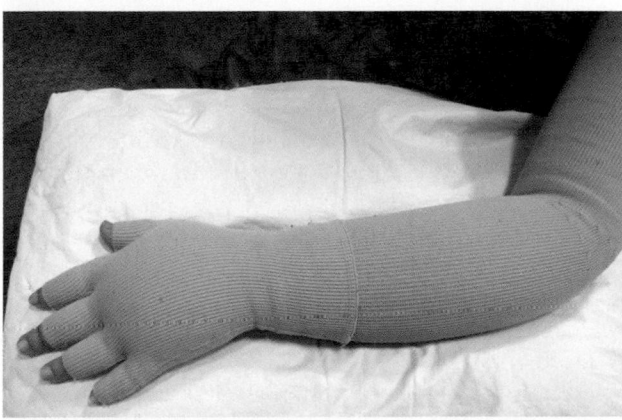

Figure 14.43 Patient wearing custom-fitted UE compression sleeve and separate glove with open fingertips.

patient's symptoms.[232-234] Currently, manufacturers are participating in clinical research supporting the use of silver in compression garments. Juzo Silver (Juzo, Cuyahoga Falls, OH 44223) adds permanently bonded silver to the textile fiber of LE garments to inhibit bacterial growth and reduce odor.

Limb Containment Systems

Another option for some individuals is a quilted compression device or limb containment system. These unique compression options may be easier to don and doff, can be worn under short stretch wraps or alone, and can be custom made to any part of the body (Figs. 14.44 and 14.45). This option may be useful for a person who is unable to apply a more fitted support garment independently or whose skin is compromised or fragile. Patients find that these options are useful as part of their home program to retain reductions they have achieved through therapy. These specialized garments can be made to support venous circulation or lymphatic drainage through altering the style and the stitching channels to complement the diagnosis. A physical therapist can consult with the leading manufacturers to get advice on how to integrate the use of this type of compression into the POC or the after-care by contacting www.jovipak.com and/or www.solarismed.com.

Compression Guidelines

Compression treatment should be customized to the characteristics of each individual. Relative contraindications for compression should be evaluated, including

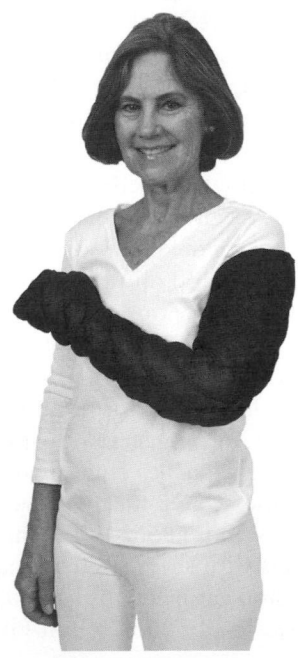

Figure 14.44 Individual wearing a custom arm garment for nighttime lymphedema management. (*Tribute*™ garment Courtesy of Solaris Inc., West Allis, WI 53214.)

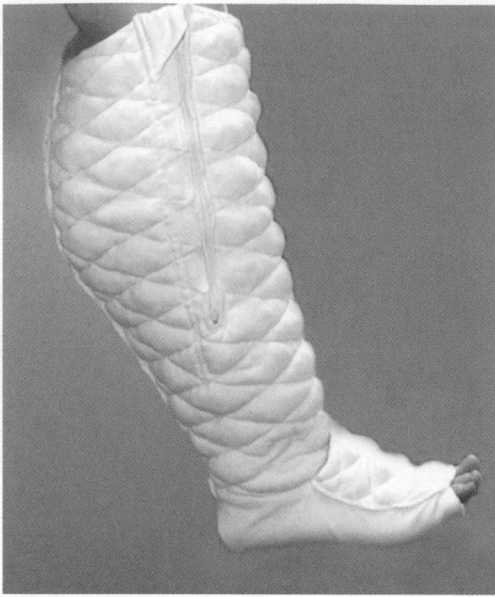

Figure 14.45 Quilted channel compression garment for venous insufficiency. *(JoviPak® garment, Courtesy of JoviPak®, Kent, WA 98032.)*

history of DVT, acute local infection, CHF, cor pulmonale, and acute dermatitis. To assist in clinical decision making, the following is a summary of general guidelines for compression bandaging and garments for edema and lymphedema:

- Arterial wounds: No compression or very light compression with close involvement of the referring practitioner. Long-stretch bandaging or off-the-shelf low compression garment (12 to 25 mm Hg) can be used. Edema will not be great and will evacuate quickly.
- Venous wounds: Compression is an essential component of treatment for wound healing and support of the venous system. Short-stretch bandaging with high working pressure and low resting pressure will facilitate the effects of the calf pump during activity. High pressure of 40 mm Hg at the ankle has been suggested.[229] Compression garments at pressures of 20 to 30 mm Hg to 30 to 40 mm Hg are used depending on location and severity of swelling, as well as ability of the patient to don and doff garments.
- Neuropathic wounds: Compression is contingent on blood flow. Fifteen percent of patients with a neuropathic condition also have an arterial component to their disease and must have an ABI checked before compression is applied. If no arterial involvement, compress with short-stretch wrap. Follow up with compression garments for long-term use at lower compression of 12 to 25 mm Hg up to 20 to 30 mm Hg.
- Lymphedema: Short-stretch compression wrap until limb reduction goal reached then moderate to high compression garments at 20 to 30 mm Hg to 30 to

40 mm Hg depending on location and severity of swelling, as well as ability of the patient to don and doff garments.[225]
- Edema: Case studies and reports from the field establish that the compression treatment for lymphedema also works well for edema.[230] Short-stretch compression bandages are worn 23 hours/day, graduating to daytime only, decreasing as edema resolves. Off-the-shelf garments at lower levels of compression provide support for skin and help to retain reductions that therapy has achieved.

Intermittent Pneumatic Compression

Until the 1990s, intermittent pneumatic compression (IPC) was one of the few clinical interventions used to treat swelling (Fig. 14.46). Since then, new information about the physiology of edema and lymphedema, as well as lymphatic system function, has limited its value in treating some edema and most lymphedema. Intermittent compression pumps can facilitate venous return and may be an important adjunct to other forms of compression for the individual with a venous disorder.[3,235] A review of the evidence provided only modest support for the use of IPC for the treatment of venous leg ulcers.[236-238] Many individuals with long-standing venous insufficiency also have lymphedema. There is even less evidence and more controversy related to the use of IPC for lymphedema.[239-242] If a trial of IPC is indicated, MLD should be delivered before and after each treatment to offset the negative effects of fluid pooling that occurs adjacent to the edge of the limb sleeves. If indicated for treatment, IPC pressure settings must be kept very low to avoid collapse of the superficial lymph capillaries. Each client should be carefully examined by an experienced health care professional before IPC is applied. Blood pressure readings should be taken before each treatment to confirm that IPC will be safe to use. Increasing total peripheral resistance with pneumatic compression will increase the work

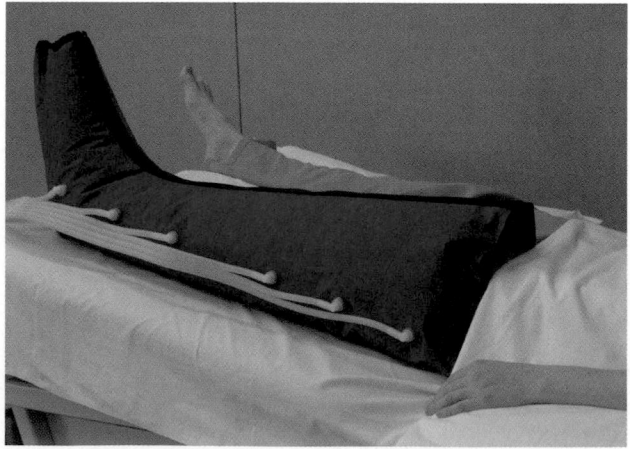

Figure 14.46 Intermittent pneumatic compression pump.

of the heart, increasing blood pressure. Pneumatic compression treatment is contraindicated for individuals with hypertension or a blood pressure reading greater than 140/90. Other contraindications to intermittent compression include acute inflammation or trauma, local infection, presence of thrombus, cardiac or kidney dysfunction, obstructed lymphatic channels, and impaired cognitive function.

Sequential Pneumatic Compression with Truncal Component

Advances in compression systems include more pneumatic chambers that inflate and deflate in a sequential pattern at very low pressures. The newest home use models include truncal decongestion and clearance in preparation for receiving lymph from affected areas. This appliance style mimics the benefits of MLD in the clinic setting (Fig. 14.47). Manual treatments clear the trunk proximally before treating more distal segments of the body. Stretch fabric is incorporated into the appliance design to further mimic the light stretch to the skin that is applied with MLD.[74,243-245]

Positioning

Positioning techniques are used to prevent or protect pressure ulcers, as well as other types of wounds, edema, lymphedema, and vascular disorders. This important aspect of intervention, as well as PRDs, should not be overlooked or underestimated during treatment planning. Devices and techniques selected for positioning should be compatible with the individual's health status. It is paramount that a personalized positioning and repositioning schedule be developed and prominently displayed for any patient who cannot position or reposition independently. The standard time intervals used for turning schedules (i.e., every 2 hours) are often too long for individuals who are frail, have fragile skin, or have existing wounds. A turning schedule could be as frequent as every 30 minutes in some cases whereas for other individuals, every 4 hours may be enough. Suggestions for patient positioning programs include the following:[246-248]

- The patient's heels should be protected and elevated off the surface of the bed.
- The head of bed should not be elevated past 30° unless medically necessary.
- An individualized turning schedule should be provided.
- PRDs should be used in conjunction with a turning schedule.
- Positioning with weight-bearing directly over the greater trochanter should be avoided.
- Positioning with full weight-bearing over an existing wound should be avoided.
- Donut-shaped devices for seating solutions should not be used.
- Pillows and wedges should be used to separate bony prominences from bed and other body parts.

Pressure-Redistributing Devices

Pressure has a direct influence on perfusion or vascularity of a wound site. PRDs should be used to prevent skin breakdown, during the wound healing phase, and during the self-management phase, for life-long protection and prevention (Fig. 14.48). Along with positioning, patients and their caregivers must be educated about pressure redistribution and prevention of pressure-related trauma.[249] Advances in support surfaces that redistribute weight have made them more sophisticated and effective (Fig. 14.49). Experts in positioning systems are readily available to advise and instruct clinicians working with special populations.[250] Groups such as the Consortium for Spinal Cord Medicine, NPUAP, and HHS have made recommendations and algorithms for positioning and pressure redistributing devices that can be used for intervention planning.[76,101,251,252]

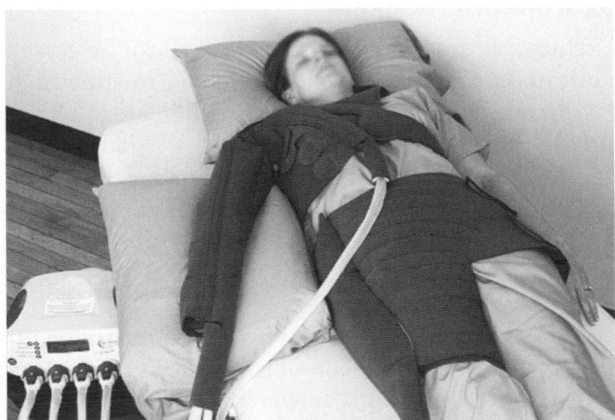

Figure 14.47 Flexitouch® system: Sequential pneumatic compression with truncal component designed to retain and support the benefits of in-clinic lymphedema therapy at home. *(Courtesy of Tactile Systems Technology, Minneapolis, MN 55413.)*

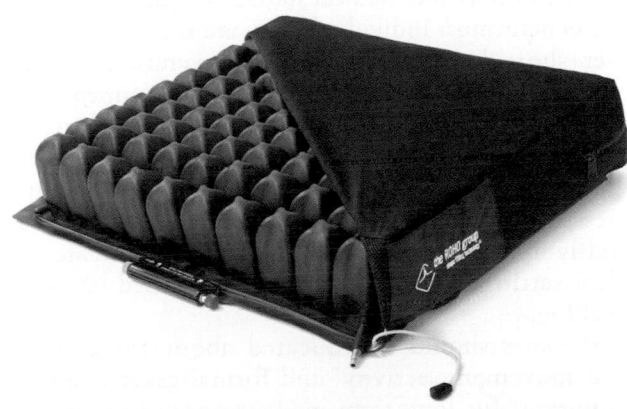

Figure 14.48 ROHO® QUADTRO SELECT® HIGH PROFILE® Cushion for pressure redistribution and skin protection. *(Courtesy of ROHO, Inc., Belleville, IL 62221.)*

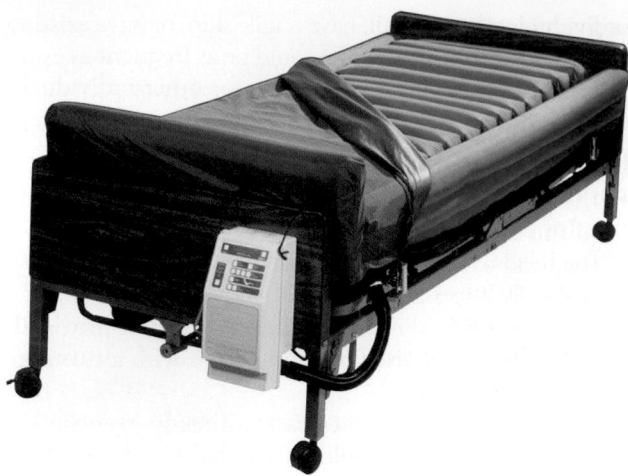

Figure 14.49 *Select*Air® MAX, a low-air-loss support system for pressure relief. *(Courtesy of The ROHO Group, Belleville, IL 62221.)*

Exercise

The physical therapist should educate patients and promote activities in the POC related to increasing activity levels as appropriate. Too often, exercise is neglected in the intervention plan for individuals with vascular, lymphatic, and integumentary disorders, especially those with wounds or edema. Exercise is indicated for a variety of reasons, including, but not limited to, the following: increase strength and joint ROM, improve quality of movement, increase ADL, improve QOL perceptions, increase blood flow to the extremities, improve calf pump activity, prevent pressure ulcers, and enhance the effects of lymphedema bandaging. Exercise might be contraindicated or planned with caution when medical issues arise such as the need to be non–weight-bearing on a foot wound, unstable cardiopulmonary conditions, or related orthopedic problems that would limit activity.

Exercise prescription should be customized to the patient's needs and medical status. A walking program can benefit most individuals who are able to ambulate even short distances. Water-based exercise programs can facilitate the transition from bed or chair to land-based exercise. Individuals with wounds can participate in water-based exercise if it is appropriate to cover the wounds with occlusive dressings. The hydrostatic pressure of water contributes to support of edematous and lymphedematous body segments and creates an ideal setting for exercise for most individuals with swelling.

Patients should be educated about the concept that movement, activity, and formal exercise are all important for long-term management of the conditions listed in this chapter. Physical therapists introduce these concepts, provide expert instruction, and develop appropriate home exercise programs. Patients are guided to accept responsibility for following the exercise prescriptions at home and for making them a part of their everyday lives.

Orthotics

Splinting

Patients who are immobile may benefit from resting splints to retain, or dynamic splints to regain, functional ROM. Splinting can also prevent skin breakdown by retaining normal positioning of joints during periods of immobility. Extra precautions (i.e., padding) must be taken to protect aging or fragile skin from breakdown when semi-rigid thermoplastic materials are used for splinting. The use of splinting to manage burn scar is an essential part of the POC for an individual with a thermal injury (see Chapter 24, Burns). Positioning and splinting pointers found there can also be applied to patients with other types of wounds.

Total Contact Casting

One method for reduction of weight-bearing stresses on the foot is the application of a *total contact cast (TCC)*. This method can be useful for the individual with a neuropathic ulcer on the plantar surface of the foot. After infection and swelling have been controlled, a plaster cast is applied from the toes to below the knee. A specially trained individual uses plaster, padding techniques, and the placement of a rubber insert on the weight-bearing part of the cast to complete the application. A TCC is usually worn for 7 to 10 days at a time, removed for skin care, and then reapplied. According to a classic article by Salsich et al,[253] TCC is effective at healing ulcers initially, but the rate of reulceration once the cast is removed is high.

Neuropathic Walker

A removable ankle-foot orthosis (AFO) can be custom fabricated or ordered prefabricated to provide weight distribution and cushioning for the individual with an insensate foot, a chronic foot ulcer, or Charcot joint (Fig. 14.50). This option is versatile in fit and allows skin checks, dressing changes, and pressure alterations as needed.

Cast Shoes

Cast shoes or post-operative (post-op) shoes can be utilized as an inexpensive, temporary alternative for wound off-loading. These shoes, however, do not provide any means of controlling foot motion and little cushioning protection for the chronic wound. This option should be considered temporary. Patients wearing cast shoes for pressure distribution should be monitored closely for signs of complications.

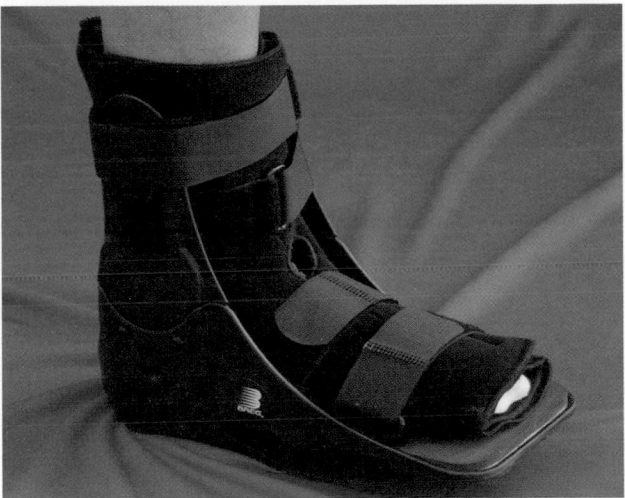

Figure 14.50 An ankle-foot orthosis specifically designed to allow distributed weight-bearing for individuals with neuropathy.

Extra-Depth Shoes

Extra-depth shoes have a roomy toe box and a deep sole to provide shock absorption and cushion. The shoes should redirect foot pressure away from bony prominences and wounds (Fig. 14.51).[254] Available in many styles, they can be purchased from an orthotist or at a specialty shoe store. Individuals with insensate feet, with or without wounds, should strongly consider wearing this type of shoe to support skin protection and ulcer prevention.

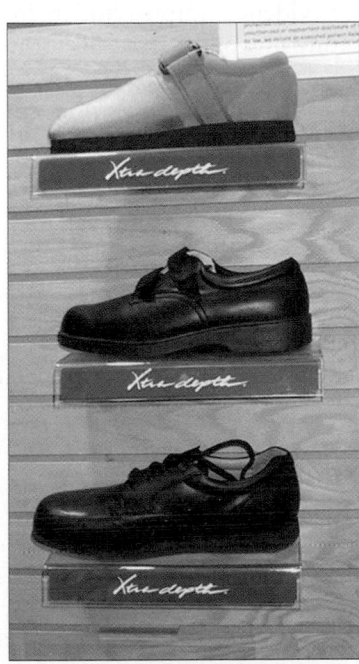

Figure 14.51 Extra-depth shoe.

Scar Management

As described earlier in this chapter, scar formation is a component of wound healing.[255] After the wound is filled with collagen, the tissue must be remodeled and shaped into the finely structured end product. Contraction of scar tissue can lead to disfigurement and loss of function, especially if the scar tissue is located over a joint surface. Issues of disfigurement and dysfunction are greatest following thermal injury (see Chapter 24, Burns). Currently, the mechanisms by which scar can be controlled are not completely understood. Although some interventions do seem to help, there is room for further investigation into how to achieve optimal control of scar formation. Most scar tissue is managed by a physical therapist using compression garments, stretching exercises, orthotics, positioning, specific types of massage, and the use of topical adjuncts such as silicone gel sheets (Fig. 14.52) and elastomer putty (Fig. 14.53). Topical creams, oils, and ointments have

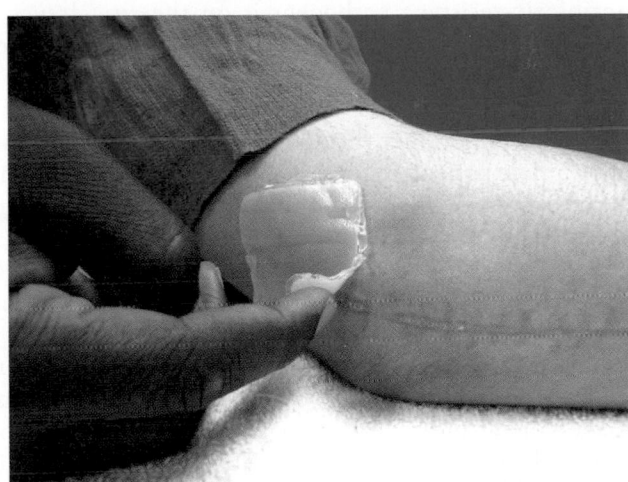

Figure 14.52 Application of a silicone gel sheet to scar tissue during the maturation phase of wound healing.

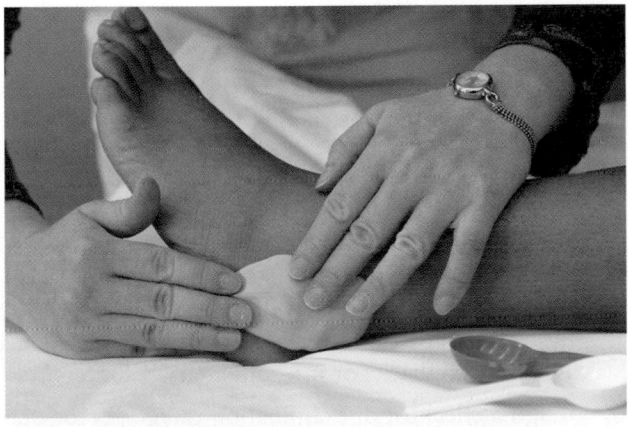

Figure 14.53 Application of elastomer putty to scar tissue during the maturation phase of wound healing.

some positive effects on scar but it is not known if the massaging actions used to apply the agents or the agents themselves provide the therapeutic effects. Early and adequate intervention can prevent most of the complications of scarring. Since the process of scar formation usually continues for 6 to 24 months, follow-up care should be part of the intervention plan. Individuals with scar tissue must learn how to safely massage the skin at home because frequent pressure applications have the greatest influence on new connective tissue orientation. When conservative measures of scar management have not controlled scarring, surgical intervention may be indicated. Following surgery, the individual will have a new wound and subsequent new scar to manage.

SUMMARY

These are exciting times for clinicians interested in the care of patients with vascular, lymphatic, and integumentary disorders. Skin and wound care practices continue to advance with clinical trials, randomized controlled studies, and empirical data all contributing to the pool of knowledge. New information about the microcirculation of blood and lymph has changed intervention strategies. The role of the skin as an organ has gained new respect. It is not surprising that there is an explosion of research, literature, and products to serve the needs of individuals with disorders affecting these systems. Current and future generations are facing healthcare challenges of a magnitude never before seen in our society, including an increase in the number of individuals with conditions related to the disorders discussed in this chapter. The incidence of diabetes, obesity, vascular and lymphatic disease, chronic wounds, and antibiotic-resistant pathogens is on the rise. Issues compounding the challenges include a growing population of older individuals, health care reimbursement challenges, and numerous ethical dilemmas in daily practice.

This chapter provides support for clinicians in their efforts to provide excellent patient care. Topics of particular importance include current strategies for wound management, the importance of adequate and appropriate patient education, pressure ulcer prevention and precautions, advanced foot care for individuals with diabetic neuropathy, optimal compression for lymphedema, the essential role of moisture in wound healing, and the importance of exercise as part of the POC.

There is great need for ongoing research to establish the level of strength of evidence for a variety of topics that may or may not be important in the world of vascular, lymphatic, and integumentary disorders. Some of the concepts that deserve a second look are the impact of bio-burden on the wound infection continuum, the preparation of the wound bed, the use of exogenous oxygen applications, noncontact US, nonthermal radiofrequency stimulation, cold laser, biosurgery, bioengineered tissue, exogenous growth factors, medical-grade honey, and topical silver preparations. In addition to expanding the evidence, improvements in the standardizing of wound care education are needed. The interdisciplinary nature of wound care calls for more communication among health care professionals. Wise clinicians must keep abreast of new information and current standards of care, approaching new entries to the field with a strong sense of clinical intuition, as well as a firm grasp of the scientific evidence.

Questions for Review

1. Discuss the differences, similarities, and relationships among the arterial, venous, and lymphatic systems. Compare anatomy, method of fluid movement, and function.

2. Outline some of the unique characteristics that can be identified clinically for disorders of the vascular, lymphatic, and integumentary systems.

3. Prepare a list of factors that contribute to abnormal wound healing. Divide the list into intrinsic, extrinsic, and iatrogenic factors.

4. Review the annotated tests and measurements included in this chapter that should be used during a physical therapy examination. Identify tests and measurements routinely performed for patients with vascular, lymphatic, or integumentary disorders.

5. Design a checklist of examination categories for examining a patient with a disorder of the vascular, lymphatic, and/or integumentary systems.

6. Create a general list of the primary components of a POC for a patient with a wound.

7. Explain how a physical therapist should respond to the knowledge that many vascular, lymphatic, and integumentary disorders have a long latency period and require a heightened level of vigilance and proactivity in order to identify symptoms and begin treatment as early as possible.

8. Explain the rationale for each of the following treatments in skin and wound care: moist wound healing, arterial wound hydration, venous wound compression, lymphedema treatment, and foot care for the individual with diabetes.

CASE STUDY

REFERRAL
A 78-year-old woman with a primary diagnosis of Alzheimer's disease has been living in a residential facility for 10 months. The physician at the facility refers her to physical therapy. Referral is for advanced wound care.

PAST MEDICAL HISTORY
Unremarkable until onset of symptoms of Alzheimer's 3 years ago.

CURRENT MEDICAL HISTORY
Health conditions include mild hypertension controlled by medication and a Stage III pressure ulcer over the right ischial tuberosity.

MEDICAL INTERVENTION PREVIOUS TO CURRENT REFERRAL
Pressure ulcer treated for 4 weeks (30 days) with bid hydrogen peroxide flushes followed by dry gauze 4 × 4s covered with gauze pad and adhesive tape. No changes in wound bed for 4 weeks. No other intervention in place.

PSYCHOSOCIAL
Husband also resident of same facility, lives in same room. Husband is frail but mobile and contributes to care for wife. No children. Patient enjoys music and trips by wheelchair to activity center in facility.

COGNITIVE
Patient disoriented to place and time. Becomes agitated during wound care. She is unable to follow weight shift and turning schedules independently and has difficulty following instructions.

PHYSICAL THERAPY EXAMINATION DATA
Body Structure/Function
- *Wound:* Stage III pressure ulcer over right ischial tuberosity. Measures 6 × 4 cm (2.36 × 1.57 in) with depth of 4 cm (1.57 in). The wound bed is 50% necrotic yellow tissue and 50% red granulation tissue. Periwound tissue is intact. Drainage is moderate, yellow-brown, and thin with minimal odor. The wound is currently contaminated but not infected (i.e., colonized bacteria are present but not to the level of clinical infection).
- *Strength and ROM:* Patient unable to follow commands consistently for examination of strength but appears to have functional strength and ROM of bilateral upper extremities (BUEs). Gross bilateral lower extremity (BLE) strength is impaired perhaps owing to declining activity levels. Active ROM appears functional in BUEs. Bilateral hip flexion contractures of 30° can be reduced to 15° with passive ROM.

Activity Limitations—Mobility
Patient is either in wheelchair or bed 24 hours/day. Patient is unable to roll independently but can often assist using BUEs when instructed. Requires maximum assist of two to pivot transfer. The patient is unable to ambulate at this time.

Participation Restrictions
Requires close supervision during social engagement due to propensity to become agitated.

GUIDING QUESTIONS
1. What are the contributing factors that have most likely led to the chronicity of this wound?

2. What other factors might contribute to the slow healing time of this wound?

3. What combination of interventions to clean and débride would allow removal of necrotic tissue while protecting granulation tissue?

4. Clinically, which electromodalities are biocompatible for the treatment of this wound (irrespective of payment) and how will they contribute to wound healing?

5. Other than local wound care, what intervention will be essential for wound closure?

6. Once progress has been made in wound healing, if the wound were to become dry, what dressing types could be used to create a moist wound environment?

7. If using an occlusive dressing, why should this patient be closely monitored?

8. Assuming this patient's wound will close, what are the expectations for the condition of her skin over the wound site?

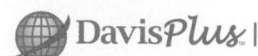 For additional resources, including answers to the questions for review and case study guiding questions, please visit **http://davisplus.fadavis.com**

References

1. Martini, FH: Fundamentals of Anatomy and Physiology, ed 4. Prentice-Hall, Upper Saddle River, NJ, 2008.
2. Kelly, DG: A Primer on Lymphedema. Prentice-Hall, Upper Saddle River, NJ, 2002.
3. McCulloch, JM: Therapeutic modalities stimulate wound management. Biomechanics 67, April 2004.
4. Eliska, O, and Eliskova, M: Are peripheral lymphatics damaged by high pressure manual massage? Lymphology 28:21, 1995.
5. Casley-Smith, JR: Varying total tissue pressures and the concentration of initial lymphatic lymph. Microvasc Res 25:369, 1983.
6. Mortimer, PS, et al: The measurement of skin lymph flow by isotope clearance—reliability, reproducibility, injection dynamics and the effect of massage. J Invest Dermatol 95(6):677, 1990.
7. Olszewski, WL, and Engeset, A: Intrinsic contractility of prenodal lymph vessels and lymph flow in human leg. Am J Physiol 239(6):H775, 1980.
8. Smith, A: Lymphatic drainage in patients after replantation of extremities. Plast Reconstr Surg 79:163, 1987.
9. Bertram, CD, Macaskill, C, and Moore, JE, Jr: Simulation of a chain of collapsible contracting lymphangions with progressive valve closure. J Biomech Eng 133(1):011008, 2011.
10. Gashev, AA: Lymphatic vessels: Pressure-and flow-dependent regulatory reactions. Ann NY Acad Sci 1131:100, 2008.
11. Campton-Johnson, S, and Wilson, J: Infected wound management: Advanced technologies, moisture-retentive dressings, and die-hard methods. Crit Care Nurs Q 24(2):64, 2001.
12. Sen, CK: The general case of redox control of wound repair. Wound Repair Regen 11(6):431, 2003.
13. Gordillo, GM, and Sen, CK: Revisiting the essential role of oxygen in wound healing. Am J Surg 186:259, 2003.
14. Grief, R, et al: Supplemental perioperative oxygen to reduce the incidence of surgical wound infection. N Eng J Med 342:161, 2000.
15. Atiyeh, BS, et al: Management of acute and chronic open wounds: The importance of moist environment to optimal wound healing. Curr Pharm Biotechnol 3:179, 2002.
16. Svensjo, T, et al: Accelerated healing of full-thickness skin wounds in a wet environment. Plast Reconstr Surg 106(3):602, 2000.
17. Bolton, L: Operational definition of moist wound healing. J Wound Ostomy Continence Nurs 34(1):23, 2007.
18. Okan, D, et al: The role of moisture balance in wound healing. Adv Skin Wound Care 20:39, 2007.
19. Schultz, GS, et al: Wound bed preparation: A systematic approach to wound management. Wound Rep Reg 11:1, 2003.
20. Lee, JE, et al: An infection-preventing bilayered collagen membrane containing antibiotic-loaded hyaluronan microparticles: Physical and biological properties. Artif Organs 26(7): 636, 2002.
21. Thomas, DW, et al: Randomized clinical trial of the effect of semi-occlusive dressings on the microflora and clinical outcome of acute facial wounds. Wound Repair Regen 8(4):258, 2000.
22. Koupil, J, et al: The influence of moisture wound healing on the incidence of bacterial infection and histological changes in healthy human skin after treatment of interactive dressings. Acta Chir Plast 45(3):89, 2003.
23. Ratliff, CR: Wound exudate: An influential factor in healing. Adv Nurs Pract 16(7):32, 2008.
24. Mechanick, JI: Practical aspects of nutritional support for wound-healing patients. Am J Surg 188(1, Suppl 1):52, 2004.
25. Shepherd, AA: Nutrition for optimum wound healing. Nurs Stand 18(6):55, 2003.
26. Gray, M: Does oral supplementation with vitamins A or E promote healing of chronic wounds? J Wound Ostom Continen Nurs 30(6):290, 2003.
27. Gray, M: Does vitamin C supplementation promote pressure ulcer healing? J Wound Osteom Continen Nurs 30(5):245, 2003.
28. Collins, N: The right mix: Using nutritional interventions and an anabolic agent to manage a Stage IV ulcer. Adv Skin Wound Care 17(1):36, 2004.
29. Collins, N: Diabetes, nutrition and wound healing. Adv Skin Wound Care 16(6):292, 2003.
30. Williams, JZ, and Barbul, A: Nutrition and wound healing. Surg Clin North Am 83:571, 2003.
31. Zulkowski, K, and Albrecht, D: How nutrition and aging affect wound healing. Nursing 33(8):70, 2003.
32. Barnes, P, Sauter, T, and Azheri, S: Subnormal prealbumin levels and wound healing. Tex Med 103(8):65, 2007.
33. Rodriguez-Key, M, and Alonzi, A: Nutrition, skin integrity, and pressure ulcer healing in chronically ill children: An overview. Ostomy Wound Manage 53(6):56, 2007.
34. Stechmiller, JK: Understanding the role of nutrition and wound healing. Nutr Clin Pract 25(1):61, 2010.
35. Zhang, XJ, et al: Enteral arginine supplementation stimulates DNA synthesis in skin donor wound. Clin Nutr, Jan 29, 2011. [Epub ahead of print.]
36. McMahon, L, et al: A randomized phase II trial of arginine butyrate with standard local therapy in refractory sickle cell leg ulcers. Br J Haematol 151(5):516, 2010.
37. Cartwright, A: Nutritional assessment as part of wound management. Nurs Times 98(44):62, 2002.
38. Bill, TJ, et al: Quantitative swab culture versus tissue biopsy: A comparison in chronic wounds. Ostomy Wound Manage 47(1):34, 2001.
39. Hardy, M: The physiology of scar formation. Phys Ther 69(22):1014, 1989.
40. Goldberg, SR, and Diegelmann, RF: Wound healing primer. Surg Clin North Am 90:1133, 2010.
41. Dunn, SL: The wound healing process. In Kloth, LC, and McCulloch, JM (eds): Wound Healing: Evidence-Based Management, ed 4. FA Davis, Philadelphia, 2010, p 9.
42. Sussman, C, and Bates-Jensen, BM: Wound healing physiology and chronic wound healing. In Sussman, C, and Bates, BM (eds): Wound Care: A Collaborative Practice Manual for Physical Therapists and Nurses, ed 3. Lippincott Williams & Wilkins, Baltimore, MD, 2007, p 21.

43. Bates-Jensen, BM, and Sussman, C: Tools to measure wound healing. In Sussman, C, and Bates, BM (eds): Wound Care: A Collaborative Practice Manual for Physical Therapists and Nurses, ed 3. Lippincott Williams & Wilkins, Baltimore, MD, 2007, p 144.

44. Weed, T, Ratliff C, and Drake DB: Quantifying bacterial bioburden during negative pressure wound therapy. Ann Plast Surg 52(3):276, 2004.

45. Lindholm, C: Pressure ulcers and infection—understanding clinical features. Ostomy Wound Manage 49(5A):4, 2003.

46. Beitz, JM, and Goldberg, E: The lived experience of having a chronic wound: A phenomenologic study. Medsurg Nurs 14(1):51, 2005.

47. Glasper, ER, and Devries, AC: Social structure influences effects of pair-housing on wound healing. Brain Behav Immun 19(1):61, 2005.

48. Detillion, CE, et al: Social facilitation of wound healing. Psychoneuroendocrinology 29(8):1004, 2005.

49. Ebrecht, M, et al: Perceived stress and cortisol levels predict speed of wound healing in healthy male adults. Psychoneuroendocrinology 29(6):798, 2004.

50. Norman, D: The effects of stress on wound healing and leg ulceration. Br J Nurs 10;12(21):1256, 2003.

51. Jones, J: Stress responses, pressure ulcer development and adaptation. Br J Nurs 12(11 Suppl):S17, 2003.

52. Worldwide Wound Management 2002–2012: Products, Technologies and Market Opportunities, Report S200, February 2003, MedMarket Diligence, LLC.

53. Hiatt, WR: Medical treatment of peripheral arterial disease and claudication. N Engl J Med 344(21):1608, 2001.

54. Valencia, IC, et al: Chronic venous insufficiency and venous leg ulceration. J Am Acad Dermatol 44(3): 401, 2001.

55. Kunimoto, B, et al: Best practices for the prevention and treatment of venous leg ulcers. Ostomy Wound Manage 47(2):34, 2001.

56. Seiggreen, MY, and Kline, RA: Vascular ulcers. In Baranoski, S, and Ayello, EA (eds): Wound Care Essentials: Practice Principles. Lippincott Williams & Wilkins, Springhouse, PA, 2004, p 271.

57. Word, R: Medical and surgical therapy for advanced chronic venous insufficiency. Surg Clin North Am 90(6):1195, 2010.

58. Kolbach, DN, et al: Severity of venous insufficiency is related to the density of microvascular deposition of PAI-1, uPA and von Willebrand factor. J Vasc Dis 33(1):19, 2004.

59. Berard, A, et al: Risk factors for the first time development of venous ulcers of the lower limbs: The influence of heredity and physical activity. Angiology 53(6):647, 2002.

60. Gloviczki, P, et al: The care of patients with varicose veins and associated chronic venous diseases: Clinical practice guidelines of the Society for Vascular Surgery and the American Venous Forum. J Vasc Surg 53(5 Suppl):2S, 2011.

61. Kelechi, TJ, et al: Skin temperature and chronic venous insufficiency. J Wound Ostomy Continence Nurs 30(1):17, 2003.

62. Strossenreuther, RHK, et al: Guidelines for the application of MLD/CDT for primary and secondary lymphedema and other selected pathologies. In Foldi, M, Foldi, E, and Kubik, S (eds): Textbook of Lymphology for Physicians and Lymphedema Therapists, ed 5. Elsevier, Munich, Germany, 2003, p 590.

63. Foldi, E, et al: Lymphostatic diseases. In Foldi, M, Foldi, E, and Kubik, S (eds): Textbook of Lymphology for Physicians and Lymphedema Therapists, ed 5. Elsevier, Munich, Germany, 2003, p 232.

64. Bunke, N, Brown, K, and Bergan, J: Phlebolymphedema, usually unrecognized, often poorly treated. Perspect Vasc Surg Endovasc Ther 21(2):65, 2009.

65. Gaber, Y: Secondary lymphoedema of the lower leg as an unusual side-effect of a liquid silicone injection in the hips and buttocks. Dermatology 208:342, 2004.

66. Halaska, MJ, et al: A prospective study of postoperative lymphedema after surgery for cervical cancer. Int J Gynecol Cancer 20(5):900, 2010.

67. Kasper, DA, and Meller, MM: Lymphedema of the hand and forearm following fracture of the distal radius. Orthopedics 31(2):172, 2008.

68. Szuba, A, et al: The third circulation: Radionuclide lymphoscintigraphy in the evaluation of lymphedema. J Nucl Med 44:43, 2003.

69. Tartaglione, G, et al: Intradermal lymphoscintigraphy at rest and after exercise: A new technique for the functional assessment of the lymphatic system in patients with lymphoedema. Nucl Med Commun 31(6):547, 2010.

70. Yuan, Z, et al: The role of radionuclide lymphoscintigraphy in extremity lymphedema. Ann Nucl Med 20(5):341, 2006.

71. Hamner, JB, and Fleming, MD: Lymphedema therapy reduces the volume of edema and pain in patients with breast cancer. Ann Surg Onc 14(6):1904, 2007.

72. Mondry, TF, Riffengurgh, RH, and Johnstone, PA: Prospective trial of complete decongestive therapy for upper extremity lymphedema after breast cancer therapy. Cancer J 10:42, 2004.

73. Koul, R, et al: Efficacy of complete decongestive therapy and manual lymphatic drainage on treatment-related lymphedema in breast cancer. Int J Radiat Oncol Biol Phys 67(3):841, 2007.

74. Mayrovitz, HN: The standard of care for lymphedema: Current concepts and physiological considerations. Lymphat Res Biol 7(2):101, 2009.

75. Baumgarten, M, et al: Pressure ulcers and the transition to long-term care. Adv Skin Wound Care 16(6):299, 2003.

76. Consortium for Spinal Cord Medicine: Pressure Ulcer Prevention and Treatment Following Spinal Cord Injury: A Clinical Practice Guideline for Health Care Professionals. Paralyzed Veterans of American, Washington, DC, 2000. Retrieved July 4, 2011, from www.pva.org.

77. Langemo, DK, Anderson, J, and Volden, C: Uncovering pressure ulcer incidence. Nurs Manage 34(10):64, 2003.

78. Scott, EM, et al: Effects of warming therapy on pressure ulcers—a randomized trial. J Periop Nurs, May 2001.

79. Reed, RL, et al: Low serum albumin levels, confusion, and fecal incontinence: Are these risk factors for pressure ulcers in mobility-impaired hospitalized adults? Gerontology 49(4):255, 2003.

80. de Souza, DM, and de Gouveia Santos, VL: Incidence of pressure ulcers in the institutionalized elderly. J Wound Ostomy 37(3):272, 2010.

81. Institute for Clinical Systems Improvement (ICSI): Pressure Ulcer Prevention and Treatment. Health Care Protocol. ICSI, Bloomington, MN, 2010.

82. Lyder, C, et al: Quality of care for hospitalized Medicare patients at risk for pressure ulcers. Arch Intern Med 161:1549, 2001.

83. Van Rijswijk, L: The question of outcomes. Ostomy Wound Manage 49(2):6, 2003.

84. Ennis, WJ, et al: Ultrasound therapy for recalcitrant diabetic foot ulcers: Results of a randomized, double-blind, controlled, multi-center study. Ostomy Wound Manage 51(8):24, 2005.

85. Centers for Disease Control and Prevention: National Diabetes Fact Sheet: National Estimates and General Information on Diabetes and Prediabetes in the United States, 2011. US Department of Health and Human Services, Centers for Disease Control and Prevention, Atlanta, 2011.

86. Cowie, CC, et al: Prevalence of diabetes and impaired fasting glucose in adults—United States, 1999–2000. MMWR Morb Mortal Wkly Rep 52(35):833, 2003.

87. Centers for Disease Control and Prevention: National Diabetes Fact Sheet: General Information and National Estimates on Diabetes in the Unites States, 2011. US Department of Health and Human Services, Centers for Disease Control and Prevention, Atlanta, 2011.

88. American Physical Therapy Association: Guide to Physical Therapist Practice, ed 2. Phys Ther 81(1):S49, 2001.

89. Ridner, SH, et al: Comparison of upper limb volume measurement techniques and arm symptoms between healthy volunteers and individuals with known lymphedema. Lymphology 40(1):35, 2007.

90. Warren, AG, et al: The use of bioimpedance analysis to evaluate lymphedema. Ann Plast Surg 58(5):541, 2007.

91. Cornish, BH, et al: Early diagnosis of lymphedema using multiple frequency bioimpedance. Lymphology 34(1):2, 2001.

92. Czerniec, SA, et al: Assessment of breast cancer–related arm lymphedema—comparison of physical measurement methods and self-report. Cancer Invest 28(1):54, 2010.

93. Brittain, A (ed): Lymphedema: Understanding and Managing Lymphedema after Cancer Treatment. American Cancer Society, Atlanta, 2006, p 59.

94. McCulloch, JM: Assessing the circulatory and neurological systems. In Kloth, LC, and McCulloch, JM (eds): Wound Healing: Evidence-Based Management, ed 4. FA Davis, Philadelphia, 2010, p 94.

95. Patterson, GK: Vascular evaluation. In Sussman, C, and Bates, BM: Wound Care: A Collaborative Practice Manual for Physical Therapists and Nurses, ed 3. Lippincott Williams & Wilkins, Baltimore, 2007, p 180.

96. Mehta, T, et al: Disease-specific quality of life assessment in intermittent claudication: Review. Eur J Endovasc Surg 25: 202, 2003.

97. Lehert, P: Quality-of-life assessment in comparative therapeutic trials and causal structure considerations in peripheral occlusive arterial disease. Pharmacoeconomics 19(2):121, 2001.

98. Marquis, P, Comte, S, and Lehert, P: International validation of the CLAUS-S Quality-of-Life Questionnaire for Use in Patients with Intermittent Claudication. Pharmacoeconomics 19(6):667, 2001.

99. Tiedjen, KU, et al: Radiological diagnostic procedures in edema of the extremities. In Foldi, M, Foldi, E, and Kubik, S (eds): Textbook of Lymphology for Physicians and Lymphedema Therapists, ed 5. Elsevier, Munich, Germany, 2003, p 434.

100. Black, J: National Pressure Ulcer Advisory Panel's updated pressure ulcer staging system. Adv Skin Wound Care 20(5): 269, 2007.

101. Bergstrom, N, et al: Pressure Ulcer Treatment, Clinical Practice Guideline, Quick Reference Guide for Clinicians, No. 15. AHRQ Pub. No. 95-0653. U.S. Department of Health and Human Services, Public Health Service Agency, Agency for Health Care Research and Quality, Rockville, MD, December 1994.

102. Hon, J, et al: A prospective, multicenter study to validate use of the PUSH in patients with diabetic, venous, and pressure ulcers. Ostomy Wound Manage 56(2):26, 2010.

103. Gul, A: Role of wound classification in predicting the outcome of diabetic foot ulcer. J Pak Med Assoc 56(10):444, 2006.

104. Schoonhoven, L, et al: Prospective cohort study of routine use of risk assessment scales for prediction of pressure ulcers. BMJ 12:325, 2002.

105. Mortenson, WB, et al: A review of scales for assessing the risk of developing a pressure ulcer in individuals with SCI. Spinal Cord 46(3):168, 2008.

106. Beeson, T, et al: Thinking about the Braden Scale. Clin Nurse Spec 24(2):49, 2010.

107. Sussman, C: Wound Care: Patient Education Resource Manual. Aspen, Gaithersburg, MD, 2000.

108. Ehrlich, A, Vinje-Harrewijn, A, and McMahon, E: Living Well with Lymphedema. Lymph Notes, San Francisco, 2005.

109. Ayello, EA: New evidence for an enduring wound-healing concept: Moisture control. J Wound Ostomy Continence Nurs 33(65):S1, 2006.

110. Sarsam, SE, Elliott, JP, and Lam, GK: Management of wound complications from cesarean delivery. Obstet Gynecol Surv 60(7):462, 2005.

111. Folkedahl, BA, and Frantz, R: Treatment of Pressure Ulcers. University of Iowa Gerontological Nursing Interventions Research Center, Research Dissemination Core, Iowa City, IA, August 2002.

112. McCulloch, JM, and Boyd, V: The effects of whirlpool and the dependent position on LE volume. J Orthop Sports Phys Ther 16:169, 1992.

113. Sussman, C: Whirlpool. In Sussman, C, and Bates, BM (eds): Wound Care: A Collaborative Practice Manual for Physical Therapists and Nurses, ed 3. Lippincott Williams & Wilkins, Baltimore, 2007, p 644.

114. Burke, DT, et al: Effects of hydrotherapy on pressure ulcer healing. Am J Phys Med Rehabil 77(5):394, 1998.

115. Hess, CL, Howard, MA, and Attinger, CE: A review of mechanical adjuncts in wound healing: Hydrotherapy, ultrasound, negative pressure therapy, hyperbaric oxygen, and electrostimulation. Ann Plast Surg 51(2):210, 2003.

116. Ho, CH, and Bogie, K: The prevention and treatment of pressure ulcers. Phys Med Rehabil Clin North Am 18:235, 2007.

117. Luedtke-Hoffmann, KA, and Schafer, DS: Pulsed lavage in wound cleansing. Phys Ther 80:292, 2000.

118. Loehne, HB, et al: Aerosolization of microorganisms during pulsatile lavage with suction. Presented at Combined Sections Meeting/American Physical Therapy Association, February 2000, New Orleans, LA.

119. Wilson, JR, et al: A toxicity index of skin and wound cleansers used on in vitro fibroblasts and keratinocytes. Adv Skin Wound Care 18(7):373, 2005.

120. Spear, M: Wet-to-dry dressings—evaluating the evidence. Plast Surg Nurs 28(2):92, 2008.

121. Cowan, LJ, and Stechmiller, J: Prevalence of wet-to-dry dressings in wound care. Adv Skin Wound Care 22(12):567, 2009.

122. Rodeheaver, G, et al: Wound healing and wound management: Focus on debridement. Adv Wound Care 7(1):22, 1994.

123. Ovington, LG: Hanging wet-to-dry dressings out to dry. Home Health Nurse 19(8):477, 2001.

124. Shinohara, T, et al: Prospective evaluation of occlusive hydrocolloid dressing versus conventional gauze dressing regarding the healing effect after abdominal operations: Randomized controlled trial. Asian J Surg 31(1):1, 2008.

125. Singh, A, et al: Meta-analysis of randomized controlled trials on hydrocolloid occlusive dressing versus conventional gauze dressing in the healing of chronic wounds. Asian J Surg 27(4):326, 2004.

126. Vermeulen, H, et al: Dressings and topical agents for surgical wounds healing by secondary intention (review). Cochrane Database Syst Rev 1; CD003554, 2004.

127. Bergstrom, N, et al: The national pressure ulcer long-term care study: Outcomes of pressure ulcer treatments in long-term care. J Am Geriatr Soc 53:1721, 2005.

128. Jones, KR, and Fennie, K: Factors influencing pressure ulcer healing in adults over 50: An exploratory study. J Am Med Dir Assoc 8:378, 2007.

129. Lawrence, JC: Dressings and wound infection. Am J Surg 167(1A):21S, 1994.

130. Lawrence, JC, Lilly, HA, and Kidson, A: Wound dressings and airborne dispersal of bacteria. Lancet 339:807, 1992.

131. Kohr, R: Moist healing versus wet to dry. Can Nurse 97(1):17, 2001.

132. Payne, WG, et al: A prospective, randomized clinical trial to assess the cost-effectiveness of a modern foam dressing versus a traditional saline gauze dressing in the treatment of Stage II pressure ulcers. Ostomy Wound Manage 55(2):50, 2009.

133. Capasso, VA, and Munro, BH: The cost and efficacy of two wound treatments. J Perioper Nurs 77(5):984, 2003.

134. Hall, S: A review of maggot debridement therapy to treat chronic wounds. Br J Nurs 19(15):S26, 2010.

135. Sherman, RA: Maggot therapy takes us back to the future of wound care: New and improved maggot therapy for the 21st century. J Diabetes Sci Technol 3(2):336, 2009.

136. Mumcuoglu, KY: Clinical applications for maggots in wound care. Am J Clin Dermatol 2(4):219, 2001.

137. Jones, M: An overview of maggot therapy used on chronic wounds in the community. Br J Community Nurs 14(3): S16, 2009.

138. Wollina, U, et al: Biosurgery in wound healing—the renaissance of maggot therapy. Eur Acad Dermatol Venereol 14: 285, 2000.

139. Allen, CS: Merit in maggots. Physical Therapy Products, p 44, May/June 2003.

140. Paul, AG, et al: Maggot debridement therapy with Lucilia cuprina: A comparison with conventional debridement in diabetic foot ulcers. Int Wound J 6(1):39, 2009.

141. Hunter, S, et al: Maggot therapy for wound management. Adv Skin Wound Care 22(1):25, 2009.

142. Gethin, G, and Cowman, S: Manuka honey vs hydrogel—a prospective, open label, mulitcentre, randomized controlled trial to compare desloughing efficacy and healing outcomes in venous ulcers. J Clin Nurs 18:466, 2009.

143. Robson, V: Leptospermum honey used as a debriding agent. Nurse 2(11):66, 2002.

144. Cutting, KF: Honey and contemporary wound care: An overview. Ostomy Wound Manage 53(11):49, 2008.

145. Molan, PC: Re-introducing honey in the management of wounds and ulcers—theory and practice. 48(11):28, 2002.

146. Kramer, SA: Effect of povidone-iodine on wound healing: A review. J Vasc Nurs 17(1):17, 1999.

147. Landis, SJ: Chronic wound infection and antimicrobial use. Adv Skin Wound Care 21:531, 2008.

148. Bates-Jensen, BM, and Ovington, LG: Management of exudate and infection. In Sussman, C, and Bates, BM (eds): Wound Care: A Collaborative Practice Manual for Physical Therapists and Nurses, ed 3. Lippincott Williams & Wilkins, Baltimore, 2007, p 215.

149. Takahashi, M, et al: Possible mechanisms underlying mammary carcinogenesis in female Wistar rats by nitrofurazone. Cancer Lett 156(2):177, 2000.

150. Popescu, A, and Salcido, R: Wound pain: A challenge for the patient and the wound care specialist. Adv Skin Wound Care 17(1):14, 2004.

151. Nagai, MK, and Embil, JM: Becaplermin: Recombinant platelet derived growth factor, a new treatment for healing diabetic foot ulcers. Expert Opin Biol Ther 2(2):211, 2002.

152. Mandracchia, VJ, Sanders, SM, and Frerichs, JA: The use of becaplermin (rhPDGF-BB) gel for chronic nonhealing ulcers. A retrospective analysis. Clin Podiatr Med Surg 18(10):189, 2001.

153. Kantor, J, and Margolis, DJ: Treatment options for diabetic neuropathic foot ulcers: A cost-effectiveness analysis. Dermatol Surg 27(4):347, 2001.

154. Edmonds, M, et al: New treatments in ulcer healing and wound infection. Diabetes/Metab Res Rev Suppl 1:S51, September-October 2000.

155. Ladin, D: Becaplermin gel (PDGF-BB) as topical wound therapy. Plastic Surgery Educational Foundation DATA Committee. Plast Reconstr Surg 105(3):1230, 2000.

156. Goldman, R: Growth factors and chronic wound healing: Past, present, and future. Adv Skin Wound Care 17(1):24, 2004.

157. Rappl, LM: Effect of platelet rich plasma gel in a physiologically relevant platelet concentration on wounds in persons with spinal cord injury. Int Wound J 8:187, 2011.

158. McCulloch, JM, and Kloth, LC: Wound Healing: Evidence-Based Management, ed 4. FA Davis, Philadelphia, 2010.

159. Sussman, C, and Bates, BM: Wound Care: A Collaborative Practice Manual for Health Professionals, ed 3. Lippincott Williams & Wilkins, Philadelphia, 2007.

160. Kloth, LC, and Niezgoda, JA: Ultrasound for wound debridement and healing. In Kloth, LC, and McCulloch, JM (eds): Wound Healing: Evidence-Based Management, ed 4. FA Davis, Philadelphia, 2010, p 545.

161. Sussman, C, and Dyson, M: Therapeutic and diagnostic ultrasound. In Sussman, C, and Bates, BM (eds): Wound Care: A Collaborative Practice Manual for Physical Therapists and Nurses, ed 3. Lippincott Williams & Wilkins, Baltimore, 2007, p 612.

162. McCulloch, J, and Kloth, L: Physical agents in wound repair: What is the evidence? Course handout. Annual Conference and Exposition of the American Physical Therapy Association, Washington, DC, 2003.

163. McCulloch, J: The integumentary system—repair and management: An overview. Physical Therapy Magazine, p 52, February 2004.

164. Baba-Akbari, SA, et al: Therapeutic ultrasound for pressure ulcers. Cochrane Database Syst Rev CD001275, 2006.

165. Serena, T, et al: The impact of noncontact, nonthermal, low-frequency ultrasound on bacterial counts in experimental and chronic wounds. Ostomy Wound Manage 55(1):22, 2009.

166. Lai, J, and Pittelkow, MR: Physiological effects of ultrasound MIST on fibroblasts. Int J Dermatol 46(6):587, 2007.

167. Cole, PS, Quisberg, J, and Melin, MM: Adjuvant use of acoustic pressure wound therapy for treatment of chronic wounds: A retrospective analysis. J WOCN 36(2):171, 2009.

168. Haan, J, and Lucich, S: A retrospective analysis of acoustic pressure wound therapy: Effects on healing progression of chronic wounds. Journal of the American College of Certified Wound Specialists 1(1):28, 2009.

169. Bell, AL, and Cavorsi, J: Noncontact ultrasound therapy for adjunctive treatment of nonhealing wounds: Retrospective analysis. Phys Ther 88(12):1517, 2008.

170. Kloth, LC: Electrical stimulation for wound healing: A review of evidence from in vitro studies, animal experiments, and clinical trials. Int J Low Extrem Wounds 4(1):23, 2005.

171. Demir, H, Balay, H, and Kirnap, M: A comparative study of the effects of electrical stimulation and laser treatment on experimental wound healing in rats. J Rehabil Res Dev 41(2):147, 2004.

172. Ojingwa, JC, and Isseroff, RR: Electrical stimulation of wound healing. J Invest Dermatol 121(1):1, 2003.

173. Houghton, PE, et al: Effect of electrical stimulation on chronic leg ulcer size and appearance. Phys Ther 83(1):17, 2003.

174. Edsberg, LE, et al: Topical hyperbaric oxygen and electrical stimulation: Exploring potential synergy. Ostomy Wound Manage 48(1):42, 2003.

175. Kloth, LC: Five questions—and answers—about electrical stimulation. Adv Skin Wound Care 14(3):156, 158, 2001.

176. Thawer, HA, and Houghton, PE: Effects of electrical stimulation on the histological properties of wounds in diabetic mice. Wound Repair Regen 9(2):107, 2001.

177. Evans, RD, Foltz, D, and Foltz, K: Electrical stimulation with bone and wound healing. Clin Podiatr Med Surg 18(1):79, 2001.

178. Kloth, LC, and Pilla, AA: Electromagnetic stimulation for wound repair. In Kloth, LC, and McCulloch, JM (eds): Wound Healing: Evidence-Based Management, ed 4. FA Davis, Philadelphia, 2010, p 514.

179. Sussman, C: Electrical stimulation for wound healing. In Sussman, C, and Bates, BM (eds): Wound Care: A Collaborative Practice Manual for Physical Therapists and Nurses, ed 3. Lippincott Williams & Wilkins, Baltimore, 2007, p 505.

180. Johnson, W, and Draper, DO: Increased range of motion and function in an individual with breast cancer and necrotizing fasciitis—manual therapy and pulsed short-wave diathermy treatment. Case Report Med 2010. [Epub July 14, 2010.]

181. Hill, J, et al: Pulsed short-wave diathermy effects on human fibroblast proliferation. Arch Phys Med Rehabil 83(6):832, 2002.

182. Al-Mandeel, MM, and Watson, T: The thermal and nonthermal effects of high and low doses of pulsed short wave therapy (PSWT). Physiother Res Int 15(4):199, 2010.

183. Conner-Kerr, T et al: Phototherapy in wound management. In Sussman, C, and Bates, BM (eds): Wound Care: A Collaborative Practice Manual for Physical Therapists and Nurses, ed 3. Lippincott Williams & Wilkins, Baltimore, 2007, p 591.

184. Rennekampff, HO: Is UV radiation beneficial in postburn wound healing? Med Hypotheses 75(5):436, 2010.

185. Ennis, WJ, Lee, C, and Meneses, P: A biochemical approach to wound healing through the use of modalities. Clin Dermatol 25(1):63, 2007.

186. Thai, T, et al: Ultraviolet light C in the treatment of chronic wounds with MRSA: A case study. Ostomy Wound Manage 48(11):52, 2002.

187. Murugan, S, et al: Prevalence and antimicrobial susceptibility patter of metallo β lactamase producing *Pseudomonas aeruginosa* in diabetic foot infection. Int J Microbiol Res 1(3):123, 2010.

188. Boykin, JV: The nitric oxide connection: Hyperbaric oxygen therapy, becaplermin and diabetic ulcer management. Adv Skin Wound Care 13:169, 2000.

189. Londahl, M, et al: Hyperbaric oxygen therapy facilitates healing of chronic foot ulcers in patients with diabetes. Diabetes Care 33(5):998, 2010.

190. Duzgun, AP, et al: Effect of hyperbaric oxygen therapy on healing of diabetic foot ulcers. J Foot Ankle Surg 47(6):515, 2008.

191. Boykin, JV, and Baylis, C: Hyperbaric oxygen therapy mediates increased nitric oxide production associated with wound healing: A preliminary study. Adv Skin Wound Care 20(7):382, 2007.

192. Kalliainen, L, et al: Topical oxygen as an adjunct to wound healing: A clinical case series. Pathophysiology 9:81, 2003.

193. Edsberg, LE, et al: Topical hyperbaric oxygen and electrical stimulation: Exploring potential synergy. Ostomy Wound Manage 48(11):42, 2002.

194. Landau, Z, and Schattner, A: Topical hyperbaric oxygen and low energy laser therapy for chronic diabetic foot ulcers resistant to conventional treatment. Yale J Biol Med 74:95, 2001.

195. Joseph, E, et al: A prospective randomized trial of vacuum-assisted closure versus standard therapy of chronic nonhealing wounds. Wounds 12(3):60, 2000.

196. Gupta, S, Gabriel, A, and Shores, J: The perioperative use of negative pressure wound therapy in skin grafting. Ostomy Wound Manage 50(4A Suppl):32, 2004.

197. Armstrong, DG, et al: Plantar pressure changes using a novel negative pressure wound therapy technique. J Am Podiatr Med Assoc 94(5):456, 2004.

198. Mendez-Eastman, S: Determining the appropriateness of negative pressure wound therapy for pressure ulcers. Ostomy Wound Manage 50(4A Suppl):13, 2004.

199. Wanner, MB, et al: Vacuum-assisted wound closure for cheaper and more comfortable healing of pressure sores: A prospective study. Scand J Plast Reconstr Surg 37(1):28, 2003.

200. Zannis, J, et al: Comparison of fasciotomy wound closures using traditional dressing changes and the vacuum-assisted closure device. Ann Plast Surg 62(4):407, 2009.

201. Borgquist, O, Ingemansson, R, and Malmsjo, M: Individualizing the use of negative pressure wound therapy for optimal wound healing: A focused review of the literature. Ostomy Wound Manage 57(4):44, 2011.

202. Vuerstaek, JD, et al: State-of-the-art treatment of chronic leg ulcers: A randomized controlled trial comparing vacuum-assisted closure (VAC) with modern wound dressings. J Vasc Surg 44(5):1029, 2006.

203. Eginton, MT, et al: A prospective randomized evaluation of negative-pressure wound dressings for diabetic foot wounds. Ann Vasc Surg 17(6):645, 2003.

204. Hunter, S, et al: The use of monochromatic infrared energy in wound management. Adv Skin Wound Care 20(5):265, 2007.

205. Kochman, AB, Carnegie, DH, and Burke, TJ: Symptomatic reversal of peripheral neuropathy in patients with diabetes. J Am Podiatr Med Assoc 92(3):125, 2002.

206. Leonard, DR, Farooqi, MH, and Myers, S: Restoration of sensation, reduced pain, and improved balance in subjects with diabetic peripheral neuropathy: A double-blind, randomized, placebo-controlled study with monochromatic near-infrared treatment. Diabetes Care 27(1):168, 2004.

207. Powell, MW, Carnegie, DE, and Burke, TJ: Reversal of diabetic peripheral neuropathy and new wound incidence: The role of MIRE. Adv Skin Wound Care 17(6):295, 2004.

208. Harkless, LB, et al: Improved foot sensitivity and pain reduction in patients with peripheral neuropathy after treatment with monochromatic infrared photo energy—MIRE. J Diabetes Complications 20(2):81, 2006.

209. Burke, TJ: Five questions—and answers—about MIRE treatment. Adv Skin Wound Care 16(7):369, 2003.

210. Prendergast, JJ, Miranda, G, and Sanchez, M: Improvement of sensory impairment in patients with peripheral neuropathy. Endocr Pract 10(1):24, 2004.

211. Carter, MJ, Tingley-Kelley, K, and Warriner, RA: Silver treatments and silver-impregnated dressings for the healing of leg wounds and ulcers: A systematic review and meta-analysis. J Am Acad Dermatol 63(4):668, 2010.

212. Cohn, S, et al: Open surgical wounds: How does Aquacel compare with wet-to-dry gauze? J Wound Care 13(1):10, 2004.

213. Bethell, E: Why gauze dressings should not be the first choice to manage most acute surgical cavity wounds. J Wound Care 12(6):237, 2003.

214. Allie, DE, et al: Novel treatment strategy for leg and sternal wound complications after coronary artery bypass graft surgery: Bioengineered Apligraf. Ann Thorac Surg 78(2):673, 2004.

215. Colletta, V, et al: A trial to assess the efficacy and tolerability of Hyalofill-F in non-healing venous leg ulcers. J Wound Care 12(9):357, 2003.

216. Taddeucci, P, et al: An evaluation of Hyalofill-F plus compression bandaging in the treatment of chronic venous ulcers. J Wound Care 13(5):202, 2004.

217. Williams, AF, et al: A randomized controlled crossover study of manual lymphatic drainage therapy in women with breast cancer–related lymphoedema. Eur J Cancer Care 11:254, 2002.

218. Williams, A: Manual lymphatic drainage: Exploring the history and the evidence base. Br J Community Nurs 15(4):S18, 2010.

219. Molski, P, et al: Patients with venous disease benefit from manual lymphatic drainage. Int Angiol 28(2):151, 2008.

220. Vairo, GI, et al: Systematic review of efficacy for manual lymphatic drainage techniques in sports medicine and rehabilitation: An evidence-based practice approach. J Man Manip Ther 17(3):80, 2009.

221. Strossenreuther, RHK, et al: Practical instructions for therapists—manual lymph drainage according to Dr. E. Vodder. In Foldi, M, Foldi, E, and Kubik, S (eds): Textbook of Lymphology for Physicians and Lymphedema Therapists, ed 2. Elsevier, Munich, Germany, 2006, p 526.

222. Robson, MC: Treating bacterial infections in chronic wounds. Contemp Surg Suppl 9, September 2000.

223. Koksal, C, and Bozkurt, AK: Combination of hydrocolloid dressing and medical compression stockings versus Unna's boot for the treatment of venous leg ulcers. Swiss Med Wkly 133(25-26):364, 2003.

224. Moffat, CJ, et al: Randomized trial comparing two four-layer bandage systems in the management of chronic leg ulceration. Phlebology 14:139, 1999.

225. Weissleder, H, and Schuchhardt, C: Lymphedema: Diagnosis and therapy. In Weissleder, H, and Schuchhardt, C (eds): Therapy Concepts, ed 4. Viavital Verlag, Essen, Germany, 2008, p 403.

226. Leduc, O, Peeters, A, and Borgeois, P: Bandages: Scintigraphic demonstration of its efficacy on colloidal protein reabsorption during muscle activity. Progress in Lymphology—XII. Elsevier, Philadelphia, 1990.

227. Johansson, K, et al: Effects of compression bandaging with or without manual lymph drainage treatment in patients with postoperative arm lymphedema. Lymphology 32:103, 1999.

228. Schmid-Schonbein, GW: Microlymphatics and lymph flow. Physiol Rev 70(4):987, 1990.

229. Simon, DA, Dix, FP, and McCollum, CN: Management of venous leg ulcers. Br Med J 328:1358, 2004.

230. Weiss, J: Treatment of leg edema and wounds in a patient with severe musculoskeletal injuries. Phys Ther 78(10):1104, 1998.

231. Asmussen, PD, and Strossenreuther, RHK: Compression therapy. In Foldi, M, Foldi, E, and Kubik, S (eds): Textbook of Lymphology for Physicians and Lymphedema Therapists, ed 5. Elsevier, Munich, Germany, 2003, p 528.

232. Yasuhara, H, Shigematsu, H, and Muto, T: A study of the advantages of elastic stocking for leg lymphedema. Int Angiology 15(3):272, 1996.

233. Harris, SR, et al: Clinical practice guidelines for the care and treatment of breast cancer: 11. Lymphedema. Can Med Assoc J 164(2):191, 2001.

234. Badger, CM, Peacock, JL, and Mortimer, PS: A randomized, controlled, parallel-group clinical trial comparing multiplayer bandaging followed by hosiery versus hosiery alone in the treatment of patients with lymphedema of the limb. Cancer 88(12):2832, 2000.

235. Apaqut, U, and Dayioglu, E: Importance and advantages of intermittent external pneumatic compression therapy in venous stasis ulceration. Angiology 56(1):19, 2005.

236. Berline, E, Ozbilgin, B, and Zarin, DA: A systematic review of pneumatic compression for treatment of chronic venous insufficiency and venous ulcers. J Vascul Surg 37(3):539, 2003.

237. Comerota, AJ: Intermittent pneumatic compression: Physiologic and clinical basis to improve management of venous leg ulcers. J Vasc Surg 53(4):1121, 2011.

238. Nelson, EA: Intermittent pneumatic compression for treating venous leg ulcers. Cochrane Database Syst Rev 16; 2:CD001899, 2011.

239. Haghighat, S, et al: Comparing two treatment methods for post mastectomy lymphedema: Complex decongestive therapy alone and in combination with intermittent pneumatic compression. Lymphology 43(1):25, 2010.

240. Partsch, H, et al: Clinical trials needed to evaluate compression therapy in breast cancer related lymphedema (BCRL). Proposals from an expert group. Int Angiol 25(5):442, 2010.

241. Devoogdt, N, et al: Different physical treatment modalities for lymphoedema developing after axillary lymph node dissection for breast cancer: A review. Eur J Obstet Gynecol Reprod Biol 149(1):3, 2010.

242. Rockson, SG: Current concepts and future directions in the diagnosis and management of lymphatic vascular disease. Vasc Med 15(3):223, 2010.

243. Adams, KE, et al: Direct evidence of lymphatic function improvement after advanced pneumatic compression device treatment of lymphedema. Biomed Opt Express 1(1):114, 2010.

244. Ridner, SH, et al: Home-based lymphedema treatment in patients with cancer-related lymphedema or noncancer-related lymphedema. Oncol Nurs Forum 35(4):671, 2008.

245. Wilburn, O, Wilburn, P, and Rockson, SG. A pilot, prospective evaluation of a novel alternative for maintenance therapy of breast cancer–associated lymphedema. BMC Cancer 6:84, 2006.

246. Van Rijswijk, L: Pressure ulcer prevention updates. Am J Nurs 109(8):S6, 2009.

247. Brienza, DM, Geyer MJ, and Sprigle, S: Seating, positioning, and support surfaces. In Baranoski, S, and Ayello, EA (eds): Wound Care Essentials: Practice Principles. Lippincott Williams & Wilkins, Philadelphia, 2004.

248. National Pressure Ulcer Advisory Panel, European Pressure Ulcer Advisory Panel: Pressure ulcer treatment recommendations. In Prevention and Treatment of Pressure Ulcers: Clinical Practice Guideline. National Pressure Ulcer Advisory Panel, Washington, DC, 2009.

249. Brienza, D, et al: A randomized clinical trial on preventing pressure ulcers with wheelchair seat cushions. J Am Geriatr Soc 58(12):2308, 2010.

250. Stockton, L, Gebhardt, KS, and Clark, M: Seating and pressure ulcers: Clinical practice guidelines. J Tissue Viability 18(4):98, 2009.

251. McInnes, E: The use of pressure-relieving devices (beds, mattresses and overlays) for the prevention of pressure ulcers in primary and secondary care. J Tissue Viability 14(1):4, 2004.

252. Stier, L, et al: Reinforcing organization-wide pressure ulcer reduction on high-risk geriatric inpatient units. Outcomes Manage 8(1):28, 2004.

253. Salsich, GB, et al: Effect of Achilles tendon lengthening on ankle muscle performance in people with diabetes mellitus and a neuropathic plantar ulcer. Phys Ther 85(1):34, 2004.

254. Cavanagh, PR, and Bus, SA: Off-loading the diabetic foot for ulcer prevention and healing. Plast Reconstr Surg 127:248S, 2011.

255. Shaw, TJ, Kishi, K, and Mori, R: Wound associated skin fibrosis: Mechanisms and treatments based on modulating the inflammatory response. Endocr Metab Immune Disord Drug Targets 10(4):320, 2010.

■ INSPECT YOUR SKIN

1. Look at your feet every day. Use a mirror, a magnifying glass, or the assistance of a family member to help you see all over your feet including between your toes and the bottoms of your feet.

2. Look for these things on your feet: blisters, sores, corns, calluses, red spots, swelling, pain, drainage from a sore, broken toenails, cracked skin, odor. Notify your health care provider if you see any of these things on your feet or if you injure either of your feet.

■ TAKE CARE OF YOUR SKIN

1. Wash your feet gently every day using lukewarm water and mild soap. Test the water temperature with your hand before you wash your feet. If your hand is not sensitive to temperature, use a thermometer. The temperature should be about 85° Fahrenheit (29.44° Celsius).

2. Dry your feet well, especially between your toes.

3. You may want to use a lanolin-based lotion or petroleum jelly to soften dry skin. Do not apply any lotion between your toes. You may use powder or cornstarch between your toes.

4. Never try to treat corns, calluses, or toenails with sharp instruments, home remedies, or store-bought foot care products. These items can all hurt your skin.

5. Cut toenails straight across; do not cut into corners. Use an emery board for sharp edges. A pumice stone can be used to treat small corns and calluses. Alert your health care provider about your foot care practices.

6. For padding and air circulation, use small bits of lamb's wool between the toes. Change the lamb's wool every day. Be sure to use new pieces after you wash your feet. Do not use cotton or cotton balls because the fibers may irritate your skin.

7. Put on a clean pair of white socks after your skin care routine.

8. Do not walk barefoot.

9. If your feet are cold at bedtime, wear cotton socks; do not use a hot water bottle or heating pad to warm your feet.

■ CHECK YOUR SHOES

1. Check your shoes every day before you put them on. Look inside for small things that could cause a sore on your foot. Alternate shoes each day to allow them to breathe and dry completely.

2. Be sure that your shoes are the right size and width.

3. Do not wear old worn-out shoes or socks.

4. Shop for shoes in the afternoon when your feet are the largest.

5. Break in your new shoes gradually.

■ SEE YOUR HEALTH CARE PROVIDER

1. Get help in controlling your diabetes.

2. Have regular appointments with your doctor.

3. Call your health care provider immediately if you find a wound on your foot.

Special Tests for Arterial and Venous Function

Special Tests	Description
Rubor of dependency	A noninvasive test to examine the lower extremity (LE) for the presence of ischemia. Following elevation of the limb, lowering of the limb should return the skin of the limb to a pink color. If the color is dark red and takes more than 30 seconds to appear, the test is positive for arterial insufficiency.
Air plethysmography (APG)	A noninvasive test of both the arterial and venous circulation. Changes in LE volume are measured using a pressure cuff that quantifies volume changes during rest, standing, and light walking. Venous obstruction and arterial inflow can be observed with this test.
Transcutaneous oxygen (TcPO$_2$)	A noninvasive examination tool for arterial circulation. A special probe and a heating element measure profusion. Measurement of oxygen at the skin level gives information about what is happening at the cellular level. Also found in the literature as *transcutaneous partial pressure of oxygen* and *transcutaneous oxygen tension measurement*. The results are predictive for healing of ulcers and amputation wounds.
Skin perfusion pressure (SPP) measurement	A noninvasive test that measures blood flow in the skin. To take the measurements, a modified laser Doppler probe is secured in the bladder of a specialized blood pressure cuff. Results are predictive for healing of ulcers and amputation wounds.
Venous filling time	The extremity is elevated and then lowered into a dependent position. The time it takes for the veins on top of the foot to refill is recorded. Normal filling time is 15 seconds. Greater than 15 seconds indicates arterial disease whereas less than 15 indicates venous disease.
Percussion test	With LE in a dependent position, the greater saphenous vein is palpated distal to the knee with one hand while it is tapped 6 in (15.2 cm) proximal to the knee with the other hand. If a wave of fluid is detected under the distal palpation site, this indicates the possibility of valvular incompetency.
Trendelenburg test	Test measures the time required to refill the veins in the dorsum of the foot. The LE is elevated to allow venous blood to empty. A tourniquet on the thigh prevents backflow. After 1 minute, the individual stands. If veins fully distend within 5 seconds before the tourniquet is released, valvular incompetence in the deep veins is suspected. If distention occurs within 5 seconds after the tourniquet is released, incompetence of superficial veins is suspected.

Sample Wound Examination Form

Name _____

B/P _____ Resp _____ HR _____ Temp _____ Weight _____

Date: Orientation to time/place/person? ( ) Yes ( ) No

Arrived: ( ) Ambulatory ( ) Cane ( ) Crutches ( ) Walker ( ) Wheelchair ( ) Stretcher ( ) N/A

( ) Initial Examination Reviewed: Changes in medicine, allergies, or health history since last visit? ( ) Yes ( ) No
(If yes, indicate changes)

Wound Number				
Wound Location				
Wound Type	Ulcer: ☐ pressure ☐ venous ☐ arterial ☐ diabetic; ☐ SDTI ☐ burn ☐ donor site ☐ Other: _____ ☐ Infected ☐ Contaminated ☐ Unknown ☐ Biopsy: ☐ Yes, Date: _____ ☐ No ☐ Other: _____	Ulcer: ☐ pressure ☐ venous ☐ arterial ☐ diabetic; ☐ SDTI ☐ burn ☐ donor site ☐ Other: _____ ☐ Infected ☐ Contaminated ☐ Unknown ☐ Biopsy: ☐ Yes, Date: _____ ☐ No ☐ Other: _____	Ulcer: ☐ pressure ☐ venous ☐ arterial ☐ diabetic; ☐ SDTI ☐ burn ☐ donor site ☐ Other: _____ ☐ Infected ☐ Contaminated ☐ Unknown ☐ Biopsy: ☐ Yes, Date: _____ ☐ No ☐ Other: _____	Ulcer: ☐ pressure ☐ venous ☐ arterial ☐ diabetic; ☐ SDTI ☐ burn ☐ donor site ☐ Other: _____ ☐ Infected ☐ Contaminated ☐ Unknown ☐ Biopsy: ☐ Yes, Date: _____ ☐ No ☐ Other: _____
Wound Stage (Circle)	I II III IV U/S	I II III IV U/S	I II III IV U/S	I II III IV U/S
Length				
Width				
Depth				
Tunnels/ Undermining	( ) Yes ( ) No	( ) Yes ( ) No	( ) Yes ( ) No	( ) Yes ( ) No
Granulation				
Slough				
Eschar	( ) Yes ( ) No	( ) Yes ( ) No	( ) Yes ( ) No	( ) Yes ( ) No

Odor	( ) Yes ( ) No	( ) Yes ( ) No	( ) Yes ( ) No	( ) Yes ( ) No
Drainage Amount	( ) None ( ) Minimal ( ) Moderate ( ) Heavy	( ) None ( ) Minimal ( ) Moderate ( ) Heavy	( ) None ( ) Minimal ( ) Moderate ( ) Heavy	( ) None ( ) Minimal ( ) Moderate ( ) Heavy
Drainage Color	( ) Serous ( ) Serosanguineous ( ) Sanguineous ( ) Purulent ( ) Yellow/Green ( ) NA	( ) Serous ( ) Serosanguineous ( ) Sanguineous ( ) Purulent ( ) Yellow/Green ( ) NA	( ) Serous ( ) Serosanguineous ( ) Sanguineous ( ) Purulent ( ) Yellow/Green ( ) NA	( ) Serous ( ) Serosanguineous ( ) Sanguineous ( ) Purulent ( ) Yellow/Green ( ) NA
Wound Margin ( ) Yes ( ) No	( ) Well Defined ( ) Poorly Defined	( ) Well Defined ( ) Poorly Defined	( ) Well Defined ( ) Poorly Defined	( ) Well Defined ( ) Poorly Defined
Exposed Bone	( ) Yes ( ) No	( ) Yes ( ) No	( ) Yes ( ) No	( ) Yes ( ) No
Exposed Muscle/ Tendon/Ligament	( ) Yes ( ) No	( ) Yes ( ) No	( ) Yes ( ) No	( ) Yes ( ) No
Periwound	( ) Maceration ( ) Intact	( ) Maceration ( ) Intact	( ) Maceration ( ) Intact	( ) Maceration ( ) Intact
Appearance	( ) Callus ( ) Necrotic ( ) Erythema	( ) Callus ( ) Necrotic ( ) Erythema	( ) Callus ( ) Necrotic ( ) Erythema	( ) Callus ( ) Necrotic ( ) Erythema

■ PAIN MANAGEMENT

Pain Scale: None   0   1   2   3   4   5   6   7   8   9   10   Severe

Locations(s):

Described as: ( ) Sharp   ( ) Dull   ( ) Burning   Relieved by: ( ) Elevation of Legs/Offloading/Rest
( ) Throbbing ( ) Radiating ( ) Constant   ( ) Medication
( ) Intermittent ( ) AM   ( ) PM   ( ) Standing/Walking ( ) Other_____
( ) Only with Dressing Change   Comments: _____

Pain Management Measures: ( ) LAT   ( ) Lidocaine   ( ) NA   ( ) Refused   ( ) Other:

Strength/ROM/ADL/Gait/Transfers/Mobility: ( ) Impaired   ( ) Not Impaired
Comments:

Other Test Results: ABI: Monofilaments:

■ PLAN OF CARE

Cleansing:

Dressing:

Modalities:

Débridement:

Exercise:	
Education:	
Pressure Relief:	
Compression:	

Other:
ABI: Ankle-Brachial Index
LAT: Lidocaine, Adrenaline, and Tetracaine
ROM: range of motion
Stage Descriptions
SDTI: suspected deep tissue injury (purple or maroon localized area of discolored intact skin)
Stage I: skin intact, light skin: nonblanchable red area; dark skin: warm, indurated, hard edema
Stage II: partial-thickness skin loss
Stage III: full-thickness skin loss
Stage IV: muscle/bone/joint(s) involved
U/S: unstageable (full thickness tissue loss/base covered by slough and/or eschar)
     Signature: _____
     Date/Time: _____

Web-Based Resources for Clinicians, Families, and Patients with Vascular, Lymphatic, and Integumentary Disorders

■ FOR CLINICIANS

American Academy of Wound Management (AAWM)	www.aawm.org
American College of Certified Wound Specialists (ACCWS)	www.accws.org
World Wide Wounds	www.worldwidewounds.com
The Wound Care Institute, Inc.	www.woundcare.org
Wound Care Net	www.woundcarenet.com
National Lymphedema Network	www.lymphnet.org
JoViPak Corporation	www.jovipak.com
Solaris Med	www.solarismed.com
Wound Expert	www.woundexpert.com
Consortium for Spinal Cord Medicine	www.scicpg.org
Boston University Wound Biotech	www.bu.edu/woundbiotech/woundcare
Wound Care Information Network (WCIN)	www.medicaledu.com
Wound Care Consultants	www.wound.com
Journal of Wound Care	www.journalofwoundcare.com
Association for the Advancement of Wound Care (AAWC)	www.aawcone.com
American Podiatric Medical Association (APMA)	www.apma.org
Medline	www.medline.com
Wound Care Associates	www.woundcareresources.com
Merck	www.merck.com
Wound, Ostomy and Continence Nurses Society (WOCN)	www.wocn.org
Medscape Reference	www.emedicine.medscape.com
US Department of Health and Human Services (HHS)	www.hhs.gov
Centers for Disease Control and Prevention (CDC)	www.cdc.gov/diabetes/pubs/factsheet.htm

■ SELECTED LIST OF PROGRAMS FOR SPECIALIZED EDUCATION IN CDT AND MLD

National Lymphedema Network	www.lymphnet.org
Academy of Lymphatic Studies	www.acols.com
Dr. Vodder School International	www.vodderschool.com
Klose Training & Consulting	www.klosetrainng.com
Norton School of Lymphatic Therapy	www.nortonschool.com
Complex Lymphatic Therapy	www.casley-smith-lymphedema-courses.org

■ FOR PATIENTS AND FAMILY MEMBERS

National Lymphedema Network	www.lymphnet.org
Veins Online	www.veinsonline.com
American Cancer Society	www.cancer.org
Lymph Notes	www.lymphnotes.org
Wound Care Caregiver Support	www.walgreens.com/pharmacy/caregivers/woundcare
The CareGiver Partnership	www.blog.caregiverpartnership.com
Strength for Caring	www.strengthforcaring.com
Kestrel Health Media	www.kestrelhealthinfo.com/catalog/caregiver education-skin-and-wound-care

Selected Wound Dressing Manufacturer Web Sites

Augustine Medical	www.augustinemedical.com
Coloplast	www.coloplast.com
ConvaTec	www.convatec.com
DeRoyal	www.deroyal.com
Healthpoint	www.healthpoint.com
Jobst	www.jobst-usa.com
Johnson & Johnson	www.jnj.com
Kendall	www.kendall.com
Smith & Nephew	www.smith-nephew.com
Spenco	www.spenco.com
3M	www.shop3M.com

Dressings by Treatment Goal (Purpose) and Wound Type (Indication)

I. Dressing by Treatment Goal

Purpose	Dressing
Space filling (cavities, undermining, tunnels, or sinuses)	Gauze Foams (some) Hydrogels (amorphous/sheets) Alginates Impregnated gauze Absorptive dressings (beads, powders, and pastes) Composite dressings (some)
Mechanical débridement	Gauze
Exudate absorption	Gauze Foams Absorptive dressings (beads, powders, and pastes) Alginates Hydrocolloids Collagen
Hydration	Hydrogels (amorphous/sheets) Saline-moistened gauze
Autolytic débridement	Transparent films Hydrocolloids Hydrogels (amorphous/sheets) Foams Alginates Impregnated gauze Absorptive dressings (beads, powders, and pastes) Composite
Protection against contamination	Transparent films Hydrocolloids Hydrogel sheets (some) Composite (some) Foams (some)
Hemostasis	Alginates Collagen
Site coverage	Transparent films Hydrocolloids Hydrogel sheets (some) Foams Composite Gauze

Friction reduction	Transparent films Hydrocolloids Hydrogels sheets (some)
Insulation	Transparent films Hydrocolloids Hydrogels (amorphous/sheet) Foams Composite (some) Gauze
Pain reduction	Transparent films Hydrocolloids Hydrogels (amorphous/sheet) Foams Alginates Composites
Odor reduction	Hydrocolloids Hydrogels (amorphous/sheets) (some) Alginates (some) Foams (charcoal) Absorptive dressings (beads, powders, and pastes) (some)
Cushioning	Hydrocolloids Hydrogel sheets (some) Foams Composite dressings (some) Gauze
Antibacterials	Silver-based dressings Iodine-based dressings Silver sulfadiazine

II. Dressings by Wound Type

Indication	Dressing
Infected wounds	Gauze Alginates Hydrogels Hydrogel sheets Impregnated gauze Foams
Burns	Alginates Hydrocolloids Hydrogels Transparent films Impregnated gauze Foams Biological dressings Collagen
Stage I pressure ulcers	Transparent films Foams

Continued

Stage II pressure ulcers	Alginates Hydrocolloids Hydrogels Transparent films Impregnated gauze Foams Collagen
Stage III pressure ulcers	Alginates Hydrocolloids Hydrogels Impregnated gauze Foams Collagen
Stage IV pressure ulcers	Alginates Hydrocolloids Hydrogels Impregnated gauze Foams Collagen
Venous ulcers	Alginates Hydrocolloids Hydrogels Foams
Arterial ulcers	Alginates Hydrogels Foams
Diabetic ulcers	Alginates Hydrocolloids Transparent films Foams
Donor sites	Alginates Hydrocolloids Hydrogels Hydrogels sheets Transparent films Impregnated gauze Collagen

LEARNING OBJECTIVES

1. Describe the epidemiology, etiology, pathophysiology, symptomatology, and sequelae of stroke.
2. Identify and describe the examination procedures used to evaluate patients with stroke to establish a diagnosis, prognosis, and plan of care.
3. Describe the role of the physical therapist in assisting the patient in recovery from stroke in terms of interventions, patient/client-related instruction, coordination, communication, and documentation.
4. Identify and describe strategies of intervention during inpatient rehabilitation.
5. Analyze and interpret patient data, formulate realistic goals and outcomes, and develop a plan of care when presented with a clinical case study.

CHAPTER OUTLINE

Stroke (cerebrovascular accident [CVA]) is the sudden loss of neurological function caused by an interruption of the blood flow to the brain. **Ischemic stroke** is the most common type, affecting about 80% of individuals with stroke, and results when a clot blocks or impairs blood flow, depriving the brain of essential oxygen and nutrients. **Hemorrhagic stroke** occurs when blood vessels rupture, causing leakage of blood in or around the brain. Clinically, a variety of focal deficits are possible, including changes in the level of consciousness and impairments of sensory, motor, cognitive, perceptual, and language functions. To be classified as stroke, neurological deficits must persist for at least 24 hours. Motor deficits are characterized by paralysis (**hemiplegia**) or weakness (**hemiparesis**), typically on the side of the body opposite the side of the lesion. The term *hemiplegia* is often used generically to refer to the wide variety of motor problems that result from stroke. The location and extent of brain injury, the amount of collateral blood flow, and early acute care management determine the severity of neurological deficits in an individual patient. Impairments may resolve spontaneously as brain swelling subsides (reversible ischemic neurological deficit), generally within 3 weeks. Residual neurological impairments are those that persist longer than 3 weeks and may lead to lasting disability. Strokes are classified by etiological categories (thrombosis, embolus, or hemorrhage), specific vascular territory (anterior cerebral artery syndrome, middle cerebral artery syndrome, and so forth), and management categories (transient ischemic attack, minor stroke, major stroke, deteriorating stroke, young stroke).

■ EPIDEMIOLOGY AND ETIOLOGY

Stroke is the fourth leading cause of death and the leading cause of long-term disability among adults in the United States. An estimated 7,000,000 Americans older than 20 years of age have experienced a stroke. Each year approximately 795,000 individuals experience a stroke; approximately 610,000 are first attacks and 185,000 are recurrent strokes. Women have a lower age-adjusted stroke incidence than men. However, this is reversed in older ages; women over 85 years of age have an elevated risk compared to men. Compared to whites, African Americans have twice the risk of first-ever stroke; rates are also higher in Mexican Americans, American Indians, and Alaska Natives. The incidence of stroke increases dramatically with age, doubling in the decade after 65 years of age. Twenty-eight percent of strokes occur in individuals younger than 65 years of age. Between 5% and 14% of persons who survive an initial stroke will experience another one within 1 year; within 5 years stroke will recur in 24% of women and 42% of men. Current data reveal that stroke incidence has been declining in recent years in a largely white adult cohort.[1]

The incidence of stroke deaths is greater than 143,000 annually, and strokes account for 1 of every 18 deaths in the United States. The type of stroke is significant in determining survival. Of patients with stroke, hemorrhagic stroke accounts for the largest number of deaths, with mortality rates of 37% to 38% at 1 month, whereas ischemic strokes have a mortality rate of only 8% to 12% at 1 month. Survival rates are dramatically lessened by increased age, hypertension, heart disease, and diabetes. Loss of consciousness at stroke onset, lesion size, persistent severe hemiplegia, multiple neurological deficits, and history of previous stroke are also important predictors of mortality.[1,2]

Stroke is the leading cause of long-term disability in the United States. Of ischemic stroke survivors 65 or older, incidences of disabilities observed at 6 months include hemiparesis (50%), unable to walk without assistance (30%), dependent in activities of daily living (ADL) (26%), aphasia (19%), and depression (35%). Stroke survivors represent the largest group admitted to rehabilitation hospitals and about a third of patients receive outpatient rehabilitation services. Another indicator of disability is the fact that approximately 26% of patients with stroke are institutionalized in a long-term care facility. Direct and indirect costs of stroke are in the billions.[1]

Atherosclerosis is a major contributory factor in cerebrovascular disease. It is characterized by plaque formation with an accumulation of lipids, fibrin, complex carbohydrates, and calcium deposits on arterial walls that leads to progressive narrowing of blood vessels. Interruption of blood flow by atherosclerotic plaques occurs at certain sites of predilection. These generally include bifurcations, constrictions, dilations, or angulations of arteries. The most common sites for lesions to occur are at the origin of the common carotid artery or at its transition into the middle cerebral artery, at the main bifurcation of the middle cerebral artery, and at the junction of the vertebral arteries with the basilar artery (Fig. 15.1).

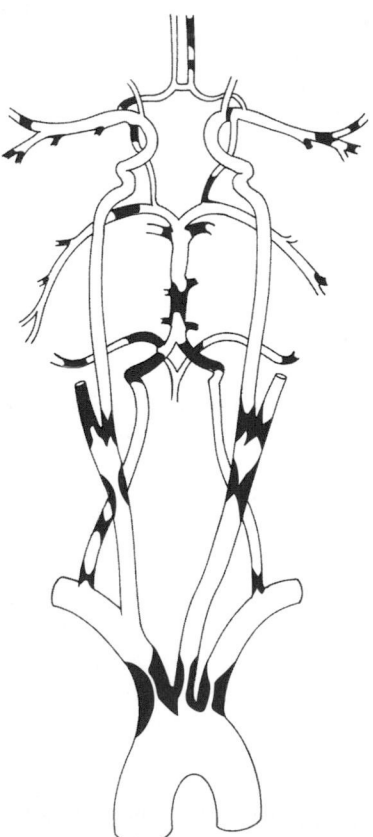

Figure 15.1 Preferred sites for atherosclerotic plaque. *(From American Heart Association: Diagnosis and Management of Stroke, 1979, p 4, with permission.)*

Ischemic strokes are the result of a thrombus, embolism, or conditions that produce low systemic perfusion pressures. The resulting lack of cerebral blood flow (CBF) deprives the brain of needed oxygen and glucose, disrupts cellular metabolism, and leads to injury and death of tissues. A thrombus results from platelet adhesion and aggregation on plaques. **Cerebral thrombosis** refers to the formation or development of a blood clot within the cerebral arteries or their branches. It should be noted that lesions of extracranial vessels (carotid or vertebral arteries) can also produce symptoms of stroke. Thrombi lead to ischemia, or occlusion of an artery with resulting **cerebral infarction** or tissue death (*atherothrombotic brain infarction [ABI]*). Thrombi can also become dislodged and travel to a more distal site in the form of an intra-artery embolus. **Cerebral embolus (CE)** is composed of bits of matter (blood clot, plaque) formed elsewhere and released into the bloodstream, traveling to the cerebral arteries where they lodge in a vessel, producing occlusion and infarction. The most common source of CE is disease of the cardiovascular system. Occasionally systemic disorders may produce septic, fat, or air emboli that affect the cerebral circulation. Ischemic strokes may also result from low systemic perfusion, the result of cardiac failure or significant blood loss with resulting systemic hypotension. The neurological deficits produced with systemic failure are global in nature with bilateral neurological deficits.

Hemorrhagic strokes, with abnormal bleeding into the extravascular areas of the brain, are the result of rupture of a cerebral vessel or trauma. Hemorrhage results in increased intracranial pressures with injury to brain tissues and restriction of distal blood flow. **Intracerebral hemorrhage (IH)** is caused by rupture of a cerebral vessel with subsequent bleeding into the brain. Primary **cerebral hemorrhage** (nontraumatic spontaneous hemorrhage) typically occurs in small blood vessels weakened by atherosclerosis producing an **aneurysm**. **Subarachnoid hemorrhage (SH)** occurs from bleeding into the subarachnoid space typically from a saccular or berry aneurysm affecting primarily large blood vessels. Congenital defects that produce weakness in the blood vessel wall are major contributing factors to the formation of an aneurysm. Hemorrhage is closely linked to chronic hypertension. **Arteriovenous malformation (AVM)** is another congenital defect that can result in stroke. AVM is characterized by a tortuous tangle of arteries and veins with agenesis of an interposing capillary system. The abnormal vessels undergo progressive dilation with age and eventually bleed in about 50% of cases. Sudden and severe cerebral bleeding can result in death within hours, because intracranial pressures rise rapidly and adjacent cortical tissues are compressed or displaced as in brainstem herniation.

■ RISK FACTORS AND STROKE PREVENTION

Cardiovascular diseases affecting the brain and heart share a number of common risk factors important to the development of atherosclerosis. Major risk factors for stroke are hypertension, heart disease (HD), disorders of heart rhythm, and diabetes mellitus (DM). In patients with ABI, approximately 70% have hypertension, 30% HD, 15% congestive heart failure (CHF), 30% peripheral arterial disease (PAD), and 15% DM.[2] This coexistence of multiple pathologies increases significantly with age. Individuals with hypertension (blood pressure [BP] (140/90 mm Hg or higher) have twice the lifetime risk of stroke. Risk is increased with elevated total blood cholesterol *(hypercholesterolemia),* defined as 240 mg/dL or greater. Lipid profiles are also important. Risk is increased with elevated low-density lipoprotein (LDL ["bad"]) cholesterol. LDL levels are defined as borderline high levels of 130 to 159 mg/dL, high levels of 160 to 189 mg/dL, and very high levels of 190 mg/dL or greater. Low levels of high-density lipoprotein (HDL ["good"]) cholesterol, defined as below 40 mg/dL in adult males and below 50 mg/dL in adult females, also increases stroke risk. Fasting triglyceride level of greater than 150 mg/dL in adults is considered elevated and a risk factor for HD and stroke. Patients with marked elevations of hematocrit are also at an increased risk of occlusive stroke owing to a generalized reduction of CBF. Cardiac disorders such as rheumatic heart valvular disease, endocarditis, or cardiac surgery (e.g., coronary artery bypass graft [CABG]) increase the risk of embolic stroke. Atrial fibrillation is a powerful risk factor for stroke with a fivefold increased risk. End-stage renal disease and chronic kidney disease also increase the risk of stroke. Sleep apnea is an independent risk factor for stroke, doubling the risk of stroke or death. Control of these chronic diseases and conditions is essential in reducing stroke risk.[1,2]

A number of stroke risk factors are specific to women. Women with early menopause (before 42 years of age) have twice the risk of ischemic stroke as women with later menopause. The use of estrogen alone or estrogen plus progestin increases the risk of ischemic stroke (up to 44% to 55% or higher). Pregnancy, birth, and the first 6 weeks postpartum can also increase risk of stroke, especially in older women and African Americans. Preeclampsia is an independent risk factor for stroke.[1]

Modifiable risk factors include cigarette smoking, physical inactivity, obesity, and diet. Current smokers have 2 to 4 times increased stroke risk compared to nonsmokers or those who have quit for more than 10 years. Physical activity (moderate to vigorous exercise) is associated with an overall 35% reduction in stroke risk whereas light exercise (walking) does not appear to have the same benefit. As with a cardiac risk profile, the more risk factors present or the greater the degree of abnormality of any one factor, the greater the risk of stroke. Stroke risk factors considered nonmodifiable include family history, age, gender, and race (African American).

Lifestyle changes can greatly reduce the risk of stroke. Recommendations include controlling BP, diet (cholesterol and lipids), weight loss, quitting smoking, and increasing physical activity, as well as effective disease management.[1,2]

Effective stroke prevention depends on improving public awareness concerning the *early warning signs of stroke.* Only about 60% of Americans can recognize even one warning sign and only 55% can identify one stroke symptom.[1] Early warning signs identified by the American Heart Association and National Stroke Association are presented in Box 15.1.[3] The significance of recognizing early warning signs rests with prompt initiation of emergency care under the rule that *"time is brain."* Patients and families are encouraged to call 911 immediately, even if these symptoms go away quickly or are not painful. Early computed tomography (CT) is used to differentiate between atherothrombotic stroke and hemorrhagic stroke. If the stroke is atherothrombotic, clot-dissolving enzymes (e.g., tissue plasminogen activator [tPA]) can be used for thrombolysis. To be effective, thrombolytic therapy such as tPA must be given within 3 hours of the onset of symptoms and cannot be given with hemorrhagic stroke because the drug may worsen bleeding. Within this window of opportunity, the patient must recognize the situation as a medical emergency, be transported to an appropriate hospital, be evaluated by emergency department(ED) staff (including a CT scan of the brain), and be treated.[4,5] Although this treatment has been available since the mid-1990s and has been shown to be safe and to dramatically reduce death and disability, fewer than half of individuals experiencing stroke arrive at the ED within 2 hours of symptoms.[6] Women are less likely than men to arrive in time. Of those arriving at the ED within 2 hours of symptoms, only 65% received imaging within 1 hour of ED arrival.[7]

In the United States, there is a developing Stroke Center Network dedicated to providing the highest quality of acute stroke care. Direct access to a Comprehensive Stroke Center (CSC) is associated with a shorter onset-to-treatment time and better outcomes for ischemic stroke treated with thrombolysis.[8] Even with policy changes that allow emergency first responders to transmit individuals directly to a CSC, still only about half of patients have timely access.[9] A significant predictor in successfully accessing emergency care is the "executive" spouse or significant other who is able to make the decision to seek treatment immediately. Patients who do receive tPA within 3 hours are at least 33% more likely to recover from their stroke with little or no disability after 3 months as compared to those who do not receive the treatment.[10] Major heart and stroke organizations currently promote the use of the term *brain attack,* comparable to heart attack, to help individuals recognize the importance of seeking immediate emergency care.

Box 15.1   Stroke Early Warning Signs

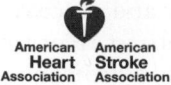

STROKE WARNING SIGNS
American Heart Association | American Stroke Association.

 SUDDEN NUMBNESS OR WEAKNESS OF THE FACE, ARM OR LEG, ESPECIALLY ON ONE SIDE OF THE BODY

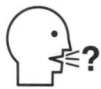 SUDDEN CONFUSION, TROUBLE SPEAKING OR UNDERSTANDING

 SUDDEN TROUBLE SEEING IN ONE OR BOTH EYES

 SUDDEN TROUBLE WALKING, DIZZINESS, LOSS OF BALANCE OR COORDINATION

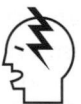 SUDDEN SEVERE HEADACHE WITH NO KNOWN CAUSE

Immediately call 9-1-1 or the emergency medical services (EMS) number so an ambulance (ideally with advanced life support) can be sent for you.

Also, check the time so you'll know when the first symptoms appeared. It's very important to take immediate action. If given within 3 hours of the start of symptoms, a clot-busting drug called tissue plasminogen activator (tPA) may reduce long-term disability for the most common type of stroke.

© 2011 American Heart Association   www.strokeassociation.org

Reprinted with permission. www.strokeassociation.org © 2011, American Heart Association, Inc.

■ PATHOPHYSIOLOGY

Sudden cessation of cerebral blood flow and oxygen-glucose deprivation sets in motion a series of pathological events. Within minutes neurons die within the ischemic core tissue, while the majority of neurons in the surrounding penumbra survive for a slightly longer time. Cell survival depends largely on the severity and the duration of the ischemic episode. For cells to survive, 20% to 25% of regular blood flow is required. Without timely reperfusion, cells in the penumbra will die, neuronal activity ceases, and the infarct expands. Ischemia triggers a number of damaging cellular events, termed **ischemic cascade**. The release of excess neurotransmitters (e.g., glutamate and aspartate) produces a progressive disturbance of energy metabolism and anoxic depolarization. This results in an inability of brain cells to produce energy, particularly adenosine triphosphate (ATP). This is followed by excess influx of calcium ions and pump failure of the neuronal membrane. Excess calcium reacts with intracellular phospholipids to form free radicals. Calcium influx also stimulates the release of nitric oxide and cytokines. Both mechanisms further damage brain cells. Research efforts are ongoing toward development of drugs that might promote angiogenesis, restore blood supply, stimulate neuroprotective genes, and reverse the metabolic changes of the ischemic penumbra area.[11]

Ischemic strokes produce **cerebral edema**, an accumulation of fluids within the brain that begins within minutes of the insult and reaches a maximum by 3 to 4 days. It is the result of tissue necrosis and widespread rupture of cell membranes with movement of fluid from the blood into brain tissues. The swelling gradually subsides and generally disappears by 2 to 3 weeks. Significant edema can elevate intracranial pressures, leading to intracranial hypertension and neurological deterioration associated with contralateral and caudal shifts of brain structures (**brainstem herniation**). Clinical signs of *elevating intracranial pressure (ICP)* include decreasing level of consciousness (stupor and coma), widened pulse pressure, increased heart rate, irregular respirations (*Cheyne-Stokes respirations*), vomiting, unreacting pupils (cranial nerve [CN] III signs), and papilledema. Cerebral edema is the most frequent cause of death in acute stroke and is characteristic of large infarcts involving the middle cerebral artery and the internal carotid artery.

Management Categories

Transient ischemic attack (TIA) refers to the temporary interruption of blood supply to the brain. Symptoms of focal neurological deficit may last for only a few minutes or for several hours, but by definition do not last longer than 24 hours. After the attack is over there is no evidence of residual brain damage or permanent neurological dysfunction. TIAs may result from a number of different etiological factors, including occlusive episodes, emboli, reduced cerebral perfusion (arrhythmias, decreased cardiac output, hypotension, overmedication with antihypertensive medications, subclavian steal syndrome), or cerebrovascular spasm. The major clinical significance of TIA is as a precursor to susceptibility for both cerebral infarction and myocardial infarction. Approximately 15% of all strokes are preceded by a TIA, with the greatest risk of occurrence within 90 days.[1]

Patients are classified as having a *major stroke* in the presence of stable, usually severe, impairments. The term *deteriorating stroke* is used to refer to the patient whose neurological status deteriorates after admission to the hospital. This change in status may be due to cerebral or systemic causes (e.g., cerebral edema, progressing thrombosis). The category of *young stroke* is used to describe a stroke affecting persons younger than age 45. Causes of stroke in children include perinatal arterial ischemic stroke, sickle cell disease, congenital HD, thrombophlebitis and trauma.[1]

Vascular Syndromes

Cerebral blood flow (CBF) varies with the patency of the vessels. Progressive narrowing secondary to atherosclerosis decreases blood flow. As in coronary heart disease,

symptomatic changes generally result from a restriction of flow greater than 80%. The severity and symptoms of stroke are dependent on a number of factors, including (1) the location of the ischemic process, (2) the size of the ischemic area, (3) the nature and functions of the structures involved, and (4) the availability of collateral blood flow. Presenting symptoms may also depend on the rapidity of the occlusion of a blood vessel because slow occlusions may allow collateral vessels to take over, whereas sudden events do not.

CBF is controlled by a number of *autoregulatory mechanisms* (cerebral) that modulate a constant rate of blood flow through the brain. These mechanisms provide homeostatic balance, counteracting fluctuations in systolic blood pressure while maintaining a normal flow of 50 to 60 mL per 100g of brain tissue per minute. The brain has high energy requirements and very little metabolic reserves. Thus, it requires a continuous, rich perfusion of blood to deliver oxygen and glucose to the tissues. Cerebral flow represents approximately 17% of available cardiac output. Chemical regulation of CBF occurs in response to changes in blood concentrations of carbon dioxide or oxygen. Vasodilation and increased CBF are produced in response to an increase in $PaCO_2$ or a decrease in PaO_2, whereas vasoconstriction and decreased CBF are produced by the opposite stimuli. Blood flow is also altered by changes in the blood pH. A fall in pH (increased acidity) produces vasodilation, and a rise in pH (increased alkalinity) produces a decrease in blood flow. Neurogenic regulation alters blood flow by vasodilating vessels in direct proportion to local function of brain tissue. Released metabolites probably act directly on the smooth muscle in local vessel walls. Changes in blood viscosity or ICP may also influence CBF. Changes in BP produce minor alterations of CBF. As pressure rises, the artery is stretched, resulting in contraction of smooth muscle in the vessel wall. Thus, the patency of the vessel is decreased, with a consequent decrease in CBF. As pressure falls, contraction lessens and CBF increases. Following stroke, autoregulatory mechanisms may be impaired.[12]

Knowledge of cerebral vascular anatomy is essential to understand the symptoms, diagnosis, and management of stroke. Extracranial blood supply to the brain is provided by the right and left internal carotid arteries and by the right and left vertebral arteries. The *internal carotid artery* begins at the bifurcation of the common carotid artery and ascends in the deep portions of the neck to the carotid canal. It turns rostromedially and ascends into the cranial cavity. It then pierces the dura mater and gives off the ophthalmic and anterior choroidal arteries before bifurcating into the middle and anterior cerebral arteries. The anterior communicating artery communicates with the anterior cerebral arteries of either side, giving rise to the rostral portion of the **circle of Willis** (Fig. 15.2). The *vertebral artery* arises as a branch off the subclavian artery. It enters the

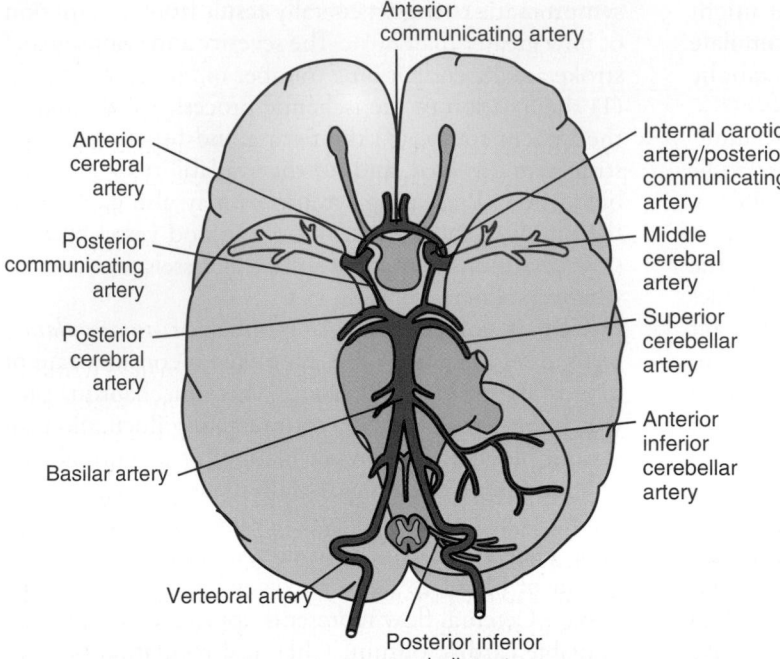

Figure 15.2 Cerebral circulation: circle of Willis.

vertebral foramen of the sixth cervical vertebra and travels through the foramina of the transverse processes of the upper six cervical vertebrae to the foramen magnum and into the brain. There it travels in the posterior cranial fossa ventrally and medially and unites with the vertebral artery from the other side to form the basilar artery at the upper border of the medulla. At the upper border of the pons, the basilar artery bifurcates to form the posterior cerebral arteries and the posterior portion of the circle of Willis. Posterior communicating arteries connect the posterior cerebral

arteries with the internal carotid arteries and complete the circle of Willis.

Anterior Cerebral Artery Syndrome

The *anterior cerebral artery (ACA)* is the first and smaller of two terminal branches of the internal carotid artery. It supplies the medial aspect of the cerebral hemisphere (frontal and parietal lobes) and subcortical structures, including the basal ganglia (anterior internal capsule, inferior caudate nucleus), anterior fornix, and anterior four-fifths of the corpus callosum (Fig. 15.3). Because

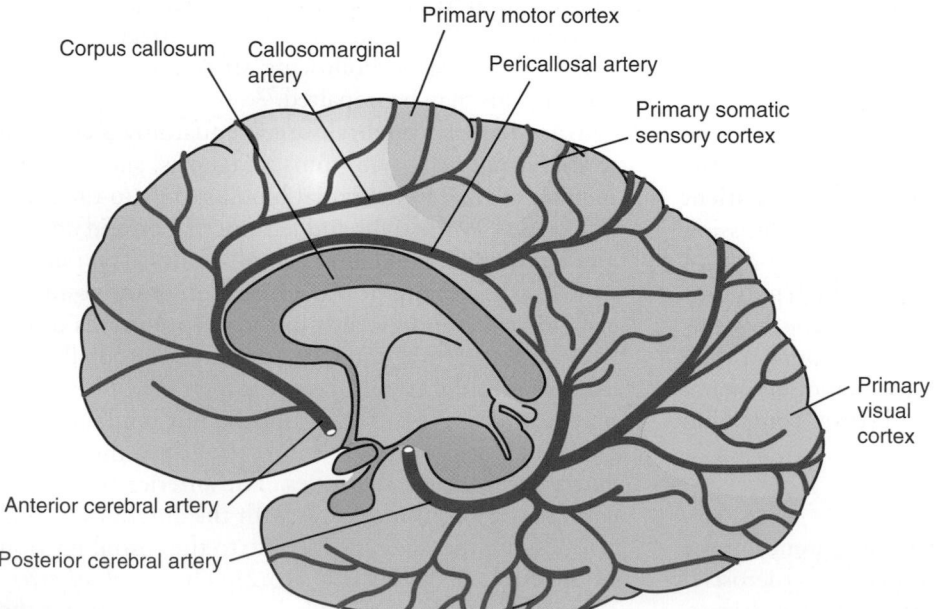

Figure 15.3 Cerebral circulation: a diagram of a midsagittal view of the brain illustrates the distribution of the anterior and posterior cerebral arteries.

the anterior communicating artery allows perfusion of the proximal ACA from either side, occlusion proximal to this point results in minimal deficit.

More distal lesions produce more significant deficits. Table 15.1 presents the clinical manifestations of *anterior cerebral artery (ACA) syndrome*. The most common characteristics of ACA syndrome include contralateral hemiparesis and sensory loss with greater involvement of the lower extremity (LE) than the upper extremity (UE) because the somatotopic organization of the medial aspect of the cortex includes the functional area for the LE.

Middle Cerebral Artery Syndrome

The *middle cerebral artery (MCA)* is the second of the two main branches of the internal carotid artery and supplies the entire lateral aspect of the cerebral hemisphere (frontal, temporal, and parietal lobes) and subcortical structures, including the internal capsule (posterior portion), corona radiata, globus pallidus (outer part), most of the caudate nucleus, and the putamen (Fig. 15.4). Occlusion of the proximal MCA produces extensive neurological damage with significant cerebral edema. Increased intracranial pressures typically lead to loss of consciousness, brain herniation, and possibly death. Table 15.2 presents the clinical manifestations of *middle cerebral artery (MCA) syndrome*. The most common characteristics of MCA syndrome are contralateral spastic hemiparesis and sensory loss of the face, UE, and LE, with the face and UE more involved than the LE. Lesions of the parieto-occipital cortex of the dominant hemisphere (usually the left hemisphere) typically produce aphasia. Lesions of the right parietal lobe of the nondominant hemisphere (usually the right hemisphere) typically produce perceptual deficits (e.g., **unilateral neglect, anosognosia, apraxia,** and **spatial disorganization**). **Homonymous hemianopsia** (a visual field defect) is also a common finding. The MCA is the most common site of occlusion in stroke.

Internal Carotid Artery Syndrome

Occlusion of the *internal carotid artery (ICA)* typically produces massive infarction in the region of the brain supplied by the middle cerebral artery. The ICA supplies both the MCA and the ACA. If collateral circulation to the ACA from the circle of Willis is absent, extensive cerebral infarction in the areas of both the ACA and MCA can occur. Significant edema is common with possible uncal herniation, coma, and death (mass effect).

Posterior Cerebral Artery Syndrome

The two posterior cerebral arteries (PCAs) arise as terminal branches of the basilar artery and each supplies the corresponding occipital lobe and medial and inferior temporal lobe (see Fig. 15.3). It also supplies the upper brainstem, midbrain, and posterior diencephalon, including most of the thalamus. Table 15.3 presents the clinical manifestations of *posterior cerebral artery (PCA) syndrome*. Occlusion proximal to the posterior communicating artery typically results in minimal deficits owing to the collateral blood supply from the posterior communicating artery (similar to ACA syndrome). Occlusion of thalamic branches may produce hemianesthesia (contralateral sensory loss) or **central post-stroke (thalamic) pain**. Occipital infarction produces homonymous hemianopsia, **visual agnosia, prosopagnosia,** or, if bilateral, cortical blindness. Temporal lobe ischemia results in amnesia (memory loss). Involvement of subthalamic branches may involve the subthalamic nucleus or its pallidal connections, producing a wide variety of deficits. Contralateral hemiplegia occurs with involvement of the cerebral peduncle.

Lacunar Strokes

Lacunar strokes are caused by small vessel disease deep in the cerebral white matter (penetrating artery disease). They are strongly associated with hypertensive hemorrhage and diabetic microvascular disease. Lacunar syndromes are consistent with specific anatomical sites. *Pure motor lacunar*

Table 15.1	Clinical Manifestations of Anterior Cerebral Artery Syndrome
Signs and Symptoms	**Structures Involved**
Contralateral hemiparesis involving mainly the LE (UE is more spared)	Primary motor area, medial aspect of cortex, internal capsule
Contralateral hemisensory loss involving mainly the LE (UE is more spared)	Primary sensory area, medial aspect of cortex
Urinary incontinence	Posteromedial aspect of superior frontal gyrus
Problems with imitation and bimanual tasks, apraxia	Corpus callosum
Abulia (akinetic mutism), slowness, delay, lack of spontaneity, motor inaction	Uncertain localization
Contralateral grasp reflex, sucking reflex Can be asymptomatic if circle of Willis is competent.	Uncertain localization

LE = lower extremity; UE = upper extremity.

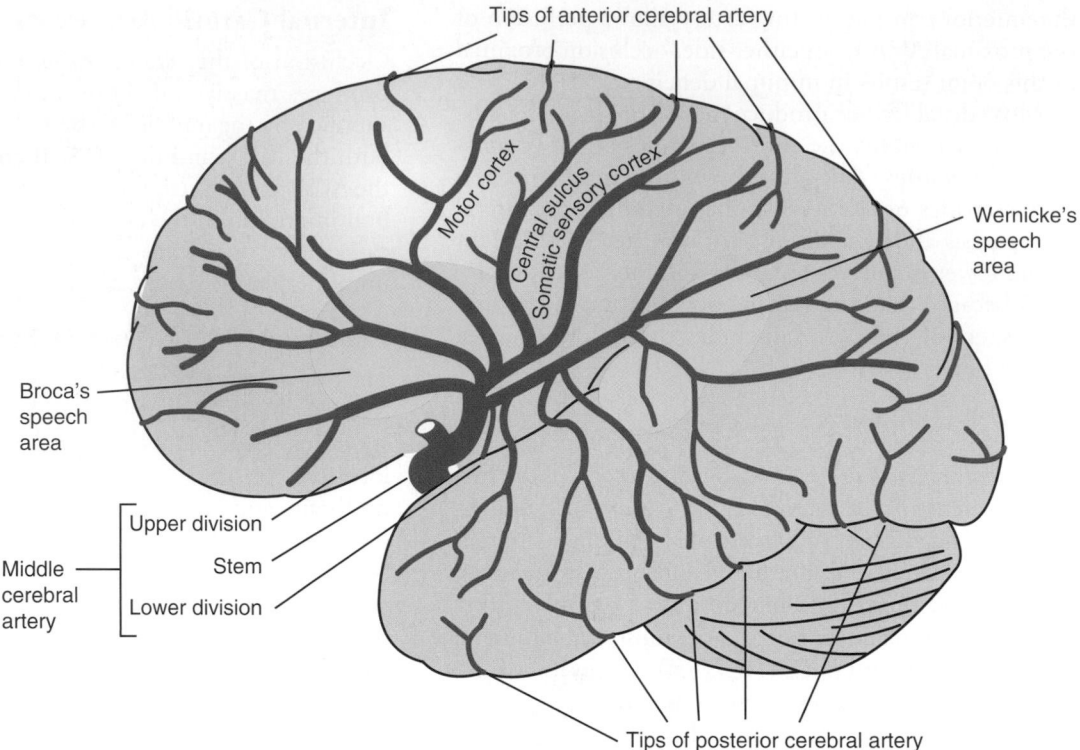

Figure 15.4 Cerebral circulation: diagram of a lateral view of the brain illustrates the distribution of the middle cerebral artery.

Table 15.2 Clinical Manifestations of Middle Cerebral Artery Syndrome	
Signs and Symptoms	Structures Involved
Contralateral hemiparesis involving mainly the UE and face (LE is more spared)	Primary motor cortex and internal capsule
Contralateral hemisensory loss involving mainly the UE and face (LE is more spared)	Primary sensory cortex and internal capsule
Motor speech impairment: Broca's or nonfluent aphasia with limited vocabulary and slow, hesitant speech	Broca's cortical area (third frontal convolution) in the dominant hemisphere, typically the left hemisphere
Receptive speech impairment: Wernicke's or fluent aphasia with impaired auditory comprehension and fluent speech with normal rate and melody	Wernicke's cortical area (posterior portion of the temporal gyrus) in the dominant hemisphere, typically the left
Global aphasia: nonfluent speech with poor comprehension	Both third frontal convolution and posterior portion of the superior temporal gyrus
Perceptual deficits: unilateral neglect, depth perception, spatial relations, agnosia	Parietal sensory association cortex in the nondominant hemisphere, typically the right
Limb-kinetic apraxia	Premotor or parietal cortex
Contralateral homonymous hemianopsia	Optic radiation in internal capsule
Loss of conjugate gaze to the opposite side	Frontal eye fields or their descending tracts
Ataxia of contralateral limb(s) (sensory ataxia)	Parietal lobe
Pure motor hemiplegia (lacunar stroke)	Upper portion of posterior limb of internal capsule

LE = lower extremity; UE = upper extremity.

Table 15.3   Clinical Manifestations of Posterior Cerebral Artery Syndrome

Signs and Symptoms	Structures Involved
Peripheral Territory	
Contralateral homonymous hemianopsia	Primary visual cortex or optic radiation
Bilateral homonymous hemianopsia with some degree of macular sparing	Calcarine cortex (macular sparing is due to occipital pole receiving collateral blood supply from MCA)
Visual agnosia	Left occipital lobe
Prosopagnosia (difficulty naming people on sight)	Visual association cortex
Dyslexia (difficulty reading) without agraphia (difficulty writing), color naming (anomia), and color discrimination problems	Dominant calcarine lesion and posterior part of corpus callosum
Memory defect	Lesion of inferomedial portions of temporal lobe bilaterally or on the dominant side only
Topographic disorientation	Nondominant primary visual area, usually bilaterally
Central Territory	
Central post-stroke (thalamic) pain Spontaneous pain and dysesthesias; sensory impairments (all modalities)	Ventral posterolateral nucleus of thalamus
Involuntary movements; choreoathetosis, intention tremor, hemiballismus	Subthalamic nucleus or its pallidal connections
Contralateral hemiplegia	Cerebral peduncle of midbrain
Weber's syndrome Oculomotor nerve palsy and contralateral hemiplegia	Third nerve and cerebral peduncle of midbrain
Paresis of vertical eye movements, slight miosis and ptosis, and sluggish pupillary light response	Supranuclear fibers to third cranial nerve

LE = lower extremity; UE = upper extremity.

stroke is associated with involvement of the posterior limb of the internal capsule, pons, and pyramids. *Pure sensory lacunar stroke* is associated with involvement of the ventrolateral thalamus or thalamocortical projections. Other lacunar syndromes include *dysarthria/clumsy hand syndrome* (involving the base of the pons, genu of anterior limb, or the internal capsule), *ataxic hemiparesis* (involving the pons, genu of internal capsule, corona radiata, or cerebellum), *sensory/motor stroke* (involving the junction of the internal capsule and thalamus), or *dystonia/involuntary movements* (choreoathetosis with lacunar infarction of the putamen or globus pallidus; hemiballismus with involvement of the subthalamic nucleus). Deficits in consciousness, language, or visual fields are not seen in lacunar strokes because the higher cortical areas are preserved. A hypertensive hemorrhage affecting the thalamus can also produce central post-stroke pain.[12]

Vertebrobasilar Artery Syndrome

The *vertebral arteries* arise from the subclavian arteries and travel into the brain along the medulla where they merge at the inferior border of the pons to form the basilar artery. The vertebral arteries supply the cerebellum (via posterior inferior cerebellar arteries) and the medulla (via the medullary arteries). The basilar artery supplies the pons (via pontine arteries), the internal ear (via labyrinthine arteries), and the cerebellum (via the anterior inferior and superior cerebellar arteries). The basilar artery then terminates at the upper border of the pons giving rise to the two posterior arteries (see Fig. 15.2). Occlusions of the vertebrobasilar system can produce a wide variety of symptoms with both ipsilateral and contralateral signs, because some of the tracts in the brainstem will have crossed and others will not. Numerous cerebellar and cranial nerve abnormalities also are present. Table 15.4 presents the clinical manifestations of *vertebrobasilar artery syndromes*.

Locked-in syndrome (LIS) occurs with basilar artery thrombosis and bilateral infarction of the ventral pons. LIS is a catastrophic event with sudden onset. Patients develop acute hemiparesis rapidly progressing to tetraplegia and lower bulbar paralysis (CNs V through XII are involved). Initially the patient is dysarthric and dysphonic but rapidly progresses to mutism (anarthria). There is preserved consciousness and sensation. Thus the patient cannot move or speak but remains alert and oriented. Horizontal eye movements are impaired but

Table 15.4   Clinical Manifestations of Vertebrobasilar Artery Syndrome

Signs and Symptoms	Structures Involved
Medial medullary syndrome	Occlusion vertebral artery, medullary branch
Ipsilateral to lesion Paralysis with atrophy of half the tongue with deviation to the paralyzed side when tongue is protruded	CN XII, hypoglossal, or nucleus
Contralateral to lesion Paralysis of UE and LE	Corticospinal tract
Impaired tactile and proprioceptive sense	Medial lemniscus
Lateral medullary (Wallenburg's) syndrome	Occlusion of posterior inferior cerebellar artery or vertebral artery
Ipsilateral to lesion Decreased pain and temperature sensation in face	Descending tract and nucleus of CN V, trigeminal
Cerebellum or inferior cerebellar peduncle	Cerebellar ataxia: gait and limbs ataxia
Vertigo, nausea, vomiting	Vestibular nuclei and connections
Nystagmus	Vestibular nuclei and connections
Horner's syndrome: miosis, ptosis, decreased sweating	Descending sympathetic tract
Dysphagia and dysphonia: paralysis of palatal and laryngeal muscles, diminished gag reflex	CN IX, glossopharyngeal, and CN X, vagus, or nuclei
Sensory impairment of ipsilateral UE, trunk, or LE	Cuneate and gracile nuclei
Contralateral to lesion Impaired pain and thermal sense over 50% of body, sometimes face	Spinal lemniscus—spinothalamic tract
Complete basilar artery syndrome (locked-in syndrome)	Basilar artery, ventral pons
Tetraplegia (quadriplegia)	Corticospinal tracts bilaterally
Bilateral cranial nerve palsy: upward gaze is spared	Long tracts to cranial nerve nuclei bilaterally
Coma	Reticular activating system
Cognition is spared	
Medial inferior pontine syndrome	Occlusion of paramedian branch of basilar artery
Ipsilateral to lesion Paralysis of conjugate gaze to side of lesion (preservation of convergence)	Pontine center for lateral gaze paramedian pentine reticular formation (PPRF)
Nystagmus	Vestibular nuclei and connections
Ataxia of limbs and gait	Middle cerebellar peduncle
Diplopia on lateral gaze	CN VI, abducens, or nucleus
Contralateral to lesion Paresis of face, UE, and LE	Corticobulbar and corticospinal tract in lower pons
Impaired tactile and proprioceptive sense over 50% of the body	Medial lemniscus
Lateral inferior pontine syndrome	Occlusion of anterior inferior cerebellar artery, a branch of the basilar artery
Ipsilateral to lesion Horizontal and vertical nystagmus, vertigo, nausea, vomiting	CN VIII, vestibular, or nucleus
Facial paralysis	CN VII, facial, or nucleus
Paralysis of conjugate gaze to side of lesion	Pontine center for lateral gaze (PPRF)
Deafness, tinnitus	CN VIII, cochlear, or nucleus

Table 15.4   Clinical Manifestations of Vertebrobasilar Artery Syndrome—cont'd

Signs and Symptoms	Structures Involved
Ataxia	Middle cerebellar peduncle and cerebellar hemisphere
Impaired sensation over face	Main sensory nucleus and descending tract of fifth nerve
Contralateral to lesion Impaired pain and thermal sense over half the body (may include face)	Spinothalamic tract
Medial midpontine syndrome	Occlusion of paramedian branch of the mid-basilar artery
Ipsilateral to lesion Ataxia of limbs and gait (more prominent in bilateral involvement)	Middle cerebellar peduncle
Contralateral to lesion Paralysis of face, UE, and LE	Corticobulbar and corticospinal tract
Deviation of eyes	Abducent nerve nucleus, medial longitudinal fasciculus
Lateral midpontine syndrome	Occlusion of short circumferential artery
Ipsilateral to lesion Ataxia of limbs	Middle cerebellar peduncle
Paralysis of muscles of mastication	Motor fibers or nucleus of CN V, trigeminal
Impaired sensation over side of face	Sensory fibers or nucleus of CN V, trigeminal
Medial superior pontine syndrome	Occlusion of paramedian branches of upper basilar artery
Cerebellar ataxia	Superior or middle cerebellar peduncle
Internuclear ophthalmoplegia	Medial longitudinal fasciculus
Contralateral to lesion Paralysis of face, UE, and LE	Corticobulbar and corticospinal tract
Lateral superior pontine syndrome (occlusion of superior cerebellar artery, a branch of the basilar artery)	
Ipsilateral to lesion Cerebellar ataxia of limbs and gait, falling to side of lesion	Middle and superior cerebellar peduncles, superior surface of cerebellum, dentate nucleus
Dizziness, nausea, vomiting	Vestibular nuclei
Horizontal nystagmus	Vestibular nuclei
Paresis of conjugate gaze (ipsilateral)	Uncertain
Loss of optokinetic nystagmus	Uncertain
Horner's syndrome: miosis, ptosis, decreased sweating on opposite side face	Descending sympathetic fibers
Contralateral to lesion Impaired pain and thermal sense of face, limbs, and trunk	Spinothalamic tract
Impaired touch, vibration, and position sense, more in LE than UE (tendency to incongruity of pain and touch deficits)	Medial lemniscus (lateral portion)

CN = cranial nerve; LE = lower extremity; UE = upper extremity.

vertical eye movements and blinking remain intact. Communication can be established via these eye movements. Mortality rates are high (59%), and those patients who do survive are left with severe impairments associated with brainstem injury.[12]

Extracranial injuries to the vertebral arteries as they travel through the cervical spine can also produce vertebrobasilar signs and symptoms. Forceful neck motions (e.g., whiplash or aggressive neck manipulations) are among the more common types of injuries.

■ NEUROLOGICAL COMPLICATIONS AND ASSOCIATED CONDITIONS

Altered Consciousness

Altered level of consciousness (coma, decreased arousal levels) may occur with extensive brain damage (e.g., large proximal MCA occlusion). The *Glasgow Coma Scale* developed by Teasdale and Jennett[13] is the gold standard used to document level of coma (see Chapter 19, Traumatic Brain Injury). Three areas of function are examined: eye opening, best motor response, and verbal responses. The therapist should document levels of consciousness using standard descriptive terms: *normal, lethargy, obtundation, stupor*, and *coma* (see Chapter 5, Examination of Motor Function: Motor Control and Motor Learning). Since the patient's behaviors can be expected to fluctuate widely, frequent repeat observations are necessary.

Disorders of Speech and Language

Patients with lesions involving the cortex of the dominant hemisphere (typically the left hemisphere) demonstrate speech and language impairments. **Aphasia** is the general term used to describe an acquired communication disorder caused by brain damage and is characterized by an impairment of language comprehension, formulation, and use. Aphasia has been estimated to occur in 30% to 36% of all patients with stroke.[2] There are many different types of aphasias; major classification categories are fluent, nonfluent, and global. In **fluent aphasia (Wernicke's/ sensory/receptive aphasia)**, speech flows smoothly with a variety of grammatical constructions and preserved melody of speech. Auditory comprehension is impaired. Thus, the patient demonstrates difficulty in comprehending spoken language and in following commands. The lesion is located in the auditory association cortex in the left lateral temporal lobe. In **nonfluent aphasia (Broca's/expressive aphasia)**, the flow of speech is slow and hesitant, vocabulary is limited, and syntax is impaired. Speech production is labored or lost completely whereas comprehension is good. The lesion is located in the premotor area of the left frontal lobe. **Global aphasia** is a severe aphasia characterized by marked impairments of both production and comprehension of language. It is often an indication of extensive brain damage. Severe problems in communication may limit the patient's ability to learn and often impede successful outcomes in rehabilitation. See Chapter 28, Neurogenic Disorders of Speech and Language, for a complete discussion of these impairments and their management.

Patients with stroke commonly present with **dysarthria** with a reported incidence ranging from 48% to 57%.[2] This term refers to a category of motor speech disorders caused by lesions in parts of the central or peripheral nervous system that mediate speech production. Respiration, articulation, phonation, resonance, and/or sensory feedback may be affected. The lesion can be located in the primary motor cortex in the frontal lobe, the primary sensory cortex in the parietal lobe, or the cerebellum. Volitional and automatic actions such as chewing and swallowing and movement of the jaw and tongue are impaired resulting in slurred speech. In patients with stroke, dysarthria can accompany aphasia, complicating the course of rehabilitation (see Chapter 28).

The patient's communication abilities should be fully ascertained before proceeding on with other examination procedures. It is not uncommon for family and staff to overestimate the patient's abilities to understand language, especially if the patient is cooperative. Close collaboration with the speech-language pathologist is important in making an accurate determination of the patient's communication impairments. Receptive language functions (auditory comprehension, reading comprehension) and expressive language function (word finding, fluency, writing) should be carefully examined. Neuromotor disorders (dysarthria) need to be clearly differentiated from aphasia. If communication is severely limited and alternate forms are required (gestures, demonstration, communication boards), therapists should be fully knowledgeable of such methods before the physical therapy examination.

Dysphagia

Dysphagia, an inability to swallow or difficulty in swallowing, occurs in about 51% of patients with stroke. It can be seen in hemispheric stroke, brainstem stroke, or pseudobulbar and suprabulbar palsy. In brainstem stroke, the reported incidence is as high as 81%. Cranial nerve involvement results in swallowing dysfunction of the oral stage (CN V [trigeminal], CN VII [facial]), the pharyngeal stage (CN IX [glossopharyngeal], CN X [vagus], and CN XI [accessory]), or oral and pharyngeal (CN XII [hypoglossal]). Dysphagia is also common in patients with multiple strokes. The most common problems seen in patients with dysphagia include delayed triggering of the swallowing reflex, reduced pharyngeal peristalsis, and reduced lingual control. Altered mental status, altered sensation, poor jaw and lip closure, impaired head control, and poor sitting posture also contribute to the patient's swallowing difficulties. Most patients demonstrate multiple problems that can include drooling, difficulty ingesting food, compromised nutritional status, and dehydration. **Aspiration**, the penetration of food, liquid, saliva, or gastric reflux into the airway, occurs in about one-third of patients with dysphagia. Aspiration is an important complication in that it can lead to acute respiratory distress within hours, aspiration pneumonia, and, if left untreated, death. Dysphagia can also lead to dehydration and compromised nutrition.[14,15]

A referral to a dysphagia specialist or multidisciplinary dysphagia team is indicated. Team members typically include the physician, nurse, occupational therapist, speech-language pathologist, and dietitian. Clinical evaluation of dysphagia includes an examination of oral-motor function, pharyngeal function, functional status (e.g., upright sitting position, use of adaptive feeding equipment), examination of abnormal reflexes, and a feeding trial. Instrumental testing can include a *modified barium swallow* (MBS), *videofluoroscopic evaluation of swallowing*, and a *fiberoptic endoscopic evaluation of swallowing* (FEES).[16] If dysphagia is severe enough, patients may be placed on nothing-by-mouth (NPO) precautions. The use of tube feeding, either a nasogastric (NG) tube for short periods of time or an invasive gastrostomy (G) tube for more long-term care, is required. Nutrition can also be provided through an intravenous route (total parenteral nutrition [TPN]).

Cognitive Dysfunction

Cognitive dysfunction may be present with lesions involving the cortex and includes impairments in alertness, attention, orientation, memory, or executive functions. Premorbid changes associated with pathological aging may also account for some of the dysfunction noted and should be carefully determined from interviews with family, significant others, or caregivers. The patient with acute stroke may be largely unaware of what is going on in the external environment, a problem of impaired alertness that results from lesions in the prefrontal cortex and reticular formation. The patient may also be disoriented and unable to provide information about self, time of day, physical or geographical location, or disability, the result of lesions affecting the prefrontal cortex, limbic system, and limbic cortex. *Attention* is the ability to select and attend to a specific stimulus while simultaneously suppressing extraneous stimuli. Attention disorders include impairments in sustained attention, selective attention, divided attention, or alternating attention. Altered attention results from lesions in the prefrontal cortex and reticular formation. *Memory* is defined as the ability to store experiences and perceptions for later recall. Immediate and short-term memory impairments are common, occurring in about 36% of patients with stroke, whereas long-term memory typically remains intact.[2] Thus, the patient cannot remember the instructions for a new task given only minutes or hours ago but can easily remember events 30 years ago. Short-term memory loss is associated with lesions of the limbic system, limbic association cortex (orbitofrontal areas), or temporal lobes. Long-term memory loss is associated with lesions of the hippocampus of the limbic system. Memory gaps may be filled with inappropriate words or fabricated stories, an impairment termed *confabulation* that also results from lesions in the prefrontal cortex. The patient may be confused, demonstrating disorientation and an inability to understand the specific context of a conversation. *Confusion* is the result of disruption of the prefrontal cortex. *Perseveration* is the continued repetition of words, thoughts, or acts not related to current context. Thus, the patient gets "stuck" and repeats words or acts without much success at stopping. Preservation results from lesions in the premotor and/or prefrontal cortex.

Executive functions, defined as those abilities that enable a person to engage in purposeful behaviors, include volition, planning, purposeful action, and effective performance. Patients with lesions of the prefrontal cortex typically demonstrate impairments in executive function including some or all of the following: impulsiveness, inflexible thinking, lack of abstract thinking, impaired organization and sequencing, decreased insight, impaired planning ability, and impaired judgment. Patients are unable to realistically appraise their environment and the people and events in it. They also demonstrate difficulty in self-monitoring and self-correcting behaviors, thereby posing safety risks.[17,18] (See Chapter 27, Cognitive and Perceptual Dysfunction, for a complete discussion of these impairments and their management.)

Multi-infarct dementia (vascular dementia) results from multiple small infarcts of the brain and is seen in 6% to 32% of patients. It is more common in individuals over age 60 and is associated with episodes of cerebral ischemia (microvascular or small vessel disease) and hypertension. Other contributing factors include arrhythmias, myocardial infarct, TIAs, diabetes, obesity, and smoking. Scattered areas of the brain are involved, evidenced by focal neurological deficits. Onset is frequently abrupt. The patient exhibits impairments in memory and cognition and may fluctuate between periods of impaired function and periods of improved function. This stepwise and paroxysmal deterioration of intellectual function is in contrast to the gradual onset and steadier, widespread decline seen in Alzheimer's dementia.[17]

Delirium, also known as *acute confusional state*, is seen more commonly in the acute care setting and results from a number of factors following acute stroke. Deprivation of oxygen to the brain, metabolic imbalance, or adverse drug reactions can all induce confusion. Additional contributory factors can include sensory and perceptual losses coupled with an unfamiliar hospital environment and inactivity. Delirium is characterized by a clouding of consciousness or dulling of cognitive processes and impaired alertness. Thus, the patient is inattentive, incoherent, and disorganized with fluctuating levels of consciousness. Hallucinations and agitation are also common. Nighttime may be particularly problematic. Patients with significant sensory loss following stroke may experience sensory deprivation problems evidenced by irritability, confusion, psychosis, delusions, and even hallucinations. These problems are more frequently seen in the acute phase, especially with patients who have been confined to a bed or whose bed is positioned to limit social interaction (e.g., with the more involved side toward the door). Some patients are equally unable to deal with a sensory overload, produced by too much stimulation. Altered arousal levels are implicated.

It is important to examine cognitive abilities early because they may affect the validity of other tests and measures. An examination of orientation (to person, place, time, and circumstance [e.g., awareness of event causing need for medical care]), attention (selective, sustained, alternating, divided), memory (immediate, short- and long-term), and ability to follow instructions (one-, two-, and three-level commands) can be made from observations of the patient's interactions and responses to specific questions. Higher cortical functions can be examined using tests of simple arithmetic and abstract reasoning (grasp of information, abstract thinking and problem solving, calculating ability, constructional ability). The *Mini-Mental Status Examination (MMSE)* provides a valid and reliable quick screen of cognitive function.[19] A determination of learning impairments (retention and generalization) usually requires repeat sessions with the patient before a complete picture can be ascertained. Difficulties arise in reaching an accurate determination of cognition when the patient presents with impairments in communication or perception. Close collaboration with the occupational therapist, speech-language pathologist, and the rest of team is essential.

Altered Emotional Status

Lesions of the brain affecting the frontal lobe, hypothalamus, and limbic system can produce a number of emotional changes. The patient with stroke may demonstrate **pseudobulbar affect** (PBA), also known as *emotional lability* or *emotional dysregulation syndrome*. PBA occurs in about 18% of cases and is characterized by emotional outbursts of uncontrolled or exaggerated laughing or crying that are inconsistent with mood. The patient quickly changes from laughing to crying with only slight provocation. The patient is typically unable to control these episodes or to inhibit the expression of spontaneous emotions. Frequent crying may also accompany depression. *Apathy* occurs in about 22% of cases and is characterized by a shallow affect and blunted emotional responses. In such patients, apathy is frequently misconstrued as depression or poor motivation. Patients can also demonstrate *euphoria* (exaggerated feelings of well-being), increased levels of irritability or frustration, and social inappropriateness. Changes in the ability to sense, move, communicate, think, or act as before are enormously frustrating by themselves and create high stress levels for the patient with stroke. Increased levels of anxiety, irritability, and frustration are the natural outcomes of high stress levels. These behaviors along with a poor perception of one's self and environment may lead to increasing isolation and social withdrawal.[18]

Depression is common, occurring in approximately 35% of stroke cases.[18] It is characterized by persistent feelings of sadness accompanied by feelings of hopelessness, worthlessness, and/or helplessness. Depressed patients may also experience a loss of energy or persistent fatigue, an inability to concentrate, and decreased interest in daily life along with changes in weight and sleep patterns, generalized anxiety, and recurrent thoughts of death or suicide. Depression is seen with lesions in the left frontal lobe (acute stage) and with lesions in the right parietal lobes (subacute stage).[20] Most patients remain significantly depressed for many months, with an average time of 7 to 8 months. The period from 6 months to 2 years after a CVA is the most likely time for depression to occur.[21] Depression occurs in both mildly and severely involved patients and thus is not significantly related to the degree of motor impairment. Patients with lesions of the left hemisphere may experience more frequent and more severe depression than patients with right hemisphere or brainstem strokes. These findings suggest that post-stroke depression is not simply a result of psychological reaction to disability but rather a direct impairment of the CVA.[22] Anxiety can coexist with depression during any phase of recovery.[20] Prolonged post-stroke depression can interfere with the success of rehabilitation and result in poorer long-term functional outcomes. The reader is referred to Chapter 26, Psychosocial Disorders, for a more complete discussion of psychosocial impairments and their management.

Hemispheric Behavioral Differences

Individuals with stroke differ widely in their approach to processing information and in their behaviors. Those with *left hemisphere lesions* (right hemiplegia) demonstrate difficulties in communication and in processing information in a sequential, linear manner. They are frequently described as cautious, anxious, and disorganized. This makes them more hesitant when trying new tasks and increases the need for feedback and support. They tend, however, to be realistic in their appraisal of their existing problems. Individuals with *right hemisphere lesions* (left hemiplegia), on the other hand, demonstrate difficulty in spatial–perceptual tasks and in grasping the whole idea of a task or activity. They are frequently described as quick and impulsive. They tend to overestimate their abilities while acting unaware of their deficits. This lack of insight and concreteness impairs the patient's ability to participate in rehabilitation. Safety is a far greater issue for patients with left hemiplegia, where poor judgment is common. These patients also require a great deal of feedback when learning a new task. The feedback should be focused on slowing down the activity, checking sequential steps, and relating them to the whole task. Patients also need help recognizing the consequences and risks of their actions. The patient with left hemiplegia frequently cannot attend to visuospatial cues effectively, especially in a cluttered or crowded environment. Table 15.5 summarizes the behavioral differences attributed to damage of the left and right hemispheres.

Table 15.5 Hemispheric Differences Commonly Seen Following Stroke	
Right Hemisphere Lesion	**Left Hemisphere Lesion**
Left-side hemiplegia/paresis	Right-side hemiplegia/paresis
Left-side sensory loss	Right-side sensory loss
Visual–perceptual impairments:	***Speech and language impairments:***
Left-side unilateral neglect	Dominant hemisphere:
Agnosias	• Nonfluent (Broca's) aphasia
Visuospatial disorders	• Fluent (Wernicke's) aphasia
Disturbances of body image and body scheme	• Global aphasia
Difficulty processing visual cues	Difficulty processing verbal cues, verbal commands
Behavioral deficits:	***Behavioral deficits:***
Quick, impulsive behavioral style	Slow, cautious behavioral style
Poor judgment, unrealistic	Disorganized
Inability to self-correct	Often very aware of impairments, extent of disability
Poor insight, awareness of impairments, denial of disability	
Increased safety risk	
Intellectual deficits:	***Intellectual deficits:***
Difficulty with abstract reasoning, problem solving	Disorganized problem solving
Difficulty synthesizing information and grasping whole idea of task	Difficulty initiating tasks, processing delays
Rigidity of thought	Highly distractible
Memory impairments, typically related to spatial-perceptual information	Memory impairments, typically related to language
	Perseveration
Emotional deficits:	***Emotional deficits:***
Difficulty with ability to perceive emotions	Difficulty with expression of positive emotions
Difficulty with expression of negative emotions	
Task performance:	***Task performance:***
Fluctuations in performance	Apraxia common: difficulty planning and sequencing movements
	• Ideational
	• Ideomotor
Deficits of either hemisphere depending on lesion location:	
Visual field defects: Homonymous hemianopsia	
Emotional abnormalities: Lability, apathy, irritability, low frustration levels, anxiety, depression	
Cognitive deficits: Confusion, short attention span, loss of memory, executive functions	

Emotional states and behavioral styles can best be examined through observation of the patient in a variety of situations over a number of sessions. It is important to correlate findings with those reported by other team members and by the family regarding premorbid behaviors and emotional characteristics. Families who report a "personality change" after stroke are likely responding to presenting emotional impairments and disinhibition. Episodes of euphoria and crying should be carefully documented and links to situational or environmental circumstances explored. Duration and frequency of these episodes should also be documented along with strategies that are successful in bringing about an end to the episode (redirecting strategies). The patient's response to new or stressful situations should also be carefully observed for evidence of anxiety (e.g., excessive worrying, restlessness, irritability). The therapist should examine

for evidence of depression. Depressed patients can also be irritable, angry, or hostile and wish to be left alone.[18] The *Beck Depression Inventory*[23] is a useful instrument for depression screening. It consists of 21 statements that are scored on a scale from 0 to 3 (the short version has 13 questions and takes 5 minutes to complete).

Perceptual Dysfunction

Stroke can produce visual–perceptual deficits, with a reported incidence ranging from 32% to 41%.[2] They are frequently the result of lesions in the right parietal cortex and seen more with left hemiplegia than right. These may include disorders of **body scheme/body image, spatial relations,** and **agnosias.** Body scheme refers to a postural model of the body including the relationship of the body parts to each other and the relationship of the body to the environment. Body image is the visual and mental image of one's body that includes feelings about one's body. Both may be distorted following stroke. Specific impairments of body scheme/body image include **unilateral neglect, anosognosia, somatoagnosia, right–left discrimination, finger agnosia,** and **anosognosia.** Spatial relations syndrome refers to a constellation of impairments that have in common a difficulty in perceiving the relationship between the self and two or more objects in the environment. It includes specific impairments in **figure–ground discrimination, form discrimination, spatial relations, position in space,** and **topographical disorientation.** Agnosia is the inability to recognize incoming information despite intact sensory capacities. Agnosias can include visual object agnosia, auditory agnosia, or tactile agnosia (asterognosis). Significant information on sensory and perceptual deficits will be gained by close collaboration with the occupational therapist. The reader is referred to Chapter 27, Cognitive and Perceptual Dysfunction, for a more complete discussion of these deficits and their management.

Because the patient with left hemiplegia may behave in ways that tend to minimize his or her disabilities, it is easy for staff to overestimate the patient's perceptual abilities. For the patient with visuospatial deficits, the use of gestures or visual cues may decrease this patient's ability to perform tasks, whereas verbal cues may increase chances for success. Equally important strategies include carefully structuring the environment to minimize clutter and activity, provide adequate lighting, and provide clear boundaries and reference points.

Problems in **unilateral neglect** (lack of awareness of part of the body or the external environment) will limit movement and use of the more involved extremities (usually the nondominant left side). The patient typically does not react to sensory stimuli (visual, auditory, or somatosensory) presented on the more involved side. Careful observation of spontaneous use of affected limbs, as well as specific responses to inquiries for movement on or toward the hemiplegic side, will provide important information about neglect. Persistent neglect may result in bruising or trauma to the hemiplegic limbs during activity and negatively affect rehabilitation outcomes.

Seizures

Seizures occur in a small percentage of patients with stroke and are slightly more common in occlusive carotid disease (17%) than in MCA disease (11%). Seizures are common right after stroke during the acute phase (e.g., in about 15% of cases with cerebral hemorrhage); late-onset seizures can also occur several months after stroke. They tend to be of the partial motor type. Seizures are potentially life threatening if not controlled. Anticonvulsant medications may be indicated (e.g., phenytoin [Dilantin], carbamazepine [Tegretol], phenobarbital [Solfoton]).[2]

Bladder and Bowel Dysfunction

Disturbances of bladder function are common during the acute phase, occurring in about 29% of cases.[2] Urinary incontinence can result from bladder hyperreflexia or hyporeflexia, disturbances of sphincter control, and/or sensory loss. A toileting schedule for prompted voiding is often implemented to reduce the incidence of incontinence and to accommodate for factors that cause functional incontinence such as inattention, mental status changes, or immobility. Generally, this problem improves quickly. Persistent incontinence is often due to a treatable medical condition (e.g., urinary tract infection). Absorbent pads and special undergarments or external collection devices may be used if incontinence proves refractory. Urinary retention can be controlled pharmacologically and with intermittent or indwelling catheterization. Early treatment is desirable to prevent further complications such as chronic urinary tract infection and skin breakdown. Patients who are incontinent often suffer embarrassment, isolation, and depression. Persistent incontinence is associated with a poor long-term prognosis for functional recovery.

Disturbances of bowel function can include incontinence and diarrhea or constipation and impaction. Patients who are constipated may require stool softeners and dietary/fluid modifications and medications to resolve this problem. Physical activity is also helpful.

Cardiovascular and Pulmonary Dysfunction

The majority of strokes are caused by vascular disease. Patients who suffer a stroke as a result of underlying coronary artery disease (CAD) may demonstrate impaired cardiac output, cardiac decompensation, and serious rhythm disorders. If these problems persist, they can directly alter cerebral perfusion and produce additional focal signs (e.g., mental confusion). Patients with stroke typically exhibit low peak VO_2 levels during exercise (about half of that achieved by age-matched healthy individuals).[24] These vary according to age, level of disability, number and severity of co-morbidities, secondary complications, and medications. Cardiac limitations in exercise tolerance may restrict rehabilitation potential and requires diligent monitoring and careful exercise prescription by the physical therapist.

Many patients with stroke are significantly deconditioned and exhibit low work capacities, the result of acute illness, bed rest, and limited activity levels. Some individuals may have been inactive before the stroke. Changes in the cardiovascular system associated with deconditioning include reduced cardiac output, decreased maximal heart rate, increased resting and exercise blood pressures, decreased maximal oxygen uptake, and decreased vital capacity. Changes in the musculoskeletal system (e.g., decreased muscle mass and strength, decreased bone mass, decreased flexibility) and decreased glucose tolerance also affect exercise tolerance and endurance levels. Decreased activity levels may also be related to depression, a common finding in stroke.

Pulmonary function is often impaired in individuals with stroke. Decreased lung volume, decreased pulmonary perfusion and vital capacity, and altered chest wall excursion are all common findings. The decreased respiratory output is accompanied by increased oxygen demands required during activity using altered and unfamiliar movement patterns. For example, walking using an orthosis and assistive device dramatically increases the energy demands of the activity. The end result for the patient with stroke is increased fatigue and decreased endurance.

Deep Venous Thrombosis and Pulmonary Embolus

Deep venous thrombosis (DVT) and pulmonary embolus (PE) are potential complications for all immobilized patients. The incidence of DVT in patients with stroke is as high as 47% with an estimated 10% of deaths attributed to PE.[2] The dangers are particularly high during the acute phase when venous stasis from immobility and prolonged bed rest, limb paralysis, hemineglect, and reduced cognitive status significantly elevate the risk. About 50% of cases do not present with clinically detectable symptoms and can be identified only by Doppler duplex ultrasonography (the gold standard for rapid screening), radiocontrast venography, or impedance plethysmography. Patients with symptoms may report calf pain and tenderness, or a tight feeling in the calf. Swelling can vary from minimal to high and typically affects the foot and ankle. Prompt diagnosis and treatment of acute DVT are necessary to reduce the risk of fatal PE. About half of patients at time of diagnosis of DVT have already had a PE. Signs and symptoms of PE include chest pain, tachypnea, tachycardia, anxiety, restlessness, and apprehension together with persistent cough. About 10% to 15% of patients with PE will die. Symptomatic treatment of DVT consists of continuous infusion or subcutaneous injections of low-molecular-weight heparin (LMWH) followed by long-term oral anticoagulants (warfarin [Coumadin]). Bed rest is instituted (up to 24 hours) until anticoagulation from medications takes effect. The patient is then mobilized out of bed and will wear compression stockings. In select cases, surgical removal of the thrombus or placement of intracaval filters is undertaken. Treatment of PE involves supplemental oxygen or intubation in severe cases, anticoagulants, and thrombolytic drugs and, in some cases, surgical intervention. Primary prevention of DVT and PE involves prophylactic administration of anticoagulants, exercising the legs to improve blood flow, early mobilization, and use of elastic support stockings.[25]

Osteoporosis and Fracture Risk

Osteoporosis, a bone disease characterized by a loss of bone mass per unit volume, is common in the elderly and results from decreased physical activity, changes in protein nutrition, hormonal deficiency, and calcium deficiency. Patients with stroke who are immobilized and restricted in weight-bearing demonstrate increased risk of osteoporosis and disuse muscle atrophy. Fall risk is also increased with incidence rates ranging between 23% and 50% for individuals with chronic stroke.[26] Risk of falls in patients with stroke is multifactorial, arising from sensorimotor deficits, impaired balance, confusion, attention deficits, perceptual deficits, visual impairments, behavioral impulsivity, depression, and communication problems.[27-29] Increased risk of fracture, especially vertebral and hip fracture, is the natural outcome of osteoporosis and falls. In patients with stroke, osteoporosis and hip fracture are more likely on the more involved side.[30]

■ MEDICAL DIAGNOSIS OF STROKE

History and Examination

An accurate history profiling the timing of neurological events is obtained from the patient or from family members in the case of the unconscious or noncommunicative patient. Of particular importance are the exact time and pattern of symptom onset. An abrupt onset with worsening symptoms and decreasing level of consciousness is suggestive of cerebral hemorrhage. Severe headache described as "the worst headache of my life" is suggestive of subarachnoid hemorrhage. An embolus also occurs rapidly, with no warning, and is frequently associated with heart disease and/or heart complications. A more variable and uneven onset is typical with thrombosis. The patient's past history, including episodes of TIAs or head trauma, presence of major or minor risk factors, and medications, pertinent family history, and any recent alterations in patient function (either transient or permanent) are thoroughly investigated.[31] Stroke can mimic a number of other conditions that must be ruled out, including seizures, space-occupying lesions (e.g., subdural hematoma, cerebral abscess/infection, tumor), syncope, somatization, and delirium secondary to sepsis.[32]

The physical examination of the patient includes an investigation of vital signs (heart rate, respiratory rate, blood pressure), signs of cardiac decompensation, and function of the cerebral hemispheres, cerebellum, cranial nerves, eyes, and sensorimotor system. The presenting symptoms will help to determine the location of the lesion, and comparison of both sides of the body will reveal the side of the lesion. Bilateral signs are suggestive of brainstem lesions or massive cerebral involvement.[31]

Tests and Measures

The *National Institutes of Health Stroke Scale (NIHSS)* is a valuable screening tool that focuses on initial and serial examination of impairments following acute stroke. The scale includes 11 items and uses a variable ordinal scale. Some items are scored 0–2 or 0–3 (level of consciousness, best gaze, visual fields, facial palsy, limb ataxia, sensory, best language, dysarthria, extinction, and inattention); other items are scored 0–4 (motor arm and motor leg). Specific descriptors are attached to each score. It was designed to be completed in 5 to 8 minutes. (The NIHSS is available at www.ninds.nih.gov/doctors/NIH_Stroke_Scale.pdf.)[33] An examination scoring service for the NIHSS is maintained by the National Stroke Association. The NIHSS has been used to discriminate between stroke subtypes.[34-36]

A number of biomarkers can be used to help identify acute cerebral ischemia. These include inflammatory mediators such as IL-6, matrix metalloproteinase [MMP-9], markers of glial activation, and so forth. Biomarker assays may play an increasing role in the diagnosis of acute stroke as more research becomes available.[32]

A standardized set of blood analyses is performed, including hematological studies, serum electrolyte levels, and renal and hepatic tests. These tests are used to rule out metabolic abnormalities, as well as blood, kidney, or liver conditions.

Cerebrovascular Imaging

Cerebrovascular imaging is the main tool to establish the diagnosis of suspected ischemic stroke and to rule out hemorrhagic stroke and other types of central nervous system (CNS) lesions (e.g., tumor or abscess). Advanced neuroimaging can rapidly identify the occluded artery and estimate the size of the core and the penumbra. It is also used to guide ischemic stroke therapy. Lack of imaging use is high in acute stroke primarily because many patients arrive beyond the strict 3-hour time window.[37]

Computed Tomography

Computed tomography (CT) scan is the most commonly used and readily available neuroimaging technique. CT resolution allows identification of large arteries and veins and venous sinuses. It demonstrates poor sensitivity for detecting small infarcts and infarction in the posterior fossa. Many times CT scans during the acute phase are negative with no clear evidence of abnormalities. However, acute bleeding and hemorrhagic transformation are visible on CT scanning (Fig. 15.5). In the subacute phase, CT scans can delineate the development of cerebral edema (within 3 days), which then fades over the next 2 to 3 weeks. Cerebral infarction (within 3 to 5 days) is visible with the addition of contrast material by showing areas of decreased density. Long-term parenchymal changes consistent with scar formation are also visible on CT. It is important to remember that the extent of CT lesion does not necessarily correlate with clinical signs or changes in function.

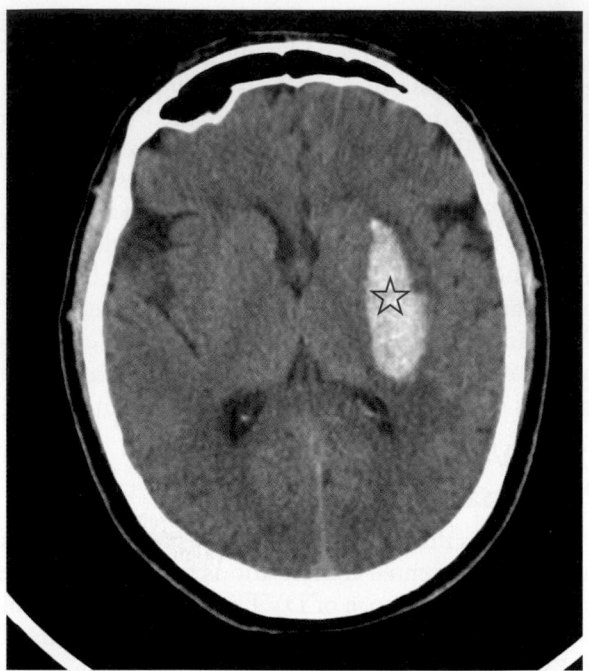

Figure 15.5 CT demonstrating an acute intracerebral hemorrhage (star). *(From Weber, E, Vilensky, J, and Fog, A: Practical Radiology: A Symptom-Based Approach. FA Davis, Philadelphia, 2013, with permission.)*

Magnetic Resonance Imaging

Magnetic resonance imaging (MRI) has evolved to become the first-line imaging in some stroke centers, whereas in other facilities it is used when CT has not provided clear evidence of lesion location. MRI measures nuclear particles as they interact with a powerful magnetic field. MRI, especially diffusion/perfusion MRI, shows greater resolution of the brain and its structural detail than with a CT scan (Fig. 15.6). MRI is more sensitive in the diagnosis of acute strokes, allowing detection of cerebral ischemia as early as 30 minutes after vascular occlusion and infarction within 2 to 6 hours. It is also able to detail the extent of infarction or hemorrhage and can detect smaller lesions than a CT scan. Use of contrast enhancement allows documentation of changes in an infarct over the first 2 to 3 weeks. MRI scans cannot be performed on individuals with certain implantable devices (e.g., pacemakers) or with patients who are claustrophobic.[37]

Magnetic Resonance Angiography

Magnetic resonance angiography (MRA) is a type of magnetic resonance image that uses special software to create an image of the arteries in the brain. It is used to identify vascular abnormalities (e.g., stenosis), and alterations in blood flow as a result of embolus or thrombosis. It provides similar information as classical angiography (x-ray of blood vessels following dye injection) with increased sensitivity of detection and with lowered risks.[37]

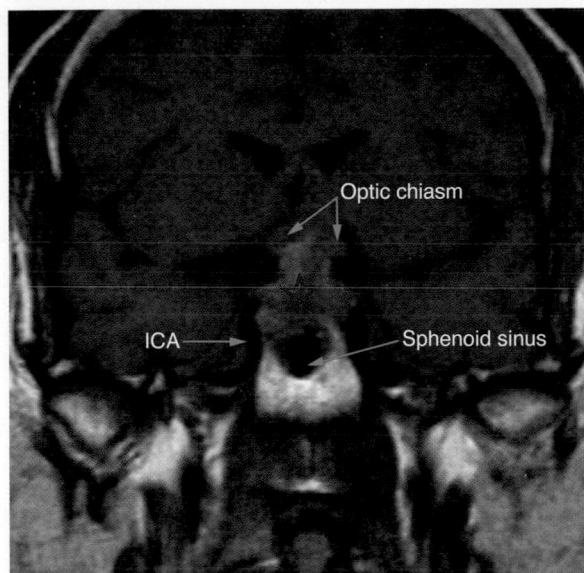

Figure 15.6 Coronal MRI without contrast enhancement on a pregnant patient with headache and visual field defect. The T1 hyperintensity of the greatly enlarged pituitary (star) indicates subacute hemorrhage. ICA = internal carotid artery. *(From Weber, E, Vilensky, J, and Fog, A: Practical Radiology: A Symptom-Based Approach. FA Davis, Philadelphia, 2013, with permission.)*

Doppler Ultrasound

Doppler ultrasound imaging is a noninvasive technique that sends sound waves into the body. Echoes bounce off the moving blood and artery and are formed into an image. Diagnostically, transcranial Doppler is used to examine the posterior circulation of the brain (the vertebrobasilar system). Carotid Doppler is used to examine the carotid arteries and typically precedes carotid endarterectomy. It is also used to examine the peripheral arteries in the diagnosis of PAD.

Arteriography and Digital Subtraction Angiography

Arteriography is an x-ray of the carotid artery with a special dye injected into an artery in the leg or arm. Digital subtraction angiography DSA is also an x-ray of the carotid artery with less dye used. These procedures are considered invasive and carry a small risk of causing a stroke.

■ MEDICAL, PHARMACOLOGICAL, AND NEUROSURGICAL MANAGEMENT OF STROKE

Medical Management

Medical management of completed stroke includes strategies to achieve the following:

- Improve cerebral perfusion by reestablishing circulation and oxygenation and assist in stopping progression of the lesion to limit deficits. Oxygen is delivered via mask or nasal cannula. Patients in a coma may require intubation or assisted ventilation and suctioning.
- Maintain adequate blood pressure. Hypotension or extreme hypertension is treated; antihypertension agents have the added risk of inducing hypotension and decreasing cerebral perfusion.
- Maintain sufficient cardiac output. If the causes of stroke are cardiac in origin, medical management focuses on control of arrhythmias and cardiac decompensation.
- Restore/maintain fluid and electrolyte balance.
- Maintain blood glucose levels within the normal range.
- Control seizures and infections.
- Control edema, intracranial pressure, and herniation using antiedema agents. Ventriculostomy may be indicated to monitor and drain cerebrospinal fluid.
- Maintain bowel and bladder function, which may include urinary catheter. Catheterization is typically short-term but may be long-term with the patient in coma.
- Maintain integrity of skin and joints by instituting protective positioning, a turning schedule every 2 hours, and early physical and occupational therapy.
- Decrease the risk of complications such as DVT, aspiration, decubitus ulcers, and so forth.

Pharmacological Management

Pharmacological interventions for completed stroke and its co-morbidities are summarized in Box 15.2.[38,39]

Neurosurgical Management

Neurosurgical interventions may include the following:[40]

- In hemorrhagic stroke, surgery may be indicated to repair a superficial ruptured aneurysm or AVM, prevent rebleeding, and evacuate a clot (hematoma). Larger, deeper intracranial or brainstem vascular lesions are generally not amenable to surgery. Surgery may also be indicated for resection of a superficial unruptured AVM when there is high risk of rupture and stroke.
- Patients who are not eligible for tPA or who do not respond to tPA may be candidates for surgical intervention using the Merci® Retriever System. This device is threaded via a catheter into a large artery just beyond the site of occlusion. It uses a tiny corkscrew-shaped device that wraps around and traps the clot. The clot is then retrieved and slowly removed from the artery. Blood flow is successfully restored. This system is not effective for smaller arteries and more distant locations.
- The Penumbra System® uses a catheter and separator that is threaded to the site of the clot. It suctions and grabs the clot and aspirates the site. This system can be used effectively within an 8-hour window of symptom onset.

Box 15.2   Medications Commonly Used to Treat Patients with Stroke[38,39]

- **Thrombolytics** (Alteplase [Activase or tPA]): Converts plasminogen to plasmin, degrades fibrin present in clots, dissolves clots and reestablishes blood flow (e.g., lysis of thrombi causing ischemic stroke; also to dissolve clots in coronary arteries, pulmonary emboli, deep vein thrombosis).
  Possible adverse effects: The most common complication is bleeding and brain hemorrhage.

- **Anticoagulants** (e.g., warfarin [Coumadin], heparin, dabigatran etexilate [Pradaxa]): Used to reduce the risk of blood clots and prevent existing clots from getting bigger by thinning the blood; indications include DVT prophylaxis, stroke prevention, peripheral vascular disease. With Coumadin, clotting times are closely monitored. Heparin is given intravenously and is faster acting.
  Possible adverse effects: Increased risk of bleeding and hemorrhage, hematomas.

- **Antiplatelet therapy** (e.g., acetylsalicylic acid [aspirin]; clopidogrel bisulfate [Plavix]; dabigatran etexilate [Pradaxa]; ticlopidine hydrochloride [Ticlid]): Prevent platelets (blood cells) from sticking together; long-term, low-dose is used to decrease the risk of thrombosis and recurrent stroke; higher doses may be used in place of anticoagulants and may be recommended for patients with atrial fibrillation.
  Possible adverse effects: Increased risk of gastric ulcers and bleeding.

- **Antihypertensive agents** (e.g., ACE inhibitors, alpha-blockers [Minipress], beta-blockers, calcium channel blockers, direct vasodilators, diuretics, postganglionic neuron inhibitors): Used to control hypertension.
  Possible adverse effects: Dizziness, hypotension, among other symptoms.

- **Angiotensin II receptor antagonists** (telmisartan [Micardis], losartan potassium [Cozaar]): Block angiotensin II, a chemical that triggers muscle contraction around blood vessels, narrowing them; enlarges blood vessels and reduces blood pressure.
  Possible adverse effects: Dizziness, hypotension, among other symptoms.

- **Anticholesterol agents/statins** (atorvastatin calcium [Lipitor], rosuvastatin calcium [Crestor], Zocor, Mevacor, Lescol): Lower cholesterol by inhibiting the enzyme in the blood that produces cholesterol in the liver; for management of hypercholesterolemia and mixed dyslipidemias.
  Possible adverse effects: Dizziness, headache, insomnia, weakness.

- **Antispasmodics/spasmolytics** (e.g., carisoprodol [Soma], chlorzoaxazone [Parafon Forte], cyclobenzaprine [Flexeril], diazepam [Valiu], methocarbamol [Robaxin], orphenadrine [Norflex/Norgesic]): Used to relax skeletal muscle and decrease muscle spasm.
  Possible adverse effects: May cause drowsiness, dizziness, dry mouth, among other symptoms.

- **Antispastics** (e.g., baclofen [Lioresal], dantrolene sodium [Dantrium], diazepam [Valium], tizanidine [Zanaflex]): Used to relax skeletal muscle and decrease muscle spasm.
  Possible adverse effects: May cause drowsiness, dizziness, confusion, weakness, among other symptoms.

- **Anticonvulsants** (e.g., carbamazepine [Tegretol], clonazepam [Klonopin], diazepam [Valium], phenobarbital [Luminal], phenytoin [Dilantin]): Used to control seizures; act as a generalized CNS depressant.
  Possible adverse effects: May cause drowsiness, ataxia, sedation, among other symptoms.

- **Antidepressants** (e.g., fluoxetine [Prozac], monoamine oxidase inhibitors, sertraline [Zoloft], tricyclics [Amitriptyline]): Used to control depression.
  Possible adverse effects: May cause anxiety, tremor, insomnia, nausea.

- Carotid endarterectomy is a surgical procedure used to remove fatty deposits from the carotid artery. It is a useful procedure to prevent recurrent strokes or the development of stroke in individuals with TIAs. Stenosis of 60% to 99% is the typical guideline used when surgery is considered and can reduce stroke risk by as much as 55%. It cannot be performed with acute stroke because altered pressures could subject ischemic areas to further damage.

■ FRAMEWORK FOR REHABILITATION

Rehabilitation has an important role in reducing disability and promoting independence. In addition, known complications of stroke can be reduced or prevented while quality of life is promoted. Optimal management involves a coordinated interdisciplinary team to oversee a *comprehensive plan of care* (POC). The team of rehabilitation specialists includes the physician, nurse, physical therapist, occupational therapist, speech-language pathologist, and social worker. Additional disciplines may include a neuropsychologist, nutritionist, and recreational therapist or vocational counselor. The patient/client, family, and caregivers are also important members of the team and should be involved in all decision making regarding the POC. Interdisciplinary communication is critical for effective team function and occurs through case conferences, informal interactions, patient care rounds, and patient/client family meetings. Effective case management also includes a coordinated education plan and accurate and effective documentation. It is critical for the team to provide a supportive environment to assist patients and their family members in their adjustment to this life-altering event.

The National Stroke Association has instituted a process to certify stroke rehabilitation specialists. The designation of *clinical stroke rehabilitation specialist (CSRS)* ensures that therapists are expert stroke clinicians through a rigorous set of four-tiered courses culminating in a written examination and nationally recognized credential, the CSRS certification. Additional information can be found at www.stroke.org.

The rehabilitation POC considers the patient's history, course, and symptoms, together with impairments, activity limitations, and participation restrictions. Of equal importance are the patient's abilities (assets), priorities, and resources, including family, home, and community resources. Interventions are *restorative* (aimed at improving impairments, activity limitations, and participation restrictions), *preventive* (aimed at minimizing potential complications and indirect impairments), and *compensatory* (aimed at modifying the task, activity, or environment to improve function). See discussion in Chapter 1, Clinical Decision Making. The overall focus for patients with moderate to severe stroke is on long-range planning, with consideration of anticipated episodes of care that typically include hospital-based care (acute care, inpatient rehabilitation), outpatient rehabilitation, and home/community-based care.

The preferred practice pattern for patients with stroke from the *Guide to Physical Therapist Practice* is 5 D, *Impaired Motor Function and Sensory Integrity Associated with Nonprogressive Disorders of the Central Nervous System—Acquired in Adolescence or Adulthood.*[41, p. 365] In this document the reader will find relevant information on patient/client diagnostic classification; ICD-9-CM codes; examination components; considerations for evaluation, diagnosis, and prognosis; and suggested interventions. Thus, the *Guide to Physical Therapist Practice* serves as a primary resource for physical therapists in designing a comprehensive POC and documenting the services provided and outcomes achieved.

A therapeutic care continuum refers to the complete range of care, services, and/or programs provided for a patient. For patients with stroke, the care continuum is based on two important factors: (1) stage of recovery; and (2) degree of disability resulting from stroke.

Acute Phase

Low-intensity rehabilitation is begun in the acute care facility as soon as the patient is medically stabilized, typically within 72 hours. The patient may be first seen in a neurological intensive care unit (ICU) or specialized stroke care unit in a facility that also provides comprehensive rehabilitation services. Evidence supports the benefits of specialized stroke units in improving functional outcomes when compared to patients not receiving specialized care. Individuals who received this care were more likely to be alive, independent, and living at home 1 year after stroke.[42,43] The therapist needs to be aware of the patient's current status by reviewing the medical record and communicating with the medical team. During acute care, the therapist assists in ongoing monitoring of the patient's recovery and is alert for significant changes in the patient's status (e.g., changes in vital signs [heart rate (HR), blood pressure (BP, or respiratory rate (RR)], drop in O_2 saturation levels, skin changes, alterations in mental status and consciousness, and so forth). Early mobilization prevents or minimizes the harmful effects of bed rest and deconditioning. It may also increase the patient's level of consciousness and foster return to independence. Functional reorganization is promoted through early stimulation and use of the hemiparetic side. *Learned nonuse* of the hemiparetic extremities and maladaptive patterns of movement are minimized. Mental deterioration, depression, and apathy can be reduced through the fostering of a positive outlook toward the rehabilitation process. Interventions include but are not limited to positioning, functional mobility training (e.g., bed mobility, sitting, transfers, locomotion), ADL training, range of motion (ROM), splinting, and positioning.

Instruction, education, and training of patients and their families/caregivers is initiated early regarding current condition (pathophysiology, impairments, activity limitations) and risk factors for disability. It includes an overview of the recovery process, the rehabilitation POC, and expected transitions across care settings. It is important to remember that this is a highly stressful time for patients and families and information needs to be graded in appropriate amounts and repeated and reinforced throughout the course of treatment. The therapist needs to establish effective communication. This includes speaking to the patient in a normal tone and volume, speaking slowly and giving the patient enough time to respond, using simple yes/no questions, and using gesture and tactile cues whenever appropriate. Controlling the environment and reducing distractions will also help to ensure the patient's attention and promote good communication. The therapist also needs to be aware of the presence of visual field defect (homonymous hemianopsia) and perceptual changes (unilateral neglect) that will influence choice of position when interacting with the patient. The therapist needs to be sensitive to the devastating nature of these changes for both the patient and family members and work to help empower patients and their families to begin the recovery process. They need to understand that the therapist will work together with them as a team.

Current trends are toward shorter acute care hospital stays (average stay is about 5 days).[1] However, early discharge has resulted in an increase in the number of serious medical complications seen during subacute rehabilitation or at home. These complications may result in delays during active rehabilitation and, for some, temporary cessation of therapy or transfer back to the acute hospital until medical complications are resolved. Therapists need to be vigilant in monitoring patients for potential risk of complications and medical emergencies (e.g., cardiac arrhythmias, DVT, uncontrolled BP, recurrent stroke, and so forth).

Subacute Phase

Patients with moderate or severe residual impairments or activity limitations may benefit from intensive inpatient rehabilitation provided in a freestanding rehabilitation facility or in a rehabilitation unit within the acute care hospital. Rehabilitation programs certified by the Commission on Accreditation of Rehabilitation Facilities (CARF) and the Joint Commission on Accreditation of Healthcare Organizations (JCAHO) can be expected to adhere to uniform standards and provide high-quality care.[2] Evidence supports the value of physical therapy in producing improved functional outcomes for patients with stroke.[43-52] Patients are referred to inpatient rehabilitation if they can tolerate an intensity of services consisting of two or more rehabilitation disciplines, 6 days a week for a minimum of 3 hours of active rehabilitation per day. If the patient requires less intensive services, transfer to a transitional care unit (TCU) within a skilled nursing facility is instituted. Here rehabilitation services are less intense, ranging from 60 to 90 minutes of therapy services 5 days per week.[2]

The timing of rehabilitation services is an important factor in predicting outcome. In general, a shorter onset-to-admission interval, within the first 20 days, has been shown to significantly improve functional outcomes when compared to longer intervals.[53] Additional factors that influence the timing of rehabilitation efforts include medical stability, severity of cognitive-perceptual deficits, motivation, patient endurance, and recovery. In an era of time-limited payment for comprehensive rehabilitation services, selecting the optimal time for rehabilitation services may prevent unnecessary patient failures and improve long-term functional outcomes.

Chronic Phase

Rehabilitation services during the chronic phase, generally defined to be more than 6 months post-stroke, are typically delivered in an outpatient rehabilitation facility, in a community setting, or at home. Outpatient services are prescribed for the patient who is discharged from inpatient rehabilitation, is in need of continuing rehabilitation, and can enter and exit the home with ease. Many of the interventions begun during inpatient rehabilitation are continued and progressed in order to sustain the gains made and improve functional performance.[44,46,48-52] Other interventions, including constraint-induced movement therapy (CIMT),[45] bilateral training,[47] virtual reality training,[53] and electromechanical-assisted walking,[54] may be implemented. Some patients with mild involvement who did not require intense inpatient rehabilitation also benefit from outpatient rehabilitation services. A complete record of past medical and rehabilitation services should be made available to these agencies. The intensity of services provided varies but is generally less than that of inpatient rehabilitation (e.g., 60 to 90 minutes per visit, two to three times per week). Outpatient intervention programs that target progressive improvements in flexibility, strength, balance, locomotion, endurance, and UE function have been shown to be effective in producing meaningful outcomes.[55] The patient and family are instructed in a home exercise program (HEP) and educated about the importance of maintaining exercise levels, health promotion, fall prevention, and safety.

The patient may receive home care rehabilitation services, typically for the patient who is unable to exit the home independently. The challenges of being home can impose additional daily stresses for the patient and family. Difficulties should be addressed promptly as they arise. The therapist needs to emphasize the development of problem solving skills to ensure successful adaptation to variable home and community environments. Fall risk factors should be eliminated or minimized as appropriate or possible. Examination of the environment and recommendations for modification of the environment are important parts of the preparation for return to home (see Chapter 9, Examination of the Environment).

Finally, the patient should be assisted in resuming participation in community and recreational activities. With increasing activity levels, it is important to monitor the patient's endurance levels carefully and provide instruction in activity pacing and energy conservation techniques as needed. Community fitness programs[51] and water-based activities[56] have been shown to improve function after stroke. A small number of stroke survivors can be evaluated and assisted in return to work. As the patient becomes successful in the home and community environments, services should be gradually phased out. Follow-up visits at periodic intervals are recommended to identify problems as they develop and to ensure long-term maintenance of function.

Note: Although there is a large body of research on the efficacy of stroke rehabilitation and more than 10 Cochrane Systematic Reviews,[43-56] the Cochrane researchers conclude that further high-quality research (i.e., randomized controlled trials) is needed to determine the most effective interventions. Additional research is also needed to investigate the effect of rehabilitation interventions on quality of life, participation, and overall cost-benefit ratios, and the differential effects of stroke severity, latency, and age.

■ EXAMINATION

The three basic components of a comprehensive physical therapy examination include patient/client history, systems review, and tests and measures. The selection of examination procedures will vary based on a number of factors including patient's age, location and severity of stroke, stage of recovery, data from initial screenings, phase of rehabilitation, and home/community/work situation, as well as other factors.

The purposes of the examination are to

- Determine the diagnosis and classification within a specific practice pattern.
- Monitor recovery from stroke.
- Identify patients who are most likely to benefit from rehabilitation services and the most appropriate choice of a care setting.
- Develop a specific POC, including anticipated goals, expected outcomes, prognosis, and interventions.
- Monitor progress toward projected goals and outcomes through periodic reevaluation.
- Determine if referral to another practitioner is indicated.
- Plan for discharge.

The comprehensive examination provides the main source of information for clinical decision making. Examination findings should be coordinated with those of the rehabilitation team in order to arrive at an integrated POC. Box 15.3 presents Elements of the Examination of the Patient with Stroke[41] and possible impairments. Many of these examination procedures, tests, and measures are discussed in earlier chapters (see Chapters 2 through 9). This section discusses relevant aspects of the examination, including tests and measures and diagnosis-specific instruments developed for the patient with stroke. The therapist must differentiate between those impairments that are a direct consequence of the stroke and those that are indirect or secondary, resulting from sequelae or complications that originate from other systems. Aspects of functional performance, including activity limitations and restrictions in participation, are equally important to ascertain.

Data obtained through interview with the patient/family and review of the medical record should include information on general demographics, medical/surgical history, social and employment history, family history, living environment, general health status

and risk factors, and social and health habits. Coexisting health problems and medications should also be identified. The older patient with stroke typically has a history of a number of cardiovascular and other co-morbidities. Data obtained from the history will help further focus the systems review and in-depth examination.

Cranial Nerve Integrity

The therapist should examine for facial sensation (CN V), facial movements (CNs V and VII), and labyrinthine/auditory function (CN VIII). The presence of swallowing difficulties and drooling necessitates an examination of the motor nuclei of the lower brainstem cranial nerves (CNs IX, X, and XII) affecting the muscles of the face, tongue, larynx, and pharynx. This includes determination of motor function of the lips, mouth, tongue, palate, pharynx, and larynx. The gag reflex should be examined because hypoactivity may lead to aspiration into the airway. Adequacy of cough mechanisms should also be carefully examined. The therapist needs to be able to recognize the presence of swallowing difficulties and initiate prompt referral.

The visual system should be carefully investigated, including tests for visual field defects (CN II, optic radiation, visual cortex), acuity (CN II), pupillary reflexes (CNs II and III), and extraocular movements (CNs III, IV, and VI). Ocular motility disturbances may be present with brainstem strokes, such as diplopia, oscillopsia, visual distortions, or paralysis of conjugate gaze. Visual field defects (homonymous hemianopsia) need to be differentiated from visual neglect, a perceptual deficit characterized by an inattention to or neglect of visual stimuli presented on the involved side. The patient with pure hemianopsia is typically aware of the deficit and may spontaneously compensate by moving the eyes or head toward the side of deficit; the patient with visual neglect will be unaware (inattentive) of the deficit (see Chapter 29). The use of prescriptive eyeglasses should be determined before any testing; the therapist should ensure that eyeglasses are worn and clean.

Sensation

Deficits in somatic sensations (touch, temperature, pain, and proprioception) are common after stroke. The type and extent of impairment are related to the location and size of the vascular lesion. Specific localized areas of dysfunction are common with cortical lesions, whereas diffuse involvement throughout one side of the body suggests deeper lesions involving the thalamus and adjacent structures. Impairment in touch sensation (64% to 94%), proprioception (17% to 52%), vibration (44%), and loss of pinprick sensation (35% to 71%) have been reported.[57-59]

Box 15.3 Elements of the Examination of the Patient with Stroke[41]

Patient/Client History

- Age, sex, race/ethnicity, primary langu.age, education
- Social history: cultural beliefs and behaviors, family and caregiver resources, social support systems
- Occupation/employment/work
- Living environment: home/work barriers
- Hand dominance
- General health status: physical, psychological, social, and role function, health habits
- Family history
- Medical/surgical history
- Current conditions/chief complaints
- Medications
- Medical/laboratory test results
- Functional activity level: premorbid

Systems Review

- Neuromuscular
- Musculoskeletal
- Cardiovascular/pulmonary
- Integumentary

Tests and Measures/Impairments

Tests and measures are selected based on their ability to quantify or describe each of the following:

- Level of consciousness, arousal, attention, and cognition: mental status, insight, motivation
  Primary impairments: impaired alertness and attention, perseveration, confabulation, confusion, disorientation, distractibility, memory deficits, impaired judgment
- Emotional status
  Primary impairments: depression, pseudobulbar affect, apathy, euphoria
- Behavioral style
  Primary impairments: impulsive or cautious behavioral styles; frustration, irritability
- Communication and language: coordinate efforts with the speech-language pathologist
  Primary impairments: fluent, nonfluent, or global aphasia, dysarthria
- Circulation; cardiovascular signs and symptoms
  Common co-morbidities: hypertension, CAD, CHF, diabetes, DVT
- Ventilation and respiration/gas exchange: pulmonary signs and symptoms
  Common co-morbidities: chronic pulmonary disease
- Anthropometric characteristics: body mass index, girth, length
  Secondary impairments: edema, common in hand and foot
- Integumentary integrity: skin condition, pressure-sensitive areas; effectiveness of protective pressure-relieving devices
  Secondary impairments: altered skin integrity, decubitus ulcers
- Pain: intensity and location
  Primary impairments: central post-stroke pain
  Secondary impairments: hemiplegic shoulder and/or hand pain

- Cranial and peripheral nerve integrity.
  Primary impairments: dysphagia
- Sensory integrity and integration
  Primary impairments: homonymous hemianopsia, tactile/proprioceptive/kinesthetic losses, astereognosis
- Perceptual function: coordinate efforts with occupational therapist
  Primary impairments: spatial relations syndrome, body scheme/body image disorders, unilateral neglect, agnosia, topographical disorientation
- Joint integrity, alignment, and mobility: ROM (active and passive); muscle length and soft tissue extensibility
  Secondary impairments: altered biomechanical alignment; loss of joint ROM, muscle and soft tissue length
- Posture: alignment and position, symmetry (static and dynamic, sitting and standing); ergonomics and body mechanics
  Secondary impairment: altered biomechanical alignment
- Motor function: motor control and motor learning
  Primary impairments:
  Altered reflex integrity: hyperreflexia, tonic reflexes, associated reactions
  Abnormal tone: flaccidity initially; spasticity: spastic posturing
  Abnormal (obligatory) synergies: flexion and extension synergy patterns
  Altered voluntary movement patterns: altered initiation, sequencing, timing of muscle contractions; altered force production
  Coordination, dexterity, agility: coordination deficits
  Motor planning: ideomotor or ideational apraxia
- Muscle performance: strength, power, and endurance
  Primary impairments: paralysis or weakness; fatigue
  Secondary impairments: disuse atrophy
- Postural control and balance: sensorimotor integration, balance strategies (static and dynamic); safety
  Primary impairments: altered balance, increased fall risk
- Gait and locomotion: gait pattern and speed, use of assistive devices/orthotic devices, safety
  Primary impairments: altered sequencing, timing, balance, endurance
- Wheelchair management and mobility: safety and endurance
- Aerobic capacity and endurance: functional activity testing, graded exercise testing
  Secondary impairments: decreased endurance
- Orthotic, protective and supportive devices: fit, alignment, function, use, safety
- Functional status and activity level: performance-based examination of functional skills (FIM level), basic and instrumental ADL; functional mobility skills; home management skills; assistive or adaptive devices: fit, alignment, function, use; safety
  Primary impairments: loss of independent function
- Work, community, and leisure activities: ability to assume/resume activities, safety

Sensory loss has also been reported in the ipsilateral, less affected limbs though to a lesser extent (12% to 25%). Symptoms of crossed anesthesia (ipsilateral facial impairments with contralateral trunk and limb involvement) typify brainstem lesions. Disturbances in cortical sensory modalities (two-point discrimination, stereognosis, kinesthesia, graphesthesia) are also found.[60,61] Profound sensory impairments will negatively affect motor performance, motor learning, and rehabilitation outcomes and contribute to unilateral neglect and *learned nonuse* of limbs. Sensory impairment is also associated with pressure sores, abrasions, and shoulder pain and subluxation.

Central post-stroke pain (CPSP) is defined as pain arising as a direct consequence of a lesion or disease affecting the central somatosensory system and occurs in about 10% of strokes.[62] It can result from lesions at any level of the somatosensory pathways including the medulla, thalamus, and cortex. The thalamus is thought to play an important part in the underlying pathophysiology of central pain. CPSP can be severe and persistent (described as "burning," "aching"), spontaneous and intermittent (described as "lacerating" or "shooting" pain), or evoked by mechanical (stroking the skin, pressure) or thermal (heat or cold) stimuli. Symptoms may be focal, affecting the hand/arm or foot/leg, or in severe cases affect half the body. Development of pain is typically within the first few months after stroke though onset may be delayed for many months. Spontaneous recovery is rare and chronic suffering common. The debilitating nature of CPSP frequently limits participation in rehabilitation programs and outcomes.[63]

A sensory examination should include testing of superficial sensations (e.g., touch, pressure, sharp or dull discrimination, temperature) and deep sensations (proprioception, kinesthesia, vibration). Combined (cortical) sensations such as stereognosis, tactile localization, two-point discrimination, and texture recognition should also be examined once the integrity of the superficial sensations of touch and pressure is established. Sensory testing procedures are described in detail in Chapter 3, Examination of Sensory Function. The quality of sensory impairments experienced can range from mild altered perception to marked changes in sensory thresholds, delayed perceptions, uncertainty of responses, altered time for sensory adaptation, and sensory persistence.[57] Impairments may be evident in one sensory modality and not in others. Differences can also be expected between upper and lower hemiplegic extremities, depending on lesion location. Comparisons with the intact side should be viewed with caution because impairments may exist in the supposedly "normal" extremities due to aging and co-morbidities. Sensory testing may be difficult or need to be deferred owing to cognitive or communication deficits.

Flexibility and Joint Integrity

An examination of joint flexibility should include passive ROM using a goniometer, joint hypermobility/hypomobility, and soft-tissue changes (swelling, inflammation, or restriction). The shoulder and wrist should be examined closely because joint malalignment problems are common. Edema of the wrist often produces malaligned carpal bones with resulting impingement during wrist extension. Problems with spasticity may result in inconsistent ROM findings, because fluctuations in tone may occur from one testing session to the next. Thus, tonal abnormalities should be noted at the time of examination. Active ROM (AROM) may be limited or impossible for the patient in early or middle recovery in the presence of paresis, spasticity, or obligatory synergies that can preclude isolated voluntary movements. ROM limitations and developing contractures should be carefully documented.

Contractures can develop anywhere but are particularly apparent in the paretic limbs. As contractures progress, edema and pain may develop and further restrict mobility. In the UE, limitations in the shoulder motions of flexion, abduction, and external rotation are common. Contractures are likely in the elbow flexors, wrist and finger flexors, and forearm pronators. In the LE, plantarflexion contractures are common.

Motor Function

Stages of Motor Recovery

Initially, flaccid paralysis is present (*stage 1*). This is replaced by the development of spasticity, hyperreflexia, and mass patterns of movement, termed **obligatory synergies**, all characteristics of upper motor neuron syndrome. Muscles involved in obligatory synergy patterns are strongly linked in a highly stereotyped, abnormal pattern; isolated joint movements outside the obligatory pattern are not possible. During *stage 2* (early synergy), facilitatory stimuli will elicit synergies with minimal voluntary movement. As recovery progresses, spasticity is marked with full strong obligatory synergies (*stage 3*). Synergy influence begins to decline in *stage 4* as some isolated out-of-synergy joint movements emerge. During *stage 5*, relative independence of synergy, spasticity continues to wane and isolated joint movements become more apparent, and during *stage 6* patterns of movement are near normal. This general pattern of recovery was initially described by Twitchell[64] and Brunnstrom[65,66] and confirmed by additional investigators[67,68] (Box 15.4). Several important points merit consideration. An overall pattern of motor recovery exists though individual recovery is highly variable. Some patients experience mild involvement with early full recovery whereas other patients demonstrate severe involvement with incomplete recovery.

Box 15.4	Sequential Motor Recovery Stages Following Stroke
STAGE 1	Recovery from hemiplegia occurs in a stereotyped sequence of events that begins with a period of *flaccidity* immediately following the acute episode. *No movement of the limbs* can be elicited.
STAGE 2	As recovery begins, the basic limb synergies or some of their components may appear as associated reactions, or *minimal voluntary movement* responses may be present. At this time, spasticity begins to develop.
STAGE 3	Thereafter, the patient gains *voluntary control of the movement synergies,* although full range of all synergy components does not necessarily develop. Spasticity has further increased and may become severe.
STAGE 4	Some *movement combinations that do not follow the paths of either synergy are mastered,* first with difficulty, then with more ease, and *spasticity begins to decline.*
STAGE 5	If progress continues, more *difficult movement combinations are learned* as the basic limb synergies lose their dominance over motor acts.
STAGE 6	With the *disappearance of spasticity, individual joint movements become possible and coordination* approaches normal. From here on, as the last recovery step, normal motor function is restored, but this last stage is not achieved by all, for the recovery process can plateau at any stage.

From Brunnstrom, S: Movement Therapy in Hemiplegia. Harper & Row, New York, 1970, with permission.

The degree of recovery depends on a number of factors, including lesion location and severity and capacity for adaptation through training. Finally, recovery differs within patients. For example, the UE may be more involved and demonstrate less complete recovery than the LE as is seen in MCA syndrome. For examination of recovery stages, see discussion of the *Fugl-Meyer Assessment of Physical Performance* later in this section and Appendix 15.A.

Tone

Flaccidity (hypotonicity) is present immediately after stroke and is due primarily to the effects of cerebral shock. It is generally short-lived, lasting a few days or weeks. Flaccidity may persist in a small number of patients with lesions restricted to the primary motor cortex or cerebellum. **Spasticity** (hypertonicity) emerges in about 90% of cases and occurs on the side of the body opposite the lesion. Spasticity in upper motor neuron syndrome occurs predominantly in antigravity muscles (see Chapter 5, Table 5.3). In the patient with stroke, UE spasticity is frequently strong in scapular retractors; shoulder adductors, depressors, and internal rotators; elbow flexors and forearm pronators; and wrist and finger flexors. In the neck and trunk, spasticity may cause increased lateral flexion to the hemiplegic side. In the LE, spasticity is often strong in the pelvic retractors, hip adductors and internal rotators, hip and knee extensors, plantarflexors and supinators, and toe flexors. Spasticity results in tight (stiff) muscles that restrict volitional movement. Posturing of the limbs (e.g., a tightly fisted hand with the elbow flexed and held tightly against the chest or a stiff extended knee with a plantarflexed foot) is common with moderate to severe spasticity. Spastic posturing can lead to development of painful spasms (similar to muscle cramping), degenerative changes, and fixed contractures. The automatic adjustment of postural muscles that occurs normally in preparation for and during a movement task is also impaired. Thus, patients with stroke may lack the ability to adjust and stabilize proximal limbs and trunk appropriately during movement, with resulting postural abnormalities, balance impairments, and increased risk for falls.

An examination of tone is essential. Passive motion testing can be used to determine the presence of hypotonicity or spasticity. Severity of spasticity can be graded on the basis of resistance to passive stretch using the *Modified Ashworth Scale (MAS)* (see Chapter 5, Table 5.4). The position of the affected limbs at rest (resting postures) and during voluntary movements should be observed for tonal influences.

Reflexes

Reflexes are altered and also vary according to the stage of recovery. Initially, stroke results in hyporeflexia with flaccidity. When spasticity and synergies emerge, hyperreflexia is seen. Deep tendon reflexes are hyperactive and patients may demonstrate clonus, clasp-knife response, and a positive Babinski, all consistent findings of upper motor neuron syndrome (see Chapter 5, Table 5.5).

Tonic reflexes may appear in a readily identifiable form similar to that seen in other types of neurological insult (e.g., traumatic brain injury [TBI], cerebral palsy [CP]). Thus, movement of the head or position of the body may elicit an obligatory change in resting tone or movement of the extremities. The most commonly seen is the asymmetrical tonic neck reflex (ATNR) in which head rotation causes elbow extension of the UE on the jaw side with elbow flexion of the opposite skull limb (see Chapter 5, Table 5.7).

Associated reactions are also typically present in patients with stroke who exhibit strong spasticity and obligatory synergies. These consist of unintentional movements of the hemiparetic limb caused by voluntary action of another limb or by other stimuli such as yawning, sneezing, or coughing. For example, the patient vigorously contracts the elbow flexors of the stronger UE; the hemiparetic elbow also flexes. Or the patient flexes the hip to lift the hemiparetic LE in sitting; the hemiparetic UE also flexes. Associated reactions can limit functional performance, especially in the UE. An examination of stretch reflexes and pathological reflexes (e.g., Babinski, tonic reflex activity, associated reactions) should be performed (see Chapter 5, Table 5.7).

Voluntary Movements

Abnormal and highly stereotyped obligatory synergies emerge with spasticity following stroke. Thus, the patient is unable to perform an isolated movement of a single limb segment without producing movements in the remainder of the limb. For example, efforts to flex the elbow also result in shoulder flexion, abduction, and external rotation. The patient is severely limited in the ability to adapt movements to varying task or environmental demands. Obligatory synergies can appear reflexively during very early recovery, or as voluntary movements. As recovery progresses they become stronger and are linked to the presence and severity of spasticity. Two distinct abnormal synergy patterns have been described for each extremity: a flexion synergy and an extension synergy (Table 15.6). An inspection of the synergy components reveals that certain muscles are not usually involved in either the flexion or extension synergy. These muscles include the (1) latissimus dorsi, (2) teres major, (3) serratus anterior, (4) finger extensors, and (5) ankle evertors. These muscles, therefore, are generally difficult to activate while the patient is exhibiting these patterns. Obligatory synergies are often incompatible with normal ADL and functional mobility skills. For example, the patient with a strong LE extensor synergy

will have difficulty walking owing to foot plantarflexion and inversion with hip and knee extension and adduction (scissoring gait pattern). As recovery progresses, spasticity and obligatory synergies begin to disappear and more normal synergies with isolated joint control become possible.

Voluntary movement patterns should be examined for synergy influence. The therapist bases the examination of synergy dominance on knowledge of the typical components of the synergies. It is possible for one limb to vary significantly from the other (e.g., the UE may demonstrate more synergistic dominance than the LE). Synergistic dominance versus isolated joint control may also vary within a limb (e.g., the shoulder may demonstrate more isolated control than the wrist and hand). During later recovery, voluntary movements demonstrate isolated joint control and appear more normal in the absence of spasticity and synergy restrictions. See discussion of the *Fugl-Meyer Assessment of Physical Performance* later in this section.

Coordination

Proprioceptive losses can result in sensory ataxia. Strokes affecting the cerebellum typically produce cerebellar ataxia (e.g., lateral medullary syndrome, basilar artery syndrome, pontine syndromes) and motor weakness. The resulting problems with timing and sequencing of muscles can significantly impair function and limit adaptability to changing task and environmental demands. Basal ganglia involvement (posterior cerebral artery syndrome) may lead to slowed movements (bradykinesia) or involuntary movements (choreoathetosis, hemiballismus).

Coordination tests can be used to examine control. The therapist focuses on elements of speed/rate control, steadiness, response orientation, and reaction and movement times. Fine motor control and dexterity should be examined using writing, dressing, and feeding tasks (see Chapter 6, Examination of Coordination and Balance). Although more significant impairments can be

Table 15.6	Obligatory Synergy Patterns Following Stroke	
	Flexion Synergy Components	Extension Synergy Components
Upper extremity	Scapular retraction/elevation or hyperextension Shoulder abduction, external rotation Elbow flexion* Forearm supination Wrist and finger Flexion	Scapular protraction Shoulder adduction,* internal rotation Elbow extension Forearm pronation* Wrist and finger flexion
Lower extremity	Hip flexion,* abduction, external rotation Knee flexion Ankle dorsiflexion, inversion Toe dorsiflexion	Hip extension, adduction,* internal rotation Knee extension* Ankle plantarflexion,* inversion Toe plantarflexion

*Generally the strongest components.

expected on the hemiparetic side, it is important to remember that subtle deficits can occur on the less involved side. Thus, it is important to examine both unilateral and bilateral movements, including symmetrical, asymmetrical, and unrelated movements. Performance may vary as the patient moves from supine to sitting to standing positions with the resultant increased postural demands and greater degrees of freedom.

Motor Programming

Motor praxis is the ability to plan and execute coordinated movement. Lesions of the premotor frontal cortex of either hemisphere, left inferior parietal lobe, and corpus callosum can produce **apraxia**. Apraxia is more evident with left hemisphere damage than right and is commonly seen with aphasia. The patient demonstrates difficulty planning and executing purposeful movements that cannot be accounted for by any other reason (i.e., impaired strength, coordination, sensation, tone, cognitive function, communication, or uncooperativeness). There are two main types of apraxia. **Ideational apraxia** is an inability of the patient to produce movement either on command or automatically and represents a complete breakdown in the conceptualization of the task. The patient has no idea how to do the movement and thus cannot formulate the required motor programs. With **ideomotor apraxia** the patient is unable to produce a movement on command but is able to move automatically. Thus, the patient can perform habitual tasks when not commanded to do so and often perseverates, repeating the activity over and over. Significant information on apraxia will be gained by close collaboration with the occupational therapist. The reader is referred to Chapter 27 for a more complete discussion of these deficits and their management.

Muscle Strength

Paresis is found in 80% to 90% of all patients after stroke and is a major factor in impaired motor function, activity limitation, and disability. Patients are unable to generate the force necessary for initiating and controlling movement. The degree of primary weakness is related to the location and size of the brain injury and varies from a complete inability to achieve any contraction (**hemiplegia**) to **hemiparesis** with measurable impairments in force production.[69] Deficits on the contralateral side typically include hemiparesis (opposite UE and LE). Owing to the high incidence of MCA strokes, the UE is frequently more affected than the LE. About 20% of individuals with MCA strokes fail to regain any functional use of the affected UE. Typically, distal muscles exhibit greater strength deficits than proximal. This can be explained by the greater facilitation of distal muscles than proximal by the corticospinal system. Mild weakness also occurs on the ipsilateral, "supposedly normal" side.[70,71] This can be explained by the fact that only 75% to 90%

of the corticospinal fibers cross in the medulla to the contralateral side. The remainder are transmitted to the spinal cord ipsilaterally in the anterior or ventral corticospinal tract. Once in the spinal cord some of these fibers cross while the rest remain uncrossed, thereby explaining bilateral weakness.[72] The amount of weakness experienced by the patient may also vary according to the extent and level of inactivity (disuse atrophy) and the specific functional tasks attempted. Thus, a patient may appear stronger in some tasks than others.[73]

Post-stroke weakness is associated with a number of changes in both the muscle and the motor unit. Changes occur in muscle composition, including atrophy of muscle fibers. There is a selective loss of type II fast-twitch fibers with subsequent increase in the percentage of type I fibers (a finding also reported in the elderly). This selective loss of type II fibers results in slowed force production, difficulty with initiation and production of rapid, high-force movements, and rapid onset of fatigue.[60,73-75] The number of functioning motor units and discharge firing rates also decrease. This is explained by the presence of transsynaptic degeneration of alpha motor neurons that occurs with loss of corticospinal innervation. Abnormal recruitment of motor units with altered timing occurs.[76-78] Thus, patients demonstrate inefficient patterns of muscle activation and higher levels of co-contraction. This opposing muscle activation can contribute to muscle weakness and incoordination. These impairments in force production and coordination have been reported in both paretic and less affected UEs after stroke.[79,80] Patients demonstrate increased effort and fatigability with frequent complaints of feelings of weakness. Denervation potentials on electromyography (EMG) are common, also the result of denervation changes in the corticospinal tracts. Overall reaction times are increased, a finding also reported in the less affected extremities and for the elderly in general. Movement times are prolonged, a timing abnormality that contributes to impairment of coordinated motor sequences.

Although an examination of strength is necessary, the traditional manual muscle test (MMT) poses problems of validity in the presence of strong spasticity, reflex, and synergy dominance. The patient who is not able to isolate specific movements should not be examined using MMT. In this situation, an estimation of strength can be made from observation of active movements during functional activities (functional strength testing). The patient's self-report can also yield important indicators of weakness and fatigue. The patient in later recovery with improving motor control and isolated movement can be examined using traditional MMT or handheld dynamometry. Use of a computerized isokinetic dynamometer can reveal important objective data regarding forces generated, peak torque, time to peak torque, and total work normalized to body weight. See Chapter 4, Musculoskeletal Examination.

Postural Control and Balance

Postural control and balance are disturbed following stroke with impairments in alignment, stability, symmetry, and dynamic balance common. Common postural alignment deviations following stroke are presented in Table 15.7.

Balance impairments may exist when reacting to a destabilizing external force (*reactive postural control*) and/or during self-initiated movements (*proactive or anticipatory postural control*). Thus, the patient may be unable to maintain stable balance in sitting or standing or to move in the posture without loss of balance. Disruptions of central sensorimotor processing contribute to an inability to recruit effective postural strategies and adapt postural movements to changing task and environmental demands. Patients with stroke typically demonstrate uneven weight distribution and increased postural sway in standing (a finding characteristic of the elderly in general). Delays in the onset of motor activity, abnormal timing and sequencing of muscle activity, and abnormal co-contraction result in disorganization of normal postural synergies. For example, proximal muscles are typically activated in advance of distal muscles or, in some patients, very late (a finding also found in many elderly). Compensatory responses typically include excessive hip and knee movements. Corrective responses to perturbations or destabilizing forces are inadequate and result in loss of balance and frequent falls. Patients with hemiplegia typically fall in the direction of weakness.[80-85]

Static and dynamic balance control should be examined in sitting and standing. The patient's ability to maintain a stable position (steadiness) and position (symmetry) within the base of support (BOS) is determined. Dynamic stability control can be examined by having the patient move within a given posture (weight shift) or reach within his or her limits of stability (LOS). The patient should be encouraged to shift weight in all directions, especially to the more involved side where greater impairments are expected. Functional tasks that utilize moving from one posture to another (e.g., supine-to-sit, sit-to-stand) can also be used to examine dynamic postural control.[86]

Performance-based tests can be used to examine postural control and balance following stroke. These tests have been examined for reliability and/or validity and are reviewed in Chapter 6.

- The *Berg Balance Scale (BBS)*
- The *Performance-Oriented Mobility Assessment (POMA, Tinetti)*
- The *Functional Reach Test (RT)* and the *Multidirectional Reach Test (MDRT)*
- The *Timed Up and Go Test (TUG)*
- The *Clinical Test for Sensory Interaction in Balance (CTSIB)*

Stroke-specific tests of postural control and balance include the following:

- The *Postural Assessment Scale for Stroke Patients (PASS)* was developed to examine the postural abilities of patients with acute stroke. It includes 12 items that examine sitting and standing without support, standing on the paretic LE, and changing posture

Table 15.7	Common Postural Alignment Deviations Associated with Stroke
Body Segment	**Postural Alignment Deviations**
Pelvis	• Asymmetrical weight-bearing with majority of weight borne on the stronger side • Reluctance (fear) of shifting weight toward the more affected side • In sitting, posterior pelvic tilt (sacral sitting) • In standing, unilateral retraction and elevation on the more affected side
Trunk	• With sacral sitting, a flattened lumbar curve with exaggerated thoracic curve and forward head • Lateral flexion with trunk shortening on more affected side
Shoulders	• Unequal height with more affected shoulder depressed • Humeral subluxation with scapular downward rotation and lateral flexion of trunk • Scapular instability (winging) may be present
Head/Neck	• Protraction with lateral trunk flexion • Lateral flexion of the head with rotation away from the more affected side
Upper Extremities	• More affected UE typically held in a flexed, adducted position, with internal rotation and elbow flexion, forearm pronation, wrist and finger flexion; limb is non–weight-bearing • Stronger UE used for postural support
Lower Extremities	• In sitting: more affected LE typically held in hip abduction and external rotation with hip and knee flexion (flexion synergy pattern) • In standing: more affected LE typically held in hip and knee extension with adduction and internal rotation (scissoring pattern); ankle plantar flexion • Unequal weight bearing on feet, similar to pelvis in sitting

(supine–to–affected side, supine–to–unaffected side, supine-to-sitting, sitting-to-standing, and standing picking a pencil off the floor). It is scored using an ordinal scale with descriptors ranging from cannot perform to perform with little help, to perform without help. It demonstrates good construct validity and high interrater and intrarater reliability (0.88 and 0.72, respectively).[87]

- The *Trunk Impairment Scale* was developed to evaluate motor impairment of the trunk after stroke. It includes 3 items of static control, 10 items of dynamic balance control, and 4 items of coordination. The items are tested in the sitting position (edge of bed or treatment table) without back or arm support. Each item is performed three times with the highest score accepted. Scores range from a minimum of 0 (unable) to a maximum of 23.[88]

- The *Function in Sitting Test (FIST)* was developed by expert consensus as a test for sitting balance deficits in adults after acute stroke. It includes 14 items that examine static and dynamic balance function. Static sitting (steady state) is examined by having the patient sit with eyes open and eyes closed. Reactive challenges are introduced using sternal nudges (anterior, posterior, and lateral). Dynamic, anticipatory (proactive) challenges are introduced using body segment motions (head turns, lifting foot up on the least involved side, turning and picking an object up placed behind the patient, forward and lateral reach, picking an object up off the floor), and scooting movements (posterior, anterior, lateral). Eleven items examine anterior/posterior control and three items examine lateral/rotational control. Scoring is based on a 5-point ordinal scale that includes the following: No Balance (0/4), Poor (1/4), Fair (2/4), Good (3/4) to Normal (4/4). Specific descriptive criteria are given for each grade for static and dynamic control. Maximum score is 56 (similar to the BBS). Initial reliability and validity of the FIST has been demonstrated; however, additional testing is indicated.[89]

Ipsilateral Pushing

Ipsilateral pushing (also known as *pusher syndrome or contraversive pushing*) is an unusual motor behavior characterized by active pushing with the stronger extremities toward the hemiparetic side with a lateral postural imbalance.[90] The end result is a tendency to fall toward the hemiparetic side. Ipsilateral pushing occurs in about 10% of patients with acute stroke and results from stroke affecting the posterolateral thalamus.[91,92] The result is an altered perception of the body's orientation in relation to gravity. Karnath et al[90] found that patients experienced a misperception of subjective postural vertical position, perceiving their body as vertical when it was actually tilted about 20° toward the hemiparetic side. They also found that the visual and vestibular input for orientation perception to vertical remained intact as patients were able to align their bodies with the help of visual cues and conscious strategies. No significant association between ipsilateral pushing and hemineglect, anosognosia, aphasia, or apraxia has been found.[91]

Functional skills are significantly impaired for patients with ipsilateral pushing. During sitting, the push results in a strong lateral lean toward the weaker side; when sitting in a wheelchair, this often thrusts the patient over onto the wheelchair arm. In standing, a strong push creates an unstable situation with a high risk of falls because the hemiparetic LE typically cannot support the body weight. The patient shows no fear even when active pushing leads to instability and strongly resists any attempts to passively correct posture to midline, symmetrical weight-bearing. This pattern is totally opposite the expected postural deficiency seen in most patients after stroke, that is, increased weight-bearing to the stronger side to compensate for deficits on the hemiparetic side. Patients also typically demonstrate severe problems in transfers and gait. During transfers to the less involved side, the patient demonstrates increased pushback away from that side.

During walking, the patient typically exhibits inadequate extension of the hemiparetic LE with inability to transfer weight toward the less involved LE. During swing, strong scissoring (adduction) of the more involved LE is typically evident. The use of a cane during ambulation is problematic because patients use the cane to increase push to the hemiplegic side. Pedersen et al[91] demonstrated that patients with ipsilateral pushing behavior have poorer rehabilitation outcomes with longer hospital stays and prolonged recovery times. They also had significantly lower functional scores on admission and discharge with increased levels of dependence at discharge. However, with training, the brain can compensate well. The syndrome is rarely still evident at 6 months.[93]

Examination of the patient with ipsilateral pushing should include a focus on several criteria of behavior, including the following: (1) spontaneous body posture with tilting toward the more paretic side, (2) an increase of pushing force by the less involved extremities evidenced by increased abduction and extension, and (3) resistance to passive correction of the posture. Broetz and Karnath[94] developed the *Clinical Assessment Scale for Contraversive Pushing (SCP)*, which scores each of these three criteria in both sitting and standing. A subjective rating scale is used. The scores for each criteria range from 0 to 1. Because the criteria are examined in both sitting and standing, the maximum for each is 2 with a maximum possible overall score of 6. Patients are diagnosed with pushing behaviors if all three criteria are present and a score of 1 or more exists in each of the three criteria. Functional examination will reveal consistent difficulties with transfers to the less affected side, and difficulties with independent sitting, standing, and walking.[95]

Gait and Locomotion

Gait is altered following stroke owing to a number of factors. Some of the more common problems in hemiplegic gait and their possible causes are summarized in Box 15.5. An examination of gait typically includes an *observational gait analysis* (OGA). The therapist examines the movements occurring at the ankle, foot, knee, hip, pelvis, and trunk during walking (kinematic gait analysis). Gait is observed from the different planes of motion and deviations are identified. Digital video recording of a patient's gait for subsequent OGA can improve identification of gait deviations, provides a visual record of performance, and offers a useful teaching tool (patient feedback) to assist with remediation of gait problems. Quantitative measures of distance and time, cadence, velocity, and stride times should also be

---

Box 15.5 Gait Deviations Commonly Seen Following Stroke

Stance Phase	Swing Phase
Trunk/pelvis	**Trunk/pelvis**
Unawareness of affected side: poor proprioception	Insufficient forward pelvic rotation (pelvic retraction): weak abdominal muscles
Forward trunk:	Inclination to sound side for foot clearance: weakness of flexor muscles
• Weak hip extension	**Hip**
• Flexion contracture	Inadequate flexion:
Hip	• Weak hip flexors
Poor hip position (typically adduction or flexion): poor proprioception	• Poor proprioception
Trendelenburg limp: weak abductors	• Spastic quadriceps
Scissoring: spastic adductors	• Abdominal weakness (hip hikers)
Knee	• Hip abductor weakness of opposite site
Flexion during forward progression:	Abnormal substitutions include circumduction, external rotation/adduction, backward leaning of trunk/dragging toes; momentum/uncontrolled swing
• Flexion contracture	Exaggerated hip flexion: strong flexor synergy
• Weak hip and knee extensors	**Knee**
• Poor proprioception	Inadequate knee flexion:
• Ankle dorsiflexion range past neutral	• Inadequate hip flexion and poor foot clearance
• Weakness in extension pattern or in selective motion of hip and knee extensors and plantarflexors	• Spastic quadriceps
Hyperextension during forward progression:	Exaggerated but delayed knee flexion: strong flexor synergy
• Plantarflexion contracture past 90°	Inadequate knee extension at weight acceptance
• Impaired proprioception: knee wobbles or snaps back into recurvatum	• Spastic hamstrings
• Severe spasticity in quadriceps	• Sustained total flexor pattern
• Weak knee extensors: compensatory locking of knee in hyperextension	Weak knee extensors or poor proprioception
Ankle/foot	**Ankle/foot**
Equinus gait (heel does not touch the ground): spasticity or contractures of gastrocnemius soleus	Persistent equinus and/or equinovarus
Varus foot (patient bears weight on the lateral surface of the foot): hyperactive or spastic anterior tibialis, post tibialis, toe flexors, and soleus	• Plantarflexor contracture or spasticity
	• Weak dorsiflexors
Unequal step lengths: hammer toes caused by spastic toe flexors prevent the patient from stepping forward onto the opposite foot because of pain/weight-bearing on flexed toes	• Delayed contraction of dorsiflexors
	• Toes drag during midswing
Lack of dorsiflexion range on the affected side (approximately 10° is needed)	Varus: spastic anterior tibialis, weak peroneals, and toe extensors
	Equinovarus: spasticity of post tibialis and/or gastrocnemius soleus
	Exaggerated dorsiflexion: strong flexor synergy pattern

Adapted from educational materials used at Rancho Los Amigos Medical Center, Downey, CA, and Spaulding Rehabilitation Hospital, Boston, MA.

obtained using measured walkways and a stopwatch (e.g., the *10-Meter Walk Test*). Kinetic gait analysis examines the forces involved in the production of movement during walking and requires sophisticated instrumentation (force plates). See Chapter 7, Examination of Gait.

Ambulation profiles and scales can be used to determine locomotor function following stroke. These tests have been examined for reliability and/or validity and are reviewed in Chapter 7.

- *Functional Ambulation Profile (FAP)* and modifications
- The *Iowa Level of Assistance Score*
- The *Community Balance and Mobility Scale*
- The *Gait Abnormality Rating Scale (GARS)* and the *Modified GARS*
- The *Dynamic Gait Index (DGI)*
- The *Functional Gait Assessment (FGA)*
- The *High-Level Mobility Assessment Tool (HiMAT)*
- The *Fast Evaluation of Mobility, Balance, and Fear*
- The *Figure-of-Eight Walk Test*
- *Dual Tasking: Walks while Talking Test*

Perry et al[96] constructed a walking ability questionnaire and surveyed a group of 147 patients with chronic stroke about the effects of their limited walking ability. They then developed the *Classification of Walking Handicap After Stroke* (Box 15.6). The use of functional categories (physiological walker, household walker, and community walker) provides a useful method of identifying customary level of walking at home and in the community. *Walking handicap,* defined as the social disadvantage as a result of limitations in walking ability, can also be identified. Factors that differentiated household from community ambulators included strength, proprioception, isolated knee control (flexion and extension), and velocity. This classification system can be used to improve communication among clinicians, treatment planning, and documentation. It also forms the basis for the *Functional Ambulation Classification Scale.*[97]

Integumentary Integrity

Ischemic damage and subsequent necrosis of the skin results in skin breakdown and pressure ulcers (decubitus ulcers). The skin breaks down typically over bony prominences from pressure, friction, shearing, and/or maceration. Intense pressure for a short time or low pressure for a long time results in pressure ulcers. Friction occurs as the skin rubs or is dragged against the supporting surface, for example, when the patient slides down in bed or is pulled up. Spasticity and contractures also contribute to increased friction. Shearing occurs from sliding of adjacent structures in opposite directions (skin vs. underlying bone), for example, during transfers from bed to wheelchair. Maceration is caused

---

Box 15.6   Functional Walking Categories

Physiological Walker

- Walks for exercise only either at home or in parallel bars during physical therapy.

Household Walker

Limited household walker:

- Relies on walking to some extent for home activities.
- Requires assistance for some walking activities, uses a wheelchair, or is unable to perform others.

Unlimited household walker:

- Able to use walking for all household activities without any reliance on a wheelchair.
- Encounters difficulty with stairs and uneven terrain.
- May not be able to enter or leave the house independently.

Community Walker

Most-limited community walker:

- Can enter and leave the home independently.
- Can ascend and descend a curb independently.
- Can manage stairs to some degree.
- Independent in at least one moderate community activity (e.g., appointments, restaurants) and needs assistance or is unable in no more than one other low-challenge activity (e.g., church, neighborhood, visiting friend).

Least-limited community walker:

- Demonstrates independent stair management.
- Independent in all moderate community activities without assistance or use of wheelchair.
- Independent in either local stores or uncrowded shopping centers.
- Independent in at least two other moderate community activities.

Community walker:

- Independent in all home and community activities.
- Can accept crowds and uneven terrain.
- Demonstrates complete independence in shopping centers.

Note: Patients in each higher category can perform all activities of the previous group as well as the additional level of challenge listed.

From Perry et al,[96 p. 985] with permission.

---

by excess moisture, for example, with urinary incontinence. Additional risk factors include reduced activity (bedfast or chairfast), immobility, decreased sensation, abnormal patterns of movement, poor nutrition, and decreased level of consciousness. The incidence of pressure sores is increased with co-morbid medical conditions such as infections, peripheral vascular disease, edema, and diabetes.

Daily systematic inspection of the skin is indicated for high-risk patients, particularly over areas prone to breakdown. The skin must be kept clean, dry, and protected from injury. Adherence to proper techniques for positioning, turning, and transferring is essential. The therapist needs to check the posted positioning schedule and time in each position. Assumption of upright postures (sitting and standing) is promoted as soon as possible. Pressure-relieving devices (PRDs) are used to minimize high concentrations of pressure. These include foam pads, alternating pressure mattress, water mattress, air-fluidized bed, sheepskin, heel and elbow protectors, multipodus boots, and wheelchair cushions. Proper use of PRDs and positioning (seating) in the wheelchair should be closely examined.

Aerobic Capacity and Endurance

A supervised exercise test with electrocardiogram (ECG) monitoring may be indicated for survivors of stroke with cardiovascular disease in the subacute phase. Performance measures include significant ECG changes, HR, BP, *Rating of Perceived Exertion (RPE)*, and other signs of ischemic intolerance. The mode of testing will depend on the individual patient and can include leg cycle ergometry, semirecumbent cycle ergometry, a combination arm-leg ergometer, treadmill (TM) walking, or a seated stepper. If balance is impaired, recumbent equipment or an overhead safety harness on a TM should be used. Test protocols are individualized and are generally submaximal with a gradual progression in intensity. An intermittent protocol with rest periods may be required for some patients. Clinical endpoints of testing are similar as for other patients with cardiovascular disease (serious dysrhythmias, greater than 2 mm ST-segment depression or elevation, systolic BP [SBP] greater than 250 mm Hg or diastolic BP [DBP] greater than 115 mm Hg, volitional fatigue).[24]

For ambulatory patients, walking endurance can be measured using a *6- or 12-minute walk test* (see discussion in Chapter 7). The time, total distance, number of rest stops, and symptoms at rest stops are recorded. Shorter distances (e.g., a 2-minute walk test) have been used for patients with acute stroke.[98]

Functional Status

Functional measures are used to determine the impact of impairments and activity limitations, inform the POC, monitor progress, ascertain efficacy of stroke rehabilitation efforts, and make recommendations for long-term care or placement. Instruments can include items to examine *functional mobility skills* (bed mobility, movement transitions, transfers, locomotion, stairs),

basic ADL (BADL) skills (feeding, hygiene, dressing), and *instrumental ADL (IADL) skills* (communication, home chores). Information on functional disability following stroke is typically gained through performance-based measures. The *Barthel Index*[99] and the *Functional Independence Measure (FIM)*[100] have been extensively tested and demonstrate excellent reliability, validity, and sensitivity. The FIM is now in widespread use in rehabilitation facilities across the United States. Higher FIM scores have been correlated to successful outcomes, discharge home, and return to the community for patients with stroke.[101] See Chapter 8, Examination of Function, for a more detailed discussion of these instruments.

Stroke-Specific Instruments

Fugl-Meyer Assessment of Physical Performance (FMA)

The pioneering work of Twitchell[64] and Brunnstrom[65,66] on motor recovery and behavior following stroke led to the development of the FMA.[102] This is an impairment-based test with items organized by sequential recovery stages. A three-point ordinal scale is used to measure impairments of volitional movement with grades ranging from 0 (item cannot be performed) to 2 (item can be fully performed). Specific descriptions for performance accompany individual test items. Subtests exist for UE function, LE function, balance, sensation, ROM, and pain. The cumulative test score for all components is 226 with availability of specific subtest scores (e.g., UE maximum score is 66, LE score 34; balance score 14). This instrument has good construct validity and high reliability (r = 0.99) for determining motor function following stroke (a gold standard instrument).[103,104] Quantifiable outcome data, standardized measurement methods, and therapist training was used to ensure high interrater reliability for documenting stage wise recovery and outcomes in a large, multicenter clinical trial research (LEAPS trials).[105] The instrument requires an estimated 30 to 40 minutes to administer (see Appendix 15.A). A shortened version consists of combining the UE and LE sections to form the *Fugl-Meyer Motor Scale*. This version has also been shown to be a useful measure of stage wise recovery and outcomes with a shortened administration time.[106]

Stroke Rehabilitation Assessment of Movement (STREAM)

The *STREAM* is a clinical measure of voluntary movements and basic mobility following stoke. It consists of 30 items (test movements) distributed equally among three subscales: upper-limb movements, lower-limb movements, and basic mobility items. Voluntary movement items explore out-of-synergy control and are scored using a 3-point ordinal scale (unable to perform, partial performance, complete performance). The basic mobility section includes a variety of items (rolling, bridging, sit-to-stand, standing, stepping, walking, and stairs) and is scored using a 4-point ordinal scale (unable, partial, complete/with aid, complete/no aid). The maximum STREAM score is 70 with each limb subscore worth 20 points and the functional mobility subscore worth 30 points.[107] The instrument has good construct validity and high reliability.[108] It has been used to document motor recovery over time and predict discharge destination following stroke.[109,110]

Chedoke-McMaster Stroke Assessment

The Chedoke-McMaster Stroke Assessment examines physical impairment and disability after stroke. It includes two components: the Impairment Inventory and the Activity Inventory.

There are 14 items scored using a 7-point scale with a 2-point score used for walking distance. The Impairment Inventory examines the presence and severity of impairments in six areas (shoulder pain, postural control, and control of the arm, hand, foot, and leg). The Activity Inventory is subdivided into the Gross Motor Function Index (with items including moving in bed and transferring to a chair) and the Walking Index (with items including walking on rough terrain and climbing stairs).[109]

Stroke Impact Scale (SIS)

The SIS is a self-report measure developed to assess function and quality of life after stroke. It includes 59 items organized into 8 subgroups: strength, memory and thinking, emotions, communication, ADL, mobility, hand function, and participation. The final item asks the person to rate perceived recovery on a scale of 0 to 100 with 100 representing full recovery and 0 representing no recovery. It takes about 30 minutes to complete. The SIS is a valid, reliable, and sensitive measure of change in this population.[111,112] Responses can also be accurately provided by proxy.[113] The form and user agreement is available at the following website: www2.kumc.edu/coa/SIS/Stroke-Impact-Scale.htm.

■ GOALS AND OUTCOMES

Examples of general goals and outcomes for patients with stroke (Preferred Practice Pattern 5D) as adapted from the *Guide to Physical Therapist Practice*[41] are presented in Box 15.7. These general goals will provide the basis for development of specific anticipated goals and expected outcomes for an individual patient.

■ PHYSICAL THERAPY INTERVENTIONS

Therapists select interventions based on an accurate examination of existing impairments, activity limitations, and goals. Functional, task-specific training is the mainstay of therapy and is designed to assist patients in regaining control of functional movement patterns. Improved motor control and strength of the trunk and limbs, with an emphasis on the more involved side, is achieved through specific reeducation strategies. Intense practice both during therapy sessions and outside of therapy is needed to effect meaningful change. The therapist needs to incorporate motor learning principles and behavioral shaping techniques to effectively support learning. It is also important to create an environment that supports learning and provides the typical challenges of everyday life. In cases of severe deficits, limited recovery, and/or multiple co-morbidities, compensatory training strategies may be necessary to promote resumption of function using the less involved extremities and alternate movement patterns. Strategies to improve motor function are discussed fully in Chapter 10.

Evidence-based practice (EBP) promotes the use of current best research evidence along with individual clinical expertise in order to reach informed decisions about patient care. EBP allows therapists to identify the best (most effective) techniques and to take responsibility for evaluating their practice on an ongoing basis. Studies designed to delineate differences between exercise approaches for the patient with stroke (e.g., neuromuscular reeducation and facilitation approaches [neurodevelopmental treatment (NDT), proprioceptive neuromuscular facilitation (PNF)], motor relearning program, functional training) have often failed to demonstrate clear superiority of one approach over another.[44,46,114–117] Conclusions from Cochrane reviewers state, "There is insufficient evidence to conclude that any one physiotherapy approach is more effective in promoting recovery of lower limb function or postural control following stroke than any other approach. We recommend that future research should concentrate on investigating the effectiveness of clearly described individual techniques and task-specific treatments, regardless of their historical or philosophical origin."[44, p. 4] Many studies are subject to methodological flaws. For example, studies used small sample sizes, failed to include a control group or to control for experimenter bias and co-interventions, and/or utilized poorly defined treatments and/or inappropriate outcome measures. There are a limited number of large, multicenter, randomized controlled trials (RCTs) that offer clinicians a higher level of confidence. Some will be discussed later in this section (e.g., STEPS trial, LEAPS trial, EXCITE trial). Evidence concerning the effectiveness of task-oriented training is presented in Chapter 10, Box 10.1, and Box 15.9 (later in this chapter). Important conclusions to be drawn from these studies are that (1) collectively they provide consistent evidence for the beneficial effects of physical therapy when compared to no treatment or placebo control; and (2) studies on

Box 15.7 Examples of General Goals and Outcomes for Patients with Stroke

Impact of pathology/pathophysiology is reduced.

- Patient/client, family, and caregiver knowledge and awareness of the disease, prognosis, and plan of care are enhanced.
- Symptom management is enhanced.
- Changes associated with recovery are monitored.
- Risk of secondary impairments and recurrence of condition is reduced.
- Intensity of care is decreased.

Impact of impairments is reduced.

- Cognitive function is improved.
- Communication is improved.
- Sensory awareness and skin integrity are improved.
- Perceptual function is improved.
- Awareness and use of the hemiplegic side is improved.
- Pain is decreased.
- Joint integrity and mobility are improved.
- Motor function (motor control and motor learning) is improved.
- Muscle performance (strength, power, and endurance) is improved.
- Postural control and balance are improved.
- Gait and locomotion are improved.
- Aerobic capacity is increased.

Ability to perform physical actions, tasks, or activities is improved.

- Independence in ADL is increased.
- Tolerance of upright postures and activities is increased.

- Problem solving and decision making skills are enhanced.
- Safety of patient/client, family, and caregivers is improved.

Disability associated with chronic illness is reduced.

- Ability to assume/resume self-care and home management is improved.
- Ability to assume work (job/school/play), community, and leisure roles is improved.
- Awareness and use of community resources are improved.

Health status and quality of life are improved.

- Sense of well-being is enhanced.
- Stressors are reduced.
- Insight, self-confidence, and self-management skills are improved.
- Health, wellness, and fitness are improved.

Patient/client satisfaction is enhanced.

- Access and availability of services are acceptable to patient/client and family.
- Quality of rehabilitation services is acceptable to patient/client and family.
- Care is coordinated with patient/client, family, caregivers, and other professionals.
- Discharge placement needs are determined.

Adapted from the *Guide to Physical Therapist Practice*.[41]

---

task-oriented training have yielded positive results in terms of improving locomotor function (post-stroke locomotor training studies) and UE function (CIMT training studies). Specificity of training and increased intensity of training are important factors in these positive results.

It is important to point out that there is no one intervention optimal for all patients with stroke. Because patients with stroke are a diverse group with variable levels of function, interventions must be carefully selected based on individual abilities and needs. Therapists need to select interventions that have the greatest chance of successfully remediating existing impairments and promoting functional recovery. The choice of interventions must also take into consideration a number of other factors, including phase of post-stroke recovery (acute, postacute, chronic), age of the patient, number of co-morbidities, social and financial resources, and potential discharge placement. Early emphasis on improving functional

independence provides an important source of motivation for both the patient and family.

Strategies to Improve Motor Learning

Motor skill learning is based on the brain's capacity for recovery through mechanisms of reorganization and adaptation. An effective rehabilitation plan capitalizes on this potential and encourages active participation—*the patient must be fully engaged*. Activities are selected that are meaningful and important to the patient. Optimal motor learning can be promoted through attention to a number of factors, most importantly, strategy development, feedback, and practice. Carr and Shepherd[118] describe many of these strategies in their book *A Motor Relearning Programme for Stroke*.

Strategy Development

The therapist first assists the patient in learning the desired task (cognitive stage). Explicit verbal instructions are used to direct the patient's attention to the task.

More specifically, critical task elements and successful outcomes are identified. The desired task is demonstrated at the ideal performance speeds. The patient then begins to practice. If the task has a number of interrelated steps, practice of component parts may precede practice of the whole task. It is important, however, not to delay practice of the integrated task because this may interfere with effective transfer of learning. The therapist should give clear, simple verbal instructions and not overload the patient with excessive or wordy instructions. There is some evidence to suggest that providing excessive information about the task can be disruptive to learning, especially for patients with MCA stroke involving the sensorimotor cortex. This interference may block formation of the implicit motor plan.[119,120] Correct performance should be reinforced and intervention provided when movement errors become consistent. Active participation is essential for learning; *there is no learning with passive movements*. Practicing the movements on the less affected side first can yield important transfer effects.

Mental practice or mental rehearsal is the systematic application of imagery techniques for improving performance and learning. The patient is instructed to visualize the movement and imagine himself or herself functionally using the affected limb. Mental practice can be facilitated through the use of audiotapes and has been successfully combined with physical practice to enhance UE recovery[121] and LE recovery and walking ability (gait speed) in patients with stroke.[122] When used in an RCT of early post-stroke patients, recovery of hand movements was not superior using motor imagery than with an equally intense conventional therapy.[123]

As practice progresses, the patient is asked to self-examine performance and identify problems, specifically, what difficulties exist, what can be done to correct the difficulties, and what movements can be eliminated or refined. If a complex task is practiced, the patient is asked to identify if the correct components were performed, how the individual components fit together, and if they were appropriately sequenced. If the patient is unable to provide an accurate assessment of problems, the therapist can prompt the patient in decision making using guiding questions and utilize demonstration to help identify problems. For example, if the patient consistently falls to the right while standing, questions can be directed toward this problem (e.g., "In what direction did you fall?" "What do you need to do to prevent yourself from falling?"). The patient is thus actively involved in developing task analysis and problem-solving skills leading to improved ability to self-correct movements. These skills are essential in ensuring independence in the home and community.

Feedback

Feedback can be intrinsic (naturally occurring as part of the movement response) or extrinsic (provided by the therapist). During early motor learning the therapist provides extrinsic feedback (e.g., verbal cueing, manual cueing), and manual guidance to shape performance. It is important to monitor performance carefully and provide accurate feedback. The patient's attention should be directed to naturally occurring intrinsic feedback. During early intervention visual inputs are critical for motor learning. This can be facilitated by having the patient look at the movement (a central concept of PNF).[124,125] During later learning (associative phase), proprioception becomes important for movement refinement. This can be encouraged by early and carefully reinforced weight-bearing (approximation) on the more affected side during upright activities. Additional proprioceptive inputs (manual contacts, tapping, stretch, light tracking resistance, antigravity postures) can be used to improve feedback and stimulate learning. The patient should be encouraged to "feel the movement" while learning to distinguish correct movement responses from incorrect ones. Surface EMG biofeedback can be used to provide augmented feedback. Exteroceptive inputs (light rubbing, stroking) may be used to provide additional sources of sensory inputs, particularly where distortions of proprioception exist. As treatment progresses, the emphasis again shifts from extrinsic to intrinsic feedback and to self-monitoring and self-correcting movement responses. Great care must be taken to avoid dependence on the therapist (i.e., the patient is only able to move with the therapist's manual or verbal assistance) by providing decreasing amounts of physical guidance and augmented feedback. This requires careful consideration during each treatment session. Therapists should allow the patient adequate time for introspection about the movements and available feedback.

The use of a mirror can be an effective adjunct for some patients to improve motor function using visual feedback. *Mirror therapy (MT)* is a therapeutic intervention that focuses on moving the less impaired limb while watching its mirror reflection. A mirror is placed in the patient's midsagittal plane, presenting the patient with the mirror image of his or her less affected limb as if it were the hemiparetic limb. It was first introduced by Ramachandran et al[126] for individuals with arm amputation. For patients with stroke, MT has been shown to improve LE recovery and ankle dorsiflexion.[127] MT has also been shown to improve UE recovery and distal motor function and recovery from hemineglect.[128,129] In these studies, both the mirror groups and the control groups also participated in a conventional stroke rehabilitation program. It is important to note that use of mirrors is contraindicated in patients with marked visuospatial perceptual impairments.

Practice

Practice, practice, and more practice is essential for motor skill learning and recovery. The therapist needs to organize the patient's therapy session to ensure optimal practice. *Blocked practice* (constant repetition of a single task) is used to improve *initial* performance and motivation, especially for patients with disorganized movements. Most hospitalized patients also initially require a *distributed practice schedule* with adequate rest periods owing to limited endurance as both physical and cognitive fatigue can result in decreased performance. The patient should be encouraged to self-monitor practice sessions and recognize when fatigue may be setting in and rest is required. The therapist needs to progress the patient to *variable practice* (practice of more than one task within a session) using a serial or random order as soon as possible. Variable practice improves performance and results in better retention of learned skills and improved ability to adapt to changing task demands. Patient, staff, and family efforts should be coordinated to ensure continued and consistent practice during off-therapy times.

Careful attention to the learning environment will also yield important therapeutic gains. Distractions should be reduced and a consistent and comfortable environment provided in which the patient can learn. For many patients with stroke and cognitive/perceptual deficits, this will initially be a *closed environment* with limited distractions. Later the environment can be varied, providing an appropriate level of *contextual interference*. Thus the patient is progressed toward performing the same skill in a more *open environment*, with variable and real-life challenges. The addition of *Easy Street Environments* to many rehabilitation centers provides an important tool to simulate community environments.

Motivation is key to successful learning. The patient should be fully involved in collaborative goal-setting from the beginning and continually reminded of the goal, the task, what progress has been made, and the expected outcomes. Treatment sessions should include positive experiences, ensuring the patient experiences success in therapy and instilling self-confidence. Beginning and ending the therapy session on a positive note (a successful activity) is a helpful strategy. Self-efficacy ratings and summary comments can be used to monitor progress (e.g., "What successes did you achieve in therapy today?"). Supportive strategies should be discussed with family and caregivers. Finally, the therapist needs to continually communicate support and encouragement. Recovery from stroke is an extremely stressful experience that will challenge the coping abilities of both patient and family.

Interventions to Improve Sensory Function

Patients who have significant sensory impairments may demonstrate impaired or absent spontaneous movement. The more the patient can be encouraged to use the affected side, the greater the chance of increased awareness and function. Conversely, the patient who refuses to use the hemiplegic side contributes to the problems imposed by lack of sensorimotor experience. Without attention during treatment, this *learned nonuse* phenomenon can contribute to further deterioration.[130]

Multiple interventions for UE sensory impairment after stroke have been described. These can be categorized into sensory retraining or sensory stimulation approaches. *Sensory retraining programs* include use of mirror therapy (previously discussed), repetitive sensory discrimination activities, bilateral simultaneous movements, and repetitive task practice (e.g., *sensorimotor integrative treatment* with its focus on normalizing tone, practice of functional activity, and use of augmented sensory cues). *Sensory stimulation intervention* includes compression techniques (weight-bearing, manual compression, inflatable pressure splints, intermittent pneumatic compression), mobilizations, electrical stimulation, thermal stimulation, or magnetic stimulation. In a review of 13 studies, Cochrane reviewers[48] found significant clinical and methodological diversity, limited RCT trials, generally small sample sizes with inadequate data, variability in outcome measures, and limited used of functional performance and participation outcome measures. They concluded there was insufficient evidence to support or refute the effectiveness of many of these interventions in improving sensory function. Limited evidence was found in support of the following:

- Mirror therapy for improving detection of light touch, pressure, and temperature pain
- Thermal stimulation intervention for improving rate of recovery of sensation
- Intermittent pneumatic compression for improving tactile and kinesthetic sensation

The results of a systematic review of sensory retraining by Schabrun and Hillier[131] were similar with additional support found for electrical stimulation interventions.

During functional training, the therapist needs to maximize weight-bearing and compression of the sensory deficient limbs. Approximation can be applied with the sensory-deficient UE weight-bearing in sitting or standing/modified plantigrade position and to the pelvis during standing activities. While sitting on a ball, the patient can practice bouncing. The compression and approximation that occur through the spine enhances activity in the postural extensors. During the application of sensory stimulation to the more involved limbs, the therapist directs the patient's attention and assists in shaping the patient's responses.[132,133]

A safety education program should be instituted early for patients, family, and caregivers to improve awareness of sensory impairments and ensure protection of anesthetic limbs. This is particularly important for preventing UE trauma during transfer and wheelchair activities.

Interventions to Improve Hemianopsia and Unilateral Neglect

Patients with hemianopsia or unilateral neglect demonstrate a lack of awareness of the contralesional side. The impairments are more pervasive in patients with neglect and in its most severe form (anosognosia) may extend to a total unawareness of the disability or the extent of the problems. These patients benefit from training strategies that encourage awareness and use of the environment on the hemiparetic side and use of the hemiparetic extremities. It is important to teach active visual scanning movements through turning of the head and axial trunk rotation to the more involved side. Cueing (e.g., visual, verbal, or motor cues) is used to direct the patient's attention. For example, a red anchor line can be taped on the floor and the patient directed to visually follow the line from one side to the other. Or a red ribbon can be attached to the patient's hemiparetic wrist and the patient directed to keep the red ribbon in sight. Scanning movements can also be stimulated using visual tracking tasks using a computer. Patients are given feedback about the success of their efforts and reinforcement for each successful performance (shaping). Imagery has also been shown to help (e.g., "Imagine you are a lighthouse beam; use your beam to sweep and scan the floor from one side to the other"). During therapy, the therapist stimulates and encourages active voluntary movements of the neglected limbs while encouraging the patient to look at his or her limbs while moving. UE exercises that involve crossing the midline toward the hemiparetic side (e.g., reaching activities or PNF chop or lift patterns) are important. Functional activities that encourage bilateral interaction are also valuable (e.g., pouring a drink and drinking from a cup; picking up an object with the more involved hand and placing it in the other; "dusting a tabletop" with a cloth held by both hands). The therapist needs to maximize the patient's attention by optimizing visual, tactile, or proprioceptive stimuli on the more affected side. These can include stroking, brushing, tapping, or vibrating the hemiparetic limbs. The therapist also needs to consistently reorient the patient as inattention develops. Patients with very low levels of arousal are likely to be less responsive to therapy efforts.[134-136]

Interventions to Improve Flexibility and Joint Integrity

Soft tissue/joint mobilization and ROM exercises are initiated early to maintain joint integrity and mobility and prevent contractures. Passive ROM (PROM), and AROM when possible, with terminal stretch should be performed daily in all motions. If a contracture is developing, more frequent ROM (twice daily or more) is necessary.

Positioning strategies are also important in maintaining soft tissue length (Box 15.8). Effective positioning of the hemiparetic extremities encourages proper joint alignment while positioning the limbs out of the abnormal

---

Box 15.8 Positioning Strategies to Reduce Common Malalignments

Supine Position

- Head/neck: Neutral and symmetrical; supported on pillow.
- Trunk: Aligned in midline.
- More affected UE: Scapular protracted, shoulder forward and slightly abducted; arm supported on a pillow; elbow extended with hand resting on a pillow; wrist neutral, fingers extended, and thumb abducted.
- More affected LE: Hip forward (pelvis protracted); knee on a small pillow or towel roll to prevent hyperextension; nothing against the soles of feet. For persistent plantarflexion, a splint can be used to position the foot and ankle in neutral position.

Side-lying on Less Affected Side

- Head/neck: Neutral and symmetrical.
- Trunk: Aligned in midline; small pillow or towel can be placed under the rib cage to elongate the hemiplegic side.
- More affected UE: Scapular protracted, shoulder forward; arm on a supporting pillow with elbow extended, wrist neutral, fingers extended, and thumb abducted.
- More affected LE: Hip forward and flexed, knee flexed and supported on a pillow.

Side-lying on More Affected Side

- Head/neck: Neutral and symmetrical.
- Trunk: Aligned in midline.
- More affected UE: Scapular protracted; shoulder forward; arm placed in slight abduction and external rotation; elbow extended, forearm supinated, wrist neutral, fingers extended, and thumb abducted.
- More affected LE: Hip extended and knee flexed and supported by pillows. An alternative position is slight hip and knee flexion with pelvic protraction.

Sitting in an Armchair or Wheelchair

- Head/neck: Neutral and symmetrical; head directly above pelvis.
- Trunk: Spine extension.
- Pelvis: Aligned in neutral with weight-bearing on both buttocks.
- More affected UE: Shoulder protracted and forward; elbow supported on an arm trough or lapboard; forearm, wrist neutral, fingers extended, and thumb abducted (resting splint as needed).
- Both LEs: Hips flexed to 90°, positioned in neutral with respect to rotation.

---

postures typically assumed. The use of protective devices such as resting splints may be necessary. Coordination with staff, family, and caregivers is essential for long-term management.

In the UE, correct PROM techniques require careful attention to external rotation and distraction of the humerus, especially as ranges approach 90° of flexion or more. The scapula should be mobilized on the thoracic wall with an emphasis on upward rotation and protraction to prevent soft tissue impingement in the subacromial space during overhead movements of the arm (Fig. 15.7) and to prepare for forward reach patterns. The use of overhead pulleys for self-ROM is contraindicated because of failure to achieve the above requirements for scapulohumeral movement. Full extension of the elbow is important because the majority of patients with stroke develop tightness in elbow flexors as a result of excess flexor spasticity. Normal length of wrist and finger extensors should also be maintained as tightness is typical in flexion. This can be achieved functionally through sitting, weight-bearing on the extended paretic UE with the wrist extended and fingers open and extended (Fig. 15.8). Edema and tonal changes may produce impingement with wrist extension. In this situation, the carpal bones should be mobilized before stretching at the wrist.

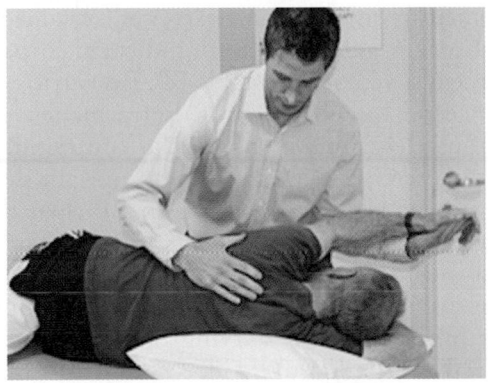

Figure 15.7 Range-of-motion exercises for the hemiparetic UE. The therapist carefully mobilizes the scapula during arm elevation.

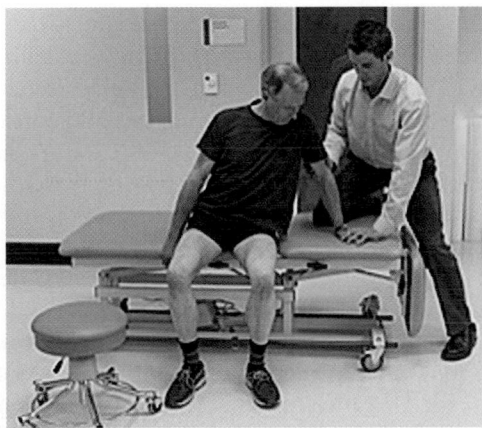

Figure 15.8 Sitting, with extended arm support. The therapist assists in stabilizing the elbow and fingers in extension.

Strategies to teach patients safe self-ROM activities should be instituted early. Suggested activities include the following:

- *Arm cradling*: The stronger UE cradles and lifts the more affected UE to 90° humeral flexion; the arm is moved into positions of horizontal abduction and adduction. Active trunk rotation is combined with the arm movements.
- *Table-top polishing*: The more affected UE is positioned in humeral flexion with scapular protraction and elbow extension; both hands are positioned on a towel. The less affected hand moves the paretic hand by pulling on the towel (forward, and side-to-side). Trunk movements and ROM are optimized by placing the chair slightly back from the table.
- Sitting, the patient leans forward and reaches both hands down to the floor. This position encourages forward flexion of the humerus with scapular protraction, and extension of the elbow, wrist, and fingers.
- Supine, hands are clasped together and placed behind the head, the elbows fall flat to the mat. This activity should be considered only if scapula upward mobility is present. Hands clasped, self-overhead movements are contraindicated if scapulohumeral rhythm is lacking.

When sitting in a wheelchair, the patient's paretic UE can be positioned on an arm trough (shallow elbow/ forearm support) attached to the armrest. The shoulder is positioned in 5° of abduction and flexion and neutral rotation; elbow in 90° flexion and slightly forward; forearm pronated; and hand in a functional resting position. Splinting the hand is also common. *A volar resting (pan) splint* positions the forearm, wrist, and fingers in a functional position (20° to 30° of wrist extension, metacarpophalangeal [MP] flexion 40° to 45°, interphalangeal [IP] flexion 10° to 20°, and thumb opposition). A resting splint is appropriate for nighttime use, allowing patients daytime use of their hand. In the presence of spasticity, tone-reducing devices can be considered (e.g., finger abduction splint, firm cone, spasticity reduction splint, or inflatable pressure splint).

As most patients regain some use of their LEs early in recovery, ROM techniques focus on individual patient needs with attention to several common areas of impairment. For many patients, voluntary movement in the foot and ankle is limited owing to plantarflexor spasticity and/or dorsiflexor weakness. Weight-shifting activities in modified plantigrade (forward shift stretches the plantarflexors) or prolonged static positioning using adaptive equipment (i.e., tilt table with toe wedges) can be used to gain range. Facilitation of active contraction of dorsiflexors can also be combined with stretching to provide reciprocal inhibition to plantarflexors. If synergistic influence is strong, the patient can be effectively positioned while supine on a mat with the paretic LE abducted off the side with knee flexed and foot flat on the floor or a stool. This position of hip abduction and extension with knee flexion serves to breakup synergistic dominance and position the limb out of the typical spastic scissoring posture. If the patient spends considerable time sitting in a wheelchair, care should be taken to stretch the hip flexors. If hip flexor contractures are allowed to develop, they can lead to increased difficulty with standing, transfers, and ambulation.

Interventions to Improve Strength

Muscle weakness is a major impairment after stroke and contributes to significant activity limitations (e.g., walking, sit-to-stand transfers, stair climbing, UE activities). Progressive resistive strength training has been shown to improve muscle strength in individuals with stroke,[137-149] with no evidence of a detrimental increase in spasticity or reduction in ROM.[137,138] Most studies have indicated improvements in function,[138,142,143,145,149] although some have failed to demonstrate carryover to improved function.[137] Specificity of training as well as variable intensities of training may explain this inconsistency.

Exercise modalities for strengthening include free weights, elastic bands or tubing, and machines (PRE, isokinetics). For patients who are very weak (less than 3/5), gravity-minimized exercises using powder boards, sling suspension, or aquatic exercise is indicated. Gravity-resisted active movements are indicated for patients who demonstrate 3/5 strength (e.g., arm lifts, leg lifts). Patients who demonstrate adequate strength in independent gravity-resisted movement (e.g., 8 to 12 repetitions) can be progressed to exercise using added resistance (e.g., free weights, bands, or machines). Ideally resistance training should occur 2 to 3 times a week; three sets of 8 to 12 repetitions per exercise should be used.[24]

Combining resistance training with task-oriented functional activities enhances carryover in terms of improving function (e.g., sit-to-stand transfers, partial wall squats [Fig. 15.9], step-ups, stair climbing while the patient is wearing weighted cuffs). Circuit training workstations can be used to maximize muscle training.[145] Lifting free weights or using elastic bands places added demands for postural stability in sitting and standing and is an important element of training to improve postural control.

Exercise Precautions

Many patients with stroke demonstrate poor hand function with no effective grasp. Specially designed gloves may be necessary to ensure maintained contact with exercise equipment (e.g., leather mitts with Velcro®, wrist cuffs). Patients with impaired sensation are at increased risk for injury and should be monitored closely. Patients with postural deficits should be safely

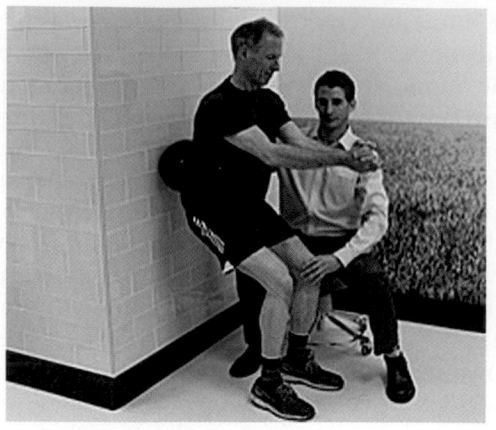

Figure 15.9 Partial wall squats using a small ball; the therapist assists in control of knee.

positioned to prevent falls (e.g., stable seat, corner standing while lifting free weights).

In determining a safe exercise prescription, it is important to remember the high incidence of hypertension and cardiac disease in patients with stroke. High-intensity strengthening exercises (sustained maximal effort) is generally contraindicated in patients with recent stroke and unstable BP. Isometric exercise that is accompanied by the Valsalva maneuver and dangerous elevations in BP is also contraindicated. Dynamic exercises performed in an upright position (sitting) produce less elevations in BP than recumbent/supine exercises. For patients at risk, submaximal protocols using low-intensity exercises (e.g., 30% to 50% of maximal voluntary contraction) are appropriate for initial exercise. Varying the exercises is also an effective strategy to reduce cardiovascular risk. The therapist needs to ensure that warm-ups and cooldowns are adequate and the overall exercise progression is gradual.

Interventions to Manage Spasticity

Patients who demonstrate spasticity can benefit from interventions designed to manage the effects of spasticity (immobility, soft-tissue contracture, and deformity). These include early mobilization and daily stretching to maintain the length of spastic muscles and soft tissues and promote optimal positioning.[150] It is important to note that the methodological quality of research studies in this area is diverse and not well controlled, and available evidence about the effectiveness of stretching is inconclusive.[151,152] The technique of *rhythmic rotation*, a manual technique that incorporates slow gentle rotations of the limb while progressively moving the limb into its lengthening range, can be effective in gaining initial range.[153] Once full range is achieved, the limb is positioned in the lengthened position. For example, the shoulder is extended, abducted, and externally rotated with the elbow, wrist, and fingers extended. The hand is positioned in weight-bearing to the patient's side (see Fig. 15.8) and maintained for several minutes. The benefits of *sustained stretching* include relaxation through mechanisms of autogenic inhibition. In sitting, slow rocking movements can be added to increase relaxation effects from influences of slow vestibular stimulation. Spasticity in the quadriceps can be similarly inhibited through prolonged positioning and weight-bearing in kneeling or quadruped positions. A reduction in truncal stiffness can be promoted using techniques of rhythmic rotation or rhythmic initiation combined with axial trunk rotation (e.g., in side-lying, sitting or hook-lying, segmental trunk rotation).[153] PNF upper trunk patterns (chopping or lifting) that emphasize rotational movements of the trunk can also be effective in maintaining range and reducing trunk stiffness.[125] Side sitting on the hemiparetic side provides sustained stretch to the spastic side flexors. The patient, family members, and caregivers should be taught safe ROM and stretching techniques.

Active exercise should focus on the activation of the weak antagonist muscles using slow, controlled movements. Local facilitation techniques (e.g., stretch, tapping, light resistance) can be added to enhance the action of very weak antagonist muscles. Contraction helps reduce agonist tone through the effects of reciprocal inhibition. Thus, in the UE, efforts are directed toward active contractions of the elbow extensors in the presence of flexor spasticity, whereas in the LE efforts are directed toward active contractions of the knee flexors with extensor spasticity. It is important to remember that reciprocal relationships may not be within normal ranges, particularly in the presence of strong spastic co-contraction. Excessive effort should be avoided because it can have a negative effect on spasticity. Soothing verbal commands and cognitive relaxation techniques (mental imagery) can be used to provide an overall calming influence and generally relax tone while pain has the opposite effect.

Modalities can be used to treat spasticity. These include the application of cold, massage, and electrical stimulation. Cold slows nerve conduction and decreases muscle spindle activity. These factors can lead to a temporary reduction of tone. Cold can be applied with ice packs or ice massage (duration 10 to 20 minutes) or using vapocoolants. The effects of cold are short-lived, generally lasting for about 20 to 30 minutes. Functional electrical stimulation (FES) can be used to target the weak antagonist muscles (e.g., peroneal nerve stimulators) and works to decrease tone through the effects of reciprocal inhibition. FES has been used with some success to decrease tone during the treatment time.[152]

Orthotic devices can be used to maintain the spastic muscle in its lengthened position and help decrease hypertonia and increase or maintain PROM. These include inflatable pressure splints,[154] static or resting splints, and serial casts.[155,156] Air splints can also help control unwanted synergistic movements and stabilize limbs during early weight-bearing activities (e.g., sitting, modified plantigrade). Patients with a flaccid, hypotonic limb may also benefit from the use of pressure splints to provide sensory input and initial stabilization. Long or full limb pressure splints also assist in controlling edema, a common problem of paralyzed limbs. Positioning the splinted limb in elevation can assist in reducing edema.

Interventions to Improve Movement Control

Activities that promote voluntary movement control, postural control, and functional use of the extremities are the primary focus of initial movement training. Patients with stroke typically present with loss of dissociated or fractionated movements with obligatory synergy patterns. For example, coordinated grasp and manipulation are lost as the fingers respond with strong flexion when lifting the arm results in elbow flexion with flexion, abduction, and external rotation of the shoulder. Interlimb and intralimb control is also abnormal with movements of one limb linked to movements of the other through associated reactions. During initial training, the therapist needs to focus on *dissociation* of different body segments (the ability to isolate and move the different parts of the body or limb separately) and *selective* (out-of-synergy) movement patterns. For example, the more affected UE is stabilized in an extended weight-bearing position while the patient practices stepping movements in modified plantigrade position.

The linking together of the proper components of movement and the refinement of isolated control requires a great deal of concentration and volitional control. Movements that are performed too quickly or with too much force will be ineffective in producing the control needed. Thus, the therapist needs to instruct the patient to avoid excessive effort during movement. The therapist should aim for as much normalcy in movement as possible and select postures that assist the desired movements through optimal biomechanical stabilization and/or use of the optimal point in the range. As control develops, postures can be changed to more difficult ones that challenge developing control. For example, initial elbow extension can be first attempted in side-lying with the shoulder flexed to 90° (e.g., the patient pushes the arm forward, extending the elbow). The posture can then be changed to sitting, and finally standing.

The therapist may need to assist (guide) initial movement attempts or use facilitation techniques (e.g., stretch, resistance, electrical stimulation). Movements should shift to active control as soon as possible. Often the resistance of gravity acting on the body or slight manual resistance is enough to initiate or facilitate correct movement responses through proprioceptive loading.

Repetitive task-specific training is the main focus of the rehabilitation program. The tasks selected should be relevant and important to the patient (e.g., reaching and manipulation, walking, stair climbing). Normal function implies variability of movements. Muscles need to be activated in varied activities using varied types of contractions. All three types—eccentric, isometric, and concentric—are important to include in an exercise program. For the patient with stroke who demonstrates very weak movements, isometric and eccentric contractions should be practiced before concentric contractions because they utilize elastic elements and muscle spindle support more efficiently. For the same amount of tension, fewer motor units are required. Practice of functional tasks that utilize variations of contractions should also be implemented. For example, the patient who practices modified wall squats in standing is utilizing a sequence of eccentric (lowering), isometric (holding), and concentric (extending) contractions of the hip and knee extensors (Fig. 15.9). Weak muscles (typically antagonistic to strong spastic muscles) should be activated first in unidirectional movements. As control develops, exercises can shift to include slow active reciprocal contractions of agonist and antagonist muscles first in limited ranges, then in full range. This emphasis on balanced interaction of both agonists and antagonists is crucial for normal coordination and function. Proprioceptive neuromuscular facilitation patterns can be effective for the patient with limited voluntary control with its emphasis on normal synergistic patterns (e.g., D1 patterns), reversals of antagonists, and proprioceptive loading through light resistance.[124,125] Excellent resources for exercise and training for patients with stroke can be found in the works of Carr and Shepherd,[157] Davies,[158,159] and Howle.[160]

Strategies to Improve Upper Extremity Function

Patients with MCA syndrome may exhibit severe sensory, motor, and functional impairments of the UE with limited recovery. These patients benefit from early mobilization, ROM, and positioning strategies, previously discussed in this chapter. Compensatory training strategies and environmental adaptations should be considered to maximize function. For patients who achieve some recovery of voluntary movement, training strategies should focus on repetitive, task-specific practice. UE training activities should be closely coordinated with the occupational therapist.

UE Weight-Bearing as a Postural Support

Postural shift toward the more affected side with weight-bearing on the extended arm and stabilized hand on a support surface is an important early activity to promote proximal stabilization and counteract the effects of excess flexor hypertonus and a dominant flexion synergy. Approximation can be used to increase activity of shoulder/scapular stabilizers and tapping can facilitate the elbow extensors. Weight-bearing activities are performed in sitting (see Fig. 15.8), modified plantigrade (Fig. 15.10), and standing positions. Control should progress from holding to dynamic stabilization activities. For example, the patient stabilizes with the more affected UE while performing weight shifts and functional tasks with the stronger UE (e.g., reaching). As previously mentioned, the more affected UE should also be recruited for postural assistance during functional training activities (e.g., pushing up from side-lying into sitting).[161]

Task-Oriented Reaching and Manipulation

Patients with stroke have difficulty regaining control of scapular upward rotation and protraction, elbow extension, and wrist and finger extension necessary for forward reach and manipulation. Reaching and manipulation also requires accurate processing and use of visual–perceptual information. Patients with limited voluntary control can practice initial reaching in a supported position (e.g., side-lying with arm supported by therapist or on a powder board, sitting with the UE resting on a tabletop). The patient is encouraged to slide the hand forward over tabletop, recruiting shoulder flexors, scapular protractors, and elbow extensors. A cloth can be used to decrease friction effects as the patient practices wiping or polishing a table. The patient can also practice reaching forward and downward touching the floor. More advanced reaching activities include independent lifting and reaching forward (e.g., UE placed into a shirt sleeve), overhead, or sideward. A PNF D1 thrust pattern can

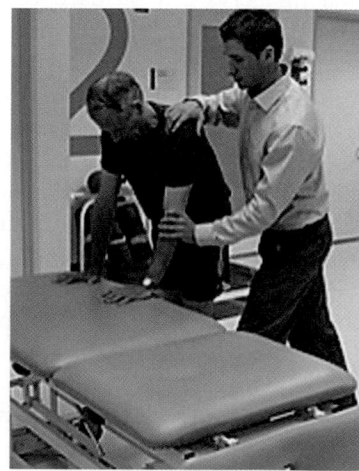

Figure 15.10 Standing in modified plantigrade, both UEs extended and weight-bearing; the therapist assists elbow extension of the hemiparetic UE while providing approximation through the shoulder.

be practiced (reverse thrust is contraindicated as the limb is moving into a flexion synergy pattern). Combining reaching with increased balance challenges in modified plantigrade or standing should also be incorporated. For example, the patient can practice pushing a ball side-to-side or forward-backward while standing in modified plantigrade (Fig. 15.11). Or in standing the patient can practice reaching to pick an object up off a shelf, a low stool, or the floor. Varying the height and distance reached, increasing the weight of objects held in the hand, or increasing the speed and accuracy requirements can increase difficulty. Substitution movements (e.g., trunk or head lateral movements) should not be allowed. Excessive shoulder elevation should also be discouraged.[161]

Meaningful task-oriented practice involving grasp and manipulation is important for stimulating recovery. Initial hand movements typically include gross grasp and release while advanced hand patterns (fine motor control) may not be present unless there is more advanced recovery. Voluntary release is generally much more difficult to achieve than voluntary grasp, and stretching/positioning and inhibitory techniques may be necessary to facilitate extension movements. Initial hand tasks can include using the more affected hand to stabilize (e.g., hand stabilizes paper while the stronger hand writes, hand stabilizes food while the stronger hand cuts) or holding a book with both hands for reading. The patient should be encouraged to use the weaker hand to assist in ADL (e.g., washing the upper body with a washcloth, bringing food to mouth). Forks, toothbrushes, and pens may need to have built-up handles for grasp. Task training should combine reach patterns with hand activity (e.g., picking sock off floor, reaching for an object off a shelf). Advanced hand activities include practice of wrist and finger extension, opposition, and manipulation of objects (e.g., using utensils to eat, drinking from a cup, writing, picking up and reorienting coins, paperclips, or other objects). Pronation often predominates while active supination without elbow and shoulder flexion is difficult to achieve. The therapist must observe movements carefully and assist in eliminating those aspects of movement patterns that interfere with effective and efficient control. Graded physical assist and use of mental practice/imagery techniques can be helpful to improve learning and performance.[157,161,162]

Constraint-Induced Movement Therapy

Constraint-induced movement therapy (CIMT) is a multifaceted intervention designed to promote increased use of the more affected UE. The patient is engaged in intense task-oriented practice of the more affected UE for up to 6 hours a day, performed on consecutive weekdays for 10 to 15 days (Fig. 15.12). The less affected UE is restrained from use by having the patient wear a safety mitt up to 90% of waking hours.[163] The therapist uses shaping techniques to modify and progress performance (e.g., an object is lifted and placed at increasing distances away from the patient). Feedback, coaching, modeling, and encouragement are provided during practice. Behavioral methods designed to ensure adherence to exercise and developing task-oriented behaviors include engaging the patient in:

- Self-monitoring of target behaviors (e.g., mode of activity, duration, frequency, perceived exertion, and overall response to activity)
- Problem-solving to identify obstacles and generate potential solutions

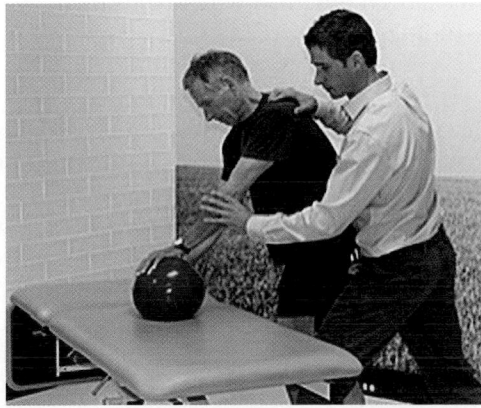

Figure 15.11 Standing in modified plantigrade with hemiparetic hand positioned on small ball; the patient practices rolling the ball from side-to-side; the therapist stabilizes the elbow and shoulder.

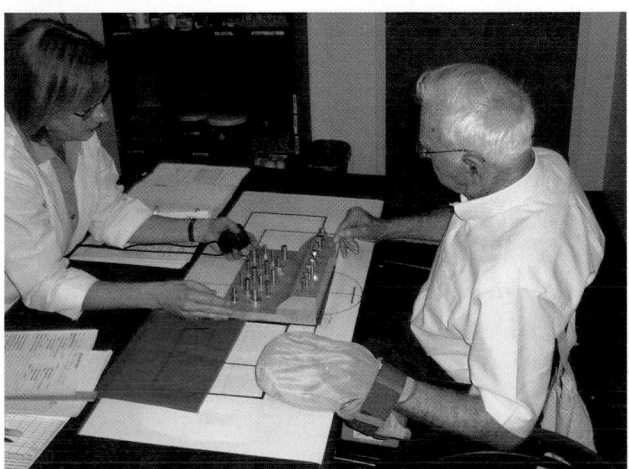

Figure 15.12 Constraint-induced movement therapy (CIMT). The patient practices a pegboard task using the hemiparetic hand while the less affected hand wears a mitt. The therapist times the activity while encouraging the patient.

- Behavioral contracting to engage the patient in carrying out behaviors throughout the day
- Social support strategies to educate and enlist caregivers in provident optimal support

The reader is referred to the work of Morris and Taub[164,165] for a more complete description of these techniques. *Modified CIMT* (mCIMT) has also been used for patients with stroke. For example, Page et al[166,167] used 30 minutes of functional task practice and shaping techniques 3 days per week, and restraint of the less affected UE for up to 5 hours per day. Training occurred over an extended 10-week period. This outpatient protocol increased the use and function of the more affected arm.[166,167]

Significant gains in motor function and a moderate reduction in disability following CIMT have been demonstrated in patients with stroke.[45,168,169] The *EXCITE trial* was a large prospective, single-blind, randomized, multisite study that included 222 patients after stroke. CIMT was compared to customary care and found to significantly improve outcomes as measured by the Wolf Motor Function test and the Motor Activity Log.[170] Associated changes in brain organization with CIMT have also been demonstrated on functional magnetic resonance imaging (fMRI), including an apparent shift in motor cortical activation toward other ipsilateral areas and the contralesional hemisphere.[171] Significant gains have also been reported in the patients receiving mCIMT.[165,166,172] It is important to note that patients were included in the studies if they had potential for recovery and some residual upper arm and hand movement (active wrist and finger extension) but tended not to use the arm. Limited pain or spasticity and absence of cognitive impairment were also inclusion criteria. Many early studies involved patients with chronic stroke (greater than 1 year). Evidence also exists for positive results with subacute stroke patients (less than 1 year)[170] and acute patients (less than 2 weeks after stroke).[173] The Cochrane researchers in their review of the literature concluded that evidence supporting maintained improvement from CIMT over 6 months is lacking.[45] The reader is referred to additional discussion in Chapter 10 and a summary of research findings presented in Box 10.1 Evidence Summary CIMT.

Simultaneous Bilateral Training

Simultaneous bilateral training involves using both arms simultaneously alone or in combination with augmented sensory feedback. Bilateral arm training with rhythmic auditory cueing (BATRAC) is an example of this intervention.[174] It is theorized that similar movement in the less affected extremity facilitates movement in the more affected extremity. Positive results have been reported in improving motor recovery after stroke.[174-176] When compared to usual or conventional care, simultaneous bilateral training was not shown to

be significantly better than other UE interventions in terms of improvements in ADL, arm or hand movements, or scores on motor impairment measures. The Cochrane reviewers cited lack of high-quality evidence in these findings.[47]

Electromyographic Biofeedback

Electromyographic biofeedback (EMG-BFB) has been used to improve motor function in patients following stroke. The technique allows patients to alter motor unit activity based on augmented audio and visual feedback information. Training can focus on voluntary inhibition of spastic muscles (e.g., reducing firing frequency of spastic finger flexors), or on increasing kinesthetic awareness and recruitment of motor units in weak, hypoactive muscles (e.g., wrist/forearm extensor muscles). Patients in late recovery for whom spontaneous recovery is more or less complete (greater than 6 months post-stroke) have demonstrated positive results that have been attributed to biofeedback therapy.[177,178] Reported benefits include improvements in ROM, voluntary control, and function. Researchers indicate that effectiveness of biofeedback neuromuscular reeducation is greatest when used as an adjunct to task-specific training.

Electrical Stimulation

Neuromuscular electrical stimulation (NMES) has been used with patients recovering from stroke to reduce spasticity, improve sensory awareness, prevent or reduce shoulder subluxation, and stimulate volitional movements.[179-182] NMES has been shown to increase the ability of muscle to exert force by preferentially activating the fast-contracting motor units. Effective treatment results have been reported for improving function in wrist extensors and the deltoid and supraspinatus muscles. In the latter example, glenohumeral alignment was improved and subluxation reduced. As with the biofeedback research, optimal results have been obtained when combined with task-specific training.[182]

Robot-Assisted Therapy

Robotic devices have been developed to assist the patient with moderate to severe motor impairments in improving UE function and recovery. They are used in conjunction with task-oriented training and motor learning principles. Robots work to restore lost motor function and can include pneumatic actuators (acting as muscles) to power the device or passive robotic systems using elastic bands or springs. Reach and grasp/release movements are typically targeted. These devices are used to augment therapist-patient interventions and enable high levels of intensive practice.[183] Limited evidence exists of treatment efficacy that can be generalized to arm and hand use during ADL. High cost of equipment limits widespread use in the clinical setting.[184]

Management of Shoulder Pain

Several causes of hemiplegic shoulder pain have been identified that can be broadly divided into flaccid and spastic presentations. In the flaccid stage, proprioceptive impairment, lack of tone, and muscle paralysis reduce the support and normal seating action of the rotator cuff muscles, particularly the supraspinatus. The ligaments and capsule thus become the shoulder's sole support. The normal orientation of the glenoid fossa is upward, outward, and forward, so that it keeps the superior capsule taut and stabilizes the humerus mechanically. In the absence of supporting musculature, any abduction or forward flexion of the humerus, or scapular depression and downward rotation, reduces this stabilization and causes the humerus to sublux. Initially the subluxation is not painful, but mechanical stresses resulting from traction and gravitational forces produce persistent malalignment and pain. Glenohumeral friction–compression stresses also occur between the humeral head and superior soft tissues during flexion or abduction movements in the absence of normal scapulohumeral rhythm (*shoulder impingement syndrome*). During the spastic stage, abnormal muscle tone may contribute to poor scapular position (depression, retraction, and downward rotation) and to subluxation and restricted movement. Secondary tightness in ligaments, tendons, and joint capsule can develop quickly. *Adhesive capsulitis* (intracapsular inflammation and "frozen shoulder") can occur. Poor handling and positioning of the more affected UE have been implicated in producing joint microtrauma and pain. Activities that traumatize the shoulder include PROM without adequate mobilization of the scapula (promoting normal scapulohumeral rhythm), traction or pulling on the UE during a transfer, or using reciprocal pulleys.[185-187] An incorrectly aligned joint can significantly impair the patient's ability to move. Additional interventions aimed at reducing subluxation can include NMES therapy, EMG biofeedback, taping, and slings.

Complex regional pain syndrome type 1 (CRPS-1), also known as shoulder-hand syndrome (SHS) or reflex sympathetic dystrophy, is caused by proximal trauma to the shoulder or neck or can occur with stroke and may be the result of autonomic nervous system (ANS) changes. Clinical factors associated with its development include motor deficits, spasticity, sensory deficits, and initial coma.[188] Early on, pain is intermittent and limited to the shoulder. During later stages pain is intense and involves the whole extremity. CRPS-1 is associated with a range of other symptoms. Stiffness and limitations in ROM occur. The wrist tends to assume a flexed position with intense pain likely during wrist extension movements.

The elbow is not typically involved. Early *stage 1* vasomotor changes include discoloration (pale pink or cool) and alterations in temperature. The skin may be hypersensitive to touch, pressure, or temperature variations. The patient typically guards against movement attempts. *Stage 2* is characterized by subsiding pain and early dystrophic changes: muscle and skin atrophy, vasospasm, hyperhidrosis (increased sweating), and coarse hair and nails. There is radiographic evidence of early osteoporosis. In *stage 3*, the atrophic phase, pain and vasomotor changes are rare. There is progressive atrophy of the skin, muscles, and bones (severe osteoporosis is evident). Pericapsular fibrosis and articular changes become pronounced. The hand typically becomes contracted in a clawed position with MP extension and IP flexion (similar to the intrinsic minus hand). There is marked atrophy of thenar and hypothenar muscles with flattening of the hand. Chances of reversal of signs and symptoms are high for stage 1 and variable for stage 2, whereas stage 3 changes are largely irreversible.[188]

Early diagnosis and identification of factors that cause CRPS is essential. Interventions are selected based on examination findings. Because of close daily contact with the patient, the physical therapist is frequently one of the first to recognize and report early signs and symptoms. A prevention protocol should be implemented.[189] In the flaccid stage, the arm should be supported at all times. Proper positioning and handling are essential. In bed, patients should be positioned so they cannot roll onto the more affected UE, compressing it. In supine and wheelchair sitting the scapula/shoulder should be supported with the arm forward in slight abduction and neutral rotation. During transfers and standing supportive devices should be considered to prevent traction injury (see section below). Interventions aimed at reducing pain and stiffness include appropriate PROM and mobilization techniques (gentle grade 1 to 2 mobilizations). PROM to the UE without scapular mobilization is *not* permitted. PROM of the shoulder should be limited to 90 degrees during flexion and abduction or to the point of pain, not beyond the pain position. The therapist needs to ensure that everyone involved in assisting the patient (e.g., family member, caregiver, nurses, and aides) has been instructed in proper handling/mobilization of the UE and recognizes the importance of avoiding trauma and traction injuries during PROM, transfers, and wheelchair activities. Active movements of the UE are encouraged to promote shoulder ROM (e.g., pushing away a tabletop therapy ball while standing). Interventions to manage edema are also a consideration. Additional considerations include no infusions into the veins of the hemiplegic hand. Persistent pain may be managed with oral analgesics or local injection techniques (corticosteroids). Repeat steroid injections are not recommended due to likely weakening of the rotator cuff. With intractable pain, surgical nerve blocks may be considered.[187]

Supportive Devices

A patient with hypotonia is at increased risk of shoulder *traction injury*. Slings can be used to prevent soft-tissue stretching (e.g., supraspinatus, capsular stretching) and relieve pressure on the neurovascular bundle (e.g., brachial plexus/brachial artery). They support the weight of the arm and protect the patient. They also free up the therapist to attend to postural/trunk control during functional activities. However, slings have a number of negative features. They do little to reduce subluxation or improve shoulder function, especially if scapular and trunk malalignment are not adequately addressed. Most slings have the additional negative feature of positioning the arm close to the body in adduction, internal rotation, and elbow flexion. With prolonged use, contractures and increased flexor tone may develop. Slings also contribute to body scheme disorders and body neglect. Prolonged use of slings blocks spontaneous use of the UE and contributes to learned nonuse. Slings may also block balance reactions involving the UE.

There are considerable differences in the effectiveness of the various types of slings. A pouch sling or single strap hemisling with two cuffs that support the elbow and wrist provides minimal mechanical support of the humerus. An alternate approach to the traditional sling is a humeral cuff sling. This device has an arm cuff on the distal humerus supported by a figure-eight harness. It provides humeral support with slight external rotation while allowing elbow extension, and may also provide some reduction of subluxation. This style of sling can be worn for longer periods because it does not restrict the elbow in a flexed position or limit distal function.[190-192]

Close collaboration with the occupational therapist is important in the appropriate selection and use of slings. Gillen[161] suggests the following guidelines:

- Therapists should minimize sling use during rehabilitation.
- Slings may be useful for initial transfer and gait training.
- Slings that position the UE in flexion are less desirable and should be used only for select upright activities and only for short time periods.
- No one sling is appropriate for all patients; selection and use should be carefully evaluated and sling effectiveness carefully reevaluated.
- Effective alternatives to use of a sling should be considered: humeral taping (strapping) to facilitate or inhibit musculature surrounding the scapula; NMES. The hand can also be positioned in a garment pocket.

The patient, family members, and caregivers should be instructed in and allowed to practice proper use of the support. As recovery progresses and spasticity and voluntary movement emerge, spontaneous reduction of shoulder subluxation may occur. Slings have no value at this point in recovery.

For patients using a wheelchair, an arm board or lap tray can provide support for the flaccid arm. A lateral elbow guard and/or straps may be necessary if the patient's arm slips off the side. Patients with decreased sensation are at risk for hand injury if the hand becomes stuck in the spokes of the wheelchair; elbow trauma can occur if the elbow slips off the side (e.g., the elbow hits as the patient is going through a doorway).

Strategies to Improve Lower Extremity Function

LE training activities essentially prepare the patient for the gait. This requires breaking up the obligatory synergy patterns. For example, during midstance hip and knee extensors need to be activated with hip abductors and dorsiflexors. Suggested activities include PNF LE D1 extension pattern; holding against elastic band resistance around the upper thighs in supine or standing positions; and standing, lateral side-steps. Hip adduction should be stressed during flexion movements of the hip and knee. Suggested activities include supine, PNF LE D1 flexion pattern; sitting, crossing, and uncrossing the more affected LE over the less affected; and standing step-ups. Hip extension with knee flexion is needed to allow for toe-off at the end of stance. Activities that can be used to promote knee flexion with hip extension include bridging (Fig. 15.13), supine hip extension with knee flexion over the side of the mat pushing down through the heel, or standing, unilateral heel rises. Pelvic control is important and can be promoted through lower trunk rotation (LTR) activities that emphasize forward pelvic rotation (protraction); post-stroke, the patient typically demonstrates a retracted and elevated pelvis. Lower trunk rotation can be practiced in

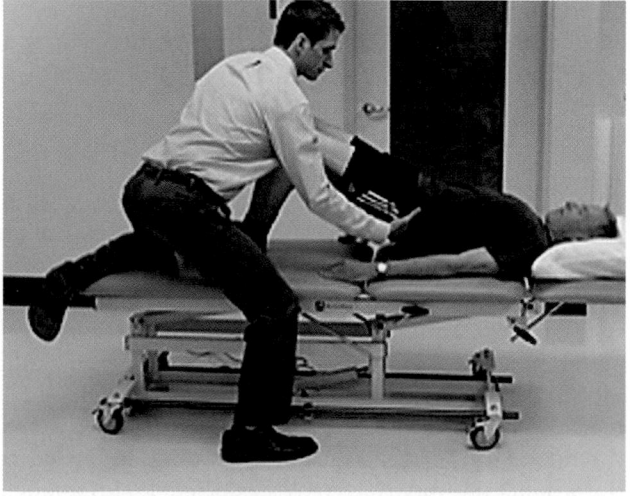

Figure 15.13 The patient practices bridging, combining hip extension with knee flexion; the therapist assists using tactile and proprioceptive cues to stimulate the hip extensors on the hemiparetic LE.

side-lying; supine, modified hook-lying; kneeling; or standing. Sitting on a therapy ball, pelvic shifting is another useful activity to promote pelvic control. Control of knee motions is often problematic; post-stroke, the patient with knee weakness typically exhibits hyperextension when standing. Reciprocal action (smooth reversals of flexion and extension movements) should be stressed early, beginning first in supine (e.g., foot slides in hook-lying), sitting (e.g., foot slides under the chair), partial sitting, or partial wall squats in standing.

An effective progression increases the challenge to the patient gradually by modifying postures while reducing synergy influence (e.g., hip abduction can be performed first in hook-lying, then supine, side-lying, modified plantigrade, and finally standing). Dorsiflexors can be activated in sitting by first having the patient hold and slowly let the forefoot move down, then pull the forefoot up. This simulates the functional expectations of the normal gait cycle as the foot goes from swing phase through stance. The sequence can then be repeated in standing, a much more difficult position in which to control dorsiflexors. Voluntary control of eversion is often the most difficult motion to achieve because these muscles do not function in either synergy. The application of stretch and resistance to these muscles during an activity that recruits dorsiflexors and evertors may be effective in initiating a response (e.g., in bridging, knee rocks side-to-side).

Interventions to Improve Functional Status

The loss of sensory and motor function on one side will present a tremendous challenge for the patient struggling to relearn postural control and functional mobility. Initial treatment strategies should focus on trunk symmetry and use of both sides of the body. Progression is from guided movements to active movements as soon as the patient is able to assume independent control. Suggested functional training activities include the following.

Bed Mobility

Rolling to both sides should be practiced; rolling onto the less affected side will prove more difficult. Extremity movement patterns (e.g., PNF D1 flexion of the LE) can be used to enhance the movement. Care must be taken to ensure the patient does not leave the more affected UE behind but rather brings it forward. This can be accomplished by having the patient clasp the hands together first. The more affected LE can be used to assist in rolling by pushing off from a flexed and adducted, hook-lying position (Fig. 15.14). Rolling onto the more affected side and into a side-lying–on–elbow position is important to promote early weight-bearing. This position also has the added benefit of elongating the lateral trunk flexors, which may be spastic.

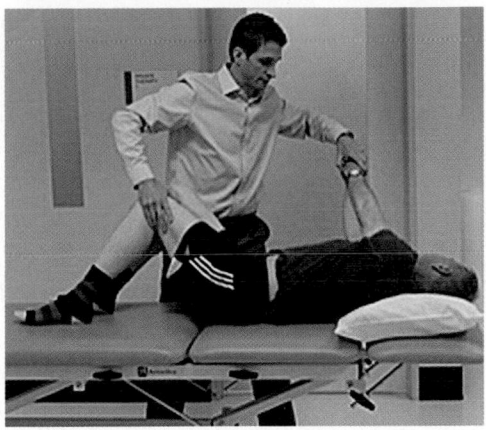

Figure 15.14 Early mobility activities: rolling onto the unaffected side. The therapist assists the movement through contacts on the knees and clasped hands.

The patient should practice moving from supine-to-sit leading from both sides, with an emphasis on rising with the more involved side leading (closest to the edge of bed or mat). The therapist can provide assistance from side-lying on the more affected side by shifting the LEs over the edge of the bed or mat while the patient pushes up into sitting using both UEs for support. Controlled lowering should also be practiced.

Bridging activities help develop trunk and hip extensor control important for use of a bedpan, pressure relief on the buttocks, initial bed mobility (scooting), and sit-to-stand transfers. It also develops advanced LE out-of-synergy control (hip extension with knee flexion) and stimulates early weight-bearing through the foot (see Fig. 15.13). Bridging activities include independent assumption of the posture, holding in the posture, and moving in the posture (lateral weight shifts, bridge-and-placing hips to one side). If the more affected LE is unable to hold in a hook-lying position, the therapist will need to assist by stabilizing the foot. Lifting the less affected foot off the surface (placing it on a small ball) while maintaining the pelvis level significantly increases the difficulty and can be used to increase demands on the more affected side. Difficulty can also be increased by varying the position of the UEs, from extended and abducted at the sides, to arms folded across the chest or hands clasped together overhead in a prayer position.

Sitting

Early training in sitting should focus on achieving a symmetrical posture with proper spine and pelvic alignment. The pelvis should be neutral, spine straight. Feet should be flat on the support surface. Typically, patients with stroke will sit asymmetrically with weight borne more on the less affected side, pelvis in a posterior tilt, and upper trunk flexed (kyphotic). Lateral flexion to the affected side is also common. The therapist can manually guide the patient into the correct sitting position and provide verbal and tactile cues. Early sitting can be assisted by having the patient use the UEs for bilateral support at sides or in front on tabletop, a large ball, or the therapist's shoulders with the therapist sitting directly in front of the patient. Sitting on a therapy ball can also be used to promote pelvic alignment and mobility (pelvic rotations) and trunk upright alignment (gentle bouncing). Sitting control should be progressed from first holding steady in the posture (stability) to moving in the posture (dynamic stability), and finally to dynamic challenges (reaching). A common problem with hemiplegia is the inability of the upper trunk to move independently of the lower trunk (dissociate). Upper trunk mobility with reciprocal flexion/extension, lateral flexion, and rotation movements should therefore be practiced. PNF lift/reverse patterns with the less involved arm leading can be used to promote upper trunk rotation and bilateral UE activity with the more involved arm moving out of synergy, and crossing the midline (important for unilateral neglect) (Fig. 15.15). Lateral weight shifts to the more affected side typically are the most difficult. Manual contacts in the direction of the movement combined with gentle resistance can provide important early learning cues. The patient should also practice scooting in sitting ("butt walking") to ensure mobility for dressing (putting pants on) and practice initial positioning for sit-to-stand transitions (coming to the edge of the seat to place the feet back and under the body).

Sit-to-Stand and Sit-Down Transfers

Sit-to-stand transfers should be practiced with a focus on symmetrical weight-bearing, coordinated muscular responses, and adequate timing. Initially the patient must actively flex the trunk and use momentum to shift the body mass forward (*flexion-momentum*

phase). The feet should be placed well back to allow ankle dorsiflexors to assist with forward rotation. The patient with stroke typically demonstrates decreased forward movement and momentum. The therapist should focus the patient's eyes on a visual target directly in front at eye level and use verbal cues to facilitate the desired movements ("move your shoulders forward and stand up"). The patient can be assisted in this phase by keeping both UEs forward with hands clasped together. Pushing off with both hands on the support surface is not effective in producing the forward weight shift and should be discouraged. The patient's movements must then be directed into the *extension phase,* which requires hip and knee extensors to produce vertical movement into the upright position. The therapist can provide tactile and proprioceptive cues to assist knee extension (Fig. 15.16). The height of the seat can be elevated at first to decrease the extensor force required. Progression is then to lower seat heights. Increased weight-bearing on the stronger LE can be achieved by varying the initial foot position, placing the stronger foot slightly behind the weaker foot. As the patient improves, the position of the feet can be reversed to focus attention on increased use of the weaker side. The patient with stroke typically accomplishes standing up very slowly. With repetitive practice, the patient should be encouraged to focus on increasing the speed of the movement and to not pause between the two phases. Using a prayer position (hands clasped together and held straight ahead with elbows extended) reduces UE push-off. The patient with stroke also demonstrates decreased control in sitting down owing to lack of eccentric control and will sit down abruptly after moving partially through the range.

Eccentric movements (small range movements) can be practiced with the patient positioned back against a

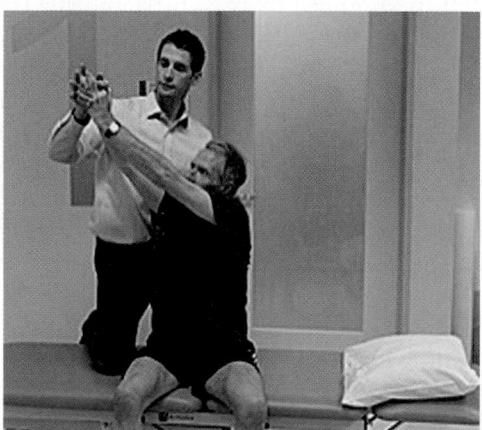

Figure 15.15 Sitting, patient practices PNF lift pattern (less affected UE leading). The pattern promotes upper trunk rotation, bilateral UE activity with the hemiparetic UE moving out of synergy, and crossing the midline.

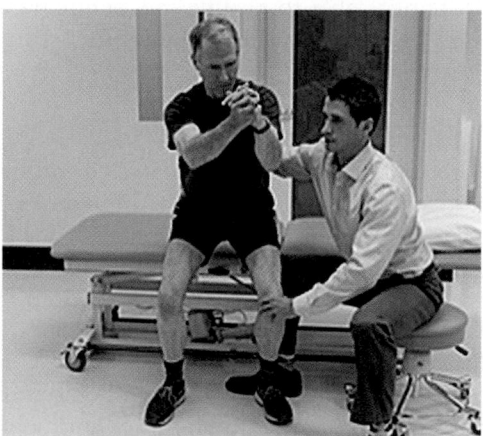

Figure 15.16 Sit-to-stand transitions. The therapist assists the patient in straightening the hemiparetic knee while bringing the center of mass forward. Hands are clasped together.

wall doing partial wall squats. Lower trunk rotation can be promoted by having the patient practice sit-to-stand using a platform mat. From standing, the patient shifts the pelvis laterally to the more affected side, and then sits down. By using this activity, the patient can move all the way around the mat alternating standing and controlled sitting, focusing on moving toward the weaker side.

Standing

Modified plantigrade is an ideal early standing posture to develop postural and extremity control. The more affected UE is extended and weight-bearing (an out-of-synergy posture), while the more affected LE is holding in extension (also an out-of-synergy pattern of hip flexion with knee extension). The forward trunk position creates an extension moment at the knee, thus assisting weak knee extensors. In addition, the posture has a wide (four-limb) BOS and is very stable (see Fig. 15.10). Progression should again be from holding in the posture to moving in the posture (weight shifts) to reaching tasks.

Initial upright standing can be enhanced using fingertip light touch-down support on a high table or wall. As soon as possible, the patient should be encouraged to practice standing with unilateral UE support (more affected side) and then free standing (no UE support). As in other postures, an appropriate progression includes first holding in the posture, to moving in the posture (weight shifts), and finally withstanding challenges to dynamic balance (e.g., reaching in all directions, stepping). The patient is instructed in proper symmetry and alignment. Gentle resistance can be applied to assist in holding, using the PNF technique of rhythmic stabilization. Weight shifts should incorporate moving forward-backward, side-to-side, and diagonally (incorporating upper trunk rotation). Lateral weight shifts to the more affected side are the most difficult. Manual contacts in the direction of the movement combined with gentle resistance can provide important early learning cues.

Transfers

During early transfers, the patient may require maximal assistance. Adjusting the hospital bed to the height of the chair or wheelchair will help to decrease the difficulty of the transfer. Staff often emphasize the sound side by placing the chair to that side and having the patient stand and pivot a quarter turn on the stronger LE before sitting down. Although this compensatory strategy promotes early transfers, it neglects the weaker side and may make subsequent training more difficult. The patient should be taught to transfer to both sides, with emphasis on moving toward the more affected side. Practice to both sides has functional significance, because most bathrooms are not large enough to allow positioning of the wheelchair on both sides of a tub or toilet. Also, the patient is not likely to be able to reposition the wheelchair once he or she transfers into bed so that a transfer toward the same side can be achieved when getting out of bed. When transferring, the patient's affected arm can be stabilized in extension and external rotation against the therapist's body. Alternatively, the patient's UEs (hands in prayer position) can be placed in front or to one side on the therapist's shoulders. The therapist can then assist by using manual contacts, either at the upper trunk or pelvis. The more affected LE may be stabilized by the therapist's knee exerting a counterforce on the patient's knee as needed. Transfer training should include practice in transferring to various different surfaces and heights (e.g., wheelchair, toilet, tub seat, car).

Functional training is begun early and continued throughout the course of rehabilitation. Training activities and postures are varied according to individual needs. Additional postures such as modified prone-on-elbows (tabletop weight-bearing), quadruped, side-sitting, kneeling, and half-kneeling may be appropriate and can be used to increase the level of difficulty and focus on specific body segments and deficiencies in control. Some postures may not be appropriate (e.g., prone-on-elbows for the patient with cardiorespiratory compromise or a flaccid, subluxed UE, or kneeling for the patient with osteoarthritis). Advanced functional training should include practice in getting down to and up from the floor in the event of a fall. See Improving Functional Outcomes in Physical Rehabilitation[150] for more complete descriptions and additional training activities.

Interventions to Improve Postural Control and Balance

Stroke results in significant changes in postural control and balance. Patients typically exhibit delayed, varied, or absent balance responses with impairments in latency, amplitude, and timing of muscle activity. Falls and fracture can occur and lead to a loss of confidence in balance and locomotor skills.[193] It is therefore important to proceed slowly in training and to select challenges appropriate for the patient's level of control. The goals of training are to progressively increase the level of difficulty (e.g., range and speed of self-initiated movements) while encouraging consistency, symmetry, and maximum use of the more affected side. Supportive devices such as a posterior leg splint, gait belt, or body-weight-support harness can be used to assist in early standing to instill confidence and prevent falls.

Once postural alignment and static stability is achieved in upright postures, the patient is ready for center-of-mass (COM) control training. In sitting and standing, the patient is instructed to explore his or her LOS through low-frequency weight shifting.

The patient learns how far in any one direction he or she can safely move and how to align the COM within the BOS to maintain upright stability. The therapist needs to stress symmetrical weight-bearing, as well as activities that promote shifting toward the more affected side. Weight-bearing on the more affected hip (sitting) and foot (standing) is encouraged while unnecessary activity of the less affected limbs (grabbing for support) is discouraged. The therapist increases the difficulty of the activity by manipulating the following:

- *Base of support:* Sitting, LEs uncrossed to crossed; standing, wide to narrow to tandem position; standing on one LE (beginning with less affected, progression to more affected LE)
- *Support surface:* Sitting on a mat to sitting on a therapy ball; standing on the floor to standing on dense foam
- *Sensory inputs:* Eyes open (EO) to eyes closed (EC); feet on firm surface or foam
- *UE position/support:* Light touch-down support; UEs extended out to the side to UEs folded across the chest
- *UE movements:* Single UE raises to bilateral UE raises (symmetrical, asymmetrical); reaching movements with emphasis to the more affected side; picking objects off table, stool, floor
- *LE movements:* Single LE support, stepping (forward-backward, side; step-ups); marching in place; foot on ball, moving ball
- *Trunk movements:* Head and trunk rotations; looking up at ceiling or down to floor
- *Destabilizing functional activities:* Sit-to-stand, sit-down, turning, floor-to-standing, lunges
- *Walking activities:* Forward, backward, sideward, crossed step
- *Dual-task training:* Standing while catching or kicking a ball; standing while talking; standing while holding a tray with a glass of water
- *Modifying environmental conditions:* Closed to open environments

Postural strategy training is an important component of intervention. Ankle strategies can be promoted through small range anterior-posterior shifts or by applying a small perturbation at the hips (forward-backward). Standing on a half-foam roller or wobble board also promotes ankle strategies, but may be too advanced for some patients during early rehabilitation. Hip strategies can be promoted through larger anterior-posterior shifts or stronger perturbations. Medial-lateral hip strategies are promoted by tandem stance (on floor or foam roller). Stepping strategies are promoted by increased displacements of the COM (e.g., forward, backward, or sideward leans that move the COM outside of the BOS). The therapist can apply an elastic band around the hips, offering resistance to the forward lean. Resistance that is quickly released once the patient achieves the desired lean will necessitate a step to control balance. Step-ups (small step to large; foam surface) should also be practiced.

The patient's full attention and concentration is required and should be directed toward completion of the task at hand. The therapist provides well-timed feedback to help the patient correct alignment and adjust postural control while minimizing hands-on support (only as needed). During balance training, the patient should be encouraged to actively problem solve. The patient is presented with challenges, identifies potential problems, and recruits safe strategies to maintain balance. Adaptability of skills needed for successful community reentry is promoted. Safety education about fall prevention is a critical factor in ensuring maintenance of the patient's hard-won functional independence.[194]

Research supports the effectiveness of balance training programs in improving balance ability for patients with stroke. Programs that demanded high frequency and duration had a high dropout rate for patients with acute stroke, largely due to medical reasons or fatigue. A reasonable exercise prescription for this group might include a frequency of 5 sessions per week for 45 to 60 minutes per session. For patients with subacute and chronic stroke, more intense individualized programs are possible. A combination of interventions that focused on static and dynamic balance was most often used. Both one-on-one training and group programs have produced positive results. Finally, there is limited evidence that balance performance may deteriorate once the intervention is stopped.[195,196]

Force Platform Biofeedback

Force platform biofeedback (center-of-pressure biofeedback) provided to the patient while standing on a computerized forceplate system can be used to improve balance. The patient practices voluntary movement shifts in response to computer generated visual feedback. Patients can also practice responding to unexpected platform tilts (perturbations) in order to improve reactive balance control. A safety harness may be required during early training; holding on with one or both hands is discouraged.

Improvements with biofeedback/forceplate training have been found in steadiness (reduced sway),[197,198] postural symmetry,[197,198] and dynamic stability.[198-200] Evidence is stronger and more consistent for the latter two parameters than for changes in steadiness.[201] There is limited evidence of carryover of improved balance during functional skills, specifically transfer skills and endurance,[200] functional reach,[202] and measures of ADL and mobility.[198] Carryover to improved locomotor performance has not been demonstrated.[197,200] Failure to find significant correlations to gait is most likely related to specificity of training, specifically a dissimilarity between training mode and outcome measure. Studies comparing conventional balance training with biofeedback/forceplate training based on improvements on functional balance measures (Berg Balance Scale, Timed Up and Go) have failed to show any significant differences between the training modes; both interventions were effective in improving balance.[203,204]

The Patient with Ipsilateral Pushing (Pusher Syndrome)

The patient with ipsilateral pushing presents with an entirely different set of postural control and balance problems. The patient sits or stands asymmetrically, but with most of the weight shifted toward the weaker side. The patient uses the stronger UE or LE to push over to the weaker side, often resulting in instability and falls. Efforts by the therapist to passively correct the patient's tilted posture often result in the patient pushing stronger. Training needs to emphasize upright positions with *active* movement shifts toward the stronger side. Use of visual stimuli is effective as patients retain the ability to correct posture with such stimuli but may not be able to do so spontaneously. Patients should be asked to look at their posture and see if they are upright. Environmental prompts can be used to assist orientation. These can include use of a mirror if visuospatial deficits are not present or vertical structures in the environment. For example, the therapist can sit on the patient's less involved side and instruct the patient to "lean over to me." Or the patient can be positioned with the stronger side next to a wall and instructed to "lean toward the wall."[95] Therapists can provide verbal and tactile cues for postural orientation. To improve sitting posture, training activities can include sitting on a therapy ball to promote symmetry and sitting. In early standing the weaker LE is often flexed and has difficulty supporting the body on that side. Extension can be assisted by the use of an air splint or a posterior leg splint or by direct tapping over the quadriceps muscle. The modified plantigrade position is effective for early supported standing; however, the therapist should focus on unilateral support using the weaker UE. Again, an air splint can be used to assist extension of the weaker arm. If a cane is used, it can be shortened to encourage weight shift to the stronger side. An environmental boundary can be used to achieve symmetrical standing (e.g., standing in a doorway or corner standing). It is important to limit pushing with the sound extremities. For example, in sitting or standing, the therapist should block the stronger limb from drifting laterally into abduction and extension and pushing.[205,206] During wheelchair sitting, the patient should be assisted to maintain upright posture and midline orientation. Motor learning strategies are very effective in reducing the effects of this disorder and enhancing recovery. In particular, the therapist should

demonstrate correct orientation to vertical, provide consistent feedback about body orientation, and practice correct orientation and weight shifts. The patient should be fully involved in problem solving. For example, the therapist should ask questions such as "what direction are you tilted?" and "what direction do you have to move in order to achieve vertical?" Karnath et al[93] indicate that the prognosis for recovery is good with effective training.

Interventions to Improve Gait and Locomotion

Task-Specific Overground Locomotor Training

An accurate analysis of a patient's walking pattern is critical to planning effective interventions (see Box 15.5). These abnormalities arise as a result of impairments in flexibility, strength, movement control, coordination, and balance. Critical areas of stance phase control that will need to be addressed include initial weight acceptance, midstance control, and forward weight advancement during stance on the more involved limb. During swing, control of knee and foot for toe clearance and foot placement are key requirements (Fig. 15.17). Finally, persistent posturing of the UE in flexion and adduction during gait should be addressed. This latter problem can be effectively controlled through positioning the hemiplegic UE in extension and abduction with the hand open.

Task-specific overground locomotor training (LT) focuses on practicing a variety of activities and on improving the quality of walking and walking endurance. Appropriate stretching, particularly of the calf muscles, and strengthening exercises for LE muscles are important preparatory interventions. Parallel bars and ambulation aids (e.g., walkers, hemiwalkers, quad

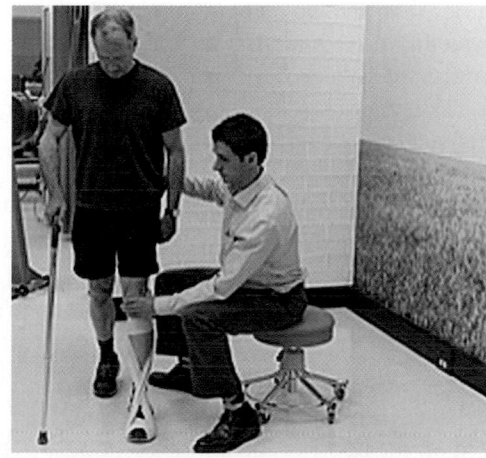

Figure 15.17 Assisted overground gait training. The therapist provides assistance in stabilizing the hemiparetic knee and weight transfer onto the more affected side.

canes) can assist in early gait stability and safety. However, prolonged use of these devices can be problematic for a patient who has the potential to walk without the device. There is increased loading on UEs and the stronger LE. With prolonged use, the patient also fails to develop appropriate balance mechanisms while asymmetry is promoted. There is an excessive weight shift toward the less affected side with the use of a hemi-walker or quad cane. Prolonged use of a walker encourages a forward trunk position with maximum loading on the UEs. Gait is typically slower with assistive devices and overall locomotor rhythm is impaired. It is important to progress patients as quickly as possible to the least restrictive device and to no device whenever possible. Gait practice with an overhead harness and partial body weight support provides the least interference with early balance and walking activities.

The patient should practice functional, task-specific skills, including the following:

- Walking forward: Focus is on moving out of synergy by combining hip and knee extension with hip abduction (scissoring is common).
- Walking backward: Focus is on moving out of synergy by combining hip extensors with knee flexors.
- Side stepping: Focus is on moving out of synergy by combining hip abductors with hip and knee extensors.
- Crossed stepping: The PNF activity of braiding combines side-stepping and cross-stepping.
- Step-up/step-down activities; lateral step-ups.
- Stair climbing, step-over-step.
- Walking in a simulated home environment: Through doorways, over and around obstacles, stairs in/out of the home.
- Walking in a community environment: Walking on ramps, curbs, uneven terrain, over and around obstacles.
- Activities that involve coincident timing: Crossing at a streetlight; stepping on and off elevators or escalators; walking through automatic doors.
- Dual-task activities: Walking while holding a ball, bouncing a ball, carrying a tray, carrying on a conversation.
- Balance activities: Tandem walking on a line, walking on/off foam.

Initially walking will be slow and deliberate. As control develops, the patient is encouraged to improve rhythm and speed of walking. Even steps can be facilitated by the use of real-time, rhythmic auditory cues (e.g., verbal cues, clapping, metronome) and foot markers placed on the floor. Progression is to longer steps and to increased overall distances with faster speeds. The patient should also practice walking in varying complex environments. This encourages the development of the patient's skills to adapt walking as needed (e.g., vary speeds, direction, navigate changing support surface). Timing and reciprocity of LE movements can be improved with the use of a motorized treadmill, cycle ergometer, and Kinetron® isokinetic training. Functional practice in real-life environments will assist the patient in developing the confidence needed for meeting the demands of community reentry.

A Cochrane Systematic Review of research on overground LT for individuals with chronic stroke included nine studies involving 499 participants. Results were mixed. Improvements in walking speed and functional performance (Timed Up and Go Test, 6-Minute Walk Test) were found in some studies. Overall, the researchers felt there was insufficient evidence to determine the benefits on broad measures of walking function. Again, lack of high-quality research (RCTs) was cited.[207] Limited data exist with subacute stroke patients.

Locomotor Training using Body Weight Support and Motorized Treadmill Training

While locomotor control is distributed across discrete regions of the CNS, walking is primarily a brainstem and spinal cord function. For example, locomotor central pattern generators (CPGs) have been identified as existing in the ventral spinal cord while integrating command centers have been identified in the medial medullary reticular formation. Thus, patients with cortical stroke may be able to regain the ability to walk. The CNS is responsive to training-induced plastic changes in locomotor function and recovery. Thus, patients with limited recovery who lack voluntary isolated control can still be trained to walk. Although sensation is normally used for walking, patients can also learn to walk with limited sensation.

Body weight support (BWS) and motorized treadmill training (TT) allows the clinician to improve recovery of walking ability after stroke using intensive task-oriented training. Normal kinematics and phase relationships of the full gait cycle are promoted, including limb loading in midstance and unweighting and stepping during swing. Initially, manual assistance can be provided by trainers to normalize gait in the presence of muscle weakness and impaired balance. For example, one therapist provides manual assistance to foot placement during stepping movements of the weaker LE while a second therapist stands behind the patient and provides manual assistance to pelvic rotation movements (Fig. 15.18). An overhead harness is used to support a portion of the patient's weight (e.g., 30% progressing down to 20%, and 10%). The harness controls the upright position of the patient in the absence of good postural stability and reduces fear of falling. The use of a harness also eliminates the need for adaptive UE support to compensate for LE weakness (e.g., as seen with the use of a walker).

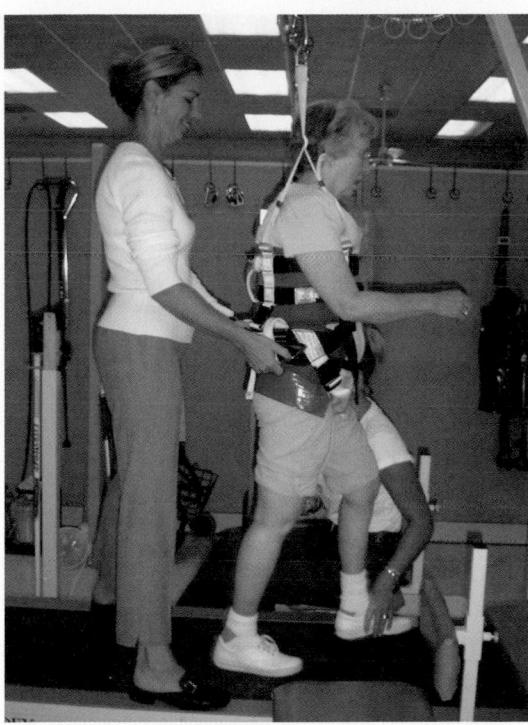

Figure 15.18 Locomotor training using body weight support and a motorized treadmill. One therapist manually assists pelvic motions while a second therapist assists stepping of the hemiparetic left LE.

As improvements in walking occur, the harness is removed and full weight-bearing is allowed. At this point, the patient is practicing supervised walking on a treadmill. Initially the treadmill speeds are slow (e.g., 0.52 mph [0.23 m/sec]) and are gradually increased as the patient's walking ability is improved (e.g., 0.95 mph [0.42 m/sec]).[101] Progression is to task-specific practice and overground walking. See Chapter 11, Locomotor Training, for additional discussion.

Treadmill training and BWS is a relatively safe task-oriented LT activity that has been extensively studied in patients recovering from stroke.[208-223] In a Cochrane Systematic Review,[49] the researchers identified 15 high-quality trials with 622 post-stroke participants. They concluded that there were no significant statistical differences between TT, with or without BWS, and other physiotherapy interventions on outcomes of walking dependency, speed, and endurance. For people who were independent walkers at the start of treatment, higher walking speeds were evident, though not significantly so. Patients with stroke who were dependent in walking at the start of treatment may benefit from TT with BWS, though data were limited to support this conclusion. Serious adverse events were uncommon. Individual studies have reported improvements in walking speed,[211-215,222] distance,[211,215,216] endurance,[211,218,219] and walking function.[211] Treadmill training is a safe intervention for

patients with acute and subacute stroke,[208,209,216-218,221] as well as for chronic stroke[210-212, 219] (see Box 15.9 Evidence Summary).

The *Locomotor Experience Applied Post-Stroke (LEAPS)* trial was a large, multicenter randomized controlled trial.[223,224] Four hundred eight participants were recruited from six inpatient rehabilitation centers and stratified according to walking impairment. Those with moderate impairment were able to walk 0.4 to less than 0.8 m per second while those in the severe group were able to walk less than 0.4 m per second. Participants were randomly assigned to one of three treatment groups: (1) early locomotor training using BWS TT 2 months after stroke, (2) late locomotor training using BWS TT 6 months after stroke, and (3) home exercise using therapist-directed exercise training 2 months after stroke. The latter group received exercises designed to improve flexibility, strength, coordination, and balance along with encouragement for daily walking. Each intervention had similar intensity and duration (36 sessions of 90 minutes each for 12 to 16 weeks). The researchers found that all participants increased in their functional walking ability. No significant differences were found between the groups in terms of improvements in walking speed, motor recovery, balance, functional status, and quality of life. Outcomes of participants in the early and late locomotor training (LT) groups also revealed no significant differences at 1 year. The researchers concluded that early intervention may accelerate gains in walking ability after stroke. The research reviewed supports the benefits of physical therapy in improving walking outcomes. There is no clear evidence of the superiority of one type of intervention over another.

Robotic-Assisted Locomotor Training

Electromechanical, robotic-assisted LT is used in rehabilitation to improve walking after stroke. In a Cochrane Systematic Database review, Mehrholz et al[54] reviewed 17 trials involving 837 participants. When combined with conventional physiotherapy, these devices were found to increase the odds of patients becoming independent walkers. Increases in gait speed or walking capacity were not found. Study differences were noted in variations of (1) initial level of patient independence in walking, (2) duration and frequency of treatment, and (3) use of electrical stimulation used in some devices. In a systematic review of 16 studies that included a total of 558 patients, Tefertiller et al found that no studies demonstrated a significantly improved functional ambulatory capacity with conventional LT or TT with BWS and manual assistance versus TT with BWS and robotic assistance.[225] Lewek et al[226] found that therapist-assisted LT when compared to robotic-assisted LT resulted in significant improvements in coordination of intralimb kinematics, lending support to the value of

Box 15.9 Evidence Summary   Post-Stroke Locomotor Training Using Body Weight Support and Motorized Treadmill Training

Reference	Subjects	Design/Intervention	Duration	Results	Comments
Richards et al[209] (1993)	27 subjects	RCT; compared early task-based PT (standing, weight-shifting, and Kinetron exercises; TT), 1.74 hr/day with conventional PT intervention groups (1.79 hr/day and 0.73 hr/day) Outcome measures: FMA, BI, BBS, gait velocity at 6-month follow-up	Daily	Significant improvement in gait velocity for task-based PT group	Small sample size One of the pioneering early studies
Visintin et al[211] (1998)	100 subjects postacute phase	RCT; TT: compared BWS (BWSTT) with no-BWS (no-BWSTT) Outcome measures: balance (BBS); motor recovery (STREAM); OG walking speed and endurance	4/wk for 6 wk	BWSTT group demonstrated significant improvement over no-BWSTT in balance, motor recovery, and OG walking speed and endurance	79% BWSTT group progressed to full weight-bearing OG walking; improvements were sustained; good sample size; one of the pioneering early studies
Nilsson et al[213] (2001)	60 subjects postacute stage	RCT; compared walking using BWSTT with OG walking training (motor relearning approach) Outcome measures: FIM, FMA, FAC, 10-m walk test, and BBS	30 min/day, 5/wk for 2 months	Both groups improved on function (FIM, FAC), balance (BBS), and walking speed	10-month follow-up Good sample size
Sullivan et al[215] (2002)	24 subjects with chronic stroke	Nonrandomized cohort design Intervention program: BWSTT, 3 groups of varying speeds (slow speeds 0.22 m/sec; variable speeds 0.22 m/sec to 0.89 m/sec; fast speeds greater than 0.89 m/sec) Outcome measures: FMA, 10-m walk; self-selected walking speed OG	12 sessions, 20-min duration, over 4–5 wk	Training at fast speeds was more effective at improving speeds of OG walking than training at slow or variable speeds	No control group Gains maintained at 3 months Small sample size
Dean et al[218] (2010) (the *MOBILIZE trial*)	12 subjects, within 4 weeks of stroke, undergoing inpatient rehab, unable to walk	RCT 2 groups: (1) BWSTT, (2) OG walking	30 min/day	At 6 months, no difference between indep walkers from both groups in terms of speed or stride; indep walkers in BWSTT group walked 57 m further (6-Minute Walk Test) and rated their walking 1 point (out of 10) higher than OG group	BWSTT is safe and feasible for patient with subacute stroke; supports better walking capacity and perception of walking compared to OG walking

Box 15.9 Evidence Summary Post-Stroke Locomotor Training Using Body Weight Support and Motorized Treadmill Training—cont'd

Reference	Subjects	Design/ Intervention	Duration	Results	Comments
Sullivan et al[222] (2007) (the *STEPS trial*)	80 subjects, ambulatory; 4 mo–5 yr post-stroke	RCT; 4 groups of combined interventions: (1) BWSTT with UE ergometry (BWSTT/UE-EX), (2) leg cycle ergometry with UE-EX (CYCLE/UE-EX), (3) BWSTT with leg cycling (BWSTT/CYCLE), and (4) BWSTT with LE progressive resistive exercise (BWSTT/LE-EX)	Exercise sessions were 4/wk for 6 wk (24 total sessions) Outcome measures: self-selected and fast walking speeds, 6-Minute Walk Test	The BWSTT/UE-EX group had significantly greater increases in walking speed compared to CYCLE/UE-EX group; both groups improved walking distance; all BWSTT groups increased walking speed and distance	Task-specific BWSTT was more effective in improving walking speed and maintaining gains at 6 mo than leg cycling (CYCLE/UE-EX) LE strength training alternated daily with BWSTT (BWSTT/LE-EX) did not provide an added benefit
Moseley et al[49] (2009) (*Cochrane Database Systematic Review*)	15 high-quality studies, 622 subjects	Meta-analysis of LT studies Outcomes: walking dependency, speed, and endurance	Variable by study	No significant statistical differences between TT, with or without BWS, and other physiotherapy interventions on outcomes; indep walkers at start of treatment tended to develop higher walking speeds; dep walkers at start of treatment may benefit from BWS; few adverse events reported	Physiotherapy, both BWSTT and conventional LT, were effective in improving walking function in patients post-stroke
Franceschini et al[221] (2009)	97 subjects, within 6 weeks of stroke onset	RCT; 2 intervention groups: (1) conventional rehab plus BWSTT, (2) conventional rehab plus OG gait training Outcome measures = Motricity Index, Trunk Control Test, Barthel Index, Functional Ambulation Categories, 10-Meter and 6-Minute Walk Tests, Walking Handicap Scale	60-min sessions every weekday for 4 weeks	After treatment, all patients were able to walk Both groups showed significant improvement on all outcome measures	In subacute patients, BWSTT is as feasible and effective as conventional gait training
Lewek et al[227] (2009)	19 subjects with chronic stroke (> 6 mo)	RCT; comparing therapist-assisted versus robotic-assisted LT Outcome measures: gait analysis (kinematic coordination), self-selected speed during OG walking	4 wk of LT, 3 sessions of LT per week for 4 weeks	LT with therapist assistance resulted in significant improvements in consistency of intralimb movements of the impaired limb	Providing consistent (fixed) kinematic assistance during robotic-assisted LT did not result in improvements in intralimb consistency Small sample size

Continued

Box 15.9 Evidence Summary Post-Stroke Locomotor Training Using Body Weight Support and Motorized Treadmill Training—cont'd

Reference	Subjects	Design/Intervention	Duration	Results	Comments
Duncan et al[224] (2011) (the *LEAPS trial*)	408 subjects with stroke (2 months; stratified into 2 groups: (1) moderate impairment (able to walk 0.4 to (0.8 m/sec); and (2) severe impairment (able to walk (0.4 m/sec)	RCT; 3 intervention groups: (1) BWSTT 2 mo after stroke (early LT), (2) BWSTT 6 mo after stroke (late LT), and (3) home-based exercise program Outcome measure: proportion of participants with improvement in walking ability at 1 yr (walking speed, motor recovery, balance, functional status, and quality of life)	36 sessions of 90 min each for 12–16 wk	52% of all participants improved in walking ability; no significant differences between groups in terms of walking function; multiple falls were more common in severe impairment group receiving early LT	LT using BWSTT was *not* found superior to progressive exercise at home managed by a physical therapist

BBS = Berg Balance Scale; BI = Barthel Index; BWS = body weight support using an overhead harness; dep = dependent; FAC = Functional Ambulation Category; FIM = Functional Independence Measure; FMA = Fugl-Meyer Assessment of Physical Performance; indep = independent; LT = locomotor training; mAS = Modified Ashworth Scale; MCA = middle cerebral artery syndrome; OG = overground; PT = physical therapy; RCT = randomized controlled trial; rehab = rehabilitation; STREAM = Stroke Rehabilitation Assessment of Movement; TT = treadmill training.

variable practice versus constant practice. In a systematic review of studies recruiting nonambulatory patients early after stroke (6 studies involving 549 participants), Ada et al[227] found that mechanically assisted LT with BWS resulted in more people walking independently at 4 weeks and at 6 months.

Functional Electrical Stimulation

Functional Electrical Stimulation (FES) can be used to stimulate dorsiflexor function and improve the gait pattern of patients with drop foot. Sufficient strength in the quadriceps muscle is needed to prevent the knee from buckling. This requirement limits the number of patients who can successfully use the device. The patient wears a small, lightweight cuff that fits just below the knee. Electrodes are positioned to stimulate the anterior tibialis and the peroneus longus muscles. A gait sensor attaches to the patients shoe and transmits a wireless signal to the stimulator. The level of stimulation can be adjusted by a handheld remote control, which also allows the patient to turn the device off and on. The device can be used as a bridge to the recovery of normal motor function or, in the absence of recovery, can be used indefinitely. FES training should be paired with a comprehensive physical therapy POC. In a systematic review of the literature (30 studies), Roche et al[228] reported that FES had a significant positive effect on gait with improvements noted in gait speed and physiological cost index (PCI) in patients with chronic stroke. FES is theorized to have a positive effect on brain plasticity with its provision of high-level sensory-motor input into

the CNS.[229] This may explain research findings of improved gait function with FES when compared to orthotic intervention.[230]

Orthotics and Assistive Devices

An orthosis may be required when persistent problems prevent safe ambulation (e.g., inadequate ankle dorsiflexion during swing, mediolateral ankle instability, and insufficient push-off during late stance). Prescription will depend on the unique problems each patient presents. The pattern of instability and weakness at the ankle and knee and the extent and severity of spasticity and sensory deficits of the limb are major considerations when prescribing an orthosis. Temporary devices (e.g., dorsiflexor assists) may be used during the early stages while recovery is proceeding to allow the patient to practice standing and walking. Use of a temporary orthosis also provides insight into the type of components that will most effectively address the patient's needs. Permanent devices are prescribed once the patient's status stabilizes. Consultation with a certified orthotist and clinic team is initiated if a permanent orthosis is needed.

- *Foot-Ankle Controls.* An *ankle-foot orthosis* (AFO) is commonly prescribed to control impaired ankle/foot function. These may include a custom-molded polypropylene AFO (*posterior leaf spring, modified AFO, or solid ankle AFO*), or *conventional double upright/dual channel AFO*. The least restrictive AFO is the posterior leaf spring (PLS) used to control drop foot. An AFO of higher-density plastic that covers more surface area can provide additional control of calcaneal and forefoot inversion and eversion. A solid ankle molded AFO provides maximum stabilization through its lateral trim lines that project more anteriorly. Movement in all planes (dorsiflexion, plantarflexion, inversion, and eversion) is limited. The conventional double upright metal AFO may be indicated for patients who cannot tolerate plastic AFOs owing to sensory impairments, girth fluctuations, or diabetic neuropathy, or who require additional controls. A posterior stop can be added to limit plantarflexion while a spring assist can be added to assist dorsiflexion (Klenzak joint). Advantages of a conventional AFO include better stabilization of the ankle, allowing improved heel-strike and push-off.[231] Disadvantages include heavier weight, less cosmetic appearance, and increased difficulty donning and doffing.

- *Knee Controls.* Knee instability following stroke can be controlled with an AFO by adjusting the position of the ankle. An ankle set in 5° dorsiflexion limits knee hyperextension, while an ankle set in 5° plantarflexion decreases the flexor moment and stabilizes the knee during midstance. A patient with knee hyperextension without foot and/or ankle instability may benefit from the application of a *Swedish Knee Cage* or strapping to protect the knee. Extensive bracing using a knee-ankle-foot orthosis (KAFO) is rarely indicated or successful. The added weight and restrictions in normal knee joint motion significantly increase energy costs and limit independent function.

The need for an orthosis or a particular type of orthosis may change with continuing recovery. The therapist may need to recommend a change in prescription or discontinuing the use of a device. With limited reimbursements, ordering a new orthosis may prove problematic and speaks to the need to anticipate changes when ordering the initial device. For example, a good option for the patient who needs a custom-molded solid AFO is to order a hinged AFO with a plantarflexion stop. As the patient regains sufficient knee and dorsiflexor control, the device can be adjusted to remove the stop and allow the hinges to work. Orthotic training includes donning and doffing, skin inspections, and education in safe use of the device during gait. See Chapter 30, Orthotics, for a more complete description of orthotic devices, examination, and training.

Wheelchairs

Most patients require the use of a wheelchair for mobility at some point during their recovery. Patients with stroke exhibit typical postural asymmetries, which need to be carefully evaluated. These include the following:

- Trunk laterally flexed to the weaker side; head may also be flexed to the weaker side.

- Pelvic posterior tilt with some obliquity (lower on the unaffected side).
- LE rolled out into abduction and external rotation; if spasticity is present, increased hip extension, adduction, and internal rotation with knee extension may occur; foot is typically plantarflexed and inverted.
- UE held flexed and adducted to the trunk with increased elbow, wrist, and finger flexion. With flaccidity, the shoulder is subluxed with the hand dangling in a dependent position.

Positioning in a wheelchair needs to correct for these postural asymmetries and ensure correct sitting posture. The reader is referred to Chapter 32, The Prescriptive Wheelchair, for a more complete discussion of general principles of prescription and wheelchair adaptations.

A patient with stroke can learn to propel a wheelchair using the stronger UE and LE. The seat-to-floor height is critical in ensuring successful use of the foot for steering and propulsion. A *hemi-height wheelchair* with a lower seat-to-floor height (17.5 in [44.45 cm]) may be required. A standard wheelchair has a seat-to-floor height of 19.5 in (49.53 cm). One-arm drive chairs in which both handrims are placed on one wheel were designed for individuals with only one functional UE. The patient with stroke is rarely successful in using this type of chair because it takes a great deal of strength and coordination to propel the wheelchair in a forward direction. It is contraindicated in patients with significant perceptual and cognitive impairments. A power wheelchair may be required for some individuals who cannot successfully use a manual wheelchair and will depend on a wheelchair as their primary means of locomotion. The therapist needs to consider individual needs and reimbursement policies when ordering a wheelchair. It is important to balance both present and future needs as providers restrict frequent reordering of a new wheelchair. It is also important to remember that prolonged used of a wheelchair contributes to learned nonuse and may limit recovery, especially if walking is a primary goal of therapy. Wheelchair training activities include patient and caregiver instruction in the use, maintenance, and safety of all parts of the wheelchair (e.g., brakes, leg rests, removable armrests). The patient needs to be instructed in methods of propulsion and given the opportunity to practice on level and varied surfaces (e.g., ramps, outdoor terrain). Transfers (to and from bed, toilet, tub, car) should also be practiced once the patient receives the prescriptive wheelchair.

Interventions to Improve Aerobic Capacity and Endurance

Patients with stroke demonstrate decreased levels of physical conditioning following periods of prolonged immobility and reduced activity. The energy costs to complete many functional tasks are higher than normal owing to the abnormal ways in which the activities are performed. Many patients also demonstrate concomitant cardiovascular disease and may experience hypertension, serious dysrhythmias, and volitional fatigue. Patients with stroke require careful determination of cardiopulmonary responses during exercise and appropriate monitoring.

Individuals recovering from stroke can benefit from endurance (aerobic) training to improve cardiovascular function. During the early acute stages, functional activity training is appropriate (e.g., overground walking). During the postacute stage, patients/clients may be able to engage in more traditional exercise training modes such as treadmill walking, cycle ergometry (upper and lower body ergometer), or seated stepper. Patients with balance impairments will benefit from treadmill training or overground walking with a safety harness, or a recumbent cycle ergometer. To ensure safety, patients should receive a thorough examination and supervised exercise test before starting a training program (e.g., symptom-limited graded exercise test). Prescriptive elements include mode (type of exercise), frequency, intensity, and duration (see Chapter 13, Heart Disease). Choice of training mode depends on the individual's abilities and interests. Intensities are typically in the range of 40% to 70% of maximal oxygen uptake. Suggested frequency is three to five days per week for 20 to 60 minutes per session. Frequency may be increased to daily if lower intensities are used. Because of the level of deconditioning, patients with stroke should begin with intermittent training protocols but can be progressed to 30 minutes of continuous exercise. The use of a training log or exercise diary is an excellent way to help the patient keep track of prescriptive elements, objective measurements (heart rate, BP), and subjective reactions (RPE, perceived enjoyment). Adequate supervision, monitoring, and safety education about warning signs for impending stroke and heart attack are critical components.[24,232]

Exercise Precautions

Careful monitoring of exercise is essential. For patients at risk, BP, heart rate (HR), and RPE should be taken initially, during, and after each exercise. As exercise progresses, less frequent monitoring can be implemented. The therapist also needs to monitor breathing rate and pattern, ensuring breath holding and Valsalva do not occur. Patients should be instructed in how to measure their own HR and RPE. They should also be taught the warning signs for when to stop exercising. These include the following:

- Lightheadedness or dizziness
- Chest heaviness, pain, or tightness; angina
- Palpitations or irregular heart beat
- Sudden shortness of breath not due to increased activity
- Volitional fatigue and exhaustion

Patients who are on medications that limit cardiac output (e.g., beta-blockers) will demonstrate reduced HR responses and lower peak HRs. Patients taking diuretics to reduce fluid volume may demonstrate altered electrolyte balance with resulting dysrhythmias. Patients taking vasodilators may require a longer cool-down period after exercise to prevent post-exercise hypotension.[24]

Patients undergoing an aerobic conditioning program demonstrate improvements in physical fitness, functional status, psychological outlook, and self-esteem. Regular exercise may also have the additional benefit of reducing risk of recurrent stroke or heart attack. Patients who participate in a regular conditioning program may be more successful in adopting continuing, life-long exercise habits and in moving beyond the disability associated with stroke. In a Cochrane Database Systematic Review, Brazzelli et al[51] reviewed 32 trials with 1,414 participants and found that cardiorespiratory fitness training after stroke can improve walking performance including maximal walking speed, preferred gait speed, and walking capacity while reducing dependence during walking. Training effects were retained at follow-up. Adverse effects including death were infrequent.

Circuit class training (CCT) for improving mobility after stroke was the subject of a Cochrane Systematic Database Review.[52] English and Hillier[52] reviewed 6 trials with 292 participants (inpatients or community-dwelling) and found that CCT was safe and effective for improving mobility for people after moderate stroke. It may also reduce inpatient length of stay. Rose et al[233] reported on the effectiveness of a circuit training physical therapy (CTPT) program in the acute rehabilitation setting. Patients received a 60-minute training session, 5 days/wk, using four task-specific stations. Activities were stratified and tailored to patients' specific mobility levels (nonambulatory, severe, moderate, and mild groups). In addition, a 30-minute daily session was dedicated to critical inpatient rehabilitation issues (family and home program education, wheelchair and orthotic prescription). When compared to standard physical therapy (SPT) of the same intensity, the CTPT groups showed significantly greater improvements in gait speed, primarily in ambulatory patients.

■ PATIENT/CLIENT-RELATED INSTRUCTION

Stroke represents a major health crisis for patients and their families. Ignorance about the cause of the illness or the recovery process and misconceptions concerning the rehabilitation program and potential outcomes can negatively influence coping responses and progress in rehabilitation. Frequently the problems seem unmanageable and overwhelming for the family, especially when faced with alterations in the patient's behavior, cognition, and emotion. Patients may feel depressed, isolated, irritable, or demanding. Families often demonstrate reactions that include initial relief and hope for full recovery, followed by feelings of entrapment, depression, anger, or guilt when complete recovery does not occur. These changes and feelings can strain even the best of relationships. Therapists can often have a dramatic influence on this situation because of the high frequency of contact and the often close relationships that develop with patients and their families. There are a number of important guidelines to follow when planning educational interventions:

- Give accurate, factual information; counsel family members about the patient's capabilities and limitations; *avoid* predictions that categorically define expected function or future recovery.
- Structure interventions carefully, giving only as much information as the patient or family need or can assimilate; provide reinforcement and repetition.
- Adapt interventions to ensure they are appropriate to the educational and cultural background of the patient and family.
- Offer a variety of educational interventions: didactic sessions, books, brochures, and videotapes, and family participation in therapy. (See Appendix 15.B.)
- Provide a forum for open discussion and communication.
- Be supportive and sensitive, and maintain a positive, hopeful manner.
- Assist patients and families in confronting alternatives and developing problem solving abilities.
- Motivate and provide positive reinforcement in therapy; enhance patient satisfaction and self-esteem.
- Refer patients and families to support and self-help groups such as the following national associations:

American Stroke Association—A Division of the American Heart Association
7272 Greenville Avenue
Dallas, TX 75231
1-800-AHA-USA1 (1-800-242-8721)

National Stroke Association
9707 East Easter Lane
Englewood, CO 80112
1-800-STROKES (1-800-787-6537)

Psychotherapy and counseling (e.g., sexual, leisure, vocational) can assist in improving overall quality of life and should be recommended as needed.

■ DISCHARGE PLANNING

Planning for discharge begins early in rehabilitation and involves the patient and family. Potential placement (safe place of residence), level of family and community support, and need for continued medical and rehabilitation services should be explored. Family members should regularly participate in therapy sessions to learn exercises and activities designed to support the patient's independence. Discharge should be considered when reasonable treatment goals/outcomes are attained.

Indication of the attainment of a functional ceiling can be considered when there is lack of evidence of progress at two successive evaluations. Home visits should be made before discharge to determine the home's physical structure and accessibility. Potential problems can be identified and corrective measures initiated. See Chapter 9 for additional discussion. Home adaptations, assistive devices, and supportive services should be in place before the patient is discharged to home. Several trial home stays may be helpful in smoothing the transition from rehabilitation center to home. A home exercise program coupled with patient and caregiver training should be instituted. Patients with residual impairments or activity limitations who will be receiving outpatient or home therapy should be given all the necessary information concerning these services. Community services should be identified and information provided to the patient and family. Long-term follow-up at regularly scheduled intervals should be initiated in order to maintain patients at their highest possible functional level.

■ RECOVERY AND OUTCOMES

Recovery from stroke is generally fastest in the first weeks and months after onset. Patients can continue to make measurable functional gains generally at a reduced rate for months or years after insult. Late recovery of function has been consistently demonstrated for patients with chronic stroke (defined as greater than 1 year post-stroke) who undergo extensive task-specific functional training that emphasizes use of the more involved extremities. Prolonged recovery with improvements occurring over a period of years is especially apparent in the areas of language and visuospatial function. Rates of motor recovery vary across management categories: patients suffering minor stroke recover rapidly with few or no residual deficits whereas severely impaired individuals demonstrate more limited and prolonged recovery. The initial grade of paresis, measured on initial hospital admission, is an important predictor of motor recovery. In the case of complete paralysis on admission, complete motor recovery occurs in less than 15% of patients. In an extensive review of the literature, Hendricks et al[234] found no significant difference in potential for motor recovery between type of stroke (hemorrhage vs. infarction) and location (brainstem vs. hemispheric infarction).

Functional mobility skills are impaired following stroke and vary considerably from individual to individual. During the acute stroke phase, 70% to 80% of patients demonstrate mobility problems in ambulation whereas 6 months to 1 year later the figures are reversed, with only 20% of patients needing help to walk independently. Basic ADL skills such as feeding, bathing, dressing, and toileting are also compromised during acute stroke, with 67% to 88% of patients demonstrating partial or complete dependence. Independence in ADL also improves with time with only 31% of survivors requiring partial or total assistance a year later.[2] The ability to recover functional tasks is influenced by a number of factors. Motor and perceptual impairments have the greatest impact on functional performance, but other limiting factors include sensory loss, disorientation, communication disorders, and decreased cardiorespiratory endurance. Enablement factors include high motivation, stable supportive family, financial resources, and intensive training with repetitive practice.[235-240]

Patients who receive inpatient stroke rehabilitation (skilled occupational, physical, and speech therapy) demonstrate improved motor recovery, functional status, and quality of life at discharge.[234-244] In a systematic review of the literature (151 studies), Van Peppen et al[243] found strong evidence in support of task-oriented exercise and intensive training. Inpatient rehabilitation admission averages a little over 2 weeks. Approximately 80% of patients are discharged home.[236]

Post-discharge outpatient treatment or home care for stroke survivors is often indicated because functional status is typically not stabilized at discharge from a rehabilitation hospital and effects diminish over time with no treatment. Patients who demonstrate less successful rehabilitation outcomes tended to include those with (1) advanced age; (2) severe motor impairments (prolonged paralysis, apraxia); (3) persistent medical problems (incontinence); (4) impaired cognitive function (decreased alertness, poor attention span, judgment, memory, learning difficulty); (5) severe language disturbances; (6) severe visuospatial hemineglect; and (7) other less well-defined social and economic problems.[241-244] Researchers who studied long-term follow-up at 2 years post-stroke (148 patients) found that only 12% demonstrated a decline in mobility. Depression was cited as the single major risk factor for mobility decline.[245]

SUMMARY

Stroke results from a number of different vascular events that interrupt cerebral circulation and impair brain function, including cerebral thrombosis, emboli, or hemorrhage. The location and size of the ischemic process, the nature and functions of the structures involved, the availability of collateral blood flow, and effectiveness of early emergency medical management all influence the symptomatology that evolves. For many patients, stroke represents a major cause of disability, with diffuse problems affecting widespread areas of function. From a practical standpoint, patients with stroke present a tremendous challenge for clinicians. Effective rehabilitation should take advantage of the brain's capacity for repair and recovery. Rehabilitation interventions seek to promote recovery and independence through neurofacilitation, functional, and compensatory training strategies. Interventions also focus on the prevention of secondary impairments. The utilization of effective motor learning strategies with task-oriented training for real-life environments is critical for the successful attainment of functional outcomes.

Questions for Review

1. Differentiate between anterior cerebral artery syndrome and middle cerebral artery syndrome in terms of expected deficits.

2. Differentiate between lesions of the right and left hemispheres in terms of expected behavioral deficits.

3. Describe the role of the CT scan in the diagnosis of acute stroke and the implementation of emergency medical measures.

4. What are the major types of aphasia that can result from stroke? Where are the lesions located?

5. Differentiate between the following stroke-specific instruments: the Fugl-Meyer Assessment of Physical Performance (FMA) and the Stroke Rehabilitation Assessment of Movement (STREAM).

6. Describe the behaviors of the patient with stroke who demonstrates ipsilateral pushing. What is the primary focus of rehabilitation intervention?

7. Describe the role of force platform biofeedback (center-of-pressure biofeedback) in promoting improve postural control and balance in patients post-stroke.

8. What are the essential elements of constraint-induced movement therapy to improve UE function post-stroke?

9. What are the elements of task-specific overground gait training to improve function post-stroke?

10. What are the required elements of locomotor training using body weight support to improve function post-stroke?

11. What important guidelines should be followed when planning an educational program for the patient with stroke and family members?

CASE STUDY

HISTORY

The patient/client is a 41-year-old man admitted to an acute care hospital with a diagnosis of CVA with R hemiparesis (L MCA). Admitted to a rehabilitation facility 7 days later.

PAST MEDICAL HISTORY

- Seizure disorder since childhood. Dilantin was discontinued 5 years ago.
- History of mild hypertension well controlled with medication.
- Smokes 1 pack/day; 20-year history.

MEDICATIONS

- Persantine 50 mg po tid
- Tenormin 25 mg po qd
- Aspirin 10 grains po bid

TESTS

- Carotid angiography: complete occlusion of left internal carotid artery.
- Cardiac ultrasound: intermittent mitral valve prolapse.
- EKG: nonspecific ST wave changes.
- CT scan: initial scan unremarkable; repeat CT scan consistent with a large left middle cerebral artery ischemic infarction.

SOCIAL HISTORY

Patient lives with his wife and three teenage children and was independent and active before CVA. He has a college education and has worked for 20 years as a computer programmer. There is a two-step access to a rented, single-family house.

COGNITION

- Mild disorientation to time and place.
- Limited attention span for up to 3 minutes on task.
- Difficult to examine further owing to language impairment; cognitive deficits likely.
- Patient has difficulty following directions for motor responses; two- or three-step commands.

LANGUAGE/COMMUNICATION

- Auditory comprehension: moderate to severe decrease in understanding words and simple concrete sentences; unreliable yes/no responses.
- Verbal expression: severely decreased to nonfunctional; limited to only occasional automatic words.
- Reading comprehension: severely decreased to nonfunctional at a word level. Unable to match word to object.
- Written expression: to be determined.
- Gestures: spontaneous use of gestures not evident.

PHYSICAL THERAPY EXAMINATION

Passive Range of Motion

- BUEs WNL; R shoulder pain at end ranges
- BLEs WNL except R dorsiflexion 0° to 5°

Sensation

- RUE: likely impaired, unable to test fully owing to communication deficits; no apparent sensation to sharp/dull stimuli.
- RLE: likely impaired, unable to test fully owing to communication deficits; few consistent responses to sharp/dull stimuli proximally.
- Patient reports pain in RUE, end ranges of shoulder motions.

Tone
- RUE increased tone (moderate to severe) in elbow flexors; shoulder adductors and internal rotators.
- RLE increased tone (moderate) in hip and knee extensors, plantar flexors.

Motor Control
- RUE: partial motion (1/2 range) in extensor synergy pattern (shoulder and elbow extension); no voluntary motion of hand; limited in flexor synergy pattern.
- RLE: full motion in both extensor and flexor synergy patterns with extensor pattern dominating; LE flexion synergy achieved with associated reaction of RUE (increased flexion).

Strength
- LUE and LLE: full isolated movement with G+ to N strength.
- RUE and RLE limited movements; unable to MMT.

Coordination
- LUE and LLE intact.
- RUE and RLE: limited movements; unable to test.

Motor Planning
- Suspected mild motor apraxia; unable to test.

Postural Control/Balance
- Head control: good.
- Sitting static control: good, able to maintain balance without support; maintains centered alignment (COM) for 5 minutes.
- Sitting dynamic control: fair, able to maintain balance; weight shifting with reduced limits of stability (LOS); shifts to R are reduced 50%; shifts to L are normal.
- Standing static control: fair, able to maintain independent standing in parallel bars for up to 1 minute with LUE handhold.
- Standing dynamic control: poor; unable to weight shift to R without loss of balance; weight shifts to L are reduced 50%.

Functional Status
- Rolls to R: independent with bed rail
- Rolls to L: min assist
- Scoots up in bed: supervision
- Supine-to-sit: min assist
- Sit-to-supine: min assist
- Transfers bed-to-chair: stand pivot transfer, mod assist (FIM 3)
- Eating: supervision (FIM 5)
- Bathing: mod assist RUE and RLE (FIM 3)
- Dressing: mod assist RUE and RLE (FIM 3)

Gait and Locomotion
- W/C mobility: propels 150 ft with supervision (FIM 5); uses LUE and L foot for propulsion.
- Locomotion: ambulates 10 ft in parallel bars with max assist of one (FIM 1).
- Requires assist in initiation of movement of RLE.
- Requires assist with R knee control for extension.
- R foot is plantarflexed and supinated during stance, foot drop during swing.
- Uses temporary dorsiflexor assist (elastic wrap); AFO ordered (solid ankle AFO).
- Stairs: unable to test.

Endurance
- Tolerates 3/4-hour treatment session with frequent rests.

PSYCHOSOCIAL
Patient is motivated and cooperative. He appears anxious about his future and exhibited a brief episode of crying during the initial therapy session. His main goal is to walk again. Family is supportive and anxious to have him home again.

GUIDING QUESTIONS
1. Identify/categorize this patient's problems in terms of:
   a. Direct impairments.
   b. Indirect impairments.

c. Activity limitations.

d. Participation restrictions.

2. Identify three anticipated goals (remediation of impairments) and three expected outcomes (remediation of activity limitations) for this patient.

3. Formulate three treatment interventions that could be used during the first 2 weeks of therapy. Provide a brief rationale that justifies your choice.

4. Identify relevant motor learning strategies appropriate for the initial physical therapy sessions with this patient.

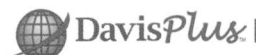 **DavisPlus** | For additional resources, including answers to the questions for review and case study guiding questions, please visit **http://davisplus.fadavis.com**

The reader is referred to the following video case studies for additional review and study:
- **Case Study 9: Patient with Right Hemorrhagic CVA**
- **Case Study 10: Patient with Left Ischemic CVA**
- **Case Study 11: Patient with Right Thalamic Ischemic Infarct and Left Lateral Medullary Ischemia**
- **Case 12: Patient with Right Basal Ganglia Intraparenchymal Hemorrhage**

A written case summary appears in the final Appendix at the end of the text. The full written case study including all tables, figures, charts, and 3 video segments (examination, intervention, and outcome) appears online at DavisPlus. The case studies pose questions for the reader's consideration with suggested answers to the case study questions, also posted online at DavisPlus.

References

1. Roger, V, et al: Heart and stroke statistical—2012 update: A report from the American Heart Association. 2012. Circulation, published online December 15, 2011. Retrieved February 25, 2012, from http://circ.ahajournals.org/content/early/2011/12/15/CIR.0b013e31823ac046.citation.

2. Post-Stroke Rehabilitation Guideline Panel: Post-Stroke Rehabilitation Clinical Practice Guideline. Aspen, Gaithersburg, MD, 1996 (formerly published as AHCPR Publication No. 95-0662, May 1995).

3. American Heart Association/American Stroke Association: Stroke Warning Signs. American Heart Association, Dallas Texas, 2011. Retrieved February 6, 2012, from www.strokeassociation.org/STROKEORG/WarningSigns/Stroke-Warning-Signs_UCM_308528_SubHomePage.jsp.

4. NINDS Group: Tissue plasminogen activator for acute ischemic stroke. N Engl J Med333:1581–1587, 1995.

5. NINDS t-PA Stroke Study Group: Generalized efficacy of t-PA for acute stroke: Subgroup analysis of the NINDS t-PA stroke trial. Stroke 28(11):2119, 1997.

6. Hertzberg V, et al: Methods and processes for the reanalysis of the NINDS tissue plasminogen activator for acute ischemic stroke. Clin Trials 5:308–315, 2008.

7. Kwan, J, et al: A systematic review of barriers to delivery of thrombolysis for acute stroke. Age Ageing 33:116, 2004.

8. De la Ossa, N, et al: Influence of direct admission to comprehensive stroke centers on the outcome of acute stroke patients treated with intravenous thrombolysis. J Neurol 256:1270, 2009.

9. Barclay, L: Acute cerebrovascular care in emergency stroke systems. Arch Neurol 67:1210, 2010.

10. Kwiatkowski, T, et al: Effects of tissue plasminogen activator or acute ischemic stroke at one year. N Engl J Med 340:1781, 1999.

11. Mitsios, N, et al: Pathophysiology of acute ischaemic stroke: An analysis of common signaling mechanisms and identification of new molecular targets. Pathobiology 73:159, 2006.

12. Kaplan, P, Cailliet, R, and Kaplan, C: Rehabilitation of Stroke. Butterworth-Heinemann, Woburn, MA, 2003.

13. Teasdale, G, and Jennett, B: Assessment of coma and impaired consciousness: A practical scale. Lancet 13:2, 1974.

14. Smithard, DG, et al: The natural history of dysphagia following stroke. Dysphagia 12(4):188, 1997.

15. Meng, N, Wang, T, and Lien, I: Dysphagia in patients with brainstem stroke: Incidence and outcome. Am J Phys Med Rehabil 79(2):170, 2000.

16. Avery, W: Dysphagia management. In Gillen, G: Stroke Rehabilitation: A Function-Based Approach. Elsevier/Mosby, St. Louis, 2011, pp 629–647.

17. Sachdev, P, et al: Clinical determinants of dementia and mild cognitive impairment following ischaemic stroke: The Sydney Stroke Study. Dement Geriatr Cogn Disord 21:275, 2006.

18. Chemerinski, E, and Robinson, R: The neuropsychiatry of stroke. Psychosomatics 41(1):5, 2000.

19. Folstein, MF, et al: Mini Mental State: A practical method for grading the cognitive state of patients for the clinician. J Psychiatr Res 12:189, 1975.

20. Barker-Collo, S: Depression and anxiety 3 months post stroke: Prevalence and correlates. Arch Clin Neuropsychol 22:519, 2007.

21. Berg, A, et al: Post stroke depression: An 18-month follow-up. Stroke 34(1):138, 2003.

22. Robinson, RG: Vascular depression and post-stroke depression: Where do we go from here? Am J Geriatr Psychiatry 13(2):85, 2005.

23. Beck, A, and Beck, R: Screening depressed patients in family practice: A rapid technique. Postgrad Med 52:81, 1972.

24. Palmer-McLean, K, and Harbst, K. Stroke and brain injury. In American College of Sports Medicine: ACSM's Exercise Management for Persons with Chronic Diseases and Disabilities, ed 3. Human Kinetics, Champaign, IL, 2009, p 287.

25. Porth, C: Pathophysiology, ed 7. Lippincott Williams & Wilkins, Philadelphia, 2005.

26. Harris, J, et al: Relationship of balance and mobility to fall incidence in people with chronic stroke. Phys Ther 85:150, 2005.

27. Teasall, R, et al: The incidence and consequences of falls in stroke patients during inpatient rehabilitation: Factors associated with high risk. Arch Phys Med Rehabil 83:329, 2002.

28. Tutuarima, J, et al: Risk factors for falls of hospitalized stroke patients. Stroke 28:297, 1997.

29. Forster, A, and Young, J: Incidence and consequences of falls due to stroke: A systematic inquiry. Br Med J 311:83, 1995.

30. Ramnemark, A, et al: Fractures after stroke. Osteoporos Int 8:92, 1998.

31. Yew, K, and Cheng, E: Acute stroke diagnosis. Am Fam Physician 80(1):33, 2009.

32. Nor, A, and Ford, G: Misdiagnosis of stroke. Expert Rev Neurotherapeutics 7(8):989, 2007.

33. National Institute of Neurological Disorders and Stroke. NIH Stroke Scale. 2003. Retrieved March 7, 2012, from www.ninds.nih.gov/doctors/NIH_Stroke_Scale.pdf.

34. Leira, E, et al: Baseline NIH Stroke Scale responses estimate the probability of each particular stroke subtype. Cerebrovasc Dis 26:573, 2008.

35. Wityk, RJ, Pessin, MS, and Kaplan, RF: Serial assessment of acute stroke using the NIH Stroke Scale. Stroke 25(2):362, 1994.

36. Goldstein, LB, and Samsa, GP: Reliability of the National Institutes of Health Stroke Scale. Stroke 28:307, 1997.

37. Hakimelahi, R, and Gonzalez, R: Neuroimaging of ischemic stroke with CT and MRI: Advancing towards physiological based diagnosis and therapy. Expert Rev Cardiovasc Ther 7(1):29, 2009.

38. National Stroke Association: Explaining Stroke-Related Medications. Retrieved March 8, 2012, from www.stroke.org/site/PageServer?pagename=med_adherence#explain.

39. Deglin, J, and Vallerand, A: Davis's Drug Guide for Nurses, ed 11. FA Davis, Philadelphia, 2007.

40. National Stroke Association: Stroke Treatment. Retrieved March 8, 2012, from http://nsa.convio.net/site/PageServer?pagename=treatment.

41. American Physical Therapy Association (APTA): Guide to Physical Therapist Practice, ed 2. APTA, Alexandria, VA, 2003.

42. Langhorne, P, et al: Do stroke units save lives? Lancet 342:395, 1993.

43. Stroke Unit Trialists Collaboration: Organised inpatient (stroke unit) care after stroke (review). Cochrane Database Syst Rev 2007, Issue 4. Art. No.: CD000197. DOI: 10.1002/14651858.CD000197.pub2.

44. Pollock, A, et al: Physiotherapy treatment approaches for recovery of postural control and lower limb function following stroke (review). Cochrane Database Syst Rev 2007, Issue 1. Art. No.: CD001920. DOI:10.1002/14651858.CD001920.pub2.

45. Sirtori, V, et al: Constraint-induced movement therapy for upper extremities in stroke patients (review). Cochrane Database Syst Rev 2009, Issue 4 Art. No.: CD004433. DOI: 10.1002/14651858.CD004433.pub2.

46. Winter, J, et al: Hands-on therapy interventions for upper limb motor dysfunction following stroke (review). Cochrane Database Syst Rev 2011, Issue 6. Art. No.: CD006609. DOI: 10.1002/14651858.CD006609.pub2.

47. Coupar, F, et al: Simultaneous bilateral training for improving arm function after stroke (review). Cochrane Database Syst Rev 2010, Issue 4. Art. No.: CD006432. DOI: 10.1002/14651858.CD006432.pub2.

48. Doyle, S, et al: Interventions for sensory impairment in the upper limb after stroke (review). Cochrane Database Syst Rev 2010, Issue 6. Art. No.: CD006331. DOI: 10.1002/14651858.CD006331.pub2.

49. Moseley, AM, et al: Treadmill training and body weight support for walking after stroke (review). Cochrane Database Syst Rev 2009, Issue 4. Art. No.: CD002840. DOI: 10.1002/14651858.CD002840.pub2.

50. French B, et al: Repetitive task training for improving functional ability after stroke (review). Cochrane Database Syst Rev 2007, Issue 4. Art. No.: CD006073. DOI: 10.1002/14651858.CD006073.pub2.

51. Brazzelli, M et al: Physical fitness training for stroke patients (review). Cochrane Database Syst Rev 2011, Issue 11. Art. No.: CD003316. DOI: 10.1002/14651858.CD003316.pub4.

52. English, C, and Hillier, SL: Circuit class therapy for improving mobility after stroke (review). Cochrane Database Syst Rev 2010, Issue 7. Art. No.: CD007513. DOI: 10.1002/14651858.CD007513.pub2.

53. Laver, KE, et al: Virtual reality for stroke rehabilitation (review). Cochrane Database Syst Rev 2011, Issue 9. Art. No.: CD008349. DOI: 10.1002/14651858.CD008349.pub2.

54. Mehrholz, J, et al: Electromechanical-assisted training for walking after stroke (review). Cochrane Database Syst Rev 2007, Issue 4. Art. No.: CD006185. DOI: 10.1002/14651858.CD006185.pub2.

55. Outpatient Service Trialists: Therapy-based rehabilitation services for stroke patients at home (review). Cochrane Database Syst Rev 2009, Issue 1. Art. No.: CD002925. DOI: 10.1002/14651858.CD002925.

56. Mehrholz, J, Kugler, J, and Pohl, M: Water-based exercises for improving activities of daily living after stroke (review). Cochrane Database Syst Rev 2011, Issue 1. Art. No.: CD008186. DOI: 10.1002/14651858.CD008186.pub2.

57. Hunter, SM, and Crome, P: Hand function and stroke. Rev Clin Gerontol 12(1):66–81, 2002

58. Tyson, SF, et al: Sensory loss of in-hospital admitted people with stroke: Characteristics, associated factors, and relationship with function. Neurorehabil Neural Repair 22:166-172, 2008.

59. Carey, L: Somatosensory loss after stroke. Crit Rev Phys Med Rehabil 7(1):51–91, 1995.

60. Rand, D, Gottlieb, D, and Weiss, P: Recovery of patients with a combined motor and proprioception deficit during the first six weeks of post stroke rehabilitation. Phys Occup Ther Geriatr 18(3):69–87, 2001.

61. Connell, LA, Lincoln, NB, and Radford, KA: Somatosensory impairment after stroke: Frequency of different deficits and their recovery. Clin Rehabil 22:758–767, 2008.

62. Canavero, S, and Bonicalzi, V: Central pain syndrome: Elucidation of genesis and treatment. Expert Rev Neurotherapeutics 7(11):1485, 2007.

63. Klit, H, Finnerup, N, and Jensen, T: Central post-stroke pain: Clinical characteristics, pathophysiology, and management. Lancet Neurol 8:857–868, 2009.

64. Twitchell, T: The restoration of motor function following hemiplegia in man. Brain 47:443, 1951.

65. Brunnstrom, S: Motor testing procedures in hemiplegia based on recovery stages. J Am Phys Ther Assoc 46:357, 1966.

66. Brunnstrom, S: Movement Therapy in Hemiplegia. Harper & Row, New York, 1970.

67. Gray, C, et al: Motor recovery following acute stroke. Age Ageing 19:179, 1990.

68. Wade, D, et al: Recovery after stroke: The first 3 months. J Neurol Neurosurg Psychiatry 48:7, 1985.

69. Patten, C, Lexell, J, and Brown, H : Weakness and strength training in persons with post-stroke hemiplegia: Rationale, method and efficacy. J Rehabil Res Dev 41:293–312, 2004.

70. Carin-Levy, G, et al: Longitudinal changes in muscle strength and mass after acute stroke. Cerebrovasc Dis 21:201, 2006.

71. Adams, R, Gandevia, S, and Skuse, N: The distribution of muscle weakness in upper motoneuron lesions affecting the lower limb. Brain 113:1459, 1990.

72. Davidoff, R: The pyramidal tract. Neurology 40:332, 1990.

73. Andrews A, and Bohannon, R: Distribution of muscle strength impairments following stroke. Clin Rehabil 14:79, 2000.

74. Canning, C, Ada, L, and O'Dwyer, N: Slowness to develop force contributes to weakness after stroke. Arch Phys Med Rehabil 80:66, 1999.

75. Eng, J: Strength training in individuals with stroke. Physiother Can 56:189, 2004.

76. Dattola, R, et al: Muscle rearrangement in patients with hemiparesis after stroke: An electrophysiological and morphological study. Eur Neurol 33:109, 1993.

77. Stoeckmann, T, Sullivan, K, and Scheidt, R: Elastic, viscous, and mass load effects on poststroke muscle recruitment and co-contraction during reaching: A pilot study. Phys Ther 89(7):665, 2008.

78. Chae, J, et al: Delay in initiation and termination of muscle contraction, motor impairment, and physical disability in upper limb hemiparesis. Muscle Nerve 2(25):568–575, 2002.

79. McCrea, PH, Eng JJ, and Hodgson, A: Time and magnitude of torque generation is impaired in both arms following stroke. Muscle Nerve 28:46–53, 2003.

80. Desrosiers, J, et al: Performance of the "unaffected" upper extremity of elderly stroke patients. Stroke 27:1564–1570, 1996.

81. Sackley, CM: The relationships between weight-bearing asymmetry after stroke and function and activities of daily living. Physiother Theory Pract 6:179–185, 1990.

82. Badke, MB, and Duncan, P: Patterns of rapid motor responses during postural adjustments when standing in healthy subjects and hemiplegic patients. Phys Ther 63:13–20, 1983.

83. Dickstein, R, and Ablaffio, N: Postural sway of the affected and nonaffected pelvis and leg in stance of hemiparetic patients. Arch Phys Med Rehabil 81:364–367, 2000.

84. DiFabio, R, and Badke, M: Relationship of sensory organization to balance function in patients with hemiplegia. Phys Ther 70:543, 1990.

85. Shumway-Cook, A, Anson, D, and Haller, S: Postural sway biofeedback: Its effect on reestablishing stance stability in hemiplegic patients. Arch Phys Med Rehabil 69:395, 1988.

86. Gustavsen, M, Aamodt, G, and Mengshoel, A: Measuring balance in subacute stroke rehabilitation. Adv Physiother 8(1): 15–22, 2006.

87. Benaim, C, et al: Validation of a standardized assessment of postural control in stroke patients: The Postural Assessment Scale for Stroke Patients (PASS). Stroke 30(9):1862, 1999.

88. Verheyden, G, et al: The Trunk Impairment Scale: A new tool to measure motor impairment of the trunk after stroke. Clin Rehabil 18(3):326, 2004.

89. Gorman, S, et al: Development and validation of the Function in Sitting Test in adults with acute stroke. J Neurol Phys Ther 34:150, 2010.

90. Karnath, H, Ferber, S, and Dichgans, J: The origin of contraversive pushing: Evidence for a second graviceptive system in humans. Neurology 55:1298, 2000.

91. Pedersen, P, et al: Ipsilateral pushing in stroke: Incidence, relation to neuropsychological symptoms, and impact on rehabilitation. The Copenhagen stroke study. Arch Phys Med 77: 25, 1996.

92. Karnath, H, Ferber, S, and Dichgans, J: The neural representation of postural control in humans. PNAS 97:13931, 2000.

93. Karnath, H, et al: Prognosis of contraversive pushing. J Neurol 249:1250, 2002.

94. Broetz, D, and Karnath, H: New aspects for the physiotherapy of pushing behavior. Neurorehabil 20:133, 2005.

95. Karnath, H, and Broetz, D: Understanding and treating "pusher syndrome." Phys Ther 83:1119, 2003.

96. Perry, J, et al: Classification of walking handicap in the stroke population. Stroke 26:982, 1995.

97. Viosca, E, et al: Proposal and validation of a new functional ambulation classification scale for clinical use. Arch Phys Med Rehabil 86:1234, 2005.

98. Miller, P, Moreland, J, and Stevenson, T: Measurement properties of a standardized version of the Two-Minute Walk Test for individuals with neurological dysfunction. Physiother Can 54(4):241, 2002.

99. Mahoney, F, and Barthel, D: Functional evaluation: Barthel Index. Md State Med J 14:61, 1965.

100. Keith, RA, et al: The Functional Independence Measure. Adv Clin Rehabil 1:6, 1987.

101. Uniform Data Service, Data Management Service: UDS Update. State University of New York at Buffalo, 1993.

102. Fugl-Meyer, A, et al: The post stroke hemiplegic patient, 1. A method for evaluation of physical performance. Scand J Rehabil Med 7:13, 1976.

103. Duncan, P, et al: Reliability of the Fugl-Meyer Assessment of Sensorimotor Recovery following cerebrovascular accident. Phys Ther 63:1606, 1983.

104. Gladstone, DJ, Danells, CJ, and Black, SE: The Fugl-Meyer assessment of motor recovery after stroke: A critical review of its measurement properties. Neurorehabil NeuralRepair 16: 232–240, 2002.

105. Sullivan, KJ, et al: Fugl-Meyer Assessment of Sensorimotor Function after stroke: Standardized training procedure for clinical practice and clinical trials. Stroke 42(2):427, 2011.

106. Crowe, J, and Harmeling-vander Wel, B: Hierarchical properties of the motor function sections of the Fugl-Meyer Assessment Scale for people after stroke: A retrospective study. PhysTher 88(12): 1555, 2008.

107. Daley, K, et al: The Stroke Rehabilitation Assessment of Movement (STREAM): Refining and validating the content. Physiother Can 49:269, 1997.

108. Daley, K, Mayo, N, and Wood-Dauphinee, S: Reliability of scores on the Stroke Rehabilitation Assessment of Movement (STREAM) measure. Phys Ther 79:8, 1999.

109. Ahmed, S, et al: The Stroke Rehabilitation Assessment of Movement (STREAM): A comparison with other measures used to evaluate effects of stroke and rehabilitation. Phys Ther 83: 617, 2003.

110. Gowland C, et al: Measuring physical impairment and disability with the Chedoke-McMaster Stroke Assessment. Stroke 24(1):58–63, 1993.

111. Duncan, PW, et al: The Stroke Impact Scale version 2.0: Evaluation of reliability, validity, and sensitivity to change. Stroke 30(10): 2131–2140, 1999.

112. Lin, K, et al: Psychometric comparisons of the Stroke Impact Scale 3.0 and the Stroke-Specific Quality of Life Scale. Qual Life Res 19:435, 2010.

113. Duncan, PW, et al: Evaluation of proxy responses to the Stroke Impact Scale. Stroke 33(11):2593, 2002.

114. Sunderland, KJ, et al: Enhanced physical therapy improves recovery of arm function after stroke: A randomized controlled trial. J Neurol Neurosurg 55(7):530, 1992.

115. Feys, HM, et al: Effect of a therapeutic intervention for the hemiplegic upper limb in the acute phase after stroke. Stroke 29(4): 785, 1998.

116. Langhammer, B, and Stanghelle, J: Bobath or motor relearning programme? A comparison of two different approaches of physiotherapy in stroke rehabilitation: A randomized controlled study. Clin Rehabil 14(4):361, 2000.

117. Mudie, M, et al: Training symmetry of weight distribution after stroke: A randomized controlled pilot study comparing task-related reach, Bobath, and feedback training approaches. Clin Rehabil 16(4):361, 2002.

118. Carr, J, and Shepherd, R: A Motor Relearning Programme for Stroke, ed 2. Aspen, Gaithersville, MD, 1987.

119. Boyd, L, and Winstein, C: Impact of explicit information on implicit motor-sequence learning following middle cerebral artery stroke. Phys Ther 83:976, 2003.

120. Orrell, A, Eves, F, and Masters, R: Motor learning of a dynamic balancing task after stroke: Implicit implications for stroke rehabilitation. Phys Ther 86:369, 2006.

121. Page, S, et al: Mental practice combined with physical practice for upper-limb motor deficit in subacute stroke. Phys Ther 81:1455, 2001.

122. Dicksten, R, Dunsky, A, and Marcovitz, E: Motor imagery for gait rehabilitation in post-stroke hemiparesis. Phys Ther 84:1167, 2004.

123. Ietswaart, M, et al: Mental practice with motor imagery in stroke recovery: Randomized controlled trial of efficacy. Brain 134:1373, 2011.

124. Voss, D, et al: Proprioceptive Neuromuscular Facilitation, ed 3. Harper & Row, Philadelphia, 1985.

125. Adler, S, et al: PNF in Practice, ed 3. Springer-Verlag, Berlin, 2008.

126. Ramachandran, VS, and Roger-Remachandran, D: Synaesthesia in phantom limbs induced with mirrors. Proc R Soc Lond B Biol Sci 263:431, 1996.

127. Subeyaz, S, et al: Mirror therapy enhances lower-extremity motor recovery and motor functioning after stroke: A randomized controlled trial. Arch Phys Med Rehabil 88:555, 2007.

128. Dohle, C, et al: Mirror therapy promotes recovery from severe hemiparesis: A randomized controlled trial. Neurorehabil Neural Repair 20:1–9, 2008.

129. Yavuzer, G, et al: Mirror therapy improves hand function in subacute stroke: A randomized controlled trial. Arch Phys Med Rehabil 89:393, 2008.

130. Taub, E: Somatosensory deafferentation research with monkeys. In Ince, L (ed): Behavioral Psychology in Rehabilitation Medicine: Clinical Applications. Williams & Wilkins, Baltimore, 1980, p 371.

131. Schabrun, SM, and Hillier, S: Evidence for the retraining of sensation after stroke: A systematic review. Clin Rehabil 23:27, 2009.

132. Dannenbaum, R, and Dykes, R: Sensory loss in the hand after sensory stroke: Therapeutic rationale. Arch Phys Med Rehabil 69:833, 1988.

133. Weinberg, J, et al: Training sensory awareness and spatial organization in people with right brain damage. Arch Phys Med Rehabil 60:491, 1979.

134. Bailey, M, Riddoch, M, and Crome, P: Treatment of visual neglect in elderly patients with stroke: A single-subject series using either a scanning and cueing strategy or a left-limb activation strategy. Phys Ther 82(8):782, 2002.

135. Bailey, M, and Riddoch, M: Hemineglect in stroke patients. Part 2. Rehabilitation techniques and strategies: A summary of recent studies. Phys Ther Rev 4:77, 1999.

136. Wiart, L, et al: Unilateral neglect syndrome rehabilitation by trunk rotation and scanning training. Arch Phys Med Rehabil 78:424, 1997.

137. Morris, S, Dodd, K, and Morris, M: Outcomes of progressive resistance strength training following stroke: A systematic review. Clin Rehabil 18:27–39, 2004.

138. Ada, L, Dorsch, S, and Canning, C: Strengthening interventions increase stroke and improve activity after stroke: A systematic review. Aust J Physiother 52:241, 2006.

139. Flansbjer, U, et al: Progressive resistance training after stroke: Effects on muscle strength, muscle tone, gait performance, and perceived participation. J Rehabil Med 40:42–48, 2008.

140. Carr, M, and Jones, J: Physiologic effects of exercise on stroke survivors. Top Stroke Rehabil 9:57, 2003.

141. Moreland, JD, et al: Progressive resistance strengthening exercises after stroke: A single-blind randomized controlled trial. Arch Phys Med Rehabil 84:1433, 2003.

142. Ouellette, M, et al: High-intensity resistance training improves muscle strength, self-reported function, and disability in long-term stroke survivors. Stroke 35:1404, 2004.

143. Weiss, A, et al: High intensity strength training improves strength and functional performance after stroke. Am J Phys Med Rehabil 79:369, 2000.

144. Badics, E, et al: Systematic muscle building exercises in the rehabilitation of stroke patients. Neuro Rehab 17:211, 2002.

145. Yang, YR, et al: Task-oriented progressive resistance strength training improves muscle strength and functional performance after stroke. Clin Rehabil 20:860, 2006.

146. Patten, C, et al: Combined functional task practice and dynamic high intensity resistance training promotes recovery of upper-extremity motor function in post-stroke hemiparesis: A case study. J Neurol Phys Ther 30:99–115, 2006.

147. Kim, CM, et al: Effects of isokinetic strength training on walking in persons with stroke: A double-blind controlled pilot study. J Stroke Cerebrovasc Dis 10:265, 2001.

148. Sharp, SA, and Brouwer, BJ: Isokinetic strength training of the hemiparetic knee: Effects on function and spasticity. Arch Phys Med Rehabil 78:1231, 1997.

149. Butefisch, C, et al: Repetitive training of isolated movements improves the outcome of motor rehabilitation of the centrally paretic hand. J Neurol Sci 130:59, 1995.

150. Gracies, JM, et al: Pathophysiology of impairment in patients with spasticity and use of stretch as a treatment of spastic hypertonia. Phys Med Rehabil Clin North Am 12(4):747, 2001.

151. Bovend'Eerdt, TJ, et al: The effects of stretching in spasticity: A systematic review. Arch Phys Med Rehabil 89(7):1395, 2008.

152. Watanabe, T: The role of therapy in spasticity management. Am J Phys Med Rehabil 83:S45, 2004.

153. O'Sullivan, S, and Schmitz, T: Improving Functional Outcomes in Physical Rehabilitation. FA Davis, Philadelphia, 2010.

154. Johnstone, M: Restoration of Normal Movement After Stroke. Churchill Livingstone, New York, 1995.

155. Singer, BJ, Singer, KP, and Allison, G: Evaluation of extensibility, passive torque and stretch reflex responses in triceps surae muscles following serial casting to correct spastic equinovarus deformity. Brain Injury 17(4):309, 2003.

156. Mortensen, P, and Eng, J: The use of casts in the management of joint mobility and hypertonia following brain injury in adults: A systematic review. Phys Ther 83:648, 2003.

157. Carr, J, and Shepherd, R: Stroke Rehabilitation—Guidelines for Exercise and Training to Optimize Motor Skill. Butterworth Heinemann, Elsevier, Philadelphia, 2003.

158. Davies, P: Steps to Follow, ed 2. Springer-Verlag, New York, 2004.

159. Davies, P: Right in the Middle. Springer-Verlag, New York, 1990.

160. Howle, J: Neuro-Developmental Treatment Approach—Theoretical Foundations and Principles of Clinical Practice. NDTA, Laguna Beach, CA, 2002.

161. Gillen, G: Upper extremity function and management. In Gillen, G, and Burkhardt, A (eds): Stroke Rehabilitation: A Function-Based Approach, ed 3. Mosby, St. Louis, 2011, p 218.

162. Woldag, H, and Hummelsheim, H: Evidence-based physiotherapeutic concepts for improving arm and hand function in stroke patients: A review. J Neurol 249(5):518, 2003.

163. Mark, V, and Taub, E: Constraint-induced movement therapy for chronic stroke hemiparesis and other disabilities. Restorative Neurol Neurosci 22:317, 2002.

164. Morris, D, and Taub, E: Constraint-induced movement therapy. In O'Sullivan, S, and Schmitz, T: Improving Functional Outcomes in Physical Rehabilitation. FA Davis, Philadelphia, 210, p 232.

165. Morris, D, Taub, E, and Mark, V: Constraint-induced movement therapy: Characterizing the intervention protocol. Eura Medicophy 42:257, 2006.

166. Page, S, et al: Efficacy of modified constraint-induced movement therapy in chronic stroke: A single-blinded randomized controlled trial. Arch Phys Med Rehabil 85:14, 2004.

167. Page, S, and Levine, P: Modified constraint-induced therapy in patients with chronic stroke exhibiting minimal movement ability in the affected arm. Phys Ther 87:872–878, 2007.

168. Bjorklund, A, and Fecht, A: The effectiveness of constraint-induced therapy as a stroke intervention: A meta-analysis. Occupational Therapy in Health Care 20:31–49, 2006.

169. Hakkennes, S, and Keating, JL: Constraint-induced movement therapy following stroke: A systematic review of randomized controlled trials. Aus J Physiother 51:221, 2005.

170. Wolf, SL, et al: Effect of constraint-induced movement therapy on upper extremity function 3 to 6 months after stroke: The EXCITE randomized clinical trial. JAMA 296(17):2095–2104, 2006.

171. Schaechter, JD, et al: Motor recovery and cortical reorganization after constraint-induced movement therapy in stroke patients: A preliminary study. Neurorehabil Neural Repair 16(4):326, 2002.

172. Richards, L, et al: Limited dose response to constraint-induced movement therapy in patients with chronic stroke. Clin Rehabil 20:1066, 2006.

173. Dromerick, A, Edwards, DF, and Hahn, M: Does the applications of constraint-induced movement therapy during acute rehabilitation reduce arm impairment after ischemic stroke? Stroke 31(12):2984, 2000.

174. Whitall, J, et al: Repetitive bilateral arm training with rhythmic auditory cueing improves motor function in chronic hemiparetic stroke. Stroke 31:2390, 2000.

175. Richards, LG, et al: Bilateral arm training with rhythmic auditory cueing in chronic stroke: Not always efficacious. Neurorehabil Neural Repair 22(2):180–184, 2008.

176. Stewart, KC, Cauraugh, J, and Summers, J: Bilateral movement training and stroke rehabilitation: A systematic review and meta-analysis. J Neurol Sci 244:89–95, 2006.

177. Armagan, O, Tascioglu, F, and Oner, C: Electromyographic biofeedback in the treatment of the hemiplegic hand: A placebo-controlled study. Am J Phys Med Rehabil 82(11):856, 2003.

178. Glantz, M, et al: Biofeedback therapy in post-stroke rehabilitation: A meta-analysis of the randomized controlled trials. Arch Phys Med Rehabil 76:508, 1995.

179. Chae, J, et al: Neuromuscular stimulation for upper extremity motor and functional recovery in acute hemiplegia. Stroke 29(5):975, 1998.

180. Hardy, J, et al: Meta-analysis examining the effectiveness of electrical stimulation in improving the functional use of the upper limb in stroke patients. Phys Occup Ther Geriatr 21(4):67–78, 2003.

181. Ada, L, and Foongchomcheay, A: Efficacy of electrical stimulation in preventing and treating subluxation of the shoulder after stroke: A meta-analysis. Aust J Physiother 48(4):257, 2002.

182. Price, C, and Pandyan, A: Electrical stimulation for preventing and treating post-stroke shoulder pain. Cochrane Database Syst Rev 2000, Issue 4. Art. No.: CD001698. DOI: 10.1002/14651858.CD00169.

183. Fasoli, S: Rehabilitation technologies to promote upper limb recovery after stroke. In Gillen, G, and Burkhardt, A (eds): Stroke Rehabilitation: A Function-Based Approach, ed 3. Mosby, St. Louis, 2011, p 280.

184. Brewer, B, McDowell, S, and Worthen-Chaudhari, L: Poststroke upper extremity rehabilitation: A review of robotic systems and clinical results. Top Stroke Rehabil 14(6):1562, 2003.

185. Jespersen, HF, et al: Shoulder pain after a stroke. Int J Rehabil Res 18A:273, 1995.

186. Turner-Stokes, L, and Jackson, D: Shoulder pain after stroke: A review of the evidence base to inform the development of an integrated care pathway. Clin Rehabil 16:276, 2002.

187. Snels, I, et al: Treating patients with hemiplegic shoulder pain. Am J Phys Med Rehabil 81(2):150, 2002.

188. Daviet, JC, et al: Clinical factors in the prognosis of complex regional pain syndrome type 1 after stroke. Am J Phys Med Rehabil 81(1):34–39, 2002.

189. Davis, J: The role of the occupational therapist in the treatment of shoulder-hand syndrome. Occup Ther Pract 1(3):30, 1990.

190. Zorowitz, R, et al: Shoulder subluxation after stroke: A comparison of four supports. Arch Phys Med Rehabil 76:763, 1995.

191. Brooke, M, et al: Shoulder subluxation in hemiplegia: Effects of three different supports. Arch Phys Med Rehabil 72:582, 1991.

192. Bernath, V: Shoulder supports in patients with hypotonicity following stroke. Centre for Clinical Effectiveness, Clayton, Australia, January 2001. Retrieved August 20, 2005, from www.med.monash.edu.au/healthservices/cce/evidence/pdf/c/470.pdf.

193. Eng, J, Pang, M, and Ashe, M: Balance, falls, and bone health: Role of exercise in reducing fracture risk after stroke. J Rehabil Res Dev 45(2):297–313, 2008.

194. Rose, D: Fall Proof: A Comprehensive Balance and Mobility Training Program, ed 2. Human Kinetics, Champaign, IL, 2010.

195. Lubetzky-Vilnai, A, and Kartin, D: The effect of balance training on balance performance in individuals poststroke: A systematic review. J Neurol Phys Ther 34:127–137, 2010.

196. Hammer, A, Nilsagard, Y, and Wallquist, M: Balance training in stroke patients—a systematic review of randomized, controlled trials. Adv Physiother 10(4):163, 2008.

197. Winstein, C, et al: Standing balance training: Effect on balance and locomotion in hemiparetic adults. Arch Phys Med Rehabil 70:755, 1989.

198. Sackley, C, and Lincoln, N: Single blind randomized controlled trial of visual feedback after stroke: Effects on stance symmetry and function. Disabil Rehabil 19:536, 1997.

199. Hamman, R, et al: Training effects during repeated therapy sessions of balance training using visual feedback. Arch Phys Med Rehabil 73:738, 1992.

200. McRae, J, et al: Rehabilitation of hemiplegia: Functional outcomes and treatment of postural control. Phys Ther 74(Suppl):S119, 1994.

201. Nichols, D: Balance retraining after stroke using force platform biofeedback. Phys Ther 77:553, 1997.

202. Fishman, M, et al: Comparison of functional upper extremity tasks and dynamic standing. Phys Ther 76(Suppl):79, 1996.

203. Walker, C, Brouwer, B, and Culham, E: Use of visual feedback in retraining balance following acute stroke. Phys Ther 80:886, 2000.

204. Geiger, R, et al: Balance and mobility following stroke: Effects of physical therapy interventions with and without biofeedback/forceplate training. Phys Ther 81:995, 2001.

205. Davies, P: Steps to Follow: The Comprehensive Treatment of Patients with Hemiplegia, ed 2. Springer-Verlag, New York, 2000.

206. Paci, M, and Nannetti, L: Physiotherapy for pusher behavior in a patient with post-stroke hemiplegia. J Rehabil Med 36:183, 2004.

207. States, R, Salem, Y, and Pappas, E: Overground gait training for individuals with chronic stroke: A Cochrane systematic review. J Neurol Phys Ther 33(4):179, 2009.

208. Malouin, F, et al: Use of an intensive task-oriented gait training program in a series of patients with acute cerebrovascular accidents. Phys Ther 72:781, 1992.

209. Richards, C, et al: Task-specific physical therapy for optimization of gait recovery in acute stroke patients. Arch Phys Med Rehabil 74(6):612, 1993.

210. Hesse, S, et al: Restoration of gait in nonambulatory hemiparetic patients by treadmill training with partial body-weight support. Arch Phys Med Rehabil 75:1087, 1994.

211. Visintin, M, et al: A new approach to retrain gait in stroke patients through body weight support and treadmill stimulation. Stroke 29:1122, 1998.

212. Barbeau, H, and Visintin, M: Optimal outcomes obtained with body-weight support combined with treadmill training in stroke subjects. Arch Phys Med Rehabil 84:1458, 2003.

213. Nilsson, L, et al: Walking training of patients with hemiparesis at an early stage after stroke: A comparison of walking training on a treadmill with body weight support and walking training on the ground. Clin Rehabil 15(5):515, 2001.

214. Pohl, M, et al: Speed-dependent treadmill training in ambulatory hemiparetic stroke patients: A randomized controlled trial. Stroke 33:553, 2002.

215. Sullivan, K, Knowlton, B, and Dobkin, BH: Step training with body weight support: effect of treadmill speed and practice paradigms on poststroke locomotor recovery. Arch Phys Med Rehabil 83:683, 2002.

216. Ada, L, et al: Randomized trial of treadmill walking with body weight support to establish walking in subacute stroke: The MOBILIZE trial. Stroke 41:1247, 2010.

217. Eich, HJ, et al: Aerobic treadmill plus Bobath walking training improves walking in subacute stroke: A randomized controlled trial. Clin Rehabil 18:640, 2004.

218. Dean, C, et al: Treadmill walking with body weight support in subacute non-ambulatory stroke improves walking capacity more than overground walking: A randomized trial. J Physiother 56(2):97, 2010.

219. Macko, RG, Ivey, FM, and Forrester, LW: Treadmill exercise rehabilitation improves ambulatory function and cardiovascular fitness in patients with chronic stroke: A randomized controlled trial. Stroke 36:2206, 2005.

220. Hesse, S: Treadmill training with partial body weight support after stroke: A review. NeuroRehabil 23:55, 2008.

221. Franceschini, M, et al: Walking after stroke: What does treadmill training with body weight support add to overground training in patients with very early stroke? A single-blind randomized controlled trial. Stroke 40:3079, 2009.

222. Sullivan, K, et al: Effects of task-specific locomotor and strength training in adults who were ambulatory after stroke: Results of the STEPS randomized clinical trial. Phys Ther 87(12):1580, 2007.

223. Duncan, PW, Sullivan, KJ, and Behrman, AL: Protocol for the Locomotor Experience Applied Post-Stroke (LEAPS) trial: A randomized controlled trial. BMC Neurol 7:39, 2007.

224. Duncan, PW, et al: Body-weight-supported treadmill rehabilitation after stroke. N Engl J Med 364:2026, 2011.

225. Tefertiller, C, et al: Efficacy of rehabilitation robotics for walking training in neurological disorders: A review. J Rehabilit Res Dev 48(4): 387, 2011.

226. Lewek, M, et al: Allowing intralimb kinematic variability during locomotor training poststroke improves kinematic consistency: A subgroup analysis from a randomized clinical trial. Phys Ther 89(8):829, 2009.

227. Ada, L, et al: Mechanically assisted walking with body weight support results in more independent walking than assisted overground walking in non-ambulatory patients early after stroke: A systematic review. J Physiother 56(3):153, 2010.

228. Roche, A, Laighin, G, and Coote, S: Surface-applied functional electrical stimulation for orthotic and therapeutic treatment of drop-foot after stroke—a systematic review. Phys Ther Rev 14(2): 63, 2009.

229. Weingarden, H, and Ring, H: Functional electrical stimulation–induced neural changes and recovery after stroke. Eur J Phys Rehabil Med 42(2):87, 2006.

230. Swigchem, R, et al: Effect of peroneal electrical stimulation versus an ankle-foot orthosis on obstacle avoidance ability in people with stroke-related drop foot. Phys Ther 92:398, 2012.

231. Gok, H, et al: Effects of ankle-foot orthoses on hemiparetic gait. Clin Rehabil 17:137, 2003.

232. Roth, EJ, et al: Physical activity and exercise recommendations for stroke survivors: An American Heart Association scientific

statement from the Council on Clinical Cardiology, Subcommittee on Exercise, Cardiac Rehabilitation and Prevention; the Council on Cardiovascular Nursing; the Council on Nutrition, Physical Activity, and Metabolism; and the Stroke Council. Circulation 109:2031, 2004.

233. Rose, D, et al: Feasibility and effectiveness of circuit training in acute stroke rehabilitation. Neurorehabil Neural Repair 20:1, 2010.

234. Hendricks, H, et al: Motor recovery after stroke: A systematic review of the literature. Arch Phys Med Rehabil 83:1629, 2002.

235. Meijer, R, et al: Prognostic factors for ambulation and activities of daily living in the subacute phase after stroke. A systematic review of the literature. Clin Rehabil 17(2):119, 2003.

236. Paolucci, S, et al: One-year follow-up in stroke patients discharged from rehabilitation hospital. Cerebrovasc Dis 10(1):25, 2000.

237. Jorgenson, H, et al: Outcome and time course of recovery. Part II: Time course of recovery. The Copenhagen Stroke Study. Arch Phys Med Rehabil 76:406, 1995.

238. Jorgensen, H, et al: Recovery of walking function in stroke patients: The Copenhagen Stroke Study. Arch Phys Med Rehabil 76:27, 1995.

239. Studenski, S, et al: Daily functioning and quality of life in a randomized controlled trial of therapeutic exercise for subacute stroke survivors. Stroke 36:1764, 2005.

240. Chen, M: Effects of exercise on quality of life in stroke survivors. Stroke 42:832–837, 2011.

241. Ottenbacher KJ, et al: Trends in length of stay, living setting, functional outcome, and mortality following medical rehabilitation. JAMA 292:1687, 2004.

242. Karges, J, and Smallfield, S: A description of outcomes, frequency, duration and intensity of occupational, physical, and speech therapy in inpatient stroke rehabilitation. J Allied Health 38:e1, 2009.

243. Van Peppen, RPS, et al: The impact of physical therapy on functional outcomes after stroke: What's the evidence? Clin Rehabil 18:833, 2004.

244. Dobkin, V: Rehabilitation after stroke. N Engl J Med 352:1677, 2005.

245. vanWijk, I, et al: Change in mobility activity in the second year after stroke in a rehabilitation population: Who is at risk for decline? Arch Phys Med Rehabil 87(1):45, 2006.

SUMMARY OF SCORES

MOTOR

Upper arm	_____	Maximum Score	36
Wrist & hand	_____ _____	Maximum Score	30
TOTAL UPPER EXTREMITY SCORE	_____	MAXIMUM SCORE	66
TOTAL LOWER EXTREMITY SCORE	_____	MAXIMUM SCORE	34

TOTAL MOTOR SCORE _____ TOTAL MAXIMUM SCORE 100 PERCENTAGE OF RECOVERY

BALANCE

TOTAL SCORE _____ MAXIMUM SCORE 14

SENSATION

TOTAL SCORE _____ MAXIMUM SCORE 24

JOINT RANGE OF MOTION

TOTAL SCORE _____ MAXIMUM SCORE 44

PAIN

TOTAL SCORE _____ MAXIMUM SCORE 44

TOTAL FUGL-MEYER SCORE _____ TOTAL MAXIMUM SCORE 226 PERCENTAGE OF RECOVERY

Area	Test	Scoring Criteria	Maximum Possible Score	Attained Score
Upper Extremity (sitting)	*Motor* I. Reflexes a. biceps _____ b. triceps _____	0—No reflex activity can be elicited. 2—Reflex activity can be elicited.	4	
	II. Flexor Synergy elevation _____ shoulder retraction _____ abduction (at least 90°) _____ external rotation _____ elbow flexion _____ forearm supination _____	0—Cannot be performed at all. 1—Performed partly. 2—Performed faultlessly.	12	
	III. Extensor Synergy shoulder adduction/internal rotation _____ elbow extension _____ forearm pronation _____	0—Cannot be performed at all. 1—Performed partly. 2—Performed faultlessly.	6	

Continued

713

Area	Test	Scoring Criteria	Maximum Possible Score	Attained Score
	IV. Movement Combining Synergies a. Hand to lumbar spine _____	a. 0—No specific action performed. 1—Hand must pass anterior superior iliac spine. 2—Action is performed faultlessly.		
	b. Shoulder flexion to 90° elbow at 0° _____	b. 0—Arm is immediately abducted or elbow flexes at start of motion. 1—Abduction or elbow flexion occurs in later phase of motion. 2—Faultless motion.		
	c. Pronation/supination of forearm with elbow at 90° and shoulder at 0° _____	c. 0—Correct position of shoulder and elbow cannot be attained, and/or pronation or supination cannot be performed at all. 1—Active pronation or supination can be performed even within a limited range of motion, and at the same time the shoulder and elbow are correctly positioned. 2—Complete pronation and supination with correct positions at elbow and shoulder.	6	
	V. Movement Out of Synergy a. Shoulder abduction to 90° elbow at 0° and forearm pronated _____	a. 0—*Initial* elbow flexion occurs or any deviation from pronated forearm occurs. 1—Motion can be performed partly, or if during motion, elbow is flexed or forearm cannot be kept in pronation. 2—Faultless motion.		
	b. Shoulder flexion, 90–180° elbow at 0° and forearm in mid position _____	b. 0—Initial flexion of elbow or shoulder abduction occurs. 1—Elbow flexion or shoulder abduction, occurs during shoulder flexion. 2—Faultless motion.		
	c. Pronation/supination of forearm elbow at 0° and shoulder between 30–90° of flexion _____	c. 0—Supination and pronation cannot be performed at all or elbow and shoulder position cannot be attained. 1—Elbow and shoulder properly positioned and pronation and supination performed in a limited range. 2—Faultless motion.	6	
Upper Extremity	VI. Normal Reflex Activity biceps and/or finger flexors and triceps _____	(This stage, which can render the score of two, is included only if the patient has a score of 6 in stage V.)		

Area	Test	Scoring Criteria	Maximum Possible Score	Attained Score
		0—At least 2 of the 3 phasic reflexes are markedly hyperactive. 1—One reflex markedly hyperactive or at least 2 reflexes are lively. 2—No more than one reflex is lively and none are hyperactive.	2	
Wrist	VII. a. Stability, elbow at 90°, shoulder at 0°	a. 1—Dorsiflexion is accomplished, but no resistance is taken. 2—Position can be maintained with some (slight) resistance.		
	b. Flexion/extension, elbow at 90°, shoulder at 0° _____	b. 0—Volitional movement does not occur. 1—Patient cannot actively move the wrist joint throughout the total ROM. 2—Faultless, smooth movement.		
	c. Stability, elbow at 0°, shoulder at 30° _____	c. Scoring is the same as for item a.		
	d. Flexion/extension, elbow at 0°, shoulder at 30° _____	d. Scoring is the same as for item b.		
	e. Circumduction _____	e. 0—Cannot be performed. 1—Jerky motion or incomplete circumduction. 2—Complete motion with smoothness.	10	
Hand	VIII. a. Finger Mass Flexion _____	a. 0—No flexion occurs. 1—Some flexion, but not full motion. 2—Complete active flexion (compared with unaffected hand).		
	b. Finger Mass Extension _____	b. 0—No extension occurs. 1—Patient can release an active mass flexion grasp. 2—Full active extension.		
	c. Grasp #1—MP joints extended and PIPS & DIPS are flexed. Grasp is tested against resistance.	c. 0—Required position cannot be acquired. 1—Grasp is weak. 2—Grasp can be maintained against relatively great resistance.		
	d. Grasp #2—Patient is instructed to adduct thumb, 1st carpometacarpophalangeal and interphalangeal joint at 0°	d. 0—Function cannot be performed. 1—Scrap of paper interposed between the thumb and index finger can be kept in place, but not against a slight tug. 2—Paper is held firmly against a tug.		

Continued

Area	Test	Scoring Criteria	Maximum Possible Score	Attained Score
	e. Grasp #3—Patient opposes the thumb pad against the pad of index finger. A pencil is interposed _____	e. Scoring procedures are the same as for Grasp #2.		
	f. Grasp #4—The patient should grasp a cylinder shaped object (small can), the volar surface of the 1st and 2nd finger against each other _____	f. Scoring procedures are the same as for Grasp #2 and #3.		
	g. Grasp #5—A spherical grasp.	g. Scoring procedures are the same as for Grasp #2, 3, and 4.	14	
Hand	IX. Coordination/Speed—Finger-to-nose (five repetitions in rapid succession). a. Tremor _____ b. Dysmetria _____ c. Speed _____	a. 0—Marked tremor. 1—Slight tremor. 2—No tremor. b. 0—Pronounced or unsystematic dysmetria. 1—Slight or systematic dysmetria. 2—No dysmetria. c. 0—Activity is more than 6 seconds longer than unaffected hand. 1—2 to 5 seconds longer than unaffected hand. 2—Less than 2 seconds difference.	6	
		TOTAL MAXIMUM UPPER EXTREMITY SCORE	66	
Lower Extremity (supine)	I. Reflex activity—tested in supine position. Achilles _____ atellar _____	0—No reflex activity 2—Reflex activity	4	
Supine	II. a. Flexor Synergy Hip flexion _____ Knee flexion _____ Ankle dorsiflexion _____ b. Extensor synergy—(motion is resisted) Hip extension _____ Adduction _____ Knee extension _____ Ankle plantarflexion _____	a. 0—Cannot be performed 1—Partial motion 2—Full motion b. 0—No motion 1—Weak motion 2—Almost full strength compared to normal	6 8	
Sitting (knees free of chair)	III. Movement Combining Synergies a. Knee flexion beyond 90° _____	a. 0—No active motion 1—From slightly extended position knee can be flexed but not beyond 90°		

Area	Test	Scoring Criteria	Maximum Possible Score	Attained Score
	b. Ankle dorsiflexion _____	b. 0—No active flexion 1—Incomplete active flexion 2—Normal dorsiflexion	4	
Standing	IV. Movement Out of Synergy Hip at 0° a. Knee flexion _____ b. Ankle dorsiflexion _____	a. 0—Knee cannot flex without hip flexion 1—Knee begins flexion without hip flexion, but doesn't get to 90°, or hip flexes during motion 2—Full motion as described b. 0—No active motion 1—Partial motion 2—Full motion	4	
Sitting	V. Normal Reflexes Knee flexors _____ Patellar _____ Achilles _____	0—2 of the 3 are markedly hyperactive 1—One reflex is hyperactive or 2 reflexes are lively 2—No more than 1 reflex lively	2	
(Supine)	VI. Coordination/Speed Heel to opposite knee (5 repetitions in rapid succession) a. Tremor _____ b. Dysmetria _____ c. Speed _____	a. 0—Marked tremor 1—Slight tremor 2—No tremor b. 0—Pronounced or unsystematic 1—Slight or systematic 2—No dysmetria c. 0—Six seconds slower than unaffected side 1—Two to 5 seconds slower 2—Less than 2 seconds difference	6	
		TOTAL MAXIMUM LOWER EXTREMITY SCORE	34	
Balance	a. Sit without support _____ b. Parachute reaction, non-affected side _____ c. Parachute reaction, affected side _____ d. Supported standing	a. 0—Cannot maintain sitting without support 1—Can sit unsupported less than 5 minutes 2—Can sit longer than 5 minutes b. 0—Does not abduct shoulder or extend elbow 1—Impaired reaction 2—Normal reaction c. Scoring is the same as #2 d. 0—Cannot stand 1—Stands with maximum support of others 2—Stands with minimum support of one for 1 minute		

Continued

Area	Test	Scoring Criteria	Maximum Possible Score	Attained Score
	e. Stand without support	e. 0—Cannot stand 1—Stands less than 1 minute or sways 2—Stands with good balance more than 1 min.		
	f. Stand on unaffected side _____	f. 0—Cannot be maintained longer than 1–2 sec. 1—Stands balanced 4–9 seconds 2—Stands balanced more than 10 sec.		
	g. Stand on affected side _____	g. 0—Scoring is the same as #6		
		MAXIMUM BALANCE SCORE	14	

Upper and Lower Extremities	*Sensation*
	I. Light Touch
	  a. Upper arm _____
	  b. Palm of hand _____
	  c. Thigh _____
	  d. Sole of foot _____
	
	II. Proprioception
	  a. Shoulder _____
	  b. Elbow _____
	  c. Wrist _____
	  d. Thumb _____
	  e. Hip _____
	  f. Knee _____
	  g. Ankle _____
	  h. Toe _____
		Light Touch Scoring
		  0—Anesthesia
		  1—Hyperaesthesia/dyesthesia
		  2—Normal
		
		Proprioception Scoring
		0—No sensation
		1—Three quarter of answers are correct, but considerable difference in sensation compared with unaffected side.
		2—All answers are correct, little or no difference
			8
			
			16	

Shoulder *Elbow* *Wrist* *Fingers* *Forearm* *Hip*	Motion/Pain Motion Pain Flexion _____ _____ Abduction to 90° _____ _____ External rotation _____ _____ Internal rotation _____ _____ Flexion _____ _____ Extension _____ _____ Flexion _____ _____ Extension _____ _____ Flexion _____ _____ Extension _____ _____ Pronation _____ _____ Supination _____ _____ Flexion _____ _____ Abduction _____ _____ External rotation _____ _____ Internal rotation _____ _____	Motion Scoring 0—Only a few degrees of motion 1—Decreased passive range of motion 2—Normal passive range of motion Pain Scoring 0—Marked pain at end of range or pain through range 1—Some pain 2—No pain	Motion 44 44	

Area	Test			Scoring Criteria	Maximum Possible Score	Attained Score
Knee	Flexion	———	———			
	Extension	———	———			
Ankle	Dorsiflexion	———	———			
	Plantarflexion	———	———			
Foot	Pronation	———	———			
	Supination	———	———			

Web-Based Resources for Clinicians, Families, and Patients with Stroke

American Heart Association	http://www.americanheart.org/
American Stroke Association—a division of the American Heart Association	http://www.strokeassociation.org/
National Stroke Association	http://www.stroke.org/
American Stroke Foundation	http://www.americanstroke.org/
International Stroke Society	http://www.internationalstroke.org
Stroke Association—UK	http://www.stroke.org.uk/
Heart and Stroke Foundation of Canada	http://www.heartandstroke.ca/
Veterans Affairs—stroke	http://www.va.gov/
Americans with Disabilities Act: ADA home page	http://www.usdoj.gov/crt/ada
Medicare information	http://www.cms.hhs.gov
Social Security Online	http://www.ssa.gov
National Institute of Neurological Disorders and Stroke	http://www.ninds.nih.gov
National Library of Medicine	http://www.nlm.nih.gov
American Association of Physical Medicine and Rehabilitation	http://www.aapmr.org/condtreat/rehab/stroke.htm
American Academy of Neurology (ANA)	http://www.aan.com/professionals
	http://www.aan.com/public (public education)
	http://www.neurology.org (Journal of Neurology)
National Rehabilitation Information Center (NARIC)	http://www.naric.com
Stroke rehab forum at Med Help	http://www.medhelp.org/forums/stroke Rehab/
Rehabilitation Research & Training Center on Stroke Rehabilitation	http://www.rrtc-stroke.org
Internet Handbook of Neurology	http://www.neuropat.dote.hu/stroke1.htm
Stroke and depression	http://www.nimh.nih.gov/publicat/depstroke.cfm
National Aphasia Association	http://www.aphasia.org
National Easter Seal Society	http://www.easter-seals.org
Disease prevention	http://www.everydaychoices.org
The Neurology Channel—stroke	http://www.neurologychannel.com/stroke/
Agency for Healthcare Research & Quality	http://www.ahrq.gov/consumer/strokecon.htm
Brain attack-stroke prevention & treatment—USFDA	http://www.fda.gov/fdac/features/2005/205_stroke.html
Stroke Information Directory	http://www.stroke-info.com
Clinical trials—National Institutes of Health (NIH)—stroke	http://www.clinicaltrials.gov/search/term=stroke
Stroke survivors	http://www.stroke-survivors.com
Resource center for clinicians and families	http://www.strokehelp.com/
The Stroke Network, Inc	http://www.strokenetwork.org
National Family Caregivers Association (NFCA)	http://www.nfcacares.org
Well Spouse Foundation	http://www.wellspouse.org
Ability Hub—assistive technology solutions	http://www.abilityhub.com
ABLEDATA—assistive technology information	http://www.abledata.com
Disabled Online	http://www.disabledonline.com

Multiple Sclerosis

Susan B. O'Sullivan, PT, EdD
Robert J. Schreyer, PT, DPT, NCS, MSCS, CSCS

Chapter 16

LEARNING OBJECTIVES

1. Describe the etiology, epidemiology, pathophysiology, signs and symptoms, diagnosis, and course of multiple sclerosis (MS).
2. Describe elements of the medical management of patients with MS.
3. Identify and describe the examination procedures used to inform the evaluation of patients with MS to establish the physical therapy diagnosis, prognosis, and plan of care.
4. Describe the role of the physical therapist in the management of patients with MS in terms of direct interventions and patient/client-related instruction to maximize function and quality of life.
5. Describe appropriate elements of the exercise prescription for patients with MS.
6. Review current research findings concerning the rehabilitation of patients with MS.
7. Identify the psychosocial impact of MS and describe appropriate interventions.
8. Analyze and interpret patient data, formulate realistic goals and outcomes, and develop a plan of care when presented with a clinical case study.

Multiple sclerosis (MS) is an autoimmune disease characterized by inflammation, selective demyelination, and gliosis. It causes both acute and chronic symptoms and can result in significant disability and impaired quality of life. MS affects approximately 400,000 persons in the United States; worldwide MS affects approximately 2.1 million people.[1] It was first defined by Dr. Jean Charcot in 1868 by its clinical and pathological characteristics: paralysis and the cardinal symptoms of intention tremor, scanning speech, and nystagmus, later termed *Charcot's triad*. Using autopsy studies he identified areas of hardened plaques and termed the disease *sclerosis in plaques*.[2]

The onset of MS typically occurs between ages 20 and 40 years. MS is rare in children, as is the onset of symptoms in adults older than age 50 years. The disease is more common in woman than in men by a ratio of 2:1 to 3:1. Although the incidence and prevalence of MS overall have increased over the last 5 decades, this increase appears to be mostly related to an increased prevalence in women.[3] There are also ethnic differences. MS affects predominantly white populations; African Americans demonstrate approximately half the risk of acquiring the disease. Low rates are also reported in Asians and Native Americans.[1]

Epidemiological studies have established a geographical pattern of MS prevalence with areas of high, medium, and low frequency. High-frequency areas include the temperate zones of the northern United States, the Scandinavian countries, northern Europe, southern Canada, New Zealand, and southern Australia. Areas of medium frequency closer to the equator include the southern United States and Europe and the rest of Australia, and low-frequency tropical areas include Asia, Africa, and South America. Migration studies indicate that the geographical risk associated with an individual's birthplace is retained if emigration occurs after age 15 years. Individuals migrating before this age assume the risk of their new location.[4,5]

ETIOLOGY

The risk of MS is increased in persons with an affected family member. The risk is 3.0% for a sibling, 5.0% for a fraternal co-twin, and rises to 25.0% for an identical co-twin. Genetic studies have revealed many interacting alleles that may contribute to MS susceptibility with mutations in the human leukocyte antigen major histocompatibility complex (MHC) gene most strongly correlated. It appears that although individuals do not inherit the disease, they may inherit a genetic susceptibility to immune system dysfunction.[1]

When persons with a genetic susceptibility are exposed to a viral agent, the immune system responds with activated myelin-reactive lymphocytes, a concept known as *molecular mimicry*. Implicated viruses in this process under investigation include the Epstein-Barr virus, measles, canine distemper, human herpesvirus-6, and *Chlamydia pneumoniae,* though none have been definitely proven to trigger MS. The viruses may be retained in the body, resulting in a self-perpetuating autoimmune process. Risk of MS may also be increased with vitamin D deficiency and smoking.[1]

PATHOPHYSIOLOGY

In patients with MS, the immune response triggers activation of immune cells (e.g., T cells, CD4+ helper T cells, B cells) that cross the blood–brain barrier. In turn, these cells activate autoantigens, producing autoimmune cytotoxic effects within the central nervous system (CNS) (this process can be viewed as a form of "friendly fire"). Phagocytic activity of macrophages may also contribute to demyelination.[1] **Myelin** serves as an insulator, speeding up the conduction along nerve fibers from one node of Ranvier to another (termed *saltatory conduction*). It also serves to conserve energy for the nerve because depolarization occurs only at the nodes. Disruption of the myelin sheath and active **demyelination** slows neural transmission and causes nerves to fatigue rapidly. With severe disruption, conduction block occurs with resulting disruption of function.

An acute inflammatory event emerges. Edema and infiltrates (e.g., monocytes, macrophages, and microglia) surround the acute lesion and can cause a *mass effect* (abnormally high pressures), further interfering with the conductivity of the nerve fiber. Conceivably, this inflammation (which gradually subsides) may, in part, account for the pattern of fluctuations in function that characterize this disease. With repeat attacks, the anti-inflammatory processes become less effective and are

unable to keep up. During the early stages of MS, *oligodendrocytes* (myelin-producing cells) survive the initial insult and can produce remyelination. This process is often incomplete and, as the disease becomes more chronic, stalls altogether. Eventually the oligodendrocytes become involved and myelin repair cannot occur. One form of MS, primary-progressive MS, appears to be associated exclusively with disease of the oligodendrocytes.[6] Demyelinated areas eventually become filled with fibrous astrocytes and undergo a process called gliosis. **Gliosis** refers to the proliferation of neuroglial tissue within the CNS and results in glial scars *(plaques)*. At this stage, the axon itself becomes interrupted and undergoes neurodegeneration. This is believed to be the main cause of permanent neurological disability. In advanced cases, there are both acute and degenerative lesions of varying size scattered throughout the CNS (brain, brainstem, cerebellum, and spinal cord). Lesions primarily affect white matter early, with lesions of gray matter evident in more advanced disease (type 1 lesions). Lesions may also include small perivascular areas of demyelination (type 2 lesions) and pial surface lesions (type 3). Brain atrophy, the loss of axons and myelin throughout the brain, is evident even in early stages of the disease and is progressive.[1] There are certain areas of predilection, such as the optic nerves, periventricular white matter, spinal cord (corticospinal tracts, posterior white columns), and cerebellar peduncles.[6]

DISEASE COURSE

MS is highly variable and unpredictable from person-to-person and within a given individual over time. At one end of the continuum, there is *benign MS,* defined as disease in which the patient remains fully functional in all neurological systems 15 years after onset. Benign MS affects fewer than 20% of cases. At the other end of the continuum, there is *malignant MS (Marburg disease),* a relatively rare disease course characterized by rapid onset and almost continual progression leading to significant disability or death within a relatively short time after onset.

There are four major disease courses (clinical subtypes) of MS. *Relapsing-remitting MS (RRMS)* is the most common course, affecting approximately 85% of patients with MS. It is characterized by discrete attacks or *relapses,* defined as periods of acute worsening of neurological function. Relapses are followed by *remissions,* defined as periods without disease progression and partial or complete abatement of signs and symptoms. Before the advent of disease-modifying medications, the majority of patients with RRMS went on to develop *secondary-progressive MS (SPMS).* SPMS begins with a relapsing-remitting course followed by progression to steady and irreversible decline with or without occasional acute attacks. *Primary-progressive MS (PPMS)* is a rare form occurring in about 10% of cases. It is characterized by a nearly continuous worsening of the disease from the onset without distinct attacks. Patients may experience modest fluctuations. *Progressive-relapsing MS (PRMS)* begins with a progressive disease course from the onset and steady deterioration (similar to PPMS), but with occasional acute attacks. It affects approximately 5% of patients with MS. Because the course of the disease may alter (RRMS to SPMS), clinicians need to be alert to changes in signs or symptoms in terms of severity, frequency, and impact on function.[1,7] Box 16.1 summarizes the clinical subtypes of multiple sclerosis.

Exacerbating Factors

MS relapses (exacerbations) are defined by new and recurrent MS symptoms lasting more than 24 hours but generally of longer duration that are unrelated to

---

Box 16.1 Four Major Clinical Subtypes of MS[1]

Relapsing-Remitting MS (RRMS)

- Characterized by discrete attacks of neurological deficits (relapse) with either full or partial recovery (remission) in subsequent weeks to months.
- The periods between relapses are characterized by lack of disease progression.
- The stable patient may have local inflammatory activity that is clinically silent.
- Affects approximately 85% of patients with MS at diagnosis.

Secondary-Progressive MS (SPMS)

- Characterized by an initial relapsing-remitting course, followed by a change in clinical course with progression to steady and irreversible decline with or without continued acute attacks.
- May be the result of progressive axonal loss rather than new lesions.
- Before newer treatments, the majority of patients with RRMS progressed to SPMS.

Primary-Progressive MS (PPMS)

- Characterized by disease progression and steady functional decline from onset; patients may experience modest fluctuations in neurological disability but discrete attacks do not occur.
- PPMS is associated with later onset (mean age 40 years) and more equal gender distribution.
- Affects approximately 10% of patients with MS.

Progressive-Relapsing MS (PRMS)

- Characterized by a steady deterioration in disease from onset (similar to PPMS) but with occasional acute attacks.
- Intervals between attacks are characterized by continuing disease progression.
- Affects approximately 5% of patients with MS.

---

another etiology. Several exacerbating factors have been identified. Avoiding these factors is important in ensuring the patient's optimal function. An individual whose overall health deteriorates is more likely to have a relapse than one who remains healthy. Viral or bacterial infections (e.g., cold, flu, urinary tract infection, sinus infection) and diseases of major organ systems (e.g., hepatitis, pancreatitis, asthma attacks) are associated with relapses of disease. There is also a modest link between stress and acute attacks. Both major life stress events (divorce, death, losing a job, trauma) and minor stresses (exhaustion, dehydration, malnutrition, and sleep deprivation) can affect the immune system and an already compromised nervous system.

Pseudoexacerbation refers to the temporary worsening of MS symptoms. The episode typically comes and goes quickly, usually within 24 hours. The overwhelming majority of individuals with MS demonstrate an adverse reaction to heat, known as *Uthoff's symptom.* Anything that raises the body temperature can bring on a pseudo-attack. External heat stressors include sun exposure, hot muggy environmental temperatures, or a hot bath. Internal elevations in temperature can be produced by fever or prolonged exercise. The effects are usually immediate and dramatic in terms of reduced function and increased fatigue. Most pseudo-attacks resolve within 24 hours of cooling off and/or the end of a fever.

■ SYMPTOMS

Symptoms of MS vary considerably, depending on the location of specific lesions. Early symptoms typically include minor visual disturbances (e.g., episodes of double vision) and paresthesias progressing to numbness, weakness, and fatigability. In more advanced stages, patients demonstrate multiple symptoms with varying involvement. Common MS symptoms are presented in Box 16.2.[8,9] The onset of symptoms can develop rapidly over a course of minutes or hours; less frequently, onset is insidious, occurring over a period of weeks or months. An early remission may lead the individual to postpone initial neurological workup for months or longer.

Sensory

Complete loss of any single sensation (anesthesia) is rare. Focal deficits can produce limited areas of diminished sensation. Altered sensations are far more common and can include *paresthesias* (pins-and-needles sensation) or numbness of the face, body, or extremities. Disturbances in position sense are also common, as are lower extremity (LE) impairments of vibratory sense.[9]

Pain

Approximately 80% of patients with MS experience pain, with clinically significant pain occurring in about 55%. Almost half experience chronic pain.[10] Patients often experience acute, paroxysmal pain characterized by sudden and spontaneous onset. The pains are described

Box 16.2   Common Symptoms in Multiple Sclerosis

Sensory Symptoms

- Hypoesthesia, numbness
- Paresthesias

Pain

- Paroxysmal limb pain, dysesthesias
- Headache
- Optic or trigeminal neuritis
- Lhermitte's sign
- Hyperpathia
- Chronic neuropathic pain

Visual Symptoms

- Blurred or double vision (diplopia)
- Diminished acuity/loss of vision
- Scotoma
- Nystagmus
- Lateral gaze palsy

Cognitive Symptoms

- Short-term memory deficits

Bowel Symptoms

- Diminished attention, concentration
- Diminished executive functions
- Diminished information processing
- Diminished visual–spatial abilities

Affective Symptoms

- Depression
- Anxiety
- Pseudobulbar affect
- Anxiety

Motor Symptoms

- Paresis or paralysis
- Fatigue
- Spasticity, spasms
- Ataxia: incoordination, intention tremor
- postural tremor
- Impaired balance and gait

Speech and Swallowing

- Dysarthria
- Diminished verbal fluency
- Dysphonia
- Dysphagia

Bladder Symptoms

- Spastic bladder
- Flaccid bladder
- Dyssynergic bladder
- Constipation
- Diarrhea and incontinence

Sexual Symptoms

- Impotence
- Decreased libido
- Impaired ability to achieve orgasm

Pattern of Symptoms

- Varies greatly from person to person
- Varies over time in each individual affected
- First symptoms usually transient; typically sensory and visual
- Diagnosis involves evidence of damage occurring in at least two separate areas of CNS and at two separate points in time at least one month apart (*dissemination of lesions in space and time*)

CNS = central nervous system.

as intense, sharp, shooting, electric shock–like, and burning. The most common types are trigeminal neuralgia, paroxysmal limb pain, and headache. *Trigeminal neuralgia* (tic douloureux) results from demyelination of the sensory division of the trigeminal nerve innervating the face, cheek, and jaw. Eating, shaving, or simply touching the face may trigger painful episodes. A common sign of posterior column damage in the spinal cord is **Lhermitte's sign** in which flexion of the neck produces an electric shock–like sensation running down the spine and into the LEs. Paroxysmal limb pain presents as abnormal burning, aching pain (dysesthesias) that can affect any part of the body but is more common in the LEs. It is the most common type of pain in MS and is worse at night and after exercise. It can be aggravated by temperature elevations. *Hyperpathia*, a hypersensitivity to minor sensory stimuli, can occur. For example, a light touch or light pressure stimulus elicits a severe pain reaction. Headache is more frequent in MS than in the general population and can be migraine or tension type. Chronic *neuropathic pain* can result from demyelinating lesions in spinothalamic tracts or in the sensory roots. It is more common in patients with minimum disability and is described as a burning pain similar to pain described by individuals with disk herniation. Musculoskeletal pain associated with muscle and ligament strain can develop from mechanical stress, abnormal postures, and immobility, often the result of weak muscles, powerful spasticity, and tonic spasms. Anxiety and fear can worsen pain symptoms.[10]

Visual

Visual symptoms are common with MS and are found in approximately 80% of patients. Involvement of the optic nerve produces altered visual acuity; blindness is rare. *Optic neuritis,* inflammation of the optic nerve, is a common problem, and produces an icepick-like pain behind the eye with blurring or graying of vision or blindness in one eye. A *scotoma* or dark spot may occur in the center of the visual field. Neuritis rarely affects both eyes and is usually self-limiting. Vision generally improves within 4 to 12 weeks. Damage to the optic nerve will also affect light reflexes. *Marcus Gunn pupil* often develops in individuals with MS who have had an episode of optic neuritis. Shining a bright light into the healthy eye will produce reflex contraction in both eyes (consensual light reflex). If the light is then shone in the affected eye only, a paradoxical widening (dilation) of both pupils occurs.

Eye movements can be disturbed in a variety of ways. *Nystagmus* is common in patients with MS and results from lesions affecting the cerebellum or central vestibular pathways. This involves involuntary cyclical movements of the eyeball (horizontal or vertical) that develop when the patient looks to the sides or vertically (gaze-induced nystagmus) or when the patient moves the head. *Internuclear ophthalmoplegia* (INO) produces incomplete eye adduction (lateral gaze palsy) on the affected side and nystagmus of the opposite abducting eye with gaze to one side. It is caused by demyelination of the pontine medial longitudinal fasciculus (MLF). Additional impairments in conjugate gaze and control of eye movements may also be present with brainstem lesions affecting cranial nerves III, IV, and VI or the MLF. *Diplopia,* double vision, occurs when the muscles that control the eyes are not well coordinated. Visual disturbances frequently remit and are seldom the primary cause of disability. The effects of impaired vision on balance and movement should be carefully examined.[11]

Motor

Patients with corticospinal lesions demonstrate signs and symptoms of upper motor neuron (UMN) syndrome. Paresis, spasticity, brisk tendon reflexes, involuntary flexor and extensor spasms, clonus, Babinski's sign, exaggerated cutaneous reflexes, and loss of precise autonomic control all characterize UMN involvement. (See discussion in Chapter 5, Examination of Motor Function: Motor Control and Motor Learning.)

Weakness

Patients with UMN syndrome demonstrate movements that are slow, stiff, and weak, the result of loss of orderly recruitment and reduced firing rate modulation of motor neurons. Reduced muscle strength, power, and endurance, along with impaired synergistic relationships, are evident. Patients with cerebellar lesions demonstrate asthenia or generalized muscle weakness along with ataxia. Patients can also experience muscle weakness secondary to inactivity. Muscle weakness can vary from a mild paresis, often transient at first, to total paralysis of the involved extremities.[9]

Spasticity

Spasticity is an extremely common problem in patients with MS, occurring in 75% of all cases. Spasticity can range from mild to severe, depending on the duration of the disease, number of relapses, and worsening symptoms in recent months. It occurs in the muscles of the upper extremities (UEs) and particularly the LEs. Clinical indications of spasticity include impaired voluntary control of movement (abnormal co-contraction); increased deep tendon reflexes (DTRs); clonus; and decreased range of motion (ROM). Spasticity also results in increased fatigue, impaired functional mobility, and impaired activities of daily living (ADL). Spasticity can cause pain, disabling contractures, abnormal posturing, problems in maintaining skin integrity, and falls. For some patients, spasticity can be beneficial to sitting and standing.[11] Spasticity fluctuates on a daily basis and can be exacerbated by certain factors, such as fatigue, stress, overheating (fever, environmental), infections, or noxious stimuli (e.g., pain, bladder, renal, bowel, skin lesions/injury).[12] Certain antidepressant agents (serotonin-reuptake inhibitors such as fluoxetine, sertraline, and paroxetine) can exacerbate spasticity.[13] Spasticity does not typically abate during spontaneous remissions. In patients with advanced disease, spasticity can be quite disabling and difficult to manage.[12]

Fatigue

Fatigue has been defined by the *Panel on Fatigue of the MS Council for Clinical Practice Guidelines* as "a subjective lack of physical and/or mental energy that is perceived by the individual or caregiver to interfere with usual and desired activities."[13, p. 1] Fatigue comes on abruptly without warning and typically worsens throughout the day. Patient complaints may include feelings of overwhelming tiredness, exhaustion, and weakness together with difficulty concentrating and mental dullness.[8] Fatigue is a daily event, experienced by 75% to 95% of individuals with the disease. Approximately 50% to 60% of patients report that fatigue is one of their most troubling symptoms. Patients consistently report that fatigue interferes with physical functioning (79% of patients), overall role performance (67% of patients), social participation, and perceived health status. Severity of disease does not seem to be related to fatigue severity; that is, individuals mildly affected by disease (ambulatory patients) report disabling fatigue as often as more severely disabled patients.[14] Fatigue is the result of central activation failure (*central fatigue*). Aggravating factors contributing to fatigue include physical exertion, exposure to heat and humidity (reported by 92% of patients), disturbed or reduced sleep, depression, low self-esteem and mood disorders, and medical conditions (e.g., respiratory infection). Side effects of medications also affect fatigue, including analgesics, anticonvulsants, antidepressants, antihistamines, antihypertensive agents, and anti-inflammatory agents.[12] Sense of mastery (control) is a strong psychosocial predictor of fatigue. Individuals with a low sense of mastery reported significantly more fatigue and fatigue-related distress.[15]

Coordination and Balance

Demyelinating lesions in the cerebellum and cerebellar tracts are common in MS, producing cerebellar symptoms. Clinical manifestations include ataxia, postural and intention tremors, hypotonia, and truncal weakness. **Ataxia** is a general term used to describe uncoordinated movements characterized by **dysmetria, dyssynergia,** and **dysdiadochokinesia.** Progressive ataxia of the trunk and LEs is often apparent. During sitting or standing, when a limb or the body must be supported against gravity, the patient typically presents with *postural tremor* (shaking, back-and-forth oscillatory movements). *Intention (action) tremors* are involuntary, rhythmic, shaking movements that occur when purposeful movement is attempted and results from the inability of the cerebellum to dampen motor movements (see Chapter 6, Examination of Coordination and Balance). Tremors vary in severity from slight, barely perceptible quivering (fine tremor) to wide oscillations (gross tremors). Severe tremors impose significant limitations in performance of functional activities, particularly in such areas as eating, speaking clearly, writing, personal hygiene, and walking. Tremor can be exacerbated by stress, excitement, and anxiety, all adrenalin-releasing conditions producing a temporary aroused condition.[9] Severe numbness of the feet can contribute to difficulty with standing balance or walking (sensory ataxia).

Lesions affecting the cerebellum (archicerebellum) or central vestibular pathways can produce vestibular dysfunction. Patients may experience symptoms of dizziness, disequilibrium, vertigo, nausea, and so forth. Symptoms are precipitated or made worse by movements of the head or eyes (see Chapter 21, Vestibular Disorders).

Gait and Mobility

Individuals with MS experience difficulty walking as a result of muscle weakness, fatigue, spasticity, impaired balance, impaired sensation, visual problems, and ataxia. Approximately half of patients with RRMS will require some form of assistance during walking within 15 years of their diagnosis. Staggering, uneven steps, poor foot placement, uncoordinated limb movements, and frequent loss of balance characterize ataxic gait. It is often mistaken for drunkenness, a finding that frequently results in the patient revealing the disease for the first time ("outing"). Severe LE extensor spasticity may produce a scissoring gait pattern. Gait and balance impairments increase the risk of falls and fall injury. Approximately half of patients with MS report recent falls. Fear of falling is associated with self-imposed restrictions in mobility and contributes to disability and social isolation.[8]

Speech and Swallowing

Speech problems are the result of muscle weakness, spasticity, tremor, or ataxia and affect as many as 40% of individuals with MS. **Dysarthria** is characterized by slurred or poorly articulated speech with low volume, unnatural emphasis, and slow rate. **Dysphonia** is characterized by changes in vocal quality including harshness, hoarseness, breathiness, or hypernasal sounds. Poor coordination of the tongue and oral muscles can also result in **dysphagia**, difficulty in swallowing. Signs of swallowing dysfunction include difficulty chewing and maintaining a lip seal, inability to swallow (ingest food), and spitting or coughing during or after meals. Aspiration pneumonia is a serious complication that can develop if foods or liquids are inhaled into the trachea. Signs of this include a wet voice quality with gurgling or sounds of congestion, and fever. The patient is also at risk for poor nutritional intake and dehydration and may experience weight loss. Poor coordination of breath control and posture contributes to speech and feeding difficulties.[16]

Cognitive

Cognitive symptoms in MS are common, with approximately 50% of patients demonstrating measurable impairments. Only 10% of patients experience problems severe enough to interfere with daily activities. Cognitive impairments are related to the specific location of the lesions rather than to the overall severity of the disease, its course, or the patient's disability status. Cognitive functions likely to be affected in MS include short-term memory, attention and concentration, information processing, executive functions (concept formation, abstract reasoning, problem solving, and planning and sequencing), visuospatial functions, and verbal fluency. Long-term memory, conversational skills, and reading comprehension are typically intact. Focal frontal lobe lesions can produce cognitive inflexibility and poor impulse control. Significant mental deterioration (global dementia) is relatively rare and may be seen in rapidly progressing disease (malignant MS) or in patients with significant cerebral lesions. Secondary factors that can influence cognition include depression, fatigue, medications, and co-morbid conditions (e.g., cardiovascular or cerebrovascular disease). Level of cognitive dysfunction is a major factor in determining quality of life, social functioning, employment status, and function.[8,17]

Depression

Clinical depression is common in patients with MS, with at least 50% of individuals experiencing a major depressive episode. Depressive symptoms can include feelings of hopelessness or despair, diminished interest or pleasure in activities, changes in appetite and significant weight loss or gain, insomnia or hypersomnia (daytime sleepiness), feelings of lethargy or worthlessness, fatigue or loss of energy, decreased concentration, and recurrent thoughts of death and suicide.[18] It can occur as a direct result of MS lesions, as a side effect of some drugs (e.g., corticosteroids, possibly interferon), or as a psychological reaction to the stresses of this far-reaching and unpredictable disease.[19] Anxiety, denial, anger, aggression, or dependency can also occur. Patients with MS face enormous issues related to the ambiguity of their health status, the unpredictable course of disease activity, unpredictable future status, and the loss of effective functioning during the prime of their lives. Feelings of learned helplessness and low self-efficacy are common and have been linked to depression.[20] Moreover, many of the symptoms of MS (tremor, scanning speech, incontinence) are socially embarrassing, causing additional emotional distress.

Emotional

Affective disorders occur in approximately 10% of cases and can include changes in mood, feelings, emotional expression, and control. **Pseudobulbar affect** (PBA), also known as *involuntary emotional expression disorder* or *emotional incontinence,* is characterized by sudden and unpredictable episodes of crying, laughing, or other emotional displays. It may occur when the disease damages the area of the brain that controls normal expression of emotion. **Euphoria** consists of an exaggerated feeling of well-being, a sense of optimism incongruent with the patient's incapacitating disability. Bipolar affective disorders (alternating periods of depression and mania) can also occur. Affective symptoms have been linked to more advanced disease and greater intellectual impairment.[21,22]

Bladder

Urinary bladder dysfunction occurs in about 80% of patients. Demyelinating lesions affecting the lateral and posterior spinal tracts unmask the sacral reflex arc producing loss in volitional and synergistic control of the micturition reflex. Types of bladder dysfunction in MS can include a small, spastic bladder (a failure to store problem), a flaccid or big bladder (a failure to empty problem), or a dyssynergic bladder. The dyssynergic or conflicting bladder represents a problem with coordination between the bladder contraction and sphincter relaxation. Common symptoms include urinary urgency, urinary frequency, hesitancy in starting urination, nocturia (frequency at night), dribbling, and incontinence. The severity of bladder symptoms is associated with severity of other neurological symptoms, particularly pyramidal tract involvement. Progressive loss of functional mobility (e.g., hand skills, sitting balance and transfer skills, ambulation) contributes to personal hygiene problems, emotional distress, and functional incontinence (inability to toilet or manage dysfunction). Emptying dysfunction with large residual urine volume increases the risk of recurrent urinary tract infections (UTIs) and kidney damage from frequent UTIs.[23]

Bowel

Constipation is the most common bowel complaint in MS and results from lesions affecting control of the gastrocolic reflex. It is associated with the presence of spasticity of the pelvic floor muscles and is also a frequent consequence of inactivity, lack of fluid intake, poor diet and bowel habits, depression, and medication side effects. Bowel impaction is a serious complication that requires immediate attention. Diarrhea and incontinence are less problematic but can also occur as a result of loss of rectal control, sphincter abnormalities, or other, secondary problems (e.g., gastroenteritis, inflammatory bowel disease).[24]

Sexual

Sexual dysfunction is common, affecting as many as 91% of men and 72% of women. In women, symptoms can include changes in sensation, vaginal dryness, trouble reaching orgasm, and loss of libido. In men, symptoms can include impotence, decreased sensation, difficulty or inability to ejaculate, and loss of libido. Sexual activity is also affected by the appearance of other symptoms such as spasticity, uncontrollable spasms, pain, weakness and fatigue, bladder or bowel incontinence, losses in functional mobility, and changes in self-image. Psychological factors have a large impact on function. Sexual dysfunction has tremendous functional and psychosocial implications for both patient and partner.[25]

■ DIAGNOSIS

The diagnosis of MS is made by the neurologist based on a careful medical history, a complete neurological examination, and supportive laboratory tests. Evidence of damage must be present in at least two separate areas of the CNS (dissemination of lesions in space) and damage must have occurred at two separate points in time at lease 1 month apart (dissemination of lesions in time). In addition, other possible diagnoses must be ruled out. The revised 2010 *McDonald Criteria of the International Panel on Diagnosis of MS* has resulted in earlier diagnosis of MS with improved specificity and sensitivity (TipSheet is available at www.nationalmssociety.org/).[26, 27]

Laboratory tests used to help confirm the diagnosis include magnetic resonance imaging (MRI), evoked potentials (EP), and lumbar puncture (LP) with cerebrospinal fluid (CSF) analysis.

MRI is highly sensitive for detecting MS plaques in the white matter of the brain and spinal cord (Fig. 16.1). New lesions with active inflammation that occur during the preceding 6 weeks or so are seen as areas of increased signal intensity, "bright spots." Contrast-enhanced T1-weighted images (gadolinium-enhanced) are used to

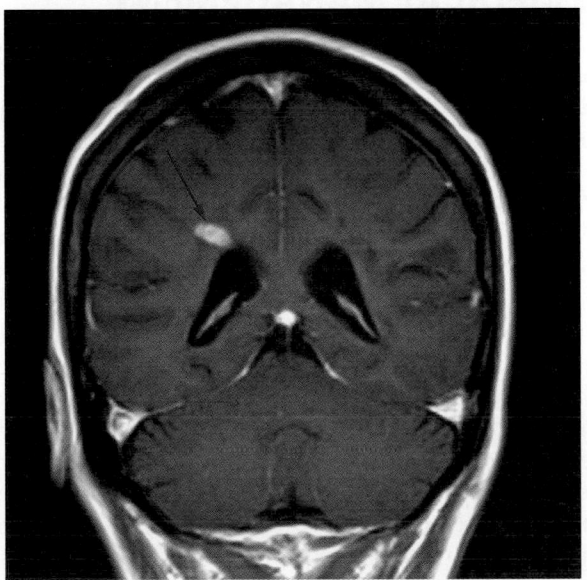

Figure 16.1 Coronal contrast-enhanced T1 MRI. The contrast enhancement of a periventricular white matter lesion (arrow) indicates that this is an active MS plaque. Other (older) plaques in this case that were T2 hyperintense showed no enhancement. *(From Weber et al,[29] with permission.)*

detect more long-term disease activity (i.e., loss of myelin and axons, gliosis). These lesions are seen as "black holes" on the MRI; the darker the lesion, the more extensive the tissue damage. Approximately 95% of patients with clinically defined MS have well-defined MRI changes. Excessive MRI activity includes three or more enhancements on repeat scans separated by at least quarterly intervals. Lesions revealed on MRI do not always correlate with clinical disability. "Silent attacks" documented by MRI changes outnumber the attacks that cause active symptoms such as paralysis or vision loss by 10:1. Misdiagnosis can occur, because 5% of individuals with confirmed MS do not exhibit MRI changes. In addition, other diseases can cause similar lesions evident on MRI (e.g., disseminated encephalomyelitis) and some healthy individuals can exhibit bright spots on MRI. Neurology guidelines call for MRIs to be performed at predefined intervals to document disease progression and response to disease-modifying medications.[28,29]

Up to 90% of individuals with MS demonstrate abnormal EP. The presence of demyelinating lesions on visual, auditory, and somatosensory pathways produces slowed conduction. Of the three, visual evoked potentials (VEPs) have been found to be the most helpful in the diagnostic process.[26]

Patients with MS show elevated total immunoglobulin (IgG) in CSF and the presence of oligoclonal IgG bands (seen in 90% to 95% of patients) in response to inflammatory demyelinating lesions. Patients with PPMS have higher levels of immunoglobulins in spinal fluid than patients with RRMS.[26]

■ MEDICAL MANAGEMENT

A number of medications are used to help treat and prevent relapses and slow the progression of neurological disability. Medications are also given to provide symptom relief.

Management of Acute Relapses

Corticosteroid therapy (methylprednisolone) is used to treat acute disease relapses (exacerbations), shortening the duration of the episode. These drugs exert powerful anti-inflammatory and immunosuppressive effects, including diminished swelling within the CNS, decreased T-cell activation, limited immune cell penetration of the CNS, and enhanced apoptosis of activated immune cells. The drugs do not modify the disease course or degree of recovery. Typically, corticosteroids are given in high doses (500 to 1,000 mg/day), administered intravenously for a brief course (e.g., 3 to 5 days), followed by tapered dosage of oral medication over a period of 1 to 3 weeks. There are a number of potential adverse side effects, including mood changes, increased blood pressure, fluid retention, hyperglycemia, acne, and insomnia. Chronic use is associated with hypertension, diabetes, aseptic femoral necrosis, osteopenia, and peptic ulcer.[30]

Plasmapheresis (plasma exchange) may be used to enhance recovery from an acute relapse in patients who fail to respond to steroids. It is used for an exacerbation of RRMS and is not recommended for PPMS or SPMS.

Disease-Modifying Therapeutic Agents

Since 1993 the U.S. Food and Drug Administration (FDA) has approved drugs to reduce disease activity in people with MS. Synthetic interferon drugs (interferon beta-1b [Betaseron, Extavia], interferon beta 1-a [Avonex and Rebif]) are first-line injectable drugs that have substantial immunomodulating properties. These are close copies of a naturally occurring human chemical, interferon beta. Interferons slow down the immune system response by reducing inflammation, swelling, and rapid proliferation of T and B cells. They also block activated T cells from crossing the blood–brain barrier and damaging myelin. Other disease-modifying drugs include glatiramer acetate (Copaxone), fingolimod (Gilenya), natalizumab (Tysabri), and mitoxantrone (Novantrone). Daily pills have also been approved by the FDA to treat MS (e.g. Aubagio, Tecfidera). Patients may show reduced relapses, reduced number of new lesions on MRI, and reduced severity of attack as evidenced by acquired neurological deficits. For patients with new and suspected MS (clinical isolated syndrome [CIS]), the medications may delay time to a second clinical episode and a confirmed diagnosis of MS. Continued, frequent relapses or excessive MRI activity may indicate the need to switch drug therapy to higher doses or combination therapies. These agents cannot, however, reverse existing deficits. All of these medications are contraindicated for women who are pregnant or trying to become pregnant, or who are breastfeeding.[20,31] Table 16.1 presents an overview of the disease-modifying drugs.

Common adverse effects of the injectable interferon drugs include injection-site skin reactions (soreness, redness, pain, bruising, or swelling) and flu-like symptoms following injection that lessen over time (fever, chills, sweating, muscle aches, and fatigue). Injection sites are varied to reduce adverse effects. Rare and more severe adverse reactions include depression, allergic reactions, and liver reactions. Copaxone can produce similar injection-site reactions and an initial flushing reaction immediately after injection (anxiety, chest pain, palpitations, shortness of breath). It has the advantage of not causing flu-like symptoms or depression. Patients receive Novantrone by intravenous (IV) infusion in a medical facility and must be closely monitored for serious heart and liver damage. Tysabri poses serious risks for a rare brain infection (progressive multifocal leukoencephalopathy [PML]). An additional disadvantage is the significant annual cost of these drugs (in the thousands of dollars) that may not be covered fully by private insurance plans.[30,31]

Problems with adherence using immunomodulating agents are well documented, especially for the injectable medications. Health professionals can have a significant impact on promoting acceptance and maintenance of

Table 16.1   Disease-Modifying Therapeutic Agents for MS

Agent	FDA-Approved Indications	Delivery System and Frequency
Interferon beta-1b	RRMS, CIS	
Betaseron		SC injections, every other day
Extavia		SC injections, every other day
Interferon beta-1a	RRMS	
Avonex		IM injection, once/week
Rebif		SC injection, 3 times/week
Glatiramer acetate (Copaxone)	RRMS, CIS	SC injection, every day
Gilenya (Fingolimod)	RRMS	Capsule, once daily
Tysabri (natalizumab)	RRMS Not used as an initial treatment	IV infusion in a medical center, monthly
Novatrone (mitoxantrone)	SPMS, PRMS, worsening RRMS Not approved for PPMS Not for use as an initial treatment or for individuals with heart dysfunction	IV infusion in a medical center, once every 3 months Maximum of 8–12 doses over 2–3 years
Tecfidere	RRMS	Oral: twice daily capsule
Aubagio (teriflunomide)	RRMS	Oral: once-daily pill

CIS = clinical isolated syndrome; FDA = Food and Drug Administration; IM = intramuscular; IV = intravenous; PPMS = primary-progressive MS; PRMS = progressive-relapsing MS; RRMS = relapsing-remitting MS; SC = subcutaneous; SPMS = secondary-progressive MS.

immunomodulating therapy. In discussions with the patient the therapist needs to determine the patient's understanding of the treatment benefits and risks, perception of his or her illness, general mood and level of self-esteem, lifestyle and daily living situation, and level of family and community support. Professionals need to support the patient's hope for a positive outcome from drug therapy and emphasize the benefits of early treatment and the importance of consistency in management.[32]

Management of Symptoms

Pharmacological agents are used for symptomatic relief of a wide range of symptoms in MS. The clinician should have a thorough understanding of the medications the patient is taking, the expected benefit, and potential adverse reactions.

Spasticity

Management of spasticity and spasms includes the use of muscle relaxants. Oral baclofen (Lioresal) is commonly used and is highly effective in reducing muscle tone and decreasing the frequency of spasms and clonus. Dosage is progressed gradually to obtain optimal effects. Other examples of oral agents include tizanidine (Zanaflex), dantrolene sodium (Dantrium), and diazepam (Valium). The reduction in spasticity must be balanced with the possibility of adverse effects from overdosing that may include sedation (drowsiness), weakness, and fatigue. The therapist must be alert to these changes and communicate with the physician to achieve optimal dosing for rehabilitation. The therapist must also recognize that at times

spasticity can be used to enhance function, substituting for lack of strength. For example, extensor spasticity can be used to assist standing during a stand-pivot transfer. Significant reduction of spasticity with medications might serve to produce loss of function. Carbamazepine (Tegretol) can be effective in reducing paroxysmal (sudden, sharp-onset) spasms. Patients who do not adequately respond to standard drug treatment (e.g., those with intractable spasticity or spasms) may benefit from intrathecal administration of baclofen directly into the CSF of the lumbar spine via a catheter. A programmable implanted pump controls the dosage. Significant reduction in spasticity and spasms has been reported in the LEs and trunk with less improvement reported in the UEs. Adverse effects can include sedation, dizziness, impaired vision, and impaired speech. Pump failure, infection, and lead displacement can also occur.[8,33]

Botulinum toxin (BT) injections are used to provide localized relief of muscle tone and spasms. Efficacy is short term and generally lasts up to 3 months. Excessive use of BT can overly weaken muscles, so it is typically reserved for patients with significant problems. Physical therapy stretching of the limb for at least 4 weeks after injection is an important adjunct. Phenol injections have also been used but are more unpredictable in degree and duration of response and are associated with sensory side effects.[8]

Surgical intervention may be considered for patients with intractable spasticity. The typical surgical candidate presents with spastic paralysis for many years resulting in a nonfunctional limb and serious complications (e.g., contractures and skin breakdown). Interventions include severing tendons (*tendonotomy*), nerves (*neurectomy*), or nerve roots (*rhizotomy*).[8]

Pain

A variety of drugs are available to manage pain and clinical decisions are based on type of pain. Tricyclic antidepressants are used to treat burning, central neuropathic pain similar to the use with peripheral neuropathic pain. Paroxysmal pain responds to carbamazepine (Tegretol), amitriptyline (Elavil), phenytoin (Dilantin), diazepam (Valium), or gabapentin (Neurontin). Dysesthesias are managed with low doses of amitriptyline (Elavil), imipramine (Tofranil), or desipramine (Norpramin). Antiepileptic drugs (carbamazepine) are used with trigeminal neuralgia. The discomfort and pain associated with spasticity and spasms may be managed with over-the-counter or prescription anti-inflammatory drugs. Sometimes pain can be managed with mild painkillers (acetaminophen or ibuprofen). Strong opioids (oxycodone, methadone, morphine) have limited effectiveness and are not typically prescribed.[10,30]

Fatigue

Amantadine (Symmetrel) and modafinil (Provigil) have demonstrated moderate benefit in managing MS-related fatigue in some patients. In patients receiving disease-modifying agents, glatiramer acetate is associated with less fatigue than interferon beta-1b.[8]

Tremor

Agents to decrease tremor have been used with varying degrees of success. Some patients respond well to a single drug, some to combinations of drugs, and some find no benefit. Medications used to decrease tremor include hydroxyzine (Atarax, Vistaril), clonazepam (Klonopin), propranolol (Inderal), buspirone (Buspar), ondansetron (Zofran), and primidone (Mysoline). Dizziness and vertigo can be managed with antinausea drugs (meclizine [Antivert]) or with scopolamine patches. Severe tremor can also be treated with deep brain stimulation, which involves implanting electrodes into the thalamus.[28]

Cognitive and Emotional Impairments

Cognitive rehabilitation training has been used to improve function in patients with MS. Compensatory training strategies (e.g., memory aids, organizational tools) can improve function in everyday activities together with modifying the home environment to limit distractions. Medications approved for the treatment of Alzheimer's disease (donepezil [Aricept]) have been shown to provide only modest benefits in memory deficits and verbal learning in some patients.[8]

Depression can be managed effectively with antidepressant medications (e.g., fluoxetine [Prozac], Paxil, sertraline [Zoloft]). Some antidepressants can also decrease fatigue. Patients with pseudobulbar affect can be effectively treated with the antidepressant medication amitriptyline (Elavil). Professional counseling and participation in support groups often help the patient cope with the stresses of this unpredictable disease. Exercise and an active lifestyle are important components to reduce depression and anxiety.

Bladder and Bowel Impairments

Urinary problems require a complete urodynamic workup to identify the specific cause of the problem and to arrive at the appropriate course of treatment. Treatment for an overactive, spastic bladder (storage dysfunction) typically involves pharmacological management with anticholinergic medications (propantheline [Pro-Banthine], oxybutynin [Ditropan], imipramine [Tofranil]) to regulate bladder emptying. Adverse effects can include dry mouth, tachycardia, blurred vision, and accommodation disturbances. Dietary recommendations include drinking 8 glasses of fluid per day (water) while limiting intake of caffeine or alcohol. A flaccid bladder (emptying dysfunction) is managed with alternate techniques for emptying, including instruction in the *Crede maneuver* (the application of manual downward pressure over the lower abdomen) or intermittent self-catheterization (ISC) performed four to five times per day. Pharmacological agents may include cholinergic stimulation with urecholine. Dietary recommendations include limiting intake of citrus juices while drinking cranberry juice daily or taking cranberry tablets. A dyssynergic bladder (combined dysfunction) is managed with alpha-adrenergic blocking agents (e.g., terazosin [Hytrin], prazosin [Minipress], tamsulosin [Flomax]) and antispasticity agents (e.g., baclofen [Lioresal], tizanidine hydrochloride [Zanaflex]). On rare occasions when bladder symptoms cannot be controlled with medication and/or ISC, continuous catheterization (indwelling or Foley catheter; condom, or Texas catheter) or surgical urinary diversion (suprapubic catheter) may be necessary. For example, the patient with advanced disease and significant ataxia of the UEs may be unable to manually perform self-catheterization. Urinary tract infections result from retention of urine in the bladder and from catheterization procedures. Antibiotic therapy is the mainstay of treatment.[8]

Constipation is a common problem and may be associated with medications that can exacerbate constipation (e.g., antihypertensives, analgesics/narcotics, tricyclic antidepressants, anticholinergics, diuretics, sedatives/tranquilizers, antacids). It is typically managed with dietary changes including increased fluid intake (six to eight glasses daily) and fiber in the diet. Bulk-forming supplements (Metamucil, FiberCon, Citrucel, Benefiber), or stool softeners (Colace [docusate], Surfak [docusate], miraLax [polyethylene glycol]) can also be used. Regular or continuous use of stimulant laxatives and enemas is not recommended. Bowel training may also include manual disimpaction. Incontinence management includes dietary changes such as avoidance of irritants (caffeine, alcohol); adjustment of medications used to reduce spasticity, which can contribute to the problem; or addition of medications to control bowel spasms (tolterodine [Detrol], propantheline [Pro-Banthine]).[34]

■ FRAMEWORK FOR REHABILITATION

The chronicity of this disease, along with its variable and unpredictable course, may lead some to view individuals with MS as poor rehabilitation candidates. Although the disease or its direct impairments cannot be altered, there is strong evidence to support rehabilitation in producing significant gains in enhancing levels of activity and participation.[35-50] In a Cochrane Database Systematic Review of multidisciplinary rehabilitation for adults with MS, researchers identified 10 trials (9 randomized controlled trials [RCTs] and 1 controlled clinical trial [CCT] with 954 participants and 73 caregivers) that met the inclusion criteria. Support was strong for producing both short- and long-term gains (up to 12 months) following rehabilitation in activity and participation for both inpatient and outpatient programs. Low-intensity programs conducted over longer time periods produced stronger evidence in improving quality of life. Evidence of benefits to caregivers was limited. The researchers concluded that suggestions for "best dose" of therapy or optimal therapy are not possible given the current level of clinical trials.[51]

According to the National MS Society's Medical Advisory Board, rehabilitation referral should be initiated whenever there is an "abrupt or gradual worsening of function or an increase in impairment that has a significant impact on the individual's mobility, safety, independence, and/or quality of life."[52, p. 1]

Individuals with neurodegenerative diseases such as MS benefit from *restorative intervention,* aimed at remediating or improving impairments, activity limitations, and participation restrictions.[53] Direct CNS impairments are not responsive to intervention whereas indirect impairments caused by evolving multisystem dysfunction from inactivity and disuse can be modified (Fig. 16.2). For example, strength training can result in meaningful improvements in balance and gait. Goals and outcome statements reflective of restorative intervention focus on remediating impairments and regaining functional independence while promoting self-management skills. As the disease progresses, important goals and outcomes also include assisting the patient in effective coping skills by promoting acceptance and adjustment to limitations and disabilities and enhancing quality of life. The enhancement of quality of life may in fact be the most meaningful outcome for patients in the face of chronic neurodegenerative disease.

Preventative intervention is aimed at minimizing potential complications, impairments, activity limitations, or disabilities as the disease progresses. Preventative interventions for the patient with MS are geared toward decreasing the duration and severity of symptoms or delaying the

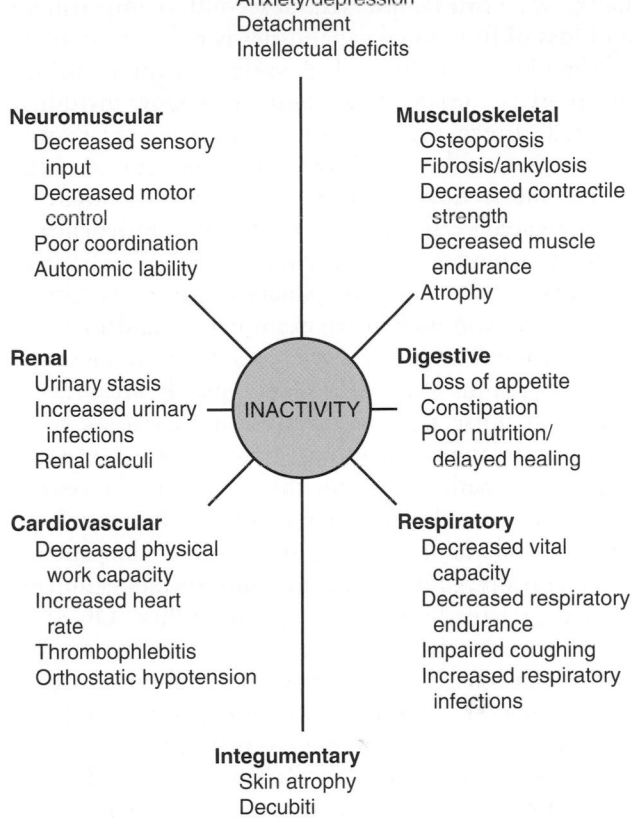

Figure 16.2 Clinical manifestations of inactivity.

emergence of disease sequelae through early detection and intervention, termed *secondary prevention.* Prevention is also aimed at minimizing the degree of disability, termed *tertiary prevention.* Goal and outcome statements reflective of preventative intervention focus on promotion of health, wellness, and fitness, and preservation of optimal function.[53]

Compensatory intervention is aimed at modifying the task, activity, or environment to maintain optimal function within the scope of existing impairments and limitations. Goal and outcome statements reflective of compensatory intervention focus on regaining/maintaining function.[53]

Maintenance therapy is defined as a series of occasional clinical, educational, and administrative services designed to maintain the patient's current level of function. Individuals with MS who benefit from maintenance therapy typically are in the late stages of the disease (Expanded Disability Status Scale [EDSS] stages 7.0 to 9.5; the EDSS is discussed later in the section titled Tests and Measures). Maintenance programs are not well funded by insurance and require careful documentation. Medicare, which covers services for the elderly and the disabled, covers maintenance therapy if the *professional skills of a therapist* (specialized knowledge and judgment) are needed to maintain a person's condition because of identified dangers.[54] For example, risk of secondary impairment and loss of functional capabilities is reduced or safety of caregivers is enhanced. A variety of interventions are used to achieve goals and outcomes, including limited direct interventions, patient/client-related instruction, and supportive counseling. The therapist tapers the frequency of the visits as the patient or family/caregivers are able to assume independent self-management of the care plan.

A coordinated interdisciplinary team is necessary to oversee the comprehensive examination and management needed to address the patient's complex and multifaceted problems. The team typically includes the physician, nurse, physical therapist, occupational therapist, speech-language pathologist, nutritionist, and social worker. As with any team, the patient is the central figure, with family and caregivers being key members. The ideal rehabilitation program considers the patient's disease history, course, and symptoms, including impairments, activity limitations, and disability. Of equal importance are the patient's abilities (assets), priorities, and resources (e.g., family, home, community). The focus is on long-range planning with anticipated episodes of care, including hospital-based, outpatient, and home/community-based care. Dal Bello-Haas[55] discusses a continuum of care based on disease stage (early, middle, and late) for individuals with neurodegenerative diseases. Considerations for the patient with MS are presented in Table 16.2.

■ PHYSICAL THERAPY EXAMINATION

Because many different areas of the CNS may be affected, it is imperative that a careful examination is performed to determine the extent of neurological and functional involvement. Subsequent reexaminations at specified intervals are used to distinguish change in status as well as effects of treatment. It may not always be possible to differentiate change in status associated with remission of symptoms from treatment outcomes. Considering the variability of symptoms of any individual patient, it is often beneficial to observe performance over a period of a few days to obtain a representative sample of baseline functioning. Fatigue and exacerbating factors should be taken into account when scheduling the examination.

Physical therapy examination data can be obtained through the patient's history and systems review and relevant tests and measures. The selection of examination procedures and level of inquiry are determined by the patient's unique status. The severity of problems, stage of disease (early/mild, middle/moderate, and late/advanced), age, setting of rehabilitation, and other factors must all be taken into account in structuring the examination.

Patient/Client History

Data obtained through interview with the patient/family and review of the medical record will provide information on general demographics, medical/surgical history, social and employment history, family history, living environment, general health status, and social and health habits. The patient's current/primary complaints and current functional status and activity level should be ascertained. Coexisting health problems and medications should also be identified.

Systems Review

Data obtained from the history and medical record will inform the systems review and help focus selection of appropriate tests and measures (Box 16.3). Review of the following systems is included: (1) cardiovascular, (2) integumentary, (3) musculoskeletal, (4) neuromuscular, and (5) cognitive, emotional, and communication.

Tests and Measures

The following are specific areas and relevant tests and measures that can be used to examine function in patients with MS (for more detailed descriptions, see earlier chapters in this text focusing on examination).

Cognition

Memory function, attention, concentration, conceptual reasoning, problem solving, and speed of information processing should be examined, as well as the effects of fatigue on cognitive performance. An expert panel convened by the Consortium of MS Centers in 2001 developed the *Minimal Examination of Cognitive Function in MS (MACFIMS)*. This 90-minute battery of seven neuropsychological tests examines processing speed/working memory, learning and memory, executive function, visual–spatial processing, and word retrieval.[56] A brief screen of cognitive function can be achieved using the *Mini-Mental Status Examination (MMSE)*.[57]

Affective and Psychosocial Function

Emotional stability should be examined. The presence of emotional lability, euphoria, emotional dysregulation, or depression (symptoms, severity, length, effect on functional performance); the level of stress and anxiety; coping strategies; and presence of sleep disorders should be documented. A useful instrument is the *Beck Depression Inventory*.[58] As previously mentioned, it is imperative that the physical therapist be familiar with the patient's medications, because numerous medications will have effects on the affective and psychosocial domain.

Sensation

Given the extent of variability in sensory deficits in individuals with MS, a detailed examination of superficial and deep sensations should be completed (see Chapter 3,

Stage of MS	Common Impairments and Activity Limitations	Intervention Strategies
Early/Mild	• Few/minimal impairments and activity limitations with independence maintained • Motor symptoms present but do not interfere with daily activities • Symptoms for RRMS are more variable and do not progress at the same rate as PPMS or PRMS • SPMS initially presents with relapsing-remitting course (RRMS) followed by a more progressive course	***Preventive and Restorative*** • Regular exercise to improve/maintain motor performance, strength, mobility, flexibility, range of motion (ROM), balance, locomotion, endurance, and perceived quality of life • Community classes to improve/maintain socialization, camaraderie, positive outlook, and life purpose ***Compensatory*** • Patient/family/caregiver education about disease process, rehabilitation, energy conservation • Determine need for adaptive or assistive devices • Determine need for environmental modification of home/workplace • Provide psychological support with early referral to support groups for patient and family/caregiver • Referral to other health care professionals as needed
Middle/Moderate	• Progressive course with increasing number and severity of impairments • Minimal to moderate activity limitations, participation restrictions • Activities of daily living (ADL) with modified dependence (assistance) • Difficulty with balance and gait, postural instability	***Preventative and Restorative*** • Regular exercise to maintain/improve motor performance, strength, mobility, flexibility, ROM, balance, locomotion, endurance, and perceived quality of life • Community classes to improve/maintain socialization, camaraderie, positive outlook and life purpose ***Compensatory*** • Assistive devices to maintain function • Motorized wheelchair or scooter for community mobility • Environmental modifications to home • Patient/family/caregiver education and training • Psychological support for patient and family/caregiver • Referral to other health care professionals as needed

Late/Advanced	• Progressive course with numerous impairments with increasing severity
	• Severe activity limitations with dependence in most activities
	• Great difficulty walking; typically in wheelchair or bed most of the day
	• Assistance needed with all ADL
	• Severe participation restrictions:
	  • Not able to live alone
	  • Typically requires full-time assistance or placement in chronic care facility
	• Social interactions restricted
	• Cognitive problems may be prominent, including dementia, hallucinations, and delusions
		Preventive
		• Maximize upright posture, out-of-bed time
		• Maximize participation in ADL
		• Prevention of contractures, pressure wounds, pneumonia, and so forth
		Compensatory
		• Family/caregiver education and training: safety education, transfers, positioning, turning, skin care
		• Pressure-relieving devices
		• Hospital bed, wheelchair, mechanical lift
		• Psychological support for patient and family/caregiver
		• Referral to other health care professionals as needed

Adapted from Dal Bello-Haas.[55]
PPMS = primary-progressive multiple sclerosis; PRMS = progressive-relapsing multiple sclerosis; RRMS = relapsing-remitting multiple sclerosis; SPMS = secondary-progressive multiple sclerosis.

Box 16.3   Elements of the Examination of the Patient with Multiple Sclerosis[53]

Patient/Client History

- Age, sex, race/ethnicity, primary language, education
- Social history: cultural beliefs and behaviors, family and caregiver resources, social support systems
- Occupation/employment/work
- Living environment: home/work barriers
- Hand dominance
- General health status: physical, psychological, social, and role function, health habits
- Family history
- Medical/surgical history
- Current conditions/chief complaints
- Medications
- Medical/laboratory test results
- Functional status and activity level: premorbid and current

Systems Review

- Neuromuscular
- Musculoskeletal
- Cardiovascular/pulmonary
- Integumentary

Tests and Measures/Impairments

- Cognition: mental status, memory
- Communication
- Anthropometric characteristics: body mass index, girth, length
- Circulation: response to position change/degree of orthostatic hypotension
- Aerobic capacity and endurance: during functional activities and standardized exercise protocols; cardiovascular signs and symptoms in response to exercise and activity; pulmonary signs and symptoms in response to exercise and activity
- Ventilation and gas exchange
- Integumentary integrity: skin condition, pressure sensitive areas; activities, positioning, and postures to relieve pressure
- Sensory integrity and integration
- Pain: intensity and location
- Perceptual function: visuospatial skills
- Joint integrity, alignment, and mobility: range of motion (active and passive); muscle length and soft tissue extensibility
- Posture: alignment and position, symmetry (static and dynamic, sitting and standing); ergonomics, and body mechanics
- Muscle performance: strength, power, and endurance
- Motor function: motor control and motor learning
- Postural control and balance: degree of postural instability, balance strategies; safety
- Gait and locomotion: gait pattern and speed, safety
- Functional status and activity level: performance-based examination of functional skills (FIM level), basic and instrumental ADL; functional mobility skills; home management skills
- Psychosocial function: motivation
- Assistive or adaptive devices: fit, alignment, function, use; safety
- Environment, home, and work barriers
- Work, community, and leisure activities: ability to participate in activities, safety

Examination of Sensory Function). Additionally, sensory deficits and their effects on quality of life (QOL) in individuals with MS can be quantified by using the *Nottingham Sensory Assessment*[59] or *Guy's Neurological Disability Scale*.[60] The latter is a comprehensive multidimensional scale designed to assess the wide range of disability in patients with MS. It is a questionnaire driven by patient interview and can be administered by any health care personnel.[61]

Pain

The presence of acute, paroxysmal pain (Lhermitte's sign, dysesthesias) and chronic pain including pain behaviors and reactions during specific movements and provoking stimuli should be documented. The *McGill Pain Questionnaire*[62] or the *Neuropathic Pain Scale,*[63] developed to assess distinct pain qualities associated with neuropathic pain, can be used. (See discussion in Chapter 25, Chronic Pain.)

Visual Acuity

Acuity, tracking, and accommodation should be examined; the presence of visual deficits (blurred vision, field defects [scotoma], diplopia) should be documented.

Cranial Nerve Integrity

Motor and sensory cranial nerve function should be examined; the presence of deficits (optic pain [optic neuritis], oculomotor dyscontrol, dysphagia, impaired gag reflex, trigeminal neuralgia) should be documented.

Range of Motion

Passive range of motion (PROM) and active range of motion (AROM) should be examined; the presence of specific range of motion (ROM) impairments should be documented.

Muscle Performance

Functional strength using manual muscle testing (MMT) and dynamometers (isokinetic, grasp and pinch dynamometers) should be examined; strong spasticity may be a contraindication to standard MMT positions.

Fatigue

The frequency, duration, and severity of fatigue should be examined; precipitating factors, activity levels, and efficacy of rest attempts should be documented.[64] The *Modified Fatigue Impact Scale (MFIS)* developed by Fisk et al[65,66] is a structured, self-report, 21-item questionnaire addressing the effects of fatigue on cognitive, physical, and psychosocial function using a 5-point ordinal scale with 0 equal to never and 4 equal to almost always. Each area (subscale) can be scored separately; the total MFIS score range is from 0 to 84 (see Appendix 16.A). The MFIS can be downloaded in PDF format (www.nationalmssociety.org/MUCS_fatigue.asp). An abbreviated version of the MFIS has five items (the *MFIS-5*). Additionally, the *Fatigue Scale for Motor and Cognitive Functions (FSMC)* is a 20-item scale developed as a measure of cognitive and motor fatigue for people with MS.[67] To measure fatigue during the examination and treatment process, the Visual Analog Scale—Fatigue can be used as a single-item self-report of fatigue.[68]

Temperature Sensitivity

The degree of temperature sensitivity and its effect on fatigue and weakness should be examined. A tympanic membrane thermometer (ear thermometer) can be used before, during, and after moderate-intensity exercise. A determination of the correlation between temperature

changes and worsening of neurological symptoms can be made. This transient increase in symptoms following a raise in core temperature has been more accurately termed a *pseudoexacerbation*, and occurs due to transient increased blockade of nerve conduction in demyelinated fibers.[69,70]

Motor Function

The therapist should examine for the presence of corticospinal signs (paresis, spasticity, hyperactive DTRs, positive Babinski's sign, and involuntary spasms [flexor or extensor]). The *Amended Motor Club Examination (AMCA)* was developed to examine the nature and degree of motor and functional deficits in patients with MS.[71]

Spasticity can be examined using a subjective rating scale. The *Ashworth Spasticity Scale*[72] led to the more widely used *Modified Ashworth Scale.*[73] These are ordinal scales designed to measure tone intensity; the modified Ashworth has an additional grade at the lower end allowing for more discrete rating. A determination should be made of the differences between lower limbs versus upper limbs; right and left sides; and factors that influence tone.

The therapist should examine for the presence of cerebellar signs (ataxia, intention tremor, nystagmus, dysarthria). The effects of position change (e.g., sitting-to-standing) may produce an increase in ataxic movements with increased demands for postural stability and should be documented.

The therapist should examine for the presence of vestibular dysfunction (dizziness, vertigo, nystagmus, blurred vision with head and body movements, and postural imbalance; see Chapter 21, Vestibular Disorders).

Posture

Static and dynamic postural control in various different positions (e.g., sitting, standing) should be examined. The presence of postural abnormalities and postural tremor should be documented. Instruments can include posture grids, plumb lines, and still photography with light-emitting diodes.

Balance, Gait, and Locomotion

The therapist should examine static and dynamic balance, reactive and anticipatory control, sensory interaction, and synergistic strategies. Useful instruments include the *Clinical Test for Sensory Interaction in Balance,*[74] dynamic posturography,[75,76] the *Berg Balance Scale,*[77,78] the *Tinetti Performance Oriented Mobility Examination (POMA),*[79] and the *Balance Evaluation Systems Test* (BESTest).[80]

Gait parameters and characteristics should be examined including gait speed, kinematics, stability, safety, and endurance. Examination of patients with significant ataxia can be enhanced by use of videotaped performance.

Useful tests include timed walk tests (10-Meter Walk Test or 6-Minute Walk Test); the *Dynamic Gait Index;* [81] and the *Ambulation Index (AI).*[82] The *Rivermead Visual Gait Examination (RVGA)* was developed to examine gait in patients with MS.[83]

Alignment and fit, safety, practicality, and ease of use of orthotic and assistive devices should be examined along with energy conservation and expenditure. Wheelchair skills, including functional mobility, management, safety, transfers, and energy conservation and expenditure, should be examined.

Aerobic Capacity and Endurance

Vital signs (heart rate, blood pressure, respiratory rate) and breathing patterns should be examined at rest and during exercise. Exertional symptoms (dyspnea; elevated blood pressure, heart rate, respiratory rate) and perceived exertion during and after activity should be documented. Useful scales include the *Rating of Perceived Exertion Scale (the Borg RPE Scale)*[84] and the *Dyspnea Scale.*[85]

Skin Integrity and Condition

Skin integrity and condition should be examined. Areas of insensitivity, bruising, moisture buildup, and skin breakdown should be examined and documented, along with level of urinary continence; bed and wheelchair positioning; effectiveness of pressure-relieving compensatory strategies and pressure-relieving devices (PRDs); and cognitive status and safety awareness.

Functional Status

An examination of functional mobility skills (FMS), basic activities of daily living (BADL), and instrumental activities of daily living (IADL) is indicated, together with social functioning and community and work adaptive skills. A commonly used instrument for patients undergoing active rehabilitation is the *Functional Independence Measure (FIM)*[86,87] (see Chapter 8, Examination of Function).

Environment (Home, Community, and Work)

Physical space for barriers, access, and safety should be examined; a specific task-analysis (patient performance-based examination) in relevant environments (home, work) may be included (see Chapter 9, Examination of the Environment).

General Health Measures

General health measures are used to examine outcomes across a broad spectrum of global or long-term health outcomes. Instruments involve self-report of the patient's perceptions of limitations and quality of life (e.g., physical and social function, general health and vitality, emotional well-being, bodily pain, and so forth). The *Health Status Questionnaire (SF-36)*[88] is widely acknowledged as the gold standard of generic measures of health status. The properties of this instrument have been investigated in patients with MS. Freeman et al[89] found limitations in evaluating change in moderate to severely disabled patients participating in inpatient rehabilitation with significant floor and ceiling effects in four of eight SF-36 dimensions. The *Sickness Impact Profile*[90] and the *Examination of Motor and Process Skills*[91] are also general health measures.

Disease-Specific Measures

Disease-specific measures are designed to examine attributes common in a specific disease entity. Items are included to provide information about the disease process and outcomes, and ideally document clinically meaningful change over time. Thus, the instruments have greater responsiveness or sensitivity to change than general health measures.

Expanded Disability Status Scale (EDSS) for Patients with Multiple Sclerosis

In 1955, Kurtzke developed a 10-point scale for rating overall disability in MS (the Disability Status Scale or DSS).[92] This scale was expanded in 1983 to increase its clinical sensitivity by including half-point increments, becoming the EDSS (Appendix 16.B).[93] This scale has been widely adopted by clinicians and has been used as a standard in MS research. Based on a standard neurological examination, patients are first graded on presenting symptoms in seven specific functional systems (pyramidal, cerebellar, brainstem, sensory, bowel and bladder, visual, mental), plus other functions. Functional system scores (FSS) are obtained using an ordinal clinical rating scale ranging from 0 to 5 or 6. The EDSS is based on the grades obtained from the FSS and uses a 0 to 10 ordinal scale graded in half-point increments, with 0 equal to normal neurological function and 10.0 equal to death owing to MS. For example, patients classified in EDSS step 2.5 demonstrate minimal disability in two FSS (two FSS grade 2, others 0 or 1). The EDSS focuses on ambulation as the primary indicator of disability (see scores 3.0 through 6.5 for levels of ambulation; patients with scores 7.0 or greater are unable to walk). Criticisms of the EDSS include its lack of sensitivity to changes that do not include functional mobility (ambulation) and problems in interrater reliability with patients whose performance is less impaired (scores in the lower ranges, ambulation less impaired).[94] Copies of the EDSS can be obtained from the National Multiple Sclerosis Society at www.nationalmssociety.org/MUCS_FSS.asp.

The Minimum Record of Disability (MRD)

The Minimum Record of Disability (MRD) was developed by the International Federation of Multiple Sclerosis Societies in 1985.[95] This instrument has three subscales: the EDSS with FSS, the *Incapacity Status Scale (ISS),* and the *Environmental Status Scale (ESS).* It is widely used and includes classification of dysfunction according to World Health Organization (WHO) terminology. Thus, the instrument addresses impairments (the FS and EDSS), disability (ISS), and handicap (ESS). The ISS includes 16 items that address functional disability in ADL. The ESS measures social performance, including work status, financial status, and economic status, and place of residence, personal assistance, transportation, community assistance, and social activity. Solari et al[96] examined the validity of the self-administered version of the MRD and found that determination of ambulatory ability, ADL skills, and social activities was both accurate and cost-effective.

MS Functional Composite (MSFC)

The MS Functional Composite (MSFC) is a 21-item test that includes 3 different functional subtests: the Timed 25-Foot Walk (T25FW), the 9-Hole Peg Test (9HPT), and the Paced Auditory Serial Addition Test (PASAT). The *MSFC Administration and Scoring Manual* can be obtained from the National Multiple Sclerosis Society at www.nationalmssociety.org/search-results/index.aspx?q=MSFC&x=28&y=14&start=0&num=20.

Multiple Sclerosis Quality of Life—54 (MSQOL-54)

The Multiple Sclerosis Quality of Life—54 (MSQOL-54) is a multidimensional health-related quality-of-life measure that combines both generic and MS-specific items into a single instrument.[97] The generic items are from the SF-36 to which 18 items were added to provide more information regarding MS-specific issues.[98] No overall summary score is used: the MSQOL-54 consists of 12 subscales, 2 combined summary scores, and 2 single-item measures. The subscales are physical function, role limitations—physical, role limitations—emotional, pain, emotional well-being, energy, health perceptions, social function, cognitive function, health distress, overall quality of life, and sexual function. The summary scores are the physical health composite summary and the mental health composite summary. The single-item measures are satisfaction with sexual function and change in health.

MS Quality of Life Inventory (MSQLI)

The Consortium of Multiple Sclerosis Centers, Health Science Research Subcommittee, developed the MS Quality of Life Inventory (MSQLI) as a comprehensive outcomes examination package.[99] It includes a battery of 10 self-report scales (138 items) that provide information about health-related quality of life in MS, including the Health Status Questionnaire (SF-36), Modified Fatigue Impact Scale (MFIS), MOS Pain Effects Scale (PES), Sexual Satisfaction Scale (SSS), Bladder Control Scale (BLCS), Bowel Control Scale (BWCS), Impact of Visual Impairment Scale (IVIS), Perceived Deficits Questionnaire (PDQ), Mental Health

Inventory (MHI), and MOS Modified Social Support Survey (MSSS). The battery can be administered in approximately 45 minutes in most cases. Abbreviated versions of some of the scales can reduce the set to 81 items requiring approximately 30 minutes to administer. A *User's Manual* can be obtained from www.nationalmssociety.org/for-professionals/researchers/clinical-study-measures/msqli/indcx.aspx.

Functional Examination of Multiple Sclerosis (FAMS)

The Functional Examination of MS (FAMS) is a 59-item index of health-related quality-of-life measures developed by Cella et al.[100] There are six subscales (mobility, symptoms, emotional well-being [depression], general contentment, thinking/fatigue, and family/social well-being). The mobility subscale strongly correlates with the EDSS.

Multiple Sclerosis Impact Scale (MSIS-29)

The MS Impact Scale (MSIS-29) measures the physical and psychological impact of MS.[101] The scale was primarily developed for community-based populations though testing with hospital-based populations (patients admitted for inpatient rehabilitation, IV corticosteroid treatment for MS relapses, and patients admitted with PPMS) revealed consistency of psychometric properties.[102]

The *Neurology Section Multiple Sclerosis Outcome Measures Taskforce* of the American Physical Therapy Association (APTA) has compiled a list of measures for each relevant International Classification of Functioning, Disability, and Health (ICF) category together with instrument analysis, recommendations for use, and relevant references. The document can be found at www.neuropt.org/files/FINAL_EDGE_DOCUMENT.pdf.

Goals and Outcomes

The general goals and outcomes for patients with progressive disorders of the CNS, adapted from the *Guide to Physical Therapist Practice*,[53] are presented in Box 16.4. These general goals will provide the basis for development of specific anticipated goals and expected outcomes for an individual patient.

The preferred practice pattern for patients with MS from the *Guide to Physical Therapist Practice* is 5E, *Impaired Motor Function and Sensory Integrity Associated with Progressive Disorders of the Central Nervous System.*[53] In this document the reader will find relevant information on patient/client diagnostic classification; ICD-9-CM codes; examination components; considerations for evaluation, diagnosis, and prognosis; and suggested interventions. Thus the *Guide to Physical Therapist Practice* serves as a primary resource to help physical therapists design an appropriate plan of care (POC) and document the services provided and outcomes achieved.

Box 16.4   Examples of General Goals and Outcomes for Patients with Progressive Disorders of the Central Nervous System[53]

Impact of pathology/pathophysiology is reduced.

- Patient/client, family, and caregiver knowledge and awareness of the disease, prognosis, and plan of care is enhanced.
- Symptom management is enhanced.
- Risk of secondary impairment is reduced.
- Intensity of care is decreased.

Impact of impairments is reduced.

- Cognitive function is improved.
- Joint integrity and mobility are improved.
- Sensory awareness and skin integrity are improved.
- Pain is decreased.
- Motor function is improved.
- Muscle performance (strength, power, and endurance) is improved.
- Postural control and balance are improved.
- Gait and locomotion are improved.
- Management of fatigue is enhanced.
- Aerobic capacity is increased.

Ability to perform physical actions, tasks, or activities is improved.

- Independence in activities of daily living is increased.
- Tolerance of positions and activities is increased.
- Activity pacing and energy conservation are enhanced.
- Problem solving and decision making skills are enhanced.
- Safety of patient/client, family, and caregivers is improved.

Disability associated with chronic illness is reduced.

- Ability to assume/resume self-care and home management is improved.
- Ability to assume work (job/school/play), community, and leisure roles is improved.
- Patient/client and family knowledge and awareness of personal and environmental factors associated with worsening of the condition is enhanced.
- Awareness and use of community resources are improved.

Health status and quality of life are improved.

- Sense of well-being is enhanced.
- Stressors are reduced.
- Insight, self-confidence, and self-management skills are improved.
- Health, wellness, and fitness are improved.

Patient/client satisfaction is enhanced.

- Access and availability of services are acceptable to patient/client and family.
- Quality of rehabilitation services is acceptable to patient/client and family.
- Care is coordinated with patient/client, family, caregivers, and other professionals.

Adapted from the *Guide to Physical Therapist Practice.*[53]

■ PHYSICAL THERAPY INTERVENTIONS

Management of Sensory Deficits and Skin Care

In patients with MS, inflammation causes a disruption in neuronal signaling, causing a variety of sensory symptoms.[103] Strategies should be instituted to increase awareness of sensory deficits, compensate for sensory loss, and promote safety.[104] It is important to remember that sensory deficits may remit, so ongoing examination is necessary. The success of compensatory training strategies depends on the availability of other intact sensory systems. For example, visual compensation techniques can be instituted when deficits in proprioception produce imbalance and place the patient at risk for falls.

If multiple sensory systems are involved (e.g., vision is also impaired), sensory compensatory strategies are not likely to be successful.

Patients with proprioceptive losses demonstrate impairments in movement control and motor learning. They require increased use of other sensory systems, especially vision. Tapping, verbal cueing, and/or biofeedback can all be effective forms of augmented feedback. Proprioceptive loading through exercise, light tracking resistance, resistance bands or weights, and the use of a pool may heighten residual proprioceptive function and improve movement awareness.

Visual loss will interfere with movement and postural control. Blurred vision, especially at night or in low light situations, can occur after episodes of optic neuritis. When individuals with MS have to stand in an upright position in the dark, the likelihood of falls increases.[105] It is therefore important to instruct the patient to maintain adequate lighting at all times (e.g., use of a bright light at night) and reducing clutter to improve safety. Adding color contrast between items in the environment (e.g., stair markings) can also improve safety. Double vision is frequently the result of impaired coordination and weak eye muscles. It can be controlled by placing a patch over one eye and is an important strategy for improving reading, driving, or watching television. However, eye patching should not be used all the time, because it will prevent possible adaptation of the CNS. Eye patching also interferes with depth perception. The symptoms of visual blurring and double vision also fluctuate and can be heightened with fatigue, an increase in temperature, stress, and infection. Management of these symptoms is important to improve vision.[104] If low vision persists, the patient should be referred to a low-vision specialist or one of the national service organizations that provide help to individuals with vision impairments (*National Association for Visually Handicapped, National Federation of the Blind, American Foundation for the Blind*).

One of the most common early sensory symptoms of MS is decreased sensitivity to touch.[103] Patients with MS face an increased risk of developing pressure ulcers owing to the symptoms of MS, including loss of sensation, immobility, loss of bowel and bladder control, and a catabolic nutritional state.[104] Changes in skin turgor, static posturing, and prolonged pressure over bony prominences increase the likelihood of skin breakdown. Approximately 20% of patients with MS will develop a pressure ulcer during the course of the disease.[8] Patients may not feel the discomfort of a prolonged position or may be unable to shift position because of weakness or spasticity. In addition, spasticity and/or spasms may cause friction effects between the skin and supporting surfaces. Awareness, protection, and care of desensitized parts should be taught early in the rehabilitation process and consistently

reinforced by all members of the team. It has been demonstrated that patient education programs result in 50% reductions in pressure sore incidence.[106] The patient/family/caregiver should be educated in the following principles of skin care:

- The skin should be kept clean and dry. Soiled skin should be cleansed and dried promptly.
- The skin should be inspected regularly (at least once a day) and carefully, with particular attention to persistent areas of redness and over bony prominences.
- Clothing should be breathable and comfortable (soft, not too loose or wrinkled, or too tight). Seams, buttons, and pockets should not press on the skin, particularly in weight-bearing areas.
- Regular pressure relief is essential. Patients should be instructed to change their position or be changed frequently, typically every 2 hours in bed and every 15 to 30 minutes when sitting in a wheelchair.[107]

Pressure-relieving devices (PRDs) may be necessary to protect insensitive areas and should be implemented as appropriate. These can include mattresses (water, gel, air, or alternating pressure) to distribute body weight and reduce shear and friction in bed. Sheepskins, air or foam cushions, cuffs, and/or boots may be necessary to protect body areas prone to breakdown (shoulder blades, elbows, ischial tuberosities, sacrum, trochanters, knees, malleoli, or heels). Cushions (foam; fluid or air pressure–relieving cushions) are necessary for patients who spend prolonged periods of time sitting in their wheelchair. When evaluating a PRD it is imperative that a pressure mapping system be used to determine its effectiveness and to ensure that the areas of high pressure are adequately protected.[107-109]

Prevention is the best strategy. Important measures for maintaining skin integrity and function include maintaining good nutrition and drinking plenty of fluids. Studies suggest that for patients with MS with pressure sores, there are increased requirements for specific nutrients; particularly zinc and iron supplementation should be considered.[110] The patient must be cautioned against activities that might traumatize the skin. Dragging, bumping, or scraping body parts during a transfer or bed mobility activities can injure the skin. Thermal injury can result from contact with hot water or hot objects. If nonblanchable skin redness develops (lasting longer than 30 minutes), patients should be instructed to stay off the area until the redness disappears. If the redness does not disappear within 24 hours, the individual should seek medical attention. Blisters, blue areas, or open sores indicate more serious injury and require immediate attention. This may include systemic antibiotic therapy for infection and wound management techniques (cleansing and débridement, topical antibiotic agents, and protective dressings).[8]

Management of Pain

Pain can be classified into four categories: pain directly from MS, pain secondary to other symptoms of MS, pain as a result of drug treatment for MS, and pain independent of MS. The management of pain depends on an accurate determination of its causes. Musculoskeletal strain or joint malalignment from chronically weakened muscles are important considerations and are responsive to physical therapy intervention. Patients may experience relief of pain with regular stretching or exercise, massage, and ultrasound. Postural retraining and correction of faulty movement patterns along with orthotic and/or adaptive seating devices can reduce malalignment and pain. Stabbing pain from Lhermitte's sign may be relieved with a soft cervical collar to limit neck flexion. Hydrotherapy or pool therapy using *lukewarm* water may have a beneficial effect on painful dysesthesias. Pressure stockings or gloves can also be used to relieve pain, converting the sensation of pain to one of pressure. Neutral warmth may be an additional factor in the pain relief experienced with stockings or gloves. Patients with chronic pain may benefit from referral to a total management approach for chronic pain, for example, the *multidisciplinary pain clinic* (see Chapter 25, Chronic Pain). Stress management techniques, relaxation training, biofeedback, and meditation are often helpful in reducing both anxiety and pain. The use of transcutaneous electrical nerve stimulation (TENS) to modulate pain in patients with MS has had conflicting results, with some patients experiencing improvement and some a worsening of symptoms.[9,10]

Exercise Training

Muscle weakness and decreased endurance are common findings in patients with MS. In addition, patients with MS often adopt a sedentary lifestyle and limit their physical activity. The benefits of exercise have been firmly established in terms of producing meaningful physiological and psychological changes, improving function while lessening disability, and enhancing quality of life.[111-128] In a Cochrane Database Systematic Review of Exercise Therapy for MS, researchers identified nine high-quality RCTs (260 participants).[128] Six trials compared exercise versus no exercise while three trials compared two types of exercise therapy. The researchers found strong evidence in favor of exercise therapy for improving muscle power, exercise tolerance, and mobility-related activities. Moderate evidence was found for improving emotional mood. There were no adverse effects on fatigue and perception of handicap. The researchers found no evidence that a specific exercise therapy program was more successful in improving level of activity and participation than another. Individuals with minimal to moderate impairments (i.e., EDSS scores between 1 and 6) demonstrate the best exercise tolerance. This speaks to the need to institute exercises early in the course of the disease. Exercise responses of the patient with MS are influenced by a host of factors that require careful attention during exercise, including fatigue, spasticity, incoordination, impaired balance, sensory loss (numbness), tremor, and heat intolerance. Depression may affect adherence to an exercise program. Therapists therefore need to provide constant reinforcement and a positive environment.

Individuals with MS will vary greatly in their responses to exercise. The focus and pace of therapy must be readjusted according to the patient's specific abilities and needs at that time. Patients with RRMS who are experiencing an exacerbation should not exercise until remission is evident. Exercise therapy can be reinstituted when the deterioration has stabilized and no new symptoms are appearing. Patients with PPMS can exercise within the limits of their capabilities as exercise may slow further deterioration and optimize remaining function.[129,130] Box 16.5 Evidence Summary presents a summary of selected research on exercise and MS.

Strength and Conditioning

Maximal muscle force during sustained isometric or isokinetic exercise is lower for persons with MS secondary to reduced ability to activate muscles (reduced force/unit muscle mass), reduced muscle metabolic responses, and muscle weakness secondary to muscle fiber atrophy, spasticity, and disuse.[129] Determining an appropriate exercise prescription to improve strength and endurance is challenging and needs to be carefully individualized for each patient. Prescription is based on four interrelated elements: frequency of exercise, intensity of exercise, type of exercise, and time or duration (the *FITT equation*). The following guidelines can be used:[130]

- Exercise sessions should be scheduled on alternate (non-endurance) days and during optimal times, such as in the morning, when body core temperatures tend to be lowest and before fatigue sets in. Patients with greater neurological involvement may require more frequent exercise (e.g., daily exercise time).
- Resistance training modes can include weight machines, free or pulley weights, latex resistance bands, or isokinetic machines.
- Circuit training, in which improved work capacity is developed through the use of various different stations that alternate work between UEs and LEs, distributes the load among muscles and may prove beneficial for reducing the likelihood of fatigue.
- Sessions should involve discontinuous work, carefully balancing exercise with adequate rest periods.
- Progression is generally slower than with healthy individuals.
- Precautions should be taken to prevent the deleterious effects of overwork. Exercising to the point of fatigue is contraindicated and can result in worsening of symptoms, most notably increased weakness.

Box 16.5 Evidence Summary Exercise and Multiple Sclerosis

Reference	Subjects	Design/Intervention	Duration	Results	Comments
Andreasen et al[122] (2011)	Identified 21 studies	Systematic review of studies evaluating the effect of exercise on MS fatigue; studies included endurance training, resistance training, combined training, or other training modalities		Heterogeneous results; only a few studies evaluated MS fatigue as the primary outcome; many studies applied nonfatigued study populations; those studies that included fatigued patients with MS show positive results	Exercise has the potential to have a positive effect on MS fatigue; remains unclear whether any exercise modalities are superior to others; high-quality studies are needed regarding the different exercise interventions, using fatigue as a primary endpoint
Cakit et al[124] (2010)	45 subjects, in 2 exercise groups, 1 control group; relapsing-remitting or secondary progressive MS, mild-mod MS, no exacerbation, able to stand indep	RCT Exer group 1: PRT on bicycle ergometer and balance exer Exer group 2: home-based LE strengthening and balance exer Control group: home-based LE strengthening and balance exer Outcome measures: duration of exercise; TMW; TUG; DGI, FR, FES; 10-mWT, FSS, Beck Depression Inventory, SF-36	8 weeks, 2×/wk 15 repetitions of high resistance (40% TMW) 2 min followed by low resistance or rest 2 min	Exer group 1: significant improvement in all outcome measures Exer group 2: significant improvement in FES, TMW, and duration of exer Control group: no improvements	PRT results in improved balance, decreased fear of falling, and decreased depression; there were no injuries or increases in MS symptoms
Dalgas et al[123] (2010)	45 subjects with RRMS, EDSS, 3.0–5.5, able to walk > 100 m, age > 18	RCT, crossover design; 5 min warm-up followed by PRT (loads and volume increased every 2 weeks); control group participated in same intervention after 12 weeks Outcome measures: FSS, MDI, SF-36, muscle strength (MVC), functional capacity	12 weeks, 2×/wk; post-study follow-up period of 12 weeks	Significant improvements in strength, fatigue, and functional capacity score; significant changes in mental but not physical components of SF-36	Resistance training well tolerated; improved scores for strength, fatigue, mood, QOL, and ambulatory function; at follow-up no significant deterioration in scores
Rampello et al[125] (2007)	19 subjects with mild to mod MS, score of 6 or less on EDSS, no recent relapse	RTC, crossover design AT group: leg cycle ergometer (5 min warm-up; 30 min at 60% max work rate; 5 min cool-down) Control group: neurological rehab program (NR) Outcome measures: MFIS, MSQOL-54; 6-MWT; walking speed	3 training sessions per week for 8 weeks	With AT but not NR, walking distances and speeds, max work rate, peak O2 uptake and max work rate significantly improved; no differences on fatigue	AT improves maximum exercise capacity and walking capacity; subjects who were most disabled tended to benefit from AT; there was a high rate of subject loss (4/19 in AT group)

Continued

Box 16.5 Evidence Summary   Exercise and Multiple Sclerosis—cont'd

Reference	Subjects	Design/Intervention	Duration	Results	Comments
Rietberg et al[128] (2004)	Identified 9 studies (RCTs); 262 subjects with MS	Meta-analysis of 9 high-quality RCTs Inclusion criteria: exercise therapy for adults with MS (not currently experiencing an exacerbation) Outcome measures: activity limitation and QOL, or both	6 trials: exercise therapy versus no exercise therapy; 3 trials: compared 2 interventions of exercise therapy	Best evidence: Strong evidence in favor of exercise compared to no exercise, improvements in muscle power function, exercise tolerance functions, mobility-related activities noted; moderate evidence: for improving mood; no evidence: effect on fatigue and perception of handicap; no evidence: any specific exercise therapy better than others	No deleterious effects of exercise therapy described. Exercise therapy is beneficial for patients with MS not experiencing an exacerbation. Consensus is needed for core set of outcome measures. Better controls needed for type, intensity of training and for type of MS.
Surakka et al[112] (2004)	95 subjects with MS, mild-mod disability; EDSS scores between 1 and 5.5; exercise group = 46; non-exercise group = 48	RCT, 5 PRT and 5 AT sessions; aerobic exercises in pool (temp 82.4°F[28°C]), 65%–70% age-predicted HR_{max}; resistance training (RT) = circuit training UE and LE Ms, 50%–60% 1-RM; home exercise program (HEP): RT used elastic bands; aerobic training, walking; subjects kept daily diary Outcome measures: Ms torque (dynamometer); Fatigue (FI, FSS, AFI)		Significant decrease in motor fatigue in women ($n = 30$) but not men ($n = 17$) after 6 months of aerobic and strength exercise; exercise activity of women was 25% more than men	Long training period (6 months) may have masked disease progression, especially in men. Men more likely to have PPMS then RRMS.
Mostert and Kesselring[113] (2002)	26 subjects with MS, mild-mod disability, inpatient rehabilitation; EDSS scores between 2.5–6.5; MS-exercise group =13; MS–no intervention group = 13; healthy control group = 26	Randomized control trial Aerobic exercise training: leg cycle ergometry Outcome measures: max GXT; tests of lung function (FVC); spasticity LEs (mAS); EDSS Baecke Activity Questionnaire; SF-36 Health Survey; FSS	4 weeks, 5x/wk, 30 min sessions	MS training group increased aerobic threshold, improved health perception (vitality increased 46%, social interaction increased 36%); increased activity level (17%); tendency for less fatigue; lung function did not change	Aerobic training is safe and improves aerobic capacity; symptom exacerbation lower than expected (6%); compliance of MS training group was low (65%); stresses need for motivational setting; MS patients less fit than healthy controls; more disabled MS patients improved more than less impaired patients; small sample size.

Box 16.5 Evidence Summary   Exercise and Multiple Sclerosis—cont'd

Reference	Subjects	Design/Intervention	Duration	Results	Comments
Sutherland et al[121] (2001)	22 subjects, with MS, mild-mod disability; EDSS of 5.0 or less; no-special-activity group = 11; exercise group = 11	RCT, exercise intervention: land-based weight training; water aerobics, water jogging Outcome measures: submax GXT; HRQOL	10 weeks, 3×/wk, 45 min sessions	Exercise group increased in physical fitness (not significant); reported increased energy and vigor, mood, better social and sexual functioning; less bodily pain and fatigue	Exercise improved psychological health and quality of life; use of water-based aerobics can be effective in patients with MS who have spasticity and coordination deficits; small sample size.
Snook and Motl[127] (2009)	Meta-analysis of 22 studies of 600 patients with MS	Search included published exercise training studies from 1960 to 2007; studies measured walking mobility, using instruments identified as acceptable walking mobility constructs and outcome measures for individuals with neurological disorders, before and after an intervention that included exercise training.	22 studies over 47 years	Computed effect sizes expressed as Cohen's d. Sixty-six effect sizes were retrieved and yielded a weighted mean effect size of $g = 0.19$ (95% confidence interval, 0.09–0.28). There were larger effects associated with supervised exercise training ($g = 0.32$), exercise programs that were less than 3 months in duration ($g = 0.28$), and mixed samples of RRMS and progressive MS ($g = 0.52$).	The cumulative evidence supports that exercise training is associated with a small improvement in walking mobility among individuals with MS.
Dodd et al[126] (2006)	Seven women and two men (mean age 45.6 years, SD 10.7) with MS	Cohort study Gymnasium-based progressive resistance strengthening program: 3 exercises for the legs (leg press, knee extension, seated heel raise) and 3 exercises for the arms (lat pull down, seated chest press, and seated row)	10 weeks, 2×/wk	Positive physical, psychological, and social benefits and decreases in fatigue. Key extrinsic factors for program completion were the leaders' encouragement and knowledge of exercise and the group aspect of the program	Progressive resistance strength training is a feasible fitness option for some people with MS. Choosing encouraging leaders with knowledge of exercise and exercising in a group may contribute to program success.

AFI = Ambulatory Fatigue Index (500-m walk test); AT = aerobic training; BMI = body mass index; DGI = Dynamic Gait Index; EDSS = Expanded Disability Status Scale (Kurtzke); exer = exercise; FES = Falls Efficacy Scale; FI = Fatigue Index; FSS = Fatigue Severity Scale; FR = functional reach; GXT = Graded Exercise Test; QOL = quality of life; LE = lower extremity; mAS = Modified Ashworth Scale; MDI = Major Depression Inventory; MHR = maximal heart rate; MFIS = Modified Fatigue Impact Scale; 6MWT = 6-Minute Walk Test; MVIC = maximal voluntary isometric contraction; MSQOL-54 = Multiple Sclerosis Quality of Life–54 questionnaire; MS = multipal sclerosis; POMS = Profile of Mood States; PPMS = primary-progressive multiple sclerosis; PRT = progressive resistance training; RCT = randomized controlled trial; RRMS = relapsing-remitting multiple sclerosis; SIP = Sickness Impact Profile; 1-RM = 1-repetition maximum contraction; TMW = tolerated maximum workload; TUG = Timed Up and Go Test; UE = upper extremity; VLDL = very-low-density lipoprotein; VO$_{2max}$ = maximal oxygen uptake.

This may have additional adverse effects on the continuing motivation of the patient.

- Precautions should be taken to monitor the effects of fatigue. *Time to fatigue* varies greatly among individuals with MS and is *not* correlated with the level of physical impairment or disability.
- Precautions should be taken to manage core body temperature and prevent overheating.[131,132] Environmental temperatures should be carefully controlled. Air conditioning is a medical necessity in many climates. Additional cooling can be achieved through the use of fans, wet neck wraps, spray bottles for misting the skin with cool water, and immersion in cool water with aquatic exercises. Surface cooling devices have emerged as effective tools in managing body temperatures, controlling fatigue, and improving function. These include cooling suits or vests.[133-135]
- Precautions should be taken with certain impairments. Tactile and proprioceptive losses or incoordination and tremors may make the use of some equipment (e.g., free weights) unsafe. Visual feedback, when intact, should be used to monitor exercise performance. An alternative suggestion would be to use synchronized arm/leg ergometers to control limb movements.
- Precautions should be taken with cognitive and memory impairments. Individuals may require written or posted exercise instructions/diagrams including reminders of the number of repetitions, proper form, and correct use of equipment.
- Functional training activities (e.g., closed chain exercises) can be used to promote strength and functional endurance. Individuals with ataxia and balance problems may require the use of more stable postures (e.g., modified plantigrade, quadruped, or supported sitting).
- Group exercise classes can provide valuable motivation and social support. The therapist's primary role is one of educator and group leader. Successful management of group classes requires careful, individualized examination of group members to determine specific goals and exercises.
- Outcome measures can include isokinetic dynamometry, MMT (may be unreliable if spasticity is present), functional tests (e.g., sit-to-stand), fatigue (MFIS), and quality-of-life measures (HRQL).

Aerobic Conditioning

Individuals with MS demonstrate expected physiological responses to submaximal aerobic exercise; that is, heart rate (HR), blood pressure (BP), and oxygen uptake (VO_2) all increase in a linear fashion in response to increasing workloads. Respiratory responses (respiratory rate [RR] and minute ventilation) also increase.[129] However, HR and BP responses may be blunted if cardiovascular dysautonomia is present. A direct relationship exists between the duration and extent of disease and the likelihood of autonomic cardiovascular dysfunction. Patients with MS can also demonstrate respiratory muscle dysfunction (weakness, dyssynergia), contributing to reduced exercise tolerance.

Exercise tolerance and maximal aerobic power (VO_{2max}) are reduced in individuals with reduced cardiorespiratory fitness secondary to physical inactivity. Decreased physical work capacity, decreased vital capacity, increased HR at rest and in response to exercise, decreased muscular strength, increased fatigue, increased anxiety, and depression are common findings.

Determining an appropriate exercise prescription to improve cardiovascular conditioning needs to be carefully individualized for each patient. While predicting exercise capacity and cardiorespiratory fitness is challenging for individuals with MS, recent studies have shown that peak VO_2 and exercise capacity can be predicted through submaximal testing.[136,137] The following guidelines for *clinical exercise testing* can be used.[130]

- The preferred mode is either an upright or recumbent leg cycle ergometer. A recumbent device is indicated if sitting balance is impaired. Combination leg and arm ergometry or UE ergometry alone may be necessary in the presence of significant LE involvement. Toe clips and heel straps are recommended to control foot placement especially in patients with spasticity, tremor, or weakness.
- Performance measures include HR, ratings of perceived exertion (RPE), BP, and expired gas analysis (VO_2). Using the RPE scale, peripheral (muscles, joints) exertion is consistently rated as more stressful (higher) than central (cardiopulmonary) exertion.
- A continuous or discontinuous protocol (3- to 5-minute stages) can be used; the discontinuous protocol is indicated with symptomatic disease, especially fatigue.
- A submaximal test should be used. Most individuals with MS can achieve 70% to 85% of their age-predicted maximal heart rate (HR_{max}).
- Recommendations for increasing workloads for each stage are 12 to 25 watts for LE work and 8 to 12 watts for combined UE and LE work.
- Termination criteria include achievement of peak HR, peak VO_2, volitional fatigue, significant BP changes (systolic blood pressure [SBP] greater than 250 mm Hg or diastolic blood pressure [DPB] greater than 115 mm Hg or a hypotensive response), or a decrease in oxygen uptake with increasing work rate.
- Precautions should be taken to monitor for attenuated HR or BP responses during exercise. A category-ratio RPE scale can be used to estimate central and peripheral exertion.[84]
- Precautions should be taken to manage core body temperature and prevent overheating (e.g., use of a fan for cooling).

- Precautions should be taken to monitor the effects of fatigue.
- Precautions should be taken to prevent the deleterious effects of overwork.
- Precautions should be taken with certain medications that can affect results: amantadine hydrochloride (HCl) may temporarily reduce fatigue; baclofen and amitriptyline HCl may cause muscle weakness; prednisone can also cause muscle weakness along with reduced sweating and hypertension.
- Morning is the optimal time for testing.

Prescription is again based on the four interrelated elements of the FITT equation. Recommendations for exercise programming to improve aerobic conditioning include the following:[130]

- Recommended training frequency is 3 to 5 days/week, on alternate days. Daily exercise at lower levels of intensity is recommended for individuals with more limited exercise capacities (e.g., 3 to 5 metabolic equivalent [METs]).
- Training intensity should be limited to 60% to 85% HR_{peak} or 50% to 70% peak VO_2.
- Recommended duration is 30 minutes per session or, for more involved individuals, three 10-minute sessions per day.
- Type of exercise can include cycling, walking, swimming, or water aerobics.
- Circuit training may prove best for optimizing training.
- Individuals with balance problems or sensory loss will require non–weight-bearing activities.
- Exercise precautions: discussed in previous section.
- Outcome measures include graded exercise test results (GXT), HR (which may be difficult to monitor with dysautonomia; sensory loss in the fingers may make self-monitoring difficult), tests of lung function (forced vital capacity [FVC]), body composition, RPE, fatigue (FI, MFIS), functional status, and quality-of-life measures (HRQL).

Patient education is particularly important because the overall success of a fitness program is influenced by the individual's level of understanding of the basic principles of training, independence in self-monitoring, and skill in decision making relative to level of impairment and exercise modifications required, as well as lifestyle and general health and safety considerations.

Flexibility Exercises

Stretching and ROM exercises are necessary to ensure adequate joint motion and to counteract the effects of spasticity (Fig.16.3). Sedentary or inactive persons who are dependent on wheelchairs often develop tightness in hip flexors, adductors, hamstrings, and plantarflexors. Limited overhead ROM is seen with tightness in the pectoralis major/minor, and latissimus dorsi and is associated with a slumped, forward posture. Patients confined to bed typically present with tightness in hip/knee

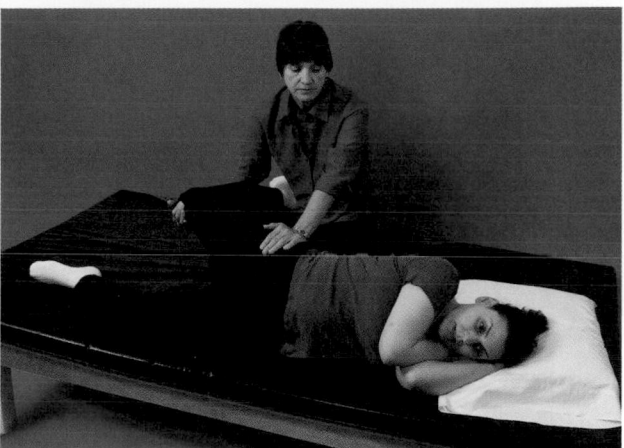

Figure 16.3 Side-lying hip flexor/rectus femoris stretch. This position allows the therapists to control the hip and ensure that excessive lumber lordosis is prevented while also modulating the amount of stretch between the iliopsoas and the rectus femoris.

extensors, adductors, and plantarflexors. Stretching and ROM exercises should be performed daily. For adequate stretching, holding at end range should be a minimum of 30 to 60 seconds repeated for a minimum of 2 repetitions. The use of orthoses or dynamic splinting is an appropriate option for prevention and in some cases reversal of contractures.[138,139] Considering the gait deviations and difficulty with transfers/bed mobility that arise from limited ROM and spasticity, it is important to also include aggressive trunk ROM to allow for full function of the core musculature, most notably the quadratus lumborum (Fig. 16.4). More active patients may benefit from Tai Chi, which provides additional important benefits of relaxation and balance training. ROM measurement using goniometry is an appropriate outcome measure.

Management of Fatigue

With approximately 75% of individuals with MS describing persistent or sporadic symptoms, fatigue is among the most debilitating. Fatigue is characterized by overwhelming sleepiness, excessive tiredness, and sense of weakness that comes on suddenly and severely. Aversion to activity for fear of bringing on fatigue is also common. The resultant lowered activity levels have important implications for diminished health status and deconditioning. Therapists are faced with a balancing act, on one hand prescribing exercise, while on the other hand avoiding overwork and the development of fatigue. Aerobic exercise training (previously discussed) and *energy effectiveness strategies (EES)* are central to any intervention plan to lessen fatigue.[13] During exercise prescription and physical therapy sessions, it is imperative that a skilled therapist recognize the difference between MS-related fatigue and the expected exercise-related fatigue. MS-related fatigue during exercise is

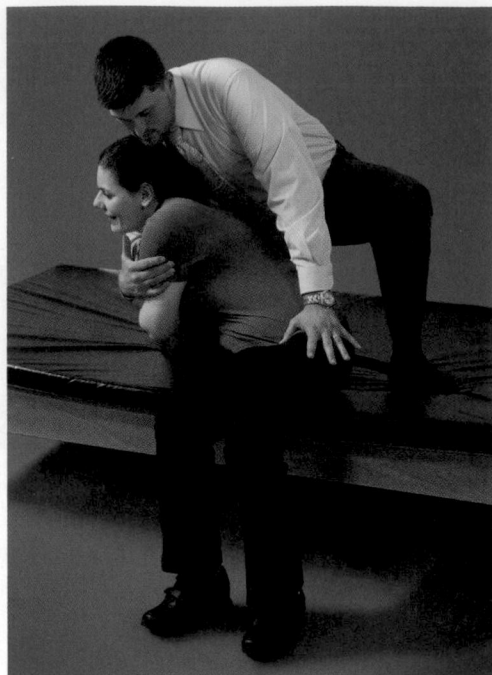

Figure 16.4 Seated trunk stretch. The pictured position allows the therapist to control the pelvis to ensure trunk stretching while maintaining control of the individual's trunk to apply the correct emphasis to the desired muscle groups.

often associated with thermal stress, which can be offset with adequate rest and the use of cooling and precooling treatments during exercise.[132-134]

Patients are instructed to keep an *activity diary* in which they record how they slept the night before, daily activities by hour, and how costly those activities were. For each activity, they can be asked to rate their level of fatigue (F), the value or importance of the activity (V), and satisfaction perceived with performance of the activity (S) by assigning a number between 1 and 10 with 1 being very low and 10 being very high. For example, the activity might be fixing lunch. Scores reported for this activity might be $F = 7$, $V = 3$, and $S = 2$. Aggravating factors associated with increasing fatigue (e.g., heat stress) and MS symptoms that appear or worsen during the day are also recorded. An *MS Daily Activity Diary* is presented in Appendix 16.C.[140]

Based on this information, therapists can initiate training sessions, teaching energy effectiveness strategies. **Energy conservation** refers to the adoption of strategies that reduce overall energy requirements of the task and overall level of fatigue. These can include modifying the task or modifying the environment to ensure successful completion of daily activities. For example, a motorized scooter or powered wheelchair can be considered for community or home mobility to help conserve energy and maintain independence. Other mobility equipment such as walkers, crutches, or orthotics can also be considered. Activities that are difficult or have high energy needs can be broken down into component parts,

requiring accurate activity analysis. **Activity pacing** refers to the balancing of activity with rest periods interspersed throughout the day. For the patient with chronic fatigue, *rest–activity ratios* are developed, with periodic rest periods planned in advance. Time-outs with complete rest should be instituted if an activity becomes exhaustive. Overall levels of energy can be improved if patients learn to set priorities and limit their activities, saving their energy for those activities that are truly important to them (e.g., activities that are enjoyable and meaningful in terms of the individual's lifestyle). The occupational therapist addresses EES and can provide valuable suggestions in terms of planning, work simplification, and developing energy-efficient activities for self-care and home management. The vocational rehabilitation counselor can provide useful strategies for behavioral modification and vocational rehabilitation. Team efforts with the physical therapist and others are important for consistency and reinforcement. Weekly review of activities and recommended modifications is used to evaluate progress. The MFIS should be administered on a regular basis to monitor ongoing fatigue status (see Appendix 16.A). Finally, stress management techniques are important components of symptom management.

The occupational and physical therapist should complete a direct environmental examination of the home and/or job site (see Chapter 9, Examination of the Environment). A number of adaptations may be considered to improve efficiency and safety, including air-conditioning, home, or work modifications, or ergonomic equipment. The patient/family/caregivers should be educated as to the importance of these recommendations for improved function. Periodic review of equipment and environmental modifications is also recommended.

Proper communication between the occupational and physical therapist and the patient's physician can ensure that the correct doses of the pharmacological treatments are in place, as the therapist has the unique opportunity of observing the patient in various circumstances and activity levels.

Management of Spasticity

Although spasticity varies greatly from person to person, muscles that typically demonstrate strong tone include the antigravity muscles. For example, in the LEs, the quadriceps, hip adductors, and plantarflexors are often spastic while in the UEs the elbow, wrist, and finger flexors together with shoulder adductors are spastic. Individuals with MS typically demonstrate stronger spasticity in the LEs than the UEs. Spasticity is functionally limiting and contributes to the development of a number of secondary impairments such as contractures, postural deformity, and decubitus ulcers.

A variety of physical therapy interventions can be used, including cryotherapy, hydrotherapy, therapeutic exercise, stretching, positioning, or any combination thereof. The responses to these interventions must be monitored closely and carefully balanced with pharmacological interventions. The therapist must closely monitor the effects of the antispasticity medications prescribed and optimize physical therapy interventions with the dosing cycle. For example, patients on baclofen will respond better to stretching techniques if they are applied in the middle of the dosing cycle rather than at the end or beginning. Physical therapists must also recognize contributing factors that affect tone and respond appropriately. For example, infection or fever that increases tone may require a referral to the physician. It is important to reduce or eliminate all factors that can aggravate spasticity (e.g., heat, humidity, stress).

Topical cold (ice packs or wraps) or hydrotherapy (cool bath) can temporarily reduce spasticity by decreasing tendon reflex excitability and clonus and by slowing conduction of impulses in nerves and muscles. The effects of cryotherapy are relatively short-lived, although some patients may experience enhanced ability to move that lasts for minutes or hours. It is important to remember that some patients, particularly those with intact sensation, may react to the unpleasant sensation of cold with *fight or flight* (autonomic nervous system) responses, such as increased HR, increased RR, or nausea. Cryotherapy is contraindicated in these patients.

Stretching and ROM exercises begun early in the course of the disease and continued daily can help patients maintain joint integrity and mobility in the presence of spasticity. Combining stretching with movements using rhythmic rotation (gentle rotation of the limb) or proprioceptive neuromuscular facilitation (PNF) stretching techniques (hold–relax active contraction [HRAC], contract–relax active contraction [CRAC]) is effective in gaining ROM.[141] See Chapter 10, Strategies to Improve Motor Function, for a discussion of these techniques. Maintained stretch, held for 30 minutes to 3 hours, also can be used to decrease stretch reflex activity. Maintained stretch can be achieved with prolonged positioning (e.g., tilt table standing with toe wedges), low-load weights applied using skin traction, or serial casts. Air splints also provide an effective mechanism to maintain limbs in lengthened, out of spasticity positions. Patients/family members/clients should be taught stretching exercises as part of a home exercise program (HEP). Fast, ballistic stretching movements are contraindicated, because spasticity is velocity sensitive. Stretching movements need to proceed slowly to gradually achieve the desired range.

Active exercises at slow or self-selected speeds should focus on expanding the available ROM. Emphasis on contracting the antagonist muscles can assist through mechanisms of reciprocal inhibition. Electrical stimulation of muscles antagonist to the spastic muscles can also be used to decrease spasticity. Movements that encourage abnormal postures should be discouraged. Patients with abnormal co-contraction may benefit from exercises focused on improving motor control (timing exercises) or biofeedback. Tai Chi, yoga, and aquatic exercises combined with cool water temperatures (less than 85°F [29.44°C]) can also be helpful in producing desired relaxation.[12]

Functional activities aimed at reducing tone should concentrate on trunk and proximal segments, because many patterns of hypertonus seem to be fixed from the action of the stronger proximal muscles. Extensor tone seems to predominate, so activities that stress LE flexion with trunk rotation are generally the most effective. For example, lower trunk rotation (LTR) in hook-lying can be effective in reducing proximal extensor tone. One very effective strategy is to position the patient in hook-lying with a therapy ball under the flexed legs and gently rock the ball back and forth. Moving from quadruped position to side-sitting can also be effective in reducing extensor tone in some patients as the activity combines LTR with prolonged inhibitory pressure on the quadriceps.[142]

For the patient with limited functional mobility (EDSS levels of 7.0 or above) positioning out of abnormal spastic postures is an important component of the management program. In general, prolonged or static positioning in any fixed posture can be deleterious to the patient with strong spasticity and should be avoided. For example, the patient who remains in bed all day with the LEs positioned in extension, adduction, and plantarflexion may be unable to flex enough at the hips and knees to sit in a wheelchair. Similarly, the feet will remain fixed in plantarflexion and cannot be positioned on the footpedals. A positioning schedule using varied positions (in bed, chair, or wheelchair) will help keep the patient from getting stuck in any one posture. Mechanical positioning devices (e.g., resting splints, toe spreader, finger spreader, ankle splint) are helpful in maintaining position and preserving joint structures.

Management of Coordination and Balance Deficits

Cerebellar deficits (ataxia, postural instability) are common in MS. Impairments in somatosensory, visual, and vestibular systems are also common and result in disordered proprioception. Spasms and muscle weakness can affect balance by changing the force and sequence of muscle contraction.[143] These combined effects result in difficulty in sustaining upright postures, walking, and other functional activities, leading to an increased risk of falls.

Interventions directed at promoting postural control should first focus on static control (holding) in weight-bearing, antigravity postures (e.g., sitting, quadruped, kneeling, modified plantigrade, and standing). Progression through a series of postures is used to gradually increase postural demands by varying the base of support (BOS), raising the center of mass (COM), and increasing the number of body segments (degrees of freedom) that must be controlled. Specific exercise techniques that can be used to promote stability include joint approximation applied through proximal joints (shoulders or hips) or spine, and rhythmic stabilization (PNF). Patients with significant ataxia will not be able to hold steady and may benefit from the application of the technique of PNF dynamic reversals (slow reversals), progressing through decrements of range.[141] Dynamic postural control can be challenged by incorporating activities such as weight shifting and UE reaching (Fig. 16.5) or LE stepping. In sitting, a resisted PNF

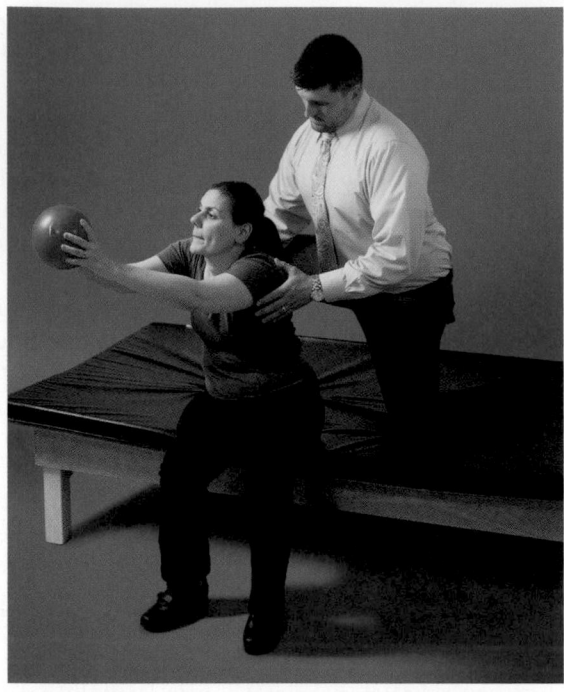

Figure 16.5 Dynamic postural control is promoted through weight shifting and upper trunk rotation to the right.

chop pattern that combines UE movements with trunk movements (flexion with rotation and extension with rotation) is an excellent activity. This can be progressed to more advanced dynamic activities with the patient sitting on a therapy (Swiss) ball as opposed to sitting on a hard flat surface (Fig. 16.6). Core musculature is engaged while the demands on ankle and knee musculature are minimized. This allows for a more focused core balance program that can be progressed to standing.[144,145]

An important goal of therapy is to promote safe and functional balance. Effective training should involve a variety of everyday functional tasks that challenge balance. Figure 16.7 demonstrates a dynamic postural control activity of combined stepping and reaching. Figure 16.8 demonstrates sit-to-stand movement transitions. As training progresses, tasks are modified (e.g., wide base to narrow base to tandem stance, stable surface to moveable surface) to promote adaptation of skills. Sensory contexts are also varied to promote adaptive control in various different perceptual contexts (e.g., eyes open to eyes closed, firm surface to thick foam surface).[142] Patients with MS and central vestibular dysfunction may benefit from vestibular rehabilitation to improve impaired balance and disability due to dizziness or disequilibrium (Fig. 16.9). See Chapter 21, Vestibular Disorders, for additional discussion.[146]

The pool is an important therapeutic medium to practice static and dynamic postural control in both sitting and standing, as well as walking. Water provides graded resistance that slows down the patient's ataxic

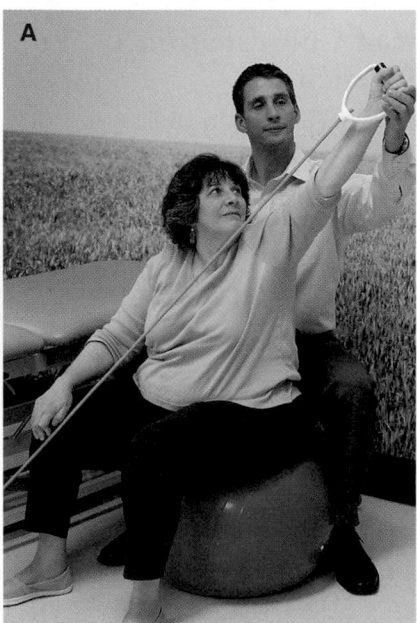 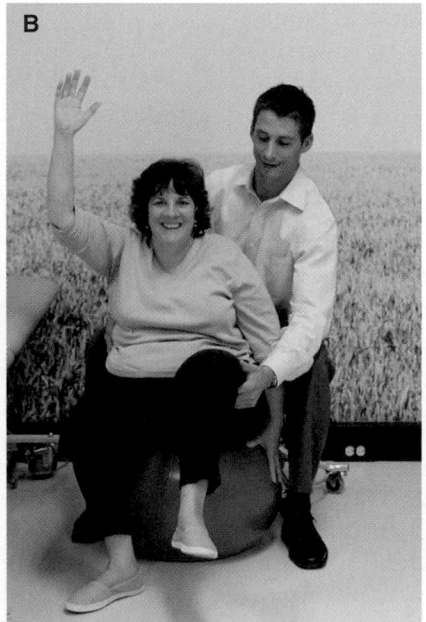 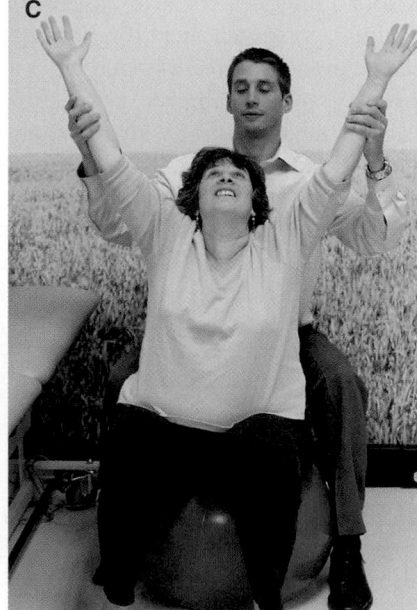

Figure 16.6 Sitting on the ball, the patient practices dynamic postural control activities: (a) unilateral resisted overhead reach, (b) reciprocal stepping and overhead arm swing, and (c) resisted bilateral symmetrical PNF D2 flexion patterns with extension.

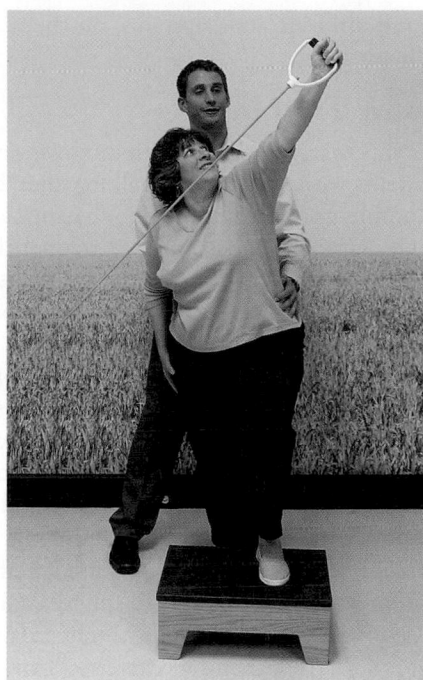

Figure 16.7 Dynamic postural control activities. This position demonstrates an advanced stepping and reaching activity with the added challenge of a resistance tube.

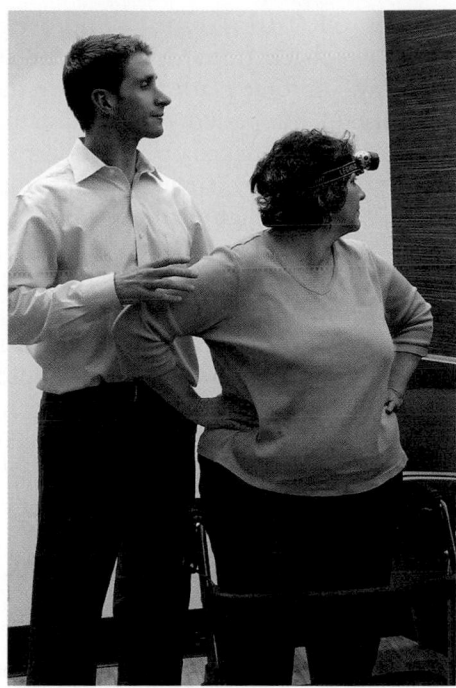

Figure 16.9 Head turns for vestibular training.

movements, while the buoyancy aids in upright balance. Water aerobics have been shown to be effective in improving strength, decreasing muscular fatigability, increasing endurance, and improving quality of life in patients with MS.[120,147] When recommending aquatic exercise programs it is imperative to assess the individual's tolerance to heat. It is commonly recommended

that persons with MS exercise in a pool that is 80° to 85°F (26.66° to 29.44°C).

Biofeedback training using augmented feedback can be used to improve balance function. Augmented visual feedback[148] and augmented proprioceptive feedback (e.g., whole body vibration platform training)[149] have been used to improve function in patients with MS. Training on a moveable force platform (e.g., SMART Balance Master® [NeuroCom International,

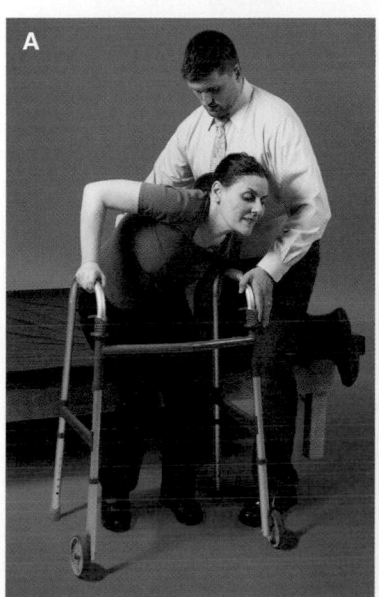
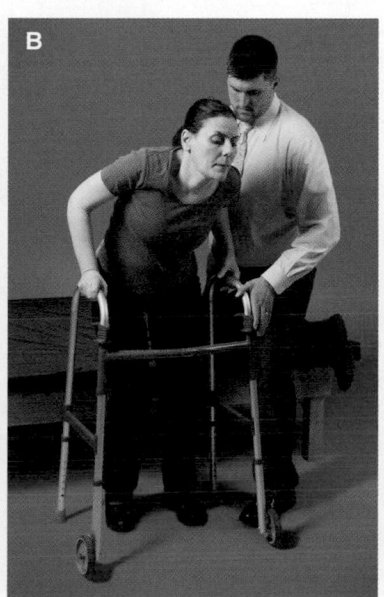
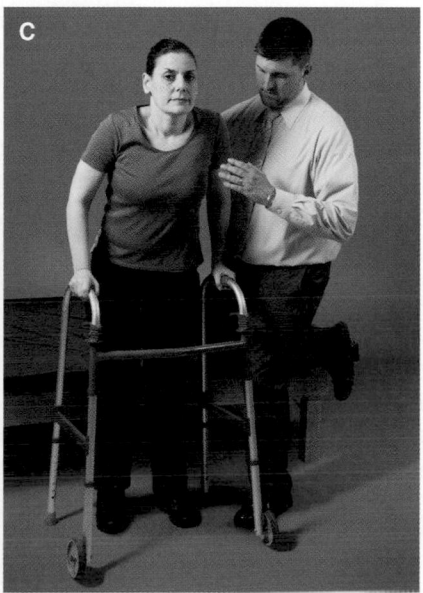

Figure 16.8 Sit-to-stand movement transition. The sit-to-stand transition is an important component of pre-gait/gait training, transfer training, and balance training.

Inc., Clackamas, OR 97015]) can also improve balance. The added biofeedback from visual and/or auditory feedback displays on force platform training machines is especially useful for patients with somatosensory deficits. The patient with ataxia needs to learn how to reduce excess postural sway (frequency and amplitude) and to control center of alignment position. Prolonged latencies (onset of responses) should be expected. Additionally, with advancements in technology, whole body vibration[150] and household video game platforms (i.e., Nintendo Wii) have become useful tools for balance training for individuals with neurological conditions.[151,152]

Control of ataxic limb movements (tremor and dysmetria) can be achieved through proprioceptive loading and light resistance. For example, the therapist can use PNF extremity patterns using the technique of dynamic reversals with light tracking resistance to modulate force output and reciprocal actions of muscles. Ataxic movements have sometimes been helped by the application of latex resistance bands or light weights to stabilize movements. Velcro® weight cuffs (wrist or ankle), weighted boots, or a weighted jacket or belt can reduce tremors of the limbs or trunk. The extra weight will also increase energy expenditure, and must therefore be carefully balanced against the increased fatigue they might cause. Weighted canes or walkers can be used to reduce ataxic UE movements that interfere with the use of an assistive device during ambulation. Weighted spoons or forks can be used to enhance eating. For patients with significant tremor, these devices may mean the difference between dependent and independent function. External devices (braces or splints) can be used to stabilize ataxic limbs but also have the undesirable effect of adding weight to limb movements. Air splints can also stabilize limb movements and should be considered, because they are lighter and less energy costly. A soft cervical collar can be used to stabilize head and neck tremors. All these strategies, however, should be viewed as temporary and compensatory. Once the devices are removed, ataxic movements will return or in some cases may actually temporarily worsen.

Unwanted movements are worse under conditions of stress, anxiety, and excitement. The increased arousal, the result of adrenalin pumping through the system, increases existing tremors while decreasing function. Stress management techniques are therefore an important component of the POC. In general, patients do better in a low-stimulus environment that allows full concentration on control of movements. They benefit from augmented feedback (verbal cueing of knowledge of results and knowledge of performance; biofeedback) and repetition to improve motor learning. The patient with MS is often restricted in practice by neuromuscular fatigue and neurological deficits that impair sensory feedback, attention, memory, and concentration. The successful therapist will need to carefully identify the patient's resources and abilities and capitalize on them to maximize motor learning.

Locomotor Training

Walking ability is frequently impaired. However, at least 65% of patients with MS are still walking after 20 years.[9] Early gait problems often include poor balance and heaviness of one or more limbs. Patients frequently report difficulty lifting their legs (hip flexor weakness). Weak dorsiflexors are also common, resulting in foot drop. Problems with foot clearance may result in a circumducted gait pattern, among other gait deviations. Later problems evolve owing to clonus, spasticity, sensory loss, and/or ataxia. Weakness generally extends to include the quadriceps and hip abductors. Quadriceps weakness typically results in hyperextension of the knee and forward flexion of the trunk with increased lumbar lordosis. Hip abductor weakness results in a Trendelenburg gait pattern with a strong lateral lean to the weak side.

A well-designed exercise program of tone management, stretching, and strengthening exercises can improve walking. Standing and walking activities should stress safety and maintaining a stable BOS; maximum weight-bearing through the LEs; and adequate weight transfer and forward progression with trunk, limb, and pelvic kinematics consistent with safe walking. Verbal and manual cueing can assist the patient in the correct mechanics of gait. A variety of functional activities should be practiced. These include walking forward and backward, side-stepping, and cross-stepping (Fig. 16.10). Braiding (a PNF activity that combines side-stepping and cross-stepping) is a complex, higher-level walking activity. Stair

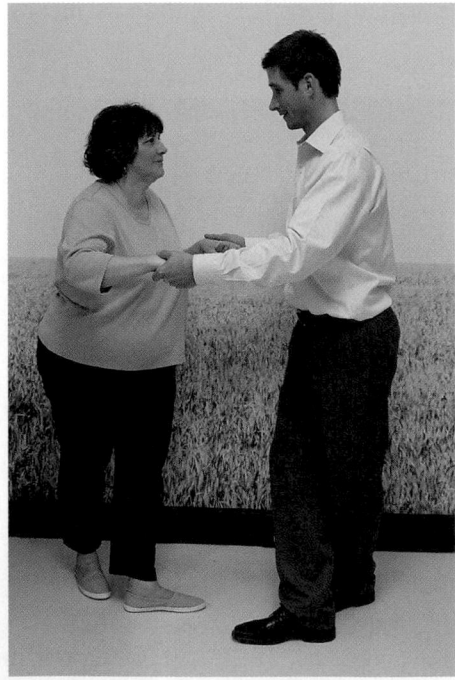

Figure 16.10 Patient practices cross-stepping. Dynamic standing activities are an integral component of an exercise program geared toward improving gait/locomotion.

climbing, negotiating curbs and ramps, navigation around obstacles, and walking on varied surfaces should also be practiced for safety in community mobility. See Chapter 11, Locomotor Training, for further discussion. As previously mentioned, the pool is an important medium that can be used to assist training of the more involved patient with ataxia while reducing tone and fatigue.

Locomotor training (LT) using an antigravity treadmill or a treadmill training (TT) with body weight support (BWS) has been the focus of increasing attention in the literature and used extensively to improve gait in patients with spinal cord injury and stroke (see discussion in Chapter 10 and Evidence Summary Boxes in Chapter 15, Stroke, and Chapter 20, Traumatic Spinal Cord Injury). In studies involving persons with MS using LT and BWS, improvements in muscle strength, spasticity, endurance, balance, walking speed, and quality of life have been reported. Level of effort was reduced while detrimental effects on fatigue are not evident.[153-155] Robot-assisted treadmill training (RATT) with BWS has also been used and when compared to conventional BWS TT, patients in both groups experienced similar improvements in outcome measures.[156,157] When RATT was compared to conventional gait training, no difference in outcomes was found between the groups.[158] In summary, LT with BWS is an activity-dependent intervention that is feasible and safe and has the potential to result in significant improvements in function for patients with MS.

Orthotics and Assistive Devices

Patients with MS typically require orthotic devices as ambulation skills decline. Ankle-foot stability can be achieved by the addition of an ankle-foot orthosis (AFO). Improvements in energy efficiency and safety are also important outcomes. AFOs are prescribed for foot drop, poor knee control (especially hyperextension), minimal to moderate spasticity, and poor somatosensation. The most common type used is the standard polypropylene AFO, which is lightweight and has the added benefit of cosmesis (Fig. 16.11). An AFO with an articulated joint can be prescribed to provide more rigid control for the ankle with the addition of a plantarflexion stop. Functional electrical stimulation (FES) devices have become prevalent in treatment and compensation for foot drop with improvements in walking performance and satisfaction reported. Patients also experienced fewer falls and reduced fatigue.[159-161] In order to effectively use any orthotic or FES device for foot drop, an individual must have adequate hip flexion strength. Relative contraindications to the prescription of these devices include severe spasticity, foot edema, and weakness (nonfunctional grades of LE muscles, especially hip flexors). Although knee-ankle-foot orthoses (KAFOs) can provide additional stabilization control of the knee, they are rarely used because of the increased energy expenditure required.

Canes, forearm crutches, or a walker may be necessary to compensate for deficits in fatigue, strength, sensory

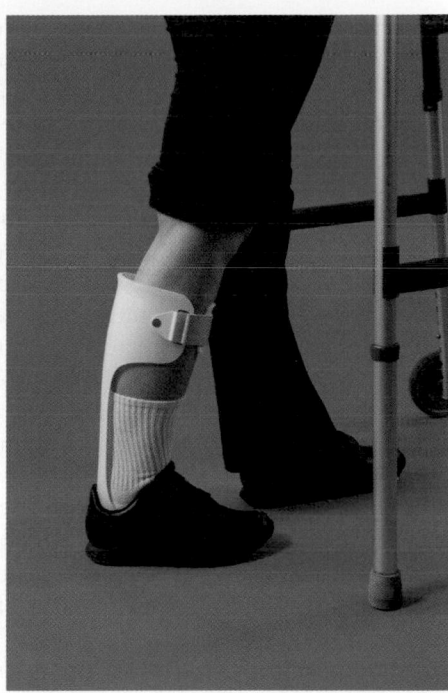

Figure 16.11 Patient is wearing an ankle-foot orthosis (AFO) to stabilize the ankle and prevent foot drop.

loss (numbness), or balance (Fig. 16.12). For many patients acceptance of an assistive device involves full recognition of their disability. They need to be convinced that use of these devices is far safer than "wall walking" or "furniture walking." Devices also provide recognition to the community at large that patients are not staggering or losing their balance because they are "drunk," a

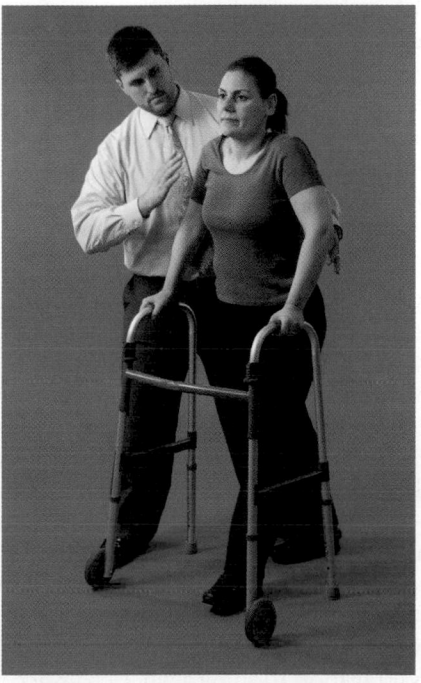

Figure 16.12 Locomotor training with a front-wheeled rolling walker.

frequent occurrence with many patients. The devices may be the difference between community participation or remaining homebound because of fear of falling. Patients should be encouraged to try out different devices to determine which works best for them. For example, the patient with significant fatigue levels may benefit from a large-wheeled walker with locking hand brakes and a seat that allows for frequent rests. Recent technological advancements have brought a new breed of mechanical upright walking devices that have integrated computer chips, sensors, and motors to aid an individual in ambulation. Cosmesis is an important factor in promoting acceptance. There are many innovations in assistive technology that make the choices easier. For example, designer canes now come in many different colors and styles, including clear Lucite. ABLEDATA (www.able-data.com) is a federally funded project that offers product information, resources, and links to manufacturers.[162]

As the disease progresses, many patients benefit from a wheeled mobility device (powered scooter or wheelchair). The course and progression of the disease and presenting symptoms should be taken into consideration when deciding on a device. For patients with adequate trunk stability, UE function, and appropriate visual, perceptual, and cognitive skills, a scooter provides needed mobility while conserving energy. Scooters also do not carry the same negative stigma as that of a wheelchair. Both three- and four-wheel scooters are available. Four-wheel scooters have superior outdoor and uneven terrain performance, but are not as easily transported. Features that should be recommended include a seat that rotates for easy mounting and dismounting, easy dismantling for loading into the car, and steering mechanisms that minimize the work of the UEs. One disadvantage of scooters is that seating cannot always be customized. They are often not designed for prolonged sitting or for patients with moderate to severe postural instability. Some new three-wheeled scooters are designed to turn in very small areas while others have a wide turning radius and may not be suitable for in-home use. The individual with MS must be adequately educated on the safety precautions of a scooter, because the trunk strength and stability requirements are significantly higher than those of a power wheelchair.

A wheelchair should be considered when postural demands necessitate increased support. A standard wheelchair requires additional energy expenditure and coordination for propulsion. When prescribing a manual wheelchair to an individual with MS it is important to include education on proper wheelchair propulsion for both preservation of shoulder strength and energy conservation. A power wheelchair should be considered when impairments prevent or limit manual propulsion or when fatigue is a major limiting factor in mobility (Fig. 16.13). However, they are more costly and require specialized transportation by a wheelchair-accessible van or bus. Most patients will navigate using a joystick. For patients with impaired hand strength and sensation, the

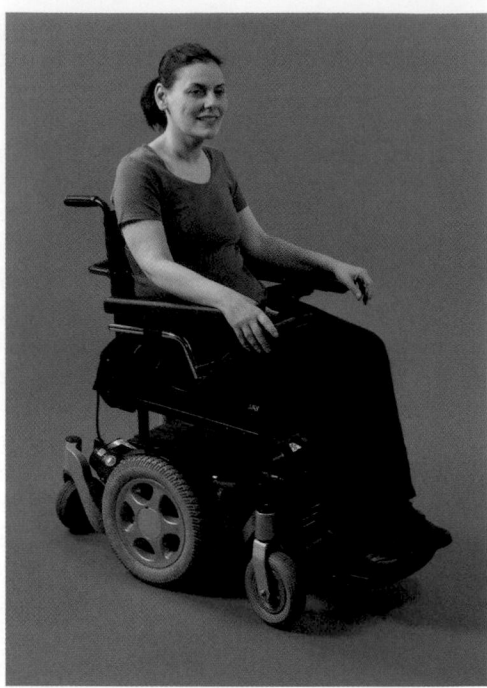

Figure 16.13 An individual with MS using a power wheelchair with joystick control for mobility. The correct power wheelchair prescription can encourage proper alignment of the pelvis, trunk, head, and limbs.

joystick can be adjusted to increase sensitivity. Wheelchair seating should ensure proper alignment of the pelvis, trunk and head, and limbs while enhancing function. Common malalignments include posterior tilting of the pelvis (sacral sitting) with kyphosis, typically the result of spasticity in the hamstring muscles. This can be improved with the addition of a seat cushion. Postural alignment can also be assisted by the addition of contoured seating (custom built). A solid back support and adjustable lateral trunk supports may be needed to enhance postural alignment and upright sitting. Footrests should be positioned to ensure that the thighs are parallel to the floor. If extensor spasms are strong, they can actually propel the patient out of the chair. A strong lap belt that secures firmly around the pelvis is necessary for safety. For patients with strong adductor spasticity, a medial knee block (pommel) may be necessary. Heel loops and straps may be required to maintain foot position on the footrests. Patients who no longer demonstrate adequate trunk and head stability require an alternate seating design. A tilt-in-space wheelchair with head/neck support is a better option than a reclining wheelchair with high back and elevating leg rests. The former maintains the normal hip sitting angle; the latter produces extension of the hips and may feed into strong extensor spasticity. Elevating leg rests tend to stretch hamstring muscles and may cause posterior pelvic tilting when spasticity is present. The reclining wheelchair with elevating leg rests also creates greater environmental access problems. Motorized control of the seat back available in tilt-in-space wheelchairs will allow the patient to make easy adjustments in position, thus preventing skin breakdown. See Chapter 32, The Prescriptive Wheelchair, for additional discussion.

Patients should be instructed in transfer and wheelchair mobility/management skills. A transfer board or hydraulic lift may be necessary as UE function deteriorates. Attention to good sitting posture and pressure-relief techniques is essential to maintain alignment and prevent skin breakdown. Patients should be encouraged to balance time in the wheelchair with other activities, such as walking or exercising, and should be extra diligent in stretching muscles that tend to contract as a result of prolonged sitting (e.g., hip and knee flexors).

One of the constraints the therapist will have to deal with is financial reimbursement for the changing mobility needs of the patient with chronic MS. Private or public insurance organizations require a statement of medical necessity for payment. Because symptoms are not static in MS but rather typically exacerbate or remit, the therapist needs to provide clear and convincing documentation of need, stressing improved function and safety. Many third-party payers will not reimburse for new wheelchairs prescribed within specified time intervals or may be hesitant to finance expensive specialty wheelchairs such as the tilt-in-space chair or a second lightweight chair for traveling. The therapist will need to provide careful documentation of potential adverse outcomes to justify the cost of the new chair. For example, a likely deleterious outcome for a patient who is denied reimbursement for a tilt-in-space chair may be skin breakdown. The costs of nursing and surgical care for decubitus ulcers can then be compared to the cost of the new wheelchair, which can be justified as a preventive measure. It is equally important to anticipate future needs as they relate to rate of disease progression when ordering equipment.

Functional Training

Functional training should focus on problem solving and the development of appropriate decision making skills required to meet the challenges of being disabled. Skills should be adapted and practiced to ensure safe performance in both the home and community environments. Training in functional mobility skills (e.g., bed mobility, transfers, locomotion) is typically directed by the physical therapist whereas ADL (e.g., dressing, personal hygiene, bathing, toileting, grooming, and feeding) and IADL (e.g., cooking, laundry, and bed making) training is directed by the occupational therapist and training in communication skills by the speech-language pathologist. Close communication and coordination among team members is necessary to ensure that training methods are consistently applied and successful. Full participation of the patient in all phases of planning and training will increase personal involvement while decreasing dependency and passivity.

The majority of patients with MS will use multiple adaptive devices. This requires careful attention to appropriate prescription of devices and environmental modifications to assist the patient in conserving energy and maintaining function. Adaptive equipment can include bed or bathroom grab bars, overhead trapeze, raised seats, transfer board, or hydraulic lift. Appropriate positional and functional splints to facilitate writing or typing and plates and cups with lips to minimize spills are often helpful in assisting with hand function. Long-handled shoehorns, reachers, button hooks, sock aids, or Velcro® closures can assist in dressing. Effective communication may require built-up writing utensils or a universal cuff for written communication or more sophisticated computerized devices. Patients with severe speech problems may require voice amplification devices, electronic aids, or computer-assisted alternative communication systems. The team must recognize when a device is indicated, and assist the patient in acceptance and in learning how to use the device *before* significant deterioration of function occurs.

Management of Speech and Swallowing

Impairments in communication and swallowing have been identified in individuals with MS.[163] The scientific literature reports that 44% of MS patients experience impairments of speech and voice in the early onset of their disease, and as many as 35% to 43% of MS patients can acquire voice, chewing, and swallowing disorders.[164] Respiratory deconditioning, characterized by reduced diaphragmatic support and shortening of the intercostal muscles, contributes to speech disorders and increases the likelihood of respiratory infections. Thus, collaborating with a speech-language pathologist to develop a *resistive breathing training* (RBT) program paired with activities to improve trunk stability, head control, and sitting balance is an important component of the POC for patients with MS. Improved respiration can be facilitated through the implementation of prolonged phonation exercises, resistive breathing exercises, and incentive spirometry. The therapist should focus on diaphragmatic and segmental chest expansion, expiratory training, and volitional and effortful coughing.[165]

When dysphagia or difficulty in swallowing occurs, physical therapists should work closely with speech-language pathologists to preserve safety of swallowing. Often a detailed examination is needed to investigate the deceptively complex swallowing mechanism. Diagnostic methods include *Videofluoroscopic Swallowing Studies (VFSS)* and *Flexible Endoscopic Evaluation of Swallowing* (FEES).[166] The role of the physical therapist is important in assisting with improving sitting position, body posture, and head control. An upright body posture with a slightly forward and downward-pointing chin position can be helpful in achieving a safe swallow and preventing aspiration.[167] Application of transcutaneous neuromuscular electric stimulation (NMES) to the submental muscles (suprahyoid triangle) to facilitate muscle reeducation was cleared by the FDA in late 2002, after the submission of data from over 800 patients (adults and children). NMES of the submental muscles paired with selected oral–motor exercises and swallowing maneuvers (e.g., Mendelsohn maneuver, effortful swallow, super-supraglottic swallow) can improve the strength, ROM, and coordination of the swallowing musculature.[165]

Thermal-tactile stimulation (TTS) is a sensory technique whereby stimulation is provided to the anterior faucial pillars to improve swallowing reflexes and the pharyngeal phase of swallowing. Anecdotally, the use of cold and icy beverages such as a shakes, fruit slushes, and ice chips provide heightened sensory input, which can improve the initiation of swallowing for many patients. Some patients also benefit from alternating small (teaspoon sized) sips of liquids with their food during mealtime. Most patients should be discouraged to engage in consecutive swallowing because it increases demand on the respiratory system and decreases airway protection. Resistive sucking through a straw can also be helpful. Thick liquids such as honey-thick and nectar-thick liquids can provide some resistance to facilitate muscle strengthening.[168] Moist foods (with sauces, broth, water, or milk) are easier to manage than dry ones. Semisolid and pureed foods are easier than regular solids. Foods that irritate the throat (e.g., vinegar) and crumbly or stringy foods (e.g., cake, cookies, potato chips, celery, cheeses) should be avoided. Patients also benefit when instructed to focus their effort on eating and never attempting to talk during active eating (mastication). Maintaining a quiet and peaceful environment during meals is helpful in improving attention and focus. Fatigue can also affect food intake. Many patients with MS benefit from reducing the size of their meals and eating smaller, more nutrient-dense meals throughout the day. Percutaneous endoscopic gastrostomy (PEG) feeding tubes and/or nasogastric tubes may become medically necessary for individuals with severe dysphagia.[169] For overall safety, it is important that family members, caregivers, and health care providers alike are educated in the use of the Heimlich maneuver in the event of an emergency.[170]

Cognitive Training

Cognitive impairments can present major difficulties for the patient and for the rehabilitation team in general. Referral to a neuropsychologist may be indicated to determine the patient's strengths and weaknesses and to assist in the adaptive process. Compensatory strategies for memory deficits can be helpful. These include the use of memory aids, timing devices, and environmental strategies. Memory can be assisted by using a memory notebook to log daily events and reminders. With the increasing availability of mobile technologies, mobile devices have proven helpful for individuals with cognitive impairment related to MS. Trials have shown that use of a personal digital assistant (PDA) device significantly improves functional performance of everyday tasks. Patients who have incorporated mobile devices into their daily routines note improvement in organization and self-efficacy that positively affected their daily lives.[171] A pill

dispenser can assist the patient in maintaining a correct medication schedule. Cueing devices such as an alarm clock, bell timer, or watch alarm can help patients remember when to do certain tasks (e.g., taking medications, performing pressure relief). Structuring and labeling the environment is also an effective strategy to assist memory (e.g., labeled drawers, cabinets). Directions for functional tasks (e.g., transfers, self-stretching techniques) should be carefully written down for both patients and caregivers. Complex tasks can be broken down with clear written directions provided for each step. Directions can be posted in different areas of the home (e.g., steps to follow for toilet or tub transfer posted in the bathroom). Additional cognitive strategies that may be helpful include mental rehearsal, requesting assistance, maximizing alertness, avoidance of difficult situations, and mental exercises. Poor follow-through should be expected among patients with severe cognitive deficits, because often there is very little insight. In this situation, the efforts of family and caregivers must be fully maximized.[17]

Cognitive-behavioral therapy (CBT) for patients with MS can yield significant improvement in the ability to deal with distress, debilitating symptoms, impairment and disease exacerbation, and progression.[172] As with healthy individuals, regular physical activity can have a positive effect on cognitive function, self-efficacy, and quality of life.[173,174] A computer-based home training program used in conjunction with other treatments has been shown to improve function in patients with MS.[175]

■ PSYCHOSOCIAL ISSUES

Individuals with MS and their families experience a variety of losses such as loss of social functioning, interpersonal relationships, employment status, independence, and functional skills. Disabilities emerge as the disease progresses over time. Various different psychosocial adaptations can be seen, including anger, denial, depression, and so forth. The unique feature of a relapsing-remitting disease course is that it requires continual readjustment every time a new set of symptoms appears. Patients who appear well adjusted at one stage may regress as the disease worsens. The uncertainty of MS produces significant cognitive and emotional stress. Patients often feel out of control and unsure of themselves. Living with MS requires not only initial acceptance, but also a tremendous flexibility to deal with this lack of closure. Patients also experience the cumulative effects of smaller, everyday stresses that are associated with fluctuating symptoms, inability to perform ADL, dependency on others, architectural barriers, and so forth. Many factors play a role in determining how an individual reacts to MS. These include the overall effect of the disease on daily life functioning, previous coping skills, perceived self-efficacy, extent of social support, and spiritual well-being. They may experience attitudes of "wait and see" or "nothing can be done." This may explain why many individuals with MS do not take medications to help control their MS despite medical guidelines recommending disease-modifying drugs. The longer they are influenced by these attitudes, the less likely they are to seek help. Learned helplessness, low self-efficacy, and lack of environmental mastery have been identified as major factors contributing to depression and fatigue.[20]

As mentioned, depression does not necessarily correlate to the severity of the disease. For example, a person with mild disease can be severely depressed, whereas the person with severe disability is not. The therapist must be alert to the signs of depression and intervene as appropriate. Chapter 26, Psychosocial Disorders, presents a complete discussion of this topic.

Despite the negative psychosocial effects of the disease, studies indicate that while initial diagnosis was met with negative reactions, over time positive changes in terms of values and outlook often occur. Interventions that target reexamination of the individual's role and identity result in an increased appreciation for life and can assist individuals with MS in better managing the disease and enjoying their lives.[176] *Self-efficacy* is the belief that an individual will be able to deal with particular situations that may contain novel, unpredictable, and stressful elements. Strategies that enhance self-efficacy and self-management (elements of CBT) empower the patient with MS.[177] Additional interventions include education, involvement in goal-setting and treatment planning, wellness forums, and support or psychotherapy groups. The use of stress reduction techniques (e.g., relaxation techniques, meditation, and exercise) can also be helpful in promoting effective coping. Family and multidisciplinary support are key elements in effective psychosocial management.[178,179]

■ PATIENT AND FAMILY/ CAREGIVER EDUCATION

The primary roles of the clinician can be categorized as caring professional, expert teacher, and competent practitioner. A positive, affirming attitude can effectively influence patients' attitudes and assist them to view rehabilitation from a more positive perspective. The development of a strong collaborative relationship with the patient and family/caregivers in which there is respect, compassion, and effective communication is key to successful rehabilitation outcomes.[177] The overall focus should be on the maintenance of *hope* and *encouragement* tempered with *realism*.

As an educator, the therapist has an important role in assisting the patient and family/caregivers in providing information on the following:

- The disease process, clinical manifestations, and their significance in terms of management

- Prevention of secondary complications, indirect impairments, and activity limitations
- The rehabilitation process, the POC, and its specific interventions
- The HEP, including interventions that can be carried out independently
- Monitoring the effects and possible adverse reactions of medications
- Use of assistive devices and adaptive equipment
- General health and stress management techniques
- Community resources

Prompt referral to community resources including a support group can provide a necessary stabilizing base for patients and their families/caregivers. Within this environment individuals can gain accurate and useful information about the disease, discuss common problems and methods of coping, and share anxieties and resources. Thus, it provides a valuable forum to assist in the continual adjustment process. The National Multiple Sclerosis Society (www.nationalmssociety.org) provides education, emotional support, and a variety of programs and services to individuals with MS and their families through their local chapters.[180] Web-based resources are provided in Appendix 16.D.

A significant number of patients with MS (one out of every two patients) will require the assistance of another person at some point in the course of their disease. This places an extra burden on family members and on the financial resources of the patient if outside caregivers must be utilized. The majority of caregivers experience moderate levels of stress associated with their caregiving duties. As the level and duration of physical care increases, caregivers can experience a variety of signs and symptoms, including physical (e.g., fatigue, headache, sleep disturbances, appetite changes), psychological (e.g., anxiety, depression, frustration), social (e.g., family conflicts, decreasing social experiences or "lack of life"), and spiritual changes (e.g., hopeless and meaningless life and work).[181] This can also put stress on relationships, as the caregiver is often a spouse and the dependency and the degree of support needed to perform certain tasks can be a source of tension.[182] The therapist will need to be sensitive to these changes and to conflicts, problems, and tensions as they develop. Considerable time and energy will be devoted to counseling and educating caregivers and coordinating home management. Attention should also be paid to the children of patients with MS, because studies have indicated that parental MS has a negative impact on children's psychological well-being. This is due, in part, to lack of understanding about the disease, and education may help ameliorate some of the negative effects.[183]

SUMMARY

Timely referral to neurorehabilitation services is the key to successful management of activity limitations, disability, and quality-of-life issues in patients with MS. Too often services are not begun until the individual becomes severely disabled. A comprehensive POC that addresses the needs of the whole patient and emphasizes meaningful functional activities, patient education, and self-management is ideal for such a complex neurodegenerative disorder. Activities that prove attainable and safe ensure patient success and build self-efficacy. Many patients with MS report that they lack the knowledge and skills needed to exercise safely. Promoting self-efficacy, self-management, and mastery can be achieved through supervised programs that focus on regular exercise, activity pacing, energy conservation, and overall healthy behaviors. Comprehensive efforts of the interdisciplinary team are needed to provide the coordinated and continuing care required with anticipated inpatient, outpatient, and home/community episodes of care.

Acknowledgment

The authors wish to thank Marissa A. Barrera, MS, MPhil, MSCS, CCC-SLP for her contributions to this chapter.

Questions for Review

1. What are the pathophysiological processes involved in MS? What are the primary areas of CNS involvement?

2. Differentiate among the various disease courses (clinical subtypes) of MS.

3. How is the diagnosis of MS established? What tests and measures are used to confirm the diagnosis?

4. What is the role of disease-modifying drugs used in the medical management of MS? What are their indications and potential adverse effects?

5. Discuss the Expanded Disability Status Scale (EDSS) for patients with MS and indications for use.

6. Discuss the guidelines for an effective exercise prescription for the patient with MS to improve strength and conditioning.

7. Discuss the guidelines for an effective exercise prescription for the patient with MS to improve aerobic performance.

8. Discuss the problem of fatigue in MS and how it influences the design of an exercise program.

9. What strategies can be used to assist in the psychosocial adjustment of the patient with relapsing-remitting MS?

CASE STUDY

HISTORY

The patient is a 27-year-old graduate student who was admitted to an acute care facility with a chief complaint of double vision for 2 weeks. She reported that both lower extremities (LEs) seemed weaker recently. Four months earlier, she had noticed persistent tingling of her fingers on the left hand and some numbness on the left side of her face.

Neurological examination showed a scotoma in the upper field of the left eye, weakness of the left medial rectus muscle, horizontal nystagmus on left lateral gaze, and mild weakness of the left central facial muscles. All other muscles had normal strength. The deep tendon reflexes were normal on the right and brisk on the left, and there was a left extensor plantar response. The sensory system was unremarkable. A diagnosis of suspected MS was made. The patient was discharged a few days later, seemingly improved after corticosteroid treatment.

The patient was readmitted to a neurological service 10 months later because she noticed increased difficulty in walking and her speech had become thickened.

NEUROLOGIST REPORT

Patient presents with wide-based ataxic gait, minor slurring of speech, bilateral tremor in the finger-to-nose test, and dysdiadochokinesia. CT scan is within normal limits. MRI scan reveals numerous white areas indicative of lesions. Lumbar puncture shows 56 mg of protein with increased level of gamma-globulin. All other CSF findings are normal. Treatment with high doses of intravenous corticosteroids seemed to improve the neurological symptoms. Patient was discharged home with a referral for outpatient rehabilitation.

Two months later, the patient's symptoms worsened and she is now admitted for intensive rehabilitation.

MEDICATIONS

Prednisone 20 mg po qid
Maalox 30 mL po qid
Valium 10 mg qid

SOCIAL HISTORY

Patient has been living on her own for several years until her recent illness. She has taken a medical leave from graduate school and had returned home to live with her parents. They are both support- ive and would like some advice as to how to modify their two-story home. There are five entry stairs with a handrail on both sides. There is a first floor bathroom, and they plan to convert the first floor study into a bedroom. Her parents are both in their early 60s, in good health, and very anxious about their daughter's rapidly deteriorating condition.

PHYSICAL THERAPY EXAMINATION FINDINGS

Mental Status

Alert, oriented
Memory: minimal impairment
At times lacks insight, seems unaware of the seriousness of her condition
Euphoric at times; other times she is depressed and cries easily

Communication

Speech is dysarthric, difficult to understand at times

Vision

Transient double vision
Gaze-evoked nystagmus to both left and right
Ocular dysmetria
Upper field defect of left eye

Endurance/Fatigue

Moderate impairment
Tolerance to activity is approximately 10 minutes before rest is required

Skin

WNL except for small bruise on right lateral malleolus

ROM

WNL except for 0° right dorsiflexion; 0° to 5° left dorsiflexion

Tone

Moderate extensor spasticity (2 on the modified Ashworth Scale) in both lower extremities (BLEs), left greater than right
Occasional extensor spasms, which are a major safety risk when they occur during transfers

Sensation

Paresthesias in BLEs with moderate proprioceptive losses, ankle joints greater than proximal joints
Both upper extremities (BUEs): mild decrease in light touch, left greater than right

Strength

Moderate weakness in BLEs; generally functional muscle grades (able to move against gravity), with the greatest weakness noted at the hips
Standard MMT positions not used owing to spasticity
BUEs 3+/5 (fair+) to 4/5 (good) strength

Coordination

BUEs: Intention tremors with mild limb ataxia; voluntary movements are hypermetric
RAM are moderately impaired
BLEs: Movements restricted by spasticity and spasms; unable to test

Balance

Sitting balance:
- *Static:* With eyes open (EO), able to maintain position independently up to 5 minutes with minimal postural tremor; with eyes closed (EC), truncal ataxia is pronounced

- *Dynamic:* With EO, able to weight shift to left and right to about 40% of limits of stability (LOS); with EC, experiences loss of balance (LOB) with minimal weight shifts

Standing balance:

- *Static:* Able to maintain standing position in parallel bars with min assist × 1 for up to 3 minutes; during standing, patient is unable to maintain centered alignment; demonstrates moderate postural tremor; with EC, sway is increased dramatically and patient quickly loses her balance
- Tends to keep her hips and knees stiff in extension/hyperextension
- *Dynamic:* Unable to weight shift or step without bilateral handhold

Functional

Functional Independence Measure (FIM):

- Eating: FIM 6; requires adaptive equipment
- Grooming: FIM 6; requires adaptive equipment
- Bathing: FIM 5; requires setup and adaptive equipment
- Dressing—upper and lower: FIM 4; minimal assist
- Toileting: FIM 4; minimal assist for balance
- Sphincter control—bladder FIM 6; bowel FIM 6
- Transfers—bed, chair, wheelchair: FIM 4, minimal contact assist for stand pivot transfers
- Transfers—toilet and tub: FIM 4; minimal contact assist
- Locomotion—walk: FIM 4; minimal contact assist, uses walker
- Locomotion—stairs: FIM 2; less than 4 to 6 stairs, maximal assist
- Locomotion—wheelchair: FIM 5; supervision, uses manual wheelchair for distances up to 150 ft; posture in wheelchair: sacral sitting
- Requires a lap belt due to extensor spasms, which can cause her to fling out of the chair
- Communication—expression: FIM 6; requires extra time, mild dysarthria
- Communication—comprehension: FIM 6; complete understanding, requires extra time for processing
- Social interaction: FIM 7
- Problem solving: FIM 6; requires extra time, slight difficulty initiating decisions
- Memory: FIM 6; slight difficulty remembering daily routines and executing requests without need for repetition

Expanded Disability Status Scale (EDSS) score: 6.5

PATIENT'S GOALS

She would like to regain ambulation skills and independent living status. She recognizes the need to live with her parents for the time being but sees this as only temporary.

GUIDING QUESTIONS

1. Develop a problem list: identify/categorize this patient's problems in terms of direct impairments, indirect impairments, functional limitations, and disability.

2. Identify two outcomes (the remediation of functional limitations and disability) and two goals (remediation of impairments) for this patient.

3. Formulate four treatment interventions that could be used at the start of therapy to achieve the stated outcomes and goals. Provide a brief rationale for each.

4. What strategies can be used to develop self-management skills and promote self-efficacy and quality of life?

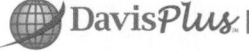 For additional resources, including answers to the questions for review and case study guiding questions, please visit **http://davisplus.fadavis.com**

References

1. Cohen, B, Zamvil, S, and Cerruto, L (eds): Neurology: Multiple Sclerosis 2011 Edition. Living Medical eTextbook. Retrieved May 23, 2012, from http://lmt.projectsinknowledge.com/Activity/index.cfm?jn=2023&sj=2023.01&i=8.

2. Rolak, LA: History of Multiple Sclerosis. National Multiple Sclerosis Society, New York, 2003.

3. Celine, J, Coyle, P, and Duquette, P: Gender issues in multiple sclerosis: An update. Women's Health 6(6):797, 2010.

4. Alter, M, et al: Migration and risk of multiple sclerosis. Neurology 28:1089, 1978.

5. Weinshenker, B: Epidemiology of multiple sclerosis. Neurol Clin 14:291, 1996.

6. Herndon, R: The pathology of multiple sclerosis and its variants. In Herdon, R (ed): Multiple Sclerosis: Immunology, Pathology and Pathophysiology. Demos Medical Publishers, New York, 2003, p 184.

7. Lublin, F, and Reingold, S: Defining the clinical course of multiple sclerosis: Results of an international survey. Neurology 46:907, 1996.

8. Cohen, B (ed): Managing symptoms in multiple sclerosis. In Neurology: Multiple Sclerosis 2011 Edition. Living Medical eTextbook. Retrieved May 23, 2012, from http://lmt.project-sinknowledge.com/Activity/index.cfm?jn=2023&sj=2023.01&i=8.

9. Shapiro, R: Managing the Symptoms of Multiple Sclerosis, ed 5. Demos Medical Publishers, New York, 2007.

10. Maloni, H: Pain in multiple sclerosis. Clinical Bulletin for Health Professionals, 2011. National Multiple Sclerosis Society, New York, 2001. Retrieved May 10, 2012, from www.nationalmssociety.org/.

11. Frohman, E: Diagnosis and management of vision problems in MS. Clinical Bulletin for Health Professionals, 2011, National Multiple Sclerosis Society, New York, 2011. Retrieved May 10, 2012, from www.nationalmssociety.org/.

12. Kushner, S, and Brandfass, K: Spasticity. Clinical Bulletin for Health Professionals. National Multiple Sclerosis Society, New York, 2011. Retrieved May 10, 2012, from www.nationalmssociety.org/.

13. National Clinical Advisory Board of the National Multiple Sclerosis Society: Management of MS-related fatigue. National Multiple Sclerosis Society, New York, 2006. Retrieved May 10, 2012, from www.nationalmssociety.org/.

14. Fisk, J, et al: The impact of fatigue on patients with multiple sclerosis. J Can Sci Neurol 21:9, 1994.

15 Schwartz, C, et al: Psychosocial correlates of fatigue in multiple sclerosis. Arch Phys Med Rehabil 77:165, 1996.

16. Logemann, J: Swallowing disorders and their management in patients with multiple sclerosis. Clinical Bulletin for Health Professionals. National Multiple Sclerosis Society, New York, NY, 2011. Retrieved May 12, 2012, from www.nationalmssociety.org/.

17. Benedict, R: Cognitive dysfunction in multiple sclerosis. Clinical Bulletin for Health Professionals. National Multiple Sclerosis Society, New York, 2011. Retrieved May 12, 2012, from www.nationalmssociety.org/.

18. Samuel, L, and Cavallo, P: Emotional issues of the person with MS. Clinical Bulletin for Health Professionals. National Multiple Sclerosis Society, New York, 2011. Retrieved May 23 2012, from www.nationalmssociety.org/.

19. Brassington, J, and Marsh, N: Neuropsychological aspects of multiple sclerosis. Neuropsychol Rev 8:43, 1998.

20. Shnek, Z, et al: Helplessness, self-efficacy, cognitive distortions and depression in multiple sclerosis and spinal cord injury. Ann Behav Med 19:287, 1997.

21. Minden, S: Pseudobulbar affect. Clinical Bulletin for Health Professionals. National Multiple Sclerosis Society, New York, 2011. Retrieved May 12 2012, from www.nationalmssociety.org/.

22. Feinstein, A, et al: Prevalence and neurobehavioral correlates of pathological laughing and crying in multiple sclerosis. Arch Neurol 54:1116, 1997.

23. Holland, N, and Reitman, N: Bladder dysfunction in multiple sclerosis. Clinical Bulletin for Health Professionals. National Multiple Sclerosis Society, New York, 2011. Retrieved May 13 2012, from www.nationalmssociety.org/.

24. Holland, N and Kennedy, P: Bowel management in multiple sclerosis. Clinical Bulletin for Health Professionals. National Multiple Sclerosis Society, New York, 2011. Retrieved May 23, 2012, from www.nationalmssociety.org/.

25. Foley, F: Assessment and treatment of sexual dysfunction in multiple sclerosis. Clinical Bulletin for Health Professionals. National Multiple Sclerosis Society, New York, 2011. Retrieved May 13, 2012, from www.nationalmssociety.org/.

26. Polman, C, et al: Diagnostic criteria for multiple sclerosis: 2010 revisions to the McDonald criteria. Ann Neurol 69(2):292, 2011.

27. McDonald, W, et al: Recommended diagnostic criteria for multiple sclerosis: Guidelines from the International Panel on the Diagnosis of Multiple Sclerosis. Ann Neurol 50(1):121, 2001.

28. Cohen, B, and Pelletier, D (eds): MRI and new imaging technologies in multiple sclerosis. In Neurology: Multiple Sclerosis 2011 Edition. Living Medical eTextbook. Retrieved May 10, 2012, from http://lmt.projectsinknowledge.com/Activity/index.cfm?jn=2023&sj=2023.01&i=8.

29. Weber, E, Vilensky, J, and Fog, A: Practical Radiology: A Symptom-Based Approach. FA Davis, Philadelphia, 2013.

30. Cohen, B (ed): Currently available treatments for multiple sclerosis. In Neurology: Multiple Sclerosis 2011 Edition. Living Medical eTextbook. Retrieved May 13, 2012, from http://lmt.projectsinknowledge.com/Activity/index.cfm?jn=2023&sj=2023.01&i=8

31. Kalb, R, and Reitman, N: Overview of multiple sclerosis. National Multiple Sclerosis Society, New York, 2011. Retrieved May 13 2012, from www.nationalmssociety.org/.

32. Holland, N: Improving adherence to therapy with immunomodulating agents. National Multiple Sclerosis Society, New York, 2011. Retrieved May 5, 2012, from www.nationalmssociety.org/.

33. Orsnes, G, et al: The effect of baclofen on the transmission in spinal pathways in spastic multiple sclerosis patients. Clin Neurophysiol 111:1372, 2000.

34. Holland, N, and Kennedy, P: Bowel management in multiple sclerosis. In Neurology: Multiple Sclerosis 2011 Edition. Living Medical eTextbook. Retrieved May 13, 2012, from http://lmt.projectsinknowledge.com/Activity/index.cfm?jn=2023&sj=2023.01&i=8.

35. Thompson, A: The effectiveness of neurological rehabilitation in multiple sclerosis. J Rehabil Res Dev 37(4):455, 2000.

36. Baker, N, and Tickle-Degnen, L: The effectiveness of physical, psychological, and functional interventions in treating clients with multiple sclerosis: A meta-analysis. Am J Occup Ther 55(3):324, 2001.

37. Craig, J, et al: A randomized controlled trial comparing rehabilitation against standard therapy in multiple sclerosis patients receiving steroid treatment. J Neurol Neurosurg Psychiatry 74:1225, 2003.

38. Di Fabio, R, et al: Health-related quality of life for persons with progressive multiple sclerosis: Influence of rehabilitation. Phys Ther 77(12):1704, 1997.

39. DiFabio, R, et al: Extended outpatient rehabilitation: Its influence on symptom frequency, fatigue, and functional status for persons with progressive multiple sclerosis. Arch Phys Med Rehabil 79:141, 1998.

40. Freeman, J, et al: The impact of inpatient rehabilitation on progressive multiple sclerosis. Ann Neurol 42(2):236, 1997.

41. Liu, C, Playford, E, and Thompson, A: Does neurorehabilitation have a role in relapsing remitting multiple sclerosis? J Neurol 250(10):1214, 2003.

42. Patti, F, et al: Effects of a short outpatient rehabilitation treatment on disability of multiple sclerosis patients—a randomized controlled trial. J Neurol 250(7):861, 2003.

43. Slade, A, Tennant, A, and Chamberlain, M: A randomized controlled trial to determine the effect of intensity of therapy upon length of stay in a neurological rehabilitation setting. J Rehabil Med 34(6):260, 2002.

44. Guagenti-Tax, EM, et al: Impact of a comprehensive long-term care program on caregivers and persons with multiple sclerosis. Int J M S Care 2(1):5, 2000.

45. Khan, F, et al: Effectiveness of rehabilitation intervention in person with multiple sclerosis. J Neurol Neurosurg Psychiatry 79:1230, 2008.

46. Patti, F, et al: Effects of a short outpatient rehabilitation treatment on disability of multiple sclerosis patients: A randomised controlled trial. J Neurol 250(7):861, 2003.

47. Pozzilli, C, et al: Home based management in multiple sclerosis: Results of a randomised controlled trial. J Neurol Neurosurg Psychiatry 73:250, 2002.

48. Storr, LK, Sorensen, PS, and Ravnborg, M: The efficacy of multidisciplinary rehabilitation in stable multiple sclerosis patients. Mult Scler 12:235, 2006.

49. Stuifbergen, AK, et al: A randomized clinical trial of a wellness intervention for women with multiple sclerosis. Arch Phys Med Rehabil 84(4):467, 2003.

50. Wiles, C, et al: Controlled randomized crossover trial of the effects of physiotherapy on mobility in chronic multiple sclerosis. J Neurol Neurosurg Psychiatry 70:174, 2001.

51. Khan, F, et al: Multidisciplinary rehabilitation for adults with multiple sclerosis (review). Cochrane Database of Systematic Reviews 2007, Issue 2. Art. No.: CD006036. DOI: 10.1002/14651858.CD006036.pub2.

52. Kraft, G, and Schapiro, R (Co-Chairs) National MS Society's Medical Advisory Board: Rehabilitation: Recommendations for Persons with Multiple Sclerosis. National Multiple Sclerosis

Society, New York, 2004 Retrieved June 10, 2012, from www.nationalmssociety.org.

53. American Physical Therapy Association (APTA): Guide to Physical Therapist Practice, ed 2. APTA, Alexandria, VA, 2003.

54. Medicare Benefit Policy Manual, Chapter 15, Covered Medical and Other Health Services, Rev. 151, 11-18-11. Retrieved June 10, 2012, from www.cms/gov/Regulations-and-Guidance.

55. Dal Bello-Haas, V: A framework for rehabilitation of neurodegenerative diseases: Planning care and maximizing quality of life. Neurology Report (now JNPT) 26(2):115, 2002.

56. Benedict, R, et al: Minimal neuropsychological examination of MS patients: A consensus approach. Clin Neuropsychol 16(3): 381, 2002.

57. Folstein, M: Mini-Mental State: A practical method for grading the cognitive state of patients for the clinician. J Psychiatr Res 12:189, 1975.

58. Beck, A, and Beck, R: Screening depressed patients in family practice: A rapid technique. Postgrad Med 52:81, 1972.

59. Lincoln, NB, Jackson, JM, and Adams, SA: Reliability and revision of the Nottingham Sensory Assessment for stroke patients. Physiother 84(8):358, 1998.

60. Sharrack, B, and Hughes, R: The Guy's Neurological Disability Scale (GNDS): A new disability measure for multiple sclerosis. Mult Scler 5(4):223, 1999.

61. Hoogervorst, E, et al: Comparisons of patient self-report, neurologic examination, and functional impairment in MS. Neurology 56(7):934–937, 2001.

62. Melzack, R: The McGill Pain Questionnaire: Major properties and scoring methods. Pain 1:227, 1975.

63. Rog, DJ, et al: Validation and reliability of the Neuropathic Pain Scale (NPS) in multiple sclerosis. Clin J Pain 23(6):473, 2007.

64. Flachenecker, P, et al: Fatigue in multiple sclerosis: A comparison of different rating scales and correlation to clinical parameters. Mult Scler 8(6):523, 2002.

65. Fisk, JD, et al: The impact of fatigue on patients with multiple sclerosis. Can J Neurol Sci 21(1):9, 1994.

66. Fisk, JD, et al: Measuring the functional impact of fatigue: Initial validation of the fatigue impact scale. Clin Infect Dis Suppl 1:S79, 1994.

67. Penner, IK, et al: The Fatigue Scale for Motor and Cognitive Functions (FSMC): Validation of a new instrument to assess multiple sclerosis related fatigue. Mult Scler 15(12):1509, 2009.

68. APTA Multiple Sclerosis Outcome Measures Taskforce: Multiple Sclerosis Outcome Measures. Retrieved from www.neuropt.org/files/FINAL_EDGE_DOCUMENT.pdf.

69. Karpatkin, HI: Multiple sclerosis and exercise: A review of the evidence. Int J MS Care 7(2):36, 2005.

70. Vukusic, S, and Confavreux, C: The natural history of multiple sclerosis. In Cook, SD (ed): Handbook of Multiple Sclerosis. Marcel Dekker, New York, 2001, p 443.

71. De Souza, L, and Ashburn, A: Examination of motor function in people with multiple sclerosis. Physiother Res Int 1:98, 1996.

72. Lee, K, et al: The Ashworth Scale: A reliable and reproducible method of measuring spasticity. J Neuro Rehab 3:205, 1989.

73. Bohannon, R, and Smith, M: Interrater reliability of a modified Ashworth scale of muscle spasticity. Phys Ther 67:206, 1987.

74. Shumway-Cook, A, and Horak, F: Assessing the influence of sensory interaction on balance. Phys Ther 66:1548, 1986.

75. Nelson, S, et al: Vestibular and sensory interaction deficits assessed by dynamic platform posturography in patients with multiple sclerosis. Ann Otol Rhinol Laryngol 104:62, 1995.

76. Jackson, R, et al: Abnormalities in posturography and estimations of visual vertical and horizontal in multiple sclerosis. Am J Otol 16:88, 1995.

77. Berg, K, et al: Measuring balance in the elderly: Preliminary development of an instrument. Physiother Can 41:304, 1989.

78. Berg, K, et al: Measuring balance in the elderly: Validation of an instrument. Can J Public Health Suppl 2(Jul-Aug):S7–11, 1992.

79. Tinetti, M: Performance-oriented examination of mobility problems in elderly patients. J Am Geriatr Soc 34:119, 1986.

80. Horak, FB, Wrisley, DM, and Frank, J: The Balance Evaluation Systems Test (BESTest) to differentiate balance deficits. Phys Ther 89(5):484, 2009.

81. Shumway-Cook, A, et al: Predicting the probability of falls in community dwelling older adults. Phys Ther 77:812, 1997.

82. Schwid, S, et al: The measurement of ambulatory impairment in multiple sclerosis. Neurology 49:1419, 1997.

83. Lord, SE, et al: Visual gait analysis: The development of a clinical examination and scale. Clin Rehabil 12:107, 1998.

84. Borg, G: Psychophysical bases of perceived exertion. Med Sci Sports Exerc 14:377, 1982.

85. American College of Sports Medicine: ACSM's Guidelines for Exercise Testing and Prescription, ed 8. Lippincott Williams & Wilkins, Philadelphia, 2010.

86. Guide for the Uniform Data Set for Medical Rehabilitation including the FIM instrument, Version 5.0. State University of New York at Buffalo, Buffalo, 1996.

87. Granger, C, et al: Functional examination scales: A study of persons with multiple sclerosis. Arch Phys Med Rehabil 71:870, 1990.

88. Stewart, A, Hays, R, and Ware, J: The MOS short-form general health survey. Reliability and validity in a patient population. Med Care 26(7):724, 1988.

89. Freeman, JA, et al: Clinical appropriateness: A key factor in outcome measure selection: The 36 item short form health survey in multiple sclerosis. J Neurol 68(2):150, 2000.

90. Gilson, B, et al: The Sickness Impact Profile: Development of an outcome measure of health care. Am J Public Health 65:1304, 1975.

91. Doble, S, et al: Functional competence of community-dwelling persons with multiple sclerosis using the Examination of Motor and Process Skills. Arch Phys Med Rehabil 75:843, 1994.

92. Kurtzke, J: On the evaluation of disability in multiple sclerosis. Neurology 11:686, 1961.

93. Kurtzke, J: Rating neurological impairment in multiple sclerosis: An expanded disability status scale (EDSS). Neurology 33:1444, 1983.

94. Noseworthy, J, et al, and Canadian Cooperative MS Study Group: Interrater variability with the Expanded Disability Status Scale (EDSS) and Functional Systems (FS) in a multiple sclerosis clinical trial. Neurology 40:971, 1990.

95. Haber, A, and LaRocca, N (eds): MRD Minimal Record of Disability for Multiple Sclerosis. National Multiple Sclerosis Society, New York, 1985.

96. Solari, A, et al: Accuracy of self-examination of the minimal record of disability in patients with multiple sclerosis. Acta Neurol Scand 87:43, 1993.

97. Vickrey, BG, et al: A health-related quality of life measure for multiple sclerosis. Qual Life Res 4:187, 1995.

98. Vickrey, BG, et al: Comparison of a generic to disease-targeted health-related quality of life measure for multiple sclerosis. J Clin Epidemiol 50:557, 1997.

99. Consortium of Multiple Sclerosis Centers, Health Science Research Subcommittee: Multiple Sclerosis Quality of Life Inventory: A User's Manual. National Multiple Sclerosis Society, New York, 1997.

100. Cella, DF, et al: Validation of the Functional Examination of Multiple Sclerosis quality of life instrument. Neurology 47(1):129, 1996.

101. Hobart, JC, et al: The Multiple Sclerosis Impact Scale (MSIS-29): A new patient-based outcome measure. Brain 124:962, 2001.

102. Riazi, A, et al: Multiple Sclerosis Impact Scale (MSIS-29): Reliability and validity in hospital based samples. J Neurol Neurosurg Psychiatry 73(6):701, 2002.

103. Sloane, E, et al: Anti-inflammatory cytokine gene therapy decreases sensory and motor dysfunction in experimental MS: MOG-EAE behavioral and anatomical symptom treatment with cytokine gene therapy. Brain Behav Immun 23:92, 2009.

104. Bitton, L, and Fred, D: Palliative care in patients with MS. Neurol Clin 19:801, 2001.

105. Cattaneo, D, and Jonsdottir, J: Sensory impairments in quiet standing in subjects with MS. Mult Scler 15(1):59, 2009.

106. Cramp, A, et al: The incidence of pressure ulcers in people with MS and persons responsible for their management. Int J M S Care 6(2):52, 2004.

107. Shelley, A, et al: Impact of sitting time on seat-interface pressure and on pressure mapping with MS patients. Arch Phys Med Rehabil 86:1221, 2005.

108. Taylor, V: Pressure mapping clinical protocol. Proceedings of Canadian Seating and Mobility Conference, Toronto, ON, September 22–24, 1999.

109. Yang, Y, et al: Remote monitoring of sitting behaviors for community-dwelling manual wheelchair users with spinal cord injury. Spinal Cord 47(1):67, 2009.

110. Williams, C, et al: Iron and zinc status in MS patients with pressure sores. Eur J Clin Nutr 42(4):321, 1988.

111. White, LJ, et al: Resistance training improves strength and functional capacity in persons with multiple sclerosis. Mult Scler 10:668, 2004.

112. Surakka, J, et al: Effects of aerobic and strength exercise on motor fatigue in men and women with multiple sclerosis: A randomized control trial. Clin Rehabil 18:737, 2004.

113. Mostert, S, and Kesselring, J: Effects of a short-term exercise training program on aerobic fitness, fatigue, health perception, and activity level of subjects with multiple sclerosis. Mult Scler 8:161, 2002.

114. Petajan, J, et al: Impact of aerobic training on fitness and quality of life in multiple sclerosis. Ann Neurol 39:432, 1996.

115. DeBolt, LS, and McCubbin, JA: The effects of home-based resistance exercise on balance, power, and mobility in adults with multiple sclerosis. Arch Phys Med Rehabil 85(2):290, 2004.

116. Jones, R, Davies-Smith, A, and Harvey, L: The effect of weighted leg raises and quadriceps strength, EMG and functional activities in people with multiple sclerosis. Physiother 85(3):154, 1999.

117. Lord, SE, Wade, DT, and Halligan, PW: A comparison of two physiotherapy treatment approaches to improve walking in multiple sclerosis: A pilot randomized controlled study. Clin Rehabil 2(6):477, 1998.

118. Solari, A, et al: Physical rehabilitation has a positive effect on disability in multiple sclerosis patients. Neurology 52(1):57, 1999.

119. Wiles, CM, et al: Controlled randomised crossover trial of the effects of physiotherapy on mobility in chronic multiple sclerosis. J Neurol Neurosurg Psychiatry 70(2):174, 2001.

120. Patti, F, et al: Effects of a short outpatient rehabilitation treatment on disability of multiple sclerosis patients. J Neurol 250:861, 2003.

121. Sutherland, G, Andersen, M, and Stoove, M: Can aerobic exercise training affect health-related quality of life for people with multiple sclerosis? J Sport Exerc Psychol 23:122, 2001.

122. Andreasen, AK, Stenager, E, and Dalgas, U: The effect of exercise therapy on fatigue in multiple sclerosis. Mult Scler 17(9):1041, 2011.

123. Dalgas, U, et al: Fatigue, mood and quality of life improve in MS patients after progressive resistance training. Mult Scler 16(4):480, 2010.

124. Cakit, BD, et al: Cycling progressive resistance training for people with multiple sclerosis—a randomized controlled study. Am J Phys Med Rehabil 89:446, 2010.

125. Rampello, A, et al: Effect of aerobic training on walking capacity and maximal exercise tolerance in patients with multiple sclerosis: A randomized crossover controlled study. Phys Ther 87(5) 545, 2007.

126. Dodd, K, et al: A qualitative analysis of a progressive resistance exercise programme for people with multiple sclerosis. Disabil Rehabil 28(18):1127, 2006.

127. Snook, NM, and Motl, RW: Effect of exercise training on walking mobility in multiple sclerosis: A meta-analysis. Neurorehabil Neural Repair 23(2):108, 2009.

128. Rietberg, MB, et al: Exercise therapy for multiple sclerosis (review). Cochrane Database of Systematic Reviews 2004, Issue 3. Art. No.: CD003980. DOI: 10.1002/14651858.CD003980.pub2.

129. Mulcare, J, and Petajan, J: Multiple sclerosis. In American College of Sports Medicine: ACSM's Resources for Clinical Exercise Physiology: Musculoskeletal, Neuromuscular, Neoplastic, Immunologic, and Hematologic Conditions. Lippincott Williams & Wilkins, Philadelphia, 2002, p 29.

130. Jackson, K, and Mulcare, J: Multiple sclerosis. In American College of Sports Medicine: ACSM's Exercise Management for Persons with Chronic Diseases and Disabilities, ed 3. Human Kinetics, Champaign, IL, 2009, p 321.

131. Ku, YE, et al: Physiologic and functional responses of MS patients to body cooling. Am J Phys Med Rehabil 79:427, 2000.

132. Davis, SL, et al: Thermoregulation in multiple sclerosis. J Appl Physiol 109(5):1531, 2010.

133. Meyer-Heim, A, et al: Advanced lightweight cooling-garment technology: Functional improvements in thermosensitive patients with multiple sclerosis. Mult Scler 13(2):232, 2007.

134. White, AT, et al: Effect of precooling on physical performance in multiple sclerosis. Mult Scler 6:176, 2000.

135. Flensner, G, and Lindencrona, C: The cooling-suit: Case studies on its influence on fatigue among eight individuals with multiple sclerosis. J Adv Nurs 37(6):541, 2002.

136. Motl, RW: Accurate prediction of cardiorespiratory fitness using cycle ergometry in minimally disabled persons with relapsing-remitting multiple sclerosis. Arch Phys Med Rehabil 93(3):490, 2012.

137. Kuspinar, A, et al: Predicting exercise capacity through submaximal fitness tests in persons with multiple sclerosis. Arch Phys Med Rehabil 91(9):1410, 2010.

138. Curran, SA, and Willis, FB: Chronic ankle contracture reduced: A case series. Foot Ankle Online J 4(7):2, July 2011.

139. Harvey, L, Herbert, R, and Crosbie, J: Does stretching induce lasting increases in joint ROM? A systematic review. Physiother Res Int 7(1):1, 2002.

140. Multiple Sclerosis Council for Clinical Practice Guidelines: Fatigue and Multiple Sclerosis: Evidence-Based Management Strategies for Fatigue in Multiple Sclerosis. Paralyzed Veterans of America, New York, 1998.

141. Adler, S, Beckers, D, and Buck, M: PNF in Practice, ed 3. Springer, New York, 2008.

142. O'Sullivan, S, and Schmitz, T: Improving Functional Outcomes in Physical Rehabilitation. FA Davis, Philadelphia, 2010.

143. Kelleher, K, et al: Ambulatory rehabilitation in multiple sclerosis. Disabil Rehabil 31(20):1625, 2009.

144. Vera-Garcia, FJ, Grenier, SG, and McGill, SM: Abdominal muscle response during curl-ups on both stable and labile surfaces. Phys Ther 80:564, 2000.

145. Freeman, JA, et al: The effect of core stability training on balance and mobility in ambulant individuals with multiple sclerosis: A multi-center series of single case studies. Mult Scler 16(11): 1377, 2010.

146. Hebert, J, et al: Effects of vestibular rehabilitation on multiple sclerosis–related fatigue, upright postural control: A randomized controlled trial. Phys Ther 91(8):1166, 2011.

147. Roehrs, T, and Karst, G: Effects of an aquatics exercise program on quality of life measures for individuals with progressive multiple sclerosis. JNPT 28(2):63, 2004.

148. Cattaneo, D, et al: Effects of balance exercises on people with multiple sclerosis: A pilot study. Clin Rehabil 21:771, 2007.

149. Prosperini, L, et al: Visuo-proprioceptive training reduces risk of falls in patients with multiple sclerosis. Mult Scler 16(4):491, 2010.

150. Claerbout, M, et al: Effects of 3 weeks' whole body vibration training on muscle strength and functional mobility in hospitalized persons with multiple sclerosis. Mult Scler J 18(4):498, 2012.

151. Taylor, D: Can Wii improve balance? N Z J Physiother 39(3): 131, 2011.

152. Taylor, M, et al: Activity-promoting gaming systems in exercise and rehabilitation. J Rehab Research Dev 48(10):1171, 2011.

153. Giesser, B, et al: Locomotor training using body weight support on a treadmill improves mobility in persons with multiple sclerosis: A pilot study. Mult Scler 13:224, 2007.

154. Newman, MA: Can aerobic treadmill training reduce the effort of walking and fatigue in people with multiple sclerosis? A pilot study. Mult Scler 13:113, 2007.

155. Fulk, G: Locomotor training and virtual reality-based balance training for an individual with multiple sclerosis: A case report. JNPT 29(1):34, 2005.

156. Wier, LM, et al: Effect of robot-assisted versus conventional body-weight-supported treadmill training on quality of life for people with multiple sclerosis. J Rehabil Res Dev 48(4):483, 2011.

157. Lo, AC, and Triche, EW: Improving gait in multiple sclerosis using robot-assisted, body weight supported treadmill training. Neurorehabil Neural Repair 22(6):661, 2008.

158. Schwartz, I, et al: Robot-assisted gait training in multiple sclerosis: A randomized trial. Mult Scler 18(6):881, 2012.

159. Esnouf, JE, et al: Impact on activities of daily living using a functional electrical stimulation device to improve dropped foot in people with multiple sclerosis, measured by the Canadian Occupational Performance Measure. Mult Scler 16(9):1141, 2010.

160. Paul, L, et al: The effect of functional electrical stimulation on the physiological cost of gait in people with multiple sclerosis. Mult Scler 14:954, 2008.

161. Chag, Y, et al: Decreased central fatigue in multiple sclerosis patients after 8 weeks of surface functional electrical stimulation. J Rehabil Res Dev 48(5):555, 2011.

162. Provance, P: Physical therapy in multiple sclerosis rehabilitation. Clinical Bulletin for Health Professionals. National Multiple Sclerosis Society, New York. Retrieved May 15, 2012, from www.nationalmssociety.org/.

163. Achiron, A, et al: Aphasia in multiple sclerosis: clinical and radiologic correlations. Neurology 42: 2195, 1992.

164. Beukelman, DR, Kraft, GH, and Freal, J: Expressive communication disorders in persons with multiple sclerosis. Arch Phys Med Rehabil 66:675, 1985.

165. Blumenfeld, L, et al: Transcutaneous electrical stimulation versus traditional dysphagia therapy: A nonconcurrent cohort study. Otolaryngol Head Neck Surg 135:754, 2006.

166. Mari, F, et al: Predictive value of clinical indices in detecting aspiration in patients with neurological disorders. J Neurol Neurosurg Psychiatry 63(4):456, 1997.

167. Calcagno, P, et al: Dysphagia in multiple sclerosis—prevalence and prognostic factors. Acta Neurol Scand 105(1):40, 2002.

168. Regan, J, Walshe, M, and Tobin, WO: Immediate effects of thermal-tactile stimulation on timing of swallow in idiopathic Parkinson's disease. Dysphagia 25(3):207, 2010.

169. Thomas, FJ, et al: Dysphagia and nutritional status in multiple sclerosis. J Neurol 246(8):677, 1999.

170. Duffy, JR: Motor Speech Disorders: Substrates, Differential Diagnosis, and Management, ed 2. Mosby, St Louis, 2005.

171. Gentry, T: Handheld Computers as Assistive Technology for Individuals with Cognitive Impairment Related to Multiple Sclerosis [e-book]. UMI Dissertation Services, ProQuest Information and Learning, Ann Arbor, MI, 2006. Retrieved May 22, 2012, from www.proquest.com/products_umi/dissertations/.

172. Dennison, L, and Moss-Morris, R: Cognitive-behavioral therapy: What benefits can it offer people with multiple sclerosis? Expert Rev Neurother 10(9):1383, 2010.

173. Motl, R: Physical activity and cognitive function in multiple sclerosis. J Sport Exerc Psychol 33(5):734, 2011.

174. Motl, R, and Snook, E: Physical activity, self-efficacy, and quality of life. Ann Behav Med 35:111, 2008.

175. Shatil, E, et al: Home-based personalized cognitive training in MS patients: A study of adherence and cognitive performance. Neurorehabil 26(2):143, 2010.

176. Irvine, H: Psychosocial adjustment to multiple sclerosis: Exploration of identity redefinition. Disabil Rehabil 31(8):599, 2009.

177. Leino-Kilpi, H, et al: Elements of empowerment and MS patients. J Neurosci Nurs 30:116, 1998.

178. Malcomson, KS, Dunwoody, L, and Lowe-Strong, AS: Psychosocial interventions in people with multiple sclerosis—a review. J Neurol 254:1, 2007.

179. Plow, M, Mathiowetz, V, and Resnik, L: Multiple sclerosis: Impact of physical activity on psychosocial constructs. Am J Health Behav 32(6):614, 2008.

180. Hertz, D, and Holland, N: Community Resources for Your Patients with MS (Resource Bulletin, Information for Health Professionals). National Multiple Sclerosis Society, New York, 2004.

181. Bello-Hass, V, Bene, M, and Mitsumoto, H: End of life: Challenges and strategies for the rehabilitation professional. Neurology Report (now JNPT) 26(4):174, 2002.

182. Irvine, H, et al: Psychosocial adjustment to multiple sclerosis: exploration of identity redefinition. Disabil Rehabil 31(8):599, 2009.

183. Bogosian, A, Moss-Morris, R, and Hadwin, J: Psychosocial adjustment in children and adolescents with a parent with multiple sclerosis: A systematic review. Clin Rehabil 24(9):789, 2010.

Supplemental Readings

Blackstone, M: First Year—Multiple Sclerosis: An Essential Guide for the Newly Diagnosed, ed 2. Marlow & Co., New York, 2007.

Compston, A, et al: McAlpine's Multiple Sclerosis, ed 4. Churchill Livingstone/Elsevier, St Louis, 2005.

Coyle, PK, and Halper, J: Living with Progressive Multiple Sclerosis: Overcoming Challenges, ed 2. Demos Medical Publishers, New York, 2008.

Holland, NJ, Murray, TJ, and Reingold, SC: Multiple Sclerosis: A Guide for the Newly Diagnosed, ed 3. Demos Medical Publishing, New York, 2007.

Kalb, R (ed): Multiple Sclerosis: A Guide for Families, ed 3. Demos Medical Publishing, New York, 2006.

Kesselring, J, Comi, G, and Thompson, A (eds): Multiple Sclerosis: Recovery of Function and Neurorehabilitation. Cambridge University Press, Cambridge, 2010.

Raine, C, McFarland, H, and Hohlfeld, R: Multiple Sclerosis: A Comprehensive Text. Saunders/Elsevier, St Louis, 2008.

Shapiro, R: Managing the Symptoms of Multiple Sclerosis, ed 4. Demos Medical Publishing, New York, 2007.

Weiner, L, and Stankiewicz, J: Multiple Sclerosis: Diagnosis and Therapy. Wiley-Blackwell, West Sussex, UK, 2012.

Fatigue is a feeling of physical tiredness and lack of energy that many people experience from time to time. But people who have medical conditions like MS experience stronger feelings of fatigue more often and with greater impact than others.

Following is a list of statements that describe the effects of fatigue. Please read each statement carefully, then *circle the one number* that best indicates how often fatigue has affected you in this way during the *past 4 weeks*. (If you need help in marking your responses, *tell the interviewer the number* of the best response.) *Please answer every question.* If you are not sure which answer to select, choose the one answer that comes closest to describing you. Ask the interviewer to explain any words or phrases that you do not understand.

Name: _____   Date: _____ / _____ / _____

ID#: _____   Test: 1   2   3   4

Because of my fatigue during the past 4 weeks. . .

	Never	Rarely	Sometimes	Often	Almost always
1. I have been less alert.	0	1	2	3	4
2. I have had difficulty paying attention for long periods of time.	0	1	2	3	4
3. I have been unable to think clearly.	0	1	2	3	4
4. I have been clumsy and uncoordinated.	0	1	2	3	4
5. I have been forgetful.	0	1	2	3	4
6. I have had to pace myself in my physical activities.	0	1	2	3	4
7. I have been less motivated to do anything that requires physical effort.	0	1	2	3	4
8. I have been less motivated to participate in social activities.	0	1	2	3	4
9. I have been limited in my ability to do things away from home.	0	1	2	3	4
10. I have trouble maintaining physical effort for long periods.	0	1	2	3	4
11. I have had difficulty making decisions.	0	1	2	3	4
12. I have been less motivated to do anything that requires thinking.	0	1	2	3	4
13. My muscles have felt weak.	0	1	2	3	4
14. I have been physically uncomfortable.	0	1	2	3	4
15. I have had trouble finishing tasks that require thinking.	0	1	2	3	4
16. I have had difficulty organizing my thoughts when doing things at home or at work.	0	1	2	3	4
17. I have been less able to complete tasks that require physical effort.	0	1	2	3	4
18. My thinking has been slowed down.	0	1	2	3	4

	Never	Rarely	Sometimes	Often	Almost always
19. I have had trouble concentrating.	0	1	2	3	4
20. I have limited my physical activities.	0	1	2	3	4
21. I have needed to rest more often or for longer periods.	0	1	2	3	4

Instructions for Scoring the MFIS

Items on the MFIS can be aggregated into three sub-scales (physical, cognitive, and psychosocial), as well as into a total MFIS score. All items are scaled so that higher scores indicate a greater impact of fatigue on a person's activities.

Physical Subscale

This scale can range from 0 to 36. It is computed by adding raw scores on the following items: 4 + 6 + 7 + 10 + 13 + 14 + 17 + 20 + 21.

Cognitive Subscale

This scale can range from 0 to 40. It is computed by adding raw scores on the following items: 1 + 2 + 3 + 5 + 11 + 12 + 15 + 16 + 18 + 19.

Psychosocial Subscale

This scale can range from 0 to 8. It is computed by adding raw scores on the following items: 8 + 9.

Total MFIS Score

The total MFIS score can range from 0 to 84. It is computed by adding scores on the physical, cognitive, and psychosocial subscales.

From Multiple Sclerosis Council for Clinical Practice Guidelines,[140] with permission.

An Expanded Disability Status Scale (EDSS) for Patients with Multiple Sclerosis

■ FUNCTIONAL SYSTEMS

Pyramidal Functions

0. Normal.
1. Abnormal signs without disability.
2. Minimal disability.
3. Mild or moderate paraparesis or hemiparesis; severe monoparesis.
4. Marked paraparesis or hemiparesis; moderate quadriparesis; or monoplegia.
5. Paraplegia, hemiplegia, or marked quadriparesis.
6. Quadriplegia.
V. Unknown.

Cerebellar Functions

0. Normal.
1. Abnormal signs without disability.
2. Mild ataxia.
3. Moderate truncal or limb ataxia.
4. Severe ataxia, all limbs.
5. Unable to perform coordinated movements due to ataxia.
V. Unknown.
X. Is used throughout after each number when weakness (grade 3 or more on pyramidal) interferes with testing.

Brainstem Functions

0. Normal.
1. Signs only.
2. Moderate nystagmus or other mild disability.
3. Severe nystagmus, marked extraocular weakness, or moderate disability of other cranial nerves.
4. Marked dysarthria or other marked disability.
5. Inability to swallow or speak.
V. Unknown.

Sensory Functions (revised 1982)

0. Normal.
1. Vibration or figure-writing decrease only, in one or two limbs.
2. Mild decrease in touch or pain or position sense, and/or moderate decrease in vibration in one or two limbs; or vibratory decrease alone in three or four limbs.
3. Moderate decrease in touch or pain or position sense, and/or essentially lost vibration in one or two limbs; or mild decrease in touch or pain and/or moderate decrease in all proprioceptive tests in three or four limbs.
4. Marked decrease in touch or pain or loss of proprioception, alone or combined, in one or two limbs; or moderate decrease in touch or pain and/or severe proprioceptive decrease in more than two limbs.
5. Loss (essentially) of sensation in one or two limbs; or moderate decrease in touch or pain and/or loss of proprioception for most of the body below the head.
6. Sensation essentially lost below the head.
V. Unknown.

Bowel and Bladder Functions (revised 1982)

0. Normal.
1. Mild urinary hesitancy, urgency, or retention.
2. Moderate hesitancy, urgency, retention of bowel or bladder, or rare urinary incontinence.
3. Frequent urinary incontinence.
4. In need of almost constant catheterization.
5. Loss of bladder function.
6. Loss of bowel and bladder function.
V. Unknown.

Visual (or Optic) Functions

0. Normal.
1. Scotoma with visual acuity (corrected) better than 20/30.
2. Worse eye with scotoma with maximal visual acuity (corrected) of 20/30 to 20/59.
3. Worse eye with large scotoma, or moderate decrease in fields, but with maximal visual acuity (corrected) of 20/60 to 20/99.
4. Worse eye with marked decrease of fields and maximal visual acuity (corrected) of 20/100 to 20/200; grade 3 plus maximal acuity of better eye of 20/60 or less.
5. Worse eye with maximal visual acuity (corrected) less than 20/200; grade 4 plus maximal acuity of better eye of 20/60 or less.
6. Grade 5 plus maximal visual acuity of better eye of 20/60 or less.
V. Unknown.
X. Is added to grades 0 to 6 for presence of temporal pallor.

Cerebral (or Mental) Functions

0. Normal.
1. Mood alteration only (does not affect DSS score).
2. Mild decrease in mentation.
3. Moderate decrease in mentation.
4. Marked decrease in mentation; chronic brain syndrome: moderate.
5. Dementia or chronic brain syndrome: severe or incompetent.
V. Unknown.

Other Functions

0. None.
1. Any other neurological findings attributed to MS (specify).
V. Unknown.

■ EXPANDED DISABILITY STATUS SCALE (EDSS)

0 = Normal neurological examination (all grade 0 in functional systems [FS]; cerebral grade 1 acceptable).

1.0 = No disability, minimal signs in one FS (i.e., grade 1 excluding cerebral grade 1).

1.5 = No disability, minimal signs in more than one FS (more than one grade 1 excluding cerebral grade 1).

2.0 = Minimal disability in one FS (one FS grade 2, others 0 or 1).

2.5 = Minimal disability in two FS (two FS grade 2, others 0 or 1).

3.0 = Moderate disability in one FS (one FS grade 3, others 0 or 1), or mild disability in three or four FS (three/four FS grade 2, others 0 or 1) though fully ambulatory.

3.5 = Fully ambulatory but with moderate disability in one FS (one grade 3) and one or two FS grade 2; or two FS grade 3; or five FS grade 2 (others 0 or 1).

4.0 = Fully ambulatory without aid, self-sufficient, up and about some 12 hours a day despite relatively severe disability consisting of one FS grade 4 (others 0 or 1), or combinations of lesser grades exceeding limits of previous steps. Able to walk without aid or rest some 500 meters.

4.5 = Fully ambulatory without aid, up and about much of the day, able to work a full day, may otherwise have some limitation of full activity or require minimal assistance; characterized by relatively severe disability, usually consisting of one FS grade 4 (others 0 or 1) or combinations of lesser grades exceeding limits of previous steps. Able to walk without aid or rest for some 300 meters.

5.0 = Ambulatory without aid or rest for about 200 meters; disability severe enough to impair full daily activities (e.g., to work full day without special provisions). (Usual FS equivalents are one grade 5 alone, others 0 or 1; or combinations of lesser grades usually exceeding specifications for step 4.0.)

5.5 = Ambulatory without aid or rest for about 100 meters; disability severe enough to preclude full daily activities. (Usual FS equivalents are one grade 5 alone, others 0 or 1; or combinations of lesser grades usually exceeding those for step 4.0.)

6.0 = Intermittent or unilateral constant assistance (cane, crutch, or brace) required to walk about 100 meters with or without resting. (Usual FS equivalents are combinations with more than two FS grade 3+.)

6.5 = Constant bilateral assistance (canes, crutches, or braces) required to walk about 20 meters without resting. (Usual FS equivalents are combinations with more than two FS grade 3+.)

7.0 = Unable to walk beyond about 5 meters even with aid, essentially restricted to wheelchair; wheels self in standard-wheelchair and transfers alone; up and about in wheelchair some 12 hours a day. (Usual FS equivalents are combinations with more than one FS grade 4+; very rarely, pyramidal grade 5 alone.)

7.5 = Unable to take more than a few steps; restricted to wheelchair; may need aid in transfer, wheels self but cannot carry on in standard wheelchair a full day; may require motorized wheelchair. (Usual FS equivalents are combinations with more than one FS grade 4+.)

8.0 = Essentially restricted to bed or chair or ambulated in wheelchair, but may be out of bed itself much of the day; retains many self-care functions; generally has effective uses of arms. (Usual FS equivalents are combinations, generally grade 4+ in several systems.)

8.5 = Essentially restricted to bed much of the day; has some effective use of arm(s); retains some self-care functions. (Usual FS equivalents are combinations, generally 4+ in several systems.)

9.0 = Helpless bed patient; can communicate and eat. (Usual FS equivalents are combinations, mostly grade 4+.)

9.5 = Totally helpless bed patient; unable to communicate effectively or eat/swallow. (Usual FS equivalents are combinations, almost all grade 4+.)

10.0 = Death due to MS.

From Kurtzke,[93] with permission.

Multiple Sclerosis Daily Activity Diary

■ INSTRUCTIONS

1. At the top of the day's diary, describe how you slept the night before.

2. Assign a number value from **1 to 10** (1 being very low and 10 being very high) for:
- Your level of fatigue (**F**)
- The value or importance of the activity you are doing (**V**)
- The satisfaction you feel with your performance of the activity (**S**)

You can compute the "value" of an activity by comparing it to other activities you would like to do during the course of the day.

For example:

1 PM: F = 7   V = 3   S = 2 Activity: Fixing lunch standing 15 minutes (hot);

Comment: Blurred vision

3. Always describe the physical work done in the **Activity** section (e.g., stood to shower 10 minutes, went up 20 stairs, walked 200 feet).

4. Note the **external temperature** of the environment under Activity.

5. List under **Comment** all MS symptoms as they appear or worsen during the day, including cognitive problems, visual problems, weakness, dizziness, dragging foot, pain, numbness, burning, and so forth.

6. Make notes **every hour.**

Name: _____ Date: _____

Describe sleep last night: _____

Time	F	V	S	Activity	Comment
6:00 AM					
7:00					
8:00					
9:00					
10:00					
11:00					
12:00 PM					
1:00					
2:00					
3:00					
4:00					
5:00					
6:00					
7:00					
8:00					
9:00					
10:00					
11:00					

Web-Based Resources for Clinicians and Patients/Families Living with Multiple Sclerosis

National Multiple Sclerosis Society	www.nationalmssociety.org
Americans with Disabilities Act: ADA home page	www.usdoj.gov/crt/ada
Medicare information	http://cms.hhs.gov
Social Security Online	www.ssa.gov
National Institute of Neurological Disorders and Stroke	www.ninds.nih.gov
National Library of Medicine	www.nim.nih.gov
Archives of Neurology	http://archneur.ama-assn.org
Neurology	www.neurology.org
CenterWatch Clinical Trials Listing Service	www.centerwatch.com
Veterans Affairs MS Centers of Excellence	www.va.gov/ms
CLAMS: Computer Literate Advocates for Multiple Sclerosis	www.clams.org
Consortium of Multiple Sclerosis Centers	www.mscare.org
The Heuga Center—MS Can Do program	www.heuga.org
Multiple Sclerosis International Federation	www.msif.org
Amgen—drug manufacturer of Novantrone	www.amgen.com
	www.novantrone.com
Biogen—drug manufacturer of Avonex	www.msactivesource.com
	www.biogen.com
	www.avonex.com
Berlex—drug manufacturer of Betaseron	www.berlex.com
	www.betaseron.com
Teva Neurosciences—drug manufacturer of Copaxone	www.tevaneuroscience.com
	www.mswatch.com
Serono Group—drug manufacturer of Rebif	www.serono.com
	www.rebif.com
MSWorld	www.msworld.org/communications.htm
The Myelin Project—MS research	www.myelin.org
Rocky Mountain MS Center	www.mscenter.org
National Family Caregivers Association (NFCA)	www.nfcacares.org
Well Spouse Foundation	www.wellspouse.org
American Academy of Neurology (ANA)	www.aan.com (ANA members, professionals)
	www.aan.com/public (public education)
National Rehabilitation Information Center (NARIC)	www.naric.com
Paralyzed Veterans of America (PVA)	www.pva.org
Ability Hub—assistive technology	www.abilityhub.com
ABLEDATA—assistive technology	www.abledata.com
Disabled Online	www.disabledonline.com
Apple Computer Accessibility	www.apple.com/accessibility
IBM Accessibility	www.306.ibm.com/able
Microsoft Accessibility Technology for Everyone	www.microsoft.com/enable

Amyotrophic Lateral Sclerosis

Vanina Dal Bello-Haas, PT, PhD

Chapter 17

LEARNING OBJECTIVES

1. Describe the epidemiology, risk factors, etiology, pathogenesis, diagnosis, and general prognosis of amyotrophic lateral sclerosis (ALS).
2. Compare and contrast the El Escorial diagnostic criteria for ALS.
3. Differentiate among impairments related to lower motor neuron pathology, upper motor neuron pathology, and bulbar impairments.
4. Discuss the medical and health care management of individuals with ALS.
5. Outline a framework for rehabilitation for individuals with ALS.
6. Describe the components of the physical therapy examination for individuals with ALS.
7. Describe the role of the physical therapist in the management of an individual with ALS and the factors that influence intervention options.
8. Compare and contrast overwork damage and disuse atrophy as it relates to ALS.
9. Summarize the literature related to exercise and ALS.
10. Describe considerations that must be taken into account when designing an exercise program for the individual with ALS.
11. Discuss problems commonly seen in individuals with ALS and the physical therapy interventions for these common problems.
12. Determine the anticipated goals and expected outcomes for an individual with ALS based on physical therapist examination findings.
13. Design an intervention program for the individual with ALS based on the physical therapist examination findings.

CHAPTER OUTLINE

Motor neuron diseases (MND) include a heterogeneous spectrum of inherited and sporadic (no family history) clinical disorders of the upper motor neurons (UMNs), lower motor neurons (LMNs), or a combination of both[1] (Table 17.1). **Amyotrophic lateral sclerosis** (ALS),* commonly known as Lou Gehrig's disease, is the most common and devastatingly fatal MND among adults. ALS is characterized by the degeneration and loss of motor neurons in the spinal cord, brainstem, and brain, resulting in a variety of UMN and LMN clinical signs and symptoms.[2]

■ EPIDEMIOLOGY

It is estimated that 30,000 individuals in the United States have ALS at any one time and 15 cases are diagnosed every day. Except in a very few high-incidence areas, such as Guam and the Kii Peninsula of Japan (geographical foci, Western Pacific form of ALS), the overall incidence of ALS has been reported to be in the range of 0.4 to 2.4 cases per 100,000, with the incidence increasing with each decade of life, until at least the seventh decade. The prevalence of ALS has been reported to be 4 to 10 cases per 100,000.[3-7]

Although ALS can occur at any age, the average age at onset is the mid-to-late 50s.[4,5,7,8] Most studies have found that the disease affects men slightly more than women, with an approximate ratio of 1.7:1;[3,5,6] however, after age 65, this gender-related incidence is less pronounced.[3] In about 5% to 10% of individuals the disease is inherited as an autosomal dominant trait (*familial ALS [FALS]*),[3,9,10] although rare cases of juvenile-onset ALS are inherited in an autosomal recessive pattern.[11] Of the hereditary adult ALS cases,

approximately 20% are a result of one of more than 100 mutations in superoxide dismutase 1 (SOD1),[12,13] a gene that encodes the copper-zinc superoxide dismutase enzyme. The very large majority of adult individuals with ALS have no family history of the disease (*sporadic ALS*), although a very small percentage of individuals with sporadic ALS do have a mutation in *SOD1*.[14,15]

Approximately 70% to 80% of individuals develop *limb-onset ALS*, with initial involvement in the extremities; 20% to 30% develop *bulbar-onset ALS*, with initial involvement in the bulbar muscles.[6,16,17] Bulbar-onset ALS is more common in middle-aged women, and initial symptoms may include difficulty speaking, chewing, or swallowing.[2,6]

■ ETIOLOGY

Epidemiologic evidence has identified several known and possible risk factors for ALS (Fig. 17.1). However, other than the small percentage of hereditary (FALS) cases, etiology for the most part is unknown. It is thought that no one single mechanism but rather multiple or cumulative mechanisms, including oxidative stress, exogenous neurotoxicity, excitotoxicity, impaired axonal transportation, protein aggregation, **apoptosis** (programmed cell death), and lifestyle factors, may be responsible for neuron degeneration in ALS:[13]

1. *Superoxide dismutases* are a group of enzymes that eliminate oxygen free radicals that, although products of normal cell metabolism, have been implicated in neurodegeneration. There are three isoforms of SOD in humans: *cytosolic copper-zinc superoxide dismutase (CuZnSOD), mitochondrial manganese superoxide dismutase (MnSOD),* and *extracellular superoxide dismutase (ECSOD).* SOD1, a gene on chromosome 21, encodes CuZnSOD. Genetic studies of individuals with adult-onset FALS have determined that about 20% of these individuals have mutations in SOD1; however, the primary gene defect is unknown. When the SOD enzyme activity is decreased, as has been observed in individuals with FALS with SOD1 mutations, free radicals may accumulate causing damage.[13,18,19] Most mutations identified in FALS show modest loss in enzyme activity,[20] suggesting the mutant SOD-1 protein may have toxic properties that cause motor neurons to die. However, the mechanism has yet to be determined.[13]

2. *Glutamate,* an excitatory neurotransmitter, has also been implicated in neurodegeneration. Excess glutamate triggers a cascade of events leading to cell death.[13] Increased levels of glutamate in the cerebrospinal fluid (CSF), plasma, and in postmortem tissue of individuals with ALS have been reported.[21,22] A deficiency in excitatory amino acid transporters 2 (EAAT2), a specific glutamate transporter protein, in the motor cortex and spinal cord of postmortem ALS tissue was reported and lends support to the theory of excitotoxicity causing neurodegeneration.[23,24]

Table 17.1	Motor Neuron Disorders
Subtype	Nervous System Pathology
Amyotrophic lateral sclerosis	Degeneration of the corticospinal tracts, neurons in the motor cortex and brainstem, and anterior horn cells in the spinal cord
Primary lateral sclerosis	Degeneration of upper motor neurons
Progressive bulbar palsy	Degeneration of motor neurons of cranial nerves IX to XII
Progressive muscular atrophy	Loss or chromatolysis of motor neurons of the spinal cord and brainstem

Adapted in part from Rowland.[1]

---

*The term MND is used to describe the disease in the United Kingdom, whereas the term ALS is used in North America and Europe. In Europe, ALS is also called Charcot's disease.

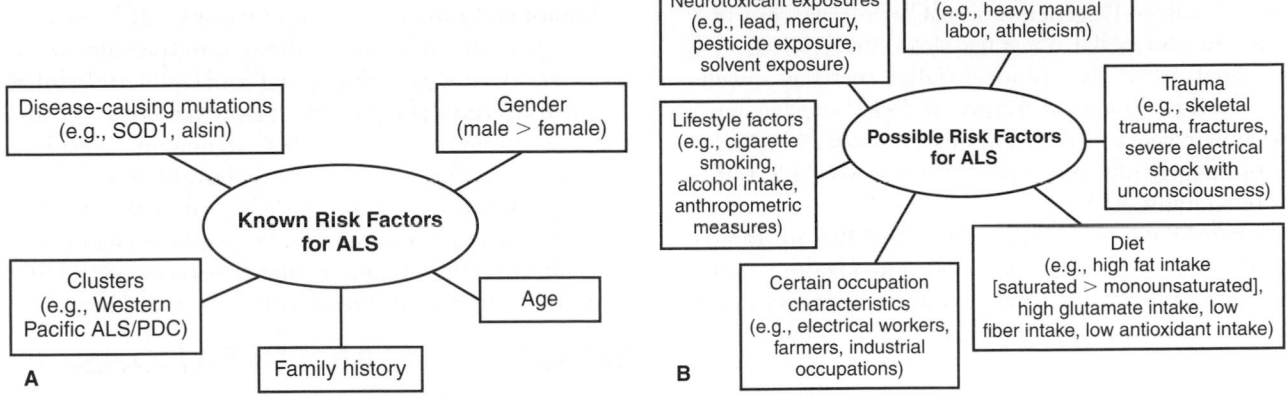

Figure 17.1 **(A)** Known risk factors for ALS. **(B)** Possible risk factors for ALS. ALS/PDC = amyotrophic lateral sclerosis and parkinsonism dementia complex.

3. Clumping of neurofilament proteins into spheroids in the cell body and proximal axon is one of the histopathological characteristics of ALS.[13,25,26] Whether or not abnormal accumulation is secondary to the pathology or contributes to motor neuron degeneration has yet to be determined.[13]

4. Several studies have implicated an autoimmune reaction in the etiology of ALS.[7,27-29] For example, serum factors toxic to anterior horn motor neurons in individuals with ALS have been reported,[27] and antibodies to calcium channels have been identified in individuals with ALS.[29]

5. It has been hypothesized that a lack of neurotrophic factors could contribute to the development of ALS and other neurodegenerative disorders.[30] In vivo experiments and experiments with isolated motor neurons in cell culture have shown that neurotrophic factors are important in motor neuron survival.[31,32] However, factor deficits in ALS have not been conclusive. For example, a postmortem study found decreased amounts of ciliary neurotrophic factor (CNTF) in the ventral horn of the spinal cord, but not in the motor cortex; nerve growth factors were decreased in the motor cortex, but increased in the lateral column of the spinal cord.[33]

6. Other potential theories thought to contribute to neurodegeneration in ALS, which have anecdotal, limited, or indirect evidence, include exogenous or environmental factors,[34] apoptosis,[35] and viral infections.[36]

■ PATHOPHYSIOLOGY

Amyotrophic lateral sclerosis is characterized by a progressive degeneration and loss of motor neurons in the spinal cord, brainstem, and motor cortex (Fig. 17.2). UMNs in the cortex are affected, as are the corticospinal tracts. Brainstem nuclei for cranial nerves V (trigeminal), VII (facial), IX (glossopharyngeal), X (vagus), and XII (hypoglossal) and anterior horn cells in the spinal cord are also involved.[2] Brainstem nuclei for cranial nerves controlling external ocular muscles (III: oculomotor,

IV: trochlear, and VI: abducens) are usually spared; if degeneration occurs, it does so late in the course of the disease.[37] Motor neurons of the *Onufrowicz nucleus (Onuf's nucleus),* located in the ventral margin of the anterior horn in the second sacral spinal level, are also generally spared; if they are affected, it is to a very limited extent.[38,39] These neurons control striated muscles in the pelvic floor, including anal and external urethral sphincters.[40]

The sensory system and spinocerebellar tracts are also generally spared in ALS. Some studies suggest that sensory neurons may be involved in ALS, but to a much lesser extent than the motor neurons. Morphological studies have found that peripheral sensory nerves exhibit axonal atrophy, demyelination, and degeneration.[41,42]

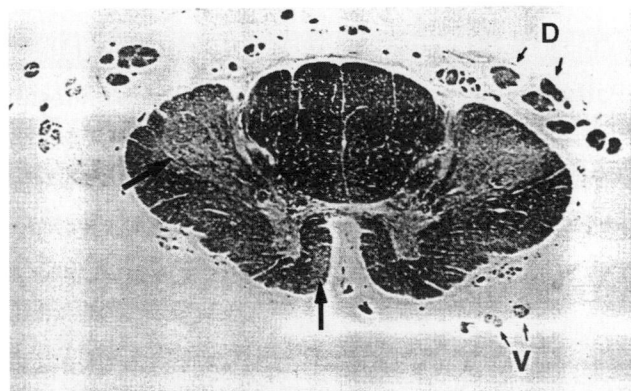

Figure 17.2 Luxol Fast B stained cross section of spinal cord at the high cervical level from a patient with classical ALS. Marked pallor, secondary to degeneration of the lateral and anterior corticospinal tracts, can be seen (large arrows). The ventral roots (V, small arrows) are atrophied, especially compared to the dorsal roots (D, small arrows). *(From King, PH, and Mitsumoto, H: Neuropathology of amyotrophic lateral sclerosis. In Belsh, JM, and Schiffman, PL [eds]: Amyotrophic Lateral Sclerosis: Diagnosis and Management for the Clinician. Blackwell Publishing, Oxford, UK, 1996, p 205, with permission.)*

and dorsal root ganglia cells at autopsy reveal loss of large ganglion cells.[43] Degeneration of Clarke's neurons and of the spinocerebellar tracts has also been reported.[44-46] Degeneration of the spinocerebellar tracts is a well-recognized pathological feature of FALS and has been described in sporadic ALS, although it is rare.[44] Posterior column degeneration is more common in FALS, but is rare in sporadic ALS.[47]

As motor neurons degenerate, they can no longer control the muscle fibers they innervate. Healthy, intact surrounding axons can sprout and reinnervate the partially denervated muscle[48] (Fig. 17.3), in essence assuming the role of the degenerated motor neuron and preserving strength and function early in the disease; however, the surviving motor units undergo enlargement.[49,50] Reinnervation can compensate for the progressive degeneration until motor unit loss is about 50%,[49,50] and electromyography (EMG) studies have found evidence of motor unit reinnervation in individuals with ALS.[51,52] As the disease progresses, reinnervation cannot compensate for the rate of degeneration,[51] and a variety of impairments develop (Table 17.2).

The progression of ALS is thought to spread in a *contiguous* manner, e.g., within spinal cord segments (cervical segments to cervical segments), before developing rostral or caudal symptoms.[17,53] Thus, signs and symptoms spread locally within a region (e.g., bulbar, cervical, thoracic, lumbosacral) before moving to other regions. Caudal-to-rostral spread within the spinal cord and spread from the cervical to bulbar region appears to occur faster than rostral-to-caudal spread within the spinal cord.[17,53]

■ CLINICAL MANIFESTATIONS

Clinical manifestations of ALS vary depending on the localization and extent of motor neuron loss, the degree and combination of LMN and UMN loss, pattern of onset and progression, body region(s) affected, and stage of the disease. At onset, signs or symptoms are usually asymmetrical and focal.[2] Progression of the disease leads to increasing numbers and severity of impairments.

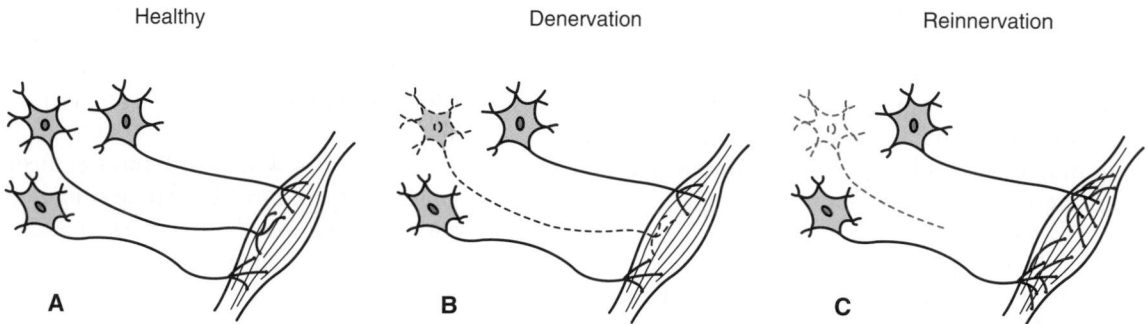

Figure 17.3 Sprouting: **(A)** normal motor neurons; **(B)** denervation; **(C)** reinnervation.

Table 17.2	Common Impairments Associated with Amyotrophic Lateral Sclerosis
Pathology/System Affected	**Clinical Manifestations/Impairments**
LMN pathology	Muscle weakness, hyporeflexia, hypotonicity, atrophy, muscle cramps, fasciculations
UMN pathology	Spasticity, pathological reflexes, hyperreflexia, muscle weakness
Bulbar	Bulbar muscle weakness, dysphagia, dysarthria, sialorrhea, pseudobulbar affect
Respiratory	Respiratory muscle weakness (inspiratory and expiratory), dyspnea, exertional dyspnea, nocturnal respiratory difficulty, orthopnea, hypoventilation, secretion retention, ineffective cough
ALS-FTD, ALSci, ALSbi	Frontotemporal dementia–related impairments (e.g., loss of insight, emotional blunting), cognitive impairments (e.g., attention deficits, deficits in cognitive flexibility), behavioral impairments (e.g., irritability, social disinhibition)
Other	*Rare impairments:* sensory impairments, bowel and bladder dysfunction, ocular palsy *Indirect and composite impairments:* Fatigue, weight loss, cachexia, decreased range of motion, tendon shortening, joint contracture, joint subluxation, adhesive capsulitis, pain, balance and postural control impairments, gait disturbances, deconditioning, depression, anxiety

Adapted in part from Swash.[2]

ALS = amyotrophic lateral sclerosis; ALSbi = ALS with behavioral impairment; ALSci = ALS with cognitive impairment;
　ALS-FTD = ALS with frontotemporal dementia; LMN = lower motor neuron; UMN = upper motor neuron.

Impairments Related to LMN Pathology

The most frequent presenting impairment, occurring in the majority of patients, is focal, asymmetrical muscle weakness beginning in the lower extremity (LE) or upper extremity (UE), or weakness of the bulbar muscles.[3,7] Muscle weakness is considered the cardinal sign of ALS and may be caused by LMN or UMN loss. The weakness associated with LMN loss causes more significant dysfunction than the weakness from UMN loss.[54] Initial muscle weakness usually occurs in isolated muscles, most often distally, and is followed by progressive weakness and activity limitations.[2,54] For example, at onset an individual may notice difficulty with fine motor movements, such as buttoning, pinching, or writing, or may notice foot "slapping" or increased frequency of tripping while walking. Individuals with bulbar onset may notice changes in their voice, difficulty moving the tongue, or decreased ability to move the lips or open or close the mouth.

In people with ALS, cervical extensor weakness is typical.[2,54] Individuals may initially notice neck stiffness, feel "heavy-headed" after reading or writing, or may have difficulties stabilizing the head with unanticipated movements, such as in an accelerating car. As weakness progresses, the head may begin to fall forward, and in more advanced stages the neck becomes completely flexed with the head dropped forward, causing cervical pain and impairments in ambulation and feeding (Fig. 17.4).

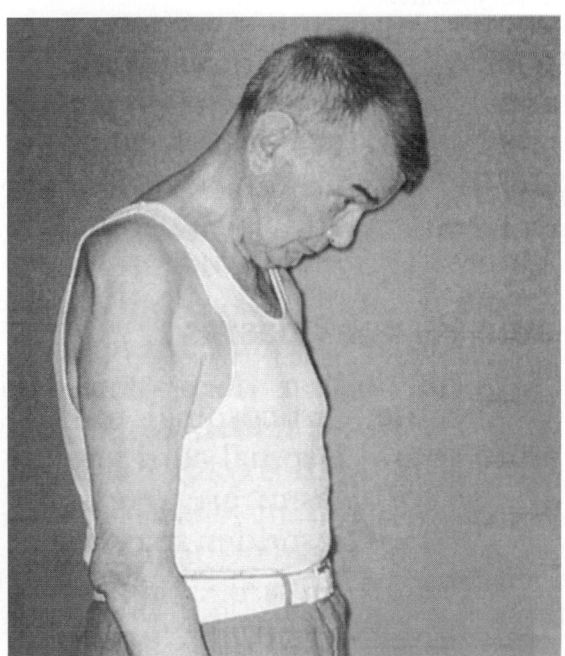

Figure 17.4 Marked head droop in a 65-year-old man with ALS who first developed progressive weakness in both upper extremities. *(From Mitsumoto, H, Chad, DA, and Pioro, EK: Clinical features: Signs and symptoms. In Mitsumoto, H, Chad, DA, and Pioro, EK (eds): Amyotrophic Lateral Sclerosis. F.A. Davis, Philadelphia, 1998, p 47, with permission.)*

Muscle weakness leads to secondary impairments, including decreased range of motion (ROM), predisposing the patient to joint subluxation (e.g., shoulder), tendon shortening (e.g., Achilles), joint contractures (commonly claw-hand deformity), and adhesive capsulitis. Weakness also results in ambulation difficulties, deconditioning, and impaired postural control and balance. Foot drop, secondary to distal weakness, and instability, secondary to proximal weakness, are common. The pattern and progression of LE weakness are characterized by greater losses of muscle force in distal muscles compared to proximal muscles.[55,56] A retrospective study found that decreases in walking ability from independent walking, to walking in the community with assistance, to walking only at home, to being unable to walk were precipitated by relatively small changes in muscle force.[56] Falls are also common, reported to occur in 46% of individuals with ALS.[57]

Several factors affect fatigue levels in patients with ALS. As motor neurons die, the remaining neurons or sprouted neurons are overburdened. Weak muscles must work at a higher percentage of their maximal strength to perform the same activity. This hastens muscle fatigue.[58] Fatigue may also be related to sleep disturbances, respiratory impairments, hypoxia, and depression. Sanjak et al[59] demonstrated that individuals with ALS have abnormal physiological and metabolic responses to single bouts of exercise. Sharma et al[60] found that in individuals with ALS, tetanic and maximal voluntary force during sustained contraction were decreased compared to controls. No impairment was found in the muscular membrane or neuromuscular transmission, suggesting that muscle fatigue in ALS, in part, is due to impaired contraction activation.[60]

As muscle fibers progressively denervate, their volume decreases resulting in atrophy. *Fasciculations*, random spontaneous twitching of muscle fibers often seen through the skin, are common in individuals with ALS, although they are rarely an initial symptom. The etiology of fasciculations remains unclear and is thought to be related to hyperexcitability of motor axons.[54]

Other LMN signs include hyporeflexia, decreased or absent reflexes, decreased muscle tone or flaccidity, and muscle cramping.[2,54] The etiology of muscle cramping is not well understood and is also thought to be related to hyperexcitability of motor axons. In individuals with ALS, muscle cramps can occur in uncommon sites such as the tongue, jaw, neck, or abdomen, as well as in the UEs, hands, and calf or thigh.[2]

Sensory pathways are spared for the most part in people with ALS; however, some patients may complain of ill-defined paresthesia or pain in the limbs. Pain can occur, especially when muscle weakness and spasticity lead to immobility, adhesive capsulitis, or contractures. Cramps and spasticity are other sources of pain, as is increased pressure on the skin, bones, and joints owing to immobility.[2,54]

Impairments Related to UMN Pathology

UMN loss is characterized by spasticity, hyperflexia, clonus, and pathological reflexes, such as a Babinski or Hoffmann sign, and may also cause muscle weakness. As the disease progresses, UMN signs may decrease.[2,54]

Spasticity can eventually lead to contractures and deformities, as well as cause dyssynergic movement patterns, abnormal timing, loss of dexterity, and fatigue, all of which affect motor control and function.[61,62] For example, difficulties with the swing phase of gait secondary to distal spasticity and decreased balance owing to generalized spasticity are often seen in individuals with ALS.

Impairments Related to Bulbar Pathology

As bulbar UMNs and LMNs degenerate, *spastic bulbar palsy* or *flaccid bulbar palsy* (respectively) develops. In individuals with ALS a mixed palsy, which includes both flaccid and spastic components, is common.[54]

Dysarthria, impaired speech, can occur with either spastic or flaccid palsy, owing to weakness of the tongue and muscles of the lip, jaw, larynx, and pharynx. Initial symptoms include the inability to project the voice (e.g., shouting, singing) and problems with enunciation. With spastic dysarthria, the voice sounds forced, as more effort is needed to move air through the upper airway; whereas in flaccid dysarthria, the voice sounds hoarse or breathy. With pharyngeal weakness, air in the mouth leaks into the nose during enunciation, resulting in a nasal tone. As the disease progresses, speech becomes more difficult and unintelligible, and eventually the individual becomes **anarthric**.[2,54]

Dysphagia, impaired chewing or swallowing, can also occur with either spastic or flaccid palsy. Manipulating food inside the mouth or moving food into the esophagus is difficult, and swallowing is impaired. With flaccid bulbar palsy, liquids may regurgitate into the nose because of pharyngeal weakness and the cough reflex may be weak or absent, greatly increasing the risk of aspiration. Individuals with spastic bulbar palsy will have uncoordinated closure of the epiglottis, which may allow liquids or solids to pass to the larynx.[2,54] Choking and slowed eating pattern are associated with dysphagia, placing the patient at risk for less than optimal fluid and caloric intake that results in weight loss and potentially cachexia.[54]

Individuals with ALS frequently experience **sialorrhea**, excessive saliva and drooling, because of an absence of automatic, spontaneous swallowing to clear excessive saliva, or because the lower facial muscles are too weak to close the lips tightly to prevent leakage.[54] Individuals with bulbar onset will experience this symptom relatively early. Initially, the individual may begin to notice drooling at night (e.g., the pillow is wet in the morning); this eventually leads to needing to use a tissue repeatedly to wipe away the saliva.

Pseudobulbar affect is a term used to describe poor or pathological emotional control.[63] Spontaneous crying or laughter occurs in the absence of emotional triggers or emotional responses are exaggerated and not related to the context.[63] This symptom is commonly seen in individuals with spastic bulbar palsy,[2,54] and can occur in as many as 50% of individuals.[64]

Respiratory Impairments

Respiratory impairments in people with ALS are related to loss of respiratory muscle strength and a decrease in vital capacity (VC). A VC reduced to 50% of predicted is often associated with respiratory symptoms.[65] Early signs and symptoms of respiratory muscle weakness may include fatigue, dyspnea on exertion, difficulty sleeping in supine, frequent awakening at night, recurrent sighing, excessive daytime sleepiness, and morning headaches due to hypoxia.[66,67] Patients experiencing a gradual increase in respiratory muscle weakness will not complain of respiratory symptoms because they tend to decrease their overall level of physical activity owing to muscle weakness in the extremities.[68] Although the decline of respiratory muscle strength differs among individuals, for the most part it tends to progress at a linear rate.[69] As weakness progresses, truncated speech, orthopnea, dyspnea at rest, paradoxical breathing, accessory muscle use, and a weak cough are typically evident. A VC of less than 25% to 30% of predicted indicates significant risk of impending respiratory failure or death.[65] If an individual does not receive ventilatory support, eventual CO_2 retention will lead to acidosis, coma, and respiratory failure.[68]

Cognitive Impairments

Although once considered rare outside the western Pacific region, cognitive impairments ranging from mild deficits[70] to severe *frontotemporal dementia (FTD)*[71] are now considered part of the ALS disease spectrum.[72] A large prospective study found that 35.6% of patients with ALS showed clinically significant cognitive impairment.[73] ALS-associated FTD has been characterized by cognitive decline; executive functioning impairments; difficulties with planning, organization, and concept abstraction; and personality and behavior changes.[71,74-76] Individuals with ALS, without FTD, have been reported to have a variety of cognitive impairments, including difficulties with verbal fluency, language comprehension, memory, abstract reasoning, and generalized impairments in intellectual function.[73,76-78] Studies have found that patients with bulbar-onset ALS are more likely to have cognitive impairments than patients with limb-onset disease.[76,77]

Rare Impairments

Sensory pathways are spared, for the most part, in people with ALS. Some individuals may complain of vague, ill-defined sensory symptoms of paresthesia or focal pain in the limbs.[54] External ocular muscles are usually spared in people with ALS; if degeneration occurs, it does so late in the course of the disease.[37] Patients who have been maintained on ventilators for long periods of time may develop the inability to voluntarily close the eyes or *ophthalmoplegia,* complete ocular paralysis.[37]

Motor neurons controlling the anal and vesicourethral sphincter muscles and muscles of the pelvic floor are generally spared. Urinary symptoms, such as urgency, obstructive micturition, or both, have been reported, suggesting that supranuclear control over sympathetic, parasympathetic, and somatic neurons may be abnormal in ALS.[54]

■ DIAGNOSIS

With the exception of one genetic test, no definitive diagnostic test or diagnostic biological marker exists for ALS. For individuals with a clinical presentation of ALS, laboratory studies, EMG, nerve conduction velocity (NCV) studies, muscle and nerve biopsies, and neuroimaging studies are used to support the diagnosis of ALS and to exclude other diagnoses.

The diagnosis of ALS requires the *presence* of (1) LMN signs by clinical, electrophysiological, or neuropathological examination; (2) UMN signs by clinical examination; and (3) progression of the disease within a region or to other regions by clinical examination or via the medical history. The *absence* of (1) electrophysiological and pathological evidence of other diseases that may explain the UMN and LMN signs; and (2) neuroimaging evidence of other disease processes that may explain the observed clinical and electrophysiological signs are also evaluated.[79]

Because of the variability in clinical findings in the early stages of ALS and the lack of absolute biological diagnostic markers, the *World Federation of Neurology Research Group on Motor Neuron Diseases* established the *El Escorial criteria* in 1994, and these were revised in 1998.[79] These widely accepted criteria are considered standard for the diagnosis of ALS for clinical practice, therapeutic trials, and other research purposes. In the absence of pathological evidence, the diagnosis of ALS is classified into *clinically definite, clinically probable, clinically probable with laboratory support,* and *clinically possible* categories (Fig. 17.5).[79] A diagnosis of *clinically definite ALS* is defined as both UMN and LMN findings in at least three of four regions (bulbar, cervical, thoracic, or lumbosacral) or UMN and LMN signs in the bulbar region and at least two spinal regions. *Clinically probable* ALS is defined as UMN and LMN signs in two regions, with at least one UMN finding rostral to the LMN findings. *Clinically probable, laboratory-supported* ALS is defined as UMN and LMN clinical signs in one region only, or UMN signs alone present in one region and LMN signs defined by EMG criteria present in at least two regions. The EMG criteria include signs of active denervation, such as fibrillation potentials and positive sharp waves; and signs of chronic denervation, such as large motor unit potentials (increased duration, increased proportion of polyphasic potentials, increased amplitude) and unstable motor unit potentials. *Clinically*

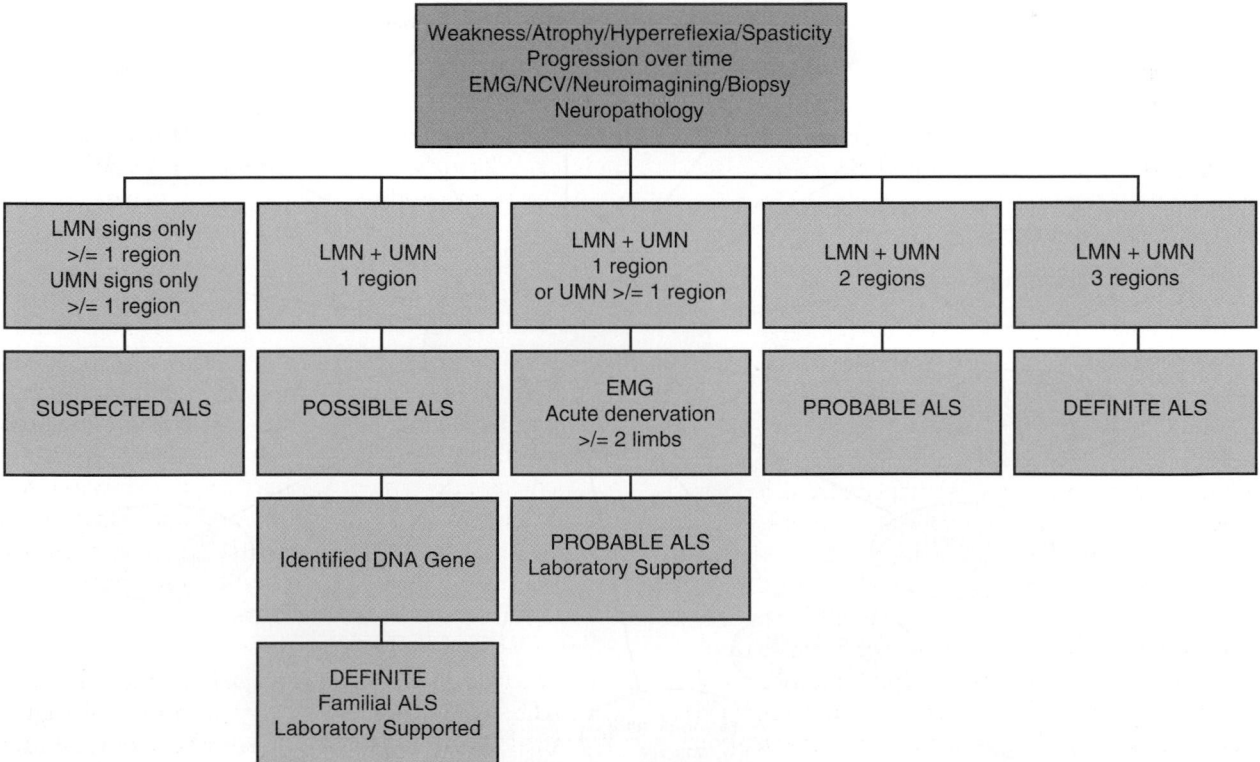

Figure 17.5 El Escorial Criteria for the Diagnosis of ALS. *(Note: The Suspected ALS category was removed when the El Escorial criteria were revised.)*

possible ALS is defined as UMN and LMN signs found together in only one region, or UMN signs found alone in two or more regions, or LMN signs found rostral to UMN signs and the inability to establish a diagnosis of clinically probable, laboratory-supported ALS.[79]

■ DISEASE COURSE

ALS has a progressive and deteriorating disease trajectory, and the progression from pathology to impairments to activity limitations to participation restrictions is inevitable. Although the disease course varies among individuals, with time from onset to death ranging from several months to 20 years, studies have found the average duration of ALS to be between 27 and 43 months, and the median duration to be between 23 and 52 months.[3,5,7,80,81] Five-year and ten-year survival rates range from 9% to 40% and 8% to 16%, respectively.[7,80,82,83] A 50% survival probability after the first symptom of ALS appears is slightly greater than 3 years, unless mechanical ventilation is used to sustain breathing.[6] In most patients, death occurs within 3 to 5 years after diagnosis and usually results from respiratory failure.[5]

■ PROGNOSIS

Age at time of onset has the strongest relationship to prognosis. Studies have found that patients less than 35 to 40 years of age at onset had better 5-year survival rates than older individuals.[5,6,81,84,85] Individuals with limb-onset ALS have a better prognosis than those with bulbar-onset ALS; 5-year survival rates were reported to be 37% and 44%, compared to survival rates of 9% and 16% for patients with bulbar-onset ALS.[84,85] Less severe involvement at the time of diagnosis, a longer interval between onset and diagnosis, and no symptoms of dyspnea at onset are other factors associated with a better prognosis.[5,6,86]

A study of 144 individuals with ALS found that those individuals with psychological well-being had significantly longer survival times compared to those with psychological distress. Mortality rates were found to be 6.8 times greater in those experiencing psychological distress, and the relationship was independent of age, disease severity, and length of time from diagnosis.[87] These findings were confirmed in a later study that found degree of physical disability, disease progression, and survival could be predicted by the patient's psychological status.[88]

■ MANAGEMENT

Patients with ALS may receive care in a variety of health care settings. Care via specialized centers or clinics that provide a comprehensive and multidisciplinary approach is considered the most advantageous owing to the progressive nature of the disease and continually changing patient status (Fig. 17.6). A study comparing a cohort of patients attending a multidisciplinary clinic versus

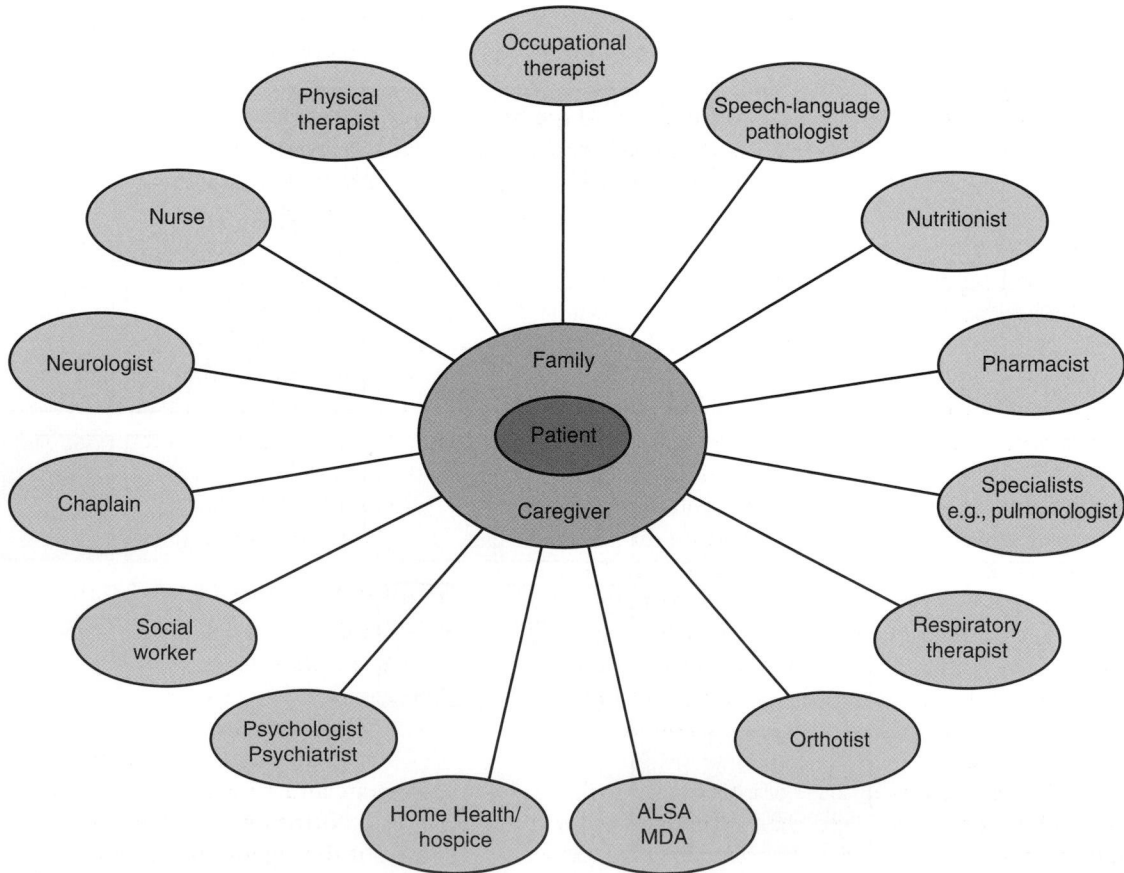

Figure 17.6 Multidisciplinary approach to the care of the individual with ALS. ALSA = Amyotrophic Lateral Sclerosis Foundation; MDA = Muscular Dystrophy Association.

those attending a general neurology practice found the median survival of the ALS clinic cohort was 7.5 months longer than for patients in the general neurology cohort. The findings indicated that attendance at the ALS clinic was an independent covariate of survival, suggesting that active and aggressive management enhances survival.[89]

The *Amyotrophic Lateral Sclerosis Association (ALSA)* and the *Muscular Dystrophy Association (MDA)*, nonprofit voluntary health agencies, have developed standards for ALS clinics and centers. Clinics and centers that meet ALSA's standards and pass a rigorous application and site visit are certified as ALSA Centers. MDA centers that conduct ALS research and have staff with expertise in dealing with ALS earn special designations as MDA ALS Research and Clinical Centers.

Disease-Modifying Agents

Currently, there is no cure for ALS, although a number of clinical drug trials are ongoing. In 1995, the Food and Drug Administration approved riluzole (Rilutek), a glutamate inhibitor, for the treatment of ALS. The standard dose of riluzole is one 50 mg tablet two times a day, and side effects include liver toxicity (which requires discontinuation), asthenia, nausea, vomiting, and dizziness. Evidence suggests the effects of riluzole to be modest, extending survival for 2 to 3 months.[90,91]

Symptomatic Management

Disease-modifying agents currently available are not curative and may extend survival for a very short time. Because the pathological process cannot be reversed and is progressive in nature, the context of medical management for individuals with ALS may be considered palliative. As defined by the World Health Organization, palliative care is "an approach that improves the quality of life of patients and their families facing the problem associated with life-threatening illness, through the prevention and relief of suffering by means of early identification and impeccable assessment and treatment of pain and other problems, physical, psychosocial and spiritual."[92, p. 1]

Although there is no cure for ALS, it is still considered a "treatable disease" and rehabilitation plays an integral role in the overall comprehensive care of the patient. Medical management is symptomatic and individualized and involves supportive care to address impairments as they arise. Medical management may include the prescription of anti-cramping and antispasticity agents, drying agents for sialorrhea, and antidepressants; recommendations and referrals for *percutaneous endoscopic gastrostomy* tubes and ventilatory support (noninvasive ventilation, tracheostomy); and discussion of advanced care directives.[2,54,93]

In 1999 a multidisciplinary task force was established to develop consensus-based recommendations for the management of people with ALS and these recommendations were recently updated.[94,95] Research and clinical evidence related to the care of individuals with ALS in several keys areas were examined: (1) informing the patient and family about the diagnosis and prognosis; (2) management of communication problems, insomnia, anxiety, depression, spasticity, fatigue, cramps, *sialorrhea, and pseudobulbar affect;* (3) nutrition management and percutaneous endoscopic gastrostomy (PEG) decisions; (4) management of respiratory insufficiency and ventilation decisions; (5) diagnosis and management of cognitive and behavioral impairments; (6) drug therapies; and (7) multidisciplinary management and palliative care. Clinical decision making algorithms (practice parameters) for the management of nutrition and respiratory signs and symptoms are presented in Figures 17.7 and 17.8. Full guidelines for other recommendations and information regarding definitions of the levels of recommendations and classifications of evidence can be found at the *American Academy of Neurology* website (www.aan.com).

Management of Sialorrhea and Pseudobulbar Affect

Management of *sialorrhea* in people with ALS and other diseases is often directed toward prescription of anticholinergic medications that decrease saliva production. Examples include glycopyrrolate (Robinul), benztropine (Cogentin), transdermal hyoscine (scopolamine), atropine, and trihexyphenidyl hydrochloride (Artane).[93] For patients with associated thick mucus production, beta-blockers such as propranolol (Inderal) or metoprolol (Toprol) are often prescribed. Botulinum type injections into the parotid and submandibular glands and low-dose radiation have been found to be effective for individuals with ALS with medically refractory sialorrhea.[96] Use of mechanical suction to remove oropharyngeal secretions and nonpharmacological treatments that are used for clearing respiratory secretions (see section below titled Management of Respiratory Impairments) may also be useful.

For patients with pseudobulbar affect, tricyclic antidepressants, such as amitriptyline (Elavil), or selective serotonin reuptake inhibitors (SSRIs), such as fluvoxamine (Luvox), are often prescribed.[93] Research has found that a fixed-dose combination of dextromethorphan/quinidine reduced the severity and frequency of crying and laughing behaviors. However, side effects, including somnolence, dizziness, and nausea, were common.[96]

Management of Dysphagia

Early, mild **dysphagia** is addressed by a nutritionist or registered dietitian together with a speech-language pathologist (SLP). Speech-language pathologists conduct swallowing examinations such as video fluoroscopy to determine the degree and nature of the swallowing impairment and to assist in formulating a plan of care (POC). Nutritionists provide counseling and diet management throughout the course of the disease.

Nutrition status has been identified as a prognostic factor for survival and disease complications.[96] A study of 1,600 hospitalized patients with ALS found the most

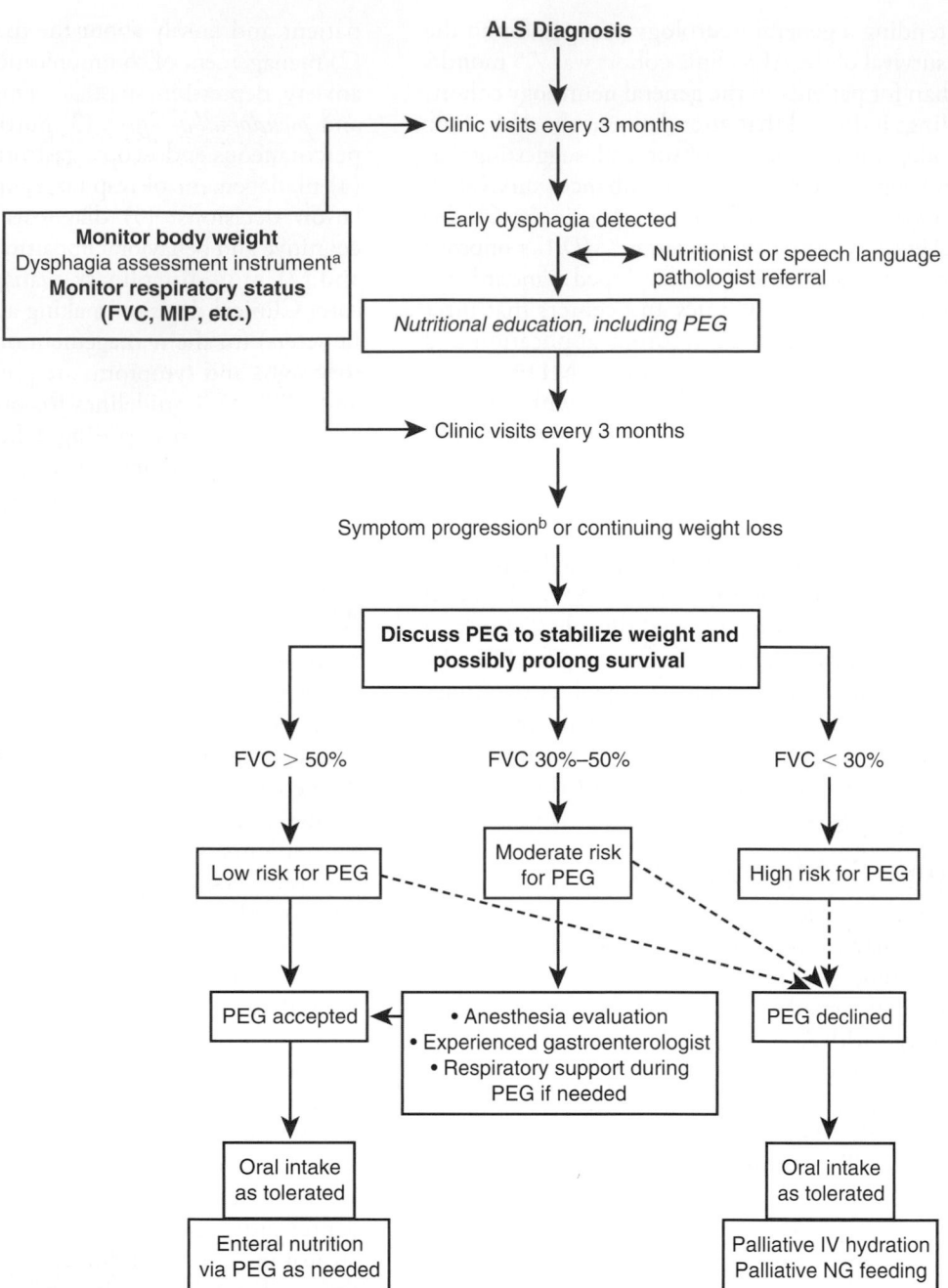

Figure 17.7 Algorithm for nutrition management. Note that **bolded text represents evidence-based information;** *text in italics denotes consensus-based information.*[a]
For example, Questions #1 to 3 (bulbar questions) from the Amyotrophic Lateral Sclerosis Functional Rating Scale—Revised (ALSFRS-R), or other instrument.[b]
For example, prolonged mealtime, ending meal prematurely because of fatigue, accelerated weight loss due to poor caloric intake, family concern about feeding difficulties.
FVC = forced vital capacity (supine or erect); IV = intravenous; MIP = maximum inspiratory pressure; NG = nasogastric; PEG = percutaneous endoscopic gastrostomy. *(From Miller, RG, et al (ALS Practice Parameters Task Force): The care of the patient with amyotrophic lateral sclerosis (an evidence-based review). Report of the quality Standards Subcommittee of the American Academy of Neurology. Neurology 52(7):1311, 1999, p 1316, with permission.)*

common concurrent diagnosis was dehydration and malnutrition, present in 36% of patients.[97] Regardless of whether poor nutritional status results from dysphagia, hypermetabolism, or inability to eat due to UE muscle weakness, research findings emphasize the need for careful attention to nutritional and hydration status, in particular with individuals with impaired oral intake or arm or hand weakness limiting self-feeding.

Initial treatment of dysphagia is directed toward (1) dietary modifications, such as adapting foods and

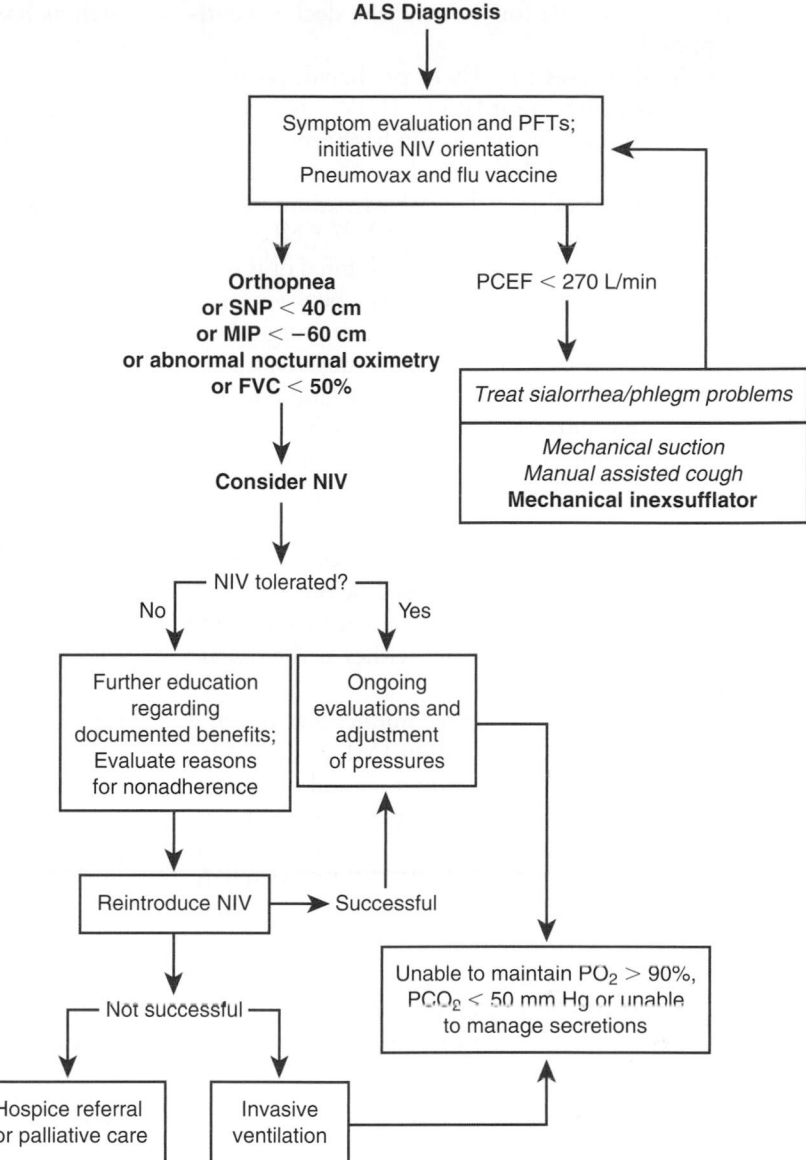

Figure 17.8 Algorithm for respiratory management. Note that **bolded text represents evidence-based information;** *text in italics denotes consensus-based information.* FVC = forced vital capacity (supine or erect); MIP = maximal inspiratory pressure; NIV = noninvasive ventilation; PCEF = peak cough expiratory flow; PFT = pulmonary function tests; SNP = sniff nasal pressure. *(From Miller, RG, et al (ALS Practice Parameters Task Force): The care of the patient with amyotrophic lateral sclerosis (an evidence-based review). Report of the quality Standards Subcommittee of the American Academy of Neurology. Neurology 52(7):1311, 1999, p 1317, with permission.)*

fluid consistencies for easier and safer swallowing; (2) patient education regarding dietary strategies for maximizing calories and nutrients and maintaining adequate hydration; and (3) adaptations to promote swallowing such as tucking the chin down during swallowing or performing a clearing cough after each swallow.[98]

As dysphagia progresses, the time required to consume a meal gradually increases owing to fatigue, increased difficulty chewing, and frequent choking. It is not uncommon for these eating difficulties to cause an accelerated weight loss. In these circumstances a PEG may be recommended. A PEG is a type of gastrostomy tube inserted via endoscopic surgery that creates a permanent opening into the stomach for the introduction of food. A PEG is useful for stabilizing body weight/mass.[94] Although there is no firm evidence, for optimal safety and efficacy the PEG procedure should be offered to the patient and completed before the individual's VC falls below 50% of predicted at the time of

the procedure.[99] Studies have found that PEG insertion may prolong survival. Patients with PEG were found to live 1 to 4 months longer than those individuals who refused PEG or were deemed ineligible for the procedure. Survival was greatest for patients with a VC greater than 50% predicted at the time of the procedure.[100,101] It is important for physical therapists to be aware that a PEG does not prevent the risk of aspiration.[102,103]

Management of Respiratory Impairments

Respiratory impairments place the patient at risk for respiratory tract infections. Important management considerations include (1) pneumococcal and yearly influenza vaccinations;[68] (2) prevention of aspiration; and (3) effective oral and pulmonary secretion management. Supplemental oxygen must be used with caution because it can suppress respiratory drive, exacerbate hypoventilation, and ultimately lead to hypercarbia and respiratory arrest. Typically, supplemental oxygen is recommended only for individuals with concomitant pulmonary disease or as a comfort measure for patients who decline ventilatory support.[68]

When VC decreases to 50% of predicted, positive-pressure noninvasive ventilation (NIV) is recommended.[68,99] Noninvasive ventilation has been shown to decrease symptoms of hypoventilation and increase survival time by several months.[104-107] In addition, improvement in cognition has been noted after NIV initiation.[89] When NIV can no longer be tolerated or it is no longer effective, a decision must be made between invasion ventilation (IV) with tracheostomy via surgical intervention or hospice care to address late-stage respiratory symptoms. Owing to the emotional, social, and financial burden of IV, patients and families must be carefully informed of the multiple costs and benefits of the intervention. No controlled studies of specific strategies for ventilation withdrawal have been published, although case studies provide practical advice.[94] Conditions for withdrawal of ventilation are discussed before, or at the time of, instituting IV because the patient may become unable to communicate his or her wishes as the disease progresses.[68,99]

Manually assisted coughing techniques and use of a mechanical insufflation–exsufflation (MI-E) device are used to facilitate clearance of respiratory and oral secretions[94] (Fig. 17.9). The MI-E device is designed to inflate the lung with positive pressure and assist cough with negative pressure through the flip of a switch. A positive-pressure breath of 30 to 50 cm H_2O over a 1- to 3-second period via an oral–nasal mask or tracheal airway is provided. The airway pressure is then reversed abruptly to –30 to –50 cm H_2O and maintained for 2 to 3 seconds. A peak expiratory "cough" flow within normal range is achieved, thereby assisting with the clearance of secretions.[108]

Management of Dysarthria

Dysarthria impairments are managed primarily by a speech-language pathologist. Initial speech changes are usually managed with intelligibility strategies,

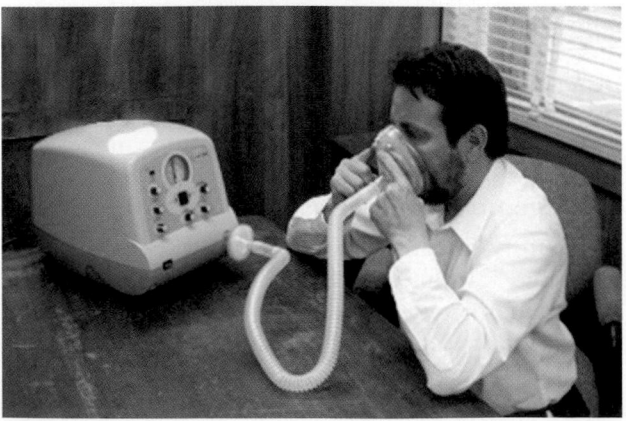

Figure 17.9 Mechanical insufflation-exsufflation (MI-E) device. *(Courtesy of JH Emerson Co., Cambridge, MA 02140.)*

such as having the individual exaggerate articulation or decrease the rate of speech; and environmental modifications, such as decreasing background noise. As the severity of dysarthria progresses, management will focus on decreasing the patient's dependence on speech as the primary method of communication. Interventions first include "low-tech" devices, such as using a writing board or pad and pen for patients with adequate hand function or using an alphabet board. A progression is then made to more "high-tech" devices, such as computers with voice synthesizers or single-switch, scanning computerized communication systems.[109,110]

A *palatal lift prosthesis* may be prescribed for individuals with good articulation but who have a breathy voice quality or decreased loudness because of excessive air loss through the nose. The device, a dental appliance designed to attach to the existing teeth and to elevate the soft palate, is custom-made by a prosthodontist. It allows the soft palate to close around the surrounding structures such as the pharynx, making verbal communication more understandable by reducing or eliminating hypernasal speech. The device also lowers the hard palate, which reduces tongue movement allowing speech to be less fatiguing.[110] Findings from a retrospective study of 25 patients with ALS treated with a palatal lift indicated 21 patients showed improvement in their dysarthria, specifically in reduction of hypernasality, with 19 patients benefiting at least moderately for 6 months.[111]

Management of Muscle Cramps, Spasticity, Fasciculations, and Pain

Anticonvulsant medication such as phenytoin (Dilantin) and carbamazepine (Atretol, Tegretol) may be prescribed for muscle cramps, if they are not relieved with a program of muscle stretching and adequate hydration and nutrition. Both of these medications can cause gastrointestinal upset and rash, and carbamazepine can cause sedation. Benzodiazepines, such as diazepam (Valium), clonazepam (Klonopin), or lorazepam (Ativan), can also be prescribed for muscle cramps, and side effects may include sedation, dizziness, respiratory depression, and increased weakness. Benzodiazepines, especially diazepam, may be prescribed for spasticity, although baclofen (Lioresal) and tizanidine (Zanaflex) are more commonly used. Side effects include weakness, fatigue, sedation, and hypotension.[54,111]

Patients with brisk, widespread fasciculations are generally instructed to avoid or minimize caffeine and nicotine. Lorazepam (Ativan) may be prescribed to decrease the intensity of the fasciculations.[54] Depending on the etiology of pain, a variety of management strategies may be utilized. Mild pain or pain associated with joint discomfort is usually addressed with analgesics, such as acetaminophen or nonsteroidal anti-inflammatory drugs (NSAIDs). For more severe refractory pain, narcotics such as codeine, hydrocodone, or methadone may be prescribed. In the terminal stages of ALS, morphine may be administered to provide analgesia, sedation, and relief from respiratory distress.[54,111]

Management of Anxiety and Depression

Anxiety and depression can greatly affect a patient's and his or her family's quality of life, as well as the ability to cope with and adapt to the progressive changes and losses of the disease. Thus, pharmacotherapy and psychological counseling are important management strategies for addressing the anxiety and depression that can develop. Individuals with depression may be prescribed an SSRI, such as fluoxetine (Prozac) or sertraline (Zoloft). It is important to note that antidepressant effects may not occur for several weeks after initiation of the medications, and side effects may include agitation and insomnia. If the patient presents with depression and insomnia or agitation, a tricyclic antidepressant, such as amitriptyline (Elavil) or imipramine (Tofranil), is preferred.[54,93]

Benzodiazepines, such as chlordiazepoxide (Librium), clorazepate, diazepam, and flurazepam (Dalmane), may be prescribed for anxiety or for patients with depression and insomnia. For patients whose respiratory status is affected, a non-benzodiazepine anxiolytic, such as buspirone (BuSpar), is preferred.[54,93,111]

■ FRAMEWORK FOR REHABILITATION

As previously described, the course of ALS cannot be altered and eventually the individual will become dependent in essentially all aspects of mobility and self-care. However, appropriate rehabilitation programs should be designed and implemented to allow the individual to maintain his or her independence and function for as long as possible, within the context of his or her goals and resources, throughout the disease and across health care settings. Because of the progressive nature of ALS, it is imperative that the physical therapist not only addresses an individual's current problems, but also plans ahead for future problems.[112,113]

A large body of evidence to help guide physical therapy decision making is currently unavailable. As identified earlier, ALS has a progressive and deteriorating disease trajectory, with inevitable progression to disability. However, there is great variability among individuals across the disease trajectory. Staging ALS into *early, middle* (early-middle and late-middle), and *late* stages based on impairments, activity limitations, and participation restrictions may assist the therapist in designing appropriate and realistic interventions throughout the disease process, as well as anticipate the evolving needs of individual patients[113] (Fig. 17.10).

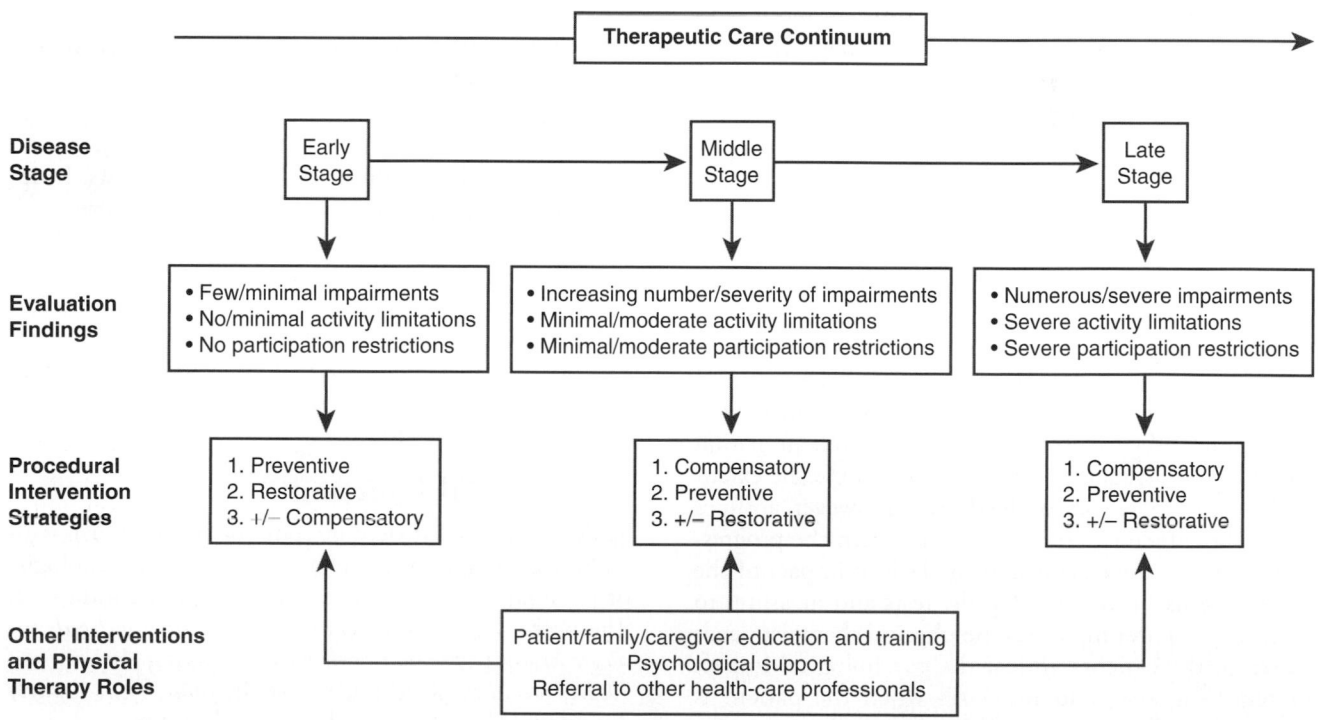

+ denotes may include; – denotes may not include

Figure 17.10 Framework for rehabilitation for individuals with ALS. *(From Dal Bello-Haas, V: A framework for rehabilitation in degenerative diseases: Planning care and maximizing quality of life. Neurology Report (now JNPT) 26(3):115, 2002, p 116, with permission.)*

In the *early* stage of the disease, ALS will manifest as a variety of signs and symptoms recognized by the patient as abnormal. The resultant impairments may or may not cause minor activity limitations and no participation restrictions are present. In the *middle* stage of ALS, the patient experiences increasing signs and symptoms, and develops an increase in the number of impairments and the severity of impairments. Minimal to moderate activity limitations will be noted and participation restrictions will develop. In the *late* stage of ALS, disease progression leads to numerous and increasingly more severe impairments. The patient becomes increasingly more functionally limited owing to lack of voluntary motor control and numerous participation restrictions ensue. The patient becomes dependent in essentially all aspects of mobility and self-care, and may require mechanical ventilation to address respiratory compromise, if not already ventilated.[113]

Within this framework, impairments, activity limitations, and participation restrictions are managed through restorative, compensatory, or preventative physical therapy interventions. These interventions should be tailored to the stage of the disease, keeping in mind individual variability throughout disease course (e.g., presence of cognitive impairments or respiratory signs and symptoms) and disease progression (e.g., slowly progressing versus fast progressing), and grounded in evidence-based research whenever possible. The patient's goals are paramount, and psychosocial factors that may influence the patient's decision making, such as acceptance of the diagnosis, and social and financial resources must be considered.[113]

■ PHYSICAL THERAPY EXAMINATION

At any one time, a variety of body regions can be affected by ALS and in various combinations. Impairments may occur as a direct result of the pathology (*direct impairment*), as sequelae to the pathology (*indirect impairment*), or may be the result of multiple underlying origins (*composite impairments*). Therefore, a careful and comprehensive examination is required to determine the extent of involvement and the impact of involvement on activity limitations and participation restrictions. Reexamination at regular intervals is necessary to determine the extent and rate of progression of the disease. However, at times it may be difficult to differentiate between the progressive course of the disease and the lack of impact of the interventions. In considering the tests and measures to include in a reexamination, the physical therapist needs to weigh the benefits against the psychological impact of repeating tests and measures when the patient is progressively deteriorating. This is especially true in the late-middle and late stage of the disease. It is important for the physical therapist to reexamine, monitor, and evaluate changes, because some medical decision making may be based on the physical therapist's findings, for

example, the patient's percent predicted VC and the timing of PEG placement.

The patient's goals and individual psychosocial factors, rate of disease progression, extent and area of involvement, stage of the disease, and respiratory and bulbar involvement that may affect the patient's ability to participate all need to be taken into account when structuring the initial examination. The types of data generated from the patient history and interview are presented in Chapter 1, Clinical Decision Making. When collecting these data, determining what is important, relevant, and valued by the individual patient is key. By understanding what is most meaningful to a patient, the physical therapist can narrow the gap between a patient's expectations and hopes and actual experiences through realistic and appropriate interventions. For example, a young mother with ALS may inform the physical therapist her priority is caring for her children rather than maintaining employment. Thus, the initial examination would be structured around abilities and activities related to home, rather than work.

Many of the tests and measures described in this text are generally appropriate components of a comprehensive examination for an individual with ALS. However, selection is always based on specific patient need. The tests and measures frequently applicable to patients with ALS include examination of sensory function, muscle performance, motor function, coordination and balance, gait, functional status, the environment, respiratory function, and cognitive function (see Chapters 3, 5, 6, 7, 8, 9, 12, and 27). The following section presents areas that typically warrant emphasis during the examination.

Cognition

No ALS-specific cognitive test or measure exists. If dementia or cognitive impairments are suspected, executive function, language comprehension, memory, and abstract reasoning should be examined. The *Mini-Mental State Examination*[114] has been used in clinical studies, although it may not be sensitive to frontotemporal function impairments. Referral for a neuropsychological evaluation may also be indicated to identify specific cognitive impairments.

Psychosocial Function

As depression and anxiety are common in individuals with ALS, screening is important and referral to a psychologist or psychiatrist for further evaluation may be indicated. The *Beck's Depression Inventory,*[115] the *Center of Epidemiologic Study Depression Scale,*[116] the *Hospital Anxiety and Depression Scale* (HADS),[117] and the *State-Trait Anxiety Inventory*[118] have been used in clinical studies.

Pain

Pain is common in individuals with ALS and should be examined subjectively and objectively, using a *Visual*

Analogue Scale (VAS) for example. Pain is not necessarily a direct impairment of ALS, but rather an indirect (decreased ROM, adhesive capsulitis) or a composite impairment (joint malalignment secondary to spasticity and faulty posture). Further examination of underlying causes of pain is often required.

Joint Integrity, Range of Motion, and Muscle Length

Functional ROM, active, active-assisted, and passive range ROM, muscle length, and soft tissue flexibility and extensibility should be examined using standard methods.

Muscle Performance

Specific deficits of muscle strength, power and endurance, and muscle performance during functional activities should be determined. Specific deficits can be measured with manual muscle testing (MMT), isokinetic muscle strength testing, or handheld dynamometry. In clinical trials, muscle strength has been examined as *maximum voluntary isometric contraction* (MVIC) using a strain gauge tensiometer system.[119] This method eliminates muscle length and velocity as factors in testing and produces reliable, valid, interval data.[119-122] MVIC is considered the most direct technique for investigating motor unit loss, and has been used extensively for examining muscle strength in individuals with ALS for the past 10 years. Its range and sensitivity have been validated by several natural history studies.[5,17,123] However, MVIC testing requires specialized equipment and training in its use.

Test reliability of MMT and MVIC scores among uniformly trained physical therapists at several institutions has been examined. Reproducibility between MMT and MVIC was found to be equivalent. Sensitivity to detect progressive muscle strength changes in individuals with ALS favored MMT. However, 6 muscles were tested with MVIC and 34 muscles were tested with MMT; thus, the difference in detecting change was largely accounted for by the number of muscles sampled by MMT versus MVIC.[124]

Motor Function

Impairments in dexterity, coordination of large movement patterns, as well as gross and fine motor control may be evident owing to spasticity and muscle weakness. Hand function and initiation, modification, and control of movement patterns should be examined.

Tone and Reflexes

Muscle tone may be examined using the *Modified Ashworth Scale*.[125] Deep tendon and pathological reflexes should be tested to distinguish between UMN and LMN involvement.

Cranial Nerve Integrity

The cranial nerves commonly affected by ALS include V, VII, IX, X, and XII. Cranial nerves should be tested to determine the extent of bulbar involvement. Screening for oral motor function, phonation, and speech production can be accomplished through the interview and observation. Referral to a speech-language pathologist is recommended.

Sensation

If the patient complains of sensory symptoms or if sensory involvement is suspected, sensory testing should be completed.

Postural Alignment, Control, and Balance

Static and dynamic postural alignment and body mechanics during self-care, functional mobility skills, functional activities, and work conditions and activities should be examined. Postural stability, reactive control, anticipatory control, and adaptive postural control should also be determined. No ALS-specific balance test or measure exists. A variety of balance status measures, originally designed for use with other patient populations, including the *Tinetti Performance Oriented Mobility Assessment* (POMA),[126] the *Berg Balance Scale*,[127] the *Timed Up and Go Test* (TUG),[128] and the *Functional Reach Test*,[129] can be used. Low total *Tinetti Balance Test* scores, indicating impaired balance, were found to be moderately to strongly related to LE muscle weakness and disability in individuals with ALS.[130,131] Kloos et al[130] suggest that the POMA is a reliable measure for individuals in the early or early-middle stages of ALS. A study of 31 individuals with ALS who underwent monthly TUG, Amyotrophic Lateral Sclerosis Functional Rating Scale—Revised (ALSFRS-R), forced vital capacity (FVC), MMT, and quality-of-life assessments for 6 months found that the TUG was significantly associated with the chance of falling.[132]

Gait

No ALS-specific gait test or measure exists. Documentation of gait within a particular time period (e.g., within 15 seconds) or over a certain distance (e.g., 10 feet [3 meters]) has been measured in clinical trials. Gait stability, safety, and endurance should be examined. Energy expenditure, alignment, fit, practicality, safety, and ease of use of orthotic and assistive devices should also be examined at regular intervals.

Respiratory Function

Determination of respiratory status and function includes examination of respiratory symptoms and muscle function, breathing pattern, chest expansion, respiratory sounds, cough effectiveness, and VC or forced vital capacity (FVC) using a handheld spirometer. Supine FVC may be a better indicator of diaphragm weakness than erect FVC, and maximal inspiratory pressure (MIP) may also be useful in respiratory function monitoring because it can detect early respiratory insufficiency.[94] Sniff nasal pressure (SNP) may be effective in detecting hypercapnia, and peak cough expiratory flow (PCEF) is the most widely used measure of cough effectiveness.[94] Aerobic capacity and cardiovascular–pulmonary endurance may be tested in the early stages of ALS using standardized, modified protocols to evaluate and monitor responses to aerobic conditioning.

Integument

In general, even in the late stage of ALS skin integrity is rarely a problem. Skin inspection should be used to examine contact points between the body and assistive, adaptive, orthotic, protective, and supportive devices, mobility devices, and the sleeping surface. Such inspection is especially important when the patient's mobility becomes increasingly more dependent. If present, swelling should also be examined and monitored. Swelling of the distal limb may develop owing to lack of muscle pumping action in a weakened extremity.

Functional Status

Functional mobility skills, safety, and energy expenditure are important considerations. Basic and instrumental activities of daily living and the need for adaptive equipment should be examined. The *Functional Independence Measure* (FIM)[133] has been used to document functional status in clinical trials.

The *Schwab and England Activities of Daily Living Scale*[134] is an 11-point global measure of functioning that asks the rater to report activities of daily living (ADL) function from 100% (normal) to 0% (vegetative functions only), and has been used to examine function in individuals with ALS (Appendix 17.A). The ALS Ciliary Neurotrophic Factor (CNTF) Treatment Study Group found the scale to have excellent test-retest reliability, to correlate well with qualitative and quantitative changes in function, and to be sensitive to changes over time.[135]

Environmental Barriers

The patient's home and work environments should be examined for current and potential barriers, access, and safety.

Fatigue

Fatigue is very common in individuals with ALS. No ALS-specific measures exist; the *Fatigue Severity Scale*[136] has been used in clinical trials.

■ DISEASE-SPECIFIC AND QUALITY-OF-LIFE MEASURES

Disease-Specific Measures

The *ALS Functional Rating Scale* (ALSFRS)[135] and the revised version, ALSFRS-R[137] (Appendix 17.B) examine the functional status of patients with ALS. The patient is asked to rate his or her function using a scale from 4 (normal function) to 0 (unable to attempt the task). The original scale, the ALSFRS, correlated positively with objective measures of UE and LE strength and was found to be valid and reliable for measuring the decline in function that results from loss of muscular strength.[135] The ALSFRS-R was expanded to include additional respiratory items, and was found to have internal consistency and construct validity, and to have retained the properties of the original scale.[137] Telephone administration of the ALSFRS-R has also been found to be reliable.[138] Other disease-specific scales include the *Appel ALS Scale* (AALS),[139] the *ALS Severity Scale* (ALSSS),[140] and the *Norris Scale*.[141]

Quality-of-Life Measures

Quality of life in individuals with ALS has been examined with generic measures, such as the SF-36,[142] the *Schedule for Evaluation of Individual Quality of Life—Direct Weighting* (SEIQoL-DW),[143] and the *Sickness Impact Profile* (SIP).[144]

The *Amyotrophic Lateral Sclerosis Assessment Questionnaire* (ALSAQ-40),[145] an ALS-specific quality of life measure, contains 40 items that represent five distinct areas of health: mobility (10 items), ADL (10 items), eating and drinking (3 items), communication (7 items), and emotional functioning (10 items). The questions refer to the patient's condition during the past 2 weeks and responses are given on a five-point Likert scale. The ALSAQ-40 measures health status in each domain using a summary score from 0 (best health status) to 100 (worst health status). The validity and reliability of this instrument have been examined and reported.[145,146] The *ALSAQ-40* has been shortened to 11 items and also appears to be valid and reliable.[147]

■ PHYSICAL THERAPY INTERVENTIONS

The role of the physical therapist in management of individuals with ALS and the extent of interventions provided vary depending on whether or not the therapist is working as a member of a team specialized in ALS care or as an independent or clinic-based therapist. Additional variables include the availability of other health care professionals in the practice setting and the reason the individual is seeking physical therapy (e.g., specific ALS-related problem versus a co-morbidity problem such as arthritis).

Restorative intervention is directed toward remediating or improving impairments and activity limitations. In the early and middle stages of ALS, restorative interventions are temporary at best because disease progression is expected and permanent loss of function and disability is likely. Restorative interventions in the late stage of ALS are for the most part directed solely toward remediation of impairments that result from other systems pathology (e.g., pressure sores, edema, pneumonia, atelectasis, adhesive capsulitis).

Compensatory intervention is directed toward modifying activities, tasks, or the environment to minimize activity limitations and participation restrictions. In the early and middle stages of ALS, tasks or activities may be adapted to achieve function. As the disease progresses, increasing environmental adaptations will be necessary to maintain and promote function.[113]

In the early and early-middle stages of ALS, **preventative intervention** is directed toward minimizing potential impairments such as loss of ROM, aerobic capacity, or strength, preventing pneumonia or atelectasis, and activity limitations. Beginning an early prevention program may alter impairments and maintain physical function temporarily, and may also improve well-being and decrease fatigue, as well as the secondary effects of immobility. In the late-middle and late stages, the pathology is more advanced and mobility becomes progressively restricted. In these stages, it may be extremely difficult or impossible to prevent impairments and activity limitations that are directly related to the nervous system pathology. Thus, the role of prevention is *tertiary,* in order to mitigate the effects of the pathology that lead to impairments in other systems (e.g., educating caregivers about a passive ROM exercise program to prevent adhesive capsulitis in the shoulder).[113] In general, the role of the physical therapist includes the following:

- Promoting independence and maximizing function throughout the stages of the disease, through restorative and compensatory interventions that address impairments, activity limitations, and participation restrictions
- Promoting health and wellness in the early and early-middle stages of the disease through restorative and preventative interventions
- Providing alternative means of carrying out functional activities with adaptive equipment and alternate methods for performing tasks and activities through compensatory interventions as the disease progresses
- Minimizing or preventing complications through preventative interventions throughout the course of the disease
- Providing education, psychological support, and recommendations for equipment and community resources to assist in adapting to the disease progression[113]

Owing to the individual variability of the disease onset, disease course, and disease progression, patients with ALS will present with unique and different sets of problems; thus, interventions will vary. As described earlier, interventions are directed mainly toward addressing activity limitations and participation restrictions, because often the impairments causing the limitations and restrictions cannot be altered. However, in the early and early-middle stages of ALS, it may be possible to direct treatment toward the underlying CNS impairments, and perhaps postpone the onset of particular activity limitations. For example, a study of patients in the early stages of ALS (FVC ≥90% predicted and ALSFRS ≥30) who engaged in moderate load, moderate resistance exercises were found to have higher ALSFRS scores and SF-36 Physical Function scores compared to a matched control group who performed stretching exercises.[148] Patients and therapists must understand that any beneficial effects of an early prevention program will be short term and will not have an impact on the overall course of the disease. Much more research into the effectiveness of interventions for individuals with ALS is needed.

In developing a POC, in addition to the patient's goals, the therapist must also consider the rate of disease progression, the extent and area of involvement, stage of the disease, respiratory and bulbar factors that may affect participation, timing of the intervention, patient acceptance and motivation, life support choices, availability of psychosocial support, and resources.

Some patients may view the need to use adaptive equipment, such as an ambulatory assistive device or wheelchair, as a definitive marker for disease progression and impending death. This may cause the patient to be hesitant to accept the recommended aid or device as a means of maintaining some aspect of control over the disease. The physical therapist will be required to maintain a balance between being realistic about what can be achieved and providing a sense of hope, not helplessness, when discussing intervention options. An overview of ALS disease stages and general intervention strategies is presented in Table 17.3. Common impairments and activity limitations associated with ALS and their respective interventions are described below.

Cervical Muscle Weakness

Progressive cervical extensor weakness will cause the head to fall forward, resulting in overstretching of the posterior musculature and soft tissues. This may cause bouts of acute pain or develop into anterior muscle tightness or a chronic cervical syndrome. Some patients will compensate for the forward head position by increasing lordosis, as they attempt to maintain their posture during ambulation.

For mild to moderate cervical weakness, a soft foam collar may be worn during specific activities. Soft collars are comfortable and usually well tolerated. However, wear-induced compressibility requires that they be replaced frequently. For moderate to severe weakness, a semirigid or rigid collar is prescribed. These are usually made of padded rigid plastic or leather and provide very firm support. Patients may find the collars very warm; may experience discomfort at points of body contact, such as the chin, mandible, sternum, or over clavicles; may feel pressure on the trachea; and may feel confined. Several types of collars are presented in Figures 17.11 and 17.12, and the pros and cons of individual collar types are summarized in Table 17.4.

Table 17.3 Amyotrophic Lateral Sclerosis Disease Stages and Common Intervention Strategies: Framework for Rehabilitation for Individuals with ALS

Stage	Common Impairments and Activity Limitations	Interventions
Early	Mild to moderate weakness in specific muscle groups Difficulty with ADL and mobility toward the end of this stage	**Restorative/Preventative** • Strengthening exercises*[147,178,179] • Endurance exercises[180] • Active ROM,[181] active-assisted ROM, stretching exercises **Compensatory** • Determine potential need for adaptive or assistive devices • Determine potential need for ergonomic modifications of home/workplace • Energy conservation • Educate the patient about the disease process, energy conservation, and support groups
Middle	Progressive decrease in mobility throughout stage Wheelchair needed for long distances; increased wheelchair use toward end of stage Severe muscle weakness in some groups; mild to moderate weakness in other groups Progressive decrease in ADL skills throughout stage Pain	**Compensatory** • Support weak muscles (assistive and supportive devices, adaptive equipment, slings, orthoses) • Modifications to workplace/home (e.g., install ramp, move bedroom to first floor) • Wheelchair prescription • Education of caregivers regarding functional training **Preventative** • Active,[181] active-assistive, and passive ROM, stretching exercises • Strengthening exercises[147,178,179] (early middle) • Endurance exercises[180] (early middle) • Determine need for pressure-relieving devices (e.g., pressure distributing mattress)
Late	Wheelchair dependent or restricted to bed Complete dependence with ADL Severe weakness of UE, LE, neck and trunk muscles Dysarthria, dysphagia Respiratory compromise Pain	**Preventative** • Passive ROM • Pulmonary care* • Hospital bed and pressure-relieving devices • Skin care, hygiene* **Compensatory** • Caregiver education regarding transfers, positioning, turning, skin care • Mechanical lift

Adapted from Dal Bello-Haas,[113 p 123] with permission.
*May be restorative.
ADL = activities of daily living; LE = lower extremity; ROM = range of motion; UE = upper extremity.

Some patients with combined cervical and upper thoracic weakness may benefit from a cervical-thoracic orthosis, or a Sternal Occipital Mandibular Immobilizer (SOMI). These devices provide greater support, but are more expensive and heavy and may be difficult to don and doff. For severe or intractable neck weakness, referral to an orthotist for a custom-made device may be necessary.

In addition to wearing collars, individuals with cervical weakness may also benefit from taking frequent rest periods; supportive seating, such as high-back chairs or recliners; tilt-in-space or reclining wheelchairs; elevating reading material; and education about good arm support for prolonged sitting, proper use of head rest when riding in a car, and ergonomic changes for work stations. It is important to note that when trunk weakness accompanies neck weakness, positioning for head support becomes more challenging.

Dysarthria and Dysphagia

In collaboration with the SLP and nutritionist, the physical therapist can play a role in managing dysarthria and dysphagia by addressing the patient's head and trunk control and position in sitting. In addition, the physical therapist can reinforce the use of strategies for eating and swallowing (e.g., chin tuck), the use of prescribed communication devices, and the need for food consistency modifications. Because patients are at

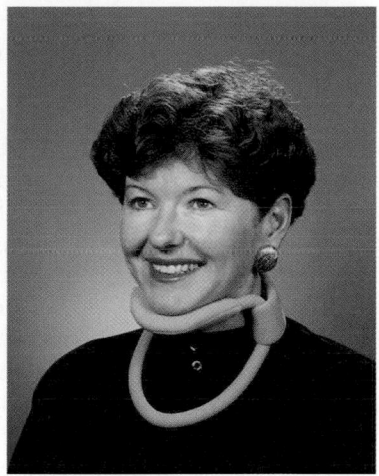

Figure 17.11 The Headmaster Collar. *(Courtesy of Symmetric Designs, Salt Spring Island, BC, Canada, V8K 1C9.)*

risk for aspiration, education of the patient, family, and caregiver is imperative (see section below titled Respiratory Muscle Weakness).

UE Muscle Weakness

Weakness of the UEs greatly affects the patient's ability to carry out ADL. There is a large variety of adaptive equipment available that may help the patient prolong function for as long as possible (see section below titled Activities of Daily Living).

Patients with a painful shoulder due to subluxation may benefit from a sling, similar to those used with patients following stroke with decreased tone, although subluxation cannot be corrected completely. Splinting of the wrist or hand may be indicated to prevent contractures or to improve the patient's function, such as the ability to grasp.

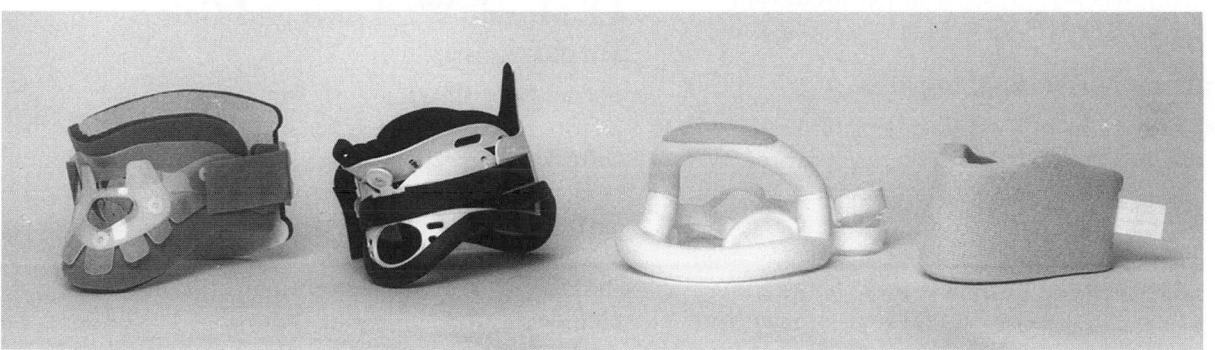

Figure 17.12 Types of collars. From left to right: Aspen Collar, Miami-J Collar, Executive Collar, and Soft Collar.

Table 17.4 Types of Semirigid and Rigid Cervical Collars

Type	Examples	Advantages	Disadvantages
Collars without anterior neck access	Philadelphia® Collar[a]	Offers good support	Patient may feel confined May cause pressure on trachea Patient may experience difficulty breathing or swallowing Can be uncomfortably warm
Collars with anterior neck access (for tracheostomy)	Miami-J® Collar[b] Aspen Collar[c] Malibu Collar[d]	Padding absorbs and wicks moisture away from skin Suitable for individuals with cervical weakness in all 3 planes	Patient may feel confined May be uncomfortably warm More expensive
	Canadian Collar[e] Headmaster Collar[e]	Open design allows for circulation of air Lightweight No pressure on trachea Some patients consider collar more cosmetically appealing	May put pressure on chin and sternum Some models more expensive Some models require custom cutting Not adequate if rotation and lateral flexion weakness is also present

[a]Philadelphia® Cervical Collar Co, Thorofare, NJ 08086.
[b]Jerome Medical, Moorestown, NJ 08057-3239.
[c]Aspen Medical Products Inc., CA, 92618-5202.
[d]Seattle Systems, Poulsbo, WA 98370.
[e]Symmetric Designs Ltd., Salt Spring Island, BC, Canada V8K 1C9.

Shoulder Pain

Individuals with ALS may develop shoulder pain and present with capsular patterns of restriction. Pain may be caused by several factors: abnormal scapulohumeral rhythm secondary to spasticity or weakness causing imbalance that may lead to impingement; overuse of strong muscles; muscle strain; faulty resting position; glenohumeral subluxation secondary to weakness; or a fall. Depending on the cause of the shoulder pain, interventions may include modalities, ROM exercises, passive stretching, joint mobilizations, and education about proper joint support and protection.

A 20% incidence of adhesive capsulitis in individuals with ALS has been found. Recommendations for managing the pain and decreased ROM included a protocol of an intra-articular analgesic and anti-inflammatory cocktail injection, followed by a course of aggressive ROM exercises. Some patients reported an acute resolution of pain, whereas others reported improvements over 2 to 3 weeks.[149]

Respiratory Muscle Weakness

Education is extremely important. Patients and caregivers must be taught how to balance activity and rest and educated about energy conservation techniques. Patients and caregivers should also be educated about signs and symptoms of aspiration; positioning to avoid aspiration, such as upper cervical spine flexion during eating; causes and signs of respiratory infection; and strategies for managing oral secretions (use of oral suction device) or choking episodes (Heimlich maneuver). Specific breathing exercises and positioning to optimize ventilation/perfusion matching may also be incorporated, although their effectiveness in ALS has not been determined. A small sample size double-blind study randomly assigned 9 people with ALS to an inspiratory muscle training (IMT) group. Subjects completed daily IMT training sessions (10 minutes per session) three times per day. After 12 weeks of training, subjects in the IMT group demonstrated trends toward improvement in FVC, VC, MIP, and SNP, compared to a control group who completed sham training (n = 10), and gains in inspiratory muscle strength were partially reversed after an 8-week period of training cessation.[150]

Airway clearance techniques may be necessary when conditions that cause secretion retention, such as pneumonia or atelectasis, arise. To compensate for a weakened cough, the patient and caregiver may be instructed in the use of manually assisted coughing techniques or MI-E. Again, the effectiveness of these techniques or device has not been demonstrated in ALS, but case reports have described the benefits from regular use of a mechanical insufflation device.[151,152] Studies of cough flows and pressures during cough augmentation have found that manual assistance increased flow 11% in those with bulbar ALS and 13% in those with nonbulbar ALS. MI-E increased flow by 26% in those with bulbar ALS and 28% in those with nonbulbar ALS. The greatest improvements were in patients with the weakest coughs.[153]

High-frequency chest wall oscillation (HF-CWO) has garnered some interest in terms of its applicability to the ALS population. HF-CWO is an external noninvasive modality that transmits high-frequency oscillatory pressures through the chest wall, thereby mobilizing secretions from the small peripheral airways and enhancing secretion clearance and gas exchange. HF-CWO has been effectively used in patient populations in which secretion retention and hypersecretion are issues (e.g., cystic fibrosis).[154,155] A study comparing 19 people with ALS who used HF-CWO to 16 who were not treated found that after 6 months, those using the device had significantly less breathlessness. In addition, those users with an FVC between 40% and 70% predicted had significantly less mean decrease in FVC and less breathlessness and fatigue.[156]

LE Muscle Weakness and Gait Impairments

Orthoses may be recommended to improve function by offering support to weakened muscles and the joints they surround, decrease the stress on remaining functioning or compensatory muscles, conserve energy, or minimize local or general muscle fatigue. Controlling knee impairments can often be achieved through an ankle-foot orthosis (AFO); as such, addressing the ankle should be considered first. It is also important to consider the weight of the orthosis as individuals with ALS will have energy expenditure issues, and it may be more fatiguing for the patient to ambulate with a heavy orthosis than to ambulate without the impairment being corrected. For this reason, a knee-ankle-foot orthosis (KAFO) is not recommended.

Deciding between a commercially manufactured versus a custom-made orthosis is certainly dependent on the patient's resources, but the rate of disease progression should also be considered. For an individual with rapidly progressive ALS and who is likely to use the orthosis for a limited time, a commercially manufactured orthosis may suffice. Solid AFOs are a good choice for patients who have medial/lateral instability of the ankle with quadriceps weakness. The fixed ankle position, combined with the quadriceps weakness, may make it difficult for sit-to-stand transfers, climbing stairs, and negotiating inclines. Hinged AFOs allow dorsiflexion and may be appropriate for the patient with adequate knee extensor strength with mild ankle strength loss.

The type of ambulatory assistive device prescribed is dependent on the degree of proximal muscle strength or instability; function of the UEs; the pattern, extent, and rate of disease progression; acceptance by the patient; and financial constraints. Again, weight of the device is an important factor to consider in decision making, while also taking into account which device will ensure optimal function and safety. Wheeled walkers, which do not require the patient to lift the device, are usually recommended. In general, individuals with ALS are rarely prescribed crutches. If crutches are warranted, Loftstrand (Canadian) crutches are preferred.

Activities of Daily Living

A large variety of adaptive equipment is available to assist individuals with muscle weakness perform everyday tasks. However, the benefits and effectiveness of adaptive equipment for people with ALS have not been evaluated systematically. No one type of device is suitable for every patient or for every stage of the disease. Reimbursement for the equipment is variable and although a piece of adaptive equipment can help the patient maintain independence, limited financial resources may prevent recommending or purchasing the item. For example, in the early stages of ALS a universal cuff with a pocket for writing or feeding utensils may be beneficial. As the disease progresses and proximal shoulder weakness increases, a mobile arm support may be incorporated to allow the patient to maintain independence in eating. In the late stage of ALS when the patient is dependent on the caregiver for eating, a long straw and straw holder may be recommended to assist the caregiver with the activity. Examples of adaptive equipment that may be beneficial for performing ADL are presented in Table 17.5.

Decreased Mobility

Patients with LE weakness may have difficulty with sit-to-stand or car transfers. Simple interventions include placing a firm cushion 2 to 3 in (5 to 7.6 cm) thick under the buttocks in the chair or elevating the chair by placing the legs in prefabricated blocks (Fig. 17.13). Self-powered lifting cushions are relatively inexpensive and portable, but the individual needs adequate trunk control and balance in order to use the device safely (Fig. 17.14). Upholstered reclining chairs with powered seat lifts may also be recommended, but are more expensive. All these interventions increase the biomechanical advantage and make it easier for the patient to rise from a sitting position.

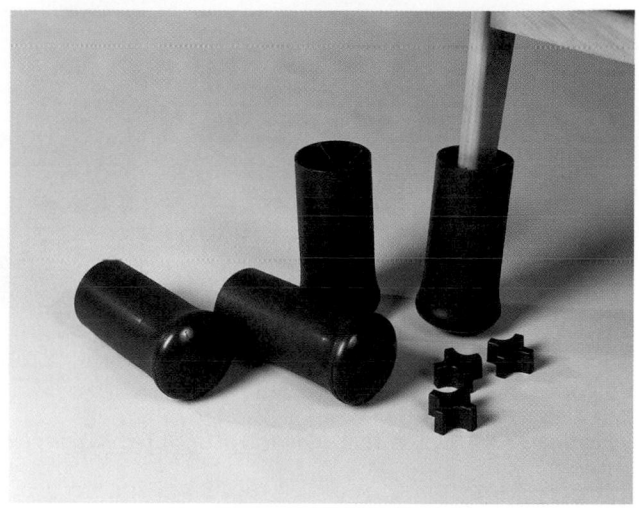

Figure 17.13 Prefabricated blocks. *(Courtesy of Homecraft AbilityOne, Kirkby-in-Ashfield, Nottinghamshire, England NG17 7ET.)*

Caregivers will need to be educated regarding assisting the patient with transitional movements. Transfer boards may be used for transfers once the individual is unable to stand, either alone if the person has adequate arm strength and good sitting balance, or the caregiver can be instructed in how to assist the patient. Other useful devices to assist the patient's mobility are transfer belts and swivel cushions or seats. Transfer belts ease the burden of the transfer for the caregiver and prevent potential pulling on the patient's UEs. Swivel cushions are lightweight, cushioned seats that swivel in both directions and make getting in and out of a car easier (Fig. 17.15).

Once an individual cannot perform transfers, even with the assistance of a caregiver, a hydraulic or mechanical lift is required. Commonly recommended lifts devices include the Easy Pivot™ (Rand-Scot Inc., Fort Collins, CO 80524), and the Hoyer Lift® (Sunrise Medical, Longmont, CO 80503). Use of an electric hospital bed may facilitate bed mobility and transfers both for the patient and caregiver, and, depending on resources,

Table 17.5	Common Types of Adaptive Equipment
Feeding and eating	Foam tubing to increase the size of utensil handles; utensils and cups with modified handles or holders; long-levered jar opener; plate guard; serrated or rocker knife; wrist splint/adapted cuff (for holding tools and instruments); mobile arm support; Dycem®
Self-care and bathing	Bathing benches; bath tub seats; shower commode; handheld shower head; grab bars; raised toilet seat; long handled sponge; electric toothbrush or shaver; strap-fitted hairbrushes
Dressing	Zipper pulls or hooks; button hooks; long-handled shoehorn; Velcro® clothing closures; elastic shoelaces
Writing and reading	Foam tubing to increase the size of the pen or pencil; triangular pencil grip; pen holders; book holders; automatic page turner; adjustable angle table
Other	Key holders; doorknob adapters; lamp extension switch; personal alarm system; switch-operated environmental controls; speaker phone with automatic dialing; telephone holder; use of telecommunication devices for the deaf (TDD)

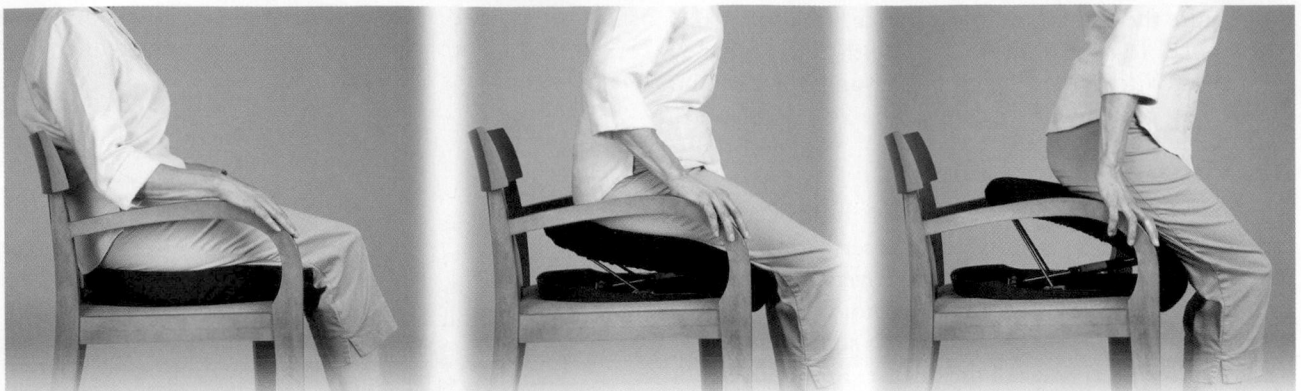

Figure 17.14 UpLift Seat. *(Courtesy of Uplift Technologies Inc., Dartmouth, NS, Canada, B3B 1M2.)*

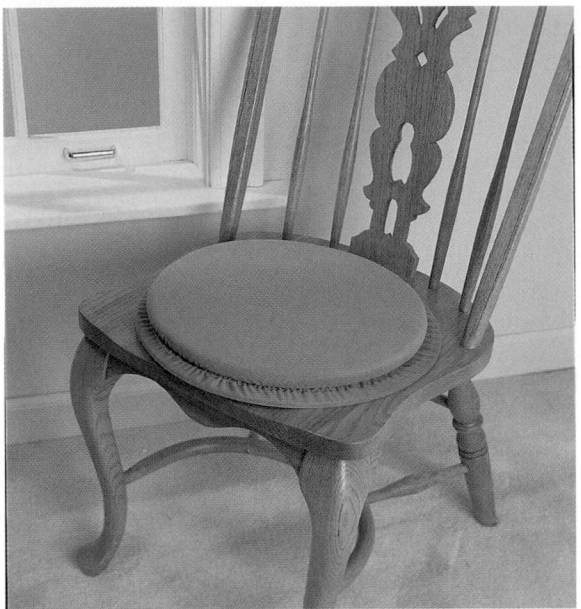

Figure 17.15 Swivel cushion. *(Courtesy of Sammons Preston Rolyan Canada, Mississauga, Ontario, Canada, L4Y 4C5.)*

home modifications and automobile adaptations may also be considered.

Chair glides or stairway lifts can be suggested for those individuals who live in multilevel homes, but who cannot or should not climb stairs (see Chapter 9, Examination of the Environment). These lifts are measured and custom-made for individual staircases and are very expensive. Insurance companies usually do not reimburse for stairway lifts, but some medical supply companies offer "rent-to-own" options. In addition, local ALSA or MDA chapters may have lifts that have been recycled.

At some time point as the disease progresses, the extent of muscle weakness or the energy requirements for ambulation will necessitate wheelchair use for mobility. In the early or early-middle stage of ALS a manual wheelchair, preferably lightweight, may be used for traveling long distances as an energy conservation technique. This wheelchair should be rented on a short-term basis

or loaned from a local ALSA or MDA chapter or other source, because most insurance companies will reimburse for only one wheelchair purchase. As the disease progresses, a power wheelchair system tailored to the patient's current needs and potential future needs will be necessary. Numerous customized wheelchair features and options are available that can assist the individual in maintaining a maximum level of independence and comfort. A referral to a wheelchair and seating clinic may be the best option owing to the numerous, specialized, and evolving needs of the individual with ALS.

Trail et al[157] surveyed 42 patients with ALS and moderate disability, as documented on the AALS, about the wheelchair features they found most beneficial. Sixty-one percent of patients reported that their wheelchairs allowed them to maintain their previous activity levels. In order of priority, manual wheelchair users cited a lightweight frame, small turning radius, high reclining back and supports for the head, trunk, and extremities as most desirable; undesirable features included low, sling, nonreclining back; nonmotorized; static, nonadjustable leg rests; heaviness or large size; and nonremovable armrests. Desirable features for patients who used powered wheelchairs included independent mobility, maneuverability, overall comfort and tilt-in-space/recline features; undesirable features included low, nonreclining back, heaviness or large size, uncomfortable seat, nonadjustable leg rests, and general discomfort.[157]

Although power scooters may be suitable for a patient with adequate UE and trunk strength in the earlier stages of ALS, the vehicle becomes limiting as the disease progresses and should not be prescribed. If the patient has already been reimbursed for a scooter, most insurance companies will not pay for a power wheelchair, because the scooter is considered a power mobility device. If a scooter is to be recommended at all, the patient should rent or borrow the device for short-term use.

Muscle Cramps and Spasticity

Muscle cramps may be alleviated with massage and a stretching program. Cold can temporarily decrease spasticity. Physical therapists can perform and instruct caregivers in slow prolonged stretches and passive ROM exercises to address spasticity. In addition, postural and positioning techniques can be incorporated to decrease spasticity and splinting may be necessary to prevent contractures. A published Cochrane review identified one randomized, controlled study that found patients with ALS who engaged in a 15-minute, twice-daily, moderate-intensity exercise had decreased spasticity, as measured by the *Modified Ashworth Scale,* compared to a control group who engaged in usual daily activities.[158]

Psychosocial Issues

A diagnosis of ALS is devastating for both the patient and family-caregiver unit. Because of the progressive nature of the disease, impairments readily lead to activity limitations and participation restrictions, which may affect quality of life. The emotional responses of the person experiencing the disease, family members, and individuals caring for the patient are multifaceted and may fluctuate throughout the stages of the disease. Much is lost when living with a terminal, progressive disease: physical health and abilities, body image, work and family roles, identity, family and social networks, lifestyle, independence, control, hope, meaning, and the anticipated future.[159,160] The physical therapist must be able to recognize the patient's ability to cope and adapt, and his or her psychological reactions, level of acceptance, and willingness and ability to integrate therapeutic recommendations. It is also imperative that the physical therapist be able to differentiate between normal reactionary grief to losses or a change in physical function and the presence of clinical anxiety and depression, and refer the patient to the appropriate health care team member, when necessary.[161]

When pervasive, anxiety and depressive symptoms need to be treated aggressively with pyschopharmacological medications, because left untreated these psychosocial impairments can adversely affect an individual's ability to adapt, cope, and participate in the POC. Depression may also lead to suicide. In addition, anxiety and depression may also be prevalent among family members or caregivers.[161]

■ EXERCISE AND ALS

Despite the high incidence of muscle weakness in individuals with ALS, the effects of exercise programs have not been extensively studied and, thus, are not well understood. Often physical therapy programs involve ROM and stretching exercises only. Despite the lack of research evidence, some discourage exercise programs because of fear of overuse weakness and believe that no exercise other than everyday activities is indicated.

Studies of individuals with other neuromuscular diseases such as poliomyelitis, Duchenne's muscular dystrophy, myotonic dystrophy, hereditary motor and sensory neuropathy, spinal muscular atrophy, and limb-girdle, Becker, and fascioscapulohumeral dystrophy have found that exercise programs are beneficial and do not produce overuse weakness.[162-169] The research evidence[162-169] from these patient populations suggests the following:

- Overuse weakness does not occur in muscles with an MMT grade of 3 (fair) or greater out of 5 (normal).
- Moderate resistance exercises can increase strength in muscles with an MMT grade of 3 or greater out of 5.
- Strength gains are proportional to initial muscle strength.
- Heavy eccentric exercise should be avoided.
- Exercise may produce functional benefits.
- Psychological benefits have yet to be determined.

When prescribed appropriately, exercise may be beneficial, especially in the early stages of the disease. Exercise may not improve the strength of muscles already weakened by ALS, certainly not those below grade 3. However, general active ROM and stretching of affected joints, resistive strengthening exercises of unaffected muscles with low to moderate weights, and aerobic activities, such as swimming, walking, and bicycling, at submaximal levels, may be prescribed.

When designing a strengthening exercise program for a patient with ALS, the physical therapist must take into consideration the balance between overuse fatigue and disuse atrophy. Evidence from patients with other neuromuscular diseases suggests that highly repetitive or heavy resistance exercise can cause prolonged loss of muscle strength in weakened, denervated muscle.[170,171] Some animal studies have found that neuromuscular activity has inhibitory effects on sprouting in partially denervated muscle,[172-174] whereas other studies have reported no effect[175,176] or that activity can promote sprouting or reinnervation.[177,178]

On the other hand, a marked reduction in activity level secondary to ALS can lead to cardiovascular deconditioning and disuse weakness beyond the amount caused by the disease itself. Therefore, the type and intensity of the exercise program should be carefully monitored and adjusted by the physical therapist in order to prevent excessive fatigue, while at the same time promoting optimal use of intact muscle groups. Patients should be advised not to carry out any activities to the point of extreme fatigue, and should keep track of *symptoms of overuse,* such as the inability to perform daily activities following exercise due to exhaustion or pain, increased fasciculations, or increased muscle cramping. They may also be advised to exercise for several brief periods throughout the day, with sufficient rest in between.

Disuse Atrophy

Reduced physical activity, particularly if prolonged, reduces function of the neuromuscular system, in addition to the skeletal and other organ systems. With insufficient activity, disuse atrophy develops when muscle contractions are less than 20% of the total tension a muscle is capable of producing. As contractile proteins are lost, the muscle weakness progresses at a rate of 3% per day.[179] Strength loss through inactivity and disuse can significantly debilitate individuals with ALS, making them highly susceptible to deconditioning, and muscle and joint tightness leading to contractures and pain.

Overuse Fatigue

The potential for inducing overwork damage in individuals with ALS through excessive exercise is a common concern. Sanjak et al[59] found that individuals with ALS demonstrate abnormal physiological and metabolic responses to single bouts of exercise. Oxygen consumption during submaximal exercise was increased in individuals with ALS compared to controls, and VO_{2max} and work capacity were decreased. In addition, it was found that several metabolic substrates of plasma and muscle compartments did not increase to the same level as untrained control subjects, indicating that the availability of substrate for energy production is affected.[59]

In individuals with ALS, the safe range for therapeutic exercise narrows, and the degree to which the range narrows is dependent on the extent of disease involvement and the rate of disease progression. A weak or denervated muscle is more susceptible to overwork damage because it is already functioning close to its maximal limits. Activities of daily living alone may cause impaired muscles to act as though in training and exercise that would improve normal muscles may actually cause overwork damage in impaired muscles. The remaining motor units will respond to training, and these motor units must work harder to handle a given amount of exercise stress.[179] Thus, special attention must be paid to developing an exercise program for patients with ALS, and physical therapists should prescribe exercise training at moderate to low intensities.

The literature related to exercise in individuals with ALS is limited. Two early case studies demonstrated positive effects of specific strengthening and endurance exercises.[180,181] More recently, the effects of exercise in individuals with ALS have been evaluated with larger samples. Both of these studies found significantly less decline in function scores and other outcome measures[182,183] in the exercise group. Two animal studies found that endurance exercise training at moderate intensities slowed disease progression;[184,185] a third study found that high-endurance exercise training had detrimental effects on male mice only.[186] The evidence related to exercise and ALS is presented in Box 17.1 Evidence Summary (human studies) and Box 17.2 Evidence Summary (animal studies).[187-188]

■ PATIENT/CLIENT-RELATED INSTRUCTION

A diagnosis of ALS is devastating for individuals and their families. They are faced with continual, multiple changes and losses, and eventual death. Assisting the individual and his or her family and caregivers to come to terms with the impact of the disease is an important role for the physical therapist, and providing psychological support and opportunities for expression of feelings,

---

Box 17.1 Evidence Summary Exercise and ALS: The Evidence from Human Studies

Reference	Subject(s)	Methods	Duration	Results
Sanjak et al[181] (1987)	46-year-old man	Case study Air-Dyne bicycle ergometer Prospective, controlled single blind	6 weeks	Isokinetic strength and cardiopulmonary responses to exercise improved in the UEs, but not in the LEs
Pinto et al[182] (1999)	20 Ss, E = 8 Mean age E: 62 ± 14 years C: 64 ± 16 years	E: Bruce or Naughton treadmill protocol, while using BiPAP; exercise to anaerobic threshold until stop parameters reached C: No endurance protocol	12 months	E: Significantly greater FIM scores ($p < 0.03$); slower Spinal Norris Score* decline ($p < 0.02$); significant difference in the slope of FVC decline ($p < 0.008$)
Drory et al[183] (2001)	25 Ss, E = 14 Mean age E: 58.0 ± 13.2 years C: 60.7 ± 16.4 years	Randomly assigned to 2 groups: E: Limb and trunk exercises against modest loads C: No endurance protocol	2 times per day for 15 minutes; 12 months	At 3 months, E: significantly less decline in ALSFRS ($p < 0.001$) and Ashworth Spasticity Scale scores ($p = 0.005$); no significant differences in MMT, FSS, pain, SF-36 scores; at 6 months, no significant differences between groups

Box 17.1 Evidence Summary   Exercise and ALS: The Evidence from Human Studies—cont'd

Reference	Subject(s)	Methods	Duration	Results
Dal Bello-Haas et al[148] (2007)	27 Ss, E = 13 Mean age E: 56.0 ± 7.3 years C: 51.8 ± 12.7 years	Randomly assigned to 2 groups: E: Moderate load, moderate intensity resistance exercises C: Stretching exercises	E: 3 times per week for 6 months	At 6 months, E: significantly greater ALSFRS ($p = 0.02$) and SF-36 Physical Function scores ALSFRS ($p < 0.02$), less decline in MVIC LE megascore ($p = 0.03$); no significant differences in FSS, other SF-36 subscale scores

ALSFRS = Amyotrophic Lateral Sclerosis Functional Rating Scale; BiPAP = bidirectional positive airway pressure ventilation; C = control; E = experimental; FIM = Functional Independence Measure; FSS = Fatigue Severity Scale; FVC = forced vital capacity; LE = lower extremity; MVIC = maximum voluntary isometric contraction; Ss = subjects; UE = upper extremity.

*The Norris Scale, a 100-point scale, examines muscle strength, reflexes, fasciculations, and muscle atrophy. Subscales include bulbar, respiratory, trunk, and limb function. Higher scores denote "better function."

Box 17.2 Evidence Summary   Exercise and ALS: The Evidence from Animal Studies

Reference	Animals	Methods	Duration	Results
Kirkinezos et al[184] (2003)	7-week-old G93A-SOD1 transgenic mice	E: Running on a treadmill (30 min at 13 m/min [42 ft/min] initially; speed and duration decreased stepwise) C: Sedentary	5 days/wk until unable to keep up with a speed of 7 m/min (23 ft/min)	E: Overall, significant increase in life span of G93A-SOD1 mice ($p = 0.007$); significant increase in male mice life span ($p = 0.02$); trend toward increase in female mice life span, but not significant ($p = 0.1$)
Veldink et al[185] (2003)	8-week-old transgenic low-copy hSOD1 mice and wild-type littermates	E: Running on a treadmill (45 min at 16 m/min [52.5 ft/min]) C: Sedentary	Until too ill to run	E: Exercise delayed onset of disease in female, but not male hSOD1 mice; exercise prolonged survival in female mice
Mahoney et al[186] (2004)	40-day-old G93A and wild-type littermate control mice	E: Running on a treadmill (20 min/day at 9 m/min [29.5 ft/min] for week 1; 25 min/day for week 2; 30 min/day for week 3; progressive increase in intensity week 2 and 3; 45 min/day at 22 m/min [72 ft/min]) C: Sedentary	3 days/wk for first 3 weeks; 5 days/wk for remainder	E: Onset of disease not affected in female and male mice; exercise hastened death in male, but not female mice ($p < 0.0001$)

Continued

Box 17.2 Evidence Summary Exercise and ALS: The Evidence from Animal Studies—cont'd

Reference	Animals	Methods	Duration	Results
Liebetanz et al[187] (2004)	3-week-old G93A-SOD1 transgenic mice; two experimental and one control group	E: Vigorous PA on motor-driven running wheel (3.4 m/min [11 ft/min] after 2 week adaptation period) E-PA: Motor-driven running wheel (0.1 m/min [32 ft/min] after 2 week adaptation period) C: Untreated	400 min daily until animal could no longer exceed motor drive speed	No differences in disease onset E: Vigorous PA: non-significant 6-day improvement in survival compared to E-PA and 4-day improvement in survival compared to C
Deforges D, et al[188] 2009	70 day old SOD1 transgenic mice	E-running: Running on a treadmill (max 13 m/min [42 ft/min]) E-swimming: Training in an adjustable-flow swimming pool (max 5 L/min) C-running: Treadmill without speed C-swimming: Floating at water surface in pool without flow	30 min/day 5 days/wk	E-swimming: Significant 16-day delay in symptom appearance ($p < 0.001$); significantly increased survival ($p < 0.01$)
Carreras et al[189] (2010)	30-day-old SOD1 transgenic mice	E-Moderate-level EX: motorized treadmill 30 min/day at 10 m/min [32.8 ft/min] after 2 week training protocol (20 min of running, 3 days/wk at 5 m/min [16.4 ft/min] for week 1 and 10 m/min [32.8 ft/min] for week 2) E-High-level EX: 60 min/days at 20 m/min (65.6 ft/min) after 2 week training period as above C: Walking around cage and climbing food grid	3 days/wk	E-Moderate-level EX: significant delay in onset of motor deficits compared to other groups ($p < 0.05$); significantly higher motor neuron density compared to C ($p < 0.05$) E-High-level EX: slight, but significant increase in time to onset of motor deficits ($p < 0.05$)

C = control; E = experimental; min = minutes; PA = physical activity; EX = exercise.

frustrations, and concerns is imperative. Collaborating with and educating the patient, family, and caregivers in an open and encouraging environment may empower patients in their efforts to cope with their disease, foster a sense of purpose and self-efficacy, and enhance the overall effectiveness of the intervention by increasing adherence with recommendations.[113]

Patient and family/caregiver education is integral throughout the stages of the disease. The scope of education can include, but is not limited to, the following:

- Providing accurate, factual information about the disease process and clinical manifestations, and their significance in terms of management. Give only as much information as the patient, family, and caregivers need; information should be provided in a manner appropriate to their understanding.

- Instructing patients, family members, and caregivers regarding interventions that can be carried out independently such as monitoring the effects and side effects of medications, use of assistive devices and adaptive equipment, and preventing secondary complications.
- Advising the patient about methods to promote general health. Instruction regarding energy conservation, balancing rest and activity, and relaxation techniques may be beneficial in assisting the patient to cope with the daily constraints of the disease.
- Counseling regarding care and life decisions, if the patient asks about these issues.
- Referring patients to support groups or psychological counseling.
- Providing information on health and available social and support services.[113]

The ALSA and the MDA are two national voluntary organizations that provide many functions and programs for individuals with ALS and their families and caregivers, including the provision of written and video educational materials, local education programs, patient and caregiver support groups, equipment loan programs, respite programs, transportation programs, advocacy programs, and ALS Awareness Programs. Patients and families can contact the ALSA and MDA for information and can explore available resources on the websites:

Amyotrophic Lateral Sclerosis Association (Operations)
27001 Agoura Road, Suite 150
Calabasas Hills, CA 91301-5104
818-880-9007
www.alsa.org
The Muscular Dystrophy Association
3300 East Sunrise Drive
Tucson, AZ 85718-3208
800-572-1717
www.mdausa.org

In addition, there are numerous international organizations whose websites provide a variety of resources, including information about ALS, information about clinical trials, evidence-based reviews, evidence-based practice guidelines, and publications about living with ALS (see Appendix 17.C for Web-based resources).

SUMMARY

Amyotrophic lateral sclerosis, the most common and devastatingly fatal motor neuron disease among adults, causes a progressive increase in the number and severity of impairments, activity limitations, and participation restrictions. Other than a small percentage of cases, etiology for the most part is unknown, and it is hypothesized that multiple mechanisms may be responsible for the disease. Although there is no cure for ALS and its course cannot be altered, it should be considered a "treatable disease." Medical management is primarily symptomatic, and a team approach to care is considered optimal. Rehabilitation management is focused on maximizing function and promoting independence to the highest level possible, and ensuring optimal quality of life throughout the course of the disease and across health care settings.

The physical therapist plays an integral role in designing and implementing therapeutic interventions for individuals with ALS that will allow them to maintain independence and function for as long as possible. The selection of interventions, grounded in evidence-based research whenever possible, is based on the stage and progression of the disease and may be restorative, compensatory, or preventative. These interventions should take into consideration the individual's goals and psychosocial factors that may affect decision making, such as the individual's acceptance of the diagnosis and the individual's social and financial resources. Because of the progressive nature of the ALS, the physical therapist must not only address the patient's current problems, but also plan for the patient's future needs.

Acknowledgments

Special thanks to Ashley Chapman, Tasha Kravchenko, and Gabi Watson for their assistance with the editorial and administrative aspects of the manuscript, and sincerest thanks to Peggy Ingels-Allred for her thoughtful and critical review of earlier editions of this chapter.

Questions for Review

1. Describe the clinical manifestations of ALS. Differentiate among impairments associated with upper and lower motor neuron pathology, bulbar pathology, and respiratory system pathology. What cognitive, rare, indirect, and composite impairments might you see in an individual with ALS?

2. What examination procedures are used to help support the diagnosis of ALS?

3. Identify and define the major classifications of ALS included in the El Escorial criteria developed by the World Federation of Neurology Research Group on Motor Neuron Diseases.

4. Describe the disease course of ALS. What factors have shown a relationship to prognosis?

5. Considering the variety of impairments associated with ALS, what factors does a physical therapist need to consider when deciding on which tests and measures should be included in a comprehensive examination?

6. Differentiate among *restorative, compensatory,* and *preventive* interventions.

7. When designing an exercise program for a patient with ALS, what factors need to be taken into consideration?

8. What information should be considered and included when developing a plan for patient and family education following the diagnosis of ALS?

CASE STUDY

The patient is a right-handed 36-year old male recently diagnosed with amyotrophic lateral sclerosis (ALS). Seven months ago, the patient experienced cramping in his left calf and a few months later noted that his left foot slapped and that he "caught his toes" and tripped while playing basketball or walking on the golf course. He also noticed painless twitching of the muscles in his right hand, forearm, and upper arm and reported difficulty fastening the snaps on his youngest son's pajamas.

PAST MEDICAL HISTORY

No significant past medical history.

SOCIAL HISTORY

The patient has been married for 10 years. He has a 3-year-old and a 9-month-old son, and his wife is pregnant with their third child. He lives in a two-story house with 4 steps up to the front door (no railing), 12 stairs between levels (bilateral railing), and 10 stairs to the basement with a railing on the right.

He stopped playing basketball and baseball because he is embarrassed about the frequent tripping, but continues to play golf on the weekend. He uses a golf cart because he is unable to keep up with his friends on the golf course. He would like to be more active.

OCCUPATION

He is a manager at a computer graphics business and reports his voice becomes hoarse on occasion after long presentations. He reports significant fatigue if he works on the computer for long periods of time or if he has to stand for long periods for presentations. He attributes this to "getting older."

DIAGNOSTIC TESTS

Electromyographic studies showed (1) low compound motor action potentials in all extremities; (2) normal sensory nerve conduction; (3) fibrillations and fasciculations in all extremities; and (4) widespread neurogenic changes in motor unit action potentials, abnormal recruitment patterns in the distal leg musculature, and mild to moderate changes in the upper extremities.

PHYSICAL EXAMINATION FINDINGS

• Observation: Marked wasting of the interossei regions bilaterally.
• Speech: No abnormalities noted.
• ROM: Within normal limits (WNL) for all joints, except the thumbs and the L ankle. Patient was only able to oppose thumbs to the third digits. He lacks 5° of L dorsiflexion.

- Strength: Bilateral LE strength graded as 5/5, except for the hip flexor group (R = 4/5; L = 4+/5) and the L ankle dorsiflexors (3–/5). Shoulder muscle strength graded as 4+/5 (R) and 4/5 (L); elbow muscle strength graded as 4/4 (R) and 4+/5 (L).
- Hand strength: R = 12 lb; L = 24 lb (handheld dynamometer).
- Pinch strength: R-tripod = 2 lb; lateral = 3 lb; L-tripod = 5 lb; lateral = 3 lb (see below for normative data on grip and pinch strength). *Note:* Tripod pinch is a component of manual dexterity that involves opposition of the thumb and the first two fingers as a "tripod." Pinch strength measures are obtained using a pinch gauge.
- Manual coordination: Purdue Pegboard Testing, R—6 peg holes in 30 seconds; L—3 peg holes in 30 seconds.
- Tone: 1 for both UEs and 1+ for both LEs (Modified Ashworth spasticity scores).
- Reflexes: A clonic jaw reflex is evident; hyperreflexia in both UEs; hyporeflexia in both LEs; positive Babinski reflex bilaterally.
- Gait: Independent of assistive devices; positive for L foot drop and hip hiking; 15-ft walk test = 3.6 seconds.
- Balance (standing): Unilateral stance/eyes open, R = 25 seconds; L = 6 seconds.
- Respiratory: Forced vital capacity (FVC) and maximum inspiratory pressure (MIP) are within normal limits.
- Functional status: The patient rated himself at 90% on the Schwab and England Rating Scale (see Appendix 17.A). ALSFRS-R scores (see Appendix 17.B):

ALSFRS-R Scores

Item	Score
Speech	4
Salivation	3
Swallowing	3
Handwriting (pre-ALS dominant hand)	3
Cutting food and handling utensils (patients without gastrostomy)	3
Dressing and hygiene	3
Turning in bed; adjusting bed clothes	4
Walking	3
Climbing stairs	3
Dyspnea	3
Orthopnea	4
Respiratory insufficiency	4

Grip and Pinch Strength Values (Pounds) for Men 35 to 39 (n = 25)

	Hand	Mean	SD	SE	Low	High
Grip	R	119.7	24.0	4.8	76	176
	L	112.9	21.7	4.4	73	157
Tip	R	18.0	3.6	.73	12	27
	L	17.7	3.8	.76	10	24
Palmar	R	26.1	3.2	.65	21	32
	L	25.6	3.9	.77	18	32
Lateral (Key)	R	26.2	4.1	.83	19	36
	L	25.9	5.4	1.17	14	40

From Mathiowetz, V, et al: Grip and pinch strength: Normative data for adults. Arch Phys Med Rehabil 66:69, 1984.

GUIDING QUESTIONS

1. What El Escorial diagnostic criteria would you anticipate documented in the patient's medical record?

2. Identify the patient's problems in terms of direct, indirect, and composite impairments.

3. What impact do the impairments have on the patient's ability to function (i.e., activity limitations)?

4. What additional tests and measurements should be conducted; what consultations should be recommended?

5. At present, what are the key areas of patient education that should be addressed initially?

6. Identify the general elements of a physical therapy plan of care for the patient.

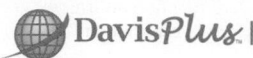 | For additional resources, including answers to the questions for review and case study guiding questions, please visit **http://davisplus.fadavis.com**

References

1. Rowland, LP: Diverse forms of motor neuron diseases. Adv Neurol 36:1, 1982.
2. Swash, M: Clinical features and diagnosis of amyotrophic lateral sclerosis. In Brown, R, Jr, Meininger, V, and Swash, M (eds): Amyotrophic Lateral Sclerosis. Martin Dunitz Ltd, London, 2000, p 3.
3. Norris, F, et al: Onset, natural history and outcome in idiopathic adult motor neuron disease. J Neurol Sci 118(1):48, 1993.
4. Pradas, J, et al: The natural history of amyotrophic lateral sclerosis and the use of natural history controls in therapeutic trials. Neurology 43(4):751, 1993.
5. Ringel, SP, et al: The natural history of amyotrophic lateral sclerosis. Neurology 43(7):1316, 1993.
6. Haverkamp, LJ, Appel, V, and Appel, SH: Natural history of amyotrophic lateral sclerosis in a database population: Validation of a scoring system and a model for survival prediction. Brain 118:707, 1995.
7. Gubbay, SS, et al: Amyotrophic lateral sclerosis. A study of its presentation and prognosis. J Neurol 232(5):295, 1985.
8. Appel, SH, et al: Amyotrophic lateral sclerosis. Associated clinical disorders and immunological evaluations. Arch Neurol 43(3):234, 1986.
9. Mulder, DW, et al: Familial adult motor neuron disease: Amyotrophic lateral sclerosis. Neurology 36(4):511, 1986.
10. Strong, MJ, Hudson, AJ, and Alvord, WG: Familial amyotrophic lateral sclerosis, 1850–1989: A statistical analysis of the world literature. Can J Neurol Sci 18:45, 1991.
11. Hamida, MB, and Hentati, F: Juvenile amyotrophic lateral sclerosis. In Brown, R, Jr, Meininger, V, and Swash, M (eds): Amyotrophic Lateral Sclerosis. Martin Dunitz Ltd, London, 2000, p 59.
12. Rosen, DR: Mutations in Cu/Zn superoxide dismutase gene are associated with familial amyotrophic lateral sclerosis. Nature 362:59, 1993.
13. Jackson, M, and Rothstein, JD: Amyotrophic lateral sclerosis. In Marcoux, FW, and Choi, DW (eds): Central Nervous System Neuroprotection. Springer, New York, 2002, p 423.
14. Jackson, M, et al: Analysis of chromosome 5q13 genes in amyotrophic lateral sclerosis: Homozygous NAIP deletion in a sporadic case. Ann Neurol 39(6):796, 1996.
15. Robberecht, W, et al: D90A heterozygosity in the SOD1 gene is associated with familial and apparently sporadic amyotrophic lateral sclerosis. Neurology 47(5):1336, 1996.
16. Caroscio, JT, Calhoun, WF, and Yahr, MD: Prognostic factors in motor neuron disease: A prospective study of longevity. In Rose, FC (ed): Research Progress in Motor Neuron Disease. Pitman, London, 1984, p 34.
17. Brooks, BR: The natural history of amyotrophic lateral sclerosis. In Williams, AC (ed): Motor Neurone Disease. Chapman & Hall, London, 1994, p 121.
18. Hosler, BA, and Brown, RH, Jr: Copper/zinc superoxide dismutase mutations and free radical damage in amyotrophic lateral sclerosis. Adv Neurol 68:41, 1995.
19. Rothstein, JD, et al: Chronic inhibition of superoxide dismutase produces apoptotic death of spinal neurons. Proc Natl Acad Sci USA 91(10):4155, 1994.
20. Borchelt, DR, et al: Superoxide dismutase 1 with mutations linked to familial amyotrophic lateral sclerosis possesses significant activity. Proc Natl Acad Sci USA 91(17):8292, 1994.
21. Plaitakis, A, and Caroscio, JT: Abnormal glutamate metabolism in amyotrophic lateral sclerosis. Ann Neurol 22(5):575, 1987.
22. Rothstein, JD, et al: Abnormal excitatory amino acid metabolism in amyotrophic lateral sclerosis. Ann Neurol 28(1):18, 1990.
23. Rothstein, JD, Martin, LJ, and Kuncl, RW: Decreased glutamate transport by the brain and spinal cord in amyotrophic lateral sclerosis. N Engl J Med 326(22):1464, 1992.
24. Rothstein, JD, et al: Selective loss of glial glutamate transporter GLT-1 in amyotrophic lateral sclerosis. Ann Neurol 38(1):73, 1995.
25. Carpenter, S: Proximal axonal enlargement in motor neuron disease. Neurology 18:841, 1968.
26. Hirano, A, et al: Fine structural study of neurofibrillary changes in a family with amyotrophic lateral sclerosis. J Neuropathol Exp Neurol 43(5):471, 1984.
27. Wolfgang, F, and Myers, L: Amyotrophic lateral sclerosis: Effect of serum on anterior horn cells in tissue culture. Science 179:579, 1973.
28. Troost, D, Van den Oord, JJ, and Vianney de Jong, JM: Immuno-histochemical characterization of the inflammatory infiltrate in amyotrophic lateral sclerosis. Neuropathol Appl Neurobiol 16(5):401, 1990.
29. Smith, RG, et al: Serum antibodies to L-type calcium channels in patients with amyotrophic lateral sclerosis. N Engl J Med 24(327):1721, 1992.
30. Appel, SH: A unifying hypothesis for the cause of amyotrophic lateral sclerosis, parkinsonism, and Alzheimer disease. Ann Neurol 10(6):499, 1981.
31. Lindsay, RM: Brain-derived neurotrophic factor: an NGF-related neurotrophin. In Loughlin, SE, and Fallon, JH (eds): Neurotrophic Factors. Academic Press, San Diego, 1993, p 257.
32. Thoenen, H, Hughes, RA, and Sendtner, M: Trophic support of motoneurons: Physiological, pathophysiological, and therapeutic implications. Exp Neurol 124(1):47, 1993.
33. Anand, P, et al: Regional changes of ciliary neurotrophic factor and nerve growth factor levels in post mortem spinal cord and cerebral cortex from patients with motor disease. Nat Med 1(2):168, 1995.
34. Strong, MJ: Exogenous neurotoxins. In Brown, R, Jr, Meininger, V, and Swash, M (eds): Amyotrophic Lateral Sclerosis. Martin Dunitz Ltd, London, 2000, p 279.
35. Brown, R, Jr: Apoptosis in amyotrophic lateral sclerosis: A review. In Brown, R, Jr, Meininger, V, and Swash, M (eds): Amyotrophic Lateral Sclerosis. Martin Dunitz Ltd, London, 2000, p 363.
36. Mitsumoto, H, Chad, DA, and Pioro, EK: Hypotheses for viral and other transmissable agents in amyotrophic lateral sclerosis. In Mitsumoto, H, Chad, DA, and Pioro, EK (eds): Amyotrophic Lateral Sclerosis. FA Davis, Philadelphia, 1998, p 239.

37. Mizutani, T, et al: Amyotrophic lateral sclerosis with ophthalmoplegia and multisystem degeneration in patients on long-term use of respirators. Acta Neuropathol 84(4):372, 1992.

38. Iwata, M, and Hirano, A: Sparing of the Onufrowicz nucleus in sacral anterior horn lesions. Ann Neurol 4(3):245, 1978.

39. Mannen, T, and et al: Preservation of certain motorneurone group of the sacral cord in amyotrophic lateral sclerosis: Its clinical significance. J Neuropathol Exp Neurol 47:642, 1988.

40. Barr, ML, and Kiernan, JA: The Human Nervous System: An Anatomical Viewpoint, ed 6. JB Lippincott, Philadelphia, 1993.

41. Bradley, WG, et al: Morphometric and biochemical studies of peripheral nerves in amyotrophic lateral sclerosis. Ann Neurol 14(3):267, 1983.

42. Heads, T, et al: Sensory nerve pathology in amyotrophic lateral sclerosis. Acta Neuropathol 82(4):316, 1991.

43. Kawamura, Y, et al: Morphometric comparison in the vulnerability of peripheral motor and sensory neurons in amyotrophic lateral sclerosis. J Neuropathol Exp Neurol 40(6):667, 1988.

44. Swash, M, et al: Selective and asymmetric vulnerability of corticospinal and spinocerebellar tracts in motor neuron disease. J Neurol Neurosurg Psychiatry 51(6):785, 1988.

45. Averback, P, and Crocker, P: Regular involvement of Clarke's nucleus in sporadic amyotrophic lateral sclerosis. Arch Neurol 39(3):155, 1982.

46. Takahaski, H, et al: Clarke's column in sporadic amyotrophic lateral sclerosis. Acta Neuropathol 84(5):465, 1992.

47. Hudson, AJ: Amyotrophic lateral sclerosis and its association with dementia, parkinsonism and other neurological disorders: A review. Brain 104(2):217, 1981.

48. Wohlfart, G: Collateral regeneration in partially denervated muscles. Neurology 8(3):175, 1958.

49. Hansen, S, and Ballantyne, JP: A quantitative electrophysiological study of motor neurone disease. J Neurol Neurosurg Psychiatry 41(9):773, 1978.

50. McComas, AJ, et al: Functional compensation in partially denervated muscles. J Neurol Neurosurg Psychiatry 34(4):453, 1971.

51. Swash, M, and Schwartz, MS: A longitudinal study of changes in motor units in motor neuron disease. J Neurol Sci 56(2–3): 185, 1982.

52. Swash, M, and Schwartz, MS: Staging motor neurone disease: Single fibre EMG studies of asymmetry, progression and compensatory reinnervation. In Rose, FC (ed): Research Progress in Motor Neuron Disease. Pitman, London, 1984, p 123.

53. Brooks, BR, et al: Natural history of amyotrophic lateral sclerosis: Quantification of symptoms, signs, strength and function. In Serratrice, G, and Munsat, TL (eds): Advances in Neurology: Pathogenesis and Therapy of Amyotrophic Lateral Sclerosis. Lippincott-Raven, Philadelphia, 1995, p 163.

54. Mitsumoto, H, Chad, DA, and Pioro, EK: Clinical features: Signs and symptoms. In Mitsumoto, H, Chad, DA, and Pioro, EK (eds): Amyotrophic Lateral Sclerosis. FA Davis, Philadelphia, 1998, p 47.

55. Brooks, BR: Natural history of ALS: Symptoms, strength, pulmonary function, and disability. Neurology 47(Suppl): S71, 1996.

56. Jette, DU, et al: The relationship of lower-limb muscle force to walking ability in patients with amyotrophic lateral sclerosis. Phys Ther 79(7):672, 1999.

57. Dal Bello-Haas, V, et al: Development, analysis, refinement, and utility of an interdisciplinary amyotrophic lateral sclerosis database. Amyotroph Lateral Scler Other Motor Neuron Disord 2(1):39, 2001.

58. Kilmer, DD: The role of exercise in neuromuscular disease. Phys Med Rehabil Clin North Am 9(1):115, 1998.

59. Sanjak, M, et al: Physiologic and metabolic response to progressive and prolonged exercise in amyotrophic lateral sclerosis. Neurology 37(7):1217, 1987.

60. Sharma, KR, et al: Physiology of fatigue in amyotrophic lateral sclerosis. Neurology 45(4):733, 1995.

61. Sahrmann, SA, and Norton, BJ: The relationship of voluntary movement to spasticity in the upper motor neuron syndrome. Ann Neurol 2(6):460, 1977.

62. Mayer, NH: Clinicophysiologic concepts of spasticity and motor dysfunction in adults with an upper motoneuron lesion. Muscle Nerve Suppl 6:S1, 1997.

63. Schiffer, RB, Cash, J, and Herndon, RM: Treatment of emotional lability with low-dosage tricyclic antidepressants. Psychosomatics 24(12):1094, 1983.

64. Gallagher, JP: Pathologic laughter and crying in ALS: A search for their origin. Acta Neurol Scand 80(2):114, 1989.

65. Fallat, RJ, et al: Spirometry in amyotrophic lateral sclerosis. Arch Neurol 36(2):74, 1979.

66. Rochester, DF, and Esau, SA: Assessment of ventilatory function in patients with neuromuscular disease. Clin Chest Med 15(4):751, 1994.

67. Vitacca, M, et al: Breathing pattern and respiratory mechanics in patients with amyotrophic lateral sclerosis. Eur Respir J 10(7):1614, 1997.

68. Krivickas, L: Pulmonary function and respiratory failure. In Mitsumoto, H, Chad, DA, and Pioro, EK (eds): Amyotrophic Lateral Sclerosis. FA Davis, Philadelphia, 1998, p 382.

69. Schiffman, PL, and Belsh, JM: Pulmonary function at diagnosis of amyotrophic lateral sclerosis. Rate of deterioration. Chest 103(2):508, 1993.

70. Abe, K, et al: Cognitive function in amyotrophic lateral sclerosis. J Neurol Sci 148(1):95, 1997.

71. Kew, JJM, et al: The relationship between abnormalities of cognitive function and cerebral activation in amyotrophic lateral sclerosis. A neuropsychological and positron emission tomography study. Brain 116:1399, 1993.

72. Wilson, CM, et al: Cognitive impairment in sporadic ALS: A pathologic continuum underlying a multisystem disorder. Neurology 57(4):651, 2001.

73. Massman, PJ, et al: Prevalence and correlates of neuropsychological deficits in amyotrophic lateral sclerosis. J Neurol Neurosurg Psychiatry 61(5):450, 1996.

74. Lomen-Hoerth, C, et al: Are amyotrophic lateral sclerosis patients cognitively normal? Neurology 60(7):1094, 2003.

75. Neary, D, et al: Frontal lobe dementia and motor neuron disease. J Neurol Neurosurg Psychiatry 53(1):23, 1990.

76. Strong, MJ, et al: A prospective study of cognitive impairment in ALS. Neurology 53(8):1665, 1999.

77. Abrahams, S, et al: Verbal fluency and executive dysfunction in amyotrophic lateral sclerosis (ALS). Neuropsychologia 38(6):734, 2000.

78. Abrahams, S, et al: Relation between cognitive dysfunction and pseudobulbar palsy in amyotrophic lateral sclerosis. J Neurol Neurosurg Psychiatry 62(5):464, 1997.

79. Brooks, BR, et al: El Escorial revisited: Revised criteria for the diagnosis of amyotrophic lateral sclerosis. Amyotroph Lateral Scler Other Motor Neuron Disord 1(5):293, 2000.

80. Juergens, SM, et al: ALS in Rochester, Minnesota. Neurology 30(5):463, 1980.

81. Caroscio, JT, et al: Amyotrophic lateral sclerosis: Its natural history. Neurol Clin 5(1):1, 1987.

82. Kristensen, O, and Melgaard, B: Motor neuron disease: Prognosis and epidemiology. Acta Neurol Scand 56(4):299, 1977.

83. Granieri, E, et al: Motor neuron disease in the province of Ferrara, Italy, in 1964–1982. Neurology 38(10):1604, 1988.

84. Tysnes, OB, Vollset, SE, and Aarli, JA: Epidemiology of amyotrophic lateral sclerosis in Hordaland county, western Norway. Acta Neurol Scand 83(5):280, 1991.

85. Rosen, AD: Amyotrophic lateral sclerosis. Clinical features and prognosis. Arch Neurol 35(10):638, 1978.

86. Tysnes, OB, et al: Prognostic factors and survival in amyotrophic lateral sclerosis. Neuroepidemiology 13(5):226, 1994.

87. McDonald, ER, et al: Survival in amyotrophic lateral sclerosis: The role of psychological factors. Arch Neurol 51(1):17, 1994.

88. Johnston, M, et al: Mood as a predictor of disability and survival in patients diagnosed with ALS/MND. Br J Health Psych 4(2):1999, 1999.

89. Traynor, BJ, et al: Effect of a multidisciplinary amyotrophic lateral sclerosis (ALS) clinic on ALS survival: A population based study, 1996–2000. J Neurol Neurosurg Psychiatry 74(9):1258, 2003.

90. Bensimon, G, Lacomblez, L, and Meininger, V: A controlled trial of riluzole in amyotrophic lateral sclerosis. ALS/Riluzole Study Group. N Engl J Med 330(9):585, 1994.

91. Lacomblez, L, et al: Dose-ranging study of riluzole in amyotrophic lateral sclerosis. Amyotrophic Lateral Sclerosis/Riluzole Study Group II. Lancet 347(9013):1425, 1996.

92. World Health Organization (WHO): Cancer—Definition of Palliative Care. 2012. WHO, Geneva, Switzerland. Retrieved August 22, 2012, from www.who.int/cancer/palliative/definition/en/.

93. Gordon, PH: Amyotrophic lateral sclerosis: Pathophysiology, diagnosis and management. CNS Drugs 25(1):1, 2011.

94. Miller, RG, et al: Practice parameter update: The care of the patient with amyotrophic lateral sclerosis: Drug, nutritional, and respiratory therapies (an evidence-based review): Report of the Quality Standards Subcommittee of the American Academy of Neurology. Neurology 73(15):1218, 2009.

95. Miller, RG, et al: Practice parameter update: The care of the patient with amyotrophic lateral sclerosis: Multidisciplinary care, symptom management, and cognitive/behavioral impairment (an evidence-based review): Report of the Quality Standards Subcommittee of the American Academy of Neurology. Neurology 73(15):1227, 2009.

96. Desport, JC, et al: Nutritional status is a prognostic factor for survival in ALS patients. Neurology 53(5):1059, 1999.

97. Lechtzin, N, et al: Hospitalization in amyotrophic lateral sclerosis: Causes, costs, and outcomes. Neurology 56(6):753, 2001.

98. Hillel, AD, and Miller, R: Bulbar amyotrophic lateral sclerosis: Patterns of progression and clinical management. Head Neck 11(1):51, 1989.

99. Miller, RG, et al (ALS Practice Parameters Task Force): The care of the patient with amyotrophic lateral sclerosis (an evidence-based review): Report of the Quality Standards Subcommittee of the American Academy of Neurology. Neurology 52(7):1311, 1999.

100. Mathus-Vliegen, LMH, et al: Percutaneous endoscopic gastrostomy in patients with amyotrophic lateral sclerosis and impaired pulmonary function. Gastrointest Endosc 40(4):463, 1994.

101. Mazzini, L, et al: Percutaneous endoscopic gastrostomy and enteral nutrition in amyotrophic lateral sclerosis. Neurology 242(10):695, 1995.

102. Jarnagin, WR, et al: The efficacy and limitations of percutaneous endoscopic gastrostomy. Arch Surg 127(3):261, 1992.

103. Kadakia, SC, Sullivan, HO, and Starnes, E: Percutaneous endoscopic gastrostomy or jejunostomy and the incidence of aspiration in 79 patients. Am J Surg 164(2):114, 1992.

104. Piper, AJ, and Sullivan, CE: Effects of long-term nocturnal nasal ventilation on spontaneous breathing during sleep in neuromuscular and chest wall disorders. Eur Respir J 9(7):1515, 1996.

105. Cazzolli, PA, and Oppenheimer, EA: Home mechanical ventilation for amyotrophic lateral sclerosis: Nasal compared to tracheostomy-intermittent positive pressure ventilation. J Neurol Sci 139(Suppl):123, 1996.

106. Pinto, AC, et al: Respiratory assistance with a non-invasive ventilator (BiPAP) in MND/ALS patients: Survival rates in a controlled trial. J Neurol Sci 129(Suppl):19, 1995.

107. Aboussouan, LS, et al: Effect of noninvasive positive-pressure ventilation on survival in amyotrophic lateral sclerosis. Ann Intern Med 127(6):450, 1997.

108. Bach, JR: Respiratory muscle aids for the prevention of pulmonary morbidity and mortality. Semin Neurol 15(1):72, 1995.

109. Yorkston, KM, et al: Speech deterioration in amyotrophic lateral sclerosis: Implications for the timing of intervention. J Med Speech-Language Pathol 1:35, 1993.

110. Adams, L, and Kazandjian, M: Managing communication and swallowing difficulties. In Mitsumoto, M, and Munsat, T (eds): Amyotrophic Lateral Sclerosis: A Guide for Patients and Families. Demos Medical Publishing, New York, 2001, p 133.

111. Esposito, SJ, Mitsumoto, H, and Shanks, M: Use of palatal lift and palatal augmentation prostheses to improve dysarthria in patients with amyotrophic lateral sclerosis: A case series. J Prosthet Dent 83(1):90, 2000.

112. Gelinas, DF, and Miller, RG: A treatable disease: A guide to management of amyotrophic lateral sclerosis. In Brown, R, Jr, Meininger, V, and Swash, M (eds): Amyotrophic Lateral Sclerosis. Martin Dunitz Ltd, London, 2000, p 405.

113. Dal Bello-Haas, V: A framework for rehabilitation in degenerative diseases: Planning care and maximizing quality of life. Neurology Report (now JNPT) 26(3):115, 2002.

114. Folstein, M, Folstein, SE, and McHugh, PR: Mini Mental State: A practical guide for grading the cognitive state of patients for the clinician. J Psychiatr Res 12(3):189, 1975.

115. Beck, AT, et al: An inventory for measuring depression. Arch Gen Psychiatry 4:561, 1961.

116. Radloff, LS: CES-D scale: A self-report depression scale for research in the general population. Appl Psychol Meas 1(3):385, 1977.

117. Zigmond, AS, and Snaith, RP: The hospital anxiety and depression scale. Acta Psychiatr Scand 67(6):361, 1983.

118. Spielberger, CS, Gorsuch, RL, and Lushene, RE: Manual for the State Trait Anxiety Inventory. Consulting Psychologists Press, Palo Alto, CA, 1970.

119. Andres, PL, et al: Quantitative motor assessment in amyotrophic lateral sclerosis. Neurology 36(7):937, 1986.

120. deBoer, A, Boukes, RJ, and Sterk, JC: Reliability of dynamometry in patients with neuromuscular disorders. N Engl J Med 11(11):169, 1982.

121. Scott, OM, et al: Quantification of muscle function in children: A prospective study in Duchenne muscular dystrophy. Muscle Nerve 5(4):291, 1982.

122. Munsat, TL, Andres, P, and Skerry, L: Therapeutic trials in amyotrophic lateral sclerosis: Measurement of clinical deficit. In Rose, C (ed): Amyotrophic Lateral Sclerosis. Demos, New York, 1990, p 65.

123. Brooks, BR, et al: Design of clinical therapeutic trials in amyotrophic lateral sclerosis. Adv Neurol 56:521, 1991.

124. Great Lakes ALS Study Group: A comparison of muscle strength testing techniques in amyotrophic lateral sclerosis. Neurology 61(11):1503, 2003.

125. Bohannon, RW, and Smith, MB: Interrater reliability of a modified Ashworth scale of muscle spasticity. Phys Ther 67(2):206, 1987.

126. Tinetti, ME: Performance-oriented assessment of mobility problems in elderly patients. J Am Geriatr Soc 34(2):119, 1986.

127. Berg, KO, et al: Measuring balance in the elderly: Validation of an instrument. Can J Public Health 83(2 Suppl):S7, 1992.

128. Podsiadlo, D, and Richardson, S: The timed "Up and Go": A test of basic functional mobility for frail elderly persons. J Am Geriatr Soc 39(2):142, 1991.

129. Duncan, PW, et al: Functional reach: A new clinical measure of balance. J Gerontol 45(6):M192, 1990.

130. Kloos, A, et al: Interrater and intrarater reliability of the Tinetti Balance Test for individuals with amyotrophic lateral sclerosis. JNPT 28(1):12, 2004.

131. Kloos, A, et al: Validity of the Tinetti Balance Assessment in individuals with amyotrophic lateral sclerosis. Proceedings of the 9th International Symposium on ALS/MND, Munich, Germany.

132. Montes, J, et al: The Timed Up and Go test: Predicting falls in ALS. Amyotroph Lateral Scler 8(5):292, 2007.

133. Guide for the Uniform Data Set for Medical Rehabilitation (including the FIM instrument), Version 5.0. State University of New York, Buffalo, 1996.

134. Schwab, R, and England, A: Projection technique for evaluating surgery in Parkinson's disease. In Gillingham, J, and Donaldson, I (eds): Third Symposium on Parkinson's Disease. Livingstone, Edinburgh, Scotland, 1969.

135. The ALS CNTF Treatment Study (ACTS) Phase I–II Study Group: The amyotrophic sclerosis functional rating scale: Assessment of daily living in patients with amyotrophic lateral sclerosis. Arch Neurol 53:141, 1996.

136. Krupp, LB, et al: The fatigue severity scale. Application to patients with multiple sclerosis and systemic lupus erythematosus. Arch Neurol 46(10):1121, 1989.

137. Cedarbaum, JM, et al: The ALSFRS-R: A revised ALS functional rating scale that incorporates assessments of respiratory function. J Neurol Sci 169:13, 1999.

138. Kaufmann, P, et al: Excellent inter-rater, intra-rater, and telephone-administered reliability of the ALSFRS-R in a multicenter clinical trial. Amyotroph Lateral Scler 8(1):42, 2007.

139. Appel, V, et al: A rating scale for amyotrophic lateral sclerosis: Description and preliminary experience. Ann Neurol 22(3):328, 1987.

140. Hillel, AD, et al: Amyotrophic Lateral Sclerosis Severity Scale. Neuroepidemiology 8(3):142, 1989.

141. Norris, F, et al: The administration of guanidine in amyotrophic lateral sclerosis. Neurology 24(8):721, 1974.

142. Ware, JE, et al: SF-36 Health Survey: Manual and Interpretation Guide. Health Institute, New England Medical Center, Boston, 1993.

143. Hickey, AM, et al: A new short form individual quality of life measure (SEIQoL-DW): Application in a cohort of individuals with HIV/AIDS. Br Med J 313(7048):29, 1996.

144. Bergner, M, et al: The Sickness Impact Profile: Development and final revision of a health status measure. Med Care 19(8):787, 1981.

145. Jenkinson, C, et al: Development and validation of a short measure of health status for individuals with amyotrophic lateral sclerosis/motor neuron disease: The ALSAQ-40. J Neurol 246:16, 1999.

146. Jenkinson, C, et al: Evidence for the validity and reliability of the ALS assessment questionnaire: the ALSAQ-40. Amyotroph Lateral Scler Other Motor Neuron Disord 1(1):33, 1999.

147. Jenkinson, C, and Fitzpatrick, R: Reduced item set for the amyotrophic lateral sclerosis assessment questionnaire: Development and validation of the ALSAQ-5. J Neurol Neurosurg Psychiatry 70(1):70, 2001.

148. Dal Bello-Haas, V, et al: A randomized controlled trial of resistance exercise in individuals with ALS. Neurology 68(23):2003, 2007.

149. Ingels, PL, et al: Adhesive capsulitis: A common occurrence in patients with ALS. Amyotroph Lateral Scler Other Motor Neuron Disord 2(S2):60, 2001.

150. Cheah, BC, et al: INSPIRATIonAL—INSPIRAtory muscle training in amyotrophic lateral sclerosis. Amyotroph Lateral Scler 10(5-6):384, 2009.

151. Lahrmann, H, et al: Expiratory muscle weakness and assisted cough in ALS. Amyotroph Lateral Scler Other Motor Neuron Disord 4(1):49, 2003.

152. Hanayama, K, Ishikawa, Y, and Bach, JR: Amyotrophic lateral sclerosis: Successful treatment of mucous plugging by mechanical insufflation-exsufflation. Am J Phys Med Rehabil 76(4):338, 1997.

153. Mustfa, N, et al: Cough augmentation in amyotrophic lateral sclerosis. Neurology 61(9):1285, 2003.

154. Scherer, TA, et al: Effect of high-frequency oral airway and chest wall oscillation and conventional chest physical therapy on expectoration in patients with stable cystic fibrosis. Chest 113(4):1019, 1998.

155. Arens, R, et al: Comparison of high frequency chest compression and conventional chest physiotherapy in hospitalized patients with cystic fibrosis. Am J Respir Crit Care Med 150(4):1154, 1994.

156. Lange, DJ, et al: High-frequency chest wall oscillation in ALS: An exploratory randomized, controlled trial. Neurology 67(6):991, 2006.

157. Trail, M, et al: Wheelchair use by patients with amyotrophic lateral sclerosis: A survey of user characteristics and selection preferences. Arch Phys Med Rehabil 82(1):98, 2001.

158. Ashworth, NL, Satkunam, LE, and Deforge, D: Treatment for spasticity in amyotrophic lateral sclerosis/motor neuron disease (Cochrane review). The Cochrane Library, Issue 4. Jon Wiley & Sons, Chichester, UK, 2004.

159. Kemp, C: Psychosocial needs, problems, and interventions: The individual. In Terminal Illness: A Guide to Nursing Care. Lippincott, Philadelphia, 1999, p 17.

160. Doka, KJ: Mourning psychosocial loss: Anticipatory mourning in Alzheimer's, ALS, and irreversible coma. In Rando, TA (ed): Clinical Dimensions of Anticipatory Mourning: Theory and Practice in Working with the Dying, Their Loved Ones, and Their Caregivers. Research Press, Champaign, IL, 2000, p 477.

161. Dal Bello-Haas, V, Delbene, M, and Mitsumoto, H: End of life: Challenges and strategies for the rehabilitation professional. Neurological Report (now JNPT) 26(4):174, 2002.

162. Kilmer, DD, et al: The effect of a high resistance exercise program in slowly progressive neuromuscular disease. Arch Phys Med Rehabil 75(5):560, 1994.

163. Lindeman, E, et al: Strength training in patients with myotonic dystrophy and hereditary motor and sensory neuropathy: A randomized clinical trial. Arch Phys Med Rehabil 76(7):612, 1995.

164. Aitkens, SG, et al: Moderate resistance exercise program: Its effect in slowly progressive neuromuscular disease. Arch Phys Med Rehabil 74(7):711, 1993.

165. Milner-Brown, HS, and Miller, RG: Muscle strengthening through high-resistance weight training in patients with neuromuscular disorders. Arch Phys Med Rehabil 69(1):14, 1988.

166. Florence, JM, and Hagberg, JM: Effect of training on the exercise responses of neuromuscular disease patients. Med Sci Sports Exerc 16(5):460, 1984.

167. Vignos, PJJ: Physical models of rehabilitation in neuromuscular disease. Muscle Nerve 6(5):323, 1983.

168. Einarsson, G: Muscle conditioning in late poliomyelitis. Arch Phys Med Rehabil 72(1):11, 1991.

169. McCartney, N, et al: The effects of strength training in patients with selected neuromuscular disorders. Med Sci Sports Exerc 20(4):362, 1988.

170. Bennett, RL, and Knowlton, GC: Overwork weakness in partially denervated skeletal muscle. Clin Orthop 12:22, 1958.

171. Johnson, EW, and Braddom, R: Over-work weakness in facioscapulohumeral muscular dystrophy. Arch Phys Med Rehabil 52(7):333, 1971.

172. Tam, SL, et al: Increased neuromuscular activity reduces sprouting in partially denervated muscles. J Neurosci 21(2):654, 2001.

173. Gardiner, PF, Michel, R, and Iadeluca, G: Previous exercise training influences functional sprouting of rat hind limb motoneurons in response to partial denervation. Neurosci Lett 45(2):123, 1984.

174. Rafuse, VF, Gordon, T, and Orozco, R: Proportional enlargement of motor units after partial denervation of cat triceps surae muscles. J Neurophysiol 68(4):1261, 1992.

175. Michel, RN, and Gardiner, PF: Influence of overload on recovery of rat plantaris from partial denervation. J Appl Physiol 66(2): 732, 1989.

176. Seburn, KL, and Gardiner, PF: Properties of sprouted rat motor units: Effects of period of enlargement and activity level. Muscle Nerve 19(9):1100, 1996.

177. Ribchester, RR: Activity-dependent and independent synaptic interactions during reinnervation of partially denervated rat muscle. J Physiol (Lond) 401:53, 1988.

178. Einsiedel, LJ, and Luff, AR: Activity and motor unit size in partially denervated rat medial gastrocnemius. J Appl Physiol 76(6):2663, 1994.

179. Coble, NO, and Maloney, FP: Effects of exercise in neuromuscular disease. In Maloney, FP, Burks, JS, and Ringel, SP (eds): Interdisciplinary Rehabilitation of Multiple Sclerosis and Neuromuscular Disorders. Lippincott, New York, 1985, p 228.

180. Bohanon, RW: Results of resistance exercise on a patient with amyotrophic lateral sclerosis. Phys Ther 63(6):965, 1983.

181. Sanjak, M, Reddan, W, and Brooks, BR: Role of muscular exercise in amyotrophic lateral sclerosis. Neurol Clin 5(2):251, 1987.

182. Pinto, AC, et al: Can amyotrophic lateral sclerosis patients with respiratory insufficiency exercise? J Neurol Sci 169:69, 1999.

183. Drory, VE, et al: The value of muscle exercise in patients with amyotrophic lateral sclerosis. J Neurol Sci 191(1-2):133, 2001.

184. Kirkinezos, IG, et al: Regular exercise is beneficial to a mouse model of amyotrophic lateral sclerosis. Ann Neurol 53(6):804, 2003.

185. Veldink, JH, et al: Sexual differences in onset of disease and response to exercise in a transgenic model of ALS. Neuromusc Disord 13(9):737, 2003.

186. Mahoney, DJ, et al: Effects of high-intensity endurance exercise training in the G93A mouse model of amyotrophic lateral sclerosis. Muscle Nerve 29(5):656, 2004.

187. Liebetanz, D, et al: Extensive exercise is not harmful in amyotrophic lateral sclerosis. Eur J Neurosci 20(11):3115, 2004.

188. Deforges, S, et al: Motoneuron survival is promoted by specific exercise in a mouse model of amyotrophic lateral sclerosis. J Physiol (Lond) 587(14):3561, 2009.

189. Carreras, I, et al: Moderate exercise delays the motor performance decline in a transgenic model of ALS. Brain Res 1313: 192, 2010.

Supplemental Readings

Albom, M: Tuesdays with Morrie—an Old Man, a Young Man, and Life's Greatest Lesson. Bantam Doubleday Dell, New York, 1997.

Andersen, PM, et al: EFNS guidelines on the clinical management of amyotrophic lateral sclerosis (MALS)—revised report of an EFNS task force. Eur J Neurol 19(3):360, 2012.

Atassi, N, et al: Depression in amyotrophic lateral sclerosis. Amyotroph Lateral Scler 12(2):109, 2011.

Blackhall, LJ: Amyotrophic lateral sclerosis and palliative care: Where we are, and the road ahead. Muscle Nerve 45(3):311, 2012.

Dal Bello-Haas, V, Kloos, A, and Mitsumoto, H: Physical therapy for the stages of amyotrophic lateral sclerosis: A case report. Phys Ther 78(12):1312, 1998.

Dal Bello-Haas, V, and Krivickas, L: Amyotrophic lateral sclerosis. In Durstine, JL, Moore, GE, and Painter, PL (eds): ACSM's Exercise Management for Persons with Chronic Diseases and Disabilities, ed 3. Human Kinetics, Champaign, IL, 2008, pp 336–341.

Feigenbaum, D (ed): Journeys with ALS: Personal Tales of Courage and Coping with Lou Gehrig's Disease. DLRC Press, Virginia Beach, 1998.

Gardner, DD: Amyotrophic lateral sclerosis in the older adult. AARC Times 35(11):22, 2011.

Genton, L, et al: Nutritional state, energy intakes and energy expenditure of amyotrophic lateral sclerosis (ALS) patients. Clin Nutr 30(5):553, 2011.

Kiernan, MC, et al: Amyotrophic lateral sclerosis. Lancet 377(9769):942, 2011.

Lancioni, GE, et al: Technology-aided programs for assisting communication and leisure engagement of persons with amyotrophic lateral sclerosis: Two single-case studies. Res Dev Disabil 33(5):1605, 2012.

Mitsumoto, H (ed): Amyotrophic Lateral Sclerosis: A Guide for Patients and Families, ed 3. Demos Medical Publishing, New York, 2009.

Mitsumoto, H, Przedborski, S, and Gordon, PH (eds): Amyotrophic Lateral Sclerosis. Marcel Dekker, New York, 2006.

Pagnini, F, et al: Respiratory function of people with amyotrophic lateral sclerosis and caregiver distress level: A correlational study. Biopsychosoc Med 6(1):14, 2012.

Rodrigues, MC, et al: Neurovascular aspects of amyotrophic lateral sclerosis. Int Rev Neurobiol 102:91, 2012.

Thonhoff, JR, Ojeda, L, and Wu, P: Stem cell–derived motor neurons: Applications and challenges in amyotrophic lateral sclerosis. Curr Stem Cell Res Ther 4(3):178, 2009.

van Groenestijn, AC, et al: Effects of aerobic exercise therapy and cognitive behavioural therapy on functioning and quality of life in amyotrophic lateral sclerosis: Protocol of the FACTS-2-ALS trial. BMC Neurol 11:70, 2011.

Yorkston, KM, et al: Management of Speech and Swallowing in Degenerative Diseases, ed 2. Pro Ed, Austin, 2004.

Schwab and England Activities of Daily Living Scale

100% =	Completely independent; able to do all chores without slowness, difficulty, or impairment; essentially normal; unaware of any difficulty
90% =	Completely independent; able to do all chores with some degree of slowness, difficulty, and impairment; may take twice as long as usual; beginning to be aware of difficulty
80% =	Completely independent in most chores; takes twice as long as normal; conscious of difficulty and slowness
70% =	Not completely independent; more difficulty with some chores; takes three to four times as long as normal in some; must spend a large part of the day with some chores
60% =	Some dependency; can do most chores, but exceedingly slowly and with considerable effort and errors; some chores impossible
50% =	More dependent; needs help with half the chores, slower, and so forth; difficulty with everything
40% =	Very dependent; can assist with all chores but does few alone
30% =	With effort, now and then does a few chores alone or begins alone; much help needed
20% =	Does nothing alone; can be a slight help with some chores; severe invalid
10% =	Totally dependent and helpless; complete invalid
0% =	Vegetative functions such as swallowing, bladder, and bowels are not functioning; bedridden

From Schwab and England,[134] with permission.

1. Speech

4 Normal speech processes.
3 Detectable speech disturbance.
2 Intelligible with repeating.
1 Speech combined with nonvocal communication.
0 Loss of useful speech.

2. Salivation

4 Normal.
3 Slight but definite excess of saliva in mouth; may have nighttime drooling.
2 Moderately excessive saliva; may have minimal drooling.
1 Marked excess of saliva with some drooling.
0 Marked drooling; requires constant tissue or handkerchief.

3. Swallowing

4 Normal eating habits.
3 Early eating problems—occasional choking.
2 Dietary consistency changes.
1 Needs supplemental tube feeding.
0 NPO (exclusively parenteral or enteral feeding).

4. Handwriting

4 Normal.
3 Slow or sloppy; all words are legible.
2 Not all words are legible.
1 Able to grip pen but unable to write.
0 Unable to grip pen.

5a. Cutting Food and Handling Utensils (Patients without Gastrostomy)

4 Normal.
3 Somewhat slow and clumsy, but no help needed.
2 Can cut most foods, although clumsy and slow; some help needed.
1 Food must be cut by someone, but can still feed slowly.
0 Needs to be fed.

OR

5b. Cutting Food and Handling Utensils (Alternate Scale for Patients with Gastrostomy)

4 Normal.
3 Clumsy but able to perform all manipulations independently.
2 Some help needed with closures and fasteners.
1 Provides minimal assistance to caregiver.
0 Unable to perform any aspect of task.

6. Dressing and Hygiene

4 Normal function.
3 Independent and complete self-care with effort or decreased efficiency.
2 Intermittent assistance or substitute methods.
1 Needs attendant for self.
0 Total dependence.

7. Turning in Bed and Adjusting Bed Clothes

4 Normal.
3 Somewhat slow and clumsy, but no help needed.
2 Can turn alone or adjust sheets, but with great difficulty.
1 Can initiate, but not turn or adjust sheets alone.
0 Helpless.

8. Walking

4 Normal.
3 Early ambulation difficulties.
2 Walks with assistance.
1 Nonambulatory functional movement only.
0 No purposeful leg movement.

9. Climbing Stairs

4 Normal.
3 Slow.
2 Mild unsteadiness or fatigue.
1 Needs assistance.
0 Cannot do.

10. Dyspnea

> 4 None.
> 3 Occurs when walking.
> 2 Occurs with one or more of the following: eating, bathing, dressing (ADL).
> 1 Occurs at rest, difficulty breathing when either sitting or lying.
> 0 Significant difficulty, considering using mechanical respiratory support.

11. Orthopnea

> 4 None.
> 3 Some difficulty sleeping at night due to shortness of breath, does not routinely use more than two pillows.
> 2 Needs extra pillows in order to sleep (more than two).
> 1 Can only sleep sitting up.
> 0 Unable to sleep.

[a] Original ALSFRS consists of items 1 through 9 and the original item 10 below:

10. Breathing

> 4 Normal.
> 3 Shortness of breath with minimal exertion (e.g., walking, talking).
> 2 Shortness of breath at rest.
> 1 Intermittent (e.g., nocturnal) ventilatory assistance.
> 0 Ventilator dependent.

BiPAP = bidirectional positive airway pressure; NPO = *non per os*, nothing by mouth.

12. Respiratory Insufficiency

> 4 None.
> 3 Intermittent use of BiPAP.
> 2 Continuous use of BiPAP during the night.
> 1 Continuous use of BiPAP during the night and day.
> 0 Invasive mechanical ventilation by intubation or tracheostomy.

From Cedarbaum, JM, et al,[137] with permission.

Organization/Resource	Website
American Academy of Neurology	www.aan.org*
Amyotrophic Lateral Sclerosis Association • Living with ALS Manuals and Videos	www.alsa.org www.alsa.org/als-care/resources
Amyotrophic Lateral Sclerosis Society of Canada • A Manual for People Living with ALS	www.als.ca www.als.ca/als_manuals.aspx
European Federation of Neurological Societies	www.efns.org
International Alliance of ALS/MND Associations' Resources Site • Full List of Documents Held	www.mndallianceresources.org www.mndallianceresources.org/contents/full_list_of_documents_held.asp
Muscular Dystrophy Association	www.mdausa.org*
National Health Services Evidence	www.evidence.nhs.uk†
National Institute of Neurological Disorders and Stroke	www.ninds.nih.gov*
National Institute of Clinical Excellence	www.nice.org.uk†
World Federation of Neurology Amyotrophic Lateral Sclerosis (WFN-ALS)	www.wfnals.org

*Search term: Amyotrophic lateral sclerosis (ALS)
†Search term: Motor neuron disease
ALS = amyotrophic lateral sclerosis; ALS/MND = amyotrophic lateral sclerosis and motor neuron disease.

Parkinson's Disease

Susan B. O'Sullivan, PT, EdD
Edward W. Bezkor, PT, DPT, OCS, MTC

Chapter 18

Parkinson's disease (PD) is a progressive disorder of the central nervous system (CNS) with both motor and nonmotor symptoms. Motor symptoms include the *cardinal features* of **rigidity**, **bradykinesia**, **tremor**, and, in later stages, postural instability. Nonmotor symptoms may precede the onset of motor symptoms by years. Early symptoms can include loss of sense of smell, constipation, rapid eye movement (REM) sleep behavior disorder, mood disorders, and orthostatic hypotension. Other nonmotor symptoms include altered bladder function, excessive saliva, integumentary changes, difficulty speaking and swallowing, and cognitive problems (slowed thinking, confusion, and in some cases dementia). Onset is insidious with a slow rate of progression. Disruptions in daily functions, roles, and activities, as well as depression, are common in individuals with PD.

■ INCIDENCE

PD is a common disease that affects an estimated 1 million Americans and an estimated 7 to 10 million people worldwide. More than 2% of people older than 65 years of age have PD, second only to Alzheimer's disease among neurodegenerative disorders. The prevalence of the disease is expected to increase substantially in the coming years due to the aging of the population. The average age of onset is 50 to 60 years. Only 4% to 10% of patients are diagnosed with early-onset PD (less than

40 years of age). Young-onset PD is classified as beginning between 21 and 40 years of age, and juvenile-onset PD affects individuals less than 21 years of age. Men are affected 1.2 to 1.5 times more frequently than women.[1,2]

ETIOLOGY

The term **parkinsonism** is a generic term used to describe a group of disorders with primary disturbances in the dopamine systems of basal ganglia (BG). Both genetic and environmental influences have been identified. Parkinson's disease, or idiopathic parkinsonism, is the most common form, affecting approximately 78% of patients. *Secondary parkinsonism* results from a number of different identifiable causes, including viruses, toxins, drugs, tumors, and so forth (Box 18.1). The term *parkinsonism-plus syndromes* refers to those conditions that mimic PD in some respects, but the symptoms are caused by other neurodegenerative disorders.[3]

Parkinson's Disease

Parkinson's disease was first described as "the shaking palsy" by James Parkinson in 1817[4] and refers to those cases where the etiology is idiopathic (unknown) or genetically determined. Two distinct clinical subgroups have been identified. One group includes individuals whose dominant symptoms include postural instability and gait disturbances (*postural instability gait disturbed [PIGD]*). Another group includes individuals with tremor as the main feature (*tremor predominant*). Patients who are tremor predominant typically demonstrate few problems with bradykinesia or postural instability.[3]

Genetic forms of PD represent less than 10% of cases overall. In a small number of families, several gene mutations have been identified (e.g., PARK1, PINK1, LRRK2, DJ-1, and glucocerebrosidase, among others).[1] Genes have been grouped into two categories: (1) causal genes, which actually produce the disease; and (2) associated genes that do not cause PD but increase the risk of developing it.

Secondary Parkinsonism

Postencephalitic Parkinsonism

The influenza epidemics of encephalitis lethargica that occurred from 1917 to 1926 affected large numbers of individuals. The onset of parkinsonian symptoms typically occurred after many years, giving rise to the theory that a slow virus infected the brain. In the absence of a recent outbreak, this type of parkinsonism is no longer seen. Moving case histories are portrayed in the book *Awakenings* by Oliver Sacks.[5]

Toxic Parkinsonism

Parkinsonian symptoms occur in individuals exposed to certain environmental toxins, including pesticides (e.g., permethrin, beta-HCH, paraquat, maneb, Agent Orange) and industrial chemicals (e.g., manganese,

---

Box 18.1   Classification of Parkinsonism

Idiopathic Parkinson's Disease

Late-onset (>40 years; generally sporadic)
Early-onset (<40 years; often familial)
 • Young-onset (>21 years)
 • Juvenile (<21 years)

Parkinsonism Due to Identifiable Causes

Virus (e.g., encephalitis lethargica)
Toxins (e.g., carbon monoxide, manganese, methylphenyltetrahydropyridine [MPTP])
Drugs (e.g., phenothiazines, reserpine, butyrophenones, metoclopramide)
Vascular disease (multi-infarct)
Tumors of basal ganglia
Normal pressure hydrocephalus
Hemiparkinsonism, hemiatrophy
Metabolic
 • Wilson's disease
 • Hepatocerebral degeneration
 • Hallervorden-Spatz disease
 • Hypoparathyroidism

Parkinsonism in Other Neurodegenerative Disorders

Progressive supranuclear palsy
Cortical–basal ganglionic degeneration
Disorders with cerebellar/autonomic/pyramidal manifestation:
 • Multiple-system atrophy
 • Striatonigral degeneration
 • Shy-Drager syndrome
 • Olivopontocerebellar atrophy
 • Machado-Joseph disease

Disorders with prominent and often early dementia:
 • Diffuse cortical Lewy body disease
 • Alzheimer's disease with parkinsonism

Parkinsonism–dementia–ALS complex of Guam
 • Pallidopontonigral degeneration/disinhibition–dementia–parkinsonism–amyotrophy complex

From Pal, P, et al: Cardinal features of early Parkinson's disease. In Factor, S, and Weiner, W (eds): Parkinson's Disease—Diagnosis and Clinical Management. Demos Medical Publishing, New York, 2002, p 42, with permission.

---

carbon disulfide, carbon monoxide, cyanide, methanol). The most common of these toxins is manganese, which represents a serious occupational hazard to many miners from prolonged exposure.[6,7] Severe and permanent parkinsonism has been inadvertently produced in individuals who injected a synthetic heroin containing the chemical MPTP (1-methyl-4-phenyl-1,2,3,6- tetra/hydropyridine).[8] It is important to note that simple exposure is never enough to cause the disease.

Drug-Induced Parkinsonism (DIP)

A variety of drugs can produce extrapyramidal dysfunction that mimics the signs of PD. These drugs are thought to interfere with dopaminergic mechanisms either presynaptically or postsynaptically. They include (1) *neuroleptic drugs* such as chlorpromazine (Thorazine), haloperidol (Haldol), thioridazine (Mellaril), and thiothixene (Navane); (2) *antidepressant drugs* such as amitriptyline (Triavil), amoxapine (Asendin), and trazodone (Desyrel); and (3) *antihypertensive drugs* such as methyldopa (Aldomet) and reserpine. High doses of these medications are particularly problematic in the elderly. Withdrawal of these agents usually reverses the symptoms within a few weeks, although in some cases the effects can persist and may be related to subclinical PD.[9]

Parkinsonism can be caused in rare cases by metabolic conditions, including disorders of calcium metabolism that result in BG calcification. These include hypothyroidism, hyperparathyroidism, hypoparathyroidism, and Wilson's disease.[9]

Parkinson-Plus Syndromes

A group of neurodegenerative diseases can affect the substantia nigra and produce parkinsonian symptoms along with other neurological signs. These diseases include striatonigral degeneration (SND), Shy-Drager syndrome, progressive supranuclear palsy (PSPO), olivopontocerebellar atrophy (OPCA), and cortical–basal ganglionic degeneration (CBGD). In addition, parkinsonian symptoms can be exhibited in patients with multi-infarct vascular disease, Alzheimer's disease, diffuse Lewy body disease (DLBD), normal pressure hydrocephalus (NPH), Creutzfeldt-Jakob disease (CJD), Wilson's disease (WD), and juvenile Huntington's disease. Many of these conditions are rare and affect relatively small numbers of individuals. Early in their course, these diseases may present with rigidity and bradykinesia indistinguishable from PD. However, other diagnostic symptoms eventually appear (e.g., cognitive impairment in Alzheimer's disease). Another diagnostic feature is that Parkinson-plus syndromes typically do not show measurable improvement from the administration of anti-Parkinson medications such as levodopa (L-dopa) therapy (termed the *apomorphine test*).[9]

■ PATHOPHYSIOLOGY

The BG is a network of subcortical nuclei consisting of the *caudate nucleus*, the *putamen*, the *globus pallidus*, and the *subthalamic nucleus* along with the *substantia nigra*. The caudate and the putamen together are called the *striatum* (Fig. 18.1). The BG engages in a number of parallel circuits or loops, only a few of which are motor. The *direct motor loop* through the BG consists of signals transmitted from the cortex to putamen to globus pallidus, to ventrolateral (VL) nucleus of the thalamus, and back to cortex (supplementary motor area [SMA]) (Fig. 18.2). This VL-SMA connection is excitatory and facilitates discharge of cells in the SMA. The BG thus serves to activate the cortex via a positive-feedback loop and assists in the initiation of voluntary movement. Inhibition of the thalamus by the BG is thought to underlie the hypokinesia seen in PD. An *indirect loop* through the BG involves the subthalamic nucleus, the globus pallidus interna, and substantia nigra pars reticulata to the superior colliculus and midbrain tegmentum (Fig. 18.3). This indirect loop serves to decrease thalamocortical activation. The BG projection to the superior colliculus assists in regulation of saccadic eye movements. The BG projection to the reticular formation assists in the regulation of trunk and limb musculature (via extrapyramidal pathways), sleep and wakefulness, and arousal. Other circuits in the BG are involved with memory and cognitive functions.[10]

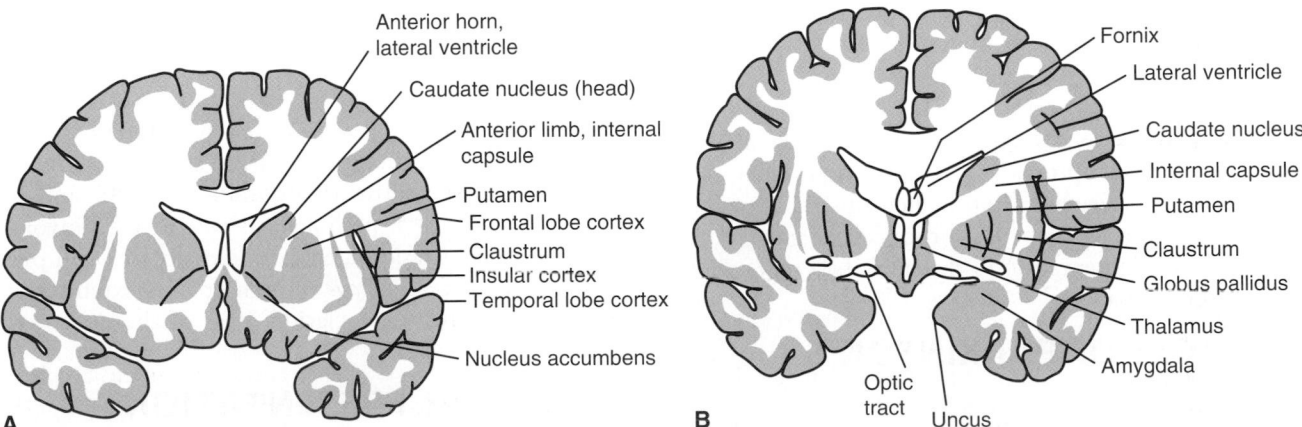

Figure 18.1 The major structures of the basal ganglia. **(A)** Coronal section through the rostral part of the frontal lobe showing the relation of the caudate nucleus, putamen, and nucleus accumbens to the surrounding telencephalic structures. **(B)** Coronal section through the caudal part of the front lobe showing the location of the lentiform nucleus later to, and the body of the caudate nucleus dorsal to, the diencephalon.

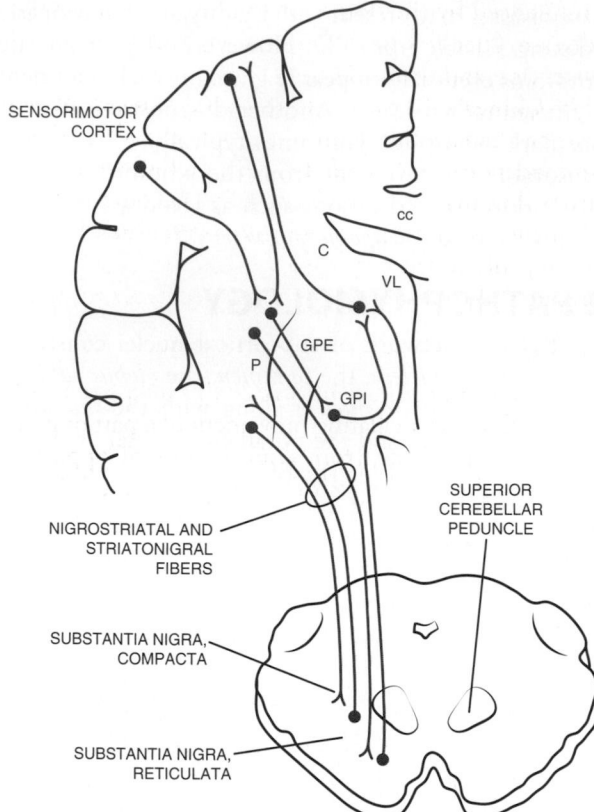

Figure 18.2 The direct loop through the putamen and the connections of the striatum with the substantia nigra pars compacta. The striatonigral fibers represented in this diagram arise in the putamen. However, most striatonigral fibers arise from the caudate. C = caudate nucleus; cc = corpus callosum; GPe = globus pallidus pars externa; GPi = glogus pallidus pars interna; P = putamen; VL = ventral lateral nucleus of the thalamus. *(From Gilman, S and Newman S, 2003,*[10, p. 151] *with permission.)*

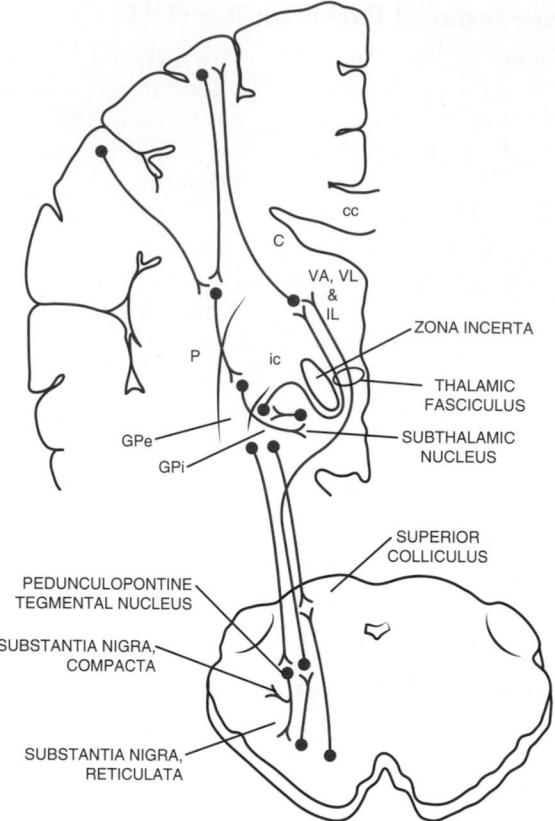

Figure 18.3 The indirect loop through the subthalamic nucleus; also represented are the efferents from the globus pallidus interna and substantia nigra pars reticulata to the superior colliculus and midbrain tegmentum. C = caudate nucleus; GPe = globus pallidus pars externa; GPi = globus pallidus pars interna; ic = internal capsule; IL = intralaminar nuclei of the thalamus; P = putamen; VA = ventral anterior nucleus of the thalamus; VL = ventral lateral nucleus of the thalamus. *(From Gilman and Newman, 2003,*[10, p. 152] *with permission.)*

Parkinson's disease is defined by (1) degeneration of dopaminergic neurons in the BG in the pars compactus of the substantia nigra that produce *dopamine* and (2) as the disease progresses and neurons degenerate, the presence of cytoplasmic inclusion bodies, called *Lewy bodies.* Substantial neurodegeneration occurs in PD before the onset of motor symptoms with clinical signs emerging at 30% to 60% degeneration of neurons. Loss of the melanin-containing neurons produces characteristic changes in depigmentation in the substantia nigra with a characteristic pallor.[11]

■ STAGES OF PARKINSON'S DISEASE

Postmortem studies by Braak and colleagues have yielded evidence supporting the view that PD is a widely dispersed neurodegenerative disease that demonstrates a progression through different stages. Early on (*stage 1*) lesions are found in the medulla oblongata (dorsal IX/X nucleus or intermediate reticular zone).

In *stage 2*, pathology is expanded to involve lesions of the caudal raphe nuclei, the gigantocellular reticular nucleus, and coeruleus-subcoeruleus complex. In *stage 3*, involvement of the nigrostriatal system is apparent (pars compacta of the substantia nigra). In *stage 4*, lesions are also found in the cortex (temporal mesocortex and allocortex). In *stage 5*, pathology is extended to involve the sensory association areas of the neocortex and prefrontal neocortex. In *stage 6*, pathology is extended to involve the sensory association areas of the neocortex and premotor areas.[12-14]

■ CLINICAL PRESENTATION
Primary Motor Symptoms
Rigidity

Rigidity is one of the clinical hallmarks of PD and is defined as increased resistance to passive motion. Patients frequently complain of "heaviness" and "stiffness" of their limbs. It is felt uniformly in both agonist and antagonist muscles and in movements in both directions. Spinal stretch reflexes are normal. Rigidity is fairly constant regardless of the task, amplitude, or speed of movement. Two types are identified: cogwheel or lead pipe. **Cogwheel rigidity** is a jerky, ratchet-like resistance to passive movement as muscles alternately tense and relax. It occurs when tremor coexists with rigidity. **Lead pipe rigidity** is a sustained resistance to passive movement, with no fluctuations. Rigidity is often asymmetrical, especially in the early stages of PD. It typically affects proximal muscles first, especially the shoulders and neck, and it progresses to involve muscles of the face and extremities. Rigidity may initially affect the left or right side, eventually spreading to involve the whole body. As the disease progresses, rigidity becomes more severe. Rigidity decreases the ability to move easily. For example, loss of bed mobility or lack of reciprocal arm swing during gait is often related to the degree of truncal rigidity. Active movement, mental concentration, or emotional stress may all increase rigidity. Prolonged rigidity results in decreased range of motion (ROM) and serious secondary complications of contracture and postural deformity. Rigidity also has a direct impact on increasing resting energy expenditure and fatigue levels.[9,10]

Bradykinesia

Bradykinesia refers to slowness of movement and is one of the cardinal features of PD. Weakness, tremor, and rigidity may contribute to bradykinesia but do not fully explain it. The principle deficit is the result of insufficient recruitment of muscle force during initiation of movement. Patients underscale movement commands in internally generated movements. The introduction of external cues (e.g., vision, sound) can partially ameliorate this and is used in treatment to guide movement. It is one of the most disabling symptoms of PD, with prolonged movement and reaction times resulting in increased time on task and dependence in daily activities. Slowness of thought, **bradyphrenia**, can contribute to bradykinesia.[15]

Akinesia refers to a poverty of spontaneous movement. For example, the patient with PD demonstrates **hypomimia** or masked facial expression, with significant social consequences. The absence of associated movements (e.g., arm swing during walking) or **freezing** (e.g., sudden stops in movement as in *freezing of gait [FOG]*) are other examples. Freezing episodes can be triggered by confrontation of competing stimuli. For example, the patient slows and stops walking (FOG) when exposed to a narrowed space or an obstacle. Freezing episodes are typically short-lived and usually can be overcome by attentional strategies or "behavioral tricks" using external cues (e.g., dropping a tissue initiates a stepping response). Stress can exacerbate freezing episodes. In advanced PD, freezing episodes can severely limit function and increase risk of falling. Akinesia can

be influenced by the degree of rigidity, as well as stage of disease, fluctuations in drug action, and disturbances in attention and depression.[9]

Hypokinesia refers to slowed and reduced movements and can also be seen in PD. For example, patients with moderate or severe PD typically present with handwriting that may start out strong but becomes smaller and smaller as writing proceeds (**micrographia**). During walking, rotational movements of the trunk with arm swing may also start out strong and decrease over time.

Tremor

Tremor, a third cardinal feature of PD, involves involuntary shaking or oscillating movement of a part or parts of the body resulting from contractions of opposing muscles. In the early stages of the disease, about 70% of patients experience a slight tremor of the hand or foot on one side of the body, or less commonly in the jaw or tongue. It tends to be mild and occurs for only short periods. The tremor is known as a *resting tremor* because it is present at rest, suppressed briefly by voluntary movement, and disappears with sleep. Tremor in the lower limbs is most apparent while the patient is supine. Tremor of the head and trunk, **postural tremor**, can be seen when muscles are used to maintain an upright posture against gravity. *Action tremor*, tremor that continues with movement, can occur in patients with advanced disease. Tremor tends to be less severe when the patient is relaxed and unoccupied. It is aggravated by emotional stress or excitement. In later stages tremor can become severe, spread to the other side, and interfere with activities of daily living (ADL). Fluctuations in frequency and intensity are common.[9]

Postural Instability

Individuals with PD demonstrate abnormalities of posture and balance, resulting in postural instability. These changes are rare in the early years (i.e., the first 5 years after diagnosis). As the disease progresses, a number of problems become evident across a broad spectrum of movement control. Patients demonstrate abnormal and inflexible postural responses controlling their center of mass (COM) within their base of support (BOS). Narrowing of the BOS (tandem stance or single-limb stance) or competing attentional demands (divided attention situations) increases postural instability. Patients also experience increased difficulty during dynamic destabilizing activities such as self-initiated movements (e.g., functional reach, walking, turning) and perform poorly under conditions of perturbed balance.[16] The response to instability is an abnormal pattern of coactivation, resulting in a rigid body and an inability to utilize normal postural synergies to recover balance.[17,18] Patients also demonstrate difficulty in regulating feed-forward, anticipatory adjustments of postural muscles during voluntary movements. Sensorimotor integration is impaired as evidenced by difficulty in adapting movement strategies to changing sensory conditions.[17] Visuospatial impairment has been identified in patients with advanced PD and correlates with lower scores in mobility.[19] Some patients are unable to perceive the upright or vertical position, which may indicate an abnormality in processing of vestibular, visual, and proprioceptive information contributing to balance. Contributing factors to postural instability include rigidity, decreased muscle torque production and weakness, loss of available ROM particularly of trunk motions, and axial rigidity. Medication side effects (e.g., postural hypotension and dyskinesias) also contribute.

Progressive development of postural deformity occurs. Weakness of antigravity muscles contributes to the adoption of a flexed, stooped posture with increased flexion of the neck, trunk, hips, and knees.[20] This results in a significant change in the center-of-alignment position, positioning the individual at the forward limits of stability. In the lower extremities (LEs), *contractures* develop in hip and knee flexors, hip rotators and adductors, and plantarflexors. In the spine, dorsal spine and neck flexors are involved, and in the upper extremities (UEs), shoulder adductors and internal rotators and elbow flexors are involved. Function becomes progressively more limited by these musculoskeletal constraints. Older individuals with reduced activity levels and poor diet are likely to develop *osteoporosis.*

Frequent falls and fall injury are the result of progressive disease. Falls are initially absent early in the disease, then become increasingly prevalent during the middle portion of disease progression, and as the patient becomes progressively immobile, disappear during late disease. About 70% of patients with PD report experiencing falls within the past year and 50% report recurrent falls. The rate of fall injury is about 40%. Although most injuries are not severe, some lead to hospitalization. Within 10 years of diagnosis, approximately 25% of patients will have developed a hip fracture. Disease severity, postural instability, and gait impairment including freezing are clearly linked to increased risk for falls.[21] Other risk factors include dementia, depression, postural hypotension, and involuntary movements associated with long-term use of anti-parkinsonian medication (dyskinesias).[22] Falls can lead to "fear of falling" with increasing levels of immobility and dependency with a deteriorating quality of life.[23]

Secondary Motor Symptoms
Muscle Performance

A reduction in strength is evident in patients with PD. Torque production is decreased at all speeds resulting in activity limitations and muscle weakness.[24-26] Changes in strength may be dopamine related as patients on dopamine replacement ("on" state) demonstrate increases in strength when compared to testing the same muscles during an "off" state.[27] Electromyography (EMG) studies reveal that motor unit recruitment is delayed with under-recruitment of muscles. Once initiated, contraction is characterized by multiple bursts and *asynchronization*, that is, pauses and an inability to smoothly increase firing rate as contraction continues.[28,29] These difficulties are compounded during the production of complex movements. As the disease progresses, disuse weakness evolves from inactivity and increases movement difficulties.

In patients with PD, *fatigue* is among the most common symptoms reported. The patient has difficulty in sustaining activity and experiences increasing weakness and lethargy as the day progresses. Repetitive motor acts may start out strong but decrease in strength and amplitude as the activity progresses. Performance decreases dramatically with great physical effort or stress. Rest or sleep may restore mobility. When L-dopa therapy is initiated, the patient may notice a dramatic improvement initially and feel significantly less fatigued. In long-standing disease and drug therapy, fatigue typically reappears. A common perception among patients is an increased sense of effort associated with movement that is manifested by difficulty activating and sustaining responses.

Motor Function

The striatum of the BG (caudate nucleus, putamen, and nucleus accumbens) receive input from all cortical areas and project throughout the thalamus to frontal lobe areas (prefrontal, premotor, and supplementary motor areas) concerned with motor planning. In PD, motor planning deficits are evident, involving a loss regulatory control of both automatic and voluntary movement responses directed through the pyramidal system.[30] Paucity of movement occurs with less accurate movements overall. This deficit in accuracy becomes more pronounced as the patient attempts to increase the speed of movement (**speed-accuracy trade-off**). This is a commonly observed problem in the elderly in general. Patients experience difficulty performing complex, sequential, or simultaneous movements (*dual-task control*). The difficulties combining tasks or shifting attentional sets from one to another can also be seen with cognitive tasks or when combining cognitive and motor tasks. Movement preparation (i.e., the when, where, and how to initiate movement) is significantly prolonged (a finding also seen with advancing age). This *start hesitation* is especially evident as the disease progresses.[31] For example, the patient is slow and hesitant in initiating movement during a transfer sequence.

Motor learning deficits are seen in patients with PD but are not universal. Learning of a new motor skills and fine-tuning of skills are intact at the early stage of PD for non-demented, medicated individuals. Retention tests may yield poorer performance but this is most likely due to problems in motor initiation than in actual retention. Deficits in motor skill learning have been demonstrated in advanced disease and for complex and sequential tasks. Thus, the processing requirements of the procedural task are critical in determining the degree of expected learning.

Learning is impaired with random presentations of stimulus conditions (random practice order) whereas blocked practice order reduces learning difficulty. Thus context interference degrades learning in patients with PD. Learning deficits can be expected to be severe if multiple motor programs are required either simultaneously or sequentially (i.e., switching among tasks). For example, the patient freezes up when asked to carry out another motor task while walking (*dual tasking*). Compounding variables that degrade learning include the severity of disease, dementia, and visual–perceptual deficits. Differences in learning can also be expected based on medication levels as motor learning is degraded when patients are in the "off" state of medication.[31-35]

Gait

Approximately 13% to 33% of patients present with postural instability and gait disturbances as their initial motor symptom and comprise a PIGD group. Gait disturbances are also a common feature of late-onset or advanced PD.[36] The patient with PD demonstrates a number of significant gait changes resulting from impoverished movement. There is a reduction in arm swing with asymmetry. An abnormal stooped posture contributes to development of a **festinating gait** pattern, characterized by a progressive increase in speed with a shortening of stride. Thus, the patient takes multiple short steps to catch up with his or her COM to avoid falling, and may eventually break into a run or trot. Gait can be *anteropulsive* (a forward festinating gait) or less commonly *retropulsive* (a backward festinating gait). Some patients are able to stop only when they come in contact with an object or a wall. Patients who are toe-walkers owing to plantarflexion contractures exhibit an additional postural instability from narrowing of their BOS. Turning or changing direction is particularly difficult and typically accomplished by taking multiple small steps. Problems with controlling posture and balance limit independence, community ambulation, and safety.[37-41] In early disease FOG is generally short in duration and rarely leads to falls. With disease progression FOG becomes more common and disabling, often leading to falls. Patients who are in the "off" state experience increased FOG and deterioration in gait performance whereas gait patterns improve when peak medication prevails.[42] Most patients with mild gait deficits can compensate at least partially using external cues and attentional strategies.

Nonmotor Symptoms

Sensory Symptoms

Patients with PD do not suffer from primary sensory loss. However, as many as 50% experience paresthesias and pain, including sensations of numbness, tingling, cold, aching pain, and burning. Pain may be due to the disease's effect on central nociception. Symptoms are typically intermittent, and vary in intensity and location. Some patients report their pain is linked to the motor fluctuations experienced during L-dopa therapy (e.g., pain is more intense in an "off" state). Pain may also be increased in patients experiencing depression.[43] It is also important to remember that some of the discomfort and pain can result from **postural stress syndrome** secondary to faulty posture, ligamentous strain, lack of movement, and muscle rigidity. For example, back pain may accompany a prolonged, stooped, kyphotic posture.

Proprioceptive regulation of voluntary movement may also be impaired. Patients with PD perform significantly worse than control subjects on tests of kinesthesia and proprioceptive position sense. Without visual guidance, patients demonstrate increased difficulty in accurately perceiving the extent of movement, consistently underscaling their movements. Deficits in visuospatial skills may also occur. Patients demonstrate significantly more errors than normal on visual perception tasks involving spatial organization.[44,45]

Olfactory dysfunction is common, with some studies showing up to 100% of patients affected. Most patients with PD report a decline or loss of sense of smell (**anosmia**), often years before motor symptoms develop. Loss of smell therefore has important implications for diagnosis of early disease. It also increases the difficulty individuals have in maintaining a healthy diet and adequate nutrition.[46]

Conventional drugs (e.g., anticholinergic drugs) used in PD can cause visual disturbances (e.g., blurred vision and sensitivity to light [photophobia]). These drugs can also worsen the normal visual changes associated with aging (presbyopia). Conjugate gaze and saccadic eye movements may also be impaired. Eye pursuit movements may have a jerky, cogwheeling quality. Decreased blinking can produce bloodshot, irritated eyes that burn and itch.

Dysphagia

Dysphagia, impaired swallowing, is present in as many as 95% of patients and is the result of rigidity, reduced mobility, and restricted range of movement.[47] It is often an early symptom of the disease though it is present in all stages. Individuals with PD experience problems in all four phases of swallowing: oral preparatory, oral, pharyngeal, and esophageal. Thus, the patient demonstrates abnormal tongue control and problems with chewing, bolus formation, delayed swallow response, and peristalsis. Dysphagia can lead to choking or aspiration pneumonia and impaired nutrition with significant weight loss. Nutritional inadequacy can contribute to the fatigue and exhaustion typically experienced by patients with PD.[48] Patients also typically experience excessive drooling (**sialorrhea**) as a result of increased saliva production and decreased spontaneous swallowing. Drooling is particularly problematic while sleeping or initiating speech and in advanced cases increases the risk of aspiration. Excessive drooling has important negative social implications.

Speech Disorders

Speech is impaired in 75% to 89% of patients and is the result of primary symptoms of PD (rigidity, bradykinesia, hypokinesia, and tremor).[47] Patients with PD experience **hypokinetic dysarthria**, which is characterized by decreased voice volume, monotone/monopitch speech, imprecise or distorted articulation, and uncontrolled speech rate. Vocal quality is degraded with speech described as hoarse, breathy, and harsh. In addition, patients experience timing difficulty of vocal onsets and offsets. Reduced mobility, restricted range, and uncontrolled rate of movement of muscles controlling respiration, phonation, resonation, and articulation are present. Reduced vital capacity results in reduced air expended during phonation. In advanced cases, the patient may speak in whispers or not at all, demonstrating **mutism**. Sensory problems may also contribute to speech difficulties. Patients who are instructed to upscale their speech sounds to produce increased volume consistently describe their speech as "too loud." Speech difficulties contribute to social isolation and impaired activity participation.[47,48]

Cognitive Dysfunction

Impairments in cognitive function can be mild (e.g., mildly impaired memory) or severe (e.g., psychosis). PD dementia occurs in approximately 20% to 40% of the patients. Older patients appear to be at greatest risk for dementia, with reported rates 4.4 times higher for individuals 80 years of age or older.[49] Dementia is associated with increased mortality rates. Coexisting Alzheimer's disease and multi-infarct dementia secondary to atherosclerotic disease are also common in the elderly and may be contributory factors in some patients. Dementia associated with PD is characterized by loss of executive functions (planning, reasoning, abstract thinking, judgment, and so forth) and changes in visuospatial skills, memory, and verbal fluency. **Bradyphrenia**, slowed thinking, is seen in patients with PD and may be one of the early nonspecific features of the disease. Cognitive performance is degraded in the "off" state. Hallucinations, delusions, and psychosis are common complications owing to L-dopa toxicity.

Depression and Anxiety

Depression is common in patients with PD. Major depression is reported to occur in approximately 40% of patients.[50] A significant number of patients develop depression before or just after onset of motor symptoms, suggesting an endogenous cause that may be related to underlying deficiencies of dopamine, serotonin, and norepinephrine. Patients demonstrate a variety of symptoms, including feelings of guilt, hopelessness, and worthlessness; loss of energy; poor concentration; deficits in short-term memory; loss of ambition or enthusiasm; and disturbances in appetite and sleep. Suicidal thoughts may also be present. **Hypomimia**, a reduction in facial expressiveness, can give the appearance of depression. Patients can also demonstrate **dysthymic disorder** characterized by chronic depression and dysphoric mood, resulting in poor appetite or overeating, insomnia or hypersomnia, low energy, low self-esteem, and poor concentration.

Anxiety is a common symptom in PD, occurring in up to 38% of patients. Clinically patients may present with symptoms of a panic attack (e.g., palpitations, sweating, trembling, shortness of breath, and so forth) as well as social phobia (social withdrawal), agoraphobia, obsessive-compulsive disorder, or panic disorder. Anxiety symptoms may not be simply related to the psychological or social difficulties patients experience, but due to specific neurobiological processes associated with the disease. Patients who are in the "off" medication state experience significant worsening of depression and anxiety.[51]

Autonomic Dysfunction

Autonomic dysfunction occurs with PD and is a direct manifestation of the disease, as evidenced by the presence of Lewy bodies found in the autonomic nervous system.[52] Thermoregulatory dysfunction includes excessive sweating and abnormal or uncomfortable sensations of warmth and coldness. Patients in the "off" state experience impaired peripheral vasodilation with difficulty dissipating body heat. *Seborrhea* (increased oil secretion of the sebaceous glands of the skin) and *seborrheic dermatitis* (oily, chafing, and reddened skin) are also common. Patients with PD exhibit abnormally slow pupillary responses to light and pain and reduced overall response to changes in light.[53]

Gastrointestinal disorders include poor motility, changes in appetite, inadequate hydration, sialorrhea, and weight loss. *Constipation* is a common problem for most patients and typically occurs early in PD. *Urinary incontinence* occurs with associated symptoms of urinary frequency, urgency, and nocturia. Many of these problems occur in the aging population in general and in men with benign prostatic hypertrophy. *Erectile dysfunction* is often present in males, including impotence and reduced rates of sexual activity.[53]

Early and progressive sympathetic denervation of the heart occurs in the majority of patients with PD. This results in diminished heart function, which may be a contributory factor to the fatigue that most patients experience.[53] Patients with advanced PD exhibit altered heart rate (HR) and blood pressure (BP) during exercise with decreased exercise efficiency.[54] Patients with mild to moderate PD do not appear to demonstrate significantly different exercise capacity (maximal HR, maximal oxygen consumption) when compared to age-matched controls. However, these patients did demonstrate decreased peak power and higher submaximal HRs and oxygen consumption rates than controls.[55-57]

Orthostatic hypotension (OH) is common in middle and late PD and is caused by a sharp drop in BP that occurs with position changes (e.g., supine-to-sit or sit-to-stand). Typical symptoms include lightheadedness or dizziness. Patients can also experience pallor, diaphoresis, weakness, trembling, nausea, difficulty thinking, or syncope. The condition puts individuals at risk for loss of balance, falls, and fall injury. Medications (e.g., levodopa/carbidopa, bromocriptine) can contribute to orthostatic hypotension.[53]

Patients with PD demonstrate respiratory impairments, reported in as many as 84% of patients. *Airway obstruction* (e.g., air trapping, lung insufflation) is the most frequently reported pulmonary problem and has been linked to episodes of pulmonary failure. The etiology remains unknown but may be linked to bradykinetic disorganization of respiratory movements. *Restrictive lung dysfunction* is common and is linked to the decreased chest expansion that occurs as a result of rigidity of the trunk muscles, loss of musculoskeletal flexibility, and kyphotic posture. Patients with PD demonstrate lower forced vital capacity (FVC), lower forced expiratory volume in 1 second (FEV$_1$), and higher residual volume (RV) and residual airway resistance (RAW) values when compared to age-matched controls. Daily function and activity participation are reduced in patients with pulmonary dysfunction.[58,59] A sedentary lifestyle with decreased activity levels contributes to cardiopulmonary deconditioning.

In long-standing disease, the LEs may exhibit circulatory changes owing to venous pooling as a result of decreased mobility and prolonged sitting. Thus, patients can present with mild to moderate edema of the feet and ankles, which usually subsides during sleep.

Sleep Disorders

Individuals with PD can experience *excessive daytime somnolence* (sleepiness). At night, *insomnia* (disturbed sleep pattern) may occur. This includes problems in falling asleep, staying asleep, and good quality of sleep. REM sleep behavior disorder (RBD) occurs early in PD and affects as many as 50% to 60% of patients. In a person with RBD, the paralysis that normally occurs during REM sleep is incomplete or absent, allowing the person to "act out" his or her dreams that are vivid, intense, and violent. Dream-enacting behaviors include agitation and physical activity during sleep (e.g., talking, yelling, punching, kicking, arm flailing, and grabbing).[60,61] Box 18.2 provides a summary of the cardinal features and clinical manifestations of PD.

■ MEDICAL DIAGNOSIS

Diagnosis at onset of PD is difficult with accurate diagnosis possible only with continued observation of evolving clinical signs and symptoms. There is no single definitive test or group of tests used to diagnose the disease. The diagnosis is made on the basis of history and clinical examination.

Handwriting samples, speech analysis, interview questions that focus on developing symptoms, and physical examination are used. In the preclinical stage, nonmotor symptoms predominate. There is an increasing focus on use of questionnaires and tests (e.g., olfactory testing, imaging of cardiac sympathetic innervation) that focus on emerging nonmotor symptoms.[62-64] Often symptoms of loss of smell, sleep disturbances, vivid dreams with REM alterations, foot dystonia and foot cramping similar to restless legs syndrome, orthostatic hypotension, and constipation are symptoms that are present many years before an official diagnoses of PD is made. A diagnosis of PD is typically made if at least two of the four cardinal motor features are present. Exclusion of Parkinson-plus syndromes is necessary. The presence of extrapyramidal signs that are bilaterally symmetrical and do not respond to L-dopa and dopamine agonists (apomorphine test) is suggestive of these syndromes, not PD. Imaging can be used to rule out other pathologies. In vivo functional imaging (magnetic resonance imaging [MRI]) using chemical markers to identify dopaminergic deficits in PD and related disorders identifies dopamine deficiency but does not discriminate between PD and other causes of parkinsonism.[65]

■ CLINICAL COURSE

The disease is progressive, with a long subclinical period (without apparent clinical manifestations) estimated to be at least 5 years. Mean PD duration is approximately 13 years. There is variability of the rate of progression. Patients with a young age at onset or who are tremor predominant typically demonstrate a more benign progression. Patients with PD who present with postural instability and gait disturbances (the PIGD group) tend to have more pronounced deterioration with a more rapid disease progression. Neurobehavioral disturbances and dementia are also more common in this group. With L-dopa therapy, progression is generally slower with an overall improvement in mortality rates. The most common causes of death are cardiovascular disease and pneumonia.[65]

Hoehn-Yahr Classification of Disability Scale

An estimate of the stage and severity of the disease can be made using a staging scale. The most widely used in clinical practice and research trials is the *Hoehn-Yahr Classification of Disability Scale* (Table 18.1).[66] It provides a broad measure for charting the progression of the disease using motor signs and elements of functional status. Stage I is used to indicate minimal disease involvement, whereas stage V is indicative of severe deterioration in which the patient is confined to bed or a wheelchair.[67]

Unified Parkinson's Disease Rating Scale (UPDRS)

The *Unified Parkinson's Disease Rating Scale (UPDRS)* has been the "gold standard" for measuring the progression

Box 18.2 Cardinal Features and Clinical Manifestations of Parkinson's Disease

Cardinal Features

Rigidity
Bradykinesia
Tremor
Postural instability

Clinical Manifestations

Motor Performance
Decreased torque production
Fatigue
Contractures and deformity common
Masked face
Micrographia

Motor Planning
Start hesitation
Freezing episodes
Poverty of movement

Motor Learning
Slower learning rates, reduced efficiency
Increased context-specificity of learning.
Procedural learning deficits for complex and sequential
   tasks

Gait
Reduced stride length; increased step-to-step variability
Reduced speed of walking
Cadence (steps per minute) typically intact; may be
   reduced in advanced PD
Increased time: double-limb support
Insufficient hip, knee, and ankle flexion: shuffling steps
Insufficient heel strike with increased forefoot loading
Reduced trunk rotation: decreased or absent arm swing
Festinating gait: anteropulsion common
Freezing of gait (FOG)
Difficulty turning: increased steps per turn
Difficulty with dual tasking: simultaneous motor and/or
   cognitive tasks
Difficulty with attentional demands of complex
   environments

Posture
Kyphosis with forward head
Leaning to one side with tonal asymmetries
Increased fall risk

Sensation
Paresthesias
Pain
Akathisia

Speech, Voice, and Swallowing Disorders
Hypokinetic dysarthria
Dysphagia

Cognition Function and Behavior
Dementia
Bradyphrenia
Visuospatial deficits
Depression
Dysphoric mood

Autonomic Nervous System
Excessive sweating
Abnormal sensations of heat and cold
Seborrhea
Sialorrhea
Constipation
Urinary bladder dysfunction

Cardiopulmonary Function
Low resting blood pressure (BP)
Compromised cardiovascular response to exercise
Impaired respiratory function

---

of PD since 1987.[68] The original UPDRS was composed of four parts: Part I, Mentation, Behavior, and Mood; Part II, Activities of Daily Living; Part III, Motor Examination; and Part IV, Complications of Therapy. Goetz and colleagues reported on a modification of this scale renamed the Movement Disorder Society–sponsored revision of the Unified Parkinson's Disease Rating Scale (MDS-UPDRS).[69-71] The goals of the revision were to improve ability to detect slower and smaller changes in mildly disabled patients and increase focus on nonmotor symptoms. It retains the 4-part structure with substantial reworking of questions and an additional 6 items (most on nonmotor aspects of PD),

bringing the total to 48. A four-point scale is used for all items (as opposed to some items graded as 0, no, or 1, yes, in the original scale). A score of 0 means normal or no problems; 1, minimal problems; 2, mild problems; 3, moderate problems; and 4, severe problems. Descriptors are added for each question. Parts I and II have been renamed: Part I is now *Non-motor Aspects of Experiences of Daily Living* and Part II is now *Motor Experiences of Daily Living*. Part III is *Motor Examination* (same title) and Part IV is renamed *Motor Complications*.[70] The total time to administer the test is an estimated 30 minutes, with Parts I and II designed to be self-administered by the patient. See Appendix 18.A.

Table 18.1	Hoehn-Yahr Classification of Disability
Stage	**Character of Disability**
I	Minimal or absent; unilateral if present.
II	Minimal bilateral or midline involvement. Balance not impaired.
III	Impaired righting reflexes. Unsteadiness when turning or rising from chair. Some activities are restricted, but patient can live independently and continue some forms of employment.
IV	All symptoms present and severe. Standing and walking possible only with assistance.
V	Confined to bed or wheelchair.

From Hoehn and Yahr,[66, p. 433] with permission.

■ MEDICAL MANAGEMENT

Medical management is directed at slowing disease progression using neuroprotective strategies, and symptomatic treatment of motor and nonmotor symptoms. Management becomes increasingly more challenging over time for patients with moderate and advanced disease (i.e., Stage III or higher on the Hoehn-Yahr Classification of Disability Scale).[72-76]

Pharmacological Management

A number of agents are available as first-line neuroprotective and symptomatic therapy. Selection is individualized according to the patient's characteristics with the benefits and risks of adverse side effects carefully weighed. Starting medication early has been shown to be beneficial in slowing the progression of the disease. Drug delivery should be as close to constant as possible to avoid large peaks and valleys. The importance of taking the medication on a fixed schedule should be stressed to patients, family members, and caregivers. When patients with PD are hospitalized it is important that they continue to receive their medication on schedule.[77] Currently three out of four patients with PD do not receive their medications on time when they are in a hospital setting. Sixty-one percent of patients who did not receive their medications on time had serious complications.[78] The *Aware in Care kit* from the National Parkinson Foundation can be helpful in avoiding these complications (www.awareincare.org).

Levodopa/Carbidopa

Levodopa/carbidopa (Sinemet) is the gold standard drug therapy for PD. Levodopa (L-dopa) was first introduced in 1961 as an experimental drug and came into widespread clinical use in the late 1960s. It is a dopamine precursor that is metabolized to dopamine in the brain.

Thus, administration of the drug represents an attempt to correct the essential neurochemical imbalance. Most of L-dopa (almost 99%) is metabolized before reaching the brain, requiring administration of high doses that can produce numerous side effects. Today, L-dopa is commonly administered with carbidopa, a decarboxylase inhibitor that allows a higher percentage of L-dopa to enter the brain. Thus, lower doses of L-dopa can be used with fewer adverse side effects. Sinemet is available in immediate-release (IR) and controlled-release (CR) formulations. The IR form has a short half-life requiring multiple oral dosing throughout the day. The CR form is a long-acting, sustained-release preparation. Both are equally effective.[79,80]

The primary benefits of dopamine replacement include controlling the PD motor symptoms of bradykinesia and rigidity. Increased movement velocity, initial burst of motor activity, and increased strength are all positive outcomes.[80] The effects on reduction of tremor are more varied. Some individuals demonstrate little or no response whereas others demonstrate a positive reduction in tremor amplitude. It does not appear to have a direct impact on postural instability. The decision about when to start levodopa/carbidopa is determined by the neurologist and is different for every person. Initial dosing improves low levels of levodopa often with dramatic improvements in functional status. This is sometimes referred to as the *honeymoon period,* in which there is clear-cut drug effectiveness.

There are numerous *adverse effects* of dopamine replacement therapy. For many patients the typical therapeutic window is 4 to 6 years before optimal benefit wears off (termed *wearing-off state*). At this point, a significant number of patients experience disabling dyskinesias, dystonia, and motor fluctuations. **Dyskinesias** are dynamic uncontrolled or involuntary movements that occur typically at peak L-dopa dose or when the patient is transitioning between "on" and "off" states. The movements are choreo-athetotic in quality and may initially appear as facial grimacing with twitching of the lips and tongue protrusion. With time the involuntary movements become more prevalent, vigorous, and more extensive, involving the limbs, trunk, and neck. Dyskinesias are estimated to develop and increase at a rate of 10% per year following start of dopamine therapy. **Dystonia,** a prolonged involuntary contraction that causes twisting or torsion of body segments, can also occur. The patient typically complains of clawing of the toes or fingers, or cramping of the calf, neck, face, or paraspinal muscles. Dystonia is associated with pain and occurs typically during "off" periods. Motor fluctuations include both the "on–off" phenomenon and wearing-off. The term **"on–off" phenomenon** refers to abrupt, random fluctuations in motor performance and responses. Production of movement errors is common. *Wearing-off* refers to

end-of-dose deterioration, a worsening of symptoms toward the end of the expected timeframe of medication effectiveness.[79] Patients may experience **akathisia**, a motor restlessness. In general, they experience an intolerance of inactivity (sitting still) and experience significant disruptions in sleep and relaxation. This affects as many as 25% of patients and is relieved with movement (e.g., walking). Akathisia is associated with advanced PD and is more commonly seen in the "off" state.

Deprenyl can be administered with levodopa/carbidopa to control mild wearing-off phenomena. Unsupervised reduction or sudden discontinuation of levodopa/carbidopa is contraindicated and may produce dangerous, life-threatening adverse effects. Adverse interactions can occur with several medications, including antacids, antiseizure drugs, antihypertensives, and antidepressants.[80]

Patients may also experience other changes that are dose related and may indicate the need for drug modification. These include (1) disabling psychiatric toxicity (visual hallucinations, delusions, and paranoia); (2) depression; (3) gastrointestinal changes (nausea, dry mouth); (4) cardiovascular changes (hypotension, dizziness, arrhythmias); (5) genitourinary changes (dysuria); and (6) sleep disturbances (insomnia, sleep fragmentation).[79,80]

Dopamine Agonists

Dopamine agonists (DAs) are a class of drugs designed to directly stimulate postsynaptic dopamine receptors. They are administered alone as a first-line monotherapy or along with levodopa/carbidopa, allowing lower doses to be administered with prolonged effectiveness (i.e., L-dopa–sparing therapy). Patients with moderate to advanced PD who demonstrate declining responses to levodopa/carbidopa therapy may benefit. The most commonly prescribed DA drugs include ropinirole (Requip) and pramipexole (Mirapex); bromocriptine (Parlodel) is less commonly used. The greatest benefit of these drugs is reducing rigidity, bradykinesia, and motor fluctuations. Adverse effects are similar to those of L-dopa with nausea, sedation, dizziness, constipation, and hallucinations being the most common. These medications have also been linked to an increased risk of impulse control disorders (e.g., pathological gambling, compulsive shopping, hypersexuality, overeating).[80]

Anticholinergics

Anticholinergic agents may be used in early PD or as an adjunct for patients on carbidopa/levodopa. They block cholinergic function and have the most benefit moderating tremor and the dystonia that may accompany the wearing-off; they have little or no effect on other PD symptoms. The drugs commonly prescribed in this group include trihexyphenidyl (Artane) and benztropine mesylate (Cogentin). Anticholinergic adverse effects include blurred vision, dry mouth,

dizziness, and urinary retention. Central toxicity is indicated by impaired memory, confusion, hallucinations, and delusions.[80]

Monoamine Oxidase B Inhibitors

Monoamine oxidase B (MAO-B) is the major enzyme that acts to degrade dopamine in the brain. MAO-B inhibitors include selegiline, also called deprenyl (Eldepryl) and rasagiline (Azilect). Patients in the early stages of PD may be given MAO-B inhibitors to enhance levels of dopamine. Clinically, early monotherapy treatment with selegiline has been shown to have a modest effect in slowing, but not halting, disease progression. Once L-dopa therapy is started, selegiline in combination improves symptom control and permits a lower dose to be used. MAO-B inhibitors have a low risk of dyskinesias. There are few adverse effects, including mild nausea, dry mouth, dizziness, orthostatic hypotension, confusion, hallucinations, and insomnia.[80]

Implications for the Physical Therapist

The therapist needs to be fully aware of each of the medications the patient is taking and potential adverse effects. It is important to remember that patients on dopamine replacement will develop motor complications at some point. Optimal performance can be expected at peak dosage whereas worsening performance is associated with end-of-dose cycle and medication depletion.[81] Timing of physical therapy examination and intervention should be consistent and occur whenever possible during optimal dosing cycle. Therapists are involved in monitoring drug effectiveness on motor performance, function, and activity participation. As the disease progresses, patients may develop an intolerance for a particular medication, necessitating a change in prescription. Often, it is the therapist who first notices a change in functional status as the patient's system adapts to either the amount or type of drug prescribed. Accurate observation, examination, and reporting of these changes greatly assists the physician in modifying a drug prescription. Therapists may also be involved with clinical drug trials as new medications or combinations are developed. Table 18.2 presents an overview of the pharmacology of PD.

Nutritional Management

A high-protein diet can block the effectiveness of L-dopa. The dietary amino acids in protein compete with L-dopa absorption. This is particularly problematic in patients with chronic disease who exhibit fluctuations in motor performance. Thus, patients are generally advised to follow a high-calorie, low-protein diet. Generally no more than 15% of calories should come from protein. Dietary recommendations may also include shifting the intake of daily protein to the evening meal when patients are less active. These modifications

Table 18.2   Pharmacology of Parkinson's Disease[80]

Drug Class	Example	Average Dosage	Possible Adverse Effects
Anticholinergics	Trihexyphenidyl	2 mg tid	Dry mouth, dizziness, blurred vision
	Bentropin	1 mg bid	Tachycardia, dry mouth, nausea, vomiting, confusion
Dopamine replacement	Levodopa/carbidopa (generic)	10 mg /100 mg tid/qid	Dystonia
		25 mg/100 mg tid/qid	Abnormal, involuntary movements
	Sinemet	25 mg/250 mg tid	Nausea, vomiting
	Sinemet CR (controlled release)	25 mg/100 mg tid	Confusion
		25 mg/200 mg bid	Dreams, hallucinations
Dopamine agonists	Pergolide	1 mg tid	Nervousness, dyskinesias, insomnia, hallucinations, nausea, confusion, erythromelalgia
	Bromocriptine	5 mg bid	Nausea, headache, dizziness, fatigue, cramps/constipation, confusion, pulmonary/peritoneal fibrosis
Amantadine	Symadine	100 mg bid	Lightheadedness, livedo reticularis, edema

bid = twice a day; mg = milligram; tid = three times a day; qid = four times a day.

minimize motor fluctuations and maximize responsiveness to L-dopa therapy. The patient is encouraged to eat a variety of foods and may be advised to take dietary supplements to ensure adequate intake of vitamins and minerals. Patients are also advised to increase their daily intake of water and dietary fiber to help control problems of constipation.[76]

Rigidity and bradykinesia can limit upright posture and UE feeding movements. Learned motor plans, for example, using a cup or eating utensils, may also be difficult. Occupational therapy intervention to improve feeding and recommend adaptive eating devices is of considerable importance in helping to maintain nutrition and general health status. The speech-language pathologist also has an important role in the evaluation of dysphagia and the recommendation of strategies to assist with swallowing dysfunction. Patient, family, and caregiver education should focus on the importance of maintaining good nutritional intake. Percutaneous endoscopic gastrostomy (PEG) is reserved for advanced disease when all other strategies for dysphagia fail.

Deep Brain Stimulation

Deep brain stimulation (DBS) involves the implantation of electrodes into the brain where they block nerve signals that cause symptoms. Brain electrodes are placed in the subthalamic nucleus (STN) or less frequently the globus pallidus (GPi). An impulse generator (IPG), similar to a pacemaker, is implanted in the subclavicular area and a thin wire goes under the skin to connect to the brain electrodes. High-frequency stimulation is provided. The patient can control the pacemaker's "on–off" switch using a controller while the physician determines the

amount of stimulation it delivers, tailoring it to the individual's needs.[82]

DBS is effective for the treatment of advanced PD. Improvement of tremor that is refractory to pharmacological therapy is seen in approximately 90% of patients with one-third to one-half of patients experiencing total suppression with DBS of the STN. DBS has been shown to successfully control PD symptoms of motor overactivity (dyskinesias), substantially increase "on" time, and improve ADL scores. DBS has also been shown to reduce the medication requirements and is a treatment of choice in patients with medication-resistant motor fluctuations and dyskinesia. Other motor symptoms of akinesia, rigidity, weakness, and reduced walking speed may improve with DBS though the responses are more variable. Possible adverse effects include confusion, headache, speech problems, gait disturbances, and falling. Most of the complications are temporary and resolve within 6 months. Surgical risks (intracerebral hemorrhage, infection) and mechanical problems with the device (lead breakage, generator malfunction) are also possible. Deep brain stimulation has largely replaced stereotaxic surgical procedures of the brain (thalamotomy and pallidotomy).[82-86]

■ FRAMEWORK FOR REHABILITATION

Rehabilitation has an important role in reducing activity limitations while promoting activity participation and independence. In addition, known complications of PD can be reduced or prevented while quality of life is promoted. Optimal management involves a coordinated interdisciplinary team to oversee a comprehensive plan of care to address the patient's individual clinical problems, concerns, and needs. The team typically includes the physician, nurse, physical therapist, occupational therapist, speech-language pathologist, and social worker. Referral to other specialists may also be necessary, for example, psychologist, nutritionist, gastroenterologist, urologist, pulmonologist, and so forth. As with any team, the patient is the central figure with family and caregivers being key members.

The ideal rehabilitation program considers the patient's disease history, course, and symptoms, together with impairments, activity limitations, and participation restrictions. Of equal importance are the patient's abilities (assets), priorities, and resources, including family, home, and community resources. Deterioration of condition and medication-induced fluctuations in performance should be expected. Depression and anxiety are common and should be carefully monitored. The overall focus is on long-range planning, with anticipated episodes of care including hospital-based, outpatient, and home/community-based care.

Therapeutic Care Continuum

A therapeutic care continuum based on disease stage (early, middle, late) is an effective way to organize care. Interventions are restorative (aimed at improving impairments, activity limitations, and participation restrictions), preventative (aimed at minimizing potential complications and indirect impairments), and compensatory (aimed at modifying the task, activity, or environment to improve function) (see discussion in Chapter 1). It is critical for the whole team to provide a supportive environment to assist patients and their family members in the difficult adjustment to living with a chronic and progressive disease.

In the *early* stage of the disease, patients are functional and independent with minimal impairments. A referral for physical therapy is often delayed at this stage, although benefits could clearly be obtained in improving fitness levels and delaying or preventing indirect impairments. Patients are typically seen on an outpatient basis.

During the *middle* stage of the disease, symptoms are more readily apparent and activity limitations emerge. The patient may still be independent in gait and ADL, although performance is slowed and less efficient. Some assistance may be required. The patient may be seen as an outpatient, during home care, or during a brief inpatient admission. There are numerous benefits to rehabilitation services. Exercise training programs have been shown to be effective for patients with mild to moderate PD in improving motor performance.[87-93] Perceived quality of life and subjective well-being are also improved.[94] Family and caregiver instruction is intensified to assist the patient in remaining as functionally independent as possible.

In the *late* stage, disease progression leads to increased and more severe impairments and complications. Patients are dependent in many or most of their daily functional

mobility skills and ADL and are typically wheelchair bound or bedridden. Family and community resources are vital in maintaining the patient in the home. Some patients may require placement in a chronic care facility. These changes can be a source of great anxiety and frustration to the patient and family. Goals need to be restructured. The therapist needs to focus on preventative care to avoid secondary complications that may be life threatening (e.g., pneumonia, pressure ulcers, and so forth). Compensatory training focuses on maintaining function, including being upright and out of bed as much as possible. Safety for both the caregiver and the patient becomes a primary concern as maximal assist dependent transfers become the norm. Often, environmental adaptations may mean the difference between total dependence and modified dependence. The rehabilitation team should be supportive of the patient's efforts no matter how small they may be. Patients in late-stage PD demonstrate extremely limited skills to interact with their environment, with increasing social isolation and withdrawal. Families also suffer from the increasing demands of care, burnout, and social isolation. Therapists need to maximize psychosocial support and be readily available for consultation. Table 18.3 presents an overview of Parkinson's disease stages and intervention strategies.

The preferred practice pattern for patients with PD from the *Guide to Physical Therapist Practice* is 5E, *Impaired Motor Function and Sensory Integrity Associated with Progressive Disorders of the Central Nervous System—Acquired in Adolescence or Adulthood.*[97, p. 375] In this document the reader will find relevant information on patient/client diagnostic classification; ICD-9-CM codes; examination components; considerations for evaluation, diagnosis, and prognosis; and suggested interventions. Thus, the *Guide to Physical Therapist Practice* serves as a primary resource in designing an appropriate plan of care (POC) and documenting the services provided and outcomes achieved.

■ PHYSICAL THERAPY EXAMINATION AND EVALUATION

A comprehensive examination is required to determine the level of impairments and degree of function. Subsequent reexamination at specified intervals is used to distinguish change in status as well as effects of treatment. Data are obtained from the history, systems review, and relevant tests and measures (Box 18.3).[97] The selection of examination procedures and instruments is determined by the patient's unique status. The severity of problems, stage of disease, age, phase and setting of rehabilitation, and other factors must all be taken into account in structuring the examination and evaluating data. During the early and middle stages of PD, measures of impairment and physical performance are relatively stable. During late stages of the disease and under conditions of fluctuating symptoms with pharmacological instability, measures can be expected to be less stable.[98]

Table 18.3   Parkinson's Disease Stages, Common Impairments and Activity Limitations, and Intervention Strategies

Stage	Common Impairments and Activity Limitations	Intervention Strategies
Early/Mild PD	• Few/minimal impairments and activity limitations with independence maintained • Movement symptoms present but do not interfere with daily activities • Movement symptoms, often tremor, occur on one side of the body • Changes noted in posture, walking ability, or facial expression • Parkinson's medications effectively suppress movement symptoms	***Preventative and Restorative*** • Regular exercise to improve/maintain motor performance, strength, mobility, flexibility, range of motion (ROM), balance, locomotion, endurance, and perceived quality of life • Community classes to improve/maintain socialization, camaraderie, positive outlook and life purpose ***Compensatory*** • Patient/family/caregiver education about disease process, rehabilitation, energy conservation • Determine need for adaptive or assistive devices • Determine need for environmental modification of home/workplace • Provide psychological support with early referral to support groups for patient and family/caregiver • Referral to other health care professionals as needed
Middle/ Moderate PD	• Increasing number and severity of impairments • Minimal to moderate activity limitations, participation restrictions • Movement symptoms occur on both sides of the body • The body moves more slowly against increasing stiffness • ADL with modified dependence (assistance) • Difficulty with balance, postural instability; stooped posture; increasing number of falls • Gait impairments evident; freezing episodes may occur • Locomotion with modified dependence (assistance) • Parkinson's medications may "wear off" between doses • Parkinson's medications may cause side effects, including dyskinesias	***Preventative and Restorative*** • Regular exercise to maintain/improve motor performance, strength, mobility, flexibility, ROM, balance, locomotion, endurance, and perceived quality of life • Community classes to improve/maintain socialization, camaraderie, positive outlook and life purpose ***Compensatory*** • Assistive devices to maintain function • Wheelchair for community mobility • Environmental modifications to home • Patient/family/caregiver education and training • Psychological support for patient and family/caregiver • Referral to other healthcare professionals as needed; occupational therapy may provide strategies for maintaining independence

Late/ Advanced PD	• Numerous impairments with increasing severity
	• Severe activity limitations with dependence in most activities:
	• Great difficulty walking; typically in wheelchair or bed most of the day
	• Assistance needed with all ADL
	• Severe participation restrictions:
	  • Not able to live alone
	  • Typically requires full time assistance or placement in chronic care facility
	• Social interactions restricted
	• Cognitive problems may be prominent, including dementia, hallucinations and delusions
	• Increasing medication intolerance with dyskinesias
	• Balancing the benefits of medications with their side effects becomes more challenging
		Preventive
		• Maximize upright posture, out-of-bed time
		• Maximize participation in activities of daily living
		• Prevention of contractures, pressure wounds, pneumonia, and so forth
		Compensatory
		• Family/caregiver education and training: safety education, transfers, positioning, turning, skin care
		• Pressure relieving devices
		• Hospital bed, wheelchair, mechanical lift
		• Psychological support for patient and family/caregiver
		• Referral to other healthcare professionals as needed

Adapted from Dal Bello-Haas[95] and Cutson et al.[96]

Box 18.3   Elements of the Examination for a Patient with Parkinson's Disease[97]

Patient/Client History

- Age, sex, race/ethnicity, primary language, education
- Social history: cultural beliefs and behaviors, family and caregiver resources, social support systems
- Occupation/employment/work
- Living environment: home/work barriers
- Hand dominance
- General health status: physical, psychological, social, and role function, health habits
- Family history
- Medical/surgical history
- Current conditions/chief complaints
- Medications
- Medical/laboratory test results
- Functional status and activity level: premorbid and current

Systems Review

- Neuromuscular
- Musculoskeletal
- Cardiovascular/pulmonary
- Integumentary

Tests and Measures/Impairments

- Cognition: mental status, memory: hesitation, slowness of thought processes
- Oromotor function: communication (fluctuations, reduced volume), swallowing
- Psychosocial function: motivation, anxiety, depression
- Anthropometric characteristics: body mass index, girth, length; edema
- Circulation: response to position change, orthostatic hypotension
- Aerobic capacity and endurance: during functional activities and standardized exercise protocols including cardiovascular and pulmonary signs and symptoms
- Ventilation and gas exchange
- Integumentary integrity: skin condition, pressure-sensitive areas; activities, positioning, and postures to relieve pressure
- Autonomic nervous system integrity: thermal responses, sweating
- Sensory integrity and integration
- Pain: intensity and location
- Perceptual function: visuospatial skills
- Joint integrity, alignment, and mobility: range of motion (active and passive); muscle length, and soft tissue extensibility
- Posture: alignment and position, symmetry (static and dynamic); ergonomics, and body mechanics
- Muscle performance: strength, power, and endurance
- Motor function: motor control and motor learning: tone, voluntary movement patterns; involuntary movements; hesitation, slowness, arrests of movements; poverty of movements
- Procedural learning for complex and sequential tasks
- Postural control and balance: degree of postural instability, balance strategies; safety
- Gait and locomotion: gait pattern and speed, safety
- Functional status and activity level: performance-based examination of functional skills (FIM level), basic and instrumental ADL; functional mobility skills; home management skills
- Assistive or adaptive devices: fit, alignment, function, use; safety
- Environment, home, and work barriers
- Work, community, and leisure activities: ability to participate in activities, safety

---

This section presents strategies for examination as well as relevant tests and measures. Complete descriptions of many of the tests and measures identified are provided in earlier chapters focusing on examination.

Cognitive Function

Memory, orientation, conceptual reasoning, problem solving, and judgment should be examined. Speed of information processing, attention, and concentration are particularly important to determine if bradyphrenia is suspected. A brief screen of cognitive function can be obtained using the *Mini-Mental Status Examination (MMSE).*[99]

Psychosocial Function

The therapist should determine overall levels of depression, stress and anxiety, and available coping strategies. It is important to ask the patient about the presence of depressive symptoms such as sadness, apathy, passivity, insomnia, anorexia, weight loss, inactivity and dependency, inability to concentrate and impaired memory, or suicidal ideation. Useful instruments include the *Geriatric Depression Scale*[100] and the *Beck Depression Inventory.*[101] Anxiety is prevalent and disabling in this patient population. The *Hospital Anxiety and Depression Scale* is reliable in detecting and grading the severity of depression and anxiety in the hospital setting.[102,103]

Sensory Function

A screening examination of sensation is indicated (superficial and deep sensations, combined cortical sensations). Sensory changes can be expected with aging (blunting of touch sensations and proprioception with greater losses in LEs than UEs, and distal more than proximal). Specific areas of sensory loss may be indicative of co-morbid pathology, for example, stroke, diabetic neuropathy, and so forth. The patient with PD should be asked about the presence of paresthesias (sensations of numbness or tingling) and pain. Mild aching and cramplike sensations are common and are often poorly localized. It is important to examine for musculoskeletal aches and pains linked to lack of movement, faulty movements or posture, and ligamentous strain.

An examination of vision should include a determination of acuity, peripheral vision, tracking, accommodation, light and dark adaptation, and depth perception. Visual changes can be expected with aging such as loss of visual acuity, inability to focus on printed word (presbyopia), decreased adaptation to light, sensitivity to light and glare, and loss of color discrimination. Patients with PD may experience blurring of vision and difficulty reading not improved by corrective lenses, as well as problems with eye pursuit (cogwheeling). Specific deficits may be indicative of co-morbid pathologies that are common in the elderly, such as cataracts (clouding of central vision first, then peripheral), glaucoma (early loss of peripheral vision), senile macular degeneration or diabetic retinopathy (early loss of central vision), and cerebrovascular accident (homonymous hemianopsia). Medications may also produce impaired or fuzzy vision, for example, antidepressants and anticholinergics.

Musculoskeletal Function
Joint Flexibility and Posture

An examination of musculoskeletal ROM and flexibility is important. The therapist can document specific active range of motion (AROM) and passive range of motion (PROM) impairments using goniometric measurement. Patients with PD are likely to present with losses in hip and knee extension, dorsiflexion, shoulder flexion, elbow extension, dorsal spine and neck extension, and axial rotation. To a lesser extent, these impairments are also generalizable to the geriatric population.

It is particularly important to examine spinal ROM (ability to rotate, flex, and extend the spine) because patients with PD have been shown to exhibit impairments in this area.[104] All segments of the spine should be examined, including cervical, thoracic, and lumbar segments. Spinal inclinometers such as the Back Range of Motion II™ (BROM II) and Cervical Range of Motion™ (CROM) instruments have been shown to be valid and reliable in measuring spinal ROM and forward head posture (www.spineproducts.com).[105] The use of a head-mounted laser and wall measurements is a novel way to assess transverse plane spine ROM. Standing with feet stationary, the patient rotates as far as possible to one side. An objective measurement of full body (trunk) rotation is obtained by measuring the distance that the laser moves along the wall. This multisegmental measurement may be a better predictor of functional trunk mobility than isolated measurements of cervical and lumbar ROM. The mobility of the spine can also be examined using a series of functional movements, such as axial rotation (looking behind) in sitting and standing and walking. Hamstring length can be determined using a straight leg test.

An examination of resting posture and changes in posture that occur with movement is indicated. The therapist can use posture grids, plumb lines, still photography, or videotape to document changes. A flexible ruler contoured to the patient's spine in standing and then traced onto graph paper can be used to record static sagittal plane posture. This technique is affordable, with good intratester and intertester reliability, and was shown to have a high correlation to radiographic measurements of the lumbar and thoracic spine.[106-108] In standing, patients with PD typically assume a flexed, stooped posture (kyphosis with forward head) with the COM placed forward within the limits of stability (LOS) (Fig. 18.4). In supine, the flexed posture with forward head is still evident (shadow pillow posture) (Fig. 18.5).

Muscle Performance

An examination of strength and endurance is indicated. The therapist can measure strength using manual muscle testing (MMT). Handheld and isokinetic dynamometry can be used to quantify peak force (torque output). Patients with PD have been shown to exhibit impairments in the rate of force development and in maximum torque production capability. Isokinetic dynamometry can also be used to document muscle endurance and has been suggested for documenting tremor, using slow speeds of movement (25 mm/sec) and low torques.[26]

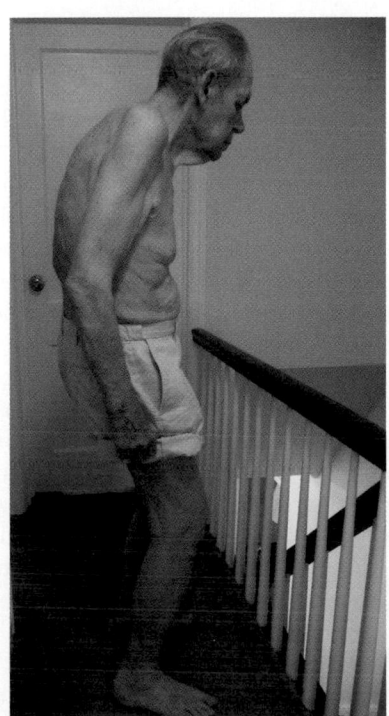

Figure 18.4 In standing, patient with PD demonstrates the typical flexed, stooped posture with kyphosis, forward head, and hip and knee flexion.

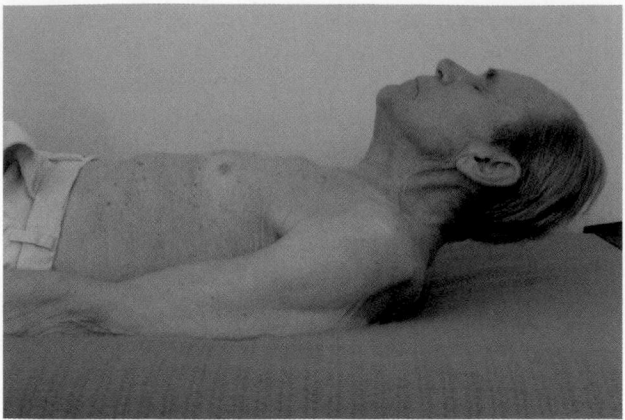

Figure 18.5 In supine, the patient with PD demonstrates the typical flexed posture (shadow pillow posture).

Motor Function

Rigidity

Rigidity is usually equal in both agonist and antagonist muscle groups. As mentioned earlier, it can be sustained (lead pipe) or intermittent (cogwheel). Distribution of rigidity is often asymmetrical especially in the early stages of the disease and can vary during the course of the day, point in the medication cycle, and with stress. It is therefore important to determine which body segments are affected and the severity of involvement. The patient should be seated or supine in a relaxed position. The therapist moves each extremity through full PROM. For head and neck and spinal PROM the patient can be seated on a mat or at the edge of a chair, perch sitting, to allow for excursion of spinal motions (flexion, extension, rotation). A determination of severity of rigidity can be made based on the level of resistance to passive movement and availability of ROM. For example, a determination of severe rigidity is made if full PROM can only be achieved with difficulty. Tone changes in the neck and shoulders are suggestive of early disease, whereas tone changes in the trunk and extremities are typically present with moderate and extensive disease. Deficits in functional mobility and postural reactions should be suspected in the presence of significant trunk rigidity. The patient should also be examined for facial mobility (e.g., hypomimia or masked face) including ability to produce spontaneous expressions and part the lips; the ability to smile or use the muscles of facial expression should also be examined. An inspection of voluntary repetitive movements should be performed to determine active limitations imposed by rigidity.

Bradykinesia

Initially movements are slowed, then movements decrease in amplitude (hypokinesia); in later stages, movements become arrhythmic with frequent start hesitations and arrests (akinesia). A stopwatch can be used to quantify

detectable slowing of movement (*movement time*) and start hesitancy or *reaction time* (elapsed time between the patient's desire to move and the actual movement response). The therapist should examine overall amplitude of movement and fluctuations in amplitude. For example, impaired coordination and asymmetry of arm swing during walking is a common finding in early PD. As the disease progresses, movements are characterized by marked slowness, poverty, and reduced amplitude. Timed tests for rapid alternating movements (RAM) can be used to determine the effects of bradykinesia. Examples of RAM include repeated opposition of the forefinger and thumb, alternating between pronation and supination, opening and closing of hands, and tapping (finger or foot tapping). Dexterity in complex motor tasks (e.g., writing, dressing, skilled object manipulation) can be expected to be impaired and should be examined. This is also true for motor tasks involving simultaneous use of both sides (e.g., bilateral RAM between pronation and supination). See Chapter 6, Examination of Coordination and Balance, for additional test examples.

More sophisticated methods have been used to study movement in patients with PD, largely in the research setting. EMG has been used to quantify the effects of rigidity and bradykinesia on motor performance. Long-latency EMG responses (50 to 120 msec) have been observed when muscles are subjected to sudden stretch. Abnormal patterns of motor unit recruitment have also been observed.[109]

Tremor

The location, persistence, and severity (amplitude) of tremor should be recorded. The therapist should determine if tremor is present at rest (initial typical pattern) or present with action and interferes with function. This latter pattern may occur in severe, long-standing disease. UE functional skills such as drinking from a cup, feeding, dressing, and writing can be used to test for the effects of tremor during movement. With severe tremor, the patient will be unable to complete the functional task. Stress can increase tremor. The use of simultaneous cognitive tasks such as serial seven subtractions (i.e., counting backward from 100 by 7) can be used to test the impact of dual-task performance.[110]

Postural Control and Balance

A thorough examination of postural control and balance is indicated. The therapist should first observe the patient's resting posture in sitting and standing. The patient's perception of vertical may be impaired, as some patients with advanced disease will perceive themselves as fully upright when they are actually leaning forward.

Clinical measures of balance performance have been shown to be reliable and sensitive in the examination of functional performance and balance in patients with Parkinson's disease.[111-120] These include the *Berg Balance Scale* (BBS),[121] the *Functional Reach Test* (FRT),[122] the *Timed Up and Go test* (TUG),[123] the *Cognitive Timed Up and Go* (CTUG),[124] and the *Dynamic Gait Index* (DGI).[125] These tests are discussed in Chapter 6, Examination of Coordination and Balance. The BBS correlates well with the UPDRS and has been found to be a good overall measure of function in this population.[111,112] Dibble and Lange[113] demonstrated that each of these tests has the ability to discriminate among people with PD who had a history of falls from those without a history of falls and suggested cutoff scores to maximize sensitivity and minimize false negatives. False negatives can also be reduced when interpretation is based on the collective interpretation of multiple balance tests. A clinical decision making algorithm that involves the serial use of clinical balance tests has been proposed.[114] Leddy et al[115] examined the BBS, the Functional Gait Assessment (FGA),[126] and the *Balance Evaluation Systems Test (BESTest)*[127] and found that all three demonstrated high reliability scores and that the BESTest was most sensitive for identifying fallers. Steffen and Seney[118] also found high reliability scores for the BBS, the 6-Minute Walk Test (6-MWT), and gait speed. Minimal detectable change (MDC) values were identified with MDC for the BBS = 5/56, the 6-MWT = 82 m, comfortable gait speed = 0.18 m/sec, and fast gait speed = 0.24 m/sec. In contrast, the *Tinetti Gait Assessment (TGA)* was not sensitive for detecting change in gait impairments in people with moderately disabling PD.[128] Strong stability of measurements on balance tests occurs during the "on" phase of the medication cycle while stability of measurements is not maintained during the "off" period.[129]

Reduced postural control is evident during quiet standing (static control), with increased oscillations in both medial-lateral and anterior-posterior planes.[130] During dynamic posturographic tests, postural restabilization strategies are often inadequate to maintain balance. Available postural strategies and reactions should be carefully documented (e.g., use of ankle, hip, and stepping strategies). Healthy individuals typically respond initially using an ankle strategy with small shifts in their COM, followed by hip and stepping strategies with larger shifts in the COM. Persons with PD and the elderly population in general typically respond to destabilizing forces with postural strategies involving more the hip joints than ankle joints. Start hesitation, abnormal coactivation patterns (rigid body) with an inability to recover a stable posture, is common. An absence of postural strategies (i.e., patient would fall if not for overhead body support harness) is also seen in advanced disease. During complex postural situations involving sensory conflict (e.g., the Sensory Organization Test), persons with advanced PD typically demonstrate reduced postural performance, suggesting inadequate sensory organization.[131] Balance control can also be expected to degrade under conditions of reduced cognitive monitoring. Patients with PD especially in the early stages of the disease may not demonstrate balance

impairments in response to steady standing with normal BOS or self-initiated movements as along as their attention is fully directed to the task at hand. However, if competing attentional demands are instituted (i.e., *dual-task interference* such as talking while balancing), instability can be seen.[132] Balance confidence is also related to functional mobility and falls in people with PD.[133]

Gait

Parameters and characteristics of gait that should be examined during unobstructed walking on level surfaces include start time or gait initiation, speed of walking, stride length, cadence, stability, variability, and safety. The *10-Meter Walk Test* can be used to determine speed, average stride, and cadence or more sophisticated kinetic analysis can be obtained from embedded force plates, body markers, and computerized equipment (motion analysis systems typically seen in the laboratory setting). Persons with PD frequently demonstrate decreased step length and trunk rotation, difficulty initiating gait, and difficulty attaining increased walking speed. When instructed to walk as fast as possible, the movements produced are smaller and more variable when compared to healthy elders.[134,135]

Gait should be examined for kinematic or qualitative changes, including reductions in hip, knee, and ankle motions that result in a short-stepped, shuffling (festinating) gait pattern with reduced trunk rotation and arm swing. Postural abnormalities that contribute to the development of a festinating gait pattern should be documented (i.e., flexed, stooped posture). Gait should be examined in all movement directions: forward, backward, and sideward. A complex gait pattern such as cross-stepping or braiding can be used to examine deficits in motor planning. Patients with advanced PD typically experience difficulty with adaptability and cannot easily vary walking or walk in complex confined areas such as narrow doorways or open environments. Walking should be examined in varied environments (e.g., community environment) or negotiating an obstacle course. Increased difficulty in walking is also experienced in response to varying attentional demands and dual-task interference. Changes in gait speed, stride length, and cadence can be observed while simultaneously performing a secondary cognitive task (e.g., *Walkie-Talkie Test)* or walking while simultaneously performing a secondary motor task (e.g., carrying objects on a tray). The degree of change was not significantly different with regard to type of dual task interference.[132] Clinical measures of locomotor performance shown to be reliable and sensitive for people with PD include the DGI, the FGA, and the TUG (all previously discussed). Huang et al[136] identified the minimal detectable change values for both the TUG and the DGI.

Freezing of Gait

Freezing of gait, an episodic inability to generate effective stepping in the absence of any known cause, has a dramatic effect on quality of life and risk of falls for patients with PD.[137,138] Assessment is often difficult due to the unpredictable nature of the episodes. The therapist needs to document triggers or provoking factors. Common triggers for FOG include initiating gait, walking through narrow passages (e.g., doorway) or turning in tight spaces, a change in the environment or attentional demands, and walking under time pressure, anxiety, or stress. In the early stages of the disease, episodes are levodopa sensitive and more common in the "off" time. In advanced stages, FOG can occur during the "on" time.[139] The *New Freezing of Gait Questionnaire (NFOG-Q)* is a reliable three-part questionnaire and short video to detect and rate FOG severity and impact.[140]

Fall Risk

A determination of fall history and fall injuries is an important component of the examination of balance and gait function. There is a strong association between duration and severity of PD with increased risk of falls. Of particular significance is balance and walking impairments including FOG, anterior displacement of COM, decreased postural righting reactions, and the presence of dyskinesias. Other linked factors include postural hypotension, dementia, depression, and prior history of falls.[112-115] A *fall risk diary* can be used to assist the patient and family/caregivers in accurately recording a fall event and the context of daily life in which the fall occurred. For example, activity at the time of the fall, relation to timing of medication and food intake, type of footwear, degree of fatigue and injury, and other risk factors all should be documented. The need for assisted gait and frequency of contact guarding from family members or caregivers during walking should also be documented.

Fatigue

Fatigue is a common impairment associated with PD. As the disease process progresses so does the prevalence of fatigue and its impact on quality of life.[141,142] The Movement Disorders Society (www.movementdisorders.org) created a task force to evaluate and make recommendations on available fatigue rating scales.[143] Following the systematic review, the task force recommended the *Multidimensional Fatigue Inventory (MFI)* and the *Fatigue Severity Scale (FSS)* for assessment of fatigue in patients with PD. The MFI is a 20-item self-report scale that measures general fatigue, physical fatigue, mental fatigue, reduced motivation, and reduced activity.[144] The FSS is a self-administered 9-item rating scale that emphasizes the functional impact of fatigue.[145]

Dyskinesias

Drug-induced dyskinesias have a profound effect on physical and social functioning. Risk factors include high total dosage of dopaminergic drugs, young age at onset of PD, and extended duration of the disease process.[146,147] The *Rush Dyskinesia Scale* assesses functional disability by

grading the subject walking, drinking from a cup, and putting on and buttoning a coat. The scale is recommended by the Movement Disorders Society (MDS) Task Force on scales to assess dyskinesia in PD and has been used extensively in clinical trials and patient care, and has undergone extensive clinimetric testing.[148]

The therapist can explore the impact of motor fluctuations using questions that address changes in performance during the day. Sample questions might include the following:

- Do you experience increasing difficulties with your functional activities during certain times of the day?
- What time of day do you experience the greatest difficulty?
- How long after you take your medications do you start to move better?
- Do you experience increasing difficulties as your medications wear off?

Swallowing and Speech

An examination of swallowing function, feeding, and speech is important. Referral to a speech-language pathologist may be indicated if the patient demonstrates significant limitations in any of these areas.

Autonomic Function

The therapist should examine for problems with autonomic dysfunction. Excessive drooling (salivation) or sweating, greasy skin, and abnormalities in thermoregulation should be noted. Excessive sweating and flushing during the "on" state is linked to the presence of dyskinesias.

Cardiorespiratory Function

Endurance may be reduced as a result of impaired cardiorespiratory function and long-standing inactivity, both common problems in PD. An examination of respiratory function should include inspection of rib cage compliance, chest wall mobility, and thoracic expansion. Visual inspection of breathing patterns and an examination of the influence of posture and activity on breathing should be performed. Objective measurements include respiratory rate (RR) and circumferential measurements of the chest. Specific ventilation parameters may be determined in patients with significant respiratory compromise. These can include FVC, FEV_1, maximal expiratory flow (MEF), maximal inspiratory flow (MIF), total lung capacity (TLC), residual volume (RV), and RAW.

Individuals with mild PD (Hoehn-Yahr Classification Stages I and II) can demonstrate aerobic exercise capacities similar to healthy adults. Individuals with more advanced disease (Hoehn-Yahr Classification Stages III and IV) demonstrate greater variability and lower aerobic capacities compared to healthy adults. It is important to remember that many older adults are at high risk for latent cardiovascular disease. Exercise testing can be used to determine the patient's level of fitness before commencing an exercise program. Patients who have balance deficits or freezing episodes should not be tested on a treadmill without the use of a safety harness. Cycle ergometry (arm or leg) may be an acceptable alternative. A *6- or 12-Minute Walk Test* can be used to determine endurance capacity and walking velocity. The therapist should document vital signs (HR, RR, BP), exertional symptoms (dyspnea, dizziness or confusion, excessive fatigue, pallor, and so forth), time, distance, and number of rest stops.[54] For patients with advanced PD (Hoehn-Yahr Classification Stages III and IV), Light et al[149] used a *2-Minute Walk Test* to evaluate walking endurance and found it to be a sensitive and feasible test. Perceived exertion can be documented using Borg's Rating of Perceived Exertion Scale (RPE Scale).[150]

Orthostatic Hypotension

Orthostatic hypotension (OH) with positional change should be examined. Subjective signs and symptoms of OH on sitting up and standing up are documented (e.g., dizziness, light-headedness, pallor, diaphoresis, or syncope). A drop in systolic blood pressure (SBP) of 20 mm Hg, or a drop of 10 mm Hg in diastolic blood pressure (DBP), *and* a 10% to 20% increase in pulse rate is diagnostic of the condition. The examination begins with the patient resting in supine for 2 to 3 minutes. Resting BP and HR are taken. The patient is then asked to move from supine-to-sitting. After at least 1 minute, BP and HR are taken. If the patient is stable after at least 3 minutes (no symptoms), testing can be performed in the standing position. The patient is asked to move from sitting-to-standing with BP and HR again taken after at least 1 minute and repeated between 3 and 5 minutes. BP that continues to drop after at least 1 minute of standing is problematic and is evident in advanced PD.[151]

Integumentary Integrity

Sympathetic skin responses may be abnormal. For example, the skin may become oily (e.g., on face). Seborrhea or seborrheic dermatitis occurs frequently in patients with PD. The therapist should examine the patient closely for areas of bruising and skin breakdown. Patients who are severely disabled (Hoehn-Yahr Classification Stage V) are restricted to bed, wheelchair, or both. Incontinence may occur during late-stage disease. The effect of these problems on skin integrity should be carefully documented. Use and effectiveness of pressure-relieving strategies and devices should also be documented.

Functional Status

An examination of functional status is indicated, including performance of functional mobility skills, basic activities of daily living (BADL), and instrumental activities of daily living (IADL). For patients undergoing inpatient rehabilitation, the *Functional Independence Measure (FIM)* is commonly administered[152] (see Chapter 8, Examination of Function). Need for and appropriate use of protective and supportive devices is an important component of the functional status examination. Close collaboration with the occupational therapist is essential.

During functional performance tests, each skill should be analyzed to determine the impact of direct and indirect impairments on performance. For example, sit-to-stand transfers typically present a significant challenge for patients with moderate to severe PD as evidenced by increased time and increased falls. These changes have been attributed to hypokinesia, decreased rates of force production, and changes in distal muscle timing.[153,154] The *Five Times Sit-to-Stand Test (FTSTS)* is a timed test that has been used to determine performance in patients with PD at different disease stages and to discriminate between fallers and nonfallers with PD. In one study the average time for FTSTS performance for community-dwelling individuals with PD was 20 seconds with a cutoff time of 16 seconds discriminating between fallers and nonfallers.[155] Timed performance can also be used for other functional tasks such as rolling over in bed or moving from supine-to-sitting that are likely to prove difficult. These activities have a large rotational component of the trunk, typically lacking in many patients with PD.

Functional testing should be balanced with adequate rest to ensure that fatigue does not degrade performance with resultant fluctuations. Repeat testing should be undertaken at the same time of day and importantly at the same time in the medication cycle. Filming task activities can provide an objective record of functional performance. This is particularly useful to document motor fluctuations and dyskinesias. An examination of functional performance in the home (or work) environment is also indicated. The patient's physical environment is examined for barriers, access, and safety.

Profile of Function and Impairment Level Experience with Parkinson's Disease

The *Profile of Function and Impairment Level Experience with Parkinson's Disease (Profile PD)* was developed to assist the physical therapist's examination and evaluation of individuals with PD in the early and middle stages of disease. It uses a 0 to 4 scale with 0 = no problem and 4 = severe or marked difficulty with descriptive anchors for each score. Approximately 50% of the test relates to deficits in body systems and cognitive/emotional factors. These include questions on tremor (with activity and at rest), rigidity, posture, postural stability, dyskinesia, dystonia, clinical fluctuations, falling, FOG, bradykinesia, speech, depression, memory, and involvement (routine daily/leisure/social activities). The remaining 50% of items focus on functional activities that are typically difficult for individuals with PD (e.g., dressing, hygiene, mealtime activities, transfers, bed mobility, chair rise, gait, fine and gross motor performance). Initial testing revealed it to be a reliable and valid scale with an interrater reliability of 0.97 and construct validity with the UPDRS of 0.86. It has an estimated administration time of 15 minutes.[156]

Global Health Measures

Global health measures can be used to determine individual outcomes across a broad spectrum of populations. Instruments typically include items that examine ability to perform routine daily activities and quality of life (e.g., physical and social function, general health and vitality, emotional well-being, bodily pain, and so forth). General health measures have been used to study large populations and are most useful in determining long-term health outcomes. They lack the sensitivity needed to document short-term outcomes of treatment. Commonly used measures of general health status include the *Rand 36-Item Health Survey SF-36*[157] and the *Sickness Impact Profile.*[158]

Disease-Specific Measures

Disease-specific measures are designed to determine attributes unique to a specific disease entity. Items are included that provide information about the disease process and outcomes, and ideally document clinically meaningful change over time. Thus, these instruments have greater responsiveness or sensitivity to change than general health measures. The *Parkinson's Disease Questionnaire (PDQ-39)* is a 39-item questionnaire developed from in-depth interviews with patients with PD.[159] It focuses on the subjective report of the impact of PD on daily life and addresses eight health-related quality-of-life dimensions (mobility, ADL, emotional well-being, stigma, social support, cognition, communication, and bodily discomfort). The PDQ-39 produces a profile of scores on the eight individual dimensions. A summary score using the *Parkinson's Disease Summary Index* (PDSI) can also be determined, with scores that range from 0 (perfect health) to 100 (worst health). It provides a useful indication of the global impact of PD on health status. Internal and test–retest reliability were found to be moderate to high with reported ranges from 0.68 to 0.96. Construct validity was examined by comparing the PDSI with other measures of health. Significant and high correlations were found between the PDQ-39 and the SF-36 and the Hoehn and Yahr staging score.[160]

A determination of goals and outcomes is based on careful examination and evaluation of the patient's individual abilities, impairments, activity limitations, and disability. Box 18.4 provides examples of general goals

---

Box 18.4 Examples of General Goals and Outcomes for Patients with Progressive Disorders of the Central Nervous System,* adapted from the *Guide to Physical Therapist Practice*[97]

Impact of pathology/pathophysiology is reduced.

- Patient/client, family, and caregiver knowledge and awareness of the disease, prognosis, and plan of care is enhanced.
- Symptom management is enhanced.
- Risk of secondary impairment is reduced.
- Intensity of care is decreased.

Impact of impairments is reduced.

- Cognitive function is improved.
- Joint integrity and mobility are improved.
- Sensory awareness and skin integrity are improved.
- Pain is decreased.
- Motor function is improved.
- Muscle performance (strength, power, and endurance) is improved.
- Postural control and balance are improved.
- Gait and locomotion are improved.
- Management of fatigue is enhanced.
- Aerobic capacity is increased.

Ability to perform physical actions, tasks, or activities is improved.

- Independence in activities of daily living is increased.
- Tolerance of positions and activities is increased.
- Activity pacing and energy conservation skills are enhanced.

- Problem solving and decision making skills are enhanced.
- Safety of patient/client, family, and caregivers is improved.

Disability associated with chronic illness is reduced.

- Ability to assume/resume self-care and home management is improved.
- Ability to assume work (job/school/play), community, and leisure roles is improved.
- Patient/client and family knowledge and awareness of personal and environmental factors associated with worsening of the condition are enhanced.
- Awareness and use of community resources are improved.

Health status and quality of life are improved.

- Sense of well-being is enhanced.
- Stressors are reduced.
- Insight, self-confidence, and self-management skills are improved.
- Health, wellness, and fitness are improved.

Patient/client satisfaction is enhanced.

- Access to and availability of services are acceptable to patient/client and family.
- Quality of rehabilitation services is acceptable to patient/client and family.
- Care is coordinated with patient/client, family, caregivers, and other professionals.

*Anticipated goals and expected outcomes are specific to the individual patient.

and outcomes for patients with progressive disorders of the CNS and is adapted from the *Guide to Physical Therapist Practice.*[97]

■ PHYSICAL THERAPY INTERVENTION

A combined approach of physical therapy and pharmacological intervention plays a key role in the management of the patient with PD. Despite best efforts, progressive disability develops and affects the patient's quality of life. A variety of interventions to maximize functional ability and minimize secondary complications are used to achieve goals and outcomes, including direct interventions, supervision of assistive personnel, patient/family/caregiver instruction, environmental modification, and supportive counseling. Early intervention is critical in preventing the devastating musculoskeletal impairments these patients are so prone to develop. Interventions also focus on improvement of motor function, exercise capacity, functional performance, and activity participation. Education and support of patients, family members, and caregivers at each stage of the disease is critical to attaining optimal outcomes. The research team for the Cochrane Database of Systematic Reviews found that there was insufficient evidence to support or refute the efficacy of any given form of physical therapy over another in PD. The researchers stressed the need for improved research in this area, including large well-designed placebo-controlled randomized controlled trials (RCTs) to demonstrate the efficacy and effectiveness of "best practice" physical therapy in PD.[161,162]

Motor Learning Strategies

Patients with PD typically demonstrate motor learning deficits, including slower learning rates reduced efficiency, and increased context-specificity of learning. Learning complex movement sequences and movements dependent on internally generated cues are more difficult than those dependent on external cues. In the early and middle stages of the disease, patients can improve their performance through practice and by using additional sensory information. The amount and persistence of learning are variable and can be expected to be lower than in healthy age-matched people. In more advanced stages and in the presence of pronounced cognitive deficits, training will likely be less successful.[163-165] The therapist needs to structure treatment sessions to optimize motor learning.

Critical elements of practice include a large number of repetitions to develop procedural skills. The therapist should instruct the patient to deliberately focus his or her full attention on the desired movement. The environment should also be modified to reduce clutter and competing attentional demands that may trigger freezing episodes. The task should be modified to minimize competing cognitive demands (e.g., dual tasking). Long and complex movement sequences should be avoided or broken down into component parts. Initially, *random*

practice order (i.e., practice in which the patient switches back and forth between tasks) should be avoided in favor of a *blocked practice order*, thereby reducing the effects of contextual interference. Use of *structured instructional sets* has been shown to improve movement speed and consistency.[166] For example, walking patterns can be improved with focused instructions of "swing your arms," "walk fast," or "take large steps." For the patient with advanced disease and cognitive deficits, repetitive drill-like practice should be used together with an increased focus on caregiver training to ensure safety.

External cues have been shown to be effective in triggering sequential movements and improving movement characteristics in individuals with mild to moderate PD.[167] Box 18.5 Evidence Summary presents a review of selected research in this area. *Visual cues* include stationary floor markings (e.g., brightly colored lines on the floor placed perpendicular to the gait path and spaced about one step length apart) and dynamic transportable cues (e.g., laser light signals). A laser light that projects a line onto the floor in front of the patient can be mounted on an assistive device (cane or walker) or on a subject's chest harness.[168] Visual cues have been shown to improve stride length and velocity while cadence was relatively unchanged. Freezing episodes are also reduced.[169] *Rhythmic auditory stimulation (RAS)* includes use of a metronome beat or a steady beat from a musical listening device. RAS has been shown to improve gait speed, cadence, and stride length.[170-172] The beat is typically set 25% faster than the patient's preferred pace. Auditory cues such as "Big step" have also been shown to improve gait. Examples include "1, 2, 3 stand, ready set go, big first step." Cues should be consistent, not rushed and have a rhythmical quality to them. Auditory cues appear to have a greater influence on the temporal components of movement (e.g., gait cadence, stride synchronization) rather than on spatial components. *Multisensory cueing* (use of both visual and auditory cueing) has been used for patients with PD. When sensory enhanced therapy using multisensory cueing was compared with conventional therapy, significant improvements were found in the sensory training group.[173-182]

External cues appear to facilitate movement by utilizing different brain areas. For example, the premotor cortex is active in the generation of movement in response to visual or auditory stimuli. Normally the supplementary motor area (SMA) with inputs from the BG is involved in the initiation of self-generated movements and the performance of well-learned, repetitive movement sequences. External cues heighten patient attention through a common mode of action, that is, to bypass the diminished internal cueing of the BG. Thus, focus is shifted to less automatic movement using alternative, more conscious motor control pathways. This is supported by the finding that when patients were requested to carry out a secondary task while walking (dual-tasking), the beneficial effects of visual and attentional cues was reduced.[183]

Box 18.5 Evidence Summary Effect of Visual and Auditory Cues on Gait in Individuals with Parkinson's Disease

Reference	Subjects	Design Intervention	Results	Comments
Frazzitta et al[182] (2009)	40 subjects with PD, randomly assigned to 2 groups	Cohort study that examined difference between conventional and treadmill (TM) locomotor training using cues. Group 1: TM training with RAS and visual cues. Group 2: rehabilitation protocol with RAS and visual cues and no TM. *Outcome measures:* UPDRS III, FOGQ, 6-MWT, gait speed, and stride cycle.	Both groups had significant improvement in all variables; TM group had more improvement in most functional indicators (FOGQ, 6-MWT, gait speed, stride cycle); most striking change was in 6-MWT.	TM training using auditory and visual cues might give better results than more conventional treatments; the TM may act as a supplemental external cue.
Nieuwboer et al[181] (2009)	133 subjects with PD (part of RESCUE trial), able to walk independently; freezing episodes were identified using FOGQ	Cohort study that examined the effect of 3 different cue modalities on a turning task. *Procedure:* Subjects walked at preferred speed, completing a functional task and synchronizing each step to external cueing (auditory, visual, somatosensory); order of cueing was varied. *Duration:* Test repeated 8 times: 1 baseline, 6 cueing trials, and 1 post trial. *Outcome measures:* Functional test consisting of walking 6 m, picking up a tray, turning 180°, carrying tray back to start position, and stop; using an activity; FOGQ.	Cueing, all types, increased the speed of turn in all subjects; no difference in turn performance between freezers and nonfreezers in cued and no cued conditions; auditory cueing made turning significantly faster than visual cues. Short carryover was evident in noncued trial.	Researchers used 3 types of cueing. Rhythmic cueing resulted in faster performance of a functional turn in both freezers and nonfreezers. May be explained by enhanced attention mechanisms.
Arias and Cudeiro[178] (2008)	25 subjects with PD grouped into mild (n = 16) and severe (n = 9) disease and 10 age-matched controls	Cohort, repeated measures study; examined kinematic parameters of gait (cadence, step length, velocity, coefficient of variability [CV]) at rest and in response to RAS and visual stimulation.	Patients with mild PD demonstrated altered step length, velocity and CV. Those with severe PD (III-IV Hoehn and Yahr) showed greater changes; RAS at preferred walking speed led to a dec. in CV and an inc. in step length. Visual stimulation did not modify any of the kinematic parameters for either group.	RAS is effective in facilitating gait in patients with PD. A decrease in CV may reduce risk of falling.

Box 18.5 Evidence Summary		Effect of Visual and Auditory Cues on Gait in Individuals with Parkinson's Disease—cont'd		
Reference	Subjects	Design Intervention	Results	Comments
Jiang et al[175] (2006)	14 subjects with PD	Cohort, repeated measures study. Analysis of first 2 steps of gait initiation with RAS and visual cues (transverse lines). *Duration*: 1 time visit. *Outcome measures*: Computerized gait way/force platform (velocity, step length, push-off force).	Visual cue condition resulted in inc. push-off force and velocity compared to baseline; no significant effect of RAS on these measures.	RAS does not appear to influence the first 2 steps of gait initiation whereas visual cues do.
Lim et al[167] (2005)	24 studies identified (total number of patients = 626) out of 159 screened studies	Systematic review of literature.	Best evidence synthesis showed strong evidence for improving walking speed with the help of RAS. Insufficient evidence was found for the effectiveness of visual and somatosensory cues.	More high-quality research is needed. Unclear whether positive effects found in the laboratory can be generalized to improved ADL and reduced frequency of falls. The sustainability of a cueing training program remains uncertain.
Rochester et al[179] (2005)	20 subjects with PD and 10 age-matched controls	Cohort, repeated measures study, examined effect of cues on walking in home. *Procedure:* Walking while performing simple task (dual-motor task); performed with and without RAS and visual cues. *Outcome measures:* Walking speed, step length, and step frequency.	Use of auditory cues was useful in reducing interference and maintaining gait performance during dual-tasking, with significant inc. in step length.	RAS may be useful in counteracting the effects of interference during more complicated functional activities.
Del Olmo and Cudeiro[172] (2005)	15 subjects with PD and 15 age-matched controls	Cohort, repeated measures study. *Procedure:* Program of RAS and walking with and without secondary UE tasks. *Duration:* 1 hr/day 5(/wk for 4 wk. *Outcome measures:* Computerized walkway (gait velocity, step length, cadence, CV).	PD group improved temporal stability of walking; no significant difference from controls.	RAS is a valuable method of improving gait in patients with PD.
Lehman et al[173] (2005)	Part 1: 5 subjects, no controls Part 2: 11 subjects with early stage,	Cohort, repeated measures study. *Procedure:* PD group: walked 30 feet using verbal cueing ("take long steps") 10 times/	Significant inc. in gait velocity and step length; reduced cadence.	Significant effects noted in both groups but more pronounced in PD group.

Continued

Box 18.5 Evidence Summary Effect of Visual and Auditory Cues on Gait in Individuals with Parkinson's Disease—cont'd

Reference	Subjects	Design Intervention	Results	Comments
	stable PD (Hoehn and Yahr Stage 2–2.5); within 1–2 hours on PD meds Training group = 6 Control group = 5	session; control group: walking with no verbal cueing. *Duration*: 3 training sets/day for 10 days. *Outcome measures*: Step length, velocity, and cadence, preferred walking speed (GaitRite® electronic walkway).		
Mak and Hue-Chan[177] (2004)	30 subjects: 15 subjects with PD (Hoehn and Yahr Stage 2.5) Patients stable, within 1 hour on PD medication: 15 healthy controls matched for age, gender, weight, height (no PD)	Cohort, repeated measures study. *Procedure*: 2 conditions STS: (1) self-initiated; (2) with auditory cues (verbal) and visual cues (circular light at eye level). *Duration*: 2 test trials: self-initiated and cue-initiated STS. *Outcome measures*: Force through feet (force plate); kinematic analysis of movements (reflective markers, high-speed video camera).	PD group: STS self-initiated; significant dec. in hip flex and ankle DF torques; dec. velocities; prolonged MT to complete STS STS cued: Significant inc. all torque values; time to peak torque reduced by 23%–27%; no improvement in peak velocity; significant dec. in MT. Control group—STS cued: Small but significant inc. knee ext torque.	Verbal and visual cueing significantly improved performance in STS.
Suteerawattananon et al[176] (2004)	24 subjects with PD	Cohort study that examined effect of cues on gait. *Procedure*: 2 trials for each of 4 conditions (random order) that included walking: without cues; with a visual cue; with an auditory cue (25% faster speed); and with both cues. *Outcome measures*: Gait speed, cadence, stride length.	Significantly improved velocity, cadence, and stride length when cues were used; auditory cues improved cadence and speed more; visual cues improved stride length more.	The combined condition did not improve gait significantly over using each cue alone; cueing may be used to reduce gait difficulties.
Freedland et al[174] (2002)	16 subjects with PD, able to walk independently without assistive device	Cohort study, examined \effect of pulsed auditory stimulation on gait. *Procedure*: Pre-test/post-test; walking using ASM set 10% above baseline cadence. *Outcome measures*: Functional Ambulation Profile (FAP); electronic walkway (GaitRite system): footfall data, velocity; heart rate.	With ASM: FAP scores inc.; dec. in cycle time and double support; inc. in step length and step-extremity ratio.	Results confirm prior findings that ASM positively influences gait of persons with PD.

COM = center of mass; COP = center of pressure; dec. = decrease; DF = dorsiflexion; f = female; flex = flexion; FOGQ = Freezing of Gait Questionnaire; inc. = increase; indep = independent; m = male; meds = medications; MMSE = Mini-Mental State Examination; MT = movement time; PD = Parkinson's disease; RAS = rhythmic auditory stimulation; 6-MWT = 6-Minute Walk Test; STS = sit-to-stand; UPDRS = Unified Parkinson Disease Rating Scale.

Selection of the type of cue and successful use will depend on the individual patient with predicted long-term benefit of a particular type of cue linked to its initial success. External cues are clearly not effective for all patients with PD. For patients with advanced disease and severe reductions in stride length, cueing is not effective. When cueing is withheld, performance can be expected to deteriorate. Focused attention with cueing requires constant vigilance and is cognitively demanding. Thus, cueing is not suitable for patients with dementia.

Cueing may also not be effective when medication instability and disease fluctuations are present. However, for many patients, use of external cues is a valid treatment strategy and one in which improved performance can be anticipated.

Exercise Training

Amplitude-based behavioral intervention is a concept that can be applied in different contexts in the treatment of PD.[184] The "Training Big" program, also known as the Lee Silverman Voice Treatment (LSVT) Big program, is based on the concept that repetitive high-amplitude movements yield greater improvements in motor performance and possibly have a neuroprotective effect.[185] Patients are guided by a physical therapist to exercise at a high intensity (8/10 Borg's RPE Scale) for 1 hour 4 times a week for 4 weeks with large amplitude, multiple repetitions, and whole body movements that increase in complexity (Fig. 18.6). Examples of the exercises and patient directions include the following:

- "Reach left arm across the body to opposite side, keep hand open, palm up, right leg fully extended, toe pushing into the floor. Repeat on other leg and alternate."
- "Step out and land 'Big,' pushing the left foot into the floor while reaching with bilateral 'Big arms,' open hands, palms up (Fig. 18.7). Return the foot

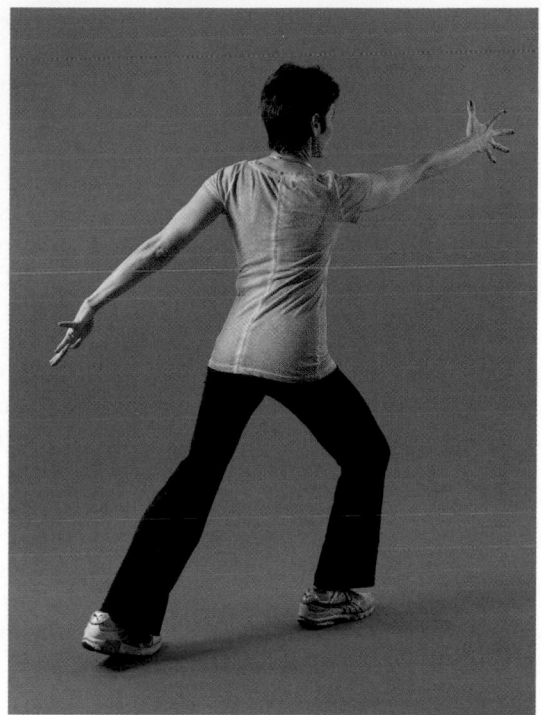

Figure 18.7 The patient with young-onset PD steps out and lands "Big," pushing the left foot into the floor while reaching with bilateral "Big arms," hands open.

back to the start, end 'Big.' Repeat on other leg and alternate."[186]

These vigorous large movements of the trunk and extremities are counter to the paucity of movement normally associated with PD. After a 4-week program of LSVT "Big" training the subjects had significant improvements in UPDRS motor scores, TUG, and timed 10-m walking.[187]

Relaxation Exercises

Gentle rocking can be used to produce generalized relaxation of excessive muscle tension owing to rigidity. Professor Charcot, who noted dramatic improvement in patients with PD following rides in bumpy, horse-drawn carriages, first described this effect almost 100 years ago in Paris. Following this observation he constructed a vibrating chair to use with his patients.[188] Although the exact mechanism underlying rigidity has not been identified, the beneficial effects of slow rocking on excess tone have been demonstrated.[189] Following Charcot's lead, a rocking chair can be used to temporarily relax the patient and enhance sit-to-stand transfers. During therapy, slow, rhythmic, rotational movements of the extremities and trunk can precede interventions such as ROM and stretching, and functional training. For example, hook-lying, lower trunk rotation, or side-lying rolling can be used to promote relaxation. The proprioceptive neuromuscular facilitation (PNF) technique of *rhythmic initiation (RI),* in which movement progresses from passive to active-assistive to lightly resisted or active

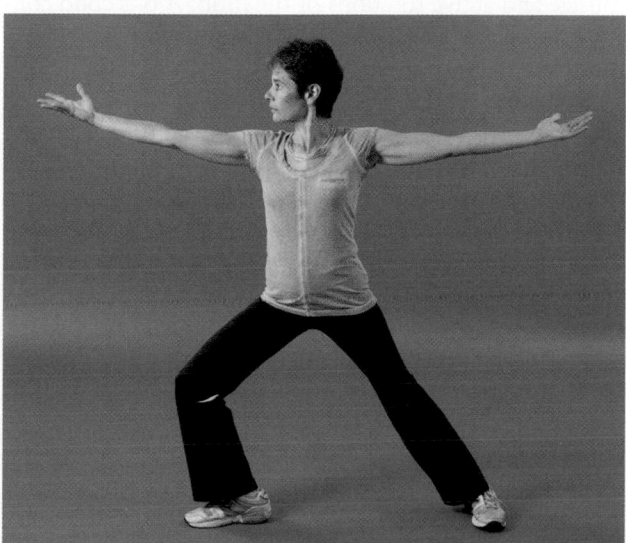

Figure 18.6 The patient with young-onset PD steps "Big" to the side with bilateral "Big arms" and hands open, palms up.

movement, was specifically designed to help overcome the effects of rigidity in PD.[190,191]

Another strategy to promote relaxation is emphasis on diaphragmatic breathing during exercise. For example, bilateral symmetrical PNF D2 flexion patterns are important patterns that can be used to expand the restricted chest and promote shoulder ROM (Fig. 18.8). The patient's attention can be focused on deep inspiration during D2F ("breathe in deeply") while during D2E patterns attention is focused on expiration ("breathe out deeply").[191] Patients may also benefit from cognitive imaging or meditation techniques (e.g., the relaxation response of Benson[192]). Relaxation audiotapes can be used at home as part of the home exercise program (HEP). Stress management techniques are an important adjunct to relaxation training. A daily schedule needs to be planned to accommodate the restrictions of the disease and the functional needs of the patient. Lifestyle modifications and time management strategies reduce anxiety associated with movement difficulties and prolonged times required to complete basic functional tasks.

Flexibility Exercise

The purpose of flexibility exercise (stretching) is to improve ROM and physical function. A combination of static (PROM), dynamic (AROM), and facilitated PNF exercises is used to achieve maximum ROM. Flexibility exercises should be performed a minimum 2 to 3 days per week and ideally 5 to 7 days per week. A minimum

of 4 repetitions per stretch held for 15 to 60 seconds is recommended.[54] Special consideration should be given to stretching common areas of limitation (Table 18.4). Stretching can be combined with joint mobilization techniques to reduce tightness of the joint capsule or of ligaments around a joint (Fig. 18.9). By using selected grades of accessory movement, both improved ROM and decreased pain can be achieved. The stretching will be more effective if the muscles have been warmed with active exercise or with an external heating modality. Stretching exercises are an important component of the HEP. The patient and caregiver should be instructed in the appropriate stretching exercises.

A yoga sequence can be used effectively to focus attention on developmental postures, core stability, and stretching of structures that are traditionally restricted with PD, as well as to promote relaxation (Appendix 18.B).

Patients with PD have a minimum of energy to expend and multiple clinical problems. They may benefit from ROM exercises in physiological patterns of motion. For example, PNF patterns combine several motions at once while emphasizing rotation, a movement component typically lost early in PD. In the UEs, bilateral symmetrical D2 flexion patterns are ideal in promoting upper trunk extension and in counteracting kyphosis. Unilateral bridging with trunk rotation, bilateral bridging, and high-kneeling with anterior pelvis translation can all be used to stretch tight hip flexors and strengthen spinal and hip extensors. In the LEs, hip and knee extension should be emphasized, ideally in a D1 extension pattern (hip extension, abduction, internal rotation) to counteract the typical flexed, adducted position of the LEs. Muscle contractures typically respond well to PNF facilitated stretching techniques such as the *hold–relax (HR)* or *contract–relax (CR) techniques*.[191,192] Of the two, CR is the preferred technique because it combines autogenic inhibition from isometric contraction of the tight agonist muscle and active rotations of the limb. A 6-second contraction followed by a 10- to 30-second assisted stretch is recommended for these PNF techniques.[54]

Patients with PD benefit from additional attention and cueing strategies during active stretching exercises. Patients are instructed to "Think BIG, and move through the whole range" and maintain full focus and attention during each repetition. Additional tactile or visual cueing can assist in maximizing range during active motions. For example, during active trunk rotation and reaching movements in sitting, the patient can be cued to touch an object or target. Ballistic stretches (high-intensity bouncing stretches) should be avoided because they are linked to increased injury. Muscle tears or ruptures of weakened tissues are especially prevalent in elderly, sedentary individuals. Vigorous stretching can stimulate pain receptors and cause rebound muscle contraction. Patients with PD who are elderly and have long-standing disease must be considered at risk for osteoporosis and therefore

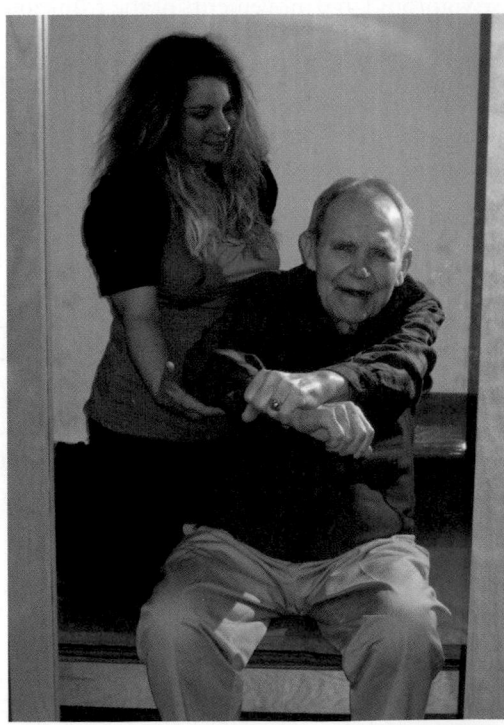

Figure 18.8 The patient with PD performs bilateral symmetrical PNF D2 flexion patterns while sitting (note the difficulty in achieving full shoulder flexion with the LUE).

Table 18.4 Common Areas of Limitation and Suggested Stretching Exercises

Areas of Limitation	Suggested Stretching Exercises
Cervical retraction	• Sitting, back against wall (or supine), head retractions (chin tuck position)
Cervical rotation	• Sit (or supine), with head retracted, head turns side-to-side
Shoulder flexion with trunk extension	• Sitting, hands clasped together, overhead arm lifts with thoracic extension • Supine, pillow under thoracic spine, hands clasp together, overhead arm lifts with thoracic extension
Elbow extension	• Sitting (or standing, modified plantigrade) weight-bearing with both upper extremities (UEs), elbows extended
Trunk extension	• Sitting, thoracic extension over the back of a chair with elbows bent and shoulders retracted • Prone lying, prone push-ups (press-ups) • Standing trunk extension, hands positioned on hips
Trunk rotation	• Supine, upper trunk rotation, hands clasped together (or holding a small ball), arms move with trunk rotation side-to-side • Hook-lying, lower trunk rotation, knees move with trunk rotation side-to-side • Sitting or standing, both arms out to one side (clasped together or holding a small ball), arms move with trunk rotation side-to-side
Hip extension	• Supine with one lower extremity (LE) over edge of mat (hip extended, knee flexed), other knee held to chest • Supine, hips and knees extended • Hook-lying bridging • Standing, active hip extension or forward lunge • High-kneeling with hips extended
Hip abduction	• Supine, one LE extended and abducted, other LE in hook-lying
Knee extension	• Standing, forward lean with wall push-ups
Ankle dorsiflexion	• Standing, both forefeet on edge of step or block, heels off step, lower heels down with light touch-down support of both hands • Standing, forward lean with wall push-ups

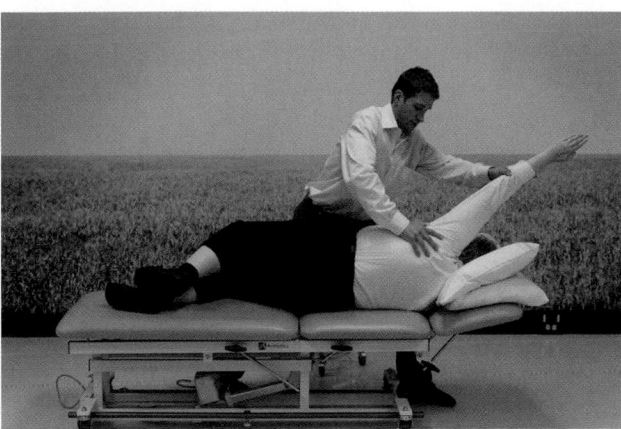

Figure 18.9 Shoulder ROM with scapular mobilization performed in the side-lying position.

must be stretched accordingly. The therapist should also use caution when stretching edematous tissue, a common LE problem associated with prolonged immobility, because risk of injury is also increased in this situation.

Positioning can also be used to stretch tight muscles and soft tissues. Patients in late-stage PD are likely to demonstrate severe flexion contractures of the trunk and limbs. Early on, the patient may benefit from daily positioning in prone-lying. As the disease progresses and significant postural deformity and cardiorespiratory impairments develop, the patient may not tolerate this position. The patient with a developing lateral curvature can be positioned in side-lying with a small pillow under the lateral trunk. Positional stretching is prolonged, with times typically ranging from 20 to 30 minutes. Additional mechanical stretching can be achieved through the use of a tilt table, for example, the patient is positioned with fixed leg straps to reduce hip and knee flexion contractures and toe wedges to reduce plantarflexion contractures.

Resistance Training

Resistance training is indicated for patients with PD who demonstrate primary muscle weakness with impaired motor unit recruitment and rate of force development and disuse weakness associated with prolonged inactivity. Specific areas of weakness are targeted, such as the antigravity extensor muscles. Weakness of these muscles is associated with poor posture (e.g., a flexed, stooped posture) and functional deficits (e.g., inability to get out of a chair, limitations in gait function).[193-195] Weakness also contributes to postural instability, falls, and fall injury, as well as increased sense of effort.[196] The benefits of strength training in the frail elderly have been well documented by the *Frailty and Injuries: Cooperative Studies of Intervention Techniques (FICSIT) trials.*[197] Collectively these studies have shown that the frail elderly improve on measures of strength, functional mobility, balance, gait, fall risk, and quality of life following interventions that include strength training.[198,199] Strength training has also been shown to improve muscle force, bradykinesia, and quality of life in patients with PD.[200] Hirsch et al[201] compared two different exercise training programs for patients with PD. They found significantly greater improvements in balance and strength using a combined program of balance training and high-intensity resistance training for knee extensors and flexors and ankle plantarflexors as compared to balance training alone.

Resistance training is based on the *progressive overload principle.* The amount of resistance is increased during training. Load can be applied using resistance machines, free weights, elastic resistance bands, or manually. With older adults the recommendation is to begin at a lower intensity (e.g., using an RPE Scale of somewhat hard, 5 to 6 on a 10-point scale), ensuring that a set of 10 to 12 repetitions per set can be completed.[202] Progression is as tolerated. Each repetition should be held for 10 seconds. Strength training can be performed 2 days per week on nonconsecutive days. Exercise machines may be safer than free weights for patients with more advanced disease because the movements are more controlled, especially for the patient who demonstrates dyskinesias at peak dose or cognitive changes.[54] Because patients with PD already demonstrate too much stiffness and coactivation, isometric training is generally contraindicated. Functional training activities (see next section) can also be effective interventions to improve strength.

Corcos et al[24] found a significant interaction between medication and strength. Withdrawal of L-dopa during an "off" state period caused a decrease in strength and rate of force development. Exercise training should therefore optimally be timed for "on" periods when the patient is at his or her best (i.e., 45 minutes to 1 hour after medication has been taken). Exercising during an "off" period may not be possible or pose great difficulty for the patient. The patient should consistently exercise at the same time during a medication cycle.

Functional Training

An exercise program should be based on focused practice of functional skills. The overall emphasis is on improving functional mobility with specific emphasis on improving mobility of axial structures, the head, trunk, hips, and shoulders. Progression to more difficult motor activities should be gradual. The more severely involved patient

may benefit initially from assisted movements progressing to active movements (e.g., the PNF technique of RI) to improve initial motor performance.[203]

Bed mobility skills (i.e., rolling, bridging, supine-to-sit transitions) are essential skills that are often very difficult owing to truncal rigidity and bradykinesia. Side-lying rolling activities that emphasize segmental rotation patterns (i.e., isolated upper and lower trunk rotations) should be practiced rather than a log-rolling pattern. Patients with very stiff trunks may benefit from compensatory rolling strategies using the UE or LE to reach over and initiate the movement (e.g., D1F patterns of the UE or LE). Rolling should be practiced on different surfaces progressing from firm to soft and finally simulating the patient's bed surface at home. Bridging is an important activity that improves scooting in bed as well as sit-to-stand transfers (Fig. 18.10).

Sitting can be enhanced through exercises designed to improve pelvic mobility as the patient with PD typically sits with a stiff and posteriorly tilted pelvis (i.e., sacral sitting position) along with a flexed upper trunk. Anterior and posterior tilts, side-to-side tilts, and pelvic clock exercises can be practiced while sitting on a therapy ball, which enhances ease of movement (Fig. 18.11). These activities can then be progressed to sitting on a stationary surface such as a mat table using an inflatable disc to finally no apparatus. Sitting activities should include weight shifting emphasizing upper trunk rotations and reaching. PNF extremity patterns in sitting can be used to enhance trunk mobility. For example, bilateral symmetrical UE D2F and D2E patterns are ideal to promote upper trunk extension. Or a lift/reverse lift pattern can be used to promote upper trunk extension with rotation.

Sit-to-stand (STS) is a difficult activity for many patients with PD, especially with moderate or advanced disease or when in the "off" state. Issues in poor dynamic stability and inadequate limb support contribute to falls. Patients demonstrate poor timing in controlling their COM forward velocity, which tends to be slower. Insufficient upward momentum (LE extension torques) in

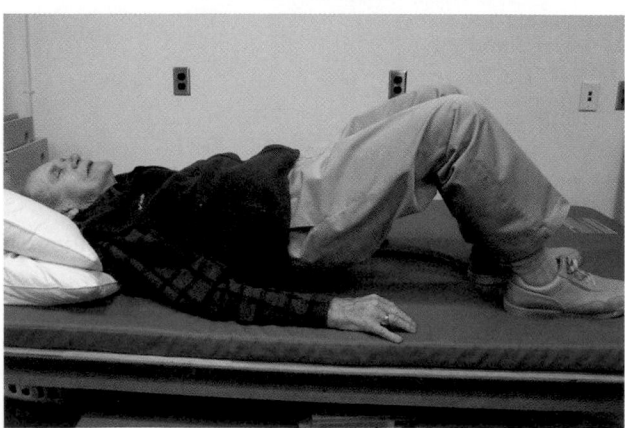

Figure 18.10 The patient with PD practices bridging (note the difficulty in achieving full hip extension).

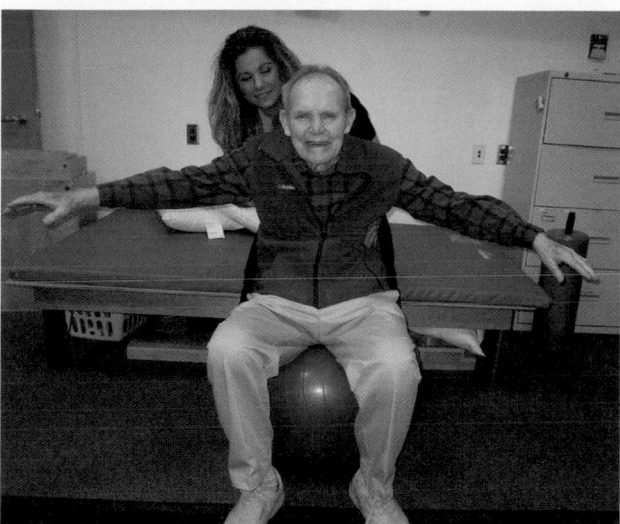

Figure 18.11 The patient with PD practices sitting on ball with UEs abducted to the sides, hands open.

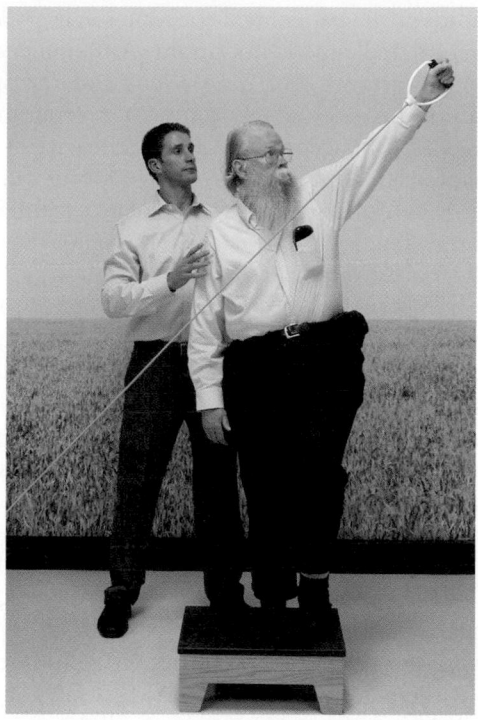

Figure 18.12 The patient with PD practices maintaining a step-up position while performing resisted UE shoulder abduction and flexion using elastic band resistance. The patient is encouraged to turn and look at the hand.

standing up is also problematic.[194] Other factors include level of agonist-antagonist coactivation and rigidity. STS training begins with the patient scooting to the edge of the mat and placing both feet under the knees and apart. Forward trunk flexion can be enhanced through initial rocking, which encourages relaxation. Cueing strategies (e.g., counting, placing one hand between the patient's shoulder blades) can be used to assist the forward lean. Sitting on an inflated disc can also assist in the forward weight shift and seat-off. Standing-up is enhanced by improved LE muscle strength. Strengthening of the hip and knee extensors can be achieved using modified wall squats. Practice standing up from a firm *raised* seat decreases the total excursion and work of extensor muscles and promotes ease of rise. Once control is achieved, progression is then to lower, standard height seats. Standing directly in front of the patient should be avoided, because this may block initial standing attempts. Instead, the therapist or caregiver should stand to the patient's side. If safety issues are apparent, a safety gait belt should be used. The more involved patient can practice STS from a chair with both hands on armrests.[193]

Standing activities can model the progression used in sitting. The patient needs to first gain the fully upright position with symmetrical weight-bearing over the BOS. Tactile cueing or light resistance can be used on the anterior pelvis to encourage movement of the hips forward into full extension. Once standing, weight shifts and rotational movements of the trunk should be practiced (e.g., reciprocal arm swings or reaching movements). Step-ups using a low platform step (forward, lateral) should be practiced. Backward stepping can be used to strengthen hip and spinal extensors and promote upright posturing. To increase the challenge during stepping, elastic resistive bands can be used (Fig. 18.12). The patient can also practice standing with UEs extended and hands weight-bearing on a wall to promote upper trunk extension.

Patients with PD typically experience a high number of falls and should be taught how to get up after a fall. To that end, skills in quadruped creeping should be practiced so the patient is able to move to a nearby stable chair or couch at home. The patient should also practice transitions moving from quadruped to kneeling to half-kneeling and finally to standing using UE support.

Mobilizing facial muscles is another important component of the exercise program because the patient will have limited social interaction and poor feeding skills in the presence of marked facial rigidity and bradykinesia. These factors can greatly influence the patient's overall psychological state, motivation, and social participation. Massage, stretch, manual contacts, and verbal cueing can be used to enhance facial movements. The patient can be instructed to practice lip pursing, movements of the tongue, swallowing, and facial movements such as smiling, frowning, and so forth. A mirror can be used to provide visual feedback. In cases where eating is impaired by immobility, the movements of opening and closing the mouth and chewing should be combined with neck stabilization in a neutral position. Verbal skills should be practiced in association with breath control.

Balance Training

It is important to recall that learning is task and context specific. Thus, a balance training program should include a variety of activities that alter task demands and expose the patient to varying environmental conditions. Whenever possible the therapist should try to duplicate the conditions the patient will encounter in everyday life. The level of challenge is important. A therapist should know the limitations of the patient and the specific demands of the task and environment in order to select and progress tasks accordingly and ensure patient safety. See Chapter 10, Strategies to Improve Motor Function, for a more complete discussion of balance training.

An important focus of balance training for the patient with PD is COM and LOS control training. Patients should be instructed in how COM influences balance and how to improve posture in sitting, in standing, and during dynamic movement tasks. Patients should also explore their LOS and practice working toward expanding them in both sitting and standing. In standing, patients with PD typically demonstrate restricted LOS with forward displacement of center of foot pressure. Patients should be instructed in how to improve postural alignment and in ways to avoid postural disturbances and falls. The therapist can assist with postural and safety awareness by using appropriate verbal, tactile, or proprioceptive cues to facilitate the desired responses. For example, the patient is instructed to "sit tall" or "stand tall" and a mirror is used to provide feedback concerning upright posture. A standing platform training device (i.e., posturography system) can be valuable in providing COM position and LOS biofeedback. The patient is instructed in weight shifting that expands the LOS. The Nintendo Wii Balance Board is a widely available and economical force platform and biofeedback system. When compared to a laboratory-grade force platform the Nintendo Wii Balance Board was valid in quantifying center of pressure, an important component of standing balance.[204] Subjects with poor positional awareness who trained on the Wii Balance Board with real-time visual biofeedback demonstrated significant improvements in weight-bearing symmetry.[205] Elderly subjects who trained with this device over a 4-week period improved on average 9.14 points on the BBS.[206]

Balance training should emphasize practice of dynamic stability tasks (e.g., weight shifts, alternating unilateral weight-bearing, reaching, axial rotation of the head and trunk, axial rotation combined with reaching, and so forth). Seated activities can include sitting on a compliant surface (inflatable disc) or a therapy ball. Challenges to balance can also be introduced in quadruped (Fig. 18.13), kneeling (Fig. 18.14), half-kneeling (Fig. 18.15), and standing on a disc (Figs. 18.16 and 18.17). Altering arm positions (e.g., arms out to side, arms folded across chest, reaching); altering foot/leg positions (e.g., feet apart, feet together); or adding voluntary movements (e.g., overhead arm clapping, head and trunk rotations, single leg raises, stepping or marching in place) can all be used to increase difficulty of the activity. Training should focus on achieving faster initiation and execution movement times supported by the use of appropriate cueing strategies.[166] Externally induced perturbations in the form of gentle manual displacements of the patient's COM are generally contraindicated for many patients with PD because they

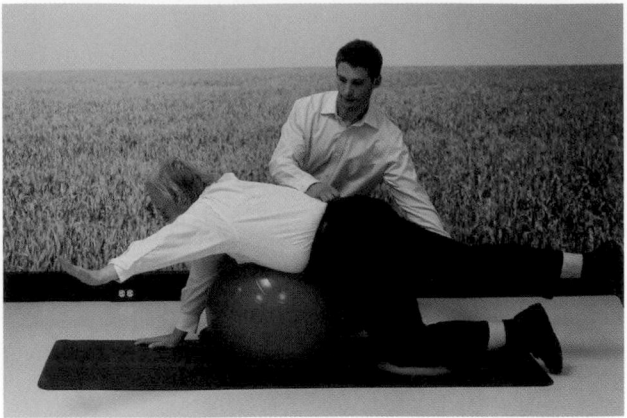

Figure 18.13 The patient with PD practices contralateral UE/LE lifts in quadruped over a ball.

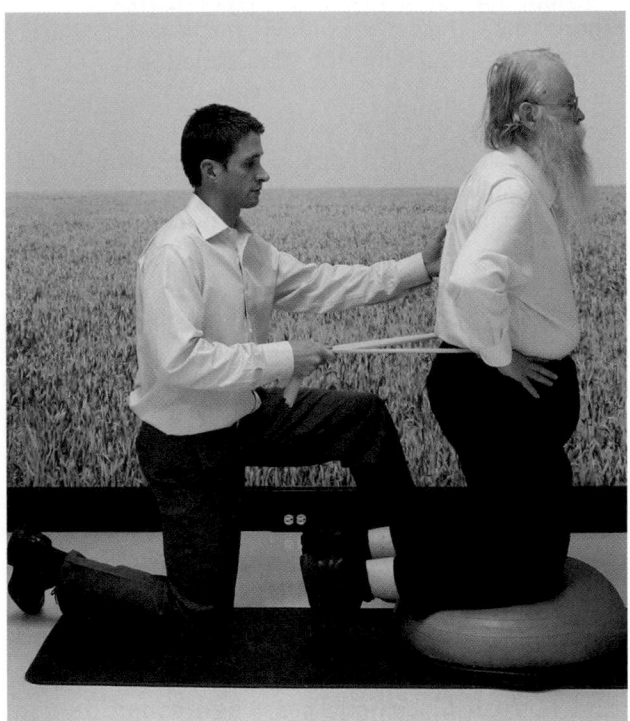

Figure 18.14 The patient with PD practices kneeling on a BOSU™ disc. The therapist provides resistance using an elastic band to promote full hip extension.

can produce an increase in postural stiffness and fixation. Strategies for varying environmental demands include altering the support surface (e.g., standing on foam), visual inputs (e.g., reduced lighting, eyes closed), or challenging the patient with a variable open environment (e.g., busy clinic setting).

Adequate strength and ROM are important components needed to withstand the challenges of balance. The patient can be instructed in standing exercises to enhance balance, including heel-rises and toe-offs, partial wall squats and chair rises, single-limb stance with side-kicks or back-kicks, and marching in place. Collectively these exercises are sometimes referred to as the *"kitchen sink exercises"* and are important components of the HEP

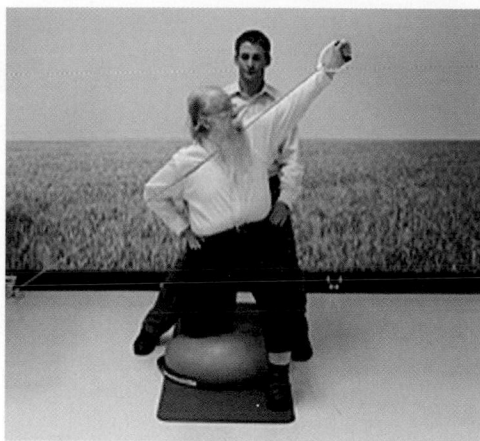

Figure 18.15 The patient with PD practices half-kneeling on a BOSU™ disc while performing resisted UE shoulder abduction and flexion using elastic band resistance.

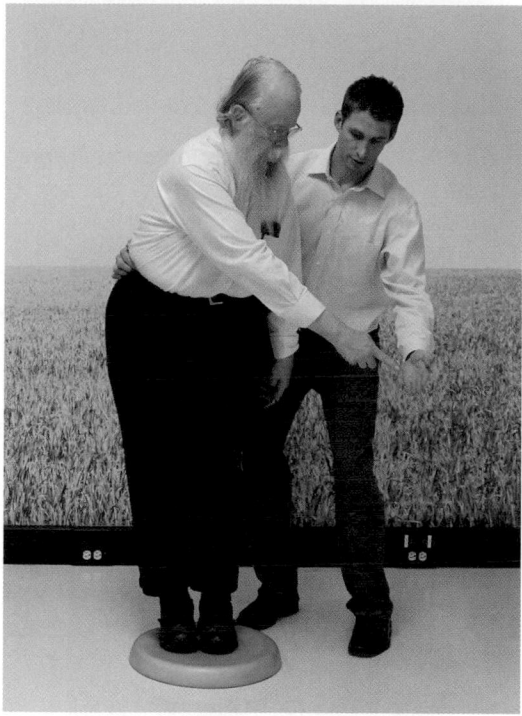

Figure 18.16 The patient with PD practices standing on an inflated disc while reaching across, promoting upper trunk rotation.

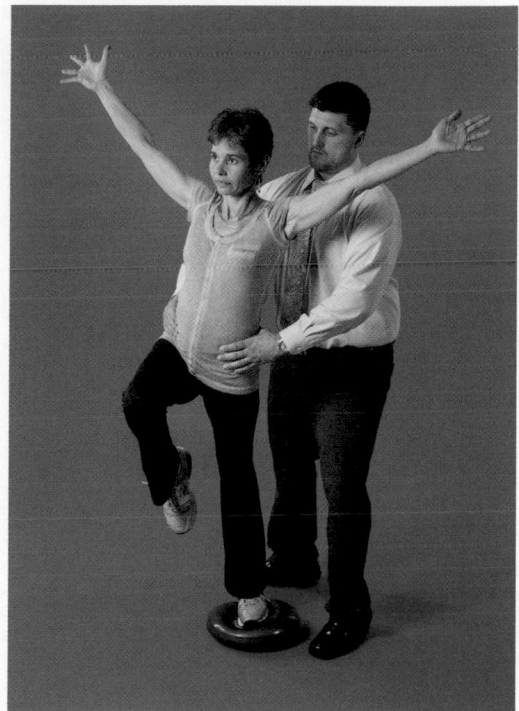

Figure 18.17 The patient with young-onset PD practices standing with one foot on an inflated disc with bilateral "Big arms" and hands open, palms up.

for patients with balance deficiencies. The patient may require light touch-down support of the hands to start in order to stabilize; progression should be to no support as soon as possible.

Whole body vibration (WBV) is gaining popularity as a treatment for patients with neurological diseases. It is theorized that the seesaw-like displacement of the platform mimics human gait[207] and that postural responses are induced by vibration of the foot soles.[208,209] It is also believed that WBV increases efficiency of agonist/antagonist pairs.[210,211] Systematic literature reviews reveal insufficient high-quality studies and only minor evidence from the current literature that WBV improves strength, proprioception, gait, and balance.[212,213] For people with PD, WBV seated in a physioacoustic chair resulted in improved gait, UPDRS scores, and upper limb control and significant reductions in tremor and rigidity.[214] Another study examined the effect of treatment standing on a random multidirectional vibrating platform. After WBV, subjects presented with significantly improved scores on the UPDRS with reductions in tremor and rigidity.[215] Additional quality research examining the efficacy of WBV in the treatment of people with PD is needed.

Locomotor Training

Locomotor training goals focus on reducing primary gait impairments, which typically include slowed speed, decreased stride length, lack of a heel-toe sequence with forward progression characterized by a shuffling (festinating) gait pattern, diminished contralateral trunk movement and arm swing, and an overall attitude of flexion while walking. Goals also focus on increasing the patient's ability to safely perform functional mobility activities and prevent falls.[216] Effective strategies for improving upright alignment and safety include having the patient walk with vertical poles (pole walking) (Fig. 18.18). Strategies to enhance posture, step length, velocity, and arm swing include the use of *verbal instructional sets* (e.g., "Walk tall," "Walk fast," "Take large steps," "Swing both arms"). Behrman et al[217] found that commands for large step and arm swing were more effective instructional strategies than the command to walk

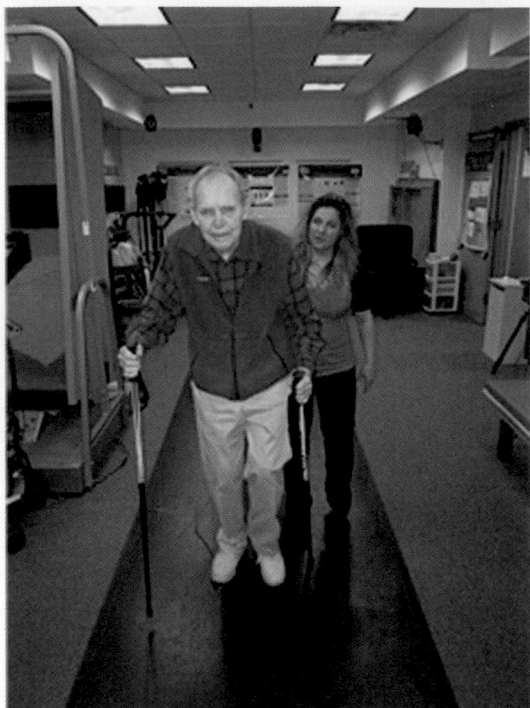

Figure 18.18 The patient with PD practices walking using two vertical poles.

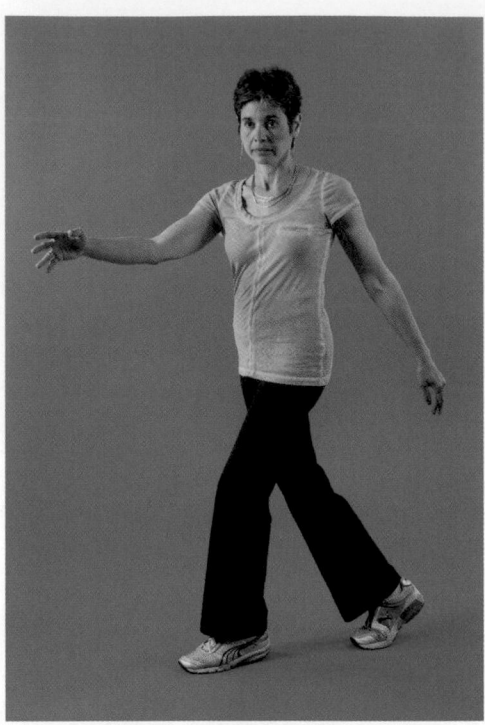

Figure 18.19 The patient with young-onset PD practices cross-step walking.

fast. As previously discussed, visual and auditory cues are also effective in improving gait speed and step length. Transverse visual–spatial cues (across the gait path) were more beneficial than parallel visual cues (alongside the gait path) in improving gait velocity, stride length, and percentage of leg stance time.[218] Strategies to improve foot placement can include use of floor markers or footprints on the floor. Strategies to improve step height include practice marching in place progressing to walking using an exaggerated high stepping pattern. Brisk marching music can be used to enhance pace. Sidestepping and crossed-step walking can be practiced (Fig. 18.19). The PNF activity of braiding, which combines side-stepping with alternate crossed-stepping, is an ideal training activity for the patient with early PD because it emphasizes lower trunk rotation with stepping and side-stepping movements. It can be practiced with the patient holding on lightly to a dowel held jointly with therapist or as a free walking pattern. Advanced stepping and balancing can be achieved by having the patient practice juggling scarves (Fig. 18.20). Reciprocal arm swing during gait can be enhanced by having the patient and therapist hold onto a set of two dowels (one in each hand). The therapist walks behind the patient and uses his or her arm swing to assist the patient's.

Patients with PD who practiced locomotor training on a motorized treadmill with an overhead harness demonstrated improvements in postural stability, gait (e.g., walking speed, step and stride length), motor function, and quality of life.[219-227] Both body weight support (e.g., up to 20%)[220] and no body support have been

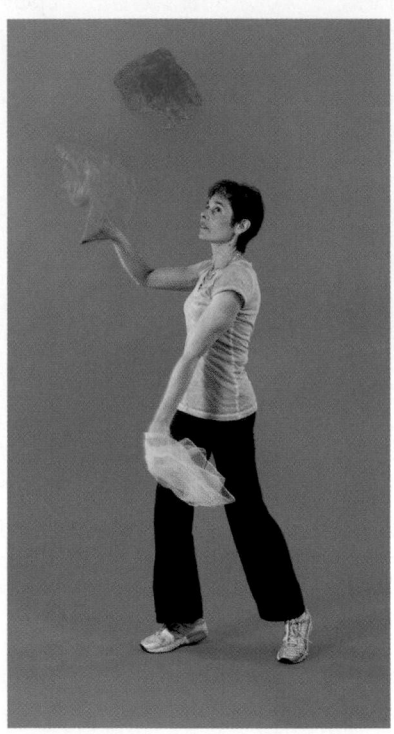

Figure 18.20 The patient with young-onset PD practices stepping and juggling a set of scarves.

used.[219] In a long-term study, Miyai et al[221] found that gains in walking speed and number of steps following this type of training were maintained at 4 months. The researchers stated that attentional strategies were not used and speculate that the enhancement of gait might be due to activation of central pattern generators as is thought the case in stroke and spinal cord injury (SCI) studies. The treadmill may be acting as an external cue to enhance gait rhythmicity and reduce gait variability.[224] The benefits of treadmill training, as with exercise training in general, are dose dependent. More pronounced improvements are noted with high-intensity practice and incremental increases in treadmill speed.[225,226] High-intensity treadmill training has been shown to normalize corticomotor excitability in early PD.[226] The motorized treadmill has also been used for step training in people with PD. While supported in a safety harness, patients practiced stepping in all four directions in response to suddenly turning the treadmill on and off.[228]

Locomotor training should also include task-specific training designed to promote full participation in social roles pertaining to family life, leisure, and community participation. This includes varying the walking task (e.g., walking on a tile floor, on carpet, outdoors on sidewalks and grassy terrain). Additional challenges include walking in the community (e.g., variable open environments), stair climbing, up and down curbs, and ramp walking. Patients with PD often demonstrate difficulties in obstacle stepping due to minimized foot clearance. Foot clearance can be improved with repeated practice of stepping over horizontal floor markers or laser light signals.

Patients in the advanced stage of the disease will be limited in terms of walking and variations that can be utilized. The overall goal at this stage is to promote regular walking while maintaining safety and preventing falls. Compensatory training strategies are indicated. Caregiver instruction regarding assisted walking and safety is imperative. Freezing episodes are common and are often resistant to drug therapy. The therapist and patient should identify and practice strategies for unfreezing gait.[229] For example, cueing or "trick" movements such as dropping a tissue that the patient must step over can be successful in reducing freezing. Some patients, especially those in the postural instability gait disturbed group, can benefit from walking with a therapy dog. The dog provides an assist in balance and momentum, and a source of external cueing of stepping movements (Fig. 18.21).

Spinal Orthotics

Spinal bracing may be an appropriate adjunct to therapy for patients with postural deformities common to PD (e.g., increased thoracic kyphosis, decreased costal expansion, and forward head posture). The Spinomed thoracolumbar orthosis is unique in that it not only corrects faulty posture but also has been shown to increase trunk stability, increase respiratory vital capacity, and improve a patient's self-report of well-being.[230,231] When the brace was worn for 6 months the subjects had a 73% increase in back extensor strength and a 58% increase in

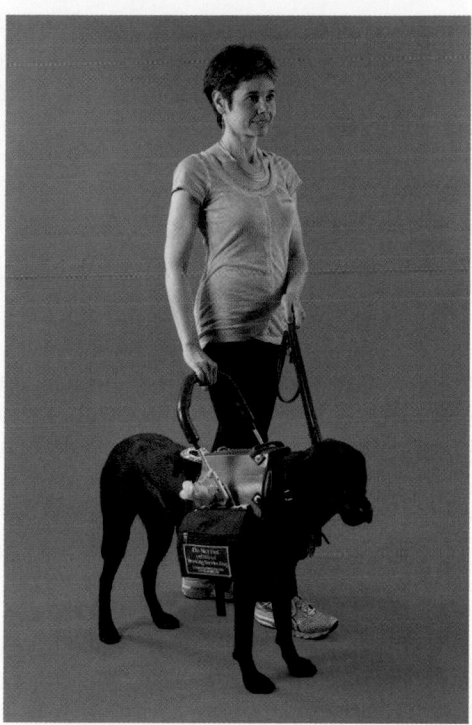

Figure 18.21 The patient with young-onset PD and primary impairments in postural stability and gait walks with the assist of canine partner.

abdominal flexor strength. These strength gains are attributed to increased muscular activity in response to the proprioceptive biofeedback of the brace.[232] A study investigating gait stability and physical functioning in women with postmenopausal osteoporosis demonstrated decreased double limb stance time associated with a beneficial impact on gait stability.[233] Further research is warranted to determine if this type of orthotic intervention holds potential for patients with PD.

Pulmonary Rehabilitation

The four main classifications of respiratory disorders in patients with PD are medication complications, upper airway obstructions, restrictive disorders, and aspiration pneumonia.[234] Since respiratory dysfunction in the neurological movement disorders population is linked to a high rate of disability and mortality, it is critical that the prevention and treatment of these dysfunctions take priority. Components include diaphragmatic breathing exercises, air-shifting techniques, and exercises that recruit neck, shoulder, and trunk muscles. Manual techniques such as vibration and shaking can be used to ensure complete exhalation, distal alveoli opening, and to assist with secretion clearance. The patient should be instructed in deep-breathing exercises to improve chest wall mobility and vital capacity. Air shifts are promoted to lesser-ventilated areas of the lung. For example, basal expansion can be promoted using side-lying recumbent positioning, manual stretch, and resistance to those segments. Upper body resistance training exercises are indicated. These can include raising and lowering a dowel with light weights added to increase resistance (e.g., 1 lb [453.5 g]). Weights are increased as function improves. As previously mentioned, chest wall mobility can be improved by using PNF UE bilateral symmetrical D2 flexion and extension patterns. Light weights (wrist cuffs) can also be added to these exercises. Patients are encouraged to coordinate breathing with UE movement. Exercises are performed in unsupported sitting to promote trunk stabilization. A focus on improving trunk extension is especially important in improving breathing patterns in patients with postural kyphosis. Pulmonary rehabilitation programs have been shown to be safe and effective for patients with PD in improving pulmonary function (i.e., oxygen consumption [VO_2], minute ventilation [VE], respiratory rate, inspiratory muscle strength)[235,236] and perception of dyspnea.[237]

Speech Therapy

The quality of speech in patients with PD is often a breathy monotone, soft voice that is perceived by the patient to be of normal loudness. Hypophonia is caused by a bradykinetic bellows mechanism (chest wall and diaphragm) and patients' inaccurate perception of their own speech effort. Speech deficits are seen in 80% of patients with PD and have a dramatic effect on function with 30% reporting it as the most disabling part of the disease.[239] As mentioned earlier, the Lee Silverman Voice Treatment (LSVT) was designed specifically for patients with PD.[239] It focuses on intensive high-effort exercise with a single functionally relevant target (loudness) and a recalibration of self-perception of vocal loudness. This technique effectively increases vocal loudness and improves facial expressions in patients with PD.[240-242]

Aerobic Exercise

An individualized exercise prescription is developed based on the ACSM guidelines for frequency, intensity, duration, and progression.[54] Intensities will be less than normal training intensities or submaximal (i.e., 60% to 80% of maximum HR), based on the patient's level of disease, fitness, and lifestyle. When lower intensities are used, longer-duration or more frequent exercise sessions are necessary to improve fitness. Careful monitoring is indicated, because autonomic dysfunction is common. Long-term L-dopa use can produce arrhythmias and OH along with dyskinesias. The therapist should monitor vital signs (HR, RR, BP), RPE, fatigue levels, and symptoms of exertional intolerance (e.g., significant dyspnea, hypotensive response, and so forth).

Training modes can include leg and arm ergometry and walking. Selection will depend on the specific abilities of the patient; for example, postural instability and increased risk of falls may rule out use of a treadmill without an overhead harness. Recumbent or seated LE ergometry is a suitable alternative. For most patients a program of regular walking is recommended. The duration, speed, and terrain covered can be modified, based on individual ability. Accessibility to a supervised walking program using an indoor walking track is important for some to ensure safety. A shopping mall can provide an acceptable environment for community walkers in case of inclement or extremes of weather. A supervised aerobic pool program can also provide an acceptable mode of exercise for some patients. The warmth of the water may be relaxing and the buoyancy may enhance stepping movements. The minimum recommended aerobic exercise frequency is 3 sessions per week. Daily walking with short multiple bouts (20 to 30 minutes) spaced throughout the day is recommended for individuals with lower functional capacity. Intermittent exercise with adequate rest intervals is indicated for those patients who are elderly and deconditioned, and who present with restrictive pulmonary dysfunction. Aerobic training programs have been shown to be safe and effective for patients with PD in improving aerobic capacity.[243,244]

Group and Home Exercises

Community-based group exercise classes can be valuable for patients with PD. Patients benefit from the positive support, camaraderie, and communication the group situation offers.[245,246] Careful evaluation of each patient before admission into a group is essential. Patients should be able to perform the therapeutic core of the class. Selecting patients with similar levels of disability is often advisable because the sense of competition can frequently be a key factor in motivating groups. The ratio of staff to patients should be kept small (ideally 1:8 or 1:10), and extra staff should be added if patients are unable to work on their own. A variety of activities can be used to stimulate and motivate patients. The patients can begin in the seated position and progress to standing, using light, touch-down support of the back of the chair. Stretching exercises or calisthenics involving large muscle groups and multijoint compound movements can be used as an initial warm-up activity. Progression is to combination movements (UEs and LEs with axial trunk rotation). Well-structured, low-impact aerobics are an appropriate focus for a group class. For example, patients can march in place, first in sitting, then in standing. The group can then practice walking with an emphasis on taking large, high steps. Music is used to provide necessary stimulation to movement and movement pacing. Exercise stations (e.g., stationary bicycle, mats, pulleys, and so forth) can also be used. Exercises done by the whole group together should focus on important exercise goals (e.g., improving ROM, mobility, and so forth). Recreational activities can follow the aerobic portion, such as line dancing, ball activities, beanbag toss, and so forth. The activities selected should be interesting and varied. A relaxation segment should be incorporated into each class. Yoga and Tai Chi group classes effectively address multiple components of PD by improving posture, flexibility, core stability, functional mobility, balance, relaxation, and socialization.[247-251] King and Horak[252] recommend incorporating Tai Chi with other agility exercises (e.g., kayaking, boxing, lunges, agility training, and Pilates exercises) to delay loss of mobility in people with PD.[252]

The home-based exercises include exercises designed to improve relaxation, flexibility, strength, and cardiopulmonary function (all previously discussed). A key element is stressing the importance of regular daily exercise and avoidance of prolonged periods of inactivity. The HEP should be realistic and of moderate duration and intensity. The patient should be cautioned against overdoing activity, which could result in excessive fatigue. Early morning warm-up calisthenics are often helpful in reducing the increased stiffness patients may experience on arising. Stretching and strengthening exercises are performed in supine, sitting, and standing positions. Home ROM exercises can often be assisted by use of adaptive equipment. For example, to reduce the effects of forward head and kyphotic posture, the patient can be instructed to hang by the hands using an overhead bar. Standing, corner wall stretches can also be used to provide a maintained stretch on the upper trunk flexors. Use of a wand or cane can be effective in promoting overhead motions. In standing, a countertop or back of a sturdy chair can be used to assist in stabilization during standing calisthenics and balance activities. Home-based exercise programs have been found to be effective in improving postural control and mobility in people with PD.[253,254]

ADAPTIVE AND SUPPORTIVE DEVICES

Attention should be directed toward needs for adaptive and supportive devices that can improve function. To promote bed mobility, the patient can be helped to assume a sitting position by elevating the head of an electronic hospital bed or with commercially available blocks approximately 4 in (10 cm) high (furniture legs fit into a recess in the block). A simpler solution might include attaching a knotted rope or canvas "ladder" to the end of the bed to pull on. The bed should be stable and the mattress firm to facilitate mobility. Satin sheets and pajamas have sometimes been helpful to enhance bed mobility. Patients should be instructed to select firm chairs with armrests and avoid soft, low seats such as a low sofa. The chair can be raised (i.e., 4 in [10 cm] and secured with blocks, or tilted forward by elevating only the back legs about 2 in [5 cm]). Some patients benefit from the use of a rocking chair to facilitate independent sit-to-stand transfers. Chairs that have spring-loaded seats that push the patient into standing are heavily marketed to the geriatric population but should be used with caution. The patient is propelled into standing but may have difficulty stopping the movement and/or getting his or her balance within an appropriate time frame when first reaching the standing position. A raised toilet seat and toilet rails are also essential devices to facilitate ease of sit-to-stand transitions in the bathroom.

Loose-fitting clothing and sneakers with hook and loop closures can be used to facilitate dressing. If the patient demonstrates a shuffling gait, shoes should have leather or hard composition soles, because shoes with crepe or rubber soles will not slide easily and can result in falls. A festinating gait can sometimes be alleviated by the addition of modified heel or shoe wedges. A flat heel or toe wedge may slow down a propulsive gait. The use of assistive devices can be problematic owing to movement difficulties. A cane can be helpful for patients with mild to moderate disease to assist in balance or cue stepping (inverted walking stick). It is important that the height of the device not promote increased flexion of the trunk. Vertical poles (previously mentioned) can also be helpful to improve upright posture, trunk rotation, and arm swing during walking. Patients with more pronounced movement difficulties and poor balance are not likely to benefit from assistive devices. Walkers with wheels are particularly hazardous and are likely to increase a festinating gait; hand brakes are an essential requirement.

Most patients use adaptive devices to assist in ADL. Reachers can be used to provide assistance in dressing as well as for other activities. Eating can be facilitated in a number of ways. The patient should be seated properly, close to the table, with good posture. Specially adapted utensils, plate guards, and enlarged handles can aid the patient's efforts. Because eating time will be prolonged, heated plates or pads may help keep food warm and palatable. Drooling and/or spills should be anticipated and clothing protected. Extra time should be planned, and the patient should not feel rushed.

PSYCHOSOCIAL ISSUES

The progressive nature of PD necessitates frequent personal and social adjustments, and affects all aspects of life for both the patient and family. Disruptions in daily functions, roles, and activities are experienced. Some of the changes associated with PD are socially isolating (masked face, progressive immobility, and unintelligible speech) whereas other changes (increased salivation, perspiration, decreased sexual function) are distressing and can be socially embarrassing. The patient may feel increasingly isolated and family relationships may suffer. The principal goal for team members is to assist the patient and family in their understanding of the disease and in developing insights and adjustments that lead to more effective self-management. Some individuals are able to successfully deal with the changes associated with the disease; others are not. Coping skills can be facilitated. First and foremost, education is the key to assisting patients and family members assume responsibility. Feelings of hopelessness and dependency are reduced as the patient develops a sense of control over his or her own life. Self-management skills that should be promoted include advanced planning of activities, effective time management strategies, and stress management techniques. It is equally important to ensure that patients do not become isolated and that appropriate services are available. Team members must be vigilant regarding their assumptions and expectations. A condescending or pessimistic and limiting attitude can become a self-fulfilling prophecy. Patients and family members need reassurances and encouragement. An overall emphasis on what patients *can do* rather than what they cannot do helps to empower patients. Therapists need to provide a message of *hope tempered with realism*.

PATIENT, FAMILY, AND CAREGIVER EDUCATION

The interdisciplinary team provides information about a variety of topics related to living with PD. These are presented in Box 18.6. Interventions can take the form of direct one-on-one instruction, group sessions, printed materials, and video or computer presentations. The therapist's overall approach needs to be positive and supportive.

Community support groups are available for patients and their families. They disseminate information and offer a chance to discuss common issues, problems, and management tips. They also can provide a stabilizing influence, assisting patients and families to focus on healthy behaviors, coping skills, and effective self-management. For some patients in the early stages of the disease, participation in a support group may increase levels of anxiety as they observe more disabled patients. Groups particularly targeted to patients with early-stage disease and similar ages may be more helpful.

Educational pamphlets, newsletters, and location of support groups can be obtained through national PD associations.

National Parkinson Foundation (NPF)
1501 Northwest 9th Street (Bob Hope Road)
Miami, FL 33136-1407
Website: www.parkinson.org

Box 18.6   Elements of a Patient, Family, and Caregiver Education Program

- Parkinson's disease: clinical presentation, strategies to manage symptoms
- Medications: purpose, dosage, possible adverse side effects, signs of either overmedication or undermedication
- Preventative measures to minimize the secondary complications and impairments
- Impact of PD on movement and effective strategies to manage movement problems
- Barriers to exercise and effective solutions to regular exercise participation
- Impact of PD on function and effective strategies to maintain independent function in home, community, or work environments
- Strategies for energy conservation and activity pacing
- Strategies for ensuring activity participation in valued leisure and family activities
- Community resources for patients: support groups, in-home interventions, community training programs, day programs
- Community resources for caregivers: counseling, support groups, exercise programs, respite care

---

Phone: 800-327-4545
E-mail: mailbox@parkinson.org
Parkinson's Disease Foundation (PDF)
1359 Broadway, Suite 1509
New York, NY 10018
Website: www.pdf.org
Phone: 800-457-6676
E-mail: info@pdf.org

Web-based resources for clinicians and patients/families living with PD are presented in Appendix 18.C. A listing of sample educational and video materials can be found in Supplemental Readings and Materials.

SUMMARY

PD is a chronic, progressive disorder of the BG characterized by the cardinal features of rigidity, bradykinesia, tremor, and postural instability. Additional impairments include the development of abnormal fixed postures, poverty of movement, fatigue, masked face, contractures, a festinating gait pattern, swallowing and communication difficulties, visual and sensorimotor disturbances, cognitive and behavioral dysfunction, autonomic dysfunction, and cardiopulmonary changes. Pharmacological interventions have become the mainstay of treatment and provide protective and symptomatic treatment. Effective rehabilitation focuses on the patient's stage of disease and symptoms, activity limitations, and residual abilities and assets. Interventions are restorative; that is, rehabilitation is focused on the improvement of strength, ROM, functional skills, endurance, and so forth. Individuals with PD also benefit from functional maintenance programs designed to manage the effects of progressive disease. Strategies are developed to prevent or reduce indirect impairments and promote regular exercise, good health, and self-management skills. A comprehensive team approach including active involvement of patient and family provides optimal benefits. Team members need to be active during all stages of the disease, assisting the patient and family in maintenance of function and providing psychosocial support as needed.

Questions for Review

1. What are the major CNS structures involved in Parkinson's disease and what are the pathophysiological changes associated with the disease?

2. Differentiate between cogwheel rigidity and lead pipe rigidity.

3. What impairments in postural stability are typically seen in patients with PD?

4. What are the nonmotor impairments in cognition associated with PD?

5. What are the major adverse effects associated with long-term use of levodopa/carbidopa?

6. How might the goals/outcomes and interventions vary by stage of disease?

7. Orthostatic hypotension is a common problem in patients with PD. How should it be examined?

8. Identify appropriate motor learning strategies for the patient with PD in terms of practice and feedback.

9. Describe the gait impairments common in patients with PD. What interventions can be used to improve locomotor function?

10. What guidelines for aerobic training are appropriate for the patient with early- to middle-stage PD?

CASE STUDY

The patient is a 60-year-old woman with a 7-year history of PD. Lately she has experienced increasing severity of symptoms and is referred for outpatient physical therapy and a home exercise program (HEP).

HISTORY

The patient first presented with tremor of her left hand that progressed to include stiffness and awkwardness of her left UE and LE. Her family physician referred her to a neurologist who found moderate tremor and rigidity on the left side. He prescribed Artane, which was helpful for a while. Eventually the tremor became worse, especially under conditions of stress when she was unable to use her left UE at all. She was then started on Sinemet and referred for an initial episode of physical therapy as an outpatient. Once Sinemet began to work and her symptoms dramatically lessened, she stopped physical therapy and her HEP. Over the next few years as her symptoms increased, her dose of Sinemet was increased.

CURRENT STATUS

The patient is currently taking Sinemet and bromocriptine. She reports bouts of dyskinesia about 45 minutes into taking her Sinemet that involve involuntary writhing movements of her LUE. Her chief complaints are:

- Difficulty walking, especially when she has to go through a narrow doorway, or walk in a crowded place.
- Episodes of gait blocks (freezing of gait); if she tries to do something while walking, such as take a tissue out of her pocket, she stops abruptly in her tracks. The harder she tries to move, the worse it gets. Episodes of freezing have lasted up to 20 minutes.
- Postural instability: over the past few years she has experienced increasing bouts of uncontrolled or unsteady balance. This is particularly disturbing to her because if it occurs while she is walking, it causes her to fall. She has fallen seven times in the past month, with no residual fall injury. Because of her increased fear of falling, she has stopped going out by herself.
- Experiences increased difficulty rolling over in bed, getting out of bed, and standing up from a chair independently. Her husband now has to provide assistance 90% of the time to accomplish these activities.
- Reports having trouble sleeping at night. She has stopped drinking coffee but this has not helped. She wakes four to five times a night, and requires assistance from her husband to go to the bathroom at night. She also has hallucinated at night, claiming to see bugs on the wall. During these periods she becomes extremely frightened.
- Complains her medication seems to be helping less and less. If she plans to go out, she takes an extra Sinemet. She revisited her neurologist in hopes that he would increase her dosage. Instead he told her the symptoms were most likely the result of excess medication. He instructed her not to take the extra Sinemet and adjusted her dosage.

EXAMINATION FINDINGS
Cognition
Alert, oriented × 3; she is displaying mild impairments in short-term memory.
Psychosocial
She is showing signs of depression; she is less interested in going out and socializing; she reports "it is just too much effort."
Speech
Mild dysarthria, hypophonia.
Sensation
Slightly decreased proprioception bilaterally in both ankles; otherwise intact.
Tone
Rigidity (cogwheel type) moderate in all extremities L > R.
   Marked rigidity throughout neck and trunk.
   Masklike face.
Range of Motion
Decreased due to moderate rigidity; with limitations in:
- Bilateral elbow extension (10° to 140°)
- Bilateral hip extension (0° to 10°)
- Bilateral knee extension (10° to 120°)
- Bilateral ankle dorsiflexion (0° to 15° RLE; 0° to 10° LLE).
Strength
Generally fair (3/5) to good minus (4–/5).
   Poor (2/5) dorsiflexor muscle grades in both ankles.
Motor Function
Moderate to severe resting tremors, L hand > R hand.
   Bradykinesia: marked slowness, poverty of movement.
   Hesitation on initiation of movement; frequent arrests of ongoing movement.
   Dyskinesias: LUE
Posture
Forward head position; flexed; kyphotic spine.
   Stands with flexion of elbows, hips, and knees.
Balance
Decreased limits of stability.
   Patient's forward alignment position increases her tendency to fall forward.
   Sitting static control: good (able to maintain balance without handhold).
   Sitting dynamic control: fair (accepts minimal challenge; able to lift both arms).
   Standing static control: good (able to maintain balance without handhold).
   Standing dynamic control: poor (unable to accept minimal challenge without handhold).
   She has slowed reactions to loss of balance with decreased rotational movements of head/trunk and ineffective use of stepping strategies.
   Timed Up and Go score is 36 seconds.
   Patient is fearful of falling.
Functional Mobility
Generally decreased.
   Requires moderate assist: rolling in bed, supine-to-sit and sit-to-stand transfers.
   Unable to bridge secondary to hip flexion contractures.
   Patient has good safety awareness.
Locomotion
Ambulates independently with a shuffling gait pattern with decreased step length and arm, trunk, hip, and knee motions; tendency for propulsive gait.
   Afraid to walk outside alone for fear of falling.
   Frequent freezing of gait.
Self-Care
Requires minimal assistance to supervision for feeding.
   Requires minimal to moderate assist for dressing/bathing.
Cardiopulmonary Function/Endurance
Shallow (upper respiratory) breathing pattern.

Generally decreased functional capacity (estimated functional work capacity [FWC] is 6 metabolic equivalents [METs]).

Patient fatigues easily and requires frequent rest periods.

Mild edema both ankles.

Skin

Intact, no areas of breakdown.

Experiences bouts of increased perspiration.

GUIDING QUESTIONS

1. Identify/categorize this patient's problems in terms of:

a. Direct impairments

b. Indirect impairments

c. Activity limitations

d. Participation restrictions/disability

2. Identify two outcomes (the remediation of activity limitations and disability) and two goals (remediation of impairments) for this patient.

3. Determine four interventions that could be used at the start of therapy to achieve the outcomes and goals provided for question 2. Provide a brief rationale for each.

4. What motor learning strategies will assist in improving her motor function?

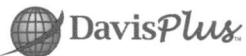 | For additional resources, including answers to the questions for review and case study guiding questions, please visit **http://davisplus.fadavis.com**

 The reader is referred to video **Case Study 6: Patient with Parkinson's Disease** for additional review and study. The full written case study, including tables, figures, charts, and three video segments (examination, intervention, and outcome), appears online at *DavisPlus*. The case study poses questions for the reader's consideration with suggested answers to the case study questions, also posted online at *DavisPlus*.

References

1. Parkinson's Disease Foundation: Statistics on Parkinson's. Retrieved April 22, 2012, from www.pdf.org/en/Parkinson_statistics.
2. Van Den Eeden, SK, et al: Incidence of Parkinson's disease: Variation by age, gender, and race/ethnicity. Am J Epidemiol 157:1015, 2003.
3. Rajput, M, and Rajput, A: Epidemiology of Parkinsonism. In Factor, S, and Weiner, W (eds): Parkinson's Disease—Diagnosis and Clinical Management. Demos Medical Publishing, New York, 2002, p 31.
4. Parkinson, J: An Essay on the Shaking Palsy. Originally published by Sherwood, Neely, and Jones, London, 1817. [Available from Classic Pieces Series (Parkinson's Disease): J Neuropsychiatry Clin Neurosci 14(2):223, 2002. Retrieved April 23, 2012, from http://neuro.psychiatryonline.org/article.aspx?volume=14&page=223.]
5. Sacks, O: Awakenings. Harper Collins, New York, 1990.
6. Wright, JM, and Keller-Byme, J: Environmental determinants of Parkinson's disease. Arch Environ Occup Health 60:32–38, 2005.
7. Koller, W, et al: Environmental risk factors in Parkinson's disease. Neurology 40:1218–1221, 1990.
8. Langston, JW, and Ballard, P: Chronic parkinsonism in humans due to a product of meperidine-analog synthesis. Science 219: 976, 1983.
9. Pal, P, Samii, A, and Calne, D: Cardinal features of early Parkinson's disease. In Factor, S, and Weiner, W (eds): Parkinson's Disease—Diagnosis and Clinical Management. Demos Medical Publishing, New York, 2002, p 41.
10. Gilman, S and Newman S: Manter and Gatz's Essentials of Clinical Neuroanatomy and Neurophysiology 10th ed. F A Davis, Philadelphia, 2003. Davie, CA: A review of Parkinson's disease. Br Med Bull 86:109–127, 2008.
11. Barron, K: Pathology. In Factor, S, and Weiner, W (eds): Parkinson's Disease—Diagnosis and Clinical Management. Demos Medical Publishing, New York, 2002, p 183.
12. Braak, H, et al: Staging of brain pathology related to sporadic Parkinson's disease. Neurobiol Aging 24:197–211, 2003.
13. Braak, H, Ghebremedhin, E, and Rub, U: Stages in the development of Parkinson's disease–related pathology. Cell Tissue Res 318: 121–134, 2004.
14. Dickson, DW, et al: Evidence in favor of Braak staging of Parkinson's disease. Mov Disord 25(Suppl 1):S78–S82, 2010.
15. Berardelli, A, et al: Pathophysiology of bradykinesia in Parkinson's disease. Brain 124(11):2131–2146, 2001.
16. Smithson, F, et al: Performance on clinical tests of balance in Parkinson's disease. Phys Ther 78:577, 1998.
17. Horak, F, Dimitrova, D, and Nutt, J: Direction-specific postural instability in subjects with Parkinson's disease. Exp Neurol 193:504, 2005.
18. Bloem, B, et al: Postural reflexes in Parkinson's disease during "resist" and "yield" tasks. J Neurol Sci 129:109, 1995.
19. Maeshima, S, et al: Visuospatial impairment and activities of daily living in patients with Parkinson's disease. Am J Phys Med Rehabil 76:383, 1997.
20. Bridgewater, K, and Sharpe, M: Trunk muscle performance in early Parkinson's disease. Phys Ther 78:566, 1998.
21. Bloem B, et al: Falls and freezing of gait in Parkinson's disease: A review of two interconnected, episodic phenomena. Mov Disord 19:871, 2004.
22. Gray, P, and Hildebrand, K: Fall risk factors in Parkinson's disease. J Neurosci Nurs 32:222, 2000.
23. Bloem, BR, van Vugt, JP, and Beckley, DJ: Postural instability and falls in Parkinson's disease. Adv Neurol 87:209, 2001.
24. Corcos, D, et al: Strength in Parkinson's disease: Relationship to rate of force generation and clinical status. Ann Neurol 39:79, 1996.
25. Pedersen, S, and Oberg, B: Dynamic strength in Parkinson's disease: Quantitative measurements following withdrawal of medication. Eur Neurol 33:97, 1993.

26. Stelmach, G, et al: Force production characteristics in Parkinson's disease. Exp Brain Res 76:165, 1989.

27. Yanagawa, S, et al: Muscular weakness in Parkinson's disease. Adv Neurol 53:259, 1990.

28. Berardelli A, et al: Scaling of the size of the first agonist EMG burst during rapid wrist movements in patients with Parkinson's disease. J Neurol Neurosurg Psychiatry 49:1273, 1986.

29. Dengler R, et al: Behavior of motor units in parkinsonism. Adv Neurol 53:167, 1990.

30. Herrero, MT, Barcia, C, and Navarro, JM: Functional anatomy of the thalamus and basal ganglia. Childs Nerv Sust 18(8):386, 2002.

31. Pendt, L, Reuter, I, and Muller, H: Motor skill learning, retention, and control deficits in Parkinson's disease. PLoS ONE 6(7):e21669, 2011. DOI:10.1371/journal.pone.0021669. Retrieved April 23, 2012, from www.plosone.org/article/info%3Adoi%2F10.1371%2Fjournal.pone.0021669.

32. Marsden, C: What do the basal ganglia tell premotor cortical areas? Ciba Found Symp 132:282, 1997.

33. Agostino, R, Sanes, J, and Hallett, M: Motor skill learning in Parkinson's disease. J Neurol Sci 139:218, 1996.

34. Fattapposta, F, et al: Preprogramming and control activity of bimanual self-paced motor task in Parkinson's disease. Clin Neurophys 111:873, 2000.

35. Haaland, K, et al: Cognitive-motor learning in Parkinson's disease. Neuropsychology 11:180, 1997.

36. Giladi, N: Gait disturbances. In Factor, S, and Weiner, W (eds): Parkinson's Disease—Diagnosis and Clinical Management. Demos Medical Publishing, New York, 2002, p 57.

37. Pederson, S, et al: Gait analysis, isokinetic muscle strength measurement in patients with Parkinson's disease. Scand J Rehabil Med 29:67, 1997.

38. Morris, M, et al: The biomechanics and motor control of gait in Parkinson disease. Clin Biomech 16:459, 2001.

39. Melnick, M, Radtka, S, and Piper, M: Gait analysis and Parkinson's disease. Rehab Manage p 48, Aug/Sept 2002.

40. Morris, M, et al: Temporal stability of gait in Parkinson's disease. Phys Ther 76:763, 1996.

41. Boonstra, TA, et al: Gait disorders and balance disturbances in Parkinson's disease: Clinical update and pathophysiology. Curr Opin Neurol 21:461, 2008.

42. Bloem, B, et al: Falls and freezing of gait in Parkinson's disease: A review of two interconnected, episodic phenomena. Mov Disord 19:871, 2004.

43. Zewig, R: Sensory symptoms. In Factor, S, and Weiner, W (eds): Parkinson's Disease—Diagnosis and Clinical Management. Demos Medical Publishing, New York, 2002, p 67.

44. Jobst, E, et al: Sensory perception in Parkinson disease. Arch Neurol 54:450, 1997.

45. Demirci, M, et al: A mismatch between kinesthetic and visual perception in Parkinson's disease. Ann Neurol 41:781, 1997.

46. Langston, JW: PD: More than a movement disorder. Parkinson's Disease Foundation. Retrieved April 23, 2012, from www.pdf.org/en/fall06_PD_More_than_a_Movement_Disorder.

47. Ramig, L, et al: Speech, voice, and swallowing disorders. In Factor, S, and Weiner, W (eds): Parkinson's Disease—Diagnosis and Clinical Management. Demos Medical Publishing, New York, 2002, p 75.

48. Robbins, J, et al: Swallowing and speech production in Parkinson's disease. Ann Neurol 19:282, 1986.

49. Marder, K, and Jacobs, D: Dementia. In Factor, S, and Weiner, W (eds): Parkinson's Disease—Diagnosis and Clinical Management. Demos Medical Publishing, New York, 2002, p 125.

50. Chow, T, Masterman, D, and Cummings, J: Depression. In Factor, S, and Weiner, W (eds): Parkinson's Disease—Diagnosis and Clinical Management. Demos Medical Publishing, New York, 2002, p 145.

51. Richard, I, and Kurlan, R: Anxiety and panic. In Factor, S, and Weiner, W (eds): Parkinson's Disease—Diagnosis and Clinical Management. Demos Medical Publishing, New York, 2002, p 161.

52. Marras, C, and Lang, A: Changing concepts in Parkinson disease. Neurology 70:1996, 2008.

53. Hubble, J, and Weeks, C: Autonomic nervous system dysfunction. In Factor, S, and Weiner, W (eds): Parkinson's Disease—Diagnosis and Clinical Management. Demos Medical Publishing, New York, 2002, p 95.

54. Protas, E, Stanley, R, and Jankovic, J: Parkinson's disease. In Durstine, JL, et al (eds): ACSM's Exercise Management for Persons with Chronic Diseases and Disabilities, ed 3. Human Kinetics, Champaign, IL, 2009.

55. Canning, C, et al: Parkinson's disease: An investigation of exercise capacity, respiratory function, and gait. Arch Phys Med Rehabil 78:199, 1997.

56. Protas, E, et al: Cardiovascular and metabolic responses to upper- and lower-extremity exercise in men with idiopathic Parkinson's disease. Phys Ther 76:34, 1996.

57. Stanley, R, Protas, E, and Jankovic, J: Exercise performance in those having Parkinson's disease and healthy normals. Med Sci Sports Exerc 31(6):761, 1999.

58. Hovestadt, A, et al: Pulmonary function in Parkinson's disease. J Neurol Neurosurg Psychiatry 52:329, 1989.

59. Sabate, M, et al: Obstructive and restrictive pulmonary dysfunction increases disability in Parkinson disease. Arch Phys Med Rehabil 77:29, 1996.

60. Comella, C: Sleep disorders. In Factor, S, and Weiner, W (eds): Parkinson's Disease—Diagnosis and Clinical Management. Demos Medical Publishing, New York, 2002, p 101.

61. Hauser, R (ed): Parkinson's disease: Early diagnosis. In Living Medical eTextbook. Neurology—Parkinson's Disease Edition: Early Diagnosis and Comprehensive Management. Retrieved April 23, 2012, from http://lmt.projectsinknowledge.com/neurology/2027.

62. Chaudhuri, KR, et al: International multicenter pilot study of the first comprehensive self-completed nonmotor symptoms questionnaire for Parkinson's disease: The NMSQuest study. Mov Disord 21:916, 2006.

63. Martinez-Martin, P, et al (NMSS Validation Group): The impact of non-motor symptoms on health-related quality of life of patients with Parkinson's disease. Mov Disord 26:399, 2011.

64. Suchowersky, O, et al: Practice parameter: Diagnosis and prognosis of new onset Parkinson disease (an evidence-based review). Report of the Quality Standards Subcommittee of the American Academy of Neurology. Neurology 66:968, 2006.

65. Feigin, A, and Eidelberg, D: Natural history. In Factor, S, and Weiner, W (eds): Parkinson's Disease—Diagnosis and Clinical Management. Demos Medical Publishing, New York, 2002, p 109.

66. Hoehn, M, and Yahr, M: Parkinsonism: Onset, progression and mortality. Neurology 17:427, 1967.

67. Gancher, S: Quantitative Measures and Rating Scales. In Factor, S, and Weiner, W (eds): Parkinson's Disease—Diagnosis and Clinical Management. Demos Medical Publishing, New York, 2002, p 115.

68. Fahn, S, and Elton, R: Unified Parkinson's disease rating scale. In Fahn, S, et al (eds): Recent Developments in Parkinson's Disease, Vol 2. Macmillan Health Care Information, Florham Park, NJ, 1987.

69. Goetz, CG, et al: Movement Disorder Society–sponsored revision of the Unified Parkinson's Disease Rating Scale (MDS-UPDRS): Process, format, and clinimetric testing plan. Mov Disord 22(1): 41, 2007.

70. Goetz, CG, et al: Movement Disorder Society–sponsored revision of the Unified Parkinson's Disease Rating Scale (MDS-UPDRS): Scale presentation and clinimetric testing results. Mov Disord 23(15):2129, 2008.

71. Goetz, C: New scale for measuring PD increases role of patients and caregivers. Parkinson's Disease Foundation, Newsletter, Spring 2007. Retrieved April 23, 2012, from www.pdf.org/en/spring07_new_scale_for_measuring_pd.

72. Pahwar, R et al: Practice parameter: Treatment of Parkinson disease with motor fluctuations and dyskinesia (an evidence-based review). Report of the Quality Standards Subcommittee of the American Academy of Neurology. Neurology 66:983, 2006.

73. Suchowersky, O, et al: Practice parameter: Neuroprotective strategies and alternative therapies for Parkinson disease (an evidence-based review). Report of the Quality Standards Subcommittee of the American Academy of Neurology. Neurology 66:976, 2006.

74. Hauser, R (ed): Management of early-stage Parkinson's disease. In Living Medical eTextbook. Neurology—Parkinson's Disease Edition: Early Diagnosis and Comprehensive Management. Retrieved April 23, 2012, from http://lmt.projectsinknowledge.com/neurology/2027.

75. Hauser, R (ed): Management of moderate to advanced-stage Parkinson's disease. In Living Medical eTextbook. Neurology—Parkinson's Disease Edition: Early Diagnosis and Comprehensive Management. Retrieved April 23, 2012, from http://lmt.projectsinknowledge.com/neurology/2027.

76. Hauser, R (ed): Management of nonmotor symptoms of Parkinson's disease. In Living Medical eTextbook. Neurology—Parkinson's Disease Edition: Early Diagnosis and Comprehensive Management. Retrieved April 23, 2012, from http://lmt.projectsinknowledge. com/neurology/2027.

77. Aminoff, MJ, et al: Management of the hospitalized patient with Parkinson's disease: Current state of the field and need for guidelines. Parkinsonism Relat Disord 17(3):139, 2011.

78. Magdalinou, K, Martin, A, and Kessel, B: Prescribing medications in Parkinson's disease (PD) patients during acute admissions to a district general hospital. Parkinsonism Relat Disord 13(8):539j, 2007.

79. Simuni, T, and Hurtig, H: Levodopa: 30 years of progress. In Factor, S, and Weiner, W (eds): Parkinson's Disease—Diagnosis and Clinical Management. Demos Medical Publishing, New York, 2002, p 339.

80. Parkinson's Disease Foundation: Medications and Treatments. Retrieved April 23, 2012, from www.pdf.org/en/meds_treatments.

81. Dibble, L: Motor effects of dopamine replacement: Taking the positive with the negative. JNPT 27:109, 2003.

82. Hammerstad, J: Pallidal and subthalamic stimulation. In Factor, S, and Weiner, W (eds): Parkinson's Disease—Diagnosis and Clinical Management. Demos Medical Publishing, New York, 2002, p 553.

83. Koller, W: Thalamic stimulation. In Factor, S, and Weiner, W (eds): Parkinson's Disease—Diagnosis and Clinical Management. Demos Medical Publishing, New York, 2002, p 553.

84. Liu, W, et al: Quantitative assessments of the effect of bilateral subthalamic stimulation on multiple aspects of sensorimotor function for patients with Parkinson's disease. Parkinsonism Relat Disord 11:503, 2005.

85. Ferrarin, M, et al: Effects of bilateral subthalamic stimulation on gait kinematics and kinetics in Parkinson's disease. Exp Brain Res 160:571, 2005.

86. Kelly, V, et al: Gait changes in response to subthalamic nucleus stimulation in people with Parkinson disease: A case series report. JNPT 30:184, 2006.

87. Hirsch, M, et al: The effects of balance training and high-intensity resistance training on persons with idiopathic Parkinson's disease. Arch Phys Med Rehabil 84:1109, 2003.

88. Reuter, I, et al: Therapeutic value of exercise training in Parkinson's disease. Med Sci Sports Exerc 31:1544, 1999.

89. de Goede, C, et al: The effects of physical therapy in Parkinson's disease: A research synthesis. Arch Phys Med Rehabil 82:509, 2001.

90. Schenkman, M, et al: Exercise to improve spinal flexibility and function for people with Parkinson's disease: A randomized, controlled trial. J Am Geriatr Soc 46:1207, 1998.

91. Melnick, ME, et al: Effects of rhythmic exercise on balance, gait, and depression in patients with Parkinson's disease. Gerontol 39:293, 2000.

92. Ellis, T, et al: Efficacy of a physical therapy program in patients with Parkinson's disease: A randomized controlled trial. Arch Phys Med Rehabil 86:626, 2005.

93. Ellis, T, et al: Effectiveness of an inpatient multidisciplinary rehabilitation program for people with Parkinson disease. Phys Ther 88(7):812, 2008.

94. Baatile, J, et al: Effect of exercise on perceived quality of life of individuals with Parkinson's disease. J Rehabil Res Dev 37:529, 2000.

95. Dal Bello-Haas V: A framework for rehabilitation in degenerative diseases: Planning care and maximizing quality of life. Neurology Report (now JNPT) 26(3):115, 2002.

96. Cutson, T, et al. Pharmacological and nonpharmacological interventions in the treatment of Parkinson's disease. Phys Ther 75:363, 1995.

97. American Physical Therapy Association (APTA): Guide to Physical Therapist Practice, ed 2. APTA, Alexandria, VA, 2003.

98. Schenkman, M, et al: Reliability of impairment and physical performance measures for persons with Parkinson's disease. Phys Ther 77:19, 1997.

99. Folstein, M, et al: Mini-Mental Status: A practical method for grading the cognitive state of patients for the clinician. J Psychiatr Res 12:189, 1975.

100. Yesavage, J, and Brink, T: Development and validation of a geriatric depression screening scale: A preliminary report. J Psychiatr Res 17:41, 1983.

101. Gallagher, D: The Beck Depression Inventory and older adults review of its development and utility. In Brink, T (ed): Clinical Gerontology: A Guide to Examination and Intervention. Haworth Press, New York, 1986, p 149.

102. Zigmund, AS, and Snaith, RP: The Hospital Anxiety and Depression Scale. Acta Psychiatr Scand 67:361, 1983.

103. Spinhoven, P, et al: A validation study of the Hospital Anxiety and Depression Scale (HADS) in different groups of Dutch subjects. Psychol Med 27(2):363, 1997.

104. Bridgewater, K, and Sharpe, M: Trunk muscle performance in early Parkinson's disease. Phys Ther 78:566, 1998.

105. Breum, J, Wiberg, J, and Bolton, JE: Reliability and concurrent validity of the BROM II for measuring lumbar mobility. J Manipul Physio Therapeutics 18(8):497, 1995.

106. Lundon, K, Li, A, and Bibershtein, S: Interrater and intrarater reliability in the measurement of kyphosis in postmenopausal women with osteoporosis. Spine 23(18), 1998.

107. Dunleavy, K, et al: Reliability and minimal detectable change of spinal length and width measurements using the Flexicurve for usual standing posture in healthy young adults. J Back Musculoskel Rehabil 23(4):209, 2010.

108. Youdas, JW, Suman, VJ, and Garrett, TR: Reliability of measurements of lumbar spine sagittal mobility obtained with the flexible curve. J Orthop Sports Phys Ther 21(1):13, 1995.

109. Dengler, R, et al: Behavior of motor units in parkinsonism. Adv Neurol 53:167, 1990.

110. Bohannon, R: Documentation of tremor in patients with central nervous system lesions. Phys Ther 66:229, 1986.

111. Brusse, K, et al: Testing functional performance in people with Parkinson disease. Phys Ther 85(2):134, 2005.

112. Landers, M, et al: Postural instability in idiopathic Parkinson's disease: Discriminating fallers from nonfallers based on standardized clinical measures. JNPT 32:56, 2008.

113. Dibble, L, and Lange, M: Predicting falls in individuals in Parkinson disease: A reconsideration of clinical balance measures. JNPT 30(2):60, 2006.

114. Dibble, L, et al: Diagnosis of fall risk in Parkinson disease: An analysis of individual and collective clinical balance test interpretation. Phys Ther 88(3):323, 2008.

115. Leddy, A, Crowner, B, and Earhart, G: Functional gait assessment and balance evaluation system test: Reliability, validity, sensitivity, and specificity for identifying individuals with Parkinson disease who fall. Phys Ther 91:102, 2011.

116. Morris, S, Morris, M, and Iansek, R: Reliability of measurements obtained with the Timed Up and Go test in people with Parkinson's disease. Phys Ther 81:810, 2001.

117. Huang, SL: Minimal detectable change of the Timed Up and Go test and the Dynamic Gait Index in people with Parkinson's disease. Phys Ther 91:114, 2011.

118. Steffen, T, and Seney, M: Test-retest reliability and minimal detectable change on balance and ambulation tests, the 36-item Short Form Health Survey, and the Unified Parkinson Disease Rating Scale in people with parkinsonism. Phys Ther 88:733, 2008.

119. Smithson, F, Morris, M, and Iansek, R: Performance on clinical tests of balance in Parkinson's disease. Phys Ther 78:577, 1998.

120. Matinolli M, et al: Mobility and balance in Parkinson's disease: A population-based study. Eur J Neurol 16:105, 2009.

121. Berg, K, et al: Measuring balance in the elderly: Preliminary development of an instrument. Physiother Can 41:304, 1989.

122. Duncan, P, et al: Functional reach: A new clinical measure of balance. J Gerontol 45:M192, 1990.

123. Podsiadlo, D, and Richardson, S: The Timed "Up and Go": A test of basic functional mobility for frail elderly patients. J Am Geriatr Soc 39:142, 1991.

124. Campbell, C, et al: The effect of cognitive demand on Timed Up and Go performance in older adults with and without Parkinson disease. Neurol Rep 27:2, 2003.

125. Shumway-Cook, A, et al: Predicting the probability for falls in community-dwelling older adults. Phys Ther 77(8):812, 1997.

126. Wrisley, DM, et al: Reliability, internal consistency and validity of data obtained with the Functional Gait Assessment. Phys Ther 84:906, 2004.

127. Horak, FB, Wrisley, DM, and Frank, J: The Balance Evaluation Systems Test (BESTest) to differentiate balance deficits. Phys Ther 89:484, 2009.

128. Behrman, A, Light, K, and Miller, G: Sensitivity of the Tinetti Gait Assessment in detecting change in individuals with Parkinson disease. Clin Rehabil 16:399, 2002.

129. Moore, S, et al: Locomotor responses to levodopa in fluctuating Parkinson's disease. Exp Brain Res 184:469, 2008.

130. Bloem, B: Clinimetrics of postural instability in Parkinson's disease. J Neurol 245:669, 1998.

131. Colnat-Coulbois, S, et al: Management of postural sensory conflict and dynamic balance control in late-stage Parkinson's disease. Neuroscience 193:363, 2011.

132. O'Shea, S, Morris, M, and Iansek, R: Dual task interference during gait in people with Parkinson's disease: Effects of motor versus cognitive secondary tasks. Phys Ther 82:888, 2002.

133. Mak, MK, and Pang, MY: Balance confidence and functional mobility are independently associated with falls in people with Parkinson's disease. J Neurol 256(5):742, 2009.

134. Dibble, L, et al: Maximal speed gait initiation of healthy elderly individuals and persons with Parkinson's disease. JNPT 28:2, 2004.

135. Morris, M, and Iansek, R: Gait disorders in Parkinson's disease: A framework for physical therapy practice. Neurology Report (now JNPT) 21:125, 1997.

136. Huang, S, et al: Minimal detectable change of the Timed "Up and Go" test and the Dynamic Gait Index in people with Parkinson disease. Phys Ther 91(1):113, 2011.

137. Bloem, B, et al: Falls and freezing of gait in Parkinson's disease: A review of two interconnected, episodic phenomena. Mov Disord 19(8):871, 2004.

138. Giladi, N: Freezing of gait. Clinical overview. Adv Neurol 87:191, 2001.

139. Browner, N, and Giladi, N: What can we learn from freezing of gait in Parkinson's disease? Curr Neurol Neurosci Rep 10:345, 2010.

140. Nieuwboer, A, et al: Reliability of the new freezing of gait questionnaire: Agreement between patients with Parkinson's disease and their carers. Gait Posture 30(4):459, 2009.

141. Friedman, JH, et al: Fatigue in Parkinson's disease: A review. Mov Disord 22(3):297, 2007.

142. Lou, JS, et al: Exacerbated physical fatigue and mental fatigue in Parkinson's disease. Mov Disord 16(2):190, 2001.

143. Friedman, JH, et al: Fatigue rating scales and recommendations by the Movement Disorders Task Force on rating scales for Parkinson's disease. Mov Disord 25(7):805, 2010.

144. Smets, EM, et al: The Multidimensional Fatigue Inventory (MFI), psychometric qualities of an instrument to assess fatigue. J Psychosom Res 39:315, 1995.

145. Krupp, LB, et al: The Fatigue Severity Scale. Application to patients with multiple sclerosis and systemic lupus erythematosus. Arch Neurol 46(10):1121, 1989.

146. Fabbrini, G, et al: Levodopa-induced dyskinesias. Mov Disord 22(10):1379, 2007.

147. Mones, RJ, Elizan, TS, and Siegel, GJ: Analysis of L-dopa induced dyskinesias in 51 patients with Parkinsonism. J Neurol Neurosurg Psychiatry 34(6):668–673, 1971.

148. Colosimo, C, et al: Task force report on scales to assess dyskinesia in Parkinson's disease: Critique and recommendations. Mov Disord 25(9):1131, 2010.

149. Light, K, et al: The 2-Minute Walk Test: A tool for evaluating walking endurance in clients with Parkinson's disease. Neurology Report (now JNPT) 21:136, 1997.

150. Borg, G: Psychophysical bases of perceived exertion. Med Sci Sports Exerc 14:377, 1982.

151. Parkinson's Disease Foundation: Orthostatic hypotension (low blood pressure) and Parkinson's. PDF News and Review pp 4-5, Fall 2011.

152. Guide for the Uniform Data Set for Medical Rehabilitation including the FIM Instrument, Version 5.0. State University of New York at Buffalo, Buffalo, 1996.

153. Bishop, M, et al: Changes in distal muscle timing may contribute to slowness during sit to stand in Parkinson's disease. Clin Biomech 20:112, 2005.

154. Ramsey, V, Miszko, T, and Horvat, M: Muscle activation and force production in Parkinson's patients during sit to stand transfers. Clin Biomech 19:377, 2004.

155. Duncan, R, Leddy, A, and Gammon, E: Five times sit-to-stand performance in Parkinson's disease. Arch Phys Med Rehabil 92:1431, 2011.

156. Schenkman, M, McFann, K, and Baron, A: Profile PD: Profile of function and impairment level experience with Parkinson's disease—clinimetric properties of a rating scale for physical therapist practice. JNPT 34:182, 2010.

157. McHorney, C, et al: The MOS 36-Item Short-Form Health Survey (SF-36) II. Psychometric and chemical and clinical tests of validity in measuring physical and mental health constructs. Med Care 31:247, 1993.

158. Gilson, B, et al: The Sickness Impact Profile: Development of an outcome measure of health care. Am J Publ Health 65:1304, 1975.

159. Petro, V, et al: The development and validation of a short measure of functioning and well being for individuals with Parkinson's disease. Qual Life Res 4:241, 1995.

160. Jenkinson, C, et al: Self-reported functioning and well-being in patients with Parkinson's disease: Comparison of the Short-Form Health Survey (SF-36) and the Parkinson's Disease Questionnaire (PDQ-39). Age Ageing 24:505, 1995.

161. Dean, K, et al: Physiotherapy for Parkinson's disease: A comparison of techniques. Cochrane Database of Systematic Reviews, 2001, Issue 1, Art. No.: CD002815. DOI: 10.1002/14651858.

162. Dean, K et al: Physiotherapy versus placebo or no intervention in Parkinson's disease. Cochrane Database of Systematic Reviews, 2001, Issue 3, Art. No.: CD002817. DOI: 10.1002/14651858.

163. Nieuwboer, A, et al Motor learning in Parkinson's disease: limitations and potential for rehabilitation. Parkinsonism Relat Disord 15(Suppl. 3), S53–58.

164. Abbruzzese, G, Trompetto, C, Marinell L: The rationale for motor learning in Parkinson's disease. Eur J Phys Rehabil Med 45(2):209, 2009.

165. Muslimovic, D, et al : Motor procedural learning in Parkinson's disease. Brain 130:2887, 2007.

166. Behrman, A, Cauraugh, J, and Light, K: Practice as an intervention to improve speeded motor performance and motor learning in Parkinson's disease. J Neurol Sci 174:127, 2000.

167. Lim, I, et al: Effects of external rhythmical cueing on gait in patients with Parkinson's disease: A systematic review. Clin Rehabil 19:695, 2005.

168. Donovan, S, et al: Laserlight cues for gait freezing in Parkinson's disease: An open-label study. Parkinsonism Relat Disord 17(4):240, 2011.

169. Lewis, G, Byblow, W, and Walt, S: Stride length regulation in Parkinson's disease: The use of extrinsic visual cues. Brain 123:2077, 2000.

170. Bryant, MS, et al: An evaluation of self-administration of auditory cueing to improve gait in people with Parkinson's disease. Clin Rehabil 23(12):1078, 2009.

171. Lowry, KA, et al: Use of harmonic ratios to examine the effect of cueing strategies on gait stability in persons with Parkinson's disease. Arch Phys Med Rehabil 91(4):632, 2010.

172. Del Olmo, M, and Cudeiro, J: Temporal variability of gait in Parkinson disease: Effects of a rehabilitation programme based on rhythmic sound cues. Parkinsonism Relat Disord 11:25, 2005.

173. Lehman, D, et al: Training with verbal instructional cues results in near-term improvement of gait in people with Parkinson disease. JNPT 29:2, 2005.

174. Freedland, R, et al: The effects of pulsed auditory stimulation on various gait measurements in persons with Parkinson's disease. Neuro Rehabil 17:81, 2002.

175. Jiang, Y, et al: Effects of visual and auditory cues on gait initiation in people with Parkinson's disease. Clin Rehabil 20:36, 2006.

176. Suteerawattananon, M, et al: Effects of visual and auditory cues on gait in individuals with Parkinson's disease. J Neurol Sci 219: 63, 2004.

177. Mak, M, and Hue-Chan, C: Audiovisual cues can enhance sit-to-stand in patients with Parkinson's disease. Mov Disord 19:1012, 2004.

178. Arias, P, and Cudeiro, J: Effects of rhythmic sensory stimulation (auditory, visual) on gait in Parkinson's disease patients. Exp Brain Res 186:589, 2008.

179. Rochester, L, et al: The effect of external rhythmic cues (auditory and visual) on walking during a functional task in homes of people with Parkinson's disease. Arch Phys Med Rehabil 86:999, 2005.

180. Morris, M, et al: Stride length regulation in Parkinson's disease. Normalization strategies and underlying mechanisms. Brain 119:551, 1996.

181. Nieuwboer, A, et al: The short-term effects of different cueing modalities on turn speed in people with Parkinson's disease. Neurorehabil Neural Repair 23(8):831, 2009.

182. Frazzitta, G, et al: Rehabilitation treatment of gait in patients with Parkinson's disease with freezing: A comparison between two physical therapy protocols using visual and auditory cues with and without treadmill training. Mov Disord 24:1139, 2009.

183. Lewis, G, Byblow, W, and Walt, S: Stride length regulation in Parkinson's disease: The use of extrinsic visual cues. Brain 123:2077, 2000.

184. Farley, BG: Intensive amplitude-specific therapeutic approaches for Parkinson's disease: Toward a neuroplasticity-principled rehabilitation model. Topics Geriatr Rehabil 24(2):99, 2008.

185. Farley, BG, and Koshland, GF: Training BIG to move faster: The application of the speed-amplitude relation as a rehabilitation strategy for people with Parkinson's disease. Exp Brain Res 167(3):462, 2005.

186. Brooks, M: "Training BIG" improves motor performance in Parkinson's disease. Medscape Medical News. Retrieved April 13, 2012, from www.medscape.com/viewarticle/723803.

187. Ebersbach, G, et al: Comparing exercise in Parkinson's disease—the Berlin LSVT(R)BIG study. Mov Disord 25(12):1902, 2010.

188. Louis, E: Paralysis agitans in the nineteenth century. In Factor, S, and Weiner, W: Parkinson's Disease—Diagnosis and Clinical Management. Demos, New York, 2002, p 13.

189. Peterson, B, et al: Changes in response of medial pontomedullary reticular neurons during repetitive cutaneous, vestibular, cortical and rectal stimulation. J Neurophysiol 39:564, 1976.

190. Voss, D, et al: Proprioceptive Neuromuscular Facilitation, ed 3. Harper & Row, New York, 1985.

191. Adler, S, Beckers, D, and Buck, M: PNF in Practice, ed 3. Heidelberg, Springer, 2008.

192. Benson, H: The Relaxation Response. Avon, New York, 1975.

193. Boelen, M: Health Professionals Guide to Physical Management of Parkinson's Disease. Human Kinetics, Champaign, IL, 2009.

194. Mak, M, Yang, F, and Pai, Y: Limb collapse, rather than instability, causes failure in sit-to stand performance among patients with Parkinson disease. Phys Ther 91:381, 2011.

195. Scandalis, T, et al: Resistance training and gait function in patients with Parkinson's disease. Am J Phys Med Rehabil 80:38, 2001.

196. Glendinning, D: A rationale for strength training in patients with Parkinson's disease. Neurology Report (now JNPT) 21:132, 1997.

197. Fiatarone, M, et al: High-intensity strength training in nonagenarians. Effects on skeletal muscle. JAMA 263:3029, 1990.

198. Judge, J, et al: Effects of resistive and balance exercises on isokinetic strength in older persons. J Am Geriatr Soc 42:937, 1994.

199. Wolfson, L, et al: Balance and strength training in older adults: Intervention gains and Tai Chi maintenance. J Am Geriatr Soc 44:498, 1996.

200. Dibble, L, et al: High intensity eccentric resistance training decreases bradykinesia and improves quality of life in persons with Parkinson's disease: A preliminary study. Parkinsonism Relat Disord 15(10):752, 2009.

201. Hirsch, M, et al: The effects of balance training and high-intensity resistance training on persons with idiopathic Parkinson's disease. Arch Phys Med Rehabil 84:1109, 2003.

202. American College of Sports Medicine: ACSM's Guidelines for Exercise Testing and Prescription, ed 8. Lippincott Williams & Wilkins, Philadelphia, 2010.

203. O'Sullivan, S, and Schmitz, T: Improving Functional Outcomes in Physical Rehabilitation. FA Davis, Philadelphia, 2010.

204. Clark, RA, et al: Validity and reliability of the Nintendo Wii Balance Board for assessment of standing balance. Gait Posture 31(3):307, 2010.

205. McGough, R, et al: Improving lower limb weight distribution asymmetry during the squat using Nintendo Wii Balance Boards and real-time feedback. J Strength Cond Res 26(1):47, 2012.

206. Williams, B, et al: The effect of Nintendo Wii on balance: A pilot study supporting the use of the Wii in occupational therapy for the well elderly. Occupat Ther Health Care 25(2/3):131, 2011.

207. Schyns, F, et al: Vibration therapy in multiple sclerosis: A pilot study exploring its effects on tone, muscle force, sensation and functional performance. Clin Rehabil 23(9):771, 2009.

208. Kavounoudias, A, Roll, R, and Roll, J: The plantar sole is a "dynamometric map" for human balance control. Neuroreport 9(14):3247, 1998.

209. Kavounoudias, A, Roll, R, and Roll, J: Specific whole-body shifts induced by frequency-modulated vibrations of human plantar soles. Neurosci Lett 266(3):181, 1999.

210. Cardinale, M, and Bosco, C: The use of vibration as an exercise intervention. Exerc Sport Sci Rev 31(1):3, 2003.

211. Kossev, A, et al: Crossed effects of muscle vibration on motor-evoked potentials. Clin Neurophysiol 112(3):453, 2001.

212. Pozo-Cruz, B, et al: Using whole-body vibration training in patients affected with common neurological diseases: A systematic literature review. J Alternat Complem Med 18(1):29–41, 2012.

213. Lau, R, et al: Effects of whole-body vibration on sensorimotor performance in people with Parkinson disease: A systematic review. Phys Ther 91(2):198, 2011.

214. King, L, Almeida, Q, and Ahonen, H: Short-term effects of vibration therapy on motor impairments in Parkinson's disease. NeuroRehabilitation 25(4):297, 2009.

215. Haas, C, et al: The effects of random whole-body-vibration on motor symptoms in Parkinson's disease. NeuroRehabilitation 21(1):29, 2006.

216. Morris, M: Locomotor training in people with Parkinson disease. Phys Ther 86(10):1426, 2006.

217. Behrman, A, Teitelbaum, P, and Cauraugh, J: Verbal instructional sets to normalize the temporal and spatial gait variables in Parkinson's disease. J Neurol Neurosurg Psychiatry 65:580, 1998.

218. Roberta, W: Analysis of parallel and transverse visual cues on the gait of individuals with idiopathic Parkinson's disease. Int J Rehabil Res 34(4):343, 2011.

219. Pohl, M, et al: Immediate effects of speed-dependent treadmill training on gait parameters in early Parkinson's disease. Arch Phys Med Rehabil 84:1760, 2000.

220. Miyai, I, et al: Treadmill training with body weight support: Its effect on Parkinson's disease. Arch Phys Med Rehabil 81:849, 2000.

221. Miyai, I, et al: Long-term effect of body weight–supported treadmill training in Parkinson's disease: A randomized controlled trial. Arch Phys Med Rehabil 83:1370, 2002.

222. Toole, T, et al: The effects of loading and unloading treadmill walking on balance, gait, fall risk, and daily function in parkinsonism. NeuroRehabilitation 20:307, 2005.

223. Herman, T, et al: Six weeks of intensive treadmill training improves gait and quality of life in patients with Parkinson's disease: A pilot study. Arch Phys Med Rehabil 88(9):1154, 2007.

224. Frenkel-Toledo, S, et al: Treadmill walking as an external pacemaker to improve gait rhythm and stability in Parkinson's disease. Mov Disord 20(9):1109, 2005.

225. Cakit, B, et al: The effects of incremental speed-dependent treadmill training on postural instability and fear of falling in Parkinson's disease. Clin Rehabil 21:698, 2007.

226. Fisher, B, et al: The effect of exercise training in improving motor performance and corticomotor excitability in people with early Parkinson's disease. Arch Phys Med Rehabil 89:1221, 2008.

227. Kurtais, Y, et al: Does treadmill training improve lower-extremity tasks in Parkinson disease? A randomized controlled trial. Clin J Sport Med 18(3):289, 2008.

228. Protas, E, et al: Gait and step training to reduce falls in Parkinson's disease. NeuroRehabilitation 20:183, 2005.

229. Ford, MP, et al: Gait training with progressive external auditory cueing in person's with Parkinson's disease. Arch Phys Med Rehabil 91(8):1255, 2010.

230. Pfeifer, M, Begerow, B, and Minne, H: Effects of a new spinal orthosis on posture, trunk strength, and quality of life in women with postmenopausal osteoporosis: A randomized trial. Am J Phys Med Rehabil 83(3):177, 2004.

231. Pfeifer, M, et al: Effects of two newly developed spinal orthoses on trunk muscle strength, posture, and quality-of-life in women with postmenopausal osteoporosis: A randomized trial. Am J Phys Med Rehabil 90(10):805, 2011.

232. Lantz, SA, and Schultz, AB: Lumbar spine orthosis wearing. II. Effect on trunk muscle myoelectric activity. Spine 11(8):838, 1986.

233. Schmidt, K, et al: Influence of spinal orthosis on gait and physical functioning in women with postmenopausal osteoporosis. Orthopade 41(3):200, 2012.

234. Mehanna, R, and Jankovic, J: Respiratory problems in neurologic movement disorders. Parkinsonism Relat Disord 16(10):628, 2010.

235. Koseoglu, F, et al: The effects of a pulmonary rehabilitation program on pulmonary function tests and exercise tolerance in patients with Parkinson's disease. Funct Neurol 12:319, 1997.

236. Inzelberg, R, et al: Inspiratory muscle training and the perception of dyspnea in Parkinson's disease. Can J Neurol Sci 32:213, 2005.

237. Bergen, J, et al: Aerobic exercise intervention improves aerobic capacity and movement initiation in Parkinson's disease patients. NeuroRehabilitation 17:161, 2002.

238. Meyer, TK: The larynx for neurologists. Neurologist 15(6):313, 2009.

239. Fox, CM, et al: The science and practice of LSVT/LOUD: Neural plasticity-principled approach to treating individuals with Parkinson disease and other neurological disorders. Semin Speech Lang 27(4): 283, 2006.

240. Baumgartner, CA, Sapir, S, and Ramig, TO: Voice quality changes following phonatory-respiratory effort treatment (LSVT) versus respiratory effort treatment for individuals with Parkinson disease. J Voice 15(1):105, 2001.

241. Liotti, M, et al: Hypophonia in Parkinson's disease: Neural correlates of voice treatment revealed by PET. Neurology 60(3):432, 2003.

242. Spielman, JL, Borod, JC, and Ramig, L: The effects of intensive voice treatment on facial expressiveness in Parkinson disease: Preliminary data. Cogn Behav Neurol 16(3):177, 2003.

243. Bergen, J, et al: Aerobic exercise intervention improves aerobic capacity and movement initiation in Parkinson's disease patients. NeuroRehabilitation 17:161, 2002.

244. Schenkman, M, et al: Endurance training to improve economy of movement of people with Parkinson disease: Three case reports. Phys Ther 88:63, 2008.

245. Pedersen, S, et al: Group training in parkinsonism: Quantitative measurements of treatment. Scand J Rehabil Med 22:207, 1990.

246. States, R, Spierer, D, and Salem, Y: Long-term group exercise for people with Parkinson's disease: A feasibility study. JNPT 35:122, 2011.

247. Taylor, M: Yoga therapeutics in neurologic physical therapy: Application to a patient with Parkinson's disease. Neurology Report (now JNPT) 25(2):55–62, 2001.

248. Taylor, M: Yoga therapeutics in neurologic physical therapy: Application to a patient with Parkinson's disease. Neurology Report (now JNPT) 25(2):55, 2001.

249. Lee, MS, Lam, P, and Ernst, E: Effectiveness of Tai Chi for Parkinson's disease: A critical review. Parkin Relat Disord 14: 589, 2008.

250. Fuzhong, L, et al: Tai Chi–based exercise for older adults with Parkinson's disease: A pilot-program evaluation. J Aging Phys Act 15(2):139, 2007.

251. Hackney, ME, and Earhart, GM: Tai Chi improves balance and mobility in people with Parkinson disease. Gait Posture 28(3):456, 2008.

252. King, L, and Horak, F: Delaying mobility disability in people with Parkinson disease using a sensorimotor agility exercise program. Phys Ther 89:384, 2009.

253. Lun, V, et al: Comparison of the effects of a self-supervised home exercise program with a physiotherapist-supervised exercise program on the motor symptoms of Parkinson's disease. Mov Disord 20:971, 2005.

254. Nocera, J, Horvat, M, and Ray, CT: Effects of home-based exercise on postural control and sensory organization in individuals with Parkinson disease. Parkinsonism Relat Disord 15(10):742, 2009.

Supplemental Readings and Materials

PDF Exercise Program. Available from the Parkinson Disease Foundation, New York, www.pdf.org. For the clinician.

Toolkit.Parkinson.org. Contains information on symptoms, diagnosis, evaluation, treatment, and referral resources to find specialists in the patient's area. For clinicians, patients, and caregivers.

Motivating Moves for People with Parkinson's (video divided into three sections: "How to Do Motivating Moves" [45 min], "The Exercise Class" [36 min], and "Practical Tips for Daily Living" [4 min]). Available from the Parkinson Disease Foundation, New York, www.pdf.org.

MDS UPDRS Score Sheet

Patient Name or Subject ID	Site ID	(mm-dd-yyyy) Assessment Date	Investigator's Initials

MDS UPDRS Score Sheet

1.A	Source of information	☐ Patient ☐ Caregiver ☐ Patient + Caregiver	3.3b	Rigidity– RUE	
			3.3c	Rigidity– LUE	
Part I			3.3d	Rigidity– RLE	
1.1	Cognitive impairment		3.3e	Rigidity– LLE	
1.2	Hallucinations and psychosis		3.4a	Finger tapping– Right hand	
1.3	Depressed mood		3.4b	Finger tapping– Left hand	
1.4	Anxious mood		3.5a	Hand movements– Right hand	
1.5	Apathy		3.5b	Hand movements– Left hand	
1.6	Features of DDS		3.6a	Pronation- supination movements– Right hand	
1.6a	Who is filling out questionnaire	☐ Patient ☐ Caregiver ☐ Patient + Caregiver	3.6b	Pronation- supination movements– Left hand	
			3.7a	Toe tapping–Right foot	
1.7	Sleep problems		3.7b	Toe tapping– Left foot	
1.8	Daytime sleepiness		3.8a	Leg agility– Right leg	
1.9	Pain and other sensations		3.8b	Leg agility– Left leg	
1.10	Urinary problems		3.9	Arising from chair	
1.11	Constipation problems		3.10	Gait	
1.12	Light headedness on standing		3.11	Freezing of gait	
1.13	Fatigue		3.12	Postural stability	
Part II			3.13	Posture	
2.1	Speech		3.14	Global spontaneity of movement	
2.2	Saliva and drooling		3.15a	Postural tremor– Right hand	
2.3	Chewing and swallowing		3.15b	Postural tremor– Left hand	
2.4	Eating tasks		3.16a	Kinetic tremor– Right hand	
2.5	Dressing		3.16b	Kinetic tremor– Left hand	
2.6	Hygiene		3.17a	Rest tremor amplitude– RUE	
2.7	Handwriting		3.17b	Rest tremor amplitude– LUE	
2.8	Doing hobbies and other activities		3.17c	Rest tremor amplitude– RLE	
2.9	Turning in bed		3.17d	Rest tremor amplitude– LLE	
2.10	Tremor		3.17e	Rest tremor amplitude– Lip/jaw	
2.11	Getting out of bed		3.18	Constancy of rest	
2.12	Walking and balance			Were dyskinesias presen	☐ No ☐ Yes
2.13	Freezing			Did these movements interfere with ratings?	☐ No ☐ Yes
3a	Is the patient on medication?	☐ No ☐ Yes		Hoehn and Yahr Stage	
3b	Patient's clinical state	☐ Off ☐ On	**Part IV**		
3c	Is the patient on Levodopa?	☐ No ☐ Yes	4.1	Time spent with dyskinesias	
3.C1	If yes, minutes since last dose:		4.2	Functional impact of dyskinesias	
Part III			4.3	Time spent in the OFF state	
3.1	Speech		4.4	Functional impact of fluctuations	
3.2	Facial expression		4.5	Complexity of motor fluctuations	
3.3a	Rigidity– Neck		4.6	Painful OFF-state dystonia	

July 1, 2008

Movement Disorder Society-Unified Parkinson's Disease Rating Scale (MDS-UPDRS), Score Sheet, 2008 version. Used with permission of the MDS.

Yoga Sequence for Early/Mild Parkinson's Disease

Marjaryasana (Cat Pose)

1. Start on your hands and knees. Tabletop position.
2. As you exhale round your spine toward the ceiling. Hold for 5 seconds.

Bitilasana (Cow Pose)

1. As you inhale lift your sitting bones and chest toward the ceiling. Hold for 5 seconds.

Bhujanga (Cobra Pose)

1. Lie on your stomach with your hands under your shoulders.
2. As you inhale press the shoulders and torso off the mat and look up. Hold for 5 seconds.

Adho Mukha Svanasana (Downward-Facing Dog)

1. Start in the tabletop position.
2. As you exhale lift your knees and torso from the ground forming an inverted "V."
3. Push your shoulder blades against your back and heels to the ground.
4. Hold for 5 seconds.

Anjaneyasana (Low Lunge)

1. Step your right foot forward and maintain your left knee on the ground.
2. As you inhale raise your arms to the sky and stretch your torso forward.

Virabhadrasana II (Warrior II Pose)

1. Rise up from low lunge maintaining the right knee bent and the left knee straight.
2. Right foot should be straight ahead and the left foot should be turned out 90 degrees.
3. Ensure that outside border of the left foot stays on the ground.
4. With the right arm straight forward and the left arm straight back sink into the pose looking over the fingers of your right hand.

Yoga Sequence for Late Parkinson's Disease

Marjaryasana (Chair Cat Pose)

1. Start perch sitting (body at front of chair), sitting tall and hands on the side of your head.
2. As you exhale round your spine toward the back of the chair, bring your shoulders and head forward while bringing your elbows together. Hold for 5 seconds.

Bitilasana (Chair Cow Pose)

1. As you inhale arch your back and look up to the sky. Open your chest and spread your elbows wide. Hold for 5 seconds.

Parighasana (Chair Gate Pose)

1. Start sitting tall with your right hand on the chair and left arm raised to the sky palm facing in.
2. Inhale deeply.
3. As you exhale side bend your torso to the right and look up to your left hand. Hold for 5 seconds.
4. Repeat on the opposite side.

Ardha Matsyendrasana (Chair Spinal Twist)

1. Start sitting tall with your hands on the side of your head.
2. Inhale deeply.
3. As you exhale rotate to one side. Hold for 5 seconds.
4. Repeat on the opposite side.

Eka Pada Rajakapotasana (Chair Pigeon Pose)

1. Start sitting tall with your legs crossed, right ankle on top of left knee.
2. As you exhale lean forward from the hips keeping your spine long. Hold for 5 seconds.
3. Repeat on the opposite side.

Anjaneyasana (Modified Low Lunge)
Variation A (Advanced)
Variation B (Beginner)

Variation A:
1. Stand holding onto a stable surface for stability.
2. Left foot supported on chair behind you.
3. With a tall upright spine exhale, and bend the right knee while moving the pelvis forward. Hold for 5 seconds.
4. Repeat on the opposite side.

Continued

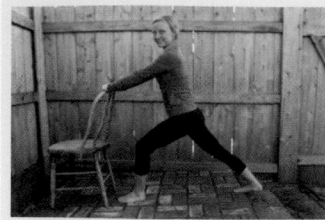

Variation B:
1. Stand holding onto a stable surface for stability. Left foot forward and right foot back.
2. With a tall upright spine exhale while bending the left knee and maintaining the right leg straight. Hold for 5 seconds.
3. Repeat on the opposite side.

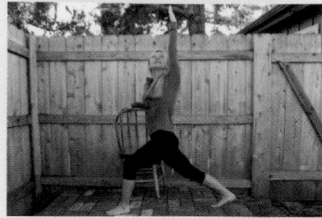

Utthita Parsvakonasana (Modified Extended Side Angle Pose)

1. Hold on to a stable surface with your right hand, left foot forward and right foot back.
2. While maintaining a long spine bend the left knee moving the pelvis forward and keeping the right knee straight.
3. As you exhale raise the left arm to the sky and turn your head to the left looking up to your left hand. Hold for 5 seconds.
4. Repeat on the opposite side.

Web-Based Resources for Clinicians and Patients/Families Living with Parkinson's Disease

National Parkinson Foundation (NPF)	www.parkinson.org www.parkinson.org/books (free publications available for download) www.parkinson.org/library (broader library resources for professionals) www.parkinson.org/search (registry of health professionals or support groups by local area) helpline@parkinson.org: provides dialogue for outreach and education www.toolkit.parkinson.org (Aware in Care kit for patients to bring with them for hospital stays)
Parkinson's Disease Foundation (PDF)	www.pdf.org
American Parkinson Disease Association (APDA)	www.apdaparkinson.org
World Parkinson Disease Association (WPDA)	www.wpda.org
Parkinson Society Canada	www.parkinson.ca
Young Onset Parkinson's Association	www.yopa.org
Young Parkinson's Information and Referral Center	www.youngparkinsons.org
Michael J. Fox Foundation for Parkinson's Research	www.michaeljfox.org
The Parkinson Alliance	www.parkinsonalliance.net
Parkinson's Action Network	www.ParkActNet@AOLcom
The Parkinson's Institute	www.parkinsoninstitute.org
People Living with Parkinson's	www.plwp.org
Understanding Parkinson's	www.understandingparkinson's.com
Americans with Disabilities Act: ADA home page	www.usdoj.gov/crt/ada
Medicare information	http://cms.hhs.gov
Social Security Online	www.ssa.gov
National Institute of Neurologic Disorders and Stroke (Parkinson's Disease Information Page)	www.ninds.nih.gov/disorders/parkinsons_disease/parkinsons_disease.htm
National Library of Medicine	www.nim.nih.gov
Archives of Neurology	http://archneur.ama-assn.org
Neurology	www.neurology.org
Veterans Affairs	www.va.gov
National Family Caregivers Association (NFCA)	www.nfcacares.org
Parkinson's Disease Caregiver Information	www.myparkinsons.org
Well Spouse Foundation	www.wellspouse.org

Continued

American Academy of Neurology (AAN)	www.aan.com (AAN members, professionals)
	www.aan.com/public (public education)
National Rehabilitation Information Center (NARIC)	www.naric.com
Ability Hub-assistive technology	www.abilityhub.com
ABLEDATA—assistive technology	www.abledata.com
Disabled Online	www.disabledonline.com
Canine Partners for Life	www.k94life.org

Traumatic Brain Injury

George D. Fulk, PT, PhD
Coby D. Nirider, PT, DPT

Chapter **19**

LEARNING OBJECTIVES

1. Describe the pathophysiology of traumatic brain injury.
2. Analyze the impact of cognitive, neurobehavioral, and neuromuscular impairments on outcomes of people with traumatic brain injury.
3. Identify the different team members and settings in the management of the patient with traumatic brain injury.
4. Compare and contrast persistent vegetative state and minimally conscious state.
5. Identify key components of the physical therapy examination during the acute stage of recovery in patients with severe to moderate traumatic brain injury.
6. Create a plan of care for a patient with a severe to moderate traumatic brain injury in the acute stage of recovery.
7. Select evidence-based outcome measures to use during the physical therapy examination of a patient with moderate to severe traumatic brain injury during the active rehabilitation stage of recovery.
8. Explain the impact of cognitive and neurobehavioral impairments on the physical therapy plan of care in the active rehabilitation stage of recovery.
9. Create a plan of care for a patient with a severe to moderate traumatic brain injury in the active rehabilitation stage of recovery.
10. Select evidence-based outcome measures to use during the physical therapy examination of a patient with a mild traumatic brain injury.
11. Outline a return to play timeline for a patient with a mild traumatic brain injury.
12. Create a plan of care for a patient with a mild traumatic brain injury.

CHAPTER OUTLINE

A traumatic brain injury (TBI) is defined as "an alteration in brain function, or other evidence of brain pathology, caused by an external force."[1] The TBI population is one of the most challenging that a physical therapist is likely to encounter.

Because of the multiple body systems affected by a brain injury and the strong likelihood of secondary impairments, a physical therapist must be proficient in a wide variety of examination procedures and intervention techniques. Owing to behavioral difficulties

859

encountered during recovery, a physical therapist working with this population must also possess strong communication and interpersonal skills, be able to react quickly and effectively to suddenly changing situations, and have keen observation skills. These factors and others can make working with this population challenging and exhausting, both emotionally and physically. However, the rewards of assisting a patient with a severe brain injury to return home or to school vastly outweigh the challenges of rehabilitation.

The patient with a brain injury is treated across a wide continuum of care, which includes the intensive care unit, acute hospitalization, rehabilitation centers, community reentry programs, outpatient therapy, schools, vocational rehabilitation, and assisted living centers. Because of the wide variety of presenting impairments and complications, rehabilitation for the patient with TBI requires a strong interdisciplinary team. A physical therapist is an important member of this team. It is crucial that there be open communication between and among all team members to ensure safe, timely, and consistent treatment. Regardless of the setting, it is important to remember that the patient is the central member of the team.

■ PREVALENCE AND IMPACT

Traumatic brain injury is the leading cause of injury-related death and disability in the United States. Approximately 1.7 million people in the United States are admitted to emergency departments with TBI each year.[2-4] Of these, 50,000 people die as a result of the injury and 300,000 require hospitalization.[3] In all likelihood these numbers underrepresent the true incidence of TBI. They do not take into account military personnel, people who seek medical attention in settings other than emergency departments, and many sports-related brain injuries that often go unrecognized.[2]

Falls are the leading cause of TBI (32%) followed by motor vehicle/traffic accidents (19%), struck by/against events (18%), and assaults (10%).[3,4] Children, older adolescents/young adults (less than 25 years old), and older adults are most at risk for experiencing TBI. Traumatic brain injuries are most common in young children (0 to 4 years old). However, hospitalization and death as a result of TBI is most common in older adults (65 years old and over).[3,4]

The long-term consequences of TBI on the health care system, society, and the individual are high. There are approximately 5.3 million people living in the United States who are disabled as a result of TBI.[5] Four out of ten are not working 1 year after injury and one-third have difficulty with social integration.[6] One quarter of people with severe to moderate TBI require assistance with activities of daily living (ADL), and approximately 40% report poor mental and physical health.[6]

■ MECHANISM OF INJURY AND PATHOPHYSIOLOGY

Traumatic brain injury is a heterogenous injury, with a wide variety of pathophysiological mechanisms.[7] The brain damage results from external forces that cause brain tissue to make direct contact with an object (bony skull or penetrating object), rapid acceleration or deceleration forces, or blast waves from an explosion.[8] Generally speaking, brain tissue damage can be categorized as either *primary injury* that is due to direct trauma to the parenchyma or *secondary injury* that results from a cascade of biochemical, cellular, and molecular events that evolve over time due to the initial injury and injury-related hypoxia, edema, and elevated intracranial pressure (ICP).[7,9]

Primary Injury

Primary TBI results from either brain tissue coming into contact with an object (e.g., bony skull or external object such as a bullet or sharp instrument creating a penetrating injury) or rapid acceleration/deceleration of the brain. Contact injuries often result in contusions, lacerations, and intracerebral hematomas. This damage is generally focal in nature as the brain comes into contact with bony protuberances on the inside surface of the skull or damage from the penetrating object. Common areas of focal injury are the anterior temporal poles, frontal poles, lateral and inferior temporal cortices, and orbital frontal cortices.

Acceleration and deceleration cause shear, tensile, and compression forces within the brain, which causes **diffuse axonal injury (DAI)**, tissue tearing, and intracerebral hemorrhages.[9] Diffuse axonal injury is the predominant mechanism of injury in most individuals with severe to moderate TBI.[10] It is common in high-speed motor vehicle accidents (MVAs) and can be seen in some sports-related TBIs.[11,12] The term *diffuse* is somewhat misleading because DAI most often occurs in discrete areas: the parasagittal white matter of the cerebral cortex, the corpus callosum, and the pontine-mesencephalic junction adjacent to the superior cerebellar peduncles.[13] The mechanism of DAI is microscopic, so often there are minimal initial findings on computed tomography (CT) and magnetic resonance imaging (MRI). The acceleration/deceleration forces cause disruption of neurofilaments within the axon leading to Wallerian-type axonal degeneration.[13]

Blast Injury

Blast injury is considered a signature injury of the U.S. military conflicts in the Middle East.[14,15] When an explosive device detonates a transient shock wave is produced, which can cause brain damage.[15,16] Primary blast injury results from the direct effect of blast overpressure on organs (in this case the brain), secondary injury results from shrapnel and other objects being hurled at the individual, and tertiary injury occurs when the victim is flung backward and strikes an object. Although the exact mechanisms are not fully understood, there appear to be three mechanisms by which primary blast brain injury may occur: (1) direct transcranial blast wave propagation; (2) the transfer of kinetic energy from the blast wave through the vasculature, which triggers pressure oscillations in the blood vessels leading to the brain; and (3) elevations in cerebrospinal fluid (CSF) or venous pressure caused by compression of the thorax and abdomen and by propagation of a shock wave through the blood vessels or CSF.[15,16] Blast-related brain injury can result in edema, contusion, DAI, hematomas, and hemorrhage.[17,18] A wide spectrum of injury severities ranging from mild (blast concussion) to severe and fatal can result from blast TBI.

Secondary Injury

Secondary cell death occurs as a result of a chain of cellular events that follow tissue damage in addition to the secondary effects of hypoxemia, hypotension, ischemia, edema, and elevated ICP. Secondary processes develop over hours and days, and include glutamate neurotoxicity, influx of calcium and other ions, free radical release, cytokines, and inflammatory responses that can lead to cell death.[8,9] The release of glutamate and other excitatory neurotransmitters exacerbates ion-channel leakage and contributes to brain swelling and raised ICP.[8] Hypoxic-ischemic injury results from a lack of oxygenated blood flow to the brain tissue. It can be caused by systemic hypotension, anoxia, or damage to specific vascular territories of the brain. Because the rigid skull surrounds the brain, swelling, abnormal brain fluid dynamics, or hematoma can result in elevated ICP. Hematomas are usually classified according to their site (epidural, subdural, or intracerebral). Normal ICP is 5 to 20 cm H_2O.[19] Severely increased ICP typically results in herniation of the brain, requiring prompt emergency treatment. Common types of herniations are uncal, central, and tonsillar.

It is important to keep in mind that both primary and secondary mechanisms of injury are not mutually exclusive and often do not occur in isolation. This is one reason that the impact of TBI is so widespread across the International Classification of Functioning, Disability, and Health (ICF) spectrum.

■ SEQUELAE OF TRAUMATIC BRAIN INJURY

Traumatic brain injury is associated with a wide spectrum of neuromuscular, cognitive, and behavioral impairments that can lead to limitations in activity, restrictions in social participation, and diminished quality of life.[20] Box 19.1 identifies some of the prevalent body structure/function impairments associated with TBI. Although physical therapy interventions primarily address physical limitations related to mobility, the cognitive and behavioral changes associated with TBI are often more disabling.

Box 19.1   Impairments Commonly Associated With Traumatic Brain Injury

Neuromuscular
- Paresis
- Abnormal tone
- Motor function
- Postural control

Cognitive
- Arousal level
- Attention
- Concentration
- Memory
- Learning
- Executive functions

Neurobehavioral
- Agitation/Aggression
- Disinhibition
- Apathy
- Emotional lability
- Mental inflexibility
- Impulsivity
- Irritability

Communication

Swallowing

Neuromuscular Impairments

Individuals with TBI commonly exhibit impaired motor function.[21] Upper extremity (UE) and lower extremity (LE) paresis,[21,22] impaired coordination,[21-23] impaired postural control,[21,22,24-28] abnormal tone,[22] and abnormal gait[21,27] may be present as life-long impairments.[21] Abnormal, involuntary movements such as tremor and chorea form and dystonic movements are less common.[21] Patients may also present with impaired somatosensory function, depending on the location of the lesion.

Cognitive Impairments

Cognition is the mental process of knowing and applying information. Owing to the complex nature of many cognitive processes it is difficult to localize the exact neuroanatomical structures responsible for many different cognitive functions. However, many cognitive functions are controlled in the frontal lobes. This makes people with TBI particularly susceptible to cognitive impairments. Cognition includes many complex neural processes, including arousal, attention, concentration, memory, learning, and executive functions.[29-31] Executive functions can be categorized into the following main areas: planning, cognitive flexibility, initiation and self-generation, response inhibition, and serial ordering and sequencing.[31] Chapter 27, Cognitive and Perceptual Dysfunction, provides an in-depth discussion.

Altered levels of consciousness are commonly seen. Between 10% and 15% of patients with severe TBI are discharged from the acute hospital in a *vegetative state*,[32] and the prevalence of *minimally conscious state* is greater than that of vegetative state.[33] **Coma, vegetative state, and minimally conscious state** are disordered arousal states seen after severe brain injury. It can be difficult to distinguish among the disordered arousal states. Many severe injuries begin with coma. In a coma the arousal system is not functioning. The patient's eyes are closed, there are no sleep/wake cycles, and the patient is ventilator dependent. There is no auditory or visual function and no cognitive or communicative function.[33,34] Abnormal motor and postural reflexes may be present. A coma is usually not permanent. Patients may become brain dead, enter a vegetative or minimally conscious state, or go onto full recovery.

In a vegetative state there is disassociation between wakefulness and awareness.[34] The higher central nervous system (CNS) centers are not integrated with the brainstem. The brainstem is able to manage basic cardiac, respiratory, and other vegetative functions and the patient can be weaned off the ventilator. Sleep/wake cycles are present. The eyes may be open though awareness of surroundings is absent, and sleep/wake cycle is present. Patients may startle to visual or auditory stimuli and briefly orient to sound or visual stimuli. Meaningful cognitive and communication function is absent. Reflexive smiling/crying may be present.[33,34] A withdraw response to noxious stimuli is present. Although patients in a vegetative state may appear to have purposeful movement, these movements are nonpurposeful and reflexive in response to external stimuli. Movement will also not be reproducible. Patients in a permanent vegetative state may have no meaningful motor or cognitive function and a complete absence of awareness of self or the environment for a period greater than 1 year after TBI and greater than 3 months after anoxic brain injury.[35,36]

In a minimally conscious state there is minimal evidence of self or environmental awareness. Cognitively mediated behaviors occur inconsistently and are reproducible or sustained such that they can be differentiated from reflexive behaviors.[33] Similar to a vegetative state, sleep/wake cycles are present. However, instead of withdrawing or posturing to noxious stimuli, patients in a minimally conscious state will localize to noxious stimuli and may inconsistently reach for objects.[33,34] Patients may localize to sound location and demonstrate sustained visual fixation and visual pursuit.[33]

Commonly used terms to describe other altered levels of consciousness are *stupor* and *obtunded*. Stupor is an unresponsive state from which the patient can be aroused only briefly with vigorous, repeated sensory stimulation. The patient in an obtunded state sleeps often and when aroused exhibits decreased alertness and interest in the environment and delayed reactions.

Neurobehavioral Impairments

Patients can exhibit profound behavioral changes as they progress through recovery. These impairments can be closely linked to cognitive impairments and are often more debilitating in the long run than physical disability. Common behavioral sequelae include low frustration tolerance, agitation, disinhibition, apathy, emotional lability, mental inflexibility, aggression, impulsivity, and irritability.[31]

Communication

Language and communication deficits after brain injury are generally nonaphasic in nature[37] and are related to cognitive impairment. Common language and communication deficits include disorganized and tangential oral or written communication, imprecise language, word retrieval difficulties, and disinhibited and socially inappropriate language. Patients may also exhibit difficulties communicating in distracting environments, reading social cues, and adjusting communication to meet the demands of the situation.[38] These communication deficits can affect employability, social integration, and quality of life.[39,40] Chapter 28, Neurogenic Disorders of Speech and Language, provides more detail on communication deficits and intervention strategies.

Dysautonomia

Elevated sympathetic nervous system activity occurs as a normal response to trauma; following TBI this response may become overactive. Increased sympathetic activity results in increased heart rate, respiratory rate, and blood pressure; diaphoresis; and hyperthermia.[41,42] Other symptoms of dysautonomia include decerebrate and decorticate posturing, hypertonia, and teeth grinding.[42] The term *paroxysmal sympathetic hyperactivity* accurately describes this phenomenon.[41] The incidence of paroxysmal sympathetic hyperactivity ranges from 8% to 33% in patients with TBI in the intensive care unit.[42]

Post-traumatic Seizures

Between 12% and 50% of people with severe TBI develop post-traumatic seizures.[43-45] For adults with severe injury, phenytoin (an anticonvulsant) is effective in decreasing the risk of early post-traumatic seizures.[46]

Secondary Impairments and Medical Complications

Due to the high potential of prolonged immobility and concomitant injury, patients with TBI are at risk of developing a number of secondary impairments and other medical issues. Up to 50% of patients with severe brain injury develop gastrointestinal difficulties, 45% develop genitourinary problems, 34% develop respiratory problems, 32% develop cardiovascular problems, and 21% develop dermatological complications.[47] Box 19.2 lists some of the more common secondary impairments

---

Box 19.2   Secondary Impairments and Concomitant Injuries

- Deep vein thrombosis
- Heterotopic ossification
- Pressure ulcer
- Pneumonia
- Chronic pain
- Contractures
- Decreased endurance
- Muscle atrophy
- Fracture
- Peripheral nerve damage

---

and concomitant injuries associated with TBI,[45,48-50] including urinary and bowel incontinence, deep vein thrombosis (DVT), heterotopic ossification, pressure ulcer, pneumonia, and chronic pain.

■ DIAGNOSIS AND PROGNOSIS

Traumatic brain injury is generally categorized as severe, moderate, or mild using the *Glasgow Coma Scale* (GCS) (Fig. 19.1).[51] The GCS, developed by Teasdale and Jennett,[51] is the most widely used clinical scale that measures level of consciousness and helps define and classify the severity of injury. The GCS is comprised of three response scores: motor response, verbal response, and eye opening. The scores from the separate responses are summed to provide a score between 3 and 15. Scores

Glasgow Coma Scale	
Activity	**Score**
Eye Opening	
Spontaneous	4
To speech	3
To pain	2
No response	1
Best Motor Response	
Follows motor commands	6
Localizes	5
Withdraws	4
Abnormal flexion	3
Extensor response	2
No response	1
Verbal Response	
Oriented	5
Confused conversation	4
Inappropriate words	3
Incomprehensible sounds	2
No response	1

Figure 19.1 Glasgow Coma Scale. *(From Teasdale and Jennett,[51] with permission.)*

of 8 or less are classified as severe, scores between 9 and 12 are defined as moderate, and scores of 13 to 15 are classified as mild brain injury. Table 19.1 provides an overview of some of the characteristics that distinguish mild, moderate, and severe brain injury. However, these categorizations can be somewhat misleading in that a mild TBI can have a profound impact across the ICF spectrum.

Owing to the wide range of cognitive, motor, and neurobehavioral impairments that accompany brain injury, it can be difficult to establish and predict long-term outcomes and set goals for these patients, even for an experienced clinician. However, researchers have identified some factors that can be useful in estimating future outcomes. Low initial scores on the GCS, particularly motor score and pupillary reactivity, have been identified by a number of studies as a predictor of poor recovery in patients with moderate to severe TBI.[52-56] Other factors associated with poor outcomes are age, race, and lower education level.[52,53,55,57] Petechial hemorrhages, subarachnoid bleed, obliteration of 3rd ventricle or basal cisterns, midline shift, and subdural hematoma findings on initial CT scan are also predictive of poor outcomes.[52,55,56]

The *Medical Research Council* (MRC) CRASH (corticosteroid randomization after significant head injury) study provides a Web-based calculator (www.crash2. lshtm.ac.uk/Risk%20calculator/index.html) that allows clinicians to enter demographic and prognostic information (country, age, GCS score, pupil reactivity to light, presence of major extra cranial injury, and CT findings if available); it calculates the 14 day mortality risk and unfavorable outcome at 6 months, along with the 95% confidence interval.[52] Unfavorable outcome is defined as dead, vegetative state, or severe disability as measured by the *Glasgow Outcome Scale* (GOS).

Duration of **post-traumatic amnesia** (PTA), the length of time between the injury and the time at which the patient is able to consistently remember ongoing events, is also an important factor in predicting recovery. Brown et al[58] found that duration of PTA as measured

Table 19.1	Characteristics of Mild, Moderate, and Severe Traumatic Brain Injury		
Mild TBI		**Moderate TBI**	**Severe TBI**
LOC: 0–30 min		>30 min and <24 hr	>24 hr
AOC: brief >24 hr		>24 hr	>24 hr
PTA: 0–1 day		>1 and <7 days	>7 days
GCS: 13–15		9–12	<9
Neuroimaging: normal		Normal or abnormal	Normal or abnormal

TBI = traumatic brain injury, LOC = loss of consciousness, AOC = alteration of consciousness, PTA = post-traumatic amnesia, GCS = Glasgow Coma Scale.

by the *Galveston Orientation and Amnesia Test* (GOAT), the revised GOAT, or the *Orientation Log* (O-Log) during inpatient rehabilitation is able to predict functional independence, employment, good overall recovery, and independent living 1 year after injury. Patients with PTA less than 48.5 days are likely to have higher *Functional Independence Measure* (FIM) scores at discharge from inpatient rehabilitation; patients with PTA less than 27 days are likely to be employed; patients with PTA less than 34 days are likely to have a good overall recovery (as measured by the GOS); and those with PTA less than 53 days are likely to be living without assistance.[58]

■ CONTINUUM OF CARE AND INTERDISCIPLINARY TEAM

The rehabilitation of patients with TBI occurs across a continuum of care in a variety of settings (Fig. 19.2). Patients who are in a persistent vegetative state may receive ongoing therapy in a nursing home or other long-term care facility once they are medically stable. Patients who are beginning to recover from coma with moderate to severe cognitive, behavioral, and physical impairments often continue rehabilitation in either an acute or subacute inpatient rehabilitation facility. As patients progress in recovery, they will be discharged to other community-based settings depending on the needs of the individual patient.

The foundation for successful rehabilitation following TBI is an *interdisciplinary team*. An interdisciplinary team approach is essential to providing the most comprehensive care that will lead to maximizing functional recovery. An interdisciplinary approach to rehabilitation for this population has been shown to be effective for improving activity levels and participation in society.[59-61]

Within the context of the team, individual members collaborate, contributing their expertise in a specific area, thereby enhancing the team's overall effectiveness. Communication and open mindedness are key to any team.

The different members must share their skills and findings with the whole team and be willing to learn from other team members to promote optimal recovery. The physical therapist must be willing to share a unique knowledge of movement and motor control, but be open to learning from other team members such as the speech-language pathologist (SLP) about cognitive deficits. Each team member should develop an approach to treatment that considers information obtained from all other participating disciplines. This will lead to a consistent and comprehensive approach to care.

Some members may play more prominent roles depending on the setting and stage of recovery. For example, a recreational therapist will not likely be involved with a patient in the acute hospital, but would play a vital role in a community reentry setting. The following subsections identify some of the team members involved in the care of individuals with brain injury and their roles in an acute rehabilitation hospital.

Patient and Family

The patient and family are at the center of the team. The lives of both the patient and family members are likely to be dramatically changed as a result of the injury. Familial roles often change. The patient who previously took care of the children may now be on the receiving end of care. The team must garner information regarding the patient's work, school, financial status, and social history. Family members should be interviewed to obtain information about the patient's lifestyle (work/school/leisure), favorite social and recreational activities, and so forth. Information about the family dynamics should be ascertained. What is the patient's role in the family (e.g., head of the household, primary wage earner)? Is the patient responsible for taking care of children? Is the patient in school? What level? Is the patient working? All of these and many other similar questions should be answered to develop a comprehensive plan of care (POC).

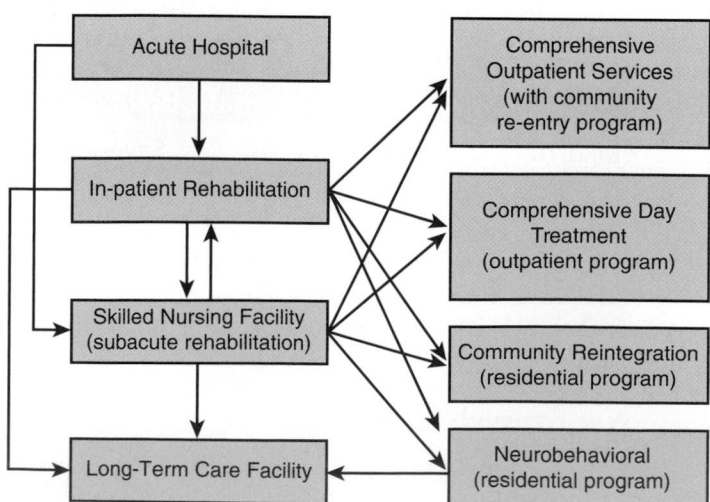

Figure 19.2 Rehabilitation settings for individuals with TBI across the continuum of care.

Physician

In the acute rehabilitation hospital, the physician overseeing the care of the patient with a brain injury is usually a physiatrist or neurologist. The physiatrist has expertise and training in physical medicine and rehabilitation. A neurologist's skills lie in the realm of the brain and nervous system. A neurologist will have particular knowledge related to how the brain may recover, and what impairments and activity limitations are likely to be seen given the location and the extent of the injury. Both a physiatrist and neurologist have vast knowledge in neuropharmacology, an extremely important part of management with this patient population. Certain medications may have harmful side effects that may not be readily apparent. For example, the physician may be able to prescribe a less sedating drug than would normally be used to treat a certain clinical problem in other patient populations.

Speech-Language Pathologist

Owing to the nature of a brain injury, the SLP plays an important and diverse role in rehabilitation. The SLP examines, evaluates, and treats communication, swallowing, and cognitive impairments. As can be seen from the cognitive and communication impairments described above, this can be a challenging task. It is important for the physical therapist to be in close communication with the SLP to provide consistency of care in relation to cognitive, swallowing, and communication impairments. With the guidance of the SLP, the team will be able to devise the most effective and consistent way to communicate with the patient. He or she will also be able to instruct the team in how the patient's cognitive impairments may impede new learning, which in turn will affect everyone's interactions with the patient and their approach to treatment.

Occupational Therapist

The occupational therapist (OT) examines, evaluates, and treats the patient's diminished ability to perform ADL, visual/perceptual impairments, UE functional loss, and sensory integration problems, and will often work with the SLP in treating cognitive impairments. **Basic ADL** (BADL) includes dressing, self-feeding, bathing, and grooming. **Instrumental ADL** (IADL) includes home management, housekeeping, grocery shopping, driving, and telephone use. In the rehabilitation hospital, the occupational and physical therapists often work very closely together. A useful treatment approach is co-treatments with the OT. Having two trained professionals working at the same time with the patient can be very productive. This is especially true with patients who have severe motor control and cognitive deficits. The OT will also work closely with the nursing staff to educate them on the best ways to assist the patient with ADL.

Rehabilitation Nurse

In a rehabilitation hospital, the nurse is responsible for dispensing medications and closely monitoring their effects. The nurse will initiate a bowel and bladder retraining program to assist the patient in learning to become continent again. Bowel and bladder control is extremely important for self-esteem and is related to discharge placement. The nurse performs daily monitoring of vital signs to make sure the patient remains medically stable. The nurse will inspect the patient's skin daily to ensure there are no signs of skin breakdown. The nurse also has the difficult task of consistently following through with the team's treatment plan throughout the day. For example, each shift of nursing staff must follow splinting schedules established by the physical and occupational therapists. The nurse often has the most interaction on a regular basis with the patient's family.

Case Manager/Team Coordinator

The case manager acts as the coordinator for the team. The case manager is often a nurse, social worker, or other health professional. The case manager will direct team meetings, schedule family conferences, and act as a liaison with third-party payers. He or she must promote good communication among all team members to ensure that the rehabilitation care being provided is truly team oriented. The case manager will also be in constant communication with the patient and family to ensure that their needs are being met and that questions and concerns are adequately addressed. The case manager will coordinate payment and insurance benefit issues with the case manager from the patient's insurance company. In addition, the case manager is responsible for setting up follow-up and discharge services for the patient and family.

Social Worker

The social worker provides much needed support to both the patient and family. During the first few days after the initial injury, the family is often in a state of crisis. They are thrown into a world that they, most likely, never knew existed. The social worker can support the family with education and counseling. As the patient progresses with recovery, the social worker will also provide counseling for the patient. This is particularly important as the patient begins to develop greater awareness and insight into his or her deficits. If the patient has behavioral impairments, the social worker can be pivotal in assisting both the patient and family. By providing counseling to both the patient and family, the social worker assists in the development of coping strategies for what may be a life-long disability.

Neuropsychologist

The neuropsychologist plays an important role on the team. He or she will often perform neuropsychological testing when appropriate to determine the patient's baseline cognitive functioning. He or she will also assist the team in developing a behavioral management program. When the patient with a brain injury has severe behavioral impairments, the neuropsychologist may assume the role of the team leader.

Other Team Members

Many patients with severe brain injury may require ventilatory support. The respiratory care practitioner is a vital participant in the evaluation and treatment of respiratory impairments. In the rehabilitation hospital, the respiratory therapist contributes to monitoring the patient's pulmonary status and providing appropriate treatment.

A recreational therapist assists the patient's return to activities enjoyed before the accident, or in helping identify new activities that the patient will find rewarding. Therapeutic recreation is an extremely important part of rehabilitation. Being able to participate in some type of leisure or recreational activities is a significant step in returning to a fulfilling lifestyle.

■ EARLY MEDICAL MANAGEMENT

Medical treatment following brain injury starts at the scene of the accident. Early resuscitation with the goal of stabilizing the cardiovascular and respiratory systems is important to maintain sufficient blood flow and oxygen to the brain.[62,63] Once the patient arrives at the medical center the primary goals are to minimize secondary brain injury by optimizing cerebral blood flow and oxygenation, stabilize vital signs, perform a complete examination, identify and treat any nonneurological injuries, and continuously monitor the patient.[62,63] Systolic blood pressure should be kept above 90 mm Hg and oxygen saturation above 90%.[62] Patients with severe injury and some with moderate injury will need to be intubated. The patient's neck should be stabilized with a collar and the head elevated 30 degrees.[62] This is done to protect the spine in case of instability, as well as avoid an increase in ICP. The GCS is used to determine the severity of the brain injury. A complete neurological examination is also done. Additional information about the extent of the injury is obtained through x-ray films and neuroimaging studies such as CT and MRI. This is done to determine if neurosurgery is warranted. Large intracranial hematomas or other mass lesions may need to be surgically evacuated.

The patient is monitored continuously. For patients with a GCS of 8 or less, any acute abnormality on CT, a systolic pressure of less than 90 mm Hg, or age greater than 40 years, ICP monitoring is recommended.[62] An external ventricular drain provides the most accurate and reliable data and also provides a means to control ICP by cerebrospinal fluid removal. Other monitoring options that are less invasive include the subdural bolt and a fiberoptic catheter. Elevated ICP can be treated with the use of sedating medications, moderate head-up positioning (head elevated to 30°), osmotherapy, hypothermia, surgical decompression, and barbiturates.[62,63] Intracranial pressure should be less than 20 mm Hg and the cerebral perfusion pressure (CPP) greater than 60 mm Hg.[62] If ICP cannot be treated successfully, inducing a pharmacologic coma or surgical decompression may be necessary.

■ PHYSICAL THERAPY MANAGEMENT OF MODERATE TO SEVERE TRAUMATIC BRAIN INJURY IN THE ACUTE STAGE

The remainder of this chapter is divided into three main sections: (1) physical therapy management of patients with severe to moderate TBI during the early stages of recovery, (2) physical therapy management of patients with severe to moderate TBI during active rehabilitation, and (3) physical therapy management of patients with mild TBI. Patients in the early stage of recovery after severe to moderate TBI often demonstrate low levels of arousal. The primary goal of physical therapy is to prevent secondary complications due to the TBI and prolonged bedrest/immobilization, begin early mobilization when medical clearance is received, and initiate patient and family education. Depending on the patient's presentation, some of the examination and intervention procedures described in the section on physical therapy management during active rehabilitation can be used in the early stage of recovery as well.

Examination

The first step in beginning an examination at this early stage of recovery is to conduct a complete medical record review. Because the patient may not be medically stable and will likely have various precautions and complications, it is important to obtain all critical information from the medical record before actually seeing the patient. The patient may be on a ventilator with ongoing monitoring of ICP. He or she may have weight-bearing precautions and range of motion (ROM) restrictions owing to musculoskeletal injuries and/or interventions, and open wounds. A thorough medical record review provides a comprehensive perspective about the patient's condition, as well as a complete understanding of the precautions and contraindications that must be observed during the examination and subsequent treatment. Because the patient's medical status may be dynamic at these stages, it is important to check with the patient's primary nurse before beginning any session. Team members should always observe universal precautions and may need to wear gowns, gloves, and/or masks or other personal protective equipment when treating the patient.

After reviewing the medical record and receiving an update on the patient's status from the nursing staff, the physical therapist is ready to begin the examination. Key areas to examine include the following:

- Arousal, attention, and cognition
- Integument integrity
- Sensory integrity
- Motor function
- Range of motion
- Reflex integrity
- Ventilation and respiration/gas exchange

Patients with severe TBI who are in low arousal state (coma, vegetative, or minimally conscious) may present with abnormal tone and posturing. Primitive postures may include those associated with **decorticate or decerebrate rigidity.** In decorticate rigidity, the upper extremities are in a flexed posture and the lower extremities are extended. With decerebrate rigidity, both the upper and lower extremities are positioned in extension. Abnormal tone may take the form of spastic hypertonia. This may range from spasticity that severely affects the entire body and greatly inhibits normal, functional movement, to lesser levels of tone that affect individual muscle groups.

If not medically contraindicated, the examination should include sitting on the side of the bed with assistance. The therapist should monitor vital signs and document any changes in tone or head and trunk control. When appropriate, the patient should be transferred into a wheelchair. The patient may require the assistance of two to three people to transfer at this stage. In most cases, a reclining or tilt-in-space wheelchair is the best option for positioning, with a specialized pressure-reducing cushion. Often it may require several treatment sessions to complete the entire examination. Because early patient status is often dynamic, any signs of progress or regression should be carefully monitored and documented.

Outcome Measures

Arousal, Attention, and Cognition

The *Coma Recovery Scale–Revised* (CRS-R) is recommended to assess patients with disordered consciousness.[64] The CRS-R is a valid and reliable 23-item measure with six subscales: auditory, visual, motor, oromotor, communication, and arousal.[65,66] Scores range from 0 to 23. Data are useful in distinguishing between different states of consciousness (vegetative state, minimally conscious state, and emerging), determining the prognosis, and informing treatment planning.[65]

The *Disorders of Consciousness Scale* (DOCS) is a valid and reliable scale also designed to measure arousal and neurobehavioral recovery in patients with disorders of consciousness.[67,68] It consists of 23 items, which assess social knowledge, taste/swallowing, olfactory function, proprioception, tactile sensation, auditory function, and visual function. Scoring is based on patient response and includes no response, generalized response, or localized response. The DOCS can be used to differentiate states of consciousness (i.e., vegetative state and minimally conscious state) and assist in determining prognosis for recovery.[64,67-70] A manual and video training are available for the DOCS at www.queri.research.va.gov/ptbri/docs_training/default.cfm.

The *Rancho Los Amigos Levels of Cognitive Functioning* (LOCF) scale is a descriptive scale used to examine cognitive and behavioral recovery in individuals with TBI (Box 19.3) as they emerge from coma.[71] This scale does not address specific cognitive deficits, but is useful for communicating general cognitive and/or behavioral status and for treatment planning. The eight categories describe typical cognitive and behavioral progress after a brain injury. Patients may plateau at any level. The LOCF has been shown to be a reliable and valid measure of cognitive and behavioral function for individuals with brain injury.[72]

Plan of Care
Outcomes/Goals

A list of general goals and outcomes anticipated for patients in Levels I, II, and III (LOCF) adapted from the American Physical Therapy Association's *Guide to Physical Therapist Practice*[73] are presented in Box 19.4. They can be used to guide the development of specific anticipated goals and expected outcomes for an individual patient.

Interventions
Preventing Secondary Impairments

Because of the patient's inability to move at these levels, he or she is susceptible to indirect impairments such as contractures, decubiti, pneumonia, and DVT.[47] If prevention is not addressed early in rehabilitation, these impairments are likely to impede future progress, and can be life threatening. Proper positioning both in bed and in a wheelchair is essential. Appropriate positioning will assist in preventing skin breakdown and contractures, improve pulmonary hygiene and circulation, and may modify muscle tone. When the patient is in bed, the head should be kept in neutral. The hips and knees should be slightly flexed, but ROM should be monitored to ensure that contractures do not develop. Splints may be used to assist in positioning. Special boots can be used to position the foot to prevent foot drop and skin breakdown on the heel (Fig. 19.3). Turning will help prevent skin breakdown and pneumonia. Patients should be repositioned every 2 hours when in bed. Specialized air mattresses are another effective way to assist with the prevention of pressure sores.

Serial casting may be used to maintain or improve ROM.[74-77] Serial casting is often used for plantarflexor or biceps contractures resulting from either increased tone or prolonged shortening of the muscle. With a

Box 19.3   Rancho Los Amigos Levels of Cognitive Functioning (LOCF)[a]

I.	No Response

Patient appears to be in a deep sleep and is completely unresponsive to any stimuli.

II.	Generalized Response

Patient reacts inconsistently and nonpurposefully to stimuli in a nonspecific manner. Responses are limited and often the same regardless of stimulus presented. Responses may be physiological changes, gross body movements, and/or vocalization.

III.	Localized Response

Patient reacts specifically but inconsistently to stimuli. Responses are directly related to the type of stimulus presented. May follow simple commands such as closing eyes or squeezing hand in an inconsistent, delayed manner.

IV.	Confused-Agitated

Patient is in a heightened state of activity. Behavior is bizarre and nonpurposeful relative to immediate environment. Does not discriminate among persons or objects; is unable to cooperate directly with treatment efforts. Verbalizations frequently are incoherent and/or inappropriate to the environment; confabulation may be present. Gross attention to environment is very brief; selective attention is often nonexistent. Patient lacks short- and long-term recall.

V.	Confused-Inappropriate

Patient is able to respond to simple commands fairly consistently. However, with increased complexity of commands or lack of any external structure, responses are nonpurposeful, random, or fragmented. Demonstrates gross attention to the environment but is highly distractible and lacks ability to focus attention on a specific task. With structure, may be able to converse on a social automatic level for short periods of time. Verbalization is often inappropriate and confabulatory. Memory is severely impaired; often shows inappropriate use of objects; may perform previously learned tasks with structure but is unable to learn new information.

VI.	Confused-Appropriate

Patient shows goal-directed behavior but is dependent on external input or direction. Follows simple directions consistently and shows carryover for relearned tasks such as self-care. Responses may be incorrect due to memory problems, but they are appropriate to the situation. Past memories show more depth and detail than recent memory.

VII.	Automatic-Appropriate

Patient appears appropriate and oriented within the hospital and home settings; goes through daily routine automatically, but frequently robot-like. Patient shows minimal to no confusion and has shallow recall of activities. Shows carryover for new learning but at a decreased rate. With structure is able to initiate social or recreational activities; judgment remains impaired.

VIII.	Purposeful-Appropriate

Patient is able to recall and integrate past and recent events and is aware of and responsive to environment. Shows carryover for new learning and needs no supervision once activities are learned. May continue to show a decreased ability relative to premorbid abilities, abstract reasoning, tolerance for stress, and judgment in emergencies or unusual circumstances.

[a]Condensed form. From Professional Staff Association, Ranchos Los Amigos Hospital, with permission.[71]

Box 19.4   General Goals and Outcomes Anticipated for Patients With Severe to Moderate Traumatic Brain Injury in the Acute Stage

- Physical function and level of alertness are increased.
- The risk of secondary impairments is reduced.
- Motor control is improved.
- The effects of tone are managed.
- Postural control is improved.
- Tolerance of activities and positions is increased.
- Joint integrity and mobility are improved or remain functional.
- Family and caregivers are educated on patient's diagnosis, physical therapy interventions, goals, and outcomes.
- Care is coordinated among all team members.

plantarflexion contracture, the ankle is stretched into as much dorsiflexion as possible and then a short leg cast is applied. In approximately 2 to 5 days the cast is removed. The muscle is stretched again and another cast is applied (Figs. 19.4, 19.5, and 19.6). This procedure is repeated until satisfactory gains in ROM have been achieved, or no further progress is made. Because the individual with brain injury is likely to have impaired sensation and communication, as well as behavioral deficits, there is a risk of skin breakdown or the patient hurting himself or herself or others with the cast. The decision to use casts should be made carefully. The benefits and possible side effects should be thoroughly discussed with input from appropriate team members. It is also important to monitor the patient after the cast is applied. Hands-on experience under the supervision

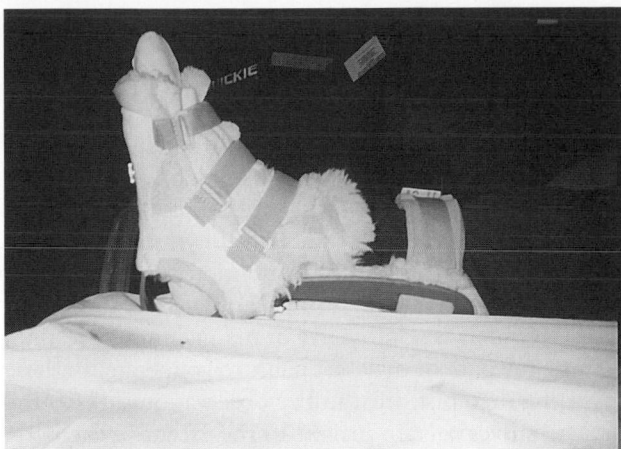

Figure 19.3 Multi-podus boot used for ankle and foot positioning and to prevent skin breakdown on the heel. This type of positioning device may not be beneficial for the patient with moderate to severe tone at the ankle; it is not strong enough to prevent the ankle from plantarflexing.

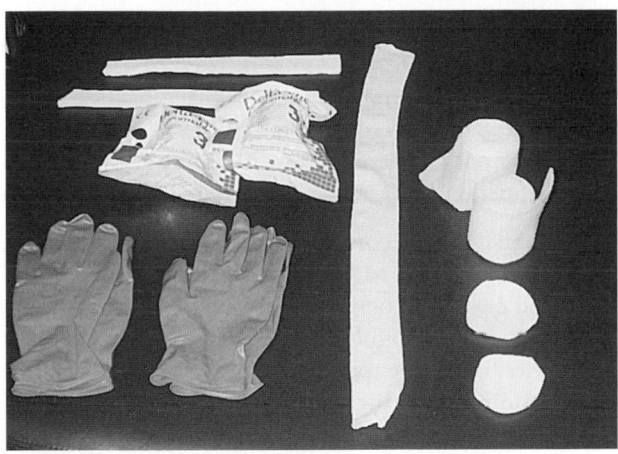

Figure 19.4 Materials used for serial casting: fiberglass casting material, rubber gloves, stockinette, a layer of padding to wrap around the lower leg and foot, and padding for the malleoli and proximal and distal ends of the cast.

of a skilled clinician is recommended before attempting cast applications.

Proper wheelchair positioning is important.[78] Because of reduced postural control at these levels, a reclining wheelchair or a tilt-in-space wheelchair is typically required. Proper pelvic positioning and head positioning are key elements in promoting good posture in a wheelchair. Refer to Chapter 32, The Prescriptive Wheelchair, for further discussion of this topic.

Respiratory care practitioners, physical therapists, and nurses often use postural drainage, percussion, vibration, and positioning to prevent pulmonary complications and improve pulmonary function.[79] Irwin and Tecklin[80] provide in-depth coverage of different interventions to improve ventilation and respiration.

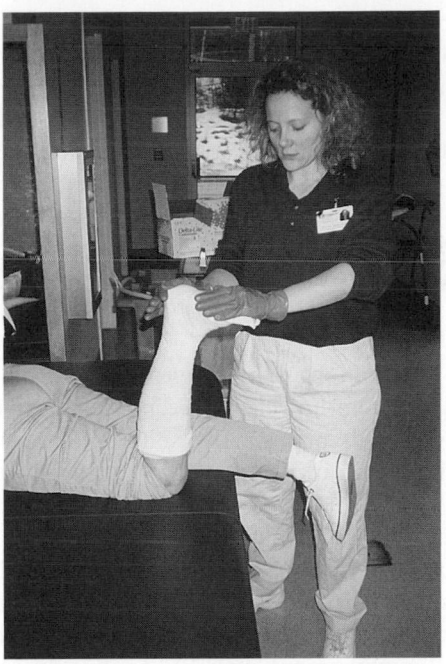

Figure 19.5 Serial casting: first a layer of padding is wrapped around the lower leg and foot.

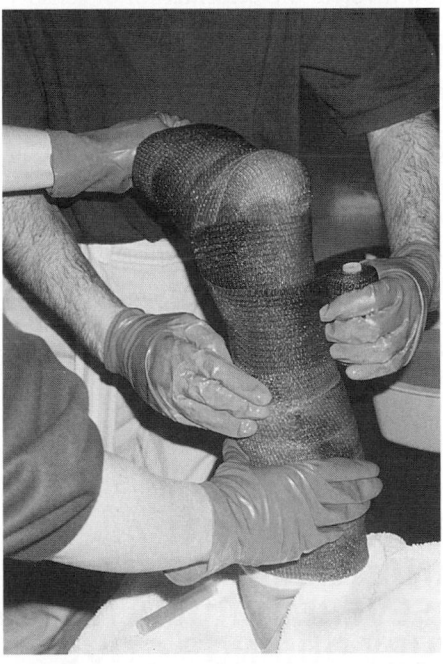

Figure 19.6 Serial casting: then the fiberglass casting material is wrapped around the lower leg and foot. One clinician does the wrapping, while another holds the leg and foot in the proper position.

Early Mobility

Upright sitting is extremely important because it addresses elements of treatment goals for the early levels of recovery. As soon as medically stable, the patient should be transferred to a sitting position and out of bed to a wheelchair. All precautions should be observed. The head should be properly supported, because the patient is not likely to have adequate neck and head control to maintain an upright posture without support. Co-treatment with an occupational therapist provides two skilled professionals to assist the patient, because maximal assistance is often required. Use of a tilt table is also advantageous because it allows early weight-bearing through the LEs. The upright position, both on a tilt table and in a wheelchair, may improve overall level of alertness.

Sensory Stimulation

Sensory stimulation is an intervention used to increase the level of arousal and elicit movement in individuals in a coma or persistent vegetative state. The theory is that by providing stimulation in a controlled, multisensory manner, with a balance of stimulation and rest, the reticular activating system may be stimulated causing a general increase in arousal. Theoretical support for such programs comes from research in four areas: (1) effects of sensory deprivation on neurological recovery; (2) effects of "enriched" environments on behavior and nervous system structure and function; (3) nervous system plasticity; and (4) effects of environmental input during sensitive periods of neurodevelopment.[81] In general, multisensory stimulation involves the presentation of sensory stimulation in a highly structured and consistent manner. The following sensory systems are systematically stimulated: auditory, olfactory, gustatory, visual, tactile, kinesthetic, and vestibular.[82,83] During this type of intervention, the patient should be closely monitored for any changes in behavior.

The value of sensory stimulation for patients who are slow to recover remains unproven. A systematic review published by the Cochrane library suggests that there is no reliable evidence to support or rule out the effectiveness of sensory stimulation programs for this patient population.[84]

Not all patients with severe TBI recover fully. Some may remain in a state of low arousal. In these cases, the interventions described above may need to be continued by caregivers.

■ PHYSICAL THERAPY MANAGEMENT OF MODERATE TO SEVERE TRAUMATIC BRAIN INJURY DURING ACTIVE REHABILITATION

As patients with severe to moderate TBI recover, they require extensive and protracted rehabilitation across a variety of settings throughout the continuum of care. This may include acute and subacute inpatient rehabilitation, postacute rehabilitation, day treatment program, and outpatient or home care. The many cognitive, physical, and/or behavioral impairments that affect activity levels and social participation often necessitate multiple episodes of physical therapy care over the patient's lifetime. Goals and interventions should be focused on the patient's abilities and personal goals regardless of the setting.

Examination

Irrespective of injury chronicity, some patients with TBI will have cognitive and behavioral impairments that pose barriers to the examination process. These barriers may include disorientation, confusion, physical aggression, memory deficits, and limited attention span. It may be difficult to gather data using standardized tests and measures, such as goniometry or manual muscle testing, because the patient may be unable to cooperate. In these cases, the therapist must utilize observation skills as the patient moves to gain insight to the extent of the body structure/function impairments and activity restrictions. The physical therapist should determine the patient's cognitive abilities, because these will affect the ability to relearn motor skills. This will include orientation, attention span, memory, insight, safety awareness, and alertness. Key initial questions that warrant consideration include the following:

- Is the patient able to follow commands: one-step, two-step, or multistep commands?
- Is the patient oriented to person, place, and/or time?
- Does the patient recognize family members?
- Does the patient demonstrate any insight into what has happened?

It is beneficial to consult with other team members, especially the SLP, to obtain additional information about the patient's cognitive status.

As the patient's cognitive and behavioral impairments become less obtrusive to the process, the physical therapy examination should include the elements and outcome measures found in Box 19.5.[73]

Depending on the status of the individual patient, some of these areas may be screened whereas others require more in-depth examination. Determination of the patient's functional abilities should be done in a variety of environments, because some patients may perform well in the closed environment of a private room, but performance may deteriorate in an open environment with multiple distractions. Section One of this book (Chapters 1 through 9 on clinical decision making and examination) provides a detailed description of procedures, tests and measures, and specific outcome measures for examining the above-mentioned areas. A brief description of some of the more clinically useful outcome measures for individuals with TBI follows.

Outcome Measures: Body/Structure Function
Balance

The Berg Balance Scale (see Chapter 5) is a valid and clinically useful measure of balance in individuals with TBI.[85,86] The Berg Balance Scale, together with functional status measured using the Functional Independence Measure (FIM), may assist predicting inpatient

---

> **Box 19.5** Elements of the Examination and Outcome Measures
>
> - Aerobic capacity/endurance
> - Arousal, attention, and cognition
>   - *Coma Recovery Scale–Revised, Disorders of Consciousness Scale, Rancho Los Amigos Levels of Cognitive Functioning, Moss Attention Rating Scale, Test of Everyday Attention, Trail Making Test Part B, Galveston Orientation and Amnesia Test, Orientation Log*
> - Behavioral status
>   - *Supervision Rating Scale, Neurobehavioral Rating Scale– Revised, Agitated Behavior Scale*
> - Cranial nerve integrity
> - Gait, locomotion, and balance
>   - *Berg Balance Scale, Community Balance and Mobility Scale, High-Level Mobility Assessment Tool, Rancho Los Amigos (RLA) OGA System, 10-Meter Walk Test, 6-Minute Walk Test, Modified Walking and Remembering Test*
> - Integumentary integrity
> - Joint integrity and mobility
> - Motor function (motor control and motor learning)
> - Muscle performance, including strength, power, and endurance
> - Neuromotor development and sensory integration
> - Pain
> - Posture
> - Range of motion
> - Reflex integrity
> - Self-care and ADL skills
>   - *Functional Independence Measure, Functional Assessment Measure*
> - Sensory integrity
> - Ventilation and respiration/gas exchange
> - Work/leisure/community reintegration
>   - *Mayo-Portland Adaptability Inventory, Community Integration Questionnaire*

rehabilitation length of stay, falls during rehabilitation stay, and functional gains during rehabilitation.[85,86] However, as patients improve the Berg Balance Scale may exhibit a ceiling effect.[87]

The *Community Balance and Mobility Scale* (CB&M) by Howe et al[88] is an instrument developed specifically for patients with persistent balance deficits following TBI. The CB&M is a reliable and valid tool that assesses higher-level balance abilities typically associated with community mobility. This tool shares similarities to the *High-Level Mobility Assessment Tool* (HiMAT) developed by Williams et al.[89,90] This is a unidimensional measure of higher-level motor performance for individuals with TBI. The test items are more difficult than general measures of balance and functional mobility and are intended to quantify abilities required of physically demanding vocational and social roles, as well as sporting activities.

A revised version of the HiMAT has a minimal detectable change score of 2 points.[91]

Attention and Cognition

The *Moss Attention Rating Scale* (MARS) is an observational rating scale that provides a reliable and valid measure of attention-related behavior after TBI. The scale allows the therapist to rate a patient's behavior on a 5-point scale across 22 items that capture the effects of impaired attention on cognitive and motor performance.[92] Other measures of attention most often employed by neuropsychologists include the *Test of Everyday Attention*[93] and the *Trail Making Test Part B*.[94] Though all three of these measures capture attentional deficits and may serve as useful global outcome measures, they will be less helpful in measuring changes in attention behavior attributable to physical therapy interventions.

The *Galveston Orientation and Amnesia Test* is a measure of PTA.[95] The GOAT is administered by asking a series of standardized questions related to orientation and the ability to recall events before and after the injury. Scores between 100 and 76 are considered normal and patients with scores below are considered to have PTA. The GOAT has high interrater reliability and is a valid measure of PTA.[95,96] The *Orientation Log* (O-Log) measures orientation to time, place, and circumstance.[97] The O-Log can be used for serial assessment of orientation to document improvements during rehabilitation.[98] It is reliable, is valid, and can be used to predict outcome.[96,97,99] Measures of dual-task performance (see later discussion) are more specific to physical therapy practice.

Behavior and Safety

Rehabilitation teams often use an outcome measure that captures the impact of behavior and safety on overall independence. The *Supervision Rating Scale*[100] provides a one-step method for rating a patient's current level of supervision ranging from independent to full-time direct supervision. The *Neurobehavioral Rating Scale–Revised* (NRS-R) is a 29-item multidimensional, clinician-based assessment instrument designed to measure neurobehavioral disturbances.[101] The items cover numerous cognitive and behavioral constructs such as memory, attention, communication, mood, and agitation. The *Agitated Behavior Scale* (ABS) measures the type and degree of agitation after TBI.[102]

Outcome Measures: Activity and Participation

Global Functioning

The *Functional Independence Measure*[103,104] is a commonly used measure of functional mobility, ADL function, cognition, and communication. The FIM was designed to measure level of disability and burden of care in individuals undergoing inpatient rehabilitation, and is useful for monitoring patient progress and evaluating outcomes. The *Functional Assessment Measure (FAM)*[105,106] was developed as an adjunct to the FIM. It includes functional areas not addressed in the FIM that are important for individuals with TBI and stroke. The other items include community access, reading, writing, safety, employability, and adjustment to limitations. The FIM, in combination with the FAM, is a valid and reliable measure of disability after TBI.[107] In addition to measuring the amount of physical assistance required to perform a functional task, the therapist should also analyze how the patient performs the task. A thorough movement analysis of how the FIM items and other functional tasks are performed will aid the therapist in identifying the motor function and other impairments that underlie specific activity limitations.

Community Reintegration

Rehabilitation teams commonly employ the use of a participation-level measure that quantifies the extent of reintegrate into social, familial, and vocational roles. One such measure is the *Mayo-Portland Adaptability Inventory* (MPAI-4),[108,109] which is frequently used in postacute TBI rehabilitation. Another, similar measure is the *Community Integration Questionnaire* (CIQ).[110] The CIQ consists of 15 items relevant to home integration, social integration, and productive activities.

Locomotion

Spatiotemporal gait deficits are common following TBI, yet, to date, no classification system of gait disorders exists for this population.[111] There are many different methods of examining gait and walking ability. Physical therapists use *observational gait analysis* (OGA) as a preferred method in the clinic.[112] One instrument used clinically is the *Rancho Los Amigos (RLA) OGA System*. Refer to Chapter 7, Examination of Gait, for further discussion of this instrument. The RLA OGA instrument gathers data on the cyclical movements of walking that occur from one stride cycle to the next. The gait cycle is divided into stance and swing phases. The physical therapist visually analyzes a patient's walking pattern, looking for asymmetries and deviations from normal. Based on these observations, the physical therapist gains insight into which impairments may be the cause of the deviations. Specific interventions are then designed to address the possible causes of the gait deviations. However, caution should be used when interpreting OGA findings. Some gait abnormalities identified by quantitative gait analysis may not be detected by OGA.[113] Chapter 7 reviews instrumented walkways and other methods of more precisely and accurately measuring specific kinematics and kinetics associated with gait.

Gait speed is also an important measure of walking ability. The *10-Meter Walk Test* (10MWT) is a reliable measure of both fast-paced and self-paced gait speed in patients with TBI.[114,115] Caution should be used when interpreting gait speed measured with the 10MWT, because there is evidence suggesting that the 10MWT may not fully reflect the many different demands of walking in the community (e.g., crossing a busy street, walking in a crowded mall, walking on uneven surfaces, and so forth).[114]

Fatigue and deconditioning are common following TBI.[116,117] As such, measuring walking endurance is clinically useful. The *6-Minute Walk Test* (6MWT) is a common, reliable, and valid way to measure this aspect of walking ability.[118,119] Normative values from healthy adults are available for this test.[120] Other methods of assessing cardiorespiratory fitness have also been validated for patients with TBI, including the *graded exercise test*[121] and a *modified shuttle test*.[122]

Several tests of dynamic balance (see above) and walking ability are appropriate for this population; however, they do not offer insight into how walking and balance are affected by the addition of a cognitive load. Measures of *dual-task performance* allow the therapist to examine the extent to which deficits in attention and memory affect gait speed and safety. These two cognitive abilities (attention and memory) are strongly associated with dual-task performance and also commonly impaired in persons with TBI.[123,124] There are a variety of clinical tests of dual-task performance that can be used for clients with acquired brain injury. A review of several dual-task performance measures is available.[125] One such measure is the *Modified Walking and Remembering Test* (WART) developed by McCulloch et al.[123] The WART involves a single-task condition (simple walking task) and a dual-task condition (walking task and cognitive task).

Further information on these and other outcome measures specifically used in TBI rehabilitation can be found at the *Center for Outcome Measurement in Brain Injury (COMBI)* website (www.tbims.org/combi/index.html).

Plan of Care
Goals/Outcomes

Persons with moderate to severe TBI present with a wide variety and degree of physical, cognitive, and behavioral limitations. As the patient progresses in these areas, anticipated goals and expected outcomes will move from basic mobility and self-care, toward skills that facilitate community inclusion and social participation. The American Physical Therapy Association's *Guide to Physical Therapist Practice*[73] offers examples of general anticipated goals and expected outcomes pertinent to patients with TBI. Examples include the following:

- The risk of secondary impairments is reduced.
- Performance of functional mobility and ADL skills is increased.
- Ability to assume or resume self-care and home management roles is improved.

These can be used to guide the development of specific anticipated goals and expected outcomes tailored to each individual patient. Refer to Chapter 15, Box 15.6, for more examples of goals and outcomes for patients with impaired motor function and sensory integrity associated with nonprogressive disorders of the CNS—stroke and TBI (Practice Pattern 5 D).[73]

Interventions

Motor (Re)Learning Strategies

Treatment sessions should be thoughtfully planned to maximize the patient's motor learning capabilities. Practice should be *distributed*, with frequent rest periods. Owing to cognitive impairments, patients may experience mental as well as physical fatigue during treatment sessions. Signs of mental fatigue may include increased irritability, decreased attention and concentration, deterioration in performance of physical skills, and delayed initiation. Treatment sessions should include sufficient rest periods to minimize both physical and mental fatigue and maximize motor relearning.

The impact of manipulating motor learning variables on motor skill acquisition and generalizability has not been thoroughly studied in patients with TBI. Refer to Chapter 10, Strategies to Improve Motor Function, for an in-depth discussion of motor learning principles. There are a few studies with a limited number of subjects, however, that suggest the use of *video self-modeling*,[126] and the *concept of self-generation*[127] may be beneficial to the relearning of functional tasks. With video self-modeling the patient watches himself or herself engaging in skillful behavior on edited videotapes. The self-generation concept is a phenomenon whereby items that are self-generated are better learned and remembered compared to information that is provided. As the cognitive and behavioral barriers to treatment become less intrusive, sessions can be progressively more challenging both mentally and physically. A *random practice schedule* may be more beneficial to learning,[128] although this schedule can be employed only after the patient has demonstrated some initial learning of the task's dynamics.[129] Feedback is also very important. Owing to cognitive, sensory, and perceptual impairments, *explicit or augmented feedback* may be more beneficial in the early stages of motor learning as opposed to intrinsic feedback. However, care should be taken not to overwhelm the patient with feedback.

Restorative Versus Compensatory-Based Interventions

As discussed earlier, an early, interdisciplinary approach to rehabilitation after TBI has been shown to be beneficial. There are many intervention approaches available to the physical therapist that can promote functional recovery following brain injury. Two basic treatment strategies are a *compensatory* and a *restorative* (recovery) approach.

The compensatory approach seeks to improve functional skills by compensating for the lost ability. A simple example of this would be teaching one-handed dressing techniques to a patient with UE hemiparesis resulting from a TBI. A restorative approach seeks to restore the "normal" use of the affected UE. Both approaches seek to reinstitute functional independence, and the exact definition of each approach is a subject of ongoing debate.

Compensation is commonly defined as the resumption of the ability to complete a task using alternative motor patterns and strategies. The definition of recovery varies. Some feel that it refers to the resumption of the ability to complete a task using the same motor patterns and strategies as before. Another, more liberal, definition is completing a task using similar strategies despite inferior efficiency, speed, and/or accuracy. Levin et al[130] addressed this topic and proposed explicit definitions for recovery and compensation. The authors argue that the definitions of recovery and compensation will change based on whether performance or function is measured. To make this point clearer, the authors used the framework of the *World Health Organization's ICF Model*. Refer to Table 19.2 for more details.

In most cases involving moderate to severe TBI, clinical management will likely require a balance between both restorative and compensatory approaches. As an example, a therapist may determine that a restorative approach to gait training is indicated but may also choose to ensure that the client and caregiver have adequate training in the use of an assistive device for safety during the earlier stages of recovery should it be needed. Current literature offers little guidance for the practitioner attempting to choose between approaches. Table 19.3 offers questions that can guide this aspect of clinical decision making. After a thorough examination and consideration of the patient's unique personal and environment barriers and facilitators, these questions can help lead the clinician and patient to a shared agreement about which approach will be used.

The last decade of translational and applied research in the areas of neural plasticity, motor learning, and neurological rehabilitation has heightened awareness that (re)learning is directly related to the rehabilitative experiences patients are exposed to. Using the example above, interventions that seek compensation will result not only in learning how to use the less affected UE but also learning "not" to use the more affected UE. (See the discussion of "learned nonuse" in Chapter 15.) Alternatively, a restorative rehabilitative experience that allows the patient to practice using the affected arm for everyday tasks will result in greater functional independence and affected UE use. This knowledge is useful in clinical decision making when developing the POC.

Restorative Interventions and Neural Plasticity

No studies to date have identified what types of restorative interventions are the most beneficial to persons with

Table 19.2	Motor Recovery and Compensation Across Three Levels of the ICF	
Level	**Recovery**	**Compensation**
ICF: Health Condition (neuronal)	*Restoring function in neural tissue that was initially lost after injury.* May be seen as reactivation in brain areas previously inactivated by the circulatory event. Although this is not expected to occur in the area of the primary brain lesion, it may occur in areas surrounding the lesion (penumbra) and in the diaschisis.	*Neural tissue acquires a function that it did not have prior to injury.* May be seen as activation in alternative brain areas not normally observed in nondisabled individuals.
ICF: Body Functions/ Structure (performance)	*Restoring the ability to perform a movement in the same manner as it was performed before injury.* This may occur through the reappearance of premorbid movement patterns during task accomplishment (voluntary joint range of motion, temporal and spatial interjoint coordination, etc).	*Performing an old movement in a new manner.* May be seen as the appearance of alternative movement patterns (i.e., recruitment of additional or different degrees of freedom, changes in muscle activation patterns such as increased agonist/antagonist coactivation, delays in timing between movements of adjacent joints, etc.) during the accomplishment of a task.
ICF: Activity (functional)	*Successful task accomplishment using limbs or end effectors typically used by nondisabled individuals.*[a]	*Successful task accomplishment using alternate limbs or end effectors.* For example, opening a package of chips using one hand and the mouth instead of two hands.

ICF = World Health Organization International Classification of Functioning.
[a]Note that task performance may be successful using compensatory motor strategies and movement patterns.
Levin, MF, Kleim, JA, and Wolf, SL: What do motor "recovery" and "compensation" mean in patients following stroke?
Neurorehabilitation and Neural Repair 23(4):313–319, 2009.[130] Reprinted by permission of SAGE Publications.

Table 19.3	Compensation Versus Restoration: Guiding Questions to Consider
Injury Severity Motor Learning Resources	• Are sensorimotor deficits so severe that restorative approaches are not possible or appropriate? • Do secondary complications or co-morbidities exist that pose barriers to recovery (e.g., contractures, fractures)? • Is an appropriate motor recovery program (specificity, intensity, frequency, duration, difficulty) feasible? • How chronic is the injury? • What strengths and weaknesses does the patient have relative to his or her ability to learning motor tasks? • Are there significant cognitive, behavioral, or medical barriers? • Does the patient have any financial or support barriers? • Will funding lapse before functional recovery occurs? • Do financial resources suggest that a more rapid approach be used? • What impact will discharge destination have on the prescribed treatment approach?

TBI. Current research has demonstrated that task-specific interventions with large amounts of practice can induce beneficial neuroplastic changes in the CNS and restore function.[131-133] Studies involving monkey and rat models of brain injury have demonstrated the importance of intensive, task-oriented training on neuroplastic changes in the motor cortex and functional recovery.[134,135] This line of research was extended to include human models with neurological deficits and later the sum of these findings was translated into tangible principles of experience-dependent neural plasticity.[131,136,137] Table 19.4 provides examples of several of these principles. Current evidence suggests that treatment interventions that are most beneficial will be specific to the function/task being retrained, meaningful to the client, and challenging to the cortical systems involved in the activity.

Task-Oriented Approach

Also in line with these principles, current theories of motor control and motor learning advocate for a task-oriented approach to interventions for individuals with neurological deficits.[129] The majority of research on the principles that underpin effective, task-oriented interventions for clients with neurological disorders has been done with persons with stroke. Despite this, these same principles will serve the physical therapist well in selecting and applying appropriate interventions for persons

Table 19.4	Principles of Experience-Dependent Neuroplasticity
Principle	**Description**
Use It or Lose It	Failure to drive specific brain functions can lead to functional degradation.
Use It and Improve It	Training that drives a specific brain function can lead to an enhancement of that function.
Specificity	The nature of the training experience dictates the nature of the plasticity.
Repetition Matters	Induction of plasticity requires sufficient repetition.
Intensity Matters	Induction of plasticity requires sufficient training intensity.
Time Matters	Different forms of plasticity occur at different times during training.
Salience Matters	The training experience must be sufficiently salient to induce plasticity.
Age Matters	Training-induced plasticity occurs more readily in younger brains.
Transference	Plasticity in response to one training experience can enhance the acquisition of similar behaviors.
Interference	Plasticity in response to one experience can interfere with the acquisition of other behaviors.

From Kleim, JA, and Jones, TA: Principles of experience-dependent neural plasticity: Implications for rehabilitation after brain damage. J Speech Lang Hear Res 51(1):S225–239, 2008, with permission.[136]

with TBI.[138] Locomotor training, utilizing body weight support (BWS) and a treadmill,[139-141] and constraint-induced movement therapy (CIMT) for improving UE function[142,143] are two interventions that have shown potential. See additional discussion in Chapter 15, Stroke, and Chapter 20, Traumatic Spinal Cord Injury.

Another task-oriented approach for improving mobility skills such as walking and running was developed by Williams and Schache.[144] They used a conceptual framework based on the hierarchical ordering of high-level mobility tasks based on the HiMAT (see above) and biomechanical parameters associated with normal walking and running as the basis for the specific interventions. Easier items on the HiMAT are set as goals and mastered before moving on to more difficult tasks.

For example, once a patient can walk backwards, the next, more difficult tasks (walking on toes and walking over obstacles) are set as goals. Important biomechanical aspects of walking and running, such as the generation of ankle and hip flexion power at push-off, are targeted through the specific interventions.

An important consideration for these and other task-oriented strategies is treatment dosing. Although not well researched for persons with TBI, literature on UE rehabilitation and locomotor training after stroke suggest that these interventions are commonly underdosed[145-147] and that there is a dose-response relationship.[148]

Locomotor Training with Body Weight Support

Locomotor training with BWS and a treadmill involves suspending the client in a parachute-like overhead harness that allows for a percentage of body weight to be relieved. Therapists assist the patient by providing trunk/pelvic stabilization, assistance with weight shifting, and advancing the LEs. Locomotor training with BWS is commonly combined with treadmill ambulation (Fig. 19.7), but can be done overground as well. Locomotor training with BWS and a treadmill allows for repetitive training throughout a complete gait cycle. Progressively decreasing the amount of BWS and increasing the treadmill speed allows the physical therapist to gradually increase the difficulty of the task as walking ability improves. Locomotor training with BWS and a treadmill has a solid theoretical basis. However, it is not clear what the optimal parameters for treatment should be for

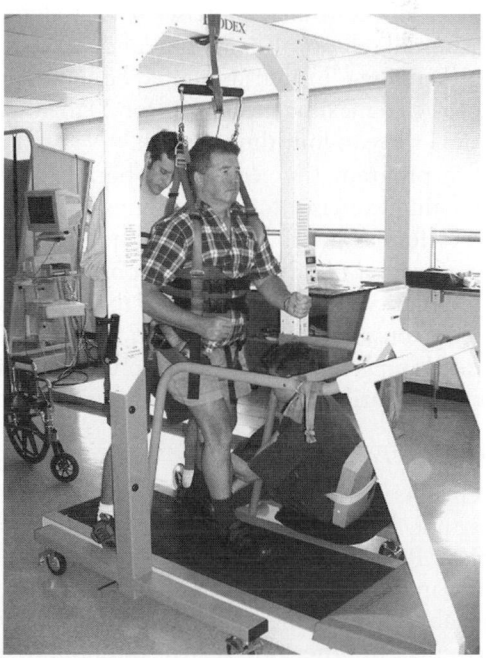

Figure 19.7 Locomotor training utilizing a body weight support system and treadmill. One trainer is assisting with the trunk and pelvic stability and weight shifting, while another trainer is facilitating stepping at the left LE.

patients with TBI, and it has not been demonstrated that it is more effective than conventional gait training (see Chapter 20, Traumatic Spinal Cord Injury).

Constraint-Induced Therapy

Constraint-induced movement therapy involves promoting the use of the more affected UE for up to 90% of waking hours and reducing the use of the least affected UE. Intensive, task-oriented training is provided for the affected UE for up to 6 hours per day over a 2- to 3-week period.[149] Most of the research published on CIMT has been done in people with stroke (see Evidence Summary Box 10.1 in Chapter 10). However, this same intervention may also be useful for people with TBI.[142,143] Given the frequency of behavioral and cognitive impairments after TBI, patients undergoing CIMT may require greater structure and caregiver support outside of therapy to maximize their adherence to the protocol.

Aerobic and Endurance Conditioning

Fatigue and cardiopulmonary pathology are common after TBI.[116] The severity of deconditioning found in persons with TBI is significantly greater than that found in sedentary persons without disabilities.[117] Aerobic training is effective for persons with TBI.[138,150] Appropriately dosed aerobic exercise has the potential to not only reduce long-term cardiovascular risks, but also may improve sleep hygiene and reduce both depression and reports of fatigue.[150]

There are many options when developing an endurance-training program. The mode of training can vary from traditional exercises (e.g., walking, jogging, treadmill, elliptical machines, and ergometers)[150] to circuit training.[151] Intensity should be at 60% to 90% of age predicted maximal heart rate, for 20 to 40 minutes per session, three to four times a week.[150] Hassett et al[152] studied a program that combined both aerobic and strengthening exercises for 62 participants with severe TBI. They found that the program, whether performed in a fitness center or at home, had a positive impact on cardiorespiratory fitness. The physical therapist will need to carefully consider both cognitive and physical abilities when developing an aerobic conditioning program for an individual patient.

Resistance Training

Interventions aimed at improving force-production capacity may be beneficial supplements to the physical therapist's POC.[153,154] There is currently a dearth of literature investigating the role of strength training in TBI rehabilitation. There is, however, evidence of a positive effect in other progressive and nonprogressive neurological disorders. A recent review by Pak and Patten[155] suggest that for persons with stroke, resistance training is associated with improved force production, functional abilities, and quality of life. Similar findings have been demonstrated for persons with Parkinson's disease,[156] and it is plausible that patients with TBI might also achieve similar benefits. Strength training should be done 2 to 3 days a week at an intensity of 3 sets of 8 to 12 repetitions at 10 repetition max.[157] Postural and balance impairments require modification of positions used.

Electrical Stimulation

The application of *functional electrical stimulation* (FES) to motor rehabilitation has increased significantly in the last decade. Several manufactures have developed various types of FES foot-drop stimulators. All rely on peroneal nerve stimulation to increase active dorsiflexion during the swing phase of gait. The devices range from traditional electrical stimulation devices with manual stimulation triggers to cuff-type units that employ inclinometers or pressure sensors. Similar units can be used to augment active wrist extension during UE reaching tasks. Little research exists on use of this modality with patients with TBI,[158] and there is limited evidence as to their long-term efficacy in other populations.[158] These devices, however, can be used to increase both the quality and number of repetitions of a desired task (e.g., steps or reaching) and can be an effective addition to early, task-oriented training sessions.

Dual-Task Performance

As mentioned above, many patients make significant improvements in physical function at this stage of rehabilitation. Many will demonstrate independence with basic ambulation as examined with measures of gait speed and dynamic balance. Most will also have persisting cognitive deficits. Beyond basic locomotor recovery, another important consideration is how these ongoing cognitive deficits affect mobility and community reentry. As discussed in the examination section, a dual-task paradigm can give valuable insight into how safely and efficiently patients will ambulate when also performing secondary, cognitive tasks. Research suggests that dual-task decrements, such as reduced walking speed and postural stability, are common after brain injury.[125]

Like many other interventions, improvements in dual-task performance are training specific. This should be taken into consideration when designing and progressing a dual-task training regimen. The tasks and environments used in training should match those that the patient is anticipated to return to. Progressing this type of training can involve manipulation of the training environment, motor task (type and difficulty), and also the cognitive demands of the secondary task. A training program to improve dual-task performance can coincide with the achievement of independence in walking across different terrains. For example, once independent with walking down a corridor, progressively more challenging cognitive tasks such as serial subtraction or visual scanning tasks can be added. Furthering this example, the client might be asked to ambulate in a parking lot and scan for vehicles with certain characters in their license plate or walk the aisle of a busy grocery store and find specific items. Training speed can also be varied to add challenge. Walking on a treadmill while reading is one example of a dual-task intervention.

Patient/Family/Caregiver Education

Patient/family/caregiver education and training are important goals across each level of rehabilitation. The goals of this education and training will vary based on the cognitive and behavioral abilities of the patient.

Clients in the early phase of recovery may go through a period where they are significantly confused and agitated. It is difficult to provide education for the patient at this level; the patient has very little, if any, ability for new learning. However, it is extremely important to provide education for the patient's family. Above all, the family should understand that the patient does not have control of his or her behavior. The patient is not striking out or cursing because of intent to hurt others, but because of agitation and confusion. Many times families do not understand why a patient is performing these behaviors. They should be educated that these behaviors are a symptom of the brain injury just as the patient's inability to walk or eat is. It is important to educate the family that entering this level of recovery is a good sign because it indicates the patient is moving toward the next level of recovery. Aggressive behaviors are usually short lived, typically lasting only a few weeks at most. Family members should also be taught to use specific behavioral strategies (see below) when interacting with their loved one. Consistency is important for everyone, including family members. If a behavioral plan is being implemented, the family should be a part of devising it and carrying it out.

It is important to emphasize safety awareness education with the patient and caregivers. The individual is beginning to exhibit improved mobility skills at these levels, but may lack the insight to recognize that he or she may not yet be safe to ambulate or transfer alone. Family members and caregivers should learn how to safely assist the patient with functional mobility. This typically includes training in bed mobility, transfers, ambulation, and wheelchair mobility skills. They should be instructed in proper body mechanics when assisting with functional mobility, so as to avoid risking injury to the patient or themselves. Family members/caregivers should be educated about how to assist the patient with strengthening exercises, passive ROM, and other elements of the exercise program. They should also be made aware of methods to enhance the patient's decision making skills and safety awareness. Family members typically become the primary caregiver for the patient upon discharge to home.

Behavioral Factors

Therapists may encounter a variety of behavioral barriers to examining and treating patients with moderate to severe TBI. As the patient begins to emerge from coma, he or she often experiences a period of acute post-traumatic agitation.[31,159,160] The confusion, amnesia, and disorientation during this phase of recovery often result in agitation, aggression, noncompliance, and combative behavior.[31,160] The therapist should incorporate creativity and flexibility when designing and providing interventions. This is particularly true with individuals who are in the confused and agitated stage of recovery. At this stage, the therapist should work near the patient's physical level of function using familiar activities, rather than progress to more challenging skills that require new learning, because the patient does not have the capacity for new learning at this level of recovery. The neuropsychologist can assist the team by providing insight into different ways to manage the patient's agitated behavior and may set up a behavioral modification program. Behavioral modification techniques such as positive reinforcement using a point or reward system, redirection, and compliance training are useful in managing these inappropriate behaviors and improving participation in therapy.[159] Different medications may be effective in helping the patient manage behavior as well.[160] Table 19.5 summarizes special considerations for the management of patients who display significant cognitive and/or neurobehavioral impairments.

Professionals who frequently encounter aggressive and disruptive behaviors from patients with TBI may benefit from further training in managing these events. *Nonviolent Crisis Intervention® Training* and *Brain Injury Specialist Training* through the Brain Injury Association of America are two such training programs.

Community Reentry Programs

Many clients will make significant progress in the early phase of rehabilitation. Before discharge, it is crucial to begin to wean the patient from the external structure provided by the hospital setting that was so important in the early stages of recovery. As the patient becomes better able to control himself or herself, external control provided by the environment should be lessened. Doing so will prepare the patient for the challenges of the next level of rehabilitation, postacute, community reentry programming.

This level of therapy is often delivered in a comprehensive day treatment setting, with an interdisciplinary emphasis on community reentry, return to work or school, and cognitive, behavioral, and psychosocial issues.[161,162] In this setting, the patient goes to therapy throughout the day for 4 to 5 days a week and returns home in the late afternoon. Individuals with more severe physical impairments may continue their rehabilitation in a residential-based community reentry program, whereas those with continued, severe behavioral issues may require a residential neurobehavioral program.

Table 19.5   Special Considerations for Confused and Agitated Patients

Strategy	Rationale and Clinical Application
Consistency	• Consistency is important. All team members, including family members, should interact and address inappropriate behaviors in a consistent manner. • Remember that the patient is confused. To help decrease confusion, the patient should be seen by the same person at the same time and in the same location every day. • Establishing a daily routine is very important. It is calming and reassuring to have a sense of familiarity. Additionally, orientation (i.e., person, place, and time) should be provided frequently and in a nonthreatening manner. At this level, it is often better to provide orientation information than to challenge the patient to provide it, particularly if the patient is not expected to succeed.
Expect No Carryover	• Teaching new skills at this level is unrealistic. The patient may begin to perform a functional task, such as brushing teeth or ambulating. However, this does not indicate a general learning ability, because brushing one's teeth and especially walking are automatic skills with an ingrained neural network. • The use of charts or graphs may be useful to help the patient progress each day. Without the use of such aids, the patient is likely to have no recall of the previous day's performance.
Model Calm Behavior	• The patient is likely to perceive, and may reflect, the demeanor of the caregiver. Therefore, it is important for the therapist to assume a calm and focused affect. • The patient may not be able to control his or her behavior and may not feel safe. To help the patient feel safe, it is important for the therapist to be perceived as in control of his or her emotions and behavior.
Expect Egocentricity	• At this level of recovery, the patient cannot be expected to see another's point of view. He or she will tend to think only of himself or herself and, at this point, it is unwise to stress the patient with attempts to do otherwise.
Flexibility/Options	• The patient will have a limited attention span and may not be able to concentrate on any given activity for a very long time. It is important to be prepared with numerous activities. If the patient cannot be redirected to the selected task, it is appropriate to attempt to engage him or her in another. For example, it may be difficult for a client to tolerate a full constraint-induced therapy protocol. You might, however, be able to engage the client in a variety of UE reaching tasks in various environments allowing the patient's level of attention and tolerance to dictate the duration of each. • Treat the patient at an appropriate age level. • Give control to the patient when it is safe and appropriate. Control can be given while maintaining focus on therapeutic goals by phrasing questions as, "Would you rather play ball or go for a walk?" This prevents situations where the patient chooses an undesirable or unrealistic activity if asked, "What would you like to do?" or the case where the patient simply answers "No" when asked, "Would you like to . . . ?" • Provide safe choices for the patient. This allows the patient to feel that he or she has some control over the situation. This is important, because the patient typically feels considerable loss of control during prolonged hospitalization.
Safety	• Owing to the patient's often unpredictable and inappropriate behaviors, it is important to keep the patient and those interacting with him or her safe. • In addition to utilizing some of the above-mentioned behavioral strategies, patients in this level of recovery may be kept on a locked unit of the hospital. Patients may require one-to-one staff supervision and assistance throughout the day.

The major goal of treatment at this level is to assist the patient in integrating the cognitive, physical, and emotional skills necessary to function in the community. Skills in judgment, problem solving, planning, self-awareness, health and wellness, and social interaction are emphasized. For the demands of treatment to approximate the demands of the real world, treatment focuses on advanced activities such as community skills, social skills, and daily living skills. Examples of these skills are presented in Table 19.6. The interdisciplinary team emphasizes patient assumption of self-responsibility. Because the patient now has some insight into his or her own strengths and weaknesses, it is important to involve the individual in decision making.

Table 19.6	Components of Community Skills, Social Skills, and Daily Living Skills Programs	
Daily Living	**Social Skills**	**Community Skills**
Food preparation	Introductions	Shopping
Housekeeping	Nonverbal communication	Public transport
Money management	Assertiveness	Map reading
Meal planning	Listening skills	Leisure planning
Telephone use	Giving/receiving feedback	Community resources
Time management		

Independent as well as cooperative work with others is encouraged. Group treatment sessions are often the basis of interventions. Honest feedback from the therapist and support group is crucial for the patient to learn how to function in society with his or her present abilities and limitations. Trial periods of independent living and supported work are important. Adaptations are often required by the family, work, and school to accommodate to the needs of the individual.

■ MILD TRAUMATIC BRAIN INJURY

The military conflicts in the Middle East and increased media attention to sports-related concussion has highlighted the impact of *mild TBI* (mTBI) or postconcussion injury and the need for appropriate assessment and management. Between 1.6 and 3.8 million sports-related mTBIs occur annually in the United States,[2,163] and approximately 12% of military personnel report symptoms consistent with blast-related mTBI.[164] There are varying definitions of mTBI.[165] As mentioned above, the GCS defines mTBI as a score between 13 and 15. Generally speaking, mTBI is characterized by varying degrees of loss of consciousness (0 to 30 minutes; it is important to recognize that no loss of consciousness may occur) and PTA and altered mental state for up to 24 hours. Individuals with mTBI often experience a combination of neurocognitive deficits, postural control and balance impairments, and self-report symptoms such as blurred vision, nausea, light sensitivity, sleep disturbance, and ringing in the ears. It is also important to keep in mind that the appearance of symptoms may be delayed several hours.

Mild TBI often results in a functional injury of the CNS rather than a structural one, which is thought to be due to metabolic dysfunction.[166] Fortunately, most individuals with mTBI fully recover in approximately 3 months.[167] However, up to 10% to 20% of people with mTBI experience postconcussive syndrome and have deficits months to years after the initial injury.[168-170]

Physical Therapy Management of mTBI

The Proponency Office for Rehabilitation and Reintegration, Office of the Surgeon General, and the United States Army developed physical therapy guidelines for assessment and intervention of working service members with mTBI.[171] The main areas recommended to assess and provide intervention for are patient education, activity intolerance, vestibular dysfunction, high-level balance dysfunction, post-traumatic headache, temporomandibular disorder, attention and dual-task performance, and participation in exercise (Box 19.6).[171] A full guide to mTBI developed by the Department of Defense and Veterans Affairs is available online at www.healthquality.va.gov/mtbi/concussion_mtbi_full_1_0.pdf. Although there are differences between sports- and blast-related mTBI, these guidelines can also be applied to those with sports-related mTBI.

Return to Play/Activity

Cognitive and physical rest until symptoms resolve followed by a graded exercise program is recommended.[172] It is important to recognize that not only physical activity, but activities that require attention and concentration (e.g., school work), can exacerbate symptoms and prolong recovery. Return to play or activity after an mTBI should follow a graduated, stepwise progression of increasing activity levels (Table 19.7).[172] Each step should take 24 hours, so that it will take approximately 1 week to return to full active duty or full-contact sports activity. If any postconcussive symptoms return during the progressive increase in activity, the patient should step back to the previous stage and attempt to progress again after a 24-hour period of rest.[172] Results from baseline neurocognitive tests, balance tests, and self-report symptoms should all be used in the return to play/activity decision. No one test should be used by itself. If the medical professional has any doubts about whether or not the patient experienced an mTBI or is ready to return to play/activity, the patient should be removed from the game and return to activity delayed until a full recovery is achieved.

Box 19.6	Areas for Physical Therapist to Examine and Intervene in Patients With Mild Traumatic Brain Injury

- Patient education
- Activity intolerance
- Vestibular dysfunction
- High-level balance dysfunction
- Post-traumatic headache
- Temporomandibular disorder
- Attention and dual-task performance
- Participation in exercise

Table 19.7   Graduated Return-to-Play Protocol

Rehabilitation Stage	Functional Exercise at Each Stage of Rehabilitation	Objective of Each Stage
1. No activity	Complete physical and cognitive rest.	Recovery.
2. Light aerobic exercise	Walking, swimming, or stationary cycling keeping intensity at 70% of maximum predicted heart rate. No resistance training.	Increase heart rate.
3. Sport-specific exercise	Skating drills in ice hockey, running drills in soccer. No head-impact activities.	Add movement.
4. Noncontact training drills	Progression to more complex training drills (e.g., passing drills in football and ice hockey). May start progressive resistance.	Exercise, coordination, and cognitive load.
5. Full-contact practice	Following medical clearance, participate in normal training activities.	Restore confidence and assess functional skills by coaching staff.
6. Return to play	Normal game play.	

From McCrory, P, et al: Consensus Statement on Concussion in Sport: The 3rd International Conference on Concussion in Sport held in Zurich, November 2008. British Journal of Sports Medicine 43(Suppl 1):i76–90, 2009, with permission.[172]

Examination

Ideally, there should be a baseline assessment of cognition and balance, which can be used for comparison as the patient recovers to assist in the return to play/activity decision.

Arousal, Attention, and Cognition

Computerized tests have been developed to assess cognition after mTBI. One such test is the *Immediate Post-Concussion Assessment and Cognitive Testing* (ImPACT). The ImPACT assesses attention span, working memory, sustained and selective attention time, response variability, nonverbal problem solving, and reaction time. The ImPACT can be used to track recovery and assist in the return-to-play decision after mTBI.[173-175]

The *Standardized Assessment of Concussion* (SAC) is a short test that can be completed on the sideline of a sports event within minutes of injury to assess mental status.[176-178] The instrument is intended as a supplement to other methods of mTBI assessment (e.g., neuropsychological evaluation, postural stability testing). It should not be used as the only means of determining the severity of the injury and return to play.

Vestibular and Balance

The incidence of vestibular-related symptoms (e.g., dizziness, vertigo, imbalance) after blast mTBI range from 24% to 83%, and is seen in the acute (1 to 3 days), subacute (3 to 30 days), and chronic (30 to 360 days) stage.[179] Vestibular and postural control deficits are also seen in sports-related mTBI.[180] Vestibular dysfunction after blast-related mTBI includes benign paroxysmal positional vertigo (BPPV) of the posterior or lateral canals and unilateral vestibular hypofunction of central origin.[181] Positional tests such as the Dix-Hallpike test and supine roll test and dynamic visual acuity testing should be performed.[171] Chapter 21, Vestibular Disorders, provides detailed information on these and other tests of vestibular function.

The *NeuroCom Sensory Organization Test* (SOT) is a computerized dynamic posturography test that assesses the ability to use and integrate sensory information from the visual, somatosensory, and vestibular systems to maintain balance.[180,182] The *Balance Error Scoring System* (BESS) is a clinical analog to the SOT. Both of these measures (SOT and BESS) have been used to demonstrate impaired postural control in people with sports-related mTBI.[180,183] It also appears that balance deficits as measured with the SOT or BESS generally resolve within 3 to 7 days after injury.[180,182,184] Other measures of high-level balance activity such as the HiMAT[89,90] (see above), *Dynamic Gait Index*,[185,186] *Functional Gait Assessment*,[187, 188] and *Balance Evaluation Systems Test*[189] can also be used to assess balance.

Self-Report

There are many self-report symptom scales.[190] These scales ask patients to rate the severity of postconcussion symptoms such as headache, dizziness, blurred vision, difficulty concentrating, fatigue, and sensitivity to light. The *Post-Concussion Scale* (revised)[191] is a 21-item checklist that is commonly used. The *Sport Concussion Assessment Tool Post-Concussion Symptom Scale* (SCAT) is another.[192] The SCAT scale contains 18 items used to screen for an acute concussion and another 7 items to gather information at a follow-up visit. Self-report measures specific to the impact of impaired balance include the *Dizziness Handicap Inventory*[193] and the *Activities-specific Balance Confidence* scale.[194]

Other

Post-traumatic headache and temporomandibular disorder can be assessed using a standard musculoskeletal examination of the neck, shoulders, and jaw along with standardized pain questionnaires.[171] Dual-task performance should be assessed as described above. Box 19.7 lists some of the more commonly used outcome measures and tests and measures.

Intervention

As mentioned above, physical and cognitive rest is critical for recovery. Patients should be carefully monitored during treatment sessions to determine if the intervention exacerbates any symptoms. If so the intensity, duration, and frequency should be reduced. The evidence supporting physical therapy for patients with mTBI consists mostly of case studies, case series, and retrospective reviews.[195-198] Box 19.8 Evidence Summary summarizes some of these studies.

Vestibular, Balance, and Dual Task

If the patient has BPPV, canalith repositioning treatment can be performed for the posterior semicircular canals, anterior semicircular canals, or horizontal semicircular canals. These treatment techniques involve moving the patient's head into different positions in a specific sequence to move the debris out of the involved semicircular canal back into the vestibule. Gaze stabilization exercises should be done in patients with unilateral vestibular hypofunction. See Chapter 21, Vestibular Disorders, for specifics on these interventions.

High-level, task-oriented balance and gait training as described above in the section on interventions for persons with moderate to severe TBI can be performed. Activities that are challenging to the vestibular system such as walking with head turns and on uneven, varied surfaces are recommended, as well as sport-specific skill training.[171] Balance training that incorporates the use of different sensory modalities such as standing on dense foam with eyes open and eyes closed can be performed. Balance training using computerized dynamic posturography can also be performed. Dual-task training as described above is another important intervention. See additional discussion in Chapter 10, Strategies to Improve Motor Function.

Other

Musculoskeletal-based interventions such as stretching, strengthening, and manual therapy and modalities can be used when appropriate for patients with post-traumatic headache or temporomandibular disorder.[171]

Patient Education

Patients should be provided with educational material about the symptoms of mTBI, informed that in most cases symptoms will resolve in days to a few months, and informed about the dangers of second impact syndrome. If appropriate, depending on the patient's symptoms and status, patients can be taught how to perform neck ROM and isometric strengthening exercises, appropriate sleep posture, vestibular positional techniques, gaze stabilization exercises, and balance exercises. Patients can also be instructed to begin an aerobic and strengthening exercise program.

Box 19.7 Tests and Measures/Outcome Measures Commonly Used in Patients With Mild Traumatic Brain Injury

- Immediate post-concussion assessment and cognitive testing
- Standardized Assessment of Concussion
- Vestibular positional tests
- Sensory Organization Test
- Balance Error Scoring System
- Dynamic Gait Index
- Functional Gait Assessment
- High-Level Mobility Assessment Tool
- Post-Concussion Scale–Revised
- Sport Concussion Assessment Tool Post-Concussion Symptom scale
- Dizziness Handicap Inventory
- Activities-specific Balance Confidence scale

Box 19.8 Evidence Summary Evidence-Based Summary of Selected Studies of Physical Therapy for Patients With Mild Traumatic Brain Injury

Reference	Subjects	Methods/Procedure	Results	Comments
Gurr and Moffat (2001)[196]	18 subjects with complaints of vertigo and balance deficits after mTBI	Vestibular rehabilitation × 1/week for 6 weeks. Intervention consisted of education, "vertigo exercises," graded exposure to movement and activity, anxiety management, and coping strategies.	Significant decrease in self-reported vertigo symptoms and anxiety, as well as less postural sway on unstable surface with eyes open.	Pre-test/post-test design with no comparison group. The authors do not provide sufficient detail on the characteristics and etiology of the mTBI of the subjects.

Continued

Box 19.8 Evidence Summary   Evidence-Based Summary of Selected Studies of Physical Therapy for Patients With Mild Traumatic Brain Injury—cont'd

Reference	Subjects	Methods/Procedure	Results	Comments
Gagnon et al (2009)[197]	16 children/adolescents ages 8–17 who sustained a concussion, with postconcussive symptoms >4 weeks after injury	Graded rehabilitation consisting of submaximal aerobic conditioning for up to 15 minutes; coordination exercises tailored to subject's sport for up to 10 minutes; sports-related visualization; and home program of the same activities. Subjects were closely monitored, and any increase in symptoms and the activities were stopped. Mean duration of intervention was 4.4 weeks.	Decrease in Post-Concussion Scale–Revised, all subjects were able to resume normal physical activity participation.	Retrospective review of the program, lack of standardized outcome measures presented.
Hoffer et al (2004)[198]	58 active duty or retired military personnel within 1–3 days post-mTBI; subjects subdivided into 3 groups: post-traumatic positional vertigo, PTMAD, and post-traumatic spatial disorientation	6–8 weeks of vestibular rehabilitation for the PTMAD and post-traumatic spatial disorientation groups consisting of VOR exercises, COR exercises, somatosensory exercises, and aerobic activity.	84% of PTMAD group and 27% of post-traumatic spatial disorientation group demonstrated improvement in VOR tests. Significantly shorter time to return to work and resolution of symptoms in the PTMAD group compared to post-traumatic spatial disorientation group.	Specific results of VOR tests and subject self-report measures (DHI and ABC) not presented.
Alsalaheen et al (2010)[195]	114 children (≤18 years old) and adults (>18 years old) referred for vestibular rehabilitation after concussion; 96 days median time from concussion to evaluation	30 subjects came for only one session, 84 returned for a median of 4 visits (range 2–13) over a median of 33 days (range 7–181). Vestibular rehabilitation consisted of gaze stabilization exercises (VOR × 1 in sitting and standing), standing balance on foam surface with EO and EC, walking with balance challenges, and canalith repositioning maneuvers when indicated.	Significant improvement in all self-report measures and performance measures: ABC, DHI, DGI, FGA, gait speed, TUG, FTST, and SOT. Only three measures demonstrated significantly greater improvement in children compared to adults: DHI, FGA, and FTST.	Retrospective review.

PTMAD = post-traumatic migraine-associated dizziness, VOR = vestibular-ocular reflex, COR = cervico-ocular reflex, DHI = Dizziness Handicap Inventory, ABC = Activities-specific Balance Confidence scale, EO = eyes open, EC = eyes closed, DGI = Dynamic Gait Index, FGA = Functional Gait Assessment, TUG = Timed Up and Go, FTST = Five Time Sit to Stand, and SOT = Sensory Organization Test.

SUMMARY

A TBI is a devastating and life-changing event for the individual and his or her family. The resulting impairments make working with the patient with brain injury extremely rewarding and challenging. There are a multitude of issues to consider. The physical therapist must adapt traditional physical therapy examination procedures and interventions to the unique motor function, cognitive, and behavioral challenges presented. The interdisciplinary team offers a unique opportunity for the physical therapist to learn and collaborate with experienced professionals. By working together with a team, the physical therapist is able to provide appropriate care that will help the individual with a TBI to maximize performance of activities and enhance social participation.

Questions for Review

1. List primary and secondary mechanisms of TBI.

2. Identify common neuromuscular, cognitive, and neurobehavioral impairments that result from TBI.

3. Contrast persistent vegetative state and minimally conscious state.

4. Identify key prognostic factors for individuals with TBI.

5. Identify and describe the roles of the interdisciplinary team members working with a patient with TBI.

6. Discuss the primary goals of physical therapy during the early stage of recovery in patients with severe to moderate TBI.

7. Select key outcome measures to use during the active rehabilitation stage in patients with severe to moderate TBI.

8. Describe strategies that should be taken into account when designing a plan of care for a patient with a severe to moderate TBI with cognitive and neurobehavioral deficits.

9. Contrast recovery- versus compensation-based interventions.

10. Develop a physical therapy plan of care for a patient with a severe to moderate TBI, which incorporates key elements of neuroplasticity.

11. Outline a graduated return to play for a patient that has experienced a mild TBI.

12. Develop a physical therapy plan of care for a patient with a mild TBI.

CASE STUDY

The patient is a 22-year-old male who was involved in a motor vehicle accident (MVA). He was struck by another car as he exited his car. The patient suffered a severe closed brain injury, GCS score of 7 at the emergency department, and both pupils were reactive to light. He was taken to a local hospital. CT scan revealed a left parietal subarachnoid hemorrhage. He also experienced a fracture of his right scapula. Two weeks after his injury, the patient is now transferred to an acute rehabilitation hospital.

MEDICATIONS
Ritalin, tegretol, zanaflex, and ativan prn.

SOCIAL HISTORY
Patient is a graduate student in a computer science program at a local college. His parents live approximately 2 hours away. They are very supportive, and his mother has taken a leave of absence from her job in order to be with the patient and assist in his rehabilitation. He has private insurance through his parents, which covers inpatient and outpatient rehabilitation.

PHYSICAL THERAPY EXAMINATION
I. Screening: cardiopulmonary: HR 78, BP 110/76; integumentary: intact; musculoskeletal: see below; neuromuscular: see below.

II. Arousal, attention and cognition: Rancho Los Amigos Levels of Cognitive Functioning: Level V. Easily distracted.

A. Agitated behavior scale: 26/56

B. Galveston Orientation and Amnesia Test: 66

C. Moss Attention Rating Scale:

1. Total Raw Score: 84

2. Average MARS Item Score: 3.82

3. Factor 1 (Restlessness/Distractibility) Score: 4.60

4. Factor 2 (Initiation) Score: 4.00

5. Factor 3 (Consistent/Sustained Attention) Score: 3.67

III. Assistive and adaptive devices: currently uses a standard wheelchair in the hospital environment with gel cushion and solid back.

IV. Gait, locomotion, and balance:

A. Able to ambulate with small based quad cane (SBCQ) with minimal assistance for 150 feet using 3-point step to/through pattern

B. Gait speed: 0.44 m/s

C. Observational gait assessment: difficulty clearing right foot in swing, right knee in extension throughout swing phase, circumducts and hip hikes right hip to clear foot, initial contact with mid foot on right

D. Sitting balance: able to sit on edge of bed or mat with supervision

E. Standing balance: able to stand with close supervision, decreased WB on right LE, Berg Balance Scale score: 36/56

V. Joint mobility: decreased posterior and inferior glide R glenohumeral joint.

VI. Motor function: tone: increased extensor tone in right hip and knee and ankle, 2 on Modified Ashworth Scale, increased flexor tone in right UE, 2 on MAS. Able to isolate movement in left UE and LE, not able to isolate movement in right UE or LE. However, he does exhibit active right dorsiflexion, wrist, and finger extension.

VII. Orthotic, protective, and supportive devices:

A. Has a bivalve cast at ankle and elbow from the acute care hospital for positioning ankle into dorsiflexion and elbow into extension.

VIII. Range of motion: passive WNL except:

A. Right LE

1. Dorsiflexion: has 5 degree plantar flexion contracture

2. Knee extension: has 5 degree flexion contracture

B. Right UE

C. Shoulder flexion: 95, abduction: 90, external rotation: 65, internal rotation: 80, extension: 45

D. Elbow extension: has a 10 degree flexion contracture

E. Wrist extension: 0 degrees

IX. Self-care and home management:

A. FIM score:

Self-Care	Score	Self-Care	Score	Self-Care	Score
Eating	4	Bowel	4	Cognition	4
Grooming	4	Transfers	4	Comprehension	4
Bathing	3	Toilet	3	Expression	4
Dressing UE	3	Tub/shower	3	Problem solving	3
Dressing LE	2	Bed/wheelchair	4	Memory	2
Toileting	3	Locomotion	4	Social interaction	3
Sphincter control	4	Walk/wheelchair	4	Total	75
Bladder	4	Stairs	2		

X. Sensory integrity:

A. Proprioception, light touch, and sharp/dull discrimination intact right and left extremities

CASE STUDY GUIDING QUESTIONS

1. List factors that support a good prognosis for this patient, as well as factors that support a poor prognosis.

2. What factors make a restorative intervention approach appropriate for this patient? What factors make a compensatory approach appropriate for this patient?

3. List three long-term goals for this patient related to balance, walking ability, and transfer ability that are appropriate for discharge from the acute rehabilitation hospital.

4. Describe interventions to improve his walking ability.

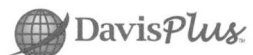 For additional resources, including answers to the questions for review and case study guiding questions, please visit **http://davisplus.fadavis.com**

For this chapter, see also:
Web-Based Resources for Clinicians, Families, and Patients with Traumatic Brain Injury in Appendix A p. 1447.

 The reader is referred to the following video case studies for additional review and study.
- **Case Study 7: Patient with Traumatic Brain Injury and Shoulder Amputation**
- **Case Study 8: Patient with Traumatic Brain Injury**

The full written case study including all tables, figures, charts and 3 video segments (examination, intervention, and outcome) appear online at *DavisPlus*. The case studies poses= questions for the reader's consideration with suggested answers to the case study questions, also posted online at *DavisPlus*.

References

1. Menon, DK, et al: Position statement: Definition of traumatic brain injury. Arch Phys Med Rehabil 91(11):1637, 2010.
2. Langlois, JA, Rutland-Brown, W, and Wald, MM: The epidemiology and impact of traumatic brain injury: A brief overview. J Head Trauma Rehabil 21(5):375, 2006.
3. Faul, M, et al: Traumatic Brain Injury in the United States: Emergency Department Visits, Hospitalizations and Deaths, 2002–2006. Centers for Disease Control and Prevention, National Center for Injury Prevention and Control, 2010.
4. Rutland-Brown, W, et al: Incidence of traumatic brain injury in the United States, 2003. J Head Trauma Rehabil 21(6):544, 2006.
5. Finkelstein, EA, Corso, PS, and Miller, TR: The Incidence and Economic Burden of Injuries in the United States. Oxford University Press, New York, 2006.
6. Andelic, N, et al: Disability, physical health and mental health 1 year after traumatic brain injury. Disabil Rehabil 32(13):1122, 2010.
7. Povlishock, JT, and Katz, DI: Update of neuropathology and neurological recovery after traumatic brain injury. J Head Trauma Rehabil 20(1):76, 2005.
8. Maas, AI, Stocchetti, N, and Bullock, R: Moderate and severe traumatic brain injury in adults. Lancet Neurol 7(8):728, 2008.
9. Kochanek, PM, Clark, RSB, and Jenkins, LW: TBI: Pathobiology. In Zasler, ND, Katz, DI, and Zafonte, RD (eds): Brain Injury Medicine: Principles and Practice, Demos Medical Publishing, New York, 2007.
10. Bennett, M, et al: Clinicopathologic observations in 100 consecutive patients with fatal head injury admitted to a neurosurgical unit. Ir Med J 88(2):60, 59, 1995.
11. Powell, JW, and Barber-Foss, KD: Traumatic brain injury in high school athletes. JAMA 282(10):958, 1999.
12. Tegner, Y, and Lorentzon, R: Concussion among Swedish elite ice hockey players. Br J Sports Med 30(3):251, 1996.
13. Meythaler, JM, et al: Current concepts: Diffuse axonal injury–associated traumatic brain injury. Arch Phys Med Rehabil 82(10):1461–1471, 2001.
14. Warden, D: Military TBI during the Iraq and Afghanistan wars. J Head Trauma Rehabil 21(5):398, 2006.
15. Hicks, RR, et al: Neurological effects of blast injury. J Trauma 68(5):1257, 2010.
16. Kocsis, JD, and Tessler, A: Pathology of blast-related brain injury. J Rehabil Res Dev 46(6):667, 2009.
17. Levi, L, et al: Wartime neurosurgical experience in Lebanon, 1982–85. II: Closed craniocerebral injuries. Isr J Med Sci 26(10):555, 1990.
18. Schwartz, I, et al: Cognitive and functional outcomes of terror victims who suffered from traumatic brain injury. Brain Injury 22(3):255, 2008.
19. Pleasure, SJ, and Fishman, RA: Ventricular volume and transmural pressure gradient in normal pressure hydrocephalus. Arch Neurol 56(10):1199, 1999.
20. Lippert-Gruner, M, et al: Health-related quality of life during the first year after severe brain trauma with and without polytrauma. Brain Injury 21(5):451, 2007.
21. Walker, WC, and Pickett, TC: Motor impairment after severe traumatic brain injury: A longitudinal multicenter study. J Rehabil Res Dev 44(7):975, 2007.
22. Brown, AW, et al: Impairment at rehabilitation admission and 1 year after moderate-to-severe traumatic brain injury: A prospective multicentre analysis. Brain Injury 21(7):673, 2007.
23. Haaland, KY, et al: Recovery of simple motor skills after head injury. J Clin Exp Neuropsychol 16(3):448, 1994.
24. Lehmann, JF, et al: Quantitative evaluation of sway as an indicator of functional balance in post-traumatic brain injury. Arch Phys Med Rehabil 71(12):955–962, 1990.
25. Newton, RA: Balance abilities in individuals with moderate and severe traumatic brain injury. Brain Injury 9(5):445, 1995.
26. Wober, C, et al: Posturographic measurement of body sway in survivors of severe closed head injury. Arch Phys Med Rehabil 74(11):1151, 1993.
27. Basford, JR, et al: An assessment of gait and balance deficits after traumatic brain injury. Arch Phys Med Rehabil 84(3):343, 2003.
28. Campbell, M, and Parry, A: Balance disorder and traumatic brain injury: Preliminary findings of a multi-factorial observational study. Brain Injury 19(13):1095, 2005.
29. Anderson, CA, and Arciniegas, DB: Cognitive sequelae of hypoxic-ischemic brain injury: A review. Neuro Rehabil 26(1):47, 2010.
30. Vogenthaler, DR: An overview of head injury: Its consequences and rehabilitation. Brain Injury 1(1):113, 1987.
31. Riggio, S, and Wong, M: Neurobehavioral sequelae of traumatic brain injury. Mt Sinai J Med 76(2):163, 2009.
32. Levin, HS, et al: Vegetative state after closed-head injury. A Traumatic Coma Data Bank Report. Arch Neurol 48(6):580, 1991.
33. Giacino, JT, et al: The minimally conscious state: Definition and diagnostic criteria. Neurology 58(3):349, 2002.
34. Fine, RL: From Quinlan to Schiavo: Medical, ethical, and legal issues in severe brain injury. Proc Bayl Univ Med Cent 18(4):303, 2005.
35. The Multi-Society Task Force on PVS: Medical aspects of the persistent vegetative state (1). N Engl J Med 330(21):1499, 1994.
36. The Multi-Society Task Force on PVS: Medical aspects of the persistent vegetative state (2). N Engl J Med 330(22):1572, 1994.
37. Ylvisaker, M: Communication outcomes following traumatic brain injury. Seminars in Speech and Language 13:239, 1992.
38. Leblanc, J, et al: Early prediction of language impairment following traumatic brain injury. Brain Injury 20(13-14):1391, 2006.
39. Galski, T, Tompkins, C, and Johnston, MV: Competence in discourse as a measure of social integration and quality of life in persons with traumatic brain injury. Brain Injury 12(9):769, 1998.
40. Wehman, P, et al: Critical factors associated with the successful supported employment placement of patients with severe traumatic brain injury. Brain Injury 7(1):31, 1993.

41. Rabinstein, AA: Paroxysmal sympathetic hyperactivity in the neurological intensive care unit. Neurol Res 29(7):680, 2007.

42. Bower, RS, et al: Paroxysmal sympathetic hyperactivity after traumatic brain injury. Neurocrit Care 13(2):233, 2010.

43. Annegers, JF, et al: A population-based study of seizures after traumatic brain injuries. N Engl J Med 338(1):20, 1998.

44. Salazar, AM, et al: Epilepsy after penetrating head injury. I. Clinical correlates: A report of the Vietnam Head Injury Study. Neurology 35(10):1406, 1985.

45. Safaz, I, et al: Medical complications, physical function and communication skills in patients with traumatic brain injury: A single centre 5-year experience. Brain Injury 22(10):733, 2008.

46. Chang, BS, and Lowenstein, DH: Practice parameter: Antiepileptic drug prophylaxis in severe traumatic brain injury: Report of the Quality Standards Subcommittee of the American Academy of Neurology. Neurology 60(1):10, 2003.

47. Kalisky, Z, et al: Medical problems encountered during rehabilitation of patients with head injury. Arch Phys Med Rehabil 66(1):25, 1985.

48. Vitaz, TW, et al: Outcome following moderate traumatic brain injury. Surg Neurol 60(4):285, discussion 291, 2003.

49. Hammond, FM, and Meighen, MJ: Venous thromboembolism in the patient with acute traumatic brain injury: Screening, diagnosis, prophylaxis, and treatment issues. J Head Trauma Rehabil 13(1):36, 1998.

50. Nampiaparampil, DE: Prevalence of chronic pain after traumatic brain injury: A systematic review. JAMA 300(6):711, 2008.

51. Teasdale, G, and Jennett, B: Assessment of coma and impaired consciousness. A practical scale. Lancet 2(7872):81, 1974.

52. Perel, P, et al: Predicting outcome after traumatic brain injury: Practical prognostic models based on large cohort of international patients. BMJ 336(7641):425, 2008.

53. Steyerberg, EW, et al: Predicting outcome after traumatic brain injury: Development and international validation of prognostic scores based on admission characteristics. PLoS Med 5(8):e165, 2008.

54. Marmarou, A, et al: Prognostic value of the Glasgow Coma Scale and pupil reactivity in traumatic brain injury assessed pre-hospital and on enrollment: An IMPACT analysis. J Neurotrauma 24(2):270, 2007.

55. Murray, GD, et al: Multivariable prognostic analysis in traumatic brain injury: Results from the IMPACT study. J Neurotrauma 24(2):329, 2007.

56. Husson, EC, et al: Prognosis of six-month functioning after moderate to severe traumatic brain injury: A systematic review of prospective cohort studies. J Rehabil Med 42(5):425, 2010.

57. Mushkudiani, NA, et al: Prognostic value of demographic characteristics in traumatic brain injury: Results from the IMPACT study. J Neurotrauma 24(2):259, 2007.

58. Brown, AW, et al: Predictive utility of weekly post-traumatic amnesia assessments after brain injury: A multicentre analysis. Brain Injury 24(3):472, 2010.

59. Semlyen, JK, Summers, SJ, and Barnes, MP: Traumatic brain injury: Efficacy of multidisciplinary rehabilitation. Arch Phys Med Rehabil 79(6):678, 1998.

60. Malec, JF: Impact of comprehensive day treatment on societal participation for persons with acquired brain injury. Arch Phys Med Rehabil 82(7):885, 2001.

61. Braverman, SE, et al: A multidisciplinary TBI inpatient rehabilitation programme for active duty service members as part of a randomized clinical trial. Brain Injury 13(6):405, 1999.

62. Ling, GS, and Marshall, SA: Management of traumatic brain injury in the intensive care unit. Neurol Clin 26(2):409, 2008.

63. Clausen, T, and Bullock, R: Medical treatment and neuroprotection in traumatic brain injury. Curr Pharm Des 7(15):1517, 2001.

64. Seel, RT, et al: Assessment scales for disorders of consciousness: Evidence-based recommendations for clinical practice and research. Arch Phys Med Rehabil 91(12):1795, 2010.

65. Giacino, JT, Kalmar, K, and Whyte, J: The JFK Coma Recovery Scale–Revised: Measurement characteristics and diagnostic utility. Arch Phys Med Rehabil 85(12):2020, 2004.

66. Schnakers, C, et al: A French validation study of the Coma Recovery Scale–Revised (CRS-R). Brain Injury 22(10):786, 2008.

67. Pape, TL, et al: A measure of neurobehavioral functioning after coma. Part I: Theory, reliability, and validity of Disorders of Consciousness Scale. J Rehabil Res Dev 42(1):1–17, 2005.

68. Pape, TL, et al: A measure of neurobehavioral functioning after coma. Part II: Clinical and scientific implementation. J Rehabil Res Dev 42(1):19, 2005.

69. Pape, TL, et al: Establishing a prognosis for functional outcome during coma recovery. Brain Injury 20(7):743, 2006.

70. Pape, TL, et al: Predictive value of the Disorders of Consciousness Scale (DOCS). PM&R 1(2):152, 2009.

71. Hagen, C, Malkmus, D, and Durham, P: Levels of Cognitive Functioning. Rancho Los Amigos Hospital, Downey, CA, 1972.

72. Gouvier, WD, et al: Reliability and validity of the Disability Rating Scale and the Levels of Cognitive Functioning Scale in monitoring recovery from severe head injury. Arch Phys Med Rehabil 68(2):94, 1987.

73. Guide to Physical Therapist Practice. Second Edition. American Physical Therapy Association. Phys Ther 81(1):9, 2001.

74. Lannin, NA, et al: Splinting the hand in the functional position after brain impairment: A randomized, controlled trial. Arch Phys Med Rehabil 84(2):297–302, 2003.

75. Moseley, AM: The effect of casting combined with stretching on passive ankle dorsiflexion in adults with traumatic head injuries. Phys Ther 77(3):240, 1997.

76. Hill, J: The effects of casting on upper extremity motor disorders after brain injury. Am J Occup Ther 48(3):219, 1994.

77. Mortenson, PA, and Eng, JJ: The use of casts in the management of joint mobility and hypertonia following brain injury in adults: A systematic review. Phys Ther 83(7):648, 2003.

78. Kanyer, B: Meeting the seating and mobility needs of the client with traumatic brain injury. J Head Trauma Rehabil 7(3):81, 1992.

79. Ciesla, ND: Chest physical therapy for patients in the intensive care unit. Phys Ther 76(6):609, 1996.

80. Irwin, S, and Tecklin, JS: Cardiopulmonary Physical Therapy, ed 4. Mosby, St. Louis, 2004.

81. Ansell, BJ: Slow-to-recover brain-injured patients: Rationale for treatment. J Speech Hear Res 34(5):1017, 1991.

82. Mitchell, S, et al: Coma arousal procedure: A therapeutic intervention in the treatment of head injury. Brain Injury 4(3):273, 1990.

83. Gruner, ML, and Terhaag, D: Multimodal early onset stimulation (MEOS) in rehabilitation after brain injury. Brain Injury 14(6):585, 2000.

84. Lombardi, F, et al: Sensory stimulation for brain injured individuals in coma or vegetative state. Cochrane Database Syst Rev (2):CD001427, 2002.

85. Feld, JA, et al: Berg balance scale and outcome measures in acquired brain injury. Neurorehabil Neural Repair 15(3):239, 2001.

86. Juneja, G, Czyrny, JJ, and Linn, RT: Admission balance and outcomes of patients admitted for acute inpatient rehabilitation. Am J Phys Med Rehabil 77(5):388, 1998.

87. Inness, EL, et al: Measuring balance and mobility after traumatic brain injury: Validation of the Community Balance and Mobility Scale (CB&M). Physiother Can 63(2):199, 2011.

88. Howe, JA, et al: The Community Balance and Mobility Scale—a balance measure for individuals with traumatic brain injury. Clin Rehabil 20(10):885, 2006.

89. Williams, G, et al: The High-Level Mobility Assessment Tool (HiMAT) for traumatic brain injury. Part 1: Item generation. Brain Injury 19(11):925–932, 2005.

90. Williams, G, et al: The High-Level Mobility Assessment Tool (HiMAT) for traumatic brain injury. Part 2: Content validity and discriminability. Brain Injury 19(10):833, 2005.

91. Williams, G, Pallant, J, and Greenwood, K: Further development of the High-Level Mobility Assessment Tool (HiMAT). Brain Injury 24(7-8):1027, 2010.

92. Whyte, J, et al: The Moss Attention Rating Scale for traumatic brain injury: Initial psychometric assessment. Arch Phys Med Rehabil 84(2):268, 2003.

93. Robertson, IH, et al: The structure of normal human attention: The Test of Everyday Attention. J Int Neuropsychol Soc 2(6):525, 1996.

94. Gaudino, EA, Geisler, MW, and Squires, NK: Construct validity in the Trail Making Test: What makes Part B harder? J Clin Exp Neuropsychol 17(4):529, 1995.

95. Levin, HS, O'Donnell, VM, and Grossman, RG: The Galveston Orientation and Amnesia Test. A practical scale to assess cognition after head injury. J Nerv Ment Dis 167(11):675, 1979.

96. Bode, RK, Heinemann, AW, and Semik, P: Measurement properties of the Galveston Orientation and Amnesia Test (GOAT) and improvement patterns during inpatient rehabilitation. J Head Trauma Rehabil 15(1):637, 2000.

97. Novack, TA, et al: Validity of the Orientation Log, relative to the Galveston Orientation and Amnesia Test. J Head Trauma Rehabil 15(3):957, 2000.

98. Alderso, AL, and Novack, TA: Measuring recovery of orientation during acute rehabilitation for traumatic brain injury: Value and expectations of recovery. J Head Trauma Rehabil 17(3):210, 2002.

99. Jackson, WT, Novack, TA, and Dowler, RN: Effective serial measurement of cognitive orientation in rehabilitation: The Orientation Log. Arch Phys Med Rehabil 79(6):718, 1998.

100. Boake, C: Supervision rating scale: A measure of functional outcome from brain injury. Arch Phys Med Rehabil 77(8):765, 1996.

101. McCauley, SR, et al: The neurobehavioural rating scale–revised: Sensitivity and validity in closed head injury assessment. J Neurol Neurosurg Psychiatry 71(5):643, 2001.

102. Corrigan, JD: Development of a scale for assessment of agitation following traumatic brain injury. J Clin Exp Neuropsychol 11(2): 261, 1989.

103. Dodds, TA, et al: A validation of the functional independence measurement and its performance among rehabilitation inpatients. Arch Phys Med Rehabil 74(5):531, 1993.

104. Stineman, MG, et al: The Functional Independence Measure: Tests of scaling assumptions, structure, and reliability across 20 diverse impairment categories. Arch Phys Med Rehabil 77(11):1101, 1996.

105. Gurka, JA, et al: Utility of the functional assessment measure after discharge from inpatient rehabilitation. J Head Trauma Rehabil 14(3):247, 1999.

106. Hall, KM: The Functional Assessment Measure (FAM). J Rehabil Outcomes 1(3):63, 1997.

107. Hawley, CA, et al: Use of the functional assessment measure (FIM + FAM) in head injury rehabilitation: A psychometric analysis. J Neurol Neurosurg Psychiatry 67(6):749, 1999.

108. Malec, JF: The Mayo-Portland Participation Index: A brief and psychometrically sound measure of brain injury outcome. Arch Phys Med Rehabil 85(12):1989, 2004.

109. Kean, J, et al: Rasch measurement analysis of the Mayo-Portland Adaptability Inventory (MPAI-4) in a community-based rehabilitation sample. J Neurotrauma 28(5):745, 2011.

110. Willer, B, Ottenbacher, KJ, and Coad, ML: The community integration questionnaire. A comparative examination. Am J Phys Med Rehabil 73(2):103, 1994.

111. Williams, G, et al: Spatiotemporal deficits and kinematic classification of gait following a traumatic brain injury: A systematic review. J Head Trauma Rehabil 25(5):366, 2010.

112. Krebs, DE, Edelstein, JE, and Fishman, S: Reliability of observational kinematic gait analysis. Phys Ther 65(7):1027, 1985.

113. Williams, G, et al: Observational gait analysis in traumatic brain injury: Accuracy of clinical judgment. Gait and Posture 29(3): 454, 2009.

114. Moseley, AM, et al: Ecological validity of walking speed assessment after traumatic brain injury: A pilot study. J Head Trauma Rehabil 19(4):341, 2004.

115. van Loo, MA, et al: Inter-rater reliability and concurrent validity of walking speed measurement after traumatic brain injury. Clin Rehabil 17(7):775, 2003.

116. Englander, J, et al: Fatigue after traumatic brain injury: Association with neuroendocrine, sleep, depression and other factors. Brain Injury 24(12):1379, 2010.

117. Mossberg, KA, et al: Aerobic capacity after traumatic brain injury: Comparison with a nondisabled cohort. Arch Phys Med Rehabil 88(3):315, 2007.

118. Mossberg, KA, and Fortini, E: Responsiveness and validity of the six-minute walk test in individuals with traumatic brain injury. Phys Ther 92(5):726, 2012.

119. van Loo, MA, et al: Test–re-test reliability of walking speed, step length and step width measurement after traumatic brain injury: A pilot study. Brain Injury 18(10):1041, 2004.

120. Gibbons, WJ, et al: Reference values for a multiple repetition 6-minute walk test in healthy adults older than 20 years. J Cardiopulm Rehabil 21(2):87, 2001.

121. Mossberg, KA, and Greene, BP: Reliability of graded exercise testing after traumatic brain injury: Submaximal and peak responses. Am J Phys Med Rehabil 84(7):492, 2005.

122. Hassett, LM, et al: Validity of the modified 20-metre shuttle test: Assessment of cardiorespiratory fitness in people who have sustained a traumatic brain injury. Brain Injury 21(10):1069, 2007.

123. McCulloch, KL, et al: Balance, attention, and dual-task performance during walking after brain injury: Associations with falls history. J Head Trauma Rehabil 25(3):155, 2010.

124. McFadyen, BJ, et al: Modality-specific, multitask locomotor deficits persist despite good recovery after a traumatic brain injury. Arch Phys Med Rehabil 90(9):1596, 2009.

125. McCulloch, K: Attention and dual-task conditions: Physical therapy implications for individuals with acquired brain injury. J Neuro Phys Ther 31(3):104, 2007.

126. McGraw-Hunter, M, Faw, GD, and Davis, PK: The use of video self-modelling and feedback to teach cooking skills to individuals with traumatic brain injury: A pilot study. Brain Injury 20(10): 1061, 2006.

127. Goverover, Y, Chiaravalloti, N, and DeLuca, J: Pilot study to examine the use of self-generation to improve learning and memory in people with traumatic brain injury. Am J Occup Ther 64(4):540, 2010.

128. Giuffrida, CG, et al: Functional skill learning in men with traumatic brain injury. Am J Occup Ther 63(4):398, 2009.

129. Shumway-Cook, A, and Woollacott, MH: Motor Control: Translating Research into Clinical Practice, ed 4. Lippincott Williams & Wilkins, Philadelphia, 2012.

130. Levin, MF, Kleim, JA, and Wolf, SL: What do motor "recovery" and "compensation" mean in patients following stroke? Neurorehabil Neural Repair 23(4):313, 2009.

131. Nudo, RJ: Neural bases of recovery after brain injury. J Commun Disord 44(5):515, 2011.

132. Birkenmeier, RL, Prager, EM, and Lang, CE: Translating animal doses of task-specific training to people with chronic stroke in 1-hour therapy sessions: A proof-of-concept study. Neurorehabil Neural Repair 24(7):620, 2010.

133. Wolf, SL, et al: Effect of constraint-induced movement therapy on upper extremity function 3 to 9 months after stroke: The EXCITE randomized clinical trial. JAMA 296(17):2095, 2006.

134. Nudo, RJ: Functional and structural plasticity in motor cortex: Implications for stroke recovery. Phys Med Rehabil Clin North Am 14(1 Suppl):S57, 2003.

135. Kolb, B: Overview of cortical plasticity and recovery from brain injury. Phys Med Rehabil Clin North Am 14(1 Suppl): S7, 2003.

136. Kleim, JA, and Jones, TA: Principles of experience-dependent neural plasticity: implications for rehabilitation after brain damage. J Speech Lang Hear Res 51(1):S225, 2008.

137. Fisher, BE, and Sullivan, KJ: Activity-dependent factors affecting poststroke functional outcomes. Top Stroke Rehabil 8(3):31, 2001.

138. Hellweg, S, and Johannes, S: Physiotherapy after traumatic brain injury: A systematic review of the literature. Brain Injury 22(5):365, 2008.

139. Brown, TH, et al: Body weight–supported treadmill training versus conventional gait training for people with chronic traumatic brain injury. J Head Trauma Rehabil 20(5):402, 2005.

140. Mossberg, KA, Orlander, EE, and Norcross, JL: Cardiorespiratory capacity after weight-supported treadmill training in patients with traumatic brain injury. Phys Ther 88(1):77, 2008.

141. Wilson, DJ, and Swaboda, JL: Partial weight-bearing gait retraining for persons following traumatic brain injury: Preliminary report and proposed assessment scale. Brain Injury 16(3):259, 2002.

142. Shaw, SE, et al: Constraint-induced movement therapy for recovery of upper-limb function following traumatic brain injury. J Rehabil Res Dev 42(6):769, 2005.

143. Karman, N, et al: Constraint-induced movement therapy for hemiplegic children with acquired brain injuries. J Head Trauma Rehabil 18(3):259, 2003.

144. Williams, GP, and Schache, AG: Evaluation of a conceptual framework for retraining high-level mobility following traumatic brain injury: Two case reports. J Head Trauma Rehabil 25(3): 164, 2010.

145. Lang, CE, MacDonald, JR, and Gnip, C: Counting repetitions: An observational study of outpatient therapy for people with hemiparesis post-stroke. J Neuro Phys Ther 31(1):3, 2007.

146. Kimberley, TJ, et al: Comparison of amounts and types of practice during rehabilitation for traumatic brain injury and stroke. J Rehabil Res Dev 47(9):851, 2010.

147. Lang, CE, et al: Observation of amounts of movement practice provided during stroke rehabilitation. Arch Phys Med Rehabil 90(10):1692, 2009.

148. Moore, JL, et al: Locomotor training improves daily stepping activity and gait efficiency in individuals poststroke who have reached a "plateau" in recovery. Stroke 41(1):129, 2010.

149. Morris, DM, Taub, E, and Mark, VW: Constraint-induced movement therapy: Characterizing the intervention protocol. Eura Medicophys 42(3):257, 2006.

150. Mossberg, KA, Amonette, WE, and Masel, BE: Endurance training and cardiorespiratory conditioning after traumatic brain injury. J Head Trauma Rehabil 25(3):173, 2010.

151. Bhambhani, Y, Rowland, G, and Farag, M: Effects of circuit training on body composition and peak cardiorespiratory responses in patients with moderate to severe traumatic brain injury. Arch Phys Med Rehabil 86(2):268, 2005.

152. Hassett, LM, et al: Efficacy of a fitness centre–based exercise programme compared with a home-based exercise programme in traumatic brain injury: A randomized controlled trial. J Rehabil Med 41(4):247, 2009.

153. Killington, MJ, Mackintosh, SF, and Ayres, M: An isokinetic muscle strengthening program for adults with an acquired brain injury leads to meaningful improvements in physical function. Brain Injury 24(7-8):970, 2010.

154. Killington, MJ, Mackintosh, SF, and Ayres, MB: Isokinetic strength training of lower limb muscles following acquired brain injury. Brain Injury 24(12):1399, 2010.

155. Pak, S, and Patten, C: Strengthening to promote functional recovery poststroke: An evidence-based review. Top Stroke Rehabil 15(3):177, 2008.

156. Scandalis, TA, et al: Resistance training and gait function in patients with Parkinson's disease. Am J Phys Med Rehabil 80(1):38, 2001.

157. Palmer-McLean, K, and Harbst, KB: Stroke and brain injury. In Durstine, JL, and Moore, GE (eds): ACSM's Exercise Management for Persons with Chronic Diseases and Disabilities. American College of Sports Medicine, Champaign, IL, 2003.

158. Stein, RB, et al: Long-term therapeutic and orthotic effects of a foot drop stimulator on walking performance in progressive and nonprogressive neurological disorders. Neurorehabil Neural Repair 24(2):152, 2010.

159. Slifer, KJ, et al: Antecedent management and compliance training improve adolescents' participation in early brain injury rehabilitation. Brain Injury 11(12):877, 1997.

160. Kim, E: Agitation, aggression, and disinhibition syndromes after traumatic brain injury. Neuro Rehabil 17(4):297, 2002.

161. Cicerone, KD, et al: A randomized controlled trial of holistic neuropsychologic rehabilitation after traumatic brain injury. Arch Phys Med Rehabil 89(12):2239, 2008.

162. Klonoff, PS, Lamb, DG, and Henderson, SW: Outcomes from milieu-based neurorehabilitation at up to 11 years post-discharge. Brain Injury 15(5):413, 2001.

163. Centers for Disease Control and Prevention: Sports-related recurrent brain injuries—United States. Int J Trauma Nurs 3(3):88, 1997.

164. Schneiderman, AI, Braver, ER, and Kang, HK: Understanding sequelae of injury mechanisms and mild traumatic brain injury incurred during the conflicts in Iraq and Afghanistan: Persistent postconcussive symptoms and posttraumatic stress disorder. Am J Epidemiol 167(12):1446, 2008.

165. Carroll, LJ, et al: Prognosis for mild traumatic brain injury: Results of the WHO Collaborating Centre Task Force on Mild Traumatic Brain Injury. J Rehabil Med 43(Suppl):84, 2004.

166. Inverson, GL, Zasler, N, and Lange, RT: Post concussive disorder. In Zasler, N, Katz, DI, and Zafonte, R (eds): Brain Injury Medicine: Principles and Practice. Demos Medical Publishing, New York, 2007.

167. Ruff, R: Two decades of advances in understanding of mild traumatic brain injury. J Head Trauma Rehabil 20(1):5, 2005.

168. Hartlage, LC, Durant-Wilson, D, and Patch, PC: Persistent neurobehavioral problems following mild traumatic brain injury. Arch Clin Neuropsychol 16(6):561, 2001.

169. Vanderploeg, RD, et al: Long-term morbidities following self-reported mild traumatic brain injury. J Clin Exp Neuropsychol 29(6):585, 2007.

170. Sosnoff, JJ, et al: Previous mild traumatic brain injury and postural-control dynamics. J Athl Train 46(1):85, 2011.

171. Weightman, MM, et al: Physical therapy recommendations for service members with mild traumatic brain injury. J Head Trauma Rehabil 25(3):206, 2010.

172. McCrory, P, et al: Consensus Statement on Concussion in Sport: The 3rd International Conference on Concussion in Sport held in Zurich, November 2008. Br J Sports Med 43(Suppl 1):76, 2009.

173. Iverson, GL, et al: Tracking neuropsychological recovery following concussion in sport. Brain Injury 20(3):245, 2006.

174. Iverson, GL, Lovell, MR, and Collins, MW: Interpreting change on ImPACT following sport concussion. Clin Neuropsychol 17(4):460, 2003.

175. Schatz, P, et al: Sensitivity and specificity of the ImPACT Test Battery for concussion in athletes. Arch Clin Neuropsychol 21(1):91, 2006.

176. McCrea, M, et al: Standardized assessment of concussion (SAC): On-site mental status evaluation of the athlete. J Head Trauma Rehabil 13(2):27, 1998.

177. McCrea, M: Standardized mental status testing on the sideline after sport-related concussion. J Athl Train 36(3):274, 2001.

178. Valovich McLeod, TC, et al: Psychometric and measurement properties of concussion assessment tools in youth sports. J Athl Train 41(4):399, 2006.

179. Hoffer, ME, et al: Blast exposure: Vestibular consequences and associated characteristics. Otol Neurotol 31(2):232, 2010.

180. Guskiewicz, KM, et al: Alternative approaches to the assessment of mild head injury in athletes. Med Sci Sports Exerc 29(7 Suppl): S213, 1997.

181. Scherer, MR, et al: Evidence of central and peripheral vestibular pathology in blast-related traumatic brain injury. Otol Neurotol 32(4):571, 2011.

182. Guskiewicz, KM: Balance assessment in the management of sport-related concussion. Clin Sports Med 30(1):89, 2011.

183. Riemann, BL, and Guskiewicz, KM: Effects of mild head injury on postural stability as measured through clinical balance testing. J Athl Train 35(1):19, 2000.

184. Broglio, SP, and Puetz, TW: The effect of sport concussion on neurocognitive function, self-report symptoms and postural control: A meta-analysis. Sports Med 38(1):53, 2008.

185. Whitney, S, Wrisley, D, and Furman, J: Concurrent validity of the Berg Balance Scale and the Dynamic Gait Index in people with vestibular dysfunction. Physiother Res Int 8(4):178, 2003.

186. Kleffelgaard, I, et al: Associations among self-reported balance problems, post-concussion symptoms and performance-based tests: A longitudinal follow-up study. Disabil Rehabil 34(9):788, 2012.

187. Wrisley, DM, et al: Reliability, internal consistency, and validity of data obtained with the functional gait assessment. Phys Ther 84(10):906, 2004.

188. Wrisley, DM, and Kumar, NA: Functional gait assessment: Concurrent, discriminative, and predictive validity in community-dwelling older adults. Phys Ther 90(5):761, 2010.

189. Horak, FB, Wrisley, DM, and Frank, J: The Balance Evaluation Systems Test (BESTest) to differentiate balance deficits. Phys Ther 89(5):484, 2009.

190. Alla, S, et al: Self-report scales/checklists for the measurement of concussion symptoms: A systematic review. Br J Sports Med 43(Suppl 1):12, 2009.

191. Lovell, MR, and Collins, MW: Neuropsychological assessment of the college football player. J Head Trauma Rehabil 13(2):9–26, 1998.

192. McCrory, P, et al: Summary and agreement statement of the 2nd International Conference on Concussion in Sport, Prague 2004. Br J Sports Med 39(4):196, 2005.

193. Whitney, SL, Marchetti, GF, and Morris, LO: Usefulness of the dizziness handicap inventory in the screening for benign paroxysmal positional vertigo. Otol Neurotol 26(5):1027, 2005.

194. Powell, LE, and Myers, AM: The Activities-specific Balance Confidence (ABC) Scale. J Gerontol A Biol Sci Med Sci 50A(1): M28, 1995.

195. Alsalaheen, BA, et al: Vestibular rehabilitation for dizziness and balance disorders after concussion. J Neurol Phys Ther 34(2):87, 2010.

196. Gurr, B, and Moffat, N: Psychological consequences of vertigo and the effectiveness of vestibular rehabilitation for brain injury patients. Brain Injury 15(5):387, 2001.

197. Gagnon, I, et al: Active rehabilitation for children who are slow to recover following sport-related concussion. Brain Injury 23(12):956, 2009.

198. Hoffer, ME, et al: Characterizing and treating dizziness after mild head trauma. Otol Neurotol 25(2):135, 2004.

Traumatic Spinal Cord Injury

George D. Fulk, PT, PhD
Andrea L. Behrman, PT, PhD, FAPTA
Thomas J. Schmitz, PT, PhD

Chapter 20

LEARNING OBJECTIVES

1. Identify the major etiological factors associated with traumatic spinal cord injury.
2. Describe the clinical presentation following damage to the spinal cord.
3. Given a patient with a spinal cord injury, identify the motor and sensory level of injury and the American Spinal Injury Association impairment scale classification.
4. Analyze the impact of complications associated with spinal cord injury on the physical therapy plan of care and outcomes.
5. Identify the expected functional outcomes for patients with spinal cord injury at various lesion levels.
6. Explain how common precautions will affect physical therapy interventions.
7. Evaluate different outcome measures commonly used in people with spinal cord injury.
8. Analyze and interpret patient data, formulate anticipated goals and expected outcomes, and develop a plan of care when presented with a clinical case study.
9. Justify the selection of different interventions for the acute and active rehabilitation stages of recovery.
10. Discuss the use of neurotechnologies for people with spinal cord injury.

CHAPTER OUTLINE

Spinal cord injury (SCI) is a relatively low-incidence, high-cost injury that results in tremendous change in an individual's life. Paralysis of the muscles below the level of the injury can lead to limited and altered mobility, self-care, and ability to participate in valued social activities. In addition to the musculoskeletal system, many other body systems are impaired after a SCI, including the cardiopulmonary, integumentary, gastrointestinal, genitourinary, and sensory systems. The psychosocial impact of SCI can be just as great as the physical impact. Changes in body image and sexual function, incontinence, and having to rely on others to complete everyday tasks that were previously done without thought or effort can profoundly influence a person's identity. Rehabilitation is an important element toward achieving a fulfilling and active life after SCI. Physical therapists play a key role in the rehabilitation process.

■ DEMOGRAPHICS AND ETIOLOGY

It is estimated that approximately 11,000 new cases of SCI occur in the United States annually. Between 225,000 and 288,000 individuals with SCI are currently living in the United States.[1] Spinal cord injury is generally thought to primarily affect young adults. However, the age at injury has steadily increased. During the 1970s the average age at the time of injury was 28.7 years old. Between 2005 and 2008 this increased to 37.1 years old.[1] This may be due to the aging of the U.S. population and an increase in falls as a cause of injury. The majority of persons with SCI are male (78.3% male vs. 21.7% female). Ethnic distributions indicate that whites represent 66.5% of those with SCI, followed by African Americans (26.8%), Hispanics (8.3%), and Asians (2.0%).[2]

Spinal cord injuries can be grossly divided into two broad etiological categories: *traumatic* injuries and *nontraumatic* damage. Trauma is the most frequent cause of injury in adult rehabilitation populations. Injury results from damage caused by traumatic events such as motor vehicle accidents (40.4%), falls (27.9%), violence (15.0%), and sports (8.0%).[2] Nontraumatic damage in adult populations generally results from disease or pathological influence. Conditions that may damage the spinal cord are vascular dysfunction (arteriovenous malformation [AVM], thrombosis, embolus, or hemorrhage); vertebral subluxations secondary to rheumatoid arthritis or degenerative joint disease; spinal neoplasms; syringomyelia; abscess of the spinal cord; infections, such as syphilis or transverse myelitis; and neurological diseases, such as multiple sclerosis and amyotrophic lateral sclerosis. Nontraumatic etiologies account for approximately 39% of all SCIs.[3]

Fifty-six percent of patients experience cervical lesions resulting in tetraplegia, whereas 43% of SCIs result in paraplegia from thoracic, lumbar, or sacral lesions. The number of people with neurologically incomplete lesions has increased since the 1970s from 43.9% to 52.7% in 2008. The most common type of injury is incomplete tetraplegia (39.5%), followed by complete paraplegia (22.1%), incomplete paraplegia (21.7%), and complete tetraplegia (16.3%). This trend may be partially attributed to improved emergency medical services delivered at the scene of the injury. The length of hospital stay, both in acute care and inpatient rehabilitation, has also changed considerably since the 1970s. The median length of stay in the acute care hospital has decreased from 24 days in the 1970s to 12 days in 2005. This trend is true for length of stay of inpatient rehabilitation as well, 98 days in the 1970s compared to 37 days in 2005.[2]

Life expectancy has increased over the years but is still less than that for individuals without a SCI. Factors that influence life expectancy are age at onset and level and extent of neurological injury. Individuals with an incomplete neurological SCI have a longer life expectancy than those with a complete injury, and individuals with more caudal injuries also have a greater life expectancy. A 20-year-old healthy individual without a SCI has a life expectancy of an additional 58.6 years (total life expectancy of 78.6 years). A person who experiences a SCI at age 20 with a neurologically incomplete injury has a life expectancy of an additional 52.6 years, a person with complete paraplegia an additional 45.2 years, low tetraplegia (C5–C8) an additional 40.0 years, and a person with high tetraplegia (C1–C4) an additional 35.7 years. Mortality rate is also significantly higher during the first year after injury.

The financial impact of SCI is extremely high. Spinal cord injury is characterized by lengthy hospitalization, medical complications, extensive follow-up care, and recurrent hospitalizations. The costs of medical care in 2009 during the first year after injury were approximately $986,000 for high tetraplegia (C1–C4), $712,000 for low tetraplegia (C5–C8), and $480,000 for paraplegia. Average lifetime costs for an individual injured at 25 years of age are $3.5 million for high tetraplegia (C1–C4), $2.5 million for low tetraplegia (C5–C8), and $1.6 million for paraplegia.[4] These numbers do not take into account lost wages, fringe benefits, and productivity.

This brief presentation of demographic information provides some important general perspectives on characteristics of SCI. It is a relatively low-incidence disability affecting predominantly younger males, although more older adults are experiencing SCI likely due to falls, and SCI is associated with lengthy and costly care.

■ CLASSIFICATION OF SPINAL CORD INJURIES

Spinal cord injuries typically are divided into two broad functional categories: tetraplegia and paraplegia. **Tetraplegia** refers to complete paralysis of all four extremities and trunk, including the respiratory muscles, and results from lesions of the cervical cord. **Paraplegia** refers to complete paralysis of all or part of the trunk and both lower extremities (LEs), resulting from lesions of the thoracic or lumbar spinal cord or cauda equina.

Neuroanatomical Organization and Structure

Before considering designation of spinal cord lesions, it is useful to review briefly the anatomy of the spinal cord and its relationship with nerve roots to the vertebral bodies. The spinal cord exits the foramen magnum and extends to approximately the L1 vertebral level. It contains white matter, which consists of ascending sensory tracts, descending motor tracts, and an H-shaped central area of grey matter. The primary ascending tracts are the dorsal column (conveys proprioception, vibratory sensation, deep touch, and discriminative touch); anterolateral system consisting of the spinothalamic, spinoreticular, and spinotectal tracts (conveys pain, temperature, and crude touch); and the dorsal and ventral spinocerebellar tracts (conveys unconscious proprioception) (Fig. 20.1). The primary descending tracts are the lateral corticospinal (voluntary movement); anterior corticospinal (voluntary movement of axial muscles, minimal clinical significance due to small size); medial vestibulospinal (positioning of head and neck); lateral and medial vestibulospinal (posture and balance); lateral and medial reticulospinal (posture, balance, automatic gait-related movements);

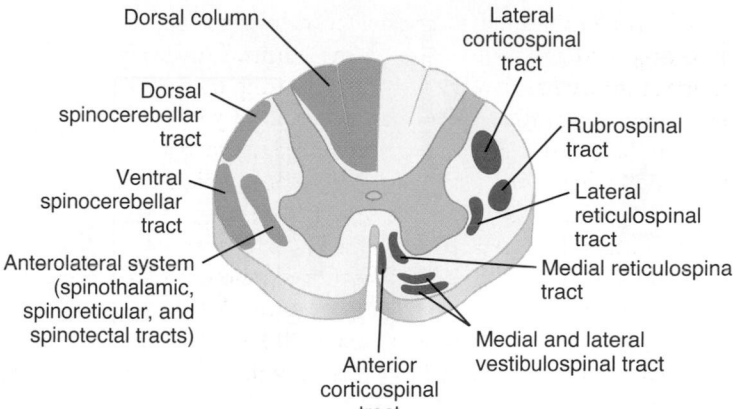

Figure 20.1 Main ascending sensor tracts: dorsal column, spinothalamic, spinoreticular, spinotectal, and dorsal and ventral spinocerebellar tracts. Main descending motor tracts: lateral corticospinal, anterior corticospinal, lateral and medial vestibulospinal, lateral and medial reticulospinal, and rubrospinal tracts.

and rubrospinal (movement of limbs) (see Fig. 20.1). In addition to these long tracts, the white matter contains axons of interneurons, which convey information between spinal cord segments. The H-shaped grey matter is arranged such that the dorsal section in each half contains neurons involved in sensory function, the middle portion contains interneurons, and the ventral section contains neurons involved in motor function (anterior horn cells) that project to the peripheral muscles.[5]

There are 31 pairs of spinal nerves: 8 cervical, 12 thoracic, 5 lumbar, 5 sacral, and 1 coccygeal (Fig. 20.2). The cervical nerves are relatively horizontal as they exit the intervertebral foramina. The nerve roots for C1–C7 exit above the corresponding vertebrae. C8 exits below the C7 vertebrae. The remaining nerves exit in a downward direction and do not emerge at the corresponding vertebral level. During fetal development the cord fills the entire length of the vertebral canal and the spinal nerves run in a horizontal direction. As the vertebral column elongates with growth, the spinal cord, which does not elongate at the same rate or as much, is drawn upward. In adults the spinal cord ends in the conus medullaris at the L1 vertebral level. The nerve roots assume an increasingly oblique and downward direction, running in an almost vertical direction in the lumbar area, giving the appearance of a "horse's tail" (cauda equina) (see Fig. 20.2). Because of this, in more caudal injuries the vertebral level of injury does not correspond directly to the spinal cord segment level of injury.

Designation of Lesion Level

It is extremely important for clinicians and researchers to be able to accurately determine the extent of neurological impairment in terms of motor and sensory loss when working with individuals with SCI. The extent of motor and sensory function after injury has a large impact on the medical and rehabilitation needs of the individual. The American Spinal Injury Association (ASIA) created the *International Standards for Neurological Classification of Spinal Cord Injury* (ISNCSCI)[6,7] (Fig. 20.3) in an effort to standardize the way in which severity of injury is determined and documented.

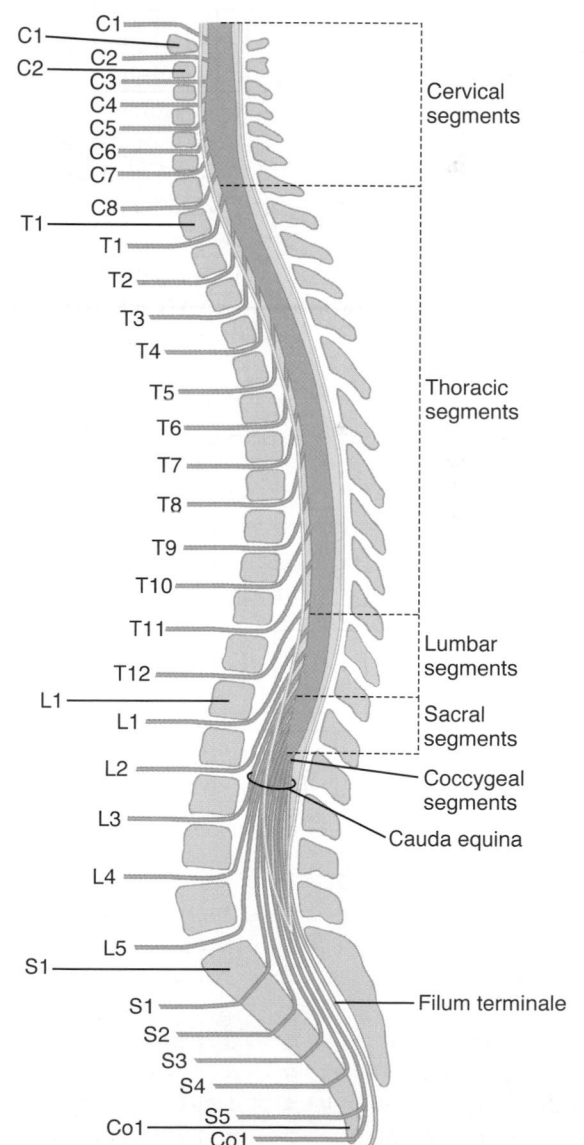

Figure 20.2 Relationship between spinal cord and nerve roots to vertebral bodies.

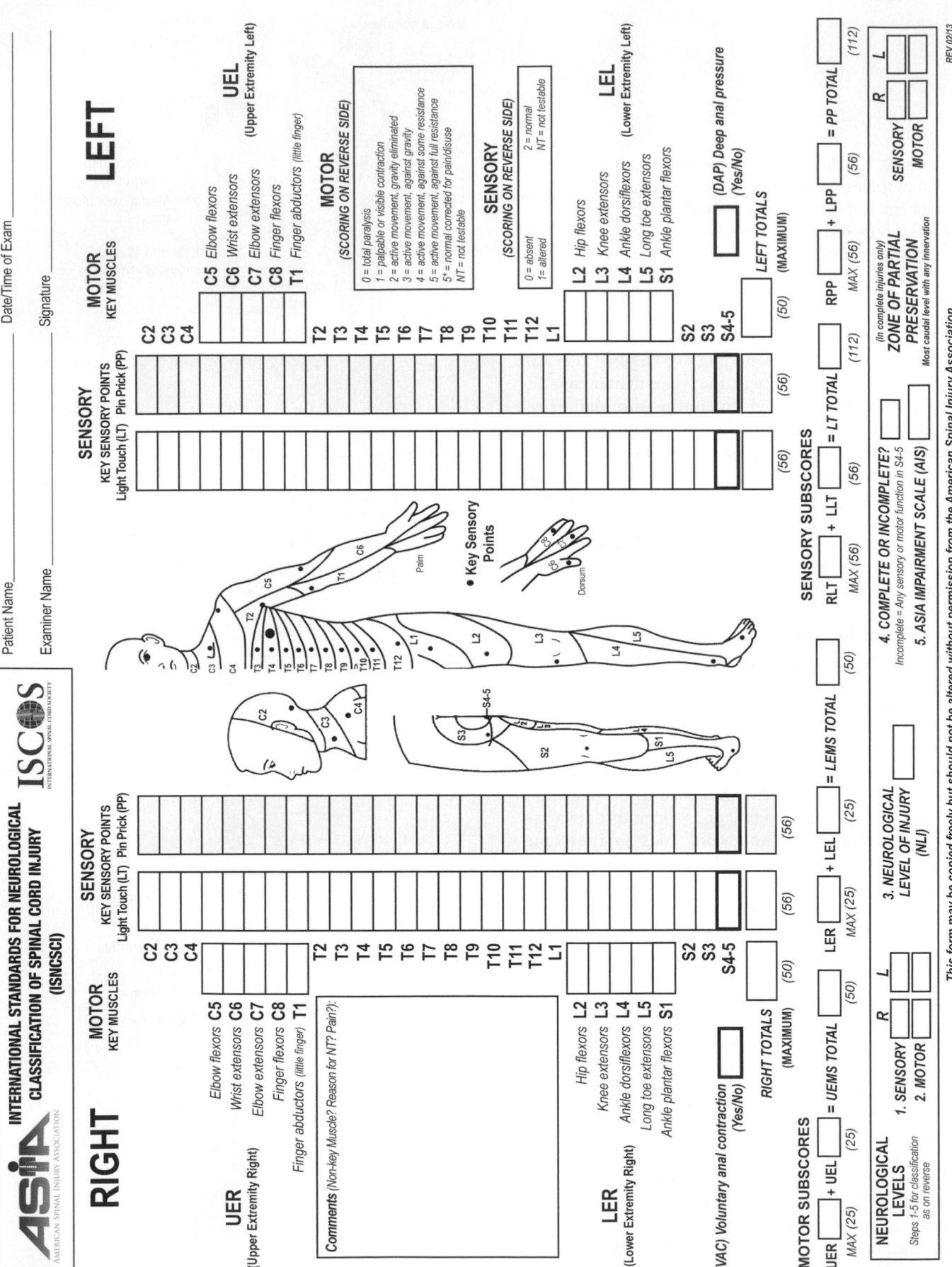

Figure 20.3 International Standards for Classification of Spinal Cord Injury. *(With permission from American Spinal Injury Association: International Standards for Neurological Classification of Spinal Cord*

The ISNCSCI provides a standardized examination method to determine the extent of motor and sensory function loss after a SCI. It promotes better communication between and among professionals, provides guidance for establishing the prognosis, and is an important tool for clinical research trials.

The **neurological level** is defined as the most caudal level of the spinal cord with normal motor and sensory function on both the left and right sides of the body. **Motor level** is referred to as the most caudal segment of the spinal cord with normal motor function bilaterally. **Sensory level** is defined in the same way except in terms of sensory function. Sensory level is determined by testing the patient's sensitivity to light touch and pinprick on the left and right side of the body at key dermatomes (see Fig. 20.3). Scoring of sensation is based on a 3-point ordinal scale where 0 = absent, 1 = impaired, and 2 = normal. Motor level is determined by testing the strength of a key muscle on the right and left side of the body at myotomes adjacent to the suspected level of impairment (see Fig. 20.3 for key muscles). Key muscle strength is scored using the 6-point ordinal scale commonly used for manual muscle testing.

Assigning a single muscle to represent one myotome is a generalization. Most muscles are innervated by more than one segmental nerve root; usually two nerve roots innervate each muscle. For example, the extensor carpi radialis longus receives innervation from the C6 and C7 spinal nerve roots. For the purpose of determining motor and neurological level, the key muscle is defined as having intact innervation if it has a manual muscle test score of at least 3/5 (fair) and the next most rostral key muscle exhibits 5/5 (normal) strength on the manual muscle test. If the rostral key muscle does not demonstrate 5/5 strength, but the therapist feels that the muscle would test normally except for factors that would impede normal testing (e.g., pain with testing or difficulty with positioning), then this information should be carefully documented. For myotomes that are not clinically testable (i.e., C1–C4, T2–L1, and S2–S5) the motor level is defined as the same as the sensory level.[6,7]

In determining neurological level there may be differences in terms of level of sensory and motor function and between the left and right sides of the body. For example, a patient's sensory level may be at C5 on the left and C8 on the right, and the motor level may be C5 on the left and T1 on the right. In these cases, it is not appropriate to assign a single neurological level, because this can be misleading. Each of the sensory and motor levels on the right and left sides of the body should be documented separately.[6]

Complete Injuries, Incomplete Injuries, and Zone of Partial Preservation

A complete anatomical transection of the spinal cord is rare. However, even if the injury is not anatomically complete, it may present as clinically complete.

The ISNCSCI defines a **complete injury** as having no sensory or motor function in the lowest sacral segments (S4 and S5). Sensory and motor function at S4 and S5 are determined by anal sensation and voluntary external anal sphincter contraction. An **incomplete injury** is classified as having motor and/or sensory function below the neurological level including sensory and/or motor function at S4 and S5. If an individual has motor and/or sensory function below the neurological level but does not have function at S4 and S5, then the areas of intact motor and/or sensory function below the neurological level are termed **zones of partial preservation**.[6]

ASIA Impairment Scale

Individuals with incomplete injuries may have variable clinical presentations in terms of motor and/or sensory function below the neurological level. For example, one patient may have close to normal sensory and motor function below the level of the lesion whereas another with the same lesion level may have impaired sensation and no motor function below the neurological level. The ASIA impairment scale (Table 20.1)[6] was created so that clinicians and researchers could better communicate the degree of motor and sensory impairment of individuals with SCIs.

Clinical Syndromes

Despite the disparity associated with incomplete lesions, several syndromes have emerged with consistent clinical features. Approximately one-fifth of all SCIs result in an

Table 20.1 ASIA Impairment Scale
☐ **A = Complete:** No motor or sensory function is preserved in the sacral segments S4 to S5.
☐ **B = Incomplete:** Sensory but not motor function is preserved below the neurological level and includes the sacral segments S4 to S5.
☐ **C = Incomplete:** Motor function is preserved below the neurological level, and more than half of key muscles below the neurological level have a muscle grade less than 3.
☐ **D = Incomplete:** Motor function is preserved below the neurological level, and at least half of key muscles below the neurological level have a muscle grade of 3 or more.
☐ **E = Normal:** Motor and sensory function is normal.
Clinical Syndromes   ☐ Central cord   ☐ Brown-Sequard   ☐ Anterior cord   ☐ Conus medullaris   ☐ Cauda equina

From American Spinal Injury Association,[6, p 28,] with permission.

injury pattern similar to clinical SCI syndromes.[8] Information related to the anticipated sensory and motor functions of these syndromes is useful in establishing anticipated goals, expected outcomes, and plan of care (POC). The area of cord damage of each syndrome is presented in Figure 20.4. The corresponding clinical features of the different syndromes are explained by the anatomical organization of the motor and sensory pathways described earlier.

Brown-Sequard Syndrome

Brown-Sequard syndrome occurs from hemisection of the spinal cord (damage to one side) and is typically caused by penetration wounds, that is, gunshot or stab. Partial lesions (termed *Brown-Sequard plus syndrome*) occur more frequently; true hemisections are rare. The clinical features of this syndrome are asymmetrical. On the *ipsilateral* (same) side as the lesion, there is paralysis and sensory loss. The ipsilateral loss of proprioception, light touch, and vibratory sense is due to damage to the dorsal column; paralysis results from damage to the lateral corticospinal tract. On the side *contralateral* (opposite) to the lesion, damage to the spinothalamic tracts results in loss of sense of pain and temperature.[8] This loss begins several dermatome segments below the level of injury.[9] This discrepancy in levels occurs because the lateral spinothalamic tracts ascend two to four segments on the same side before crossing.[5,10,11] Individuals with Brown-Sequard syndrome typically achieve good functional gains during inpatient rehabilitation.[8]

Anterior Cord Syndrome

Anterior cord syndrome is frequently related to flexion injuries of the cervical region with resultant damage to the anterior portion of the cord and/or its vascular supply from the anterior spinal artery. There is typically compression of the anterior cord from fracture, dislocation, or cervical disk protrusion. This syndrome is characterized by loss of motor function (corticospinal tract damage) and loss of the sense of pain and temperature (spinothalamic tract damage) below the level of the lesion. Proprioception, light touch, and vibratory sense are generally preserved, because they are mediated by the dorsal columns with a separate vascular supply from the posterior spinal arteries.[5,8,10,11] Individuals with anterior cord syndrome often require a longer length of stay during inpatient rehabilitation compared to people with other types of SCI clinical syndromes.[8]

Central Cord Syndrome

Central cord syndrome is the most common SCI syndrome.[8,12] It generally occurs from hyperextension injuries to the cervical region.[13] It also has been associated with congenital or degenerative narrowing of the spinal canal. The resultant compressive forces give rise to hemorrhage and edema, producing damage to the most central aspects of the cord. There is characteristically more severe neurological involvement of the upper extremities (UEs) (cervical tracts are more centrally located) than of the LEs (lumbar and sacral tracts are located more peripherally).[8] Varying degrees of sensory impairment occur but tend to be less severe than motor deficits. With complete preservation of sacral tracts, normal sexual, bowel, and bladder function may be retained. Patients with central cord syndrome typically recover the ability to ambulate. Some distal UE weakness and loss of fine motor control remain, which can result in moderate to severe limitations in the ability to perform functional tasks.[12]

Cauda Equina Injuries

The spinal cord tapers distally to form the conus medullaris at the lower border of the first lumbar vertebra. Although some anatomical variations exist, this is the typical termination point of the spinal cord. Below this level is the collection of long nerve roots known as the *cauda equina*. Complete transections in this area are rare. **Cauda equina lesions** are frequently anatomically incomplete owing to the great number of nerve roots involved and the comparatively large surface area they encompass (i.e., it would be unlikely that an injury to this region would involve the entire surface area and all the nerve roots).

Individuals with cauda equina injuries exhibit areflexic bowel and bladder and saddle anesthesia. Lower extremity paralysis and paresis is variable depending on the extent of the injury to the cauda equina.[8] Cauda equina lesions are peripheral nerve (**lower motor neuron [LMN]**) injuries. As such, they have the same potential to regenerate as peripheral nerves elsewhere in the body. However, full return of innervation is not common because (1) there is a large distance between the lesion and the point of innervation; (2) axonal regeneration may not occur along the original distribution of the nerve; (3) axonal regeneration may be blocked by glial-collagen

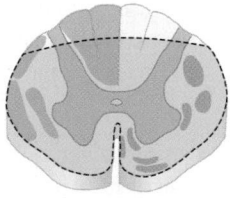
Anterior cord syndrome

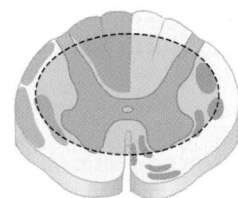
Central cord syndrome

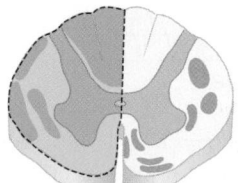
Brown-Sequard syndrome

Figure 20.4 Areas of spinal cord damage in clinical syndromes.

scarring; (4) the end organ may no longer be functioning once reinnervation occurs; and (5) the rate of regeneration slows and finally stops after about 1 year.

■ NEUROLOGICAL COMPLICATIONS AND ASSOCIATED CONDITIONS

Spinal cord injury results in a disruption of communication from higher centers in the central nervous system to the periphery. This disruption results in loss of motor and sensory function, as well as impaired autonomic function.

Spinal Shock

Immediately following SCI there is a period of areflexia that is part of **spinal shock**. This period of transient reflex depression is not clearly understood.[14] It is believed to result from the very abrupt withdrawal of connections between higher centers and the spinal cord.[5,10] It is characterized initially by an absence of all reflex activity, impairment of autonomic regulation resulting in hypotension and loss of control of sweating and piloerection.[10] In addition to the loss of deep tendon reflexes, there is a loss of the bulbocavernosus reflex, the cremasteric reflex, a Babinski response, and a delayed plantar response.

Spinal shock evolves over time. The initial period of total areflexia lasts approximately 24 hours. This is followed by a gradual return of reflexes 1 to 3 days after injury, a period of increasing hyperreflexia lasting 1 to 4 weeks, and final hyperreflexia 1 to 6 months after injury.[14]

Motor and Sensory Impairments

Following SCI there will be either complete (paralysis) or partial (paresis) loss of muscle function below the level of the lesion. Disruption of the ascending sensory fibers following SCI results in impaired or absent sensation below the level of the lesion.

The clinical presentation of motor and sensory impairments depends on the specific features of the lesion. These include the neurological level and the completeness of the lesion.

Autonomic Dysreflexia

Autonomic dysreflexia (AD, also referred to autonomic hyperreflexia) is a pathological autonomic reflex that can be life threatening. Typically AD occurs in lesions above T6 (above sympathetic splanchnic outflow).[15] However, it has been reported in patients with lower injuries. Incidence of this problem varies. One study found a 48% occurrence in a group of 213 patients.[16] Although AD is more common in the chronic stage of recovery (more than 3 to 6 months after injury), it may also occur in the early stages after SCI.[17] It is more common with complete injury, but it may also occur with an incomplete SCI.[18]

This clinical syndrome produces an acute onset of autonomic activity from noxious stimuli below the level of the lesion. Afferent input from these stimuli reach the lower spinal cord (lower thoracic and sacral areas) and initiate a mass reflex response resulting in elevation of blood pressure. Normally, the impulses stimulate the receptors in the carotid sinus and aorta, which signal the vasomotor center to readjust peripheral resistance. Following SCI, however, impulses from the vasomotor center cannot pass the site of the lesion to counteract the hypertension by vasodilation.[19] This is a critical, emergency situation. Owing to the lack of inhibition from higher centers, hypertension will persist if not treated promptly. Hypertension triggered by AD can result in seizures, cardiac arrest, subarachnoid hemorrhage, stroke, or even death.

Initiating Stimuli

The most common cause of this pathological reflex is bladder and bowel distention/irritation.[19] Common bladder issues that may trigger AD are distended bladder, blocked catheter, urinary tract infection, kidney stones, and irritation of bladder or urethra during catheterization or other procedures. Other precipitating stimuli include pressure sores, noxious cutaneous stimuli below the level of the lesion, kidney malfunction, electrical stimulation below the level of the lesion, sexual activity, labor, and skeletal fracture below the level of the lesion.[19] Table 20.2 summarizes stimuli that may trigger an onset of AD, as well as common associated signs and symptoms.

Symptoms

The symptoms of AD include hypertension, bradycardia, headache (often severe and pounding), profuse sweating, increased spasticity, restlessness, vasoconstriction below the level of lesion, vasodilation (flushing) above the level of the lesion, constricted pupils, nasal congestion, piloerection (goose bumps), and blurred vision.[19] Less commonly, AD may also present as asymptomatic. A rise in systolic blood pressure of 20 to 30 mm Hg is diagnostic of an episode of AD[15] (such a rise may appear to be within normal range for a person without SCI). People with SCI typically have lower than normal resting blood pressure; systolic may be in the range of 90 to 110 mm Hg for those with neurological level above T6. During an episode of AD, systolic blood pressure may rise to 250 to 300 mm Hg and diastolic to 200 to 220 mm Hg.

Intervention

The onset of symptoms should be treated as a medical emergency. If lying flat, the patient should be brought to an upright position, inasmuch as blood pressure will be lowered in this position, and loosen any tight clothing or restrictive devices. Blood pressure and pulse should be monitored. The individual should be questioned as to possible triggers, starting with urinary system. Because bladder

Table 20.2   Initiating Stimuli and Signs and Symptoms of Autonomic Dysreflexia

Initiating Stimuli	Signs and Symptoms
Bladder distention/irritation*	Hypertension (rise in systolic BP 20–30 mm Hg)
Bowel distention/irritation*	Bradycardia
Stimuli that would normally be painful below level of lesion	Severe headache
Gastrointestinal irritation	Feeling of anxiety
Sexual activity	Constricted pupils
Labor	Blurred vision
Skeletal fracture below level of injury	Flushing and piloerection above level of lesion
Electrical stimulation below level of lesion	Dry, pale skin below level of lesion (due to vasoconstriction)
	Nasal congestion
	Increased spasticity
	May be asymptomatic

*Most common triggers of AD.

distention is a primary cause of AD, the drainage system should be examined first. If the patient is using an indwelling catheter it should be checked to make sure it is not blocked. If any type of blockage is found it should be removed immediately. If the patient catheterizes intermittently, a catheter should be placed and the bladder drained. The patient should then be questioned about when the last bowel movement occurred and checked for an impaction. The patient's body should be examined for triggering stimuli such as tight clothing, restricting catheter straps, abdominal binders, or anything that may be a noxious stimulus.[20,21]

If hypertension and other symptoms do not subside with the identification and elimination of specific triggers, medical and/or nursing assistance should be sought emergently. Pharmacological intervention may be required to lower blood pressure. Nifedipine, nitrates, and captopril are commonly used antihypertensive medications.[22]

Education related to triggers, signs and symptoms, and management of AD is critical. A recent study found that 41% of people with SCI above T6 reported never having heard about AD, and 22% of those who did know about it did not know how to respond to an episode of AD.[23] Because, in most cases, AD is not manifested until the chronic stages of recovery, people with SCI may no longer be in a health care setting when they first experience an episode. People with SCI who are at risk of experiencing AD should be educated on initiating stimuli, symptoms, and management.

Spastic Hypertonia

Individuals with SCI and other central nervous system disorders such as traumatic brain injury, multiple sclerosis, and stroke often present with spastic hypertonia. Approximately 65% of people with SCI have spasticity, and it is more common in people with cervical-level

injuries.[24] Spastic hypertonia is part of upper motor neuron (UMN) syndrome, which encompasses a range of conditions including spasticity, muscle spasms, abnormally high muscle tone, hyperactive stretch reflexes, and clonus.[25] These terms are sometimes used interchangeably in the literature. The classic definition of spasticity is a velocity-dependent increase in resistance to passive stretch.[26] Spastic hypertonia is thought to be a result of altered input at the spinal segmental level, which causes an imbalance between excitation and inhibition of the spinal motor neurons. Descending, suprasegmental signals are altered or eliminated following SCI, the anterior horn cell may become hyperexcitable, and there are changes in afferent input.[25]

Spastic hypertonia typically emerges below the level of lesion after spinal shock evolves. There is a gradual increase in spastic hypertonia during the first 6 months and a plateau is usually reached 1 year after injury. Various stimuli including positional changes, cutaneous stimuli, environmental temperatures, tight clothing, bladder or kidney stones, fecal impactions, catheter blockage, urinary tract infections, decubitus ulcers, and emotional stress may trigger or increase spasticity and muscle spasms.

Spasticity varies in the degree of severity. Approximately 50% of people with SCI report that their spasticity is problematic.[24,27] Patients with minimal to moderate involvement may learn to trigger the spasticity or muscle spasm at appropriate times to assist in functional activities. However, strong spasticity can be a deterrent to independent function. For example, severe spasms during transfers may cause loss of balance and a fall. The management of spasticity must balance the potential benefits against the negative effects.

Spasticity is generally managed through a variety of methods including stretch, modalities, and medications.[28-30] Although stretch is commonly used in the clinic,[28] a recent systematic review found that stretch had no clinically important impact on spasticity in people with neurological conditions.[31] This may be due to the differences in how spasticity was measured and length of time and force used while providing the stretch between studies.

Medications typically used include muscle relaxants and spasmolytic agents such as baclofen,[30,32] tizanidine,[33] diazepam,[34] and dantrolene sodium.[34] Intrathecal baclofen (where an implanted pump delivers small amounts of baclofen directly at the spinal cord level to minimize side effects) can be used in cases of severe spasticity when individuals do not respond well to oral administration.[35] Intramuscular injection of botulinum neurotoxin can be used to manage focal spasticity.[36] Pharmacological management is usually not completely successful in alleviating spasticity, and its benefits must be weighed against potentially adverse side effects (e.g., weakness, dizziness, drowsiness). In addition, patients may develop a tolerance to prolonged use of individual drugs. Despite the widespread use of pharmacological agents to treat spasticity, few clinical trials directly support their use in people with SCI.[37]

Surgical approaches also have been used to combat spasticity in more severe cases and are only considered after all other alternative interventions have been tried.[30] Surgical procedures used include myotomy, a sectioning or release of a muscle; tenotomy, a sectioning of a tendon that allows subsequent lengthening (e.g., heel cords); and a dorsal rhizotomy (cutting of the posterior nerve roots to disrupt the stretch reflex arc).[30]

Cardiovascular Impairment

In healthy individuals with an intact spinal cord, cardiovascular function is regulated by the brainstem and hypothalamus via the sympathetic and parasympathetic nervous systems.[5,38] Parasympathetic signals to the heart arise from the vagus nerve, decreasing heart rate and contractility. Sympathetic input comes from spinal segments T1 to L2 through the sympathetic trunk, which runs parallel to the spinal cord. Sympathetic input increases heart rate and contractility and peripheral vasoconstriction.[5]

A rostral SCI will result in a loss of sympathetic communication between the brainstem and the heart, while parasympathetic input remains intact. This causes bradycardia and dilation of the peripheral vasculature below the level of the lesion. Because of the disrupted balance between sympathetic and parasympathetic input, as well as a lack of or decrease in active muscle contraction and prolonged time in bed, orthostatic hypotension is often experienced during early transitions to a more upright posture. Symptoms of orthostatic hypotension include blurred vision, ringing in the ears, light-headedness, and fainting. Orthostatic hypotension is usually only significant in people with SCI above T6. Although the exact mechanism is not clearly understood, the cardiovascular

system, over time, gradually reestablishes sufficient vasomotor tone to allow assumption of the vertical position.[39]

To minimize these effects when mobilizing patients early after SCI, the cardiovascular system should be allowed to adapt gradually by a slow progression to the vertical position. This frequently begins with elevation of the head of the bed and progresses to a reclining wheelchair with elevating leg rests and use of a tilt table. Vital signs should be monitored carefully, and the patient should always be moved very slowly. Use of compressive stockings and an abdominal binder may further minimize these effects.[40] Pharmacological therapy may be indicated (e.g., ephedrine to increase blood pressure or low-dose diuretics to relieve persistent edema of legs, ankles, or feet). As vasomotor stability returns, tolerance to the vertical position will gradually improve.

Past the acute stage of injury, people with SCI below or within the thoracolumbar sympathetic output will exhibit a reduced exercise tolerance, lower stroke volume, and reduced cardiac output.[41,42] Deconditioning often occurs due to physical inactivity and an impaired cardiovascular system. A regular cardiovascular fitness exercise program is an important component of rehabilitation. Programs should be designed based on the level of injury and include careful patient monitoring.[42]

Impaired Temperature Control

After damage to the spinal cord the hypothalamus can no longer control cutaneous blood flow or level of sweating. This autonomic (sympathetic) dysfunction results in loss of internal thermoregulatory responses. The ability to shiver below the level of the injury is also lost. The degree of impaired thermoregulation will vary depending on the level of the injury and whether the injury is complete or incomplete. Individuals with cervical-level injuries and complete injuries demonstrate more impairment. Initially after injury hypothermia may occur due to peripheral vasodilation. Later, hyperthermia is more likely due to the lack of sympathetic control of sweat glands. Although some improvement in thermoregulatory responses occurs over time, patients with tetraplegia typically experience long-term impairment of body temperature regulation, especially in response to extreme environmental changes.

Pulmonary Impairment

Ventilatory and respiratory function varies considerably, depending on the level of lesion. In people with high cervical injuries, pulmonary problems are the leading cause of death both in the early and late stages of recovery.[43,44] Individuals with injuries below T10 are likely to have near-normal ventilatory and respiratory function. Paralysis or paresis of the muscles of respiration leads to poor ventilation, which may then cause impaired respiration leading to atelectasis and pneumonia. Ten percent of people with complete tetraplegia develop pneumonia or atelectasis 1 year after injury.[45]

With high spinal cord lesions at C1 and C2, phrenic nerve innervation and spontaneous respiration are lost. The only muscles of respiration that are intact are accessory muscles: sternocleidomastoid, upper trapezius, and cervical extensors. An artificial ventilator or phrenic nerve stimulator is required to sustain life. Expiration is passive; as a result, individuals with SCI at these levels require assistance for airway clearance. C3- and C4-level injuries have partial diaphragm innervation, as well as scalenes, levator scapulae, and trapezius. In the acute stage of recovery individuals with an injury at these levels will require mechanical ventilation. With recovery and training they will likely be able to breathe on their own.[46] However, they may need part-time ventilatory support, especially individuals with C3-level injury. Because they do not have abdominal or intercostal muscle innervation, these individuals will also need assistance for airway clearance. Patients with mid to lower cervical level injuries have better pulmonary function than those with higher cervical level injuries. Injuries at C5–C8 have a fully innervated diaphragm, as well as many accessory muscles. Some cough ability is preserved; however, it is usually weak. Although individuals with paraplegia have better respiratory function than people with tetraplegia, they still have impaired respiratory function compared to healthy individuals without a SCI.[47] Pulmonary impairment increases with the more rostral the injury. Individuals with weak or absent abdominal and intercostal musculature will have impaired airway clearance ability and be at a greater risk for developing pneumonia and atelectasis.

The primary muscles of expiration are the abdominals and internal intercostals. Normally, relaxed expiration is essentially a passive process that occurs through elastic recoil of the lungs and thorax. However, the abdominals and internal intercostals contribute several important functions related to movement of air out of the lungs. Loss of these muscles significantly decreases expiratory efficiency. Control of the abdominal muscles originates from T5–T12. When fully innervated, they play an important role in maintaining intrathoracic pressure for effective respiration. They support the abdominal viscera and assist in maintaining the position of the diaphragm. They also function to push the diaphragm upward during forced expiration. With paralysis of the abdominals this support is lost, causing the diaphragm to assume an unusually low position in the chest. This lowered position and lack of abdominal pressure to move the diaphragm upward during forced expiration results in a decreased expiratory reserve volume. This subsequently decreases cough effectiveness and the ability to expel secretions. Table 20.3 summarizes respiratory muscle function by level of SCI.[48]

Paralysis or paresis of the scalenes and intercostal muscles also results in the development of an altered breathing pattern, called *paradoxical breathing pattern*.[49] This pattern is characterized by flattening of the upper

Table 20.3	Neurological Level of Spinal Cord Injury and Muscles of Respiration
Level of Injury	**Respiratory Muscles***
C1–C2	Sternocleidomastoid, upper trapezius, cervical extensors
C3–C4	Partial diaphragm, scalenes, levator scapulae
C5–C8	Diaphragm, pectoralis major and minor, serratus anterior, rhomboids, latissimus dorsi
T1–T5	Some intercostals, erector spinae
T6–T10	Intercostals and abdominals
T11 and below	All of the muscles above

*Each successive level has the muscles of the more rostral levels.

chest wall, decreased chest wall expansion, and a dominant epigastric rise during inspiration. This breathing pattern is inefficient, requiring more energy to breathe, and as a result patients can become fatigued quickly.

Other factors may further impair respiratory status. Additional trauma sustained at the time of injury, premorbid respiratory problems, age, weight, and smoking history can all further compromise respiratory function.[47,50]

Bladder and Bowel Dysfunction
Bladder Dysfunction

The effects of bladder dysfunction following SCI pose a serious medical complication requiring consistent and long-term management. Urinary tract infections (UTIs) are a major cause of mortality and morbidity in people with SCI. Spinal cord injury alters the complex reflexive and voluntary control of **micturition**. As a result, people with SCI often require a catheter to drain the bladder.

Spinal control for micturition originates from the sacral segments of S2, S3, and S4.[5] The level of the SCI dictates the type of bladder dysfunction. Patients with lesions that occur above the conus medullaris and sacral segments develop a *spastic* or *hyperreflexic bladder*.[5] This is also termed a *UMN bladder*. Following a lesion of the sacral segments or conus medullaris, a *flaccid* or *areflexic bladder* develops.[5] This is also termed a *LMN bladder*.

A spastic or hyperreflexic bladder (UMN lesion) contracts and reflexively empties in response to a certain level of filling pressure. The reflex arc is intact with this type of injury. The detrusor muscle is generally hyperreflexive. There can be increased tone of the sphincter, contraction of the detrusor with small urine volumes, and lack of coordination between detrusor and sphincters (dyssynergia). A flaccid or areflexive bladder (LMN lesion) is essentially flaccid because there is no reflex action of the detrusor muscle.

There are generally two types of bladder dysfunction: failure to store urine and failure to empty urine.[51]

These can be due to detrusor muscle or sphincter impairment. Inability to store urine may be due to an areflexive sphincter or spastic detrusor muscle. Inability to empty the bladder sufficiently may be due to an areflexive bladder or a sphincter that is unable to relax. Dyssynergia between the detrusor and sphincter can also cause incomplete drainage of the bladder.[51]

Bladder Management

The primary goal of bladder management is to prevent or minimize urinary tract complications. These include UTIs, *hydronephrosis* (swelling of kidney due to backup of urine), renal calculi, bladder calculi, and *vesicoureteral reflux* (backward flow of urine up the ureter).[51] Because urinary incontinence has very strong psychosocial implications for the patient, a coordinated approach to this problem is particularly important. Knowledge of and participation in the bladder management program is an important consideration for the physical therapist.

In the early stage of recovery, while the patient is still in spinal shock, the bladder is flaccid and an indwelling catheter is inserted. After the patient is stable during rehabilitation, the most frequently used method of bladder management is *intermittent catheterization*.[51,52] Briefly stated, the program involves establishing a fluid intake pattern of approximately 2000 mL/day. Intake is stopped late in the day to reduce the need for catheterization during the night. Initially, the patient is catheterized every 4 hours. A record is maintained of voided and residual urine. While in the hospital, sterile intermittent catheterization should be done; after discharge, a clean technique can be used.

Although intermittent catheterization is the most common method of bladder management after discharge from the rehabilitation hospital, many males switch to the use of an external, condom catheter.[52] Other methods of bladder management include suprapubic tapping and the Valsalva maneuver. *Suprapubic tapping* involves tapping directly over the bladder with fingertips, causing a reflexive emptying of the bladder. This technique only works for individuals with an UMN bladder without dyssynergia between the detrusor and sphincter, because the sphincter must open for the bladder to reflexively drain.[51,52] Individuals with an areflexive bladder can use the *Valsalva maneuver*, which is done by straining.[51,52] In some individuals a suprapubic catheter may need to be surgically inserted.

The exact method or combination of methods used for bladder management will depend on a variety factors: type of bladder dysfunction, level of injury, functional ability, and personal preference. Whichever method(s) is used, the goal is for the patient to be catheter free, have low postvoid residual volume of urine in the bladder, and be without high bladder pressure during voiding.[53] Urodynamic testing is done after spinal shock resolves, approximately 3 months after injury, to help diagnose the specific type of bladder dysfunction and guide the selection of management strategies.

Because of impaired bladder function almost 50% people with SCI will develop UTIs.[54] Further urinary system complications linked to chronic UTIs are development of bladder and kidney stones and kidney dysfunction.

Bowel Dysfunction

As with bladder dysfunction, bowel dysfunction is a major concern after SCI. Over 98% of people with SCI report problems with bowel care and 34% require some level of assistance with bowel care.[55] People with SCI report that bowel function has a greater impact on daily life than many other impairments after SCI, including sexual function, bladder function, pain, spasticity, and skin integrity.[55-57] Bowel function also has a large impact on social activities and quality of life.[56] Neurogenic bowel conditions that develop after spinal shock subsides are of two main types. In spinal cord lesions above S2 there is a *spastic or reflex bowel* (UMN lesion). Because the parasympathetic and internal sphincter connections from S2–S4 are intact, reflex defecation can occur when the rectum fills with stool. In S2–S4 or cauda equina (peripheral nerves) lesions a *flaccid or areflexive bowel* (LMN lesion) develops. With an areflexive bowel the parasympathetic connections from S2–S4 are not intact so the bowel will not reflexively empty. This can cause feces to become impacted and, because the external sphincter is flaccid, incontinence can occur.[5,51]

Bowel Management

Safety and an appropriate, well-timed bowel care routine are common goals for bowel management. Safety includes continence in order to maintain intact and healthy skin, prevent damage to colorectal structures, and prevent AD due to bowel dysfunction.[53] In addition to type of neurogenic bowel (UMN or LMN), the bowel care program will also depend on presence of other health conditions that may affect gastrointestinal function, medications, dietary habits, fluid intake, and functional ability.[51] A typical bowel program involves establishing a daily (or every other day) pattern of eliciting a bowel movement. The exact time of day is chosen by the patient based on lifestyle needs and should be done consistently at the same time of day. This is usually in the morning or late evening. People with a reflex bowel require the use of suppositories and digital stimulation techniques to cause a reflex defecation. Digital stimulation involves manual stretch of the anal sphincter, either with a lubricated gloved finger or an orthotic digital stimulator. This stretch stimulates peristalsis of the colon and evacuation of the rectum (mediated by S2, S3, and S4).[51] Valsalva maneuver and abdominal massage may also be performed. Nonreflex bowel management relies on manual evacuation techniques and gentle Valsalva.[51] Other factors that can play a role in maintaining a consistent, safe bowel program include eating a diet with appropriate amount of fiber, fluid intake, physical activity, stool softeners, laxatives, and bulking agents.

Sexual Dysfunction

Sexuality encompasses much more than just the physical ability to have sexual intercourse. It is an important part of an individual's makeup and sense of self-esteem. Spinal cord injury not only affects the physiological ability to have intercourse but the psychosocial aspect of sexuality as well. People with paraplegia report that improved sexual function is the primary factor that would improve their quality of life. For people with tetraplegia it is the second most important after regaining hand function.[57] Education so that the patient can fully understand the impact of SCI on sexual function and support so the patient can become confident in his or her new sexuality are an important part of rehabilitation.

Male Response

Sexual response is directly related to level and completeness of injury. As with bowel and bladder function, sexual capabilities are broadly divided between UMN (damage to the cord above S2–S4) and LMN lesions. Generally speaking, erectile capacity is greater in UMN lesions than in LMN lesions and greater in incomplete lesions than in complete lesions. There are two types of erections: reflexogenic and psychogenic. *Reflexogenic erections* occur in response to external physical stimulation of the genitals or perineum. An intact reflex arc is required (mediated through S2, S3, and S4). *Psychogenic erections* occur through cognitive activity such as erotic fantasy. They are mediated from the cerebral cortex either through the thoracolumbar or sacral cord centers.[5,51] Medications such as Viagra, Levitra, and Cialis; injectable medications that relax penile smooth muscle; topical agents; and mechanical devices can also be used to improve erectile function.[51,58,59]

There is a higher incidence of ability to ejaculate with LMN lesions than with UMN lesions and incomplete as compared with complete lesions.[51] Historically, relatively few patients with SCI were able to sire children. This low level of fertility was associated with impaired spermatogenesis and an inability to ejaculate. However, vibratory stimulation and electroejaculation may improve ejaculatory response and promote higher semen quality for fertility purposes.[51,59]

Orgasm and ejaculation are two separate events. *Orgasm* is a cognitive, psychogenic event, whereas *ejaculation* is a physical occurrence. Relatively little information is available related to the effects of SCI on orgasm. This likely relates to inherent difficulties in collecting such data. From self-report surveys, approximately 45% of men with SCI report achieving orgasm.[60,61]

Female Response

Female sexual responses also follow a pattern related to location of lesion. In patients with UMN lesions, the reflex arc remains intact. Therefore, components of sexual arousal (vaginal lubrication, engorgement of the labia, and clitoral erection) will likely occur through reflexogenic stimulation, but psychogenic response will be lost. Conversely, with LMN lesions, psychogenic responses will most likely be preserved and reflex responses lost.[51]

Fertility is not affected as severely in women as men with SCI. The menstrual cycle typically is interrupted for a period of 4 to 5 months following injury. After this time, normal menses return and the potential for conception remains unimpaired.[51] Women with SCI who want to bear children should be closely supervised during pregnancy. They are more likely to encounter complications during pregnancy and childbirth than woman without SCI. Problems include UTIs, anemia, and venous thrombosis.[62] Labor and delivery must be monitored. Depending on the neurological level of injury the woman may not feel labor. There is a risk of AD during labor. See reviews by Baker and Cardenas[62] and Smeltzer and Wetzel-Effinger[63] for in-depth reviews of pregnancy in women with SCI.

As with men with SCI, there is little information available on the impact of SCI on orgasm in women. Women with SCI appear to be less likely to achieve orgasm than women without SCI and those with LMN are less likely to achieve orgasm than those with UMN.[51]

A major consideration for the physical therapist regarding sexual dysfunction is that a patient will often direct questions to the individuals with whom he or she feels most comfortable. It is not uncommon for such a discussion to arise during a physical therapy session. These questions or issues should be addressed openly and honestly. In addition, the therapist must anticipate and be prepared for these situations by (1) obtaining accurate information about the patient's physiological state and anticipated sexual function, and (2) having knowledge of referral options and support services available to the patient for appropriate examination and counseling.

Secondary Medical Complications

Individuals with SCI are at great risk for secondary medical complications throughout their life because of prolonged immobilization and the wide-ranging effects of the SCI on multiple body systems. During rehabilitation 82% of patients develop secondary medical complications. One year after injury, the three most common secondary complications are **pressure ulcers** (15%), **pneumonia** (4%), and **deep vein thrombosis** (2.5%). Twenty-five years after injury, 25% of people with SCI develop pressure ulcers[64] (Box 20.1).

Box 20.1 Common Complications Following Spinal Cord Injury

Pressure ulcer
Deep vein thrombosis
Pain
Contractures
Heterotopic ossification
Fracture/osteoporosis
Syringomyelia

Pressure Sores

Pressure sores (decubitus ulcers) are ulcerations of soft tissue (skin or subcutaneous tissue) caused by unrelieved pressure and shearing forces. They are subject to infection, which can migrate to bone. Pressure sores are a serious medical complication, are a major cause of delayed rehabilitation, and may even lead to death. Pressures sores are among the more frequent medical complications following SCI and are an important factor in increasing duration and subsequently cost of hospital stay. Up to 36% of people with SCI develop pressure sores during inpatient rehabilitation.[65]

Impaired sensory function and the inability to make appropriate and timely positional changes are influential factors in the development of pressure sores. Individuals with complete SCI are more likely to develop a pressure ulcer than patients with incomplete SCI (iSCI). Other important factors associated with the development of pressure ulcers are (1) tetraplegia; (2) spasticity; (3) bladder or bowel incontinence; (4) limited mobility and self-care; (5) nutritional deficiencies; (6) prolonged immobilization during recovery; (7) smoking; and (8) noncompliance with skin care.[65-67]

Pressure sores will develop over any bony prominence subjected to excessive pressure. The most common sites of involvement are the sacrum, heels, and ischium.[65] Other areas susceptible to skin breakdown are the greater trochanter, scapula, elbows, anterior iliac spines, and knees.

Deep Vein Thrombosis

Deep venous thrombosis (DVT) results from development of a thrombus within a vein. People with SCI are at risk of developing DVT due to lack of mobility and active muscle contraction of the LEs, which leads to stasis and hypercoagulability. The occurrence of such a clot is a dangerous medical complication. It has the potential to break free of its attachment and float freely within the venous bloodstream. Such mobile clots are known as *emboli*. They are particularly likely to block pulmonary vessels (pulmonary emboli), which can result in death. Reports of DVT vary widely and range from 0% to 100%.[68] Deep vein thrombosis is most likely to occur during the acute stage of recovery.[69]

The formation of a thrombus results in inflammation (thrombophlebitis) with characteristic clinical features of local swelling, erythema, and heat. These signs are similar to those of early ectopic bone formation and long bone fractures. Differential diagnosis is made on the basis of venous flow studies and venography.

Management of this secondary complication focuses on prevention. Nonpharmacological interventions include early mobilization, compression stockings and boots, and pneumatic compression sleeves. For people at high risk (motor complete, LE fracture, previous thrombosis, heart failure, and greater than 70 years of age), an inferior vena cava filter may be placed to prevent a pulmonary embolism.[69] Prophylactic anticoagulant drug therapy (heparin) is typically initiated following the acute onset of injury and routinely continued for 2 to 3 months.

Pain

Pain is a common occurrence following SCI both in the acute and chronic stages of recovery.[27,70-72] Between 26% and 96% of people with SCI report having chronic pain.[73] Pain can limit the performance of activities of daily living (ADL), affect sleep, and contribute to a lower quality of life.[74,75] Pain can be grossly divided into two broad categories: *nociceptive pain* and *neuropathic pain*. Nociceptive pain can be musculoskeletal or visceral in origin. Neuropathic pain can be below, at, or above the level of injury.[76]

Nociceptive Pain

Shoulder pain and pain in other UE joints and soft tissue is common in people with SCI.[77,78] Musculoskeletal injuries are often due to overuse or poor posture and commonly occur in the shoulder, wrist, or elbow joints involving capsule, tendon, ligament, and muscle tissue.[79] A variety of factors can cause musculoskeletal pain: mechanical injury to soft and bony tissue structures, inflammation, and muscle spasm. Muscular imbalances in the shoulder girdle, poor seated posture in a wheelchair, decreased flexibility, incorrect positioning in bed, older age, and higher body mass index (BMI) can all contribute to shoulder pain.[78] Overuse musculoskeletal injuries can be due to repetitive stress from propelling a wheelchair while in a biomechanically poor position, increased weight-bearing on the UEs while transferring, using assistive device(s) during ambulation, and pressure relief. Specific musculoskeletal injuries that may occur are biceps tendinitis, lateral epicondylitis, shoulder impingement, rotator cuff tears, carpal tunnel syndrome, and wrist tendonitis.[79]

Neuropathic pain

Neuropathic pain is pain due to injury to the central or peripheral nervous system. Neuropathic pain can occur below, at, or above the level of the spinal cord lesion.

Neuropathic pain below the level of the lesion is due to spinal cord damage and may take the form of **allodynia** or **hyperalgesia**. Damage to nerve roots or the spinal cord may be the cause of neuropathic pain at the level of the lesion. Neuropathic pain at the level of the lesion may also take the form of allodynia or hyperalgesia. Neuropathic pain above the level of the lesion is likely to be due to peripheral nerve damage associated with nerve impingement or compression. Neuropathic pain may be burning, shooting, or sharp. This type of pain below the level of the lesion is diffuse.[76]

Neuropathic pain is particularly challenging to treat and no single intervention option has established efficacy.[80,81] Nonpharmacological options include transcutaneous electrical nerve stimulation (TENS), massage, acupuncture, and mental imagery.[82] Pharmacological interventions commonly used are anticonvulsants such as gabapentin (Neurontin), pregabalin (Lyrica), and valproic acid (Depakote, Valparin); the antidepressant amitriptyline (Elavil, Vanatrip); and analgesics such as tramadol (Rybix, Ultram).[80,83] Chapter 25, Chronic Pain, provides an in-depth discussion of different types of pain, as well as interventions for pain management.

Contractures

Contractures develop secondary to prolonged shortening of structures across and around a joint, resulting in limitation in motion. Contractures initially produce alterations in muscle tissue but progress to involve capsular and pericapsular changes. Lack of active muscle function eliminates the normal reciprocal stretching of a muscle group and surrounding structures as the opposing muscle contracts. In addition, spasticity, positioning in wheelchair or bed for prolonged periods of time, and abnormal muscle tone are all factors that place people with SCI at a high risk for developing contractures. All joints are at risk for contractures. Contractures of the ankle, knee, hip, elbow, and shoulder joints may have significant negative impact on a person's ability to perform important activities and participate in valued social roles. Contractures may also be painful, make positioning and hygiene difficult, and lead to skin breakdown. The most important management consideration related to the potential development of contractures is prevention. Once contractures have developed it is extremely difficult to reverse the process.[31] A consistent and concurrent program of range of motion (ROM) exercises, positioning, and splinting is important to maintain joint motion and prevent contracture.

Heterotopic (Ectopic) Ossification

Heterotopic ossification (HO) is osteogenesis in soft tissues, usually near joints, below the level of the lesion. The etiology of this abnormal bone growth is unknown. The incidence of HO ranges from 10% to 53%.[84] Factors associated with HO include complete injury, trauma, severe spasticity, UTI, and pressure sores.[85,86] Care should be taken while performing passive range of motion (PROM). If it is too vigorous it may cause trauma, which may be a causative factor for HO. It most often occurs in the hip and knee joints. Early symptoms of HO including swelling, joint and muscle pain, decreased ROM, erythema, and local warmth near a joint.[87] Heterotopic ossification can lead to contractures, pressure sores, and impaired mobility skills and ability to perform ADL.

Management of ectopic bone formation utilizes several approaches, including pharmacological management, physical therapy, and, with severe activity limitations, surgery. Nonsteriodal anti-inflammatory medications are effective in preventing the formation of HO. Pulse low-intensity electromagnetic field may also be an effective method to prevent HO formation. Bisphosphonates are an effective pharmacological intervention, but are most effective when used early when radiographs may still be normal.[87] Finally, surgical excision is used when HO causes extreme limitations in activities and social participation.

Osteoporosis and Skeletal Fracture

Individuals with SCI may experience significant loss of bone both early after injury and long term. There is a rapid bone mineral loss in the first 4 to 6 months after injury. Bone mineral density (BMD) continues to decrease up to 3 years after injury; however, this may continue longer.[88,89] Although the exact etiology is not clear, the reduction in bone mineral density is thought to be due primarily to combination of no (or limited) muscle action and limited (or no) weight-bearing.[88,89] It is most common in the LEs, although osteoporosis may also occur in the UEs in people with cervical SCIs.

The reduction in BMD places people with SCI at a significant risk for fracture. Fracture incidence may be as high as 46%.[88] Risk factors for fracture include female, lower BMI, complete injury, paraplegia versus tetraplegia, and longer time since injury.[88,89] Falls or a forced maneuver during a transfer, ADL such as dressing, and stretching are common activities that precipitate a fracture. The onset of fracture can also be nontraumatic.[90] Intervention strategies focus on prevention in the early stage after injury or limiting/reversing BMD loss once osteoporosis has begun. Bisphosphonate is used in the early and later stages to prevent and reduce BMD loss.[88] Rehabilitation strategies used to prevent or reduce BMD loss are functional electrical stimulation and weight-bearing activities either with a standing frame or orthotics and assistive devices. The effectiveness of these rehabilitation interventions is not fully established.[88,89] This may be associated with study designs that did not have subjects standing for long enough and/or standing without sufficient loading on the LEs.

■ PROGNOSIS

One of the most common questions that patients and families have after a SCI is how much recovery of motor function will occur. The potential for recovery from SCI is directly related to the neurological level of lesion and completeness of the injury. An incomplete lesion (ASIA B, C, or D) is a good prognostic indicator of greater likelihood of recovery of motor function.[91,92] Even with complete lesions (ASIA A), 70% patients with cervical level injuries are likely to experience one level of motor recovery below the original neurological level.[93] Preservation of pinprick sensation at 4 months after injury in the LEs or sacral region is associated with a good prognosis for motor recovery at 1 year after injury.[94] Recovery of motor function generally plateaus around 12 to 18 months after injury.[92,95] Specific factors related to prognosis of walking ability are discussed below.

■ EARLY MEDICAL AND REHABILITATION MANAGEMENT IN THE ACUTE STAGE

Emergency Care

Management of SCI begins at the location of the accident. Techniques used in stabilizing, moving, and managing the patient immediately following the trauma can influence prognosis significantly. Rescue personnel must be adept at questioning and examining for signs of SCI before moving the individual. Signs of SCI after a traumatic event include paresthesias, lack of or impaired movement or sensation in the extremities, spinal pain, and altered cognitive status or level of alertness. When an SCI is suspected, efforts should be made to avoid both active and passive movements of the spine. If the injury caused a displaced fracture, further damage to the spinal cord can occur. Movement of the spine is minimized by strapping the patient to a spinal backboard or a full-body adjustable backboard, using a supporting cervical collar, immobilizing the head, and obtaining assistance from multiple personnel in moving the patient to safety.[96] These measures assist in maintaining the spine in a neutral, anatomical position and may prevent further neurological damage.

On arrival at the emergency department, initial attention is focused on stabilizing the patient medically with a primary emphasis on ventilation and circulation. Cardiac, hemodynamic, and respiratory status are closely monitored.[96,97] Diagnosis of SCI is based on the physical examination, neurological assessment, and imaging.[97] A complete neurological examination is performed once the patient is stabilized. Imaging studies assist in determining the extent of damage and plans for medical management.[96] Attention is directed toward preventing progression of neurological impairment by restoration of vertebral alignment and early immobilization of the fracture site.[97] A urinary catheter typically is inserted, and secondary injuries are addressed.[97]

High doses of methylprednisolone may be given early after the injury. The anti-inflammatory effect of this steroid may have an effect by lessening secondary damage due to the inflammatory process. A few large clinical trials have been done giving methylprednisolone within 3 to 8 hours after injury for 24 to 48 hours, with patients demonstrating improvement in motor and sensory function.[98-101] However, these results are somewhat controversial. It is not clear that the improvements in motor and sensory function directly result in improvement in mobility and ADL. Also, there may be serious complications associated with taking high doses of steroids over a prolonged time.[102,103]

Fracture Stabilization

The goal of fracture/spinal injury site management is to stabilize the spinal column to prevent further damage to the cord. Reduction and immobilization of spinal injuries can be achieved via conservative or operative methods. Indications for surgical stabilization are unstable fracture site, gross malalignment, cord compression, and deteriorating neurological status. Animal studies have demonstrated a beneficial effect of early surgical decompression.[104] In people with acute, traumatic SCI, early (within 24 hours) surgical decompression is recommended.[96] Approximately 60% of patients with SCI admitted to model SCI system centers underwent surgical stabilization.[105] Closed reduction is indicated for patients with cervical subluxation or fracture dislocation injuries.[106] It is achieved with the use of traction devices. Patients with thoracic or lumbar injuries that are managed conservatively without surgery require immobilization by positioning in a regular or rotating bed (Fig. 20.5).

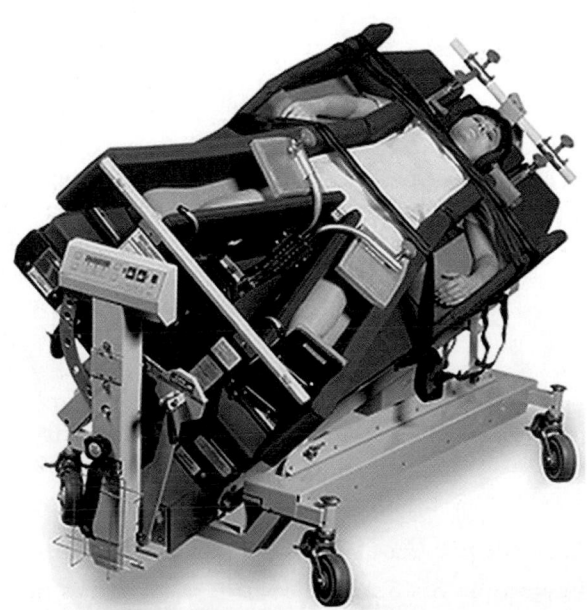

Figure 20.5 Roto rest bed. *(Courtesy of Kinetic Concepts, Inc., San Antonio, TX 78265.)*

Immobilization

Following reduction of the fracture site, through either conservative or surgical means, the spine is immobilized for a period of time through the use of spinal orthoses and recumbent positioning.

Cervical Orthoses

Halos are used commonly to immobilize cervical fractures after both open and closed reduction. This spinal orthosis (Fig. 20.6) consist of a halo ring with four steel screws that attach directly to the outer skull. The halo is attached to a body jacket or vest by four vertical steel posts. A halo is extremely effective at limiting cervical motion in all planes. The most common complication of a halo orthosis is loosening of the pin site. This can create instability at the injury site in the vertebral column or be a sign of infection. Skin breakdown may also occur under the vest portion of the halo.

Although a halo is an effective means of immobilizing and protecting the injury site, it can make learning mobility skills even more challenging. The orthosis limits shoulder motion and changes the user's center of gravity. This may cause patients to feel unstable. It can also make bed and wheelchair positioning difficult.

The **Minerva** is another type of cervical orthosis (CO) that also effectively limits motion in all planes (Fig. 20.7). Like the halo, because it provides excellent cervical stability, the Minerva allows for early mobility and rehabilitation after SCI. The sterno–occipital–mandibular immobilizer (**SOMI**) is another type of CO. It is less effective in limiting cervical ROM than either the halo or Minerva. There are a variety of cervical collars that can be used. Generally these

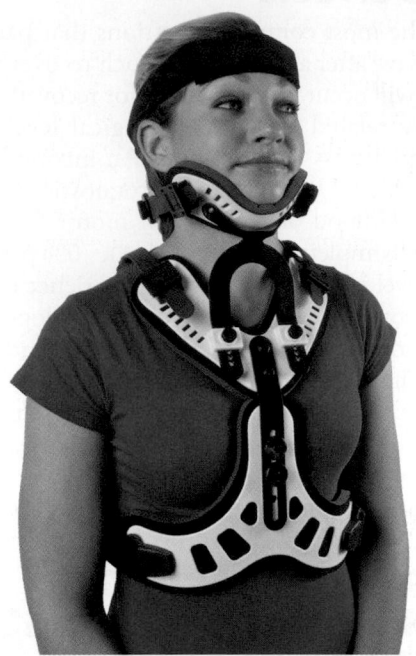

Figure 20.7 Minerva cervical orthosis. *(Courtesy of Cybertech Medical, BioCybernetics International, La Verne, CA 91750.)*

are constructed of semirigid foam and plastic and consist of two halves, which are held together with hook-and-loop closures. They do not effectively immobilize the spine. However, they may be used as transitional support following removal of a more rigid device (e.g., halo). Common types of collars include Philadelphia collar, Miami J collar, Aspen collar, and foam soft collar.

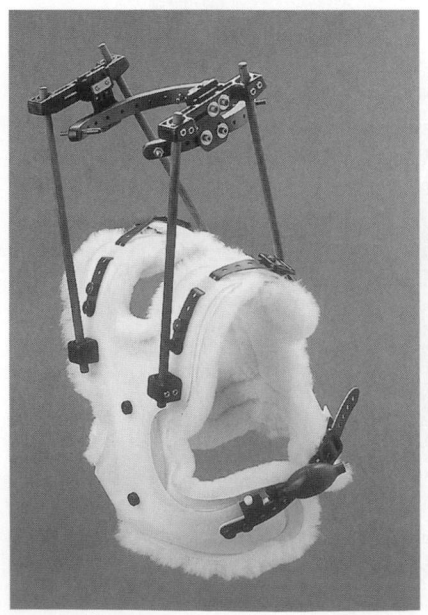
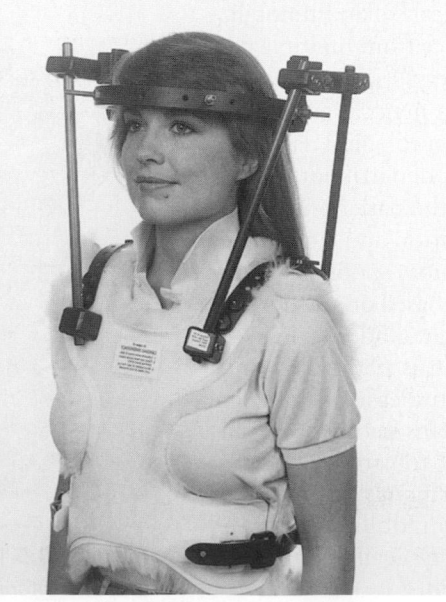

Figure 20.6 Halo orthosis. *(Courtesy of PMT Corp., Chanhassen, MN 55317.)*

Thoracolumbosacral Orthoses

A thoracolumbosacral orthosis (TLSO) is commonly used to immobilize the spine in patients with thoracic or lumbar injuries. A **TLSO** (Fig. 20.8) is made by an orthotist who takes a cast of the patient's trunk and makes the molded body jacket from the impression. Body jackets are typically bivalved and connected by hook-and-loop closures, which allows for removal during bathing and skin inspection. An extension is necessary with high thoracic injuries and low lumbar injuries in order to provide effective immobilization of the spine in these areas. A **Jewett** orthosis is a prefabricated device made of a metal frame and pads. The Jewett orthosis is not as effective for immobilizing the spine as a body jacket.

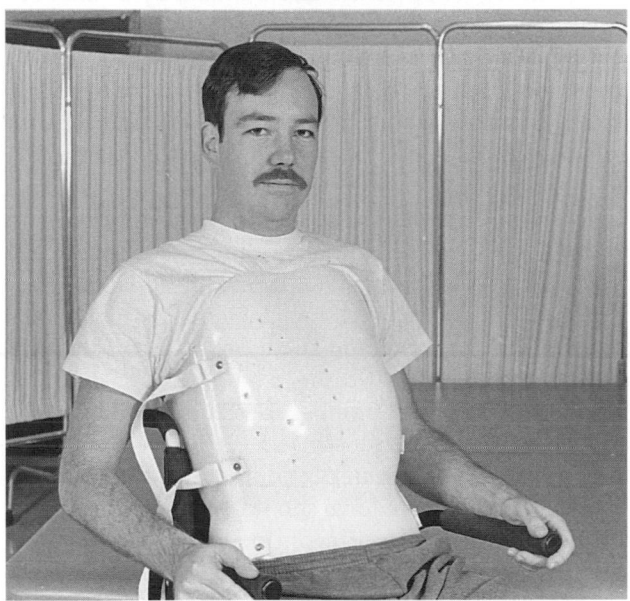

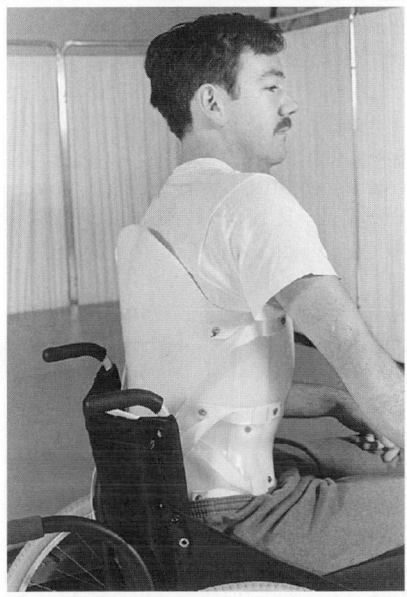

Figure 20.8 Anterior and lateral views of a thoracolumbosacral orthosis/plastic body jacket.

■ PHYSICAL THERAPY MANAGEMENT IN THE ACUTE STAGE OF RECOVERY

While hospitalized during the acute stage of recovery with immobilization in place, the patient may be on a period of bedrest. The primary goal of physical therapy is to prevent secondary complications, provide patient education, and begin early mobilization when medical clearance is received.

Physical Therapy Examination

Before beginning the initial examination, the patient must be sufficiently stable to undergo the examination and the therapist must be aware of any precautions. Spinal instability, orthotic devices, concomitant injuries, and need for medical support (e.g., ventilator) may preclude certain movements or positions. The primary areas of focus during this early stage of recovery are examination of sensory and motor function, respiratory function, skin integrity, PROM, and performance of early mobility skills.

Motor and Sensory Function

Motor and sensory function should be assessed using the ISNCSCI described earlier to determine the level of neurological injury (see Fig. 20.3). Care should be taken when performing manual muscle testing particularly if the spine is not yet stabilized or fully healed after surgery. Forceful contraction of muscles that originate from the spine may cause instability at the fracture site. Discretion should be used in applying resistance around the shoulders in tetraplegia and around the lower trunk and hips in paraplegia. In addition to testing the key muscles identified in the ISNCSCI, other muscle groups should be tested throughout the myotomes that have intact innervation. For example, if the C5 myotome is intact as indicated by normal strength in the biceps, then the strength of other muscles such as the deltoids and supraspinatus that are innervated by the C5 nerve root should also be determined. Standard techniques should be used for the manual muscle test (MMT)[107] and sensation (see Chapter 3, Examination of Sensory Function). Any alteration in testing position or procedure should be recorded.

Respiratory

The physical therapist should assess the strength of the diaphragm and intercostal muscles through observation while the patient is breathing.[49] Normally, the epigastric region should rise and the chest wall expands during inhalation while in supine. Contractions of the sternocleidomastoids and scalenes or paradoxical breathing patterns indicate weakness or lack of innervation of the diaphragm or intercostal muscles. Respiratory rate should be assessed while the patient is unaware that it is being done. Normal respiratory rate is between 12 and

20 breathes per minute.[49] To compensate for a weak diaphragm, the respiratory rate will typically increase.

Maximal chest excursion can be assessed using a tape measure with the patient supine. At both the level of the axilla and xiphoid process, the physical therapist should measure the chest's diameter at maximal exhalation and inhalation. Chest expansion measurements are the difference between chest measurements at maximal exhalation and at maximal inhalation. Normal chest expansion ranges from 2.5 to 3 in (6.35 to 7.62 cm), and negative values are an indication of paradoxical chest motions.[49]

Vital capacity (VC) should be measured often during the early stages of recovery. Vital capacity can be measured with a handheld spirometer and is strongly related to other measures of pulmonary function.[108] Forced vital capacity and volume of pulmonary secretion and gas exchange are predictive of airway management.[109] Typically, VC is approximately less than 25% of normal in individuals with high cervical lesions (above C3), 25% to 50% in mid cervical lesions, 50% to 75% in lower cervical and upper thoracic lesions, and 70% to 80% in mid to lower thoracic lesions.[49,50,110,111]

Owing to lack of full abdominal musculature innervation in many people with SCI, respiratory capability changes when the patient is sitting compared to supine. In sitting, the lack of abdominal muscle innervation causes abdominal contents to fall forward and pull down on the central tendon. This changes the motion of the diaphragm when it contracts during inspiration resulting in an inefficient breathing pattern.[112] The lack of full abdominal muscle function also impairs the ability to cough and clear the airway.

The ability to effectively cough is vital for the removal of secretions. The abdominal muscles are the major contributors to generating enough force to expel secretions or foreign objects. Cough function can be categorized into three types: functional cough, weak functional cough, and nonfunctional cough.[49,113] A *functional cough* is loud and forceful and the patient is able to generate two or more coughs with one exhalation. In this case the patient is able to clear all respiratory secretions. A *weak functional cough* is soft and the patient is only able to generate one per exhalation. The patient can clear small amounts of secretions and clear the throat. A *nonfunctional cough* is not a true cough; it is a clearing of the throat and has no expulsive force. In this case, assistance is needed to clear secretions from the airway.

Integument

During the acute phase, meticulous and regular skin inspection is a shared responsibility of the patient and the entire medical/rehabilitative team. As management progresses into the active rehabilitation phase, the patient will gradually assume greater responsibility for this activity. Patient education related to skin care is crucial and should be initiated early. The patient may view frequent position changes and skin inspection as bothersome or distracting from sleep if there is not adequate awareness of the importance and purpose of these activities.

Assessment for pressure ulcers should combine both direct skin inspection, which combines both visual observation and palpation, with assessment of risk factors. The patient's entire body should be observed regularly with particular attention to areas most susceptible to pressure (Table 20.4). Palpation is useful for identifying skin temperature changes that may be indicative of a hyperemic reaction. This is particularly important in examining individuals with dark skin, because early skin responses to pressure may not be readily apparent. Skin reactions to excess pressure include redness, local warmth, local edema, and small open or cracked skin areas. If the patient is wearing a halo, vest, or other orthotic device, contact points between the body and the appliance must also be inspected.

In addition to skin inspection, factors that increase the risk for skin breakdown should be considered. Spasticity, bladder or bowel incontinence, and nutritional deficiencies can increase the risk of developing skin ulcers. A number of specific scales can be used to assess the risk of developing a skin ulcer in people with SCI.[114] The Braden Scale is commonly used for a variety of patient groups who are at risk for developing pressure sores, including people with SCI.[114-116] The Braden Scale is more sensitive (75%) than specific (57%) and is easy to administer and has adequate validity.[114] The Spinal Cord Injury Pressure Ulcer Scale (SCIPUS) and SCIPUS-Acute were designed specifically for people

Table 20.4	**Areas Most Susceptible to Pressure in Recumbent Positions**	
Supine	**Prone**	**Side-lying**
• Occiput	• Ears (head rotated)	• Ears
• Scapulae	• Shoulders (anterior aspect)	• Shoulders (lateral aspect)
• Vertebrae	• Illiac crest	• Greater trochanter
• Elbows	• Male genital region	• Head of fibula
• Sacrum	• Patella	• Knees (medial aspect from contact between knees)
• Coccyx	• Dorsum of feet	• Lateral malleolus
• Heels		• Medial malleolus (contact between malleoli)

with SCI in acute care and in active rehabilitation.[114,117,118] The SCIPUS is more specific (84%) than sensitive (37%), whereas the SCIPUS-Acute is more sensitive (88%) than specific (59%). Both of these scales have adequate validity and are easy to administer.[114]

If a patient develops a skin ulcer there are a variety of tools that can be used to examine the wound.[119-122] The location, shape, size, and stage of the wound should be documented. A photograph of the wound on a grid is also an effective method of documenting the wound. Chapter 14, Vascular, Lymphatic, and Integumentary Disorders, provides more detailed information on wound examination.

Passive Range of Motion

Goniometry can be used to assess joint ROM. Shoulder ROM is particularly important for patients with tetraplegia. Depending on the motor level of injury, people with tetraplegia may require more than normal ROM to perform certain mobility skills,[113] and decreased shoulder ROM is associated with shoulder pain.[123] Hamstring length, hip extension, and ankle dorsiflexion are important to measure as well, due to the potential for contractures in these joints.

Early Mobility Skills

During this early phase of recovery, patients may have restrictions on certain motions and positions, as well as limited ability to tolerate an upright posture for extended periods of time (sitting or standing). A detailed, accurate, and specific determination of functional skills is usually delayed until the active rehabilitation stage when the patient is medically stable and cleared for activity. An initial screening of functional ability may be done during the early acute stage, but the therapist must be aware of any contraindications or precautions to movement necessitated by healing and potentially unstable fracture sites. Basic mobility skills that should be examined when appropriate are rolling in bed, transitioning supine to and from sitting, management of LEs, long and short sitting balance, and transfers. The section on active rehabilitation below has specific outcome measures that may be used to assess these and other mobility skills.

Physical Therapy Interventions

The extent to which the following interventions are implemented is dependent on the medical stability of the patient, stability of healing fracture and surgical sites, and status of other injuries that may have occurred during the initial event that caused the SCI. Full activity should be restricted until the fracture sites are stable and the patient receives clearance from the surgeon. The physician should be consulted regarding any rehabilitation activities that may place stress on the spine while the spine is still unstable. Although the interventions described below are usually initiated in the early stages of recovery, they should be continued throughout the rehabilitation process and be incorporated into the patient's lifestyle to manage the long-term consequences of the SCI.

Respiratory Management

Respiratory care will vary according to the level of injury and individual respiratory status. Primary goals of management include improved ventilation, increased effectiveness of cough, and prevention of chest tightness and ineffective substitute breathing patterns.[49]

Individuals with cervical injuries at and above C5 often require ventilatory support using an intermittent positive pressure ventilator (IPPV). Approximately 40% of patients with cervical injuries require mechanical ventilation, with most of these occurring in the first 3 days after injury.[43] Invasive mechanical ventilation is often done through a tracheostomy and can be provided through a stationary or portable ventilator. Noninvasive positive pressure ventilation provides an alternative to invasive mechanical ventilation.[48,124] Intubation may impair the function of the airway cilia, leading to chronic bacterial colonization and chronic inflammatory changes of the airway. Patients may also prefer noninvasive ventilation.

Deep-Breathing Exercises

Diaphragmatic breathing should be encouraged. To facilitate diaphragmatic movement and increase VC, the therapist can apply light pressure during both inspiration and expiration. Manual contacts can be made just below the sternum. This will assist the patient to concentrate on deep-breathing patterns even in the absence of thoracic and abdominal sensation. To facilitate expiration, manual contacts are made over the thorax with the hands spread wide. This creates a compressive force on the thorax, resulting in a more forceful expiration followed by a more efficient inspiration. Patients immobilized in traction devices or limited to recumbent positions may benefit from use of a mirror to provide visual feedback during these activities.

Glossopharyngeal Breathing

Glossopharyngeal breathing may be appropriate for patients with high-level cervical lesions who are dependent on a mechanical ventilator for ventilation, as well as for patients with mid to high cervical level injuries who are not dependent on mechanical ventilation.[125] Glossopharyngeal breathing utilizes the lips, pharyngeal muscles, and the tongue to inhale air.[125,126] The patient is instructed to take in small amounts of air, using a "gulping" pattern, thus utilizing available facial and pharyngeal muscles.[125] The patient repeats this 6 to 10 times. By using this technique, enough air is gradually inspired. Exhalation occurs due to the elastic recoil of the lungs. Glossopharyngeal breathing provides a method for individuals with high cervical lesions who are dependent on mechanical ventilation to breathe independently for a period of time in emergency situations[125] and as a way to increase vital capacity in people with cervical lesions who are not dependent on a mechanical ventilator.[127] Teaching a patient to perform glossopharyngeal breathing requires specialized skills and experience.[113]

Air Shift Maneuver

This technique provides the patient with an independent method of chest expansion. It involves closing the glottis after a maximum inhalation, relaxing the diaphragm, and allowing air to shift from the lower to upper thorax.[128] Air shifts can maintain and increase chest wall expansion. This technique may cause the patient to hyperventilate. The physical therapist should monitor the patient for dizziness and other signs of hyperventilation and allow for periods of rest as needed.[128]

Respiratory Muscle Strengthening

Similar to other muscles, strength training can improve respiratory muscle strength and endurance. Inspiratory muscles can be trained using relatively inexpensive handheld devices, which increase the resistive or threshold inspiratory load on muscles of inspiration (Fig. 20.9). There are generally two types of handheld inspiratory muscle

training devices: resistive or threshold trainers. Breathing through these devices increases the resistive or threshold inspiratory load on the muscles. The load can be progressively increased as the patient progresses. Inspiratory muscle training can improve pulmonary function, reduce dyspnea, and improve cough function.[129-131]

Coughing

Patients who are not able to produce a functional cough should be taught to perform a self-assisted cough. Those who cannot perform a self-assisted cough may benefit from a manually assisted cough to help remove secretions (Fig. 20.10).[132] To assist with coughing and movement of secretions, manual contacts are placed over the epigastric area. The therapist pushes quickly in an inward and upward direction as the patient attempts to cough.

Abdominal Binder

An abdominal binder may improve respiratory function[40,133,134] and cough ability[135] in patients with high thoracic and cervical lesions. An abdominal binder may improve respiratory mechanics by compensating for nonfunctioning abdominal muscles. The binder compresses abdominal contents to increase intra-abdominal pressure, and elevate the diaphragm into a more optimal position for breathing. In addition, abdominal binders may provide the secondary benefits of maintaining intrathoracic pressure and decreasing postural hypotension.

Manual Stretching

Mobility and compliance of the thoracic wall can be facilitated by manual stretching chest wall muscles in supine.[49,128] This is done by placing one hand around the side of the chest wall with the fingertips on the transverse processes and the other hand on top of the chest with the heel on the edge of the sternum. The hands are moved in a wringing motion. Pressure should be distributed across the surface of the hands.[128]

Wetzel[126] and Tecklin[128] provide an in-depth discussion of interventions to enhance respiratory function.

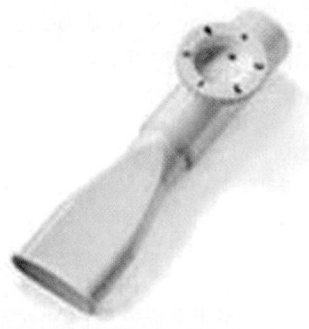

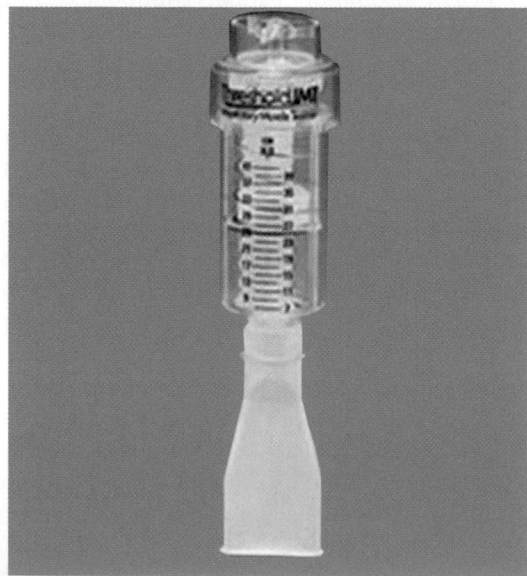

Figure 20.9 Inspiratory muscle trainers. *(Courtesy of Respironics, Inc., Murrysville, PA 15668-8525.)*

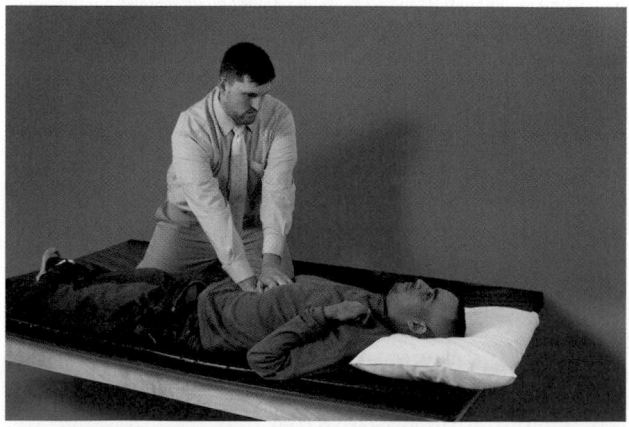

Figure 20.10 Assisted cough using abdominal thrust maneuver to clear secretions.

Skin Care

Prevention is the most effective intervention for skin care; this entails positioning, consistent and effective pressure relief, skin inspection, and education. Areas that are susceptible to skin breakdown (see Table 20.4) should be adequately protected when the patient is in bed by using pillows, foam, and positioning devices (Fig. 20.11). Positioning should also be used to prevent development of joint contractures and secondary pulmonary complications. Specific positioning of the UEs and LEs to prevent contractures will depend on the level of the SCI. Certain joints may be more prone to contracture depending on which muscles surrounding the joint are innervated. For example, a patient with a C5-level injury may tend to position the shoulder in adduction and the elbow in flexion. When positioning this patient the shoulders should be abducted and elbows extended when possible.

When in bed, patients should be repositioned at least every 2 hours.[136] Increased and consistent pressure over bony prominences, shear forces, heat, and moisture should be minimized. A variety of special beds, mattresses, and overlays can assist in the prevention of skin breakdown and aid with healing: foam, air, low air loss, air fluidized, and rotating (Fig. 20.12).

The wheelchair and seating system should also assist in promoting optimal positioning for reducing pressure

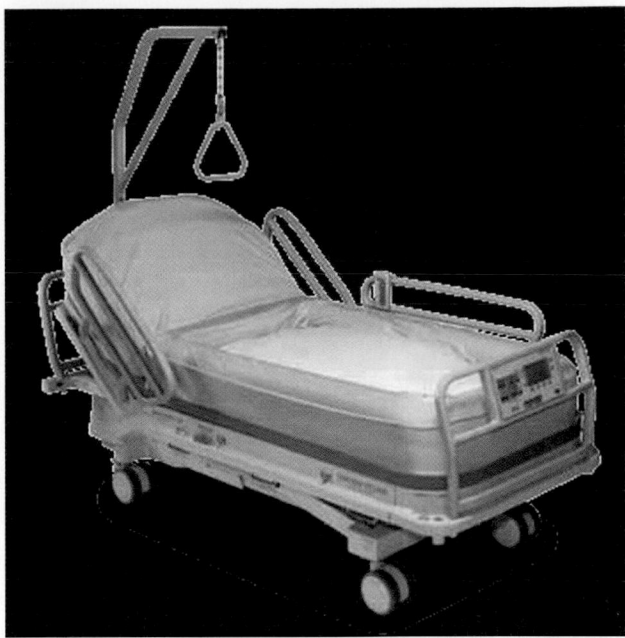

Figure 20.12 Air fluidized bed. *(Courtesy of Hill-Rom, Inc., Batesville, IN 47006.)*

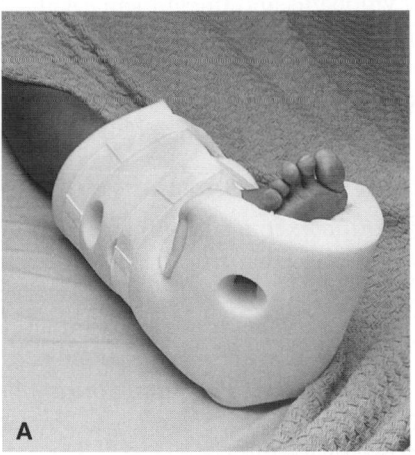

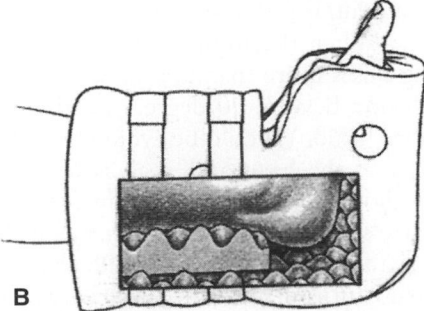

Figure 20.11 Ankle/foot positioning to prevent skin breakdown and contracture. *(Courtesy of DM Systems, Inc., Evanston, IL 60201.)*

and shear forces on susceptible areas. The pelvis should be positioned in a neutral position or slightly tilted anteriorly and be symmetrical (i.e., left anterior-superior iliac spine [ASIS] even with the right ASIS). A variety of wheelchair cushion types are designed to assist with positioning and redistribution of pressure. The main types of cushions are foam, gel, air, and flexible matrix. Cushions are often contoured to further assist in the redistribution of pressure and to reduce shear. No one type of cushion is the most effective. The exact type of cushion selected should be based on the individual patient. Chapter 32, The Prescriptive Wheelchair, provides more detail about different types of cushions, as well as their advantages and indications for use.

Patients should perform a pressure relief maneuver every 15 minutes when in the wheelchair, either with assistance or independently.[137] From the seated position, this can be done by using a push-up maneuver (Fig. 20.13), leaning to the side, or leaning forward (Fig. 20.14). If using a forward lean, the lean should be greater than 45 degrees.[138] Patients who are not able to perform these maneuvers initially can be assisted or their wheelchair can be tilted back. If tilting the entire wheelchair back, it should be tilted to at least 65 degrees.[138] All pressure relief maneuvers should be maintained for at least 2 minutes to be effective.[139] A tilt-in-space or reclining wheelchair can also be used to redistribute pressure.

The patient's skin should be routinely inspected to ensure there is no developing skin breakdown. Enhanced education on the prevention and management of pressure sores with consistent follow-up can reduce the development of skin breakdown and reduce the incidence recurrence.[140] As the rehabilitation program progresses,

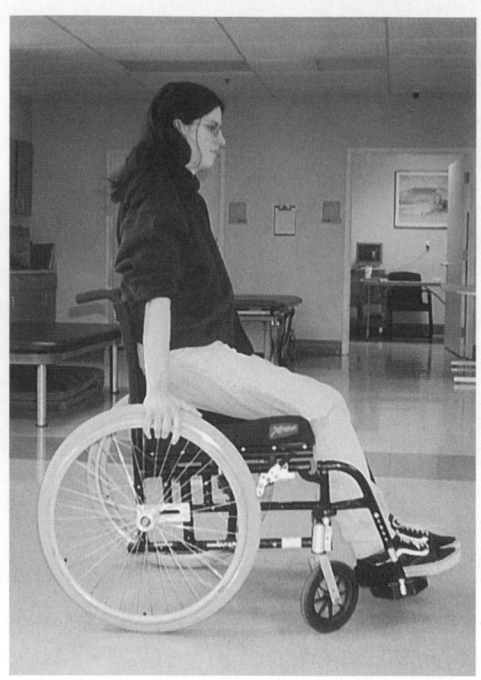

Figure 20.13 Push-up in wheelchair for pressure relief.

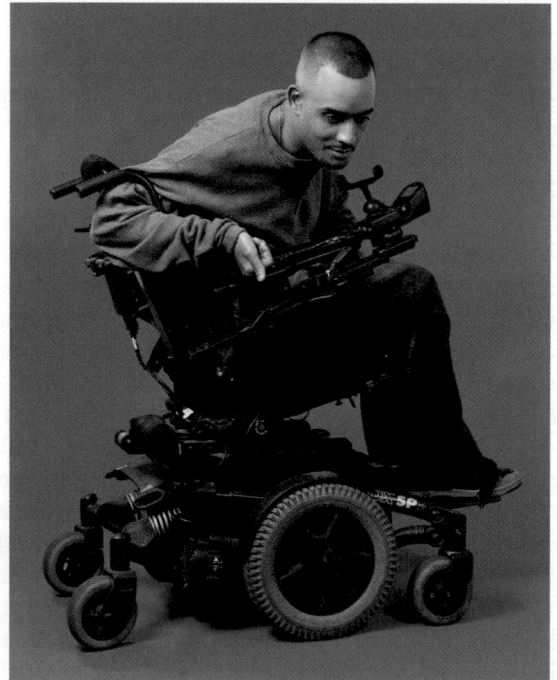

Figure 20.14 Lateral lean in wheelchair for pressure relief.

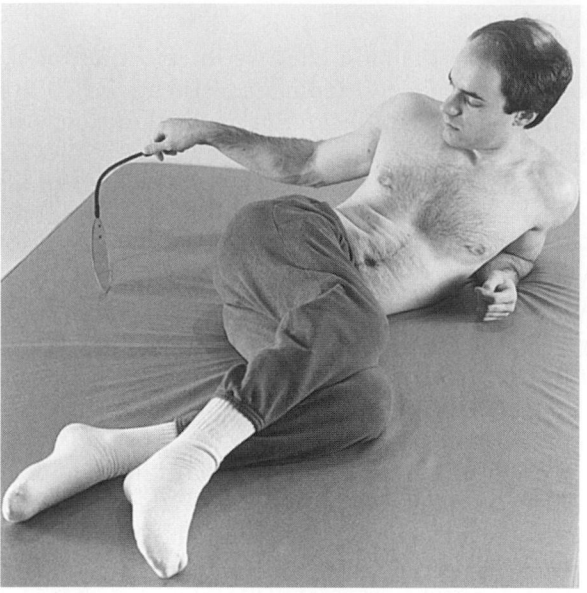

Figure 20.15 Skin inspection using a long-handled mirror.

the patient gradually assumes responsibility for skin care. Preparation for assumption of this responsibility will include patient education about the potential risks of pressure sores, the importance of hygiene, instruction in skin inspection techniques (Fig. 20.15), the use of pressure relief equipment and procedures, and what to do if a pressure ulcer develops.

If the patient develops a skin ulcer, the preventive measures described above should continue to be employed. Various therapies directed at wound healing should be initiated. Electrical stimulation,[141,142] hydrocolloid dressings,[143] and occlusive hydrogel dressings[144] can be used to facilitate the healing process. Chapter 14, Vascular, Lymphatic, and Integumentary Disorders, provides a comprehensive perspective on these and other specific wound healing interventions. The work of Sussman and Bates-Jensen[145] is also recommended for further information on wound care principles and management.

Early Strengthening and Range of Motion

Range of motion exercises should be completed daily except in those areas that are contraindicated or require selective stretching. In this early stage of recovery, ROM or strengthening exercises that are too intense may place increased pressure and stress on vertebral sites that may be unstable and are still healing. Motion of the trunk and some motions of the hip may be contraindicated depending on the location of the SCI. The pelvis should remain in a neutral position when ROM is performed on the LEs. When the injury is in the lumbar spine, straight leg raises more than approximately 60 degrees and hip flexion beyond 90 degrees (during combined hip and knee flexion) should be avoided. With tetraplegia, motion of the head and neck is contraindicated pending orthopedic clearance. Extreme caution should be used when stretching the shoulders. Generally, shoulder flexion and abduction beyond 90 degrees is contraindicated until orthopedic clearance is received indicating the spine is fully healed and stable.

Patients with SCIs do not require full ROM in all joints. Some joints benefit from allowing tightness to develop in certain muscles to enhance function.

For example, with tetraplegia, tightness of the lower trunk musculature may improve sitting posture by increasing trunk stability; tightness in the long finger flexors will provide an improved tenodesis grasp. Conversely, some muscles require a fully lengthened range. After the acute phase, the hamstrings will require stretching to achieve a straight leg raise of approximately 100 degrees. This ROM is required for many functional activities such as long sitting and LE dressing. Care should be taken not to overstretch the hamstring muscles because some tightness in this muscle group provides passive pelvic stabilization in sitting. This process of under-stretching some muscles and full stretching of others to improve function is referred to as *selective stretching*.

Positioning of the wrist, hands, and fingers is an important early consideration. Alignment of the fingers, thumb, and wrist must be maintained for functional activities or possible future splinting. Individuals with functional, active wrist extension can learn to use a tenodesis grasp to use the hand and fingers to perform ADL, manipulate objects, and hold objects without active finger control. The tenodesis grasp occurs through the biomechanics of the wrist and finger joints. When the wrist is actively extended, the tendons of the fingers are shortened causing the fingers to passively flex and grasp. When the wrist is flexed, the tension on the tendons is released and the hand opens providing release (Fig. 20.16) An *intrinsic-plus splint* can be used to position the wrist (20 degrees of extension), metacarpal phalangeal joints (80 to 90 degrees of flexion), interphalangeal joints (full extension or slight flexion), and the thumb (natural opposition) to maintain the joints in optimal intrinsic-plus position[146] (Fig. 20.17). This position helps reduce edema, preserve tenodesis function, and prevent contractures. As with any splint, the user's skin should be inspected for redness, irritation, or open areas and a progressive schedule should be used to slowly build up the wearing time to prevent skin irritation.

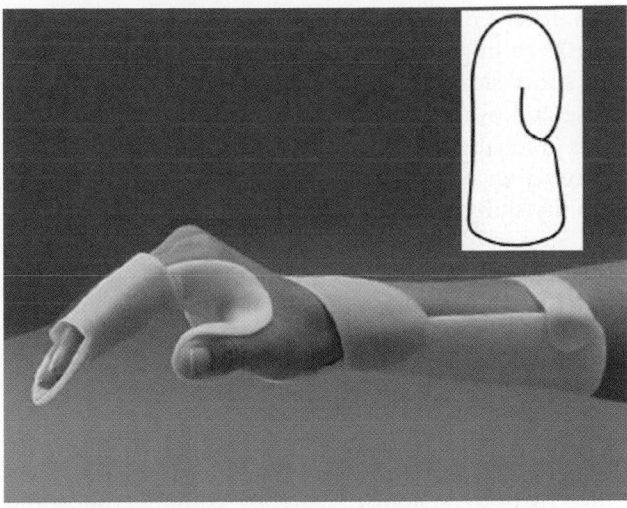

Figure 20.17 Intrinsic-plus splint. *(Courtesy 3Tailer, Charlotte, NC.)*

During the course of rehabilitation, all innervated musculature is strengthened maximally. However, during the acute phase certain muscles must be strengthened very cautiously to avoid stress at the fracture site. During the first few weeks following injury, application of resistance may be contraindicated to (1) musculature of the scapula and shoulders in people with tetraplegia and (2) musculature of the pelvis and trunk in those with paraplegia. Key muscles and strengthening techniques are discussed below.

Early Mobility Interventions

Once radiographic findings have established stability of the fracture site, or early fracture stabilization methods are complete, the patient is cleared for upright, functional activities. The patient typically will experience symptoms of postural hypotension (dizziness, nausea, ringing in ears, loss of vision, or loss of consciousness) when initially assuming sitting and standing (if able). A gradual acclimation to upright postures is necessary. The use of an abdominal binder and elastic stockings may reduce venous pooling and prevent orthostatic hypotension. During early upright positioning, elastic wraps may also be used in combination with (placed over) the elastic stockings.

Initially, upright activities can be initiated by slowly elevating the head of the bed and progressing to a reclining or tilt-in-space wheelchair with elevating leg rests. Use of the tilt-table provides another option for orienting the patient to a vertical position. Vital signs should be monitored carefully and documented during this acclimation period. If a patient experiences any of the signs or symptoms of orthostatic hypotension during sitting activities, the patient's legs can be elevated and the trunk reclined.

When the patient is cleared to participate more actively in therapy and is more acclimated to upright postures, specific training can begin on basic mobility

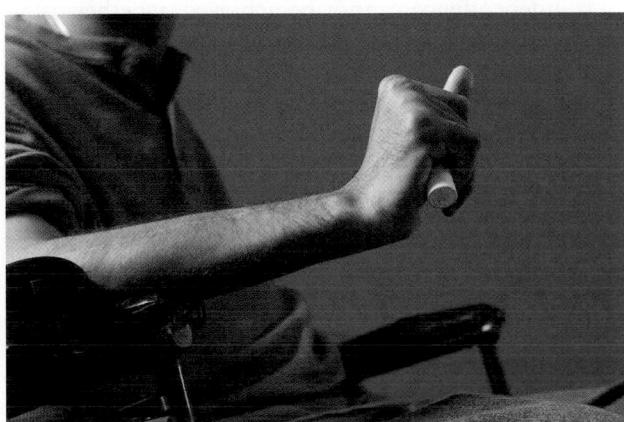

Figure 20.16 Patient extends the wrist, which causes the shortened long finger flexors to passively flex allowing a grasp.

skills. Interventions designed to teach bed mobility skills such as rolling and transitioning supine to/from long and short sitting and transfer skills can be initiated. These and other functional mobility skills become the focus of rehabilitation once the patient is stable. Specific intervention techniques on these and other functional mobility skills are discussed below.

Education

Living with a SCI requires significant adaptations and changes on the part of the patient and his or her family. In order to meet the challenges presented by a SCI, patients must fully understand all the consequences of the injury. Patient and family/caregiver education should begin early after injury about the impact of SCI on the different body systems, secondary complications, and prognosis. Later in the recovery process it may be particularly helpful to have the patient meet individuals with long-standing SCI who have completed rehabilitation and are functioning in the community to gain an appreciation of the impact of the injury on day-to-day life.

◼ ACTIVE REHABILITATION

The overarching goal of physical rehabilitation is for the patient to become as independent as possible and to achieve the functional mobility necessary for everyday living, work, and recreation. Independent mobility can be achieved in a way that (1) either uses new movement strategies to compensate for neuromuscular impairments; or (2) uses the neuromuscular system to accomplish the task with a movement pattern similar to that before the injury.[147,148] **Compensation** refers to use of an alternative or new movement strategy, or technology to compensate for neuromuscular deficits to accomplish a daily task.[149,150] **Recovery of function** refers to the restoration of the neuromuscular system so that the motor task is performed in the same manner as it was before the SCI.[147,149,150]

For instance, if a patient cannot actively flex the fingers to grasp a bottle due to weakness or paralysis of finger flexor muscles, use of wrist "tenodesis" is often taught as a compensatory strategy (Fig. 20.16). Active wrist extension simultaneously produces passive finger flexion and can be used to achieve a functional grasp. Knee-ankle-foot orthoses (KAFOs) may help a patient achieve the goal of standing, but do not have a therapeutic effect on retraining the neuromuscular system in the once familiar task of standing. Once the KAFOs are removed, the LEs cannot perform the task of standing. The braces compensate for the inability to activate antigravity LE muscles due to weakness or paralysis. The task of moving from sitting to standing with KAFOs entails the use of assistive devices and weight-bearing through the arms, further altering the preinjury movement pattern to accomplish the task. Transfers from a wheelchair to a bed that also incorporate weight-bearing through the arms and a *head-hips* movement strategy (the head

moves in one direction to move the hips in the opposite direction; see below) is another example of a compensatory behavior using a biomechanical advantage to achieve a functional goal in a new way. Focusing on recovery of the once familiar task of sit-to-stand would require a movement pattern including weight shift from the buttocks forward over the feet, a powerful activation of antigravity muscles to lift the body off of the chair, the head moving up and forward, and then full extension of the limbs and trunk to achieve standing without the arms weight-bearing.

How a goal is achieved (or expected to be achieved) is thus important in treatment planning and goal-setting. Historically, rehabilitation for persons after SCI has employed compensation strategies using muscles spared above the level of the lesion, substitution, novel movement patterns, and assistive devices/braces as the primary means for achieving independent functional mobility skills. Recent advances in our understanding of the neurobiological control of walking and in activity-dependent plasticity have provided the basis for new, alternative therapies that generate activity below the level of the lesion with the goal of recovery.[147] Our assumption that the spinal cord was simply a conduit for neural signals from the brain was incorrect. In fact, the spinal cord is quite responsive to the ensemble of sensorimotor information provided during task execution to generate a motor output. Activity elicited through such therapies (e.g., locomotor training, task-specific practice) is used to retrain the neuromuscular control required for function, then used in everyday activities, and finally integrated into daily use.[151-153]

Although both compensation and recovery-based approaches (activity-based therapies) are used in rehabilitation for SCI, compensation dominates current clinical practice. However, a large and expanding body of literature is providing new insights about integration of activity-based therapies into the clinic,[154-156] the potential for improving outcomes with combinatorial approaches,[154,157,158] and the impact on functional outcomes advancing recovery and quality of life.

If independence cannot be achieved, whether using compensation or recovery-based strategies, then the patient may be interdependent on others for assistance in accomplishing certain tasks of daily life (e.g., the patient with a complete high cervical lesion). The patient, family, friends, and caregivers receive thorough instructions and training in the knowledge and skills required for care of the individual's daily needs.

Physical Therapy Examination

All the examination procedures completed during the acute phase are continued during the active rehabilitation phase. Inasmuch as greater patient mobility is now allowed, more complete testing of muscle strength, ROM, and functional skills can be performed. However, the physical therapist should confirm that the patient is no longer on any movement restrictions (if so, the same precautions described earlier should be observed). A variety of standardized outcome measures and tests and measures are available to the physical therapist (Box 20.2). Some of the more frequently used tests and measures are discussed here.

Box 20.2 Commonly Used Outcome Measures and Tests and Measures Categories

Aerobic Capacity/Endurance

• A 6-minute arm test

Arousal, Attention, Cognition

• Mini Mental State Exam and the Montreal Cognitive Assessment

Environmental or Work Barriers
Gait, Locomotion, and Balance

• Wheelchair Skills Test, Wheelchair Circuit, Modified Functional Reach Test, Berg Balance Scale, Walking Index for Spinal Cord Injury, Spinal Cord Injury Functional Ambulation Inventory, 10-Meter Walk Test, 6-Minute Walk Test, Neuromuscular Recovery Scale

Integument

• Braden Scale
• Spinal Cord Injury Pressure Ulcer Scale
• Spinal Cord Injury Pressure Ulcer Scale–Acute

Motor Function

• Modified Ashworth Scale, Spinal Cord Injury Spasticity Evaluation Tool

Muscle Performance

• ASIA ISNCSCI, manual muscle test, handheld dynamometer

Pain

• Visual analog scale, International Spinal Cord Injury Basic Pain Data Set, Wheelchair User's Shoulder Pain Index

Range of Motion

• Goniometer

Self-Care and Home Management

• Functional Independence Measure, Spinal Cord Injury Independence Measure, Quadriplegia Index of Function, Capabilities of Upper Extremity Instrument

Ventilation

• Chest circumference with measuring tape
• Vital capacity with handheld dynamometer
• Respiratory rate

Work, Community, and Leisure Integration or Reintegration

• Craig Handicap Assessment and Reporting Technique, Assessment of Life Habits, and Reintegration to Normal Living Index

---

Aerobic Capacity/Endurance

A *6-minute arm test (6MAT)* can be used to assess aerobic capacity and cardiovascular endurance.[159] The 6MAT requires the patient to perform 6 minutes of submaximal cycling on an arm ergometer at a single, steady-state power output. It is a valid and reliable measure for people with either tetraplegia or paraplegia. Steady-state power output for clients with tetraplegia should be set between 10 and 30 watts depending on use of manual versus power wheelchair and activity level. For clients with paraplegia the power output should be set between 30 and 60 watts depending on gender and activity level.[159]

Arousal, Attention, Cognition

It is particularly important to screen patients for cognitive impairment because up to 60% of people who experience a traumatic SCI may also have a concomitant traumatic brain injury (TBI).[160] Although they have not been validated in people with SCI, the *Mini Mental State Exam* and the *Montreal Cognitive Assessment* are tools that could be used to screen for cognitive impairment.[161,162] If the physical therapist suspects that the patient has a TBI, the patient should be referred to a neuropsychologist or psychiatrist.

Environmental or Work Barriers

Because many people who experience a SCI will use a wheelchair as their primary means of mobility, it is essential that the physical therapist examine the patient's home and work environments to determine accessibility. Because structural modifications and/or additions to the home may be required to ensure patient safety and access, the rehabilitation team should perform a home evaluation early in the rehabilitation process (see Chapter 9, Examination of the Environment). Some general guidelines to allow wheelchair access are presented in Box 20.3.[113,163,164]

Gait, Locomotion, and Balance

Most individuals with SCI will rely on a wheelchair as their primary means of locomotion in the home and community. As such, it is important to examine the patient's ability to perform wheelchair skills. This includes setting and releasing the wheel locks, removing footrests and armrests, propelling the wheelchair on level surfaces, performing wheelies, ascending and descending curbs, and various other wheelchair skills necessary for independent mobility in the community. The *Wheelchair Skills Test* (Fig. 20.18) examines a wheelchair user's skills in performing 32 representative wheelchair skills.[165-167] The skills are categorized according to three levels that reflect difficulty and setting in which they will be performed: indoor, community, and advanced. The Wheelchair Skills Test can be used as a diagnostic measure to determine which wheelchair skills need to be addressed in therapy and to document improvement

---

Box 20.3   General Guidelines for Wheelchair Accessibility in the Home

- Ramp slope: 12:1 (12 ft [3.7 m] of horizontal distance for every 1 ft [0.31 m] of rise)
- Ramp width: 36 in (0.91 m)
- Ramp landings every 30 ft (9.1 m)
- No thresholds through doorways
- Lever-type door handles
- Door width at least 32 in (0.81 m)
- Open floor plan
- Tile or hardwood floors
- Wheelchair access to bathroom
- Toilet seat height same as wheelchair seat height
- Adequate clearance under sinks
- Insulated pipes
- Roll-in shower

---

during rehabilitation. The *Wheelchair Circuit* is another outcome measure that is designed to assess three aspects of manual wheelchair mobility: tempo, technical skill, and physical capacity.[168,169]

Sitting balance can be examined using the *Modified Functional Reach Test*.[170] For patients with iSCI who have some capability to stand and walk, balance can be assessed using the *Berg Balance Scale (BBS)*. See Chapter 6, Examination of Coordination and Balance, for a complete description of this instrument. Although originally developed for patients with acute stroke, it has been used extensively with older adults,[171] and the BBS has been validated in people with iSCI.[172,173]

Gait and walking ability should also be examined in patients with iSCI who maintain some ability to stand and walk. An observational gait analysis tool such as the *Rancho Los Amigos Observational Gait Analysis*[174] form can be used to identify gait deviations. See Chapter 7, Examination of Gait, for a complete description of this instrument. Identifying abnormal gait patterns will inform selection of additional tests and measures needed to determine the underlying impairments that may be causing the abnormal movements. This will also guide development of the POC.

The *Walking Index for Spinal Cord Injury (WISCI)* examines level of physical assistance, type of assistive device, and amount of bracing required to ambulate 10 meters.[175-178] Scores range from 0 (unable to stand or walk with assistance) to 20 (ambulates with no assistance, no braces, and no assistive device). The *Spinal Cord Injury Functional Ambulation Inventory (SCI-FAI)* (Fig. 20.19) is another outcome measure used to assess walking ability in people with iSCI.[179] It involves a 2-minute observational gait analysis performed using the patient's usual assistive device. Documentation includes the frequency and distances the patient typically walks in the home and community.

The *10-Meter Walk Test*[177,178,180] and *6-Minute Walk Test*[177,178,180] are reliable, valid, and responsive to change in people with iSCI. A change of 0.13 m/sec in gait speed is an indication that real change in walking speed has occurred. Gait speed is also able to distinguish between (predict) level of functional walking ability. People with iSCI who walk at 0.09 m/sec are likely to be supervised ambulators. Walking speed of 0.15 m/sec is an indication that the person can likely walk indoor but use a wheelchair outside the home. Walking speed of 0.44 m/sec is an indication that the person will likely use an assistive device or orthotic to walk in and outside the home. Finally, a walking speed of 0.70 m/sec indicates the person can walk in and outside the home without an assistive device or orthotic.[181] The minimal detectable change of the 6-Minute Walk Test is 46 meters.[180]

Motor Function

As described earlier, the ASIA ISNCSCI standards should be used to determine the level of lesion and intact motor function. The presence of spastic hypertonia should be assessed as part of the motor function examination. The *modified Ashworth Scale (MAS)* is commonly used to assess tone. The MAS is a 6-point ordinal scale that rates the amount of resistance to passive movement of the joint.[182] (See Chapter 5, Examination of Motor Function: Motor Control and Motor Learning, for a complete description of the MAS.) The *Spinal Cord Injury Spasticity Evaluation Tool (SCI-SET)* is a self-report measure of the impact of spasticity on everyday life activities. The individual rates how spasticity has affected 35 different areas on a 7-point ordinal scale that ranges from (3 (extremely problematic) to +3 (extremely helpful). Items include eating, sleeping, dressing, transferring, wheelchair use, social impact, ability to concentrate, and falls.[183]

Muscle Performance

Further MMT should be performed for all muscle groups that are innervated based on findings from the ASIA ISNCSCI. For example, if the biceps muscle is intact, then other muscles that are innervated by C5 such as the deltoids and rotator cuff muscles should be tested. Handheld dynamometry could also be used to examine muscle strength, including trunk strength.[184,185] There are several unique considerations when performing MMT for people with SCI. Patients often learn to functionally move joints by substituting intact muscle contraction for weak or paralyzed muscles. For example, supination of the forearm allows gravity to extend the wrist and lower abdominal muscles can substitute for hip flexion by causing the pelvis to tilt posteriorly. The physical therapist should carefully stabilize the proximal area to reduce substitution and palpate to ensure that the test muscle is contracting. Abnormal muscle tone

Wheelchair Skills Test 4.1
Manual Wheelchair - Wheelchair User

Name: _____

Date: _____ Tester: _____

Time start: _____ Time finish: _____

Scoring Guide	(see over for details)
✓	= pass, safe
✗	= fail, unsafe
NP	= no part (only for indicated skills)
TE	= testing error

Type of Test
❑ Objective - Capacity
❑ Questionnaire - Capacity
❑ Questionnaire - Performance

	Individual Skills	Capacity/ Performance	Safety	Comments
1.	Rolls forward 10m			
2.	Rolls forward 10m in 30s			
3.	Rolls backward 5m			
4.	Turns 90° while moving forward $^{L\&R}$			
5.	Turns 90° while moving backward $^{L\&R}$			
6.	Turns 180°in place $^{L\&R}$			
7.	Maneuvers sideways $^{L\&R}$			
8.	Gets through hinged door in both directions			
9.	Reaches 1.5m high object			
10.	Picks object from floor			
11.	Relieves weight from buttocks			
12.	Transfers from WC to bench and back			
13.	Folds and unfolds wheelchair			
14.	Rolls 100m			
15.	Avoids moving obstacles $^{L\&R}$			
16.	Ascends 5° incline			
17.	Descends 5° incline			
18.	Ascends 10° incline			
19.	Descends 10° incline			
20.	Rolls 2m across 5° side-slope $^{L\&R}$			
21.	Rolls 2m on soft surface			
22.	Gets over 15cm pot-hole			
23.	Gets over 2cm threshold			
24.	Ascends 5cm level change			
25.	Descends 5cm level change			
26.	Ascends 15cm curb			
27.	Descends 15cm curb			
28.	Performs 30s stationary wheelie			
29.	Turns 180° in place in wheelie position $^{L\&R}$			
30.	Gets from ground into wheelchair			
31.	Ascends stairs			
32.	Descends stairs			
	Total Percentage Scores			

Additional comments: _____

WST_M_WCU 4.1.15
February 15, 2012

Figure 20.18 Wheelchair Skills Test (WST) Version 4.1 Manual. *(Kirby, RL, et al. Retrieved October 25, 2012, from www.wheelchairskillsprogram.ca/eng/documents/FORM_WST_M_WCU_4.1.15.pdf, with permission.)*

SCI Functional Ambulation Inventory (SCI-FAI)

Name: Session: Date:

PARAMETER	CRITERION	L	R
A. Weight shift	Shifts weight to stance limb.	1	1
	Weight shift absent or only onto assistive device.	0	0
B. Step width	Swing foot clears stance foot on limb advancement.	1	1
	Stance foot obstructs swing foot on limb advancement.	0	0
	Final foot placement does not obstruct swing limb.	1	1
	Final foot placement obstructs swing limb.	0	0
C. Step rhythm (relative time needed to advance swing limb)	At heel strike of stance limb, the swing limb: begins to advance in <1 second *or*	2	2
	requires 1–3 seconds to begin advancing *or*	1	1
	requires >3 seconds to begin advancing	0	0
D. Step height	Toe clears floor throughout swing phase *or*	2	2
	Toe drags at initiation of swing phase only *or*	1	1
	Toe drags throughout swing phase	0	0
E. Foot contact	Heel contacts floor before forefoot *or*	1	1
	Forefoot or foot flat first contact with floor.	0	0
F. Step length	Swing heel placed forward of stance toe *or*	2	2
	Swing toe placed forward of stance toe *or*	1	1
	Swing toe placed rearward of stance toe.	0	0
	Parameter total		Sum /20

ASSISTIVE DEVICES		L	R
Upper extremity balance/weightbearing devices	None	4	4
	Cane(s)	3	3
	Quad cane(s), Crutch(es) (forearm/axillary)	2	2
	Walker	2	
	Parallel bars	0	
Lower extremity assistive devices	None	3	3
	AFO	2	2
	KAFO	1	1
	RGO	0	0
	Assistive device total		Sum /14

TEMPORAL/DISTANCE MEASURES			
Walking mobility (typical walking practice as opposed to W/C use)	Walks...		
	regularly in community (rarely/never use W/C)	5	
	regularly in home/occasionally in community	4	
	occasionally in home/rarely in community	3	
	rarely in home/never in community	2	
	for exercise only	1	
	does not walk	0	
	Walking mobility score		Sum/5
Two-minute walk test (distance walked in 2 minutes)	Distance walked in 2 minutes = ...	feet/ minute	meters/ minute

AFO: ankle-foot orthosis; KAFO: knee-ankle-foot orthosis; RGO: reciprocal gait orthosis; W/C: wheelchair.

Figure 20.19 Spinal Cord Injury Functional Ambulation Inventory,[179] with permission.

and spasms can cause involuntary muscle contractions or a muscle to appear stronger than it really is. Orthoses and spinal precautions may preclude the patient from assuming a recommended test position or forcefully contract certain muscles. The use of alternate (nonstandard) test positions should be documented.

Pain

Pain should be examined continually. A *visual analog scale* can be used to identify the intensity of pain. The patient rates pain on a scale from 0 to 10, where 0 is no pain and 10 is severe, disabling pain. There are also self-report measures of pain designed specifically for people with SCI. The *International Spinal Cord Injury Basic Pain Data Set* items have been modified for self-report use.[186] This self-report measure poses a series of questions related to impact of pain on various aspects of daily activities and life satisfaction, location of pain, intensity of pain, and duration of pain. The *Wheelchair User's Shoulder Pain Index* measures the impact of shoulder pain on transfers, self-care, wheelchair mobility, and general activities.[187,188] Wheelchair users rate the amount of pain they experience while performing different activities on a scale from 0 to 10. Total score ranges from 0 to 150, with higher scores indicating a greater impact of pain.

Self-Care and Home Management

One of the main goals of rehabilitation is to promote independence in functional mobility skills and self-care. In addition to wheelchair propulsion skills and possibly gait (discussed above), it is important to carefully examine the patient's ability to perform other mobility skills such as transfers, bed mobility, and ability to perform pressure relief. The amount of physical assistance, method of performing the task, verbal cues required, use of adaptive/assistive devices, environment, and degree of safety should all be carefully documented. In order to be truly independent with a task the patient must be able to complete the task safely, in a timely manner, without undue effort, in an open environment, in different environments, and consistently. It may be tempting to provide a small amount of assistance such as stabilizing the wheelchair while the patient transfers (to prevent sliding) and still document that the patient was independent with the bed-to-wheelchair transfer. However, in this case the patient was not truly independent with the task. The patient should be able to complete the task without the physical therapist present. However, the physical therapist must actually observe the patient performing the task because patients may overestimate their own ability.

The amount of assistance required to complete a task is commonly documented using definitions from the *Functional Independence Measure (FIM)*.[189-191] The amount of assistance is scored on an 8-point ordinal scale where 1 = total assistance (patient performs less

than 25% of the effort), 2 = maximal assistance (patient performs 25% to 49% of the effort), 3 = moderate assistance (patient performs 50% to 74% of the effort), 4 = minimal assistance (patient performs greater than 75% of the effort), 5 = supervision (patient requires verbal cues, setup, or stand by), 6 = modified independent (patient requires assistive or adaptive device), and 7 = independent. More information on the FIM is provided in Chapter 8, Examination of Function.

Several other SCI-specific outcome measures are available to examine self-care and home management. The *Spinal Cord Injury Independence Measure (SCIM)* was specifically created to assess function in people with SCI (Fig. 20.20). It is made up of 19 items divided into 3 subcategories: self-care, respiration and sphincter management, and mobility. Total scores range from 0 to 100, where higher scores indicate greater independence. The SCIM is valid, is reliable, and may be more responsive than the FIM.[192-194]

The *Quadriplegia Index of Function (QIF)* was developed to measure small but significant improvement in function in people with tetraplegia that are missed by other measures.[195] The QIF consists of 10 ADL items (transfers, grooming, bathing, feeding, dressing, wheelchair mobility, bed activities, bladder program, bowel program, and personal care). The last item, personal care, is a series of questions that examines knowledge of personal care areas such as skin, medication, and AD. The QIF is reliable, valid, and responsive to change.[194-196]

The *Capabilities of Upper Extremity Instrument (CUE)* is a questionnaire that assesses the ability to grasp, release, and lift, and wrist and finger actions, unilaterally and bilaterally.[197] Each item is scored on a 7-point ordinal scale where 1 is totally limited, cannot do at all and 7 is not at all limited. Total scores range from 32 to 224, where higher scores indicate better UE function. The CUE is reliable, valid, and responsive.[197,198]

Work, Community, and Leisure Integration or Reintegration

The ultimate goal of rehabilitation is to allow the individual to return to his or her normal roles and fully participate in society. Measures of participation provide insight into how the individual is functioning in the home and community. Some commonly used outcome measures are the *Craig Handicap Assessment and Reporting Technique*,[199] *Assessment of Life Habits*,[200,201] and *Reintegration to Normal Living Index*.[202]

Neuromuscular Recovery Scale

The *Neuromuscular Recovery Scale (NRS)* is an outcome measure used to assess the ability to perform a functional goal in the manner used by the intact neuromuscular system before injury and without compensation.[148,153] In comparison, the FIM assesses whether a functional task can be accomplished and how much assistance is required

Spinal Cord Independence Measure (SCIM)

LOEWENSTEIN HOSPITAL REHABILITATION CENTER
Affiliated with the Sackler Faculty of Medicine, Tel-Aviv University

Department IV, Medical Director: Dr. Amiram Catz

Patient Name:_____**ID:**_____ **Examiner Name:**_____

(Enter the score for each function in the adjacent square, below the date. The form may be used for up to 6 examinations.)

SCIM–SPINAL CORD INDEPENDENCE MEASURE   Version III, Sept 14, 2002

Self-Care   DATE

Exam 1 2 3 4 5 6

1. Feeding (cutting, opening containers, pouring, bringing food to mouth, holding cup with fluid)
  0. Needs parenteral, gastrostomy, or fully assisted oral feeding
  1. Needs partial assistance for eating and/or drinking, or for wearing adaptive devices
  2. Eats independently; needs adaptive devices or assistance only for cutting food and/or pouring and/or opening containers
  3. Eats and drinks independently; does not require assistance or adaptive devices

2. Bathing (soaping, washing, drying body and head, manipulating water tap.) **A–upper body; B–lower body**
  A. 0. Requires total assistance
  1. Requires partial assistance
  2. Washes independently with adaptive devices or in a specific setting (e.g., bars, chair)
  3. Washes independently; does not require **a**daptive **d**evices or **s**pecific **s**etting (not customary for healthy people) (adss)
  B. 0. Requires total assistance
  1. Requires partial assistance
  2. Washes independently with **a**daptive **d**evices or in a **s**pecific **s**etting (adss)
  3. Washes independently; does not require adaptive devices (adss) or specific setting

3. Dressing (clothes, shoes, permanent orthoses: dressing, wearing, undressing). **A–upper body; B–lower body**
  A. 0. Requires total assistance
  1. Requires partial assistance with **c**lothes **w**ithout **b**uttons, **z**ippers or **l**aces (cwobzl)
  2. Independent with cwobzl; requires **a**daptive **d**evices or in a **s**pecific **s**etting (adss)
  3. Independent with cwobzl; does not require adss; needs assistance or adss only for bzl
  4. Desses (any cloth) independently; does not require adaptive devices or specific setting
  B. 0. Requires total assistance
  1. Requires partial assistance with **c**lothes **w**ithout **b**uttons, **z**ippers or **l**aces (cwobzl)
  2. Independent with cwobzl; requires **a**daptive **d**evices or in a **s**pecific **s**etting (adss)
  3. Independent with cwobzl; does not require adss; needs assistance or adss only for bzl
  4. Desses (any cloth) independently; does not require adaptive devices or specific setting

4. Grooming (washing hands and face, brushing teeth, combing hair, shaving, applying makeup)
  0. Requires total assistance
  1. Requires partial assistance
  2. Grooms independently with adaptive devices
  3. Grooms independently without adaptive devices

SUBTOTAL (0–20)

Respiration and Sphincter Management

5. Respiration
  0. Requires tracheal tube (IT) and permanent or intermittent assisted ventilation (IAV)
  2. Breathes indpendently with TT; requires oxygen, much assistance in coughing or TT management
  4. Breathes independently with TT; requires little assistance in coughing or TT management
  6. Breathes independently without TT; requires oxygen, much assistance in coughing, a mask (e.g., peep) or IAV (bipap)
  8. Breathes independently without TT; requires little assistance or stimulation for coughing
  10. Breathes independently without assistance or device

6. Sphincter Management—Bladder
  0. Indwelling catheter
  3. Residual urine volume (RUV) >100cc; no regular catheterization or assisted intermittent catheterization
  6. RUV <100cc or intermittent self-catheterization; needs assistance for applying drainage instrument
  9. Intermittent self-catheterization; uses external drainage instrument; does not need assistance for applying
  11. Intermittent self-catheterization; continent between catheterizations; does not use external drainage instrument
  13. RUV <100cc; needs only external urine drainage; no assistance is reequired for drainage
  15. RUV <100cc; continent; does not use external drainage instrument

7. Sphincter Management—Bowel
  0. Irregular timing or very low frequency (less than once on 3 days) of bowel movements
  5. Regular timing, but requires assistance (e.g., for applying suppository); rare accidents (less than twice a month)
  8. Regular bowel movements, without assistance; rare accidents (less than twice a month)
  10. Regular bowel movements, without assistance; no accidents

8. Use of Toilet (perineal hygiene, adjustment of clothes before/after, use of napkins or diapers).
  0. Requires total assistance
  1. Requires partial assistance; does not clean self
  2. Requires partial assistance; cleans self independently
  4. Uses toilet independently in all tasks but needs adaptive devices or special setting (e.g., bars)
  5. Uses toilet independently; does not require adaptive devices or special setting

SUBTOTAL (0–40)

Figure 20.20 Spinal Cord Injury Independence Measure,[192-194] with permission. *(From Topics in Spinal Cord Injury Rehabilitation 4(1):20, 1998. Thomas Land Publishers. Available at www.thomasland.com.)*

DATE — Exam 1 2 3 4 5 6

Mobility (room and toilet)

9. Mobility in Bed and Action to Prevent Pressure Sores
- 0. Needs assistance in all activities: turning upper body in bed, turning lower body in bed, sitting up in bed, doing push-ups in wheelchair, with or without adaptive devices, but not with electric aids
- 2. Performs one of the activities without assistance
- 4. Performs two or three of the activities without assistance
- 6. Performs all the bed mobility and pressure release activities independently

10. Transfers: bed-wheelchair (locking wheelchair, lifting footrests, removing and adjusting arm rests, transferring, lifting feet).
- 0. Requires total assistance
- 1. Needs partial assistance and/or supervision, and/or adaptive devices (e.g., sliding board)
- 2. Independent (or does not require wheelchair)

11. Transfers: wheelchair-toilet-tub (if uses toilet wheelchair: transfers to and from; if uses regular wheelchair: locking wheelchair, lifting footrests, removing and adjusting armrests, transferring, lifting feet)
- 0. Requires total assistance
- 1. Needs partial assistance and/or supervision, and/or adaptive devices (e.g., grab-bars)
- 2. Independent (or does not require wheelchair)

Mobility (indoors and outdoors, on even surface)

12. Mobility indoors
- 0. Requires total assistance
- 1. Needs electric wheelchair or partial assistance to operate manual wheelchair
- 2. Moves independently in manual wheelchair
- 3. Requires supervision while walking (with or without devices)
- 4. Walks with a walking frame or crutches (swing)
- 5. Walks with crutches or two canes (reciprocal walking)
- 6. Walks with one cane
- 7. Needs leg orthosis only
- 8. Walks without walking aids

13. Mobility for Moderate Distances (10–100 meters)
- 0. Requires total assistance
- 1. Needs electric wheelchair or partial assistance to operate manual wheelchair
- 2. Moves independently in manual wheelchair
- 3. Requires supervision while walking (with or without devices)
- 4. Walks with a walking frame or crutches (swing)
- 5. Walks with crutches or two canes (reciprocal walking)
- 6. Walks with one cane
- 7. Needs leg orthosis only
- 8. Walks without walking aids

14. Mobility Outdoors (more than 100 meters)
- 0. Requires total assistance
- 1. Needs electric wheelchair or partial assistance to operate manual wheelchair
- 2. Moves independently in manual wheelchair
- 3. Requires supervision while walking (with or without devices)
- 4. Walks with a walking frame or crutches (swing)
- 5. Walks with crutches or two canes (reciprocal walking)
- 6. Walks with one cane
- 7. Needs leg orthosis only
- 8. Walks without walking aids

15. Stair Management
- 0. Unable to ascend or descend stairs
- 1. Ascends and descends at least 3 steps with support or supervision of another person
- 2. Ascends and descends at least 3 steps with support of handrail and/or crutch or cane
- 3. Ascends and descends at least 3 steps without any support or supervision

16. Transfers: wheelchair-car (approaching car, locking wheelchair, removing arm and footrests, transferring to and from car, bringing wheelchair into and out of car)
- 0. Requires total assistance
- 1. Needs partial assistance and/or supervision and/or adaptive devices
- 2. Transfers independent; does not require adaptive devices (or does not require wheelchair)

17. Transfers: ground-wheelchair
- 0. Requires assistance
- 1. Transfers independent with or without adaptive devices (or does not require wheelchair)

SUBTOTAL (0–40)

TOTAL SCIM SCORE (0–100)

Figure 20.20—cont'd

(i.e., burden of care). Other measures are used to examine the time to perform a task (e.g., 10-Meter Walk Test for walking speed). The FIM and 10-Meter Walk Test allow compensation as a movement strategy and only address whether a goal is achieved, but not how it is accomplished. Compensation may include the use of one's own body in an alternative manner, an assistive device or brace, or physical assistance to achieve a goal. The NRS uniquely examines how a goal is attempted (or achieved) and does not allow the use of compensation strategies during task performance. Thus, the gold standard for recovery is not whether a goal is achieved, but whether it is accomplished in the manner (i.e., behavioral pattern) used before injury. This scale is particularly important because therapeutic interventions for rehabilitation after SCI are now targeting recovery to preinjury status as opposed to compensation for injury-related impairments.

The need to examine recovery is further supported by the introduction of combinatorial approaches targeting restoration of function below the level of the lesion. Such approaches may combine a surgical, stem cell, or pharmacological intervention with a behavioral intervention to enhance the potential for neural plasticity. For instance, in a recent case study, an epidural stimulator was surgically implanted on the spinal cord and paired with locomotor training to activate the neuromuscular system below the lesion.[154] Neuromuscular recovery was the goal and thus could aptly be examined using the NRS.

The NRS (version 2011) is comprised of 14 motor tasks: 4 items are tested on the treadmill (TM) and 10 items are tested overground. The TM-based items include stand retraining, stand adaptability, step retraining, and step adaptability. These items are tested with the use of partial body weight support (BWS) and TM to afford an environment in which the capacity of the neuromuscular system to stand and generate steps can be determined in a safe environment. The capacity of the neuromuscular system is examined by noting the amount of BWS, TM speed, and manual facilitation required to achieve optimal standing and stepping (stand and step retraining) and independence from manual facilitation (stand and step adaptability).

Items tested overground include sit, reverse sit-up, sit-up, forward reach and grasp, overhead press, door pull and open, trunk extension in sitting, sit to stand, stand, and walking. Each item is evaluated along a continuum of performance from an inability to perform the task to full recovery by executing the task in the manner performed before injury. Each item is individually scored and a phase of recovery identified. An overall composite score of recovery is calculated based on several individual scores at the lower end of the continuum. Phase 1 is the earliest stage of recovery with the patient requiring use of a wheelchair and dependent on others for assistance. Phase 2 is the mid-stage of recovery with initiation of independent standing. Phase 3 is a later stage, and independent standing is observed and walking achieved, though with

compensation. Phase 4 is the final stage of recovery in which the patient demonstrates increasing endurance, speed, and adaptability to environmental challenges during walking while returning to preinjury activities without compensation. Therapists may use the NRS to identify specific goals for rehabilitation based on the patient's current phase of recovery for each task. The lagging items, the items least recovered (lowest on the continuum), may serve as a focal point for rehabilitation efforts.

Using "sit" as an example from the NRS, the goal is to assess the level of recovery of this specific functional task. Sitting entails no UE support and good posture of the head, shoulders, trunk, and pelvis. The continuum of recovery is from the inability to achieve good sitting posture without UE support to reaching greater than 10 in (25 cm) in forward and lateral directions with appropriate sitting posture and trunk/pelvis kinematics. Interim phases of recovery between the lowest and highest levels of recovery assess the ability to maintain sitting, sit with inappropriate posture, attain sitting, sustain sitting with appropriate kinematics, sit appropriately for at least 1 minute, sit appropriately indefinitely, sit appropriately while maintaining the arms at 90 degrees of flexion, sitting with forward and lateral reach less than 5 in (12.7 cm), sitting with forward and lateral reach 5 to 10 in (12.7 to 25 cm), and sitting with forward and lateral reach greater than 10 in (25 cm). Thus, with the NRS the therapist rates recovery of sitting via incremental advances in task difficulty with full recovery being the aim.

Prognosis and Goals

Functional outcome after SCI is dependent on many factors; primary among these, especially for individuals with complete injuries, is level of motor function. With complete lower-level lesions (i.e., more musculature intact), there is greater potential for independence in mobility tasks and ADL. With incomplete lesions (ASIA B, C, or D) there is greater functional potential as compared to ASIA A injuries; ASIA D injuries represent greater functional independence than that of ASIA B or C injuries. See Box 20.4 for other factors that can affect functional outcomes.[12,203-206] Table 20.5 provides a guide to expected functional outcomes for people with complete SCI based on level of injury. The physical therapist,

---

Box 20.4 Factors That Affect Functional Outcomes

- Motor level
- Age
- Concomitant injury
- Preexisting health conditions
- Secondary complications
- Body type
- Psychosocial support

Table 20.5 Functional Expectations for Patients With Spinal Cord Injury*

Motor Level and Key Muscles	Available Movements	Functional Capabilities	Equipment and Assistance Required
C1, C2, C3, C4			
Face and neck muscles, cranial nerve innervation, diaphragm (partial innervation at C3 and C4)	Talking Mastication Sipping Blowing Scapular elevation	Activities of daily living (ADL) Dependence in basic ADL (BADL) Activation of computer, light switches, page turners, call buttons, electrical appliances, and speaker phones	Dependent Environmental control units (ECU) Brain-computer interface (BCI) Adaptive equipment such as head or mouth stick *Full-time attendant required, directs care provided by attendants*
		Bowel and bladder	Dependent, directs care provided by attendants
		Wheelchair mobility and pressure relief in wheelchair	Independent with power wheelchair Typical components include adaptive controls such as head, chin, tongue, or sip-and-puff control Electronically controlled seating system (tilt and/or recline) Wheelchair cushion and head/trunk support Portable ventilator (depending on innervation of diaphragm) Dependent with positioning in wheelchair
		Bed mobility	Dependent Adjustable bed with pressure reducing mattress Directs care provided by attendants
		Transfers	Dependent, attendants use mechanical lift Directs care provided by attendants
		Ambulation	Unable
		Driving	Unable
C5			
Biceps Brachialis Brachioradialis Deltoid Infraspinatus Rhomboid (major and minor) Supinator	Elbow flexion and supination Shoulder external rotation Shoulder abduction and flexion to ~90°	ADL Feeding Grooming, washing face, and oral hygiene Bathing and dressing (dependent) Activation of computer, light switches, page turners, call buttons, electrical appliances, and speaker phones	Some assistance and/or setup required depending on the activity Mobile arm supports, deltoid aid Adapted utensils and splinting Adapted equipment (wash mitt, adapted toothbrush, and so forth) Dependent Adapted computer keyboard Hand splints Adapted typing sticks ECU *Part-time attendant required, directs care provided by attendants*
		Bowel and bladder	Dependent, directs care provided by attendants

Continued

Table 20.5 Functional Expectations for Patients With Spinal Cord Injury—cont'd

Motor Level and Key Muscles	Available Movements	Functional Capabilities	Equipment and Assistance Required
		Wheelchair mobility and pressure relief in wheelchair	Independent to some assist with manual wheelchair on level surfaces
			Requires plastic-coated hand rims/extensions
			Benefit from power-assist wheelchair
			Independent with power wheelchair using handheld joystick
			An electronically controlled seating system (tilt and/or recline)
			Wheelchair cushion and trunk support, dependent with positioning in wheelchair
		Bed mobility	Assistance to dependent
			Adjustable bed with pressure reducing mattress
			Bed rails and loops
			Directs care provided by attendants
		Transfers	Dependent, attendants use mechanical lift
			Directs care provided by attendants
			May be able to perform with assistance and transfer board
		Ambulation	Unable
		Driving	Independent with van with adaptive controls
C6			
Extensor carpi radialis	Shoulder flexion, extension, internal rotation, and adduction	ADL	Assistance to independent with setup and/or equipment
Infraspinatus		Feeding	Universal cuff, adaptive utensils
Latissimus dorsi	Scapular abduction, protraction, and upward rotation	Grooming, washing face, and oral hygiene	Adaptive equipment, universal cuff
Pectoralis major (clavicular portion)		Dressing	Upper body: independent with adaptive equipment
Pronator teres	Forearm pronation	Bathing	Lower body: assistance with adaptive equipment
Serratus anterior	Wrist extension	Home management	Assistance with adaptive equipment
Teres minor	(tenodesis grasp)		Assistance, may be independent with certain tasks with adaptive equipment (e.g., light meal prep)
			Part-time attendant required
		Bowel and bladder care	May be able to be independent with adaptive equipment, likely to require assistance/dependent
		Wheelchair mobility and pressure relief in wheelchair	Independent with manual wheelchair on level surfaces
			May require power wheelchair in community
			Requires plastic coated hand rims/extensions
			Benefit from power-assist wheelchair
			Independent with pressure relief in wheelchair

Table 20.5   Functional Expectations for Patients With Spinal Cord Injury—cont'd

Motor Level and Key Muscles	Available Movements	Functional Capabilities	Equipment and Assistance Required
		Bed mobility	Independent to some assistance with adaptive equipment (e.g., bed rails, loops, and so forth)
		Transfers	Independent to some assistance with transfer board
			Assistance with uneven transfers
		Ambulation	Unable
		Driving	Independent with car/van with adaptive controls
C7			
Extensor pollicus longus and brevis	Elbow extension	ADL	Independent
	Wrist flexion	Feeding	Independent with most ADL with adaptive equipment (e.g. shower chair, hand rails, button hook, adaptive utensils) and wheelchair-accessible environment
Extrinsic finger extensors	Finger extension	Grooming, washing face, and oral hygiene	
Flexor carpi radialis		Dressing	
Triceps		Bathing	
		Home management	Likely to require assistance with heavy household tasks
		Bowel and bladder care	Independent with adaptive equipment
		Wheelchair mobility and pressure relief in wheelchair	Independent with manual wheelchair in home and community with plastic-coated hand rims
			May need some assist with ramps, curbs, and uneven terrain
			May benefit from power assist
			Independent with pressure relief
		Bed mobility	Independent, may require adaptive equipment (i.e., bed rails, leg loops)
		Transfers	Independent, may require assistance between uneven surfaces
		Ambulation	Unable
		Driving	Independent with car with adaptive controls
C8			
Extrinsic finger flexors	Finger flexion	ADL	Independent
Flexor carpi ulnaris		Feeding	Independent in all ADL, may require adaptive equipment (e.g., shower chair, hand rails, reacher, adaptive utensils) for some tasks and wheelchair-accessible environment
Flexor pollicis longus and brevis		Grooming, washing face, and oral hygiene	
		Dressing	
Intrinsic finger flexor		Bathing	
		Home management	Better able to perform with less need for adaptive equipment due to improved hand function compared to higher cervical level injuries
		Bowel and bladder care	Independent with adaptive equipment

Continued

Table 20.5   Functional Expectations for Patients With Spinal Cord Injury—cont'd

Motor Level and Key Muscles	Available Movements	Functional Capabilities	Equipment and Assistance Required
		Wheelchair mobility and pressure relief in wheelchair	Independent with manual wheelchair in home and community
			Better able to propel on ramps, curbs, and uneven terrain due to improved hand function compared to higher cervical level injuries
			May benefit from power assist
			Independent with pressure relief
		Bed mobility	Independent, may require adaptive equipment (i.e., bed rails, leg loops)
		Transfers	Independent, may require assistance between uneven surfaces
			May be able to transfer from floor into wheelchair
		Ambulation	Unable
		Driving	Independent with car with adaptive controls
T1 to T12			
Intercostals Long muscles of back (sacrospinalis and semispinalis) Abdominal musculature (~T7 and below)	Improved trunk control with more caudal SCI Increased respiratory reserve Pectoral girdle stabilized for lifting objects	ADL	Independent
			Independent in all areas
			Generally tasks become easier and require less adaptive equipment to perform with improved trunk control with more caudal SCI
		Bowel and bladder care	Independent with adaptive equipment
		Wheelchair mobility and pressure relief in wheelchair	Independent with manual wheelchair in home and community
			Independent on ramps, curbs, and uneven terrain
			Independent with pressure relief
			Wheelchair mobility becomes easier and more efficient with improved trunk control with more caudal SCI
		Bed mobility	Bed mobility skills become easier and more efficient with improved trunk control with more caudal SCI
		Transfers	Independent
			Able to transfer from floor into wheelchair
			Transfers become easier and more efficient with improved trunk control with more caudal SCI
		Ambulation	Independent with physiological standing and ambulation for exercise over short distance in the home
			Assistive devices (e.g., forearm crutches)
			Orthoses: hip-knee-ankle-foot-orthosis (HKAFO), knee-ankle-foot orthosis (KAFO)

Table 20.5	Functional Expectations for Patients With Spinal Cord Injury—cont'd		
Motor Level and Key Muscles	**Available Movements**	**Functional Capabilities**	**Equipment and Assistance Required**
		Driving	Independent with car with adaptive controls
L1, L2, L3			
Gracilis	Hip flexion	Ambulation	Independent short distances in home and possibly community
Iliopsoas	Hip adduction		Many choose to use wheelchair in the community due to high energy demands of community ambulation
Quadratus lumborum	Knee extension		
Rectus femoris			
Sartorius			Assistive devices (e.g., forearm crutches)
			Orthoses: HKAFO, KAFO, AFO (depending on which muscles are innervated)
L4, L5, SI			
Quadriceps (L4)	Strong hip flexion	Ambulation	Independent ambulation in home and community (L4-level injury may elect to use wheelchair for long distances)
Anterior tibialis (L5)	Strong knee extension		
Hamstrings (L5–S1)	Knee flexion		
Gastrocnemius (S1)	Ankle dorsiflexion		Assistive devices (e.g., forearm crutches, canes)
Gluteus medius and maximus (L5–S1)	Ankle plantarflexion		
	Ankle eversion		Orthoses: AFO
Extensor digitorum, posterior tibialis, peroneals, flexor digitorum (L5, S1)	Toe extension		Less supportive assistive device and orthoses the more caudal the SCI

*This table presents general functional expectations at various lesion levels. Each progressively lower motor includes the muscles from the previous levels. Although the key muscles listed frequently receive innervation from several spinal levels, they are listed here at the key neurological levels where they add to functional outcomes. Although intact musculature plays a main role in determining functional capability, many other factors influence function, including concomitant injuries, premorbid health status, age, body type, and psychosocial factors. Individuals with an incomplete injury will likely have greater functional abilities.

rehabilitation team, and patient can use these expected outcomes to establish goals and outcomes. However, as mentioned above, factors other than motor level may affect functional recovery.

Goals should reflect what is important and meaningful to the patient. This will increase motivation, promote achievement of goals, and enhance patient autonomy. Early after injury patients are not likely to fully understand the consequences of a SCI and are still in the process of adjusting to the injury. It is important to educate patients on the impact of SCI and review the findings of the initial examination and all reexaminations. Potential functional goals should be discussed and the patient encouraged to suggest his or her own goals as well. Long-term goals should focus on activity and social participation, not body structure and function impairments. Goals should be specific in what the patient will achieve. The level of assistance, the environment/conditions, and the length of time to achieve the goal should all be documented.

Examples of general goals and outcomes for patients with SCI (Practice Pattern 5H) as adapted from the *Guide to Physical Therapist Practice*[207] are presented in Box 20.5.

For patients with high cervical SCI who may not be able to physically perform certain functional mobility tasks, goals should be directed toward the patient being able to independently direct an attendant caregiver to perform the task appropriately.

Recovery of Walking Ability

Recovery of walking ability is one of the most common goals expressed by people with SCI.[208] Individuals with complete (ASIA A) UMN injuries are not likely to regain the functional LE strength required to become independent ambulators.[209] In patients with iSCI (ASIA B, C, and D) the prognosis for recovery of walking ability is more complex. For individuals with ASIA B (sensory incomplete) the preservation of pinprick sensation is an important prognostic indicator of the recovery of

---

Box 20.5 Examples of General Goals and Outcomes for Patients With SCI

- Airway clearance is improved.
- Aerobic capacity is increased.
- Integumentary integrity is improved.
- Muscle performance is increased.
- Risk of secondary impairments is reduced.
- Tolerates upright sitting posture.
- Independence in ADL.
- Independence transfers.
- Independence in wheelchair propulsion.
- Independence in self-directing care.
- Independence with pressure relief.

---

walking ability.[94,210] Most patients with ASIA D and C SCI will regain some ability to walk.[211,212] Lower extremity ASIA motor score, quadriceps strength in particular, can be a useful predictor of functional walking ability in people with motor incomplete injuries.[213,214]

In 2011 the *European Multicenter Study on Human Spinal Cord Injury* published a clinical prediction rule for predicting ambulation after SCI.[215] In a cohort of almost 500 patients, findings indicated that age, motor scores of quadriceps and gastrocnemius, and light touch sensory scores at L3 and S1 were able to accurately distinguish between independent home ambulators (as scored on the SCIM) and those who require assistance or cannot ambulate. The clinical prediction rule was 96% accurate.[215]

As with any clinical prediction guide it is important to keep in mind that these factors should only be used as a *guide* to assist in the development of goals and the POC. Other factors such as psychosocial support, insurance coverage, and patient psychological status and motivation can affect outcomes. Additionally, new therapies may be developed that improve neurological recovery.

Physical Therapy Interventions

Improvements in body structure/function impairments, the ability to perform activities that are important to the individual, and a return to participating in normal, desired social roles can be achieved through interventions that are based on compensatory strategies, restorative strategies, or a combination of the two. In people with SCI the intervention strategy selected is largely based on the amount of preserved motor function. Independence in functional skills in patients with complete motor SCI (ASIA A and B) is largely achieved through compensatory mechanisms and interventions are developed accordingly. For example, a person with a C6 ASIA A injury is taught to transfer from bed-to-wheelchair using a sit pivot method. Patients with ASIA C or D SCI, depending on the degree of motor return, may relearn how to perform functional tasks using more normal movement strategies.

For example, a person with an ASIA D SCI may relearn how to walk through locomotor training using a BWS and TM system, an intervention that promotes normal movement patterns during gait training. This restorative approach attempts to minimize compensatory movement strategies and promote normal movement patterns to drive beneficial neuroplastic changes within the central nervous system.[216]

There are some common principles and precautions that can be applied to many interventions. Because SCI affects many different body systems, certain precautions must be considered when performing interventions (Box 20.6). Common principles used across compensatory intervention strategies to promote functional independence in mobility tasks are momentum, head–hips relationship, and muscle substitution. These strategies allow performance of functional mobility tasks through compensatory mechanisms that the patient may not be able to otherwise perform owing to loss of motor function and muscle strength below the lesion level. For example, a patient with a T1 ASIA A SCI will use momentum by swinging the arms across the body multiple times to roll from supine to side-lying to compensate for lost trunk or LE muscles that would normally assist in performing the task.

Motor learning concepts should be incorporated into the POC. In the early stages of motor learning, when the patient is not skillful and cannot perform the task independently, extrinsic feedback regarding task performance may be useful. For example, the physical therapist may provide tactile and verbal cues on correct hand placement on the hand rim when the patient is practicing and learning how to perform wheelies. Extrinsic feedback provided on a faded schedule promotes motor learning. In later stages of motor learning it is beneficial to have the patient use intrinsic feedback and rely less on extrinsic feedback. The practice schedule and environment can also be set up to promote motor learning. A random practice schedule is more beneficial to learning than a blocked practice schedule. The environment should be varied as the patient develops more skill in performing the task. For example, the patient should practice transferring to and from a

---

Box 20.6 Common Precautions to Take Into Account When Performing Interventions With People With Spinal Cord Injury

- Orthopedic/stress at the fracture site
- Skin integrity
- Blood pressure
- Fall risk
- Overstretching
- Overuse/stress

variety of different surfaces (e.g., wheelchair to/from mat, bed, chair, car, sofa, and so forth) once basic competence in the skill has been achieved. See Chapter 10, Strategies to Improve Motor Function, for a discussion of motor learning strategies.

For certain mobility tasks it may be beneficial to break down the task into component parts and practice parts of the task along with the integrated whole. For example, when learning how to move from supine to long sitting, practice can first focus on a component part such as transitioning to supine on elbows. The task can also be modified so that it is easier to perform initially. When first learning to roll from supine to prone, pillows can be placed along the patient's back so the starting position is already halfway toward side-lying. As the patient's ability improves the pillows can be removed. Assistive and adaptive equipment can be used to promote independence in functional tasks as well. A patient with a C5 ASIA A injury may be able to rise to long sitting using a trapeze or loop system suspended from the ceiling or foot of the bed.

Strengthening

As described above, strengthening innervated musculature is an important component of the physical therapy POC. Key UE muscles to strengthen include serratus anterior, latissimus dorsi, pectoralis major, rotator cuff muscles, and triceps brachii.[217-219] These muscles are important for independent transfers. Strengthening exercises should be performed 2 to 4 times a week, performing 2 to 3 sets of 8 to 12 repetitions at 60% to 80% of one repetition max.[220] Initially, strengthening exercises may be done daily during early rehabilitation. A variety of methods can be used to implement strengthening exercises: pulley systems, free weights, elastic bands, and weight cuffs. With very weak muscles (grade ≤2) strengthening can be performed in gravity-reduced positions on a powder board or with active assistive ROM. Strengthening can be done in functional postures as well. For example, push-ups can be performed in prone-on-elbows and supine-on-elbows.

Cardiovascular/Endurance Training

As with able-bodied people, cardiovascular training has important health benefits for people with SCI. A number of research studies have shown that endurance training can improve aerobic fitness.[221-224] Upper extremity–based exercises such as arm ergometry, wheelchair propulsion, and swimming are the most common method of aerobic training. In people with iSCI with sufficient walking capacity locomotor training on a TM with or without BWS is another method of endurance training.[225,226] The American College of Sports Medicine (ACSM) recommends endurance training 3 to 5 days a week, with a total duration per day of 20 to 60 minutes at 50% to 80% of peak heart rate.[220] The duration and intensity of the training should be gradually increased for those not able to initially tolerate these training levels. Surface Functional Electrical Stimulation (FES)–induced cycling or walking is also an effective means of improving cardiovascular fitness.[227-229] Surface electrodes are attached bilaterally to the hamstrings, quadriceps, and gluteal muscles; a computer controls the intensity of the muscle stimulation and cadence based on the position of the pedals (Fig. 20.21).[42]

Bed Mobility Skills

Bed mobility skills are necessary to promote independence in functional mobility. Bed mobility skills include rolling, transitioning supine to/from sitting on the edge of the bed, and LE management. Independence in these skills is also necessary for dressing, positioning in bed, and skin inspection. The degree to which these skills can be performed independently varies depending on the individual's level of injury and other factors (see Box 20.3). The exact method of performing the task will vary with the individual. The skills and intervention techniques described below provide a general guide; however, these may need to be adapted depending on the unique presentation of the patient. Also, as mentioned above, certain precautions need to be observed when teaching patients these techniques. For example, excessive friction on the elbows while weight shifting in prone-on-elbows may result in skin breakdown. Patients may begin training wearing protective elbow pads.

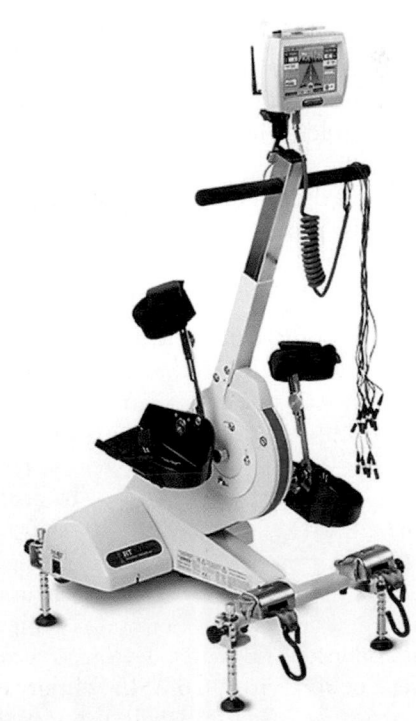

Figure 20.21 Functional Electrical Stimulation powered lower extremity ergometer. *(Courtesy of Restorative Therapies, Baltimore, MD 21224.)*

At first bed mobility skills are learned and practiced on an exercise mat, which is firmer and larger than a typical bed. However, as skill improves they should be practiced on a bed similar to that used at home. A patient may be independent performing these skills on a mat, but still require more practice to become independent performing the same task on a bed due to the softer and smaller surface.

Individuals with complete SCI will need to use compensatory movement strategies (e.g., momentum, muscle substitution, and head-hips principle) to move the entire body. For example, a patient with a T1 ASIA A injury will use momentum by swinging the arms up and across the body to generate momentum that will cause the trunk and legs to roll to the side-lying position from supine. A patient with a T10 ASIA A injury will use muscle substitution by using the UEs to lift the legs up onto the mat from a short sitting position when transitioning to supine from sitting. Individuals with iSCI may be able to use more normal movement strategies to perform these tasks. This will depend on the extent of motor recovery. Regardless of whether the injury is complete or incomplete, the recovery of normal movement patterns should be attempted and assessed (e.g., Neuromuscular Recovery Scale).

Rolling

Rolling is a frequent starting point of mat programs, and it is also a prerequisite skill for other bed mobility tasks and provides an early lesson in developing functional patterns of movement. It requires the patient to learn to use the head, neck, and UEs, as well as momentum, to move the trunk and/or LEs. It is usually easiest to begin rolling activities from the supine position, working toward the prone position. If asymmetric involvement exists, rolling should be initiated with movement toward the weaker side.

To develop maximum independence adaptive devices such as bed rails, ropes, canvas "ladders," or overhead devices such as trapezes should be avoided, if possible. However, if these adaptive devices allow more efficient or independent task performance or when the task cannot be otherwise accomplished, they should be incorporated into the overall POC. In addition, the patient should work toward achieving independent rolling when covered by sheets and blankets. To begin training and facilitate rolling, several strategies can be used:

- Flexion of the head and neck with rotation may be used to assist movement from supine to prone positions.
- Extension of the head and neck with rotation may be used to assist movement from prone to supine positions.
- Bilateral, symmetrical UE rocking with outstretched arms produces a pendular motion when moving from supine to prone positions. The patient rhythmically rocks the outstretched arms and head from side-to-side and then forcefully "tosses" them to the side to which the patient is rolling. The trunk and hips will follow (Fig. 20.22). The head and arms should be synchronized. Use of wrist cuff weights (2 to 3 lb) may be used initially to increase kinesthetic awareness and momentum. The number of rocking motions necessary will depend on the patient's skill, level of SCI, and body type.
- Crossing the ankles will also facilitate rolling initially (see Fig. 20.22). The therapist crosses the patient's ankles so that the upper limb is toward the direction of the roll (e.g., the right ankle would be crossed over the left when rolling toward the left). When first learning, flexing the hip and knee of the top LE and placing it over the opposite limb (e.g., the hip and knee of the right LE would be flexed and placed over the left when rolling toward the left) can assist.
- In moving from the supine position to the prone position, pillows may be placed under one side of the pelvis (or scapula, if needed) to create initial rotation

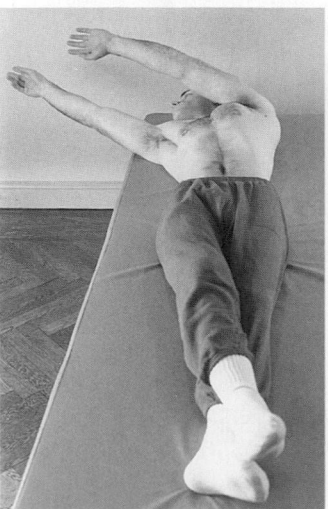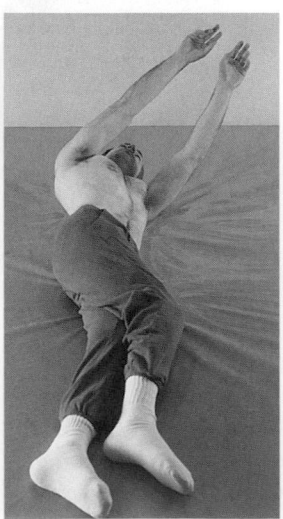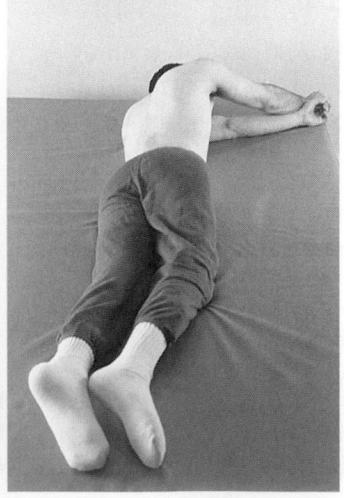

Figure 20.22 Rolling from supine to prone using UE momentum and crossing the ankles.

in the direction of the roll. The activity can be started with two pillows, progress to one, and then to rolling without the use of pillows. If difficulty is encountered in initiating the roll, the activity can be started from a side-lying position. To facilitate movement from prone to supine positions, pillows may be placed under one side of the chest and/or pelvis. Again, the number and height of pillows should be reduced gradually and eventually eliminated.

- Several *Proprioceptive Neuromuscular Facilitation* (PNF) patterns are useful during early rolling activities. The UE patterns of D1 flexion, D2 extension, and reverse chop will facilitate rolling toward the prone position. The UE lift pattern will facilitate rolling toward the supine position from side-lying.

Transitioning Supine to/from Sitting

The ability to transition from supine in bed to sitting on the edge of the bed is a critical skill necessary for independent mobility. Before a person can transfer out of bed to a wheelchair, the ability to sit up on the edge of the bed must be first achieved. There are two basic methods (with variations) to transition from supine to sitting: (1) "walking" onto elbows from prone or side-lying and (2) coming straight up from supine. Both of these methods transition the patient from supine to long sitting. The patient then must learn to manage the LEs to move into short sitting on the edge of the bed. In addition to rolling, two important prerequisite skills/postures that are necessary to come to long sitting from supine are the ability to assume and move within prone-on-elbows and supine-on-elbows.

Prone on Elbows

Prone-on-elbows can be assumed from either prone or side-lying. In prone, the shoulders can be either abducted (elbows out away from the body) or adducted (elbows at the side of the trunk) and the patient weight shifts from side to side while moving the unweighted arm to eventually position both elbows directly underneath the shoulder joints (Fig. 20.23A and B). From side-lying the patient pushes the elbow that is on the mat down into the mat by extending the shoulder, then swings the top arm forward while rolling to prone so the elbow comes onto mat in the prone-on-elbows position.

Transitioning into prone-on-elbows is a challenging skill, particularly for individuals without functioning triceps. The patient can be assisted into the position and practice stability and controlled mobility interventions initially.

- Weight-bearing in the prone-on-elbows position will improve strength stability at the upper trunk, neck, and shoulders.
- The PNF technique of rhythmic stabilization may be used to increase stability and strength at the head, neck, shoulders, and scapula.

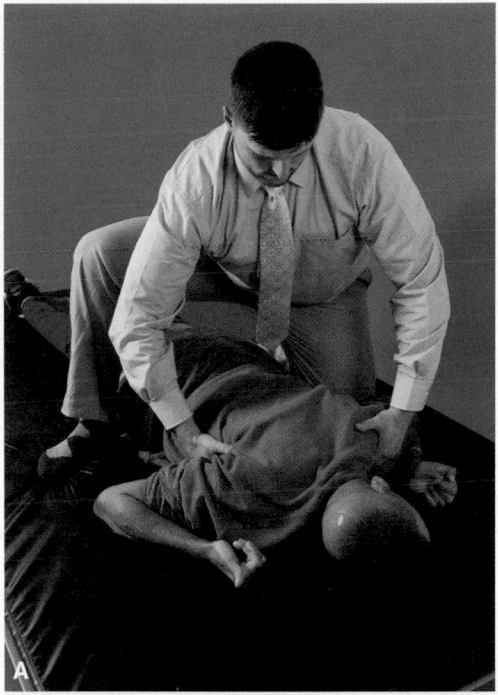

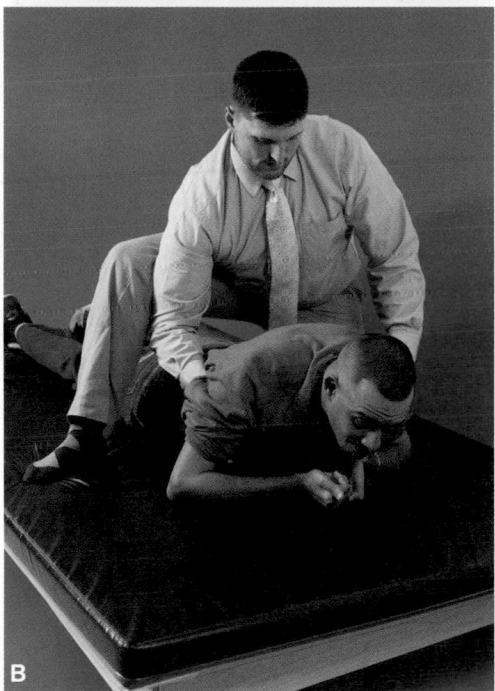

Figure 20.23 Transitioning from prone **(A)** to prone on elbows **(B)** with shoulders initially abducted and weight shifting.

- Weight shifting assists with development of controlled mobility and is usually easiest in a lateral direction with a progression to anterior or posterior movements.
- Unilateral weight-bearing on one elbow can be achieved in the prone-on-elbows position by having the patient lift one arm. This further facilitates co-contraction in the weight-bearing limb.

- Movement within this posture can be achieved by walking on elbows to both sides, up toward the head of the mat, and backward toward the foot of the mat.
- Strengthening of the serratus anterior and other scapular muscles can be achieved with prone-on-elbows push-ups. This is accomplished by having the patient push the elbows down into the mat and tuck in the chin while lifting and rounding out the shoulders and upper thorax (Fig. 20.24). This is similar to the "cat/camel" maneuver used in the quadruped position. The patient lowers the upper chest to the mat again by allowing the scapula to adduct.

Supine-on-Elbows

There are several approaches to assuming the supine-on-elbows position. If control of abdominal muscles is present, the patient may have sufficient strength to achieve the position by pushing the elbows into the mat and lifting into the position. A common technique is for the patient to "wedge" the hands under the hips or to hook the thumbs into pants pockets or belt loops. By contracting the biceps and/or wrist extensors, the patient can pull up partially into the posture. By shifting weight from side-to-side, the elbows can then be positioned under the shoulders (Fig. 20.25A, B, and C).

Some patients may find it easiest to assume this position from side-lying. The lower elbow is first positioned and pushed into the mat. The patient then rolls toward the supine position and quickly extends the upper arm, landing on the elbow as close to the shoulder as possible. By weight shifting, placement of the elbows can then be adjusted.

Much of the inherent benefit of this activity is achieved in learning to assume the posture and then move into long sitting. In addition to its direct functional significance, this activity is also an important strengthening exercise for shoulder extensors and scapular adductors.

- Rhythmic stabilization may be used to increase stability and strength at the head, neck, shoulder, and scapula.
- Lateral weight shifting can be practiced in this position.
- Side-to-side movement in this posture will enhance the patient's ability to align the trunk with the LEs when in bed or in preparation for positional changes.
- Precautions should be taken with this posture because it may cause increased shoulder pain due to the pressure exerted on the anterior shoulder joint capsule.

Walking on Elbows to Assume Long Sitting

From prone the patient walks on elbows toward one side into a "C" position. The patient then unweights the elbow closest to the legs and hooks it around the knees and pulls the trunk toward the legs. At a certain point the patient can then shift weight off the weight-bearing elbow to the palm and push with one arm while pulling with the other up to a long sitting position (Fig. 20.26A, B, C, and D).

This method of coming to long sitting does not require as much ROM in the shoulders as coming to sitting straight up from supine (see below). Practicing parts of the entire task, for example, walking on elbows or pulling up with one arm once in the "C" position, is a way to learn to the skill.

Coming Straight to Long Sitting From Supine

To come to long sitting from supine requires a more than normal amount of shoulder extension and strong elbow flexors. From supine the hands are placed under the hips or in pants pockets. By flexing the elbows from this position, the upper trunk is lifted off the mat. The shoulders are extended and the elbows placed in weight-bearing so that the patient is then in supine on elbows. From this position the patient unweights one elbow by shifting onto the opposite elbow. For the patient with a midlevel cervical SCI, the unweighted UE is thrown back into hyperextension and external rotation with the elbow extended so that the palm is on the mat. The patient then rotates the upper trunk onto the UE that was just thrown back in order to unweight the other UE. The unweighted UE upper extremity is now thrown back in a similar manner so that the patient is now weight-bearing on both hands, then weight shifts side-to-side and walks the hands up to assume a long sitting position (Fig. 20.27A, B, and C). Again, it is useful to practice parts of the task to assist in learning how to perform the entire skill.

Patients without sufficient strength or ROM, or due to other factors, may use adaptive equipment such as bed rails, loop ladder, suspended trapeze, or suspended loops to assist in coming to long sitting.

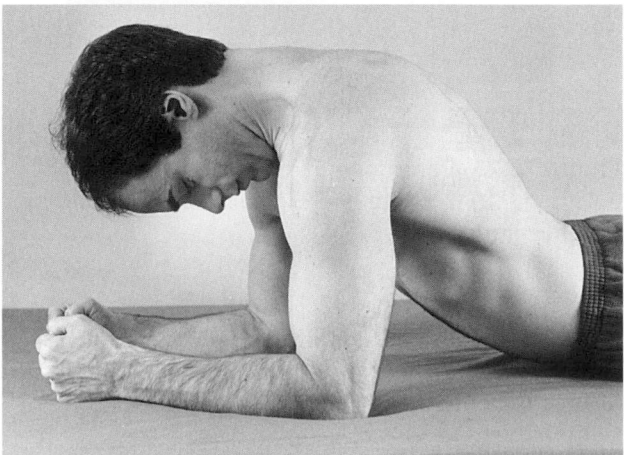

Figure 20.24 The prone-on-elbows position can be used to strengthen the serratus anterior and other scapular muscles.

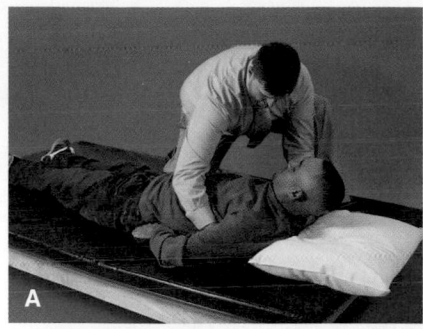
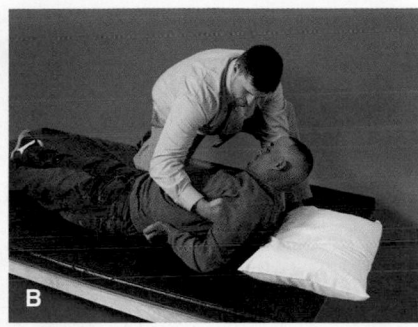
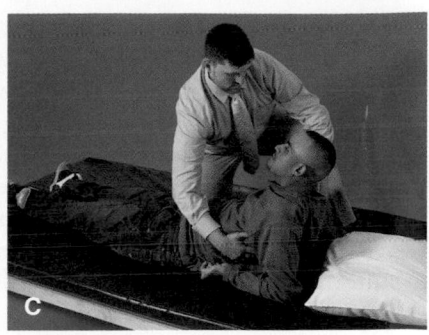

Figure 20.25 Patient transitioning from supine **(A)** to supine-on-elbows **(B)** by stabilizing hands under pelvis, forcefully pulling up by contracting the biceps, weight shifting side to side, and placing elbows further underneath the shoulder joints **(C)**.

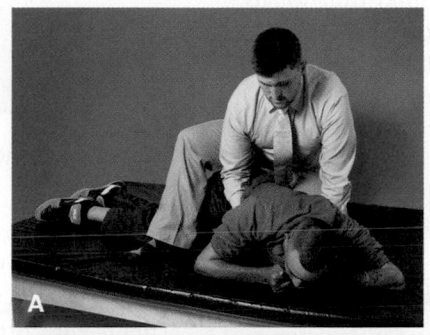
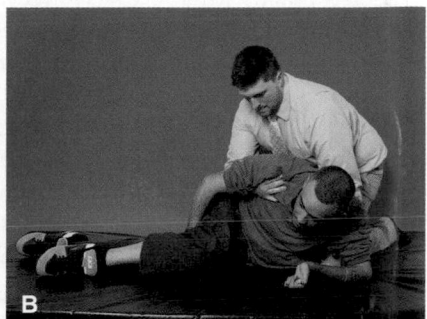
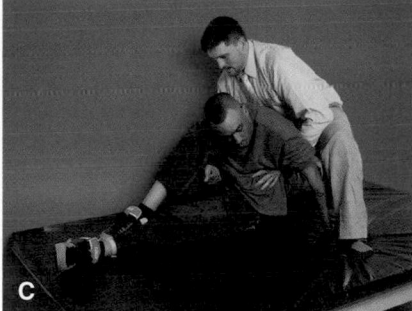
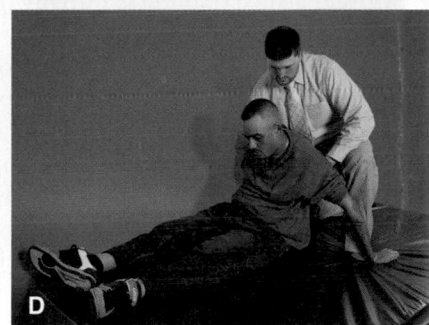

Figure 20.26 Patient transitioning from prone-on-elbows **(A)** to long sitting **(B)**; walks into a "C" position **(C)**, pulls trunk up to long sitting position **(D)**.

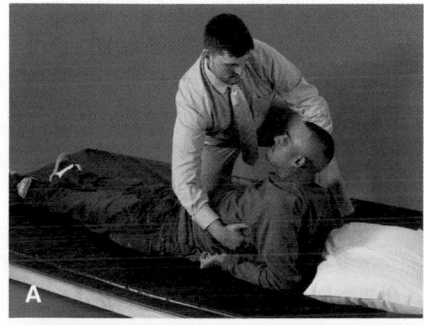
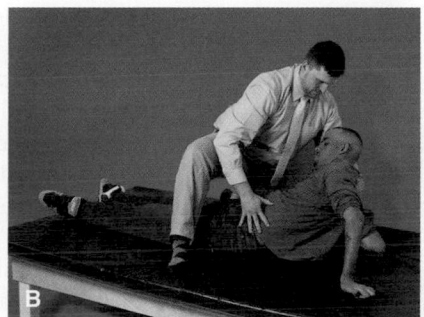
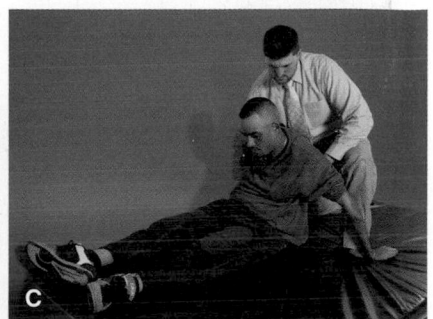

Figure 20.27 Patient transitioning to long sitting from supine-on-elbows **(A)**. Bears weight on one elbow while the other UE is thrown back into shoulder extension with the elbow extended to bear weight on the other UE **(B)**, then weight shifts onto the other UE and throws other UE back into shoulder extension with elbow extended to come into long sitting **(C)**.

Once in long sitting, patients must learn to move the LEs off the edge of the bed to come to short sitting, back onto the bed when moving from short sitting to supine, and to position themselves in bed using their UEs. Patients who do not have full finger and hand musculature innervation can slide the wrist under a leg so that the palm of the hand is facing the mat and extend the wrist to help move the legs. Alternatively, leg loops can be placed around the thighs to slide the hand in and extend the wrist to lift the leg.

Sitting Balance

Independent sitting balance, both in short sitting and long sitting, is an important skill for many different functional tasks such as transfers, dressing, and wheelchair mobility. Sitting posture will vary considerably with lesion level. Patients with low thoracic lesions can be expected to sit with a relatively erect trunk. Individuals with low cervical and high thoracic lesions maintain sitting balance by forward head displacement and trunk flexion (Figs. 20.28 and 20.29).

Due to the varying degrees of sensory and motor impairment patients need to relearn their center of balance, the limits of stability, and how to maintain postural control. The following are some suggestions that can be incorporated to improve sitting balance, both in long and short sitting.

- Sitting balance training is initially done by assisting the patient into a balanced short or long sitting position. In short sitting the patient should initially be positioned with the feet firmly supported on the floor and the hips and knees flexed to 90 degrees. In long sitting patients should have approximately 90 to 100 degrees of straight leg raise ROM to avoid overstretching the low back muscles. Initially, it is easier to maintain balance in long sitting due to the larger BOS. The LEs can be placed with the hips in external rotation and slight abduction to allow knee flexion to avoid overstretching the low back muscles.

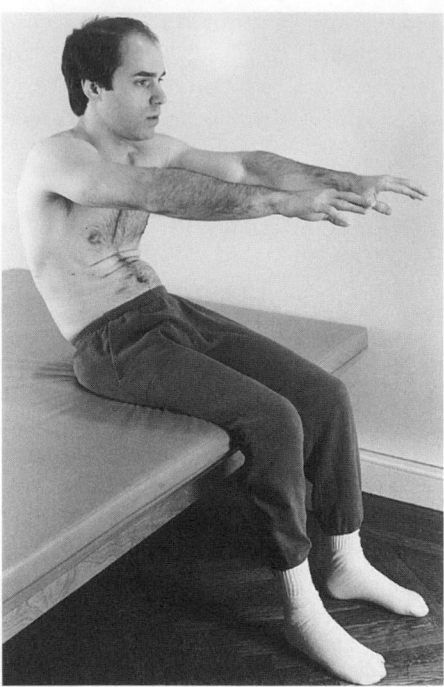

Figure 20.29 Individual with a T4 ASIA A injury in short sitting.

- Patients may initially need to bear weight through the UEs to maintain the sitting position. For patients with cervical level lesions who utilize a tenodesis grasp to hold and manipulate objects, the fingers should be flexed at the proximal and distal interphalangeal joints when the wrist is in full extension to prevent overstretching the finger flexor tendons. Patients who do not have triceps innervation need to learn to keep the elbows extended through muscle substitution. The patient throws back the shoulder into full shoulder extension while externally rotating the shoulder and supinating the forearm. When the UE is weight-bearing in this position the patient can contract the anterior deltoids to flex the shoulder in a closed chain, which will extend the elbow.
- Stability in sitting can be enhanced by providing manual resistance to the upper trunk using PNF techniques of alternating isometrics and rhythmic stabilization.
- Sitting practice should include altering UE support (bilateral, unilateral, with progression to no support). Reaching for objects with one and both UEs can improve anticipatory balance reactions. Patients should also practice maintaining postural control while manipulating objects and performing ADL in sitting.
- Patients should safely learn their new limits of stability. This can be accomplished by weight shifting until the point is reached where balance can no longer be maintained; close supervision/assistance is warranted.
- Providing unexpected perturbations in a safe manner can be used to practice reactive postural control.

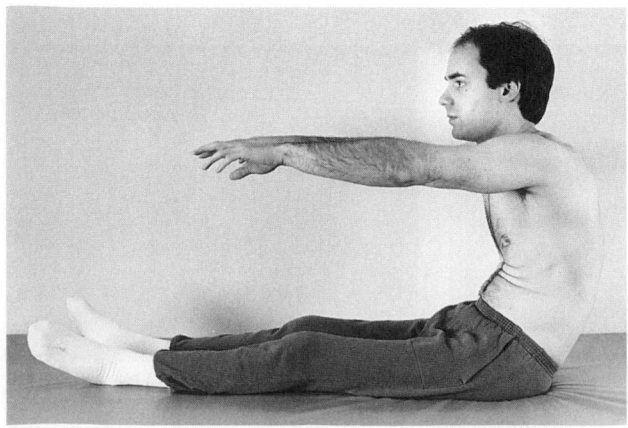

Figure 20.28 Individual with a T4 ASIA A injury in long sitting.

- Balance interventions should be practiced on a variety of surfaces: firm mat, bed, dense foam, sofa cushion, and so forth. Balance interventions should also be practiced while sitting in the patient's wheelchair.

Transfers

There are three components to the sit-pivot transfer (e.g., bed to/from wheelchair in a seated position): preparatory phase, lift phase, and descent phase.[230] During the *preparatory phase,* the trunk flexes forward, leans laterally, and rotates toward the trailing arm (Fig. 20.30A). The *lift phase* starts when the buttocks lift off the sitting surface and continues while the trunk is lifted halfway between the two surfaces (Fig. 20.30B). The *descent phase* denotes the period when the trunk is lowered to the other seated surface, from the halfway point until the buttocks are on the other surface (Fig. 20.30C).

The following are key components and intervention strategies to improve transfer ability:

- Provide support and assistance so the patient feels safe and comfortable while learning transfers.
- Confidence and skill in maintaining sitting balance is critical (see above strategies).
- The head–hips relationship is important. Moving the head and upper trunk in one direction causes the lower trunk and buttocks to move in the opposite direction. For example, if the patient wants to transfer from bed to the wheelchair, which is positioned to the patient's right, the patient rocks the head and upper trunk forward/downward and to the left. In combination with protracting the scapulae to lift the buttocks,

this will cause the lower trunk and buttocks to lift upward and swing to the right into the wheelchair.

- For patients without innervated triceps the strategies described above can be used to place and maintain the elbows in extension. For patients without full finger function, overstretching the finger flexors as described above should be avoided.
- Hand position is important. The hands should be positioned forward of the hips to form a tripod with the buttocks. Greater force is generated in the trailing UE[230,231] (UE furthest from the surface transferring to); if one UE is weaker or more painful it should be the lead UE. The lead UE should be further from the trunk/buttocks and the trailing UE closer to the trunk/buttocks.
- Using the head–hips relationship described above (leaning head and upper trunk forward and down), protracting the scapulae should be practiced to lift the buttocks off the sitting surface. The physical therapist can assist by placing his or her hands under the patient's hips and assisting the lift or by placing one hand on the front of the chest and the other between the scapulae to guide and assist the forward/downward lean and lift. Push-up blocks or wrist cuffs can be used initially to provide assistance to achieve a greater lift.
- Again using the head–hips relationship, practice should include lifting the buttocks and shifting laterally to the left and right. The patient should lean the head/upper trunk forward and downward, then twist to left or right to lift and shift the hips in the opposite direction. Patients may initially lift the hips and then twist the upper trunk to shift the lower trunk and buttocks in the opposite direction

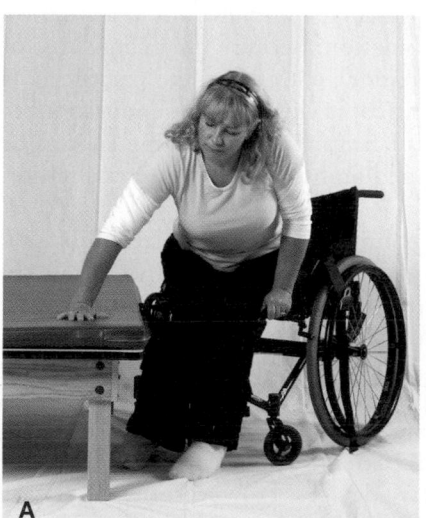 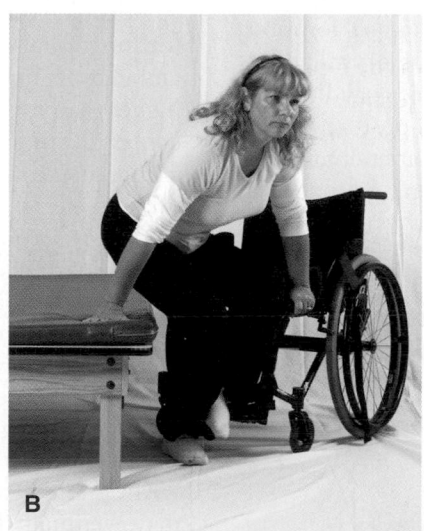 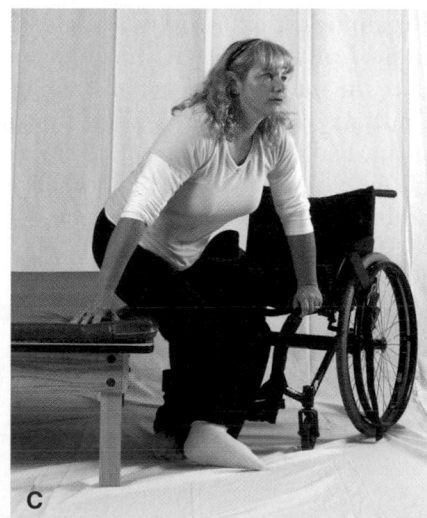

Figure 20.30 (A) Preparatory phase of the transfer; trunk is flexed forward and laterally away from surface transferring to. **(B)** Lift phase; buttocks are lifted off the seating surface as the trunk rotates. **(C)** End of the descent phase when the buttocks are on the other sitting surface. *(From O'Sullivan, S, and Schmitz, T: Improving Functional Outcomes in Physical Rehabilitation. FA Davis, Philadelphia, 2010, with permission.)*

in two motions. As the patient improves, these two movements should be performed as a single motion.

- Lower extremities should be positioned with the feet supported and the hips and knees at approximately 90 degrees of flexion or slightly more at the hips. The legs should be midway between the two surfaces so they do not block the movement of the trunk and body toward the transfer surface.
- Emphasis should be placed on lifting and shifting laterally instead of sliding/scooting to the side to avoid shearing of the skin. Control of movement should be promoted during the descent phase to avoid trauma to the skin. A transfer board may be used initially until the patient gains more skill with the task. Some patients with mid-cervical SCI may always require a transfer board.
- Transfer training should include a variety of surfaces from the wheelchair (bed, sofa, toilet, car, and so forth) and to varying heights (higher and lower than the wheelchair surface).

There are important complementary skills that patients need to perform to be fully independent with transfers (Box 20.7).

Floor-to-Wheelchair Transfers

There are three basic floor-to-wheelchair techniques: backward approach, forward approach, and sideways approach (Figs. 20.31A-C, 20.32A-D, and 20.33A-C). *Improving Functional Outcomes in Physical Rehabilitation*[232] and *Spinal Cord Injury: Functional Rehabilitation*[113] provide more detail on how to perform these transfers and other interventions to improve transfer ability.

Locomotor Training

Regaining the ability to walk is a common goal for most individuals following SCI. A number of factors will influence the success or failure in attaining this goal. Patients must possess adequate muscle strength, postural alignment, ROM, and sufficient cardiovascular endurance to become functional ambulators. Becoming a functional ambulator following a complete SCI is very difficult.

Box 20.7 Complementary Skills Necessary for Independence With Transfers

- Position wheelchair
- Set wheel locks
- Remove and replace arm rests on wheelchair
- Remove and replace leg rests on wheelchair
- Manage transfer board
- Manage lower extremities
- Manage body position in wheelchair

Walking with orthoses and assistive devices is slower and requires considerably more energy than walking before the injury. Many individuals with motor complete SCI who learn to walk with these devices may not continue walking once they stop rehabilitation. Patients with motor iSCI (ASIA C and D) are more likely to regain functional ambulation skills than those with complete or sensory incomplete injuries.[209,211,212]

This section on locomotor training is divided into two sections. The first deals with gait retraining using a compensatory-based approach for people with motor complete SCI. The second section highlights a recovery and activity-based approach for people with motor iSCI.

Locomotor Training for Individuals with Motor Complete SCI

When initiating a locomotor training (LT) program for complete SCI, therapists should be realistic and provide a clear picture of the costs and potential benefits. Patients who wish to relearn to ambulate following SCI should be given this option even if their potential for functional ambulation is limited. Although some patients may not become functional ambulators, standing alone may provide other important benefits such as improved circulation, skin integrity, bowel and bladder function, sleep, and a sense of well-being.[233]

Individuals with complete SCI rely on orthotic and assistive devices, adequate ROM, and maximizing strengthen of neurologically intact musculature for standing and walking. Full ROM in hip extension is essential in attaining balance in the upright position. The patient learns to lean into the anterior ligaments of the hip to stabilize the trunk and pelvis. The absence of knee flexion and plantarflexion contractures is also important in attaining upright standing balance.

Adequate cardiovascular endurance also is a criterion for functional ambulation. Because the energy cost of ambulation for a patient with complete paraplegia is higher than it is for people without SCI, endurance becomes an important factor in determining success or failure and continued ambulation once rehabilitation is complete.

Other factors that may restrict ambulation include severe spasticity, loss of proprioception (particularly at the hips and knees), pain, obesity, and the presence of secondary complications such as decubitus ulcers, heterotopic bone formation at the hips, or deformity. In addition, the patient's motivation plays a key role in determining success or failure in ambulation. A highly motivated patient can learn to walk using KAFOs and assistive devices. However, these patients may eventually find that the energy cost of ambulation is too great.

Follow-up studies of long-term continuation of ambulation have not been extensive. Mikelberg and Reid[234] surveyed 60 individuals with SCI for whom orthotics had been prescribed. From this group, 60% used

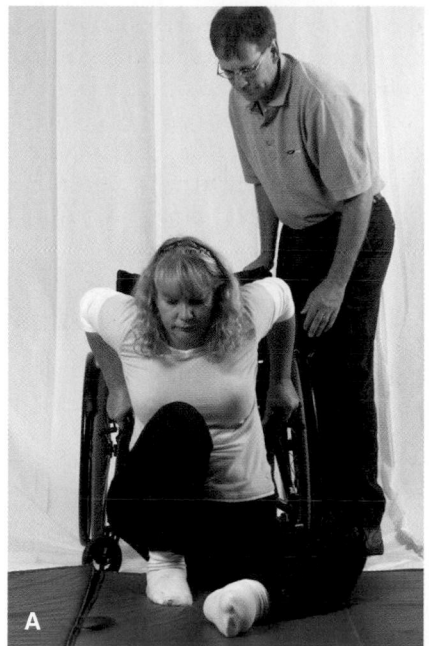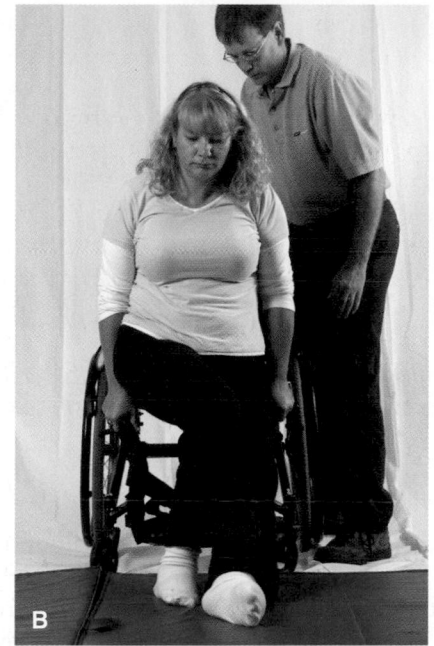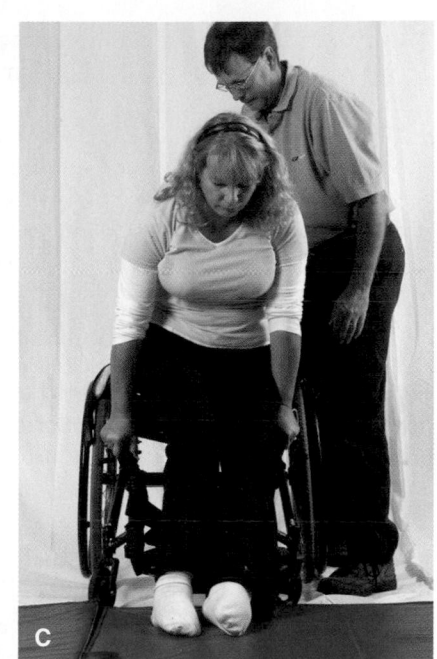

Figure 20.31 (A-C) Floor to wheelchair transfer using a backward approach. *(From O'Sullivan, S, and Schmitz, T: Improving Functional Outcomes in Physical Rehabilitation. FA Davis, Philadelphia, 2010, with permission.)*

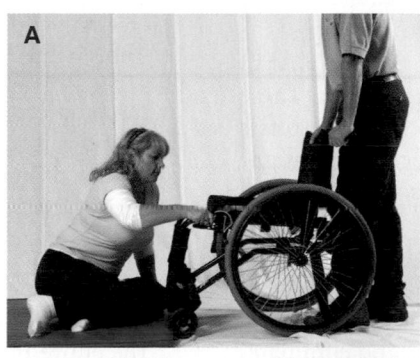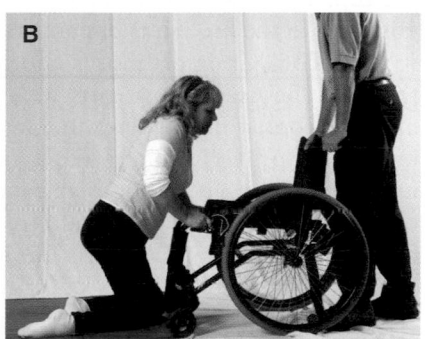

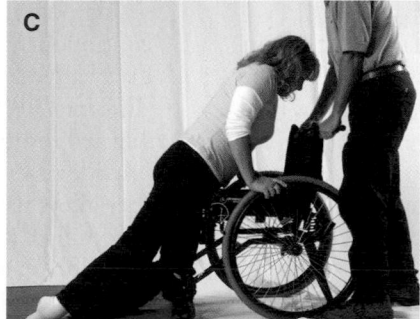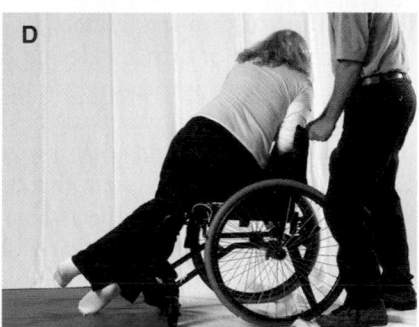

Figure 20.32 (A-D) Floor to wheelchair transfer using a frontward approach. *(From O'Sullivan, S, and Schmitz, T: Improving Functional Outcomes in Physical Rehabilitation. FA Davis, Philadelphia, 2010, with permission.)*

their wheelchairs as the primary means of mobility. Thirty-one percent completely discarded their orthoses. Those who did use their orthoses reserved them primarily for standing and exercise activities.

For patients with complete SCI, training emphasis is on strengthening available musculature; using assistive devices and orthoses to support weak or denervated muscles; and learning new, compensatory methods of walking.

Orthotic Prescription

The orthotic prescription varies according to the lesion level. Ankle and/or knee control bracing is often necessary. Patients with complete thoracic lesions will require

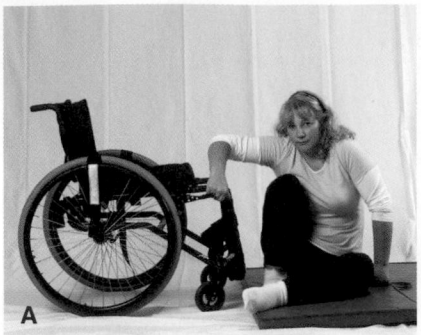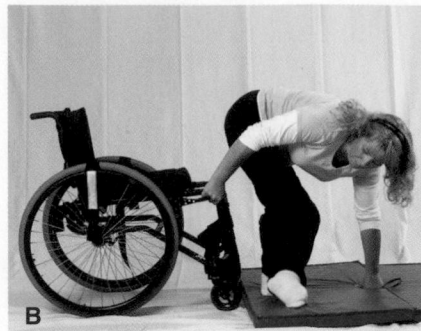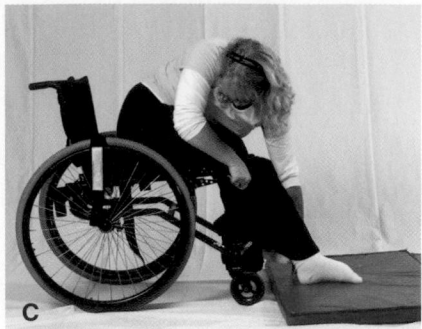

Figure 20.33 (A-C) Floor to wheelchair transfer using a sideways approach. *(From O'Sullivan, S, and Schmitz, T: Improving Functional Outcomes in Physical Rehabilitation. FA Davis, Philadelphia, 2010, with permission.)*

KAFOs. Conventional KAFOs include bilateral metal uprights, posterior thigh and calf bands, an anterior knee flexion pad, drop-ring or bail locks, adjustable locked ankle joints, a heavy-duty stirrup, and a cushion heel. The ankle joints are usually locked in 5 to 10 degrees of dorsiflexion to assist hip extension at heel strike. Orthotic hip control is not necessary, because the braces allow the patient to balance weight over the feet with the hips hyperextended. The center of gravity is kept posterior to the hip joints but anterior to the ankles.

The Scott–Craig orthosis is another type of KAFO that may be used by patients with paraplegia. These orthoses consist of standard double uprights, an offset knee joint providing improved biomechanical alignment, bail locks, a posterior thigh band, an anterior tibial band, adjustable ankle joint, and a sole plate that extends beyond the metatarsal heads. The orthosis may also include a plastic solid ankle section in place of the metal ankle joint and sole plate. This change decreases overall weight of the orthosis, improves cosmesis, and eliminates the need for custom-made shoes.

Another type of orthotic device available to patients with SCI is the reciprocating gait orthosis (RGO). The RGO is composed of two plastic KAFOs that are joined by a molded pelvic band with thoracic extensions. The RGO has a dual-cable system that runs posteriorly and attaches at the hip joints. These cable attachments transmit forces between LEs and provide reciprocal movement. Movement at the hip in one direction facilitates movement in the opposite direction on the contralateral hip. For example, as weight is shifted onto the left LE the right is moved forward. The dual-cable system allows control of both flexion and extension. These cables function to "coordinate" action between the two extremities during ambulation. As the advancing leg is unloaded, it is assisted into flexion while the stance leg is simultaneously pushed into extension. Thus, the orthosis allows for unilateral leg advancement and a reciprocating gait pattern. With this orthosis, a two- or four-point gait pattern can be used in combination with crutches or a reciprocating walker. Movement to a

seated position is accomplished by unlocking the drop lock at the knee joint.

Ankle-foot orthoses (AFOs) are often appropriate for patients with lower-level lesions (e.g., L3 and below). Either a conventional metal-upright or plastic AFO may be indicated. Chapter 30, Orthotics, provides a detailed discussion of these different types of orthoses.

Locomotor Training Strategies

Swing-through (Fig. 20.34) and 4-point gait patterns are two common walking patterns learned by patients with complete SCI using KAFOs. Initial standing balance and gait training should be done in the parallel bars and then progressed to the appropriate assistive device when the patient is ready. Relevant training activities include those described below.

- *Putting on and removing orthoses.* The patient is first taught the correct way to don and doff the orthoses. The entire procedure is usually done in the supine or sitting position. The patient must be cautioned to continuously monitor skin for pressure areas, particularly after brace removal.
- *Assistive device.* Forearm crutches are most often selected for patients with paraplegia. These crutches provide several advantages. They are lightweight; they allow use of the hand without the crutch becoming disengaged; they fit more easily into an automobile; and, most important, they improve function in ambulation and stair climbing by allowing full hip extension and unrestricted movement at the shoulders.
- *Sit-to-stand activities.* These activities should be practiced in the parallel bars using a wheelchair, then progressed to using the forearm crutches. The patient must learn to slide to the edge of the chair and unlock and lock the orthoses. Initially the patient is taught to pull to standing, using the parallel bars (a progression is made to using the wheelchair armrests to push to standing). Once in an upright position, the patient pushes down on the hands and tilts

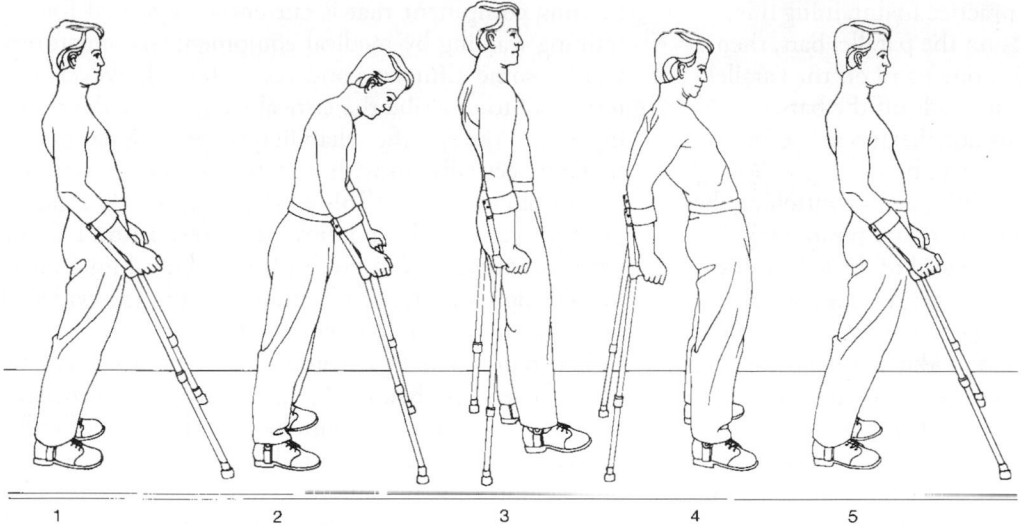

Figure 20.34 Swing-through gait pattern.

the pelvis forward in front of the shoulders. Return to sitting is a reversal of this procedure. To begin this activity with crutches the patient first places the crutches behind the chair, leaning against the push handle(s). To assume a standing position with crutches, the patient moves forward in the chair, locks both knee joints, crosses one leg over the other, and then rotates the trunk and pelvis (Fig. 20.35).

Hand placements on the armrest are reversed and the patient pushes to standing by pivoting around to face the chair. The reverse of this technique is used to return to the chair.

- *Static standing balance.* The patient learns to balance in standing with the hips in hyperextension and the upper trunk, head, feet, and arms behind the pelvis. The feet are 3 to 5 in (7.6 to 12.7 cm) apart.

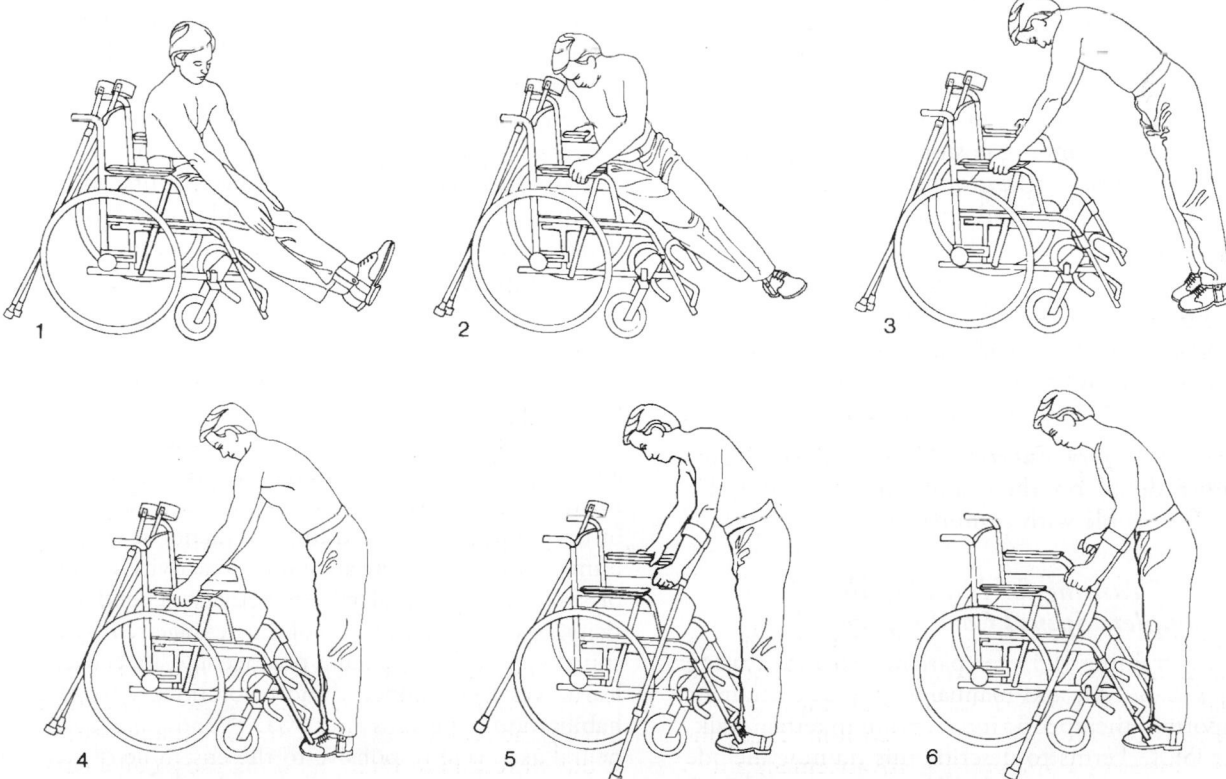

Figure 20.35 Standing from wheelchair using forearm crutches and KAFOs. The reverse sequences is used to return to sitting in the wheelchair.

The patient should first practice maintaining this position with both hands on the parallel bars, then progress to balancing with one hand off the parallel bars, and finally with both hands off the bars. The greater the amount of dorsiflexion at the ankle, the more anterior the pelvis can be.

- *Weight shifting in standing.* This entails controlling the pelvic position using UE support and positioning the head and shoulders forward ahead of the pelvis. The head hips relationship applied in transfers also applies in standing. The patient must be taught recovery to overcome and/or to prevent jackknifing from happening during ambulation. Jackknifing occurs when the patient's center of mass (COM) falls anterior to the hips causing the patient to flex forward suddenly.
- *Push-ups.* This includes lifting the body off the floor using elbow extension and scapulae depression and protraction, tucking the head to gain added height, and controlled lowering of the body.
- *Swing-through pattern.* From a balanced standing position with the hands posterior to the pelvis, the patient moves the hands forward causing the trunk to flex. Then the patient lifts up by extending the elbows and protracting/depressing the scapula and tucking the head. Gravity will cause the trunk and legs to swing forward. When the heels strike the ground the patient quickly extends the upper trunk and head, and pushes the pelvis forward to come back to the starting position (Fig. 20.34).
- *Four-point pattern.* This gait pattern is slower but safer than a swing-through pattern; three points are always in contact with the ground, as opposed to a swing-through pattern, in which there are times when only two points are in contact with the ground. From a standing position with the pelvis forward, both feet on the ground, and hands posterior to the pelvis, one hand/crutch is lifted up and placed forward. Weight is shifted away from the contralateral LE so it can swing forward as the hip is hiked and the head is moved down and away from the swing leg. This unweighting and hip hiking allows gravity to assist the forward swing. This process is repeated on the opposite side.

Spinal Cord Injury: Functional Rehabilitation[113] provides more detail on these and other gait training activities for people with complete SCI.

Locomotor Training for Individuals with Incomplete Spinal Cord Injury

Locomotor training (LT) for patients with iSCI using partial BWS, a TM, and manual assistance by trainers is an important therapeutic intervention to retrain walking after iSCI. Terms to describe this training include *body weight supported treadmill training, partial body weight supported treadmill training,* or *weight supported treadmill training.* These terms emphasize the exercise or

training equipment that is currently advocated for retraining walking by medical equipment manufacturers and by some clinicians and researchers; however, the terms fail to describe the critical elements of the training[235] and the specific rehabilitation goal. What does a therapist actually do with a patient to retrain walking using this equipment? This section provides (1) a global perspective on LT and how it differs from LT for persons with complete SCI; (2) the clinical guidelines for selection and use of LT strategies; and (3) evidence regarding use of LT following SCI.

Locomotor training is a product of *translational research* or *bridge research.* Knowledge gained by basic science researchers concerning the neurobiological control of walking laid the foundation for developing a therapeutic intervention with application to human, clinical populations. Basic scientists seeking to understand the role and contribution of the spinal cord to the control of walking used an animal model of complete SCI for their inquiries. They discovered that when mid-thoracic spinalized cats (i.e., cats that had a complete transaction of the spinal cord) were placed on a TM, suspended by a sling, and repetitively trained for hind-limb stepping with assistance of trainers for loading and limb placement, the animals learned to hind-limb step (on the TM) independent of supraspinal input. With continued training the cats were ultimately able to step on the TM independent of manual assistance.[236,237] Furthermore, this intense training was task-specific in that the spinalized cats could be trained to stand, or to step, but that training to perform one task did not transfer to performance of the other task.[238] Seminal research in this arena provided the impetus for Hugues Barbeau, a neuroscientist and physical therapist, to attempt the same strategy for retraining walking in humans after traumatic SCI: translational research.

Barbeau and co-workers published the first studies in which humans were partially suspended with a BWS apparatus over a TM to examine its impact on gait[239,240] and then provided training similar to that experienced by the cats for persons with SCI.[241] Though a suspension system and TM appear to be strong common denominators of the training, the equipment is likely not the dominant, critical component. The equipment provides an effective and controlled environment for consistent and intense practice of walking that can closely approximate the sensory experience of walking. The successes of the spinalized cats and improvements in walking by humans after iSCI were attributed to activity-dependent plasticity of the neural axis.[242] Activity-dependent plasticity, or the responsiveness of the neural circuitry of the spinal cord to task-specific practice and its capacity to learn, was a new concept and revolutionary for the rehabilitation of persons after SCI.[243] The spinal cord and neural axis were responsive to the ensemble of sensory information specific to walking and generated a motor response for stepping below the level of the lesion. Many researchers and clinicians, including Barbeau, continue to translate knowledge from basic science into developing a rehabilitation intervention to retrain walking after neurologic injury or disease.[154,244-247] In parallel, other researchers have focused on testing the efficacy of this intervention and effectiveness for the recovery of walking after SCI.[155,248-252]

Historically, rehabilitation for ambulation after SCI has been built on the premise that the spinal cord is neither "plastic" (adaptable), nor can it can learn or repair itself. After SCI, clinicians thus set goals to maximize use and strength of the musculature remaining under voluntary control and to substitute for weak or paralyzed muscles with braces and/or assistive devices. Thus, therapists taught alternative strategies for ambulation that incorporated braces and assistive devices and compensatory gait patterns. Locomotor training is a means of intensely practicing the distinct and specific task of walking (providing the sensory experience of walking) with the aim of tapping into the intrinsic neural pathways responsible for generating steps. This strategy may be viewed as a relative "bottom-up" approach, emphasizing the sensory experience of walking to drive the motor response of walking. In contrast, teaching new strategies to walk, such as "brace-walking," is a relative "top-down" approach requiring the development of a new skill with which to be upright and to ambulate. Certainly, sensory and cognitive processing is required for learning both strategies; however, the relative emphasis on recovery of preinjury movement patterns versus the introduction of alternative compensatory behaviors to achieve mobility differs.

Locomotor training occurs across three environments: (1) on the TM with use of BWS and manual facilitation; (2) assessment of the patient's ability to apply new skills, and control occurs overground (e.g., use of NRS); and (3) community integration. Retraining the neuromuscular system occurs most effectively in the TM environment with ease in control of BWS, speed, and manual facilitation by the trainers to optimize afferent input. Transfer of skills learned in the TM environment is assessed off the TM (overground) and limitations to independence assessed here and in community integration (home and community-based activities).

The focus of LT is to "*train like you walk.*" The task of walking, its kinematics, kinetics, spatial-temporal pattern, posture, balance, and adaptability as accomplished before injury, is the aim and reference point for progress. Retraining neuromuscular control for the task of walking involves (1) reciprocal stepping, (2) balance during propulsion, and (3) the ability to adapt the locomotor pattern to behavioral goals (e.g., carry a grocery bag) and environmental conditions (e.g., walk on carpet). Locomotor training is conducted in environments to experience the specific task of walking during intense practice, with progression toward independence in walking for home and community mobility.

Figure 20.36 contains a series of photos of a person walking with a rolling walker and a right AFO at a walking speed of 0.13 m/sec (0.43 ft/sec) using a traditional approach to gait retraining after SCI. Is this individual effectively practicing the task of walking? What elements are consistent with the task of walking and what elements are inconsistent with the task of walking? For instance, moving from point A to point B while upright is consistent with the aim of achieving walking. However, a forward-flexed trunk and head aimed at the ground, weight-bearing through the arms, hip extension only to neutral, uneven step lengths, hiking the right hip, vaulting on the left toe, no knee flexion on the right, and the slow walking speed are not consistent with the task of walking and its known typical pattern. Moving from point A to B while using a walker is certainly a form of mobility. However, the walker has become an inherent component to a new task of mobility and is not aligned with the known critical elements (e.g., kinematics, muscle activation) that define "walking."

Train like you walk translates into the following practical LT guidelines:

- The LEs are maximally loaded for weight-bearing, minimizing or eliminating loading of the arms.
- Sensory cues provided are consistent with the task of walking (e.g., TM speed, manual cues to facilitate flexor or extensor muscle activation).

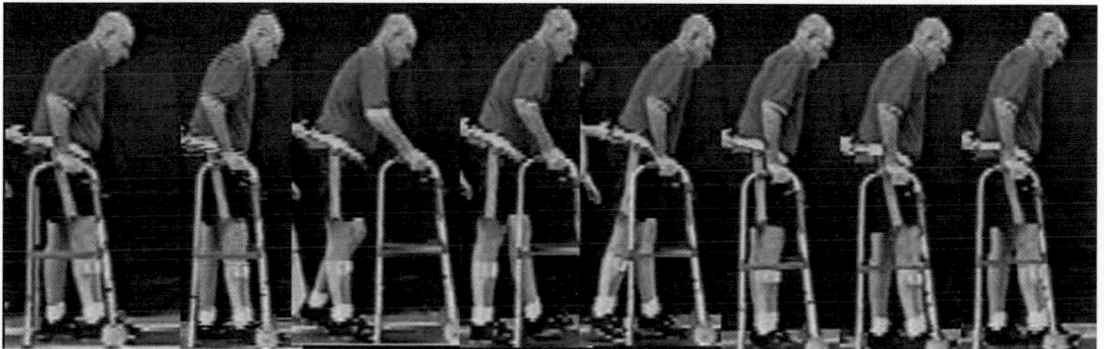

Figure 20.36 Gait pattern of a person with an incomplete spinal cord injury using a rolling walker and a right ankle-foot orthosis. *(From Behrman et al,[216] with permission.)*

- The posture, trunk, pelvis, and limb kinematics are coordinated and specific to the task of walking.
- Compensatory strategies for movement (i.e., hip hiking) are minimized or eliminated with recovery of preinjury movement patterns as the goal.[153,253]

These principles were derived from scientific evidence with animal models of SCI and from humans with and without SCI demonstrating the role of sensory input in generating a motor output.[153,243] As with learning any skill, practice and repetition are important and carryover beyond the clinic is critical. Persons with iSCI may exhibit compromised balance; weakness in the trunk, UEs, and LEs; increased or decreased muscle activity in flexors or extensors; symmetrical or asymmetrical impairments; and, in some, an inability to stand without lower or upper limb support.[254] To practice the specific task of walking for this population, a training environment must afford safety, support, task-specific repetition of walking, and a means to challenge and progress abilities.

An appropriate BWS system and TM provide such an opportunity within a controlled and safe environment. The patient wearing a trunk/pelvis harness is supported by an overhead and adjustable suspension system over a TM. Trainers require access to the trunk/pelvis and lower limbs to facilitate upright posture, weight shift, and limb movements. This environment allows control of the amount of lower limb loading, assists in upright posture and balance, and

allows control of the speed of walking (Fig. 20.37).[216] With 35% BWS, manual assistance at the trunk and pelvis to promote upright posture and minimize hip hiking, and lower limb trainers promoting step symmetry, hip extension, and hip/knee flexion on the right, the individual is able to walk at a speed of 0.8 to 1.0 m/sec. The therapist must determine what elements of practice are consistent with the task of walking and what elements are inconsistent with the task of walking. If the aim is task-specific training, then this is perhaps a good starting point for training. Each of these parameters then becomes a means of progression[216] by adjusting load, TM speed, and amount of manual assistance. As with any training protocol, intensity is required; thus, achieving 20 to 30 minutes of total stepping time is recommended, with increasing duration of each training bout. Frequency of training will depend somewhat on the setting; patients in inpatient rehabilitation may be able to train daily, whereas those in an outpatient setting may train 3 to 5 days a week. Goals must also be set to address adaptability for negotiating the environment and for meeting the behavioral demands of the individual for walking.[254]

The same training principles should be applied outside of the BWS-TM system overground in the clinic, home, and community. Adaptations can be made for advancing skills for walking when off the TM and should be consistent with LT principles. In the

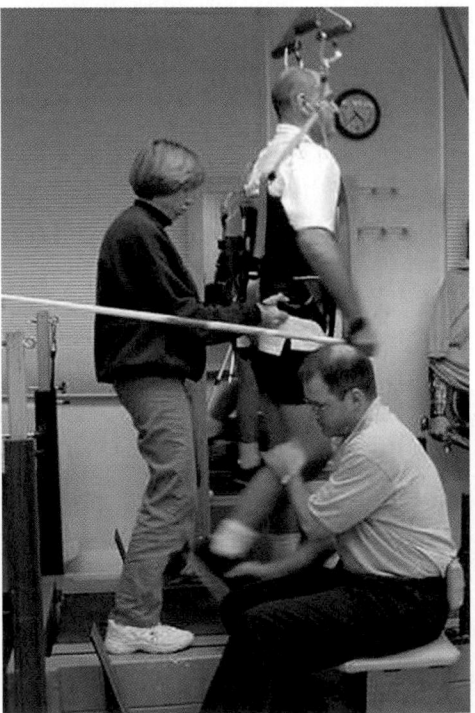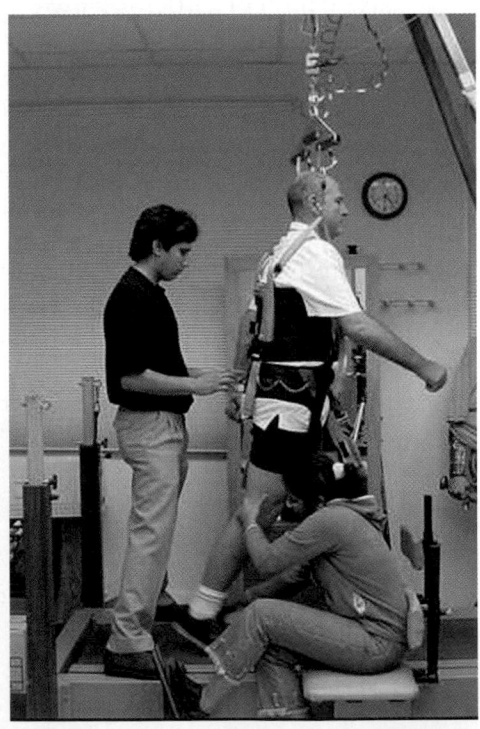

Figure 20.37 Locomotor training for a person with an incomplete spinal cord injury using body weight support, treadmill, and manual assistance by trainers. *(From Behrman et al,[216] with permission.)*

example from Fig. 20.36, the rolling walker may permit a faster walking speed; however, this individual's posture and inability to flex the right knee preclude any faster speed. The lack of upright posture also limits hip extension range and loading, likely necessary precursors to initiating swing. Several suggestions for treatment are to have this individual practice upright standing with his back to a wall using the walker to load his legs as opposed to his arms (Fig. 20.38), to have him stand weight-bearing solely on the left LE and with the right leg flexed on a stool or chair (Fig. 20.39A and B), and to elevate the height of the walker to encourage upright posture.[216] A posterior walker may also encourage a more upright posture. Certainly, use of the BWS system and TM has advantages and may be the optimal environment for consistent practice and retraining the neuromuscular system, but the transition and application to community ambulation is critical (Fig. 20.40).

Locomotor training principles can thus be applied both while on the TM with a BWS system and continued overground for community ambulation (see Fig. 20.40). Transferring skills acquired in one environment to another is an important element for learning and can be reinforced by a daily examination of the walking abilities overground and on the TM with BWS.[216] Modifying the parameters of training in both environments will challenge the use of new skills,

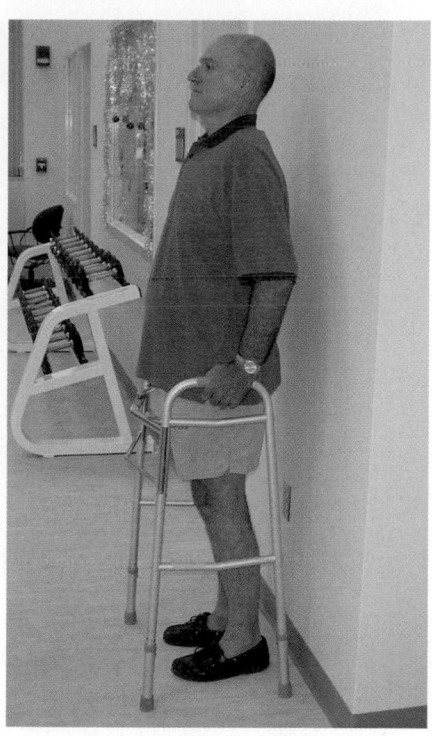

Figure 20.38 Locomotor training principles applied to the task of standing with upright posture for a person with an incomplete spinal cord injury. *(From Behrman et al,[216] with permission.)*

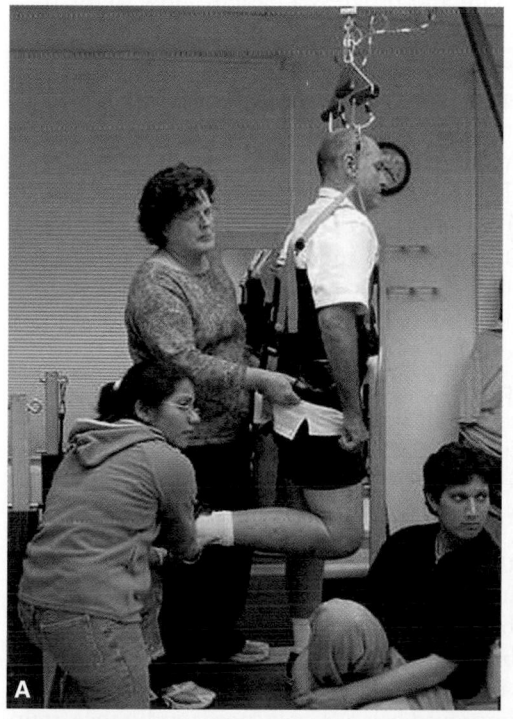 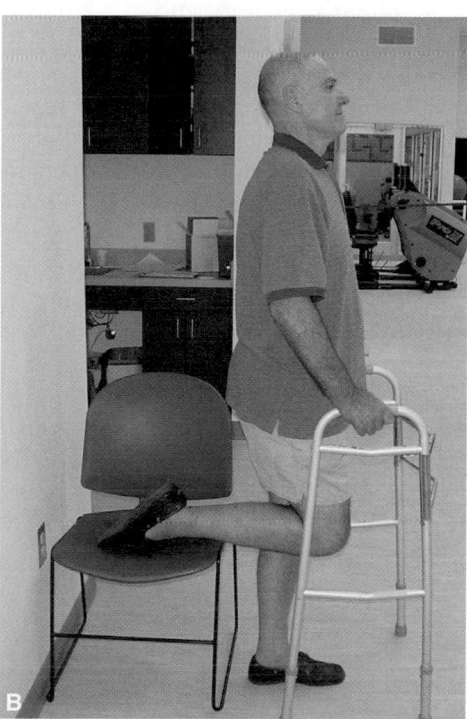

Figure 20.39 Locomotor training principles applied to standing upright while practicing loading and extension on the left lower limb while the right lower limb is unloaded and flexed on the treadmill with body weight support **(A)** and overground with a walker **(B)**. *(From Behrman et al,[216] with permission.)*

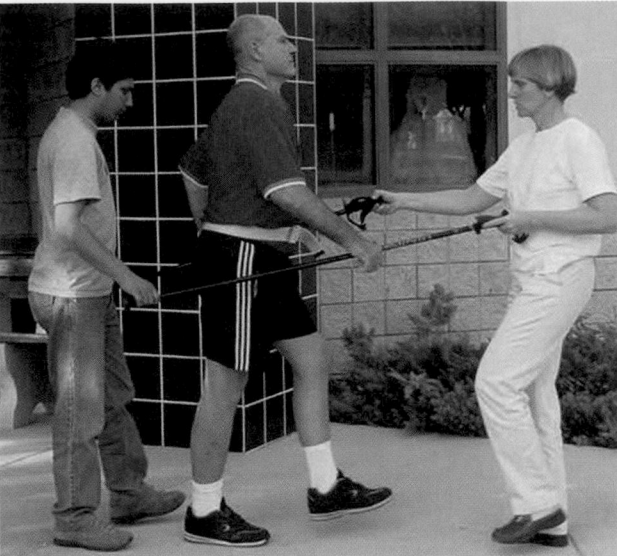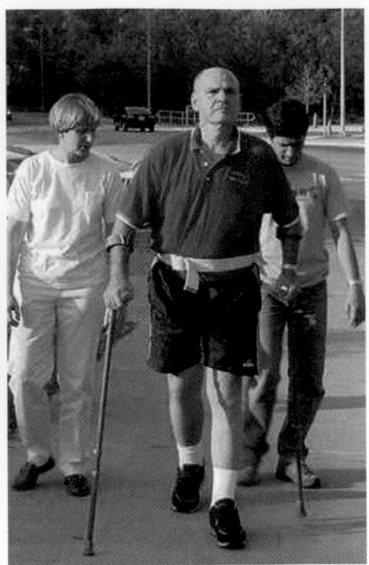

Figure 20.40 Translation of skills acquired on the treadmill to walking overground and community ambulation. *(From Behrman et al,[216] with permission.)*

reinforce new patterns and independence, and inform goal setting across environments.

Engaging the client in each aspect of goal setting and understanding of the LT principles empowers the client to extend "training" beyond the time in the clinic to the rest of the day. The choices that the therapist and client make on a daily basis may significantly affect the rate and magnitude of the client's recovery and achievement of goals. For instance, a client's choice to walk using a grocery cart instead of shopping from a wheelchair reinforces the principle of maximizing weight-bearing through the LE. If the individual walks with an upright posture, the goal is further enhanced with increased load-bearing on the LE versus the arms and achievement of hip extension during loading. This simple choice will advance the individual's recovery. Many more choices can be made by the client to support recovery regardless of where one is on a continuum of recovery.

Clinical guidelines for LT and for safe and effective use of therapeutic equipment are essential to the practice of evidence-based physical therapy for rehabilitation following SCI. As research findings are published, clinicians should seek information to guide their decision making and practice. Such information may identify the following:

- Who will benefit from LT with the aim of improving the ability to walk? Persons classified according to ASIA A, B, C, or D impairments or persons classified according to the NRS; persons who already walk, but not well; persons who have a particular clinical motor or sensory presentation; or persons at a particular neurological level of injury (i.e., severity of injury)?[254]

- When is the best time after injury to provide an intervention for optimal recovery of walking? In the acute stage of rehabilitation, after discharge from rehabilitation, or at some other point after SCI (and if so, what is the appropriate time after injury)?
- What is the optimal dose of therapy (i.e., intensity, frequency, and duration of the training)?
- How to train and progress a patient, how to use the BWS system and TM equipment, how to examine new training equipment as it reaches the market (e.g., suspension systems, robotic devices, and so forth), and how to monitor the trainers' body ergonomics during training?
- Any medical precautions and safety issues for persons with SCI and their effect on LT locomotor training (e.g., AD, skin, bowel and bladder, falling, osteoporosis, spasticity, cardiovascular health, and so forth).
- What therapies may augment LT or what combined therapies enhance the recovery of walking (e.g., strengthening, FES)?[155,255,256]
- The cost–benefit ratio (i.e., cost to provide this intervention in the clinic, including equipment and personnel; reimbursement policies; and outcomes and value to the patient and community).

Currently, the literature (case studies, small *n*, efficacy studies, clinical evaluation, and clinical trials) indicates that LT that incorporated use of a BWS system and TM in subacute and postacute rehabilitation with persons with iSCI (ASIA Impairment Scale classification C and D) improved balance, gait speed, endurance, stairclimbing, and independence[155,248,249,253,257] (Box 20.8 Evidence Summary).[155,251,257-263]

The Christopher and Dana Reeve Foundation *NeuroRecovery Network* (NRN) utilizes a standardized protocol

Box 20.8 Evidence Summary   Selected Studies Examining the Use of Locomotor Training

Created by Jayakrishnan Nair, PT, Rehabilitation Science PhD student, University of Florida, Gainesville, FL.

Reference	Participants		Methods/Procedure		Results and Comments
Field-Fote and Tepavac (2002)[258]	Ss	Total N = 14 iSCI (5 women and 9 men) and 3 healthy controls	**Design**	Pre-post design	Mean OG and TM speed improved (84% and 158%, respectively). The interlimb coordination also improved after intervention. Note: Testing speeds differed for pre and post training conditions.
	Level of injury and AIS	At or above T10 neurological level and C	**Intervention**	BWSTT with electrical stimulation: 36 sessions (3 times/wk for 12 wk). ES set at 500–750 msec train, 50–80 pulses per second, 1.0 to 1.5 msec pulse duration and 60 to 150 V. The treadmill speed and BWS was adjusted to participants' capacity to optimally walk.	
	Time after injury	70 months			
Dobkin et al (2006)[251]	Ss	Total N = 146 (BWSTT, n = 75 with 57 UMN and 18 LMN) along with OG step training (CONT; n = 71 with 54 UMN and 17 LMN)	**Design**	Single-blinded multicenter randomized clinical trial	No difference in primary outcome (walking speed) between BWSTT and control group; however, both groups exceeded expectations by achievement of near-normal walking speed, 1.1 m/sec. AIS C group showed better prognosis irrespective of the treatment they received. Individuals with ASIA B score at 8 weeks after SCI had a low probability of achieving functional walking with FIM-L score ≥4 when treated with BWSTT or CONT. Note: First study to demonstrate feasibility and safety to provide LT within the period of acute, inpatient rehabilitation and to patients wearing external stabilization devices (e.g., halo). Control group received an additional hour of therapy per day to be consistent with the experimental group.
	Level of injury and AIS	C5–L3 and B, C, D	**Intervention**	12 wk, 5 times/wk of either (1) BWSTT and OG step training or (2) control received only OG usual care stand/walking training (CONT). BWSTT = 1 hr/day of step and stand training (20–30 min BWSTT) and 10–20 min translation to OG walking. Treadmill speed > 0.72 m/sec with target training speed = 1.07 m/sec. BWS set to allow treadmill speed > 0/72 m/sec. CONT = Standing accomplished via braces or standing frame. Walking practiced with braces and assistive devices overground.	
	Time after injury	8 weeks			

Continued

Box 20.8 Evidence Summary   Selected Studies Examining the Use of Locomotor Training—cont'd

Reference	Participants		Methods/Procedure		Results and Comments
Jayaraman et al (2008)[259]	Ss	5 participants (male = 4 and female = 1)	**Design**	Longitudinal prospective case series	Plantar flexors muscle cross-section area increased by 6.8% to 21.8%, but no meaningful change in knee extensor cross-section area was observed except in 1 participant. Improvement in voluntary activation and in ability to generate both peak torque about the knee and ankle joints. Though LT had limited impact on changes in muscle size, increases in voluntary activation occurred. Note: Specific muscle resistance training may have greater impact on change in muscle size and torque generation.
	Level of injury and AIS	C4–T12 with C and D	**Intervention**	45 sessions, 5 times/wk, 30 min of step training over treadmill with manual assistance at near-normal walking speed (2.0–2.8 mph). BWS set at 30%–40% progressing to 5%–15%.	
	Time after injury	8–20 months			
Musselman et al (2009)[260]	Ss	4	**Design**	Single-blind A–B crossover design with BWSTT and OG skill training.	Modified Emory functional ambulation profile, 10-MWT, 6-MWT, BBS, ABC scales were used to measure clinically meaningful improvement in walking performance. Walking speed endurance, obstacle clearance, and stair climbing ability improved following OG skill training intervention when compared to BWSTT. 3 out of 4 participants retained their gains at follow-up.

	Level of injury and AIS	C5–L1 and C	**Intervention**	Training 1 hr/day, 5 times/wk for 3 months of either (1) BWSTT with manual assistance or (2) OG skill training, then crossover to the other intervention. BWS was the lowest amount possible to prevent knee and hips collapsing into flexion during stance at a speed selected for at least 3 min.
				
				    Braces were worn for both interventions. Side rails were allowed, but positioned at chest height to minimize weight-bearing through the arms.
				
				    Maximum treadmill speed was 1.0 m/sec. OG skill training included walking balance; skilled walking tasks (e.g., obstacle avoidance, negotiating different environmental challenges, walking with secondary task, endurance and speed increases). Borg scale was used to monitor exertion during training.	

	Time after injury	Mean time since injury = 2.7 years			

Box 20.8 Evidence Summary Selected Studies Examining the Use of Locomotor Training—cont'd

Reference	Participants		Methods/Procedure		Results and Comments
Field-Forte and Roach (2011)[155]	Ss	Total N =74 treadmill-based training with manual assistance (TM, n = 19), treadmill-based training with stimulation (TS, n = 22), overground training with electrical stimulation (OG, n = 18), treadmill-based training with robotic assistance (LR, n = 15).	**Design**	Single-blinded, randomized controlled clinical trial	Primary outcomes measures (10-MWT and distance covered in 2 min) were collected before, immediately after, and 6 months after the intervention with subjects using assistive and/or orthotic devices. Secondary outcome measure was LEMS. OG training showed the greatest improvement in the walking distance. The effect size was greater for speed and distance covered for OG than observed for any of the treadmill-based training. However, the TS group had more severely impaired subjects and the OG group had the least impaired subjects. The greater voluntary effort needed to walk during OG training was speculated as increasing the supraspinal drive for overground locomotion. The other possible factor identified was the difference in the motor strategy used for treadmill walking and OG walking. In the 6 months follow-up the amount of improvement in walking seen at immediate post time point declined but was still higher than the pre-training stage.
	Level of injury and AIS	At or above T 10, C and D			
	Time after injury	≥ 1 year	**Intervention**	5 times/wk for 12 wk using 4 types of locomotor training approaches all with BWS. (1) TM, (2) TS, (3) OG, (4) LR. The BWS was set to maintain upright posture and minimize knee flexion and progressing to ≤ 30%. In the OG condition greater BWS was used to accommodate for the increased effort needed for forward progression.	
	Age	25–58 years			Note: The amount of increase in walking speed post-intervention (0.04–0.05 m/sec) may be within measurement error and/or not clinically significant. The difference in the testing environment (overground) and the training environments (treadmill-based) may have contributed to differences in outcomes. Transfer of locomotor skills acquired on the treadmill to overground may be a necessary step.

Continued

Box 20.8 Evidence Summary   Selected Studies Examining the Use of Locomotor Training—cont'd

Reference	Participants		Methods/Procedure		Results and Comments
Harkema et al (2012)[257]	Ss	n = 196	**Design**	Prospective observational cohort	The outcome measures (BBS, 6-MWT, 10-MWT) were assessed at baseline, after every 20 sessions, and after intervention. The intensive activity-based therapy produced functional improvements in individuals with chronic iSCI. 86% of the patients had less than 45 score in BBS at enrollment out of which 27% improved their scores to beyond the value reflecting minimal risk of fall. At baseline, 69 patients were unable to complete the 6-MWT and 10-MWT, out of which 41% were able to complete the tests by the intervention end. The 6-MWT and 10-MWT speed improved by an average of 63 m and 0.20 m/sec. Significant improvement occurred in balance and walking measures for patients with AIS grades C and D. The magnitude of improvement, however, differed based on AIS grades. The chronicity of the injury was not significantly associated with the outcome measures at enrollment, but was inversely related to the level of improvement. 12% (n = 24) of the total patients failed to respond to LT.
	Level of injury and AIS	Above T11 and AIS C and D			
	Time after injury	Months to > 2 decades	**Intervention**	Median of 47 treatment sessions (minimum of 20 and maximum of 251) with 1 hour of step training with BWS and manual facilitation on treadmill followed by 30 minutes of OG assessment and community integration. TM speed was set from 0.5–10 mph. BWS was set to optimize kinematics and progressively reduced.	
	Age	Age ± SD = 41 ± 15 years			

Box 20.8 Evidence Summary   Selected Studies Examining the Use of Locomotor Training—cont'd

Reference	Participants		Methods/Procedure		Results and Comments
Studies in Children					
Prosser (2007)[261]	Ss	1	**Design**	Case study	After intervention the child ambulated independently in the community with a forward rolling walker and articulated ankle-foot orthosis. Significant improvement in strength (LEMS), ambulatory capacity (WeeFIM II scores, WISCI II scores), and participation in community occurred.
	Level of injury and AIS	C4 and C	**Intervention**	LT with BWS and manual assistance for 20–30 min/day, 3–4 times/wk for 6 months at near-normal walking speed. Ankle orthotics were used during training on the treadmill. OG training was initiated at 10 wk when independent stepping was initiated with the right leg. Least amount of BWS was used, which was enough to achieve knee extension independently starting with 80% BWS and gradually reducing to 10% by training end.	
	Time after injury	4–5 months			
	Age	5 years and 10 months			
Behrman et al (2008)[262]	Ss	1	**Design**	Case report	The child progressed from nonambulatory to first, nonexternally (sensory)-cued step at session 29 of LT. At session 33, the child took 7 consecutive, independent steps overground. The next session, he initiated 24 to 35 steps without cueing. From 51 session onward, he used a reverse rolling walker independently. After session 76, he was a community ambulator with a self-selected speed of 0.29 m/sec, fastest speed of 0.48 m/sec, and averaged 2,488 steps/day.
	Level of injury and AIS	C 6 on the left and C 8 on the right and AIS C	**Intervention**	76 sessions, 5 times/wk. Locomotor training with BWST with manual assistance for 20–30 min of step training interspaced every 5 min with stand training. This was followed by 10–20 min of overground training. Treadmill speed was set at 0.8–1.2 m/sec with emphasis on normal trunk and limb kinematics during stepping. BWS was set initially at 30%–40% and reduced to 15%–20% by training completion.	
	Time after injury	16 months			
	Age	4.5 years			

Continued

Box 20.8 Evidence Summary Selected Studies Examining the Use of Locomotor Training—cont'd

Reference	Participants		Methods/Procedure		Results and Comments
Fox, E, et al, 2010[263]	Ss	1	**Design**	This study was a 2-year follow-up to the Behrman et al (2008) case study. The age of the child was 6.5 years and the time since injury was 3 years, 6 months.	Follow-up tests were conducted at 1 month (baseline), 1 year after LT, and 2 years after LT. No change occurred in the WISCI scores as the child continued to use reverse rolling walker for ambulation. The child's fastest walking speed increased from 0.45 m/sec to 0.67 m/sec in 2 years. The number of home and community-based stepping bouts increased from 31 at baseline to 88/day at 2 years. Trunk compensation and frequency of leg crossing midline while walking decreased. The number of steps per day increased from 1,600 to 3,000 at 1 year and remained at 2 years. He showed normal musculoskeletal growth (90th–95th percentile of age and normal body weight) with no reports of secondary complications (e.g., scoliosis or hip dysplasia).

ABC = Activity Balance Confidence measure; AIS = ASIA Impairment Scale; ASIA = American Spinal Injury Association; BBS = Berg Balance Scale; BWS = body weight support; BWSTT = body weight supported treadmill training; ES = electrical stimulation; FIM = Functional Independence Measure; LT = locomotor training; LEMS = lower extremity motor score; OG = overground; Ss = subject characteristics; 10-MWT = 10-Meter Walk Test; 6-MWT: 6-Minute Walk Test; WISCI II = Walking Index for Spinal Cord Injury II; WeeFIM II = Functional Independence Measure for pediatrics.

of LT with standardized outcomes across seven outpatient clinical sites in the United States to persons with ASIA C and D injuries.[264] The NRN currently has the largest database (over 350 persons) who have received a minimum of 20 sessions of LT and is being used to evaluate the LT program and inform practice. Inclusion of persons with ASIA A and B injuries will further advance our understanding of the clinical impact of LT.

Safety and feasibility for providing LT to persons with iSCI during acute rehabilitation have also been established.[265] Clinical adaptations were required to safely train persons having a halo, a catheter and drainage bag or bladder/bowel impairments, sensory impairment, and susceptibility to orthostatic hypotension or AD. The question of whether providing LT has benefit during the acute rehabilitation phase warrants further investigation.

LT also has been provided to persons with motor complete SCI (ASIA A and B) in both research and clinical settings. Although independent walking has not been achieved, other potential benefits may be considered valuable and important to a person's quality of life after SCI.[266,267]

Another important area for research is the benefits of LT to a person's health after SCI, whether an incomplete or a complete injury. Additional questions that need to be answered include the following: Does LT decrease the risk of pressure sores or bladder infections; reduce bone loss or muscle atrophy? Do benefits for health warrant increased access to LT? Can robotic devices provide an avenue to cost-effectively provide this service? What is the impact of LT outcomes on the quality of life of the person with SCI and the impact on the family or caregiver(s)?

The advent of LT represents a new era in spinal cord rehabilitation. This era, brought forth by partnership among basic scientists, rehabilitation scientists, physicians, and clinicians, encompasses knowledge of the neurobiological control of walking and the physiological promise of activity-dependent plasticity as bases for developing new interventions and advancing the potential for recovery after SCI. Whereas LT alone may provide a means for recovery of preinjury abilities and fostering neuromuscular activity below the level of the lesion, the next generation of physical rehabilitation may employ combinatorial approaches. Such approaches may include advancing technology, epidural stimulation, stem cell transplants, and pharmacological approaches to bolster the neuroplasticity of the neural environment. Locomotor training in combination with these approaches or others may be an essential component and catalyst to achieve an effective therapeutic outcome.[154,158,268]

Activity-Based Upper Extremity Training

For people with a cervical SCI the recovery of UE function is a primary goal.[269] Interventions aimed at improving functional use of the UE have primarily been compensatory in nature. For example, patients with active wrist extension are taught how to manipulate and pick up objects using a tenodesis grasp, use the hand as a hook, and use different types of orthoses to feed themselves. More recently, researchers have begun to explore the use of massed practice interventions to promote functional recovery and corticomotor and spinal reorganization.[270,271]

Based on massed practice principles used in constraint-induced movement therapy[272] (see Chapter 10, Evidence Summary Box 10-1, and discussion in Chapter 15, Stroke), Field-Fote and colleagues[270,271,273] applied similar training techniques by having patients practice unimanual[270,271,273] or bimanual[271] UE activities 2 hour per day 5 days a week for 3 weeks. Patients did not have a UE constrained. Applying sensory electrical stimulation to the volar surface of the wrist over the median nerve while the patients performed the different tasks augmented the massed practice. Patients with cervical iSCI practiced four main types of unimanual or bimanual UE activities: finger isolation, grasp, grasps with rotation, pinch, and pinch with rotation. Finger isolation activities included activities such as typing on a keyboard, dialing phone numbers, and playing piano notes. Grasp activities included squeezing a spray bottle, cutting paper with scissors, and building with Legos. Grasp with rotation activities included pouring liquid from one container to another and opening containers. Pinch activities included picking up objects, threading a large needle, and writing. Pinch with rotation activities included screwing nuts on bolts, locking and unlocking a lock with a key, and turning a doorknob. The researchers found significant improvements in hand and arm function after the intervention.[270,271,273]

Health and Wellness

Just as with people without SCI, regular exercise is an important part of a healthy lifestyle. Patients should be provided a comprehensive home exercise program (HEP) that incorporates stretching, balance, aerobic, and strengthening exercises. Aerobic exercises such as UE ergometer should be done 3 to 5 days a week for a total of 20 to 60 minutes per session at an intensity of 50% to 80% of maximum heart rate. Strengthening exercises should be done 2 to 4 days a week at an intensity of 8 to 10 repetitions at 60% to 80% of one repetition maximum.[220] When developing the exercise program, attention should be paid to the unique precautions associated with people with SCI such as the possibility of overuse injuries (particularly in the shoulders), AD, thermal dysregulation, and exaggerated heart rate response to exercise.[42]

Patient/Client-Related Education

Because SCI can affect many different body systems and drastically change an individual's life, ongoing education about the consequences of SCI is critical. Education should begin early after injury and continue throughout rehabilitation and cover the extensive impact of SCI discussed above (e.g., skin care, AD, self-directing care, wheelchair mobility and maintenance, sexuality, and so forth). Without education patients will not be able to make informed decisions regarding their care or informed choices regarding community reintegration.

Peer mentoring with others who have experienced an SCI and are living in the community can be an effective method of providing education, support, and assistance with the rehabilitation process.[274] For example, a person with an ASIA A T2 SCI will be able to realistically demonstrate how to transfer from the bed to a wheelchair to a person recently injured who is undergoing rehabilitation. This person may also be able to discuss the impact of SCI on everyday life in a way a physical therapist could not.

An important aspect of rehabilitation involves planning for discharge and community reintegration. Consideration must be given to multiple issues, including accessible housing, nutrition, transportation, finances, maintaining functional skills and level of physical fitness, employment or further education, and methods for involvement in desired social or recreational activities. Each of these issues must be addressed early and continued throughout the course of rehabilitation in consultation with the patient, family, and appropriate team members. Educating the patient will allow him or her to make informed decisions regarding medical care and lifestyle choices throughout the life span. A plethora of resources are available on the Internet. Patients should be encouraged to contact and to explore the available resources. Appendix 20.A lists some of the many resources available for patients, families, and clinicians.

■ PRESCRIPTIVE WHEELCHAIR AND WHEELCHAIR SKILLS TRAINING

Many people with SCI will use a wheelchair as their primary means of mobility. A wheelchair both acts as a mobility base and serves to provide postural support. Because patients with SCI will have varying degrees of trunk, hip, and shoulder girdle paralysis, the wheelchair and accompanying seating system provides postural support to keep the pelvis, spine, and extremities in optimal alignment. Postural alignment affects a variety of areas, including respiration, bowel and bladder function, skin integrity, and mobility. Poor posture in the wheelchair can negatively affect all of these areas. Because most patients will be using a wheelchair exclusively, it should be custom-ordered (prescribed) for each individual. When prescribing a wheelchair consideration should be given to the patient's goals and characteristics, as well as the activities and environment in which it will be used.

The first choice is between a power and manual wheelchair. Generally, individuals with intact triceps function are able to independently propel a manual wheelchair. Individuals with a C6- or C5-level injury may also be able to independently propel a manual wheelchair, but may not have the endurance or strength for community wheelchair mobility. The selection of a manual or power wheelchair in these cases should be done on an individual basis. Individuals with higher cervical injuries generally rely on a power wheelchair for their mobility needs (see Table 20.5). Before prescribing a wheelchair a series of trials with different types of chairs with different components will assist with making an informed decision on what specific type of wheelchair to obtain.

There are two basic frames for manual wheelchairs, a *folding* or a *rigid* frame, and three weights, standard, lightweight, and ultralight. Folding chairs are an important consideration for patients who plan to transfer into a car because they can be folded compactly for storage without having to remove as many parts. Folding frames typically incorporate a below-seat crossbar and generally provide a smoother ride on uneven surfaces. Potential drawbacks include heavier and more moveable parts causing it to be less energy efficient during propulsion than rigid frames.

A rigid frame is generally lighter, is more energy efficient, and often has an adjustable seat-to-back angle. This type of frame may be more difficult to store in a car. Both wheels must be removed for storage. A rigid frame is often more durable than a folding frame.

A variety of different components and options can be selected for a manual wheelchair. There are benefits and drawbacks to the different options. For example, the wheel locks can be mounted high or low on some wheelchair frames. High-mounted wheel locks are easier to access, but can be an obstacle to transfers. Conversely, low-mounted wheel locks are more difficult to access but are not in the way of transfers or during propulsion.

Advances in rehabilitation technologies have created a new class of wheelchairs that fall between manual and power wheelchairs, *pushrim-activated power-assist wheelchairs* (PAPAWs). A PAPAW is a manual wheelchair to which power-assist wheels have been added. When the user applies force to the pushrims the motor is activated, which provides assist to the wheels. Propelling a PAPAW requires less energy, lower stroke frequency, and less shoulder ROM than a manual wheelchair.[275-277] A PAPAW may be beneficial for individuals with mid to lower level cervical injuries (C5–C6) who may not have the endurance or strength to use a manual wheelchair full time.[278]

Power wheelchairs are indicated for all patients with C4 lesions and above. Patients with C5-level lesions may also elect to use power wheelchairs, particularly for community mobility. A tilt-in-space or reclining seating system provides improved postural control and allows the user to independently perform pressure relief. There are various types of controls. They range from a hand-operated joystick to a sip-and-puff control.

A wheelchair prescription will vary according to the level and extent of injury. Some general considerations follow:

- Seat depth should be approximately 1 to 2 in (2.5 to 5.1 cm) back from the popliteal space to allow an even weight distribution on the thighs and to prevent excessive pressure on the ischial tuberosities.
- Floor-to-seat height is important. The type and dimensions of the cushion or custom-made seat must be known so that seat height can be measured accurately, allowing adequate (2 in [5.1 cm]) clearance from the floor to the foot pedals and provide slightly greater than a 90° angle at the hips.
- Back height is important. If the patient will not be pushing the wheelchair, a high back may be desired for added comfort and stability. A patient with tetraplegia who will be pushing the wheelchair requires a back height that is below the inferior angle of the scapula so that the axilla is free of the handles during functional activities. Most patients with paraplegia prefer a lower back height, especially if they have intact abdominal muscles.
- Seat width and depth are variable and should be fitted to the anthropometric characteristics of the

patient. The patient should be fitted in the narrowest chair possible, but have adequate space between the lateral edges of the thighs and wheelchair armrests or wheels to avoid skin irritation. The patient's previous weight should be considered, especially if there has been a significant loss since the initial injury, and potential exists to regain the weight. If orthoses or thick clothing in cold climates are worn, they must also be included in the consideration of width.

- Removable armrests and detachable swing-away leg rests are important components of wheelchairs used by many patients with SCI. On some chairs, the leg rests do not detach and the armrests are of a "flip-up" design. The suitability of these features must be considered with respect to the transfer capabilities and techniques used by the individual patient.

- Additional wheelchair accessories may be required to meet specific patient needs. Several features that warrant consideration include enlarged release mechanisms on the leg rests, a friction surface on the hand rims, brake extensions, anti-tipping devices, and grade aids (which decrease backward movement of the chair while ascending inclined surfaces).

Configuring the wheelchair to provide optimal postural support is an important consideration when selecting a wheelchair, seating system, and different components.[279] The wheelchair can assist in providing postural support to keep the pelvis and spine in alignment with trunk and pelvic muscle paralysis or paresis. Optimal postural support allows the patient to effectively use UEs to perform ADL and to propel the wheelchair. Configuring the wheelchair so that the seat slope is higher in the front than the rear (i.e., seat to floor height at the front of the cushion approximately 2 in. higher than at the back of the cushion) with the backrest perpendicular to the floor and relatively low may help keep the pelvis in a neutral alignment and maintain the natural curves of the spine (as opposed to a sitting posture of a posterior pelvic tilt with a C curve throughout the lumbar and thoracic spine).[280]

Some patients may require more than one wheelchair. Many lightweight "everyday" chairs are not suitable for sport and recreational activities. Depending on the interests of the patient, a second chair specifically designed for a particular sport such as tennis or racing may be desired.

The customized seating system includes a wheelchair cushion to assist in preventing skin breakdown and providing postural support. Selection of a cushion should be individualized. Patients should try different types of cushions to determine their impact on postural support, comfort, and pressure distribution. Pressure mapping can be done during the evaluation process with different types of cushions to select the cushion that provides the optimal pressure redistribution. A large variety of cushion styles are commercially available. Cushions generally are designed to redistribute pressure across the entire surface or take pressure off high-risk, bony areas. Cushions are made of different types of materials, including elastomer gel, open cell foam, closed cell foam, and air. These materials are often used in combination to provide reduced or redistributed pressure.

Chapter 32, The Prescriptive Wheelchair, provides more detail on the wheelchair and seating evaluation, drawbacks, and benefits of different wheelchair components, cushion types, and a variety of other issues associated with selecting a wheelchair. "Seating and Wheelchair Prescription" by Hastings and Betz is another excellent resource on this topic.[281]

Wheelchair Skills

For individuals who use a manual wheelchair, the ability to propel and maneuver over and around various obstacles and terrains in their home and community is essential for functional independence. In order to propel a manual wheelchair independently in the home and community environments, patients need to be able to perform certain basic wheelchair mobility skills: forward and backward propulsion, turning, ascend and descend inclines, assume and maintain a wheelie, and propulsion on uneven terrain.

Propulsion on Even Surfaces

To propel the wheelchair forward, the patient reaches back and grasps the wheelchair hand rims (Fig. 20.41) then pushes forward, releasing the hand rims after the hands have passed in front of the hips. Patients should practice reaching far back on the hand rims to initiate the stroke and pushing far forward before releasing the hand rims. A longer pushing stroke is more efficient. Patients who do not have the ability to grasp the hand rims propel the wheelchair by pressing their palms against the lateral aspect of the hand rims and then pushing forward. These patients will often use hand rim projections or have plastic-coated hand rims.

The technique used to turn depends on how quickly the patient needs to turn, as well as the size of the turning radius. To make a large radius or slow turn, the patient just pushes harder with one arm (e.g., if turning to the right the patient pushes harder with the left arm). To make a tight and/or quick turn, the patient pushes forward with one hand while pulling back with the other (e.g., if turning to the right quickly, the patient pushes forward with the left arm while pulling back with the right arm).

Inclines

There are a variety of surfaces with inclines that wheelchair users need to negotiate to be independent in their home and community. These include ramps, curb

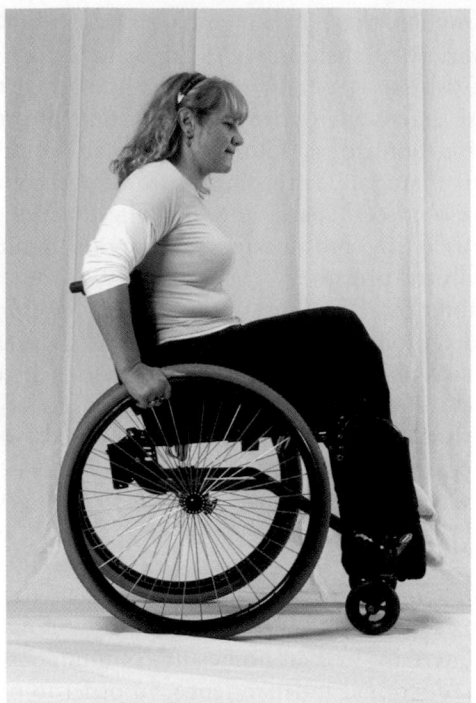

Figure 20.41 Propelling wheelchair forward. *(From O'Sullivan, S, and Schmitz, T: Improving Functional Outcomes in Physical Rehabilitation. FA Davis, Philadelphia, 2010, with permission.)*

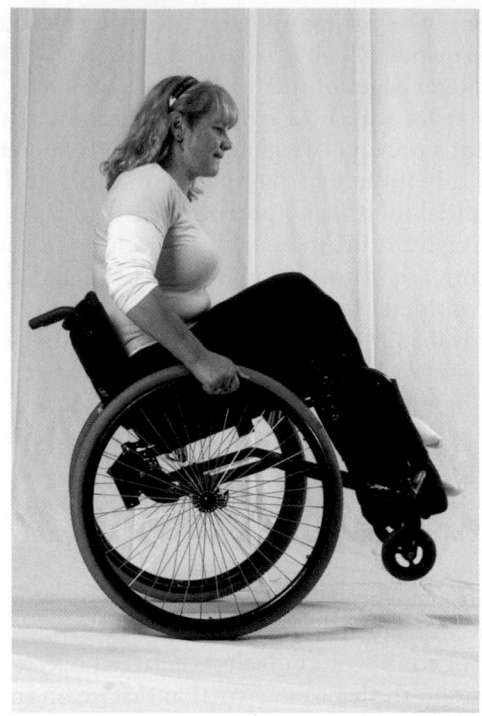

Figure 20.42 Performing a wheelie. *(From O'Sullivan, S, and Schmitz, T: Improving Functional Outcomes in Physical Rehabilitation. FA Davis, Philadelphia, 2010, with permission.)*

cutouts, slopes, and hills. The basic techniques used to ascend and descend these inclines are the same. To ascend an incline the patient takes shorter and quicker strokes and pushes on the hand rims more forcefully. If possible, the patient should lean forward with the head and trunk while pushing forward to prevent the chair from tipping backward.

Gripping the hand rim and slowly releasing the grip in a controlled manner to slow the descent of the wheelchair controls the speed of descent. Patients without full hand function control the descent of the wheelchair by applying pressure to the hand rims with the palms of the hands and slowly release the pressure to control the descent of the wheelchair.

Wheelies

The ability to perform a wheelie (Fig. 20.42) is an essential skill in order to negotiate curbs, steep declines, uneven terrain, and other areas of the community. To attain a wheelie, the patient reaches back on the hand rim and forcefully pushes forward to lift the front casters off the ground (as if attempting to tip the wheelchair over backward). When first learning any skill that involves a wheelie or there is a risk of the wheelchair tipping over, the patient should always be closely supervised and guarded. To ensure safety while practicing wheelies, a gait belt is looped through the frame of the wheelchair. The therapist is positioned behind the wheelchair, holding the gait belt in one hand with the other hand placed on the patient's shoulder or push handle of the wheelchair (Fig. 20.43).

The type of wheelchair and its configuration have an impact on how easy or difficult it is to attain a wheelie. Achieving a wheelie in a heavier wheelchair and one with the axle plate that is posterior is more difficult. An axle that is more forward, so that the user's COM is behind the axle, causes the wheelchair to be less stable and more "tippy." This makes it easier to assume a wheelie.

The ability to maintain a wheelie should be learned in conjunction with attaining a wheelie. Both of these skills are important lead-up activities to more advanced wheelie skills such as ascending and descending curbs and propulsion on uneven terrain. The therapist should assist the patient into the *balance point* in which the front casters are off the ground with the wheelchair in equilibrium. The patient's hands should lightly grip the hand rim in a position near the hips. Pushing forward on the hand rims causes the chair to tip backward and pulling backward causes the wheelchair to tip forward onto the casters back into a stable position. The patient should practice lightly pushing and pulling on the hand rim to learn the balance point; the hand rim should slide through the patient's grip as he or she does this. The patient should not keep the hand firmly grasped at the same point on the hand rim.

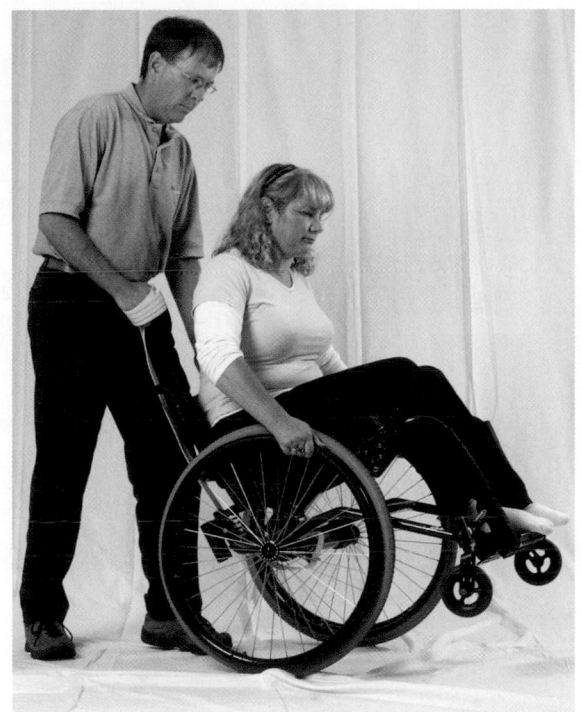

Figure 20.43 Technique to safely spot a patient while she practices performing wheelies. *(From O'Sullivan, S, and Schmitz, T: Improving Functional Outcomes in Physical Rehabilitation. FA Davis, Philadelphia, 2010, with permission.)*

When propelling a wheelchair on uneven surfaces (e.g., gravel, grass) there is a possibility of the front casters catching, causing the wheelchair to tip over in a forward direction. Being able to propel the wheelchair forward while maintaining a wheelie can minimize this risk and allow the patient to propel the wheelchair independently over a variety of terrains. When learning to propel the wheelchair forward and backward and while turning in a wheelie position, the patient should be instructed again not to use a firm grip but to allow the hand rims to slide within his or her grip.

On some uneven surfaces it may be easier to "pop up" into a wheelie for only a brief time (not maintain the wheelie) and push forward. The patient then crosses the surface in a series of short wheelies while pushing forward.

Wheelies are also used to ascend and descend curbs. To ascend a curb while moving, the patient pops a wheelie while moving forward just before reaching the curb. This lifts the front casters so they are up on top of the curb. As the wheels make contact with the curb, the patient pushes forward on the hand rims and leans his or her head and trunk forward (Fig. 20.44A-C). To descend a curb the patient pushes the wheelchair forward and just as the casters approach the edge of the curb the patient pops a wheelie. The wheelie is maintained as momentum carries the back wheels off the curb. The patient maintains the wheelie so the back wheels land first, then the casters land (Fig. 20.45A-C).

Other wheelchair skills that patients should learn include falling from a wheelchair, picking up objects off the floor, opening and closing doors, and negotiating obstacles. Patients should also learn how to manage the parts of the wheelchair: putting wheel locks on and off, removing and returning leg rests, folding the wheelchair, removing the cushion, moving arm rests, and removing and putting the wheels back on.

In addition to developing the Wheelchair Skills Test described earlier, Kirby and colleagues also developed the *Wheelchair Skills Training Program.* Based on the skills of the Wheelchair Skills Test and principles of motor learning, the Wheelchair Skills Training Program was designed to improve manual wheelchair user performance and safety. Research studies have shown it to be a safe and effective training method for new wheelchair users,[282] community-based wheelchair users,[283] occupational therapy students,[284] and caregivers.[285] Detailed information on both the Wheelchair Skills Test and Wheelchair Skills Training Program can be obtained on the Internet at www.wheelchairskillsprogram.ca/. *Spinal*

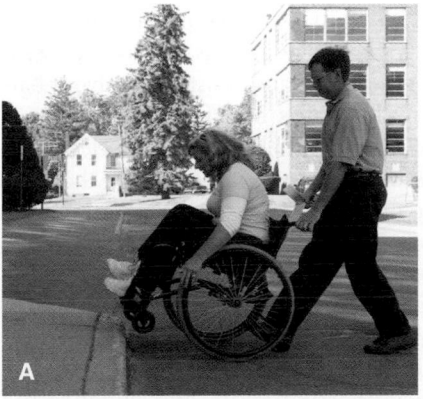
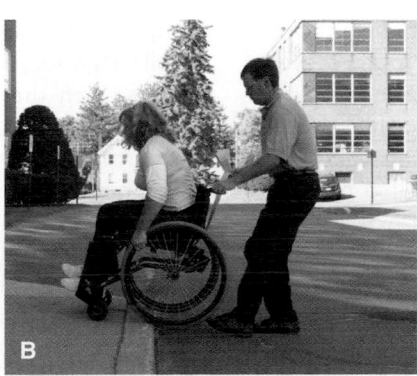
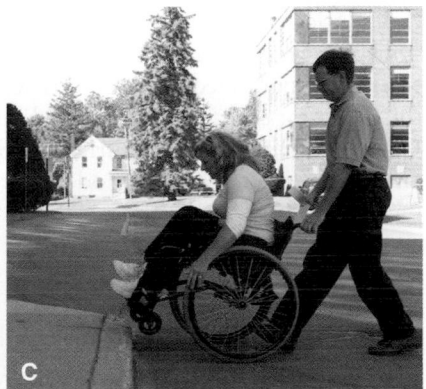

Figure 20.44 (A-C) Ascending a curb in a wheelie. *(From O'Sullivan, S, and Schmitz, T: Improving Functional Outcomes in Physical Rehabilitation. FA Davis, Philadelphia, 2010, with permission.)*

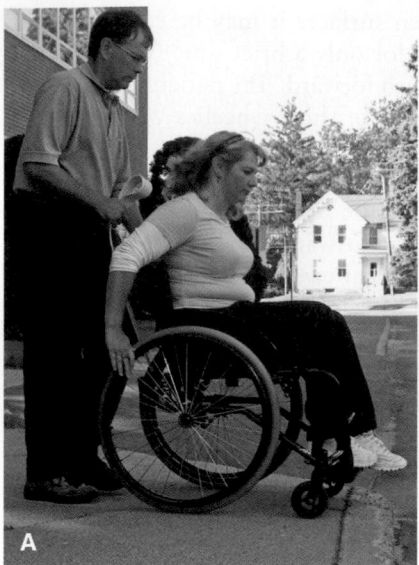
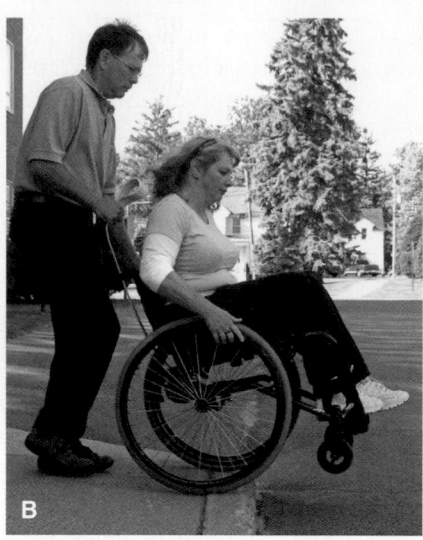
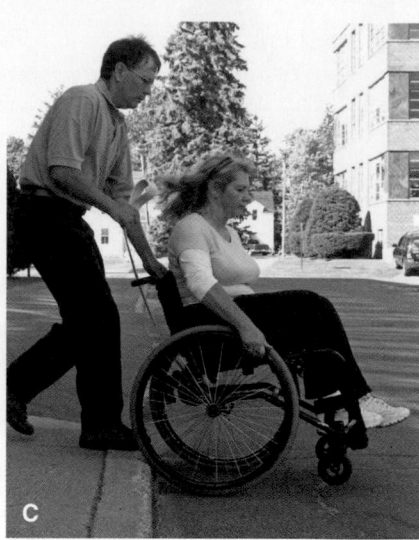

Figure 20.45 (A-C) Descending a curb in a wheelie. *(From O'Sullivan, S, and Schmitz, T: Improving Functional Outcomes in Physical Rehabilitation. FA Davis, Philadelphia, 2010, with permission.)*

Cord Injury: Functional Rehabilitation[113] and *Improving Functional Outcomes in Physical Rehabilitation*[232] are other resources that provide more detail on interventions to improve the above-mentioned and other wheelchair skills.

■ NEUROTECHNOLOGIES

People with SCI also benefit from recent advances in neurotechnologies designed to improve function and quality of life. Neurotechnologies can fall into four main areas: neuromodulation (use of electrical stimulation to improve control of an intact portion of the nervous system), neural prosthesis (use of electrical stimulation to replace or improve function of a paralyzed or weak limb), neurorehabilitation (applying technologies to promote normal recovery of impaired body functions), and neurosensing and diagnostics (technologies to monitor the nervous system or diagnose a condition).

Electrical stimulation can be used in a variety of ways. One of the most common is to use FES to cause the contraction of paralyzed or weak muscles below the level of the lesion for exercise, walking, and functional use of the UEs. As discussed above, surface FES can be used with an LE ergometer as a method of cardiovascular training.[227,228] Surface FES can also be applied to LEs to allow standing and walking in people with SCI.[286] Surface electromyography (EMG) has been paired with FES to provide patients with a method of triggering the FES to produce a more normal walking pattern than FES alone.[287] Implanted FES systems allow people with SCI to stand and walk,[288] as well as those with high cervical SCI to use their hand to grasp and manipulate

objects.[289] Implanted FES systems can also be used for phrenic nerve stimulation to allow patients with high cervical SCI to breathe without a ventilator[290] and to provide patients with bladder control.[291,292]

Brain-computer interface devices (BCIs) acquire brain signals (electroencephalogram [EEG]) and translate them into commands that are relayed to output devices that perform an action such as control a mouse on the computer screen.[293] People with high cervical SCI with little motor function are able to use BCIs to use a computer, play video games, potentially drive a power wheelchair, and control a robot.[294-297]

Robotic devices can be used during LT to move the LEs in a stepping pattern to promote recovery of walking ability.[155,298] Exoskeleton robots are being developed that will allow people with complete SCI to walk with assistance from the robot.[299]

Harkema and colleagues[154] combined epidural spinal electrical stimulation with LT on a TM with BWS and stand training in an individual with a chronic ASIA B C7 injury. After training, the individual was able to stand with full weight-bearing on the LEs and assistance only for balance when the stimulator was on. The individual was also able to voluntarily activate some LE muscles when the stimulator was on. The authors speculate that this combination therapy (epidural electrical stimulation with task-specific locomotor and stand training) may be a viable method to improve function after SCI.

These examples offer existing ways of how technology is being used and glimpses of the future of rehabilitation that provide exciting opportunities to increase activity levels, improve social participation, and enhance the quality of life for people with SCI.

SUMMARY

Spinal cord injury has a profound impact on many different body systems, which can greatly affect a person's ability to move, perform everyday tasks, and participate in expected social roles. This chapter has reviewed the impact of SCI on different body systems, common impairments that result from SCI, classification of different types of SCI, and secondary complications associated with SCI. Physical therapists play a role across the continuum of care from the acute care hospital through rehabilitation to community reintegration. Physical therapists should use standardized outcome measures as part of their examination and evaluation process. The POC should be individually tailored to the patient's presentation, concerns, and goals. Rehabilitation interventions may be compensatory or recovery based depending on the presentation of the patient. Education is a critical component, and patients who can no longer perform certain activities should be able to self-direct their care. Rehabilitation is an important cornerstone of recovery. People with SCI, no matter at what level, can lead a productive, healthy, and high-quality life.

Questions for Review

1. Identify the clinical features of Brown-Sequard, anterior, central, and posterior cord syndromes.

2. Define *spinal shock*.

3. Describe complications associated with spinal cord injury.

4. What is autonomic dysreflexia? Describe the initiating stimuli and symptoms of this syndrome. What action would you take if a patient experienced an onset of symptoms during a physical therapy treatment?

5. Identify two primary factors affecting prognosis following spinal cord injury.

6. What is included in a physical therapy examination during the acute phase of recovery? How might some of the standard examination techniques need to be modified?

7. What is meant by the term *selective stretching*?

8. Describe potential goals and interventions to improve respiratory function during the acute phase of management.

9. Identify tests and measures and outcome measures used during the active rehabilitation phase of management.

10. List factors that will have an impact on the prognosis for recovery of walking ability.

11. Outline interventions to improve transfers for a patient with C6 and ASIA A tetraplegia. Describe the specific activities you would include. What type of progressive strengthening and endurance training activities would you suggest for each patient as an adjunct to the mat program?

12. Describe how you would modify training parameters when performing LT using a BWS and TM system for an individual with an incomplete SCI.

CASE STUDY

HISTORY

The patient is a 21-year-old white man who was transferred to a rehabilitation hospital yesterday. He suffered a traumatic cervical spinal cord injury 8 days ago. He was given methylprednisolone in the emergency department. He had surgery to stabilize the fracture site, internal fixation, and decompression using a right iliac bone graft. He was discharged to your facility yesterday and is currently wearing a Philadelphia collar. He is able to extend his elbows but cannot flex his fingers in either hand. He is a senior at college, computer science major. Lives in on-campus apartment, not wheelchair accessible. His parents live in the next state.

MEDICATIONS

Lovenox, midodrine, amitriptyline, OxyContin, and Dulcolax.

PHYSICAL THERAPY EXAMINATION

Cardiopulmonary
HR: 75

BP: supine: 110/72; sitting: 100/66 (only able to tolerate sitting for about 10 minutes, then blood pressure drops due to orthostatic hypotension)

Forced vital capacity: 2.2 liters

Weak functional cough

Communication/Cognition
Alert, oriented ×3, able to follow multistep commands; MMSE: 30/30

Muscle Performance
Bilateral: biceps: 5/5, wrist extensors: 5/5, triceps: 4/5, no active contraction below C7

Sensory Integrity
Intact pinprick and light touch bilaterally C2–T4, absent below T4

Intact anal sensation

Functional Mobility
Bed mobility: moderate assistance to roll to the left and right

Supine ↔ short sit: maximal assistance

Supine ↔ long sit: maximal assistance

Transfer wheelchair ↔ bed: FIM score 2 (requires maximal assistance with transfer board)

Transfer wheelchair ↔ toilet: FIM score 2 (requires maximal assistance with transfer board)

Locomotion
Unable to ambulate.

Able to propel wheelchair 150 ft on level surface with minimal assistance.

Wheelchair Skills
Requires assistance with locking wheel locks, removing footrests and armrests, and to perform pressure relief. Wheelchair Skills Test score: 4%.

Currently uses a lightweight, folding wheelchair with hand rim projections.

Gel cushion.

Tolerates sitting in wheelchair for 20 to 30 minutes.

Balance
Long sitting: able to maintain balance on mat for 1 minute with UEs in weight-bearing position with supervision.

Short sitting: able to maintain balance on edge of mat for 1 minute with UEs in weight-bearing position with minimal assistance, 0 inches for modified functional reach.

Motor Function
Increased spasticity in bilateral hip flexors, 1+ on modified Ashworth Scale.

Passive ROM
WNL except bilateral ankle dorsiflexion is 5° from neutral.

Skin Integrity
Stage 1 wound on right heel.

Self-Care
Dressing upper body: FIM score 2 (requires maximal assistance)

Dressing lower body: FIM score 1 (dependent)

Bathing: FIM score 1 (dependent using shower chair)

Feeding: FIM score 3 (moderate assistance with adapted utensils)

Grooming: FIM score 3 (moderate assistance with adapted utensils)

Toileting: FIM score 2 (maximal assistance)

Bowel and Bladder
Bladder: FIM score 1 (just began intermittent catheterization program and requires total assist to manage)

Bowel: FIM score 1 (just began bowel training program with nursing, has been incontinent of bowel during the past day)

CASE STUDY GUIDING QUESTIONS

1. What is the patient's neurological level of injury, motor level of injury, and sensory level of injury? What is the patient's ASIA impairment classification?

2. Identify/categorize this patient's problems in terms of

   a. Body structure/function impairments

   b. Activity limitations

   c. Restrictions in social participation

3. Identify three anticipated goals and three expected outcomes for this patient.

4. Formulate three interventions with one progression that could be used during the first 3 weeks of therapy to improve bed mobility skills.

 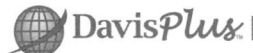 | For additional resources, including answers to the questions for review and case study guiding questions, please visit **http://davisplus.fadavis.com**

> The reader is referred to the following video case studies for additional review and study:
> - **Case Study 4: Patient with Spinal Cord Injury, T12/L1 Complete**
> - **Case Study 5: Patient with Spinal Cord Injury, C5/6 Incomplete**
>
> The full written case study, including all tables, figures, charts, and three video segments (examination, intervention, and outcome), appears online at *DavisPlus*. The case studies pose questions for the reader's consideration with suggested answers to the case study questions, also posted online at *DavisPlus*.

References

1. DeVivo, MJ, and Chen, Y: Trends in new injuries, prevalent cases, and aging with spinal cord injury. Arch Phys Med Rehabil 92(3):332, 2011.
2. National Spinal Cord Injury Statistical Center: Spinal Cord Injury: Facts and Figures at a Glance. Retrieved July 22, 2011, from www.nscisc.uab.edu.
3. McKinley, WO, Seel, RT, and Hardman, JT: Nontraumatic spinal cord injury: Incidence, epidemiology, and functional outcome. Arch Phys Med Rehabil 80(6):619, 1999.
4. Cao, Y, Chen, Y, and DeVivo, MJ: Lifetime direct costs after spinal cord injury. Topics Spinal Cord Rehabil 16(4):10, 2011.
5. Blumenfeld, H: Neuroanatomy Through Clinical Cases, ed 2. Sinauer Associates, Sunderland, MA, 2010.
6. American Spinal Injury Association: Reference Manual for the International Standards for Neurological Classification of Spinal Cord Injury. American Spinal Injury Association, Chicago, 2003.
7. Waring, WP, et al: 2009 review and revisions of the international standards for the neurological classification of spinal cord injury. J Spinal Cord Med 33(4):346, 2010.
8. McKinley, W, et al: Incidence and outcomes of spinal cord injury clinical syndromes. J Spinal Cord Med 30(3):215, 2007.
9. Tattersall, R, and Turner, B: Brown-Sequard and his syndrome. Lancet 356(9223):61, 2000.
10. Lundy-Ekman, L: Neuroscience: Fundamentals for Rehabilitation, ed 3. Saunders, Philadelphia, 2007.
11. Gilman, S, and Newman, SW: Maner and Gatz's Essentials of Clinical Neuroanatomy and Neurophysiology, ed 10. FA Davis, Philadelphia, 2003.
12. Roth, EJ, Lawler, MH, and Yarkony, GM: Traumatic central cord syndrome: Clinical features and functional outcomes. Arch Phys Med Rehabil 71(1):18, 1990.
13. Yadla, S, Klimo, P, and Harrop, JS: Traumatic central cord syndrome: Etiology, management, and outcomes. Topics Spinal Cord Rehabil 15(5):73, 2010.
14. Ditunno, JF, et al: Spinal shock revisited: A four-phase model. Spinal Cord 42(7):383, 2004.
15. Teasell, RW, et al: Cardiovascular consequences of loss of supraspinal control of the sympathetic nervous system after spinal cord injury. Arch Phys Med Rehabil 81(4):506, 2000.
16. Lindan, R, et al: Incidence and clinical features of autonomic dysreflexia in patients with spinal cord injury. Paraplegia 18(5):285, 1980.
17. Krassioukov, AV, Furlan, JC, and Fehlings, MG: Autonomic dysreflexia in acute spinal cord injury: An under-recognized clinical entity. J Neurotrauma 20(8):707, 2003.
18. Curt, A, et al: Assessment of autonomic dysreflexia in patients with spinal cord injury. J Neurol Neurosurg Psychiatry 62(5):473, 1997.
19. Karlsson, AK: Autonomic dysreflexia. Spinal Cord 37(6):383, 1999.
20. Consortium for Spinal Cord Medicine: Acute management of autonomic dysreflexia: Individuals with spinal cord injury presenting to health-care facilities. J Spinal Cord Med 25(Suppl 1):S67, 2002.
21. Consortium for Spinal Cord Medicine: Acute management of autonomic dysreflexia: Individuals with spinal cord injury presenting to health-care facilities. Retrieved May 31, 2012, from www.pva.org/site/c.ajIRK9NJLcJ2E/b.6305831/k.986B/Guidelines_and_Publications.htm.
22. Krassioukov, A, et al: A systematic review of the management of autonomic dysreflexia after spinal cord injury. Arch Phys Med Rehabil 90(4):682, 2009.
23. McGillivray, CF, et al: Evaluating knowledge of autonomic dysreflexia among individuals with spinal cord injury and their families. J Spinal Cord Med 32(1):54, 2009.
24. Skold, C, Levi, R, and Seiger, A: Spasticity after traumatic spinal cord injury: Nature, severity, and location. Arch Phys Med Rehabil 80(12):1548, 1999.
25. Meythaler, JM: Concept of spastic hypertonia. Phys Med Rehabil Clin North Am 12(4):725, 2001.
26. Young, RR, and Delwaide, PJ: Drug therapy: Spasticity (second of two parts). N Engl J Med 304(2):96, 1981.
27. Walter, JS, et al: A database of self-reported secondary medical problems among VA spinal cord injury patients: Its role in clinical care and management. J Rehabil Res Dev 39(1):53, 2002.

28. Gracies, JM: Pathophysiology of impairment in patients with spasticity and use of stretch as a treatment of spastic hypertonia. Phys Med Rehabil Clin North Am 12(4):747, vi, 2001.

29. Gracies, JM: Physical modalities other than stretch in spastic hypertonia. Phys Med Rehabil Clin North Am 12(4):769, vi, 2001.

30. Adams, MM, and Hicks, AL: Spasticity after spinal cord injury. Spinal Cord 43(10):577, 2005.

31. Katalinic, OM, Harvey, LA, and Herbert, RD: Effectiveness of stretch for the treatment and prevention of contractures in people with neurological conditions: A systematic review. Phys Ther 91(1):11, 2011.

32. Francisco, GE, Kothari, S, and Huls, C: GABA agonists and gabapentin for spastic hypertonia. Phys Med Rehabil Clin North Am 12(4):875, viii, 2001.

33. Kamen, L, Henney, HR, 3rd, and Runyan, JD: A practical overview of tizanidine use for spasticity secondary to multiple sclerosis, stroke, and spinal cord injury. Curr Med Res Opin 24(2):425, 2008.

34. Elovic, E: Principles of pharmaceutical management of spastic hypertonia. Phys Med Rehabil Clin North Am 12(4):793, vii, 2001.

35. Ivanhoe, CB, Tilton, AH, and Francisco, GE: Intrathecal baclofen therapy for spastic hypertonia. Phys Med Rehabil Clin North Am 12(4):923, 2001.

36. Yablon, SA: Botulinum neurotoxin intramuscular chemodenervation. Role in the management of spastic hypertonia and related motor disorders. Phys Med Rehabil Clin North Am 12(4):833, 2001.

37. Taricco, M, et al: Pharmacological interventions for spasticity following spinal cord injury. Cochrane Database Syst Rev 2: CD001131, 2000.

38. Martin, JH: Neuroanatomy Text and Atlas, ed 2. Appleton & Lange, Stamford, CT, 1996.

39. Naso, F: Cardiovascular problems in patients with spinal cord injury. Phys Med Rehabil Clin North Am 3(4):741, 1992.

40. Wadsworth, BM, et al: Abdominal binder use in people with spinal cord injuries: A systematic review and meta-analysis. Spinal Cord 47(4):274, 2009.

41. Gondim, FA, et al: Cardiovascular control after spinal cord injury. Curr Vasc Pharmacol 2(1):71, 2004.

42. Jacobs, PL, and Nash, MS: Exercise recommendations for individuals with spinal cord injury. Sports Med 34(11):727, 2004.

43. Claxton, AR, et al: Predictors of hospital mortality and mechanical ventilation in patients with cervical spinal cord injury. Can J Anaesth 45(2):144, 1998.

44. Jackson, AB, and Groomes, TE: Incidence of respiratory complications following spinal cord injury. Arch Phys Med Rehabil 75(3):270, 1994.

45. McKinley, WO, et al: Long-term medical complications after traumatic spinal cord injury: A regional model systems analysis. Arch Phys Med Rehabil 80(11):1402, 1999.

46. Wallbom, AS, Naran, B, and Thomas, E: Acute ventilator management and weaning in individuals with high tetraplegia. Topics Spinal Cord Rehabil 10(3):1, 2005.

47. Jain, NB, et al: Determinants of forced expiratory volume in 1 second (FEV_1), forced vital capacity (FVC), and FEV_1/FVC in chronic spinal cord injury. Arch Phys Med Rehabil 87(10):1327, 2006.

48. Berly, M, and Shem, K: Respiratory management during the first five days after spinal cord injury. J Spinal Cord Med 30(4):309, 2007.

49. Alvarez, SE, Peterson, M, and Lunsford, BR: Respiratory treatment of the adult patient with spinal cord injury. Phys Ther 61(12):1737, 1981.

50. Stolzmann, KL, et al: Longitudinal change in FEV_1 and FVC in chronic spinal cord injury. Am J Respir Crit Care Med 177(7):781, 2008.

51. Benevento, BT, and Sipski, ML: Neurogenic bladder, neurogenic bowel, and sexual dysfunction in people with spinal cord injury. Phys Ther 82(6):601, 2002.

52. Garcia Leoni, ME, and Esclarin De Ruz, A: Management of urinary tract infection in patients with spinal cord injuries. Clin Microbiol Infect 9(8):780, 2003.

53. Warms, C, et al: Bowel and bladder function and management. In Field-Fote, EC (ed): Spinal Cord Injury Rehabilitation. FA Davis, Philadelphia, 2009.

54. Waites, KB, Canupp, KC, and DeVivo, MJ: Epidemiology and risk factors for urinary tract infection following spinal cord injury. Arch Phys Med Rehabil 74(7):691, 1993.

55. Coggrave, M, Norton, C, and Wilson-Barnett, J: Management of neurogenic bowel dysfunction in the community after spinal cord injury: A postal survey in the United Kingdom. Spinal Cord 47(4):323–330, quiz 331, 2009.

56. Liu, CW, et al: Relationship between neurogenic bowel dysfunction and health-related quality of life in persons with spinal cord injury. J Rehabil Med 41(1):35–40, 2009.

57. Anderson, KD, et al: The impact of spinal cord injury on sexual function: Concerns of the general population. Spinal Cord 45(5):328, 2007.

58. Watanabe, T, et al: Epidemiology of current treatment for sexual dysfunction in spinal cord injured men in the USA model spinal cord injury centers. J Spinal Cord Med 19(3):186, 1996.

59. Elliott, S: Sexuality after spinal cord injury. In Field-Fote, EC (ed): Spinal Cord Injury Rehabilitation. FA Davis, Philadelphia, 2009.

60. Phelps, G, et al: Sexual experience and plasma testosterone levels in male veterans after spinal cord injury. Arch Phys Med Rehabil 64(2):47, 1983.

61. Alexander, CJ, Sipski, ML, and Findley, TW: Sexual activities, desire, and satisfaction in males pre- and post-spinal cord injury. Arch Sex Behav 22(3):217, 1993.

62. Baker, ER, and Cardenas, DD: Pregnancy in spinal cord injured women. Arch Phys Med Rehabil 77(5):501, 1996.

63. Smeltzer, SC, and Wetzel-Effinger, L: Pregnancy in women with spinal cord injury. Topics Spinal Cord Rehabil 15(1):29, 2009.

64. National Spinal Cord Injury Statistical Center: The 2004 Annual Statistical Report for the Model Spinal Cord Injury Care Systems. Retrieved May 31, 2012, from http://images.main.uab.edu/spinalcord/pdffiles/2004StatReport.pdf.

65. Verschueren, JH, et al: Occurrence and predictors of pressure ulcers during primary in-patient spinal cord injury rehabilitation. Spinal Cord 49(1):106, 2011.

66. Gelis, A, et al: Pressure ulcer risk factors in persons with SCI: Part I: Acute and rehabilitation stages. Spinal Cord 47(2):99, 2009.

67. Gelis, A, et al: Pressure ulcer risk factors in persons with spinal cord injury part 2: The chronic stage. Spinal Cord 47(9):651, 2009.

68. Agarwal, NK, and Mathur, N: Deep vein thrombosis in acute spinal cord injury. Spinal Cord 47(10):769, 2009.

69. Chen, D: Treatment and prevention of thromboembolism after spinal cord injury. Topics Spinal Cord Rehabil 9(1):14, 2009.

70. Demirel, G, et al: Pain following spinal cord injury. Spinal Cord 36(1):25, 1998.

71. Finnerup, NB, et al: Pain and dysesthesia in patients with spinal cord injury: A postal survey. Spinal Cord 39(5):256, 2001.

72. Widerstrom-Noga, EG, et al: Perceived difficulty in dealing with consequences of spinal cord injury. Arch Phys Med Rehabil 80(5):580, 1999.

73. Dijkers, M, Bryce, T, and Zanca, J: Prevalence of chronic pain after traumatic spinal cord injury: A systematic review. J Rehabil Res Dev 46(1):13, 2009.

74. Widerstrom-Noga, EG, Felipe-Cuervo, E, and Yezierski, RP: Chronic pain after spinal injury: Interference with sleep and daily activities. Arch Phys Med Rehabil 82(11):1571, 2001.

75. Westgren, N, and Levi, R: Quality of life and traumatic spinal cord injury. Arch Phys Med Rehabil 79(11):1433, 1998.

76. Widerstrom-Noga, EG: Pain after spinal cord injury: Etiology and management. In Field-Fote, EC (ed): Spinal Cord Injury Rehabilitation. FA Davis, Philadelphia, 2009.

77. MacKay-Lyons, M: Shoulder pain in patients with acute quadriplegia: A retrospective study. Physiother Can 46(4):255, 1994.

78. Dyson-Hudson, TA, and Kirshblum, SC: Shoulder pain in chronic spinal cord injury. Part I: Epidemiology, etiology, and pathomechanics. J Spinal Cord Med 27(1):4, 2004.

79. Irwin, RW, Restrepo, JA, and Sherman, A: Musculoskeletal pain in persons with spinal cord injury. Topics Spinal Cord Rehabil 13(2):43, 2007.

80. Teasell, RW, et al: A systematic review of pharmacologic treatments of pain after spinal cord injury. Arch Phys Med Rehabil 91(5):816, 2010.

81. Cardenas, DD, and Jensen, MP: Treatments for chronic pain in persons with spinal cord injury: A survey study. J Spinal Cord Med 29(2):109, 2006.
82. Fattal, C, et al: What is the efficacy of physical therapeutics for treating neuropathic pain in spinal cord injury patients? Ann Phys Rehabil Med 52(2):149, 2009.
83. Attal, N, et al: Chronic neuropathic pain management in spinal cord injury patients. What is the efficacy of pharmacological treatments with a general mode of administration? (oral, transdermal, intravenous). Ann Phys Rehabil Med 52(2):124, 2009.
84. van Kuijk, AA, Geurts, AC, and van Kuppevelt, HJ: Neurogenic heterotopic ossification in spinal cord injury. Spinal Cord 40(7):313, 2002.
85. Lal, S, et al: Risk factors for heterotopic ossification in spinal cord injury. Arch Phys Med Rehabil 70(5):387, 1989.
86. Bravo-Payno, P, et al: Incidence and risk factors in the appearance of heterotopic ossification in spinal cord injury. Paraplegia 30(10):740, 1992.
87. Teasell, RW, et al: A systematic review of the therapeutic interventions for heterotopic ossification after spinal cord injury. Spinal Cord 48(7):512, 2010.
88. Ashe, MC, et al: Prevention and treatment of bone loss after a spinal cord injury: A systematic review. Topics Spinal Cord Rehabil 13(1):123, 2007.
89. Giangregorio, L, and McCartney, N: Bone loss and muscle atrophy in spinal cord injury: Epidemiology, fracture prediction, and rehabilitation strategies. J Spinal Cord Med 29(5):489, 2006.
90. Fattal, C, et al: Osteoporosis in persons with spinal cord injury: The need for a targeted therapeutic education. Arch Phys Med Rehabil 92(1):59, 2011.
91. Waters, RL, et al: Motor and sensory recovery following incomplete tetraplegia. Arch Phys Med Rehabil 75(3):306, 1994.
92. Waters, RL, et al: Motor and sensory recovery following incomplete paraplegia. Arch Phys Med Rehabil 75(1):67, 1994.
93. Steeves, JD, et al: Extent of spontaneous motor recovery after traumatic cervical sensorimotor complete spinal cord injury. Spinal Cord 49(2):257, 2011.
94. Oleson, CV, et al: Prognostic value of pinprick preservation in motor complete, sensory incomplete spinal cord injury. Arch Phys Med Rehabil 86(5):988, 2005.
95. Waters, RL, et al: Motor and sensory recovery following complete tetraplegia. Arch Phys Med Rehabil 74(3):242, 1993.
96. Fehlings, MG, Cadotte, DW, and Fehlings, LN: A series of systematic reviews on the treatment of acute spinal cord injury: A foundation for best medical practice. J Neurotrauma 28(8):1329–1333, 2011.
97. Sheerin, F: Spinal cord injury: Acute care management. Emerg Nurse 12(10):26, 2005.
98. Bracken, MB, et al: A randomized, controlled trial of methylprednisolone or naloxone in the treatment of acute spinal-cord injury. Results of the Second National Acute Spinal Cord Injury Study. N Engl J Med 322(20):1405, 1990.
99. Bracken, MB, et al: Administration of methylprednisolone for 24 or 48 hours or tirilazad mesylate for 48 hours in the treatment of acute spinal cord injury. Results of the Third National Acute Spinal Cord Injury Randomized Controlled Trial. National Acute Spinal Cord Injury Study. JAMA 277(20):1597, 1997.
100. Bracken, MB, et al: Methylprednisolone or tirilazad mesylate administration after acute spinal cord injury: 1-year follow up. Results of the third National Acute Spinal Cord Injury randomized controlled trial. J Neurosurg 89(5):699, 1998.
101. Bracken, MB: Steroids for acute spinal cord injury. Cochrane Database Syst Rev 1(CD001046), 2012.
102. Qian, T, Campagnolo, D, and Kirshblum, S: High-dose methylprednisolone may do more harm for spinal cord injury. Med Hypotheses 55(5):452, 2000.
103. Gerndt, SJ, et al: Consequences of high-dose steroid therapy for acute spinal cord injury. J Trauma 42(2):279, 1997.
104. Fehlings, MG, and Tator, CH: An evidence-based review of decompressive surgery in acute spinal cord injury: Rationale, indications, and timing based on experimental and clinical studies. J Neurosurg 91(1 Suppl):1, 1999.
105. Waters, RL, et al: Emergency, acute, and surgical management of spine trauma. Arch Phys Med Rehabil 80(11):1383, 1999.
106. Initial closed reduction of cervical spine fracture-dislocation injuries. Neurosurgery 50(3 Suppl):S44, 2002.
107. Hislop, H, and Montgomery, J: Daniels and Worthingham's Muscle Testing: Techniques of Manual Examination, ed 8. Saunders, Philadelphia, 2007.
108. Roth, EJ, et al: Pulmonary function testing in spinal cord injury: Correlation with vital capacity. Paraplegia 33(8):454, 1995.
109. Berney, SC, et al: A classification and regression tree to assist clinical decision making in airway management for patients with cervical spinal cord injury. Spinal Cord 49(2):244, 2011.
110. Anke, A, et al: Lung volumes in tetraplegic patients according to cervical spinal cord injury level. Scand J Rehabil Med 25(2):73–77, 1993.
111. Roth, EJ, et al: Ventilatory function in cervical and high thoracic spinal cord injury. Relationship to level of injury and tone. Am J Phys Med Rehabil 76(4):262–267, 1997.
112. Manning, H, et al: Oxygen cost of resistive-loaded breathing in quadriplegia. J Appl Physiol 73(3):825, 1992.
113. Somers, MF: Spinal Cord Injury: Functional Rehabilitation, ed 2. Pearson Education, Upper Saddle River, NJ, 2010.
114. Mortenson, WB, and Miller, WC: A review of scales for assessing the risk of developing a pressure ulcer in individuals with SCI. Spinal Cord 46(3):168, 2008.
115. Pancorbo-Hidalgo, PL, et al: Risk assessment scales for pressure ulcer prevention: A systematic review. J Adv Nurs 54(1):94, 2006.
116. Wellard, S, and Lo, SK: Comparing Norton, Braden and Waterlow risk assessment scales for pressure ulcers in spinal cord injuries. Contemp Nurse 9(2):155, 2000.
117. Salzberg, CA, et al: A new pressure ulcer risk assessment scale for individuals with spinal cord injury. Am J Phys Med Rehabil 75(2):96, 1996.
118. Salzberg, CA, et al: Predicting pressure ulcers during initial hospitalisation for acute spinal cord injury. Wounds 11:45, 1999.
119. van Lis, MS, van Asbeck, FW, and Post, MW: Monitoring healing of pressure ulcers: A review of assessment instruments for use in the spinal cord unit. Spinal Cord 48(2):92, 2010.
120. Sussman, C, and Swanson, G: Utility of the Sussman Wound Healing Tool in predicting wound healing outcomes in physical therapy. Adv Wound Care 10(5):74–77, 1997.
121. Thomas, DR, et al: Pressure ulcer scale for healing: Derivation and validation of the PUSH tool. The PUSH Task Force. Adv Wound Care 10(5):96, 1997.
122. Ferrell, BA: The Sessing Scale for measurement of pressure ulcer healing. Adv Wound Care 10(5):78, 1997.
123. Eriks-Hoogland, IE, et al: Passive shoulder range of motion impairment in spinal cord injury during and one year after rehabilitation. J Rehabil Med 41(6):438, 2009.
124. Bach, JR: Noninvasive alternatives to tracheostomy for managing respiratory muscle dysfunction in spinal cord injury. Topics Spinal Cord Rehabil 2:49, 1997.
125. Warren, VC: Glossopharyngeal and neck accessory muscle breathing in a young adult with C2 complete tetraplegia resulting in ventilator dependency. Phys Ther 82(6):590, 2002.
126. Wetzel, JL: Management of respiratory dysfunction. In Field-Fote, EC (ed): Spinal Cord Injury Rehabilitation. FA Davis, Philadelphia, 2009.
127. Montero, JC, Feldman, DJ, and Montero, D: Effects of glossopharyngeal breathing on respiratory function after cervical cord transection. Arch Phys Med Rehabil 48(12):650, 1967.
128. Tecklin, JS: The patient with ventilatory pump dysfunction/failure—preferred practice pattern 6E. In Irwin, S, and Tecklin, JS (eds): Cardiopulmonary Physical Therapy, ed 4. Mosby, St. Louis, 2004.
129. Sheel, AW, et al: Effects of exercise training and inspiratory muscle training in spinal cord injury: A systematic review. J Spinal Cord Med 31(5):500, 2008.
130. Liaw, MY, et al: Resistive inspiratory muscle training: Its effectiveness in patients with acute complete cervical cord injury. Arch Phys Med Rehabil 81(6):752, 2000.
131. Cruzado, D, et al: Resistive inspiratory muscle training improves inspiratory muscle strength in subjects with cervical spinal cord injury. Neurol Rep 26(1):3, 2002.
132. Reid, WD, et al: Physiotherapy secretion removal techniques in people with spinal cord injury: A systematic review. J Spinal Cord Med 33(4):353, 2010.

133. Boaventura, CD, et al: Effect of abdominal binder on the efficacy of respiratory muscles in seated and supine tetraplegic patients. Physiotherapy 89(5):290, 2003.

134. McCool, FD, et al: Changes in lung volume and rib cage configuration with abdominal binding in quadriplegia. J Appl Physiol 60(4):1198, 1986.

135. Julia, PE, Sa'ari, MY, and Hasnan, N: Benefit of triple-strap abdominal binder on voluntary cough in patients with spinal cord injury. Spinal Cord 49(11):1138, 2011.

136. Royster, RA, Barboi, C, and Peruzzi, WT: Critical care in acute cervical spinal cord injury. Topics Spinal Cord Rehabil 9(3):11, 2004.

137. Gittler, MS: Acute rehabilitation in cervical spinal cord injury. Topics Spinal Cord Rehabil 9(3):60, 2004.

138. Henderson, JL, et al: Efficacy of three measures to relieve pressure in seated persons with spinal cord injury. Arch Phys Med Rehabil 75(5):535, 1994.

139. Coggrave, MJ, and Rose, LS: A specialist seating assessment clinic: Changing pressure relief practice. Spinal Cord 41(12):692, 2003.

140. Rintala, DH, et al: Preventing recurrent pressure ulcers in veterans with spinal cord injury: Impact of a structured education and follow-up intervention. Arch Phys Med Rehabil 89(8):1429, 2008.

141. Griffin, JW, et al: Efficacy of high voltage pulsed current for healing of pressure ulcers in patients with spinal cord injury. Phys Ther 71(6):433, discussion 442, 1991.

142. Adegoke, BO, and Badmos, KA: Acceleration of pressure ulcer healing in spinal cord injured patients using interrupted direct current. Afr J Med Med Sci 30(3):195, 2001.

143. Hollisaz, MT, Khedmat, H, and Yari, F: A randomized clinical trial comparing hydrocolloid, phenytoin and simple dressings for the treatment of pressure ulcers [ISRCTN33429693]. BMC Dermatol 4(1):18, 2004.

144. Whittle, H, et al: Nursing management of pressure ulcers using a hydrogel dressing protocol: Four case studies. Rehabil Nurs 21(5):239, 1996.

145. Sussman, C, and Bates-Jensen, B: Wound Care: A Collaborative Practice Manual of Health Professionals. Lippincott Williams & Wilkins, Philadelphia, 2007.

146. Bohn, AS, and Peljovich, AE: Upper extremity orthotic and postsurgical management. In Field-Fote, EC (ed): Spinal Cord Injury Rehabilitation. FA Davis, Philadelphia, 2009.

147. Behrman, AL, and Harkema, SJ: Physical rehabilitation as an agent for recovery after spinal cord injury. Phys Med Rehabil Clin North Am 18(2):183, v, 2007.

148. Behrman, A, et al: Assessment of functional improvement without compensation reduces variability of outcome measures after human spinal cord injury. Arch Phys Med Rehabil 93(9):1518, 2012.

149. Barbeau, H, Nadeau, S, and Garneau, C: Physical determinants, emerging concepts, and training approaches in gait of individuals with spinal cord injury. J Neurotrauma 23(3-4):571, 2006.

150. Levin, MF, Kleim, JA, and Wolf, SL: What do motor "recovery" and "compensation" mean in patients following stroke? Neurorehabil Neural Repair 23(4):313, 2009.

151. Harkema, SJ: Neural plasticity after human spinal cord injury: Application of locomotor training to the rehabilitation of walking. Neuroscientist 7(5):455, 2001.

152. Dietz, V, and Harkema, SJ: Locomotor activity in spinal cord-injured persons. J Appl Physiol 96(5):1954, 2004.

153. Harkema, S, Behrman, A, and Barbeau, H: Locomotor Training: Principles and Practice. Oxford University Press, 2011.

154. Harkema, S, et al: Effect of epidural stimulation of the lumbosacral spinal cord on voluntary movement, standing, and assisted stepping after motor complete paraplegia: A case study. Lancet 377(9781):1938, 2011.

155. Field-Fote, EC, and Roach, KE: Influence of a locomotor training approach on walking speed and distance in people with chronic spinal cord injury: A randomized clinical trial. Phys Ther 91(1):48, 2011.

156. Alexeeva, N, et al: Comparison of training methods to improve walking in persons with chronic spinal cord injury: A randomized clinical trial. J Spinal Cord Med 34(4):362–379, 2011.

157. Edgerton, VR, and Harkema, S: Epidural stimulation of the spinal cord in spinal cord injury: Current status and future challenges. Expert Rev Neurother 11(10):1351, 2011.

158. Musienko, P, et al: Multi-system neurorehabilitative strategies to restore motor functions following severe spinal cord injury. Exp Neurol 235(1):100, 2012. (Epub September 7, 2011.)

159. Hol, AT, et al: Reliability and validity of the six-minute arm test for the evaluation of cardiovascular fitness in people with spinal cord injury. Arch Phys Med Rehabil 88(4):489, 2007.

160. Macciocchi, S, et al: Spinal cord injury and co-occurring traumatic brain injury: Assessment and incidence. Arch Phys Med Rehabil 89(7):1350, 2008.

161. Nasreddine, ZS, et al: The Montreal Cognitive Assessment, MoCA: A brief screening tool for mild cognitive impairment. J Am Geriatr Soc 53(4):695, 2005.

162. Folstein, MF, Folstein SE and McHugh PR: "Mini-mental state." A practical method for grading the cognitive state of patients for the clinician. J Psychiatr Res 12(3):189, 1975.

163. Americans with Disabilities Act and Architectural Barriers Act Accessibility Guidelines. United States Access Board, Washington D.C. USA, 2004.

164. Davies, TD, and Lopez, CP: Accessible Home Design: Architectural Solutions for the Wheelchair User. Paralyzed Veterans of American, Washington D.C., 2006.

165. Kirby, RL, et al: The Wheelchair Skills Test (Version 2.4): Measurement properties. Arch Phys Med Rehabil 85(5):794, 2004.

166. Kirby, RL, et al: The Wheelchair Skills Test: A pilot study of a new outcome measure. Arch Phys Med Rehabil 83(1):10, 2002.

167. Lindquist, NJ, et al: Reliability of the performance and safety scores of the Wheelchair Skills Test Version 4.1 for manual wheelchair users. Arch Phys Med Rehabil 91(11):1752, 2010.

168. Kilkens, OJ, et al: The Wheelchair Circuit: Construct validity and responsiveness of a test to assess manual wheelchair mobility in persons with spinal cord injury. Arch Phys Med Rehabil 85(3):424, 2004.

169. Kilkens, OJ, et al: The Wheelchair Circuit: Reliability of a test to assess mobility in persons with spinal cord injuries. Arch Phys Med Rehabil 83(12):1783, 2002.

170. Lynch, SM, Leahy, P, and Barker, SP: Reliability of measurements obtained with a modified functional reach test in subjects with spinal cord injury. Phys Ther 78(2):128, 1998.

171. Berg, KO, et al: Measuring balance in the elderly: Validation of an instrument. Can J Public Health 83(Suppl 2):S7, 1992.

172. Lemay, JF, and Nadeau, S: Standing balance assessment in ASIA D paraplegic and tetraplegic participants: Concurrent validity of the Berg Balance Scale. Spinal Cord 48(3):245, 2010.

173. Wirz, M, Muller, R, and Bastiaenen, C: Falls in persons with spinal cord injury: Validity and reliability of the Berg Balance Scale. Neurorehabil Neural Repair 24(1):70, 2010.

174. The Pathokinesiology Laboratory and The Physical Therapy Department, Ranchos Los Amigos: Observational Gait Analysis. Ranchos Los Amigos National Rehabilitation Center, 2001.

175. Ditunno, JF, Jr., et al: Walking index for spinal cord injury (WISCI): An international multicenter validity and reliability study. Spinal Cord 38(4):234–243, 2000.

176. Ditunno, JF, et al: Validation of the walking index for spinal cord injury in a US and European clinical population. Spinal Cord 46(3):181, 2008.

177. Jackson, AB, et al: Outcome measures for gait and ambulation in the spinal cord injury population. J Spinal Cord Med 31(5):487, 2008.

178. van Hedel, HJ, Wirz, M, and Dietz, V: Assessing walking ability in subjects with spinal cord injury: Validity and reliability of three walking tests. Arch Phys Med Rehabil 86(2):190, 2005.

179. Field-Fote, EC: The Spinal Cord Injury Functional Ambulation Inventory (SCI-FAI). J Rehabil Med 33(4):177, 2001.

180. Lam, T, Noonan, VK, and Eng, JJ: A systematic review of functional ambulation outcome measures in spinal cord injury. Spinal Cord 46(4):246, 2008.

181. van Hedel, HJ: Gait speed in relation to categories of functional ambulation after spinal cord injury. Neurorehabil Neural Repair 23(4):343, 2009.

182. Haas, BM, et al: The inter rater reliability of the original and of the modified Ashworth scale for the assessment of spasticity in patients with spinal cord injury. Spinal Cord 34(9):560, 1996.

183. Adams, MM, Ginis, KA, and Hicks, AL: The Spinal Cord Injury Spasticity Evaluation Tool: Development and evaluation. Arch Phys Med Rehabil 88(9):1185, 2007.

184. Sisto, SA, and Dyson-Hudson, T: Dynamometry testing in spinal cord injury. J Rehabil Res Dev 44(1):123, 2007.

185. Larson, CA, et al: Assessment of postural muscle strength in sitting: Reliability of measures obtained with hand-held dynamometry in individuals with spinal cord injury. J Neurol Phys Ther 34(1):24, 2010.

186. Jensen, MP, et al: Reliability and validity of the International Spinal Cord Injury Basic Pain Data Set items as self-report measures. Spinal Cord 48(3):230, 2010.

187. Curtis, KA, et al: Reliability and validity of the Wheelchair User's Shoulder Pain Index (WUSPI). Paraplegia 33(10):595, 1995.

188. Curtis, KA, et al: Development of the Wheelchair User's Shoulder Pain Index (WUSPI). Paraplegia 33(5):290, 1995.

189. Dodds, TA, et al: A validation of the functional independence measurement and its performance among rehabilitation inpatients. Arch Phys Med Rehabil 74(5):531, 1993.

190. Hamilton, BB, et al: Relation of disability costs to function: Spinal cord injury. Arch Phys Med Rehabil 80(4):385, 1999.

191. Heinemann, AW, et al: Relationships between disability measures and nursing effort during medical rehabilitation for patients with traumatic brain and spinal cord injury. Arch Phys Med Rehabil 78(2):143, 1997.

192. Catz, A, et al: SCIM—Spinal Cord Independence Measure: A new disability scale for patients with spinal cord lesions. Spinal Cord 35(12):850, 1997.

193. Rudhe, C, and van Hedel, HJ: Upper extremity function in persons with tetraplegia: Relationships between strength, capacity, and the spinal cord independence measure. Neurorehabil Neural Repair 23(5):413, 2009.

194. Dawson, J, Shamley, D, and Jamous, MA: A structured review of outcome measures used for the assessment of rehabilitation interventions for spinal cord injury. Spinal Cord 46(12):768, 2008.

195. Gresham, GE, et al: The Quadriplegia Index of Function (QIF): Sensitivity and reliability demonstrated in a study of thirty quadriplegic patients. Paraplegia 24(1):38, 1986.

196. Yavuz, N, Tezyurek, M, and Akyuz, M: A comparison of two functional tests in quadriplegia: The Quadriplegia Index of Function and the Functional Independence Measure. Spinal Cord 36(12):832, 1998.

197. Marino, RJ, Shea, JA, and Stineman, MG: The Capabilities of Upper Extremity instrument: Reliability and validity of a measure of functional limitation in tetraplegia. Arch Phys Med Rehabil 79(12):1512, 1998.

198. Mulcahey, MJ, Smith, BT, and Betz, RR: Psychometric rigor of the Grasp and Release Test for measuring functional limitation of persons with tetraplegia: A preliminary analysis. J Spinal Cord Med 27(1):41, 2004.

199. Whiteneck, GG, et al: Quantifying handicap: A new measure of long-term rehabilitation outcomes. Arch Phys Med Rehabil 73(6):519, 1992.

200. Fougeyrollas, P, et al: Social consequences of long term impairments and disabilities: Conceptual approach and assessment of handicap. Int J Rehabil Res 21(2):127, 1998.

201. Noreau, L, Fougeyrollas, P, and Vincent, C: The LIFE-H: Assessment of the quality of social participation. Technol Disabil (14):113, 2002.

202. May, LA, and Warren, S: Measuring quality of life of persons with spinal cord injury: External and structural validity. Spinal Cord 40(7):341, 2002.

203. Consortium for Spinal Cord Injury Medicine Clinical Practice Guidelines: Outcomes Following Traumatic Spinal Cord Injury: Clinical Practice Guidelines for Health-Care Professionals. Paralyzed Veterans of American, Washington D.C., 1999.

204. Al-Habib, AF, et al: Clinical predictors of recovery after blunt spinal cord trauma: systematic review. J Neurotrauma 28(8): 1431, 2011.

205. Bombardier, CH, et al: Do preinjury alcohol problems predict poorer rehabilitation progress in persons with spinal cord injury? Arch Phys Med Rehabil 85(9):1488, 2004.

206. Grover, J, Gellman, H, and Waters, RL: The effect of a flexion contracture of the elbow on the ability to transfer in patients who have quadriplegia at the sixth cervical level. J Bone Joint Surg Am 78(9):1397, 1996.

207. Guide to Physical Therapist Practice, Second Edition. American Physical Therapy Association. Phys Ther 81(1):9, 2001.

208. Ditunno, PL, et al: Who wants to walk? Preferences for recovery after SCI: A longitudinal and cross-sectional study. Spinal Cord 46(7):500, 2008.

209. Waters, RL: Functional prognosis of spinal cord injuries. J Spinal Cord Med 19(2):89, 1996.

210. Crozier, KS, et al: Spinal cord injury: Prognosis for ambulation based on sensory examination in patients who are initially motor complete. Arch Phys Med Rehabil 72(2):119, 1991.

211. Burns, SP, et al: Recovery of ambulation in motor-incomplete tetraplegia. Arch Phys Med Rehabil 78(11):1169, 1997.

212. Alander, DH, Parker, J, and Stauffer, ES: Intermediate-term outcome of cervical spinal cord–injured patients older than 50 years of age. Spine 22(11):1189, 1997.

213. Crozier, KS, et al: Spinal cord injury: Prognosis for ambulation based on quadriceps recovery. Paraplegia 30(11):762, 1992.

214. Waters, RL, et al: Prediction of ambulatory performance based on motor scores derived from standards of the American Spinal Injury Association. Arch Phys Med Rehabil 75(7):756, 1994.

215. van Middendorp, JJ, et al: A clinical prediction rule for ambulation outcomes after traumatic spinal cord injury: A longitudinal cohort study. Lancet 377(9770):1004, 2011.

216. Behrman, AL, et al: Locomotor training progression and outcomes after incomplete spinal cord injury. Phys Ther 85(12):1356, 2005.

217. Nyland, J, et al: Preserving transfer independence among individuals with spinal cord injury. Spinal Cord 38(11):649, 2000.

218. Hicks, AL, et al: Long-term exercise training in persons with spinal cord injury: Effects on strength, arm ergometry performance and psychological well-being. Spinal Cord 41(1):34, 2003.

219. Mulroy, SJ, et al: Strengthening and Optimal Movements for Painful Shoulders (STOMPS) in chronic spinal cord injury: A randomized controlled trial. Phys Ther 91(3):305, 2011.

220. Figoni, SF: Spinal cord disabilities: Paraplegia and tetraplegia. In Durstine, JL, and Moore, GE (eds): ACSM's Exercise Management for Persons with Chronic Diseases and Disabilities. American College of Sports Medicine, Champaign, IL, 2003.

221. de Groot, PC, et al: Effect of training intensity on physical capacity, lipid profile and insulin sensitivity in early rehabilitation of spinal cord injured individuals. Spinal Cord 41(12):673, 2003.

222. Davis, G, Plyley, MJ, and Shephard, RJ: Gains of cardiorespiratory fitness with arm-crank training in spinally disabled men. Can J Sport Sci 16(1).64, 1991.

223. Hooker, SP, and Wells, CL: Effects of low- and moderate-intensity training in spinal cord–injured persons. Med Sci Sports Exerc 21(1):18, 1989.

224. Valent, LJ, et al: Effects of hand cycle training on physical capacity in individuals with tetraplegia: A clinical trial. Phys Ther 89(10):1051, 2009.

225. Carvalho, DC, et al: Effect of treadmill gait on bone markers and bone mineral density of quadriplegic subjects. Braz J Med Biol Res 39(10):1357, 2006.

226. Soyupek, F, et al: Effects of body weight supported treadmill training on cardiac and pulmonary functions in the patients with incomplete spinal cord injury. J Back Musculoskelet Rehabil 22(4):213, 2009.

227. Janssen, TW, and Pringle, DD: Effects of modified electrical stimulation–induced leg cycle ergometer training for individuals with spinal cord injury. J Rehabil Research Dev 45(6):819, 2008.

228. Mohr, T, et al: Long-term adaptation to electrically induced cycle training in severe spinal cord injured individuals. Spinal Cord 35(1):1, 1997.

229. Hooker, SP, et al: Physiologic effects of electrical stimulation leg cycle exercise training in spinal cord injured persons. Arch Phys Med Rehabil 73(5):470, 1992.

230. Perry, J, et al: Electromyographic analysis of the shoulder muscles during depression transfers in subjects with low-level paraplegia. Arch Phys Med Rehabil 77(4):350, 1996.

231. Forslund, EB, et al: Transfer from table to wheelchair in men and women with spinal cord injury: Coordination of body movement and arm forces. Spinal Cord 45(1):41, 2007.

232. Fulk, G: Interventions to improve transfers and wheelchair skills. In O'Sullivan, S, and Schmitz, T (eds): Improving Functional Outcomes in Physical Rehabilitation. FA Davis, Philadelphia, 2010.

233. Eng, JJ, et al: Use of prolonged standing for individuals with spinal cord injuries. Phys Ther 81(8):1392, 2001.

234. Mikelberg, R, and Reid, S: Spinal cord lesions and lower extremity bracing: An overview and follow-up study. Paraplegia 19(6):379, 1981.

235. Behrman, AL, and Plummer-D'Amato, P: "What's in a name?" revisited. Phys Ther 88(1):6, 2008.

236. Barbeau, H, and Rossignol, S: Recovery of locomotion after chronic spinalization in the adult cat. Brain Res 412(1):84, 1987.

237. Lovely, RG, et al: Effects of training on the recovery of full-weight-bearing stepping in the adult spinal cat. Exp Neurol 92(2):421, 1986.

238. Edgerton, VR, et al: Use-dependent plasticity in spinal stepping and standing. Adv Neurol (72):233, 1997.

239. Barbeau, H, Wainberg, M, and Finch, L: Description and application of a system for locomotor rehabilitation. Med Biol Eng Comput 25(3):341, 1987.

240. Finch, L, Barbeau, H, and Arsenault, B: Influence of body weight support on normal human gait: Development of a gait retraining strategy. Phys Ther 71(11):842, 1991.

241. Barbeau, H, Danakas, M, and Arsenault, B: The effects of locomotor training in spinal cord injured subjects: A preliminary study. Restor Neurol Neurosci 5(1):81, 1993.

242. Hodgson, JA, et al: Can the mammalian lumbar spinal cord learn a motor task? Med Sci Sports Exerc 26(12):1491, 1994.

243. Edgerton, VR, et al: A physiological basis for the development of rehabilitative strategies for spinally injured patients. J Am Paraplegia Soc 14(4):150, 1991.

244. Visintin, M, and Barbeau, H: The effects of body weight support on the locomotor pattern of spastic paretic patients. Can J Neurol Sci 16(3):315, 1989.

245. Harkema, SJ, et al: Human lumbosacral spinal cord interprets loading during stepping. J Neurophysiol 77(2):797, 1997.

246. Beres-Jones, JA, and Harkema, SJ: The human spinal cord interprets velocity-dependent afferent input during stepping. Brain 127(pt 10):2232, 2004.

247. Ferris, DP, et al: Muscle activation during unilateral stepping occurs in the nonstepping limb of humans with clinically complete spinal cord injury. Spinal Cord 42(1):14, 2004.

248. Wernig, A, Nanassy, A, and Muller, S: Laufband (treadmill) therapy in incomplete paraplegia and tetraplegia. J Neurotrauma 16(8):719, 1999.

249. Protas, EJ, et al: Supported treadmill ambulation training after spinal cord injury: A pilot study. Arch Phys Med Rehabil 82(6):825, 2001.

250. Field-Fote, EC, Lindley, SD, and Sherman, AL: Locomotor training approaches for individuals with spinal cord injury: A preliminary report of walking-related outcomes. J Neurol Phys Ther 29(3):127, 2005.

251. Dobkin, B, et al: Weight-supported treadmill vs over-ground training for walking after acute incomplete SCI. Neurology 66(4):484, 2006.

252. Dobkin, B, et al: The evolution of walking-related outcomes over the first 12 weeks of rehabilitation for incomplete traumatic spinal cord injury: The multicenter randomized Spinal Cord Injury Locomotor Trial. Neurorehabil Neural Repair 21(1):25, 2007.

253. Behrman, AL, and Harkema, SJ: Locomotor training after human spinal cord injury: A series of case studies. Phys Ther 80(7):688, 2000.

254. Barbeau, H, et al: Walking after spinal cord injury: Evaluation, treatment, and functional recovery. Arch Phys Med Rehabil 80(2):225, 1999.

255. Field-Fote, EC: Combined use of body weight support, functional electric stimulation, and treadmill training to improve walking ability in individuals with chronic incomplete spinal cord injury. Arch Phys Med Rehabil 82(6):818, 2001.

256. Barbeau, H, et al: The effect of locomotor training combined with functional electrical stimulation in chronic spinal cord injured subjects: Walking and reflex studies. Brain Res Brain Res Rev 40(1-3):274, 2002.

257. Harkema, SJ, et al: Balance and ambulation improvements in individuals with chronic incomplete spinal cord injury using locomotor training-based rehabilitation. Arch Phys Med Rehabil 93(9):1508, 2012.

258. Field-Fote, EC and Tepavac: Improved intralimb coordination in people with incomplete spinal cord injury following training with body weight support and electrical stimulation. Phys Ther 82(7):707, 2002

259. Jayaraman, A, et al: Locomotor training and muscle function after incomplete spinal cord injury: Case series. J Spinal Cord Med 31(2):185, 2008.

260. Musselman, KE, et al: Training of walking skills overground and on the treadmill: Case series on individuals with incomplete spinal cord injury. Phys Ther 89(6):601, 2009.

261. Prosser, LA: Locomotor training within an inpatient rehabilitation program after pediatric incomplete spinal cord injury. Phys Ther 87(9):1224, 2007.

262. Behrman, AL, et al: Locomotor training restores walking in a nonambulatory child with chronic, severe, incomplete cervical spinal cord injury. Phys Ther 88(5):580, 2008.

263. Fox, EJ, et al: Ongoing walking recovery 2 years after locomotor training in a child with severe incomplete spinal cord injury. Phys Ther 90(5):793, 2010.

264. Harkema, SJ, et al: Establishing the NeuroRecovery Network: Multisite rehabilitation centers that provide activity-based therapies and assessments for neurologic disorders. Arch Phys Med Rehabil 93(9):1498, 2012.

265. Dobkin, BH, et al: Methods for a randomized trial of weight-supported treadmill training versus conventional training for walking during inpatient rehabilitation after incomplete traumatic spinal cord injury. Neurorehabil Neural Repair 17(3):153, 2003.

266. Forrest, GF, et al: Neuromotor and musculoskeletal responses to locomotor training for an individual with chronic motor complete AIS-B spinal cord injury. J Spinal Cord Med 31(5):509, 2008.

267. Manella, KJ, Torres, J, and Field-Fote, EC: Restoration of walking function in an individual with chronic complete (AIS A) spinal cord injury. J Rehabil Med 42(8):795, 2010.

268. Fong, AJ, et al: Recovery of control of posture and locomotion after a spinal cord injury: Solutions staring us in the face. Prog Brain Res (175):393, 2009.

269. Snoek, GJ, et al: Survey of the needs of patients with spinal cord injury: Impact and priority for improvement in hand function in tetraplegics. Spinal Cord 42(9):526, 2004.

270. Beekhuizen, KS, and Field-Fote, EC: Massed practice versus massed practice with stimulation: Effects on upper extremity function and cortical plasticity in individuals with incomplete cervical spinal cord injury. Neurorehabil Neural Repair 19(1):33, 2005.

271. Hoffman, LR, and Field-Fote, EC: Functional and corticomotor changes in individuals with tetraplegia following unimanual or bimanual massed practice training with somatosensory stimulation: A pilot study. J Neurol Phys Ther 34(4):193, 2010.

272. Morris, DM, Taub, E, and Mark, VW: Constraint-induced movement therapy: Characterizing the intervention protocol. Eura Medicophys 42(3):257, 2006.

273. Beekhuizen, KS, and Field-Fote, EC: Sensory stimulation augments the effects of massed practice training in persons with tetraplegia. Arch Phys Med Rehabil 89(4):602, 2008.

274. Ljungberg, I, et al: Using peer mentoring for people with spinal cord injury to enhance self-efficacy beliefs and prevent medical complications. J Clin Nurs 20(3-4):351, 2011.

275. Cooper, RA, et al: Evaluation of a pushrim-activated, power-assisted wheelchair. Arch Phys Med Rehabil 82(5):702, 2001.

276. Arva, J, et al: Mechanical efficiency and user power requirement with a pushrim activated power assisted wheelchair. Med Eng Phys 23(10):699, 2001.

277. Algood, SD, et al: Impact of a pushrim-activated power-assisted wheelchair on the metabolic demands, stroke frequency, and range of motion among subjects with tetraplegia. Arch Phys Med Rehabil 85(11):1865, 2004.

278. Somers, MF, and Wlodarczyk, S: Use of a pushrim-activated, power-assisted wheelchair enhanced mobility for an individual with cervical 5/6 tetraplegia. Neurol Rep 27:22, 2001.

279. Hastings, JD: Seating assessment and planning. Phys Med Rehabil Clin North Am 11(1):183, 2000.

280. Hastings, JD, Fanucchi, ER, and Burns, SP: Wheelchair configuration and postural alignment in persons with spinal cord injury. Arch Phys Med Rehabil 84(4):528, 2003.

281. Hastings, JD, and Betz, KL: Seating and wheelchair prescription. In Field-Fote, EC (ed): Spinal Cord Injury Rehabilitation. FA Davis, Philadelphia, 2009.

282. MacPhee, AH, et al: Wheelchair skills training program: A randomized clinical trial of wheelchair users undergoing initial rehabilitation. Arch Phys Med Rehabil 85(1):41, 2004.

283. Best, KL, et al: Wheelchair skills training for community-based manual wheelchair users: A randomized controlled trial. Arch Phys Med Rehabil 86(12):2316, 2005.

284. Coolen, AL, et al: Wheelchair skills training program for clinicians: A randomized controlled trial with occupational therapy students. Arch Phys Med Rehabil 85(7):1160, 2004.

285. Kirby, RL, et al: The manual wheelchair-handling skills of caregivers and the effect of training. Arch Phys Med Rehabil 85(12):2011–2019, 2004.

286. Mushahwar, VK, et al: New functional electrical stimulation approaches to standing and walking. J Neural Eng 4(3):S181, 2007.

287. Dutta, A, Kobetic, R, and Triolo, RJ: Gait initiation with electromyographically triggered electrical stimulation in people with partial paralysis. J Biomech Eng 131(8):812, 2009.

288. Johnston, TE, et al: Implanted functional electrical stimulation: An alternative for standing and walking in pediatric spinal cord injury. Spinal Cord 41(3):144, 2003.

289. Kilgore, KL, et al: An implanted upper-extremity neuroprosthesis using myoelectric control. J Hand Surg Am 33(4):539, 2008.

290. DiMarco, AF, Takaoka, Y, and Kowalski, KE: Combined intercostal and diaphragm pacing to provide artificial ventilation in patients with tetraplegia. Arch Phys Med Rehabil 86(6):1200, 2005.

291. Kutzenberger, J, Domurath, B, and Sauerwein, D: Spastic bladder and spinal cord injury: Seventeen years of experience with sacral deafferentation and implantation of an anterior root stimulator. Artif Organs 29(3):239, 2005.

292. Jezernik, S, et al: Electrical stimulation for the treatment of bladder dysfunction: Current status and future possibilities. Neurol Res 24(5):413, 2002.

293. Shih, JJ, Krusienski, DJ, and Wolpaw, JR: Brain-computer interfaces in medicine. Mayo Clin Proc, 2012.

294. Machado, S, et al: EEG-based brain-computer interfaces: An overview of basic concepts and clinical applications in neurorehabilitation. Rev Neurosci 21(6):451, 2010.

295. Mason, SG, et al: Real-time control of a video game with a direct brain-computer interface. J Clin Neurophysiol 21(6):404, 2004.

296. McFarland, DJ, et al: Emulation of computer mouse control with a noninvasive brain-computer interface. J Neural Eng 5(2):101, 2008.

297. Millan, JD, et al: Combining brain-computer interfaces and assistive technologies: State-of-the-art and challenges. Front Neurosci 4:2010.

298. Tefertiller, C, et al: Efficacy of rehabilitation robotics for walking training in neurological disorders: A review. J Rehabil Res Dev 48(4):387, 2011.

299. Ferris, DP: The exoskeletons are here. J Neuroeng Rehabil 6:17, 2009.

Spinal Cord Injury Information Network
www.spinalcord.uab.edu

Christopher and Dana Reeve Paralysis Foundation
www.christopherreeve.org/index.cfm

Model Spinal Cord Injury System Dissemination Center
www.mscisdisseminationcenter.org

WheelchairNet
www.wheelchairnet.org

Wheelchair Skills Program
www.wheelchairskillsprogram.ca

Disability Resources
www.disabilityresources.org

National Council on Independent Living
www.ncil.org

Paralyzed Veterans Association
www.pva.org

American Spinal Injury Association
www.asia-spinalinjury.org

National Spinal Cord Injury Association
www.spinalcord.org

NeurotechNetwork
www.neurotechnetwork.org

Think First
www.thinkfirst.org

Sports'n Spokes
www.pvamagazines.com/sns

New Mobility
www.newmobility.com

Shake-A-Leg
www.shakealeg.org

The Cleveland Center
http://fescenter.case.edu

The Miami Project to Cure Paralysis
www.miamiproject.miami.edu

disABILITY Information and Resources
www.makoa.org

Spinal Cord Injury Rehabilitation Evidence
www.scireproject.com

Rehabilitation Measures Database
www.rehabmeasures.org

Physiotherapy Exercises for People With Spinal Cord Injury and Other Neurological Conditions
www.physiotherapyexercises.com

Vestibular Disorders

Michael C. Schubert, PT, PhD | **Chapter 21**

LEARNING OBJECTIVES

1. Differentiate vestibular symptom pathology from other manifestations of vertigo, dizziness, and dysequilibrium.
2. Identify the examination procedures used to evaluate patients with vestibular dysfunction to establish a diagnosis, prognosis, and plan of care.
3. When presented with a clinical case study, analyze and interpret examination data and determine appropriate interventions for the clinical problems presented.
4. Determine appropriate elements of the rehabilitation program for patients with vestibular dysfunction.

CHAPTER OUTLINE

Physical therapists are likely to encounter patients with vestibular disorders in a variety of clinical settings. At an incidence of 5.5%, dizziness in the United States affects more than 15 million people each year.[1] The reported prevalence of dizziness as a medical symptom in community-dwelling adults varies based on subjects' age, gender, and definition of the complaint (1% to 35%).[2-6] Dizziness is one of the most common complaints adults report to their physicians and prevalence increases with age.[7,8] A cross-sectional study of emergency department visits for dizziness found that otologic/vestibular pathology was the number one cause (32%).[9] Patients who experience dizziness report a significant disability that reduces their quality of life.[10-12] Furthermore, it has been reported that greater than 70% of patients with initial complaints of dizziness will not have a resolution of symptoms at a 2-week follow-up. Of patients with persistent dizziness, 63% reported recurrent symptoms continuing beyond 3 months.[13]

Cawthorne[14] and Cooksey[15] were the first clinicians to advocate exercises for persons suffering from dizziness and vertigo. It has only been within the last two decades, however, that our knowledge of vestibular function and related disorders has profoundly changed rehabilitation approaches. Once an accurate diagnosis involving the vestibular pathways has been made, activity limitations are minimized and progression toward disability can be prevented. Evidence suggests that an individualized approach to vestibular rehabilitation is important for a better outcome.

The peripheral vestibular system serves as the primary focus of this chapter because it is the most common origin for patient signs and symptoms. The physical therapist, however, must recognize patterns of signs and symptoms from a central pathology as well. With an appreciation of the complexity of the vestibular system coupled with an understanding of tests to measure its function, the reader will be able to discern anomalies of the system and begin to formulate effective rehabilitation strategies.

■ ANATOMY

Peripheral Vestibular System

The three primary functions of the peripheral vestibular system are (1) stabilizing visual images on the fovea of the retina during head movement to allow clear vision; (2) maintaining postural stability, especially during movement of the head; and (3) providing information used for spatial orientation.

Semicircular Canals

Within the petrous portion of each temporal bone (base of the skull between the sphenoid and occipital bones) lies the membranous vestibular labyrinth. Each labyrinth contains five neural structures that detect head acceleration: three *semicircular canals* and two *otolith* organs (Fig. 21.1). The three semicircular canals (SCCs) (*horizontal, posterior* [inferior], and *anterior* [superior]) respond to angular acceleration and are orthogonal (at right angles) with respect to one another. Alignment of the SCCs in the temporal bone is such that each canal has a contralateral coplanar mate. The horizontal canals form a coplanar pair while the posterior and contralateral anterior SCCs form coplanar pairs. The anterior aspect of the horizontal SCC is inclined 30° upward from a plane connecting the external auditory canal to the lateral canthus. The posterior and anterior SCCs are inclined about 92° and 90°, respectively, from the plane of the horizontal SCC.[16] Angular head rotation stimulates each canal to varying degrees.[17]

The SCCs are filled with *endolymph* (fluid) that has a density slightly greater than water.[18] Endolymph moves freely within each canal in response to the direction of the angular head rotation. The SCCs enlarge at one end to form the *ampulla*. Within the ampulla lies the *cupula*, a gelatinous barrier that contains the sensory hair cells (Fig. 21.2). The *kinocilia* (mechanosensing cilia involved in the sense of movement) and *stereocilia* (mechanosensing organelles) of the hair cells are seated in the *crista ampullaris* (sensory organ of angular rotation). Deflection of the stereocilia caused by motion of the endolymph results in an opening (or closing) of the transduction channels of hair cells, which results in changes in the membrane potential of the hair cells. Deflection of the stereocilia toward the kinocilia in each hair cell leads to excitation (*depolarization*) and deflection of the stereocilia away from the kinocilia leads to inhibition (*hyperpolarization*).

Each of the SCCs responds best to motion in its own plane with coplanar pairs exhibiting a *push–pull dynamic*. For example, as the head is turned to the right, the hair cells in the right horizontal SCC are excited, while hair cells in the left horizontal SCC are inhibited. The brain detects the direction of head movement by comparing input from the coplanar labyrinthine mates.

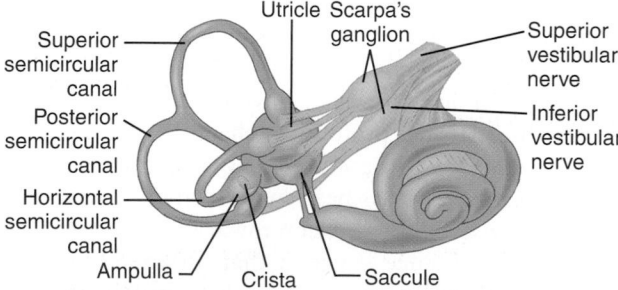

Figure 21.1 Anatomy of the vestibular labyrinth. Structures include the utricle, sacculus, superior semicircular canal, posterior semicircular canal, and the horizontal semicircular canal. The three semicircular canals (SCCs) are orthogonal with each other. Note the superior vestibular nerve innervating the superior (anterior) and horizontal semicircular canals as well as the utricle. The inferior vestibular nerve innervates the posterior semicircular canal and the saccule. The cell bodies of the vestibular nerves are located in Scarpa's ganglion (Gangl. Scarpae). Also note that the semicircular canals enlarge at one end to form the ampulla.

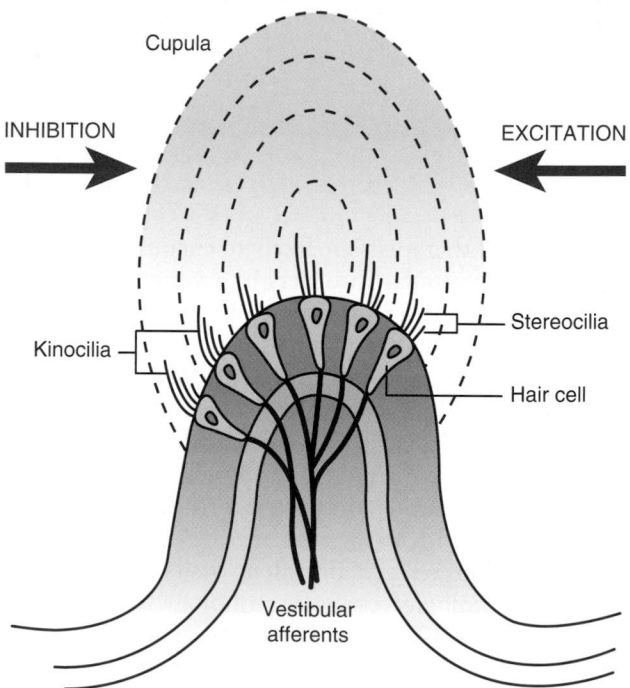

Figure 21.2 The cupula of the ampulla is a flexible, gelatinous barrier that partitions the canal. The crista ampullaris contains the kinocilia and stereocilia sensory hair cells. The hair cells generate action potentials in response to cupular deflection. Deflection of the stereocilia toward the kinocilia causes excitation; deflection in the opposite direction causes inhibition.

Otolith Organs

The saccule and utricle make up the otolith organs of the membranous labyrinth and respond to linear acceleration and static head tilt. Sensory hair cells project into a gelatinous material that has calcium carbonate crystalline-structure material (otoconia) embedded in it, which provides the otolith organs with an inertial mass (Fig. 21.3). Similar to the SCCs, motion toward the kinocilia causes excitation, while motion away leads to inhibition. Utricular excitation occurs during horizontal linear acceleration and/or static head tilt and saccular excitation occurs during vertical linear acceleration.

Central Vestibular System

Brainstem processes provide primary control of many vestibular reflexes. Tracing techniques, used to follow axonal projections from their source to point of termination, have identified extensive connections between the vestibular nuclei and the reticular formation, thalamus, and cerebellum[19-21] (Fig. 21.4). In addition, vestibular pathways appear to terminate in a unique cortical area. Primate studies have identified the junction of the parietal and insular lobes as the location for a vestibular cortex.[22-24] Recent evidence in human studies using functional magnetic resonance imaging (fMRI) appears to confirm the parietal and insular regions as the cortical location for processing vestibular information.[25] Connections with the vestibular cortex, thalamus, and reticular formation enable the vestibular system to contribute to the integration of arousal and conscious awareness of the body, as well as to discriminate between movement of self and the environment.[26,27] The cerebellar connections help maintain calibration of the vestibulo-ocular reflex (VOR), which stabilizes images on the retina during head

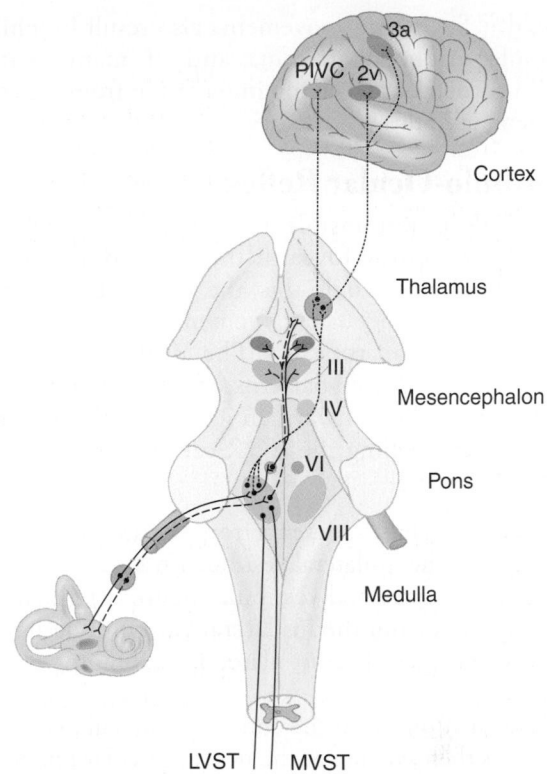

Figure 21.4 The semicircular canal (angular) and otolith (linear) input is sent to the vestibular nuclei. From the vestibular nuclei, the input travels to the ocular motor nuclei (III, IV, VI) for mediation of the vestibulo-ocular reflex. For arousal and conscious awareness of the head and body in space, information proceeds further to the thalamus and cortex. For maintenance of postural control, the peripheral vestibular input is sent distally as the medial and lateral vestibulo-spinal tracts (MVST, LVST). PIVC = Parieto-insular vestibular cortex.

movements, contributes to posture during static and dynamic activities, and influences the coordination of limb movements.

■ PHYSIOLOGY AND MOTOR CONTROL

Foundational knowledge of vestibular neurophysiology is important for understanding the signs and symptoms of vestibular dysfunction. Important principles of the vestibular system include the *tonic-firing rate, VOR, push–pull mechanism, inhibitory cutoff,* and *velocity storage system.*

Tonic Firing Rate

In primates, primary vestibular afferents of the healthy vestibular system have a resting firing rate that is typically 70 to 100 spikes/sec.[28,29] The presence of the high tonic firing rate means each vestibular system can detect head motion through excitation or inhibition. During angular head rotations, ipsilateral vestibular afferents and ipsilateral central vestibular neurons are

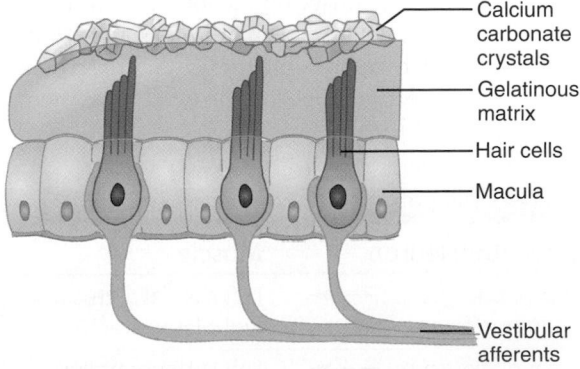

Figure 21.3 Otoconia are calcium carbonate crystals that are embedded in a gelatinous matrix which provides an inertial mass. Linear acceleration shifts the gelatinous matrix and excites or inhibits the vestibular afferents depending on the direction in which the stereocilia are deflected.

excited.[28] Such head movements also result in inhibition of peripheral afferents and of many central vestibular neurons receiving innervation from the contralateral labyrinth.

Vestibulo-Ocular Reflex

The VOR is responsible for maintaining stability of an image on the fovea of the retina during rapid head movements. To do this, the VOR must generate rapid compensatory eye movements in the direction opposite the head rotation. The VOR achieves this with relatively simple patterns of connectivity in the central vestibular pathways. In its most basic form, the pathways controlling the VOR can be described as a three-neuron arc.

- Primary vestibular afferents from the anterior SCC synapse in the ipsilateral vestibular nuclei.
- Secondary ipsilateral vestibular neurons receiving innervation from the ipsilateral labyrinth decussate and synapse in the contralateral oculomotor nucleus.
- Motor neurons from the contralateral oculomotor nucleus then synapse at the neuromuscular junction of the ipsilateral superior rectus and the contralateral inferior oblique muscles, respectively (Fig. 21.5).

Similar patterns of connectivity exist for each SCC and the eye muscles that receive innervations from them (Table 21.1). See Figure 21.6 for insertions of the ocular muscles.

VOR Gain and Phase

Normally, as the head moves in one direction, the eyes move in the opposite direction with equal velocity. This relationship of eye velocity to head velocity is expressed as the gain (*VOR gain*) of the vestibular system (eye velocity/head velocity = −1). For example, when the head is moved down, the anterior SCCs are stimulated. Excitation of the anterior SCC afferents rotates both eyes in the direction opposite the angular head movement, or up (see Fig. 21.5). *VOR phase* is a second useful measure of the vestibular system and represents the amplitude relationship between the eye and head. VOR phase

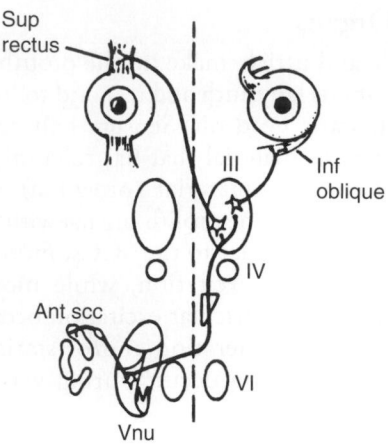

Figure 21.5 From the anterior semicircular canal (Ant Scc), afferent input travels to the vestibular nuclei (Vnu). The signal continues to the contralateral oculomotor nuclei (III). From there, motoneurons synapse with the superior rectus muscle that moves the eye upward, and the inferior oblique muscle that moves the eye upward and torsionally. Also shown are the oculomotor nuclei IV, and VI. *Adapted from Baloh and Honrubia,[30, p. 52] with permission.*

should represent an equal but opposite head and eye position relationship. Therefore, if the head moves 10 degrees to the right, the eyes should be positioned 10 degrees to the left. When the head and eyes are equally positioned but oppositely directed, this is described as a zero phase shift. *Note*: VOR phase is not equivalent with VOR gain, which examines the difference between head and eye velocity.

In individuals with healthy oculomotor function, for head velocities below 60°/sec *gaze stability* can be maintained fairly well using *smooth pursuit* (the ability to move the eyes with smooth, continuous motions in order to follow the movement of a target of interest and maintain the moving image on the fovea).[30] In situations where head velocity is greater than 60°/sec the vestibular system is primarily responsible for generating eye movement (in the direction opposite the head movement) to

Table 21.1 Innervation Pattern of Excitatory Input from the Semicircular Canals			
Primary Afferent	**Secondary Neuron**[a]	**Extraocular Motor Neuron**	**Muscle**
Horizontal (left)	Medial vestibular nucleus	Left oculomotor nucleus[b] ⟶	Left medial rectus
		Right abducens nucleus ⟶	Right lateral rectus
Posterior (left)	Medial vestibular nucleus	Right trochlear nucleus ⟶	Left superior oblique
		Right oculomotor nucleus ⟶	Right inferior rectus
Anterior/Superior (left)	Lateral vestibular nucleus	Right oculomotor nucleus ⟶	Left superior rectus
			Right inferior oblique

[a]Ascending secondary neurons travel in the medial longitudinal fasciculus.
[b]In the horizontal semicircular canal, secondary neurons also travel in the ascending tract of Dieters.

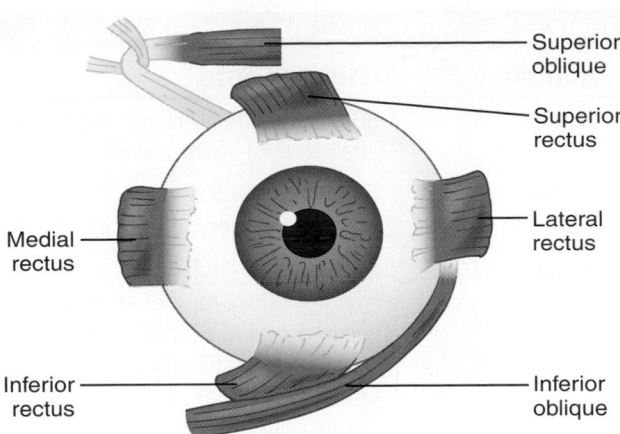

Figure 21.6 Muscle insertions of the left eye. Six extraocular muscles insert into the sclera and can be considered as complementary pairs. The medial and lateral rectus muscles rotate the eyes horizontally, the superior and inferior rectus muscles rotate the eyes vertically, and the superior and inferior oblique muscles rotate the eyes torsionally with some vertical component. By convention, the torsional rotation is noted as it relates to the superior poles of the eyes. The superior oblique muscle rotates the eye downward and toward the nose, whereas the inferior oblique muscle rotates the eye upward and away from the nose. The superior oblique muscle travels through the fibrous trochlea, which attaches to the anteromedial superior wall of the orbit.

maintain *gaze* on the target.[31] The VOR operates at head velocities as great as 350 to 400°/sec.[32]

Push–Pull Mechanism

The brain detects head movement and direction through comparison of inputs between the two vestibular systems. The SCCs each work in coplanar fashion as mentioned earlier; as the head is turned to the right, the right horizontal SCC will have an increased firing rate while the left horizontal SCC has a decreased firing rate. This is called the *push–pull mechanism* (Fig. 21.7). The brain is then responsible for recognizing the difference and interpreting movement. A faulty interpretation will lead to difficulties with gaze stabilization, postural stability, and motion perception.

Inhibitory Cutoff

Recall that during angular head rotations (rotations about an axis) ipsilateral vestibular afferents can be excited up to 400 spikes/sec.[32] A simultaneous hyperpolarization (spontaneous firing rate reduction) of the opposite labyrinth also occurs. However, the inhibition of the hair cells in the opposite labyrinth can only reduce the firing rate to zero, at which point the inhibition is cut off (*inhibitory cutoff*). Thus, for ipsilateral rapid head rotations, the contralateral vestibular afferents cannot detect head rotation when the head velocity is greater than the inhibitory cutoff

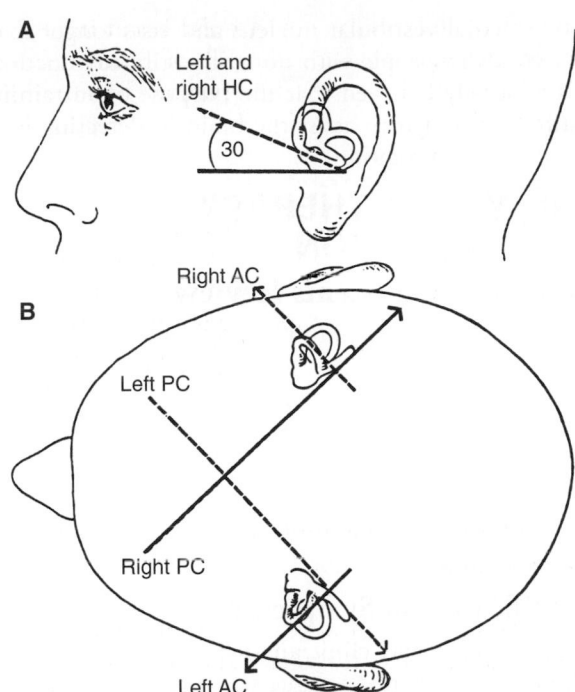

Figure 21.7 (A) Orientation of the horizontal semicircular canals (HC) in situ, with the head neutrally aligned. **(B)** The semicircular canals (ipsilateral anterior and contralateral posterior, and each horizontal) work in pairs. The arrows indicate the angular pitch direction of individual SCC stimulation. The dashed and continuous lines illustrate each SCC has an equally opposing SCC, sensitive to the opposite angular pitch direction of the head, for example, the left anterior canal (left AC) is paired with the right posterior canal (right PC) an collectively recognized as the left anterior right posterior (LARP) plane. *Adapted from Baloh and Honrubia,[30, p. 52] with permission.*

of those contralateral afferents. The response to head movements that hyperpolarize the hair cells is therefore limited to a velocity range up to 70 to 100°/sec. For example, if the tonic firing rates of the vestibular afferents are 80 spikes/sec, with a rotation to the right of 120°/sec the vestibular afferents increase their firing rate from 80 to 200 spikes/sec (tonic firing rate + rotational velocity). In contrast, the left ear will decrease from 80 to 0 (zero), not to negative 40 (–40), which limits the afferents from the left ear from adequately detecting the head velocity. (It is generally accepted that a 1:1 ratio exists between head velocity and spikes per second neuronal firing rate.) Because the resting discharge rate of these afferents and central vestibular neurons averages 70 to 100 spikes/sec, inhibitory cutoff is more likely to occur than is excitation saturation.

Velocity Storage System

The signal generated by movement of the cupula is brief, lasting only as long as the cupula is deflected.[33] The response is sustained, however, by a circuit of neurons in the medial vestibular nucleus and lasts longer than 10 seconds in people with normal vestibular function. It is generally believed that the purpose of sustaining vestibular input is to assist the brain in detecting low-frequency head rotation.

PHYSICAL THERAPY EXAMINATION

History and Systems Review

Physical therapists examining people who report dizziness and imbalance have the difficult task of sorting through potential causes. Capturing a thorough history and performing a systems review are critical components of the process. Key elements of taking the history are identification of symptoms, as well as their duration and the circumstances under which the symptoms occur.

Identification of Symptoms

Many patients and clinicians use the imprecise term "dizziness" to describe a vague sensation of lightheadedness or a feeling that they have a tendency to fall. The imprecision of the term can entangle clinical management decisions. It is essential to determine what the patient is experiencing when the term **dizziness** is used. Most complaints of being "dizzy" can be categorized as vertigo, lightheadedness, dysequilibrium, or oscillopsia (targets in visual field appear to move during head motion). Generally, dizziness is vaguely defined as the sensation of whirling or feeling a tendency to fall. Ideally, patients should be directed away from using the word and to use more precise terms that will help the clinician develop more direct treatment approaches.

Vertigo is defined as an illusion of movement. Many patients use the term "vertigo" incorrectly and thus the clinician must be certain to inform patients of the true definition, as well as identify their unique experience. Patients may describe that they sense their environment is moving or that they see the environment moving (spinning). Vertigo tends to be episodic and to indicate pathology at one or more locations along the vestibular pathways. It is most common during the acute stage of unilateral vestibular hypofunction (UVH), but may also manifest itself via displaced otoconia (benign paroxysmal positional vertigo), or an acute unilateral brainstem lesion affecting the root entry zone of the peripheral vestibular neurons or the vestibular nuclei.

Lightheadedness is often defined as a feeling that fainting is about to occur and can be caused by nonvestibular factors such as hypotension, hypoglycemia, or anxiety.[34] Lightheadedness is vague and less localizing than vertigo.

Dysequilibrium is defined as the sensation of being off balance. Typically, acute and chronic vestibular lesions will produce dysequilibrium. Often, however, this symptom is associated with nonvestibular problems such as decreased somatosensation or weakness in the lower extremities (LEs) (Table 21.2).

Table 21.2	Symptoms and Possible Causes
Symptom	Possible Cause
Vertigo	BPPV, UVH, unilateral central lesion affecting the vestibular nuclei
Lightheadedness	Orthostatic hypotension, hypoglycemia, anxiety, panic disorder
Dysequilibrium	BVH, chronic unilateral vestibular hypofunction, lower extremity somatosensation loss, upper brainstem/vestibular cortex lesion, cerebellar and motor pathway lesions

BPPV = benign paroxysmal positional vertigo; BVH = bilateral vestibular hypofunction; UVH = unilateral vestibular hypofunction.

Oscillopsia is the subjective experience of motion of objects in the visual environment that are known to be stationary. Oscillopsia can occur with head movements in patients with vestibular hypofunction since the vestibular system is not generating an adequate compensatory eye velocity during the head motion. Such a deficit in the VOR results in motion of images on the fovea and in a decline in visual acuity. The severity of gaze instability, however, varies across individuals with vestibular hypofunction.[35-38]

Duration and Circumstances of Symptoms

The physical therapist must determine how recently the patient has had an acute attack of vertigo, lightheadedness, dysequilibruim, or oscillopsia and whether the symptom is constant or episodic. If the symptom is episodic, the clinician must attempt to determine the average duration of the episodes in seconds, minutes, or hours. For example, vertigo lasting seconds to minutes commonly suggests benign paroxysmal positional vertigo. In contrast, vertigo lasting minutes to hours suggest Ménière's disease, and vertigo lasting for days implies vestibular neuronitis or migraine-associated dizziness.

The physical therapist must also determine under what circumstances the patient experiences symptoms. It is important to discern whether the patient experiences symptoms with particular movements, positions, or at rest. For example, is the patient sensitive to motion as the passenger in a moving car? Or does the patient experience a vigorous vertigo when the head is moved into certain positions?

Tests and Measures

Visual Analogue Scale

Use of a *visual analogue scale (VAS)* is an effective technique to obtain subjective intensity ratings of vertigo, lightheadedness, dysequilibrium, and oscillopsia.[39,40] The patient is asked to answer a question (e.g., *How intense are your symptoms?*) and mark on a 10-cm line (on a continuum from "none" to "worst possible intensity") where the symptoms exist at that moment. The clinician then measures the line and obtains a quantified value.

Dizziness Handicap Inventory

The *Dizziness Handicap Inventory (DHI)* is a popular tool used to measure a patient's self-perceived handicap as a result of vestibular disorders (Table 21.3).[41] The DHI has excellent test–retest reliability (r = 0.97) and good internal consistency reliability (r = 0.89). Patients respond to 25 questions, subgrouped into functional, emotional, and physical components. The DHI provides quantification of the patient's perception of dysequilibrium and its impact on daily activities. It is useful to establish subjective improvement. Measures of subjective impairment and physiological improvement are often

not correlated;[42,43] therefore, it is likely that factors other than organic recovery of vestibular function are responsible for subjective impairment.

Functional Disability Scale

The Vestibular Rehabilitation Benefit Questionnaire (VRBQ) was developed to specify the benefit from vestibular physical therapy and includes questions that address avoidance behavior, which is often absent in similar measures.[44] The VRBQ is a 22-item questionnaire that uses seven unique choices (word descriptors) to answer questions from one of four subscales: Dizziness, Anxiety, Motion-Provoked Dizziness, and Quality of Life. The VRBQ has excellent test–retest reliability (r = 0.92) and is moderately correlated with the DHI (0.59).

Table 21.3   Sample of the Types of Questions Included in the Dizziness Handicap Inventory, Based on the Three Sub-Components

Physical Domain

Does looking up increase your problem?
Does walking down the aisle of a supermarket increase your problem?
Does performing more ambitious activities like sports, dancing, or household chores (such as sweeping or putting dishes away) increase your problem?
Does bending over increase your problem?

Emotional Domain

Because of your problem, do you feel frustrated?
Because of your problem, are you afraid to leave your home without having someone accompany you?
Has your problem placed stress on your relationships with members of your family or friends?
Because of your problem, are you afraid to stay home alone?

Functional Domain

Because of your problem, do you restrict your travel for business or recreation?
Because of your problem, do you have difficulty getting into or out of bed?
Does your problem significantly restrict your participation in social activities such as going out to dinner, going to the movies, dancing, or to parties?
Because of your problem, is it difficult for you to walk around the house in the dark?

The patient instructions are as follows: The purpose of these questions is to identify difficulties that you may be experiencing because of your dizziness. Please answer "yes", "no", or "sometimes" to each question. Answer each question as it pertains to your dizziness or balance problem only.

Motion Sensitivity Quotient

The *Motion Sensitivity Quotient (MSQ)* was developed to provide a subjective score of an individual's sensitivity to motion.[45] The test involves placing patients into positions incorporating head or entire body motion to determine whether the movement reproduces dizziness (Fig. 21.8). If the patient reports an increased symptom intensity moving into a provoking position, the intensity is assigned a point, graded by the patient between 1 (mild) and 5 (severe). The duration of symptoms is also assigned points from 0 to 3 (0 to 4 seconds = 0; 5 to 10 seconds = 1; 11 to 30 seconds = 2; greater than 30 seconds = 3). The symptom intensity and duration values are then added together for a score. The MSQ is calculated by multiplying the number of positions that provoked symptoms by the score. This number is then divided by 2,048. An MSQ score of 0 indicates no symptoms whereas a score of 100 means severe dizziness in all positions.

Examination of Eye Movements

Owing to the direct relationship between vestibular receptors in the inner ear and eye movements produced by the VOR, the examination of eye movements is critical for defining and localizing vestibular pathology. The key tests include observation for nystagmus, the Head Impulse Test (examination of the VOR at high acceleration), the Head-Shaking Induced Nystagmus (HSN) test, positional testing, and the Dynamic Visual Acuity (DVA) test.

Name: _____   Age: _____   Gender: _____   Date: _____

Baseline Symptoms	INTENSITY	DURATION	SCORE
1. Sitting-to-supine			
2. Supine-to-left side			
3. Supine-to-right side			
4. Supine-to-sit			
5. Left Hallpike-Dix test			
6. Return from Hallpike-Dix test			
7. Right Hallpike-Dix test			
8. Return from Hallpike-Dix test			
9. Sitting: nose toward left knee			
10. Return to sitting			
11. Sitting: nose toward right knee			
12. Return to sitting			
13. Sitting: head rotation 5×			
14. Sitting: head flexion and extension 5×			
15. Standing: turn right (180°)			
16. Standing: turn left (180°)			
Intensity: rated from 0 to 5 (0 = no symptoms; 5 = severe symptoms)			
Duration: rated from 0 to 3 (5-10 sec = 1 point, 11-30 sec = 2 points, ≥30 sec = 3 points)			

Motion sensitivity quotient: $\dfrac{\text{\#Provoking positions} \times \text{score} \times 100}{2048}$ = _____ Total

Note: An MSQ score of zero means no symptoms and 100 means severe dizziness in all positions.

Figure 21.8 Motion sensitivity quotient. *Adapted from Smith-Wheelock et al,[45, p. 221] with permission.*

Observation for Nystagmus

Nystagmus is the primary diagnostic indicator used in identifying most peripheral and central vestibular lesions. An involuntary eye movement, nystagmus due to a *peripheral vestibular lesion* is composed of both slow and fast components. The direction of the nystagmus is named by the direction of the fast component. For individuals with a unilateral vestibular lesion, the slow component is due to relative excitation of one side of the vestibular system. The fast component is generated from the parapontine reticular formation in the brainstem and repositions the eye to the center of the orbit. For example, in left-beating nystagmus, the eyes move slowly to the right (VOR), and the resetting eye movement is to the left (fast component). Therefore, the direction opposite the quick component of the nystagmus localizes the side of the vestibular reduced firing rate (possible hypofunction).

Nystagmus due to a vestibular lesion is most commonly seen after an acute unilateral insult, *spontaneous* (at rest) *nystagmus*. This type of nystagmus occurs in the absence of motion because of the asymmetry between the healthy functioning and reduced/absent functioning vestibular systems. The brain perceives the asymmetry as active stimulation from the more neutrally active (i.e., healthy) ear. Resolution of spontaneous nystagmus in the light typically occurs within 3 to 7 days but may vary, and it can last as long as 2 months.[46,47] Spontaneous nystagmus may always be present in the dark after a unilateral loss of vestibular function. Regardless, resolution of spontaneous nystagmus in the light or dark occurs when symmetry between the resting firing rates of both vestibular systems is reestablished.[48]

Vestibular nystagmus can be suppressed in light and when a person visually fixates on a target.[49] As a result, the observation of nystagmus should be performed under conditions in which the person cannot see. This can be achieved with Frenzel lenses or an infrared camera system. Frenzel lenses look like large goggles with magnifying lenses that enable the clinician to observe for nystagmus while preventing the patient from fixating on a target. An infrared camera uses infrared light to illuminate the eyes while the patient remains in complete darkness.

Head Impulse Test (Examination of the VOR at High Acceleration)

The head impulse test (HIT) is a widely accepted clinical tool used to examine semicircular canal function.[50-54] Cervical range of motion (ROM) should be determined before performing the head impulse test and the physical therapist should explain why the head must be moved quickly. The head impulse test is performed by having the patient first fixate on a near target (e.g., the clinician's nose). When testing the horizontal SCC, the head is flexed 30°. Patients are asked to keep their eyes focused on a target while their head is manually rotated in an unpredictable direction using a small-amplitude (5° to 15°), moderate-velocity (approximately 200°/sec), and

high-acceleration (3,000 to 4,000°/sec²) angular impulse (Figs. 21.9 and 21.10). When the VOR is functioning normally, the eyes move in the direction opposite to the head movement and gaze will remain on the target. In a patient with a loss of vestibular function, the VOR will not move the eyes as quickly as the head rotation and the eyes move off the target. The patient will then make a corrective saccade to reposition the eyes (fovea) on the target. A corrective **saccade** is a rapid eye movement used to reposition the eyes to the target of interest. The appearance of corrective saccades indicates vestibular hypofunction as determined by the HIT and occurs because inhibition of vestibular afferents and central vestibular neurons on the intact side (persons with unilateral vestibular hypofunction) are less effective in encoding the amplitude of a head movement than excitation. A patient who has a unilateral peripheral lesion or pathology of the central vestibular neurons will not be able to maintain gaze when the head is rotated quickly toward the side of the lesion. A patient with a bilateral loss of vestibular function will make corrective saccades after a head impulse to either side. The HIT provides a sensitive indication of vestibular hypofunction in patients with complete loss of function in the affected labyrinth that occurs following ablative surgical procedures, such as labyrinthectomy.[50,53-55] The test is less sensitive in detecting hypofunction in patients with incomplete loss of function.[56-59]

Head-Shaking Induced Nystagmus Test

The **head-shaking induced nystagmus** (HSN) test is a useful aid in the diagnosis of a unilateral peripheral vestibular defect. During this test vision is occluded. The patient is instructed to close his or her eyes. The clinician flexes the head 30° before oscillating horizontally for 20 cycles at a frequency of 2 repetitions per second (2 Hz). On stopping the oscillation, the patient opens the eyes and the clinician checks for nystagmus. In subjects with normal vestibular function, nystagmus will not be present. An asymmetry between the peripheral vestibular inputs to central vestibular nuclei, however, may result in HSN. Typically, a person with a UVH will manifest a horizontal HSN, with the quick phases of the nystagmus directed toward the healthy ear and the slow phases directed toward the lesioned ear.[60] Not all patients with a UVH will have HSN. Patients with a complete loss of vestibular function bilaterally will not have HSN because neither system is functioning. As a result, there is no asymmetry between the tonic firing rates. The presence of vertical nystagmus after either horizontal or vertical head shaking suggests a central lesion.

Positional Testing

Positional testing is commonly used to identify whether otoconia have been displaced into the SCC, causing a condition referred to as **benign paroxysmal positional vertigo (BPPV)**. The addition of the otoconia into the

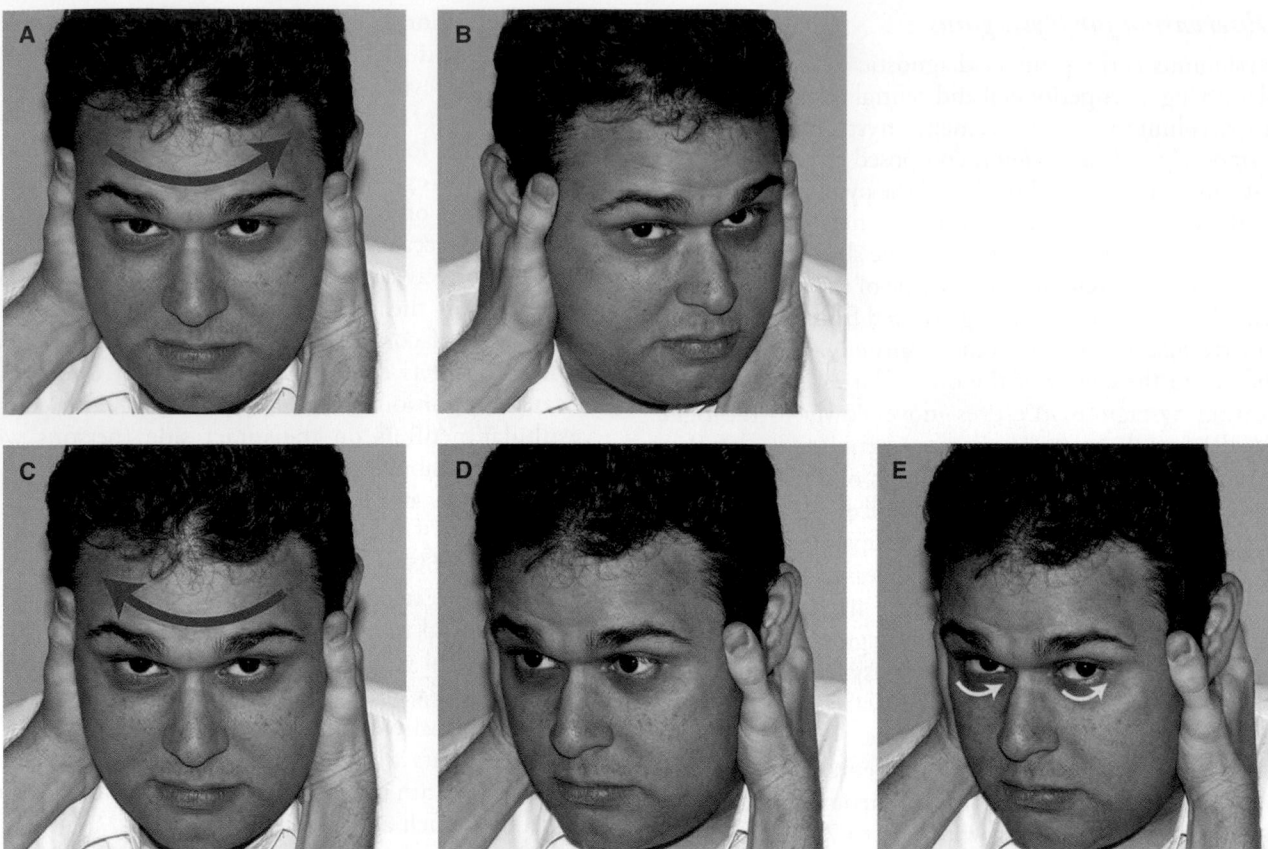

Figure 21.9 Normal horizontal canal head impulse test to the left **(A, B)**, abnormal to the right **(C–E)**. The examiner applies the head impulse test (HIT) to the patient. Large arrow denotes direction the head will be turned. **(A)** Initial starting position places subject's head into cervical flexion; eyes are focused on the target. **(B)** On stopping the head turn, the eyes are still on target and no corrective saccade is observed. In photographs **A** and **B,** the subject's eyes stay fixed on the examiner's nose throughout the test. **(C)** Initial starting position places subject's head into cervical flexion; eyes are focused on the target. **(D)** As the head is turned rapidly to the right, the eyes fall off the target and move with the head. **(E)** The subject must make a corrective saccade (small arrows) to bring the eyes back to the target of interest. For patients with cervical spine pathology, the clinician may choose to perform the horizontal canal HIT by first positioning the head in 15 degrees of rotation and then returning the head to center. *From Schubert et al,[59, p. 153] with permission of the American Physical Therapy Association.*

endolymph makes the semicircular canals sensitive to changes in head position. The **Dix-Hallpike test** is the most common positional test used to examine for BPPV.[61] The patient is moved from a long-sitting position with the head rotated 45° to one side, to a supine position with the head extended 30° beyond horizontal, head still rotated 45° (Fig. 21.11). The maneuver places each of the SCCs in a gravity-dependent position and the physical therapist should observe the eyes for nystagmus. The direction of the nystagmus is unique to the involved SCC. The direction and duration of the resultant nystagmus can help determine whether the patient has BPPV or a central lesion. An alternative form of the Dix-Hallpike test asks the patient to move into a side-lying position (Fig. 21.12). In both versions illustrated, the ear toward the ground is the labyrinth being tested. If horizontal SCC BPPV is suspected, the roll test can be used instead (Fig. 21.13). In this test, the patient is positioned

supine with the head flexed 20°. Rapid rotations to the sides are done separately and the clinician observes for nystagmus and vertigo. To prevent neck injury, the patient may move his or her own head in rotation.

Dynamic Visual Acuity Test

Dynamic visual acuity (DVA) is the measurement of visual acuity during horizontal motion of the head. A "bedside" and computerized form of the test can be used to identify the functional significance of the vestibular hypofunction.[62,63] Head velocities need to be greater than 100°/sec at the time DVA is measured to ensure that the vestibular afferents from the contralateral side are driven into inhibition and the letters (acuity chart) are not identified with a **smooth pursuit** eye movement. To perform the test, static visual acuity is determined first. The patient is asked to "Read the lowest line you can see" on a wall-mounted acuity chart. Lighthouse ETDRS (Early

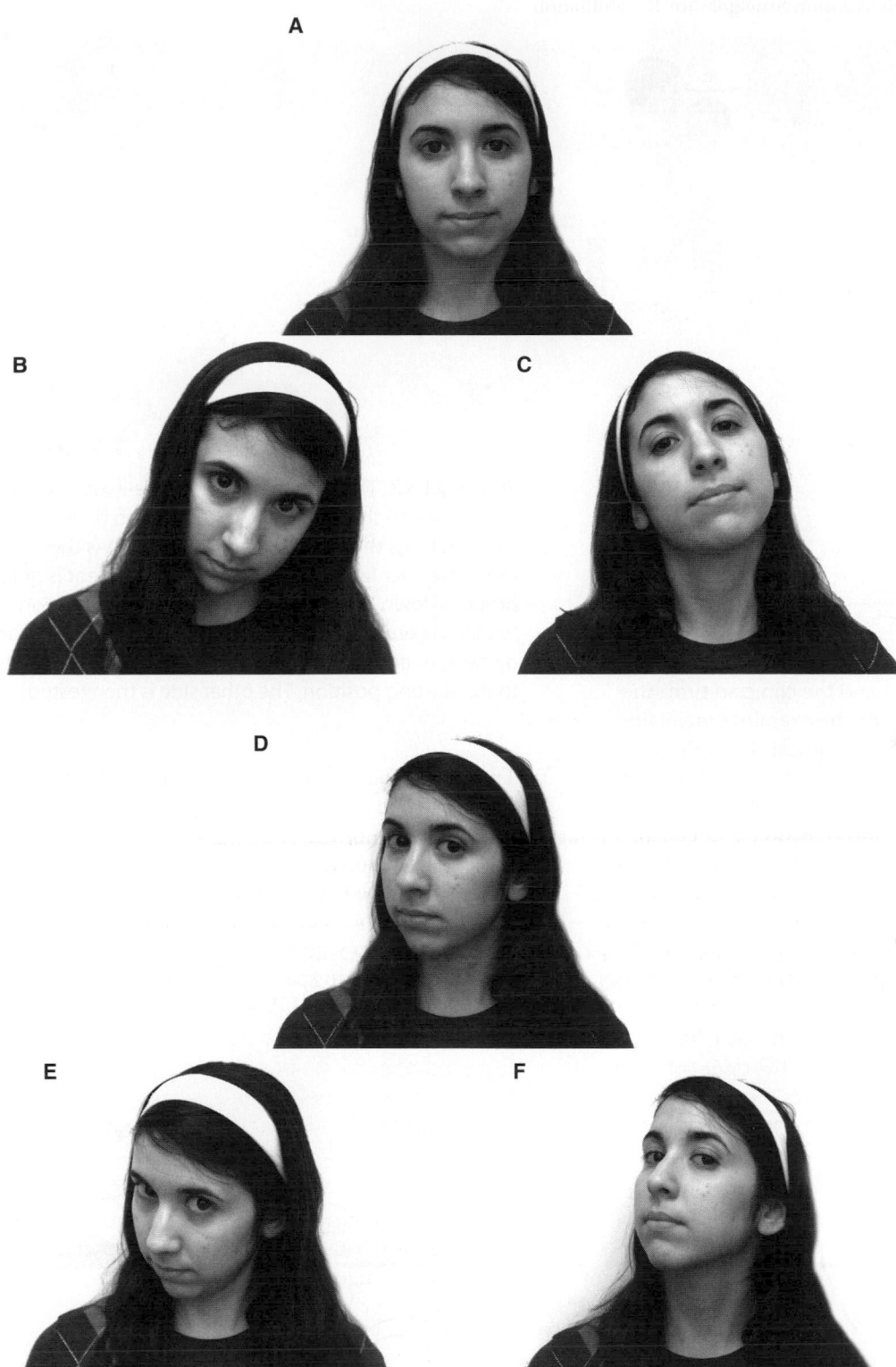

Figure 21.10 Vertical semicircular canal head impulse test (HIT), examiner's hands not shown here. There are two ways to investigate the VOR from each coplanar pair; methods **A–C** and **D–F** illustrate the two methods for the left anterior right posterior (LARP) VOR. **(A)** The head is placed in a neck neutral position. Next the head is rapidly moved pitch down while being rolled to the left **(B)** as if the head were moving diagonally. This examines the VOR from the left anterior SCC. From here, the clinician should return to **(A)** before rapidly moving the head pitch up and rolled to the right **(C)**. This examines the VOR from the right posterior canal. Alternatively, the head is rotated 45° to the right **(D)**. From this static position, the head is rapidly pitched down **(E)** examining the left anterior SCC. The head should be returned to the start position **(D)** and then the head rapidly moved pitch up to examine the right posterior SCC **(F)**. In this figure, the HIT is normal for the LARP plane, since the eyes remain gazing straight ahead.

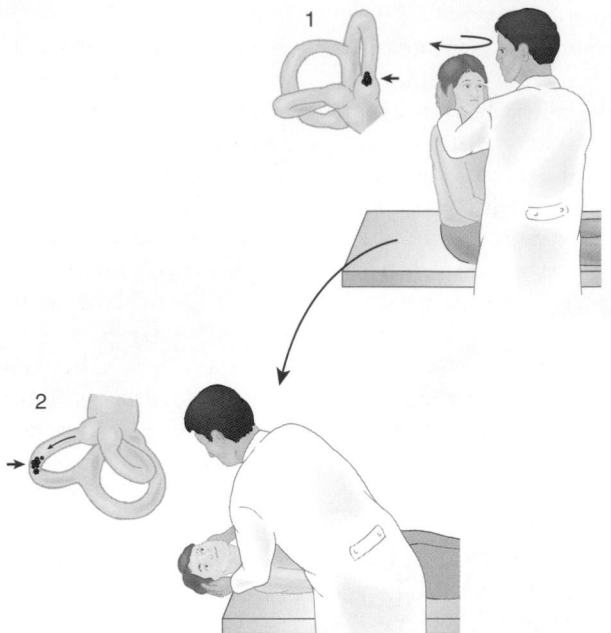

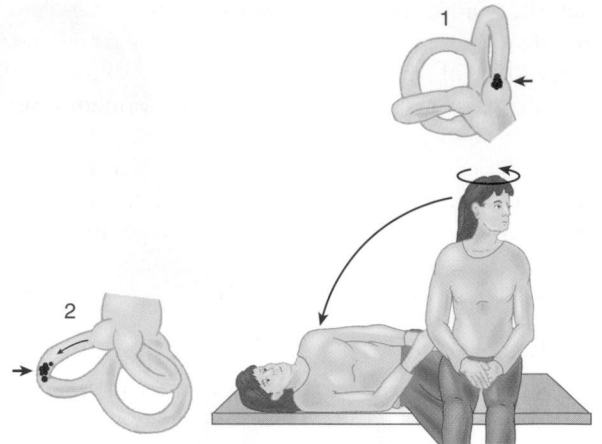

Figure 21.11 The Dix-Hallpike test. (1) The patient sits on the examination table and the clinician turns the head horizontally 45°. (2) As the examiner maintains the 45° rotation, the patient is quickly brought to a supine position with the neck extended 30° beyond the horizontal. The examiner must look for nystagmus and ask the patient if vertigo is being experienced. The patient is then slowly brought back to the starting position, and the other side is tested. The side that reproduces nystagmus and vertigo is the side that has the benign paroxysmal positional vertigo (BPPV). Shown here for testing right posterior or right anterior semicircular canal BPPV.

Figure 21.12 The Dix-Hallpike test (side-lying). (1) The patient sits on the edge of the examination table. The clinician turns the head horizontally 45°. (2) As the examiner maintains the 45° rotation, the patient is quickly brought down to the side opposite the head rotation (pictured here as the right side). The examiner checks for nystagmus and vertigo, and then slowly brings the patient to the starting position. The other side is then tested.

Treatment Diabetic Retinopathy Study) wall charts are recommended because they provide uniform light luminance for each of the letters. The patient then attempts to read the chart while the clinician horizontally oscillates the patient's head at a frequency of 2 Hz. A metronome can be useful to ensure correct frequency of the oscillation. For patients with loss of vestibular function, the eyes will not be stable in space during head movements. This causes a decrement in DVA compared with visual acuity

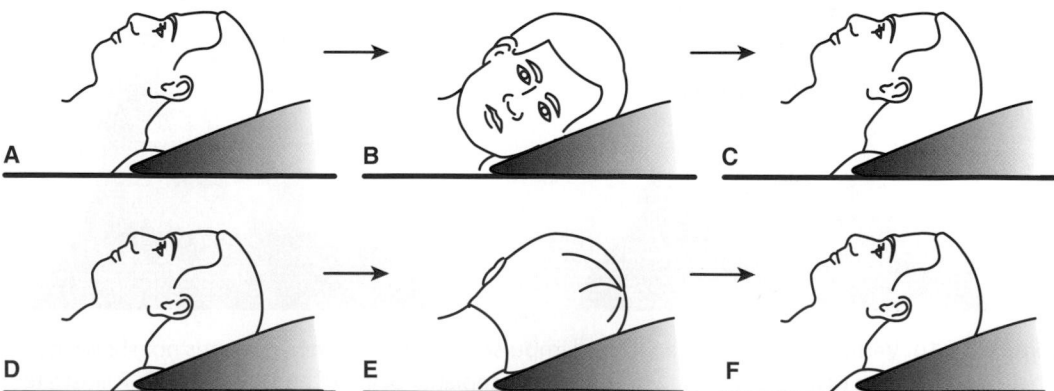

Figure 21.13 Roll test for horizontal semicircular canal BPPV. The patient is positioned in supine. **(A)** Initially, the patient's head should be placed in 20° cervical flexion. **(B)** The head is quickly turned 90° to the left side. The clinician then checks for nystagmus and vertigo. **(C)** The head is then gently returned to the neutral starting position. **(D–F)** The test is repeated to the other side (head is quickly turned 90° to the right side). The therapist again must check for nystagmus and vertigo. The head is then returned to the neutral starting position.

when the head is still. Using the acuity chart, a 3-line or more decrement in visual acuity during head movement is suggestive of vestibular hypofunction.[63] For people with normal vestibular function, head movement results in little or no change of visual acuity compared with the head still (less than 1 line difference). Computerized DVA has been found to correctly identify the side of lesion in patients with unilateral hypofunction for self-generated and unpredictable head motion[63,64] and can be used to identify single SCC lesions.[65]

Examination of Gait and Balance

Examination of gait and balance problems is important for determination of a patient's functional status. Testing should address both static and dynamic balance (e.g., weight shifting, automatic postural responses, and ambulation). Gait and balance tests *cannot* uniquely identify pathology within the vestibular system. Table 21.4 includes common balance tests and expected results.

Vestibular Function Tests
Semicircular Canal Tests

The more common SCC tests include *electro* or *videonystagmography* (ENG, VNG) testing and *rotational chair tests* and are commonly performed in a clinical vestibular function test laboratory. ENG includes a battery of tests that measure *oculomotor* and *inner ear* function. The test also examines for nystagmus in different head positions. The ENG oculomotor tests typically examine saccadic and smooth pursuit including velocity, latency, and gain. The inner ear test is known as the *caloric test* and infuses the external auditory canal with separate cold and warm air or water. This stimulus introduces a temperature gradient. In the presence of gravity, this temperature gradient results

in the convective flow of endolymph that deflects the cupula and generates nystagmus from the horizontal SCC. This test is particularly useful for determining the side of the deficit, because each labyrinth is stimulated separately. A variation with ice water is useful to determine whether minimal function exists in the vestibular system for patients with severe loss. However, the caloric test provides limited information since only the horizontal SCCs can be stimulated and that stimulation corresponds to a frequency (0.025 Hz) that is much lower than the natural frequencies of head movement (1 to 20 Hz).[66]

The rotational chair test stimulates each SCC by rotating subjects in the dark. In subjects with normal vestibular function, nystagmus should be generated by the rotation. In the presence of a vestibular disorder, the extent of pathology can be determined by comparing VOR gain and phase from rotations toward one ear with rotations toward the opposite ear. In addition, VOR gain and phase of people with normal vestibular function can be compared with that of people with suspected vestibular hypofunction. The rotational chair test is considered the standard test for bilateral vestibular hypofunction. Rotational chair testing is limited because only the horizontal SCCs are routinely tested to determine extent of pathology.

Otolith Tests

Advances in vestibular diagnostic testing have extended the region of identifiable pathology to include the otolith organs.[67-69] The *vestibular-evoked myogenic potential (VEMP)* test is a laboratory test that has gained broad clinical use and includes two subtypes: *cervical* and *ocular* VEMP. Both types use threshold and amplitude of a muscle contraction (electromyography [EMG]) to classify pathology. The cervical VEMP test exposes patients

Table 21.4	Common Balance Tests and Expected Results Related to Specific Diagnosis			
Test	BPPV	UVH	BVH	Central Lesion
Romberg	Negative	Acute: positive Chronic: negative	Acute: positive Chronic: negative	Often negative
Tandem Romberg	Negative	Positive, eyes closed	Positive	Positive
Single-legged stance	Negative	May be positive	Acute: positive Chronic: negative	May be unable to perform
Gait	Normal	Acute: wide-based, slow, decreased arm swing and trunk rotation Compensated: normal	Acute: wide-based, slow, decreased arm swing and trunk rotation Compensated: mild gait deviation	May have pronounced ataxia
Turn head while walking	May produce slight unsteadiness	Acute: may not keep balance Compensated: normal	May not keep balance or slows cadence	May not keep balance, increased ataxia

BPPV = benign paroxysmal postural vertigo; BVH = bilateral vestibular hypofunction; UVH = unilateral vestibular hypofunction.

to aural stimuli in the form of a series of ipsilateral loud (95-decibel [dB]) clicks. During the sound application, the ipsilateral sternocleidomastoid (SCM) muscle is tested for myogenic potentials. In people with healthy vestibular function, an initial inhibitory potential (occurring at a latency of 13 milliseconds [msec] after the click) is followed by an excitatory potential (occurring at a latency of 21 msec after the click). For patients with vestibular hypofunction, the VEMPs are absent on the side of the lesion. The saccule has been implicated as the site of afferent stimulation during cervical VEMP testing because saccular afferents provide ipsilateral inhibitory disynaptic input to the SCM muscle,[70] are responsive to click noise,[71-73] and are positioned close to the footplate of the stapes (inner most auditory ossicle) and therefore are subject to mechanical stimulation.[68,71]

The ocular VEMP exposes subjects to loud clicks (aural stimuli) or bone vibration applied to the central forehead, at the hairline. During the stimulus, EMG is measured from the inferior oblique muscle while subjects look upward to bring the muscle belly closer to the surface electrode. The ocular VEMP is a crossed, excitatory otolith-oculomotor response and in patients with UVH will be absent from the contralateral superior oblique.[74] The ocular VEMP is considered a test of the utricle and the superior vestibular nerve based on its absence in patients with abnormal caloric but preserved cervical VEMP.[74]

The *subjective visual vertical (SVV)* and *subjective visual horizontal (SVH)* tests are used to examine otolith function, though they cannot be used to uniquely detect saccular or utricular pathology. During the SVV test, patients are asked to align a dimly lit luminous bar (in an otherwise darkened room) with what they perceive as being vertical. The SVH test asks patients to align a bar with what they perceive as being horizontal. In the absence of vestibular problems, subjects typically align the bar within 1.5° of true or horizontal. Patients with UVH generally align the bar more than 2° from true vertical or horizontal with the bar tilted toward the lesioned side.[69,75]

■ VESTIBULAR SYSTEM DYSFUNCTION

Peripheral Pathology

Mechanical

The most common cause of vertigo, BPPV, is a biomechanical disorder. Symptoms of BPPV include nystagmus and vertigo with change in head position, and occasionally nausea with or without vomiting, and dysequilibrium. In the most common form, latency to onset of the vertigo and nystagmus occurs within 15 seconds once the head is in the provoking position. The duration is usually less than 60 seconds. The vertigo and nystagmus are direct impairments caused by the misplaced otoconia. BPPV is believed to occur via one of two mechanisms: *cupulolithiasis* and *canalithiasis*. Both of the theories involve the otoliths

becoming dislodged from the utricle and falling into the SCCs. Schuknecht[76] first theorized that fragments of otoconia break away and adhere to the cupula of one of the SCCs (cupulolithiasis). When the head is moved into certain positions, the weighted cupula is deflected by the pull of gravity. This abnormal signal results in vertigo and nystagmus, which persists as long as the patient is in the provoking position. Cupulolithiasis, therefore, does not explain the brief duration of the vertigo common in BPPV.[77] A second theory was proposed, canalithiasis, in which the otoconia are floating freely in one of the SCCs.[78] When a patient changes head position, the pull of gravity causes the freely floating otoconia to move inside the SCC resulting in endolymph movement and deflection of the cupula. Figure 21.14 illustrates BPPV occurring from cupulolithiasis or canalithiasis.

Decreased Receptor Input

The most common causes of UVH leading to decreased or eliminated receptor input are viral insults, trauma, and vascular events.[79,80] Patients who sustain a UVH will experience direct impairments of vertigo, spontaneous nystagmus, oscillopsia during head movements, postural instability, and dysequilibrium. Initially, the patient will experience the vertigo and nystagmus impairments due to the asymmetry created when one vestibular system is no longer functioning. This resolves within 3 to 7 days assuming the patient is exposed to common daylight conditions.[81] Spontaneous nystagmus in room light, beyond this time period, should alert the clinician to a possible central lesion or an unstable peripheral vestibular lesion. The direct impairments of visual blurring, postural instability, and dysequilibrium respond to physical therapy intervention. Because vertigo owing to asymmetry typically resolves within 7 days, persistent symptoms of vertigo beyond 2 weeks should be considered chronic, also necessitating vestibular rehabilitation.

The most common cause of a bilateral vestibular hypofunction (BVH) is **ototoxicity**. Certain classes of antibiotics such as aminoglycosides (e.g., gentamicin, streptomycin) are readily taken up by the hair cells of the vestibular apparatus and continue to build in this system even after the person has stopped using the antibiotic. Less common causes of BVH include meningitis, autoimmune disorders, head trauma, tumors on each eighth cranial nerve (including bilateral vestibular schwannoma), transient ischemic episodes of vessels supplying the vestibular system, and sequential unilateral vestibular neuronitis.[82-84] The primary complaint is dysequilibrium though oscillopsia and gait ataxia are common clinical signs with a BVH diagnosis, all direct impairments. Unless the BVH is asymmetrical, the patient will not experience nausea, vertigo, or nystagmus because there is no asymmetry in the tonic firing rate of the vestibular neurons. Halmagyi et al[85] reported that patients with gentamicin ototoxicity have posture and gait abnormalities, decreased visual acuity with head movement, and

Figure 21.14 Illustrated is benign paroxysmal positional vertigo (BPPV) of the posterior SCC. **(A)** Canalithiasis indicates free-floating otoconia within the SCC. When the head is moved into a position that places the SCC parallel to the pull of gravity (e.g., Dix-Hallpike position), the free-floating otoconia move to the dependent position within the canal. The movement of the free-floating otoconia results in deflection of the cupula. **(B)** Cupulolithiasis indicates otoconia adhering to the cupula. When the head is moved to a position placing one of the SCCs parallel to the pull of gravity (e.g., Dix-Hallpike position), the cupula is continually displaced. Illustrated is BPPV of the posterior SCC; also note the cupular deflection. Note that the cupula is drawn with the superior aspect detached from the ampulla.

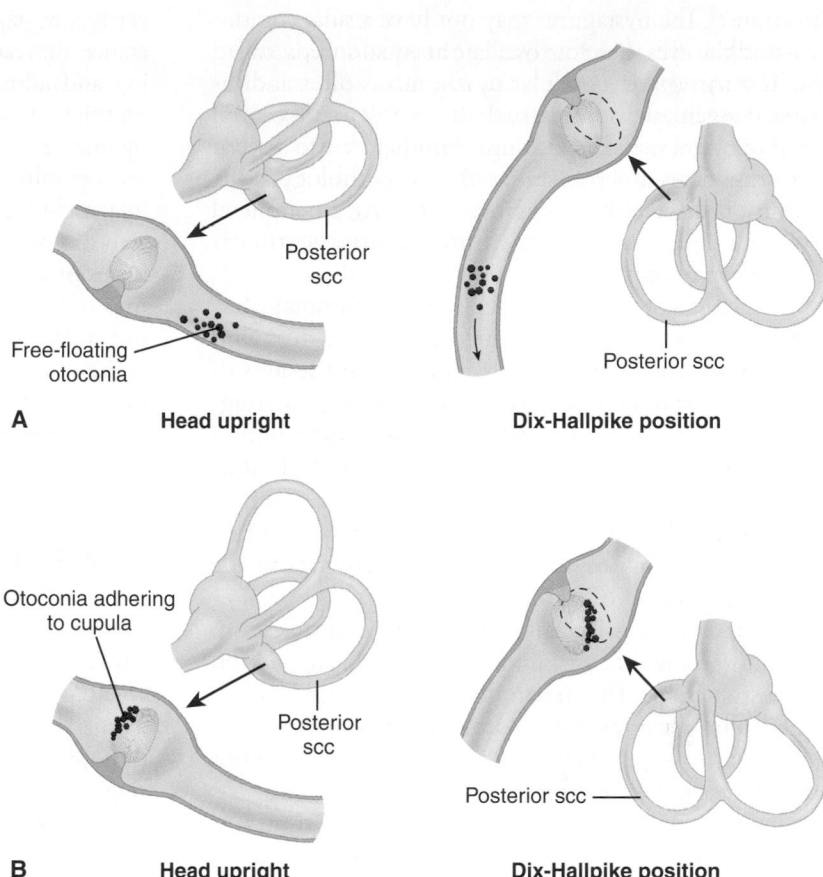

reduced VOR gains resulting in a positive head impulse test. These impairments are likely permanent though patients with BVH can return to high levels of activity.

Central Nervous System Pathology

Various central nervous system (CNS) injuries can affect the vestibular system.[86] Cerebrovascular insults involving the *anterior-inferior cerebellar artery (AICA), posterior-inferior cerebellar artery (PICA),* and *vertebral artery* may cause vertigo, though other signs associated with these infarcts are present and help clarify the site of pathology. Signs and symptoms between an AICA and PICA infarct can be difficult to distinguish though hearing loss is usually more common with AICA infarcts. Lesions of the vertebral artery may affect the cerebellum only and can mimic a peripheral vestibular hypofunction in its clinical presentation. Most patients with cerebellar lesions however, will have associated signs such as dysdiadochokinesia or past pointing.[87] Individuals with transient ischemic attacks may present with sudden vertigo that lasts minutes and also include complaint of hearing loss. For more thorough reading discerning types of central vestibular pathology, see Brandt and Dieterich[86] and Delaney.[87]

Signs and symptoms associated with *vertebrobasilar insufficiency* (VBI) typically do not involve the classic signs and symptoms of vestibular pathology. The most common cause of VBI is motor vehicle accident (MVA).[88] A recent study identified the most common symptoms of VBI as visual field cuts,[89] whereas an older study reported visual dysfunction, drop attacks (sudden, spontaneous falls), and unsteadiness/incoordination as the three most common symptoms.[90] Another cause of VBI is cervical spondylosis. In these patients, vertigo and decreased blood flow velocity through vertebral arteries after head rotation has been reported.[91]

Patients who have sustained a traumatic brain injury (TBI) due to labyrinthine or skull fractures may complain of vertigo.[92] As much as 78% of patients sustaining a mild head injury had acute complaints of vertigo, and 20% to 37% still experienced the vertigo 6 months to 5 years later.[93,94] Abnormal central processing as well as reduced receptor input may cause the perseveration of the vertigo reported in patients with TBI.

Demyelinating diseases such as multiple sclerosis (MS) can affect cranial nerve VIII where it enters the brainstem. In such a case, signs and symptoms may be identical to a UVH. A magnetic resonance image scan will need to be performed to ensure an accurate diagnosis of MS.

Discerning Peripheral Vestibular Pathology from Central Vestibular Pathology

Observation of nystagmus is a useful tool for assisting in determining a diagnosis of CNS pathology. Nystagmus from a cerebellar lesion may be in a pure vertical direction.[95] The nystagmus may not have a slow component and the eyes therefore oscillate at equal speeds, called *pendular nystagmus*. Pendular nystagmus is often indicative of congenital disorders, such as the absence of central vision (cortical visual processing). Another clue to discern a central versus a peripheral vestibular pathology is the recovery time. Unlike nystagmus following a peripheral vestibular lesion, nystagmus from a central vestibular lesion often never resolves.

Vertigo can be a symptom with central pathology but is rare and if present, is often much less intense than with a peripheral vestibular lesion.[96] Patients with lesions of the vestibular nuclei can present with vertigo, nystagmus, and dysequilibrium similar to the patient with a peripheral vestibular lesion. However, central lesions above the level of the vestibular nuclei will manifest lateropulsion, head tilt, and visual perceptual difficulties, as well as oculomotor signs. *Lateropulsion* refers to the person's tendency to fall to one side.

Brandt et al[97] classify central vestibular syndromes from a clinical consensus of establishing perceptual, oculomotor, and postural signs. They report that the most sensitive signs of unilateral brainstem infarct are tilt of the patient's SVV and ocular torsion. Ocular torsion refers to the superior pole of the eyes moving together in a role direction.

Ocular torsion combined with head tilting and skew deviation encompass a triad of signs termed a complete *ocular tilt reaction* (OTR) (Fig. 21.15).[98] Skew deviation of the eyes appears as one eye being superiorly displaced in comparison with the other eye. Kattah, et al examined 101 subjects with symptoms that may have been due to a central pathology (acute vertigo, nystagmus, nausea/vomiting, head-motion intolerance, unsteady gait). Each subject underwent neuroimaging and admission (generally 72 hours after symptom onset). Cerebrovascular accidents (CVAs) were diagnosed by magnetic resonance imaging (MRI) or computed tomography (CT). The initial MRI diffusion-weighted imaging was falsely negative in 12% (48 hours after symptom onset) of subjects. However, the presence of normal horizontal head impulse test, direction-changing nystagmus in eccentric gaze, or skew deviation was 100% sensitive and 96% specific for stroke. Furthermore, the presence of skew deviation correctly predicted lateral pontine stroke in 2 of 3 cases in which an abnormal horizontal head impulse test erroneously suggested peripheral localization. In conclusion, skew is an important predictor of brainstem involvement and can identify CVA when an abnormal horizontal head impulse test may falsely suggest a peripheral lesion. The study recommended a 3-step bedside oculomotor examination (HINTS: Head-Impulse, Nystagmus, Test-of-Skew) as a more sensitive measure for stroke than early MRI.[99]

"Red flags" that should alert the physical therapist to a central vestibular etiology include horizontal or vertical diplopia lasting longer than 2 weeks after the onset of signs or symptoms thought to be due to UVH, persistent pure vertical *positional nystagmus* (anterior canal cupulolithiasis should be ruled out), a spontaneous up-beating nystagmus (rare), and a positive test for skew deviation. The therapist should refer a patient with these manifestations to a neurologist.

It is not within the scope of this chapter to expand on the differential diagnosis within the CNS, identifying the site of lesion. However, the physical therapist must recognize the difference between central and peripheral vestibular dysfunction because this guides the treatment strategy. Table 21.5 can be used as a guide to discern central vestibular pathology from peripheral vestibular pathology.

■ INTERVENTIONS

Benign Paroxysmal Positional Vertigo

The development of specific anticipated goals and expected outcomes for the individual patient with BPPV is based on the following general goals:

- The otoconia will be returned into the vestibule.
- The patient will demonstrate reduced vertigo associated with head motion.
- The patient will demonstrate improved balance.
- The patient will demonstrate independence in daily activity (basic activities of daily living [BADL]; instrumental activities of daily living [IADL]) involving head motion.

Because BPPV is the most common peripheral vestibular pathology, physical therapists should be familiar with treatment of this disorder. The type of nystagmus generated as result of placing the SCCs in gravity-dependent positions indicates which SCC

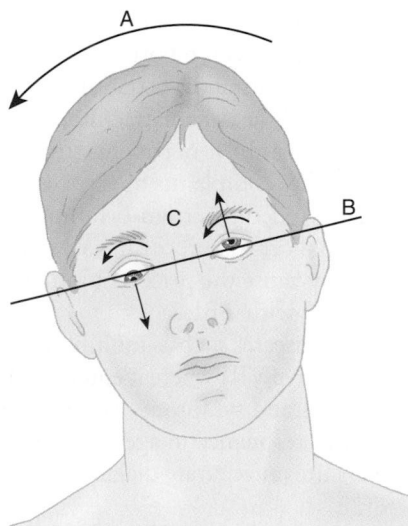

Figure 21.15 The ocular tilt reaction (OTR) consists of a triad of signs: **(A)** Head tilting to the right, indicated with the large arrow. **(B)** Skew deviation of the eyes (right eye is down, left eye is up), indicated with the bisecting line and straight arrows. **(C)** Torsion of the eyes to the right, indicated with the two smaller rounded arrows.

Table 21.5 Common Symptoms Associated with Central versus Peripheral Vestibular Pathology

Central Vestibular Pathology	Peripheral Vestibular Pathology
Ataxia often severe.	Ataxia mild.
Abnormal smooth pursuit and abnormal saccadic eye movement tests.	Smooth pursuit and saccades usually normal; positional testing may reproduce nystagmus.
SX usually do not include hearing loss; if so, it is often sudden and permanent.	SX may include hearing loss (insidious—may recover), fullness in ears, tinnitus.
SX might include diplopia, altered conscious, lateropulsion.	
SX of acute vertigo not usually suppressed by visual fixation.	SX of acute vertigo usually suppressed by visual fixation.
	SX of acute vertigo usually intense (more than central vestibular pathology).
Pendular nystagmus (eyes oscillate at equal speeds).	Nystagmus will incorporate slow and fast phases (jerk nystagmus).
Pure persistent vertical nystagmus persists regardless of positional testing (persistent downbeat nystagmus in Hallpike-Dix test may indicate anterior canal BPPV).	Spontaneous horizontal nystagmus usually resolves within 7 days in a patient with UVH.

BPPV = benign paroxysmal postural vertigo; SX = symptoms; UVH = unilateral vestibular hypofunction.

Table 21.6 Type of Nystagmus Based on SCC Location and Mechanism of BPPV

SCC[a]	Mechanism	Nystagmus[b]	Incidence (%)[10]
Right posterior	Cupulolithiasis	Persistent UBN and right torsion[c]	62
	Canalithiasis	Transient UBN and right torsion	
Left posterior	Cupulolithiasis	Persistent UBN and left torsion	
	Canalithiasis	Transient UBN and left torsion	
Horizontal[d]	Cupulolithiasis	Persistent ageotropic	35
	Canalithiasis	Transient geotropic	
Right superior	Cupulolithiasis	Persistent DBN and right torsion	3
	Canalithiasis	Persistent DBN and right torsion	
Left superior	Cupulolithiasis	Persistent DBN and left torsion	
	Canalithiasis	Persistent DBN and left torsion	

[a]Testing for BPPV in the SCC assumes the patient is in the appropriate positional test.
[b]Nystagmus is labeled by the direction of the fast component up-beat nystagmus (UBN) means the fast component of the nystagmus is beating upwards, DBN = down-beat nystagmus.
[c]The torsional rotation is noted as it relates to the superior poles of the eyes, from the perspective of the examiner.
[d]When BPPV occurs in the horizontal SCC, nystagmus will be present when the head is positioned to either side.
Ageotropic nystagmus = fast component beats away from the ground; geotropic nystagmus = fast component beats toward the ground.

is involved (Table 21.6) and directs the clinician to choose an appropriate treatment approach. Three different treatment approaches have been developed, each based on pathophysiological theories of this disorder. The techniques include the canalith repositioning maneuver, the Liberatory (Semont) maneuver, and Brandt–Daroff exercises.

The *canalith repositioning maneuver* (CRM) is based on the canalithiasis theory of free-floating debris in the SCC.[100] The patient's head is moved into different positions in a sequence that will move the debris out of the involved SCC and into the vestibule (general term

for the location of the utricle and saccule) (see Fig. 21.1). Once the debris is in the vestibule, the signs and symptoms should resolve. The positions used in the treatment of posterior and anterior SCC canalithiasis can be the same. Figure 21.16 illustrates the CRM as applied to either the left posterior or left anterior SCC. It is important to instruct the patient that horizontal movement of the head should be performed to prevent stiff neck muscles. Patients may wish to limit vertical head motion. CRM has also been adapted for application to the horizontal SCC (Fig. 21.17), although BPPV is less common in either the horizontal or anterior SCC.[101] The original

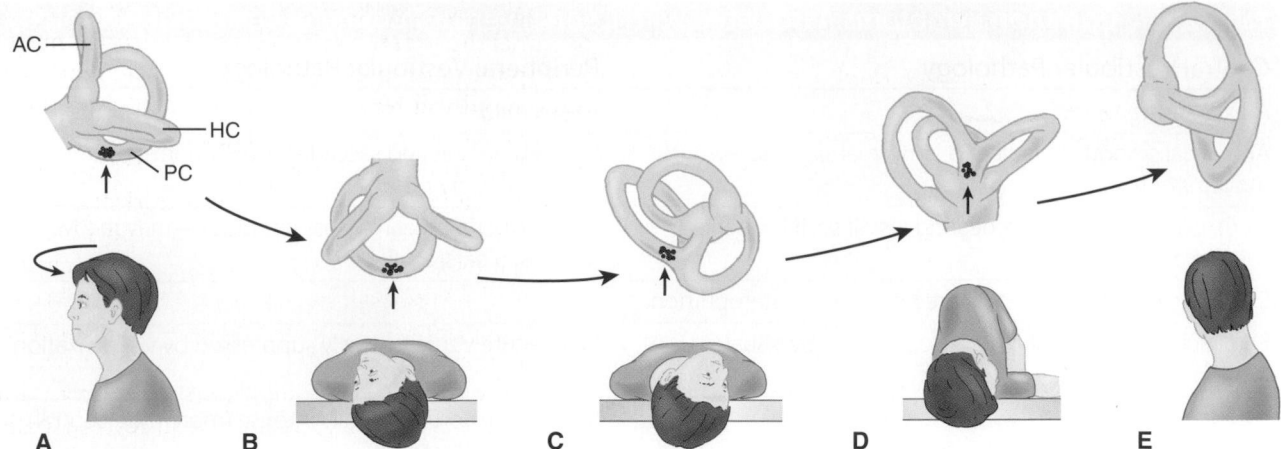

Figure 21.16 Canalith repositioning maneuver (CRM) for posterior or anterior semicircular canal BPPV. **(A)** The patient's head is first rotated 45° toward the involved side, pictured here as the left. **(B)** The patient is then moved into the Dix-Hallpike position with the affected left ear toward the ground. **(C)** Next, the head is rotated 90° to the right. It is important to maintain the 30° neck extension during this step. The head should now be positioned 45° to the right. **(D)** The patient is rolled onto the right shoulder and **(E)** slowly brought up to sitting position, head still rotated 45° to the right. The patient may then be fitted with a soft collar. Note the orientation of the labyrinth for each stage. The arrow points to the free-floating debris and shows its movement through the canal into the common crus **(D)**. AC = anterior SCC; PC = posterior SCC; HC = horizontal SCC. Between each step, the clinician should wait 1 to 2 minutes or until the vertigo and nystagmus has stopped to ensure otoconia flow through the canal.

post-CRM instructions asked patients to remain upright for one to two nights (sleep in a recliner chair) and then to avoid sleeping on the involved side for five additional nights. There is no evidence to support sleeping upright after CRM.[102] Recurrence of BPPV varies depending on the study involved.[103,104] There is no evidence that prophylactic CRM prevents recurrence.[105]

The *Liberatory (Semont) maneuver* was first offered as a treatment for posterior SCC BPPV based on the cupulolithiasis theory.[106] It involves rapidly moving the patient through positions designed to dislodge the debris from the cupula (Fig. 21.18). Data suggest it is effective as an alternative treatment for canalithiasis, though it is more difficult for the patient to tolerate.[107,108]

Brandt–Daroff exercises were originally designed to habituate the CNS to the provoking position.[109] They may also act to dislodge debris from the cupula or by causing debris to move out of the canal. Figure 21.19 illustrates the exercises. The exercise should be performed for 5 to 10 repetitions, three times a day until the patient has no vertigo for 2 consecutive days. If the patient has severe vertigo or complaints of nausea, decreasing the number of repetitions to three, performed three times a day, may render the exercises more tolerable. It is important to explain to the patient that the movements must be performed rapidly and that this will probably provoke the patient's vertigo. Patient education should also include informing the patient that it is normal to have some residual symptoms of dysequilibrium and nausea on completing the exercises.

The residual symptoms are usually temporary and patients need to continue the exercises.

The goal of performing CRM and liberatory procedures is to replace the otoconia into the vestibule, where the calcium crystals can be reabsorbed or perhaps dissolved. The Brandt–Daroff exercises, although originally designed to habituate the peripheral vestibular response, have also led to a complete remission of symptoms, sometimes after the first exercise session.[109] Physical therapy outcomes should also include teaching the patient how to use the appropriate techniques at home, in the case of recurrence. See Table 21.7 for suggested guidelines for use of the CRM, the Liberatory (Semont) maneuver, and Brandt–Daroff exercises.

Unilateral Vestibular Hypofunction

The development of specific anticipated goals and expected outcomes for the individual patient with UVH is based on the following general goals:

- The patient will demonstrate improved stability of gaze during head movement.
- The patient will demonstrate diminished sensitivity to motion.
- The patient will demonstrate improved static and dynamic postural stability.
- The patient will be independent in proper performance of a home exercise program (HEP) that includes walking.

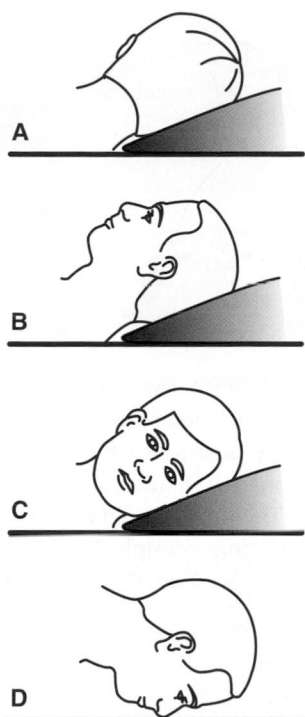

Figure 21.17 Canalith repositioning maneuver (CRM) for right horizontal semicircular canal BPPV. Initially, the patient's head should be placed in 20° cervical flexion. **(A)** For treating a right-sided horizontal canal BPPV, the patient's head is initially placed 90° to the right. **(B)** Next, the head is rotated 90° to the left. The therapist should wait in this position for 15 seconds or until the vertigo and nystagmus stops. **(C)** The head should then be rotated another 90° to the left; again the therapist must wait for 15 seconds or until the vertigo and nystagmus stops. **(D)** The patient must then roll into prone position and await the signs or symptoms to stop. The therapist must attempt to keep the head in 20° flexion during the transition from **C** to **D**. If the CRT has been successful, nystagmus and vertigo should resolve once the patient is in the prone position. The patient may need assistance to sit up from the prone position.

Patients with UVH should be informed that recovery time after initiating vestibular rehabilitation averages 6 to 8 weeks. To ensure adherence with the vestibular rehabilitation exercises, patients should be encouraged frequently and the mutually agreed on goals and outcomes regularly reinforced.

Gaze Stability Exercises

The purpose of these exercises is to improve the VOR and other systems that are used to assist gaze stability with head motion. Vestibular adaptation exercises are designed to expose patients to retinal slip. **Retinal slip** occurs when the image of an object moves off the fovea of the retina, resulting in visual blurring. Retinal slip is necessary as this is the signal used to drive vestibular adaptation within

the brain. Because the brain can tolerate small amounts of retinal slip yet see a target clearly, the patient must try to keep the target in focus. Otherwise, head motion that is too rapid will result in excessive retinal slip. The two primary paradigms of vestibular adaptation are ×1 (times 1) and ×2 (times 2) exercises.[110] In the ×1 exercise the patient is asked to move the head horizontally (and vertically if appropriate) as quickly as possible while maintaining focus on a stable target. The patient must learn to slow the head movement if the target becomes blurred. A good target to use is a business card, asking the patient to focus on a word or a letter within a word. The starting target distance should be an arm's length away. The ×2 paradigm requires the patient to move the head and target in opposite directions (Fig. 21.20). Both paradigms should be made increasingly more difficult as the patient improves. Examples of increasing difficulty include the use of a distracting background while the patient attempts to focus on the letter or word (checkerboard, venetian blinds), varying the distance from which the patient performs the exercises, moving the head more rapidly, and performing the exercise while standing or walking. The *computerized DVA* test is a useful measure of improved gaze stability for individuals with UVH and TBI.[63,111]

Postural Stability Exercises

The purpose of postural stability exercises is to improve balance by encouraging the development of balance strategies within the limitations of the patient, be they somatosensory, visual, or vestibular. The exercises should challenge the patient and be safe enough to perform independently (Table 21.8). Exercises must be updated and progressed to incorporate more challenges (Fig. 21.21). In addition, it is important to incorporate head movement into the exercises because many patients with vestibular loss tend to decrease their head movement.

Habituation Exercises (Motion Sensitivity)

Habituation exercises are warranted when a patient with a UVH has continual complaints of dizziness. *Habituation* is defined as the reduction in response to a repeatedly performed movement. These exercises were the first successful methods used to treat persons with vestibular disorders. Various investigators[45,112] have developed versions of positional tests based on the original exercises and studies by Cawthorne,[14] Cooksey,[15] Norre and DeWeerdt,[113] and Dix.[114,115] As our knowledge of the vestibular system improves, however, we are able to provide more specific exercises than what habituation offers. Clinicians should not treat all vestibular patients with habituation exercises.

To determine which habituation exercises to prescribe, the physical therapist must determine the provoking positions first (see Fig. 21.8). When a position elicits a mild to moderate dizziness, the patient remains in the provoking position for 30 seconds or until the

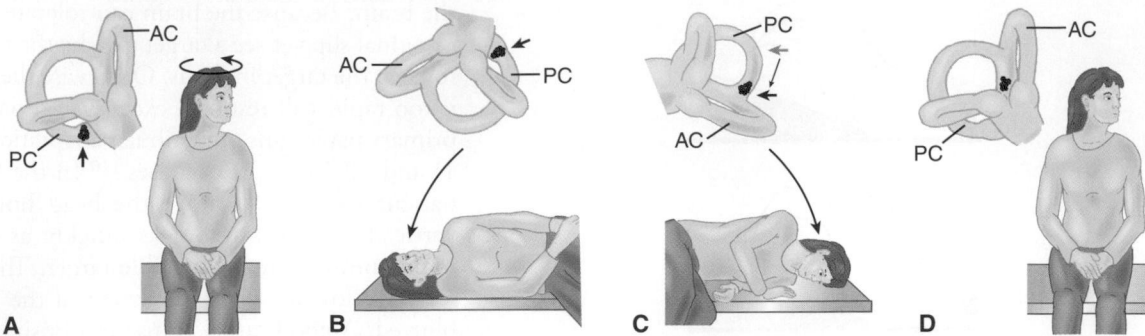

Figure 21.18 Liberatory (Semont) maneuver for right posterior SCC BPPV. The physical therapist should assist the patient through this positioning procedure. Note the otoconia adherent to the cupula in **A** and **B. (A)** The head is rotated 45° to the left side. **(B)** With assistance, the patient is then moved from sitting to right side-lying and stays in this position for 1 minute. **(C)** The patient is then rapidly moved 180°, from right side-lying to left side-lying. The head should be in the original starting position, left rotated (nose down in final position) in this example. Note that the otoconia have been dislodged from the cupula. After 1 minute in this position, **(D)** the patient returns to sitting. AC = anterior SCC; PC = posterior SCC.

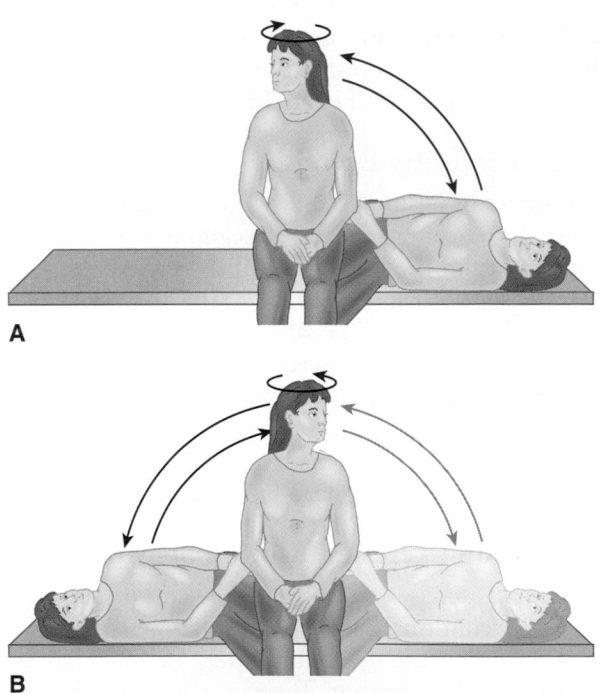

Figure 21.19 Brandt-Daroff exercises for posterior SCC BPPV. **(A)** The patient starts in a sitting position and turns the head 45° to one side (*left*) then quickly lies down on the opposite shoulder (*right*). The patient should be instructed to remain in this position for 30 seconds or until the vertigo stops. The patient then slowly returns to the starting position **(A)**, maintaining the head rotation (*left*) until sitting upright. **(B)** Next, the patient turns the head to the opposite direction (*right*) and lies down on the other shoulder (*left*), observing the similar 30-second time guidelines. The exercise should be done 10 to 20 times, three times per day until the patient is without vertigo for two consecutive days.

Table 21.7	Benign Paroxysmal Positional Vertigo Treatment Techniques
Treatment Procedure	**Diagnosis/Symptoms**
CRM	BPPV due to canalithiasis Posterior SCC canalithiasis is the most common
Liberatory maneuver	BPPV due to cupulolithiasis Posterior SCC cupulolithiasis is the most common
Brandt–Daroff exercises	Persistent/residual or mild vertigo (even after CRM) For the patient who may not tolerate CRM

BPPV = benign paroxysmal positional vertigo; CRM = canalith repositioning maneuver; SCC = semicircular canal.

symptoms abate, whichever comes first.[109] The patient is provided with a home exercise program (HEP) based on the results of the positional test.[45,109] The provoking exercises are performed from three to five times each, two to three times a day. Figure 21.22 provides an example of an HEP using vestibular habituation training. An activity diary can be a useful method to monitor response to training. The exercises are designed to reproduce the dizziness and the patient should be encouraged that the symptoms normally decrease within 2 weeks. If after 2 weeks the symptoms are no better, the habituation exercises should first be changed. If this is not helpful, the patient should be referred to either a physical therapist with special training in vestibular rehabilitation and/or a physician for further evaluation.

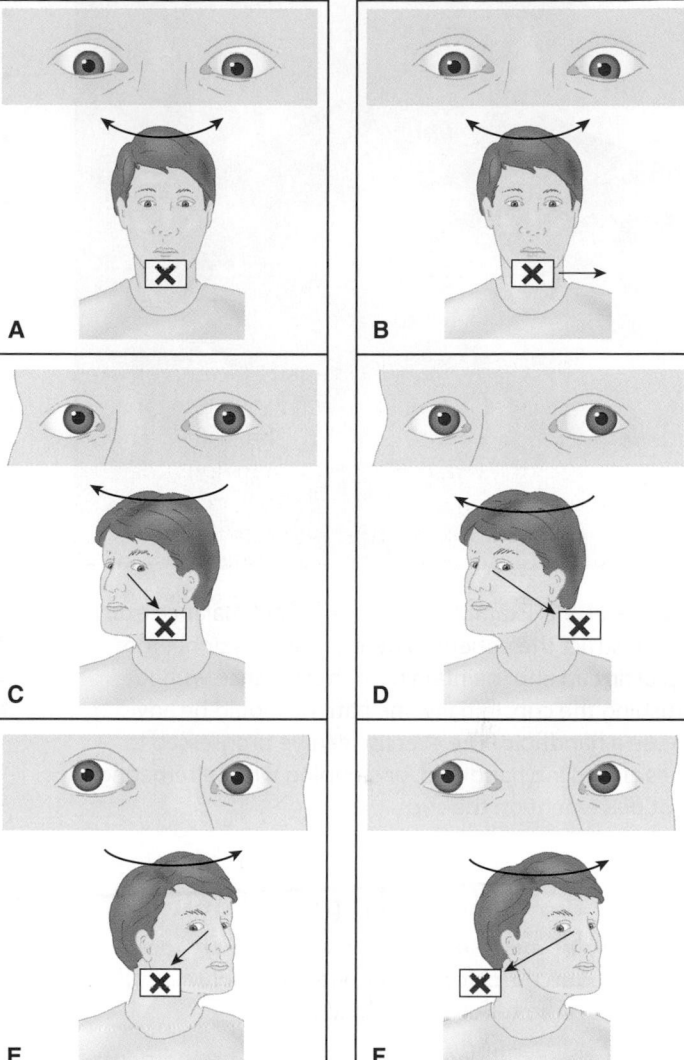

Figure 21.20 Gaze stability exercises. **(A,C,E)** ×1 paradigm: The patient is instructed to focus the eyes on a near target. While maintaining focus on the target, the patient horizontally rotates the head keeping the target still. **(B,D,F)** ×2 paradigm: The patient is instructed to focus the eyes on a near target. While the focus is maintained, the patient horizontally rotates the head and the target in *opposite* directions. Both ×1 and ×2 paradigms require vigilance of the patient to ensure clear vision during the motions. Both exercises are typically performed for 1 to 2 minutes, five times a day. It can be repeated using vertical head movements.

Table 21.8 Balance Exercises and Progressions

Begin With	Progress To	Purpose
1. Stand with feet shoulder-width apart, arms across the chest.	Bring feet closer together. Close eyes. Stand on a sofa cushion or foam.	Enhance the use of vestibular cues for balance by decreasing base of support. Eyes closed increases reliance on vestibular cues for balance.
2. Practice ankle sways: medial-lateral and anterior-posterior.	Doing circle sways. Close eyes.	Teaches the patient to use a correct ankle strategy.
3. Attempt to walk with heel touching toe on firm surface.	Do the same exercise on carpet.	Enhance the use of vestibular cues for balance by decreasing base of support. Doing the exercise on carpet alters proprioceptive input, increasing difficulty.
4. Practice walking five steps and turning 180° (left and right).	Making smaller turns. Close eyes.	Turning provides a greater challenge to the vestibular system.
5. Walk and move the head side-to-side, up and down.	Counting backward from 100 by threes.	Use distracting cognitive or motor demands to challenge balance.

Note: This table presents a limited number of exercises that are effective at improving functional balance. Each of the balance exercises should be performed three times a day for 1–2 minutes each repetition.

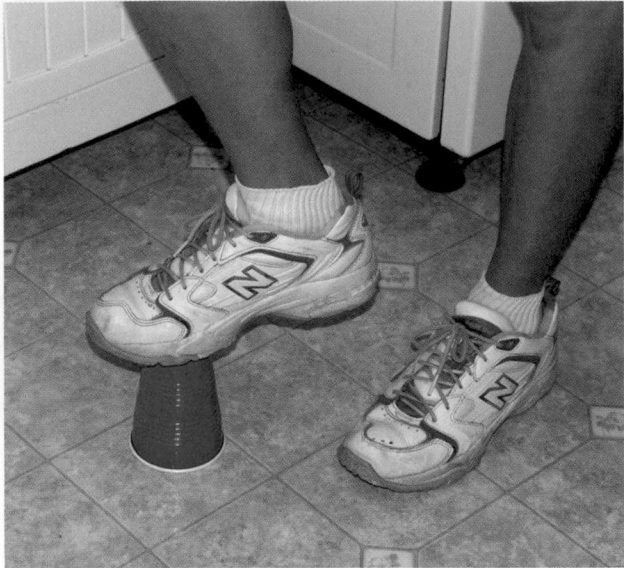

Figure 21.21 Example of a more difficult balance exercise. Instruct the patient to gently place his or her foot on a plastic cup and maintain his or her balance without crushing the cup. Initially, the patient should be advised to use a handhold. The exercise can be progressed to eyes closed, no handhold, or stepping while alternating foot placement on the cup.

Bilateral Vestibular Hypofunction

The development of specific anticipated goals and expected outcomes for the individual patient with BVH is based on the following general goals:

- The patient will demonstrate improved stability of gaze during head movement.

- The patient will demonstrate reduced subjective complaints of gaze instability.
- The patient will demonstrate improved static and dynamic balance.
- The patient will be independent in proper performance of an HEP that includes walking.
- The patient will demonstrate enhanced decision making skills regarding performance of basic and instrumental activities of daily living.

Treatment of patients with a BVH is designed to address the primary complaints of gaze instability during head motion, dysequilibrium, and gait ataxia. Gaze stability exercises can be similar to the ×1 paradigm described in treatment for UVH. Use of the ×2 paradigm is generally not recommended for a patient with a BVH because this exercise may cause excessive retinal slip. (However, many patients have an asymmetrical BVH, in which the ×2 exercise may be useful.) Instead, exercises that incorporate sequenced eye and head movements and the use of imaginary targets may improve gaze stability by enhancing central preprogramming of eye movements (Table 21.9).

Patients with BVH depend on somatosensation and/or vision to maintain postural stability. Balance exercises should enhance the use of these cues. Care must be taken that the exercises are performed safely because people with BVH are likely to fall.[116] It is imperative to begin the patient on a walking program, daily if tolerated. This can be progressed to ambulating on different surfaces (grass, gravel, sand) and in different environments (grocery store, mall). Recovery from a lesion involving both vestibular systems takes much longer than a unilateral lesion. Patients should be informed that as long as 2 years may be necessary to ensure as complete a recovery as

Instructions for the Patient:
Once in the provoking position, wait for 10 seconds to determine if the dizziness will occur. If you experience symptoms of dizziness, remain in the position for an additional 20 seconds (30 seconds total) or until the dizziness abates, whichever comes first. If you do not experience any symptoms you may return to your starting position. Now that you have returned to your starting position, remain here for 10 seconds to monitor your dizziness. If you are dizzy, remain in the return position for an additional 20 seconds (30 seconds total) or until the symptoms abate, whichever comes first. Repeat five times.

Example of Exercises:
1.) Quickly move from sitting upright to bending at the trunk as if to touch your nose to your knee.
2.) Quickly move from sitting at the edge of the bed to lying flat.
3.) In supine, roll onto your left then right side.

Guidelines for the Therapist:
Often, the patient may complain of a certain movement that provokes the symptoms which the examination does not incorporate. This movement can be adapted to be a part of the patient's home exercise program.

	Mon	Tues	Wed	Thur	Fri	Sat	Sun
Duration (0–30 seconds)							
Intensity (0–5)							

Figure 21.22 Example of a home exercise program using habituation therapy. Intensity refers to symptoms (or dizziness) on a five-point scale (0 = none; 5 = most severe).

Table 21.9	Bilateral Vestibular Lesion Exercises to Improve Central Preprogramming of Eye Movements	
Begin With		**Progress To**
1. In sitting, hold two targets at arm's length from your head (i.e., `X' and `Y'). Look with your eyes first to one of the targets (`X') and make sure your nose is pointed to the `X' as well. Now look at the `Y' with your eyes only, followed by turning your head horizontally to point your nose to the `Y'. Repeat this sequence of alternating between the two targets. Attempt to do this for 60 seconds. The patient should be instructed to always first make an eye rotation followed by a head rotation.		Progress to increasing the distance used to see the target. Use a busy background (checkerboard, venetian blinds). Progress to doing this standing.
2. In sitting perform exercise #1 above using vertical head turns.		Same as above.
3. In sitting, hold one target at arm's length from your head. Close your eyes and turn your head horizontally away from the target, attempting to keep your eyes focused on the target. Open your eyes only after having turned your head.		Progress to doing this standing. Progress to decreasing base of support.

possible. For this reason, patient education emphasizing daily activity is a high priority. Daily activity must continue beyond the course of vestibular rehabilitation. Other recommended activities include exercises in a pool and Tai Chi. A pool provides an environment of buoyancy, allowing the patient to move safely without the risk of falling quickly to the ground. Tai Chi incorporates slow, controlled motions used to improve balance, flexibility, and increase strength. In most cases, a person with a BVH will incur an activity limitation or disability. Certain activities may always be limited, such as walking in the dark, night driving, or sports involving quick movements of the head.[117] Older patients may have to use an assistive device such as a cane for safe ambulation at night or on uneven surfaces. Habituation exercises do not work for the patient with a bilateral vestibular loss.[45]

Vestibular adaptation exercises are an excellent starting point for rehabilitation of patients with vestibular hypofunction (UVH and BVH). Research supports the beneficial effects of vestibular adaptation exercises on gait, posture, and DVA (Box 21.1 Evidence Summary).[39, 118-127]

Abnormal Central Vestibular Function

The development of expected goals and anticipated outcomes for the individual patient with a central vestibular lesion is based on the following general goals:

- The patient will demonstrate enhanced decision making skill regarding fall prevention strategies and necessary safety precautions to allow safe functioning within the home and community.
- The patient will demonstrate enhanced decision making skills regarding use of compensatory strategies to assist in gaze stability.
- The patient will be independent in performance of an HEP that includes walking.

Once an accurate diagnosis of central vestibular pathology is made, the physical therapist must be careful in choosing rehabilitation strategies. Expectations for recovery should be described initially to the patient. Generally, the time to recover will be 6 months or more, and may be incomplete.[128] Many of the adaptive mechanisms thought responsible for recovery of the vestibular system are central processes that may have been damaged in the initial central lesion. Physical therapists treating patients with TBI must be careful not to be too aggressive thereby greatly exacerbating the patient's symptoms. Though vestibular rehabilitation offers promise for treating persons with TBI,[129] it may not always be the treatment of choice owing to its irritative nature.

The physical therapy intervention for a central vestibular lesion at the level of the brainstem (vestibular nuclei) likely will be similar to a UVH, with the same expectations for recovery. Vestibular cortical lesions may also recover, similar to the process in which recovery from a CVA might occur.

Because many patients with central vestibular lesions complain of dizziness, a good treatment approach is to start with habituation exercises. However, the exercises should not be too aggressive, thereby aggravating the patient's condition. In addition, gait and balance exercises designed to incorporate somatosensory, visual, and vestibular contributions are also effective with this patient population.

Patient Education

The vestibular system requires movement to recover from most lesions. This basic tenet should be thoroughly discussed when educating patients about returning to daily activity, exercising independently at home, and as a general guideline for their recovery. (Appendix 21.A includes web-based resources for clinicians, families, and patients.) The vestibular system will not improve maximally without head motion. The challenge for both outpatient and inpatient management is determining the amount of exertion the patient can tolerate and creating an effective vestibular rehabilitation strategy without causing deleterious effects.

Box 21.1 Evidence Summary   Outcome Studies Using Vestibular Adaptation Exercises to Improve Gait, Balance, and Dynamic Visual Acuity in Subjects with Vestibular Hypofunction

Reference	Subjects	Design/ Intervention	Duration	Results	Comments
Krebs et al[118] (1993)	8 subjects E (N = 4) BVH Mean age 67.3 ± 15.9 C (N = 4) BVH Mean age 61.1 ± 12.2	RCT; treatment outcome study; control group E: Vestibular adaptation and substitution exercises C: Isometric exercises and general conditioning	Each group: outpatient PT once per week and HEP 1 or 2×/day	E: quicker preferred gait velocity, reduced time in double support; tolerated COM to deviate from the COP for increased distance; no change in rotary chair test, caloric test, VOR test, or DHI scores for either E or C groups	First controlled study investigating efficacy of vestibular rehabilitation in patients with BVH
Herdman et al[119] (1995)	E: (N = 11); UVH due to AN resection; mean age 59.3 ± 10.9 years; C: (N = 8); mean age 47.9 ± 10.4 years; EC: patients with noncerebellar and/or brainstem tumor encroachment or musculoskeletal deficits	RCT; pre-test/ post-test treatment study with control group; E: Vestibular adaptation exercises, ambulation exercises C: Smooth pursuit exercises (placebo) and ambulation exercises	Exercises started on POD 3 Each group performed exercises (adaptation or smooth pursuit) for 1 minute, 5×/day for a total of 20 minutes per day	CDP main outcome measure E: less dysequilibrium; at POD 3: 64% E subjects could do RomEC vs. 25% controls; at POD 3: E had less A-P sway for conditions 4–6 of CDP; at POD 6, 80% E subjects could do RomEC vs. 57% controls	First study advocating VR as an early postoperation intervention for AN; each subject (E and C) was age-matched due to significant difference in age
Strupp et al[120] (1998)	39 patients with stable UVH due to neuritis E: (N = 19); mean age 51.7 ± 11.1 C: (N = 20); mean age 52.4 ± 9.9 EC: reduced visual acuity, diseases impairing mobilization, central vestibular disorders, prior history of vestibulopathy	RCT; pre-test/ post-test with control group; intervention: both groups received general walking program; E group also performed saccades, VOR, smooth pursuit, balance exercises, and cervico-ocular reflex enhancement	E: performed unique exercises 3×/day for 30 minutes each for 5–7 days; to be continued independently for 3 weeks via video instruction C: received walking program; encouragement	No difference in ocular torsion, subjective visual vertical, or mean slow eye velocity due to caloric irrigation; E group showed greater reduction in total sway path during stance on platform posturography	Outcome measures examined central vestibular function. Important study showing many outcome measures of static vestibular imbalance recover spontaneously.

Box 21.1 Evidence Summary   Outcome Studies Using Vestibular Adaptation Exercises to Improve Gait, Balance, and Dynamic Visual Acuity in Subjects with Vestibular Hypofunction—cont'd

Reference	Subjects	Design/ Intervention	Duration	Results	Comments
Cohen and Kimball[121] (2003)	53 subjects with chronic vestibulopathy; assigned to 1 of 3 groups EC: Ménière's disease, BPPV, acute vestibular neuritis or labyrinthitis, orthopedic limitations, head trauma, neurological disease, otologic disease, use of vestibular suppressant medication	RCT; pre-test/ post-test noncontrolled; each group performed exercises at home only (HEP); Group 1: slow head rotation while seated without visual fixation Group 2: quick head rotation with visual fixation, seated and standing Group 3: same as Group 2 with phone call follow-up for encouragement	All 3 groups: 5–10 minutes of exercise 5×/day at home (HEP); posttest after 4 weeks of HEP	No difference between 3 groups in reduction of vertigo intensity, vertigo frequency, or symptoms generated during ADL skills	HEP beneficial for patients with vestibular hypofunction; outcome measures all subjective making functional significance uncertain; difficult to discern that results are not due to natural recovery without a true control group (i.e., no treatment or no head rotation)
Krebs et al[122] (2003)	84 subjects UVH: ($N = 33$); mean age 59.42 ± 20.37 BVH: ($N = 51$); mean age 59.56 ± 18.97 EC: BPPV, Ménière's disease, unstable vestibulopathy	RCT; double blind with control; gait stability measures at baseline, 6 weeks, 12 weeks, 1 year E: Vestibular adaptation and substitution exercises; balance retraining exercises; VR HEP C: Isometric exercises and general conditioning; outpatient VR	E: outpatient PT 1×/week for 6 weeks; then 6 weeks of VR HEP C: outpatient PT 1×/week for 6 weeks; then 6 weeks of VR (1×/week)	At 6 weeks measure, only E group had significantly increased preferred gait velocity, reduced BOS, reduced double support time, reduced M-L sway, reduced lateral velocity, increased distance subjects tolerated their COM to deviate from the COP; 61% of E group demonstrated these improvements; at 1 year, significant treatment effects noted for preferred gait velocity, reduced BOS, reduced M-L sway, and reduced lateral velocity	First long-term study to document VR benefits; BVH subjects recovered by similar amounts as the UVH subjects

Continued

Box 21.1 Evidence Summary   Outcome Studies Using Vestibular Adaptation Exercises to Improve Gait, Balance, and Dynamic Visual Acuity in Subjects with Vestibular Hypofunction—cont'd

Reference	Subjects	Design/ Intervention	Duration	Results	Comments
Patten et al[123] (2003)	20 subjects E: (N = 10) patients with BVH; mean age 69 ± 13.2 C: (N = 10) healthy controls; mean age 68.9 ± 13.03; height and body mass were matched EC: CNS dysfunction, neuromusculoskeletal impairment, CVA, peripheral nerve deficit, visual impairment	RCT; pre-test/post-test with control group E: cites exercises similar to Krebs 1993 study C: no exercise	Study cites exercise duration similar to Krebs 1993	Significant improvement in head pitch coordination; comparable to healthy controls	Authors recommend VR goals include exercises to enhance head stability during gait
Herdman et al[39] (2003)	21 patients with UVH E: N = 13; mean age 65.1 ± 16.5 C: N = 8; mean age 64.9 ± 16.2. EC: normal DVA, BVH.	RCT; double blind; repeated measures with control E: VOR adaptation exercises and balance retraining C: smooth pursuit and balance exercises; DVA measured weekly for 4 weeks	E and C groups exercised 4–5×/day for 20–30 minutes in addition to 20 minutes of balance exercises	12 of 13 individuals in the E group demonstrated DVA that returned to age-matched normal values; no change in DVA for control group; only the type of exercise contributed to change in DVA	Important first study showing the beneficial effect of VOR adaptation exercises to improve gaze stability in persons with UVH as measured by the DVA
Herdman et al[124] (2007)	13 patients with BVH E: N = 8; mean age 63.6 ± 9.4 C: N = 8; mean age 63.6 ± 10.8 EC: presence of nystagmus in room light, static visual acuity with the worse than logMAR 0.500, minors/people incapable of understanding the purpose	RCT; double blind; repeated measures with control E: VOR adaptation exercises and balance retraining C: smooth pursuit and balance exercises; DVA measured weekly for 6 weeks; VAS-O measured	E and C groups exercised 4–5×/day for 20–30 minutes in addition to 20 minutes of balance exercises	7 of 8 individuals in E group only had improvement in DVA; those in C group did not. Change in VAS-O did not correlate with change in DVA	Only type of exercise was correlated with change in DVA, not age, time from onset, initial DVA, or complaints of oscillopsia and dysequilibrium
Hillier and Hollohan[125] (2007)	21 trials in the review	Cochrane review of RCT on vestibular rehabilitation in adults living in the community, diagnosed with symptomatic	Included studies addressing the effectiveness of vestibular rehabilitation against control/sham interventions,	Individual and pooled data showed a statistically significant effect in favor of the vestibular rehabilitation over	Moderate to strong evidence that vestibular rehabilitation is a safe, effective management for UVH

Box 21.1 Evidence Summary   Outcome Studies Using Vestibular Adaptation Exercises to Improve Gait, Balance, and Dynamic Visual Acuity in Subjects with Vestibular Hypofunction—cont'd

Reference	Subjects	Design/ Intervention	Duration	Results	Comments
		unilateral peripheral vestibular hypofunction	nonvestibular rehabilitation interventions, by comparing the subjects in each group who had significant resolution of symptoms and/or improved function	control or no intervention; there were no reported adverse effects	
Schubert et al[126] (2008)	E: n = 4 UVH and 1 BVH; mean age 54.4 ±8.9 years; C: n = 5 age matched healthy controls, mean 54 ± 12.8 years EC: patients with dizziness not confirmed as true vestibular hypofunction, BPPV	Age-matched control intervention study E: VOR adaptation and balance exercises 4–5×/day for 20–30 minutes C: No intervention	Mean 5.0 ± 1.4 visits; over 66 ± 24 days Outcome measures: aVOR gain and DVA	DVA improved (mean, 51% ± 25%, range 21%–81%) A VOR gain during the head rotation increased in each patient mean range, 0.7 ± 0.2 to 0.9 ± 0.2 (35%) For control subjects, aVOR gain during DVA was always near 1 Patients also increased use of compensatory saccades	First study to show mechanistic effect of exercises explaining improved DVA Saccade system also modifiable with gaze stability exercises
Giray et al[127] (2009)	E: (N = 20); chronic UVH; age 52.5 ± 14.9 years; C: (N = 22) age 50.4 ± 18.6 years EC: ambulatory problems, reduced CROM; visual or somatosensory disorder, cognitive, orthopedic, or neurologic disorder; fluctuating vertigo, BPPV, symptoms < 2 months' duration, BVH	RCT; pre-test/post-test treatment study with control group E: Custom exercises to include adaptation, habituation, visual desensitization, and balance exercises C: No intervention	4 weeks total; outpatient therapy 2×/week for 30–45 minutes; HEP 2×/day for 30–40 minutes	Only E group had improved DHI (mean 52%), BBS (mean 4.12 points), CTSIB (range 20%–33%), and VASd (mean 52%)	Patients with chronic UVH can show meaningful improvement

aVOR = angular vestibular ocular reflex; AN = acoustic neuroma; BOS = base of support; BBS = Berg Balance Scale; BPPV = benign paroxysmal positional vertigo; BVH = bilateral vestibular hypofunction; C = control group; CDP = computerized dynamic posturography; CNS = central nervous system; COM = center of mass; COP = center of pressure; CROM = cervical range of motion; CTSIB = clinical test for the sensory interaction on balance; CVA = cerebrovascular accident; DHI = Dizziness Handicap Inventory; DVA = dynamic visual acuity; E = experimental group; EC = exclusion criteria; HEP = home exercise program; M-L = medial-lateral; OKN = optokinetic nystagmus; OKS = optokinetic stimulation; POD = postoperation day; PT = physical therapy; RomEC = Romberg eyes closed; SOLEC = stand on one leg eyes closed; SOLEO = stand on one leg eyes open; UVH = unilateral vestibular hypofunction; VASd = visual analogue scale dysequilibrium; VAS-O = visual analogue scale oscillopsia; VVOR = visual vestibular interaction (visual vestibulo-ocular reflex).

■ DIAGNOSES INVOLVING THE VESTIBULAR SYSTEM

Ménière's Disease

Ménière's disease is confirmed by a documented low-frequency hearing loss and episodic vertigo. The patient may also complain of a sense of fullness in the ear and tinnitus. The symptoms gradually increase in severity and can last several hours per episode. During an episode, vestibular exercises are not recommended. Chronic Ménière's disease, however, can result in a UVH, for which rehabilitation is appropriate. The pathophysiology of Ménière's disease, in part, probably involves an increase in endolymphatic fluid causing distention of the membranous tissues.[130] Medical treatment is therefore directed toward reducing or preventing fluid buildup. Many patients can manage the symptoms well with a controlled diet. Patients with Ménière's disease are often placed on a 2 g/day or less sodium diet. This is the most important dietary restriction to follow. Other substances to be avoided are caffeine and alcohol. Sometimes medical management includes use of a diuretic to control the amount of water in the body. Surgery to either prevent the fluid buildup in the inner ear (endolymphatic shunt placement) or to stop the abnormal vestibular signal (vestibular nerve section, or chemical ablation using transtympanic gentamicin injection) may be indicated if the episodes are frequent enough to disturb daily function. Physical therapy is beneficial in treating the effects of a UVH owing to chronic Ménière's disease, although the therapy will not stop the episodes of vertigo. Gaze and postural stability exercises may be appropriate. Physical therapy is also useful in the treatment of dysequilibrium occurring after a vestibular neurectomy or chemical ablation.

Perilymphatic Fistula

Perilymphatic fistula (PLF) is most commonly caused by a rupture of the oval or round windows, membranes that separate the middle and inner ear. A rupture of these membranes results in leakage of the perilymph into the middle ear. The result is vertigo and hearing loss. Normally, perilymph bathes the SCCs and serves as a protective barrier between the bony and membranous labyrinth. PLF usually is caused from a traumatic event, such as excessive pressure changes as in deep-water diving, blunt head trauma without skull fracture, or extremely loud noise.[131] This diagnosis is much debated and the treatment for PLF is similarly ambiguous. Patients often are treated first with bedrest in hopes of allowing the membrane to heal. Surgical patches of the fistula are also performed. Physical therapy is contraindicated for most patients with PLF; however, it can be beneficial for those patients who have continual dysequilibrium or develop a vestibular hypofunction postoperatively. Medical management will likely include strict limitations on activities, warranting good communication between physical therapist and physician.

A form of PLF not debated is superior semicircular canal dehiscence. In this condition, the region of the temporal bone normally covering the superior SCC is thin or missing, rendering the membranous SCC susceptible to stimuli that it normally should not (e.g., sound, change of cranial pressure, vibrations).[132] The patient will notice a disturbing syndrome of vestibular and auditory signs that may include eye movements induced by loud noises or effort that increase intracranial pressure (e.g., coughing), sudden or progressive hearing loss, conductive hyperacusis, conductive hearing loss that can mimic otosclerosis (abnormal bone growth near middle ear), autophony (person's own voice sounds amplified), imbalance with noise, vertigo, or motion sensitivity. Some patients even report hearing their eyeballs, "as if scratching sandpaper!"

Vestibular Schwannoma

Vestibular schwannomas (VSs), historically known as **acoustic neuromas**, are benign tumors arising from the Schwann cell of the eighth cranial nerve, often in the internal auditory canal (IAC). The IAC also contains the facial nerve (cranial nerve VII) and the internal auditory artery along with the vestibulocochlear nerve. Symptom presentation is usually related to where the tumor arises. If the tumor arises in the IAC, then tinnitus and hearing loss are often the first symptoms. However, if the growth occurs in the cerebellar-pontine angle, the tumor may become quite large before symptoms of hearing loss are revealed. Thus, although unilateral hearing loss is often the initial sign of VS, the pathogenesis of the associated structures within the space can sometimes result in vestibular (i.e., vertigo, imbalance), facial, or even vascular symptoms. Generally, VS tumors grow slowly. As a result, the extent of impaired vestibular or facial nerve function is often not appreciated until the tumor is removed. This is because the tumor gradually compresses the cranial nerves, and in the case of vestibular function, allows the brain to compensate. However, as the VS enlarges, symptoms of hearing loss, tinnitus, and vestibular hypofunction worsen, resulting in the primary deficits. Treatment usually involves surgical excision of the tumor, though gamma knife radiation is also an option. On tumor removal, most unilateral vestibular afference is lost and the brain now perceives asymmetrical vestibular input. Optimally, physical therapy is initiated during the early postoperative period to help the patient resolve symptoms of dysequilibrium and oscillopsia.[119] Outpatient treatment should be considered similar to the treatment for a UVH.

Motion Sickness

Motion sickness is a normal sensation that in some people becomes debilitating. The predominant explanation for motion sickness is the *sensory conflict theory*.[133] The three sensory inputs of proprioception, vestibular, and visual information do not match stored neural patterns the brain expects to recognize. As a result, persons experience pallor, nausea, emesis, diaphoresis, and motion sensitivity. Physical therapy has been successfully used to reduce motion sensitivity.[134] Other methods reported to combat motion sickness include the use of cognitive-behavioral management, medications, biofeedback, and habituation training.[135-138]

Migraine-Related Dizziness

Migraine-related dizziness can be deceptively similar to a peripheral vestibular lesion, be it BPPV or UVH. Migraine-related symptoms include vertigo, dizziness, imbalance, and motion sickness. A recent study reported 100% of migraineurs had abnormal nystagmus during a migraine episode, if they were positionally tested as part of an oculomotor examination.[139] The prevalence of migraine is significant, affecting 6% of men and 15% to 18% of women between the ages of 25 and 55.[140] The clinical examination will often provide the differential diagnosis between vestibular pathology and migraine. The history is crucial and important questions to patients in whom migraine is suspected include asking if symptoms worsen when barometric pressure changes, and whether headache or eating certain foods are associated with any of the symptoms. If the therapist suspects migraine the patient should be referred to a neurologist, preferably one with a special interest in headache. Migraine is often well controlled with medication and diet. Migraine that is not controlled may become worse with exercises such as vestibular rehabilitation, which stimulate the peripheral vestibular end organ and central VOR pathways.[141] Vestibular rehabilitation in patients with migraine can be very helpful, but patients with both vestibular hypofunction and migraine do not respond as well.[142] Strupp et al[143] provide a thorough discussion of this topic.

Multiple Sclerosis

MS can affect cranial nerve VIII where it enters the brainstem and causes identical symptoms to a unilateral vestibular pathology. An MRI scan will ensure an accurate diagnosis of MS.

Multiple System Atrophy

Multiple system atrophy (MSA) is a progressive degenerative disease of the nervous system involving four clinical domains: cerebellar ataxia, autonomic dysfunction, Parkinson's disease–like symptoms, and corticospinal dysfunction. MSA has been found to be a cause of dizziness and imbalance.[144] The effect of physical therapy for persons with MSA has not been thoroughly investigated, though a case study has been reported.[144]

Cervicogenic Dizziness

Cervicogenic dizziness is a term meant to imply that the cause of symptoms such as dizziness or imbalance arise from pathology affecting the cervical spine or related soft tissue. Unfortunately, *cervical vertigo* is a term still often used, which implies true vertigo as a result of cervical pathology, not documented in humans. The mechanisms of involvement are believed to be from at least two sources. First, the upper cervical spine sends proprioceptive input to the contralateral vestibular nucleus.[145] Soft tissue injury and joint dysfunction might alter the afferent input contributing to spatial orientation. Vestibular rehabilitation appears to be warranted for these individuals.[146] Second, a patient might have VBI (see above section titled Central Nervous System Pathology). If VBI is suspected, vascular compromise must first be ruled out as a cause of the patient's symptoms. The VBI test can be performed while the subject is seated. The patient leans forward and extends the neck. The neck is then rotated 45° to the suspicious side. Persons suspected of having VBI should be referred to a neurologist immediately. Repeated episodes of vertigo without the associated VBI symptoms usually suggest a peripheral vestibular diagnosis.

■ CONTRAINDICATIONS TO VESTIBULAR REHABILITATION

Physical therapy is not appropriate for unstable vestibular disorders such as Ménière's disease (with the exception mentioned above), uncontrolled migraine, PLF, or an unrepaired superior semicircular canal dehiscence. Other contraindications the physical therapist should be alert to include sudden loss of hearing, increased feeling of pressure or fullness to the point of discomfort in one or both ears, and severe ringing in one or both ears. When treating patients who have had a surgical procedure, the clinician must be observant for discharge of fluid from the ears or nose, which may indicate cerebrospinal fluid leak. Patients with acute neck injuries may not be able to tolerate some components of the physical examination, the CRM, or some of the gaze stability exercises.

SUMMARY

High incidence and prevalence rates of vestibular disorders oblige the physical therapist to recognize signs and symptoms associated with inner ear disorders. It is essential to differentiate a peripheral pathology from a central one. Peripheral and central lesions have separate manifestations and may require different intervention strategies. In addition, all vestibular disorders should not be treated similarly. The most common form of vertigo, BPPV, is a biomechanical problem readily treated often with a single maneuver. This is in stark contrast to a patient with a BVH, which requires a greater rehabilitation effort. Evidence supports the use of vestibular adaptation exercises for patients with vestibular hypofunction.

Research in vestibular rehabilitation is ongoing and remains imperative to answer important questions related to dosing, recruitment of compensatory strategies to assist gaze stability, recurrence prevention for BPPV, and more. Exciting future treatments may involve virtual reality, vibrotactors to alert patients of abnormal posture, and the inclusion of computer gaming platforms. Within the next 5 years, successful implementation of a surgically implanted vestibular prosthesis for BVH is expected. Regardless of technological advances, rehabilitation will still be important in these patients.

The *Vestibular Disorders Association (VEDA)* has a list of physical therapists in each state, interested in treating patients with vestibular disorders. VEDA can be contacted via phone (800-837-8428; 24-hour voice mail), fax (503-229-8064), or through the "contact us" link on their website (www.vestibular.org) (see Appendix 21.A). The supplemental reading list contains other excellent literature for the reader interested in pursuing a greater depth of knowledge in vestibular rehabilitation.

Questions for Review

1. Why is it important to perform the head impulse test using a rapid velocity?
2. What is the name of the linear accelerometers within the vestibular labyrinth?
3. Why does the patient with an acute unilateral vestibular lesion experience spontaneous nystagmus?
4. How will cupulolithiasis present differently than canalithiasis of the posterior semicircular canal?
5. What are the key elements in taking a history for a patient with a suspected vestibular disorder?
6. Explain inhibitory cutoff.
7. Differentiate the ×1 exercise paradigm from the ×2 exercise paradigm.
8. In a patient with vestibular nystagmus, which part of the eye movement (slow or fast) is from the vestibular system? Why?
9. Describe how the Dix-Hallpike test would elicit nystagmus for posterior SCC BPPV.
10. Differentiate between adaptation and habituation training for patients with vestibular dysfunction.

CASE STUDIES

CASE STUDY 1

You are performing an initial examination of a patient with new onset of complaints of imbalance and dizziness. In a sitting position, at rest, the patient is observed to have a purely vertical and pendular nystagmus with head tilting to the left. The nystagmus is not altered with any change in head position, and the head-shaking induced nystagmus test (HSN) is negative.

GUIDING QUESTIONS

1. Do you suspect a central or peripheral pathology as a cause of the imbalance and dizziness?
2. Is physical therapy appropriate at this time?

CASE STUDY 2

On your patient's return to sitting up after you have performed the canalith-repositioning maneuver (CRM) for a left posterior canalithiasis, you notice down-beating and right torsional nystagmus. The patient is complaining of vertigo.

GUIDING QUESTIONS

1. Where is the otoconia now located?

2. How will you treat for benign paroxysmal positional vertigo (BPPV) the second time?

3. Following the second treatment for BPPV, the patient complains of dizziness and neck pain. The vertigo and nystagmus are gone. Can you prescribe any other forms of exercise for the remaining dizziness? What about the neck pain?

CASE STUDY 3

A patient with a unilateral vestibular hypofunction (UVH) complains of feeling worse after 7 days of starting a vestibular rehabilitation program. The patient has had no falls. The complaints consist of increased dizziness with head motion, nausea, and fatigue.

GUIDING QUESTIONS

1. Is your rehabilitation program making the patient worse?

2. How can you modify the program?

3. What information will you tell your patient with a UVH regarding time to recover? What will you tell patients with BPPV, BVH, or central nervous system pathology regarding times to recover?

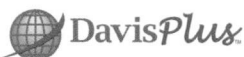 DavisPlus | For additional resources, including answers to the questions for review and case study guiding questions, please visit **http://davisplus.fadavis.com**

 The reader is referred to video **Case Study 13: Patient with Vestibular Disorder** for additional review and study. The full written case study, including tables, figures, charts, and three video segments (examination, intervention, and outcome), appears online at DavisPlus. The case study poses questions for the reader's consideration with suggested answers to the case study questions, also posted online at DavisPlus.

References

1. Kroenke, K, and Mangelsdorff, AD: Common symptoms in ambulatory care: Incidence, evaluation, therapy, and outcome. Am J Med 86(3):262, 1989.
2. Yardley, L, et al: Prevalence and presentation of dizziness in a general practice community sample of working age people. Br J Gen Pract 48(429):1131, 1998.
3. Sloane, PD: Dizziness in primary care. Results from the National Ambulatory Medical Care Survey. J Fam Pract 29(1):33, 1989.
4. Tinetti, ME, et al: Dizziness among older adults: A possible geriatric syndrome. Ann Intern Med 132(5):337, 2000.
5. Colledge, NR, et al: The prevalence and characteristics of dizziness in an elderly community. Age Ageing 23(2):117, 1994.
6. Sloane, PD, et al: Dizziness in a community elderly population. J Am Geriatr Soc 37:101, 1989.
7. Sloane, PD, et al: Dizziness: State of the science. Ann Intern Med 134:823, 2001.
8. Kroenke, K, et al: How common are various causes of dizziness? A critical review. South Med J 93:160, 2000.
9. Newman-Toker, DE, et al: Spectrum of dizziness visits to US emergency departments: Cross-sectional analysis from a nationally representative sample. Mayo Clin Proc 83(7):765, 2008.
10. Hsiao, CJ, et al: National Ambulatory Medical Care Survey: 2007 Summary Number 27, November 3, 2010. National Health Statistics Reports 2010. Retrieved August 7, 2012, from www.cdc.gov/nchs/data/nhsr/nhsr027.pdf.
11. Grimby, A, and Rosenhall, U: Health related quality of life and dizziness in old age. Gerontology 41:286, 1995.
12. Strategic Plan. National Institute on Deafness and Other Communication Disorders (NIDCD). FY 2009–2011. National Institutes of Health, Bethesda, MD. Retrieved August 7, 2012, from www.nidcd.nih.gov/staticresources/about/plans/strategic/FY2009-2011NIDCDStrategicPlan.pdf.
13. Kroenke, K, et al: Causes of persistent dizziness: A prospective study of 100 patients in ambulatory care. Ann Intern Med 117(11):898, 1992.
14. Cawthorne, T: The physiological basis for head exercises. J Charter Soc Physiother 30:106, 1944.
15. Cooksey, FS: Rehabilitation in vestibular injuries. Proc R Soc Med 39:273, 1946.
16. Della Santina, CC, et al: Orientations of human vestibular labyrinth semicircular canals. In Proceedings of the 2004 Midwinter Meeting of the Association for Research in Otolaryngology, Daytona Beach, FL (February 22–26, 2004). Association for Research in Otolaryngology, Mt Royal, NJ, 2004.
17. Cremer, PD, et al: Semicircular canal plane head impulses detect absent function of individual semicircular canals. Brain 121:699, 1998.
18. Smith, CA, et al: The electrolytes of the labyrinthine fluids. Laryngoscope 64:141, 1954.
19. Troiani, D, et al: Relations of single semicircular canals to the pontine reticular formation. Arch Ital Biol 114(4):337, 1976.
20. Buttner, U, and Henn, V: Thalamic unit activity in the alert monkey during natural vestibular stimulation. Brain Res 103(1):127, 1976.
21. Brodal, A, and Brodal, P: Observations on the secondary vestibulocerebellar projections in the macaque monkey. Exp Brain Res 58:62, 1985.
22. Buttner, U, and Buettner, UW: Parietal cortex (2v) neuronal activity in the alert monkey during natural vestibular and optokinetic stimulation. Brain Res 153:392, 1978.
23. Grusser, OJ, et al: Localization and responses of neurones in the parieto-insular vestibular cortex of awake monkeys (Macaca fascicularis). J Physiol 430:537, 1990.
24. Their, P, and Erickson, RG: Vestibular input to visual-tracking neurons in area MST of awake rhesus monkeys. Ann N Y Acad Sci 656:960, 1992.
25. Brandt, T, et al: Visual-vestibular and visuovisual cortical interaction: New insights from fMRI and PET. Ann N Y Acad Sci 956:230, 2002.

26. Dieterich, M, et al: fMRI signal increases and decreases in cortical areas during small-field optokinetic stimulation and central fixation. Exp Brain Res 148:117, 2003.

27. Brandt, T, and Dieterich, M: Vestibular syndromes in the roll plane: Topographic diagnosis from brainstem to cortex. Ann Neurol 36:337, 1994.

28. Goldberg, JM, and Fernandez, C: Physiology of peripheral neurons innervating semicircular canals of the squirrel monkey. I: Resting discharge and response to constant angular accelerations. J Neurophysiol 34:635, 1971.

29. Lysakowski, AM, et al: Physiological identification of morphologically distinct afferent classes innervating the cristae ampullares of the squirrel monkey. J Neurophysiol 73:1270, 1995.

30. Baloh, RW, and Honrubia, V: Clinical neurophysiology of the vestibular system. FA Davis, Philadelphia, 1990.

31. Meyer, CH, et al: The upper limit of human smooth pursuit velocity. Vision Res 25:561, 1985.

32. Fernandez, C, and Goldberg, JM: Physiology of peripheral neurons innervating semicircular canals of the squirrel monkey. II: Response to sinusoidal stimulation and dynamics of peripheral vestibular system. J Neurophysiol 34:661, 1971.

33. Dai, M, et al: Model-based study of the human cupular time constant. J Vestib Res 9(4):293, 1999.

34. Baloh, RW: Dizziness: Neurological emergencies. Neurol Clin 16:305, 1998.

35. Gillespie, MB, and Minor, LB: Prognosis in bilateral vestibular hypofunction. Laryngoscope 109:35, 1999.

36. Telian, SA, et al: Bilateral vestibular paresis: Diagnosis and treatment. Otolaryngol Head Neck Surg 104:67, 1991.

37. Grunfeld, EA, et al: Adaptation to oscillopsia: A psychophysical and questionnaire investigation. Brain 123(pt 2):277, 2000.

38. Bhansali, SA, et al: Oscillopsia in patients with loss of vestibular function. Otolaryngol Head Neck Surg 109:120, 1993.

39. Herdman, SJ, et al: Recovery of dynamic visual acuity in unilateral vestibular hypofunction. Arch Otolaryngol Head Neck Surg 129(8):819, 2003.

40. Dixon, JS, and Bird, HA: Reproducibility along a 10 cm vertical visual analog scale. Ann Rheum Dis 40:87, 1981.

41. Jacobson, GP, and Newman, CW: The development of the Dizziness Handicap Inventory. Arch Otolaryngol Head Neck Surg 116:424, 1990.

42. Robertson, D, and Ireland, D: Dizziness Handicap Inventory correlates of computerized dynamic posturography. J Otolaryngol 24:118, 1995.

43. Jacobson, GP, and McCaslin, DL: Agreement between functional and electrophysiologic measures in patients with unilateral peripheral vestibular system impairment. J Am Acad Audiol 14(5):231, 2003.

44. Morris, A, Lutman, ME, and Luxon, L: Measuring outcome from vestibular rehabilitation, part II: Refinement and validation of a new self-report measure. Int J Audiol 48:24–37, 2008.

45. Smith-Wheelock, M, et al: Physical therapy program for vestibular rehabilitation. Am J Otol May 12(3):218, 1991.

46. Fetter, M, and Dichgans, J: Adaptive mechanisms of VOR compensation after unilateral peripheral vestibular lesions in humans. J Vestib Res 1:9, 1990.

47. Cass, SP, et al: Patterns of vestibular function following vestibular nerve section. Laryngoscope 102:388, 1992.

48. Maioli, C, et al: Short- and long-term modifications of vestibulo-ocular response dynamics following unilateral vestibular nerve lesions in the cat. Exp Brain Res 50:259, 1983.

49. Watabe, H, Hashiba, M, and Baba, S: Voluntary suppression of caloric nystagmus under fixation of imaginary or after-image target. Acta Otolaryngol Suppl 525:155, 1996.

50. Halmagyi, GM, and Curthoys, IS: A clinical sign of canal paresis. Arch Neurol 45:737, 1998.

51. Halmagyi, GM, et al: The human horizontal vestibulo-ocular reflex in response to high-acceleration stimulation before and after unilateral vestibular neurectomy. Exp Brain Res 81:479, 1990.

52. Minor, LB, et al: Symptoms and signs in superior canal dehiscence syndrome. Ann N Y Acad Sci 942:259, 2001.

53. Aw, ST, et al: Unilateral vestibular deafferentation causes permanent impairment of the human vertical vestibulo-ocular reflex in the pitch plane. Exp Brain Res 102:121, 1994.

54. Cremer, PD, et al: Semicircular canal plane head impulses detect absent function of individual semicircular canals. Brain 121:699, 1998.

55. Foster, CA, et al: Functional loss of the horizontal doll's eye reflex following unilateral vestibular lesions. Laryngoscope 104:473, 1994.

56. Harvey, SA, and Wood, DJ: The oculocephalic response in the evaluation of the dizzy patient. Laryngoscope 106:6, 1996.

57. Harvey, SA, and Wood, DJ: Relationship of the head impulse test and head-shake nystagmus in reference to caloric testing. Am J Otolaryngol 18:207, 1997.

58. Beynon, GJ, et al: A clinical evaluation of head impulse testing. Clin Otolaryngol 23:117, 1998.

59. Schubert, MC, et al: Optimizing the sensitivity of the head thrust test for identifying vestibular hypofunction. Phys Ther 84:151, 2004.

60. Hain, TC, et al: Head-shaking nystagmus in patients with unilateral peripheral vestibular lesions. Am J Otolaryngol 8:36, 1987.

61. Dix, R, and Hallpike, CS: The pathology, symptomatology and diagnosis of certain common disorders of the vestibular system. Ann Otol Rhinol Laryngol 6:987, 1952.

62. Longridge, NS, and Mallinson, AI: The dynamic illegible E (DIE) test: a simple technique for assessing the ability of the vestibulo-ocular reflex to overcome vestibular pathology. J Otolaryngol 16:97, 1987.

63. Herdman, SJ, et al: Computerized dynamic visual acuity test in the assessment of vestibular deficits. Am J Otolaryngol 19:790, 1998.

64. Tian, JR, et al: Dynamic visual acuity during passive and self-generated transient head rotation in normal and unilaterally vestibulopathic humans. Exp Brain Res 142(4):486, 2002.

65. Schubert, MC, Migliaccio, AA, and Della Santina, CC: Dynamic visual acuity during passive head thrusts in canal planes. J Assoc Res Otolaryngol 7(4):329, 2006.

66. Grossman, GE, et al: Frequency and velocity of rotational head perturbations during locomotion. Exp Brain Res 70:470, 1988.

67. Colebatch, JG, and Halmagyi, GM: Vestibular evoked potentials in human neck muscles before and after unilateral vestibular deafferentation. Neurology 42:1635, 1992.

68. Halmagyi, GM, et al: Tapping the head activates the vestibular system: A new use for the clinical reflex hammer. Neurology 45:1927, 1995.

69. Curthoys, IS, et al: Human ocular torsional position before and after unilateral vestibular neurectomy. Exp Brain Res 85:218, 1991.

70. Kushiro, K, et al: Saccular and utricular inputs to sternocleidomastoid motoneurons of decerebrate cats. Exp Brain Res 126:410, 1999.

71. Young, ED, et al: Responses of squirrel monkey vestibular neurons to audio-frequency sound and head vibration. Acta Otolaryngol 84:352, 1977.

72. Murofushi, T, et al: Responses of guinea pig primary vestibular neurons to clicks. Exp Brain Res 103:174, 1995.

73. Murofushi, T, et al: Response of guinea pig vestibular nucleus neurons to clicks. Exp Brain Res 111:149, 1996.

74. Iwasaki, S, et al: The role of the superior vestibular nerve in generating ocular vestibular-evoked myogenic potentials to bone conducted vibration at Fz. Clin Neurophysiol 120(3):588, 2009.

75. Tabak, S, et al: Deviation of the subjective vertical in long-standing unilateral vestibular loss. Acta Otolaryngol 117:1, 1997.

76. Schuknecht, HF: Cupulolithiasis. Arch Otolaryngol 90:765, 1969.

77. Furuya, M, et al: Experimental study of speed-dependent positional nystagmus in benign paroxysmal positional vertigo. Acta Otolaryngol 123(6):709, 2003.

78. Hall, SF, et al: The mechanics of benign paroxysmal vertigo. J Otolaryngol 8(2):151, 1979.

79. Cooper, CW: Vestibular neuronitis: A review of a common cause of vertigo in general practice. Br J Gen Pract 43:164, 1993.

80. Jayarajan, V, and Rajenderkumar, D: A survey of dizziness management in general practice. J Laryngol Otol 117(8):599, 2003.

81. Fetter, M, and Dichgans, J: Adaptive mechanisms of VOR compensation after unilateral peripheral vestibular lesions in humans. J Vestib Res 1:9, 1990.

82. Baloh, RW: Vertebrobasilar insufficiency and stroke. Otolaryngol Head Neck Surg 112:114, 1995.

83. Schuknecht, HF, and Witt, RL: Acute bilateral sequential vestibular neuritis. Am J Otolaryngol 6:255, 1985.

84. Barber, HO, and Dionne, J: Vestibular findings in vertebrobasilar ischemia. Ann Otol Rhinol Laryngol 80:805, 1971.

85. Halmagyi, GM, et al: Gentamicin vestibulotoxicity. Otolaryngol Head Neck Surg 111:571, 1994.

86. Brandt, T, and Dieterich, M: Vestibular syndromes in the roll plane: Topographic diagnosis from brainstem to cortex. Ann Neurol 36:337, 1994.

87. Delaney, KA: Bedside diagnosis of vertigo: Value of the history and neurological examination. Acad Emerg Med 10(12):1388, 2003.

88. Beaudry, M, and Spence, JD: Motor vehicle accidents: The most common cause of traumatic vertebrobasilar ischemia. Can J Neurol Sci 30(4):320, 2003.

89. Purvin, V, Kawasaki, A, and Zeldes, S: Dolichoectatic arterial compression of the anterior visual pathways: Neuro-ophthalmic features and clinical course. J Neurol Neurosurg Psychiatry 75(1):27, 2004.

90. Grad, A, and Baloh, RW: Vertigo of vascular origin. Clinical and electronystagmographic features in 84 cases. Arch Neurol 46(3):281, 1989.

91. Olszewski, J, et al: The association between positional vertebral and basilar artery flow lesion and prevalence of vertigo in patients with cervical spondylosis. J Otolaryngol Head Neck Surg 134:680, 2006.

92. Berman, J, and Frederickson, J: Vertigo after head injury: A five year follow-up. J Otolaryngol 7:237, 1978.

93. Tuohimma, P: Vestibular disturbances after acute mild head injury. Acta Otolaryngol Suppl (Stockh) 359:7, 1978.

94. Masson, F, et al: Prevalence of impairments 5 years after a head injury, and their relationship with disabilities and outcome. Brain Inj 10(7):487, 1996.

95. Leigh, RJ, and Zee, DS: Diagnosis of central disorders of ocular motility. In Leigh, RJ and Zee, DS (eds): The Neurology of Eye Movements, ed 4. Oxford University Press, New York, 2006, p 598.

96. Kluge, M, et al: Epileptic vertigo: Evidence for vestibular representation in human frontal cortex. Neurology 55(12):1906, 2000.

97. Brandt, T, et al: Vestibular cortex lesions affect the perception of verticality. Ann Neurol 35:403, 1994.

98. Brandt, T, et al: Plasticity of the vestibular system: Central compensation and sensory substitution for vestibular deficits. Brain Plast Adv Neurol 73:297, 1997.

99. Kattah, JC, et al: HINTS to diagnose stroke in the acute vestibular syndrome: Three-step bedside oculomotor examination more sensitive than early MRI diffusion-weighted imaging. Stroke 40(11):3504, 2009. [Epub September 17, 2009.]

100. Epley, JM: The canalith repositioning procedure: For treatment of benign paroxysmal positional vertigo. Otolaryngol Head Neck Surg 107:399, 1992.

101. Chung, KW, et al: Incidence of horizontal canal benign paroxysmal positional vertigo as a function of the duration of symptoms. Otol Neurotol 30(2):202, 2009.

102. Fyrmpas, G, et al: Are postural restrictions after an Epley maneuver unnecessary? First results of a controlled study and review of the literature. Auris Nasus Larynx 36(6):637, 2009.

103. Simhadri, S, Freyss, G, and Vitte, E: Efficacy of particle repositioning maneuver in BPPV: A prospective study. Am J Otolaryngol 24(6):355, 2003.

104. Sakaida, M, Freyss, G, and Vitte, E: Long-term outcome of benign paroxysmal positional vertigo. Neurology 60(9):1532, 2003.

105. Helminski, JO, Janssen, I, and Hain, TC: Daily exercise does not prevent recurrence of benign paroxysmal positional vertigo. Otol Neurotol 29(7):976, 2008.

106. Semont, A, Freyss, G, and Vitte, E: Curing the BPPV with a liberatory maneuver. Adv Otorhinolaryngol 42:290, 1988.

107. Campanini, A, and Vicini, C: Semont maneuver vs. particle repositioning maneuver: Comparative study. Acta Otorhinolaryngol Ital 21(6):331, 2001.

108. Campanini, A, et al: Efficacy of the Semont maneuver in benign paroxysmal positional vertigo. Arch Otolaryngol Head Neck Surg 129(6):629, 2003.

109. Brandt, T, and Daroff, RB: Physical therapy for benign paroxysmal positional vertigo. Arch Otolaryngol 106:484, 1980.

110. Herdman, SJ, et al: Vestibular adaptation exercises and recovery: Acute stage after acoustic neuroma resection. Otolaryngol Head Neck Surg 113:77, 1995.

111. Gottshall, K, et al: Objective vestibular tests as outcome measures in head injury patients. Laryngoscope 113(10):1746, 2003.

112. Shumway-Cook, A, and Horak, FB: Vestibular rehabilitation: An exercise approach to managing symptoms of vestibular dysfunction. Semin Hearing 10:196, 1989.

113. Norre, ME, and DeWeerdt, W: Treatment of vertigo based on habituation. J Laryngol Otol 94:971, 1980.

114. Dix, MR: The rationale and technique of head exercises in the treatment of vertigo. Acta Otorhinolaryngol Belg 33:370, 1979.

115. Dix, MR: The physiological basis and practical value of head exercises in the treatment of vertigo. Practitioner 217:919, 1976.

116. Herdman, SJ, et al: Falls in patients with vestibular deficits. Am J Otol 21:847, 2000.

117. Cohen, HS, et al: Driving disability and dizziness. J Safety Res 34(4):361, 2003.

118. Krebs, DE, et al: Double-blind, placebo-controlled trial of rehabilitation for bilateral vestibular hypofunction: Preliminary report. Otolaryngol Head Neck Surg 109(4):735, 1993.

119. Herdman, SJ, et al: Vestibular adaptation exercises and recovery: Acute stage after acoustic neuroma resection. Otolaryngol Head Neck Surg 113(1):77, 1995.

120. Strupp, M, et al: Vestibular exercises improve central vestibulospinal compensation after vestibular neuritis. Neurology 51(3):838, 1998.

121. Cohen, HS, and Kimball, KT: Increased independence and decreased vertigo after vestibular rehabilitation. Otolaryngol Head Neck Surg 128(1):60, 2003.

122. Krebs, DE, et al: Vestibular rehabilitation: Useful but not universally so. Otolaryngol Head Neck Surg 128(2):240, 2003.

123. Patten, C, et al: Head and body center of gravity control strategies: Adaptations following vestibular rehabilitation. Acta Otolaryngol 123(1):32, 2003.

124. Herdman, SJ, et al: Recovery of dynamic visual acuity in bilateral vestibular hypofunction. Arch Otolaryngol Head Neck Surg 133(4):383, 2007.

125. Hillier, SL, and Hollohan, V: Vestibular rehabilitation for unilateral peripheral vestibular dysfunction. Cochrane Database Syst Rev 17(4):CD005397, 2007.

126. Schubert, MC, et al: Mechanism of dynamic visual acuity recovery with vestibular rehabilitation. Arch Phys Med Rehabil 89(3):500, 2008.

127. Giray, M, et al: Short-term effects of vestibular rehabilitation in patients with chronic unilateral vestibular dysfunction: A randomized controlled study. Arch Phys Med Rehabil 90(8):1325, 2009.

128. Shepard, NT, et al: Vestibular and balance rehabilitation therapy. Ann Otol Rhinol Laryngol 102:198, 1993.

129. Gurr, B, and Moffat, N: Psychological consequences of vertigo and the effectiveness of vestibular rehabilitation for brain injury patients. Brain Inj 15(5):387, 2001.

130. Arenberg, IK: Ménières disease: Diagnosis and management of vertigo and endolymphatic hydrops. In Arenberg, IK (ed): Dizziness and Balance Disorders. Kugler Publications, New York, 1993, p 503.

131. Bruno, E, et al: Perilymphatic fistula following trans-tympanic trauma: A clinical case presentation and review of the literature. An Otorrinolaringol Ibero Am 29(4):359, 2002.

132. Minor, LB: Superior canal dehiscence syndrome. Am J Otol 21(1):9, 2000.

133. Dobie, TG, and May, JG: Cognitive-behavioral management of motion sickness. Aviat Space Environ Med 65(Suppl 10):C1, 1994.

134. Rine, RM, et al: Visual-vestibular habituation and balance training for motion sickness. Phys Ther 79:949, 1999.

135. Reason, JT: Motion sickness adaptation: A neural mismatch model. J R Soc Med 71:819, 1978.

136. Bagshaw, M, and Stott, JR: The desensitization of chronically motion sick aircrew in the Royal Air Force. Aviat Space Environ Med 56:1144, 1985.

137. Golding, JF, and Stott, JR: Objective and subjective time courses of recovery from motion sickness assessed by repeated motion challenges. J Vestib Res 7:421, 1997.

138. Banks, RD, et al: The Canadian Forces airsickness rehabilitation program, 1981–1991. Aviat Space Environ Med 63:1098, 1992.

139. Polensek, SH, and Tusa, RJ: Nystagmus during attacks of vestibular migraine: An aid in diagnosis. Audiol Neurootol 15(4):241, 2010.

140. MacGregor, EA, et al: Migraine prevalence and treatment patterns: The global Migraine and Zolmitriptan Evaluation survey. Headache 43(1):19, 2003.

141. Murdin, L, Davies, RA, and Bronstein, AM: Vertigo as a migraine trigger. Neurology 73(8):638, 2009.

142. Wrisley, DM, Whitney, SL, and Furman, JM: Vestibular rehabilitation outcomes in patients with a history of migraine. Otol Neurotol 23(4):483, 2002.

143. Strupp, M, Versino, M, and Brandt, T: Vestibular migraine. Hand Clin Neurol 97:755, 2010.
144. Wang, SR, and Young, YI: Multiple system atrophy manifested as dizziness and imbalance: A report of two cases. Eur Arch Otorhinolayrngol 260:404, 2003.
145. Wedge, F: The impact of resistance training on balance and functional ability of a patient with multiple system atrophy. J Geriatr Phys Ther 31(2):79–83, 2008.

146. Hikosaka, O, and Maeda, M: Cervical effects on abducens motor neurons and their interaction with vestibulo-ocular reflex. Exp Brain Res 18:512, 1973.
147. Wrisley, DM, et al: Cervicogenic dizziness: A review of diagnosis and treatment. J Orthop Sports Phys Ther 30(12): 755, 2000.

Supplemental Readings

Baloh, RW, and Honrubia, V: Clinical Neurophysiology of the Vestibular System. Oxford University Press, New York, 2001.
Epley, JM: The canalith repositioning procedure: For treatment of benign paroxysmal positional vertigo. Otolaryngol Head Neck Surg 107:399, 1992.
Hain, TC: Neurophysiology of vestibular rehabilitation. NeuroRehabilitation 29(2):127, 2011.
Hall, CD, et al: Efficacy of gaze stability exercises in older adults with dizziness. J Neurol Phys Ther 34(2):64, 2010.
Herdman, SJ: Vestibular Rehabilitation, ed 3. FA Davis, Philadelphia, 2007.
Herdman, SJ, et al: Recovery of dynamic visual acuity in unilateral vestibular hypofunction. Arch Otolaryngol Head Neck Surg 129:819, 2003.

Herdman, SJ, et al: Recovery of dynamic visual acuity in bilateral vestibular hypofunction. Arch Otolaryngol Head Neck Surg. 133(4):383, 2007.
Rine, RM, et al: New portable tool to screen vestibular and visual function—National Institutes of Health Toolbox initiative. J Rehabil Res Dev 49(2):209, 2012.
Schubert, MC, et al: Mechanism of dynamic visual acuity recovery with vestibular rehabilitation. Arch Phys Med Rehabil 89(3): 500, 2008.
Schubert, MC, et al: Oculomotor strategies and their effect on reducing gaze position error. Otol Neurotol 31(2):228, 2010.
Strupp, M, et al: Vestibular migraine. Hand Clin Neurol 97:755, 2010.

Organization	Website
Vestibular Disorders Association (VEDA)	www.vestibular.org
National Institute for Deafness and Other Communication Disorders (NIDCD)	www.nidcd.nih.gov
Johns Hopkins University School of Medicine	www.hopkinsmedicine.org/otolaryngology
Micromedical Technologies	www.micromedical.com
Neurokinetics	www.neuro-kinetics.com
EquiTest	http://resourcesonbalance.com/neurocom/products/EquiTest.aspx

LEARNING OBJECTIVES

1. Discuss the role of the physical therapist in the care of any individual following lower extremity amputation.
2. Describe the major etiological factors leading to lower extremity amputation.
3. Explain the major concepts involved in lower extremity amputation surgery.
4. Develop an evaluation plan for any individual following lower extremity amputation.
   a. Prioritize data gathering for the immediate postsurgical period and the preprosthetic phase.
5. Design an effective plan of care for the immediate postsurgical period.
   a. Explain the rationale for and teach patient and caregiver proper positioning.
   b. Teach sitting and standing balance to enhance transfers and mobility.
   c. Ensure continuity of care following discharge from acute care.
6. Design an effective plan of care for the preprosthetic period.
   a. Teach proper residual limb care including bandaging as indicated.
   b. Teach standing balance to help the patient attain the highest functional level of mobility with appropriate ancillary support.
   c. Teach residual limb strengthening exercises to facilitate eventual prosthetic fitting.
   d. Teach ROM exercises to prevent/alleviate secondary contractures.
7. Respond appropriately to patient/family from an awareness of the psychological impact of lower extremity amputation.
8. Analyze and interpret patient data, formulate realistic anticipated goals and expected outcomes, and develop a plan of care when presented with a clinical case study.

The major cause of lower extremity (LE) amputation today continues to be peripheral vascular disease (PVD), particularly with associated diabetes. Two-thirds of all LE amputations in the United States today are due to complications of diabetes.[1] Approximately 16 per 1,000 individuals with diabetes over age 75 will undergo an LE amputation as compared with 1.78 of similar individuals who do not have diabetes. Major improvements in noninvasive diagnosis, revascularization, and wound healing techniques have increased the age at which individuals with diabetes may come to amputation. Perioperative mortality has been variously reported between 7% and 13% and is usually associated with other medical problems such as cardiac disease and strokes.[2-4] There are approximately 20.8 million children and adults with diabetes and about 5% of the population is affected with some form of vascular disease.[5] Many of the patients we treat in all types of settings have diabetes although we are usually treating them for some other problem. Physical therapists can help by learning more about diabetes and diabetic foot care and by making patient education an integral part of the plan of care (POC). Several studies have indicated a positive relationship between early patient education and proper foot care and a reduction in amputations.[6,7]

The second leading cause of amputation is trauma, usually from motor vehicle accidents, war, or gunshots. Individuals with traumatic amputations are often young adults, more frequently men, and have often been involved in an active lifestyle before amputation. The incidence of amputation from osteogenic sarcoma has been reduced owing to improved imaging techniques, more effective chemotherapy, and better limb salvage procedures. Amputation may be necessary if the tumor is large and cannot be resected without substantial removal of bone and tissue. However, the surgeon may choose to remove the tumor and incorporate one of several limb salvage procedures. Many factors go into this decision, including the age of the patient, the size of the tumor, and, if the patient is young, the potential for future growth.[8] Tumor excision does not affect 5-year survival rates, which have increased from about 20% in the 1970s to 60% to 70% in more recent years.[9-13] Regardless of the cause of amputation, physical therapists have a major role in rehabilitation. Early onset of appropriate treatment influences the eventual outcome of the episode of care. It is critically important, especially for the older individual, for the therapist in the acute care center to ensure continuity of care once the patient is discharged from the hospital. Too often, the patient is sent home and is not seen again for several weeks or months. By that time the patient has become debilitated and has developed contractures that interfere with prosthetic use and function.

■ LEVELS OF AMPUTATION

Traditionally, levels of amputation have been identified by anatomical considerations such as below knee and above knee. In 1974, the Task Force on Standardization of Prosthetic-Orthotic Terminology developed an international classification system to define amputation levels. Table 22.1 describes the major terms in common use today.

Table 22.1 Levels of Amputation	
Partial toe	Excision of any part of one or more toes
Toe disarticulation	Disarticulation at the metatarsal phalangeal joint
Partial foot/ray resection	Resection of the 3rd, 4th, 5th metatarsals and digits
Transmetatarsal	Amputation through the midsection of all metatarsals
Ankle disarticulation (Syme's)	Ankle disarticulation with attachment of heel pad to distal end of tibia; may include removal of malleoli and distal tibial/fibular flares
Long transtibial (below knee)	More than 50% of tibial length
Transtibial (below knee)	Between 20% and 50% of tibial length
Short transtibial (below knee)	Less than 20% of tibial length
Knee disarticulation	Amputation through the knee joint; femur intact
Long transfemoral (above knee)	More than 60% of femoral length
Transfemoral (above knee)	Between 35% and 60% of femoral length
Short transfemoral (above knee)	Less than 35% of femoral length
Hip disarticulation	Amputation through hip joint; pelvis intact
Hemipelvectomy	Resection of lower half of the pelvis
Hemicorporectomy	Amputation both lower limbs and pelvis below L4–L5 level

Traumatic amputations may be performed at any level; the surgeon tries to maintain the greatest bone length and save all possible joints. A variety of surgical techniques may be necessary to create a functional **residual limb**. Guillotine amputations (skin, muscle, and bone all transected at approximately the same level) may precede secondary closure with skin flaps; occasionally, free tissue flaps, taken from some other area of the body, may be used to cover the wound. Amputations for vascular diseases are generally performed at partial foot, transtibial, or transfemoral levels. The limited vascular supply militates against effective residual limb healing at the ankle disarticulation level in most instances.

Patients with unilateral transtibial amputations regardless of age are quite likely to become functional prosthetic users; many individuals with bilateral transtibial amputations can be successfully rehabilitated. Older adults with unilateral transfemoral amputations with good balance and coordination are also potential prosthetic users, although those who were not independently ambulatory before amputation are likely not to become independent with a prosthesis. Patients with bilateral transfemoral amputations may become prosthetic users given today's computer-driven components. Once again, good balance and coordination are a prerequisite. Hip disarticulations, hemipelvectomies, and hemicorporectomies are generally performed either for tumors or for severe trauma and represent a small percentage of the population of individuals with amputations. The most important factor in determining the prosthetic potential of an individual is her or his prior level of activity. Co-morbidities and the extent of injuries from war and trauma must be considered, but the individual who led an active life before amputation—even an individual with diabetes and related co-morbidities—is likely to become a functional prosthetic user if he or she can demonstrate good balance and coordination.[14]

■ SURGICAL PROCESS

The specific type of surgery is determined by the surgeon, whose decision depends on the status of the extremity at the time of amputation. The surgeon must allow for primary or secondary wound healing, and construct a residual limb for optimal prosthetic fitting and function. Numerous factors affect the selection of level of amputation. Conservation of residual limb length and uncomplicated wound healing, for example, are both important. Although a description of each type of surgical procedure is beyond the scope of this chapter, an understanding of the basic principles of amputation surgery is important.

Skin flaps are as broad as possible and the scar should be pliable, painless, and nonadherent. For most transfemoral and transtibial amputations without vascular impairment, equal length anterior and posterior flaps are used, placing the scar at the distal end of the bone (Figs. 22.1 and 22.2). Long posterior flaps are often used in transtibial amputations with compromised circulation

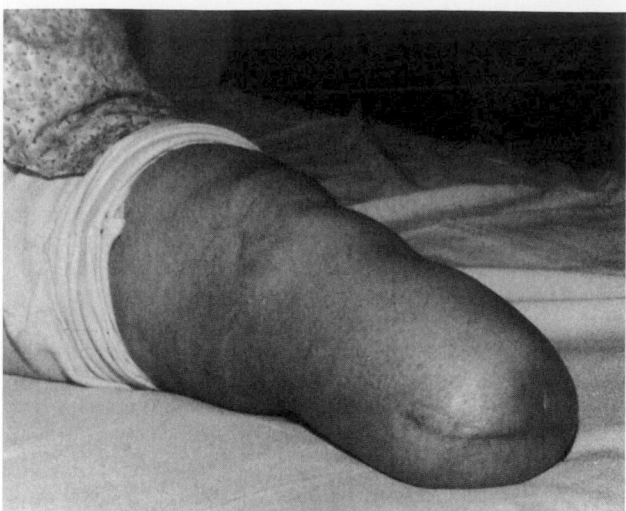

Figure 22.1 Transtibial residual limb with incision from equal-length flaps.

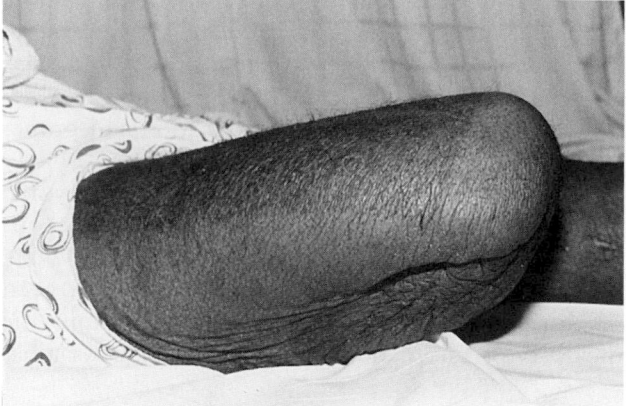

Figure 22.2 Transfemoral residual limb with incision from equal-length flaps.

because the posterior tissues have a better blood supply than anterior skin. This places the scar anteriorly over the distal end of the tibia; care must be taken to ensure that the scar does not become adherent to the bone (Fig. 22.3). In recent years, the routine use of the long posterior flap has come into question.[15] The skew flap, developed in England, is believed by some surgeons to be a better approach for individuals with severely compromised distal circulation. The skew flap is an angular medial–lateral incision that places the scar away from bony prominences, a problem with the long posterior flap. Research on the use of different skin flaps does not clearly delineate the most advantageous approach, and all indicate similar results in terms of rehabilitation.[16]

Stabilization of major muscles allows for maximum retention of function. Muscle stabilization may be achieved by myofascial closure, myoplasty, myodesis, or tenodesis. In most transtibial and transfemoral amputations, a combination of **myoplasty** (muscle to muscle

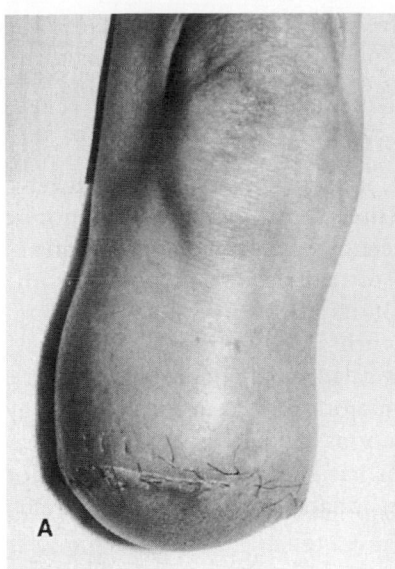
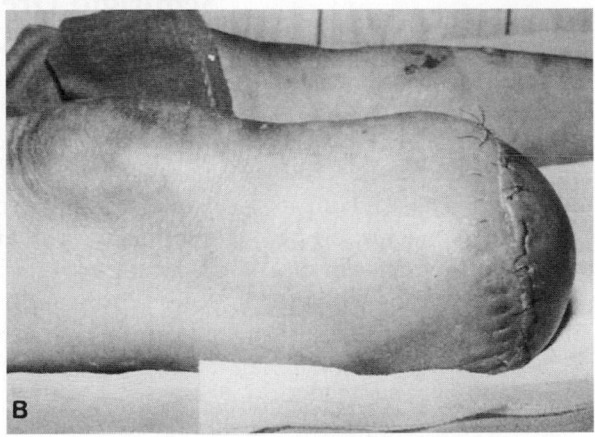

Figure 22.3 **(A)** Anterior view and **(B)** lateral view of a transtibial residual limb with anterior incision from a long posterior flap.

closure) and **myofascial** (muscle to fascial) closure is used to ensure that the muscles are properly stabilized and do not slide over the end of the bone.

In some centers, **myodesis** (muscle attached to periosteum or bone) is employed, particularly in transtibial amputations. More rarely, a **tenodesis** (tendon attached to bone) may be used for muscle stabilization. Whatever the technique, muscle stabilization under some tension is desirable at all levels where muscles must be transected.

Severed peripheral nerves form **neuromas** (a collection of nerve cell ends) in the residual limb. The neuroma must be well surrounded by soft tissue so as not to cause pain and interfere with prosthetic wear. Surgeons identify the major nerves, pull them down under some tension, and then cut them cleanly and sharply and allow them to retract into the soft tissue of the residual limb. Neuromas that form close to scar tissue or bone generally cause pain and may require later resection or revision. **Hemostasis** is achieved by ligating major veins and arteries; **cauterization** is used only for small bleeders. Care is taken not to compromise circulation to distal tissues, particularly the skin flaps, which are important to uncomplicated wound healing.

Bones are sectioned at a length to allow wound closure without excessive redundant tissue at the end of the residual limb and without placing the incision under great tension. Sharp bone ends are smoothed and rounded; in transtibial amputations, the anterior portion of the distal tibia is **beveled** to reduce the pressure between the end of the bone and the prosthetic socket. Care is taken to ensure that the bone is physiologically prepared for the pressures of prosthetic wear. Tissue layers are approximated under normal physiological tension and the incision is closed, usually with regular sutures. A drainage tube may be inserted as necessary.

In a traumatic amputation, the surgeon attempts to save as much bone length and viable skin as possible and preserve proximal joints while providing for appropriate healing of tissues without secondary complications such as infection. In potentially "dirty" (involving foreign substances) amputations, the incision may be left open with the proximal joint immobilized in a functional position for 5 to 9 days to prevent invasive infection. Secondary closure also allows the surgeon to shape the residual limb appropriately for prosthetic wear and function.

Amputation for vascular disease is generally considered an elective procedure; the surgeon determines the level of amputation by examining tissue viability through a variety of measures. Segmental limb blood pressures can be determined by Doppler systolic blood pressure measurement. Transcutaneous oxygen measurement and skin blood flow by radioisotope or plethysmography are also determined. Doppler systolic blood pressure measures have been reported to be quite accurate in predicting viable level of amputation. Improvements in noninvasive examination techniques have greatly reduced the use of arteriography to determine amputation level. Videos of actual amputation surgery at transtibial and transfemoral levels may be seen at the Amputation Surgery Education Center website (www.ampsurg.org).

■ HEALING PROCESS

Numerous factors influence the course of the healing process in each patient. One of the greatest postoperative concerns is infection, whether from external or internal sources. Individuals with contaminated wounds from injury, infected foot ulcers, or other causes are at greater risk of infection. Research indicates that smoking is a major deterrent to wound healing; one study reported that cigarette smokers had a 2.5% higher rate of infection and reamputation than nonsmokers.[17] Other factors affecting wound healing are the severity of the vascular problems, diabetes, renal disease, and other physiological problems such as cardiac disease.[15] The physical therapist can influence positive wound healing by teaching proper bed mobility and avoiding pressure on the newly amputated limb.

■ POSTSURGICAL DRESSINGS

Surgeons have several options regarding the postoperative dressing, including (1) rigid dressing, (2) semirigid dressing, or (3) soft dressing. It is important for some sort of edema control to be used because excessive edema in the residual limb can compromise healing and cause pain. Table 22.2 outlines the major postsurgical dressings in use today with their advantages and disadvantages.

Rigid Dressings

The rigid dressing, developed in the early 1960s, is generally known as an **immediate postoperative prosthesis** (IPOP).[18-20] The IPOP may be handmade from plaster of Paris by the surgeon or a prosthetist and follows the general configuration of the prosthetic socket. These are not adjustable or removable. The socket must be cut like a cast for removal and a new one applied as the residual limb heals, sutures are removed, and the limb changes shape. There are also **removable rigid dressings** (RRDs) that may be handmade from plaster or prefabricated from plastic materials and come in different sizes. Prefabricated RRDs are adjustable as the limb changes and may be removed as needed for wound inspection.[21] The addition of a pylon and foot allows for early, limited, weight-bearing ambulation.

Use of immediate postoperative rigid dressings varies greatly and is more prevalent in some areas of the country than others. Generally, orthopedic surgeons use the technique more than vascular surgeons. Rigid postsurgical dressings, whether used immediately after surgery or in the early postoperative period, have been found to be successful in reducing postoperative edema and pain and enhancing healing, even in cases of delayed healing.[15]

Semirigid Dressings

There are a number of semirigid dressings that have been reported in the literature and may or may not be used in a particular center. All provide better control of edema than the soft dressing but each has some disadvantage that limits its use. **Unna's dressing**, gauze impregnated with a compound of zinc oxide, gelatin, glycerin, and calamine, may be applied in the operating room. Its major disadvantage is that it may loosen easily and is not as rigid as the plaster of Paris dressing. However, it has been shown to be superior to the soft dressing in enhancing healing and reducing edema.[22]

Soft Dressings

The soft dressing is the oldest method of postsurgical management of the residual limb and probably the one that most physical therapists in acute care hospitals will encounter. Currently there are two forms of soft dressings: the elastic wrap and the elastic shrinker.

Elastic Wraps

The elastic wrap or elastic bandage, 4 inches wide or more, may be applied over the postsurgical dressing if care is taken to ensure proper compression. A dressing is applied to the incision followed by some form of gauze pad, then the compression wrap. The soft dressing is indicated in cases of local infection, but is not the treatment of choice for the majority of individuals. The patient or a family member should learn to apply the wrap as soon as possible after wound care is no longer necessary. Many older individuals with transfemoral amputations do not have the necessary balance and coordination to wrap effectively.

Table 22.2	Postsurgical Dressings	
Type of Dressing	**Advantages**	**Disadvantages**
Compressible soft dressing	Easy to apply Inexpensive Easy access to incision	Little edema control Minimal residual limb (RL) protection Requires frequent rewrapping
Shrinker	Easy to apply Inexpensive	Not used until sutures are removed Requires changing as RL shrinks
Semirigid dressing	Better edema control than soft dressing RL protection	Needs frequent changing Cannot be applied by patient No access to incision
IPOP	Excellent edema control Excellent RL protection Control of RL pain	No access to incision More expensive than other dressings Requires proper training for use

From May and Lockard,[26, p. 62] with permission.
IPOP = immediate postoperative prosthesis.

Some surgeons prefer delaying elastic wrap until the incision has healed and the sutures have been removed. Leaving the residual limb without any pressure wrap allows for full development of postoperative edema, which may be quite uncomfortable and interfere with circulation in the many small vessels in the skin and soft tissue, thereby potentially compromising healing. The therapist can discuss the benefits of early wrapping with the surgeon if no other form of rigid dressing is used. There is strong evidence in the literature of the benefits of either the IPOP or the RRD.[15,23-25]

One of the major drawbacks of the elastic wrap is that it needs frequent rewrapping. Movement of the residual limb against the bedclothes, bending and extending the proximal joints, and general body movements will cause slippage and changes in pressure. Covering the finished wrap with stockinet helps to reduce some of the wrinkling. However, careful and frequent rewrapping is the only effective way to prevent complications. Nursing staff, family members, and the patient, as well as the physical therapist or physical therapist assistant, need to assume responsibility for frequent inspection and rewrapping of the residual limb. Residual limb wrapping is described in detail later in this chapter.

Elastic Shrinkers

Shrinkers are sock-like garments knitted of heavy, rubber-reinforced cotton; they are conical in shape and come in a variety of sizes (Fig. 22.4). It is difficult to use a shrinker in the postoperative period because the process of donning may put unnecessary stress on the

unhealed incision. Shrinkers are best used after healing has taken place and the sutures have been removed.

■ PHASES OF CARE: POSTSURGICAL[26] AND PREPROSTHETIC

Early onset of rehabilitation produces greater potential for success. A long delay is likely to result in the development of complications such as joint contractures, general debilitation, and depressed psychological state. The rehabilitation program can be arbitrarily divided into two phases: (1) the postsurgical phase is the time between surgery and discharge from the hospital; (2) the preprosthetic phase runs from hospital discharge to prosthetic fitting or a decision that the patient is not a candidate for prosthetic fitting. These, of course, are arbitrary periods but each has different goals and emphases within the POC. The desired expected outcome of the episode of care is to help the patient regain the presurgical level of function. For some, it will mean return to gainful employment with an active recreational life. For others, it will mean independence in the home and community. For still others, it may mean living in the sheltered environment of a retirement center or nursing home. If the amputation resulted from long-standing chronic disease, the rehabilitation approach may be to help the person function at a higher level than immediately before surgery.

Postsurgical Phase

The postsurgical phase is the time between surgery and discharge from the hospital. While the primary goal of this phase of care is to get the patient discharged, it is not adequate to give the patient a walker, teach the patient to transfer, and send him or her home. Box 22.1 outlines the general goals of the postsurgical phase of care.

Box 22.2 outlines the critical data necessary to develop a POC for the hospitalized patient following amputation. Naturally, the data gathering must be prioritized according to the person's physiological status and cause of amputation; however, the information obtained on initial examination and subsequent evaluation will influence discharge planning and future care. As indicated previously, it is of critical importance for the physical therapist to act as an ombudsman for the patient and ensure continuity of care following hospital discharge. For all

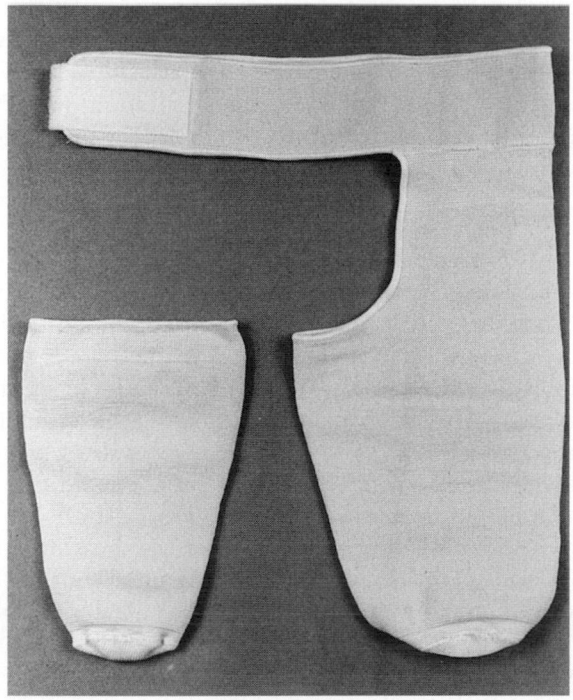

Figure 22.4 (*Left*) Transtibial shrinker. (*Right*) Transfemoral shrinker.

Box 22.1 Postsurgical General Goals
• Healing residual limb
• Protect remaining limb (if dysvascular)
• Independent in transfers and mobility
• Demonstrate proper positioning
• Begin psychological adjustment
• Understand the process of prosthetic rehabilitation

Box 22.2   Early Postsurgical Evaluation

• General systems review
• Postsurgical status
  • Cardiovascular
  • Respiratory
  • Diabetes control (if appropriate)
  • Whether out of bed
  • Infection?
• Pain
  • Incisional
  • Phantom
  • Other
• Vascularity (if appropriate)
• Functional status
  • Bed mobility, transfers, sitting, standing, balance
• Gross range of motion
  • Unamputated extremity
    • Hip, knee flexion and extension
    • Ankle dorsiflexion/plantarflexion
  • Upper extremity to note any limitations that would interfere with functional activities
  • Amputated extremity

Box 22.3   General Plan of Interventions

• Positioning to avoid contractures
• Standing balance and transfer activities
• Mobility training with crutches or a walker
• Residual limb care and protection; bandaging if appropriate
• Care of the remaining lower extremity (if circulation compromised)
• Education on amputation and prosthetics

---

patients, information on the current cardiovascular status, physiological response to surgery, presence of infection, pain level, and medication indicates to what extent the patient will be able to participate in the therapy program. Individuals amputated secondary to severe trauma, blast injuries in war, and similar problems will require a somewhat different approach from individuals with vascular disease. The type of postsurgical dressing will also influence both data gathering and interventions. The person with a rigid dressing will be able to move more easily in bed than someone with a soft dressing. At this point the physical therapy diagnosis will probably reflect an individual with limited mobility and functional capabilities. Depending on the specific findings the individual may also have compromised endurance and pain that interferes with participation in the program. The specific POC is, of course, aimed at the goals and the critical findings.

Intervention

The therapist treating a patient in the hospital has only limited time in which to achieve the goals. The intervention must be aimed at preparing for discharge from acute care and to some form of follow-up care, be it in an acute rehabilitation facility, through a home health service or agency, or an outpatient facility. Box 22.3 outlines the major components of interventions.

Positioning

Figure 22.5 illustrates the major positions for either a patient with a transtibial or transfemoral amputation. Although the figure represents someone with a transtibial

amputation, the general principles are the same. It is critical in both instances to prevent hip flexion contractures and the patient should be encouraged to spend some time in the prone position if at all possible. A pillow under the residual limb while the patient is supine is never recommended, nor is prolonged sitting. In the early days, the patient will want to avoid side-lying on the amputated side and the residual limb should be kept in extension at both hip and knee.

Balance and Transfers

Sitting balance is usually not a problem with a unilateral amputation but must be a part of the intervention program for individuals with bilateral amputations. Standing balance exercises on the remaining extremity can be quite beneficial in helping the individual regain a sense of his or her body in space. The better the person can balance on the remaining extremity the more likely he or she will be to use crutches and lead a more active life during the period before prosthetic fitting. A variety of balance exercises may be used, including balancing on a compliant surface. In the early postsurgical period the person should stand and transfer leading with the unamputated limb to protect the residual limb from possible injury against the chair or bed.

Mobility

Many physical therapists fit patients with a walker. Although this is appropriate for some individuals, trying to teach the patient safe and independent mobility with crutches is much more beneficial. While there is more stability in a walker, there is greater flexibility in accomplishing activities of daily living (ADL) on crutches. The added balance needed for crutches will also serve the individual well when it is time for prosthetic fitting.

If the patient has been fitted with an IPOP or an RRD and has good control of weight-bearing, the physician might decide to add a pylon and foot to the assembly making partial weight-bearing gait possible. In this instance, the patient must be fitted with crutches because the walker will inhibit the natural function of the prosthetic components.

When teaching mobility to someone with diabetes or any vascular compromise, it is critical that the patient

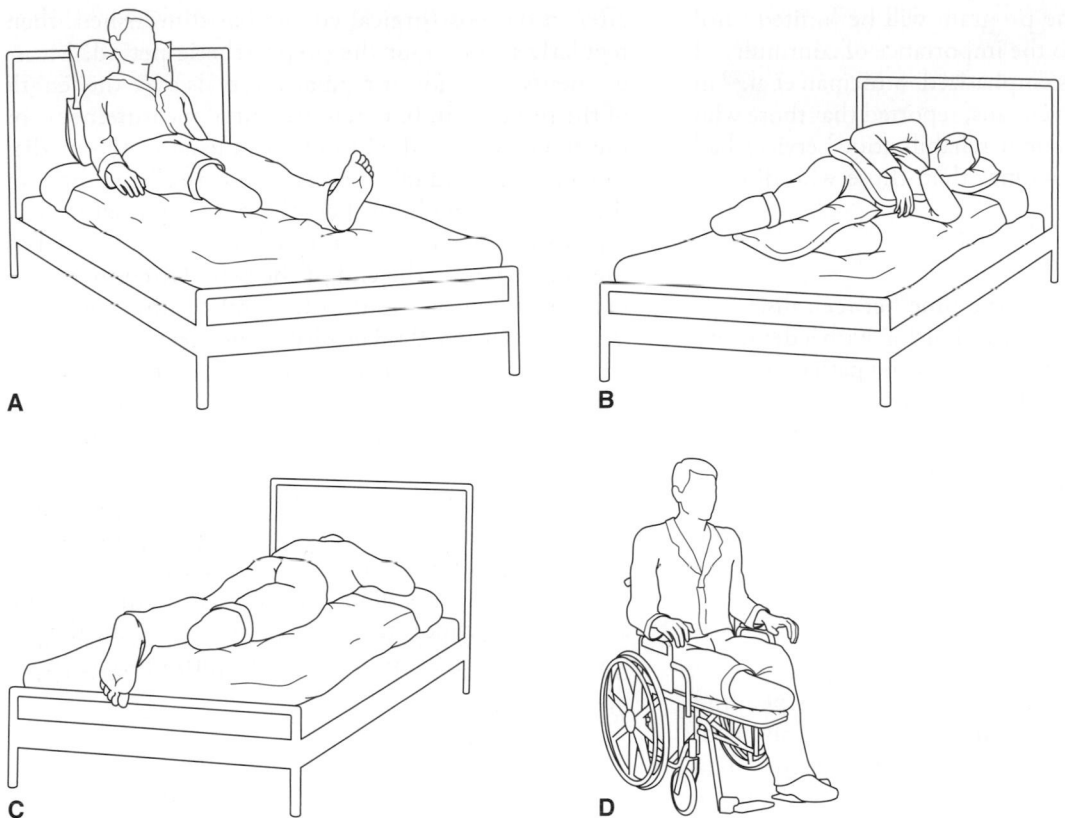

Figure 22.5 Proper transtibial position: **(A)** supine; **(B)** side-lying; **(C)** prone; **(D)** sitting. *From May and Lockard,[26, p. 67] with permission.*

wear a shoe on the remaining foot. Obviously, the remaining foot must be protected from any injury or assault, and hospital-provided slippers, or any slippers, do not provide the necessary protection. The family can bring in a regular shoe and this may be time to consider fitting the patient with an adapted shoe to prevent trauma to this foot.

Residual Limb Care

The physical therapist will need to teach the patient and family how to properly wrap the limb, and, if the patient has been fitted with an IPOP or RRD, the physical therapist needs to be alert to excessive bleeding or draining through the cast. A primary focus at this point is to teach the patient how to protect the residual limb while moving in bed, coming to sitting, and transferring. Obviously the patient should not put pressure on the limb or drag it on the bed. Slightly raising the residual limb and moving it to the side while rolling to the unamputated side is the best way to come to sitting. Careful monitoring of healing status of the residual limb is important at this point. The patient can be encouraged to move the limb gently within a pain-free range both at the knee (transtibial) and at the hip (both levels). Gentle hip extension (for transtibial amputations, with the knee straight) is an excellent exercise to teach the patient while lying on the unamputated side.

It can and should be done several times a day. Any resistive exercises for the residual limb are contraindicated at this time.

Care of the Remaining Lower Extremity

Since the majority of individuals undergoing amputation do so as a result of poor circulation, it is important to evaluate the status of the remaining extremity and teach the patient and family proper care as presented in Chapter 14, Vascular, Lymphatic, and Integumentary Disorders. As previously stated, a proper shoe must be obtained before standing and mobility activities.[27]

Patient Education

The more the patient and family understand about the amputation and rehabilitation process the better the outcome. Throughout the examination and implementation of the POC, the physical therapist continuously involves the patient and caregivers, answering questions and providing information at a level and rate commensurate with the capabilities of the individuals. The goals are to have the patient and caregivers assume responsibility for care, understand the need for continued care, and become active participants in the rehabilitation program.[28] A home program needs to be developed and the patient should be encouraged to be as mobile as possible.

By necessity, the home program will be limited until healing has occurred so the importance of continuity of physical therapy care is emphasized. Stineman et al,[29] in a study of 2,673 older veterans, reported that those who received intensive inpatient rehabilitation services had significantly better outcomes than those who did not receive such services.

Preprosthetic Phase

The preprosthetic phase is the time between discharge from the acute care hospital and fitting with a definitive prosthesis, or the decision not to fit the patient with an artificial limb. Regrettably, for many individuals this period lasts too long, does not include a regular program of physical therapy, and often results in poor outcomes. The general goals for the preprosthetic phase of care are presented in Box 22.4, and Box 22.5 provides a general preprosthetic examination guide.

Examination
Residual Limb

Approximately 7 to 12 days after surgery, depending on the condition of the residual limb, the amount of healing, and the postsurgical dressing, specific data about the residual limb and adjacent joint(s) can be gathered. Healing is, of course, of primary importance and residual limb data gathering must be deferred until the residual limb has healed enough to tolerate the stress of handling and resistance. Residual limb measurements are generally taken and reported in centimeters for uniformity with others involved in the care of individuals who have had an amputation. Circumferential measurements of the residual limb are taken after initial postsurgical edema has diminished, then regularly throughout the preprosthetic period. Measurements are made at regular intervals over the length of the residual limb. Circumferential measurements of the transtibial residual limb are started at the medial tibial plateau and taken every 5 to 8 cm depending on the length of the limb. Length of the residual limb is measured from the medial tibial plateau to the end of the bone, then to the end of the skin. Circumferential measurements of the transfemoral residual limb are started at the ischial tuberosity or the greater trochanter, whichever is most palpable, and taken every 8 to 10 cm. Length is measured from the ischial tuberosity or the greater trochanter to the end of the bone, then to the end of the skin. For accuracy of repeat measurements, exact landmarks are carefully noted. If the ischial tuberosity is used in transfemoral measurements, hip joint position is noted as well. Other information gathered about the residual limb includes its shape (conical, bulbous, or cylindrical; presence of redundant tissue), skin condition, sensation, and joint proprioception.

Range of Motion

Gross range of motion (ROM) estimations are generally adequate for examination of the uninvolved extremity but specific goniometric measurements are necessary for the amputated side, bilateral hip extension, and ankle dorsiflexion of the unamputated side. Good balance requires good ankle motion, and many older individuals have developed limited range in ankle dorsiflexion leading to stumbling and catching of toes. Hip and knee measurements are taken following transtibial amputation. Hip flexion, extension, abduction, and adduction measurements are taken following transfemoral amputation. Measurement of internal and external hip rotation is difficult to obtain and unnecessary if no gross abnormality or pathology is evident. Hip flexion contractures are particularly important to note because the patient cannot stand and bear weight properly without adequate hip extension (Fig. 22.6). Additionally, hip extension participates in prosthetic knee control for some transfemoral prostheses.

Muscle Strength

Gross manual muscle testing (MMT) of the upper extremities (UEs) and uninvolved LE is performed as part of the initial examination. MMT of the involved LE must usually wait until most healing has occurred. With a transtibial amputation, good strength in the hip extensors and abductors, as well as the knee extensors and flexors, is needed for satisfactory prosthetic ambulation. For the patient with a transfemoral amputation, good strength of the hip extensors and abductors is a requirement. The strength of these muscles should be monitored throughout the preprosthetic phase. The intervention program addresses these areas.

Box 22.4 Preprosthetic General Goals

- Independent in residual limb care
  - Bandaging or shrinker application
  - Skin care
  - Positioning
- Independent in mobility, transfers, and functional activities
  - Partial weight-bearing crutch walking if fitted with IPOP or EPOP
  - Full weight-bearing when tolerated
  - Single-leg ambulation with crutches/walker if fitted with soft dressing
- Demonstrate home exercise program accurately
  - ROM graduating to resistive exercises for all parts of residual lower extremity
  - ROM and strengthening exercises for unamputated lower extremity as needed
- Care of the remaining lower extremity if amputated for vascular reasons

Box 22.5   Preprosthetic Examination Guide

History

- Patient demographics
- Family and social data
- Preamputation status (work, activity level, independence)
- Financial status
- Other as appropriate

Systems Review

- Cause of amputation (disease, tumor, trauma, congenital)
- Associated diseases/symptoms (neuropathy, visual disturbances, cardiopulmonary disease, renal failure, congenital anomalies)
- Current physiological state (postsurgical cardiopulmonary status, vital signs, shortness of breath, pain)
- Medications

Skin

- Scar (healed, adherent, invaginated, flat)
- Other lesions (size, shape, open, scar tissue)
- Moisture (moist, dry, scaly)
- Sensation (absent, diminished, hyperesthesia)
- Grafts (location, type, healing)
- Dermatological lesions (psoriasis, eczema, cysts)

Residual Limb Length

- Bone length (transtibial limbs measured from medial tibial plateau; transfemoral limbs measured from ischial tuberosity or greater trochanter)
- Soft tissue length (note redundant tissue)

Residual Limb Shape

- Cylindrical, conical, bulbous end, and so forth
- Abnormalities ("dog ears," adductor roll)

Emotional Status

- Acceptance
- Body image

Vascularity (both limbs if amputation cause is vascular)

- Pulses (femoral, popliteal, dorsalis pedis, posterior tibial)
- Color (red, cyanotic)
- Temperature
- Edema (circumference measurement, water displacement measurement, caliper measures)
- Pain (type, location, duration, intensity)
- Trophic changes

Range of Motion

- Residual limb (specific for remaining joints)
- Other lower extremity (gross for major joints)

Muscle Strength

- Residual limb (specific for major muscle groups)
- Other extremities (gross for necessary function)

Neurological

- Pain (phantom [differentiate sensation or pain], neuroma, incisional, from other causes)
- Neuropathy
- Cognitive status (alert, oriented, confused)

Functional Status

- Transfers (bed-to-chair, to toilet, to car)
- Mobility (ancillary support, supervision)
- Home/family situation (caregiver, architectural barriers, hazards)
- Activities of daily living (bathing, dressing)
- Instrumental activities of daily living (cooking, cleaning)

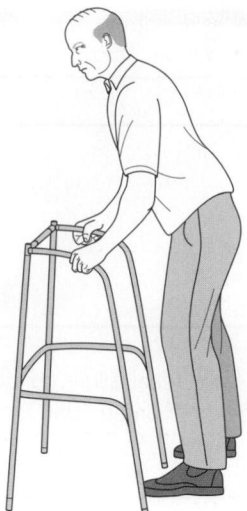

Figure 22.6 Hip flexion contractures prevent balanced standing. *From May and Lockard,[26, p. 111] with permission.*

Status of the Uninvolved Limb

The vascular status of the uninvolved LE is determined and documented. Data gathered include condition of the skin, presence of pulses, sensation, temperature, edema, pain on exercise or at rest, presence of wounds, ulceration, or other abnormalities. Chapter 14, Vascular, Lymphatic, and Integumentary Disorders, presents further information on examination and evaluation of peripheral vascular status.

Functional Status

Activities of daily living and functional mobility skills including transfer and ambulatory status are examined and documented. Balance both sitting and standing on the remaining extremity is very important and should be examined as long as the person's condition permits. Data regarding presurgical activity level and the person's own expected outcomes are obtained through interview and are often indicative of potential functional prosthetic use. An individual who had an active lifestyle before the amputation, regardless of age, is more likely to be able to learn to use a prosthesis well. Individuals with a long history of a sedentary lifestyle may encounter more difficulty, particularly if the amputation is at the transfemoral level.

Phantom Limb

The majority of individuals will encounter **phantom limb sensations** following amputation. In its simplest form, the phantom is the sensation of the limb that is no longer there. The phantom, which may occur initially immediately after surgery or as long as a year after amputation, is often described as a tingling, burning, itching, or pressure sensation, or sometimes a numbness. The distal part of the extremity is most frequently felt although, on occasion, the person will feel the whole

extremity. Phantom sensation has been around as long as individuals survived the loss of a limb; however, there has been little agreement over the centuries regarding its cause or treatment. Current researchers are investigating areas of sensory reintegration and reorganization in the somatosensory cortex.[30] A majority of individuals report phantom limb sensation and some report the feeling as noxious, yet it usually does not interfere with prosthetic rehabilitation. It is important for the patient to understand that the sensations are quite normal.[31]

Phantom limb pain is a generalized noxious sensation in the absent limb that is so strong as to interfere with prosthetic fitting. It may be localized or diffuse, continuous or intermittent, and may be triggered by some external stimuli. It may diminish over time or become a permanent and disabling condition. It occurs in only a small number of patients. It is important to differentiate phantom pain from the more common phantom sensations, residual limb pain, or neuroma pain. Sometimes, wearing a prosthesis will ease the phantom pain. On occasion, in the presence of trigger points, injection with steroids or local anesthetic has reduced the pain temporarily. Although the literature is replete with information and studies on phantom sensation, phantom pain, and residual limb pain, there is little agreement about the best approach to treatment of these phenomena.[31] In some studies, particularly of individuals who experienced considerable preoperative pain, intrathecal or epidural anesthetic drips with opioids were used both preoperatively and postoperatively with success.[32] However, others have reported no success with such treatments.[31] Noninvasive treatments such as ultrasound, icing, transcutaneous electrical nerve stimulation (TENS), and massage have been used with varying success. Mild nonnarcotic analgesics have been of limited value; biofeedback, guided imagery, psychotherapy, nerve blocks, and dorsal rhizotomies have all been used with inconsistent results. The treatment of phantom pain can be very frustrating for the clinic team as well as the patient.[31-35]

Emotional Status

Initial reaction to the traumatic loss of a limb is usually grief and depression. The person may experience insomnia and restlessness, and have difficulty concentrating. Some individuals may actually mourn the possible loss of a job or the ability to participate in a favorite sport or other activities rather than the lost limb per se. In the early stages, the person's grief may alternate with feelings of hopelessness, despondency, bitterness, and anger. Socially the patient may feel lonely, isolated, and the object of pity. Concerns about the future, about body image and sexual function, about the responses of family and friends, and about employment all affect the individual's reactions.

If the amputation was the result of vascular disease or other long-term problem, the amputation may actually come as a relief. The fight to save the limb, sometimes long and painful, is finally over. Responses vary by individuals. Some older individuals may relate the loss of the limb to the loss of independence and may become quite depressed. While not giving the individual false hope, it behooves the physical therapist to educate the patient on the rehabilitation process and the steps toward independence. Often seeing others in the treatment area with similar problems, particularly if involved in prosthetic training, may help the patient with a new amputation realize what can be achieved.

Long-term adjustment depends to a great extent on the individual's basic personality structure, sense of accomplishment, and place in the family, community, and world. In general, many individuals with amputations make a satisfactory adjustment to the loss and are reintegrated into a full and active life. In achieving final acceptance, the individual may go through a number of stages including denial, anger, euphoria, and social withdrawal. Although it is difficult to predict long-range adjustment initially, there is some evidence that early counseling and the opportunity to explore the feelings associated with amputation and rehabilitation may be beneficial for individuals in all age groups.[36]

Some individuals may try to avoid distressing thoughts of the lost limb through conscious self-control or by avoiding situations or people that remind them of the lost limb. Some may display temper tantrums or irrational resentment. Some may revert to childlike states of helplessness and dependence.

Many individuals are not fully aware of the consequences of amputation and may fear other physical limitations as a result of the surgery. Fear of impotence or sterility may lead some men to make grandiose statements or display reckless behavior to mask the fear. Thorough explanations of the amputation process and its implications by the surgeon or other rehabilitation team members may alleviate many of these fears.

Generally, people who have had an amputation may dream about themselves as having an intact limb. This image may be so vivid that they fall as they get up at night and attempt to walk to the bathroom without a prosthesis or crutches. Individuals who have lost their leg through injury may dream about the battle or accident in which they were injured. Such reenactments may lead to insomnia, trembling fits, speech impediments, and difficulty with concentration. In general, individuals with congenital amputations or acquired amputations before age 5 do not have some of the problems mentioned above because their amputation is a part of their developed self-image.

Psychological Support

The patient needs to receive reassurance and understanding from the entire rehabilitation team. Team members should create an open and receptive environment and be willing to listen. The patient should know what to expect during the entire process. The surgeon and therapists should carefully explain the steps and expectations of rehabilitation. Audiovisual media, such as films or photographs, may be helpful. The Amputee Coalition of America (ACA) is a national, nonprofit amputee consumer educational organization representing people who have experienced amputation or were born with limb differences (www.amputee-coalition.org). Members include individuals with amputations, health professionals, family members, and friends of those with amputations. The ACA supports a volunteer visitation program where individuals with amputations who have been trained to provide support will visit patients soon after surgery to help with emotional support. Therapists should be cognizant of the existence of a local ACA chapter and make use of the organization to provide support and education to their patients regardless of age or cause of amputation. The military services also have support programs for individuals with amputations, and a group of veterans organized the Wounded Warrior Project (www.woundedwarriorproject.org) as a nonprofit organization to assist severely disabled veterans.

Patients have various attitudes toward the prosthesis. Most are concerned with function and regaining the greatest level of function possible; others are concerned about its appearance, hoping that it will conceal their disability and give the illusion of an intact body. If individuals with amputations have been told that the prosthesis will replace their own limb, they may have unrealistic expectations that function will be as good as in the nonamputated extremity. Realistic adjustment will be necessary as the person learns to use the artificial substitute. Good predictors for adjustment to the prosthesis are active involvement in the postsurgical and preprosthetic program and consistent attempts to return to an active lifestyle.

The Older Adult

The older individual with a LE amputation is not content to sit in a wheelchair or limp with a walker, but seeks effective rehabilitation services and a meaningful lifestyle. Maintaining independence is a critical issue with the older adult. Any disability requiring the use of an external device, especially amputation, may be seen as the end of an independent lifestyle. To some extent, the previous level of pain and disability and the sudden or gradual onset of the disability will affect the reaction. Individuals who have suffered considerable pain may be grateful that the pain has ended. Clients who underwent extensive medical and surgical procedures may experience a sense of failure that the efforts were not successful. If preoperative attitudes are unrealistically hopeful, postoperative disturbances may be more severe. The elderly person should not be led to expect a total cure. Learning to use an artificial limb may be a slow and discouraging ordeal, and the client may not express distress or depression in front of the optimism of others. However, the physical therapist must keep in mind that the majority of older individuals, particularly those amputated at transtibial levels, make excellent adjustments to prosthetic function.[37]

Elderly individuals are subject to considerable stress from concerns about financial limitations, loss of control over their lives, and fear of becoming dependent. An elderly individual who requires an amputation must often cope with multiple physical problems. Loss is a part of normal aging—loss of physiological capabilities, loss of a spouse or friends, loss of the self-esteem related to one's career or job, and now, loss of function. It is helpful to give the client as much control over decision making as possible, to provide opportunities to be involved in goal setting and sequencing of activities. As with any client, physical therapists need to be aware of the stressors affecting the client and assist with coping by being reflective listeners and enablers.

It is a myth that elderly individuals cannot learn a new skill, have difficulty remembering, and cannot achieve at the same level as younger individuals. Some elderly individuals may have difficulty learning a new skill, but many are able to adapt successfully to a disability such as an amputation and lead a full and normal life. Although some suffer from dementia, others who are labeled as having dementia because of confusion in the acute care setting may actually only be responding to medications, metabolic imbalances, infection toxicity, insecurity in a strange environment, or the sequelae of anesthesia. It is important to remember that cognitive dysfunction does not preclude satisfactory rehabilitation. Understanding the client's cognitive capabilities will help structure learning experiences appropriately. Goal-oriented statements may be clearer than step-by-step instructions. We do many activities almost automatically—getting up from a chair, turning in bed, and walking. Most of us have developed particular patterns of movements over the years. The physical therapist can draw on such patterns while focusing on the movement goals.

Intervention
Residual Limb Care

The residual limb needs to be completely healed and have lost the postoperative edema and much of the soft tissue slackness to be ready for prosthetic fitting. The residual limb is subjected to considerable and varied pressures during prosthetic walking and is generally not fully healed and prepared for such stresses for 8 to 12 weeks. The most effective method of preparing the residual limb for prosthetic fitting is the rigid dressing, but it is more expensive than the elastic wrap and many insurers will not pay for such fitting. Individuals not fitted with a rigid dressing use elastic wrap or shrinkers to reduce the size of the residual limb. The patient, family member, or professional staff member applies the bandage, which is worn 24 hours a day, except when

bathing. Using an elastic wrap or a shrinker to reduce edema is a slow process. Edema in the residual limb may be difficult to control in individuals with diabetes, particularly if they have renal involvement.

Residual Limb Wrapping

Patients tend to wrap their own residual limb in a circular manner, often creating a tourniquet, which may compromise healing and foster the development of a bulbous end. Although the transtibial residual limb can be effectively wrapped in a sitting position, it is difficult to properly wrap and anchor the transfemoral limb while sitting. Older patients often cannot balance themselves in the standing position while wrapping. An effective bandage is smooth and wrinkle free, emphasizes angular turns, provides pressure distally, and encourages proximal joint extension. The ends of bandages are fastened with tape or safety pins, rather than clips, which can cut the skin and do not anchor well. A system of wrapping that uses mostly angular or figure-of-eight turns was developed specifically to meet the needs of the older patient.

The Transtibial Bandage

Figure 22.7 outlines the preferred methods of wrapping the transtibial residual limb. Two 4-in elastic bandages are usually enough to wrap most transtibial residual limbs. Very large residual limbs may require three bandages. The transtibial bandages should not be sewn together so that the weave of each bandage can be brought in contraposition to the other to provide more support. Although an elastic wrap does not provide as much pressure as a rigid dressing, the development of postsurgical edema must be deterred as much as possible; therefore, a firm, even pressure against all soft tissues is desirable. If the incision is placed anteriorly, an attempt should be made to bring the bandages from posterior to anterior over the distal end.

The first bandage is started at either the medial or lateral tibial condyle and brought diagonally over the anterior surface of the limb to the distal end. One edge of the bandage should just cover the midline of the incision in an anterior-posterior plane. The bandage is continued diagonally over the posterior surface, then back over the beginning turn as an anchor. At this point, there is a choice; the bandage may be brought directly over the beginning point as indicated in Figure 22.7 (step 2a), or it may be brought across the front of the residual limb in an "X" design (Fig. 22.7 [step 2b]). The latter technique is particularly useful with long residual limbs and aids in bandage suspension. An anchoring turn over the distal thigh is made making sure that the wrap is clear of the patella and is not tight around the distal thigh.

After a single anchoring turn above the knee, the bandage is brought back around the opposite tibial condyle and down to the distal end of the limb. One edge of the bandage should overlap the midline of the

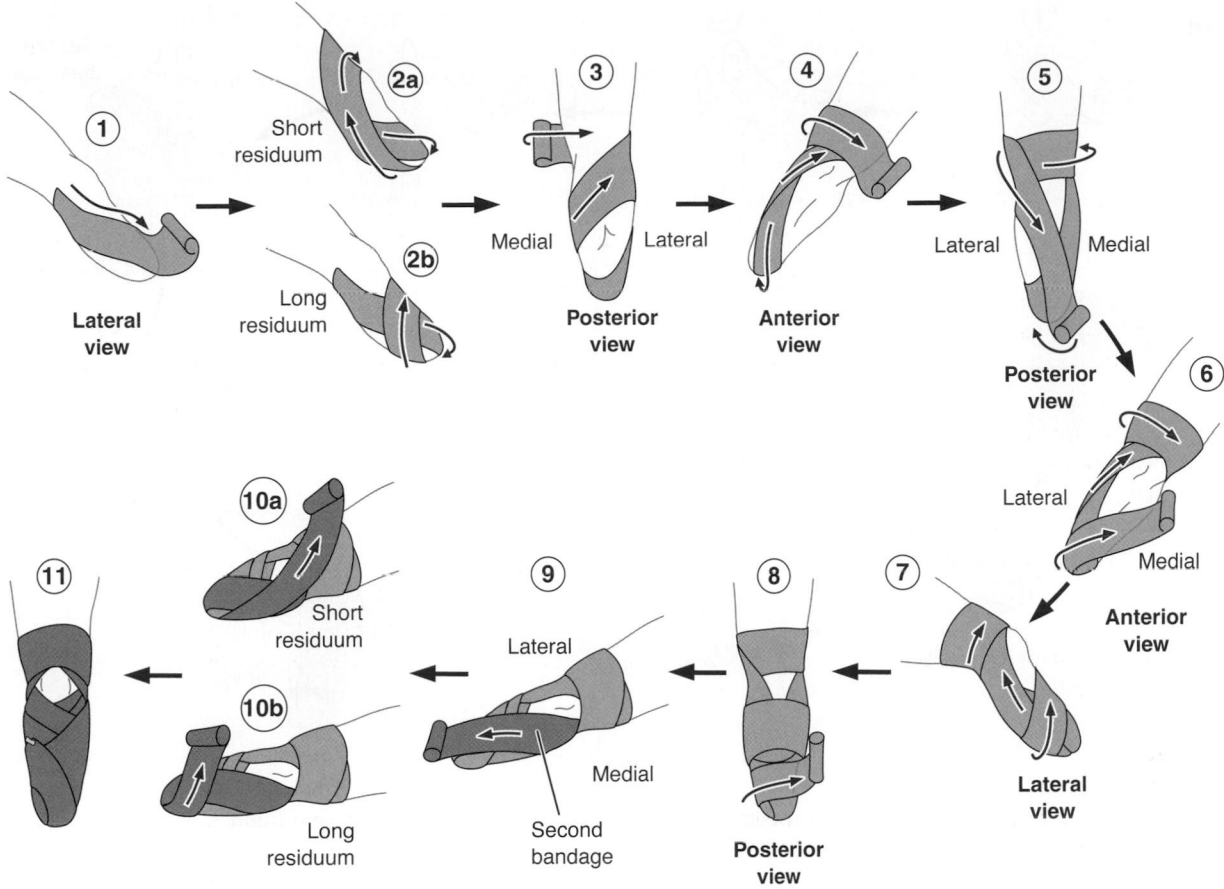

Figure 22.7 Transtibial residual limb bandaging. *From May and Lockard,[26, p. 75] with permission.*

incision and the other wrap by at least 1/2 in (1.25 cm) to ensure adequate distal end support. The figure-of-eight pattern is continued as depicted in Figure 22.7 (steps 5 through 8) until the bandage is used up. Care should be taken to completely cover the residual limb with a firm and even pressure. Semicircular turns are made posteriorly to position the bandage to cross the anterior surface in an angular line. This maneuver provides greater pressure on the posterior soft tissue while distributing pressure anteriorly where the bone is close to the skin. Each turn should partially overlap other turns so the whole residual limb is well covered. The pattern is usually from proximal to distal and back to proximal, starting at the tibial condyles and covering both condyles as well as the patellar tendon. Usually, the patella is left free to aid in knee motion, although with extremely short residual limbs, it may be necessary to cover it for better suspension.

The second bandage is wrapped like the first, except that it is started at the opposite tibial condyle from the first bandage (Fig. 22.7 [step 9]). Bringing the weave of each bandage in contraposition exerts a more even pressure. With both bandages, an effort is made to bring the angular turns across each other rather than in the same direction.

The Transfemoral Bandage

Figure 22.8 depicts the preferred method of wrapping the transfemoral residual limb with the task being done by a family member or caregiver. The side-lying position is preferred for better control of the residual limb with the hip neutral or slightly extended. Wrapping the transfemoral residual limb in the sitting position is difficult and usually leaves an area on the medial thigh uncovered. The patient with good balance on the remaining limb can bandage the residual limb in the standing position.

For most residual limbs, two 6-in bandages and one 4-in bandage will adequately cover the limb. The two 6-in bandages can be sewn together end-to-end taking care not to create a heavy seam; the 4-in bandage is used by itself. The 6-in bandages are used first. While it was noted that the transtibial wraps should not be sewn together to allow for a firmer bandage, sewing the transfemoral 6-in bandages or using a double bandage reduces the end of bandage attachments and makes for a smoother wrap. The first bandage is started in the groin and brought diagonally over the anterior surface to the distal lateral corner, around the end of the residual limb, and diagonally up the posterior side to the iliac crest and

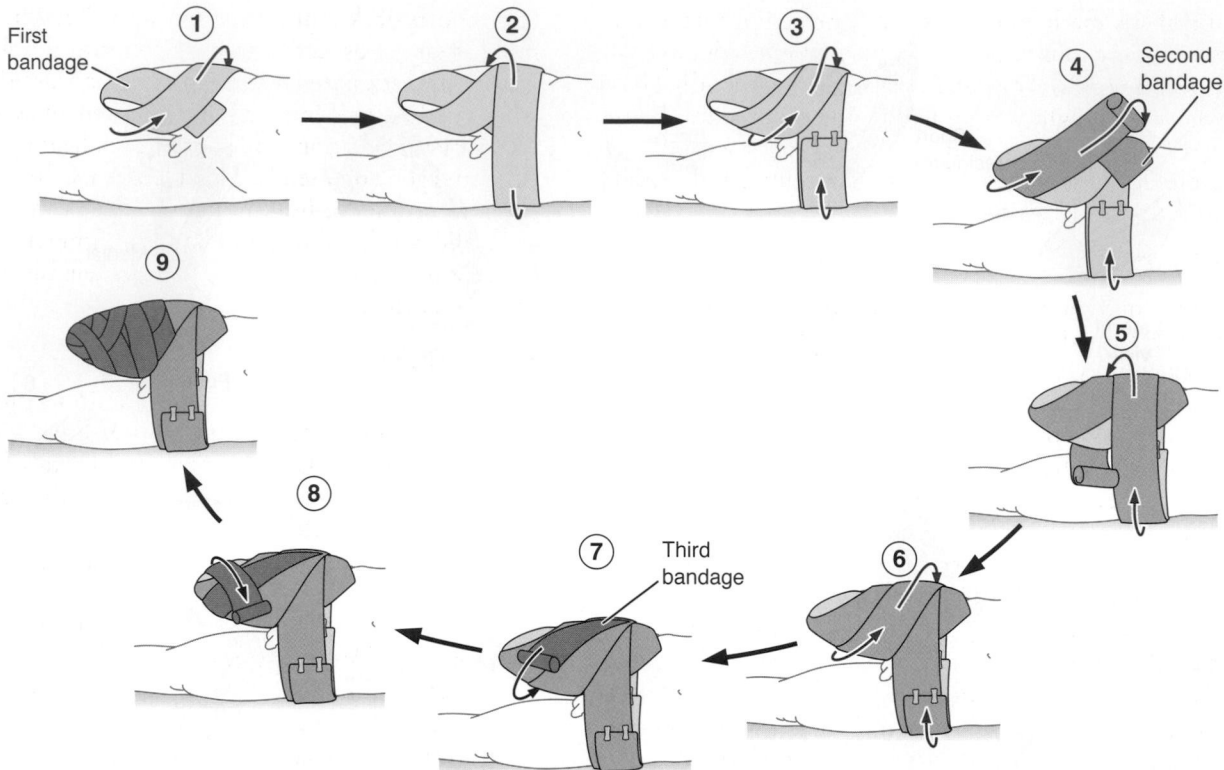

Figure 22.8 Transfemoral residual limb bandaging. *From May and Lockard,[26, p. 76] with permission.*

around the hips in a spica. The bandage is started medially so that the hip wrap (hip spica) will encourage extension. After the turn around the hips, the bandage is wrapped around the proximal portion of the residual limb high in the groin, then back around the hips. Although this is a proximal circular turn, it does not create a tourniquet as long as it is continued around the hips. Going around the medial portion of the residual limb high in the groin ensures coverage of the soft tissue in the adductor area and reduces the possibility of an adductor roll, a complication that can seriously interfere with comfortable prosthetic wear. In most instances, the first bandage ends in the second hip spica and is anchored with tape or pin.

The second 6-in bandage is wrapped like the first but is started a bit more laterally. Any areas not covered with the first bandage must be covered at this time. If a double bandage is used, this wrap can be a continuation of the first anchoring turn. The second bandage is also anchored in a hip spica after the first figure-of-eight and after the second turn high in the groin. While more of the first two bandages are used to cover the proximal residual limb, care must be taken that no tourniquet is created. Bringing the bandage directly from the proximal medial area into a hip spica helps to keep the adductor tissue covered and prevents rolling of the bandage to some degree.

The 4-in bandage is used to exert the greatest amount of pressure over middle and distal areas of the residual limb. It is usually not necessary to anchor this bandage around the hips because friction with the already applied bandages and good figure-of-eight turns limit slippage. The 4-in bandage is generally started laterally to bring the weave across the weave of previous bandages. Regular figure-of-eight turns in varied patterns to cover the entire residual limb are the most effective.

Shrinkers

The transtibial elastic shrinker is rolled over the residual limb to midthigh and is designed to be self-suspending. Individuals with heavy thighs may need additional suspension with garters or a waist belt. Currently available transfemoral shrinkers incorporate a hip spica, which provides good suspension except with obese individuals (see Fig. 22.4). Care must be taken that the patient understands the importance of proper suspension; any rolling of the edges or slipping of the shrinker can create a tourniquet around the proximal part of the residual limb. Shrinkers are easier to apply than elastic bandages and may be a better alternative, particularly for the transfemoral residual limb. Shrinkers are more expensive to use than elastic wrap; the initial cost is greater, and then new shrinkers of smaller sizes must be purchased as the limb volume decreases. However, shrinkers are a viable option for individuals who are not able to properly wrap the residual limb. Shrinkers may not be used until the incision has healed and the sutures have been removed. Sutures can be caught in the shrinker's mesh, and the distal distraction forces that accompany donning may cause wound dehiscence (splitting open). In a small study involving individuals who were taught proper bandaging techniques, Louie et al[38] found that residual limb wrapping was slightly more effective in reducing edema among individuals with transtibial amputations.

Skin Care

Proper hygiene and skin care are important. The residual limb is treated as any other part of the body; it is kept clean and dry. Individuals with dry skin may use a good skin lotion. Care must be taken to avoid abrasions, cuts, and other skin problems. Friction massage, in which layers of skin, subcutaneous tissue, and muscle are moved over the respective underlying tissue, can be used to prevent or mobilize adherent scar tissue. The massage is done gently, after the wound is healed and when no infection is present. Patients can learn to properly perform a gentle friction massage to mobilize the scar tissue and help decrease hypersensitivity of the residual limb to touch and pressure. Early handling of the residual limb by the patient is an aid to acceptance and is encouraged, particularly for individuals who may be repulsed by the limb.

The patient is taught to inspect the residual limb with a mirror each night to make sure there are no sores or impending problems, especially in areas not readily visible. If the person has diminished sensation, careful inspection is particularly important. Because the residual limb tends to become a bit edematous after bathing as a reaction to the warm water, nightly bathing is recommended, particularly once a prosthesis has been fitted. The elastic bandage, elastic shrinker, or removable rigid dressing is reapplied after bathing. If the person has been fitted with a prosthesis, the residual limb is wrapped at night and any time the prosthesis is not worn until it is fully mature (i.e., does not develop edema when not wearing a prosthesis). Patients have been known to apply a variety of "home and folk remedies" to the residual limb. Historically, it was believed that the skin had to be toughened for prosthetic wear by beating it with a towel-wrapped bottle. Various ointments and lotions have been applied; residual limbs have been immersed in substances such as vinegar, salt water, and gasoline to harden the skin. Although the skin does need to adjust to the pressures of wearing an artificial limb, there is no evidence to indicate that "toughening" techniques are beneficial. Such methods may actually be deleterious; research indicates that soft pliable skin is better able to cope with stress than tough dry skin. Patient education regarding proper skin care can reduce the use of home remedies.

The skin of the residual limb may be affected by a variety of dermatological problems such as eczema, psoriasis, or radiation burns. Some of these conditions may mitigate against fitting or wrapping. Dudek et al[39] found 528 reports of skin problems among 337 residual limbs in a 6-year retrospective study. Each skin problem was treated as a separate entity, whether it occurred in one or more than one individual. Treatment may include ultraviolet irradiation, whirlpool, reflex heating, hyperbaric oxygen, or medication. Care must be taken in using ultraviolet or heat in the presence of vascular disease. The whirlpool may not be the treatment of choice because it increases circulation and edema in the part under treatment.

Range of Motion

One of the greatest deterrents to functional prosthetic rehabilitation is contracture of hip or knee. Contractures can develop as a result of muscle imbalance or fascial tightness, from a protective withdrawal reflex into hip and knee flexion, from loss of plantar stimulation in extension, or as a result of faulty positioning such as prolonged sitting or placing the residual limb on a pillow. The patient should understand the importance of proper positioning and regular exercise in preparing for eventual prosthetic fit and ambulation. For all levels of amputation, full ROM in hip extension is critical in allowing the individual to assume a balanced upright posture.

With the transtibial amputation, full ROM in the hips and knee, particularly in extension, is needed. While sitting, the patient can keep the knee extended by using a posterior splint or a board attached to the wheelchair. The patient with a transfemoral amputation needs full ROM in the hip, particularly in extension and adduction. Prolonged sitting is to be avoided. Some time each day should be spent in the prone position.

Some individuals will present with hip or knee flexion contractures. Mild contractures may respond to manual mobilization and active exercises, but it is almost impossible to reduce moderate to severe contractures by manual stretching, especially hip flexion contractures. Some practitioners advocate holding the extremity in a stretched position with weights for a considerable length of time. There is little evidence that this traditional approach is successful. Facilitated stretching techniques (e.g., proprioceptive neuromuscular facilitation [PNF]) are more effective than passive stretching; hold–relax and hold–relax active contraction that utilizes resisted contraction of antagonist muscles may increase ROM, particularly of the knee. One of the more effective ways of reducing a knee flexion contracture is to fit the patient with a patellar-tendon-bearing (PTB) prosthesis aligned in a manner that places the hamstrings on stretch with each step. Such prosthetic alignment provides a stretch that is quite effective. Hip flexion contractures are more frequently found in persons with transfemoral amputations. It is difficult to "walk out" a hip flexion contracture with the transfemoral prosthesis. In some instances, depending on the severity of the contracture and the length of the residual limb, the contracture can be accommodated in the alignment of the prosthesis. A knee flexion contracture of less than 15° is not usually a problem. Prevention, however, continues to be the best treatment for contractures.

Exercises

The exercise program is individually designed and includes strengthening, balance, and coordination activities. The type of postsurgical dressing, degree of postoperative pain, and healing of the incision will determine when resistive exercises for the involved extremity can be started. The exercise program can take many forms and must include a home exercise program (HEP). The hip extensors and abductors and knee extensors and flexors are particularly important for prosthetic ambulation. Studies have shown a correlation between strength of the key muscle groups and ability to use a prosthesis effectively.[40-43] Figures 22.9 and 22.10 depict a series of exercises particularly well designed to strengthen key muscles around the hip and knee. These exercises can be adapted for a HEP because they are simple to perform and require no special equipment. Exercises need to be progressed with increased resistance.

A general strengthening program that includes the trunk and all extremities is often indicated, particularly for the older person who may have been quite sedentary before surgery. Proprioceptive neuromuscular facilitation exercises (PNF) are also beneficial. The exercise program needs to be individually developed and emphasize those muscles that are most active in prosthetic function. The exercises depicted in Figures 22.9 and 22.10 are particularly well suited to an HEP and combine the strengthening and coordination necessary for prosthetic ambulation. Corio et al[44] studied the effects of spinal stabilization exercises on the gait of individuals wearing a prosthesis for at least a year. Although a small sample of 34 individuals was used, the results suggest that improvement in spinal stabilization and trunk control may positively influence gait parameters.[44]

Balance and Mobility Activities

Early mobility is important to total physiological recovery. The patient needs to resume independent activities as soon as possible. Balance is a key element to effective mobility and an area too often overlooked. Poor balance and fear of falling have been found to negatively affect successful prosthetic rehabilitation.[45,46] Although individuals with unilateral amputation usually do not have a problem with sitting balance, it is important for the individual to develop good standing balance on the remaining limb. Figure 22.11 shows one type of standing balance exercise on a compliant surface. While care must be taken to protect the remaining foot from injury, particularly in patients with vascular disease, balance exercises with and without shoes as well as with eyes open and closed is an integral part of the program. Weight-bearing through the residual limb is also beneficial to future prosthetic training. This can only be

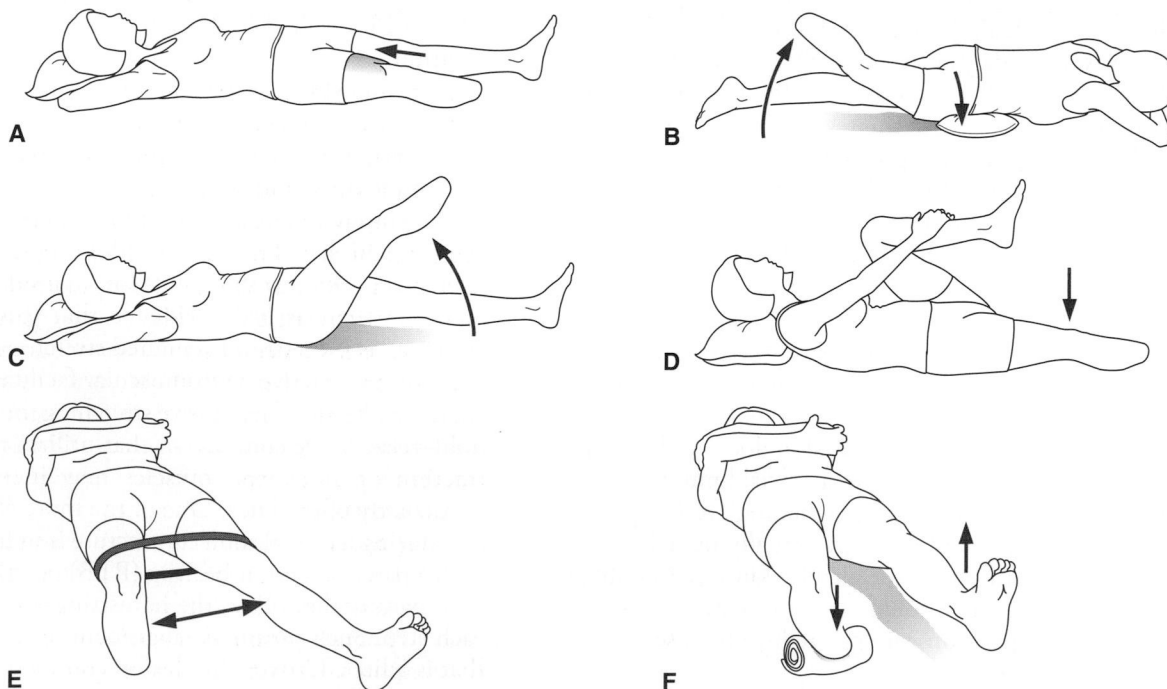

Figure 22.9 Transtibial exercises: **(A)** quad set, **(B)** hip extension with knee straight, **(C)** straight leg raise, **(D)** extension of the residual limb with the knee of the other leg against the chest, **(E)** hip abduction against resistance, and **(F)** bridging. *From May and Lockard,[26, p. 77] with permission.*

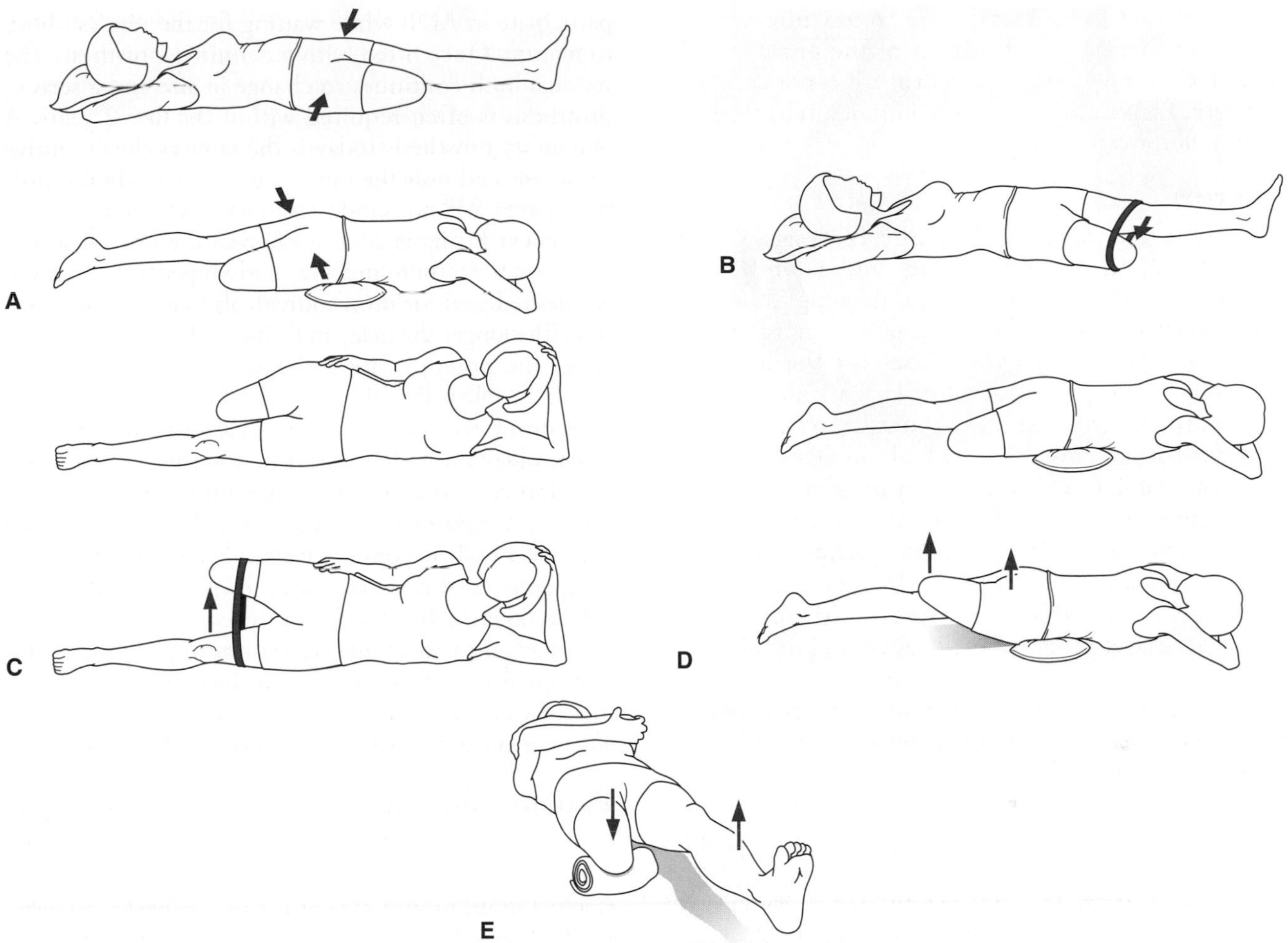

Figure 22.10 Transfemoral exercises: **(A)** gluteal sets, **(B)** hip abduction supine, **(C)** hip abduction against resistance, **(D)** hip extension prone, and **(E)** bridging. *From May and Lockard,*[26, p. 78] *with permission.*

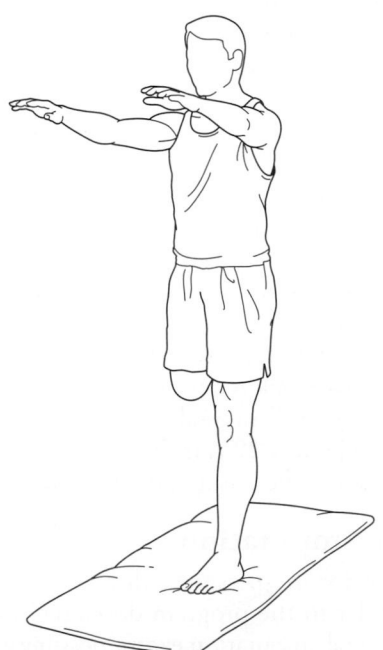

Figure 22.11 Standing balance exercise on a compliant surface. *From May and Lockard,*[26, p. 73] *with permission.*

safely achieved in patients with transtibial amputations. Figure 22.12 depicts a person kneeling on a cushion in a chair of the appropriate height and shifting her weight on and off the amputated side.

Walking is excellent exercise and necessary for independence in daily life. Gait training can start early and the person with a unilateral LE amputation can become quite independent using a three-point gait pattern on crutches. Many older individuals have difficulty learning to walk on crutches. Some are afraid, some lack the necessary balance and coordination, and others lack endurance. Walking with crutches without a prosthesis requires a greater expenditure of energy than walking with a prosthesis.

Independence in crutch walking is an outcome worthy of therapy time. The individual who can ambulate with crutches will develop a greater degree of general fitness than the person who spends most of the time in a wheelchair. Crutch walking is good preparation for prosthetic ambulation and the person who can learn to use crutches generally will not have difficulty learning to use a prosthesis. However, the individual who cannot learn to walk with crutches independently may still

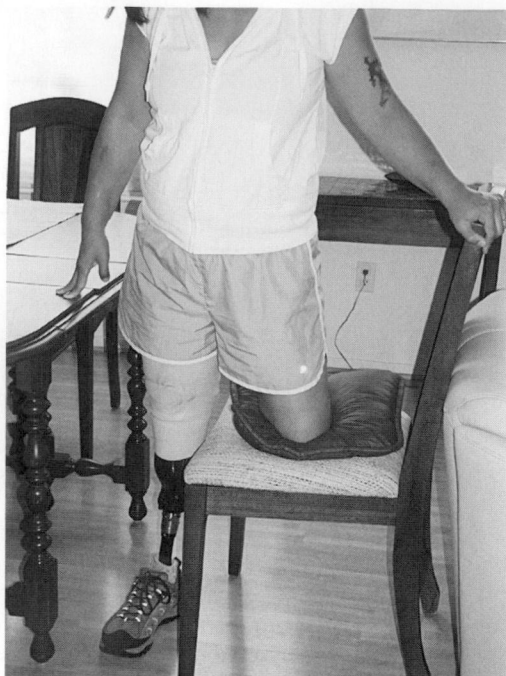

Figure 22.12 Kneeling on a pillow on a chair provides an opportunity for some weight-bearing. *From May and Lockard,[26, p. 74] with permission.*

become a very functional prosthetic user. An early graduated mobility program is also important for cardiovascular training and the development of endurance. Cardiovascular endurance is necessary for effective prosthetic ambulation, particularly at the transfemoral level.

There are advantages and disadvantages to using a walker for support. Certainly, walking with a walker is physiologically and psychologically more beneficial than sitting in a wheelchair, but it should be used only if the person cannot learn to walk with crutches. A walker is sturdier than crutches but cannot be used on stairs and curbs. It is sometimes difficult for the person who has used a walker following the amputation to switch to crutches or a cane when fitted with a prosthesis. The gait pattern used with a walker is not appropriate with a prosthesis and should not be used for any part of prosthetic training. A walker encourages a step-to gait pattern whereas efficient prosthetic use requires a step-through gait pattern. All individuals with an amputation need to learn some form of mobility without a prosthesis for use at night or when the prosthesis is not worn for some reason.

Temporary Prostheses

Many individuals are not fitted with any type of prosthetic appliance until the residual limb is free from edema and much of the soft tissue has shrunk, a process that can take many months of conscientious limb wrapping and exercises. During this period, the patient is limited to a wheelchair or to ambulation with crutches or a walker. Most individuals cannot return to work or fully participate in ADL while waiting for the residual limb to mature. Once fitted with a definitive prosthesis, the residual limb continues to change in size and a second prosthesis is often required within the first 2 years. A temporary prosthesis today is the same as the definitive prosthesis and uses the same components. Many third-party payers will not fund a temporary prosthesis, so early permanent fitting is advocated, even though the socket will be too big quite quickly. Early bipedal ambulation is a desired goal for most individuals following amputation. The longer the delay in fitting with a prosthesis, the lower the potential for effective rehabilitation. Care should be taken that the patient is fitted with optimum components for his or her expected level of function. Too often, older individuals are fitted with low-cost, low-function components when they probably could have achieved a higher level of function with more functional components. It becomes a vicious cycle with insurance companies depicting statistics showing that older individuals do not achieve independence but not considering that the components that were authorized either do not fit properly or they do not provide the necessary function. There is also a problem with insurers not providing adequate prosthetic training by a physical therapist.

Patient Education

Patient education is an integral and ongoing part of the rehabilitation program. Information on the care of the residual limb, proper care of the uninvolved extremity, positioning, exercises, and diet, if the patient has diabetes or is overweight, are necessary for the patient to be a full participant in the rehabilitation program. Discussions should also be held regarding patient goals, projected activity levels, funding, and prosthetic components. If the patient underwent the amputation for vascular problems, the education program should include information on proper footwear.

Care must be taken not to overwhelm the patient with too much information at one time; information overload leads to forgetfulness. It is more effective to prioritize the information and ask the person to remember one new thing each session rather than try to teach a complex program at one time. Written materials are necessary to supplement the teaching and help the patient remember what is required. It is also important for the program to be tailored to the individual's way of life. Involving the patient in establishing priorities enhances adherence. Appendix 22.A includes web-based resources for clinicians, families, and patients with amputation.

Bilateral Amputation

Intervention for the person with bilateral LE amputations is similar to the program developed for someone with a unilateral amputation except possibly ambulation. If the individual was fitted and ambulated after unilateral amputation, the prosthesis is useful for transfer activities and limited ambulation in the home. Some individuals may be able to use the prosthesis with external support to get around the house more easily, particularly for bathroom activities.

All individuals with bilateral amputations need a wheelchair on a permanent basis. The chair should be as narrow as possible with removable desk arms and removable leg rests. Elevating armrests are useful to assist in sit-to-stand transfers. Amputee wheelchairs with offset rear wheels and no leg rests are not recommended unless the therapist is sure that the person will never be fitted with prostheses, even cosmetically. It is easier to add anti-tipping devices to the rear of the wheelchair or attach small weights to the front uprights (counterbalance) for use when the footrests are removed.

The exercise program includes mat activities designed to help the person regain a sense of body position and balance, UE and residual limb strengthening exercises, and regular ROM exercises. Functional mobility training should stress independence in bed mobility, transfers, and wheelchair use. With bilateral amputations, individuals spend considerable time sitting and are therefore more prone to develop flexion contractures, particularly around the hip joints. The patient should be encouraged to sleep prone if possible, or at least spend some time in the prone position each day. The therapy program also emphasizes ROM of the residual limbs.

■ DETERMINING PROSTHETIC POTENTIAL

Not all people with amputations are candidates for a prosthesis, regardless of personal desire. The cost of the prosthesis and the energy demands of prosthetic training require that some judgment be used in selecting individuals for fitting.

There is no general rule that can safely be applied to all patients in making the decision to fit or not to fit. The patient is part of the decision making process, but the fact that the individual wants a prosthesis is not enough. Many people are not aware of the physiological demands of prosthetic ambulation, particularly at transfemoral levels. The development of lightweight prostheses, microprocessor knee mechanisms, stance control assistance, and energy conserving feet have made it possible to successfully fit many more individuals than in the past; however, some consideration for nonfitting is necessary. Medicare has developed a functional classification chart to guide selection of components (Box 22.6). There are several other outcome instruments that may be used to help predict functional potential for patients with amputation.[47-49]

In general, individuals who were ambulatory before amputation who sustain a unilateral transtibial amputation will be able to become independent with a properly fitted prosthesis and physical therapy intervention. Although it takes more balance, coordination, and

---

> **Box 22.6   Medicare Functional Classification Levels**
>
> - **Functional level 0:** The patient does not have the ability or potential to ambulate or transfer safely with or without assistance and a prosthesis does not enhance his or her quality of life or mobility.
> - **Functional level 1:** The patient has the ability or potential to use a prosthesis for transfers or ambulation on level surfaces at fixed cadence. Typical of the limited and unlimited household ambulator.
> - **Functional level 2:** The patient has the ability or potential for ambulation with the ability to traverse low-level environmental barriers such as curbs, stairs, or uneven surfaces. Typical of the limited community ambulator.
> - **Functional level 3:** The patient has the ability or potential for ambulation with variable cadence. Typical of the community ambulator who has the ability to traverse most environmental barriers and may have vocational, therapeutic, or exercise activity that demands prosthetic utilization beyond simple locomotion.
> - **Functional level 4:** The patient has the ability or potential for prosthetic ambulation that exceeds basic ambulation skills, exhibiting high-impact, stress, or energy levels. Typical of the prosthetic demands of the child, active adult, or athlete.

---

energy to use a transfemoral prosthesis, many individuals regardless of age can become functional following unilateral transfemoral amputation. Severe hip flexion contractures, obesity, weakness or paralysis of hip musculature, and poor balance and coordination may impede successful ambulation. The person's level of activity and participation in the postsurgical and preprosthetic programs helps in determining potential for prosthetic ambulation.

Fitting or not fitting someone with bilateral amputations is a difficult decision. Young, agile individuals are generally good candidates for prosthetic fitting regardless of level of amputations. Most patients with bilateral transtibial amputations can become quite functional with prostheses. Most older individuals with bilateral transfemoral amputations have considerable difficulty learning to use two prostheses. Patients with one transfemoral and one transtibial amputation generally can learn to use two prosthesis if the first amputation was at the transfemoral level, and if the person successfully used a transfemoral prosthesis before losing the other leg. Fitting decisions for individuals with bilateral LE amputations are individual and dependent on the person's particular capabilities. Certainly, technologically modern components including microprocessors and active components are an aid to the rehabilitation of most individuals with amputation today.

■ PROSTHETIC TRAINING

The major goal of prosthetic rehabilitation is for the client to attain a smooth, energy-efficient gait that allows the individual to perform ADL and participate in desired employment and recreational activities. Prosthetic ambulation is a skilled psychomotor activity and the person must learn to adapt well-developed patterns of movement to new situations. Box 22.7 outlines the determinants of an effective prosthetic gait. Effective gait training must guide the individual to integrate the prosthesis into all mobility activities. Table 22.3 presents the critical prosthetic training elements, starting with basic balance and progressing to ambulation. Although the table depicts training with a transfemoral prosthesis, the sequence is equally appropriate for transtibial prosthetic training other than the knee control step. It is important to do as much training as possible without the use of an external support device since many people will be able to walk more efficiently without external support. If found necessary, a cane may be added once the person has good control of weight shifting on and off the prosthesis and stepping through. A walker should never be used as part of prosthetic training unless the individual is so limited as to have used a walker before amputation. It is important for the physical therapist to know the type and function of the components of the prosthesis to appropriately plan training activities. Knee control with a microprocessor is different than with other types of transfemoral knee components.[50]

Box 22.7	Factors that Contribute to an Efficient Prosthetic Gait

- Accept the weight of the body on each leg
- Balance on one foot in single-limb support
- Advance each limb forward and prepare for the next step
- Adapt to environmental demands

Table 22.3 Critical Training Elements

Element	Activity	Details
Stability—both legs (TT/TF)	Secure standing without hand support; reaching for objects.	Hold an object a reachable distance; patient reaches and touches objects with either hand looking at object. Objects placed high/low/right/left encouraging goal-oriented weight shifting.
Knee control (TF)	Secure standing without hand support; slightly bend and straighten prosthetic knee to varying degrees.	Encourage patient to develop kinesthetic feel of knee position by socket pressures.

Table 22.3   Critical Training Elements—cont'd

Element	Activity	Details
Stability on prosthesis (TT/TF)	Secure standing without hand support; place 6–8-in stool directly in front of patient.	In a controlled manner, patient places unamputated foot on stool and back on the floor.
Stability on prosthesis (TT/TF)	Secure standing without hand support; place soccer ball in front of unamputated leg.	In a controlled manner, patient kicks the ball with the unamputated foot.
Prosthetic control (TT/TF)	Secure standing without hand support; place soccer ball in front of prosthesis.	In a controlled manner, patient kicks the ball with the prosthetic leg.

Continued

Table 22.3	Critical Training Elements—cont'd		
Element		**Activity**	**Details**
Proprioception (TT/TF) 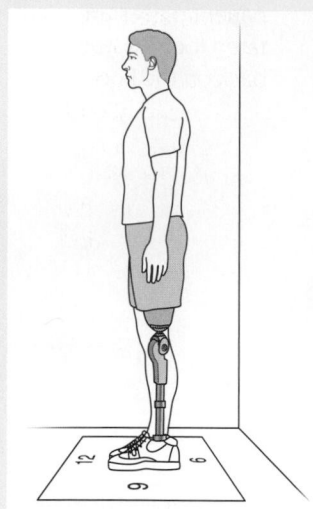		Secure standing both legs on a piece of paper with a clock face drawn and without hand support.	On command, patient shifts weight to 12, 3, 6, and 9 o'clock in random order. Learns to recognize where prosthetic foot is in relation to weight-bearing.
Pelvic control (TT/TF) 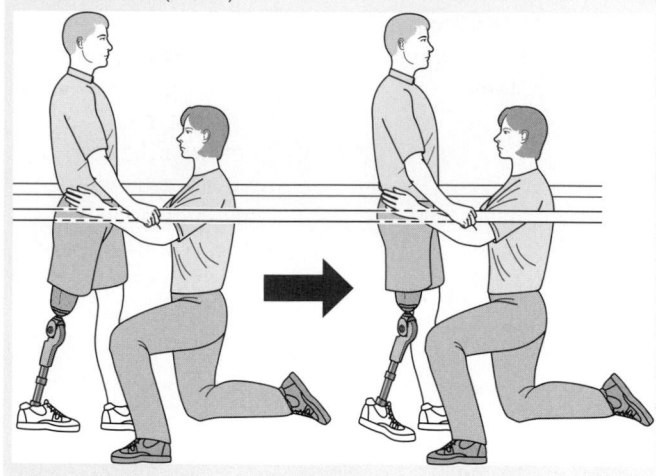		Secure standing without hand support prosthetic leg behind unamputated leg. Provide resistance to forward pelvic progression at initial contact to foot flat.	Encourage patient to transfer weight smoothly with forward and slight lateral pelvic motion by providing resistance as patient brings prosthesis forward.
Stepping with prosthesis (TT/TF) 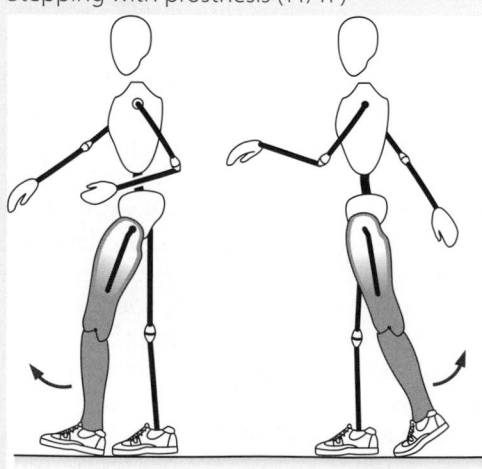		Secure standing without hand support, step forward and back with prosthesis.	Start with double leg stance, shift weight to unamputated leg and steps forward with prosthesis. Returns prosthesis to position behind sound leg. Emphasize knee control with TF.

Table 22.3 Critical Training Elements—cont'd

Element	Activity	Details
Stepping with sound leg (TT/TF) 	Secure standing without hand support, step forward and back with unamputated leg	As above but with unamputated leg. Make sure patient brings weight to forward part of foot before stepping on unamputated leg. Emphasize toe-off on TF to activate swing initiation.
Side stepping; backward stepping (TT/TF) 	Consecutive steps to the right, then to the left without hand support. Stepping backward several steps.	Side stepping, emphasize picking up the leg and placing it several inches to the side, then picking up the other leg to the first leg. TF backward stepping generally requires a larger prosthetic step than the unamputated for knee control.

From May and Lockard[26] pp. 136-141 with permission.
TT = patient with transtibial prosthesis; TF = patient with transfemoral prosthesis.

Many insurance companies, including Medicare, do not authorize very much time for gait training. Focusing the training initially on balance and integration of the prosthesis is more desirable than simply handing the patient a walker or crutches just to get him or her walking. If the patient can learn to balance on and off the prosthesis smoothly and feels a sense of control and integration of the prosthesis, he or she will progress further with less therapy than if started walking before the necessary balance was developed. Box 22.8 Evidence Summary presents studies addressing the inclusion of balance training strategies with gait training for patients with amputation.

Advanced Training

Changing the environment is an integral part of the gait training program. It is hardly functional to have the client walk only in the sheltered and simple environment of the physical therapy gym. Functional ambulation takes place in complex environments. Walking around furniture, through narrow doorways, on rugs, and around obstacles is very different from walking in the clear open space of the physical therapy gym. Placing obstacles on the floor to step around or over, walking in a busy hallway of the treatment center, picking something up from the floor, and carrying an object while walking are all more advanced activities that require balance, coordination, and the ability to shift one's weight on and off the prosthesis in different body positions. During advanced training, the client is taught to get up and down from chairs of different heights and seat resilience, especially toilet seats. An interesting obstacle course can be created using chairs, single steps, cones, and blocks to walk around, as well as different surfaces. Hofstad et al[51] studied delayed and decreased obstacle avoidance in individuals wearing one LE prosthesis. Level of amputation was not indicated but electromyography (EMG) was used to examine

Evidence Summary Box 22.8 Balance and Gait

Reference	Subjects	Design Intervention	Duration	Results	Comments
Curtze et al (2011)[a]	18 subjects with transtibial amputations and 17 matched subjects without amputation	Tracked walking on two irregular surfaces in the laboratory	4 trials on each surface	No statistically significant differences between groups.	Emphasizes importance of balance training in rehabilitation of patients with amputation.
Curtze et al (2010)[b]	17 subjects with transtibial amputation and 17 matched subjects without amputation	Forward fall was induced in laboratory setting by having subject on an inclinometer at a set angle with unexpected release	3 trials per subject leading with each leg	Statistically significant differences in response time, and knee flexion at heel strike between groups; no difference in step length, swing time of leading limb or trailing limb. Subjects with amputation used a longer step and showed less knee flexion when leading with prosthesis.	Authors emphasized the importance of incorporating balance and fall recovery activities as part of gait training following amputation.
Raya et al (2010)[c]	72 subjects with LE amputations ages 21–83 using prostheses	Tested for balance, hip strength, 6-Minute Walk Test, Amputee mobility predictor (AMP)	Strength 10 reps each motion AMP and 6-Minute Walk Test 1 time each	Hip abduction and extension strength strongest predictor of performance on 6-Min Walk Test and gait speed. Single-leg balance found important.	The 6-Minute Walk Test is useful to help identify musculoskeletal impairments. Hip strength and single-leg stance balance important.
Hlavackova et al (2009)[d]	12 elderly subjects with transfemoral amputations using prostheses	Subjects stood upright and immobile on plantar pressure data system, first in front of a wall, then in front of a mirror	Three 30-second trials for each condition	Significant decrease in pressure under sound limb when facing the mirror as compared to the wall. No concomitant significant increase in pressure under prosthetic limb.	Asymmetry in weight-bearing during quiet standing is common. Mirror feedback did somewhat increase weight-bearing on the prosthesis and could be used in training.
Vrieling et al (2008)[e]	8 subjects with amputation (3 transfemoral, 5 transtibial) and 9 subjects without amputation	CAREN balance system with anterior-posterior sway for 60 seconds (increasing for 15 sec, stable for 30 sec, decreasing for 15 sec)	3 randomized conditions: eyes open, blindfolded, and dual task with 60-second rest between	All subjects maintained balance through all tests. Subjects with amputation bore significant weight on the nonamputated limb and were more asymmetrical.	Subjects with amputations used the nonamputated limb for adjustment strategy and showed increased trunk movements. Suggests addressing asymmetry during gait training.

References:

[a]Curtze, C, et al: Over rough and smooth: Amputee gait on irregular surfaces. Gait Posture 33(2):292–296, 2011.

[b]Curtze, C, et al: Balance recovery after an evoked forward fall in unilateral transtibial amputees. Gait Posture 32(3):336–341, 2010.

[c]Raya, MA, et al: Impairment variables predicting activity limitation in individuals with lower limb amputation. Prosthet Orthot Int 34(1):73–84, 2010.

[d]Hlavackova, P, et al: Effects of mirror feedback on upright stance control in elderly transfemoral amputees. Arch Phys Med Rehabil 90(11):1960–1963, 2009.

[e]Vrieling, AH, et al: Balance control on a moving platform in unilateral lower limb amputees. Gait Posture 28(2):222–228, 2008.

responses to obstacles. Results indicated that responses to obstacles were either delayed or decreased on both limbs regardless of which limb had the prosthesis. The authors suggested that obstacle training could be useful.[51]

Steps and Ramps

Individuals wearing transtibial prostheses generally have little difficulty mastering steps and ramps once they have achieved good balance and prosthetic control. Going up step-over-step requires good quadriceps strength and a medium to long residual limb. Some gait adaption may be needed for steep ramps or hills depending on the type of prosthetic foot. The more limitation of dorsiflexion, the harder it is to go up a steep hill step-over-step. Many individuals take a long step with the prosthesis and a shorter step with the unamputated foot. Going down a steep hill again requires good quadriceps strength and prosthetic control but is accomplished by most individuals.

The technique for going up and down stairs and ramps will vary for an individual wearing a transfemoral prosthesis depending on the type of knee component. Generally, the person will ascend stairs one step at a time leading with the unamputated leg. Individuals fitted with a stance phase control knee system will have to go down steps one at a time leading with the prosthesis. All others have the potential of going down step-over-step, although, except for the C-Leg and some hydraulic units, it requires considerable balance. It is necessary for the individual to place the prosthetic heel only on the step to create a flexion moment in the knee as weight is brought forward, thereby allowing the knee to flex and the person to bring the unamputated leg down to the lower step. The process is quite easy with the C-Leg, because the computer program is designed to allow smooth flexion as the person is going down steps or a ramp. Table 22.4 presents general techniques for some advanced activities for individuals with a transfemoral prosthesis. Once good balance, prosthetic control, and gait have been achieved, most individuals will develop their own method of doing each of these activities.

Table 22.4	Advanced Activities (Transfemoral)
Activity	**Procedure**
Sitting on the floor	Place the prosthesis about half a step behind the sound foot keeping the weight on the sound foot. Bend from the waist and flex at the knees and hips, reaching for the floor with both arms outstretched and pivoting to the sound side. Then, gradually lower the body to the floor. This activity is one continuous movement.
Getting up from the floor	Get on the hands and knees; place the sound leg forward, well under the trunk, with the foot flat on the floor while balancing on the hands and the prosthetic knee. Then, extend the sound knee while maintaining the weight over the sound leg. Move to an erect position by pushing strongly with the sound leg and the arms bringing the prosthesis forward when almost erect.
Kneeling	Place the sound foot ahead of the prosthetic foot keeping the weight on the sound leg. Slowly flex the trunk, hip, and knee until the prosthetic knee can be gently placed on the floor. Clients with transfemoral limbs usually kneel on the prosthetic leg. Getting up from a kneeling position is like getting up from the floor.
Picking up an object from the floor	Place the sound foot ahead of the prosthetic foot with the body weight remaining on the sound leg. Bend forward at the waist flexing the hips and knees until the object can be reached. Care must be taken to maintain the weight on the sound leg if wearing a mechanical knee. Some individuals like to bend sideways rather than forward, whereas others find it easier to keep the prosthetic knee straight and bend the sound leg until the object can be picked up.
Clearing obstacles	Face the obstacle with the sound foot slightly in front and the body weight on the prosthesis. Step over the obstacle with the sound leg, then transfer the body weight to the sound leg. Quickly extend the prosthetic hip, and forcefully flex the prosthetic hip whipping the prosthesis forward over the obstacle. Then step forward with a normal gait pattern. An alternate method is to stand sideways to the obstacle with the sound leg closest to the obstacle. With the weight on the prosthesis, swing the sound leg over the obstacle and transfer the body weight to the sound leg. Then swing the prosthesis forward, up and over the obstacle. The "C" leg and some hydraulic units may allow enough knee flexion to clear a small obstacle.

From May and Lockard,[26] p. 147.

SUMMARY

Most individuals with LE amputations can be helped to return to a full and useful life following the loss of a limb. A program of postoperative care that includes consideration of physical and emotional needs will enable most patients to become functional prosthetic users. Many prosthetic problems can be avoided by properly preparing the individual for prosthetic wear. In this chapter, concepts related to the postoperative and pre-prosthetic management of the individual with an LE amputation have been presented. Through a process of careful evaluation and open communication, a comprehensive program designed to meet the needs of an individual patient can be achieved.

Questions for Review

1. Compare and contrast the advantages and disadvantages of the following dressings: (a) compressible soft dressing; (b) semirigid dressing; and (c) immediate postoperative prosthesis.

2. What are the general goals of the postsurgical phase of amputation care?

3. What critical information would you provide a family member about patient positioning following a transtibial amputation?

4. A 72-year-old man with a history of diabetes, cardiovascular disease, and PVD has been referred for physical therapy 24 hours post right transtibial amputation for gangrene. What examination data are needed to plan an appropriate treatment program? Which are the most critical to obtain on the first visit?

5. What are the determinants of an efficient prosthetic gait?

6. Plan three training activities that could be used to improve stability while using prosthesis.

CASE STUDY

REFERRAL

The patient is a 72-year-old female status post–right transtibial amputation yesterday secondary to arteriosclerotic gangrene.

CURRENT MEDICAL HISTORY

Diabetes type 2 since age 48 controlled by insulin 20 units bid. Arteriosclerosis; hypertension controlled by medication; treated for ulcer plantar surface of right first metatarsal area for past 3 months. Ulcer did not heal leading to amputation.

PAST MEDICAL HISTORY

Hysterectomy at age 42, otherwise unremarkable.

SOCIAL HISTORY

Widow who lives alone. Three grown children and six grandchildren in the area.

PHYSICAL THERAPY EXAMINATION (INITIAL)

Chart Review

Patient alert and awake in no apparent distress. Right residual limb wrapped in soft gauze dressing covered with an elastic wrap. Drain in place. Incision clean on dressing change.

BP: 142/70, pulse 66, respiration normal.

Respiratory therapist reports patient using spirometer properly, normal cough, and no evidence of respiratory problems.

Patient complains of some pain in residual limb (pain medication prescribed).

Patient has been sitting at the side of the bed twice/day.

Examination Data

Gross muscle strength of left lower extremity (LE) and both upper extremities (UEs) grossly within functional limits (WFL). Muscle strength of right hip flexion, abduction, and adduction grossly WFL; hip extension tested side-lying and graded a 3+/5 (Fair+). Demonstrates active motion of right knee flexion and extension with no resistance given at this time.

Residual limb measurements deferred until initial healing has taken place.

Gross range of motion of left LE and both UEs WFL. Left hip extension measurements deferred until patient can lie prone or on right side. Gross range of motion (ROM) of the right hip WFL except hip extension to 0° measured side-lying. Right knee flexion and extension grossly WFL. Specific measurement deferred until dressing can be removed.

Left LE is hairless below the ankle. Skin is warm to touch. Popliteal pulse palpable but not dorsalis pedis pulse. Toes are warm to touch. Proprioceptive sensation intact. Diminished sensation over plantar surface of left foot and dorsum of first metatarsal. No evidence of edema in left LE. Sensation testing of right residual limb deferred secondary to dressing.

FUNCTIONAL STATUS

Bed Mobility

Rolling to left: independent; rolling to right and prone: not tested.

Supine-to-sit and return: modified independent (requires use of "rope ladder" attached to foot of bed).

Transfers

Sit-to-stand with walker: moderate assistance.

Stand-to-sit in chair or bed: moderate assistance.

Locomotion

Ambulation with walker: moderate assistance for 5 feet.

Expected outcomes of physical therapy episode of care (achieved before discharge from hospital):

1. The patient will be independent in all transfers.

2. The patient will be independent in ambulation with crutches or walker for 40 feet.

3. The patient will demonstrate knowledge of proper residual limb positioning, bandaging, and care.

4. The patient will demonstrate knowledge of basic residual limb exercises.

5. The patient will demonstrate knowledge of proper care of the left lower extremity.

PREPROSTHETIC HOME CARE PHYSICAL THERAPY

On discharge from the hospital, the patient was referred to home care physical therapy.

Examination Data

Examination data obtained following discharge from hospital by home care physical therapist:

Residual limb: Sutures in place, incision healing well, no drainage; length 13.6 cm (5.4 in) from medial tibial plateau (MTP).

Circumferential measurements from MTP:

• 5 cm (2 in) below MTP = 35 cm (14 in)

• 10 cm (4 in) below MTP = 38 cm (15 in)

• 12 cm (5 in) below MTP = 37 cm (14.5 in)

Sensation intact.

ROM right knee: WFL.

ROM right hip: extension to 0° (all other motions WFL).

Expected Outcomes

Expected outcomes for physical therapy episode of care during preprosthetic home care intervention:

1. The patient will be independent in care of residual limb including bandaging or using shrinker.

2. The patient will be independent in crutch (or walker) ambulation in and around the home and community.

3. The patient will be independent in home exercise program (HEP).

4. The patient will be independent in self-care and functional activities in the home.

Three months later the patient is fitted with a transtibial prosthesis (patellar tendon bearing [PTB] prosthesis with gel liner, suction suspension, and medium energy return prosthetic foot.

GUIDING QUESTIONS

1. The patient's residual limb was wrapped in a soft dressing after amputation. Compare the advantages and disadvantages of the rigid dressing, the semirigid dressing, and soft dressings. What problems might the patient incur with a soft dressing?

2. Review the initial examination data given for the patient. What data would be important to obtain on the first postoperative visit and what can be deferred? What other data would you obtain and when?

3. How would your evaluation change if your initial contact was after hospital discharge as a home health therapist?

a. Describe your initial plan of interventions.

b. Describe your mobility program.

4. What would be the focus of a prosthetic training program for this patient?

a. Describe your initial balance training program.

b. How would you teach this person to go up and down steps?

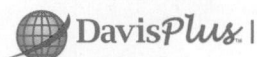 For additional resources, including answers to the questions for review and case study guiding questions, please visit **http://davisplus.fadavis.com**

> The reader is referred to video **Case Study 3: Patient with Transtibial (Below Knee) Amputation** for additional review and study. The full written case study, including tables, figures, charts, and three video segments (examination, intervention, and outcome), appears online at Davis*Plus*. The case study poses questions for the reader's consideration with suggested answers to the case study questions, also posted online at Davis*Plus*.

References

1. U.S. Department of Health and Human Services: Economics and Health Care Costs of Diabetes. Agency for Healthcare Research and Quality Outcomes, Rockville, MD, 2005. Retrieved September 24, 2011, from www.ahrq.gov/data/hcup/highlight1/high1.htm.
2. Krajewski, LP, and Olin, JW: Atherosclerosis of the aorta and lower extremities arteries. In Young, JR, et al (eds): Peripheral Vascular Diseases. Mosby–Year Book, St. Louis, 1991, p 179.
3. Wu, J, Chan, TS, and Bowring, G: Functional outcome of major lower limb amputation 1994–2006: A modern series. JPO 22(3):152–156, 2010.
4. Ebskov, LB: Relative mortality in lower limb amputees with diabetes mellitus. Prosthet Orthot Int 20:147, 1996.
5. American Diabetes Association: A column for health professionals with various data (no specific title). Resources for Health Professionals. American Diabetes Association. Retrieved from www.diabetes.org.
6. Driver, VR, Madsen J, and Goodman, RA: Reducing amputation rates in patients with diabetes at a military medical center: The limb preservation service model. Diabetes Care 28(2):248–253, 2005.
7. Dorresteijn, JA, et al: Patient education for preventing diabetic foot ulceration. Cochrane Database of Systematic Reviews 2010, Issue 5. Art. No.: CD001488. DOI: 10.1002/14651858. CD001488.pub3.
8. Nagarajan, R, et al: Limb salvage and amputation in survivors of pediatric lower-extremity bone tumors: What are the long-term implications? J Clin Oncol 20:4493, 2002.
9. Stojadinovic, A, et al: Amputation for recurrent soft tissue sarcoma of the extremity: Indications and outcome. Ann Surg Oncol 8:509, 2001.
10. Link, MP, et al: Adjuvant chemotherapy of high-grade osteosarcoma of the extremity. Clin Orthop 270:8, 1991.
11. Simon, M: Limb salvage for osteosarcoma in the 1980s. Clin Orthop 270:264, 1990.
12. Springfield, DS: Introduction to limb-salvage surgery for sarcomas. Orthop Clin North Am 22:1, 1991.
13. Yaw, KM, and Wurtz, LD: Resection and reconstruction for bone tumors in the proximal tibia. Orthop Clin North Am 22:133, 1991.
14. Stevens, P: The balancing act: Are amputees falling for it? The O&P Edge pp 5–7, May 2010. Retrieved September 24, 2011, from www.oandp.com/articles/2010-05_03.asp.
15. Smith, DG: General principles of amputation surgery. In Smith, DG, Michael, JW, and Bowker, JH: Atlas of Amputations and Limb Deficiencies: Surgical, Prosthetic, and Rehabilitation Principles, ed 3. American Academy of Orthopaedic Surgeons, Rosemont, IL, 2004, p 21.
16. Bowker, JH: Transtibial amputation: Surgical management. In Smith, DG, Michael, JW, and Bowker, JH: Atlas of Amputations and Limb Deficiencies: Surgical, Prosthetic, and Rehabilitation Principles, ed 3. American Academy of Orthopaedic Surgeons, Rosemont, IL, 2004, p 481.
17. Lind, J, et al: The influence of smoking on complications after primary amputations of the lower extremity. Clin Orthop 267:211, 1991.
18. Burgess, EM: Amputations of the lower extremities. In Nickel, VL (ed): Orthopedic Rehabilitation. Churchill Livingstone, New York, 1982, p 377.
19. Sarmiento, A, et al: Lower-extremity amputation: The impact of immediate postsurgical prosthetic fitting. Clin Orthop 68:22, 1967.
20. Harrington, IJ, et al: A plaster-pylon technique for below-knee amputation. J Bone Joint Surg (Br) 73:76, 1991.
21. Walsh, TL: Custom removable immediate postoperative prosthesis. JPO 15(4):128–161, 2003.
22. Wong, CK, and Edelstein, JE: Unna and elastic post-operative dressings: Comparisons of their effect on function of adults with amputations and vascular disease. Arch Phys Med Rehabil 81:1191, 2000.
23. Vigier, S, et al: Healing of open stump wounds after vascular below-knee amputation: Plaster cast socket with silicone sleeve versus elastic compression. Arch Phys Med Rehabil 80(10):1327, 1999.
24. Goldberg, T, Goldberg, S, and Pollak, J: Postoperative management of lower extremity amputation. Phys Med Rehabil Clin North Am 11:559, 2000.
25. Gendron, B, and Andrews, KL: The use of rigid removable dressings for juvenile amputees: A case report. JACPOC 26(1):4, 1991.
26. May, BJ, and Lockard, MA: Postsurgical management. In May, BJ, and Lockard, MA: Prosthetics and Orthotics in Clinical Practice: A Case Study Approach. FA Davis, Philadelphia, 2011, p 59.
27. Lockard, MA: Shoes and orthoses for foot impairments. In May, BJ, and Lockard, MA: Prosthetics and Orthotics in Clinical Practice: A Case Study Approach. FA Davis, Philadelphia, 2011, p 221.
28. May, BJ: Patient education past and present. J Phys Ther Educ 13(3):3–7, 1999.
29. Stineman, MG, et al: The effectiveness of inpatient rehabilitation in the acute postoperative phase of care after transtibial or trans-femoral amputation. Study of an integrated health care delivery system. Arch Phys Med Rehabil 89(10):1863–1872, 2008.
30. Ramachandran, VS, and Hirstein, WL: The perception of phantom limbs: The D. O. Hebb Lecture. Brain 9(121):1603–1630, 1998.

31. Racy, J: Psychological adaptation to amputation. In Smith, DG, Michael, JW, and Bowker, JH: Atlas of Amputations and Limb Deficiencies: Surgical, Prosthetic, and Rehabilitation, ed 3. American Academy of Orthopaedic Surgeons, Rosemont, IL, 2004, p 727.

32. Borghi, B, et al: The use of prolonged peripheral neural blockade after lower extremity amputation: The effect on symptoms associated with phantom limb syndrome. Anesth Analg 111(5):1308, 2010.

33. Silva, S, et al: Temporal analysis of regional anaesthesia-induced sensorimotor dysfunction: A model for understanding phantom limb. Br J Anaesth 105(2):208–213, 2010.

34. Mulvey, MR, et al: Transcutaneous electrical nerve stimulation (TENS) for phantom pain and stump pain following amputation in adults. Cochrane Database of Systematic Reviews 2010, Issue 5. Art. No.: CD007264. DOI: 10.1002/14651858.CD007264.pub2.

35. de Roos, C, et al: Treatment of chronic phantom limb pain using a trauma-focused psychological approach. Pain Res Manage 15(2):65–71, 2010.

36. May, BJ: Psychosocial issues. In May, BJ, and Lockard, MA: Prosthetics and Orthotics in Clinical Practice: A Case Study Approach. FA Davis, Philadelphia, 2011, p 39.

37. Gauthier-Cagnon, C, Grise, MC, and Potvin, D: Enabling factors related to prosthetic use by people with transtibial and transfemoral amputation. Arch Phys Med Rehabil 80(6):706–713, 1999.

38. Louie, WS, et al: Residual limb management for person with transtibial amputation: Comparison of bandaging technique and residual limb sock. JPO 22(3):194–201, 2010.

39. Dudek, NL, Marks, MB, and Marshall, SC: Skin problems in an amputee clinic. Am J Phys Med Rehabil 85:424–429, 2006.

40. Nadollek, H, Brauer, S, and Isles, R: Outcomes after trans-tibial amputation: The relationship between quiet stance ability, strength of hip abductor muscles and gait. Physiother Res Int 7:203, 2002.

41. Moirenfeld, I, et al: Isokinetic strength and endurance of the knee extensors and flexors in trans-tibial amputees. Prosthet Orthot Int 24:221, 2000.

42. Raya, MA, et al: Impairment variables predicting activity limitation in individuals with lower limb amputation. Prosthet Orthot Int 34(1):73–84, 2010.

43. Hlavackova, P, et al: Effects of mirror feedback on upright stance control in elderly transfemoral amputees. Arch Phys Med Rehabil 90(11):1960, 2009.

44. Corio, F, Troiano, R, and Magel, JR: The effects of spinal stabilization exercises on the spatial and temporal parameters of gait in individuals with lower limb loss. JPO 22(4):230–236, 2010.

45. Miller, WC, Speechley, M, and Deathe, AB: Balance confidence among people with lower-limb amputations. Phys Ther 82:856, 2002.

46. Miller, WC, et al: The influence of falling, fear of falling, and balance confidence on prosthetic mobility and social activity among individuals with a lower extremity amputation. Arch Phys Med Rehabil 82:1238, 2001.

47. Gailey, RS, et al: The amputee mobility predictor: An instrument to assess determinants of the lower limb amputee's ability to ambulate. Arch Phys Med Rehabil 83(5):613–627, 2002.

48. Miller, WC, Deathe, AB, and Speechley, M: Lower extremity prosthetic mobility: A comparison of 3 self report scales. Arch Phys Med Rehabil 82:1432–1440, 2001.

49. Fatiuk-Haight, ED (ed): Proceedings: Outcome measures in lower limb prosthetics. American Academy of Orthotists and Prosthetists, September 7–9, 2005.

50. May, BJ: Lower extremity prosthetic management. In May, BJ, and Lockard, MA: Prosthetics and Orthotics in Clinical Practice: A Case Study Approach. FA Davis, Philadelphia, 2011, p 105.

51. Hofstad, CJ, et al: Evidence for bilaterally delayed and decreased obstacle avoidance responses while walking with a lower limb prosthesis. Clin Neurophysiol 120(5):1009, 2009.

Supplemental Reading

May, BJ, and Lockard, MA: Prosthetics and Orthotics in Clinical Practice: A Case Study Approach. FA Davis, Philadelphia, 2011.

Smith, DG, Michael, JW, and Bowker, JH (eds): Atlas of Amputations and Limb Deficiencies: Surgical, Prosthetic, and Rehabilitation Principles, ed 3. American Academy of Orthopaedic Surgeons, Rosemont, IL, 2004.

Connects to multiple websites related to prosthesis or orthosis, including manufacturers.	www.oandp.com
Free prosthetic/orthotic-related articles and information.	www.oandp.com/edge
The website of the American Academy of Prosthetist and Orthotist and the *Journal of Prosthetics and Orthotics*. Free access to year-old journals.	www.oandp.org
Amputee Coalition of America. Largest organization for amputees, families, and clinicians.	www.amputee-coalition.org
Disabled Sports Organization. Has regional chapters as well.	www.dsusa.org
Website of the U.S. Paralympic team.	www.usparalympic.org
Website of the International Paralympic Organization.	www.paralympic.org
Website of the American Diabetes Association.	www.diabetes.org

Arthritis

Maura Daly Iversen, PT, DPT, SD, MPH

Marie D. Westby, PT, PhD **Chapter 23**

LEARNING OBJECTIVES

1. Describe the epidemiology, pathophysiology, disease course, and clinical manifestations of two common rheumatic diseases, rheumatoid arthritis and osteoarthritis, and be able to differentiate between these two conditions.

2. Identify the medical (clinical) diagnostic procedures commonly used in the examination of patients with arthritis, including laboratory tests and radiography.

3. Describe the medical management of individuals with rheumatoid arthritis and osteoarthritis.

4. Identify clinical examination and outcome measures commonly used in examining individuals with rheumatoid arthritis or osteoarthritis.

6. Discuss the rehabilitation management of individuals with arthritis.

7. Describe psychosocial, environmental, and other personal factors associated with arthritis that affect participation, achievement of anticipated goals, and expected outcomes.

8. Explain the importance of a team approach for persons with arthritis.

9. Analyze and interpret patient data, formulate realistic goals and outcomes, and develop a plan of care when presented with a clinical case study.

The terms *arthritis*, *rheumatism*, and *rheumatic disease* are generic references to an array of more than 100 diseases that are divided into 10 classification categories. Two major forms of arthritis are considered in this chapter. **Rheumatoid arthritis (RA)**, a systemic inflammatory disease, is considered in detail; **osteoarthritis (OA)**, a more localized process that has been known previously as **degenerative joint disease (DJD)**, is also discussed. Rheumatoid arthritis and osteoarthritis account for the majority of arthritis cases treated by physical therapists.

■ RHEUMATOID ARTHRITIS

RA is a major subclassification within the category of diffuse inflammatory connective tissue diseases that also includes juvenile arthritis, systemic lupus erythematosus (SLE), progressive systemic sclerosis or scleroderma, polymyositis, and dermatomyositis. Rheumatoid arthritis is primarily a disease of the **synovium**. The first clinical description of RA is attributed to A. J. Landre-Beauvais in 1800, although analysis of pictorial art of the late Renaissance suggests the existence of RA in earlier times. Early descriptions of patient symptomatology were complicated by the lack of uniform agreement about the distinguishing disease characteristics, given its wide spectrum of clinical presentations. The term *rheumatoid arthritis* was first used by Garrod in 1858, but was not accepted by the American Rheumatism Association (ARA) as the official terminology until 1941.[1] Diagnostic criteria and terminology have been developed and, in some cases, revised based on current data.[2,3]

Epidemiology

The estimated prevalence of RA among adults in the United States is approximately 1.3 million,[4] and prevalence increases with age. Women are effected two to four times more often than men. Differences in prevalence exist among certain subpopulations, which suggest a possible role for genetic or environmental factors in the etiology of the disease. For example, African Americans may have a lower prevalence of RA than whites, whereas several Native American groups demonstrate higher prevalence rates. There also is a lower prevalence of RA in native Japanese and native Chinese peoples compared to whites.[4,5]

Etiology

RA is an autoimmune disease of unknown complex etiology. RA is presently believed to have a genetic basis demonstrated by the increased disease risk and clustering in families.[6] Briefly, an **antigen** is a substance, usually foreign to the host, that provokes the immune system into action. The immune system may respond to the antigen directly (cellular immunity) or by the production of **antibodies** that circulate in the serum (humoral immunity). These responses involve two general types of lymphocytes: T cells, which are responsible for cellular immunity, and B cells, which produce circulating antibodies specific to the antigen. Antibodies are immunoglobulins, a type of serum protein.[1]

Given that individuals with RA produce antibodies to their own immunoglobulins, such as rheumatoid factor (RF) and anti–citrullinated protein antibody (ACPA), and these antibodies precede the clinical presentation of RA by years,[7,8] RA is considered an autoimmune disease.[9] It is not clear, however, whether this antibody production is a primary event or results as a response to a specific antigen from an external stimulus. Current theory and research on the cellular basis of autoimmunity suggest that aberrant functioning of cell-mediated immunity and defective T lymphocytes may trigger the autoimmune response that underlies RA.[9] A specific etiological agent for RA has not been identified, even though specific external agents may trigger disease expression.

The external agents that may initiate arthritis do so through various and differing mechanisms. For example, studies of smoking exposure suggest a strong association with tobacco smoke and manifestations of RA symptoms.[10] Bacterial organisms, including streptococcus, clostridia, diphtheroids, and mycoplasmas, have been suggested as triggers but no connections have been definitively proven. There has also been discussion of a viral etiology for RA. As with other investigations seeking to identify an etiology for RA, research remains speculative.[1]

Rheumatoid factors (RFs) are antibodies specific to immunoglobulin G (IgG) and are found in the sera of approximately 70% of all patients with RA. Current theory suggests that RFs arise as antibodies to "altered" autologous (the patient's own) IgG. Some modification of IgG changes its configuration and renders it an autoimmunogen, stimulating the production of RF. IgM is the first class of immunoglobulins formed after contact with an antigen and most RFs are of this class, although RFs may be of any immunoglobulin class.[1] The exact biological role of RF is unknown. Although RF has been implicated in the pathogenesis of RA, the disease occurs in the absence of RF in a substantial number of individuals.[10] Research indicates that the presence of RF affects disease severity, because those who have RF, or seropositive disease, have increased frequency of subcutaneous nodules, vasculitis, and polyarticular involvement.[1]

Ollier and Worthington[6] examined the literature investigating a genetic predisposition to the development of RA.[6] Human leukocyte antigens (HLAs) found on the surface of most human cells are capable of generating an **immune response** when genetically incompatible tissues are grafted to each other, for example, during organ transplants. Genes controlling these HLAs are found on the sixth chromosome. Four loci have been described: HLA-A, HLA-B, HLA-C, and HLA-D. RA has been associated with increased HLA-D and HLA-DR (D-related) antigens, suggesting that certain genes determine whether a host is more or less at risk for an immunological response that leads to RA.[6] A "rheumatoid **epitope**" has been identified through DNA typing of HLA-DR4 as a particular sequence of amino acids common among patients with RA.[11] A recent national case-control study conducted in Sweden focused on citrulline-modified proteins, proteins not normally present in healthy adults but found in about two-thirds of patients with RA, to determine if smoking and the presence of shared epitope (SE) HLA genes triggered RA. The investigators concluded that the interaction of smoking and carrying two copies of the SE gene increases the risk of developing RA by 21-fold.[12] Further studies of genomic organization of the HLA-D region specifically implicate a short sequence on the HLA-DRB1 gene and suggest that HLA-DRB1 alleles (alternate forms of a gene) modify disease expression and progression.[1] Various studies of different ethnic groups have also shown that particular variations of the HLA-DRB1 allele are overrepresented in people with RA.[1]

Pathophysiology

In early RA, synovial inflammation leads to pain, stiffness, and restricted range of motion (ROM). As the disease progresses, the joint capsule becomes inflamed and immune cells degrade the cartilage. With long-standing RA the synovium appears grossly edematous with slender villous or hair-like projections into the joint cavity (Fig. 23.1). Distinctive vascular changes, including venous distention, capillary obstruction, neutrophilic infiltration of the arterial walls, and areas of thrombosis and hemorrhage, may be evident. Synovial proliferation of vascular granulation tissue, known as **pannus**, dissolves collagen as it extends over the joint cartilage. Eventually, with disease progression, the granulation tissue leads to adhesions, **fibrosis,** or bony **ankylosis** of the joint. Chronic inflammation associated with RA weakens the joint capsule and its supporting ligamentous structures, altering joint structure and function. Tendon rupture and fraying tendon sheaths produce imbalanced muscle pull on pathologically altered joints resulting in the characteristic musculoskeletal deformities seen in advanced RA.[13]

Following alterations in blood flow, rapid changes in the cellular content and volume of the synovial fluid may result owing to low pressure in the joint space and the lack of a limiting membrane between the joint space and synovial blood vessels. High-molecular-weight substances such as macroglobulins and fibrinogens can pass through the synovial capillaries during periods of inflammation and are not easily cleared.[1] Antigen-antibody complexes may be isolated within the joint cavity and stimulate phagocytosis and further development of pannus. Although sustained **synovitis** requires the proliferation of new blood vessels, the exact mechanism of capillary growth is not understood. One hypothesis suggests that activated macrophages, responding to antigen-antibody complexes, may stimulate this development. With established synovitis, polymorphonuclear (PMN) leukocytes are drawn into the joint cavity and coupled with lysosomal enzyme activity contribute to destruction of synovial tissues.[9]

Laboratory Tests

Sensitivity and specificity are two concepts of testing that are useful in explaining the value of laboratory tests in the detection of RA. Test *sensitivity* is the proportion of truly diseased individuals who have tested positive. The clinical value of sensitive tests is particularly important when a misdiagnosis (informing the patient that he or she does not have the disease when in fact the patient does have RA) would be deleterious to the health of the patient. In research terms, sensitivity is equivalent to the laboratory test's ability to avoid a false-negative result. *Specificity,* on the other hand, refers to the proportion of truly nondiseased individuals who have a negative test. In other words, the specificity of a laboratory test is a measure of its ability to avoid false positives. A diagnostician usually uses a combination of sensitive and specific tests to confirm clinical impressions during the diagnostic process.

Elevated *erythrocyte sedimentation rate (ESR)* and *C-reactive protein (CRP)* are acute phase reactants that indicate the presence of active inflammation. Although patients with RA characteristically have active inflammation, up to 40% may have normal values for these tests despite clinical evidence of inflammation. Normal ESR and CRP values are nonspecific and alone cannot confirm or refute a diagnosis of RA. RF is the result of the binding of two immunoglobulins. The presence or absence of RF alone neither confirms nor rules out a diagnosis of RA. Nearly 25% of people with RA do not have a positive RF (seronegative RA), whereas a positive RF is seen in a number of other immunologic conditions (e.g., leprosy, tuberculosis, chronic hepatitis) and occasionally in individuals with no disease. A positive RF in combination with clinical criteria may help to confirm a clinical impression.

A *complete blood count (CBC)* is routinely ordered because a number of findings are commonly associated with RA. Red blood cell counts are often decreased, indicating the anemia of chronic disease found in approximately 20% of individuals with RA. By comparison, the white blood cell count is generally normal. *Thrombocytosis,* a high platelet count, is not uncommon in active RA.

Synovial fluid analysis can greatly enhance the process of differential diagnosis. Normal synovial fluid is transparent, yellowish, viscous, and without clots. Synovial fluid from inflamed joints is cloudy, less viscous owing to a change in hyaluronate proteins, and will clot. Significant

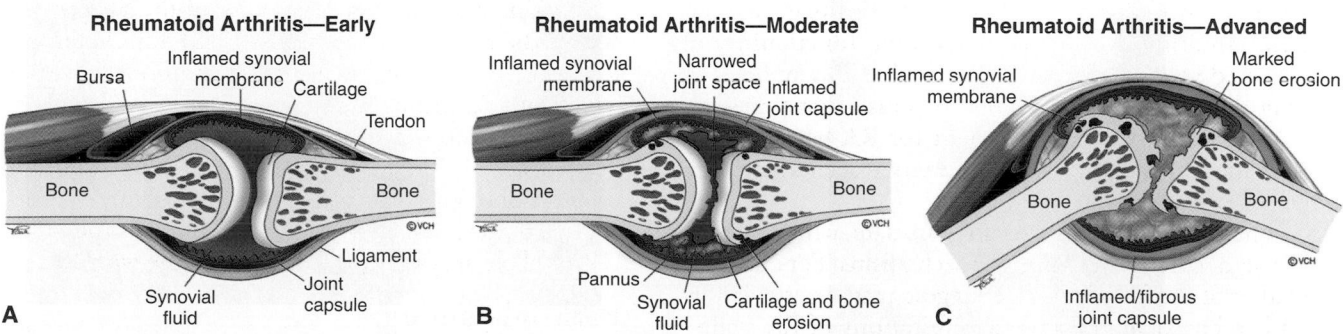

Figure 23.1 Progression of joint changes due to RA inflammation: Early to advanced disease.
From Mary Pack Arthritis Program, Vancouver Coastal Health, with permission.

inflammation also increases the number of fluid proteins. A culture can be performed to identify potential bacterial agents as the cause of joint inflammation. If the joint is inflamed, white blood cells will elevated in the fluid. Crystals are not common. If present they may confirm the diagnosis of **gout** (urate crystals) or *pseudogout* (calcium pyrophosphate crystals). A mucin clot test (a measure of viscosity) of the synovial fluid can be used to discriminate between acute infectious arthritis and inflammatory arthritis, such as RA. Poor clotting accompanies acute infectious arthritis whereas RA produces fair mucin clotting.[1]

Radiography

Radiographic study is essential in a diagnostic workup for RA. Physical therapists practicing in rheumatology should develop a basic proficiency in identifying abnormalities in joint structure and the surrounding soft tissues as these abnormalities influence the course and outcome of rehabilitation. To identify radiographic abnormalities, the therapist must be able to describe how a normal joint appears on a radiograph. Therapists can orient themselves to a radiograph by considering several parameters: alignment, bone density and surface, and cartilaginous spacing (Figs. 23.2 and 23.3). Normal alignment is present when the long axes of the proximal and distal bones of the joint are in their normal spatial relationships and the convex surface of one bone fits well with the concavity of the other. Bone density, in the absence of **osteoporosis**, should be somewhat opaque and milky and appear evenly distributed throughout. The cortices of each bone should be distinct, appropriately thick, and well defined. The joint soft tissues should conform to known anatomical shape. Soft tissue swelling and evidence of uneven spacing between joint surfaces on radiograph may suggest activity limitations. Uneven, reduced, or absent spacing suggests joint cartilage loss or joint surface erosion. A normal joint surface should be smooth and conform to known anatomical shape without osteophytes. RA progression can be characterized in four sequential stages using periodic radiographic examination (Box 23.1). Radiographic changes evident in early RA are nonspecific and usually limited to soft tissue swelling, joint effusion, and periarticular demineralization. Diagnostic confirmation is made when the disease process leads to bilateral joint space narrowing and erosions in the hands and feet.[1]

Classification and Diagnostic Criteria

The differential diagnosis of RA is predicated on the history, clinical examination of signs and symptoms, and careful exclusion of other disorders. The American College of Rheumatology (ACR) classification criteria,[2] developed using data from patients in outpatient clinics, are commonly used to confirm whether an individual's clinical presentation should be confirmed as a case of RA. Originally these criteria had four classifications of RA: classical, definite, probable, and possible. Some of these classifications were judged to be problematic. The 1987 revised criteria are presented in Table 23.1. In 2010 the ACR and the European League Against Rheumatism (EULAR) revised the 1987 classification criteria for RA[2] to help identify early RA. These criteria are based on a combination of signs, symptoms, and laboratory findings that have persisted for a specified period of time.[3] A diagnosis of definite RA is now established on the confirmed presence of synovitis in at least one joint, absence of an alternative diagnosis that better explains the synovitis, and a total score of 6 or greater (out of a possible 10) from four domains (Table 23.2). The domains are (1)*Joint Involvement,* designating the number and site of involved joints (score range 0–5); (2)*Serology,* indicating serologic abnormalities (score range 0–3);

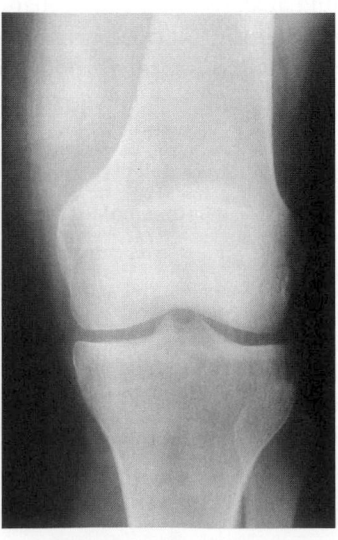

Figure 23.2 Frontal view of the normal knee. *From the American College of Rheumatology, with permission.*

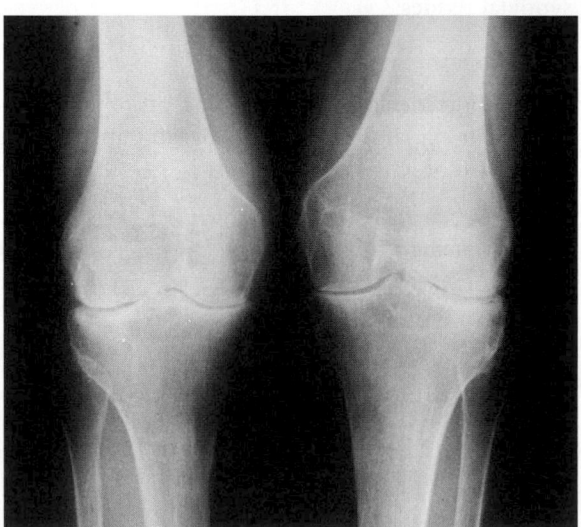

Figure 23.3 Frontal view of the knee with characteristics of rheumatoid arthritis. *From the American College of Rheumatology, with permission.*

Box 23.1   Classification of Progression of Rheumatoid Arthritis

Stage I, Early

1. No destructive changes on radiographic examination.[a]
2. Radiographic evidence of osteoporosis may be present.

Stage II, Moderate

1. Radiographic evidence of osteoporosis, with or without slight subchondral bone destruction; slight cartilage destruction may be present.[a]
2. No joint deformities, although limitation of joint mobility may be present.[a]
3. Adjacent muscle atrophy.
4. Extra-articular soft tissue lesions, such as nodules and tenosynovitis, may be present.

Stage III, Severe

1. Radiographic evidence of cartilage and bone destruction, in addition to osteoporosis.[a]
2. Joint deformity, such as subluxation, ulnar deviation, or hyperextension, without fibrous or bony ankylosis.[a]
3. Extensive muscle atrophy.
4. Extra-articular soft tissue lesions, such as nodules and tenosynovitis, may be present.

Stage IV, Terminal

1. Fibrous or bony ankylosis[a]
2. Criteria of stage III

From Schumacher, Klippel, and Robinson (eds): Primer on Rheumatic Diseases, ed 9. Arthritis Foundation, Atlanta, 1988, p 318, with permission.
[a]These criteria must be present to permit classification of a patient in any particular stage or grade.

(3)*Acute-Phase Reactants,* describing elevated acute-phase response (score range 0–1); and (4)*Duration of Symptom* (2 levels; range 0–1).[3] The inclusion of criteria for early RA may help rheumatologists to target treatment at earlier stages of the disease and decrease RA progression.

Patients with RA can also be classified based on global functional status criteria.[14] There are four functional classifications based on a person's ability to complete functional and self-care activities ranging from independence to full dependence. In addition to their clinical relevance, these functional classifications enable clinicians and researchers to classify subjects in clinical trials and inform evidence-based clinical recommendations for therapies(Table 23.3).

Disease Onset and Course

RA is commonly characterized by an exacerbating and remitting disease course. Disease onset is accompanied by complaints of generalized joint pain and stiffness, usually in multiple small joints (**polyarthritis**) though it may be localized to a single joint. Symptoms may appear spontaneously or over a prolonged period of time. Disease progression is highly variable. High titers of RF indicate a more severe disease course. Spontaneous remissions can occur. Some patients experience an intermittent course, characterized by partial to complete remissions longer than the periods of exacerbations. A third group of patients experience the full unremitting destructive process of progressive RA.[1] Comparisons of elderly-onset RA with early-onset RA revealed that abrupt onset and large joint involvement, particularly of the shoulder girdle, were more common in the older adults. The elderly-onset

Table 23.1	The 1987 Revised Criteria for the Classification of Rheumatoid Arthritis[a]
Criterion	**Definition**
1. Morning stiffness	Morning stiffness in and around the joints, lasting at least one hour before maximal improvement.
2. Arthritis of three or more joint areas	At least three joint areas simultaneously have had soft tissue swelling or fluid (not bony overgrowth alone) observed by a physician. The 14 possible areas are right or left PIP, MCP, wrist, elbow, knee, ankle, and MTP joints.
3. Arthritis of hand joints	At least one area swollen (as defined above) in a wrist, MCP, or PIP joint.
4. Symmetrical arthritis	Simultaneous involvement of the same joint areas (as defined in 2) on both sides of the body (bilateral involvement of PIPs, MCPs, or MTPs is acceptable without absolute symmetry).
5. Rheumatoid nodules	Subcutaneous nodules, over bony prominences, or extensor surfaces, or in juxta-articular regions, observed by a physician.
6. Serum rheumatoid factor	Demonstration of abnormal amounts of serum rheumatoid factor by any method for which the result has been positive in <5% of normal control subjects.
7. Radiographic changes	Radiographic changes typical of rheumatoid arthritis on posteroanterior hand and wrist radiographs, which must include erosions or unequivocal bony decalcification localized in or most marked adjacent to the involved joints (osteoarthritis changes alone do not qualify).

From Arnett et al,[2, p. 319] with permission.
[a]For classification purposes, a patient shall be said to have rheumatoid arthritis if he or she has satisfied at least four of these seven criteria. Criteria 1 through 4 must have been present for at least 6 weeks. Patients with two clinical diagnoses are not excluded. Designation as classic, definite, or probable rheumatoid arthritis is *not* to be made.

Table 23.2 The 2010 American College of Rheumatology/European League Against Rheumatism Classification Criteria for Rheumatoid Arthritis

Target population (Who should be tested?): Patients who
1. have at least 1 joint with definite clinical synovitis (swelling)*
2. with the synovitis not better explained by another disease.[†]

Classification criteria for RA (score-based algorithm: add score of categories A–D; a score of 6/10 is needed for classification of a patient as having definite RA)[‡]

	Score
A. Joint involvement[§]	
1 large joint[¶]	0
2–10 large joints	1
1–3 small joints (with or without involvement of large joints)[#]	2
4–10 small joints (with or without involvement of large joints)	3
> 10 joints (at least 1 small joint)**	5
B. Serology (at least 1 test result is needed for classification)[††]	
Negative RF and negative ACPA	0
Low-positive RF or low-positive ACPA	2
High-positive RF or high-positive ACPA	3
C. Acute-phase reactants (at least 1 test result is needed for classification)[‡‡]	
Normal CRP and normal ESR	0
Abnormal CRP or abnormal ESR	1
D. Duration of symptoms[§§]	
< 6 weeks	0
≥ 6 weeks	1

*The criteria are aimed at classification of newly presenting patients. In addition, patients with erosive disease typical of rheumatoid arthritis (RA) with a history compatible with prior fulfillment of the 2010 criteria should be classified as having RA. Patients with long-standing disease, including those whose disease is inactive (with or without treatment) who, based on retrospectively available data, have previously fulfilled the 2010 criteria should be classified as having RA.

[†]Differential diagnoses vary among patients with different presentations, but may include conditions such as systemic lupus erythematosus, psoriatic arthritis, and gout. If it is unclear about the relevant differential diagnoses to consider, an expert rheumatologist should be consulted.

[‡]Although patients with a score of 6/10 are not classifiable as having RA, their status can be reassessed and the criteria might be fulfilled cumulatively over time.

[§]Joint involvement refers to any swollen or tender joint on examination, which may be confirmed by imaging evidence of synovitis. Distal interphalangeal joints, first carpometacarpal joints, and first metatarsophalangeal joints are excluded from assessment. Categories of joint distribution are classified according to the location and number of involved joints, with placement into the highest category possible based on the pattern of joint involvement.

[¶]"Large joints" refers to shoulders, elbows, hips, knees, and ankles.

[#]"Small joints" refers to the metacarpophalangeal joints, proximal interphalangeal joints, second through fifth metatarsophalangeal joints, thumb interphalangeal joints, and wrists.

**In this category, at least 1 of the involved joints must be a small joint; the other joints can include any combination of large and additional small joints, as well as other joints not specifically listed elsewhere (e.g., temporomandibular, acromioclavicular, sternoclavicular, and so forth).

[††]Negative refers to IU values that are less than or equal to the upper limit of normal (ULN) for the laboratory and assay; low-positive refers to IU values that are higher than the ULN but 3 times the ULN for the laboratory and assay; high-positive refers to IU values that are 3 times the ULN for the laboratory and assay. Where rheumatoid factor (RF) information is only available as positive or negative, a positive result should be scored as low-positive for RF. ACPA = anti–citrullinated protein antibody.

[‡‡]Normal/abnormal is determined by local laboratory standards. CRP = C-reactive protein; ESR = erythrocyte sedimentation rate.

[§§]Duration of symptoms refers to patient self-report of the duration of signs or symptoms of synovitis (e.g., pain, swelling, tenderness) of joints that are clinically involved at the time of assessment, regardless of treatment status.

Aletaha, D, Neogi, T, Silman, AJ, et al: Rheumatoid arthritis classification criteria. Arthritis Rheum 62:2569–2581, 2010, with permission.

Table 23.3	American College of Rheumatology Revised Criteria for Classification of Functional Status in Rheumatoid Arthritis*a*	
Class I	Completely able to perform usual activities of daily living (self-care, vocational, and avocational)
Class II	Able to perform usual self-care and vocational activities, but limited in avocational activities
Class III	Able to perform usual self-care activities, but limited in vocational and avocational activities
Class IV	Limited in ability to perform usual self-care, vocational, and avocational activities

From Hochberg, MC, et al: The American College of Rheumatology 1991 revised criteria for the classification of global functional status in rheumatoid arthritis. Arthritis Rheum 35:498, 1992, with permission.
*a*Usual self-care activities include dressing, feeding, bathing, grooming, and toileting. Avocational (recreational and/or leisure) and vocational (work, school, homemaking) activities are patient-desired and age- and sex-specific.

group demonstrated clinical features more commonly associated with *polymyalgia rheumatica,* a separate and distinct disease affecting the shoulder and pelvic musculature leading to muscle inflammation.[15]

Clinical Presentation

Systemic

Systemic features of RA include weight loss, fever, and extreme fatigue. Fatigue greatly affects function and participation in daily life and is often underappreciated on physical examination.[16] A hallmark clinical feature of RA is *morning stiffness* in and around the joints lasting at least 1 hour before maximal improvement.[3] In contrast, OA-induced stiffness results from inactivity. Morning stiffness can be qualified in terms of its severity and duration, both of which are directly related to the degree of disease activity.

Joint Impairments (Articular and Nonarticular)

RA is characterized by bilateral and symmetrical synovial joint involvement. Clinically, patients present with limited mobility and signs of inflammation including pain, redness, swelling, and warm joints. The most common joints involved are the hands, feet, and cervical spine with the hands generally affected early in the disease course.[16] The term **arthralgia** refers to joint pain. The joint examination may reveal **crepitus**, an audible or palpable grating or crunching evident as the joint is moved through its ROM. Crepitus is the result of uneven degeneration of the joint surface.

Cervical Spine and Temporomandibular Joint

The cervical spine is often involved in RA and on examination ROM may be limited in all planes. The occipitoatlantal (occiput–C1) and atlantoaxial (C1–C2) joints are frequently affected due to their extensive synovial tissue. The midcervical region is also a common site of inflammation, leading to decreased ROM, particularly in rotation, accompanied by instability. Three patterns of cervical spine involvement are described: atlantoaxial subluxation (65%), atlantoaxial impaction (20% to 25%), and subaxial subluxation (10% to 15%).[17] Involvement of the C1 and C2 vertebrae may produce life-threatening situations

if the transverse ligament of the atlas should rupture or if the odontoid process should fracture or herniate through the foramen magnum, compressing the upper cervical cord. Patients presenting with cervical radiculopathy and neurological signs should be immediately referred to a physician. Magnetic resonance imaging (MRI) is the most effective tool to visualize both the spinal column and the cord.[17] **Ankylosing** (i.e., fusion) of one or more vertebrae of the spine may accompany RA and can lead to loss of ROM and function of the involved joints.

The temporomandibular joint (TMJ) is usually among the last joints involved. Inflammation of the TMJ results in pain, swelling, and limited movement and eventually to ankylosis. With juvenile RA involvement of the TMJ can lead to destruction of the condyle and potential alterations in mandibular growth and facial deformity. With early disease, TMJ x-rays are usually negative but with time and chronic inflammation can demonstrate bone destruction, which may affect the child's ability to open the mouth fully (approximately 2 in [5.08 cm]) with normal side-to-side gliding and protrusion. In resting position, the normal approximation of the upper and lower teeth may be altered following persistent inflammation.[18]

Shoulders and Elbows

Shoulder involvement may be evident in the glenohumeral, sternoclavicular, or acromioclavicular joints leading to joint surface degeneration, pain, and loss of ROM. Shoulder pain is often referred to the deltoid region. The scapulothoracic articulation may secondarily exhibit a loss of ROM as well. Chronic shoulder inflammation causes the capsule and the ligaments to become distended and thinned. As joint surfaces erode, the shoulder eventually becomes unstable. In addition, **tendinitis** and **bursitis** may complicate management.[18] Typical elbow joint findings include effusions between the lateral epicondyle and olecranon prominence, bilateral swelling of the olecranon bursa (more prevalent with severe disease), and rheumatoid nodules on the olecranon or extensor surface of the proximal ulna.[17] Inflammation, capsular and ligamentous distention, and joint erosion may lead to instability and irregular or catching movements. Flexion contractures frequently develop, due to patient posturing to reduce pain and persistent spasm.

Wrists

Early synovitis among the carpal bones and the ulna leads to a fairly rapid development of a flexion contracture, which ultimately diminishes the individual's ability to grasp. Additionally, **carpal tunnel syndrome** may occur due to compression of the median nerve in the carpal tunnel. Chronic inflammation around the ulnar styloid coupled with laxity of the radioulnar ligament produces the *piano key sign* on examination. The piano key sign is defined as an up and down movement of the styloid in response to point pressure from the examiner. Over time ulnar deviation or drift may occur from chronic inflammation causing movement of the wrist toward the ulna (Fig. 23.4). Chronic inflammation of the proximal row of carpals can lead to a volar **subluxation** of the wrist and hand on the radius, accentuating the normal 10° to 15° of volar inclination of the carpus on the distal radius (Fig. 23.5). In addition, radial deviation of the distal carpals can occur due to loss of radial ligamentous support, destruction of the extensor carpi ulnaris and the fibrocartilage on the distal side of the ulna. This allows the proximal carpals to slide down the distal radius toward the ulna, contributing to radial deviation of the distal row of carpals relative to the two bones of the forearm, where normally there is 5° to 10° of ulnar deviation.[19] Stenosing tenosynovitis of the first dorsal compartment of the wrist (*deQuervain's disease*) may also occur.

Hand Joints

Metacarpophalangeal Soft-tissue swelling around the metacarpophalangeal (MCP) joints, especially the index and long fingers, is common. The volar subluxation and **ulnar drift** of the MCPs frequently seen in RA results from exaggeration of the joints' normal structural shape that tilt the proximal phalanges in an ulnar direction.

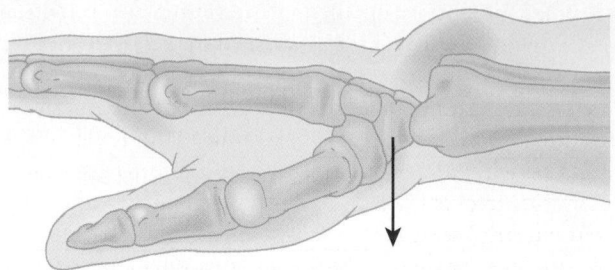

Figure 23.5 Volar subluxation of the wrist seen with rheumatoid arthritis. The chronic inflammation of the proximal carpals can eventually lead to a volar subluxation of the wrist and hand on the radius, accentuating the normal 10° to 15° of volar inclination of the carpus on the distal radius.

The anatomical placement and length of the collateral ligaments, which are most stretched during MCP flexion, and the insertions of the intrinsics, which also pull from an ulnar direction, contribute to ulnar drift at the MCPs during hand motion. Weakened ligaments cannot resist a pull toward volar subluxation during power pinch or grasp when flexor tendons bowstring across MCPs through frayed tendon sheaths damaged by long-term synovitis. The *bowstring effect* results from moving the fulcrum of the flexor tendons distally, placing an ulnar and volar pull on the proximal phalanges (Fig. 23.6). Radial deviation of the carpals further enhances MCP ulnar drift as the phalanges try to compensate for the loss of normal ulnar deviation at the wrist. This is known as the *zigzag effect,* where forces in the hand try to move the index finger back into its normal functional position in line with the radius. A **trigger finger** may be evident whereby a snapping sensation is

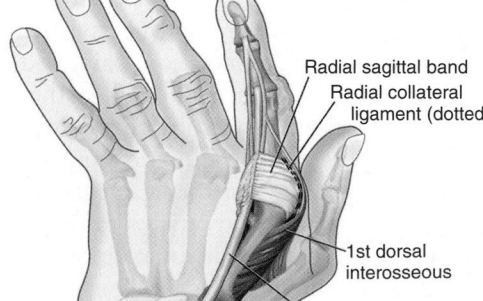

Ulnar Drift Deformity

Radial sagittal band
Radial collateral ligament (dotted)
1st dorsal interosseous
Extensor tendon
©VCH

Figure 23.4 Ulnar drift (deviation) of the fingers. This drawing depicts the impact of metacarpophalangeal joint swelling, soft tissue laxity due to synovitis, which leads to ulnar deviation of the fingers in RA.

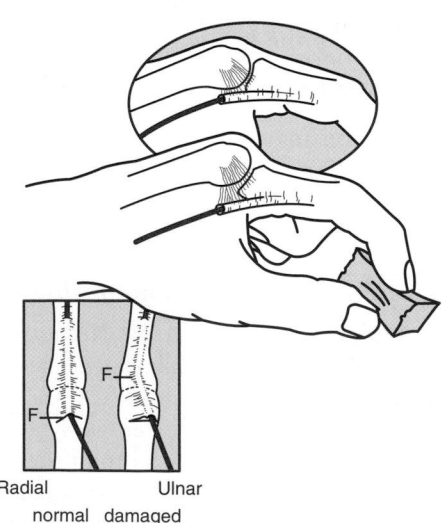

Radial   Ulnar
normal   damaged

Figure 23.6 Influence of the long flexors (F) in metacarpophalangeal drift deformity. *Adapted from Melvin,[19, p. 283] with permission.*

felt when flexing or extending the finger due to flexor tenosynovitis and resultant slippage of the tendon, friction with movement, or presence of tendon nodules.[17,20]

Proximal Interphalangeal Swelling of the proximal interphalangeal (PIP) joints is common and is easily appreciated with lateral joint palpation. There are two characteristic irreversible deformities (if not surgically repaired early) seen at the PIPs in individuals with severe RA. The first of these is known as **swan neck deformity** and consists of PIP hyperextension and distal interphalangeal (DIP) flexion (Fig. 23.7). Swan neck deformities arise in three distinct ways, depending on the site of initial involvement. Most commonly, swan neck deformity follows from initial synovitis of the MCP, where the pain of chronic synovitis leads to reflex muscle spasm of the intrinsics. The biomechanical force of the intrinsics then combines with the hypermobility found in the chronically inflamed and structurally changed PIP, resulting in volar subluxation and PIP hyperextension. Swan neck deformity may also result when the volar capsule of the PIP is stretched, the lateral bands move dorsally, and tension is placed on the flexor digitorum profundis by the PIP flexes the DIP. In these instances, a rupture of the flexor digitorum sublimus further predisposes an individual to swan neck deformity. A third mechanism for developing swan neck deformity involves a rupture of the extensor digitorum communis at its insertion on the DIP resulting in DIP flexion and PIP hyperextension owing to unrestrained pull by the flexor digitorum profundis.[17,19]

The other characteristic deformity of the PIP is known as a ***boutonniere deformity*** and consists of DIP extension with PIP flexion (Fig. 23.8). As a result of chronic synovitis, the insertion of extensor digitorum communis into the middle phalanx (known as the central slip) lengthens, and the lateral bands slide volarly to force the PIP into flexion. Bony formation or outgrowths around the end of a joint are termed ***osteophytes***. Those found at the PIP are known as ***Bouchard's nodes***, and may be seen in OA. They are unrelated to RA, although an individual may

Swan Neck Deformity

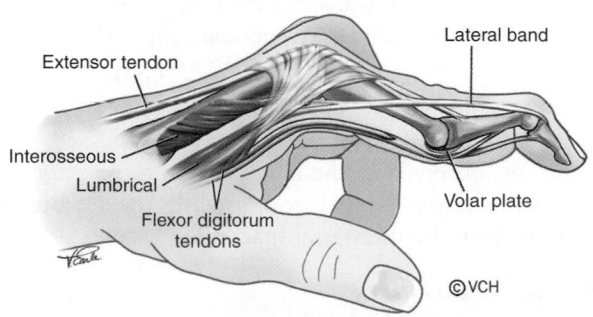

Figure 23.7 Swan neck deformity is characterized by PIP hyperextension and DIP flexion. *From Mary Pack Arthritis Program, Vancouver Coastal Health, with permission.*

Boutonniere Deformity

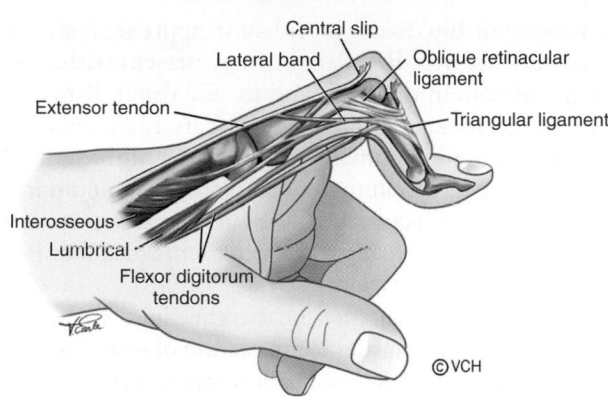

Figure 23.8 Features of a boutonniere deformity include DIP extension with PIP flexion. *From Mary Pack Arthritis Program, Vancouver Coastal Health, with permission.*

have both kinds of arthritis at the same time.[17,20]

Distal Interphalangeal The distal interphalangeal (DIP) joints are rarely affected in RA. Osteophytes are, however, common in OA and are called ***Heberden's nodes***. Occasionally, a ***mallet finger*** deformity will result from rupture of the tendon of the extensor digitorum communis, pulling the DIP into flexion as force from the flexor digitorum profundis is unopposed.[20]

Thumb A number of deformities can occur in the thumb due to synovitis. The most prevalent is a **flail IP** in which the patient loses the ability to flex the interphalangeal (IP) joint. The fibers of the dorsal hood mechanism over the MCP, the joint capsule and the collateral ligaments, and the tendons of extensor pollicis brevis and extensor pollicis longus are particularly affected. The exact mechanism of thumb deformities depends on the particular combination of affected structures. Similar to other hand deformities, the actual presentation depends on the site of initial synovitis, the direction of imbalanced muscle forces, and the integrity of the surrounding joint structures. A *type I deformity*, consisting of MCP flexion with IP hyperextension without involvement of the carpometacarpal (CMC) joint, is most commonly seen. *Type II deformity* is assigned when the CMC is subluxed and the IP is held in hyperextension. CMC subluxation and MCP hyperextension is classified as a *type III deformity*, and is more common in RA than a type II deformity.[17-20]

Mutilans Deformity (Opera-Glass Hand) Grossly unstable thumbs and severely deformed phalanges are indicative of *mutilans-type deformity*. Also known as opera-glass hand, the transverse folds of the skin of the thumb and fingers resemble a folded telescope. Radiographic study of the bones of the hand reveal severe bone resorption, erosion, and shortening of the MCP, PIP, radiocarpal, and radioulnar joints especially. The negative impact of this deformity on hand function and activities of daily living (ADL) is significant.[20]

Hips and Knees

Radiographic hip disease is evident in approximately half of all patients with RA. Patients may present with complaints of pain in the groin and medial thigh. Pain over the greater trochanter often is secondary to trochanteric bursitis. Severe inflammatory destruction of the femoral head and the acetabulum may push the acetabulum into the pelvic cavity, a condition known as *protrusio acetabuli*. With progressive hip disease, patients may require a total hip **arthroplasty**.[17]

The clinical presentation of the knee joint frequently includes synovitis, causing accumulation of relatively large amounts of fluid. The knee ballottement test is used to examine for excess fluid. The examiner presses on the patella with the index finger, resulting in a downward motion of the patella; a sensation of bogginess indicates effusion of the knee. Posterior accumulation of fluid in the knee produces a *Baker's cyst*. If a Baker's cyst ruptures it produces pain, swelling, and heat in the posterior calf similar to symptoms of a deep vein thrombosis. The bulge test is a simple procedure to examine for anterior synovitis. With this procedure the examiner strokes the medial aspect of the knee in an upward motion, then presses on the lateral aspect of the knee. A positive sign is a *wavelike* movement of fluid medially. Chronic synovitis results in distention of the joint capsule, attenuation of the collateral and cruciate ligaments, and destruction of the joint surfaces. Painful knees may be held in slightly flexed positions, ultimately resulting joint tightness or flexion contractures.[17]

Ankles and Feet

Early inflammation of the feet is often evident in the forefoot where patients note pain with compression of the forefoot on examination. Chronic synovitis accentuates the natural tendency of the talus to glide medially and plantarward, resulting in pressure on the calcaneus and leading to hindfoot pronation. The spring ligament is also stretched by these occurrences, flattening the medial longitudinal arch (Fig. 23.9). The calcaneus may erode or develop bony **exostoses** known as spurs. As synovitis weakens the transverse arch, the metatarsals spread and a splayed forefoot (*splayfoot*) may develop (Fig. 23.10). Instability of the talocalcaneal joint, if severe, can lead to the need for surgical fusion. Synovitis of the metatarsophalangeal (MTP) joints is extremely common and *metatarsalgia* (pain over the metatarsal heads) may develop. A *hallux valgus* and **bunion** (a painful bursitis over the medial aspect of the first MTP joint) may also be present. When volar subluxation of the MTP combines with flexion of the PIP and hyperextension of the DIP joints, this condition is commonly referred to as **hammer toes** (Fig. 23.11). The MTPs may also exhibit volar subluxation of the metatarsal head with flexion of the PIP and DIP joints, known as *cock-up* or *claw toes* (Fig. 23.12). As the capsule and intertarsal ligaments are weakened and stretched, the proximal phalanges move dorsally on the metatarsal head (Fig. 23.13). Similar to

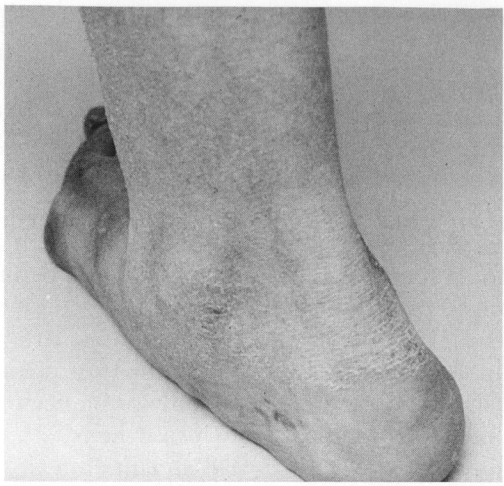

Figure 23.9 Posterior–medial view of the foot and ankle showing calcaneal valgus, pes planus (flatfoot), and hallux valgus. *Used by permission of the Arthritis Foundation.*

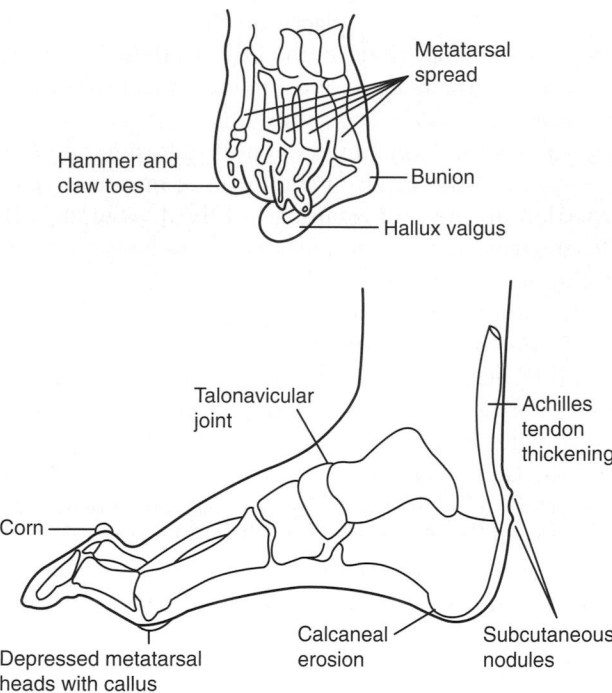

Figure 23.10 Major foot and ankle deformities seen in rheumatoid arthritis. *From Dimonte and Light,[94, p. 1149] with permission.*

conditions observed in the hand, the long toe extensors "bowstring" over the PIP joints while the flexors are displaced into the intertarsal spaces.[17]

Muscle Involvement

Muscle atrophy around affected joints may be present early. It is not definitively known, however, whether this atrophy results from disuse or selective attrition of muscles owing to some unknown mechanism specifically related to the disease process. Atrophy in the hand intrinsics and the quadriceps is particularly evident in long-standing disease, although the mechanisms for these changes may not be the same. It appears that individuals with RA experience selective attrition of Type II (phasic) muscle fibers through some unknown mechanism.[21,22] There is also some evidence that Type I (tonic) muscle fibers of the quadriceps will undergo selective atrophy following anterior cruciate ligament damage.[23] Loss of muscle bulk may also be the result of a peripheral neuropathy, **myositis**, or steroid-induced myopathy. Muscle weakness may be due to either reflex inhibition secondary to pain or atrophy.[21-23]

Tendon Involvement

Tenosynovitis, inflammation of the lining of the sheath that surrounds a tendon, may occur with active disease and interferes with the smooth gliding of the tendon through the sheath. Inflammation may directly damage the tendon, eventually leading to a tendon rupture. Common sites of tenosynovitis are wrist flexors, thumb flexors, patella, and Achilles tendons. Trigger finger and *deQuervain's disease* may occur. A patient with tendon damage or muscle weakness may exhibit a *lag phenomenon,* which refers to a substantial difference in passive versus active ROM. This is a nonspecific finding that therapists need to examine carefully to determine its cause and design appropriate treatment.[20]

Deconditioning

Deconditioning is a significant clinical feature of RA. Research assessing physical fitness in persons with RA has demonstrated diminished cardiorespiratory status, muscular strength and endurance, flexibility, and altered body composition among these individuals when compared with healthy individuals of the same age and gender without arthritis. Deconditioning results from both direct and indirect impairments.[24,25] Direct impairments of RA include loss of Type II muscle fibers, systemic fatigue, *cachexia* (wasting of lean body mass),[25] and shortening of contractile tissues. Indirect impairments of RA include deconditioning secondary to inactivity and elevated resting energy expenditure (calories required by the body during a 24-hour period under resting conditions). Immune system activity and inflammation, even in individuals with well-controlled disease, create an increased metabolism with subsequent loss of lean body tissue.[25]

Rheumatoid Nodules

Rheumatoid nodules occur in approximately 20% to 25% of patients and are associated with a positive serological test for RF. Nodules are generally tender and accompany severe disease. When nodules are present in early RA they are suggestive for a greater likelihood of severe **extra-articular** manifestations. Nodules are found in the subcutaneous or deeper connective tissues in areas

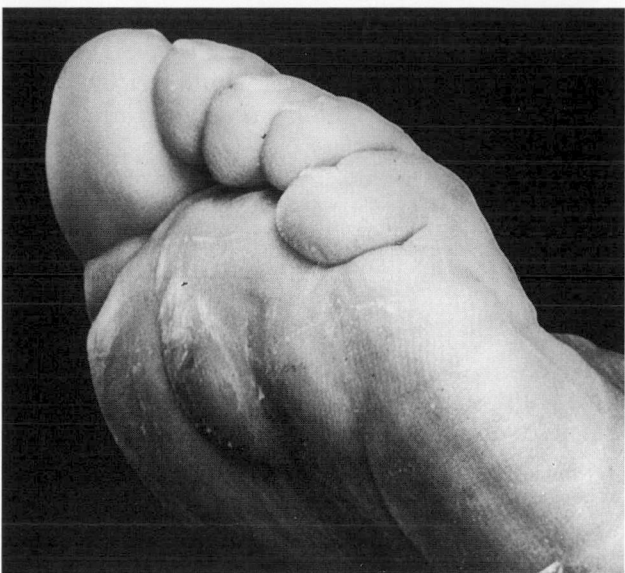

Figure 23.11 Metatarsophalangeal subluxation. *Used by permission of the American College of Rheumatology.*

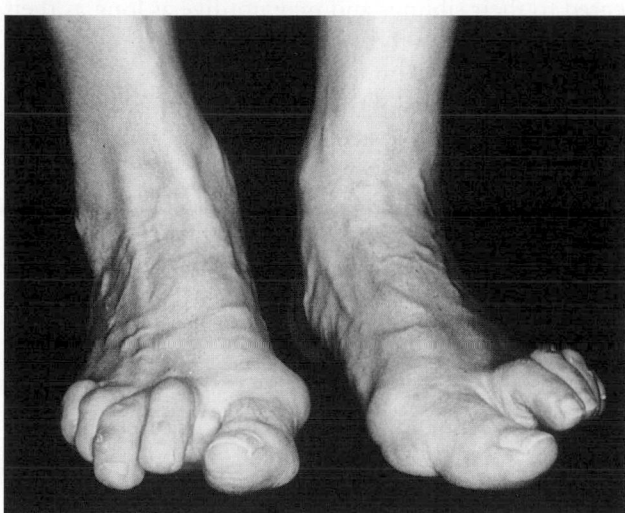

Figure 23.12 Common deformities of the rheumatoid foot. Evident in this photo are hallux valgus of the great toe, hammer toes, and cock-up toes due to metatarsophalangeal joint subluxation. *Used by permission of the American College of Rheumatology.*

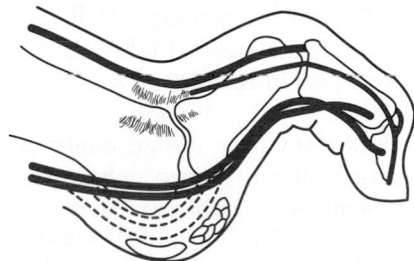

Figure 23.13 Relationship of structures to the metatarsal heads in metatarsalgia. *From Moncur, C, and Shields, M: Clinical management of metatarsalgia in the patient with arthritis. Clin Manage Phys Ther 3:7, 1983, p 10, with permission.*

subjected to repeated mechanical pressure such as the olecranon bursae, the extensor surfaces of the forearms, and the Achilles tendons. The presence of nodules on tendon mechanisms may lead to mechanical breakdown and tenosynovitis.[17,20]

Vascular and Neurologic Complications

Vasculitis, or inflammation of the blood vessels, has been found in 25% to 30% of individuals with RA on autopsy.[20] Most forms of vascular lesions associated with RA are silent and difficult to diagnose due to variability in the size of blood vessels affected. Skin vasculitis is the easiest to observe and can present as discoloration of the nail beds, purpura (red or purple discoloration), and petechiae (red or purple spots). The fulminant form of *rheumatoid arteritis* (arterial inflammation associated with a rheumatoid disorder) can be life threatening, and accompanied by malnutrition, infection, congestive heart failure (CHF), and gastrointestinal bleeding. Vasculitis of the vessels supplying nerves can lead to peripheral neuropathies such as foot or wrist drop.[1] Peripheral neuropathies may also occur secondary to mechanical compression of nerves such as carpal tunnel or tarsal tunnel syndrome. Spinal cord compression may result from inflammation in the cervical spine (see section on cervical spine and temporomandibular joint), and if clinical signs of cord compression are present, this requires immediate medical attention.[1]

Cardiopulmonary Complications

Morbidity and mortality from cardiovascular disease is elevated in persons with RA due to a greater prevalence of ischemic heart disease, secondary to accelerated atherosclerosis. Although the exact etiology of accelerated atherosclerosis is unclear, it is hypothesized that metabolic and vascular effects of chronic inflammation may be the causative factor.[24] Subclinical pericarditis may be present and has been demonstrated at autopsy. Pulmonary involvement is frequent and more prevalent in men than women. Pleuritis and pulmonary nodules may be present. Pulmonary nodules are related to presence of nodules elsewhere and found among seropositive patients with profuse synovitis. Nodules may be .40 to 3 in (1 to 8 cm) in size and affect gas exchange.[17]

Ocular Complications

Episcleritis, a benign and self-limiting process, and scleritis, a serious condition that can lead to blindness, may be present. The difference between these two is difficult to detect with clinical symptoms. Therefore, patients with RA should undergo annual eye examinations, and, if symptoms of suspected eye disease are present, they should be referred to an ophthalmologist.[20]

Activity Limitation and Participation Restriction

Patients with milder forms of RA may suffer from activity limitations and decreased participation in ADL due

to joint destruction. Almost 50% of individuals with RA will eventually have marked restrictions in ADL.[1] Late-onset RA is generally associated with better functional outcomes and less activity limitations and participation restrictions, though the cause of these findings is unclear. Table 23.3 presents a broad classification of functional status in RA that characterizes the progressive impact of the disease.[14] Loss of income is a major consequence of RA and is directly attributable to work disability. In a large international comparison study, work disability rates were high in persons with RA and disability was associated with disease factors as well as societal factors.[26]

Prognosis

RA causes increased morbidity and reduces life span. The question of mortality associated with RA is controversial. Previously, it was believed that RA itself was not usually a cause of death, although conditions such as systemic vasculitis and atlantoaxial subluxation could be fatal. There is presently a growing body of evidence that individuals with RA have decreased survival compared to their siblings and may not live as long as their counterparts without disease, especially if the early years of RA were marked by aggressive disease and poor functional status. Causes of death occurring more frequently in patients with RA as compared to the general population are infections, ischemic heart disease, and renal, respiratory, and gastrointestinal disease.[17,20,27]

Although numerous prognostic factors have been identified in the literature, there is no firm consensus regarding specific prognostic factors. Research demonstrates that individuals with a positive RF are more likely to progress to severe disease, as are those with high ESR and CRP at baseline. Baseline CRP is also associated with radiographic changes later in life.[28] Similarly, baseline radiographics are strongly associated with pattern of progression. Genetic research suggests that a shared epitope in the hypervariable region of the HLA-DR is associated with disease severity in a dose-dependent manner.[29]

Remission Criteria

In 2011, in response to the increasing ability to achieve remission with appropriate medical management, the American College of Rheumatology (ACR), the European League Against Rheumatism (EULAR), and the ACR Outcomes Measures in Rheumatology Initiatives developed a rigorous set of remission criteria. *Remission*, described as little if any active disease, can be operationally confirmed based on one of two definitions: (a) when scores on the tender joint count, swollen joint count, CRP (in mg/dL), and the Patient Global Assessment (0–10 scale rating how patient feels overall) are all less than or equal to 1, or (b) when the score on the Simplified Disease Activity Index (numerical sum of all of the above plus the score on the Physician Global Assessment) is less than or equal to 3.3.[30]

■ OSTEOARTHRITIS

Osteoarthritis (OA) is primarily confined to one or more synovial joints and its surrounding soft tissues. Two predominant, pathological features once defined OA: the progressive destruction of articular cartilage and the formation of bone at the margins of the joint.[1] OA is now recognized as a disease involving the entire joint including the periarticular musculature[31] (Fig. 23.14). Accordingly, the impairment, activity limitations, and participation restrictions related to OA extend far beyond the perimeters of the synovial joint. Data on the personal and societal impact of OA increasingly demonstrate its importance as an individual and public health issue.

Epidemiology

Osteoarthritis is the most common form of arthritis and extremely prevalent among individuals over 40 years of age. Based on data from several large population-based studies, it is estimated that approximately 12% of the U.S. population or 27 million adults age 25 and older have clinical OA of some joint.[32] It is widespread in adults older than 65, and affects men more than women before age 50, but reverses after age 50.[1] Studies concerning racial predisposition to OA have yielded conflicting data, depending on the joint studied. Data from the third National Health and Nutrition Examination Survey (NHANES) reveal that the prevalence of radiographic knee OA was highest in non-Hispanic African Americans (52.4%) compared to non-Hispanic whites (36.2%) or Mexican Americans (37.6%).[32]

Etiology

Similar to RA, no single factor that predisposes an individual to OA has been identified. Although aging is indeed strongly associated with OA, it must be emphasized that aging in itself does not cause OA, nor should OA be considered synonymous with the "normal" aging process.[1,33]

In fact, many OA-related changes seen at both a cellular and tissue level are opposite those seen with normal aging.[34] Several factors related to aging may, however, contribute to its development. Genetic factors account for between 39% and 65% of radiographic OA of the hand, hip, and knee in women and as much as 70% of OA cases of the spine.[35] Trauma before adulthood may initiate a remodeling of bone that alters joint mechanics and nutrition in a way that becomes problematic only later in life. The role of repetitive *microtrauma* in the etiology of OA has also received attention.[1] Specifically, occupational tasks involving heavy lifting are associated with the development of hip OA,[36] and those involving kneeling and heavy lifting are related to the development of knee OA.[37,38] Malalignment, including *varus* and *valgus* deformities, and leg length discrepancy are associated with greater prevalence of knee and hip OA, respectively.[38,39] The strongest predictor of disease progression in the knee is varus malalignment.[40] At the hip, there is increasing recognition of the role of *femoroacetabular impingement (FAI)* (a mechanical mismatch between the femoral head and acetabulum) in development of OA.[41] Finally, obesity has been shown to be a risk factor for the development of OA in later life; most evident in the knee joint and to a lesser extent in the hip and hands.[1,39] The relationship between obesity and incidence of OA is stronger in women than in men.[39] Risk factors for OA can be classified as either systemic or local (Box 23.2), and OA most likely results from the combined effect of multiple factors acting on a vulnerable joint that leads to disease.[39] It is imperative that physical therapists understand and are able to counsel patients on those factors that are modifiable and amenable to therapeutic interventions.

Pathophysiology

Animal models involving knee trauma have provided much of the basis for what we now know about the earliest changes associated with OA in humans. Thus, it

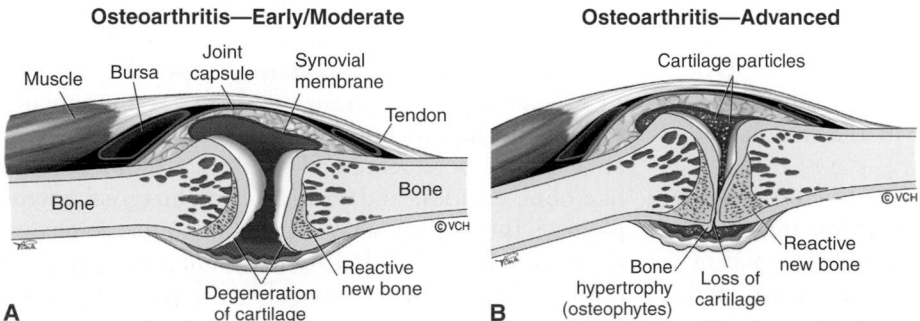

Figure 23.14 Early-advanced osteoarthritis joint changes. Early joint changes are characterized by superficial damage to articular cartilage and mild inflammation. Progression to moderate joint changes includes joint space narrowing with full-thickness damage to cartilage and thickening of the subchondral bone. Advanced joint changes are marked by bony hypertrophy (marginal osteophytes), significant joint space narrowing, and possible angulation (deformity). *From Mary Pack Arthritis Program, Vancouver Coastal Health, with permission.*

Box 23.2 Risk Factors for Osteoarthritis[1,38,39]

Systemic Factors	Local Factors
Age	Obesity
Gender	Major joint trauma (e.g., ACL rupture)
Race	
Genetics	Repetitive stress (occupation)
Metabolic/endocrine	Muscle weakness
High bone density	Altered joint biomechanics
Nutritional status (e.g., vitamin D deficiency)	Joint malalignment
	Proprioceptive impairments
Congenital/ developmental	
Obesity	

is possible that subtle, crucial, and as yet undiscovered differences in humans may alter our understanding of OA in the future.

Normal Cartilage

Healthy articular cartilage is composed of an extracellular matrix and chondrocytes. Water makes up between 65% and 80% of the matrix by weight, mostly Type II collagen contributes approximately 10%, and *proteoglycans* (molecules found in articular cartilage), noncollagenous proteins, and glycoproteins the remainder.[38,42] It is the matrix that protects the chondrocytes from damage during normal joint use.[42] *Chondrocytes*, the only cells in articular cartilage, secrete the matrix yet make up only 1% of the total volume of adult human articular cartilage.[42] Chondrocytes are dispersed throughout the extracellular matrix but most concentrated in the deep layer. The superficial layer has the highest concentration of water and collagen fibers giving this zone the greatest tensile stiffness and strength and ability to resist shearing forces.[42] Proteoglycans consist of a protein core and one or more glycosaminoglycans (GAGs), including hyaluronic acid and chondroitin sulfate. Proteoglycan concentration is highest in the middle and deep zones.[42]

Articular cartilage contains no nerves, blood vessels, or lymphatic vessels. It receives its nutrition and eliminates waste via diffusion through synovial fluid and by facilitated *imbibition* (absorption of fluid by a solid body).[38] The multiple roles of articular cartilage include decreasing friction between articulating joint surfaces, distributing static and dynamic joint forces to the underlying bone and absorbing shock.[38,43] Cartilage's shock-absorbing function is minimal (1% to 3% of load forces), however, compared to that of subchondral bone (30%)[38] and periarticular muscles (which requires timely and coordinated muscle contraction). These joint structures

together with ligaments, menisci, capsule, synovium, and synovial fluid serve to protect the joint from regular wear and tear and damaging forces. Regular forces acting on the articular cartilage include body weight, muscle contractions, and ground reaction forces that vary with the rate and duration of loading and the available load-bearing surface.[38,42] Extremes of joint loading in either direction can lead to detrimental morphological and metabolic changes in the cartilage whereas moderate, cyclic loading enhances proteoglycan synthesis and concentration.[38,42]

Joint Pathology

The first osteoarthritic change in articular cartilage, which has been confirmed in humans, is an increase in water content. This increase suggests that the proteoglycans have become swollen with water far beyond normal. This process, together with disruption of other components of the extracellular matrix, decreases the stiffness of the matrix and leads to further mechanical damage.[42] In later stages of disease progression, proteoglycans are lost, which diminishes the water content of cartilage. As proteoglycans are lost, articular cartilage loses its compressive stiffness and elasticity, which, in turn, results in the transmission of compressive forces to underlying bone. Collagen synthesis is increased initially, although there is a shift from type II collagen fibers to a larger proportion of type I collagen, the kind found in skin and fibrous tissue. Chondrocytes attempt to respond to this early tissue damage by synthesizing new matrix molecules and proliferating and forming clusters of cells.[42] As the articular cartilage is destroyed, the joint space narrows.[31] In summary, the early phases of cartilage degeneration are characterized by biosynthesis and repair as the chondrocytes attempt to restore the damaged matrix while the later phase is degradative in nature as catabolic enzyme activity digests the matrix and erodes the cartilage.

One of the first noticeable changes in cartilage is the mild fraying or "flaking" of superficial collagen fibers. Deeper fraying, or "fibrillation," of the upper third of the cartilage follows in areas of greater weight-bearing and may progress to full-thickness fissures (Fig. 23.15). As the cartilage degenerates, there are accompanying changes in the subchondral bone including increased bone density or subchondral sclerosis, creation of cyst-like bone cavities, and formation of marginal **osteophytes**.[1] The cartilage may degenerate to the point that the exposed subchondral bone becomes necrotic and *eburnated* (polished or ivory-like) (Fig. 23.16). The stiffer than normal subchondral bone further decreases the shock-absorbing properties of the joint and results in greater impact loading.[38] The traditional view of OA is that the disease process starts with an unrepaired injury to articular cartilage; however, there is also evidence that reduced compliance in subchondral bone and periarticular structures may initiate the degenerative processes.[38,42]

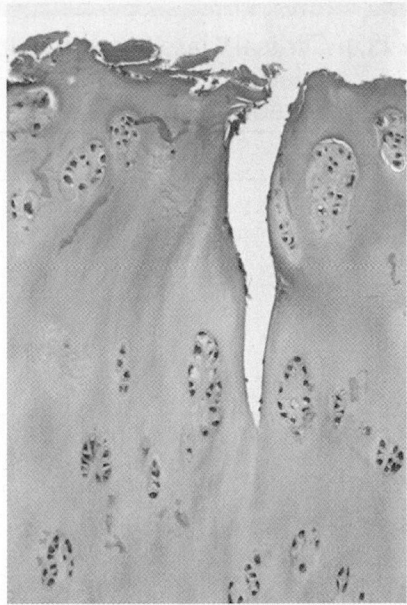

Figure 23.15 Osteoarthritis: cartilage, clefts and fibrillation (histological specimen). *Used by permission of the American College of Rheumatology.*

Osteophytes may be fibrous, cartilaginous, or bony in composition and marginal prominences are palpable and often tender in more superficial joints.[42] The process of **osteophyte** formation in OA is not well understood. Current hypotheses have implicated increased vascularity in the deepest layers of the degenerated cartilage, venous congestion from subchondral cysts and thickened subchondral trabeculae, and the

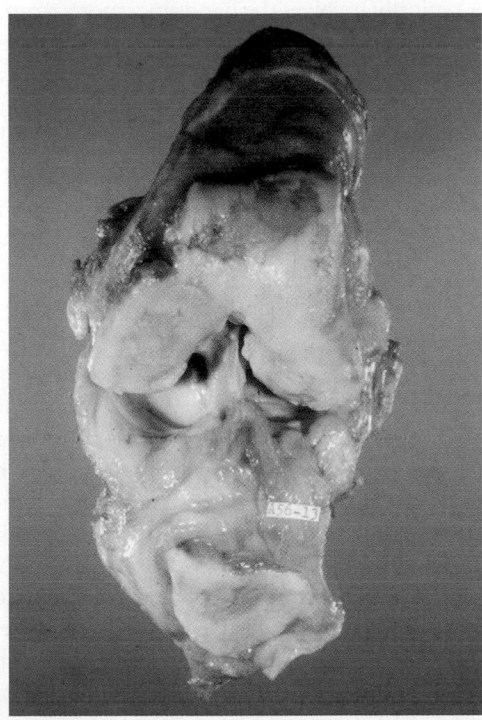

Figure 23.16 Osteoarthritis: knee, gross pathology. *Used by permission of the American College of Rheumatology.*

continued sloughing of articular cartilage.[44] Each of these hypotheses may explain how this bony growth contributes to the pain and loss of motion that accompany OA. Subchondral cysts containing **myxoid**, fibrous or cartilaginous tissue along with bone marrow lesions identified through MRI, are associated with painful knee OA.[31]

Although traditionally viewed as a non-inflammatory disease, improved detection methods suggest that inflammation does play a role and that inflammatory pathways are up-regulated (increased responsiveness).[1,43] Further inflammatory reactions occur in response to cartilage fragments in the synovial cavity and resultant low-grade synovitis.[38]

Radiography

It is widely recognized that radiographic findings are not strongly related to clinical symptoms and pain severity[39] and add little to the accuracy of the clinical diagnosis. In knee OA, muscle strength and pain are more explanatory of functional loss than radiographic findings.[45] Although the diagnosis of OA can be made through history and clinical assessment, radiographs are frequently used to confirm the extent of joint damage and disease progression and continue to be a component of the ACR diagnostic criteria.[31] The Kellgren and Lawrence 5-point classification system remains the most widely used criteria for grading radiographic changes both clinically and for purposes of research.[46]

- Grade 0: normal radiograph
- Grade 1: doubtful narrowing of the joint space and possible osteophytes
- Grade 2: definite osteophytes and absent or questionable narrowing of the joint space
- Grade 3: moderate osteophytes and joint space narrowing, some sclerosis, and possible deformity
- Grade 4: large osteophytes, marked narrowing of joint space, severe sclerosis, and definite deformity

In Figure 23.17, early OA changes of the right hip are depicted. Newer imaging techniques including high-resolution MRI are able to detect early structural changes and pathology in pain-sensitive structures well before changes are observable on radiographs.[31,47] Real-time ultrasound allows visualization of both bony and soft tissue structures and is more sensitive than clinical examination in detecting effusion, synovitis, and early osteophytes in OA.[47] Ultrasound imaging has greater potential for routine use in clinical practice than MRI.

Disease Onset and Course

OA typically starts in an insidious fashion and may progress undetected in some individuals when early, aneural articular cartilage is the only involved tissue. Pain is initially episodic and triggered by specific activity. In later disease, pain becomes a chronic, dull ache

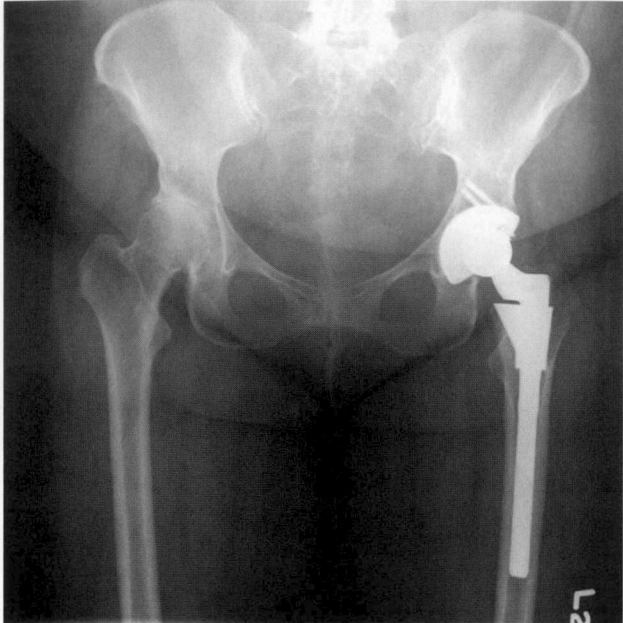

Figure 23.17 Osteoarthritis: Mild degenerative changes right hip, total hip replacement in left. *Used by permission of the American College of Rheumatology.*

---

accentuated with episodic severe pain.[31] It is pain that leads an individual to seek medical help. Unlike RA, there are no systemic features such as fatigue, fever, or malaise with the onset of OA.

OA is typically a slowly progressive condition; however, most people with radiographic evidence of joint damage in their hips or knees stabilize and do not require joint replacement surgery.[1] The pathological process involved in OA appears to be cyclical with active periods of increased matrix protein turnover interspersed with inactive phases.[48] The prognosis is variable and not necessarily bad. However, in combination with normal aging, co-morbidities often present in older adults, and high levels of inactivity in this population, OA can contribute to increasing disability.[1]

Classification and Diagnostic Criteria

Most researchers have used Kellgren and Lawrence's grade 2 definition (the presence of definite osteophytes) as the criterion for identifying disease, although a few others have required evidence of joint space narrowing (grade 3 corresponding to clinically identified disease) to designate OA.[46] Although radiographic evidence of joint space narrowing and osteophytes may help confirm the diagnosis and classify the stage of OA, the clinical criteria for hip,[49] knee,[50] and hand[51] OA are described primarily in terms of pain and limitation of motion (Box 23.3).

OA is typically differentiated in two ways: *primary* (idiopathic) and *secondary* disease.[1] When the etiology of the disease is unknown with no known prior event, it is termed *primary* or *idiopathic* OA. This category can be further divided into *localized* (one or two joints affected) or *generalized* OA (affecting three or more joints).[1] Generalized OA typically involves the hands in a more symmetrical fashion not unlike inflammatory forms of arthritis and has a stronger genetic association.[1] OA is classified as *secondary* when the etiology (e.g., trauma, biomechanical factors, congenital malformation, or other musculoskeletal disease) can be identified. There is increasing evidence that many cases categorized as idiopathic are more appropriately recognized as secondary disease as our ability to detect subtle and early biochemical, histological, morphological, and biomechanical factors improves.

Clinical Presentation

Signs and Symptoms (Impairments)

As noted above, the clinical diagnosis is often made on the basis of signs and symptoms (e.g., pain and swelling, loss of ROM, and bony deformity). Not all joints are equally affected by OA. In the upper extremity (UE), the finger DIP and PIP joints and CMC of the thumb are commonly involved. The cervical and lumbar spine, hips, knees, and MTP of the great toe are also sites for OA. The MCP joints, wrists, elbows, and shoulders are usually spared in primary OA.[1] Unlike RA, OA does not have a bilateral, symmetrical presentation (with the exception of generalized OA).[1]

A single joint or any combination of joints may be affected and of differing "etiological origins." OA is not a systemic disease, and is therefore not associated with systemic complaints such as fatigue, generalized morning stiffness, fever, or loss of appetite. Individuals with OA may experience some stiffness in particular joints on awakening that is similar to the stiffness felt when moving the same joints after inactivity during the day, but this stiffness (articular gelling) typically does not last more than 30 minutes, nor is it generalized to the entire body.[1,31] Crepitus is a common clinical finding in OA and may progress from a painless grating sensation to an extremely painful, high-pitched sound as a result of bone-on-bone articulation.

Although cartilage degeneration is the primary manifestation of OA, cartilage is aneural, and therefore not the cause of a person's pain. Pain in OA can arise from any innervated tissue and may be attributed to incongruent articulations of joint surfaces, periosteal elevation secondary to bone proliferation at the joint margin (osteophytes), vasocongestion in subchondral bone, trabecular microfractures, distention of the joint capsule, and muscle spasm or strain.[31,42] Many patients will also experience a secondary synovitis and effusion, especially when the knee is involved.[43,52]

As noted earlier, symptoms do not always match the severity of the disease on radiographs. Further, some patients with OA may have an amplified pain experience and central pain sensitization at the spinal or cortical level.[43] Unlike individuals with RA who often report more pain and stiffness at rest, the pain associated with OA is likely to occur or worsen with motion, except in the later stages of the disease when it is present at rest and with activity.[1,31]

Joints

Hands and Fingers Osteoarthritis may present differently and result in varied levels of impairment depending on the joints involved. In the hand, DIP and PIP involvement may result in reduced ROM, poor grip strength, bony nodes, and joint angulation as a result of stretched collateral ligaments or bone erosion. **Bouchard's nodes** at the PIP joints and **Heberden's nodes** at the DIP joints are often tender in the early stages and can lead to marked restrictions in finger ROM and fine motor skills later in the disease (Fig 23.18). Osteoarthritic damage in the first CMC joint results in pain or aching at the base of the thumb and can lead to decreased pinch strength and squaring of the thumb (thickening and prominence of CMC due to subluxation of first metacarpal) as a result of weakness and contracture of the thenar muscles.[53,54] This in turn affects abduction, extension, and opposition ROM of the thumb and greatly affects grip strength and hand function. In cases of generalized OA, the hands are always affected and in a more symmetrical pattern.[1] Painful inflammation with synovitis, erosive changes, cystic swellings, and osteophytes are present in this less

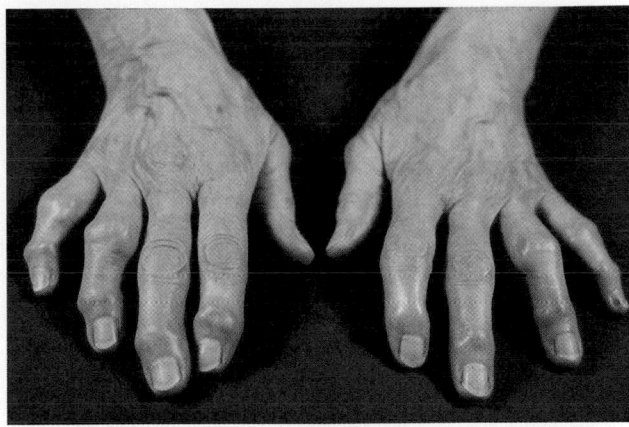

Figure 23.18 Osteoarthritis: Heberden's and Bouchard's nodes, hand. *Used by permission of the American College of Rheumatology.*

common form of OA and may lead to ankylosis of the DIP and PIP joints.[1,54]

Hips Symptoms of hip OA are usually insidious in onset and may include a limp and decreased ROM with a tendency for the hip to be held in a somewhat flexed, abducted, and externally rotated position. Internal rotation is usually restricted and painful.[55] Pain arising from the hip joint is commonly experienced in the groin, but can also be felt in the buttock, trochanteric, or knee region.[55] Decreased hip ROM is associated with decreased walking speed, decreased stride length, poor balance, and increased energy expenditure. Hip OA is also associated with increased risk of falls.[56]

Knees Early presentation of knee OA includes pain with weight-bearing activities such as climbing stairs and squatting. In later stages, both pain and stiffness are reported after prolonged sitting such as with watching a movie. Symptoms of joint locking and buckling (giving way) may also occur with damage to stabilizing menisci and ligaments[55] and lead to increased risk of falls.[31] Knee OA more commonly affects the medial joint due to the higher weight-bearing load placed on this compartment. As a result, medial joint space narrowing often results in **pseudolaxity** of the medial collateral ligament, stretching of the lateral collateral counterpart, and a genu varus deformity (Fig. 23.19). Genu valgus as a result of greater lateral compartment involvement is less common. A **flexion deformity** of several degrees can develop quickly in the painful knee and contribute to a functional leg length discrepancy, decreased step length, and quadriceps muscular fatigue or strain. Patellofemoral compartment OA, with its hallmark anterior knee pain, can occur in isolation as a result of patella malalignment, abnormal tracking and loading, and direct trauma to the patella.[55]

Feet and Toes The first MTP joint is the most common site of OA affecting the foot and may result in hallux rigidus or hallux valgus deformities. Changes in

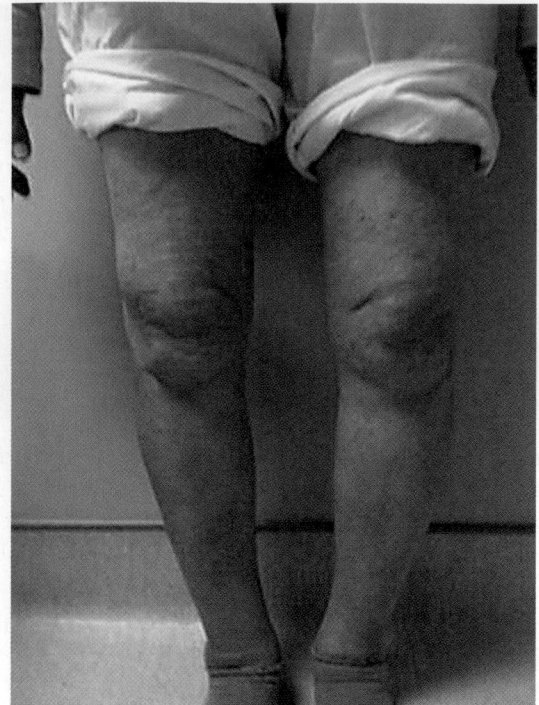

Figure 23.19 Bilateral genu varum. *Dr. Basram Masri, with permission.*

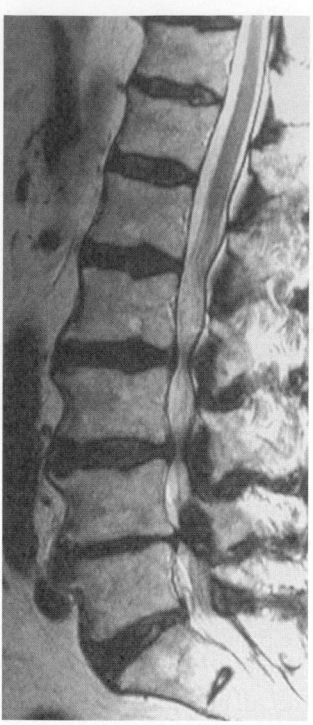

Figure 23.20 Spinal stenosis: lumbar spine, MRI image. *Used by permission of the American College of Rheumatology.*

the other MTP joints and toes as a result of OA and resultant shortening of the long extensors can lead to hammer toes. Forefoot involvement contributes to poor push-off in the terminal stance phase of gait and balance issues.[57]

Spine The lower cervical and mid to lower lumbar regions of the spine are most susceptible to OA. All spinal articulations can experience degenerative changes; however, the facet (zygapophyseal) joints are the only true synovial joints in the spine.[58] Facet joint osteophytes can contribute to lateral and central lumbar stenosis and subsequent nerve root impingement[58] (Fig. 23.20). Pain from facet joint OA can originate from the joint itself and affected nerve roots (radicular pain) and in the lumbar area, and typically increases with spinal extension, rotary motions, and when standing or sitting.[58] Lying and spinal flexion lead to pain relief.

Activity Limitations and Participation Restrictions

Overall, OA of the knee can impose functional limitations to a degree equivalent to heart disease, CHF, and chronic obstructive pulmonary disease (COPD) and accounts for a substantial proportion of the burden of disability among community-living elders.[59]

Patients with the most severe disease may not move their joints as often or in the ways that exacerbate their symptoms. Therefore, pain, disease severity, and functional disability in individuals with OA are interrelated.

Among elders, it has been shown that the functional loss associated with severe radiographic OA without pain is more likely than the loss associated with symptomatic but milder disease.[60] One explanation of this finding is that individuals with OA limit their functional activities to avoid movements that are painful. In the clinical examination it is important to determine functional status even in the absence of pain. Given that individuals with OA may reduce or eliminate their symptoms by avoiding certain activities, clinicians should explore activity limitations and physical inactivity–related symptoms in patients with OA separately from the evaluation of symptoms.

Greater self-reported disability in advanced knee OA was associated with pain, joint laxity, age, and body mass index (BMI) among Finnish adults ages 60 to 80 years while performance-based functioning was related to the self-report *Western Ontario and McMasters Universities Arthritis Index* (WOMAC) function score, pain, and obesity.[61] Of interest, the authors found no association between radiographic severity of knee OA and self-reported and performance-based function.[61] The comprehensive International Classification of Functioning, Disability, and Health (**ICF**) **Core Set** of impairments, activity limitations, and participation restrictions has been established through an international team of researchers, clinicians, and patients to identify those areas of functioning that are affected by OA, with the shorter **Brief ICF Core Set** created for clinical purposes.[62,63] OA is a leading cause of disability and major contributor to work-related disability, reduced productivity, and absenteeism.[64]

Prognosis

OA is a slow progressing disease that can be self-limiting or progress to advanced joint and soft tissue damage leading to complete failure of that joint. In such a case, joint surgery including **arthrodesis** of some joints in the foot, or arthroplasty, for example, of the knee is the final treatment option to help the patient regain function. However, rapidly progressive joint damage is uncommon and in most cases patients stabilize.[1] Increasing disability may be more related to advancing years, co-morbidities, and inactivity.

■ MEDICAL MANAGEMENT

Pharmacological Therapy in Rheumatoid Arthritis

Joint destruction and irreversible damage are most pronounced early in the disease course. Current medical management is based on the implementation of an early and aggressive approach to disease management to halt or decrease progression. Medical therapies also focus on decreasing pain and inflammation. Early aggressive

pharmacological therapy is associated with diminished joint damage and long-term maintenance of function. The major classifications of drugs used in RA management include nonsteroidal anti-inflammatory drugs (NSAIDs) and disease-modifying antirheumatic drugs (DMARDs), which include the biological response modifiers (BRMs) and corticosteroids.[65] Table 23.4 lists the most common drugs used in the management of RA.[20]

Nonsteroidal Anti-inflammatory Drugs

NSAIDs provide both *analgesic* and *anti-inflammatory* effects depending on the dose prescribed; however, they do not alter disease progression. Discontinuance of NSAIDs quickly leads to exacerbation of symptoms. Thus, NSAIDs are generally given in combination with other disease-modifying agents. At lower doses, the NSAID effect is analgesic, through the peripheral inhibition of pro-inflammatory prostaglandin synthesis. At higher doses, the effect is anti-inflammatory, probably through both prostaglandin inhibition and alterations in macrophage and neutrophil function. Due to the mechanism of action of these medications, adverse effects include gastrointestinal (GI) complaints and renal effects. Mild GI adverse effects include distress and

Table 23.4	Drugs in the Management of Osteoarthritis and Rheumatoid Arthritis		
Drug	Common Brand Names	Adverse Effects	Cautions and Contraindications
Analgesics			
Acetaminophen	Tylenol, Excedrin caplets, Panadol, Anacin-3	Potential for renal and liver toxicity, possible GI ulceration and bleeding at doses >3g/day	Not recommended with high alcohol consumption or liver disease
NSAIDs, traditional	**OTC:** Advil, Motrin IB, Nuprin, Actron, Orudis KT, Aleve **Prescription:** Voltaren, Lodine, Nalfon, Ansaid, Indocin, Motrin, Orudis, Meclomen, Relafen, Naprosyn, Anaprox, Daypro, Feldene, Clinoril, Tolectin	GI bleeding, ulcers, nausea, diarrhea, indigestion, rash, dizziness, drowsiness, slowed blood clotting, tinnitus, fluid retention	Sensitivity or allergy to similar drugs; kidney, liver, or heart disease; hypertension; asthma; ulcers; anticoagulant therapy
COX-2 inhibitors	celecoxib (Celebrex), meloxicam (Mobic), nabumetone (Relafen)	May result in serious adverse events including cardiac complications and less serious GI side effects than traditional NSAIDs; allergic reactions; elevated blood pressure	Same as above; allergy to sulfa-containing drugs for celecoxib

Continued

Table 23.4   Drugs in the Management of Osteoarthritis and Rheumatoid Arthritis—cont'd

Drug	Common Brand Names	Adverse Effects	Cautions and Contraindications
Corticosteroids			
Systemic: oral or intravenous	Prednisone, prednisolone, methylprednisolone, triamcinolone, cortisone, hydrocortisone, dexamethasone	With long-term/high-dose: Cushing syndrome, osteoporosis, cataracts, insomnia, hypertension, immune suppression, elevated blood sugar, mood changes, weight gain, altered mental status, glaucoma, restlessness, increased appetite	Diabetes, infection, hypothyroidism, hypertension, osteoporosis, gastric ulcer
Injection	Triamcinolone, prednisolone, methylprednisolone, dexamethasone, hydrocortisone, betamethasone	Post-injection flare (4–24 hours), transient systemic reaction, increased diabetic symptoms, soft tissue disruption from direct injection	Presence of infection, previous failure to respond
DMARDs			
Methotrexate	Rheumatrex	Common adverse effects: decreased appetite, abdominal discomfort, nausea, diarrhea, skin rash, itching, oral ulcers, photosensitivity, infection, unusual bleeding/bruising Serious: bone marrow suppression; liver, lung, or kidney toxicity; fetal death; congenital abnormalities	Liver or lung disease, alcoholism, immune system or bone marrow suppression, infection, pregnancy
Injectable gold	Myochrysine, Solganal	Stomach cramps/vomiting; severe allergic reactions (rash, hives, difficulty breathing, tightness in the chest, and so forth); blood in urine; cough; dark urine; metallic taste; mouth sores; nausea; pain or numbness in the hands or feet; persistent diarrhea; purple blotches or other skin spots; seizures; shortness of breath; sore throat; weakness; vision problems	Kidney disease, bone marrow suppression, colitis
Oral gold—Auranofin	Ridaura	Individual drugs may also have other specific toxicities and increase risk for other conditions	Previous adverse reaction to gold compound; kidney, liver, or inflammatory bowel disease

Table 23.4 Drugs in the Management of Osteoarthritis and Rheumatoid Arthritis—cont'd

Drug	Common Brand Names	Adverse Effects	Cautions and Contraindications
Azathioprine	Imuran	Nausea/vomiting, diarrhea, allergic reactions, chest pain or tightness; dark urine; dizziness; fever, chills, or sore throat; increased or painful urination; muscle pain or aches; pale or fatty stools; shortness of breath; unusual bleeding or bruising; unusual growths or lumps; unusual weakness or fatigue; yellowing of the eyes or skin	Kidney or liver disease, pregnancy
Cyclophosphamide	Cytoxan	Interferes with wound healing Serious: secondary malignancies, fetal harm	Kidney or liver disease, pregnancy, infection, leucopenia, thrombocytopenia
Cyclosporin	Sandimmune Neoral		Kidney or liver disease, pregnancy, infection
Hydroxychloroquine	Plaquenil		Antimalarial drug allergy, retinal abnormality, pregnancy
Penicillamine	Cuprimine Depen		Penicillin allergy, blood disease, kidney disease
Sulfasalazine	Azulfidine		Sulfa or aspirin allergy, kidney or liver disease, blood disease, bronchial asthma
Leflunomide	Arava		Liver disease
Minocycline	Minocin		Tetracycline or sun sensitivity

Biologic Response Modifiers (TNF-alpha inhibitors)

Humanized antibody Fab fragment	Etanercept (Enbrel), adalimumab (Humira), anakinra (Kineret), infliximab (Remicade), Certolizumab pegol (Cimzia), Golimumab (Simponi)	• Serious infection: increased risk of serious infection leading to hospitalization or death, including TB, bacterial sepsis, invasive fungal infections, and infections due to other opportunistic infections • Malignancy: lymphoma and other malignancies, some fatal, have been reported in children and adolescent patients treated with TNF blockers Infection at injection site, headache, rash	Serious infection Malignancies Anaphylaxis or serious allergic reactions Hepatitis B virus reactivation Demyelinating dx, exacerbation or new-onset cytopenias, pancytopenias Heart failure, worsening or new onset Lupus-like syndrome Require subcutaneous injection or intravenous infusion (infliximab); increased risk for lymphoma

Continued

Table 23.4   Drugs in the Management of Osteoarthritis and Rheumatoid Arthritis—cont'd

Drug	Common Brand Names	Adverse Effects	Cautions and Contraindications
Other Biologicals			
Fusion protein, selective T-cell costimulation modulator	Abatacept (Orencia)	Headache Upper respiratory tract infection Nasopharyngitis Nausea	Concomitant use with a TNF antagonist can increase the risk of infections and serious infections Hypersensitivity, anaphylaxis, and anaphylactoid reactions History of recurrent infections or underlying conditions predisposed to experience more infections Discontinue if serious infection develops Screen for latent TB infection before initiating therapy Patients testing positive should be treated before initiating abatacept Live vaccines should not be given concurrently or within 3 months of discontinuation
Chimeric murine/human monoclonal antibody to CD20 antigen	Rituximab (Rituxan) Tocilizumab (Actemra)	Upper respiratory tract infection Nasopharyngitis Urinary tract infection Bronchitis Infusion reactions	Infusion reactions Tumor lysis syndrome Severe mucocutaneous reactions Progressive multifocal leukoencephalopathy
Humanized anti-human IL-6 receptor monoclonal antibody		Serious infections Cardiovascular events	Cardiac arrhythmias and angina Bowel obstruction and perforation Do not administer live virus vaccines before or during rituximab Monitor CBC at regular intervals

nausea. However, approximately 2% to 4% of patients experience serious adverse effects including gastrointestinal bleeding, ulcers, and perforation. Patients are encouraged to take these medications with food, to monitor GI signs, and/or are given prophylactic therapy to decrease gastrointestinal damage. Renal and other adverse effects associated with continued use and high doses of NSAIDs include dizziness, drowsiness, headache, tinnitus (ringing in the ears), kidney dysfunction, and elevation of liver enzymes. Complete blood counts (CBCs) and stool guaiac analyses for occult blood should be conducted every 3 to 4 months to monitor for potential adverse effects.[65]

There are two primary categories of NSAIDs, based on whether they inhibit COX-1 and COX-2 enzymes or COX-2 enzymes alone. These enzymes are responsible for synthesis of prostaglandins. Traditional NSAIDs block both COX-1 and COX-2 enzymes. The main function of

the COX-1 enzyme is synthesis of prostaglandins in the endothelium and gastric mucosa, tissues present in the stomach lining and kidneys. Caution should be taken when prescribing NSAIDs to specific groups of patients at risk for GI complications such as the elderly, smokers, those taking corticosteroids, and those with severe arthritis, co-morbidities, and history of GI symptoms. The selective COX-2 inhibitors were designed to decrease the risk of GI toxicity by inhibiting only the COX-2 enzyme, which is responsible for the pain and swelling associated with inflammation. Early studies of short duration exposure supported the reduced risk of GI side effects and increased tolerability of COX-2 inhibitors.[66] However, studies of longer selective COX-2 exposure and systematic evaluation of the data from numerous trials indicate that patients on selective COX-2 inhibitors are at greater risk of acute myocardial infarction and other cardiovascular events.[67-69]

NSAIDs are an accessible and relatively inexpensive drug to manage inflammation; however, the decision to prescribe an NSAID must be based on risk factors, known toxicities, and dosing preferences. Individual response to an NSAID is extremely variable in terms of both effectiveness and tolerance. Therefore, it often requires several month-long trials to find the best product. Taking more than one NSAID increases the risk of toxicity with no increase in benefit. NSAIDs are prescribed for patients with RA at the onset of symptoms to provide rapid pain relief and control of inflammation while waiting for the slower-acting DMARD to become effective.

Disease-Modifying Antirheumatic Drugs

DMARDs are the primary class of drugs for managing disease progression in RA. An array of drugs with varying chemical structures, modes of actions, clinical indications, and toxicities are classified as DMARDs. Typical DMARDs used to manage RA include antimalarials, methotrexate, sulfasalazine, and leflumonide. Although DMARDs are effective in reducing disease progression, these medications do not provide an analgesic effect and are slow acting, taking from 3 weeks to 3 months to take effect. A drug that is classified as a DMARD must show evidence of affecting the course of RA for at least 1 year (improved function, reduced inflammation, and slowing or prevention of structural damage). DMARDs may be given alone or in combination for best effectiveness. Individuals taking DMARDs should be monitored regularly for the toxicities accompanying the specific drug. DMARDs are most often used to treat adult-onset RA; however, some are used to treat juvenile RA, ankylosing spondylitis, psoriatic arthritis, and systemic lupus erythematosus. The most commonly used DMARD to manage RA is methotrexate.[20]

Biological Response Modifiers

Biological response modifiers (BRMs) are a class of disease-modifying agents in use since 1998 that are biologically engineered to mimic the activities of targeted immune cells to reduce or block the inflammatory process. These drugs are approved to treat moderate to severe RA that is nonresponsive to traditional therapy. The mechanism of action of BRMs varies and includes inhibition of cytokine activity, by blocking either tumor necrosis factor–alpha or interleukin-1. Evidence demonstrates both inhibition of the progression of structural damage and improvement of physical function in RA and represents a significant advance in the treatment of RA. Patients who begin BRMs usually continue with their NSAIDs or corticosteroids. Adverse effects of these medications can be quite serious and patients must be monitored for signs of infection, including colds and flus, which can rapidly progress during immunosuppression. Those with a history of tuberculosis (TB) are at risk for reactivation of TB and may be excluded from this form of therapy. The number of diseases in which these agents are useful continues to expand as do the number and types of agents available.

Corticosteroids

Corticosteroids are powerful anti-inflammatory drugs creating rapid and potent suppression of inflammation. Corticosteroids are generally not given alone and may be administered orally, intravenously, or via intra-articular or periarticular injection. Unfortunately, these potent inflammatory medications also produce serious adverse effects when used long-term or in high doses. Potential adverse effects include thinning of the skin, osteoporosis, muscle wasting, adrenal suppression, increased susceptibility to infections, impaired wound healing, cataracts, glaucoma, hyperlipidemia, and aseptic bone necrosis. These drugs are generally prescribed in the presence of unremitting disease and severe extra-articular inflammation and are given in combination with other RA medications (e.g., DMARDs). Corticosteroids are often prescribed in *pulse doses* (low tapering doses over a specific time period) to reduce the risk of side effects. Patients on corticosteroids should have their blood counts, serum potassium, and glucose levels monitored and be observed for potential side effects.[20]

When inflammation is confined to a specific location, steroid injections into a joint, bursa, tendon, or tendon sheath may be administered. However, use of steroid injections is commonly limited to no more than two to four per year to reduce the risk of osteonecrosis and soft tissue damage.

Pharmacological Therapy in Osteoarthritis

To date, drug therapy in OA has no effect on disease progression and is ancillary to nonpharmacological approaches to pain management including patient education and self-management, weight loss, joint protection, and exercise.[40,70-72] The goals of drug therapy in patients with OA are to relieve pain and decrease inflammation when it is present. Oral analgesics, NSAIDs, and corticosteroid injections are the primary medications used in OA management (see Table 23.4).[1,70-72]

Acetaminophen, an oral analgesic, is usually the drug of first choice.[40,70-73] Acetaminophen-containing compounds (Tylenol, Panadol, Anacin-3) have been cited as having almost no toxicity in recommended doses (up to 4 g/day) and little or no GI side effects. However, there is no anti-inflammatory effect; acetaminophen cannot be substituted for NSAIDs in this regard. Earlier clinical studies in OA demonstrated symptom relief from acetaminophen (3 to 4 g/day) greater than that of a placebo and slightly less than that of NSAIDs.[74] However, newer evidence suggests that acetaminophen has minimal clinically important effects on pain and no significant effect on stiffness or physical function in patients with symptomatic knee OA.[73] Further, acetaminophen use can lead to liver and, less commonly, kidney toxicity, especially in individuals who drink excessive amounts of alcohol. As well, there is increasing evidence of an increased incidence of hospitalization due to GI perforation, peptic ulceration, and bleeding with acetaminophen use of more than 3 g/day compared to lower doses (less than 3g/day).[73]

NSAIDs have a place in the management of persons with OA who do not respond to acetaminophen and nonpharmacological measures.[72] NSAIDs may be used in combination with acetaminophen, and should be kept to the lowest effective dose to minimize GI toxicity. The COX-2 NSAIDs, described for RA management, had been prescribed for people who are at increased risk for GI problems until longer-term trials called their safety into question.

Intra-articular corticosteroid injections are often used for acute episodes with a moderate effect for pain relief, irrespective of the number of injections.[72] The knee is the most common site; however, soft tissue injections for subacromial, anserine, and trochanteric bursitis also may be effective.

Viscosupplementation or intra-articular injections of the knee with a form of hyaluronic acid (HA) is sometimes used. A number of synthetic forms are available (Synvisc, Hyalgan, Artzal). Hyaluronic acid is a naturally occurring polysaccharide that contributes to the thickness and viscosity of joint fluid in the healthy joint. In the OA knee, the levels of HA are lower and the joint fluid is thinner and less dense, reducing the ability of the fluid to lubricate and attenuate shock. Viscosupplementation therapy consists of a series of weekly injections. The reported effects of treatment are reduced pain and stiffness and improved function in people with mild to moderate knee OA, which may last for several months.[72] It is not clear if HA injections are more effective than corticosteroid injections, NSAIDs, or placebo injections. The injected HA does not replace normal joint fluid to achieve its effect as most is absorbed and cleared from the joint within a week. The risk of adverse effects is low. The most serious reported adverse event is an allergic reaction and less serious effects are injection site reactions and joint swelling. There is no evidence that supports increased efficacy of one product over another; however, high-molecular-weight hylan (Synvisc) may have greater efficacy.[72]

Glucosamine sulphate (GS) and glucosamine hydrochloride (GH) have been examined in placebo-controlled trials and found to be moderately effective for pain relief; however, the size of the effect diminishes when only high-quality trials are considered.[73] In one long-term follow-up study, patients who had taken GS, 1,500 mg/day for at least 12 months, were half as likely to undergo total knee replacement (TKR) at 5 years.[73] The structural-modifying effects of glucosamine products in hip and knee OA remain uncertain.

Topical agents include analgesics and anti-inflammatory preparations. Topical analgesics may be either rubifacients, which contain methyl salicylate, chemical compounds that produce a counterirritant effect, or capsaicin compounds, which reduce pain through depletion of the neurotransmitter substance P in peripheral nerves. To date, the only topical analgesic to show consistent efficacy in controlled clinical trials is capsaicin. Capsaicin is an alkaloid derived from red chili peppers and is available in topical analgesic creams in varying concentrations (Zostrix, Capsaicin-P, Dolorac). It has been shown to decrease pain approximately 33% when applied to specific joints four times daily.[72] The initial stinging or burning sensation disappears after several days of use; however, the need for frequent daily applications may limit the acceptability of this therapy for some patients.[72] Topical NSAIDs (diclofenac) are recommended as alternative or adjunctive therapy in symptomatic knee OA. Topical preparations delivered through gel, liquid, or patch formulations are absorbed through the skin with the help of an absorption enhancer are slightly less effective than oral NSAIDs with fewer adverse events.[31,72]

■ REHABILITATIVE MANAGEMENT

The chronic progressive nature of arthritis dictates a plan of care (POC) that includes patient education and self-management beyond the initial presentation. Although RA is systemic and OA is a more localized condition, both diseases can significantly affect health, function, participation, and quality of life. The rehabilitation of persons with arthritis requires comprehensive and coordinated efforts of a team of health professionals, including physical therapists, and ensures that the patient is first and foremost in treatment planning. The patient's ability to self-manage successfully is a major predictor of better health outcomes.[75] The physical therapist plays a pivotal role in helping the patient with minimal disability gain confidence and experience in using self-management skills to deal with the condition. The general goals and outcomes for persons with RA and OA are similar (see Box 23.4).

The remainder of this chapter will discuss physical therapist examination and interventions for people with RA and OA of the hip and knee. Although OA also presents at other joints, these two are the most common and disabling sites for OA and are most frequently seen by a physical therapist.

Physical Therapy Examination

A comprehensive and multisystem examination and history is an essential component of physical therapy management. Whether the patient is a direct access client or seen in a system-based clinical setting, collaboration and communication with other care providers working with the patient is imperative. As with all patient-centered care, the patient is the primary stakeholder and should be actively engaged in goal setting and in the development of the POC.

Careful observation of the patient during the initial meeting and history can help inform the process. For example, observation of the patient's gait, ability to remove outerwear, and transfer into a chair for the history will provide the therapist with a quick assessment of functional ability.

History

The medical and social history will direct and inform the examination and provide insight into the development of a POC and need for potential resources. Ascertaining the patient's understanding of the disease and the implications of the disease is an important component of the interview process. In particular, the therapist should be concerned with identifying "red flag" signs and symptoms that indicate the need for immediate medical follow up (Table 23.5).[76] Pain assessment questions should include location, duration, pattern, quality, and intensity. Specific details regarding joint inflammation such as joint heat, swelling, and erythema should be recorded and confirmed during the physical examination. A determination of joint stiffness (morning versus after prolonged static posture), previous activity level, pattern and degree of fatigue, presence of co-morbidities, and current medication is also essential. Use and effectiveness of previous therapeutic interventions and complementary approaches should be noted. Although many physical therapy tests and measures are used during the examination, specific adaptations may be made to tailor the examination to the person with RA or OA. Especially in RA, the tender and swollen joint count appears to be a sensitive measure of systemic disease activity and guides the exercise prescription.[16]

Range of Motion

Tenderness and subjective reports of pain on passive range of motion (PROM) are highly indicative of inflammation; thus, gentle pressure and appropriate hand position is paramount during examination. Goniometric measurement of PROM is indicated and necessary at all affected joints after a gross joint screening to assist in monitoring treatment effectiveness. Standardized procedures are essential for reliable and valid measures. Otherwise, potential variations in intrarater and interrater reliability will reduce the accuracy of data comparison throughout the disease course.[77] If joint pain or poor activity tolerance prohibits measurement of PROM, the therapist may consider substituting a functional ROM test by asking the patient to touch various body parts (e.g., the top of the head and small of the back) to determine the available ROM for performing self-care activities. The therapist should note any tenderness, crepitus, or pain during examination of ROM.

Regardless of whether the patient has OA and monoarticular involvement or RA with polyarticular involvement, the impact of an involved joint on the kinematic chain or on the contralateral side should not

Table 23.5	"Red Flags" Suggesting the Need for Urgent Evaluation and Management
Flag	Differential Diagnosis
History of significant trauma	Soft tissue injury, internal derangement, or fracture
Hot, swollen joint	Infection, systemic rheumatic disease, gout, pseudogout
Constitutional signs (e.g., fever, weight loss, malaise)	Infection, sepsis, systemic rheumatic disease
Weakness Focal Diffuse	 Focal nerve lesion (compartment syndrome, entrapment neuropathy, mononeuritis multiplex, motor neuron disease, radiculopathy[a]) Myositis, metabolic myopathy, paraneoplastic syndrome, degenerative neuromuscular disorder, toxin, myelopathy,[a] transverse myelitis
Neurogenic pain (burning, numbness, paresthesia) Asymmetrical Symmetrical	 Radiculopathy,[a] reflex sympathetic dystrophy, entrapment neuropathy Myelopathy,[a] peripheral neuropathy
History of significant trauma	Soft tissue injury, internal derangement, or fracture
Claudication pain pattern	Peripheral vascular disease, giant cell arteritis (jaw pain), lumbar spinal stenosis

[a]Radiculopathy and myelopathy may be due to infectious, neoplastic, or mechanical processes.

be overlooked.[78] When there is OA in a hip or knee, active motion in functional positions should be examined in all joints of both lower extremities (LEs). It is important to observe motion for symmetry and smoothness during gait, stair climbing, and rising from a chair. Ascending stairs requires the greatest amount and velocity of knee flexion and may be one of the best activities to determine knee function.[79] Decreased ROM at the hip and knee increases the risk for injury and falls. Approximately 50° hip flexion and 90° knee flexion are required to recover balance from a stumble during walking.[80]

Strength

Pain and joint effusions impede muscle contraction, limiting examination of strength. A patient may be able to generate force in the pain-free range but unable to completely contract in the painful range secondary to reflex inhibition. Traditional strength tests (e.g., manual muscle tests) are not appropriate in the presence of severely deformed and/or deranged joints. Functional strength assessments are more appropriate and will provide sufficient data to formulate treatment goals. Individuals who demonstrate a lag phenomenon will have limited active range and will not be candidates for traditional grading systems, because these are not sensitive to changes in the quality and quantity of muscle contraction. When documenting strength, it is important to include information on required modifications made to preferred testing positions, grade of strength exhibited in that arc of motion, and the method of strength testing used (e.g., break test, isometric holding at the end of range, or resistance throughout the ROM). Modifying the test protocol to include an isometric break test at midrange or most comfortable joint position generally yields higher grades than would be received if full range testing were done. Any modifications to standardized test protocols must be carefully documented. It is also important to document the time of day the patient was tested, as well as the use and timing of medications that might alter performance or exercise tolerance.

The functional threshold for LE strength has yet to be determined. However, reports from studies that have examined knee strength as a percentage of body weight suggest that isokinetic strength measured at velocities between 60° and 180° per second should be 20% to 30% body weight for knee extension and 20% to 25% for knee flexion.[78,79] Isometric knee extension below 10 kg (22 lb) of force (measured with the hip at neutral and knee at 90°) corresponded to marked disability in a study of persons with OA of the knee.[81] It is also important to perform strength testing of the muscle groups proximal to the affected joints to detect deficits that can affect function and contribute to abnormal biomechanics.

Joint Stability

Joint stability is essential for normal biomechanics, function, and independence. Inflammatory aspects of RA can lead to joint instability and eventual deformity. Intra-articular ligaments are highly susceptible to inflammatory and erosive changes in RA. Thus, ligamentous laxity of any affected joint should be fully investigated. Pseudolaxity, often detected in unicompartmental knee OA, should be differentiated from true ligamentous laxity.

Cardiovascular Status

Fatigue is one of the systemic manifestations of RA and frequently unappreciated. Individuals with OA also report fatigue. To best ascertain the impact of fatigue on patient functioning and independence, assessments should be made over the course of a single day and over several days. The increased incidence of asymptomatic cardiovascular disease, elevated risk for ischemic heart disease, and decreased cardiovascular fitness of individuals with RA demands specific attention.[24] Heart rate, respiratory rate, blood pressure and ratings of perceived exertion should all be measured during a functional activity that is reasonably stressful for the patient's current level of fitness. Excessive increases in perceived exertion may indicate the presence of inflammation or impairment of pulmonary and cardiac function that requires more extensive and formal evaluation. It is also important to determine cardiovascular fitness in individuals with OA, because cardiovascular deficits and increased risk for coronary artery disease are clearly associated with long-standing or severe disease.[24,82]

Functional Examination

Functional examination measures provide a rich and patient-centered approach to assessment. Functional measures may include ADL, work, and leisure activities (see Chapter 8, Examination of Function). The selection of a functional measure is based on the demographic features of the patient (e.g., age, gender), the level and depth of information required, and the measure's sensitivity/responsiveness in gauging the efficacy of treatment.[83-85] As with goniometric measurement, the reliability and validity are important for individual and comparative purposes. The *Functional Status Index* (FSI), a valid and reliable measure, was designed for use in outpatient rheumatologic settings to assess an individual's function in a sample of typical ADL. FSI parameters include pain, level of difficulty, and dependence (Appendix 23.A).[86,87] The *Health Assessment Questionnaire* (HAQ) is a generic measure consisting of the following five domains or subscales: disability, discomfort, pain, drug side effects (toxicity), and costs of care (Appendix 23.B).[88] The HAQ is a component of the ACR core of measures for rheumatoid arthritis[89] and has been shown to correlate highly with measures of disease progression in RA (x-ray changes).[17] The modified HAQ, an abbreviated version of the HAQ, is a quick, easy to complete and score instrument that assesses the impact of disease activity on function and disability. Both versions are available for free online. Another arthritis-specific instrument, the revised *Arthritis Impact Measurement Scales 2* (AIMS2), expands the concept of function to include performance in psychological and social domains as well as physical function. The AIMS2 also measures the patient's satisfaction with current functional status and individual preferences for outcome.[90] The AIMS2 is not well suited for program evaluation or research purposes due to its complicated scoring algorithm and associated costs. The WOMAC is a widely used, valid, and reliable self-report instrument of 24 items in three categories specific to OA of the hip and/or knee (pain, stiffness, and function). The WOMAC takes about 10 minutes to administer and is easily scored by hand. It is available in either Likert form (0–4) or visual analogue scale.[91] Both the AIMS2 and the WOMAC are sensitive to clinical intervention and provide excellent clinically feasible, standardized measures in the domains of function and disability to monitor change over time. The *Knee Injury and Osteoarthritis Outcome* (KOOS) measure was developed using the WOMAC as a base and includes sports, recreation, and leisure items. This measure is readily accessible, is relatively easy to score, and demonstrates strong validity, reliability, and responsiveness in adults.[92] A modified version of the KOOS was developed for persons with hip osteoarthritis (HOOS).[93]

Mobility, Gait, and Balance

A complete and detailed gait examination is one of the most important contributions of the physical therapist to the rehabilitation team's understanding of the individual's functional abilities and serves to identify additional areas for examination and intervention.[94,95] (See Chapter 7, Examination of Gait, for a complete discussion.) Substantial differences in fall risks,[56] knee ROM, and gait velocity between patients with either OA or RA and their peers without arthritis have been demonstrated.[95,96]

Sensory Integrity

With RA, alternations in sensation may be evident with the presence of *Raynaud's disease* or with compression of nerves due to inflammation or joint derangement. Any indication of peripheral neuropathy or nerve involvement should be investigated using standard examination procedures (see Chapter 3, Examination of Sensory Function). Sensory changes resulting from other co-morbidities or from the normal aging process should be considered when appropriate.

Psychological Status

Individuals with chronic arthritis experience years of functional and social loss that would stress any person's ability to cope and adapt.[97] Although pain is significantly correlated with self-reports of depression, no firm association with function has been identified.[98] The overall psychological status of the individual with RA is generally similar to those individuals with other chronic diseases that threaten a severe change in body image and disruption of social integration (see Chapter 26, Psychosocial Disorders). Individuals respond to these threats with various coping strategies to maintain psychological well-being. No single strategy can be deemed definitely better than another, although for individual patients some strategies will lead to better coping and more positive outcomes than others. Exploration of the patient's attitude toward rehabilitation and readiness to make health behavior changes, as well the availability of social support, can assist the therapist in shared goal setting and identifying realistic expectations of future functional ability. Persons with RA face the additional challenges of living with a chronic disease that is characterized by a fluctuating disease course and must learn to adapt their lifestyle, activity level and medication and sleep schedule according to their disease activity. Thus, it is paramount that the therapist works with the patient to set realistic, achievable goals and educate the patient about warning signs of flares to help the patient self-manage.

Anxiety and depression are also common in patients with OA and may alter the pain experience, function, and response to treatment interventions.[99] Chronic pain, fatigue, loss of function, and reduced activity levels can all contribute to emotional distress. It is therefore important to recognize the signs of anxiety and depression and, if indicated, refer to appropriate screening services and resources to help individuals manage their psychological symptoms through improved coping skills.[100] Participation in the Arthritis Self-Management Program has been shown to improve coping.

Environmental Factors

Therapists should be aware of environmental factors in the home, work, and leisure environments that might serve as facilitators or barriers to functioning and warrant specific identification, examination, and recommendations to address (see Chapter 9, Examination of Environment.) A discussion about the home and work environments may reveal conditions that threaten independence that can be addressed through ergonomic and environmental modifications and school or workplace accommodations. The costs of such changes may be a limiting factor for implementing these recommendations. The work environment affects employment and disability in more ways than the physical setting and task requirements. Acceptance and understanding by supervisors and co-workers of the disease and self-management requirements of the worker with arthritis are important determinants of maintaining employment and income. Other environmental factors common to both the RA and OA ICF Core Sets include technology and assistive devices for ADL, mobility, transportation, and employment; design and access to buildings; climate; and attitudes of family, friends, and health professionals.[62,63,101,102]

Physical Therapy Intervention

The development of specific goals and expected outcomes for the individual with arthritis is based on the following general goals and expected outcomes developed in conjunction with the patient (Box 23.4).

The specific goals and outcomes identified for each patient will depend on the type of arthritis, disease activity level, the clinical presentation, and patient preferences in line with patient-centered care. Mutual goal setting promotes patient participation in

---

Box 23.4 Examples of General Goals and Outcomes for Patients with Arthritis

Impact of impairments is reduced.

• Pain is decreased.
• ROM of all joints is maximized sufficient for functional activities.
• Muscle activation and strength is maximized sufficient for functional activities.
• Joint stability is maximized and biomechanical stress on all affected joints are decreased, deformity prevented.
• Endurance is increased for all functional activities and desired leisure activities.

Ability to perform physical actions, tasks, or activities is improved.

• Independence in ADL is promoted, including dressing, transfers, and self-care.
• Efficiency and safety of gait pattern and balance are improved.
• Patterns of adequate physical activity or exercise to maintain or improve musculoskeletal and cardiovascular fitness and general health are established.

Health status and quality of life are improved.

• Patient, family, and caregivers are educated to promote the individual's capacity for self-management, including joint protection.

Adapted from *Guide to Physical Therapist Practice*.

---

treatment. It is the physical therapist's responsibility to document the POC, implement that plan safely and effectively, and delegate responsibility appropriately to ensure that the patient's goals can be reached. The therapist should ensure that treatment goals and objectives are measurable, attainable, and documented, with specific timeframes included (e.g., increase left shoulder flexion ROM by 10° in 2 weeks, and independent ambulation with platform crutches on level surfaces for at least 250 feet without fatigue within 1 month). Failure to achieve goals within the stated timeframe indicates the need for reevaluation and reformulation of the goals. Goals and outcomes should be revised to reflect changes owing to both personal and environmental factors that may affect progress or alter the proposed time frames (see Chapter 1, Clinical Decision Making).

Modalities for Pain Relief

A variety of physical agents are available to relieve pain and prepare the patient for passive and dynamic stretching and other exercise interventions. The most common form is thermotherapy.

Heat

Superficial heat, heat that penetrates only a few millimeters, produces localized analgesia and increases circulation in the vicinity where it is applied. Types of superficial heat include moist hot packs; dry heating pads; and lamps, paraffin, and hydrotherapy. The evidence supporting the effectiveness of these modalities is weak, but patients often report that they gain comfort from moist heat. Paraffin is particularly useful in delivering superficial heat to irregularly shaped joints or to individuals who cannot tolerate the weight of a moist hot pack. Hydrotherapy allows the therapist to combine heating of tissues with exercise, and provides the patient the experience of aquatic therapy, although it is expensive. Systematic reviews of heat and cold therapy in arthritis suggest small to modest effects.[103,104]

Deep heating modalities, such as ultrasound, may affect the viscoelastic properties of collagen and increase the plastic stretch of ligaments, providing modest improvements in pain and function in individuals with knee OA.[105] However, their efficacy in RA is not demonstrated.[106] Their use in treating individuals with RA during the acute stage of inflammation is contraindicated because they may stimulate collagenase activity within the joint, furthering its destruction.[107,108] Furthermore, modalities that do not readily translate to home use foster a dependency on clinical care and do not promote self-management.

Cold

Local applications of cold will also produce local analgesia, increase superficial circulation at the site of application following an initial period of vasoconstriction, and decrease intra-articular temperature.[109] Cold is particularly useful around joints that are inflamed and swollen, a condition that usually worsens with the application of superficial heat modalities. Therapists may use either wet or dry application techniques. Superficial cold is contradicted in patients with Raynaud's phenomenon or *cryoglobulinemia,* linked to an abnormal protein (cryoglobulins) in the blood that gels at low temperatures. Both may be associated with RA.

Electrical Agents

Therapists may also wish to consider using other modalities for pain relief in treating the individual with RA, including transcutaneous electrical nerve stimulation (TENS), although the value of TENS as reported in the literature is inconsistent.[110,111] A meta-analysis of studies investigating TENS for knee OA pain concluded that the mode of TENS applied did affect results, repeated use was more effective than a single application, and use for at least 4 weeks was the most effective.[111]

Orthoses, Splints, and Braces

In RA, hand and wrist orthoses may be used to immobilize specific joints and help reduce pain and swelling by providing local rest and support. There are three primary types of splints: functional (used to restore or improve function), corrective (used to improve alignment), and resting (used to maintain joint alignment and reduce pain). Resting splints are worn at night or periodically during the day. There is evidence of small benefits for pain reduction and increased function with the use of functional splints. Hand splints may improve grip and pincher strength.[112] There is evidence that wearing functional wrist splints decreases grip strength and does not affect pain, morning stiffness, pinch grip, or quality of life with regular wear.[113] A study that investigated the effect of functional wrist splint wear on task performance reported that wearing a commercially available elastic wrist orthosis resulted in some decrement in performance speed on a number of common tasks, though pain was significantly reduced for all tasks.[114] There is consistent evidence supporting the use of splints for short- and long-term pain relief in hand OA.[115]

Foot orthoses also may be used to alleviate pain through biomechanical support or correction for individuals with knee OA. A lateral wedge insole designed to reduce medial compartment stress appears to reduce pain and NSAID use in some individuals with knee OA.[116] Other methods that show promise in treating knee OA pain are patellofemoral taping,[117] and load shifting or unloader knee braces (stress shifted away from most involved area).[116] All orthotic interventions require professional evaluation, selection, education, and monitoring of use.

Rest

Complete bed rest is rarely recommended. Adequate quality and quantity of sleep at night and short rests during the day are preferred. General recommendations include 8 to 10 hours of sleep per night and brief 30-minute rest periods during the day. Inactivity is a common problem for people with arthritis and may lead to deconditioning, depression, lower pain thresholds, diminished bone and soft tissue health, and increased risk for other serious health conditions. Thus, a major goal of therapy is to assist the person to maintain or regain adequate levels of physical activity and avoid the unnecessary consequences of inactivity.[16]

Range of Motion and Flexibility Exercise

A major factor affecting joint mobility in individuals with RA is the level of inflammation and resting position in which specific joints are maintained. For example, intra-articular pressure is reduced when the knee is slightly bent. Although helpful in reducing joint pain, this flexed position may lead to capsular and musculotendonous shortening and eventual contracture. Patients should be taught proper positioning when resting and should be encouraged to perform daily, active ROM as tolerated to maintain motion. Active-assisted, passive, and proprioceptive neuromuscular facilitation (PNF) techniques may also be applied to shortened muscles.[118] Pain should be respected at all times and should be minimal during and after exercise. Evoking a pain response during stretching may lead to a reflex contraction of the agonist muscle as opposed to creating a relaxation response. Stretching exercises to lengthen shortened muscles should be performed slowly, held for 20 to 30 seconds two to three days a week or more often if indicated. It is important to educate the patient not to do stretching exercises that involve inflamed, swollen joints because they are at risk for capsular stretching and rupture.[119] Common wisdom recommends that *exercise-induced pain should subside within 1 hour.* If the patient reports discomfort lasting longer than 1 hour, it may indicate that either the technique, intensity, or duration of the exercise was too great and should be reduced or modified at the next exercise session. Patients should be encouraged to exercise on their own during those times of the day when they feel best. Local pain relieving modalities before or immediately after exercise may be useful and increase exercise adherence.

In hip and knee OA, manual therapy may offer some additional benefit within a comprehensive treatment program that includes exercise.[118] Manual therapy is not generally recommended for individuals with RA who have joint inflammation or resultant laxity.

Strengthening Exercise

Decreased muscle function (strength, endurance, power) in persons with arthritis arises from both direct and indirect effects of the disease. These include intra-articular and extra-articular inflammatory disease elements, side effects of medication, disuse, reflex inhibition in response to pain and joint effusion, impaired proprioception, and loss of mechanical integrity around the joint. A variety of conditioning programs can be effective for improving strength, endurance, and function without exacerbation of pain or disease activity.

Initially, isometric exercise may be indicated to improve muscle tone, strength, and static endurance; to recruit or activate specific muscles; and to prepare joints for more vigorous activity. Although isometric exercise does avoid dynamic joint stress and mechanical irritation, it can produce other unwanted effects. Isometric exercise performed at more than 50% of maximal voluntary contraction constricts blood flow through the exercising muscle, leading to post-exercise muscle soreness, and the increased peripheral vascular resistance produces increased blood pressure.[119] In the knee and hip, high-intensity isometric contractions are associated with significant increases in intra-articular pressure and reduce synovial circulation.[120-122] Patients with cardiovascular disease should perform these exercises with caution and be sure to breathe during the contraction because holding one's breath can increase intra-abdominal pressure (Valsalva maneuver). Patient instructions for isometric exercise should include the cautions to (1) maintain the contraction for no more than 6 seconds; (2) avoid maximal effort because it is neither necessary nor desirable; (3) exhale during the contraction and inhale during a similar time period of relaxation; and (4) not contract more than two muscle groups at a time.

Dynamic exercise includes both shortening (concentric) and lengthening (eccentric) contractions. Strength and endurance may be improved through resistance (physiological overload) supplied by weight of the body part or external resistance in the form of free weights, elastic bands, or a variety of resistive exercise equipment. A cautious approach to resistance training is recommended to protect unstable or inflamed joints from damage.[16,119] Strengthening exercise should be performed within the pain-free range. Maximum benefit and maintenance can be achieved by incorporating functional movements and body positions in the recommended exercise routine. The use of well-controlled smooth movement toward the end part of the range is advised, and modifications to resistance, repetitions, or frequency are recommended as needed. Gradual progression of resistance and repetition is recommended. Reduce exercise intensity, frequency, or motion if increased joint swelling or pain occurs (local inflammatory response).

Individuals with RA benefit from maintaining or restoring muscular fitness. A number of well-controlled studies have reported on strengthening programs that provide overload with results indicating positive adaptations in muscle and functional performance with no exacerbation of disease symptoms. Data from selected RA exercise studies are presented in Box 23.5 Evidence Summary.[123-135] Loads of up to 70% one repetition maximum (1RM) used in a circuit training resistance program for persons with controlled RA demonstrated no exacerbation in joint symptoms and significant improvements in strength and function.[123,124,126,128]

Designing exercise interventions for individuals with RA requires careful consideration of the patient's disease activity, disease severity, and systemic disease features. Persons with RA in an active flare-up should limit their exercise to daily ROM exercises incorporated into ADLs to promote adherence to active joint movement and isometric exercises to promote strength. Walking as tolerated is encouraged together with daily periods of rest and a full night of sleep to manage fatigue. When the disease activity subsides, the exercise program can be progressed by adding dynamic strengthening exercises, with caution to avoid stress on deranged joints or cysts, and greater repetitions of isometric exercises as well as greater engagement in physical activity. When the disease is in remission, aerobic exercises and dynamic exercises with resistance should be considered to promote cardiovascular health and improve strength and conditioning.[16]

In persons with knee OA, the evidence is strong and consistent that LE exercise that includes neuromuscular and functional training reduces pain and improves function. Interventions have included isometric, isotonic, and functional exercise, as well as proprioceptive and balance training. Interventions have been tested in both clinically supervised and self-directed settings with positive results and acceptable adherence.[97,136] Evidence supporting the use of exercise in the management of knee and hip OA is presented in Box 23.6 Evidence Summary.[137-142] Physical therapists should routinely incorporate strategies to enhance patient motivation and adherence to the therapeutic exercise and home exercise programs (HEPs) including exercise booster sessions (periodic follow-up appointments), goal setting, and other self-efficacy enhancing practices.[119]

Cardiovascular Training

Individuals with RA or OA are usually deconditioned compared to their age-matched peers. A number of systematic reviews and well-controlled trials have reported improvements in aerobic capacity and activity levels through regular cardiovascular conditioning without aggravating joints and other disease symptoms.[16,24,125,130] Programs and guidelines appropriate for healthy adults or older individuals can be instituted following the

Box 23.5 Evidence Summary   Therapeutic Exercise in the Management of Rheumatoid Arthritis (RA)

Author (yr)	Design and Sample	Intervention	Adherence	Outcomes
Hakkinen et al[123] (2001)	RCT. 70 pts w/recent onset RA. 24 month study. No pt had taken glucocorticoids or DMARDs previously. Random assignment to 2 groups. Randomization performed by clustering pts according to age (<50, >50 yo) and sex to keep groups comparable.	Strength training group: all major ms @ 50-70% 1RM. 8-12 reps x 2. ~45′ per session 2x/wk. (intensity re-evaled every 6 months) Total mins/wk: 90′ ROM group: no resistance, only ROM and stretching 2x/wk. All encouraged to participate in recreational activities 2-3x/wk (30-45′ ea.) Training diaries examined @ 6-month intervals. All treated w/meds to achieve disease remission.	62 pts completed study. Strength group compliance = 1.4-1.5x/wk.	Sig incr ms strength (19-59%). Sig improvements in clinical disease activity parameters, HAQ scores, and walking speed in the strength group. Improvements in ms strength, disease activity parameters, and phys funx in control group but < strength group. *"Regular dynamic strength training combined w/endurance-type PA improves ms strength and phys funx, but not BMD*, in pts w/early RA, w/out detrimental effects on disease activity."*
Baillet et al[124] (2009)	RCT. Data collected at 1, 6, and 12 months. 50 patients. All pts treated with DMARD before enrollment. ECG performed on every pt, all had consultation w/cardiologist (pts > 45 yo, + CVD risk factors or abnorm ECG). Exclusion criteria: tx w/ >10 mg glucocorticoid/day, no/unstable DMARD regimen, disease activity score 28 variation >1.2 past 3 months, an age <18 >70 yo and global funx status RA class III or IV. Pts unable to follow the programme (complete ex, follow-ups, educational programme or complete questionnaire) excluded. Needed: 38 pts in DEP group. 76 pts in control group (conventional jt rehab). *But sample size limited to 50.*	DEP group: 1st week = educational/testing meetings 2nd week = occupational therapy – RA on ADLs 3rd week = OT skill ex and ADLs w/incr intensity (against resistance). 4th week = ex focused on office tasks. Training programme: improve ms strength, flex, endurance, balance. 5x/wk in gym (45′/day) and pool (60′/day). Cycling activity = HR 60-80% HRM. Resistance/intensity ex designed individually. Scheduled breaks and relaxation sessions for p! tolerance/psycho-soc. "warm-up" and "cool-down" for each session. Pts kept a diary. Control group: Multidisciplinary prog – 3 day intervention (~20H) designed to incr knowledge of disease, management, jt protection. Hydrotherapy (45′ @ 35°C) 1st day, relaxation 45′ 2nd day, phys ex (45 min/day) to prevent atrophy and tension.	25 randomly placed on DEP. 25 into control group. 2 individuals left after randomization. No pts lost to follow-up. 1 not assessed for NHP and AIMS2-SF @ 1 month. 3 pts not assessed @ 6 months. 4 not assessed @ 12 months.	HAQ (primary outcome) improved throughout length of trial in the DEP group** improvement > DEP than standard joint rehab group @ 1 month but not 6 months or 12. DEP improved NHP (Nottingham HealthProfile) and aerobic fitness @ 1 month but not after. DEP improved DHI, SODA, DAS 28, AIMS2-SF, but not sig.

Continued

Box 23.5 Evidence Summary Therapeutic Exercise in the Management of Rheumatoid Arthritis (RA)—cont'd

Author (yr)	Design and Sample	Intervention	Adherence	Outcomes
de Jong et al[126] (2003)	RCT. Testing effectiveness and safety of a 2-yr intensive ex program (RAPIT) w/those of PT – aka UC – usual care. 309 RA pts assigned to RAPIT or UC. Primary end points funx ability (MACTAR), Pt preference disability questionnaire, and HAQ and effects on x-ray progression in large joints.	Stratified for age (<50 and >50) and sex put into random digit generator. RAPIT: 2x/wk ex prog 1.25 hrs/session. 2.5 hrs/week. 3 parts per session: bike training (20'), ex circuit (20') and sport/game (20'). Each session had "warm-up" and "cool-down". Bike settings based on 1) HR during ride 2) RPE (0-10). HR kept @ ~70-90% HRM and RPE @ 4-5. Ex circuit: 8-10 ex for ms strength, endurance, jt mobility, ADLs. Ex: rest→ 90 sec/60 sec 1st weeks – 90 sec/30 sec after 6 months. Each ex repeated 8-15x. Sport/game section: impact-delivering sport activities. Impact loading also during "warm-up" and "ex circuit" portions. UC group: Tx by PT only if regarded as necessary by MD. All pts MDs had choice for med selection and other tx strategies (except high-intensity WB ex).	Needed 119 pts/group for statistical sig. planned to enroll @ least 150/group. Used 309 pts. RAPIT group slightly younger 45 yo vs 47 yo mean. > proportion of females – 79% vs 72%. 9 pts randomized but refused participation. Lost 5 pts in UC and 14 in RAPIT over the 2 yrs. 14 other RAPIT pts failed to attend ex classes but were reg evaled. Median % of sessions attended was 74%. 65% had high attendance rate first 6 months, 49% second 6 month period and stable thereafter.	After 2 yrs RAPIT > improvement in funx ability than UC. Mean difference in change of MACTAR was 2.6 1st year and 3.1 2nd year. 2 yr mean HAQ change -0.09. Median x-ray damage didn't incr in either group. Both groups w/considerable baseline damage showed progression in damage (more obvious in RAPIT group). RAPIT effective in improving emotional status. No detrimental effects on DA were found. *"Long-term high-intensity ex program is more effective than UC in improving funx ability of RA pts. Intensive ex does not incr x-ray damage of the lrg jts, except possibly in pts w/considerable baseline damage of the lrg jts."*
Eversden L, et al[127] (2007)	RCT. Hydrotherapy vs Land Ex. Effects on overall response to tx, phys funx, and QOL. 115 pts randomly assigned. Men and woman 18 yo+ w/RA in funx classes 1-3 in Birmingham clinics Required to understand and follow simple instructions in English. Stable dose of DMARDs for 6 weeks and NSAIDs for 2 weeks before entry. No injections of corticosteroids allowed in 4 wks before study. Excluded pts w/sx 3 months prior or scheduled, pts who'd received PT or hydrotherapy in 6 months before study. Pts w/chlorine sensitivity,	30' session 1x/wk for 6 weeks (both water and land groups). Pts allowed to default up to 3 sessions as long as 6 were completed. HEP given to all pts – not required to do ex b/n tx but could if desired. Group sizes 1-4 for hydro and 1-6 for land ex @ a time. Ex tailored to each pts ability. "Warm up" = mobilizing and stretching. Core ex focused on jt mobility, ms strength, and funx activities. Degree of difficulty reviewed weekly to ensure progress. "Cool down" phase after each session.	11 pts did not complete tx in land ex. 4 pts did not complete in hydrotherapy. Goal to recruit 60 pts into each of the groups. 115 pts were randomized. 57 pts in hydrotherapy (46 had data collection – primary outcome). 58 pts in land (40 pts had primary outcome data).	Primary outcome: self-rated global impression of change – 7pt scale. Secondary outcomes: EuroQol health related QOL, EuroQol health status valuation, HAQ, 10m walk time, p! scores – collected @ baseline, after tx, 3 months later. Hydrotherapy pts sig "much better" or "very much better" than land ex.10m walk test improved in both groups. No sig diff b/n groups in HAQ, EQ-5D utility score EQ VAS and pain VAS. *"Pts w/RA treated w/hydrotherapy are more likely to report feeling much better or very much better than those w/land ex immediately on completion of the tx programme. This perceived benefit was not reflected by differences b/n groups in 10m*

Box 23.5 Evidence Summary Therapeutic Exercise in the Management of Rheumatoid Arthritis (RA)—cont'd

Author (yr)	Design and Sample	Intervention	Adherence	Outcomes
	infected open wound, incontinence of faeces, poorly controlled epilepsy, HTN, DM, and fear of water were excluded from hydroptherapy. Excluded: pregnant women, pts w/co-morbid conditions preventing safe use of hydrotherapy, known carries of staph in the URT and weighing >102 kg b/c of safety procedures for the pool.			walk times, funx scores, QOL measures and pain scores.
Lemmey et al[128] (2009)	RCT. "Efficacy of high-intensity progressive resistive training (PRT) in restoring ms mass and funx in pts w/RA" also to "investigate the role of the insulin-like growth factor (IGF) system in ex-induced ms hypertrophy in the context of RA." 28 pts w/est controlled RA. Conducted July 2004-January 2007.	2 groups: 2x/wk PRT (n=13) or range of mvt home ex control group (n=15). Dual x-ray absorptiometry-assessed body comp; objective phys funx; disease activity; and ms IFG's assessed @ weeks 0 and 24. Stratified by age, sex and estrogen status. Assessments done @ baseline and immediately following 24 wk training period. Pts required to fast and refrained from ex for 24 hrs. PRT group: 24 wks, 2x/wk. 3x8 @ load of 80% 1RM per ex. 1-2' rest b/n ex. leg press, chest press, leg ext, seated row, leg curl, triceps ext, standing calf raises, and bicep curl. Goal to achieve hypertrophy. 1 set completed in 1st week 2 sets 2nd week 15 reps/set @ 60% of 1RM wks 1-4. 12 reps/set @ 70% 1RM 5-6 wks. 8 reps/set @ 80 % max weeks 7-24. 1RM reassessed every 4 wks. "warm up" and "cool down" periods – 10' ea. Low-intensity ROM ex. asked to perform these 2x/wk at home (ROM ex). ROM was control condition b/c most commonly prescribed for Pts w/RA. All completed training diary to check for compliance and adverse effects. Control pts phoned every 2 weeks.	Needed sample size for each group = 5 subjects. Aimed for 18 subjects to cover drop out. (36 total) 36 individuals were randomized into 2 groups. 28 attended baseline assessment and commenced training. PRT: 48 scheduled sessions – completed avg 34.6 sessions. (73%) ROM ex group: good compliance avg 25.9 sessions (54%).	PRT incr LBM and ALM (appendicular lean mass); reduced trunk fat mass by 2.5 kg (not sig); and improved training-specific strength by 119%, chair stands by 30%, knee ext strength by 25%, arm curls by 23%, and walk time by 17%. Body comp and phys funx remained unchanged in control patients. Changes in LBM and regional lean mass assoc w/changes in objective funx. Coinciding w/ms hypertrophy, previously diminished ms levels of IGF-1 and IGF binding protein 3 both incr following PRT. *"In an RCT, 24 weeks of PRT proved safe and effective in restoring lean mass and funx in pts with RA. Ms hypertrophy coincided w/sig elevations of attenuated ms IGF levels, revealing a possible contributory mechanism for rheumatoid cachexia. PRT should feature in disease management."*

Continued

Box 23.5 Evidence Summary   Therapeutic Exercise in the Management of Rheumatoid Arthritis (RA)—cont'd

Author (yr)	Design and Sample	Intervention	Adherence	Outcomes
Smidt et al[129] (2005)	Summarize available evidence on effectiveness of ex therapy for pts w/ disorders of ms, nervous, respiratory, and cv systems. *Systematic reviews.* **OA:** 7 reviews for hip/ knee OA. 3 reasonable/ good quality reviews: ex therapy, consisting of strengthening, stretching and funx ex is effective for pt with knee OA compared to no tx. Indications that ex therapy is effective for pts w/hip OA – based on 1 large RCT. Insufficient evidence to support/ refute the effectiveness of a specific type of ex therapy (individual, group, hydro tx) for pts w/knee or hip OA. *(Fransen et al 2002, McCarty and Oldham 1999, Pendleton et al 2000, Petrella 2000, Philadelphia Panel 2001a, Puett and Griffin 1994, van Baar et al 1998a, Van Baar et al 1999, van Baar et al 2001)* "Ex therapy, consisting of strengthening, stretching, and functional exercises, is effective for patients with knee OA, compared to no tx" – *Fransen, Philadelphia panel, van Baar 1998a, Van Baar 1999, and 2001.* One large RCT stated "ex therapy is effective for pts w/hip OA" – *van Baar et al 1998b.* "Insufficient evidence to support or refute the effectiveness of a specific type of exercise therapy (individual, group therapy, or hydrotherapy) for pts with knee or hip OA."	Used overview of each systematic review (>60 pts) was made. Categorized according to quality score: good (>80), reasonable quality (60-79), mod quality (40-59), poor (20-39) and very poor (<20). Used reasonable (60-70) and good (>80). Conclusions were discussed with panel of experts and categorization of conclusion based on 2 research questions: A) What is the effectiveness of ex therapy, compared to no tx, a placebo, or a wait-and-see policy? B) What is the effectiveness of ex therapy, compared to other tx (steroid injections)? Is one specific type of ex therapy more effective than others?	104 sys reviews selected. 45 = good quality. Overall inter-rater agreement for quality assessment was (86%). Most disagreements caused by differences interpretation when discussing the power of RCT and heterogeneity of RCT and outcomes. **RA:** 2 systematic reviews investigated the effectiveness of ex therapy for pts with RA. *(Augustinus et al 2000, van den Ende et al 1998, van den Ende et al 2002).* One systematic review → conclusion there is insufficient evidence to support or refute the effectiveness of ex therapy for patients w/ rheumatoid arthritis. *(van den Ende 1998 and 2002).*	Ex therapy effective for pts w/knee OA, sub-acute (6-12 wks) and chronic (>12 wks) lbp, therapy is effective for pts w/ ankylosing spony, hip OA, Parkinson's disease, pts w/stroke. *Insufficient evidence* to support/ refute effectiveness for neck pain, shld pain, repetitive strain injury, RA, asthma, and bronchiectasis. NOT effective for pts w/acute LBP. Effective for wide range of chronic disorders.

Box 23.5 Evidence Summary Therapeutic Exercise in the Management of Rheumatoid Arthritis (RA)—cont'd

Author (yr)	Design and Sample	Intervention	Adherence	Outcomes
Ottawa Panel [130] (2004)	Create guidelines for the use of ther ex and manual therapy in the management of adult patients (.18 yo) w/a dx of RA. Evidence from comparative controlled trials ID and synthesized using Cochrane Collaboration methods.	Set inclusion/exclusion criteria with a panel of 9 experts. Performed Lit search for RCTs – expanded to case-control, cohort, and non RCTs. *Rehab interventions:* IDed as specific funx strengthening ex, whole-body funx strengthening ex, and PA. comparators = placebo, untx or use of ed pamphlets or written instructions for self-management.	16 studies out of 2,280 potential articles. 862 articles for manual therapy – 4 had potential – none included. *Concluded:* ther ex – including specific funx strengthening and whole-body funx strengthening are a beneficial intervention for pts with RA – benefit may vary according to disease acuity and the time frame during which the outcomes are measured. *Clinical benefits:* pain relief, upper-limb (grip) and lower-limb force, and funx status *Other benefits:* improved overall funx, and decr number of sick leaves.	6 + recommendations clinical benefit were developed on therapeutic ex. The efficacy of manual therapy intervention could not be determined for lack of evidence. 6 + recommendations of clinical benefit were developed on ther ex. efficacy of man therapy interventions could not be determined for lack of evidence. *Panel recommends use of ther ex for RA. Further research is needed to determine efficacy of manual therapy in the management of this disease.* Recommend: knee funx strengthening, whole-body funx strengthening, general PA, and whole-body, low-intensity ex, for the management RA. Evidence is lacking for shld/hand strengthening ex and whole-body, high-intensity ex or manual therapy.
Bearne [131] (2002)	Compare quadriceps sensorimotor funx, lower limb funx performance and disability in pts w/RA and healthy subjects and to investigate the efficacy and safety of a brief rehab regime. Quad strength, voluntary activation, proprioceptive acuity and the aggregate time to perform 4 common activities – compared b/n 103 RA pts w/lower limb involvement and 25 healthy subjects.	*Quad strength/voluntary activation:* strain gauge system attached to specially constructed chair – seated w/hip/knee flex 90 deg. Used percutaneous estim on voluntary isometric contraction. Recorded 3 max voluntary contractions and analyzed. Weakest leg = "index leg". Recorded ms strength and voluntary activation using strongest MVC of the index leg for analysis.	Measured: Health Assessment Questionnaire, clinical disease activity and plasma concentration of proinflammatory cytokines were measured in the RA pts.	RA pts had weaker quads, poorer activation, and proprioceptive acuity and took longer to perform AFPT. Rehab incr quad strength and voluntary activation and subjective disability w/out exacerbating disease activity. All improvements maintained @ 6 month follow-up. No change during control period.

Continued

Box 23.5 Evidence Summary Therapeutic Exercise in the Management of Rheumatoid Arthritis (RA)—cont'd

Author (yr)	Design and Sample	Intervention	Adherence	Outcomes
		Rehabilitation: 47 pts randomized to begin immediately, 41 pts delayed. 10 ex sessions (2 x/wk x 5 wks) – simple, progressive, individually prescribed ex designed to incr quad strength, address each pt's disabilities and improve balance and coordination, using inexpensive and unsophisticated equip. Each ex session had warm-up ex (i.e., 5 mins cycling), 24 isometric MVCs (4 sets x 6 contractions – 1 min rest between each) @ 90 deg knee flex to incr quad strength, 3 individually prescribed funx ex (sit-to-stand, step-ups etc) and 3 balance ex – 1-5 min and # reps recorded. *Pts were encouraged and given feedback on performance.* Each ex session = 30-40 mins.		
Brorsson et al[132] (2009)	*"To eval the effects of hand ex in pts with RA, and to compare the results with healthy controls."* 40 women (20 w/RA and 20 healthy) performed hand ex programme. Results evaluated after 6 and 12 wks w/hand force measurements. Hand funx was evaluated with Grip Ability Test (GAT) and with patient relevant questionnaires – Disability of the arm, Shoulder, and Hand – DASH and Short Form-36. US measurements performed on EDC for analysis of ms response to ex programme.	*Study period:* 18 wks – examined @ 6 wk intervals. 2 baseline exams completed before ex regimen began. (week 0). Ex prog performed for 12 wks. Designed according to Flat (reference 12) and performed: 5x/wk, each task x 10 and position of max effort held 3-5 sec with 20 sec rest b/n reps. Ex sessions separated by @ least 1 day. *Ex program took 10 min to complete* – used therapeutic putty (85g). pts chose soft, medium, or firm putty. *Pts kept diaries during training period to declare all ex.*	40 subjects recruited – 2 control and 2 RA pts withdrew = 36 completed the study.	"The ext and flex force improved in both groups after 6 wks. Hand funx (GAT) also improved in both groups. The RA group showed improvement in the results of the DASH questionnaire. The cross-sectional area of the EDC incr significantly in both groups measured with US." Conclusion: *"A sig improvement in hand force and hand funx in pts with RA was seen after 6 weeks of hand training; the improvement was even more pronounced after 12 wks. Hand ex is thus an effective intervention for RA pts, leading to better strength and funx."*
Crowley[133] (2009)	"Review of literature....evaluate the effectiveness of HEP for pts w/RA." Searched 7 databases.		8 papers out of 18 were included. All had high risk of bias. *"Results show that HEP are effective in*	"The results of this review highlight the benefits of HEP for pts w/RA, when encompassed physical, funx, and QOL domains. Further research is needed to confirm these findings."

Box 23.5 Evidence Summary   Therapeutic Exercise in the Management of Rheumatoid Arthritis (RA)—cont'd

Author (yr)	Design and Sample	Intervention	Adherence	Outcomes
			improving ms strength, jt mobility, shld funx, and self-efficacy and reducing morning stiffness, number of tender/swollen jts, and p! w/out incr inflammation or disease activity."	
Hsieh et al [134] (2009)	"Compare the effectiveness and safety of supervised aerobic ex and home aerobic ex in female Chinese pts with RA". *Single-blind RCT.* 30 patients w/RA assigned to group. Supervised aerobic ex prog supervised by PT, home program done @ home after 1 instructional session.	1 hr ex: 3 x/wk x 8 wks. Aerobic capacity and disease-related variables, including p! intensity, funx ability, psychological status and jt funx were measured. 10 min stretching, 10 min warm-up, 30 min pool ex, 10 min cool down. Objective to allow target HR of 50-80% VO2 peak for @ least 30 mins. Multiple short sessions were allowed for total of 30 mins. Used daily logs for self-monitoring of duration intensity and freq of ex. called every 2 wks and checked ex log @ end of 8wk prog.	38 patients recruited → 30 pts randomized into 2 groups. All completed study. Most pts ACR class II.	"An 8 wk supervised aerobic ex prog induced sig improvement in aerobic capacity of female Chinese patients w/RA, and was superior to a home aerobic ex prog. Both prog of aerobic ex were safe for female Chinese pts with RA." Compliance in SAE = 100%, HAE = 52% ranging 32-75%. No sig diff in baseline data b/n groups. *Within-group:* variables of ex tolerance test (VO2, MET, work, O2 pulse, SBP @ peak CV response and VO2, MET @ ventilator threshold) = sig improvement found in SAE group but not HAE. Stat sig diff observed for b/n group comparisons b/n SAE and HAE w/changed score b/n baseline data and post-ex data in Vo2, MET, work, O2 pulse, and SBPT @ peak CV response. Sig diff b/n group comparison in changed score of VO2 and MET @ vent threshold. SAE induced mean improvements of 20%, 16%, 14% in VO2 peak, peak workload, and O2 pulse respectively. No sig difference b/n groups for disease-related measures except global self-assessment and global MD assessment. *Within group SAE* = sig diff for global p! intensity, ADL p! scale, grip strength, walking time, and global self-assessment. HAE group = sig ex effect in global p! intensity, ADL pain scale, and walking time. *No sig b/n group diff regarding changed score b/n baseline data and post-ex data for disease-related measures.*

Continued

Box 23.5 Evidence Summary Therapeutic Exercise in the Management of Rheumatoid Arthritis (RA)—cont'd

Author (yr)	Design and Sample	Intervention	Adherence	Outcomes
Kennedy[135] (2006)	Eval the outcome of intensive ex prog for pts with RA on bone mineral density and disease activity. Searched 6 databases. Included: papers investigating the effect of aerobic and/or strengthening prog on pts w/RA. 11 papers out of 30 returned were included; 4 of 11 had low risk of bias. 1999-2004.	***van den Ende et al 2000** – 20 female pts. Sample size 64. Isometric and isokinetic ms strength + bicycling for 15 min, 3x/wk @ 60% age predicted max + usual care vs usual care (ROM + isometric).* <u>Outcome measures:</u> disease activity, ms strength, jt mobility, funx ability. <u>Results:</u> Incr ms strength and physical funx w/no incr disease activity in intensive ex group. ***de Jong et al 2003** – 237 female pts, n = 309. RAPIT prog: 2x/wk: (i) bike training (20 in @ 70-90% max HR); (ii) ex circuit (20 min)p (iii) sport/game (20 min) vs usual care.* <u>Outcome measures:</u> Disease activity, funx ability, physical capacity, emotional status, radiographic damage. <u>Results:</u> No detrimental effects on disease activity. Funx ability improved more than "usual care" group. Emotional status improved in RAPIT group. Pts w/baseline jt damage showed more progression of jt damage. ***de Jong et al 2004** – 237 female, n = 309. Intervention same as above.* <u>Outcome measures:</u> Disease activity, physical capacity, funx ability, radiological damage of small and lrg jt x-rays, BMD of hip and lumbar spine. <u>Results:</u> Decr in BMD in femoral head only both groups, smaller decr in RAPIT groups. ***de Jong et al 2004** – 237 female, n = 309. Intervention per de Jong 2003.* <u>Outcome measures:</u> Rate of radiographic progression of damage in hands and feet (Larsen score) <u>Results:</u> sig less radiological damage in small jts.	30 articles = RCTs of ex in RA. Used a total of 11 papers. Only 4 studies had low level of bias. Review focused on results of the 4 low biased studies.	"Ex prog for pts w/RA don't incr disease activity, are safe, and slow down the loss of bone mineral in the hip. Results of this review highlight the safety and benefits of aerobic and dynamic strengthening ex prog for pts w/RA."

Box 23.5 Evidence Summary   Therapeutic Exercise in the Management of Rheumatoid Arthritis (RA)—cont'd

Author (yr)	Design and Sample	Intervention	Adherence	Outcomes
Williams et al 136 (2010)	"To evaluate the feasibility and gait stability and balance outcomes of a 4-month individualized HEP for women w/ arthritis." Pre-post interventional study.	Initial assessment, then all participants received home balance ex from PT based on assessment findings and ex available from commercially available kits. All measures repeated 4 months later. *Main outcome measures: Falls risk and balance measures. Intervention: Pts visited @ home by PT to start prog. Complete ex 5x/wk for 4 months. Balance, strengthening and walking ex were selected from Otago ex prog and Visual Health Information Ex Prescription Kits – Balance & Vestibular Rehab set. Participants received an ex folder including: description, graphics and dosage of each ex, ex calendar for each moth of prog. If ex weights were required = provided by PT. Given b/n 4-8 ex (~20-30 mins including rests) as well as recommendation to walk in the community @ least 3x/wk. Reviewed ex @ home on 2 occasions. 4 and 8 wk marks. Modifications made as needed.*	N = 49, females. LL OA or LL RA. Only 39 were eligible and completed study. 66.7% adherence to prog.	"At baseline, 64% of participants reported falling in the preceding 12 months, avg falls risk – Falls Risk of Older People – Community Setting – score was 14.5 w/42% rated as moderate risk. Pts achieved and improved performance on most balance and related measures after ex prog including falls risk, activity levels, fear of falling, funx reach test, rising index for sit to stand, step width in walking, and body mass index." "An individualized balance training hEP is feasible for older women with OA and RA and may improve stability during walking and other funx activities."

ADL = activities of daily living; BMD – bone mineral density; DMARDs = Disease Modifying Anti-Inflammatory Drugs; DEP = Dynamic Exercise Programme; DM = diabetes mellitus; ECG = electrocardiogram; ex = exercise; funx = functional; HAQ = Health Assessment Questionnaire (HAQ); HR = heart rate; HEP = home exercise program; HRM = heart rate max; hydro = hydrotherapy; HTN = hypertension; mins = minutes; ms = muscle; NSAIDs = nonsteroidal anti-inflammatory; OT = occupational therapy; OA = osteoarthritis; phys = physical; pts = patients; QOL = quality of life; RA = rheumatoid arthritis; RCT = Randomized Clinical Trial; RM = repetition maximum; ROM = range of motion; RPE = Ratings of Perceived Exertion; Ss = subjects Tx = treatment; WB = weight-bearing.

Centers for Disease Control and Prevention (CDC) recommendations for exercise, which suggest 30 minutes of moderate-intensity exercise five times per week[143] or the more recent guidelines to accumulate 150 minutes each week.[144] If weight-bearing is a barrier to exercise, low– or non–weight-bearing activities such as stationary cycling, pool-based aerobics, or deep water running may be options.[16,127,145] For most people, walking and stationary bicycles are a safe and effective means of aerobic exercise.[16,145] Furthermore, patients who have engaged in such a program often report an increase in self-esteem and improved emotional status.[16] Medical screening as appropriate for age and medical condition (e.g., Revised Physical Activity Readiness Questionnaire [PAR-Q]) should be performed before beginning an aerobic exercise program.

Functional Training

Functional training for the individual with arthritis proceeds in the same fashion as for other individuals with similar deficits. Therapists may choose to reduce the functional demands of an activity either temporarily, such as under conditions of acute inflammation, or permanently by incorporating a variety of adaptive equipment into ADL that substitute for lost ROM and strength. These modifications can include long-handled appliances and devices with built-up handles for easier grasp. There are aids for dressing and grooming, as well

Box 23.6 Evidence Summary Therapeutic Exercise in the Management of Knee and Hip Osteoarthritis (OA)

Reference	Subjects	Methods	Duration/Dosage	Results/Comments
Bartels et al [137] (2007)	Patients with OA in one or both knees or hips. 800 subjects in total with mean reported age ranging from 66 to 71 years.	Systematic review of 6 RCTs or quasi-experimental studies up to May 2006, compared aquatic-exercise interventions to land-based exercise.	Aquatic exercises ranged from 6 weeks to 3 months and 2 to 3 sessions/week.	Mixed findings, with small to moderate short-term improvements in function and HRQoL, and minimal to large reduction in pain immediately following intervention. No changes in stiffness or walking ability. Authors commented that aquatic exercise may be a beneficial first step in an exercise therapy program to get particularly disabled patients introduced to training.
Pisters et al [141] (2007)	Patients with OA of the hip or knee. 1721 subjects in total. No mean ages provided.	Systematic review of 11 RCTs or controlled clinical trials up to Nov 2005 in Dutch, German, or English languages. Compared long term (≥ 6 month follow-up) effects of exercise therapy compared to a control intervention.	Exercise therapy ranged from 1 to 12 months and follow-up period from 6 to 15 months.	Significant small to moderate benefits for pain that weren't maintained at long-term follow-up. Nonsignificant effects on self-reported function and conflicting evidence for performance-based function. Moderate evidence that additional post-treatment booster sessions had a positive influence on maintenance of the post-treatment effects in the long term. Authors comment that better adherence was associated with better patient outcomes and future research should focus on how exercise behavior can be stimulated and maintained in the long term.
Fransen and McConnell [138] (2008)	Adults with established diagnosis of knee OA or self-reported knee OA. 3719 subjects in total with mean age ranging from 61 to 74 years.	Systematic review of 32 RCTs up to Dec 2007, compared land-based, therapeutic exercise to non-exercise control group.	Exercise intervention ranged from 4 weeks to 12 months and <1 to 3x/week.	Small to moderate short-term beneficial treatment effects for pain and self-reported physical function. Benefits, however, are comparable to reported estimates for current simple analgesics and NSAIDs taken for knee pain. Authors also noted that it is clear that most people with knee OA need some form of ongoing monitoring or supervision to enable an exercise program to provide optimal clinical benefits.

Box 23.6 Evidence Summary Therapeutic Exercise in the Management of Knee and Hip Osteoarthritis (OA)—cont'd

Reference	Subjects	Methods	Duration/Dosage	Results/Comments
Fransen et al [139] (2009)	Adults with established hip OA. 204 subjects in total with mean age ranging from 65 to 70 years.	Systematic review of 5 RCTs up to Aug 2008, comparing some form of land-based therapeutic exercise with non-exercise control group.	Exercise intervention ranged from 6 to 12 weeks and 1 to 3x/week.	Small short-term beneficial treatment effect for pain, but no benefit for self-reported physical function. With most studies including people with either hip or knee OA, authors raise the question as to whether a non-joint specific exercise program can maximize treatment benefit.
McNair et al [140] (2009)	Patients with clinically and/or radiographic confirmed hip OA only. 356 subjects in total with mean age ranging from 66 to 72 years	Systematic review of 6 RCTs and quasi-experimental studies up to June 2008, compared a minimum of 3 weeks of exercise therapy to comparison intervention.	Exercise interventions ranged from 5 to 8 weeks and 1 to 2 sessions/week	Only 1 high quality trial, "insufficient evidence" to support exercise as treatment to reduce pain, improve function, and limited evidence for enhanced HRQoL. Exercise programs in included studies did not meet current exercise guidelines (intensity, volume, progression). Authors commented that this was insufficient description of progression of training regimens, a fundamental requirement of successful exercise programs. The authors further commented that there remains a paucity of articles addressing the effects of exercise on hip OA specifically.
Jansen et al [142] (2011)	Adults with knee OA	Systematic review of 12 RCTs; compared strength training alone, exercise therapy alone and exercise therapy plus manual therapy compared to non-exercise control.	Variable durations	Small to moderate beneficial effects of each intervention type for pain. Exercise plus manual mobilization improved pain significantly more than exercise alone. Each intervention also improved physical function significantly.

DMARDs = Disease Modifying Anti-Inflammatory Drugs; HRQoL = health-related quality of life; OT = occupational therapy; OA = osteoarthritis; RCT = randomized clinical trial;

as personal hygiene. By breaking down functional tasks, such as rising from a chair or climbing stairs, into smaller movements, the therapist can help the patient identify faulty movement patterns and address specific components of the movement that are causing difficulty.

UE involvement in RA, particularly of the wrist and hands, may complicate the choice of an ambulatory assistive device by precluding any weight-bearing on these affected joints. In these instances, platform attachments can be used to transform the forearm into a weight-bearing surface. Rearranging the home or work environment also can improve a person's functional abilities. Raising beds or chairs can reduce the effort needed to stand up. Railings placed around the bed, bath, and along stairways also can help increase an individual's independence.

Gait and Balance Training

Specific deviations will be evident throughout the gait cycle. These may include gait asymmetries, decreased velocity, cadence and stride length, prolonged period of double support, inadequate initial contact and push-off, and diminished joint excursion through both swing and stance. Gait deviations in the patient with RA, specifically owing to foot pain or deformities, may also be evident (Table 23.6).[146,147] Therapists should address the underlying joint and muscle impairments that contribute to these deviations in the gait training program with persons with any type of arthritis.

The degree to which the gait of an individual with arthritis should, or can, approximate normal is one of the most difficult questions in designing a therapeutic program. Some "abnormalities" such as antalgic limping may in fact reduce joint loading. Joint destruction may necessitate the introduction of assistive devices as simple as a standard cane or as cumbersome as platform crutches or rolling walkers with platform attachments. The gait of the individual with RA or OA should be safe, functional, and cosmetically acceptable to the patient rather than an unattainable idealized version of the norm. Use of a properly fitted, standard cane in the contralateral hand is associated with decreased joint loading and pain in individuals with both hip and knee OA.

Decreased walking speed in arthritis is common, and there is general agreement that increased speed is a meaningful measure of functional improvement. For example, a person's ability to walk fast enough to cross the street with the timing of the traffic light is important for functional and safe community locomotion. However, increased walking speed without attention to joint biomechanics may be undesirable. In a clinical trial of a nonsteroidal drug for persons with knee OA, all with a varus deformity, gait variables were included as outcome measures. The researchers found that self-reported pain diminished and walking speed increased in the active therapy group. At the same time, kinetic analysis of joint forces showed the increased speed was accompanied by increased adductor moment at the knee and greater loading of the medial compartment.[148] This additional loading of the joint and increased stress on lateral supporting tissue may not be worth the gains of increased speed. Attention to biomechanical factors thus should be considered in comprehensive management, even when drug therapy decreases pain and improves gait speed.

Decreased proprioceptive input, impaired neuromuscular reflexes, altered joint biomechanics, pain, and muscle weakness contribute to static and dynamic balance problems in the individual with LE arthritis. Balance training may include progression from static postures moving from double- to single-limb support, stable to unstable surfaces, and adding perturbations where safe. Dynamic balance activities include maintaining postural alignment while shifting weight from one limb to the other in various directions and walking on different surfaces to challenge the vestibular and proprioceptive systems (see Chapter 10, Strategies to Improve Motor Function). Table 23.7 provides a summary of outcome measures for RA and OA organized by ICF Categories.

Joint Protection

Joint protection is a key component of arthritis management, due to the impact of the disease on the joint and supportive structures. A randomized controlled trial for persons with hand OA compared the effects of a 3-month education-behavioral joint protection program to standard education (each consisting of a 20-minute session and provision of a piece of Dycem [nonslip matting] to use when opening jars). This single-blinded study demonstrated that patients in the joint protection and exercise group increased grip strength by 25% and both groups reported better hand function with the joint protection information.[16,149] Patients should be encouraged to incorporate joint care into all ADL to minimize pain and conserve energy (see Appendix 23.C, Joint Protection, Rest, and Energy Conservation).

In addition to reducing pain and improving function, orthoses also may provide support and protection for vulnerable and painful joints. Foot orthotics or specially designed shoes can serve the dual purpose of relieving biomechanical stresses and enhancing function for the person with RA foot involvement.[150,151] The cost of special shoes may not be reimbursable under many insurance programs. A good shoe will provide support and eliminate unnecessary joint motion in the talocalcaneal joint with a firm and wide heel counter. It should also help to maintain normal bony alignment and accommodate all existing foot deformities within a toe box of adequate dimensions. Pressure should be evenly distributed along the plantar surface of the foot during weight-bearing. Commercially available gel inserts may be helpful and are inexpensive; however, with more advanced biomechanical changes in the foot, the fabrication of orthoses may be required. A *rocker sole* (shoe sole that is curved at the toe) can be used to facilitate push-off with limited ankle motion. A controlled trial was conducted of the effect of off-the-shelf extra-depth orthopedic footwear for people with RA and at least 1 year of foot pain. Outcomes were measures of pain, gait, and physical function after 2 months of wearing the extra-depth shoes. The footwear group improved significantly on self-reported disability, weight-bearing and non–weight-bearing pain, and gait. In addition to extra depth in the shoe toe box, the shoes provided greater rear foot stability, an arch support, a stiff shank, and a padded heel collar above the counter for improved fit. This study reported that walking pain accounted for 75% of the variability in physical function level of the subjects.[152]

Table 23.6 Analysis of Gait Deviations, Physical Examination Findings, and Treatment Goals

Gait Deviations	Physical Examination Findings	Treatment Goals
Pronated Foot		
Shuffled progression Decreased step length Initial contact with medial border of foot Decreased single-limb balance Prolonged double-support phase Late heel rise Plantarflexion of ipsilateral ankle in swing Genu valgus with weight-bearing	Tenderness over subtalar midtarsal area Limited inversion range Weak and painful posterior tibialis muscle Pronated weight-bearing posture of foot Lax medial collateral ligament of knee	Relieve subtalar and midtarsal joint stresses Increase ankle inversion Strengthen posterior tibialis muscle Stabilize hypermobile joints with rigid orthosis Maintain neutral alignment in stance by foot positioning
Hallux Valgus		
Lateral and posterior weight shift Late heel rise Decreased single-limb balance	Lateral deviation of great toe Swelling of first MTP joint Shortening of flexor hallucis brevis muscle Tenderness of great toe Weakness of great toe abduction	Accommodate foot with wide toe box shoe Increase extension of great toe Relieve weight-bearing stresses
Metatarsophalangeal Joint Subluxation		
Diminished roll off Decreased single-limb stance Apropulsive progression Decreased single-limb balance	Painful MTP heads with weight-bearing Callus formation over MTP heads Ulcerations over MTP heads Limited MTP flexion Prominent MTP heads	Redistribute pressure with metatarsal bar Relieve pressure with soft cutout shoe insert Increase flexion mobility of MTP joints Accommodate foot with extra-depth shoe
Hammer or Claw Toes		
Diminished roll off Decreased single-limb stance Apropulsive progression Decreased single-limb balance	Posture of MTP joint hyperextension with proximal and distal interphalangeal joint flexion Posture of MTP and distal interphalangeal joint hyperextension with proximal interphalangeal flexion Callus formation at plantar tips and dorsum of proximal interphalangeal joint Limited MTP flexion	Improve toe alignment with metatarsal bar Accommodate foot with extra-depth shoe Diminish pressure with soft insert Increase toe mobility
Painful Heel		
Toe-heel pattern No heel contact in stance Decreased stride length Decreased velocity Plantarflexion of ankle in swing Increased hip flexion in swing Decreased step length of contralateral limb	Painful active plantarflexion Painful passive and active dorsiflexion Swelling and pain at Achilles insertion Tenderness over spur Decreased ankle dorsiflexion range	Decrease inflammation with steroid injection or modalities Relieve weight-bearing stress Decrease pressure over spur with soft shoe insert Maintain ankle mobility

From Dimonte and Light,[94] with permission.
MTP = metatarsal-phalangeal.

Table 23.7 Outcome Measures for RA and OA Organized by ICF Categories		
	Body Structure and Function	Activity and Participation	Quality of Life and Personal Factors
RA	• VAS or NPRS for pain • Active joint count[a] or Simplified Disease Activity Index (SDAI) • ROM (goniometry) • Strength (manual or myometry) including grip strength • Joint stability • Visual gait assessment • Multidimensional Assessment of Fatigue (MAF) • Balance (e.g., single leg stance)	• HAQ-DI or Modified HAQ • AIMS2 • Patient Specific Functional Scale (PSFS) • Arthritis Hand Function Test • Dynamic/functional balance (e.g., Berg Balance Scale, Timed Up and Go) • 6-Minute Walk Test	• EuroQoL (EQ5D) • Self-efficacy scales[a] • Readiness to Manage Arthritis Questionnaire (RMAQ) • Patient and health professional global assessment
OA	• VAS or NPRS for pain • ROM (goniometry) • Strength (manual or myometry) including grip strength • Joint stability • Visual gait assessment • Balance (e.g., single leg stance)	• Hip disability and osteoarthritis outcome score (HOOS) • Knee injury and Osteoarthritis Outcome Score (KOOS) • Lower Extremity Functional Scale (LEFS) • Patient Specific Functional Scale (PSFS) • Disabilities of the Arm, Shoulder and Hand (DASH) • Arthritis Hand Function Test • Dynamic/functional balance (e.g., Berg Balance Scale, Timed Up and Go, sit-to-stand test) • 6-Minute Walk Test	• EuroQoL (EQ5D) • Self-efficacy scales[a] • Readiness to Manage Arthritis Questionnaire (RMAQ)

[a]See Appendix 23.D, Web-Based Resources.
AIMS2 = Arthritis Impact Measure Version 2; HAQ-DI = Health Assessment Questionnaire—Disability Index; NPRS = numeric pain rating scale; ROM = range of motion; VAS = visual analogue scale.

Education and Self-Management

Patient education in the rheumatic diseases has been shown to result in positive changes in knowledge, health behaviors, beliefs, and attitudes that affect health status, quality of life, and health care utilization. A recent review of the literature documented the well-established benefits of self-management programs on mental health.[75] As in any chronic illness, education should include information needed to deal with the condition (taking medications, exercise), self-management skills necessary to carry out important social and vocational roles, and resources needed to deal with the emotional consequences of chronic illness such as depression, fear, and frustration. The evidence is overwhelming that education designed to teach self-management skills and increase client self-efficacy for these tasks is the most effective.[75,153] The *Arthritis Foundation* (1330 West Peachtree Street, Atlanta, GA 30309, www.arthritis.org) can supply the clinician or the individual with a variety of educational materials, pamphlets, and self-help courses that will increase cognitive understanding of the disease process and

self-management skills. Many local chapters of the Arthritis Foundation hold individual and family support groups to increase psychosocial adaptation, as well as conduct aquatic and land exercise programs in public facilities. The *Association of Rheumatology Health Professionals,* a division of the American College of Rheumatology (www.rheumatology.org), can provide the therapist with scientific and clinical resources for enhanced practice, as well as a network of professional colleagues who work in rheumatology. See Appendix 23.D for additional Web-based resources.

■ SURGICAL MANAGEMENT

Surgery represents one of the greatest advances in the management of arthritis in the last 50 years. Surgery is not appropriate, however, for every individual with either RA or OA, and the careful selection of the patient and the timing of the procedure are critical. The primary indications for surgery are pain, loss of function, and progression of deformity, although the last two are not always correlated. Surgical outcomes are greatly affected by personal characteristics of the individual patient, such as anxiety, depression, expectations, and motivation,[154] and external factors, such as access to quality postoperative rehabilitation. General postoperative rehabilitation goals are to restore ROM to the affected joint, promote stability within the joint, regain neuromuscular control of joint motion, restore gait and balance, and improve quality of life.

In general, there are three procedures that may be performed on soft tissues: **synovectomy**, soft tissue release, and tendon transfers. Similarly, there are three general bone and joint procedures: osteotomy, prosthetic arthroplasty, and, less frequently, arthrodesis. The choice of specific postoperative physical therapy procedures will depend on the particular surgical intervention, the extent of joint involvement before surgery, individual characteristics of the patient (including co-morbid health conditions and physical activity level), and other manifestations of the disease. It is particularly important to remember that a patient with RA, compared to a peer with OA, will have multiple joint involvement, which will ultimately affect the functional outcome of the procedure. A patient with RA is also likely to be a surgical candidate at a much younger age than a patient with OA and is at greater risk for infection following surgery due to the systemic disease process and greater use of immunosuppressive drugs.[1]

More than 800,000 total joint arthroplasty (TJA) surgeries of the hip or knee are performed in the United States annually, the majority of which are for patients with OA.[155] These highly successful procedures have revolutionized the management of disabling arthritis in the LE with significant long-term benefits,[156,157] including recovery of physical functioning.[158] The primary goals following TJA are to restore function, decrease pain, and gain muscle control to enable the individual to return to previous, or improved, levels of functioning. Immediate postoperative and rehabilitation management is shaped by a variety of factors, including the occurrence of perioperative complications, as well as surgical factors (type of prosthesis, surgical technique, and approach). Initial treatment includes therapeutic exercise, transfer and gait training, and instruction in ADL.[159,160] Once the individual has achieved an adequate level of function and is released from surgical precautions, instruction in establishing a routine of regular exercise and physical activity to support musculoskeletal and cardiovascular fitness is crucial to long-term outcomes and quality of life. A meta-analysis reviewing recovery of short- and long-term physical functioning after total hip arthroplasty (THA) found that patients had recovered between 46% and 81% of self-reported functioning compared to age-matched controls 6 to 8 months after surgery. Walking speed, daily activity in the home, and other measures of functional capacity all recovered to about 80% of that of controls 6 to 8 months after THA.[158, 161] Recovery of physical functioning and quality of life after total knee arthroplasty (TKA) is more protracted and frequently less optimal than that of THA.[156] TKA and THA improve clinical outcomes in knees and hips damaged by RA and have a positive secondary systemic effect on RA disease activity; however, there are inconsistent benefits on long-term health-related quality of life.[162]

SUMMARY

RA and OA are the two kinds of arthritis that a physical therapist is likely to see in clinical practice. The primary activity limitations and participation restrictions in the individual with RA or OA result from disease activity, musculoskeletal impairments, and cardiovascular deconditioning. Joint surface irregularities, loss of joint space and ROM, muscle weakness, and atrophy contribute directly to limitations in ADL and the ability to work. Pain secondary to changes in normal joint structure and function often limits functioning as well. Musculoskeletal impairments related to arthritis may also lead to impairments of other systems, such as decreased cardiovascular endurance for functional activities. The physical therapist is well suited to evaluate and treat these impairments, remediate the activity limitations, and educate the patient in self-management skills to avoid unnecessary participation restrictions. Rehabilitation of the individual with arthritis is most often directed toward restoring or maintaining joint mobility and strength and emphasizes functional retraining and prevention of secondary health conditions.

Questions for Review

1. What epidemiological factors are related to RA?
2. What are the major pathological changes seen in RA?
3. State two hypotheses concerning the pathogenesis of RA.
4. Describe four modifiable risk factors that may predispose an individual to OA.
5. Describe two changes in articular cartilage associated with OA.

6. Name at least two laboratory tests used in the diagnosis of RA and state their purposes.

7. Describe the parameters used in examining radiographs of arthritic joints.

8. Describe the typical joint changes seen with RA for the following joints: occipitoatlantal, atlantoaxial, temporomandibular, carpals, knees, and talocalcaneal.

9. Define the following deformities: ulnar drift, swan neck, boutonniere, hammer toes, claw toes, and hallux valgus.

10. Describe the overall goals of medical management for RA and OA.

11. What are the primary indications for surgery in RA?

12. Describe the key points in taking a history for the individual with arthritis.

13. What adaptations of standard tests and measures might be required in examining the individual with RA?

14. What are the general physical therapy goals for individuals with RA or OA?

15. Explain the goals, modifications, and progression of a typical strengthening program.

16. Discuss treatment strategies for increasing ROM.

17. Design a cardiovascular conditioning program for an individual with LE arthritic joint involvement.

18. Describe strategies to enhance patients' adherence to therapeutic exercise programs.

19. State at least four principles of joint protection and give a practical application of each.

20. What criteria guide the selection of shoes for the individual with RA?

21. What are the purposes of splints?

22. What changes in gait are commonly associated with RA? What impairments contribute to static and dynamic balance problems in the individual with LE arthritis?

CASE STUDIES

Two case studies are presented: Case 1 presents a patient with rheumatoid arthritis and Case 2 considers a patient with osteoarthritis.

CASE 1: RHEUMATOID ARTHRITIS

HISTORY

The patient is a 52-year-old married woman who has two children in high school. She is a nurse and works about 40 hours a week. She has had symptoms of joint swelling and pain, fatigue, and increasing weakness for 2 years. During initial onset of symptoms, a primary care physician diagnosed her with carpal tunnel syndrome, knee osteoarthritis, fibromyalgia, and Lyme disease. However, her symptoms continued to worsen on NSAIDs. She was also prescribed antidepressants, and she was referred to the rheumatologist 3 months ago. Based on her history, physical examination, laboratory values (Disease Activity Score [DAS] = 3.2; RF= 12.30; ESR = 26), and radiographic evidence the rheumatologist confirmed a diagnosis of seropositive RA. She began a course of methotrexate and has been referred to physical therapy.

PHYSICAL THERAPY EXAMINATION

At the initial physical therapy examination, she reports that her morning stiffness is now less than 30 minutes (previous high of 3 hours). The pain and swelling in her hands, feet, and elbows is markedly decreased, and she is feeling more energetic. Systems review of the integumentary system is unremarkable except for a slight edema and redness of the distal finger joints and wrist R > L. Her blood pressure and respiratory rate are within normal limits. Her resting heart rate is 72 but increases to 96 with modest exertion.

ROM is limited at the shoulder, elbows, wrists, and MCPs. She lacks 10° of knee extension and has no ankle dorsiflexion or hip extension beyond neutral. Bilateral strength is good minus. She exhibits a forward head, rounded shoulder posture, with the beginning of a marked kyphosis. Her pain is most prominent in her wrists, elbows, and ankles (4/10 visual analogue scale [VAS]) and indicates general fatigue. She has flat feet and moderate swelling of the metatarsal heads. She is relieved that at last she has been diagnosed with a condition for which there is effective treatment and she trusts her rheumatologist. Her immediate goals are to regain comfortable motion, strength, and stamina and to avoid deformity.

GUIDING QUESTIONS

1. Identify the general anticipated goals and expected outcomes of physical therapy for this patient.
2. What self-management strategies would you recommend and/or instruct the patient to use?
3. Describe the types of community resources you would recommend the patient explore.
4. What supportive devices might be used to decrease symptoms and increase function?
5. How would her physical therapist optimally schedule her return visits to clinic?

CASE 2: OSTEOARTHRITIS

HISTORY

The patient is a 64-year-old Caucasian woman whose low back and bilateral knee pain have increased over the past year. She is 5 ft 7 in tall and weighs 195 lb. She has hypertension and chronic renal insufficiency for which she takes prescribed medication. She works part-time as a teacher's assistant in a local elementary school and lives alone in a 3rd floor walk-up apartment. On weekends she serves as the assistant building manager, which includes both cleaning and minimal maintenance duties. She has difficulty using stairs, getting up and down from sitting, getting on and off the bus, and walking for more than 15 minutes at a time. She has had progressively greater knee pain and stiffness for the past 3 years and has recently experienced episodes of "giving way" in the right knee. Her low back pain is worse after prolonged sitting, vacuuming, and at the end of the day. She avoids over-the-counter medications due to her underlying kidney disease but reports moderate pain relief with topical diclofenac applied to both knees. The patient recently joined a local seniors' fitness club but admits to rarely attending classes.

On a recent visit to her primary care physician, she underwent radiographs of both knees, which revealed bilateral joint space narrowing, with the right knee more affected than left and greater lateral compartment involvement than medial. There is evidence of bony sclerosis, osteophytes, and mild malalignment (genu valgum) greater on the right. Her physician has suggested continued use of the topical NSAID, use of a cane, and referred her to a physical therapist for evaluation and exercise advice. The patient and her doctor have agreed to discuss surgical options for the knee if she is not satisfied with her condition in 3 to 6 months.

PHYSICAL THERAPY EXAMINATION

During the initial history and systems review, the patient reports that she is finding both of her part-time jobs difficult, and in particular her cleaning responsibilities in the apartment building. She is frequently tired and lacks the energy to go to the fitness classes despite enjoying the session she last attended about 2 months ago. She admits to not sleeping well and having to take occasional sick days from her school-based job. She is concerned about finances and feels that she needs to continue working for at least another 3 years. Her pain is intermittent during the day but wakes her up frequently during the night. Her heart rate is 82, her blood pressure is 140/85, and her respiratory rate is 16. Her skin and circulation in the lower extremities are unremarkable and sensory integrity and reflexes are intact. Her concerns are being able to keep working and to avoid knee surgery.

Selected tests and measures reveal weakness and loss of motion in hips and knees bilaterally, and an antalgic and slow gait. Her spinal ROM is restricted in extension and rotation. Anterior-posterior knee stability is good, but there is moderate pseudolaxity of the lateral collateral ligaments bilaterally. Using a numeric pain rating scale (NPRS), she rates her left knee pain as 7 out of 10 while walking and 8 out of 10 while climbing stairs, and right knee pain at 6 out of 10 for all activities. She is wearing unsupportive slip-on shoes and shows marked ankle pronation on the right and bilateral hallux valgus.

GUIDING QUESTIONS

1. What anticipated goals should the physical therapist discuss with the patient for the episode of care?
2. Formulate a home exercise program for this patient and determine an optimal schedule for follow-up by the physical therapist.
3. What kind of orthotic device(s) would reduce this patient's symptoms and increase her function?
4. What should be included in patient-related instruction to maximize this patient's function?
5. What strategies would maximize this patient's adherence to a home exercise program and regular physical activity?
6. What other health professional(s) and/or community resources would you recommend for this patient?

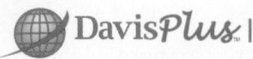 | For additional resources, including answers to the questions for review and case study guiding questions, please visit **http://davisplus.fadavis.com**

References

1. Klippel, JH (ed): Primer on the Rheumatic Diseases, ed 13. Arthritis Foundation and Springer Publishing, Atlanta, 2011.
2. Arnett, FC, et al: The American Rheumatism Association 1987 revised criteria for the classification of rheumatoid arthritis. Arthritis Rheum 31:315, 1988.
3. Aletaha, D, et al: Rheumatoid arthritis classification criteria. Arthritis Rheum 62:2569, 2010.
4. Hemlick, CG, et al: Estimates of the prevalence of arthritis and other rheumatic conditions in the United States. Arthritis Rheum 58:15, 2008.
5. Symmons, D: Epidemiological concepts and the classification of musculoskeletal conditions. In Hochberg, AJ, et al (eds): Rheumatology, ed 4. Mosby Elsevier, Philadelphia, 2008, p 3.
6. Ollier, WER, and Worthington, J: Investigation of the genetic basis of rheumatic diseases. In Hochberg, AJ, et al (eds): Rheumatology, ed 4. Mosby Elsevier, Philadelphia, 2008, p 123.
7. Nielsen, MM, et al: Specific autoantibodies precede the symptoms of rheumatoid arthritis: A study of serial measurements in blood donors. Arthritis Rheum 50:380, 2004.
8. Rantapaa-Dahlqvist, S, et al: Antibodies against cyclic citrullinated peptide and IgA rheumatoid factor predict the development of rheumatoid arthritis. Arthritis Rheum 48:2741, 2003.
9. Firestein, GS, and Zvaifler, NJ: The pathogenesis of rheumatoid arthritis. Rheum Dis Clin North Am 13:447, 1987.
10. Hutchinson, DL, et al: Heavy cigarette smoking is strongly associated with rheumatoid arthritis (RA), particularly in patients without a family history of RA. Ann Rheum Dis 60:223, 2001.
11. Carpenter, AB: Immunology and inflammation. In Robbins, L, et al (eds): Clinical Care in the Rheumatic Diseases, ed 2. American College of Rheumatology, Atlanta, 2001, p 15.
12. Klareskog, L, Gregersen, PK, and Huizinga, TW: Prevention of autoimmune rheumatic disease: State of the art and future perspectives. Ann Rheum Dis 69(12):2062, 2010.
13. Gornisiewicz, M, and Moreland, LW: Rheumatoid arthritis. In Robbins, L, et al (eds): Clinical Care in the Rheumatic Diseases, ed 2. American College of Rheumatology, Atlanta, 2001, p 89.
14. Hochberg, MC, et al: The American College of Rheumatology 1991 revised criteria for the classification of global functional status in rheumatoid arthritis. Arthritis Rheum 35:498, 1992.
15. Iversen, MD, and Kale, MK: Physical therapy management of select rheumatic conditions in older adults. In Nakasato, Y, and Yung, RL (eds): Geriatric Rheumatology. Springer, 2011, p 101.
16. Iversen, MD, Finckh, A, and Liang, MH: Exercise prescriptions for the major inflammatory and non-inflammatory arthritides. In Frontera, WR, Dawson, DM, and Slovik, DM (eds): Exercise in Rehabilitation Medicine. Human Kinetics, Champaign, IL, 2005, p 157.
17. Brasington, RD: Clinical features of rheumatic disease. In Hochberg, AJ, et al (eds): Rheumatology, ed 4. Mosby Elsevier, Philadelphia, 2008, p 766.
18. Jones, JV, and Covert, A: Diagnosis and management of arthritic conditions. In Walker, JM, and Helewa, A (eds): Physical Therapy in Arthritis. WB Saunders, Philadelphia, 1996, p 47.
19. Melvin, JL: Rheumatic Disease: Occupational Therapy and Rehabilitation, ed 3. FA Davis, Philadelphia, 1989.
20. Turkiewicz, AM, and Moreland, LW: Rheumatoid arthritis. In Bartlett, SJ, et al (eds): Clinical Care Text in the Rheumatic Diseases, ed 3. American College of Rheumatology, Atlanta, 2006, p 157.
21. Edstrom, L, and Nordemar, R: Differential changes in Type I and Type II muscle fibers in rheumatoid arthritis. Scand J Rheum 3:155, 1974.
22. Nordemar, R, et al: Changes in muscle fiber size and physical performance in patients with rheumatoid arthritis after 7 months physical training. Scand J Rheum 5:233, 1976.
23. Edstrom, L: Selective atrophy of red muscle fibers in the quadriceps in longstanding knee-joint dysfunction. J Neurol Sci 11:551, 1970.
24. Metsios, GS, et al: Rheumatoid arthritis, cardiovascular disease and physical exercise: A systematic review. Rheumatol 47:239, 2008.
25. Roubenoff, R, et al: Rheumatoid cachexia: Cytokine-driven hypermetabolism accompanying reduced body cell mass in chronic inflammation. J Clin Invest 93:2379, 1994.
26. Sokka, T, et al: Work disability remains a major problem in rheumatoid arthritis in the 2000s: Data from 32 countries in the QUEST-RA study. Arthritis Res Ther 12:R42, 2010.
27. Kumar, N, et al: Causes of death in patients with rheumatoid arthritis: Comparison with siblings and matched osteoarthritis controls. J Rheumatol 34:1695, 2007.
28. Lindqvist, E, et al: Prognostic laboratory markers of joint damage in rheumatoid arthritis. Ann Rheum Dis 64:196, 2005.
29. Gough, A, et al: Genetic typing of patients with inflammatory arthritis at presentation can be used to predict outcome. Arthritis Rheum 37:1166, 1994.
30. Felson, DT, et al: American College of Rheumatology/European League Against Rheumatism provisional definition of remission in rheumatoid arthritis for clinical trials. Arthritis Rheum 63:573, 2011.
31. Felson, DT: Developments in the clinical understanding of osteoarthritis. Arthritis Res Ther 11:203, 2009. Retrieved May 15, 2011, from http://arthritis-research.com/content/11/1/203.
32. Lawrence, RC, et al: Estimates of the prevalence of arthritis and other rheumatic conditions in the United States. Part II. Arthritis Rheum 58(1):26, 2008.
33. Loeser, RF, and Shakoor, N: Aging or osteoarthritis: Which is the problem? Rheum Dis Clin North Am 29:653, 2003.
34. Bland, JH, Melvin, JL, and Hasson, S: Osteoarthritis. In Melvin, J, and Ferrell, KM (eds): Rheumatologic Rehabilitation Series: Adult Rheumatic Diseases, vol 2. American Occupational Therapy Association, Bethesda, MD, 2000, p 81.
35. Valdes, AM, and Spector, TD: The contribution of genes to osteoarthritis. Med Clin North Am 93:45, 2009.
36. Jensen, L: Hip osteoarthritis: Influence of work with heavy lifting, climbing stairs or ladders, or combining kneeling/squatting with heavy lifting. Occup Environ Med 65:6, 2008.
37. Jensen, LK: Knee osteoarthritis: Influence of work involving heavy lifting, kneeling, climbing stairs or ladders, or knee/squatting combined with heavy lifting. Occup Environ Med 65:72, 2008.
38. Garstang, SV, and Stitik, TP: Osteoarthritis: Epidemiology, risk factors, and pathophysiology. Am J Phys Med Rehabil 85(11):S2, 2006.
39. Felson, DT: Risk factors for osteoarthritis: Understanding joint vulnerability. Clin Orthop Rel Res 427S:S16, 2004.
40. Altman, RD: Early management of osteoarthritis. Am J Manage Care 16:S41, 2010.
41. Reid, GD, et al: Femoroacetabular impingement syndrome: An underrecognized cause of hip pain and premature osteoarthritis? J Rheumatol 37(7):1395, 2010.
42. Buckwalter, JA, Mankin, HJ, and Grodzinsky, AJ: Articular cartilage and osteoarthritis. American Academy of Orthopedic Surgeons (AAOS) Instr Course Lect 54:465, 2005.
43. Dieppe, PA, and Lohmander, LS: Pathogenesis and management of pain in osteoarthritis. Lancet 365:965, 2005.
44. Guccione, AA, and Minor, MA: Arthritis. In O'Sullivan, SB, and Schmitz, TJ (eds): Physical Rehabilitation, ed 5. FA Davis, Philadelphia, 2007, p 1057.
45. McAlindon, TE, et al: Determinants of disability in osteoarthritis of the knee. Ann Rheum Dis 52:258, 1993.
46. Kellgren, JH, and Lawrence, JS: Atlas of Standard Radiographs: The Epidemiology of Chronic Rheumatism, vol 2. Blackwell Scientific, Oxford, 1963.
47. Hayashi, D, Guermaziy, A, and Hunter, DJ: Osteoarthritis year 2010 in review: Imaging. Osteoarthr Cartil 19:354, 2011.
48. Sharif, M, et al: Suggestion of nonlinear or phasic progression of knee osteoarthritis based on measurements of serum cartilage oligomeric matrix protein levels over five years. Arthritis Rheum 50(8):2479, 2004.

49. Altman, R, et al: The American College of Rheumatology criteria for the classification and reporting of osteoarthritis of the hip. Arthritis Rheum 34:505, 1991.

50. Zhang, W, et al: EULAR evidence-based recommendations for the diagnosis of knee osteoarthritis. Ann Rheum Dis 69(3):483, 2010.

51. Zhang, W, et al: EULAR evidence-based recommendations for the diagnosis of hand osteoarthritis: Report of a task force of ESCISIT. Ann Rheum Dis 68(1):8, 2009.

52. D'Agostino, MA, et al: EULAR reports on the use of ultrasonography in painful knee osteoarthritis. Part 1: Prevalence of inflammation in osteoarthritis. Ann Rheum Dis 64:1703, 2005.

53. Threlkeld, AJ: Musculoskeletal assessment. In Melvin, JL, and Jensen, GM (eds): Rheumatologic Rehabilitation Series: Assessment and Management, vol 1. American Occupational Therapy Association, Bethesda, MD, 1998, p 107.

54. Melvin, JL: Therapist's management of osteoarthritis in the hand. In Mackin, EJ, et al (eds): Rehabilitation of the Hand and Upper Extremity, ed 5. Mosby, St. Louis, 2002, p 1646.

55. Ling, SM, and Rudolph, K: Osteoarthritis. In Bartlett, SJ, et al (eds): Clinical Care in the Rheumatic Diseases, ed 3. Association of Rheumatology Health Professionals, Atlanta, 2006, p 127.

56. Arnold, CM, and Faulkner, RA: The history of falls and the association of the Timed Up and Go Test to falls and near-falls in older adults with hip osteoarthritis. BMC Geriatr 7:17, 2007.

57. Menz, HB, and Lord, SR: The contribution of foot problems to mobility impairment and falls in community-dwelling older people. J Am Geriatr Soc 49:1651, 2001.

58. Kalichman, L, and Hunter, DJ: Lumbar facet joint osteoarthritis: A review. Semin Arthritis Rheum 37:69, 2007.

59. Guccione, AA, et al: The effects of specific medical conditions on the functional limitations of elders in the Framingham Study. Am J Publ Health 84:351, 1994.

60. Guccione, AA, et al: Defining arthritis and measuring functional status in elders: Methodological issues in the study of disease and disability. Am J Publ Health 80:945, 1990.

61. Kauppila, AM, et al: Disability in end-stage knee osteoarthritis. Disabil Rehabil 31(5):370, 2009.

62. Dreinhöfer, K, et al: ICF Core Sets for osteoarthritis. J Rehabil Med 44 Suppl:75, 2004.

63. Bossmann, T, et al: Validation of the comprehensive ICF Core Set for osteoarthritis: The perspective of physical therapists. Physiotherapy 97(1):3, 2011.

64. Gignac, MAM, et al: An examination of arthritis-related workplace activity limitations and intermittent disability over four and a half years and its relationship to job modifications and outcomes. Arthritis Care Res 63(7):953, 2011.

65. American College of Rheumatology Subcommittee on Rheumatoid Arthritis Guidelines: Guidelines for the management of rheumatoid arthritis 2002 update. Arthritis Rheum 46:328, 2002.

66. Watson, DJ, et al: Gastrointestinal tolerability of the selective cyclooxygenase-2 (COX-2) inhibitor rofecoxib compared with nonselective COX-1 and COX-2 inhibitors in osteoarthritis. Arch Intern Med 160:2998, 2000.

67. Solomon, DH, et al: Relationship between selective cyclooxygenase inhibitors and acute myocardial infarction in older adults. Circulation 109:206, 2004.

68. Shaya, FT, et al: Selective cyclooxygenase inhibition and cardiovascular effects. Arch Intern Med 165:181, 2005.

69. Sowers, JR, et al: The effects of cyclooxygenase-2 inhibitors and nonsteroidal anti-inflammatory therapy on 24-hour blood pressure in patients with hypertension, osteoarthritis and type 2 diabetes mellitus. Arch Intern Med 165:161, 2005.

70. American College of Rheumatology Subcommittee on Osteoarthritis Guidelines. Recommendations for the medical management of osteoarthritis of the hip and knee: 2000 update. Arthritis Rheum 43(9):1905, 2000.

71. American Society of Orthopaedic Surgeons: Treatment of osteoarthritis of the knee (non-arthroplasty), 2008. Retrieved May 2, 2011, from www.aaos.org/research/guidelines/GuidelineOAKnee.asp, 2008.

72. Zhang, W, et al: OARSI recommendations for the management of hip and knee osteoarthritis, part II: OARSI evidence-based, expert consensus guidelines. Osteoarthr Cartil 16:137, 2008.

73. Zhang, W, et al: OARSI recommendations for the management of hip and knee osteoarthritis part III: Changes in evidence following

74. Towheed, T, et al: Acetaminophen for osteoarthritis. Cochrane Database of Systematic Reviews 2006, Issue 1. Art. No.: CD004257. DOI: 10.1002/14651858.CD004257.pub2. 2006.

75. Iversen, MD, Hammond, A, and Betteridge, N: Self-management of rheumatic diseases—state of the art and future perspectives. Ann Rheum Dis 69(6):955, 2010.

76. American College of Rheumatology Ad Hoc Committee on Clinical Guidelines: Guidelines for the initial evaluation of the adult patient with acute musculoskeletal symptoms. Arthritis Rheum 39:1, 1996.

77. Norkin, CC, and White, DJ: Measurement of Joint Motion: a Guide to Goniometry, ed 4. FA Davis, Philadelphia, 2003, p 39.

78. Messier, SP, et al: Osteoarthritis of the knee: Effects on gait, strength, and flexibility. Arch Phys Med Rehabil 73:29, 1992.

79. Jesevar, DS, et al: Knee kinematics and kinetics during locomotor activities of daily living in subjects with knee arthroplasty and in healthy controls. Phys Ther 73:229, 1993.

80. Grabiner, MD, et al: Kinematics of recovery from a stumble. J Gerontol 48:M97, 1993.

81. McAlindon, TE, et al: Determinants of disability in osteoarthritis of the knee. Ann Rheum Dis 52:258, 1993.

82. Philbin, EF, et al: Cardiovascular fitness and health in patients with end-stage osteoarthritis. Arthritis Rheum 38:799, 1995.

83. Liang, MH, et al: Comparative measurement efficiency and sensitivity of five health status instruments for arthritis research. Arthritis Rheum 28:542, 1985.

84. Guccione, AA, and Jette, AM: Assessing limitations in physical function in patients with arthritis. Arthritis Care Res 1:120, 1988.

85. Guccione, AA, and Jette, AM: Multidimensional assessment of functional limitations in patients with arthritis. Arthritis Care Res 3:44, 1990.

86. Jette, AM: Functional capacity evaluation: An empirical approach. Arch Phys Med Rehabil 61:85, 1980.

87. Jette, AM: Functional Status Index: Reliability of a chronic disease evaluation instrument. Arch Phys Med Rehabil 61:395, 1980.

88. Fries, JF, et al: Measurement of patient outcome in arthritis. Arthritis Rheum 23:137, 1980.

89. Felson, DT, et al: The American College of Rheumatology preliminary core set of disease activity measures for rheumatoid arthritis clinical trials. The Committee on Outcome Measures in Rheumatoid Arthritis Clinical Trials. Arthritis Rheum 36:729, 1993.

90. Meenan, RF, et al: AIMS2: The content and properties of a revised and expanded Arthritis Impact Measurement Scales health status questionnaire. Arthritis Rheum 35:1, 1992.

91. Katz, PP (ed): Health outcome measures. Arthritis Care Res 49 (5 Suppl):S1, 2003.

92. Roos, EM, et al: Knee injury and osteoarthritis outcome score (KOOS)—development of a self-administered outcome measure. J Orthop Sports Phys Ther 28:88, 1998.

93. Nilsdotter, AK, et al: Hip disability and osteoarthritis outcome score (HOOS)—validity and responsiveness in total hip replacement. BMC Musculoskelet Disord 4:10, 2003.

94. Dimonte, P, and Light, H: Pathomechanics, gait deviations, and treatment of the rheumatoid foot. Phys Ther 62:1148, 1982.

95. Weiss, RJ, et al: Gait pattern in rheumatoid arthritis. Gait Posture 28:229–234, 2008.

96. Brinkmann, JR, and Perry, J: Rate and range of knee motion during ambulation in healthy and arthritic subjects. Phys Ther 65:1055, 1985.

97. Parker, JC, Wright, GE, and Smarr, KL: Psychological assessment. In Robbins, L, et al (eds): Clinical Care in the Rheumatic Diseases, ed 3. American College of Rheumatology, Atlanta, 2007, p 67.

98. Bradley, LA: Psychological aspects of arthritis. Bull Rheum Dis 35:1, 1985.

99. Marks, R: Comorbid depression and anxiety impact hip osteoarthritis disability. Disabil Health J 2(1):27, 2009.

100. Keefe, FJ, Somers, TJ, and Martire, LM: Psychologic interventions and lifestyle modifications for arthritis pain management. Rheum Dis Clin North Am 34(2):351, 2008.

101. Stucki, G, et al: ICF Core Sets for rheumatoid arthritis. J Rehabil Med 44(Suppl):87, 2004.

102. Coenen, M, et al: Validation of the International Classification of Functioning, Disability and Health (ICF) Core Set for rheumatoid arthritis from the patient perspective using focus groups. Arthritis Res Ther 8(4):R84, 2006.

systematic cumulative update of research published through January 2009. Osteoarthr Cartil 18:476, 2010.

103. Robinson, V, et al: Thermotherapy for treating rheumatoid arthritis. Cochrane Database of Systematic Reviews 2002, Issue 2:CD002826.

104. Brosseau, L, et al: Thermotherapy for treatment of osteoarthritis. Cochrane Database of Systematic Reviews 2003, Issue 4. Art. No.: CD004522. DOI: 10.1002/14651858.CD004522.

105. Rutjes, AWS, Nüeshc, E, and Jüni, P: Therapeutic ultrasound for osteoarthritis of the knee or hip. Cochrane Database of Systematic Reviews 2010, Issue 1. Art. No.: CD003132. DOI: 10.1002/14651858.CD003132.pub2.

106. Casimiro, L, et al: Therapeutic ultrasound for the treatment of rheumatoid arthritis. Cochrane Database of Systematic Reviews 2002, Issue 3. Art. No.: CD003787. DOI: 10.1002/14651858.CD003787.

107. Harris, ED, Jr, and McCroskery, PA: The influence of temperature and fibril stability on degradation of cartilage collagen by rheumatoid synovial collagenase. N Engl J Med 290:1, 1974.

108. Feibel, A, and Fast, A: Deep heating of joints: A reconsideration. Arch Phys Med Rehabil 57:513, 1976.

109. Oosterveld, F, and Rasker, JJ: Effects of local heat and cold treatment on surface and articular temperature of arthritic knees. Arthritis Rheum 37(11):1578, 1994.

110. Brosseau, L, et al: Transcutaneous electrical nerve stimulation (TENS) for the treatment of rheumatoid arthritis in the hand. Cochrane Database of Systematic Reviews 2003, Issue 3. Art. No.: CD004377. DOI: 10.1002/14651858.CD004377.

111. Rutjes, AWS, et al: Transcutaneous electrostimulation for osteoarthritis of the knee. Cochrane Database of Systematic Reviews 2009, Issue 4. Art. No.: CD002823. DOI: 10.1002/14651858.CD002823.pub2.

112. Ye, L, et al: Effects of rehabilitative interventions on pain, function, and physical impairments in people with hand osteoarthritis: A systematic review. Arthritis Res Ther 13:R28, 2011.

113. Egan, M, et al: Splints/orthoses in the treatment of rheumatoid arthritis. Cochrane Database of Systematic Reviews 2003, Issue 1. Art. No.: CD004018. DOI: 10.1002/14651858.CD004018.

114. Pagnotta, A, et al: The effect of a static wrist orthosis on hand function in individuals with rheumatoid arthritis. J Rheumatol 25:879, 1998.

115. Kjeken, I, et al: Systematic review of design and effects of splints and exercise programs in hand osteoarthritis. Arthritis Care Res 63(6):834, 2011.

116. Raja, K, and Dewan, N: Efficacy of knee braces and foot orthoses in conservative management of knee osteoarthritis: A systematic review. Am J Phys Med Rehabil 90(3):247, 2011.

117. Warden, SJ, et al: Patellar taping and bracing for the treatment of chronic knee pain: A systematic review and meta-analysis. Arthritis Rheum 59(1):73, 2008.

118. Kisner, C, and Colby, LA: Therapeutic exercise. Foundations and Techniques, ed 5. FA Davis, Philadelphia, 2002.

119. Westby, M, and Minor, M: Exercise and physical activity. In Bartlett, SJ, et al (eds): Clinical Care in the Rheumatic Diseases, ed 3. Association of Rheumatology Health Professionals, Atlanta, 2006, p 211.

120. James, MJ, et al: Effect of exercise on 99mTc-DPTA clearance from knees with effusions. J Rheumatol 21:501, 1994.

121. Krebs, DE, et al: Exercise and gait effects on in vivo hip contact pressures. Phys Ther 71:301, 1990.

122. Jawed, S, Gaffney, K, and Blake, DR: Intra-articular pressure profile of the knee joint in a spectrum of inflammatory arthropathies. Ann Rheum Dis 56(11):686, 1997.

123. Hakkinen, A, et al: A randomized two year study of the effects of dynamic strength training on muscle strength, disease activity, functional capacity, and bone mineral density in early rheumatoid arthritis. Arthritis Rheum 44:515, 2001.

124. Baillet, A, et al: A dynamic exercise programme to improve patients' disability in rheumatoid arthritis: A prospective randomized controlled trial. Rheumatol 48:410, 2009.

125. Baillet, A, et al: Efficacy of cardiorespiratory aerobic exercise in rheumatoid arthritis: Meta-analysis of randomized controlled trials. Arthritis Care Res 62:984, 2010.

126. de Jong, Z, et al: Is a long-term high-intensity exercise program effective and safe in patients with rheumatoid arthritis? Arthritis Rheum 58:2415, 2003.

127. Eversden, L, et al: A pragmatic randomized controlled trial of hydrotherapy and land exercises on overall well-being and quality of life in rheumatoid arthritis. BMC Musculoskelet Disord 8:23, 2007.

128. Lemmey, AB, et al: Effects of high-intensity resistance training in patients with rheumatoid arthritis: A randomized controlled trial. Arthritis Rheum 61:1726, 2009.

129. Smidt, N, et al: Effectiveness of exercise therapy: A best-evidence summary of systematic reviews. Aust J Physiother 51:71, 2005.

130. Ottawa Panel: Ottawa Panel evidence-based clinical practice guidelines for therapeutic exercises in the management of rheumatoid arthritis in adults. Phys Ther 84:934, 2004.

131. Bearne, LM, et al: Exercise can reverse quadriceps sensorimotor dysfunction that is associated with rheumatoid arthritis without exacerbating disease activity. Rheumatol 41:157, 2002.

132. Brorsson, S, et al: A six-week hand exercise programme improves strength and hand function in patients with rheumatoid arthritis. J Rehabil Med 41:338, 2009.

133. Crowley, L: The effectiveness of home exercise programmes for patients with rheumatoid arthritis: A review of the literature. Phys Ther Rev 14:149, 2009.

134. Hsieh, LF, et al: Supervised aerobic exercise is more effective than home aerobic exercise in female Chinese patients with rheumatoid arthritis. J Rehabil Med 41:332, 2009.

135. Kennedy, N: Exercise therapy for patients with rheumatoid arthritis: Safety of intensive programmes and effects upon bone mineral density and disease activity: A literature review. Phys Ther Rev 11:263, 2006.

136. Williams, SB, et al: Feasibility and outcomes of a home-based exercise program on improving balance and gait stability in women with lower-limb osteoarthritis or rheumatoid arthritis: A pilot study. Arch Phys Med Rehabil 91:106, 2010.

137. Bartels, EM, et al: Aquatic exercise for the treatment of knee and hip osteoarthritis. Cochrane Database of Systematic Reviews 2007, Issue 4. Art. No.: CD005523. DOI: 10.1002/14651858.CD005523.pub2.

138. Fransen, M, and McConnell, S: Exercise for osteoarthritis of the knee. Cochrane Database of Systematic Reviews 2008, Issue 4. Art. No.: CD004376. DOI: 10.1002/14651858.CD004376.pub2.

139. Fransen, M, et al: Exercise for osteoarthritis of the hip. Cochrane Database of Systematic Reviews 2009, Issue 3. Art. No.: CD007912. DOI: 10.1002/14651858.CD007912.

140. McNair, PJ, et al: Exercise therapy for the management of osteoarthritis of the hip joint: A systematic review. Arthritis Res Ther 11:R98, 2009.

141. Pisters, MF, et al: Long-term effectiveness of exercise therapy in patients with osteoarthritis of the hip or knee: A systematic review. Arthritis Rheum 57:1245, 2007.

142. Jansen, MJ, et al: Strength training alone, exercise therapy alone, and exercise therapy with passive manual mobilisation each reduce pain and disability in people with knee osteoarthritis: A systematic review. J Physiother 57(1):11, 2011.

143. Centers for Disease Control and Prevention: Physical Activity for Everyone: Physical Activity Terms. Retrieved March 8, 2011, from www.cdc.gov/nccdphp/dnpa/physical/terms/index.htm.

144. US Health Department of Health and Human Services: 2008 Physical Activity Guidelines for Americans. Retrieved June 2, 2011, from www.health.gov/PAGuidelines/guidelines/default.aspx.

145. Westby, MD: A health professional's guide to exercise prescription for people with arthritis: A review of aerobic fitness activities. Arthritis Rheum 45(6):501, 2001.

146. Dimonte, P, and Light, H: Pathomechanics, gait deviations, and treatment of the rheumatoid foot. Phys Ther 62:1148, 1982.

147. Weiss, R, et al: Gait pattern in rheumatoid arthritis. Gait Posture 28(2):229, 2008.

148. Schnitzer, TJ, et al: Effect of piroxicam on gait in patients with osteoarthritis of the knee. Arthritis Rheum 36:1207, 1993.

149. Stamm, T, et al: Joint protection and home hand exercises improve hand function in patients with hand osteoarthritis: A randomized control trial. Arthritis Rheum 47(1):44, 2002.

150. Locke, M, et al: Ankle and subtalar motion during gait in arthritic patients. Phys Ther 64:504, 1984.

151. Marks, RM, and Myerson, MS: Foot and ankle issues in rheumatoid arthritis. Bull Rheum Dis 46:1, 1997.

152. Fransen, M, and Edmonds, J: Off-the-shelf footwear for people with rheumatoid arthritis. Arthritis Care Res 10:250, 1997.

153. Marks, R, Allegrante, JP, and Lorig, K: A review and synthesis of research evidence for self-efficacy-enhancing interventions for

reducing chronic disability: Implications for health education practice (part II). Health Promot Pract 6(2):148, 2005.

154. Rosenberger, PH, Jokl, P, and Ickovics, J: Psychosocial factors and surgical outcomes: An evidence-based literature review. J Am Acad Orthop Surg 14(7):397, 2006.

155. Katz, JN, Earp, BE, and Gomoll, AH: Surgical management of osteoarthritis. Arthritis Care Res 62(9):1220, 2010.

156. Ethgen, O, et al: Health-related quality of life in total hip and total knee arthroplasty: A qualitative and systematic review of the literature. J Bone Joint Surg 86:963, 2004.

157. Jones, CA, et al: Total joint arthroplasties: Current concepts of patient outcomes after surgery. Rheum Dis Clin North Am 33:71, 2007.

158. Vissers, MM, et al: Recovery of physical functioning after total hip arthroplasty: Systematic review and meta-analysis of the literature. Phys Ther 91(5):615, 2011.

159. Ganz, SB, and Viellion, G: Pre- and post-surgical management of the hip and knee. In Robbins, L, et al (eds): Clinical Care in the Rheumatic Diseases, ed 2. American College of Rheumatology, Atlanta, 2001, p 221.

160. Moncur, C: Management of persons with osteoarthritis. In Walkers, JM, and Helewa, A (eds): Physical Rehabilitation in Arthritis, ed 2. Saunders, St. Louis, 2004, p 229.

161. Westby, MD, et al: Post-acute physiotherapy for primary total hip arthroplasty. Cochrane Database of Systematic Reviews 2011, Art. No.: CD 005957. DOI: 10.1002/14651858. CD005957.

162. Momohara, S, et al: Efficacy of total joint arthroplasty in patients with established rheumatoid arthritis: improved longitudinal effects on disease activity but not on health-related quality of life. Mod Rheumatol 2011. Retrieved September 27, 2011, from www.springerlink.com/content/84g6934057p174u8/fulltext.html.

Supplemental Reading

Brosseau, L, et al: Ottawa Panel Evidence-Based Clinical Practice Guidelines for therapeutic exercises in the management of rheumatoid arthritis in adults. Phys Ther 84:934, 2004.

Brosseau, L, et al: Ottawa Panel Evidence-Based Clinical Practice Guidelines for electrotherapy and thermotherapy in the management of rheumatoid arthritis in adults. Phys Ther 84:1016, 2004.

Jordan, JL, et al: Interventions to improve adherence to exercise for chronic musculoskeletal pain in adults. Cochrane Database of Systematic Reviews 2010, Issue 1. Art. No.: CD005956. DOI: 10.1002/14651858.CD005956.pub2.

Activity	Assistance (1–5)	Pain (1–4)	Difficulty (1–4)	Comments
Mobility				
Walking inside	_____	_____	_____	_____
Climbing up stairs	_____	_____	_____	_____
Rising from a chair	_____	_____	_____	_____
Personal Care	_____	_____	_____	_____
Putting on pants	_____	_____	_____	_____
Buttoning a shirt/blouse	_____	_____	_____	_____
Washing all parts of the body	_____	_____	_____	_____
Putting on a shirt/blouse	_____	_____	_____	_____
Home Chores				
Vacuuming a rug	_____	_____	_____	_____
Reaching into low cupboards	_____	_____	_____	_____
Doing laundry	_____	_____	_____	_____
Doing yard work	_____	_____	_____	_____
Hand Activities				
Writing	_____	_____	_____	_____
Opening container	_____	_____	_____	_____
Dialing a phone	_____	_____	_____	_____
Social Activities				
Performing your job	_____	_____	_____	_____
Driving a car	_____	_____	_____	_____
Attending meetings/appointments	_____	_____	_____	_____
Visiting with friends and relatives	_____	_____	_____	_____

Used by permission of Alan M. Jette.
KEY:
ASSISTANCE: 1 = independent; 2 = uses devices; 3 = uses human assistance; 4 = uses devices and human assistance; 5 = unable or unsafe to do the activity.
PAIN: 1 = no pain; 2 = mild pain; 3 = moderate pain; 4 = severe pain.
DIFFICULTY: 1 = no difficulty; 2 = mild difficulty; 3 = moderate difficulty; 4 = severe difficulty.
TIME FRAME: On average during the past 7 days.

Health Assessment Questionnaire

© Stanford University School of Medicine

Division of Immunology and Rheumatology

Name _____ Date _____

In this section we are interested in learning how your illness affects your ability to function in daily life. Please feel free to add any comments on the back of this page.

Please check the response which best describes your usual abilities OVER THE PAST WEEK:

	Without ANY difficulty	With SOME difficulty	With MUCH difficulty	Unable to do
Dressing & Grooming				
Are you able to:				
• Dress yourself, including tying shoelaces and doing buttons?	_____	_____	_____	_____
• Shampoo your hair?	_____	_____	_____	_____
Arising				
Are you able to:				
• Stand up from a straight chair?	_____	_____	_____	_____
• Get in and out of bed?	_____	_____	_____	_____
Eating				
Are you able to:				
• Cut your meat?	_____	_____	_____	_____
• Lift a full cup or glass to your mouth?	_____	_____	_____	_____
• Open a new milk carton?	_____	_____	_____	_____
Walking				
Are you able to:				
• Walk outdoors on flat ground?	_____	_____	_____	_____
• Climb up five steps?	_____	_____	_____	_____

Please check any AIDS or DEVICES that you usually use for any of these activities:

__Cane   __Devices used for dressing (button hook, zipper, long-handled shoehorn)
__Walker   __Built-up or special utensils
__Crutches __Special or built-up chair
__Wheelchair __Other (specify) _____

Please check any categories that you usually need HELP FROM ANOTHER PERSON:

__Dressing and Grooming   __ Eating
__Arising   __ Walking

Please check the response which best describes your abilities OVER THE PAST WEEK:

	Without ANY difficulty	With SOME difficulty	With MUCH difficulty	Unable to do
Hygiene:				
Are you able to:				
• Wash and dry your body?	_____	_____	_____	_____
• Take a tub bath?	_____	_____	_____	_____
• Get on and off the toilet?	_____	_____	_____	_____
Reach:				
Are you able to:				
• Reach and get down a five-pound object (such as a bag of sugar) from just above your head?	_____	_____	_____	_____
• Bend down to pick up clothing from the floor?	_____	_____	_____	_____
Grip:				
Are you able to:				
• Open car doors?	_____	_____	_____	_____
• Open jars which have been previously opened?	_____	_____	_____	_____
Activities				
Are you able to:				
• Run errands and shop?	_____	_____	_____	_____
• Get in and out of the car?	_____	_____	_____	_____
• Do chores such as vacuuming and yard work?	_____	_____	_____	_____

Please check any AIDS or DEVICES that you usually use for any of these activities:

__Raised toilet seat   __Bathtub bar
__Bathtub seat   __Long-handled appliances for reach
__Jar opener (for previously opened jars) __Other (specify)_____

Please check any categories that you usually need HELP FROM ANOTHER PERSON:

__Hygiene   __Gripping and opening things
__Reach   __Errands and chores

We are also interested in whether or not you are affected by pain because of your illness.

How much pain have you had because of your illness IN THE PAST WEEK:

PLACE A VERTICAL (|) MARK ON THE LINE TO INDICATE THE SEVERITY OF PAIN

No Pain   Severe Pain

0   100

Joint Protection, Rest, and Energy Conservation

■ JOINT PROTECTION

Why Is Joint Protection Important?

Overuse and abuse of arthritic joints may lead to progressive deterioration of the joint and its surrounding tissues. Positive action is necessary to protect joints, conserve energy, and preserve function.

During activity, a normal joint is protected by the muscles around it that absorb the forces on the joint, preventing undue strain on the tendons, ligaments, and cartilage. A diseased joint is mechanically weak and poorly stabilized, which can contribute to the overstretching of the tendons and ligaments and damage to the cartilage. This increased stress can increase the destruction of the joint and cause increased pain.

How Can Joints Be Protected?

The main idea in joint protection is to minimize the strain on joints in daily activities. Joint protection techniques try to reduce the force on the joint, to slow down the joint damage. Good posture and positioning, changing the method of an activity, and pacing all help to protect the joint.

Which Joints Need Protection?

People with a local type of arthritis, such as osteoarthritis, need to pay close attention to the joints that are involved with the arthritis. People with a systemic or whole-body type of arthritis, such as rheumatoid arthritis, need to reduce the stress on all their joints. In addition to the joint protection principles and examples listed below, people with rheumatoid arthritis should look at the section below titled Additional Reminders for Protection of the Rheumatoid Hand.

In planning your joint protection, start by concentrating on the joints that are currently giving you the most trouble. Check off the principles that apply most strongly to you, and list several examples of how you can apply that principle to your problem joints.

Joint Protection Principles	Your Examples
☐ 1. *Respect Pain.*	
a. It is important to distinguish between discomfort and pain.	_____
b. Pain that lasts for more than 1 to 2 hours after an activity indicates that the activity is too stressful and needs to be modified.	_____
c. If there is a sharp increase in pain during activity, stop and rest, then modify the activity.	_____
d. If there is unusual pain or stiffness the next day, look back at the previous day's activities to see if they were too strenuous.	_____
☐ 2. *Avoid Positions of Deformity.*	
The foremost position of deformity for most joints is flexion, bending of the joint. Maintaining a bent position increases the possibility of deformity.	_____
a Stand erect, with weight evenly divided on both feet.	_____
b. Lay as flat as possible in bed; do not curl up or prop yourself up on several pillows.	_____
c. Work with your hands flat.	_____
d. Avoid tight grip or squeezing.	_____
☐ 3. *Avoid Awkward Positions.*	
Use each joint in its most stable and functional position. Extra strain is placed on a joint when it is twisted or rotated.	_____
a. Rise straight up from sitting, rather than leaning to one side for support.	_____
b. Reposition feet rather than twisting trunk or knees.	_____
c. Stand on a stool to reach overhead.	_____
d. Reposition yourself closer to object rather than stretch your reach.	_____
e. Sit to clean or garden, rather than squatting or kneeling down.	_____
f. Use good posture when you stand, sit, and lie down.	_____

Continued

Joint Protection Principles	Your Examples

☐ 4. *Use Strongest Joints or Distribute the Force over Several Joints.*
The stress on each individual joint is less if it is divided over several joints. The larger joints have greater muscles surrounding them to absorb the stress.

  a. Use two hands whenever possible. _____
  b. Carry packages in both arms rather than in one. _____
  c. Carry a shoulder purse or purse handle over forearm rather than in fingers. _____
  d. Use knapsack to carry packages on back. _____
  e. Lift objects from underneath, using wrist and elbow, rather than pinch gripping the sides. _____
  f. Lift objects with your knees bent, your back straight. _____
  g. Move large objects with body weight behind it, the push coming from the legs. _____
  h. Push with open palm or forearm rather than fingers. _____

☐ 5. *Use Adapted Equipment.*
Find equipment that will reduce the stress on the joint or make the job easier.
The Self-Help Manual for People with Arthritis is a catalog of adapted equipment available from the local Arthritis Foundation. _____

  a. Equipment can be modified by:
    1. Building up the handle so it is easier to grasp.
    2. Extending the handle so it is easier to reach. _____
  b. Equipment available:
Walking aids
Self-care aids
Bathroom safety
Homemaking equipment
Job modification equipment
Joints that need protection: _____

_____
Activities to be modified: _____

_____

_____

Additional Reminders for the Protection of the Rheumatoid Hand

1. Through exercise, maintain wrist extension (ability to pick hand up off table) to ensure power grip.
2. Through exercise, maintain supination (ability to turn palm up) to ensure ability to hold and to carry objects.
3. Avoid positions of deformity.
  a. Finger flexion

1. Avoid making fist or tight grip—use built-up handles.
2. Work with hand flat—use dust mitts, sponges.
3. Avoid prolonged holding of objects: pen, book, pan, needle.
4. Avoid putting any pressure on bent knuckles.
  b. Ulnar deviation (tendency of fingers to slide to little finger side)

1. Avoid pressure toward little finger side of hand.
2. Any twisting of hand, open door knobs, jars, and so forth should be turned toward thumb.
3. Grip objects parallel across palm, not diagonal; for example, hold utensil like dagger to cut food, stir with wooden spoon.

4. Avoid stress on small joints of hand.
  a. Use two hands whenever possible.
  b. Substitute larger stronger joints: for example, lift or carry with palms or forearm, not small finger joints; carry bag over elbow or shoulder, not in fingertips.
  c. Avoid activities involving pinching motions.
  d. Avoid twisting and squeezing motions with hands.

■ GETTING ADDITIONAL REST

Rest is important because it reduces the pain and fatigue that accompany arthritis. In addition, it aids the body's healing process and helps control the inflammation. Rest also may reduce the stress on joints and protect them from further damage. All of these benefits are important in managing arthritis.

Each day you need to make sure you get enough whole body rest, local joint rest, and emotional rest. There are many options: Mark off the options that may be possible for you.

☐ 1. *Plenty of Nightly Rest*
  Get the usual 8 to 10 hours of nightly rest. It is not as important that you sleep for that length of

time, but make sure you stretch out with your joints supported, so that your body can rest.

☐ **2.** *Daily Rest Periods*
Ideally, several times a day you can stretch out for 15 to 60 minutes with your joints supported. Again, it is the body rest, not sleep, that is most important.

☐ **3.** *Five-Minute "Breathers"*
Partway through a task, sit back and take it easy for a few minutes. This will allow you to finish the task almost as quickly but more comfortably and with less fatigue.

☐ **4.** *Local Joint Rest*
When a joint hurts, stop and rest. If your hip or knee hurts while walking, sit down for a few minutes with your legs supported; if your hand hurts while writing, stop and lay it flat for a few minutes. Splints can be used to rest painful wrists or fingers. If your neck hurts, lay down with just a small pillow supporting the curve of your neck. Any painful joint can be given extra rest.

☐ **5.** *Take Time for Relaxing Activities*
Listening to music, reading, playing cards, or other light leisure activities all can be a pleasant change of pace and can be restful and refreshing for you. There are unlimited options for getting additional rest. It takes creativity to find ways to fit extra rest into your schedule; then it takes self-discipline to make sure you follow through, incorporating the additional rest in your activities. Making the effort to get more rest can pay off in a reduction of pain and fatigue.
Ways to get more rest: ____
Systemic, whole body rest
Local joint rest _____
Emotional rest _____

■ ENERGY CONSERVATION TO REDUCE FATIGUE

Why Is Energy Conservation Important?

One of the major symptoms of arthritis may be fatigue—getting tired very easily. In the inflammatory types of arthritis, fatigue may be part of the disease process. In all types of arthritis, pain and difficult movement may use up energy, so you tire more easily.

It is important to avoid getting overtired. Fatigue may increase the possibility of a flare-up in inflammatory types of arthritis such as rheumatoid arthritis. In all types of arthritis, fatigue may make the pain and stiffness seem worse, and it will make activities more difficult. We hope to reduce this fatigue by conserving energy and using it carefully.

How Can You Reduce Fatigue?

Some people try to conserve energy and reduce fatigue by staying in bed all day. Others stop doing anything that is not absolutely necessary each day. Unfortunately, the activities that are usually cut out are the leisure activities—the enjoyable things people do for themselves or for fun. These are not good ideas.

You can conserve energy and reduce fatigue by modifying and simplifying your activities, pacing yourself, getting additional rest, and using adapted equipment.

Energy Conservation

By conserving your energy, you may be able to do as much or more activity with less pain and fatigue. We are trying to avoid both overactivity and underactivity. Conserving your energy and simplifying your work is *not* being lazy. It is not sensible to overtire yourself. Overwork will not keep your joints mobile, but it may damage your joints further.

It is not so much *what* you do, but *how* you do it that can help control your fatigue. An attempt should be made to modify any activities that leave you overly tired or cause pain that continues for more than 1 to 2 hours.

You will need to identify ways that your own daily activities can be simplified. As you read through the energy conservation strategies, check off strategies that may work for you, and list several of your own examples.

☐ **1.** *Plan the Task.*
Your Examples
  a. Think the task through. ____
  b. Decide when and where the job is best done. ____
  c. Plan out the simplest approach to the job. ____
  d. Gather all supplies before you begin. ____
  e. Arrange step sequence so that it moves in one direction (usually left to right). ____
  f. Use fewer, more efficient movements to complete task. ____

☐ **2.** *Eliminate Extra Trips.*
  a. Organize your shopping list according to how the store is laid out. ____
  b. Stay in the laundry room until your laundry is finished. ____
  c. Clean one area at a time. ____

☐ **3.** *Use Good Posture and Body Mechanics.*
  a. Sit to work; you will be more stable and use your strength more efficiently. ____
  b. Use large strong muscle groups, rather than straining individual muscles and joints. ____
  c. Lift with your knees bent, your back straight. ____
  d. Carry objects close to your body. ____
  e. Push objects, with body weight behind it, rather than pulling or carrying. ____
  f. Avoid awkward bending, reaching, and twisting. ____

☐ **4.** *Don't Fight Gravity.*
  a. Slide rather than lift objects. ____
  b. Use wheeled cart. ____

c. Use lightweight equipment. _____

d. Stabilize pitcher on surface and tilt
to pour, rather than picking it up. _____

☐ **5.** *Pace Yourself.*

a. Get plenty of nightly rest. _____

b. Plan several rest periods during the day. _____

c. Rest before you get tired. _____

d. Avoid a rush. _____

e. Work at a steady rate with rest period. _____

f. Develop a rhythm to your movements. _____

☐ **6.** *Use Energy-Saving Devices.*

a. Convenience foods. _____

b. Adapted equipment. _____

Strategies to be tried: Activities to be modified: ___

_____   _____

_____   _____

_____   _____

Excerpted from Brady, TJ: Home Management of Arthritis: Developing
Your Own Plan. Arthritis Foundation, Minnesota Chapter, Minneapolis,
1983. Used by permission of the author.

Web-Based Resources for Clinicians, Families, and Patients with Arthritis

Association of Rheumatology Health Professionals	www.rheumatology.org **Clinical classification and response criteria:** www.rheumatology.org/practice/clinical/classification/index.asp **Guidelines for RA management:** www.rheumatology.org/practice/clinical/guidelines/recommendations.pdf www.rheumatology.org/practice/clinical/guidelines/Prelim_definition_improve_RA.pdf www.rheumatology.org/practice/clinical/guidelines/Disease_Activity_Measures_RA_Clinical_Trials.pdf **Guidelines for OA management:** www.rheumatology.org/practice/clinical/guidelines/oa-mgmt.asp
Arthritis Foundation	www.arthritis.org **Patient Forums:** http://community.arthritis.org/forums/Forum1831-1.aspx **Support Groups Resources:** www.arthritis.org/caregiver-general-connect.php **Patient Exercise Programs:** www.arthritis.org/programs.php
The Arthritis Society	**Active joint count demonstration:** www.arthrisits.ca/saji **Tips for living well:** www.arthritis.ca/tips%20for%20living/
Stanford Patient Education Resource Center (Chronic Disease Self-Efficacy Scales)	**Chronic Disease Self-Efficacy Scales:** http://patienteducation.standford.edu/research/sec32.html **Health Assessment Questionnaire-Disability Index:** http://aramis.stanford.edu/HAQ.html
Centers for Disease Control and Prevention Exercise Guidelines for Arthritis	www.cdc.gov/arthritis/interventions.htm
OsteoArthritis Research Society International (OARSI)	www.oarsi.org/ **Guidelines for Managing OA:** www.oarsi.org/index2.cfm?section=Publications_and_Newsroom&content=OAGuidelines
The European Language Against Rheumatism (EULAR)	www.eular.org/ **Guidelines for management of OA/RA:** www.eular.org/recommendations.cfm
Orthopaedic Scores	Commercial website containing orthopedic scores and scoring systems for all regions of the musculoskeletal system www.orthopaedicscore.com

Chapter 24

Burns

Reginald L. Richard, PT, MS
R. Scott Ward, PT, PhD

LEARNING OBJECTIVES

1. Describe the anatomy and physiology of the skin as an organ in the healthy state and damaged condition that occurs with a burn injury.
2. Discuss the pathology, symptoms, and sequelae of burn injuries.
3. Compare the treatment for various depths and extent of burn injury in relation to medical, surgical, and rehabilitation management.
4. Identify the consequences of contracture formation after burn injury and the treatment of this condition.
5. Differentiate the options for management of hypertrophic scars.
6. Determine the type of skin care necessary after burn wound healing.
7. Design a physical therapy plan of care that appropriately incorporates positioning, splinting, and exercise.
8. Analyze and interpret patient data, formulate realistic goals and outcomes, and develop a plan of care when presented with a clinical case study.

CHAPTER OUTLINE

Burn injuries are one of the major health problems of the industrial world. In the United States, 450,000 to 500,000 burn injuries require medical treatment each year with an estimated 3,500 related deaths.[1] In addition, it has been estimated that burn injuries account for 45,000 hospitalizations per year, with about 25,000 patients being admitted to specialized burn treatment centers and the balance to other types of medical facilities.[1]

Although these data report the extent of the health care problem caused by burn injury, recent medical advances have significantly reduced the number of deaths from burn injuries and have improved the prognosis and functional abilities of surviving patients.[1-3] The survival rate has improved annually owing to improved resuscitation techniques, the acute medical and surgical care now practiced, and continued research into the management and care of the patient with burns. The American Burn Association (ABA) reported an overall survival rate of 94.8% from 2000 to 2009.[1] As a result of improvements in care,

treatment, and survival of patients with burns, more physical therapists will become responsible for treating these patients for a significant portion of their rehabilitation in settings other than a hospital burn center (e.g., outpatient clinics, community hospitals).

This chapter introduces the clinical presentation of different depths of burn injury and the complications that can result from thermal destruction of the skin. Current techniques used in the medical, surgical, and rehabilitative management of the patient who has been burned will be described. For more in-depth information regarding the examination and treatment of the patient with a burn injury, the reader is referred to additional sources.[4-7]

■ EPIDEMIOLOGY OF BURN INJURIES

Although the morbidity and mortality rate of patients with burns has dramatically decreased in recent years, the epidemiology of burns remains basically the same. The most common cause of burn injury in children 1 to 5 years of age is from scalds from hot liquids.[8-11] The primary cause of burn injury in adolescents and adults is accidents with hot liquids. Men, especially those between ages 16 and 40, have the highest incidence of injury.[1,8] Fires that occur in homes and other structural dwellings are the leading cause of burn injury in other age groups.[12] Most of the deaths associated with home or structure fires are due to inhalation injury. The number of burn-related accidents has decreased presumably because of better preventative measures, such as smoke detectors, education, and more stringent fire codes.[13]

A major reason for the improved prognosis and survival of patients with severe burn injury is the availability of specialized burn centers.[2] The advent of the burn center and the concentrated team care and focused research that has been generated by these facilities has improved the outcome of the most severely burned patient, as well as reduced the average hospital stay in most cases. The ABA[14] has established criteria for admission to a designated burn center as follows:

- Partial-thickness burns greater than 10% of total body surface area (TBSA)
- Full-thickness burns in any age group
- Burns that involve the hands, feet, face, perineum, genitalia, or skin overlying major joints
- Electrical burns, including lightning injury
- Chemical burns
- Inhalation injury
- Burn injury in patients with preexisting illness that could complicate management
- Patients with a burn and coexistent trauma (e.g., fractures)
- Patients who require special social, emotional, or long-term rehabilitation, including cases involving suspected child abuse
- Children with burns in hospital settings without qualified burn management personnel or equipment

Thirty-five years ago, there were only 12 specialized burn centers in the United States. Today there are over 120 specialized centers for the care of patients with burn injuries and other skin disorders. This accounts for approximately 1,700 beds.[15] Burn centers now have the opportunity to undergo a process of verification (voluntary quality assurance review) through the ABA.[16] Currently, over half of the burn centers in the United States are verified.

A burn center is staffed by specialists from multiple disciplines—physicians, nurses, physical therapists, occupational therapists, dietitians, psychiatrists, psychologists, social workers, child life therapists, chaplains, pharmacists, vocational rehabilitation specialists, and other support personnel—who direct their professional expertise toward the care, treatment, and rehabilitation of the patient with a burn injury. Each member is an integral part of the team, and the most effective burn

centers are successful because of their team approach to the care of each patient.[2] It is historically noteworthy that burn personnel, with the founding and establishment of the ABA in 1967, initiated the interdisciplinary "team" approach to patient care.

■ SKIN ANATOMY AND BURN WOUND PATHOLOGY

The skin is the largest organ of the body, comprising approximately 15% of total body weight. Anatomically, the skin consists of two distinct layers of tissue: the **epidermis**, which is the outermost layer exposed to the environment, and the deeper layer, termed the **dermis** (subdivided into the *papillary* and *reticular* dermis).[17] Although not part of the skin per se, a third layer involved in the anatomical consideration of the skin is the subcutaneous fat cell layer directly under the dermis and above muscle fascial layers. These layers are illustrated in Figure 24.1.

The epidermis, composed of multiple layers, is avascular and performs several vital functions. The layers of the epidermis include (1) the *stratum corneum,* which gives the skin its waterproof characteristic and serves the role of protection from infection; (2) the *stratum granulosum,* which is the layer responsible for water retention; (3) the *stratum spinosum,* which adds a layer of protection; and (4) the *stratum basale* layer, which contains cells that enable the epidermis to regenerate, as well as melanocytes, the cells that determine skin pigmentation. The interface between the epidermis and the dermis is termed the *rete peg region.* This area consists of an extensive series of epidermal-dermal ridges and valleys that serve to increase the surface area between the epidermis and the dermis. These ridges act as a reservoir of skin and are needed to overcome frictional forces that skin is exposed to in daily activity. Lack of these ridges in the healed burn wound will result in blisters from abrasion and poor adherence of the new epidermal tissue when it comes in contact with clothing or other surfaces.

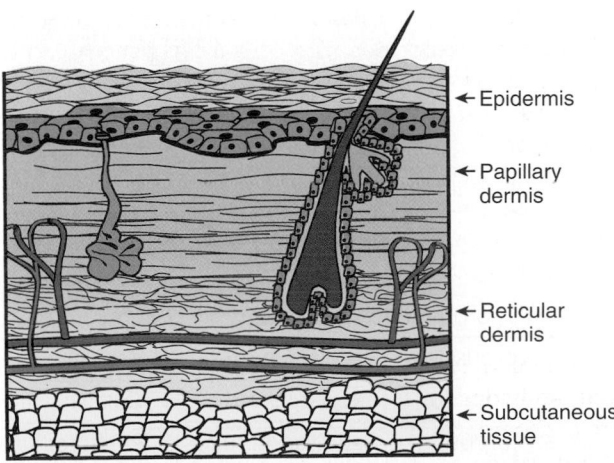

← Epidermis

← Papillary dermis

← Reticular dermis

← Subcutaneous tissue

Figure 24.1 Cross section of skin.

In earlier literature, the dermis is often referred to as the *corium* or "true skin," because it contains blood vessels, lymphatics, nerves, collagen, and elastic fibers. It also encloses the epidermal appendages (sweat ducts and sebaceous glands, and hair follicles), which provide a deep source of epidermal cells for wound healing. The dermis is 20 to 30 times thicker than the epidermis. It is comprised primarily of interwoven collagen and elastic fibers, which provide the skin with its tensile strength and elasticity to resist deformation. The predominantly parallel orientation of normal collagen in the dermis is different than the whorls of collagen typically seen in scar tissue that result from burn injury.[18] Also, the tiered location of sensory receptors in the skin is an important consideration in determining depth of burn injury (Table 24.1). The dermis is subdivided into two layers: the superficial *papillary* layer and the deep *reticular* layer.[17] The papillae of the papillary layer project upward and interlock with the epidermis. The papillae are vascular plexuses that serve, in part, to nourish the epidermis through osmosis. Morphologically, this layer is composed of a loose basket-weave network of collagen fibers. The reticular dermis lies below the papillary dermis and is composed of densely interwoven collagen fibers. The reticular dermis attaches to the subcutaneous tissue by an irregular interlacing network of fibrous connective tissue.

In addition to the functions mentioned already, the skin is important in temperature regulation through the emission of sweat and electrolytes, secretion of oils from the sebaceous glands to lubricate the skin, vitamin D synthesis, and contributes to cosmetic appearance and identity. As the result of a burn injury, some or all of these functions may be impaired and/or lost, and a patient's protective barrier defense mechanisms will be compromised.

One basic pathophysiological consideration in a burn injury is the alteration of vascular integrity, which results in the formation of edema in the interstitial spaces.

Edema formation occurs in the area of burn as well as in adjacent tissues. An initial concern of the physical therapist on the burn team is a decrease in joint range of motion (ROM) due to swelling.

The amount of skin destruction is based on temperature and length of time the tissue is exposed to heat.[19] The type of insult (i.e., flame, liquid, chemical, or electrical) also will affect the amount of tissue destruction. A tremendous amount of heat is not required to cause damage. At temperatures below 111°F (44°C), local tissue damage will not occur unless the exposure is for prolonged periods. In the temperature range between 111°F and 124°F (44°C and 51°C), the rate of cellular death doubles with each degree rise in temperature, and short exposures will lead to cell destruction.[19,20] At temperatures in excess of 124°F (51°C), exposure time needed to damage tissue is extremely brief.

■ CLASSIFICATIONS OF BURN INJURY

In the past, burn injury depth was categorized as *first*, *second*, and *third* degree. Although the lay public may use these classifications, most medical literature now classifies burn injuries by the depth of skin tissue destroyed (Table 24.2).[20] The *Guide to Physical Therapist Practice* also describes impairments of the integument in relation to the depth of the tissue injury.[21] The depth to which a burn injury causes damage depends on many factors, including the duration and intensity of heat, skin thickness of area, the distance of the area from the source of heat, the extent (percentage) of body area exposed, vascularity, and age.

The different classifications of burn wounds will present different clinical pictures, and each can change dramatically during the course of treatment. In addition to the amount of direct tissue damage from a burn, a patient's metabolic, physiological, and psychological condition can greatly affect the patient's clinical status. This section presents general clinical signs and symptoms seen in each of the burn wound classifications (see Table 24.2).

Epidermal Burn

An epidermal burn, as the name implies, causes cell damage only to the epidermis (Fig. 24.2). This depth of burns correlates to practice pattern 7B, Impaired Integumentary Integrity Associated with Superficial Skin Involvement, in the *Guide to Physical Therapist Practice*.[21] The classic "sunburn" is the best example of an epidermal burn. Clinically, the skin appears red or erythematous.[22] The erythema is a result of epidermal damage and dermal irritation, but there is no injury to the dermal tissue. There is diffusion of inflammatory mediators from sites of epidermal damage and release of vasoactive substances from mast cells. The surface of an epidermal burn is dry. Blisters will be absent, but slight edema may be apparent. After an epidermal burn, there is usually a delay in the development of pain, at which point the area becomes tender to the touch. Following epidermal damage, the injured

Table 24.1	Sensory Receptors, Location by Layer of Skin, and Sensation Mediated	
Sensory Receptor	**Location**	**Sensation Mediated**
Free nerve ending	Epidermis	Pain, itch
Free nerve ending	Dermis	Pain
Merkel's disks	Stratum spinosum	Touch
Meissner's corpuscle	Papillary dermis	Touch
Ruffini's corpuscle	Papillary dermis	Warmth
Krause's end bulb	Papillary dermis	Cold
Pacinian corpuscle	Reticular dermis	Pressure, vibration

Table 24.2 Burn Wound Classification: Differential Diagnosis

Depth of Burn	Color/Vascularity	Surface Appearance/Pain	Swelling/Healing/Scarring
Epidermal	Erythematous, pink or red; irritated dermis	No blisters, dry surface; delayed pain, tender	Minimal edema; spontaneous healing; no scars
Superficial partial-thickness	Bright pink or red, mottled red; inflamed dermis; erythematous with blanching and brisk capillary refill	Intact blisters, moist weeping, or glistening surface when blisters removed; very painful, sensitive to changes in temperature, exposure to air currents, light touch	Moderate edema; spontaneous healing; minimal scarring; discoloration
Deep partial-thickness	Mixed red, waxy white; blanching with slow capillary refill	Broken blisters, wet surface; sensitive to pressure but insensitive to light touch or soft pinprick	Marked edema; slow healing; excessive scarring
Full-thickness	White (ischemic), charred, tan, fawn, mahogany, black, red (hemoglobin fixation); no blanching; thrombosed vessels; poor distal circulation	Parchment-like, leathery, rigid, dry; anesthetic; body hairs pull out easily	Area depressed; heals with skin grafting; scarring
Subdermal	Charred	Subcutaneous tissue evident; anesthetic; muscle damage; neurological involvement	Tissue defects; heals with skin graft or flap; scarring

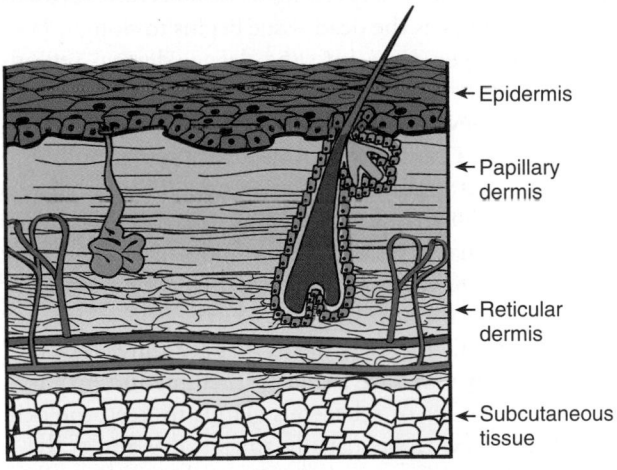

Figure 24.2 Red shading represents depth of skin involved in an epidermal burn.

epidermal layers will peel off or desquamate in 3 to 4 days. Epidermal healing is spontaneous; that is, the skin will heal by itself, and no scar tissue will form.

Superficial Partial-Thickness Burn

With a **superficial partial-thickness burn** (Fig 24.3) damage occurs through the epidermis and into the papillary layer of the dermis. The epidermal layer is destroyed completely, but the papillary dermal layer sustains only mild to moderate damage. This depth of

burn corresponds to practice pattern 7C, Impaired Integumentary Integrity Associated with Partial-Thickness Skin Involvement and Scar Formation, in the *Guide to Physical Therapist Practice*.[21] The most common sign of a superficial partial-thickness burn is the presence of intact blisters over the area that has been injured.

Although the internal environment of a blister is considered sterile, it has been shown that blister fluid contains substances that increase the inflammatory response and retard the healing process, and it is recommended that blisters be evacuated.[23-27] Healing will occur more rapidly if the damaged skin is removed and an appropriate topical agent and wound dressing applied.[28] Once blisters have been removed, the surface appearance of the burn area will be moist. The wound will be bright red because the dermis is inflamed. The wound will **blanch**, which means if pressure is exerted against the tissue with a finger, a white spot appears as a result of displacement of blood in the capillaries under pressure. On release of pressure, the white area will demonstrate brisk capillary refill. Edema can be moderate.

This type of burn is extremely painful secondary to irritation of the nerve endings contained in the dermis. When the wound is open, the patient will be highly sensitive to temperature changes, exposure to air, and light touch. In addition to pain, fever may be present if areas become infected.

Some topical antimicrobial creams will cause the wound to develop a gelatin-like film that eventually will

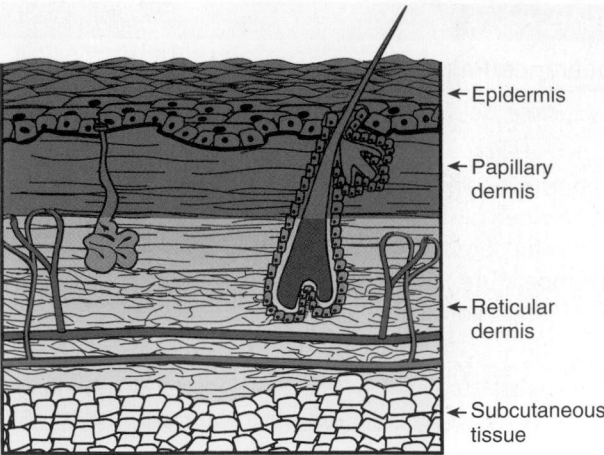

Figure 24.3 Red shading represents depth of skin involved in a superficial partial-thickness burn.

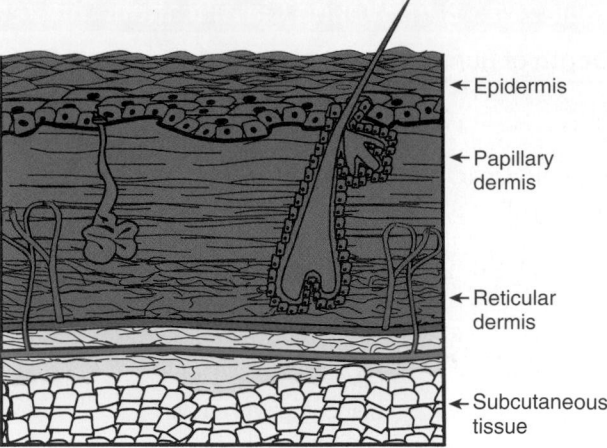

Figure 24.4 Red shading represents depth of skin involved in a deep partial-thickness burn.

peel off, similar to the **desquamation** that occurs with sunburn. This exudate is a coagulum of the topical antibiotic used to prevent infection and serum that seeps from the wound as a result of the insult to capillary integrity.

Superficial partial-thickness burns heal without surgical intervention, by means of epithelial cell production and migration from the wound's periphery and surviving skin appendages. Coverage by new epithelium resumes the barrier function of the skin, and complete healing should occur in 7 to 10 days. There may be some residual skin color change owing to destruction of melanocytes, but scarring is minimal.

Deep Partial-Thickness Burn

A **deep partial-thickness burn** (Fig. 24.4) involves destruction of the epidermis and papillary dermis with damage down into the reticular dermal layer. As this burn nears the deepest dermis it begins to resemble a full-thickness burn, and the depth best matches practice pattern 7C, Impaired Integumentary Integrity Associated with Partial-Thickness Skin Involvement and Scar Formation, in the *Guide to Physical Therapist Practice*.[21] Most of the nerve endings, hair follicles, and sweat ducts will be injured because most of the dermis is destroyed.

Deep partial-thickness burns appear as a mixed red or waxy white color. The deeper the injury, the more white it will appear. Capillary refill will be sluggish after the application of pressure on the wound. The surface usually is wet from broken blisters and alteration of the dermal vascular network, which leaks plasma fluid. Marked edema is a hallmark sign of this burn depth. There is a large amount of evaporative water loss (15 to 20 times normal) because of tissue and vascular destruction.[19,25,29] An area of deep partial-thickness burn has diminished sensation to light touch or sharp/dull discrimination but retains the sense of deep pressure due to the location of the Pacinian corpuscle deep in the

reticular dermis. Healing occurs through scar formation and re-epithelialization. By definition, the dermis is only partially destroyed; therefore, some viable epidermal cells may remain within the surviving epidermal appendages and serve as a source for new skin growth.

The depth of a deep partial-thickness injury is sometimes difficult to determine, so allowing the wound to demarcate (between normal and damaged tissue) during the first few days is necessary. Demarcation becomes evident after several days as the dead tissue begins to slough. Hair follicles that penetrate into the deeper dermal regions below the burn level remain viable. Preservation of hair follicles and new hair growth will indicate a deep partial-thickness burn rather than a full-thickness injury, and there is a corresponding greater potential for spontaneous healing. Particularly important factors that determine which epidermal structures survive and which die include the thickness of the skin in a particular location and/or the distance of the area from the source of heat.

Deep partial-thickness burns that are allowed to heal spontaneously will have a thin epithelium and may lack the usual number of sebaceous glands to keep the skin lubricated. New tissue usually appears dry and scaly, is itchy, and is easily abraded. Creams are necessary to artificially lubricate the new surface. Sensation and the number of active sweat ducts will be diminished.

A deep partial-thickness burn generally will heal in 3 to 5 weeks if it does not become infected. It is critical to keep the wound free of infection, because infection can convert a deep partial-thickness burn into a deeper injury. The development of **hypertrophic** and **keloid scars** is a frequent consequence of a deep partial-thickness burn.

Full-Thickness Burn

In a **full-thickness burn** (Fig. 24.5) all of the epidermal and dermal layers are destroyed completely. In addition, the subcutaneous fat layer may be damaged to some extent.

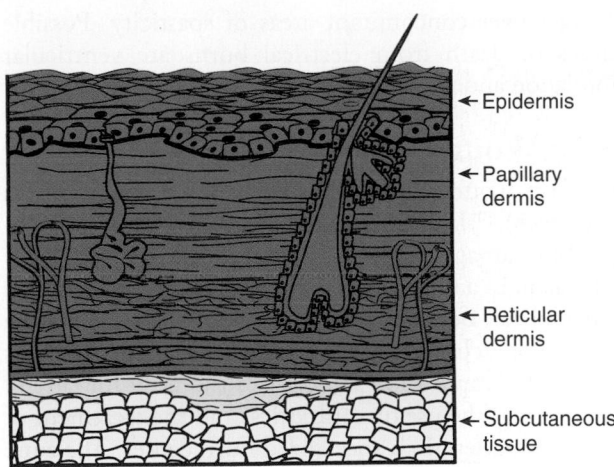

Figure 24.5 Red shading represents depth of skin involved in a full-thickness burn.

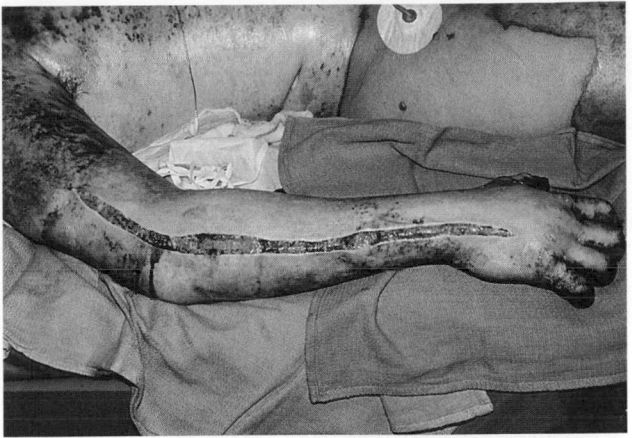

Figure 24.6 Escharotomy of the right upper extremity. *From Richard and Staley,[4, p. 113] with permission.*

This burn depth is consistent with practice pattern 7D, Impaired Integumentary Integrity Associated with Full-Thickness Skin Involvement and Scar Formation, in the *Guide to Physical Therapist Practice*.[21]

A full-thickness burn is characterized by a hard, parchment-like eschar covering the area. **Eschar** is devitalized tissue consisting of desiccated coagulum of plasma and necrotic cells. Eschar feels dry, leathery, and rigid. The color of eschar can vary from black to deep red to white; the latter indicates total ischemia of the area. Frequently, thrombosis of superficial blood vessels is apparent and no blanching of the tissue is observed. The deep red color of the tissue results from hemoglobin fixation liberated from destroyed red blood cells.

Hair follicles are completely destroyed, so body hairs pull out easily. All nerve endings in the dermal tissue are destroyed so the wound will be *insensate* (without feeling); however, a patient still may experience a significant amount of pain because adjacent areas of partial-thickness burn usually surround a full-thickness injury.

A major problem that arises from deep burns is the damage to the peripheral vascular system. Because large amounts of fluid leak into the interstitial space beneath unyielding eschar, the pressure in the extravascular space increases, potentially constricting the deep circulation to the point of occlusion (see later discussion of cardiovascular complications in the section titled Complications of Burn Injury). Because eschar does not have the elastic quality of normal skin, edema that forms in an area of a circumferential burn can cause compression of the underlying vasculature. If this compression is not relieved, it may lead to eventual occlusion with possible necrosis of tissue distal to the site of injury. To maintain vascular flow, an **escharotomy** may be necessary. An escharotomy is a midline lateral incision of the eschar the length of an extremity or chest wall.[30,31] Figure 24.6 shows an

escharotomy and the result of pressure that forces the incision to gape. Following an escharotomy, pulses are frequently examined to monitor restoration of circulation. If the escharotomy is successful, there will be an immediate improvement in the peripheral blood flow, demonstrated by normal pulses distal to the wound and by return of normal temperature and capillary refill of the distal extremity.

Although at times it may be difficult to differentiate a deep-partial from a full-thickness burn in the early postburn period, the differences will become evident after several days. With a full-thickness burn, there are no sites available for re-epithelialization of the wound. All epithelial cells have been destroyed, and skin grafting will be necessary. Grafting is discussed in detail in the section titled Surgical Management of the Burn Wound.

Subdermal Burn

An additional category of burn, the **subdermal burn**, involves complete destruction of all tissue from the epidermis down to and through the subcutaneous tissue (Fig. 24.7). This depth of injury correlates with practice pattern 7E, Impaired Integumentary Integrity Associated with Skin Involvement Extending into Fascia, Muscle, or Bone and Scar Formation, in the *Guide to Physical Therapist Practice*.[21] Muscle and bone are subject to necrosis when burned. This type of burn occurs with prolonged contact with a heat source and routinely occurs as a result of contact with electricity. Extensive surgical and therapeutic management is necessary to return a patient to some degree of function.

◾ ELECTRICAL BURN

The signs and symptoms of an **electrical burn** may vary according to the type of current, intensity of the current, and the area of the body the electric current passes

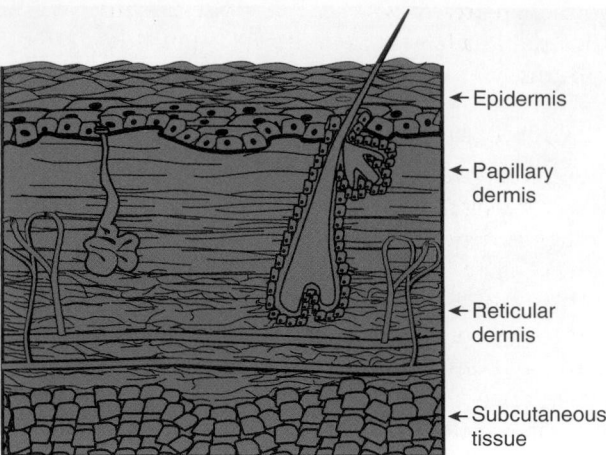

Figure 24.7 Red shading represents depth of skin involved in a subdermal burn.

through.[32] A burn results from the passage of an electric current through the body after the skin has made contact with an electrical source. Electric current follows the course of least resistance offered by various tissues. Nerves, followed by blood vessels, offer the least resistance. Bone offers the most resistance. Tissue damage results from tissue resistance to the passage of the current or by direct electrical current.[33,34]

Typically contact sites will exist where the patient first came into contact with the electricity and a second site where the patient was grounded. The wound where initial contact was made (sometimes referred to as the *entrance wound*) will appear charred and depressed, and many times, is smaller than the ground site. The skin appears yellow and ischemic. The ground site (sometimes referred to as the *exit wound*) often appears as though there was an explosion out of the tissue at the site. It is dry in appearance. Tissues along the pathway of the current may be damaged owing to heat that developed as a result of tissue resistance to current passage. An extremity or area that appears viable after an injury may become necrotic and gangrenous in a few days. Arteries may undergo spasm, and there may be necrosis of the vascular wall. The blood supply to the surrounding tissues, including muscle, may be altered. Damaged muscle will feel soft. Because the course of tissue destruction is unpredictable, there may be unequal and uneven muscle damage. Time will be required to determine which tissues will remain viable and which will not.

There can be other consequences of electricity passing through the body such as cardiac arrhythmias and acute renal failure secondary to fluid and electrolyte imbalances and release of myoglobin (protein present in muscle) into the blood. One of the most severe complications of electrical current damage is acute spinal cord damage or vertebral fracture. Clinically, these patients will have spastic paresis but may or may not have any sensory pathway changes over concomitant areas of spasticity. Possible causes of death from electrical burns are ventricular fibrillation and respiratory arrest.

Burn Wound Zones

A burn wound typically consists of three zones (Fig. 24.8).[20] In the **zone of coagulation** cells are irreversibly damaged and skin death occurs. This area is equivalent to a full-thickness burn and will require a skin graft to heal. Because of the lack of viable tissue and the amount of eschar, the risk of infection is increased. This potential complication emphasizes the need for careful monitoring, the use of antibiotics, and the treatment of a burned patient in a specialized burn center. The **zone of stasis** contains injured cells that may die within 24 to 48 hours without diligent treatment. It is in the zone of stasis that infection, drying, and/or inadequate perfusion of the wound will result in conversion of potentially salvageable tissue to completely necrotic tissue and enlargement of the zone of coagulation. Splints or compression bandages, if applied too tightly, can compromise this area. Finally, the **zone of hyperemia** is a site of minimal cell damage, and the tissue should recover within several days with no lasting effects.[35]

Extent of Burned Area

A major consideration when determining the severity of a burn is the extent of body surface involved. To calculate rapidly an estimate of the percentage of total body surface area (TBSA) burned, Pulaski and Tennison[36] developed the **Rule of Nines**. The Rule of Nines divides the body surface into areas of 9%, or multiples of 9%, of the TBSA. Figure 24.9 shows the percentages using the Rule of Nines for adults and children. Lund and Browder[37] modified the percentages of body surface area to account for a continuum of age and to accommodate for growth of different body segments. This latter method is the more accurate means of the two methods to determine the extent of burn injury. Figure 24.10 shows the relative percentages of burned area for children and adults according to the Lund and Browder formula. Although this formula provides an accurate determination of TBSA, the use of the Rule of Nines is more practical in the emergent triage of a patient with an acute burn injury.

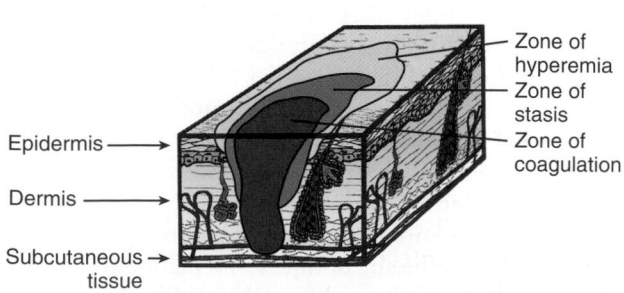

Figure 24.8 Zones of tissue damage as the result of a burn injury.

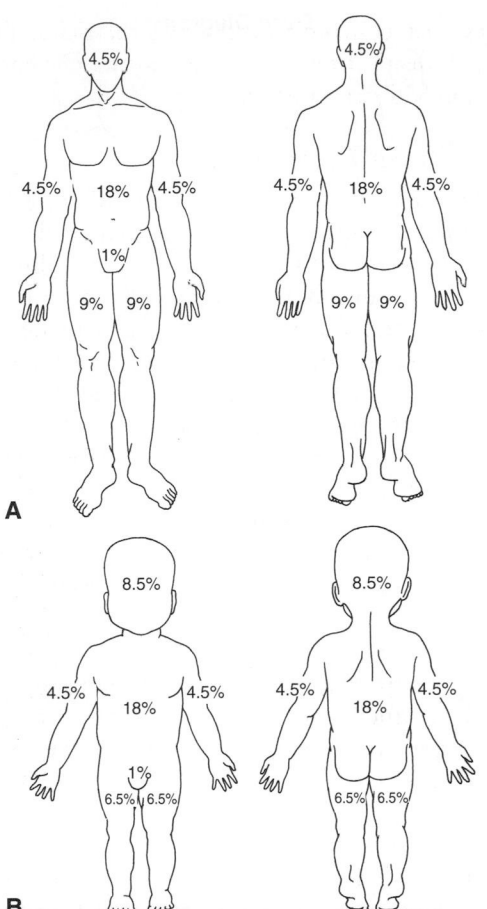

A

B

Figure 24.9 Rule of Nines to determine percentage of body surface area burn in adults (**A**) and children (**B**).

■ COMPLICATIONS OF BURN INJURY

Depending on the extent of burn injury, the depth of the burn, and the type of burn, there may be secondary systemic complications.[38] In addition, the health, age, and psychological status of a patient who is burned will affect these complications. This section will highlight selected systemic complications a patient may experience after a significant burn injury.

Infection

Infection, in conjunction with organ system failure, is a leading cause of mortality from burns.[39] Some virulent strains of *Pseudomonas aeruginosa* and *Staphylococcus aureus* are resistant to antibiotics and have been responsible for epidemic infections in burn centers.[1,39] Microbial invasion from the burn wounds to other healthy tissue can create sepsis.[40,41]

Systemic antibiotics are used to treat both burn and general system infections once they have been documented.[39,42] A bacterial count in excess of 10^5 per gram of tissue constitutes burn wound infection and levels of 10^7 to 10^9 are usually associated with lethal burns. Most wounds are treated with topical antibiotics; these will be discussed in a later section titled Medical Management of Burns.

Pulmonary Complications

Any patient who has been burned in a closed space should be suspected of having an **inhalation injury**.[43] Among patients with burns, the incidence of smoke inhalation may be in excess of 33%,[44] and this rises to 66% in patients with facial burns.[45] The incidence of pulmonary complications is extremely high after severe burns, and death due to pneumonia alone is attributed to a majority of the deaths following burn injury.[46] Direct trauma to the upper airways can also occur from the inhalation of hot gases.[47]

Signs of an inhalation injury include facial burns, singed nasal hairs, harsh cough, hoarseness, abnormal breath sounds, respiratory distress, and carbonaceous sputum and/or hypoxemia.[46]

The primary complications associated with this injury are carbon monoxide poisoning, tracheal damage, upper airway obstruction, pulmonary edema, and pneumonia. Lung damage from inhaling noxious gases and smoke may be lethal. To determine the extent of inhalation injury, several diagnostic procedures can be performed. The most helpful diagnostic procedure is bronchoscopy.[46]

Metabolic Complications

Thermal injury causes a great metabolic and catabolic challenge to the body. Most of the recent advances in burn treatment and rehabilitation have come directly from the increased understanding of the metabolic demands of a burn injury and from the ability to improve the patient's nutritional status to meet these demands.[48] Metabolic rates may increase up to 50% in a 25% TBSA burn and much more as the burn size increases.[49-51] The consequences of the increased metabolic and catabolic activity following a burn are a rapid decrease in body weight, negative nitrogen balance, and a decrease in energy stores that are vital to the healing process.[52]

As a result of the increased metabolic activity, there will be an increase of 1.8°F to 2.6°F (1°C to 2°C) in core temperature that seems to be due to a resetting of the hypothalamic temperature centers in the brain.[1] Wilmore et al[53] hypothesized that there is a significant relationship between the increased evaporative heat loss from the impaired skin barrier over a burn and the hypermetabolic state. In any event, if individuals with burns are placed in a room with normal ambient temperature, excessive heat loss will be exhibited, and this will further exaggerate the stress response seen in these patients.[1,53] Therefore, it is recommended that room temperature be kept at 86°F (30°C), which will significantly reduce the metabolic rate.

As part of the patient's altered metabolism, protein from muscle tissue is preferentially used as a source of energy. This situation, coupled with the effects of

**Burn Estimate and Diagram
Age vs Area**

Initial Examination

Cause of Burn_____

Date of Burn_____

Time of Burn_____

Age _____

Gender_____

Weight _____

Date of Admission_____

Signature _____

Date_____

Burn Diagram

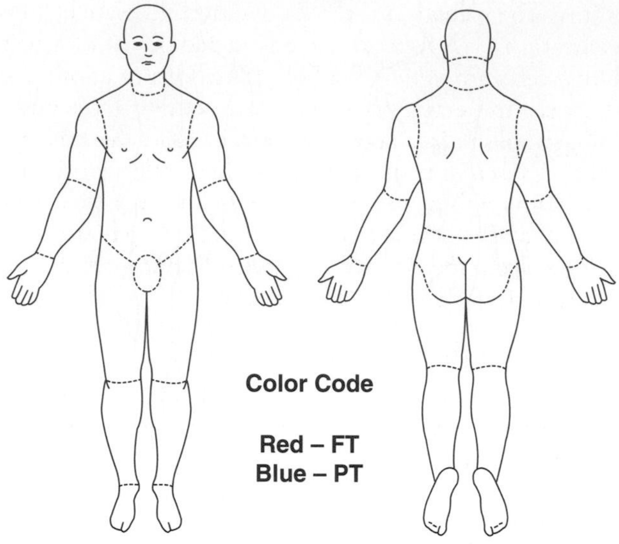

Color Code

**Red – FT
Blue – PT**

Area	Birth yr.	1–4 yrs.	5–9 yrs.	10–14 yrs.	15 yrs.	Adult	PT	FT	Total	Donor Areas
Head	19	17	13	11	9	7				
Neck	2	2	2	2	2	2				
Anterior Trunk	13	13	13	13	13	13				
Posterior Trunk	13	13	13	13	13	13				
Right Buttock	2^1/$_2$	2^1/$_2$	2^1/$_2$	2^1/$_2$	2^1/$_2$	2^1/$_2$				
Left Buttock	2^1/$_2$	2^1/$_2$	2^1/$_2$	2^1/$_2$	2^1/$_2$	2^1/$_2$				
Genitalia	1	1	1	1	1	1				
Right Upper Arm	4	4	4	4	4	4				
Left Upper Arm	4	4	4	4	4	4				
Right Lower Arm	3	3	3	3	3	3				
Left Lower Arm	3	3	3	3	3	3				
Right Hand	2^1/$_2$	2^1/$_2$	2^1/$_2$	2^1/$_2$	2^1/$_2$	2^1/$_2$				
Left Hand	2^1/$_2$	2^1/$_2$	2^1/$_2$	2^1/$_2$	2^1/$_2$	2^1/$_2$				
Right Thigh	5^1/$_2$	6^1/$_2$	8	8^1/$_2$	9	9^1/$_2$				
Left Thigh	5^1/$_2$	6^1/$_2$	8	8^1/$_2$	9	9^1/$_2$				
Right Leg	5	5	5^1/$_2$	6	6^1/$_2$	7				
Left Leg	5	5	5^1/$_2$	6	6^1/$_2$	7				
Right Foot	3^1/$_2$	3^1/$_2$	3^1/$_2$	3^1/$_2$	3^1/$_2$	3^1/$_2$				
Left Foot	3^1/$_2$	3^1/$_2$	3^1/$_2$	3^1/$_2$	3^1/$_2$	3^1/$_2$				
						Total				

Key: FT – Full Thickness
      PT – Part Thickness

Figure 24.10 Modified Lund and Browder chart for determination of percentage of body surface area burn for various ages. *Courtesy Shriners Burns Hospital, Cincinnati, OH.*

bedrest, causes muscles to atrophy and renders patients weak from both their burn injury and hospitalization.

Much of the improved management of burns has been attributed to the greater focus of research on the nutritional needs of patients. It is beyond the scope of this chapter to detail nutritional supplementation, and the interested reader is referred to several excellent reviews of advances in burn nutrition.[54-56]

Cardiovascular Complications

Hemodynamic changes result from a shift in fluid to the interstitium, which subsequently reduces the plasma and intravascular fluid volume in a patient with a burn.[57,58] The fluid shifts occur as a result of local and temporary systemic changes in capillary dynamics. This shift of fluid to the interstitium can result in significant edema. Capillary permeability returns to normal after about 24 hours. Also, with these fluid shifts, there will be a tremendous initial decrease in cardiac output, which may reach as low as 15% of normal within the first hour after injury.[59,60] Fluid replacement therapy is utilized initially to manage the loss of circulatory fluid. This additional fluid allows perfusion of vital organs but also increases the amount of tissue edema.[58,61]

Hematological changes also occur after a severe burn injury. These changes include alterations in platelet concentration and function, clotting factors, and white blood cell components; red blood cell dysfunction; and decreases in hemoglobin and hematocrit.[62] These physiological alterations, coupled with cardiac changes and injured vascular beds, will significantly affect initial resuscitation efforts and, if the patient survives, how rapidly he or she will recover. Additionally, patients will exhibit decompensation from an endurance standpoint resulting in functional deterioration.

Heterotopic Ossification

Patients with burns greater than 20% TBSA are highly susceptible to development of **heterotopic ossification (HO)**, as shown by prospective studies demonstrating a very high reported incidence.[63-66] However, the actual number of cases that progress on to become clinically problematic ranges from 1% to 3% and therefore is relatively low.[65-68] Why HO occurs in patients with burn injuries is uncertain. Suspected etiologies beyond TBSA involved include immobilization, microtrauma, high protein intake, and sepsis. The most common areas affected are the elbows, followed by the hips and shoulders; however, HO can appear anywhere throughout the body.[65,66] Usually HO occurs in areas of full-thickness injury or sites that remain unhealed for prolonged periods of time. Symptoms appear late in a patient's course of recovery and include decreased ROM, point-specific pain, and a reported quality of pain that differs from the generalized pain that patients usually report.

Neuropathy

Peripheral neuropathy in patients with burns can take two forms: **polyneuropathy** or local neuropathy.[69] The cause of polyneuropathy is unknown. As with patients with HO, patients with peripheral neuropathy generally have a large TBSA burn, and the condition may be associated with sepsis. Fortunately, most neuropathies resolve over time but some may be long-term.

Local neuropathies can be caused by a number of factors, most of which center around burn treatment issues, such as compression bandages applied too tightly, poorly fitted splints, or prolonged and inappropriate positioning.[69] The most common sites of involvement are the brachial plexus, ulnar nerve, and common peroneal nerve.

Pathological Scars

Burn scars occur in areas of deep partial-thickness burn that are allowed to heal spontaneously and in full-thickness burns that have been skin grafted, but where graft coverage is incomplete. If maturing tissue demonstrates a greater rate of collagen production than degradation, a scar becomes raised and thick.[70,71] Scars become pathological when they take on the form of **hypertrophy**, contracture, or both. Each of these scar conditions is unique and should not be viewed as synonymous. A patient can have a hypertrophic scar that does not interfere with movement or a scar contracture band that is not hypertrophied. However, both conditions can exist simultaneously, and specific treatment for each is discussed later in this chapter.

■ BURN WOUND HEALING

The burn wound has been described and the causes and complications of burn injury have been reviewed. The remaining sections of this chapter concentrate on the various types of medical and surgical interventions and physical rehabilitation of the patient with a burn. First, however, it is necessary to outline the healing process of a burn wound.[72]

The two layers of the skin—the epidermis and dermis—differ morphologically, and they heal by separate mechanisms. In the following sections, the physiology of each component is described, and the clinical implications of burns to these areas are addressed.

Epidermal Healing

When a burn injures just the epidermis, or if there are viable cells lining the skin appendages, **epithelial healing** can occur on the surface of a wound. The stimulus for epithelial growth is the presence of an open wound exposing subepithelial tissue to the environment. The intact epithelium attempts to cover an exposed wound through mitosis and the ameboid movement of cells from the basal layer of the surrounding epidermis into the wound. The epithelial cells stop migration when they are completely in contact with other epithelial cells. After this **contact inhibition**, cells can begin to differentiate to form the various epithelial layers. While epidermal cells move about the wound site, they maintain a connection with the normal epithelium at the wound margin. To continue migration and proliferation, a suitable base for the epithelial cells must be provided by adequate nutrition and blood supply, or else the new cells will die.

The process of epithelialization is most evident clinically in the partial-thickness wound that has intact hair follicles and glands. The skin appendages provide a source of epithelial cells from which the wound may heal. The cells migrate outwardly from the appendages and appear as epidermal islands from which they spread peripherally across the wound. Skin growth and coverage from these epithelial islands actually can be visualized over time.

Damage to sebaceous glands may cause dryness and itching of a healing wound. Lubrication can be a problem, and newly healed skin is characteristically dry and may split. Dryness may continue for a long time, because many of the sebaceous glands do not return to their normal function after a wound is epithelialized. Therapists need to educate patients about the type, frequency, and techniques of moisturizing cream application to lubricate newly healed tissue.

Dermal Healing

When an injury involves tissue deeper than the epidermis, **dermal healing**, or scar formation, occurs. Scar formation can be divided into three phases: *inflammatory*, *proliferative*, and *maturation*. Although these phases will be described separately, they occur on a continuum and one phase often overlaps another.

Inflammatory Phase

The primary reaction of viable tissue to a burn wound is inflammation, which prepares the wound for healing through hemostatic, vascular, and cellular events. Inflammation begins at the time of injury, ends in about 3 to 5 days, and is characterized by redness, edema, warmth, pain, and decreased ROM. Initially, when a blood vessel is ruptured, the wall of the vessel contracts to decrease blood flow. Platelets aggregate, and fibrin is deposited to form a clot over the area. Fibrin serves a threefold function: (1) to partially retain body fluids; (2) to protect the underlying cells from desiccation; and (3) to provide a firm coagulum substance from which cells can infiltrate. Therefore, fibrin can be thought of as forming a lattice network, from which cells can climb and work themselves into the healing structure.

After a transient vasoconstriction of the vasculature, which lasts about 5 to 10 minutes, vessels vasodilate to increase blood flow to the area. There is increased permeability of the blood vessels, with leaking of plasma into the interstitial space and subsequent edema formation. Leukocytes infiltrate the area and begin to rid the site of contamination. Of particular importance is the presence of macrophage cells, which are responsible for attracting fibroblasts into the area.

Proliferative Phase

During this phase, re-epithelialization is occurring at the surface of the wound, while deep within the wound, fibroblasts are migrating and proliferating. **Fibroblasts** are the cells that synthesize scar tissue, which is composed of collagen and protein polysaccharides in the form of a viscous ground substance that surrounds the collagen strands. The collagen is deposited with a random alignment and no true architectural arrangement of fibers. Stress (e.g., a force intended to elongate the scar) applied to the developing tissue during this time causes the fibers to align along the direction of force.[73] During this period of fibroplasia, the tensile strength of the wound increases at a rate proportional to the rate of collagen synthesis.

In conjunction with collagen deposition, granulation tissue is formed during this phase. Granulation tissue consists of macrophages, fibroblasts, collagen, and blood vessels.[72] Newly formed blood vessels bring a rich blood supply to the area and encourage further wound healing. However, granulation tissue formation is not necessary for skin graft adherence, and excess granulation tissue may lead to an increase in hypertrophic scarring.

During the proliferative phase, **wound contraction** occurs. Wound contraction is an active process in which the body attempts to close a wound where a loss of tissue has occurred. The amount of contraction is determined by the amount of available mobile skin around the defect. It involves movement of existing tissue at the wound edge toward the center, not formation of new tissue. Wound contraction ceases when (1) the edges of the wound meet, or (2) tension in the surrounding skin equals or exceeds the force of contraction. Skin grafting may decrease contraction, with thick grafts causing less contraction.

Maturation Phase

A wound is considered closed at the time epithelium covers the surface; however, wound healing involves remodeling of the scar tissue. During the maturation phase, there is a reduction in the number of fibroblasts, a decrease in vascularity due to a lesser metabolic demand, and remodeling of collagen, which becomes more parallel in arrangement and forms stronger bonds. The ratio of collagen breakdown to production determines the type of scar that forms. If the rate of breakdown equals or slightly *exceeds the rate of production*, maturation results in a pale, flat, and pliable scar. If the rate of collagen production *exceeds breakdown*, then a hypertrophic scar may result. This scar is characterized by a red and raised appearance with rigid texture; it stays within the boundary of the original wound. A *keloid* is a large, firm scar that overflows the boundaries of the original wound; it is more common in darkly pigmented individuals. Both of these scars take a prolonged period of time to mature. The presence and contraction of the scar can lead to both functional and cosmetic deformities. The active process of scar contraction during both this maturation phase and the proliferative phase creates a risk of contracture formation. A contracture over a joint will limit ROM and affect joint function.[74]

■ MEDICAL MANAGEMENT OF BURNS

Advances in the medical management of patients with burn injury have resulted in the survival of thousands of patients who 20 or 30 years ago would have died from their injuries.[75] Research findings and current techniques available at modern burn centers have enabled patients to receive better care through use of more sophisticated interventions for the treatment of major burn injuries. This section addresses the initial treatment of burn injuries and the surgical procedures associated with excision and grafting of new skin onto a burn wound.

Initial Management

The goals in the initial management of a patient with a burn are to address critical life-threatening problems and stabilize the patient through procedures designed to (1) establish and maintain an airway; (2) prevent cyanosis, shock, and hemorrhage; (3) establish baseline data on the patient, such as extent and depth of burn injury; (4) prevent or reduce fluid losses; (5) clean the patient and wounds; (6) examine injuries; and (7) prevent pulmonary and cardiac complications. Triage (assigning degree of urgency and order of treatment) using these procedures applies to major burn trauma.

Initially, a patient must be transported from the site of injury to a treatment facility. If possible, transportation will be directly to a burn center, rather than to a hospital emergency room. The goals of treatment in transit are to stabilize the patient and maintain an airway. During the initial transportation phase, patient history and personal data are gathered when possible. The type of agent causing the burn is noted, and initial examination of the burn injury takes place. Emergency medical personnel may use the Rule of Nines to estimate the percent of burn injury. In addition, they will prepare the individual for triage at the burn center by removing all burned clothing and jewelry and initiating the administration of fluid through an intravenous line.

One of the major advances in burn care has been in fluid volume replacement initially and throughout a patient's treatment. Research has led to an improved understanding of the physiological changes that occur in a patient after a burn injury and of the fluid volumes necessary to optimize the chance for survival.[60] Information about the physiological changes responsible for the shifts in body fluids and protein has led to the use of intravenous solutions in an amount necessary to replace vital fluids and electrolytes.[76]

After a patient arrives at a burn center and adequate fluid resuscitation (replacement) has been initiated, the burn team determines the extent and depth of injury, and begins initial wound cleansing. Wound cleansing may be performed using a variety of approaches and typically incorporates some form of hydrotherapy.[77-79] The initial wound care allows the team to establish body weight, examine the patient fully, remove hair where necessary, and start the **débridement** process by removing any loose skin. The goals of wound cleansing and debridement are to remove dead tissue, prevent infection, and promote revascularization and/or epithelialization of the area. Depending on the facility, physical therapists may be involved in the initial wound cleaning procedure.[78,80,81]

If used for wound cleansing, a large hydrotherapy tank or whirlpool tub usually will have some form of disinfectant in the water to assist in infection control.[77,82,83] Water temperature should be between 98.6°F and 104°F (37°C and 40°C). While a patient is in the water, adherent clothing or dressings applied during transport are removed. Care must be taken to ensure minimal or no bleeding. *Note*: In general, the removal of adherent material or dressings in the water is less painful than dry removal. Some burn units have converted to the use of showers, spraying, or "bed baths" for the removal of dressings and daily cleaning of wounds.[84] Regardless of the wound cleansing approach, most patients require pain medication before wound care.

Wound Care

After dressings are removed, the wound should be inspected carefully. The appearance, depth, size, exudate, and odor are noted. *Infection* is characterized by thick purulent drainage, odor, fever, a brownish-black discoloration, rapid separation of eschar, boils in adjacent tissue, or conversion of a deep partial-thickness burn to a full-thickness injury.

Wound care is carried out using clean technique and sterile instruments. If **sharp débridement** (the use of surgical scissors or scalpel and forceps to remove eschar) is performed, sloughed epidermis and loose eschar are removed and pockets of pus are drained. The procedure needs to be performed carefully so that bleeding is minimal.

After the wounds have been cleaned, the patient should be kept warm to reduce any further metabolic demand due to additional heat loss. Topical medications and/or dressings are then applied or reapplied. Table 24.3 presents common topical medications used in the treatment of burns. The technique of applying a topical cream or ointment without dressings is called the **open technique** and allows for ongoing inspection of the wound and examination of the healing process. With this technique, the topical medication must be reapplied throughout the day.

The **closed technique** consists of applying dressings over a topical agent. Dressings serve several purposes: (1) they hold topical antimicrobial agents on the wound, (2) they reduce fluid loss from the wound, and (3) they protect the wound. Dressings are changed once or twice a day, depending on the size and type of wound and the type of topical antimicrobial used.

Dressings consist of several layers. The first layer is nonadherent to protect the fragile healing surface from disruption. This may be followed by cotton padding to absorb wound drainage. The final layer consists of roll gauze or elastic bandages, which hold the other layers in place but allow movement.

Surgical Management of the Burn Wound

Primary Excision, Types of Skin Grafts, and Skin Substitutes

Primary excision is surgical removal of eschar. The excision generally includes removal of peripheral layers of eschar until vascular, viable tissue is exposed as the site for skin graft placement.[85] Much of the increased survival rate of patients with extensive burns has been due to the early primary excision of burn wounds.[86] Normally, a patient is taken to surgery after successful resuscitation, usually within 1 week of injury. As much of the eschar is removed at one time as possible. Proponents of early primary excision believe that this approach is easier on the patient than repeated débridement and that it promotes more rapid

Table 24.3 Common Topical Medications Used in Treatment of Burns

Medication	Description	Method of Application
Silver sulfadiazine	Most commonly used topical antibacterial agent; effective against *Pseudomonas* infections.	White cream applied with sterile glove 2–4 mm thick directly to wound or impregnated into fine mesh gauze.
Mafenide acetate (Sulfamylon)	Topical antibacterial agent; effective against gram-negative or gram-positive organisms; diffuses easily through eschar.	White cream applied directly to wound with thin 1–2 mm layer twice daily; may be left undressed or covered with thin layer of gauze.
Mafenide acetate solution (Sulfamylon 5% Solution) Silver nitrate	Topical solution with antimicrobial function against gram-positive and gram-negative organisms. Maintains moist environment. Antiseptic germicide and astringent; will penetrate only 1–2 mm of eschar; useful for surface bacteria; stains black.	50-gram packet of white powder that is mixed with either 1000 mL sterile water or 0.9% sodium chloride–soaked gauze. Dressings or soaks used every 2 hours; also available as small sticks to cauterize small open areas.
Bacitracin/Polysporin	Bland ointment; effective against gram-positive organisms.	Thin layer of ointment applied directly to wound and left open.
Collagenase, Accuzyme	Enzymatic debriding agent selectively debrides necrotic tissue; no antibacterial action.	Ointment applied to eschar and covered with moist occlusive dressing with or without an antimicrobial agent.

healing, reduces infection and scarring, and is more economical in terms of staff and hospital time.[86]

In many burn centers, a burn wound is closed with a skin graft at the time of primary excision. Many types of grafts can be used to close a wound. An **autograft** is a patient's own skin, taken from an unburned area and transplanted to cover a burned area. Autografts are desirable because they provide permanent coverage of the wound. An **allograft (or homograft)** is skin taken from an individual of the same species, usually cadaver skin. The skin can be kept frozen in skin banks for prolonged periods. Allografts are temporary grafts used to cover large burns when there is insufficient autograft available. **Xenograft (or heterograft)** is skin from another species, usually a pig. Allografts or xenografts are used until there is sufficient normal skin available for an autograft.

Perhaps the most progressive advancement in the care of patients with burns in recent years is the use of **skin substitutes** for coverage of an excised wound.[87-94] Skin substitutes consist of cultured autologous skin, which is grown in a laboratory from a biopsy of a patient's own tissue, the use of altered cadaver skin, or other biologically engineered tissues. Skin substitutes are used when large areas of burn exist and coverage is necessary for a patient's survival. Cultured autologous skin takes several weeks to grow and is highly susceptible to infection. Other biologically engineered tissues are more readily available and have demonstrated more reliable adherence than in the past. With the use of most skin substitutes, ROM exercises may be delayed and shearing forces must be avoided. Although skin substitutes are an expensive

intervention for wound coverage, they are useful and have proved effective in managing patients with large burn wounds. Examples of skin substitutes include the following:

- *Cultured epidermal autografts (CEAs):* A skin biopsy is obtained from a patient, and only the epidermal cells are cultured.[87,88]
- *Cultured autologous composite grafts:* A skin biopsy is obtained from a patient, and both epidermal and dermal cells are cultured. This forms a bilayer structure.
- *Allogenic skin substitute:* The epidermal layer of skin and all immune cells are removed from cadaver skin. This tissue is applied to the graft bed and once adhered, a thin epidermal autograft or CEA is applied.[95]
- *Cultured dermis (temporary):* Cultured dermal matrix is seeded with human neonatal fibroblasts and used as a temporary covering in place of cadaver skin. This substitute eventually is removed and replaced with an autograft.[92,93]
- *Cultured dermis (definitive):* This skin substitute is composed of cultured bovine collagen with a silicone outer layer. Pores in the material allow for controlled growth of a neodermis. After approximately 14 days, the silicone layer is removed and a very thin skin graft or CEA is applied.[94]

Skin Grafting Procedure

The removal of skin to graft onto a burn wound is done surgically under anesthesia. The skin used for a graft usually is removed with a **dermatome**. This instrument not only allows the surgeon to obtain a large amount of skin, but a more consistent thickness of skin can be obtained. The dermatome is adjusted to remove a predetermined thickness of skin for a **split-thickness skin graft**. A split-thickness skin graft contains epidermis and a variable amount of dermis, as opposed to a **full-thickness skin graft**, which consists of the full dermal thickness.

The site from which a skin graft is taken is called a **donor site**. Common donor sites include the thighs, buttocks, and back. These wounds heal by re-epithelialization, like a partial-thickness burn, and require appropriate care to prevent additional dermal damage with resultant scar formation. A full-thickness skin graft has the disadvantage of leaving a full-thickness wound at the donor site that will require either primary closure or grafting with a split-thickness skin graft.

Generally, the thinner the skin graft, the better the adherence, and the thicker the graft, the better the cosmetic result. Additionally, a thin graft will contract more than a thick skin graft once it has adhered to the wound bed. Selection of depth depends on many factors, including whether or not the donor site needs to be used again for another skin graft. Taking a thicker graft adversely affects the possibility of taking another graft from the same site for a prolonged period of time. Harvesting from split-thickness skin graft sites may be repeated in 10 to 14 days, depending on the amount of time the donor site takes to heal.

A **sheet graft** is a skin graft applied to a recipient bed without alteration following harvesting from a donor site (Fig. 24.11). The face, neck, and hands are covered with this type of graft for optimal cosmesis and function. When limited donor skin is available, most areas are covered with a **mesh graft** (Fig. 24.12). The meshing of a graft consists of processing the sheet graft through a device that makes tiny parallel incisions in a linear arrangement. This process permits the skin graft to be expanded before it is applied

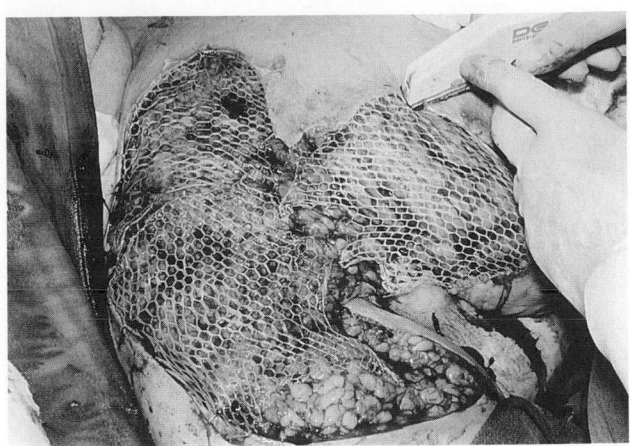

Figure 24.12 Meshed split-thickness skin graft applied to freshly excised wound and secured with staples.

to the wound bed.[96] This technique allows coverage of a larger area, and once the graft adheres, the interstices heal through re-epithelialization.

A skin graft usually is held in place with sutures, staples, or Steri-Strip™ skin closures. Once a graft is fixed in position, any blood or serum that might have become located between the graft and the recipient site should be removed. Application of a pressure dressing facilitates contact between the graft and recipient site.

A basic necessity for successful adherence of a graft is sufficient vascularity within the wound bed. Grafts will not adhere to poorly vascularized areas, such as tendon. Once a skin graft has been applied, separation of a graft from its bed must be prevented. Separation may result from shear force, mechanical trauma, or hematoma formation. Initially, an area is immobilized with a dressing that provides firm, even compression on the wound. Other reasons for graft failure include inadequate excision of necrotic tissue and infection.

Survival of a skin graft depends on several factors: (1) circulation, which provides a nutritive supply to the graft; (2) inosculation, or the process by which a direct connection is established between a graft and the host vessels; and (3) penetration of the host vessels into a graft site. Except in darkly pigmented persons, grafts are white in color at the time of transplantation and begin to show a pinkish hue within a matter of hours after their placement on an adequate vascular bed.

The reestablishment of circulation in a skin graft will take place through the formation of direct anastomosis between respective vessels, invasion from the host bed forming new channels, or both. Twenty-four hours after grafting, numerous host vessels will have penetrated the graft.[72] The invasion of new capillaries seems to be the most important consideration in vascularization. Normally, within 72 hours, inosculation has proceeded to the point where the skin graft is secure. Initially, structural connections are fibrous. Collagen is then laid down to secure the attachment of the graft.

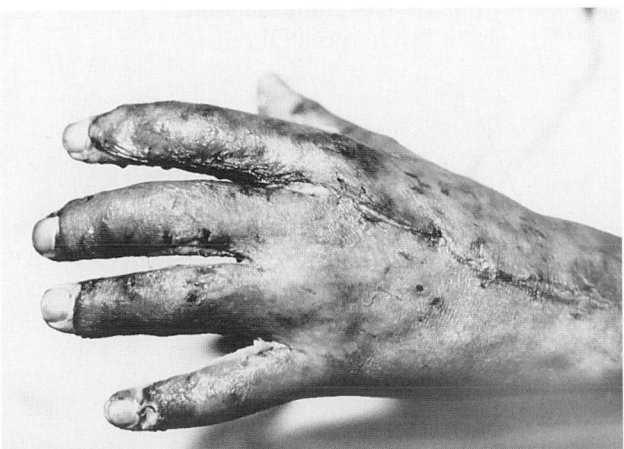

Figure 24.11 Sheet graft on dorsum of left hand, postoperative day 7. *From Richard and Staley,[4, p. 183] with permission.*

Correction of Scar Contracture

If physical therapy interventions are unsuccessful in averting scar contracture formation, and limitations are noted in ROM and function, surgery may be required. In the past, reconstructive surgery usually was postponed while a burn wound was in the active, immature phase of scar formation.[97] More recently, however, successful release of scar contractures before scar maturation has been documented.[98] Each patient's scar will require an individualized evaluation and treatment. Many surgical treatment options are available to eliminate scar contractures; among the more common procedures are skin grafts and Z-plasties.[99]

A schematic diagram of a Z-plasty is shown in Figure 24.13. The Z-plasty serves to lengthen a scar by interposing normal tissue in the line of the scar. Skin grafts are used after surgical release for more severe contractures.

■ PHYSICAL THERAPY MANAGEMENT

Rehabilitation of a patient with burns begins the moment he or she arrives at the hospital and is an evolving process that may need to be modified daily.[5-7,100] Previous sections of this chapter have discussed the pathophysiological changes and alterations of the skin that occur in the burn wound and the closure of that wound, including various types of skin graft materials. Concurrent with skin healing, is initiation of the physical therapy plan of care (POC). Commonly, physical therapy interventions are directed toward prevention of scar contracture, preservation of normal ROM, prevention or minimization of hypertrophic scar formation and cosmetic deformity, maintenance or improvement in muscular strength and cardiovascular endurance, return to pre-burn function, and performance of activities of daily living (ADL).[4] The physical therapist interacts with other members of the burn team to assist patients in obtaining these outcomes. With adherence to a well-designed treatment plan, a patient can expect to return to a normal, productive life. For many patients, the most

difficult phase of rehabilitation occurs after the wounds have healed and the scar tissue begins to contract. At this point, patient education about adherence to strategies designed to prevent or minimize contractures is particularly important. The remainder of this chapter will address the physical therapist's role in the rehabilitation program of a patient who has sustained a burn injury.

Physical Therapy Examination

After the initial examination for depth of burn and percent of TBSA involved, the physical therapist then examines the patient to determine the presence of impairments and activity limitations. The therapist needs to obtain an accurate history from the patient and family members regarding any preexisting limitations or previous injuries that may affect rehabilitation potential. The therapist must also anticipate the potential for development of indirect impairments as the burn wounds heal and mature. For example, active or passive ROM may be limited as a result of edema, restrictive eschar, or pain, and an initial baseline measure should be obtained.

Other tests and measures discussed in this text can be included in the initial examination and reexamination of a patient following burn injury (e.g., gait, functional status). Because healing of a burn wound is a dynamic process and changes may occur daily, the physical therapist needs to examine and monitor patients routinely for changes in skin integrity, ROM, and functional mobility. Frequent evaluation will keep the physical therapist and other members of the burn care team abreast of potential problems so that intervention can occur before a potential problem becomes a real one. Studies addressing assessment of burn scars are presented in Box 24.1 Evidence Summary.

In addition to the physical damage imposed by a burn, there also may be an enormous psychological impact.[101,102] The physical therapist should be cognizant of a potential problem during ongoing evaluations, because psychological trauma may affect the patient's progress and outlook toward his or her future and rehabilitation. Referral to an appropriate professional for intervention may be necessary (see Chapter 26, Psychosocial Disorders).

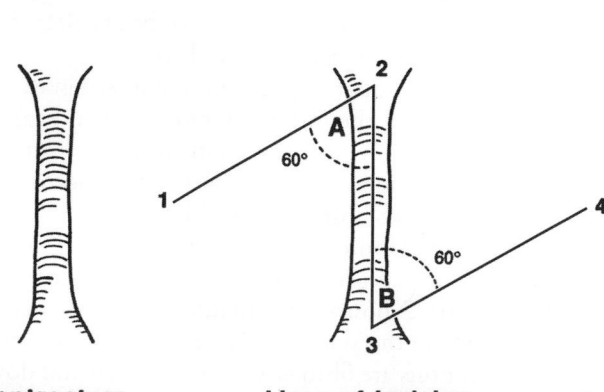

Contracture **Lines of Incision**

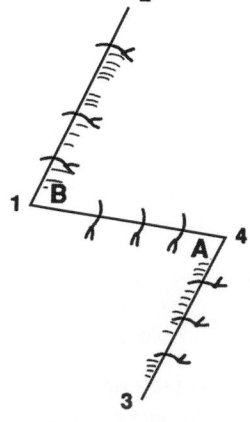

Result of Z-plasty

Figure 24.13 Schematic diagram of Z-plasty procedure. *From Richard and Staley,*[4, p. 192] *with permission.*

(Text continues on page 1109)

Box 24.1 Evidence Summary   Studies Addressing Assessment of Burn Scar

Reference	Subjects	Methods	Rating Parameters	Results	Comments
Sullivan et al (1990)[a]	73 study subjects Scars less than 1 year old A wide variety of anatomical sites were assessed	Three independent observers rated scars on the following characteristics: • Pigmentation • Vascularity • Pliability • Height	Pigmentation of the scar rated from 0 to 2 (0 = normal, 1 = hypopigmentation, 2 = hyperpigmentation); vascularity of the scar rated from 0 to 3 (0 = normal and increasing numbers represent indicators of increased vascularity). Pliability of scar rated from 0 to 5 (0 = normal and increasing numbers represent indicators of decreased pliability); height of scar was rated from 0 to 3 (0 = normal or flat, 1 = <2 mm, 2 = <5 mm, 3 = >5 mm).	Moderate reliability found between raters; reliability improved with time. No data related to intrarater reliability or validity were reported.	The study suggests the Vancouver Scar Scale (VSS) may have potential as a clinical rating of burn scars.
Baryza and Baryza (1995)[b]	No subject number was reported	Scars were rated by physical and occupational therapists using a modified version of the VSS.	A 2-mm-thick Plexiglas tool and an expanded VSS scale were developed for height measurements (0 = normal or flat, 1 = >0 to 1 mm, 2 = >1 to 2 mm, 3 = >2 to 4 mm, 4 = >4 mm). Modifications of the VSS also included expansion of the pigmentation scale with addition of a "mixed pigmentation" category.	The authors reported good interrater reliability (ICC= 0.81). Cohen's κ values were reported: $\kappa = 0.61$ for pigmentation, $\kappa = 0.73$ for vascularity, $\kappa = 0.71$ for pliability, which reflect good to excellent reliability; reliability for measurement of height was fair with a $\kappa = 0.56$.	Good reliability reported with modifications to the VSS; however, the methodology was lacking in that numbers of subjects, testers, and blinding of testers was not reported.

Continued

Box 24.1 Evidence Summary   Studies Addressing Assessment of Burn Scar—cont'd

Reference	Subjects	Methods	Rating Parameters	Results	Comments
Yeong et al (1997)[c]	A teaching set of 24 scar photographs used to train evaluators about possible scar characteristics. Ten additional photographs were used to study scar assessment.	Eight trained raters evaluated the 10 color photographs of scars using the teaching set of photographs for comparison. Assessment included the following scar characteristics: • Surface • Border height • Thickness • Pigmentation	The scale included: First, burn scar surface as smooth (-1), normal, (0), and various levels of roughness (1 to 4). Second, burn scar border height as depressed (-1), normal (0), and various levels of raised (1 to 4). Third, burn scar thickness as thinner (-1), normal (0), and various levels of thicker (1 to 4). Fourth, pigmentation of the scar as hypopigmented (-1), normal (0), and various levels of hyperpigmentation (1 to 4).	Interrater reliability was high for all areas: scar surface (0.97), border height (0.95), thickness (0.93), and pigmentation (0.85).	Provides an alternative scale to the VSS; however, the scar variables have a commonality with the VSS.
Crowe et al (1998)[d]	Ten color slide photographs of scars from 10 subjects were assessed using three different scales	Photographs of scars were evaluated by four independent raters (two were experienced clinicians and two were novice clinicians).	Scars were rated on irregularity, apparent depth or height, color, vascularity, pliability, disfigurement clothed and unclothed.	Interrater reliability ranged from 0.66 (vascularity) to 0.90 (color). Test–retest reliability ranged from 0.73 (vascularity) to 0.89 (proportion of irregular scar). Novice therapists were as reliable as expert therapists in use of the scale.	Findings suggest that the rating scale holds potential as a tool for evaluating scar surface, thickness, border height, and color. Subject and evaluator numbers were low.
Martin (2003)[e]	37 scars on 20 initial study subjects were assessed. Follow-up reassessment of scars included 17 scars on 8 subjects. A modified VSS (per Baryza and Baryza[b]) was used for rating scars both initially and on follow-up.	Scars rated were less than 6 months old. For some subjects, the same scars reassessed at approximately 1.5 years after injury. In addition to the modified VSS, a visual analogue scale (VAS) was used to obtain subject responses to two questions.	Scar assessment included pigmentation, vascularity, pliability, and height of scar. The VAS included two questions: (1) *"How would you rate your scar?"* (best possible, most attractive = 0 and worst possible, least attractive = 10); and (2) *"I feel this scar is unattractive to other people"* (completely disagree = 0, completely agree = 10).	Significant improvement in the modified VSS score from early to late assessment. The VAS scores for question 1 did not show a significant change, whereas the scores for question 2 showed significant improvement.	Findings suggest that while subjects might feel their scars improve with time, their feelings about acceptance of the scar by others may be different.

Box 24.1 Evidence Summary   Studies Addressing Assessment of Burn Scar—cont'd

Reference	Subjects	Methods	Rating Parameters	Results	Comments
Oliveira (2005)[f]	62 subjects had clinical and photographic evaluation of their scars at hospital discharge and 6, 9, 12, 18, and 24 months after injury. Observers were blinded to the subjects and the time after injury.	Assessment at each time interval included: • Photographic evaluation using VSS • Vascularity using a dermaspectrometer and a chromameter • Pliability using a pneumatonometer and a durometer • Vascularity with a laser Doppler ultrasound flow meter • Thickness with scar biopsy	Scores from the VSS; ratings from measurement instruments based on the specific variable under study. Data from VSS correlated with those from the other measurement instruments.	Photographic evaluation showed increases in scar hypertrophy between 6 and 12 months. Correlations with the VSS: VSS showed best correlation with dermaspectrometer measurements. Good correlation for pliability between VSS and both durometer and pneumatonometer. Scar heights were increased but no correlation was reported between measures. Vascularity showed significant correlation between the VSS and laser Doppler measures and significant increases in vascularity were noted at 6 to 12 months. Hypertrophic scars were associated with more itching than other scars ($p < .05$).	The correlations in this study support the use of quantitative instruments to measure some scar variables. However, the cost of the instruments may not be necessary or justifiable since these variables also appeared to correlate well with the VSS.
Forbes-Duchart et al (2007)[g]	14 pediatric subjects and 32 scars were analyzed using a modified version of the VSS. Three independent raters assessed each scar. The raters were trained together in the use of	The VSS was modified by: • Adding two color scales to address issues of variations in normal skin hue. • Two color scales were used to assist with assessment of vascularity in subjects	Two color scales were designed to assess scar based on a subject's skin tone. The two scales were labeled *"Caucasian"* and *"Aboriginal"* (described as a term used in Canada to describe Native or Indigenous Peoples).	Results indicated poor reliability with the pigmentation assessment. The vascularity subtest showed poor interrater reliability for both the Caucasian and the Aboriginal group. Reasonable reliability was reported for pliability and height.	The interrater reliability for this study was generally lower than other studies examining scar scales. A study limitation was the small sample size.

Continued

Box 24.1 Evidence Summary Studies Addressing Assessment of Burn Scar—cont'd

Reference	Subjects	Methods	Rating Parameters	Results	Comments
	the modified VSS.	with different skin tones. • Remainder of scar variables (pigmentation, pliability, and height) assessed using standard VSS scores.			
Nedelec et al (2008a)[h]	Fours skin areas evaluated (3 scar sites; 1 normal skin area) on each of 30 subjects. The four sites included: • The most severe scar • A less severe scar • A donor skin site • A normal skin site	Modified VSS used to assess scar height, pliability, and vascularity. Other measures included: • Cutometer used to assess skin elasticity. • Mexameter used to further assess scar erythema and melanin. • Dermascan used to assess scar thickness.	Each site was evaluated by the same observer using a modified VSS, a cutometer, mexameter, and dermascan. Each site was assessed on three different days within a 2-week period. The observer was blinded to any previous measurements results.	The ICC for the modified VSS for height, pliability, and vascularity subscales was adequate (0.81). The cutometer did not discriminate between normal skin and scar. The mexameter was acceptable for erythema (>0.75) and melanin index (>0.89), as was the dermascan for thickness (>0.82). *Note:* Thresholds were described for some of these measurements.	Variable sensitivity and specificity noted with some measures. Questions raised about intrarater reliability of the modified VSS with hypertrophic scar. The interrater reliabilities for the mexameter and the dermascan were acceptable, allowing consideration of these instruments for measuring the relevant scar.
Nedelec et al (2008b)[i] (*Note:* This is a companion study to the one presented above by the same authors.)	As with study above also by Nedelec et al, four skin areas evaluated (3 scar sites; 1 normal skin area) on each of 30 subjects. The four sites included: • The most severe scar • A less severe scar • A donor skin site • A normal skin site	Modified VSS used to assess scar height, pliability, and vascularity. Other measures included: • Cutometer used to assess skin elasticity. • Mexameter used to further assess scar erythema and melanin. • Dermascan used to assess scar thickness.	Each site was evaluated by the same observer by using a modified VSS, a cutometer, mexameter, and dermascan. Each site was assessed on three different days within a 2-week period. The observer was blinded to any previous measurements results.	Interrater reliabilities of all subscales of the modified VSS were not acceptable (≈0.50). Acceptable reliability was reported for the cutometer (>0.89), the mexameter, and the dermascan (0.82). Concurrent validity was significant with the VSS in every case except with the pliability subscale and the cutometer in cases of severe scar.	The interrater reliabilities of the cutometer, mexameter and dermascan and their concurrent validity with the modified VSS suggests they are objectively measuring the same scar characteristics as the modified VSS.

Box 24.1 Evidence Summary   Studies Addressing Assessment of Burn Scar—cont'd

Reference	Subjects	Methods	Rating Parameters	Results	Comments
Simons and Tyack (2011)[j]	Three-phase assessment of rating burn scars from photographs included: • Opinions from 38 health professionals about current practice in scar assessment • Opinions from 36 therapists (PTs and OTs) about what should be included in a photographic scar scale • Opinions of 10 health care consumers about scar evaluation	Opinions were gathered from health professionals using focus groups and questionnaires with instructions for assessment of scars and photographs of scars. Health care consumers received information about burn scar assessment practices, a questionnaire, and photographs of scars.	Responses and answers to open-ended questions were linked for similarity. Linked responses and answers were converted to percentages for descriptive purposes and then analyzed for significance using chi-square analysis.	Some agreement was reached that vascularity, color, contour, height, and overall opinion of the burn scar were parameters that could be assessed using color photography.	The authors suggest that a categorical scale with clear descriptors and strategies may improve photographic evaluation of burn scar.

[a]Sullivan, T, et al: Rating the burn scar. J Burn Care Rehabil 11:250, 1990.

[b]Baryza, MJ, and Baryza, G: The Vancouver Scale: An administration tool and its interrater reliability. J Burn Care Rehabil 16:535, 1995.

[c]Yeong, EK, et al: Improved burn scar assessment with use of a new scar-rating scale. J Burn Care Rehabil 18:353, 1997.

[d]Crowe, JM, et al: Reliability of photographic analysis in determining change in scar appearance. J Burn Care Rehabil 19:183, 1998.

[e]Martin, D: Changes in subjective vs. objective burn scar assessment over time: Does the patient agree with what we think? J Burn Care Rehabil 24:239, 2003.

[f]Oliveira, GV: Objective assessment of burn scar vascularity, erythema, pliability, thickness, and planimetry. Dermatol Surg 31:48, 2005.

[g]Forbes-Duchart, L, et al: Determination of inter-rater reliability in pediatric burn scar assessment using a modified version of the Vancouver Scar Scale. J Burn Care Res 28:460, 2007.

[h]Nedelec, B, et al: Quantitative measurement of hypertrophic scar: Interrater reliability, sensitivity, and specificity. J Burn Care Res 29:489, 2008a.

[i]Nedelec, B, et al: Quantitative measurement of hypertrophic scar: Interrater reliability and concurrent validity. J Burn Care Res 29:501, 2008b.

[j]Simons, M, and Tyack, Z: Health professionals' and consumers' opinion: What is considered important when rating burn scars from photographs? J Burn Care Res 32(2):275, 2011.

OT = occupational therapist; PT = physical therapist.

Anticipated Goals and Expected Outcomes

Based on evaluation of examination data with consideration to the severity of burn, and the patient's current health status, age, and physical and mental condition, the patient's prognosis can be estimated. Anticipated goals and expected outcomes are contingent on the patient's prognosis and current medical status. It is difficult to list specific goals and outcomes because of the varied nature of each burn injury; however, the *Guide to Physical Therapist Practice*[21] suggests general goals and outcomes for the physical therapy POC at which specific interventions can be directed (Box 24.2). The optimal outcome of rehabilitation is the return of a patient to normal, preinjury function and lifestyle.

Physical Therapy Intervention

Patients with burns usually begin physical therapy on the day of admission. The initial examination will determine which areas need to be addressed first. Control and resolution of edema and preserving ROM usually are the first priorities of intervention. Edema can be minimized through elevation of the extremities and active movement, especially of the hands and ankles. Prevention of scar contractures can be accomplished through positioning, splinting, exercise, and ambulation. Exercise and ambulation also will help to minimize the deleterious effects of bedrest. Following wound closure, massage and compression therapy will assist with minimizing contracture formation and management of burn scars.

The scar that forms across a joint skin crease while a burn wound is healing is composed of immature collagen. A scar will shorten as a result of the contractile or pulling forces in scar tissue.[103-106] This scar contraction can limit ROM and function unless interventions are taken against this process. Although measures to prevent a contracture are undertaken in expectation of the best result, there will be patients who develop scar contractures. There are several interventions available to address prevention and/or treatment of scar contracture.

As stated, positioning, splinting, exercise, and ambulation are interventions utilized in opposing the scar contracture process. Active exercise and patient participation in functional activities are important strategies to prevent or minimize contractures. However, owing to the relentless forces of scar tissue and pain associated with exercising a burned area, additional interventions may be necessary (e.g., skin grafts and Z-plasty). Early and ongoing patient and/or family education is needed to help these individuals understand the necessity of the burn rehabilitation process.

Positioning and Splinting

A positioning program should begin on the day of admission.[6,7,80,107] The goals of a positioning program are to (1) minimize edema; (2) prevent tissue destruction; (3) maintain soft tissues in an elongated state; and (4) preserve function.[108] Positioning strategies for common deformities are presented in Table 24.4. Examples of proper positioning of different body segments are provided in Figures 24.14 through 24.17. Burned areas should be positioned in an elongated state or neutral position of function.

Splinting can be viewed as an extension of a positioning program. There are certain "anti-deformity" positions in which patients generally are splinted; however, positioning is individualized based on the location of the burn and which movements are difficult for the patient to achieve. With the exception of splints designed to immobilize a skin graft after surgery, splints should be fabricated for patients only if ROM or function would be lost without them. General indications for the use of splints include (1) prevention of contractures, (2) maintenance of ROM achieved during an exercise session or surgical release, (3) reduction of developing contractures, (4) protection of a joint or tendon, and (5) to reduce the overall pain experience.[109,110] Splint design should be kept simple so that it is easy to apply, remove, and clean.[111] Splints are usually worn at night, when a patient is resting, or continuously for several days following skin grafting. Splints should conform to the body part, and care must be taken to ensure that there are no pressure points that may cause a breakdown in healing or normal skin. Splints should be checked routinely for proper fit and revised if necessary. Active motion is important, and splints and positioning are intended to serve as adjuncts to the therapy program until full active motion can be achieved.

Most splints used for burn injuries are static. This type of splint has no moveable parts, and maintains a position or immobilizes an area following skin grafting (Fig. 24.18). Dynamic splints also have been used successfully in the care of patients with a burn injury (Fig. 24.19).[112-114] These splints have moveable parts that allow joint movement. At the same time, dynamic splints apply a low-load, prolonged stress that can be adjusted to a patient's tolerance. They offer great potential for correcting a developing contracture and the early return of active function in areas of extensive burn and grafting.[115] The use of continuous passive motion devices also is appropriate for certain patients with burn injuries.[116-120]

Table 24.4 Positioning Strategies for Common Deformities

Joint	Common Deformity	Motions to Be Stressed	Suggested Approaches
Anterior neck	Flexion	Hyperextension	Use double mattress; position neck in extension (Fig. 24-14); with healing use rigid cervical orthosis
Shoulder-axilla	Adduction and internal rotation	Abduction, flexion, and external rotation	Position with shoulder flexed and abducted (airplane splint)
Elbow	Flexion and pronation	Extension and supination	Splint in extension
Hand	Claw hand (also called intrinsic minus position)	Wrist extension; metacarpophalangeal flexion, proximal interphalangeal and distal interphalangeal extension; thumb abduction	Wrap fingers separately. Elevate to decrease edema. Position in *intrinsic plus* position, wrist in extension, metacarpophalangeal in flexion, proximal interphalangeal and distal interphalangeal in extension, thumb in abduction with large web space
Hip and groin	Flexion and adduction	All motions, especially hip extension and abduction	Hip neutral (zero degrees of flexion/extension), with slight abduction
Knee	Flexion	Extension	Posterior knee splint
Ankle	Plantarflexion	All motions (especially dorsiflexion)	Plastic ankle-foot orthosis with cutout at Achilles tendon and ankle positioned in neutral

Therapeutic Exercise

Active and Passive Exercise

Active exercise begins on the day of admission.[5-7,80,121] Any patient who is alert and able to follow commands is encouraged to perform active exercises of involved body parts frequently throughout the day. A patient should perform active exercise of all extremities and trunk, including unburned areas. Dressing changes are an opportune time for exercise because the burn wound is visible and the therapist can monitor the wound during movement. In the presence of a recent skin graft, active and passive exercise of the area may be discontinued for a period of time to allow the graft to adhere.[100,122,123] After the surgeon determines it is safe to begin exercise again, gentle ROM—first active and then passive, if needed—is reinstituted.[124,125]

Active-assistive and passive exercise should be initiated if a patient cannot fully achieve active ROM.

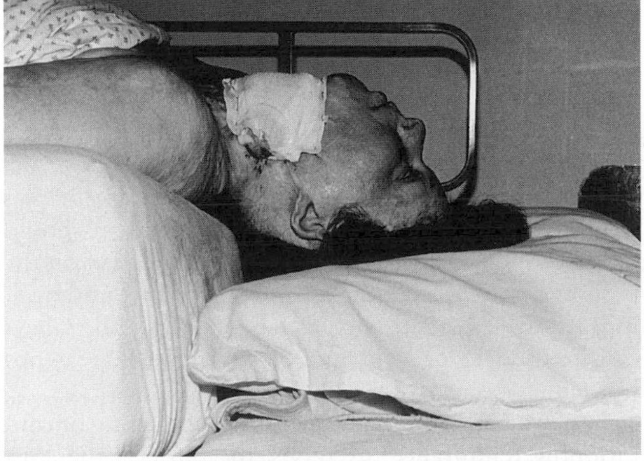

Figure 24.14 Positioning in bed of patient with burns of the anterior neck. *From Richard and Staley,[4, p. 225] with permission.*

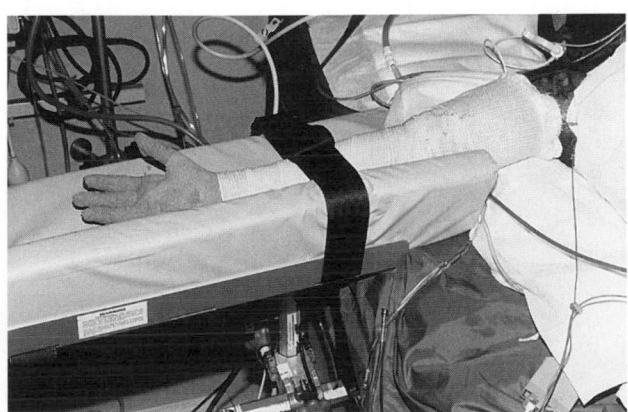

Figure 24.15 Positioning in bed of patient with burns of the axilla. *From Richard and Staley,[4, p. 228] with permission.*

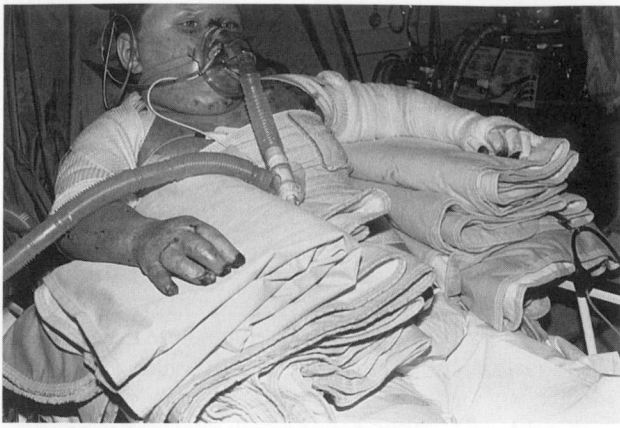

Figure 24.16 Proper positioning of upper extremities to reduce edema while seated. *From Richard and Staley,[4, p. 231] with permission.*

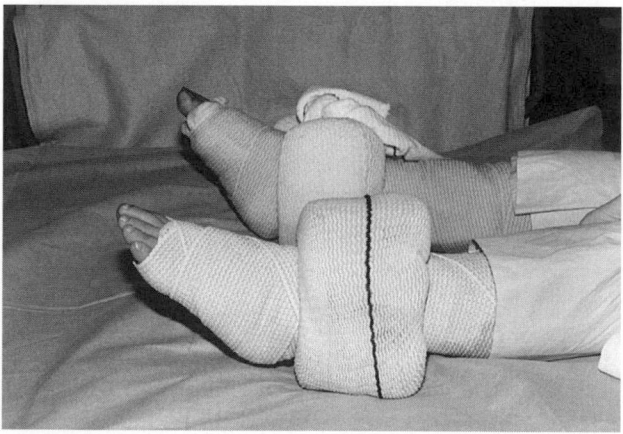

Figure 24.17 Elevation of heels off bed, with use of foam rolls encased in elastic netting. *Note:* This technique would not be used with burns to the Achilles tendon area.

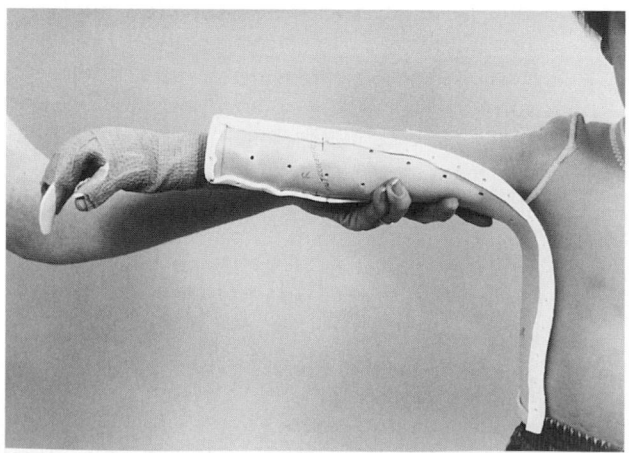

Figure 24.18 Static splint that immobilizes the shoulder in abduction and the elbow in extension.

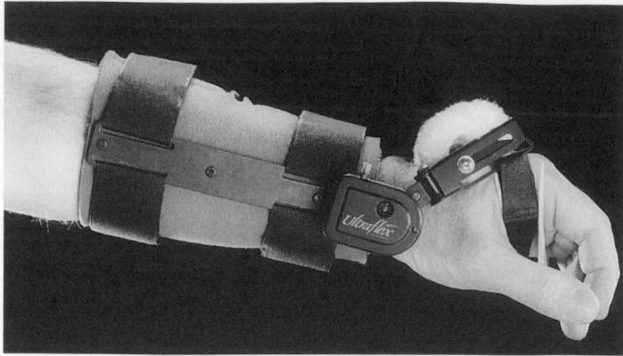

Figure 24.19 Dynamic splint used to provide a low-load, prolonged stress to scar tissue on volar aspect of forearm to gain wrist extension.

To keep the healed burned area moist, it should be lubricated before exercise is initiated. Care should be taken around areas of skin grafts, and stress should be applied in a gentle, prolonged, and gradual fashion. If the burn wounds are well healed, heating modalities (e.g., paraffin, ultrasound) may be used to increase the pliability of the tissue before exercise therapy.[126,127]

Range of motion in the area of unhealed burns can be extremely painful, and patients may voice that they would rather lose their motion than be subjected to the additional pain that occurs with movement. It usually is difficult and mentally draining on the physical therapist to push patients to exercise in and through pain, but it is critical that the therapist be persistent. Coordinating exercise activities with the administration of pain medication can lessen the painful experience for the patient.[98,121] Physical therapists should elicit the assistance of the family and caregivers in keeping the patient motivated and mobile as much as possible.

Resistive and Conditioning Exercise

As a patient continues to recover, the rehabilitation program can be progressed to include strengthening exercises.[5,80,121] Patients with major burns may lose body weight, and lean muscle mass can decrease rapidly.[128] Exercise may consist of isokinetic, isotonic, or other resistive training devices. General principles of exercise training and strength improvement should be followed, but they may need to be modified on the basis of a patient's condition and stage of wound healing. Resistive devices such as free weights and pulleys can be used to prevent loss of strength in areas not burned.

When a patient initially begins strengthening or conditioning (endurance) exercises, the physical therapist should monitor vital signs to assess cardiovascular and respiratory responses to treatment.[129] Overexertion may occur. Monitoring of pulse, blood pressure, and respiratory rate before, during, and after exercise, particularly in the recovery period after exercise, will yield valuable information as to the status of the cardiovascular and pulmonary systems (see Chapter 2, Examination of Vital Signs).

Patients should be encouraged to participate in exercises that will stress the cardiovascular system, such as walking from the burn unit to the physical therapy department. Cycling or rowing ergometry, treadmill walking, stair climbing, and other forms of aerobic exercise should be encouraged. These activities will not only increase cardiovascular endurance, but can have the added benefit of improving strength and ROM of the extremities. In addition, they introduce variety into the rehabilitation program. The physical therapist needs to be creative and innovative to motivate patients to increase their exercise capacity.

Ambulation

Ambulation activities should be initiated at the earliest appropriate time. If the lower extremities (LEs) are skin grafted, ambulation may be discontinued until it is safe to resume.[130-133] When ambulation is initiated after a skin graft, the LEs should be wrapped in elastic bandages in a figure-of-eight pattern to support the new grafts and promote venous return. If a patient cannot tolerate the upright position because of orthostatic intolerance or pain from the LEs being in a dependent position, gradual increases in tilt-table treatment time will assist in preparing the patient for standing.[134-136] Initially, a patient may require an assistive device to ambulate. However, independent ambulation without an assistive device should be achieved as soon as possible.

The physical therapist will spend a great deal of time with an individual patient during each treatment session. The rewards of a successful POC are tremendous when a patient who has suffered a life-threatening burn is able to walk out of the hospital and return to productive community involvement.

Scar Management

Following wound closure, a skin graft or healed burn wound is vascular, flat, and soft. During the following 3 to 6 months, dramatic changes may occur. The newly healed areas may become raised and firm. Pressure has been used successfully to hasten scar maturation and minimize hypertrophic scar formation.[137] However, no one study validates the mechanism by which pressure alters scar tissue. Pressure may exert control over hypertrophic scarring by (1) thinning the dermis, (2) altering the biochemical structure of scar tissue, (3) decreasing blood flow to the area, (4) reorganizing collagen bundles, or (5) decreasing tissue water content. Constant pressure dressings or garments exerting pressure

exceeding 25 mm Hg will decrease the vascularity, decrease the amount of mucopolysaccharides, decrease collagen deposition, and significantly lessen localized edema.[5,137,138] The early hypertrophic scar is readily influenced by compressive forces and thus will respond to pressure therapy. The earlier the scar tissue is exposed to pressure, the better the result.[139,140] Usually, if the scar is less than 6 months old, it will respond to pressure therapy by conforming to the pressure, remaining flat on the surface, and not developing into a hypertrophic scar.[140] If the scar is still active or shows evidence of vascularity (red color), pressure therapy may be successful, even if the scar is as much as 1 year old.

In general, if wounds heal in less than 10 to 14 days, which would be indicative of a superficial partial-thickness burn, pressure may not be needed. If wound healing takes longer than 10 to 14 days (as in a deep partial-thickness burn) or is skin grafted, pressure usually is indicated.[141]

Pressure Dressings

Elastic wraps can be used to provide vascular support of skin grafts and donor sites, as well as to control edema and scarring. Elastic wraps should be used until a patient's skin or scars can tolerate the shearing force of pressure garment application, and open areas are minimal. Elastic wraps are applied in a figure-of-eight pattern on the LEs. A spiral wrap can be used on the upper extremities (UEs) and a circular wrap on the trunk.[137]

A self-adherent elastic bandage can be used for the hand and toes.[137,142,143] This bandage adheres only to itself and can be used over dressings before the wounds have healed. It helps to minimize edema and control scar formation. It may be used before application of a customized pressure glove or as definitive pressure on an infant's hand.

Tubular support bandages come in various circumferences and garment styles. They provide a moderate amount of compression and may be used as interim garments before a custom-made garment is fitted.[137,144] The tubular support bandage is especially useful for small children who grow rapidly and require frequent alterations in garment size.

Several companies manufacture pressure garments. Some are ready made and come in several sizes to fit most patients; others are custom made for the individual patient. For custom-made garments, the physical therapist uses a tape measure to determine the periodic circumference and linear length of each limb and trunk or face so fit of the garment is exact to apply proper pressure. Garments are measured when a patient has only a few remaining open areas. The garments are very tight, and difficult to apply, but the pressure is necessary to prevent scar hypertrophy. Garments can be ordered for any or all body parts, including the face and head, and they come in many styles, options, and colors (Fig. 24.20).[137] As mentioned, garments can be worn when the skin or scars can tolerate the shearing force of application. Pantyhose may be used under waist-height pressure garments to assist with donning. Garments usually are worn 23 hours a day (removed for bathing) for as long as 12 to 18 months to assist with scar remodeling. Garments should be washed daily to prevent buildup of perspiration and moisturizing cream, which may lead to scar maceration. The patient usually receives two sets of garments, one to wear and one to wash.

Adequate pressure may not be obtained with elastic wraps or pressure garments over concave surfaces, such as the sternum or axilla. In these instances, an insert may be necessary.[145,146] Inserts can be made of many materials, including foam, silicone elastomer, elastomer putty, and gel pads.[137,144,147-149] These items also need to be removed and cleaned regularly to prevent maceration of the underlying tissue.

Early, consistent use of pressure will result in flat, pliable scars, desensitization and protection of scars, and relief of itching. Pressure is necessary until scar maturation, when the scars are pale, flat, and soft.

Silicone Gel

Silicone gel has demonstrated effectiveness in managing hypertrophic scar.[150-152] Sheets of silicone polymer gel may be applied directly over an actively maturing scar. There are varying sizes of these silicone gel sheets. The mechanism of action for the treatment outcome is unknown.[153] The only reported complication with silicone gel sheet use is a local rash with the potential, though rare, for skin breakdown. Rashes that develop are readily reversible by temporarily deferring the use of the gel sheet. Once the site is clear of the rash, the gel sheet can be reapplied.

Massage

Massage is an intervention that clinically appears useful to assist with ROM exercise by making the tissue more pliable. Deep friction massage is thought to loosen scar tissue by mobilizing cutaneous tissue from underlying tissue and acting to break up adhesions.[5,154] When massage is used in conjunction with ROM exercise, the immature scar can be elongated more easily, and a developing contracture can be corrected. Although no study has validated the use of massage for patients with burn injuries,[155] in the long term, skin pliability and texture appear to be improved by the use of massage. Firm scars that are routinely massaged tend to soften. Edges or seams of grafts or any area that is raised and firm may benefit from massage.

Camouflage Make-up

For scars of the face, neck, and hands, camouflage make-up can be used.[7,137] This type of make-up may be useful when a person has either hyperpigmentation or hypopigmentation of the skin due to the burn injury. In addition, make-up can be used before scar maturation, when the scar is still red, and a patient wants to go out in public without his or her pressure garments or devices for short periods of time. The cosmetics are opaque, color-correct burn scars, and are available in multiple shades to accommodate various skin colors. They also are waterproof and can be worn during all activities. These products can be purchased in larger department stores or where theatrical products are sold.

Follow-up Care

Well before patients are discharged from the hospital, the therapist should provide information regarding a home exercise program (HEP), a splinting and positioning program, and skin care.

An HEP should continue to stress frequent ROM exercises in combination with massaging areas involved in the burn injury. In addition, patients should be encouraged to perform as many ADL skills as possible independently. Therapists can videotape the patient's exercise program to provide the patient, family, and outpatient therapist with the actual ROM and movement pattern used in each exercise. Instructional programs (videotape, compact disc) facilitate education of those involved in the patient's rehabilitation program and will help to ensure consistency of treatment after discharge.[156]

The splinting schedule and pressure program that was followed in the hospital just before the patient's discharge should be continued at home. Before discharge,

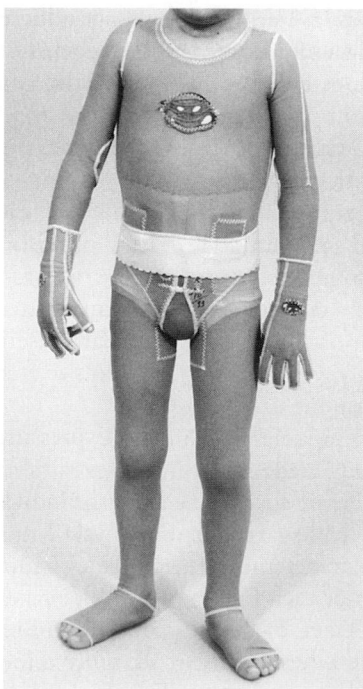

Figure 24.20 Pressure garments such as gloves, vest, and waist-height pants are worn to minimize hypertrophic scar formation.

the patient and/or his or her family members and caregivers should be able to apply and remove all splints and pressure appliances independently.

Proper skin care requires specifying the type of soap and cream a patient is to use. In general, soap should be mild without perfumes or other irritants. A moisturizing soap can be used after all open areas are healed. Moisturizing creams should be applied 2 to 3 times daily and should not contain perfumes or have a significant alcohol content. Patients should be instructed to massage the cream completely into their skin to avoid buildup on the surface. If a patient will be unavoidably exposed to the sun, a sunscreen with a skin protection factor of at least 30 should be used and reapplied frequently.[157] Patients should be cautioned to avoid the sun if at all possible and to use hats or clothing to help protect their skin against the sun's rays.

Small, superficial open areas may plague a patient for many months after wound closure because of the fragility of a healed burn wound. The patient should be instructed to wash these areas twice daily, apply a small amount of antibiotic ointment, and cover the areas with a nonadherent dressing. Avoiding shearing forces, improper fit of clothing, brisk cleansing, and soaking in water too long, or application of too much cream, can help prevent further irritation or maceration.

Itching may intensify when wounds have healed. A patient should be instructed to pat, rather than scratch, the irritated areas. Application of cream may help decrease itching; however, some patients may require oral antihistamine medication to help control this problem.

Some patients with burn injury may require outpatient therapy to supplement the HEP and monitor and adjust their splinting and pressure program. Frequency of outpatient therapy is based on each patient's needs. Regardless of whether or not a patient receives outpatient therapy, he or she should be monitored at regular intervals through an outpatient clinic. This will allow burn team members to evaluate adjustment back into society and alter the rehabilitation program according to the patient's physical abilities and extent of scar maturation. When an adult patient's burns have matured and full ROM is achieved, further follow-up care is unnecessary. However, a child will need to be monitored until he or she is fully grown, because burn scars may not keep pace with a child's growth. In these cases, surgical release of scar tissue may be necessary.[158]

■ COMMUNITY PROGRAMS

There are various community programs available to individuals who have survived a burn injury. The therapist should be aware of those in the patient's home community so an appropriate referral can be made. If programs are not available, someone in the hospital or community may want to initiate a program. Programs (see Appendix 24.A) include the following:

- Burn Prevention Programs: The American Burn Association (625 N. Michigan Ave., Chicago, IL 60611; 800-548-2876) has a Burn Prevention Committee with a myriad of printed materials.
- School Reentry Programs: Provided by the hospital staff for the students and staff in the child's school.[7,157]
- Burn Camps: Weekend- to week-long camps provide an opportunity for children to interact in a controlled, outdoor environment with peers who have sustained a similar injury.[7,157] The American Burn Association has a Burn Camp Special Interest Group with readily available information about camps throughout the United States and Canada.
- Adult Support Groups: Provide an opportunity for individuals with or without their families to share experiences and gain support from others who have had similar injuries.[157]
- Phoenix Society for Burn Survivors: This is a nonprofit organization dedicated to supporting burn survivors and families in recovery. The Phoenix Society offers many programs and resources that promote return to a meaningful life.[158]

SUMMARY

Burn injuries represent a major health problem in terms of management and care of surviving patients. Specific impairments and complications vary according to the extent and depth of thermal destruction of the skin. The classification of burn injuries is based on the depth of tissue destroyed and includes epidermal burn, superficial partial-thickness burn, deep partial-thickness burn, full-thickness burn, and subdermal burn. The Rule of Nines[30] and the Lund and Browder[31] formula were developed to assist with the initial determination of the extent of burn injury. The specific clinical signs and symptoms that result from a burn injury vary according to the different classifications. Indirect impairments can include infection, pulmonary, metabolic, skeletal, muscular, neurological, and cardiovascular and pulmonary complications. Medical management addresses life-threatening problems and stabilization of the patient. Dressings with topical medications, débridement, surgical excision, and skin grafting are primary treatment measures. Skin substitutes are slowly becoming a practical alternative to skin grafting. Physical therapy management focuses on the prevention of scar contracture, maintenance of normal ROM, development of muscular strength and endurance, improvement of cardiovascular conditioning, independence in functional activities, and prevention of hypertrophic scarring. Although burn trauma and subsequent recovery can be a devastating life occurrence, there are treatment facilities and medical professionals to assist patients with burn injuries and their families return to as normal a lifestyle as possible.

Questions for Review

1. Identify the two primary layers of skin and two functions of each.

2. Discuss the initial management of a patient with an acute burn injury.

3. Describe the differences between epidermal, superficial partial-thickness, deep partial-thickness, and full-thickness burns.

4. Explain how a deep partial-thickness burn can convert to a full-thickness burn.

5. Compare the treatments for deep partial-thickness and full-thickness burns.

6. Describe the primary involvement of the pulmonary system associated with extensive burns.

7. What is the primary metabolic complication associated with burns and how is it treated?

8. Identify and describe the three phases that occur in dermal healing of a burn wound.

9. Differentiate (1) between a split-thickness and full-thickness skin graft; and (2) between a sheet and a meshed skin graft.

10. Identify three essential factors for successful skin graft adherence.

11. For the patient with a burn injury, identify five general goals and outcomes that may be included in the physical therapy plan of care.

12. What interventions can be used to prevent (1) burn scar contractures and (2) hypertrophic scar formation?

CASE STUDY

A 29-year old male sustained a 30% total body surface area burn 6 weeks before this outpatient examination and evaluation. The patient was burned at home while he was refueling a lawnmower with gasoline, which ignited. Areas of the body affected by the burn include the right upper extremity, portions of the posterior and anterior trunk, lateral neck, right side of face, and thigh. Areas skin grafted included the right dorsal hand, forearm, and arm up to the axillary crease. The remaining wounds healed secondarily. The neck, face, and thigh burns were superficial. The patient was initially treated at a regional burn center and now is referred to the local hospital for follow-up outpatient physical therapy owing to decreased right elbow extension, decreased shoulder flexion, and inability to reach overhead. The right upper extremity lacks 15° of elbow extension (i.e., 15° to 120°) and flexion of the shoulder is limited to 0° to 155°. Scar contracture bands are noted at both locations at the end of available range with movement. The patient states that he has some difficulty donning shirts and his jacket. All other movements are within functional limits. The patient's strength overall is within functional limits. His wounds are all closed. The patient lives with his girlfriend and has medical benefits through his employer.

One week after his discharge from the hospital, the patient presented for his initial outpatient examination wearing interim pressure garments, as instructed. He also brought the static elbow splint that had been issued to him during his acute hospitalization, but which "doesn't fit right anymore." The expected outcome for this patient is to regain full right upper extremity range of motion and function.

GUIDING QUESTIONS

1. Describe how you would approach the clinical problems presented. Your answer should address positioning, splinting, exercise, and scar-management interventions.

2. (A) Identify the impairments and activity limitations you will address in determining the prognosis and the plan of care. (B) Identify the practice pattern(s) consistent with the examination findings (physical therapy diagnosis) using the *Guide to Physical Therapist Practice*.

3. Establish *general* goals (short term) and outcomes (long term) for this case. Develop one goal/ outcome that will affect each of the following areas: *impairments, muscle performance, activity limitations,* and *risk reduction/prevention.*

4. Determine the prognosis.

5. Develop a plan of care. Your response should include specific interventions, patient instruction, and required coordination, communication, and/or documentation.

6. Describe the discharge plan.

7. What is the anticipated rehabilitation potential for this patient? Your thought process should include time from burn injury and stage of healing.

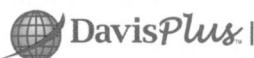 | For additional resources, including answers to the questions for review and case study guiding questions, please visit **http://davisplus.fadavis.com**

 The reader is referred to video **Case Study 2: Patient with Burns** for additional review and study. The full written case study, including tables, figures, charts, and three video segments (examination, intervention, and outcome), appears online at DavisPlus. The case study poses questions for the reader's consideration with suggested answers to the case study questions, also posted online at DavisPlus.

References

1. American Burn Association: Burn Incidence and Treatment in the US: 2011 Fact Sheet. American Burn Association, Chicago, IL 60611. Retrieved July 17, 2012, from www.ameriburn.org/resources_factsheet.php.

2. Herndon, DN, and Blakeney, PE: Teamwork for total burn care: Achievements, directions, and hopes. In Herndon, DN (ed): Total Burn Care, ed 3. Saunders/Elsevier, Philadelphia, 2007, p 9.

3. Saffle, JR, et al: Recent outcomes in the treatment of burn injury in the United States: A report from the American Burn Association patient registry. J Burn Care Rehabil 16:219, 1995.

4. Richard, RL, and Staley, MJ (eds): Burn Care and Rehabilitation: Principles and Practice. FA Davis, Philadelphia, 1994.

5. Ward, RS: Physical rehabilitation. In Carrougher, GJ (ed): Burn Care and Therapy. Mosby, St. Louis, 1998, p 293.

6. Moore, ML, Palmgren, LA, and Yenne-Laker, CJ: The burn unit. In Campbell, SK, Palisano, RJ, and Orlin, MN (eds): Physical Therapy for Children, ed 4. Elsevier/Saunders, St. Louis, 2012, p 1008.

7. Grigsby de Linde, L: Rehabilitation of the child with burns. In Tecklin, JS (ed): Pediatric Physical Therapy, ed 3. Lippincott, Philadelphia, 1999, p 468.

8. Pruitt, BA, Wolf, SE, and Mason, AD: Epidemiological, demographic, and outcome characteristics of burn injury. In Herndon, DN (ed): Total Burn Care, ed 3. Saunders/Elsevier, Philadelphia, 2007, p 14.

9. Baker, SP, et al: Fire, burns and lightning. In Baker, SP, et al: The Injury Fact Book, ed 2. Oxford University Press, New York, 1992, p 161.

10. Dissanaike, S, and Rahimi, M: Epidemiology of burn injuries: Highlighting cultural and socio-demographic aspects. Int Rev Psychiatry 21:505, 2009.

11. Guzel, A, et al: Scalds in pediatric emergency department: A 5-year experience. J Burn Care Res 30:450, 2009.

12. Renz, BM, and Sherman, R: The burn unit experience at Grady Memorial Hospital: 844 cases. J Burn Care Rehabil 13:426, 1992.

13. Shani, E, and Rosenberg, L: Are we making an impact? A review of a burn prevention program in Israeli schools. J Burn Care Rehabil 19:82, 1998.

14. Committee on Trauma: Guidelines for Operation of Burn Units. In Resources for Optimal Care of the Injured Patient. American College of Surgeons, Chicago, 2006, p 79.

15. American Burn Association: Burn Care Facilities United States. Retrieved July 18, 2012, from www.ameriburn.org/BCRDPublic.pdf.

16. Supple, KG, Fiala, SM, and Gamelli, RL: Preparation for burn center verification. J Burn Care Rehabil 18:58, 1997.

17. Holbrook, KA, and Wolff, K: The structure and development of skin. In Fitzpatrick, TB, et al (eds): Dermatology in General Medicine. McGraw-Hill, New York, 1993, p 97.

18. Lanir, Y: The fibrous structure of the skin and its relation to mechanical behavior. In Marks, R, and Payne, PA (eds): Bioengineering and the Skin. MIT Press, Massachusetts, 1981, p 93.

19. Moncrief, JA: The body's response to heat. In Artz, CP, et al (eds): Burns: A Team Approach. Saunders, Philadelphia, 1979, p 24.

20. Johnson, C: Pathologic manifestations of burn injury. In Richard, RL, and Staley, MJ (eds): Burn Care and Rehabilitation: Principles and Practice. FA Davis, Philadelphia, 1994, p 31.

21. American Physical Therapy Association (APTA): Guide to Physical Therapist Practice, ed 2. APTA, Alexandria, VA, 2001.

22. Norris, PG, et al: Acute effects of ultraviolet radiation on the skin. In Fitzpatrick, TB, et al (eds): Dermatology in General Medicine. McGraw-Hill, New York, 1993, p 1,651.

23. Heggers, JP, et al: Evaluation of burn blister fluid. Plast Reconst Surg 65:798, 1980.

24. Rockwell, WB, and Ehrlich, HP: Fibrinolysis inhibition in human burn blister fluid. J Burn Care Rehabil 11:1, 1990.

25. Garner, WL, et al: The effects of burn blister fluid on keratinocyte replication and differentiation. J Burn Care Rehabil 14:127, 1993.

26. Ono, I, et al: A study of cytokines in burn blister fluid related to wound healing. Burns 21:352, 1995.

27. Richard, R, and Johnson, RM: Managing superficial burn wounds. Adv Skin Wound Care 15:246, 2002.

28. Hermans, MH: Results of an Internet survey on the treatment of partial-thickness burns, full-thickness burns, and donor sites. J Burn Care Res 28:835, 2007.

29. Lund, T, et al: Pathogenesis of edema formation in burn injuries. World J Surg 16:2, 1992.

30. Mozingo, DW: Surgical management. In Carrougher, GJ (ed): Burn Care and Therapy. Mosby, St. Louis, 1998, p 233.

31. Miller, SF, et al: Triage and resuscitation of the burn patient. In Richard, RL, and Staley, MJ (eds): Burn Care and Rehabilitation: Principles and Practice. FA Davis, Philadelphia, 1994, p 107.

32. Wittman, MI: Electrical and chemical burns. In Richard, RL, and Staley, MJ (eds): Burn Care and Rehabilitation: Principles and Practice. FA Davis, Philadelphia, 1994, p 603.

33. Fish, RM, and Geddes, LA:. Conduction of electrical current to and through the human body: A review. Eplasty 12(9):e44, 2009.

34. Luz, DP, et al: Electrical burns: A retrospective analysis across a 5-year period. Burns 35:1015, 2009.

35. Williams, WG, and Phillips, LG: Pathophysiology of the burn wound. In Herndon, DN (ed): Total Burn Care. Saunders, Philadelphia, 1996, p 65.

36. Pulaski, GR, and Tennison, AC: Estimation of the amount of burned surface area. JAMA 103:34, 1948.
37. Lund, CC, and Browder, NC: Estimation of area of burns. Surg Gynecol Obstet 79:352, 1955.
38. Sheridan, RL, and Tompkins, RG: Etiology and prevention of multisystem organ failure. In Herndon, DN (ed): Total Burn Care, ed 3. Saunders/Elsevier, Philadelphia, 2007, p 434.
39. Gallagher, JJ, et al: Treatment of infection in burns. In Herndon, DN (ed): Total Burn Care, ed 3. Saunders/Elsevier, Philadelphia, 2007, p 136.
40. Pruitt, BAJ, et al: Burn wound infections: Current status. World J Surg 22:135, 1998.
41. Robson, MC: Burn sepsis. Crit Care Clin 4:281, 1988.
42. Weber, JM: Epidemiology of infections and strategies for control. In Carrougher, GJ (ed): Burn Care and Therapy. Mosby, St. Louis, 1998, p 185.
43. Moylan, JA: Smoke inhalation and burn injury. Surg Clin North Am 60:1530, 1980.
44. Greenberg, MI, and Walter, J: Axioms on smoke inhalation. Hosp Med 19:13, 1983.
45. Chu, CS: New concepts of pulmonary burn injury. J Trauma 21:958, 1981.
46. Cioffi, WG: Inhalation injury. In Carrougher, GJ (ed): Burn Care and Therapy. Mosby, St. Louis, 1998, p 35.
47. McCall, JE, and Cahill, TJ: Respiratory care of the burn patient. J Burn Care Res 26:200, 2005.
48. Mancusi-Ungaro, HR, et al: Caloric and nitrogen balances as predictors of nutritional outcome in patients with burns. J Burn Care Rehabil 13:695, 1992.
49. Dickerson, RN, et al: Accuracy of predictive methods to estimate resting energy expenditure of thermally-injured patients. J Parenter Enteral Nutr 26:17, 2002.
50. Deitch, EA: Nutritional support of the burn patient. Crit Care Clin 11:735, 1995.
51. Demling, RH, and Seigne, P: Metabolic management of patients with severe burns. World J Surg 24:673, 2000.
52. Demling, RH, and DeSanti, L: Increased protein intake during the recovery phase after severe burns increases body weight gain and muscle function. J Burn Care Rehabil 19:161, 1998.
53. Wilmore, DW, et al: Effect of ambient temperature on heat production and heat loss in burn patients. J Appl Physiol 38:593, 1975.
54. Prelack, K, et al: Energy and protein provisions for thermally injured children revisited: An outcome-based approach for determining requirements. Burn Care Rehabil 18:177, 1997.
55. Dominioni, L, et al: Enteral feeding in burn hypermetabolism: Nutritional and metabolic effects on different levels of calorie and protein intake. J Parenter Enteral Nutr 9:269, 1985.
56. Matsuda, T, et al: The importance of burn wound size in determining the optimal calorie: nitrogen ratio. Surgery 94:562, 1983.
57. Lund, T, Onarheim, H, and Reed, RK: Pathogenesis of edema formation in burn patients. World J Surg 16:2, 1992.
58. Latenser, BA:. Critical care of the burn patient: The first 48 hours. Crit Care Med 37:2819, 2009.
59. Demling, RH, et al: The study of burn wound edema using dichromatic absorptiometry. J Trauma 18:124, 1978.
60. Kramer, GC, Lund, T, and Beckum, OK: Pathophysiology of burn shock and burn edema. In Herndon, DN (ed): Total Burn Care, ed 3. Saunders/Elsevier, Philadelphia, 2007, p 93.
61. Alvarado, R, et al: Burn resuscitation. Burns 35:4, 2009.
62. Gordon, MD, and Winfree, JH: Fluid resuscitation after a major burn. In Carrougher, GJ (ed): Burn Care and Therapy. Mosby, St. Louis, 1998, p 107.
63. Munster, AM, et al: Heterotopic calcification following burns: A prospective study. J Trauma 12:1071, 1972.
64. Schiele, HP, et al: Radiographic changes in burns of the upper extremity. Radiology 104(1):13, 1971.
65. Rubin, MM, and Cozzi, GM: Heterotopic ossification of the temporomandibular joint in a burn patient. J Oral Maxillofac Surg 44:897, 1986.
66. Edlich, RF, et al: Heterotopic calcification and ossification in the burn patient. J Burn Care Rehabil 6:363, 1985.
67. Chen, HC, et al: Heterotopic ossification in burns: Our experience and literature reviews. Burns 235(6):857, 2009.
68. Elledge, ES, et al: Heterotopic bone formation in burned patients. J Trauma 28(5):684,1988.
69. Dutcher, K, and Johnson, C: Neuromuscular and musculoskeletal complications. In Richard, RL, and Staley, MJ (eds): Burn Care and Rehabilitation: Principles and Practice. FA Davis, Philadelphia, 1994, p 576.
70. Ladin, DA, Garner, WL, and Smith, DJ: Excessive scarring as a consequence of healing. Wound Repair Regen 3:(1)6, 1995.
71. Armour, A, Scott, PG, and Tredget, EE: Cellular and molecular pathology of HTS: Basis for treatment. Wound Repair Regen 15(Suppl 1):S6–S17, 2007.
72. Greenhalgh, DG, and Staley, MJ: Burn wound healing. In Richard, RL, and Staley, MJ (eds): Burn Care and Rehabilitation: Principles and Practice. FA Davis, Philadelphia, 1994, p 70.
73. Arem, AJ, and Madden, JW: Is there a Wolff's law for connective tissue? Surg Forum 25:512, 1974.
74. Schneider, JC, et al: Contractures in burn injury: Defining the problem. J Burn Care Res 27:(4)508, 2006.
75. Saffle, JR, et al: Recent outcomes in the treatment of burn injury in the United States: A report from the American Burn Association patient registry. J Burn Care Rehabil 16:219, 1995.
76. Warden, GD: Fluid resuscitation and early management. In Herndon, DN (ed): Total Burn Care, ed 3. Saunders/Elsevier, Philadelphia, 2007, p 107.
77. Thomson, PD, et al: A survey of burn hydrotherapy in the United States. J Burn Care Rehabil 11:151, 1990.
78. Saffle, JR, and Schnebly, WA: Burn wound care. In Richard, RL, and Staley, MJ (eds): Burn Care and Rehabilitation: Principles and Practice. FA Davis, Philadelphia, 1994, p 119.
79. Shankowsky, HA, et al: North American survey of hydrotherapy in modern burn care. J Burn Care Rehabil 15:143, 1994.
80. Ward, RS: The rehabilitation of burn patients. Crit Rev Phys Rehabil Med 2:121, 1991.
81. Neville, C, and Dimick, AR: The trauma table as an alternative to the Hubbard tank in burn care. J Burn Care Rehabil 8:574, 1987.
82. Heggers, JP, et al: Bactericidal and wound-healing properties of sodium hypochlorite solutions. J Burn Care Rehabil 12:420, 1991.
83. Richard, RL: The use of chlorine bleach as a disinfectant and antiseptic in whirlpools. Phys Ther Forum 7:7, 1988.
84. Carrougher, GJ: Burn wound assessment and topical treatment. In Carrougher, GJ (ed): Burn Care and Therapy. Mosby, St. Louis, 1998, p 142.
85. Mosier, MJ, and Gibran, NS: Surgical excision of the burn wound. Clin Plast Surg 36:617, 2009.
86. Miller, SF, et al: Surgical management of the burn patient. In Richard, RL, and Staley, MJ (eds): Burn Care and Rehabilitation: Principles and Practice. FA Davis, Philadelphia, 1994, p 180.
87. Cuono, C, et al: Use of cultured epidermal autografts and dermal allografts as skin replacement after burn injury. Lancet 8490:1123, 1986.
88. Munster, AM: Cultured epidermal autographs in the management of burn patients. J Burn Care Rehabil 13:121, 1992.
89. Sheridan, R: Closure of the excised burn wound: autografts, semipermanet skin substitutes, and permanent skin substitutes. Clin Plast Surg 36:643, 2009.
90. Chern, PL, Baum, CL, and Arpey, CJ: Biologic dressings: Current applications and limitations in dermatologic surgery. Dermatol Surg 35:891, 2009.
91. Fohn, M, and Bannasch, H: Artificial skin. Methods Mol Med 140:167, 2007.
92. Hansbrough, J, et al: Clinical trials of a biosynthetic temporary skin replacement, Dermagraft-Transitional Covering, compared with cryopreserved human cadaver skin for temporary coverage of excised burn wounds. J Burn Care Rehabil 18:43, 1997.
93. Purdue, G, et al: A multicenter clinical trial of a biosynthetic skin replacement, Dermagraft-TC, compared with cryopreserved human cadaver skin for temporary coverage of excised burn wounds. J Burn Care Rehabil 18:52, 1997.
94. Heimbach, D, et al: Artificial dermis for major burns: A multicenter, randomized clinical trial. Ann Surg 208:313, 1988.
95. Lattari, V, et al: The use of a permanent dermal allograft in full-thickness burns of the hand and foot: A report of three cases. J Burn Care Rehabil 18:147, 1997.
96. Richard, R, et al: A comparison of the Tanner and Bioplasty skin mesher systems for maximal skin graft expansion. J Burn Care Rehabil 14:690, 1993.

97. Larson, D, et al: Prevention and treatment of burn scar contracture. In Artz, CP, et al (eds): Burns: A Team Approach. Saunders, Philadelphia, 1979, p 466.

98. Greenhalgh, DG, et al: The early release of axillary contractures in pediatric patients with burns. J Burn Care Rehabil 14:39, 1993.

99. Wainwright, DJ: Burn reconstruction: The problems, the techniques, and the applications. Clin Plast Surg 36:(4)687, 2009.

100. Richard, RL, and Staley, MJ: Burn patient evaluation and treatment planning. In Richard, RL, and Staley, MJ (eds): Burn Care and Rehabilitation: Principles and Practice. FA Davis, Philadelphia, 1994, p 201.

101. Moss, BF, et al: Psychologic support and pain management of the burn patient. In Richard, RL, and Staley, MJ (eds): Burn Care and Rehabilitation: Principles and Practice. FA Davis, Philadelphia, 1994, p 475.

102. Adcock, RJ, et al: Psychologic and emotional recovery. In Carrougher, GJ (ed): Burn Care and Therapy. Mosby, St. Louis, 1998, p 329.

103. Steed, DL: Wound-healing trajectories. Surg Clin North Am 83:(3)47, 2003.

104. McHugh, AA, et al: Biomechanical alterations in normal skin and hypertrophic scar after thermal injury. J Burn Care Rehabil 18:104, 1997.

105. Li, B, and Wang, JH: Fibroblasts and myofibroblasts in wound healing: Force generation and measurement. J Tissue Viability 20:(4)108, 2011.

106. Nedelec, B, et al: Control of wound contraction: Basic and clinical features. Hand Clin 16:289, 2000.

107. Apfel, L, et al: Approaches to positioning the burn patient. In Richard, RL, and Staley, MJ (eds): Burn Care and Rehabilitation: Principles and Practice. FA Davis, Philadelphia, 1994, p 221.

108. Serghiou, M, Cowan, A, and Whitehead, C: Rehabilitation after a burn injury. Clin Plast Surg 36:675, 2009.

109. Daugherty, M, and Carr-Collins, J: Splinting techniques for the burn patient. In Richard, RL, and Staley, MJ (eds): Burn Care and Rehabilitation: Principles and Practice. FA Davis, Philadelphia, 1994, p 242.

110. Richard, R, and Ward, RS. Splinting strategies and controversies. J Burn Care Rehabil 26:392–396, 2005.

111. Kwan, M, and Ha, K: Splinting programme for patients with burnt hand. Hand Surg 7:231–241, 2002.

112. Richard, RL: Use of Dynasplint to correct elbow flexion burn contracture: A case report. J Burn Care Rehabil 7:151, 1986.

113. Richard, R, and Staley, M: Dynamic splinting: Basic science + modern technology. Phys Ther Forum 11:21, 1992.

114. Richard, RL, et al: Dynamic versus static splints: A prospective case for sustained stress. J Burn Care Rehabil 16:284, 1995.

115. Richard, R, et al: Multimodal versus progressive treatment techniques to correct burn scar contractures. J Burn Care Rehabil 21:506, 2000.

116. Covey, MH, et al: Efficacy of continuous passive motion (CPM) devices with hand burns. J Burn Care Rehabil 9:397, 1988.

117. McAllister, LP, and Salazar, CA: Case report on the use of CPM on an electrical burn. J Burn Care Rehabil 9:401, 1988.

118. McGough, CE: Introduction to CPM. J Burn Care Rehabil 9:494, 1988.

119. Covey, MH: Application of CPM devices with burn patients. J Burn Care Rehabil 9:496, 1988.

120. Richard, RL, et al: The physiologic response of a patient with critical burns to continuous passive motion. J Burn Care Rehabil 11:554, 1990.

121. Humphrey, C, et al: Soft tissue management and exercise. In Richard, RL, and Staley, MJ (eds): Burn Care and Rehabilitation: Principles and Practice. FA Davis, Philadelphia, 1994, p 324.

122. Herndon, DN, et al: Management of the pediatric patient with burns. J Burn Care Rehabil 14:3, 1993.

123. Schwanholt, C, et al: A comparison of full-thickness versus split-thickness autografts for the coverage of deep palm burns in the very young pediatric patient. J Burn Care Rehabil 14:29, 1993.

124. Richard, RL, et al: Comparison of the effect of passive exercise v static wrapping on finger range of motion in the burned hand. J Burn Care Rehabil 8(6):576, 1987.

125. Edstrom, LE, et al: Prospective randomized treatments for burned hands: Nonoperative vs. operative. Preliminary report. Scand J Plast Reconstr Surg 13(1):131, 1979.

126. Ward, RS: The use of physical agents in burn care. In Richard, RL, and Staley, MJ (eds): Burn Care and Rehabilitation: Principles and Practice. FA Davis, Philadelphia, 1994, p 419.

127. Ward, RS, et al: Evaluation of therapeutic ultrasound to improve response to physical therapy and lessen scar contracture after burn injury. J Burn Care Rehabil 15:74, 1994.

128. St-Pierre, DMM, et al: Muscle strength in individuals with healed burns. Arch Phys Med Rehabil 79:155–161, 1998.

129. Black, S, et al: Oxygen consumption for lower extremity exercises in normal subjects and burn patients. Phys Ther 60:1255, 1980.

130. Schmitt, P, et al: Lower extremity burns and ambulation. In Richard, RL, and Staley, MJ (eds): Burn Care and Rehabilitation: Principles and Practice. FA Davis, Philadelphia, 1994, p 361.

131. Schmitt, MA, et al: How soon is safe? Ambulation of the patient with burns after lower extremity skin grafting. J Burn Care Rehabil 12:33, 1991.

132. Burnsworth, B, et al: Immediate ambulation of patients with lower-extremity grafts. J Burn Care Rehabil 13:89, 1992.

133. Grube, BJ, et al: Early ambulation and discharge in 100 patients with burns of the foot treated by grafts. J Trauma 33:662, 1992.

134. Temmen, HJ, et al: Tilt table exercise guidelines for burn patients: Are cardiac exercise parameters appropriate? Proc Am Burn Assoc 30:221, 1998.

135. Boyea, BL, et al: Use of the tilt table for postural reconditioning of burn patients prior to ambulation. Proc Am Burn Assoc 30:233, 1998.

136. Trees, DW, Ketelsen, CA, and Hobbs, JA: Use of a modified tilt table for preambulation strength training as an adjunct to burn rehabilitation: A case series. J Burn Care Rehabil 24:97, 2003.

137. Staley, MJ, and Richard, RL: Scar management. In Richard, RL, and Staley, MJ (eds): Burn Care and Rehabilitation: Principles and Practice. FA Davis, Philadelphia, 1994, p 380.

138. Johnson, CL: Physical therapists as scar modifiers. Phys Ther 64:1381, 1984.

139. Kischer, CW, and Shetlar, MR: Microvasculature in hypertrophic scars and the effects of pressure. J Trauma 19:757, 1979.

140. Leung, PC, and Ng, M: Pressure treatment for hypertrophic scars. Burns 6:224, 1980.

141. Deitch, EA, et al: Hypertrophic burn scars: Analysis of variables. J Trauma 23:895, 1983.

142. Ward, RS, et al: Use of Coban self-adherent wrap in management of postburn hand grafts: Case reports. J Burn Care Rehabil 15:364, 1994.

143. Lowell, M, et al: Effect of 3M™ Coban™ self-adherent wraps on edema and function of the burned hand: A case study. J Burn Care Rehabil 24:253, 2003.

144. Kealey, GP, et al: Prospective randomized comparison of two types of pressure therapy garments. J Burn Care Rehabil 11:334, 1990.

145. Cheng, JCY, et al: Pressure therapy in the treatment of post-burn hypertrophic scar: A critical look into its usefulness and fallacies by pressure monitoring. Burns 10:154, 1984.

146. Mann, R, et al: Do custom-fitted pressure garments provide adequate pressure? J Burn Care Rehabil 18(3):247, 1997.

147. Alston, DW, et al: Materials for pressure inserts in the control of hypertrophic scar tissue. J Burn Care Rehabil 2:40, 1981.

148. Moore, ML, et al: Effectiveness of custom pressure garments in wound management: A prospective trial within wounds and with verified pressure. J Burn Care Rehabil 21:S177, 2000.

149. Perkins, K, et al: Current materials and techniques used in a burn scar management programme. Burns 13:406, 1987.

150. van der Wal, MB, et al: Topical silicone gel versus placebo in promoting the maturation of burn scars: A randomized controlled trial. Plast Reconstr Surg 126(2):524, 2010.

151. Momeni, M, et al: Effects of silicone gel on burn scars. Burns 35(1):70, 2009.

152. O'Brien, L, and Pandit, A: Silicon gel sheeting for preventing and treating hypertrophic and keloid scars. Cochrane Database Syst Rev CD003826, 2006.

153. Berman, B, et al: A review of the biologic effects, clinical efficacy, and safety of silicone elastomer sheeting for hypertrophic and keloid scar treatment and management. Dermatol Surg 33:1291, 2007.

154. Miles, WK, and Grigsby, L: Remodeling of scar tissue in the burned hand. In Hunter, JM, et al (eds): Rehabilitation of the Hand. Mosby, St. Louis, 1984, p 841.

155. Patino, O, and Novick, C: Massage on hypertrophic scars. J Burn Care Rehabil 20:268, 1999.

156. Gallagher, J, et al: Discharge videotaping: A means of augmenting occupational and physical therapy. J Burn Care Rehabil 11:470, 1990.

157. Braddom, RL, et al: The physical treatment and rehabilitation of burn patients. In Hummel, RP (ed): Clinical Burn Therapy. John Wright PSG, Boston, 1982, p 297.

158. Phoenix Society for Burn Survivors: Phoenix Society Programs and Resources. Grand Rapids, MI. Retrieved July 18, 2012, from www.phoenix-society.org/programs/.

Supplemental Readings

Alp, E, et al: Risk factors for nosocomial infection and mortality in burn patients: 10 years of experience at a university hospital. J Burn Care Res 33(3):379, 2012.

Bell, N, et al: Does direct transport to provincial burn centres improve outcomes? A spatial epidemiology of severe burn injury in British Columbia, 2001–2006. Can J Surg 55(2):110, 2012.

Butler, KL, et al: Stem cells and burns: Review and therapeutic implications. J Burn Care Res 31(6):874, 2010.

Chipp, E, Milner, CS, and Blackburn, AV: Sepsis in burns: A review of current practice and future therapies. Ann Plast Surg 65(2):228, 2010.

Ciofi-Silva, C, et al: The life impact of burns: The perspective from burn persons in Brazil during their rehabilitation phase. Disabil Rehabil 32(6):431, 2010.

Herndon, DN (ed): Total Burn Care, ed 4. Saunders/Elsevier, Philadelphia, 2012.

Hyakusoku, H, et al (eds): Color Atlas of Burn Reconstructive Surgery. Springer-Verlag, New York, 2010.

Loos, MS, Freeman, BG, and Lorenzetti, A: Zone of injury: A critical review of the literature. Ann Plast Surg 65:(6)573, 2010.

Mandell, SP, et al: Patient safety measures in burn care: Do national reporting systems accurately reflect quality of burn care? J Burn Care Res 31(1):125, 2010.

Maslow, GR, and Lobato, D: Summer camps for children with burn injuries: A literature review. J Burn Care Res 31(5):740, 2010.

Mason, ST, et al: Return to work after burn injury: A systematic review. J Burn Care Res 33(1):101, 2012.

Nedelec, B, et al: Practice guidelines for early ambulation of burn survivors after lower extremity grafts. J Burn Care Res 33(3):319, 2012.

Pan, S, et al: Deep partial thickness burn blister fluid promotes neovascularization in the early stage of burn wound healing. Wound Repair Regen 18(3):311, 2010.

Patil, V, et al: Do burn patients cost more? The intensive care unit costs of burn patients compared with controls matched for length of stay and acuity. J Burn Care Res 31(4):598, 2010.

Willebrand, M, and Kildal, M: Burn specific health up to 24 months after the burn—a prospective validation of the Simplified Model of the Burn Specific Health Scale—Brief. J Trauma 71(1):78, 2011.

Yuxiang, L, et al: Burn patients' experience of pain management: A qualitative study. Burns 38(2):180, 2012.

Web-Based Resources for Patients, Families, and Clinicians

Website Description	Web Address
National organization site for burn care in the United States	www.ameriburn.org
Informational site for therapists describing current events and description of selected splints and treatment interventions	www.burntherapist.com
Burn support information for patients and families	www.phoenix-society.org

LEARNING OBJECTIVES

1. Assess the importance of chronic pain in terms of its effect on individual activity and participation, as well as the cost to society.
2. Compare and contrast the presentation of acute, persistent, and chronic pain.
3. Apply the International Classification of Function (ICF) model to chronic pain.
4. Explain the physiology of chronic pain, contrasting chronic with acute pain.
5. Classify different types of chronic pain and provide examples of each type.
6. Propose causes and risk factors for chronic pain.
7. Relate psychosocial factors to the presentation, physiology, and risk factors for chronic pain.
8. Contrast various outcome measures for examining chronic pain and its impact on activity and participation.
9. Summarize medical management options for chronic pain.
10. Describe tests and measures appropriate for examining individuals with chronic pain.
11. Identify issues relevant in the evaluation and prognosis of individuals with chronic pain.
12. Describe intervention approaches appropriate for individuals with chronic pain.
13. Discuss complementary and alternative medicine approaches to managing chronic pain.

CHAPTER OUTLINE

■ INTRODUCTION

Pain is the most common reason why people visit health care providers and physical therapists. **Chronic pain** affects about 116 million Americans,[1-3] accounting for up to 20% of all primary care visits in the United States;[4,5] low back pain (LBP) is the second most common reason for physician visits.[6] Chronic pain affects more people than diabetes, heart disease, and cancer combined.[2] Up to 26% of American adults have had pain for more than 3 months, and one-third of those report

that this pain is disabling.[7] Internationally, chronic pain affects up to 35% of adults and 25% of children; chronic pain is almost twice as prevalent in women compared to men.[8,9] Spinal pain, headache, and arthritis are the most common sources of chronic pain: LBP affects 28%, headache and migraine affect 16%, neck pain affects 15%, and combined peripheral joint pain affects 30% of Americans.[5,10] Other conditions such as stroke, spinal cord injury (SCI), diabetes, multiple sclerosis (MS), HIV/AIDS, amputation, Guillain-Barré syndrome, cancer, and a variety of other conditions can also lead to chronic pain.[11]

Chronic pain exacts a huge toll in terms of medical care, lost workdays, and compromised quality of life. In the United States, the national economic cost of chronic pain is estimated at $560 billion to $635 billion per year with $261 billion to $300 billion per year of that due to direct medical costs.[1] Lost productivity due to pain costs $297 billion to $336 billion per year.[1] Quality of life is severely compromised for people with chronic pain, often rated even lower than among people dying of cancer.[12]

This chapter will focus on chronic neuromuscular and musculoskeletal pain most likely to present for physical therapy intervention. It is not the goal of this chapter to address cancer or visceral pain, even though those are growing specialty areas within physical therapy. Recent advances in pain physiology are presented as a foundation for understanding common chronic pain conditions and the appropriate interventions for those conditions.

Definitions of Pain

Pain is defined as an unpleasant sensory and emotional experience associated with actual or potential tissue damage, or described in terms of such damage.[13] Pain is thus more than merely the firing of **nociceptive** neurons, but also includes the *perception of pain*, the *experience of suffering*, and *pain behavior*.[14] The perception of pain may depend on the situation or mental state, such as when soldiers on the battlefield or athletes on the playing field do not feel pain when injured. In contrast, a person with post-traumatic stress disorder (PTSD) may experience significant pain without any physical stimulus. Some people experience suffering, or the affective experience of distress, with minimal tissue damage, whereas other people may have significant tissue damage and pain with minimal experience of suffering.

Acute, Persistent, and Chronic Pain

Acute pain is associated with tissue damage or the threat of such damage and typically resolves once the tissue heals or the threat resolves. Acute pain is often associated with physiological signs of distress, such as sweating, pallor, nausea, and heart rate changes. Acute pain may become persistent pain if the cause of the pain is unresolved. For example, chronic diseases such as osteoarthritis (OA) or diabetic neuropathy are associated with pain; as long as the disease remains, the pain remains. Alternatively, *pain triggers* may occur and recur, such as in a cervicogenic headache due to poor posture or LBP due to segmental instability. Although the causes of persistent pain may be difficult to resolve, the pain is nonetheless proportional to tissue damage or potential tissue damage and the nociceptive input and would resolve if the nociceptive causes could be addressed. **Recurrent pain** includes repeated episodes of acute pain, such as recurrent low back strain, or chronic pain in which the symptoms are intermittent, such as a migraine headache.

Chronic pain has been defined in a variety of ways. The simplest is to define it as any pain persisting more than a specified length of time, such as 3 or 6 months. While this definition is simple to apply, it does not reflect the psychosocial and physiological changes that occur in chronic pain.[6,15] A second definition of chronic pain is pain that is long-lasting, persistent, and of sufficient duration and intensity to adversely affect a patient's well-being, function, and quality of life.[16] While this second definition recognizes the psychosocial aspects of long-lasting pain, it still does not reflect the unique physiology that differentiates chronic pain from persistent acute pain. A third definition of chronic pain is pain that persists past the healing phase following an injury with impairment greater than anticipated based on the physical findings or injury, and occurs in the absence of observed tissue injury or damage.[6,15,17,18] Other definitions related to pain are presented in Box 25.1.[13,17,19]

The Biopsychosocial Model of Pain

The traditional biomedical model of pain correlates tissue damage to pain sensations; according to the biomedical model, if you fix the tissue damage the pain will resolve. This model works well for many types of acute pain; however, it is unable to explain many other examples of pain where no physical damage could be found.[15] Historically, pain whose physiological source could not be found was called *nonorganic pain* and was traditionally considered **psychogenic**; research now shows that chronic pain, in the absence of peripheral tissue damage, has a physiological basis and is not merely a psychological manifestation.[6,20-22] In contrast to the biomedical model, the *biopsychosocial model* of pain recognizes that physical factors interact with personal and environmental factors to affect body function and structure, activity, and participation in life activities. The biopsychosocial model provides a better framework for recent advances in the understanding of pain physiology and effective pain management.

The World Health Organization's (WHO's) *International Classification of Functioning, Disability and Health* (ICF)[23] was developed to create a consistent terminology and framework for describing, classifying, and assessing function and health. The ICF model replaces the Nagi model of disability used in early versions of the *Guide to Physical Therapist Practice.*[24] Figure 1.1 in Chapter 1, Clinical Decision Making, illustrates the interaction among different aspects of the ICF model. (*Note*: ICF terminology is defined in Chapter 1 and in the Glossary.) Within the ICF model, pain is considered an abnormal body function classified under the designation *Sensory Function and Pain*. The physiological changes observed in chronic pain may also be associated with changes in the *Structure of the Nervous System*, at the level of body structure.[25] Table 25.1 identifies the various classifications for **Body Function**, **Body Structure**, **Activities**, and **Participation** that are most relevant to patients with

Box 25.1 Pain Terminology

- **Acute pain**: Pain associated with tissue damage or the threat of such damage and typically resolves once the tissue heals or the threat resolves.[13]
- **Adjuvant medication**: Medications whose primary indication is a condition other than pain, but which have demonstrated benefit in pain management.
- **Allodynia**: Pain due to a stimulus that does not normally provoke pain.[13]
- **Analgesia**: Absence of pain in response to stimulation that would normally be painful.[13]
- **Causalgia**: A syndrome of sustained burning pain, allodynia, and hyperpathia after a traumatic nerve lesion, often combined with vasomotor and sudomotor dysfunction (such as diabetic autonomic neuropathy) and later trophic changes.[13]
- **Central pain**: Pain initiated or caused by a primary lesion or dysfunction in the central nervous system.[13]
- **Chronic pain**: Pain that persists past the healing phase following an injury; impairment is greater than anticipated based on the physical findings or injury and it occurs in the absence of observed tissue injury or damage.[19]
- **Chronic pain syndrome**: Pain that exists when individuals have developed extensive pain behaviors such as preoccupation with pain, passive approach to health care, significant life disruption, feelings of isolation, demanding, angry, or doctor-shopping.
- **Dysesthesia**: An unpleasant abnormal sensation, whether spontaneous or evoked.[13]
- **Hyperalgesia**: An increased response to a stimulus that is normally painful. Hyperalgesia reflects increased pain on suprathreshold stimulation.[13]
- **Hyperesthesia**: Increased sensitivity to stimulation, excluding the special senses. Allodynia is suggested for pain after stimulation that is not normally painful. Hyperesthesia includes both allodynia and hyperalgesia, but the more specific terms should be used wherever they are applicable.[13]
- **Hyperpathia**: A painful syndrome characterized by an abnormally painful reaction to a stimulus, especially a repetitive stimulus, as well as an increased threshold.[13]
- **Malignant pain**: Pain associated with cancer.
- **Nociceptive pain**: Pain that arises from actual or threatened damage to non-neural tissue and is due to the activation of pain receptors, nociceptors.[13]
- **Nocebo (nocebo effect)**: The opposite of a placebo or the placebo effect. A nocebo is an inert treatment or event that increases symptoms because the patient believes it will increase symptoms. The expectation of pain can result in both increased pain from painful stimuli and allodynia, pain from a normally nonpainful stimulus.
- **Pain**: An unpleasant sensory and emotional experience associated with actual or potential tissue damage, or described in terms of such damage.[13]
- **Pain neuromatrix**: A complex network of synaptic links within the central nervous system, initially determined by genetics but modified by psychological and sensory inputs both before and during the pain experience.
- **Paresthesia**: An abnormal sensation, whether spontaneous or evoked.
- **Persistent pain**: Pain related to tissue damage or the threat of such damage that persists because the causative factors persist.
- **Placebo (placebo effect)**: A placebo is an inert treatment, such as a sugar pill or fake treatment, that is beneficial because the patient believes it will be beneficial.
- **Psychogenic pain**: An older term for pain believed to be caused by psychological factors when organic factors were absent or not severe enough to explain the pain complaint.[19]
- **Recurrent pain**: Repeated episodes of acute pain.
- **Referred pain**: Spontaneous pain outside the area of injury or source of pain.[17]
- **Suffering**: Refers to the affective component of pain. Suffering includes both emotional (e.g., anxiety and anger) and cognitive (e.g., thoughts of helplessness) components, and may be due to a combination of unpleasantness and catastrophizing (making a "catastrophe" out of minor issues).

chronic pain.[23,25-28] The multidirectional nature of the ICF model is particularly pertinent to chronic pain where structure, function, activity, and participation are interrelated and can all affect one another.

Suffering refers to the affective component of pain. Suffering includes both emotional (e.g., anxiety and anger) and cognitive (e.g., thoughts of helplessness) components, and may be due to a combination of unpleasantness and *catastrophizing* (making a "catastrophe" out of minor issues).[29] Pain behavior includes verbal and nonverbal expressions of pain, activity and participation changes, fear avoidance, and treatment-seeking behavior in response to the perception of pain. As with suffering, the extent of pain behavior can be quite independent of tissue damage. **Chronic pain syndrome** exists when individuals have developed extensive pain behaviors

Table 25.1	Core Set of World Health Organization's International Classification of Functioning, Disability and Health Classifications Relevant to Patients with Chronic Pain[23,25-28]		
ICF Code	**Description**	**ICF Code**	**Description**
	Body Function		*Body Structure*
B122	Global psychosocial functions	S110	Structure of the brain
B126	Temperament and personality functions	S120	Spinal cord and related structures
B152	Emotional functions	S140	Structure of the sympathetic nervous system
B130	Energy and drive functions		
B134	Sleep functions	S199	Structure of the nervous system, unspecified
B147	Psychomotor function	S770	Additional musculoskeletal structures related to movement (bones, joints, muscles, ligaments, fascia, and so forth)
B260	Proprioceptive function		
B280	Sensation of pain		
B455	Exercise tolerance	#Needed	Structures specific to the given pathology
B710	Mobility of joint function		
B730	Muscle power functions		
B735	Muscle tone functions		
B740	Muscle endurance functions		
B760	Sensations related to muscles and motor function		
B770	Gait pattern functions		
	Activities		*Participation*
D160	Focusing attention	D230	Carrying out daily routine
D240	Difficulty handling stress and other psychological demands	D560	Unable to travel
		D620	Acquisition of goods and services
D410/5	Changing/maintaining body position	D760	Family relationships
D430	Lifting and carrying objects	D770	Intimate relationships
D450/5	Walking/moving around	D850	Remunerative employment
D530	Toileting	D910	Community life
D630	Preparing meals	D920	Recreation and leisure
D640	Doing housework		

(Box 25.2).[3] Psychosocial aspects of pain will be addressed later in this chapter.

Chronic pain can be considered a disease rather than a symptom. Just as a myocardial infarction may have many contributing factors and causes, chronic pain has multiple contributing factors and causes and has its own pathology, signs, and symptoms.[30-33] Using the disease model, treatment of chronic pain should address the secondary pathology and perpetuating factors rather than focus on a presumed initial pathology, which might no longer be present. Treatment of the disease of chronic pain should address peripheral and central sensitization, disinhibition, anxiety, catastrophizing, fear-avoidance, and so forth, as well as contributing psychosocial and behavioral factors.[30] Chronic pain affects all aspects of life just as would a chronic disease; chronic pain also needs to be managed, because it often cannot be cured.[15]

Box 25.2   Characteristic Behaviors in Chronic Pain Syndrome[3]

- Doctor-shopping
- Dependency on the health care system for multiple medical problems
- Preoccupation with pain, significant pain behavior
- Passive-dependent personality traits
- Denial of emotional or family conflicts
- Significant life disruption in many areas
- Feelings of isolation and loneliness
- Being demanding, angry, or skeptical
- Lack of insight into self-defeating behaviors
- Use of pain as a symbolic means of communication

■ PAIN PHYSIOLOGY

While a thorough discussion of pain physiology is beyond the scope of this chapter, an overview is essential to understanding how chronic and acute pain differ, both in presentation and in management. Readers can find more extensive coverage of pain physiology in one of the textbooks on pain: *Mechanisms and Management of Pain for the Physical Therapist*[34] or *Chronic Pain: An*

Integrated Biobehavioral Approach.[35] Acute pain is primarily nociceptive (peripheral nerves responding to high-intensity or harmful stimuli) including inflammatory peripheral sensitization. Mechanical, thermal, chemical, and free nociceptive nerve endings in the periphery transmit information about noxious stimuli via afferent nerves through the dorsal root into the dorsal horn.

The lightly myelinated A-δ and unmyelinated C fibers have very different features, summarized in Table 25.2. Generally, the A-δ fibers transmit detailed somatosensory information allowing localization of pain, whereas C fibers transmit more diffuse information driving the affective response to pain. The unmyelinated C fibers are approximately 10 times slower than the A-δ fibers, which are 5 to 10 times slower than other sensory receptors for touch, pressure, proprioception, muscle spindles, and Golgi tendon organs (A-γ, A-β, and A-α). Since most deep tissues such as muscles, joints, and viscera are innervated by C fibers whereas cutaneous structures are more likely innervated by A-δ fibers, pain from deep structures is perceived as slow, dull, aching, or **referred pain** whereas cutaneous structures are more likely to produce sharp, localized pain.[17] Although A-β sensory neurons do not normally transmit pain, they can produce **paresthesias** and **dysesthesias** when provoked.

Figure 25.1 shows the primary anatomical structures related to pain transmission.[33,36] Once axons enter the dorsal horn, A-δ fibers synapse with interneurons in laminae I, II, and V. Primary sensory afferents from skin, muscle, joints, and viscera may also converge on wide-dynamic-range interneurons; convergence of nociceptive and non-nociceptive input provides a mechanism for referred pain.[37] Projection fibers from A-δ and some C afferents retain a somatotopic organization, cross and ascend through the lateral spinothalamic tract to the ventral posterior lateral thalamus, then to the primary and secondary somatosensory cortex. These fibers transmit information about pain localization, intensity, duration, and quality.[37] In contrast, projection fibers from most C afferents ascend through the medial spinothalamic, spinoreticular, and spinomesencephalic tracts to the medial thalamus, reticular formation, hypothalamus, limbic system, autonomic centers, and cingulate gyrus. Pain from C fibers tends to be poorly localized and associated with affective responses to pain.

Current research suggests that different components of the brain process different aspects of the pain experience. The SI somatosensory cortex mediates the sensory-discriminatory aspect of pain whereas the SII somatosensory cortex is involved in recognition, learning, and memory of painful events. The anterior cingulate cortex processes pain unpleasantness and contributes to affect, cognition, and response selection. The insula mediates autonomic responses to noxious stimuli and the affective components of pain-related memory and learning.[29,386] Extensive crosstalk among the various pain pathways creates what Melzack called the **pain neuromatrix**, a complex network of synaptic links initially determined by genetics, but modified by psychological and sensory inputs both before and during the pain experience.[39-41] Pain is therefore not a simple cause-and-effect process, but a complex web of

Table 25.2	Features of Fast and Slow Nociceptive Pain	
Features	Fast	Slow
Nerves	A-delta (myelinated)	C (unmyelinated)
Stimulus	Pinprick, heat	Tissue damage
Sensation	Sharp, pricking, burning, dermatomal	Slow, dull, crawling, sclerotomal
Diameter	1–4 μm	0.1–1 μm
Conduction velocity	5–30 m/sec	0.4–1.4 m/sec
Distribution	Body surface	All tissues except CNS
Reflex response	Withdrawal	Muscle spasm or tone
Biological value	Avoidance of tissue damage	Enforced rest
Effect of morphine	Very little	Suppresses pain
CNS target	Thalamus, cortex	Limbic, hypothalamic
Affective response	No	Yes
Autonomic signs	No	Yes
Localized receptor field	Yes	No
Dorsal horn connection	Laminae I and V	Laminae II and III

μm = micrometer; m/sec = meters per second; CNS = central nervous system.

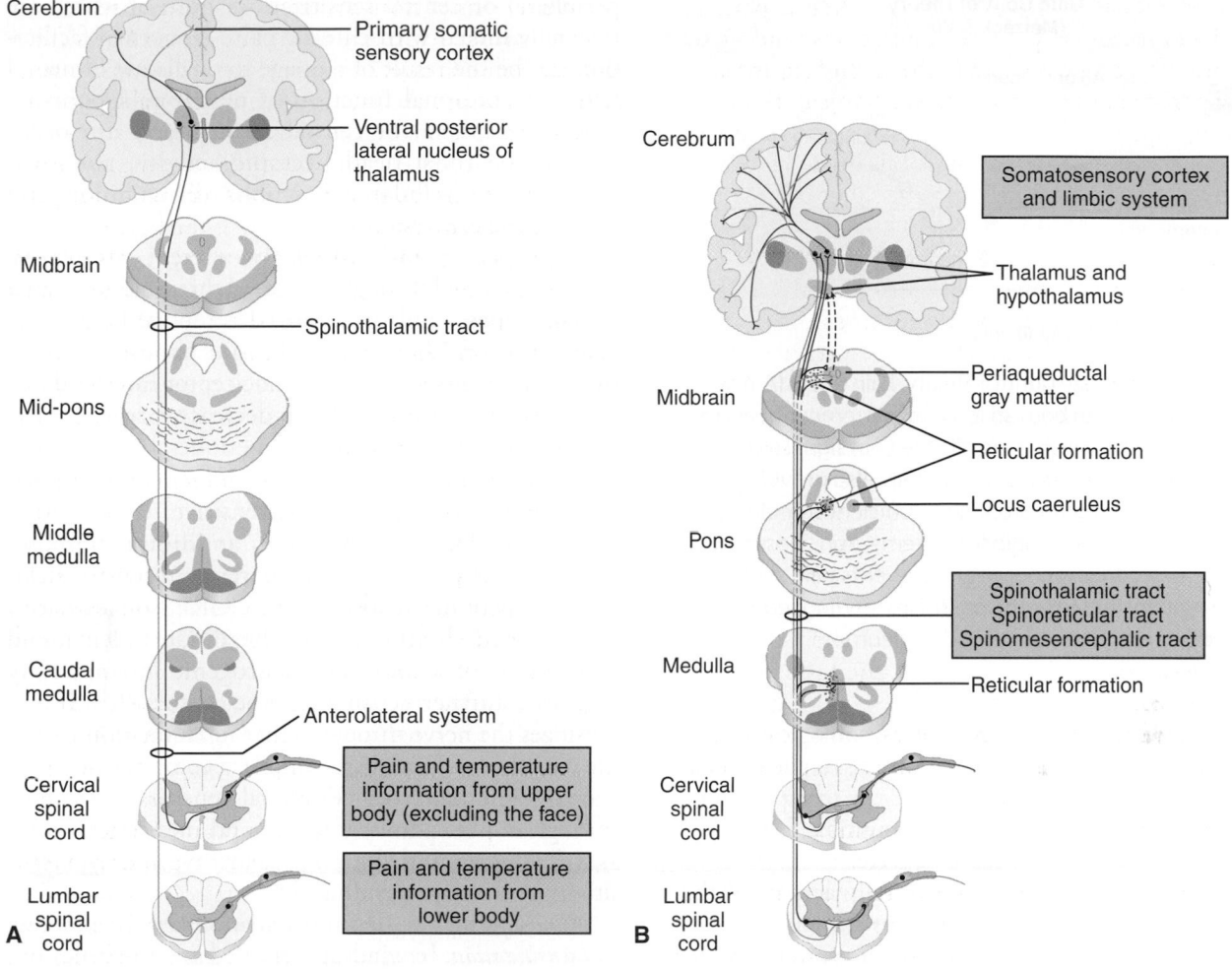

Figure 25.1 Central pain pathways. **(A)** Projection fibers from Λ-δ afferents retain a somatotopic organization, cross and ascend through the lateral spinothalamic tract to the ventral posterior lateral thalamus, then to the primary and secondary somatosensory cortex. These fibers transmit information about pain localization, intensity, duration, and quality. **(B)** Projection fibers from C afferents ascend through the medial spinothalamic, spinoreticular, and spinomesencephalic tracts to the medial thalamus, reticular formation, hypothalamus, limbic system, autonomic centers, and cingulate gyrus. The medial pain pathways contribute to the affective, autonomic, and cognitive experience of pain. *Based on diagrams from: (1) Argoff, CE, et al: Multimodal analgesia for chronic pain: Rationale and future directions. Pain Med 10(Suppl 2):S53, 2009. (2) Ford, B: Pain in Parkinson's disease. Mov Disord 25(Suppl 1):S98, 2010.*

interactions modulated by both current and previous physical and psychological states.

Pain Processing and the Evolving Gate Control Theory

Superimposed on these neuroanatomical tracts, numerous regulatory influences affect the ascending information. The Gate Control Theory, first proposed by Melzack and Wall[42] in 1965, explains a key aspect of pain regulation: how nonpainful sensory stimuli can decrease the perception of pain. Figure 25.2 shows how pain fibers synapse with an inhibitory interneuron and a secondary neuron that transmits the pain signal to the brain. Sensory nerves, such as Aα and Aβ, also provide

input into the inhibitory interneuron. With sufficient stimulus to the Aα or Aβ nerves, the inhibitory interneuron "closes the gate" on the secondary neuron and prevents pain stimuli from being transmitted to the brain. The gate control process is the basis for conventional transcutaneous electroneural stimulation (TENS).

Melzack subsequently added descending control to the model to explain how noxious stimuli might not result in pain, as when severely wounded soldiers or athletes can perceive no pain from their injuries.[39] Descending pain inhibition appears to be modulated by norepinephrine and descending noradrenergic connections.[43] Simple descending inhibition, however, fails to explain other observations such as gender differences, chronic pain in the absence of

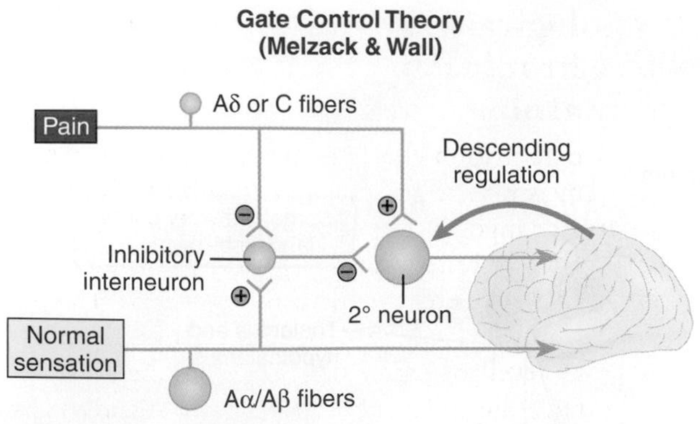

**Gate Control Theory
(Melzack & Wall)**

Figure 25.2 The Gate Control Theory. Pain fibers (A-δ or C fibers) synapse with both an inhibitory interneuron and a secondary neuron, which transmits the pain signal to the brain. Sensory nerves, such as Aα and Aβ, also provide input into the inhibitory interneuron. With sufficient stimulus to the Aα or Aβ nerves, the inhibitory interneuron "closes the gate" on the secondary neuron and prevents pain stimuli from being transmitted to the brain. Descending regulation also modifies output of the secondary neuron.

noxious stimuli, and the impact of psychological factors such as stress and previous experiences.[44] As mentioned, Melzack[39] proposed the pain neuromatrix to explain how the pain experience is modulated by multiple factors and not always proportional to tissue damage.

Descending inhibitory factors modify activity of the pain pathways at all levels of the nervous system. Descending control is opioid sensitive, and can be reversed by naloxone, the opiate antagonist. *Placebo* (use of fake treatment, especially sugar pills), antidepressants, and anticonvulsants all modulate pain through enhancing descending inhibition.[33] Descending control involves the hypothalamus, amygdala, rostral anterior cingulate cortex, periaqueductal gray (PAG) matter, rostral ventromedial medulla (RVM), projecting to the dorsal horn.[6,43] Descending inhibitory pathways travel through the dorsolateral funiculus resulting in secretion of noradrenalin, acetylcholine, serotonin, and glycine in the dorsal horn.[37,45]

Descending modulation can facilitate pain as well as inhibit it; facilitation is called the **nocebo effect**, in contrast to the placebo effect. The expectation of pain can result in both increased pain from painful stimuli but also **allodynia**, pain from normally nonpainful stimuli. Imaging studies show that the nocebo effect is mediated by a complex interplay among the ipsilateral caudal anterior cingulate cortex, the head of the caudate, the cerebellum, and the contralateral cuneiform nucleus.[43] Descending facilitation passes through the ventrolateral funiculus and is mediated in the dorsal horn by serotonin, norepinephrine, opioids, and cholecystokinin.[37,45]

Peripheral and Central Sensitization

Descending modulation of pain is a normal process. However, the facilitation process can result in abnormal peripheral or central sensitization, both of which are integrally linked with chronic pain. Abnormal facilitation can be the result of damage to or disease of neural tissue or abnormal function of neural or supporting tissues. Peripheral or central sensitization can occur through neuronal death, ectopic activity, abnormal sprouting and cellular connections, disinhibition, and altered gene expression.[20,30,31]

In *peripheral sensitization*, the afferent nociceptive input is increased through decreased threshold, increased responsiveness, and/or increased receptive field.[46] Inflammation of either peripheral tissues or neural connective tissue results in decreased nociceptor threshold as a protective response aiming to decrease further injury. The inflammatory mediators of peripheral sensitization include cytokines, prostaglandins, and serotonin; injured nerve terminals become hypersensitive to circulating norepinephine.[11] In some cases, antidromic impulses go from spinal cord to the afferent's receptive field, releasing peptides (substance P, CGRP, somatostatin) and cytokines leading to peripheral flare, edema, and stimulation of a local and neurogenic inflammatory response, further sensitizing nociceptors.[31,47] Injury sensitizes the nerve through either inflammation within the neural connective tissue or direct compromise to the axons.[20,47] Long-term peripheral sensitization occurs through modifications of the second messenger system as well as excess and abnormal branching and hypersensitivity of free nerve ending.[33,47]

Wind-up and long-term potentiations are forms of *central sensitization*. In wind-up, repeated low-frequency nociceptor stimulation results in progressively increased action potential in the dorsal horn cells.[20] Summation of C fiber action potentials causes concurrent release of substance P and glutamate, which increases postsynaptic calcium release; *N*-methyl-D-aspartate (NMDA) and other receptors are up-regulated causing a feedback loop resulting in further increased intracellular calcium.[45] Wind-up can result in long-term potentiation, in which the neural response is strengthened through increased neurogenic inflammation and altered gene expression resulting in altered nerve phenotype, with different receptors and transmitters.[45]

Central sensitization occurs through many similar mechanisms as peripheral sensitization, including changes in microglia, astrocytes, and gap junctions.[20] Glia appear to perpetuate sensitization by releasing growth hormone that stimulates an immune response.[31,48] Inflammation in the central nervous system (CNS) causes central sensitization by increasing excitability in the dorsal horn and inflammatory chemical mediators up-regulate expression of genes affecting synaptic transmission.[15] These processes result in hyperalgesia, allodynia, after-sensations, summation, and receptive field expansion.[20] **Hyperalgesia** occurs when the pain fiber synapse with the secondary neuron in the dorsal horn (see Fig. 25.1) is amplified, resulting in firing of the secondary neuron with lower peripheral stimulus. Short-term allodynia may be caused by decreased firing threshold or decreased inhibition; long-term allodynia includes sprouting of A-α and A-β fibers to synapse with nociceptor fibers in the spinal cord, causing normal sensory input to be perceived as pain. Central sensitization can be maintained by ongoing nociceptive input or may be independent of nociceptive input.[37] Central sensitization can occur in the spinal cord, rostroventral medulla, amygdala, anterior cingulate cortex, and trigeminal brainstem complex.[11]

Central sensitivity occurs in conditions such as fibromyalgia, widespread myofascial pain, chronic headache, temporomandibular joint (TMJ) disorder, and neuropathic pain. Stimulation of visceral nociceptors creates sensitization of both visceral hypersensitivity and viscera-somatic pain (i.e., hypersensitivity of musculoskeletal tissues in the referral region), leading to conditions such as irritable bowel and interstitial cystitis.[20,31] Peripheral injury can permanently alter central pain processes that can, in turn, modulate peripheral signaling mechanisms.[33] Any peripheral nociceptive stimulus can perpetuate centrally mediated pain, with joint and muscle nociceptors resulting in longer-lasting sensitization than cutaneous nociceptor stimulation. For example, muscle trigger points can generate widespread central sensitization. Chronic osteoarthritis pain may have a centrally mediated component, explaining the mismatch between radiographic signs of OA and pain. However, it appears that central sensitization does not require continued peripheral input.[20]

Peripheral and central components of the autonomic system can also abnormally perpetuate pain through a variety of mechanisms. First, sympathetic efferents can sprout synapses with nociceptors, which develop adrenergic receptors; autonomic activation then directly activates nociceptors in the spinal cord. This process is particularly important where the sympathetic efferents connect to deep somatic afferents; sympathetic stimulation can then result in somatic pain.[49] Another mechanism for autonomic amplification of pain occurs through the hypothalamic-pituitary-adrenal (HPA) axis. Physical or emotional stress activates the HPA axis, leading to a self-perpetuating cascade of events resulting in chronic sympathetic activation in chronic pain.[14,48,50] The processes are complicated, however, and some chronic pain diagnoses (e.g., fibromyalgia) actually present with elevated autonomic activity at rest but blunted responses to autonomic challenges (e.g., orthostatic).[51]

Central sensitization provides a physiological basis for pain in the absence of identifiable injury or tissue damage. It also provides a physical mechanism for pain to be exacerbated by stress or psychological state. Consequently, some or much of what used to be considered psychologically based pain (e.g., nonorganic, somatoform, psychosomatic, hysteric) may be a manifestation of central sensitization.[20,21]

Physiological Changes Occurring with Chronic Pain: Neuroplasticity and Learning

The above discussion clearly demonstrates that the nervous system is plastic and can undergo both short- and long-term changes in response to pain. Recurrent pain sensations can activate receptors, create new synapses, and alter neurotransmitter production, as well as receptor types and prevalence.[3,30,33,52] Plastic changes appear to occur at all levels of pain processing: peripheral, spinal, and central.[52] Peripheral and central sensitization may persist even when the causative factors have been removed. Within the CNS, abnormal central reorganization may include expansion of the painful area representation in the primary somatosensory cortex, S1.[53] There is also evidence of gray matter atrophy and gross changes in brain morphology with chronic pain; gray matter atrophy appears to reverse if the chronic pain resolves.[6,54] Studies show that learning related to pain is quite powerful as chronic pain provides constant reinforcement.[6]

Since prolonged pain leads to sensitization, some suggest that preemptive **analgesia** eliminating nociceptive input may prevent wind-up, peripheral, and central sensitization; however, research findings have been inconsistent for preventing acute pain and poor for preventing the transformation from acute to chronic pain.[55,56] Psychosocial factors are also critical in the transformation from acute to chronic pain. This will be discussed later in the chapter, together with other risk factors for the development of chronic pain.

Classification of Pain

Pain can be classified in several different ways and often several different classification systems can apply to a given patient. The distinction among acute, persistent, and chronic pain is described earlier in this chapter. Pain can be divided by body region affected, such as LBP or headache, or classified by pathology, such as phantom limb pain, MS, or **malignant** if cancer related. The physiological processes involved, such as nociceptive, inflammatory, neurogenic, or maladaptive, may also categorize pain.[17,57-59] The term *psychogenic pain*, once commonly used for medically unexplained pain, has been challenged with better understanding of pain physiology. Pain may also be described as having three dimensions: sensory-discriminative, motivational-discriminative, and cognitive-evaluative;[17] or four dimensions: nociception, pain cognition, suffering, and pain behavior. This section will contrast several of these classification systems. Later sections will describe special cases of chronic pain pathologies.

The three dimensions of sensory-discriminative, motivational-discriminative, and cognitive-evaluative reflect the multidimensional International Association for the Study of Pain (IASP) definition of pain as sensory, emotional, or cognitive. The *sensory-discriminative dimension* refers to localization, intensity, duration, and the nature of the pain (burning, sharp, and so forth). The *motivational-affective dimension* refers to the emotional response a person has, including physiological manifestations of that emotional response, such as nausea. The *cognitive-affective dimension* relates to how pain is interpreted in the context of past and present experience, culture, and so forth.[17]

One physiological classification system is to divide pain into nociceptive, inflammatory, and maladaptive.[57] *Nociceptive pain* is a response to an immediate noxious stimulus (mechanical, thermal, or chemical), signaling impending tissue damage; nociceptive pain typically leads to a protective withdrawal response and is therefore beneficial.[57,58] *Inflammatory pain* increases sensory sensitivity after tissue damage, discouraging use and further damage, allowing for tissue repair; the pain is due to hypersensitivity resulting from peripheral injury, pathology, or other inflammatory process. Inflammatory pain is generally a beneficial mechanism for encouraging rest of the involved tissues; however, it becomes counterproductive when severe or ongoing.[57] *Maladaptive pain* results from an abnormally functioning nervous system relaying pain signals unrelated or disproportional to tissue damage.[31] Maladaptive pain represents altered neural processing; decreased physical activity resulting from maladaptive pain does not contribute to healing and may exacerbate pain and lead to secondary problems. Examples of maladaptive pain include tension headache,

TMJ disorder, fibromyalgia, and irritable bowel syndrome.[57] Maladaptive pain is a manifestation of chronic pain that occurs in the absence of identified tissue damage.[17] A slightly different classification system could include inflammation as a type of nociceptive pain mediated by chemical stimuli or inflammation could lead to both peripheral and central neurogenic pain.

Some classification systems consider "muscle pain" distinct from nociceptive pain whereas other systems include muscle pain as a type of nociception.[16] Muscle pain is often dull, deep, aching, cramping, and difficult to localize.[60] Muscle trigger points can refer pain to other sites, as well as cause other symptoms such as tinnitus, paresthesias, and blurry vision. Trigger points may be idiopathic or associated with another disorder such as OA or rheumatoid arthritis (RA), fibromyalgia, TMJ disorder, or chronic tension-type headaches.[61] Widespread myofascial pain syndrome appears to involve central sensitization as well as peripheral nociception.[62,63]

Pain can also be divided into the following categories: nociceptive, peripheral neuropathic/neurogenic, and central neuropathic/neurogenic; some older classification systems include a category of psychogenic. Nociceptive pain can be further subdivided into superficial, deep somatic, and visceral through the different presentations; non-neurogenic inflammation, described above, is also nociceptive. Table 25.3 contrasts the different types of pain.[44,58,64]

Table 25.3 Subjective and Objective Characteristics Associated with Different Types of Pain and Tissue Sources[44,58,64]

Type of Pain	Tissue Source	Subjective	Objective
Nociceptive: Cutaneous or superficial	Skin and subcutaneous tissues (predominantly A-δ fibers)	Well-localized, stabbing, burning, cutting	Clear, consistent, proportional pain reproduced through movement or mechanical testing of target tissues
Nociceptive: Deep somatic	Bone, muscle, blood vessels, connective tissues (predominantly C fibers)	Often referred to other locations; tearing, cramping, pressing, aching	Vague, sometimes referred pain reproduced through movement or mechanical testing of deeper tissues; spasm, trigger points common
Nociceptive: Visceral	Organs and the linings of the body cavities (predominantly C fibers)	Often referred to other locations; poorly localized, diffuse, deep cramping or splitting, sharp, stabbing	Vague pain reproduction on movement or mechanical testing of visceral tissues
Peripheral neurogenic	Nerve fibers (axons or neural connective tissue)	Pain variously described as burning, shooting, sharp, aching or "electric-shock-like"	Pain or symptom provocation with movement or mechanical tests that move, load, or compress neural tissues
Central	Spinal cord and central nervous system	Disproportionate, nonmechanical, unpredictable pattern of pain provocation in response to multiple, nonspecific aggravating or easing factors	Disproportionate, inconsistent, nonmechanical or nonanatomical pattern of pain provocation in response to movement or mechanical testing

Peripheral neurogenic pain stems from mechanical or chemical damage to peripheral nerves, including inflammation of peripheral nerves. In addition to negative symptoms of hypoesthesia, anesthesia, or weakness, neurogenic pain may include positive symptoms of **paresthesia**, dysesthesia, and pain.[15,65] Peripheral neurogenic pain can be further subdivided into axonal effects versus those due to neural connective tissue. Nerves, themselves, can be the source of pain due to nociceptors and nervi nervorum in the neural connective tissue. This type of pain tends to be deep, aching, and localized with discomfort generally proportional to stimulus.[65] Pain produced by injury to the axons results in dysesthesias such as burning, prickling, tingling, searing, or crawling sensations from hyperexcitable afferents being triggered at the site of axonal injury rather than at the receptor site. Axonal pain can be quite variable and may be spontaneous or cumulative.[65] Peripheral neurogenic pain may become prolonged beyond the initial nerve injury through processes of peripheral sensitization and because of glia releasing growth factors and other substances acting on the immune system.[48] Neurogenic pain sometimes evolves into **causalgia** where vasomotor, sudomotor, or trophic changes can also occur.

Central neurogenic pain can be due to injury or disease affecting the CNS such as stroke, traumatic brain injury (TBI), MS, or fibromyalgia. Pain is often burning, aching, lancing, pricking, or pressing.[44] Both hyperalgesia and allodynia may exist. Some conditions may generate pain without any nociceptive input, whereas others appear to be mediated by centrally amplified and perpetuated peripheral nociceptive pain.[61] The HPA axis plays a central role in mediating stress-related pain syndromes, such as fibromyalgia, irritable bowel syndrome, PTSD, and burnout.[48] Central neurogenic pain appears to be mediated by glia and astrocytes altering synaptic activity[33] and synaptic connections forming between general sensory afferents and pain fibers (allodynia).[20] These various mechanisms result in descending facilitation.[43] Imaging studies show changes in both the brainstem and somatosensory cortex in response to central sensitization.[20]

■ CAUSES AND RISK FACTORS FOR CHRONIC PAIN

Chronic pain is not just a symptom; it should be considered a disease with a variety of causes and risk factors. While injury or disease often trigger the development of pain, additional risk factors include genetic predisposition, gender, psychosocial history, psychological state at the time of initial injury, and lifestyle.

Up to 50% of the variability in prevalence and severity of pain appears to be due to genetic factors. In fact, twin studies show that many chronic conditions involving central sensitization have a hereditary component.[20,66-70] This genetic predisposition may account for the high prevalence of co-morbidities among conditions involving central sensitization; the presence of any one disorder increases the likelihood of other central sensitization related conditions, with odds ratios up to 29. Common comorbid conditions include migraine, fibromyalgia, complex regional pain syndrome (CRPS), low back pain, irritable bowel syndrome, chronic tension-type headache, TMJ disorder, interstitial cystitis, depression, panic disorder, PTSD, pelvic pain, and chronic widespread pain.[20,66-68,70]

Women are more likely than men to experience most chronic pain conditions, including migraine with aura, tension headache, TMJ pain, CRPS, fibromyalgia, MS, and RA.[71-73] Munce and Stewart[73] report that in a community sample, 38.4% of women reported chronic pain compared to 27.1% of men. Women are also more likely than men to see a physician for management of pain syndromes[71] and are more likely to have co-morbid depression.[73] Increased prevalence of chronic pain in women is likely due to a combination of influences including physiological, sociocultural, and psychological factors.[72]

Psychosocial history can be a strong contributing factor in the development of chronic pain. Extensive research demonstrates relationships between past trauma and chronic pain or other central sensitization conditions. Post-traumatic stress disorder is highly correlated with chronic pain conditions. Childhood abuse and other forms of PTSD are as high as 58% among people with chronic pain conditions.[74-78] Consequently, the probability of having multiple chronic pain conditions is increased among survivors of childhood or adult abuse[70,74,77,79-85] and other psychosocial stressors.[81] There are likely to be several mechanisms by which emotional trauma leads to chronic pain. Several studies have shown physiological changes in functional magnetic resonance imaging (fMRI) patterns within the brain,[86] diurnal cortisol patterns, gene transcription, and hypothalamic-pituitary regulation.[74]

Numerous other psychosocial factors increase risk of chronic pain through both psychosocial and physiological mechanisms. These include poor social support, poor coping skills, low job security, low socioeconomic status, limited access to preventative care, external locus of control, marital/family discord, cultural background, and beliefs.[33] Work environment also affects the likelihood that acute pain will become chronic. Whether patients like their job or get along with their supervisor is highly correlated to levels of both pain and disability.[16]

Depression, psychological distress, passive coping strategies, and fear-avoidance beliefs are independently linked with poor outcome among people with chronic pain.[87,88] Recent research suggests that individuals with high levels of fear-avoidance are more likely to have successful outcomes when the intervention specifically addresses those fears.[89] Kinesiophobia, or fear of movement, is also associated with poor outcomes.[90] Maladaptive and passive coping strategies,[91,92] depression, and traumatic life events[92] all increase the likelihood of developing future chronic pain and disability due to pain.

The Effect of Lifestyle Factors

Some health habits are also risk factors for chronic pain. Smoking has a complex relationship with chronic pain; smoking has immediate analgesic effects through both central and peripheral pain receptors.[93] However, smoking is associated with greater prevalence of chronic pain disorders such as LBP,[94,95] pelvic pain,[96] and other chronic pain disorders once socioeconomic factors have been controlled.[93,97] Pain and activity restriction are also greater among smokers.[98] A high correlation exists between chronic pain and opiate or alcohol addiction, though it is difficult to determine the direction of causality.[97] Obesity and overweight are also correlated with chronic LBP[94,99] and a variety of other chronic pain conditions,[69] but it is unclear whether obesity increases the risk of chronic pain or whether chronic pain contributes to obesity.

Sleep disorders are highly correlated to chronic pain, increased disability, and suffering due to pain, and increased health care utilization.[100-102] Studies have shown that poor-quality sleep predicts onset of chronic pain 15 months later,[101] and experimental sleep deprivation can result in diffuse musculoskeletal pain.[103] The relationship between sleep disorder and chronic pain appears to be reciprocal, with each exacerbating the other,[102,104,105] and restorative sleep seems to be associated with decreases in pain.[106] Sleep disorders can be screened using the *Pittsburgh Sleep Quality Index (PSQI)*.[107]

Although there are no nutritional cures for chronic pain, nutritional deficits may exacerbate pain conditions. Research suggests that vitamin D deficiency causes dull, persistent, generalized musculoskeletal aches and pains and muscle weakness,[108,109] and may be associated with fibromyalgia, rheumatic disorders, OA, and migraine.[109,110] Studies have found vitamin D deficits in 26% to 93% of patients with diffuse bone and muscle pain responding poorly to medication.[108,111] However, studies assessing vitamin D supplements for treating chronic pain have provided inconsistent results.[112]

■ PSYCHOSOCIAL FACTORS ASSOCIATED WITH CHRONIC PAIN

The Mind-Body Relationship

The definition of pain as an unpleasant sensory and emotional experience associated with actual or potential tissue damage, or described in terms of such damage,[13] incorporates the cognitive, emotional, and social context in which pain occurs. The Cartesian concept of mind-body duality in which a problem was either in the body or in the mind is now known to be incorrect.[33,50,113-116] The spatial discrimination and affective components of

pain are equally physiological; they simply occur in different portions of the brain.[6,29,38] Autonomic and endocrine pathways relay affective, autonomic, hormonal, and immune information bidirectionally between the CNS and periphery. Pain is clearly more than somatic information transmitted from the body to the brain.[50]

Psychosocial factors have a strong impact on distress and disability outcomes, independent of chronic pain intensity. For example, catastrophization and poor coping skills are associated with increased pain intensity and greater disability.[115,117-120] Some psychosocial variables have been shown to be predictive, such as depression and past life trauma predict the transition from acute to chronic low back pain, while depression and negative pain beliefs predict greater disability.[92] Many psychosocial factors lead to vicious cycles because they both contribute to and are aggravated by chronic pain. For example, depression both contributes to chronic pain and is caused or aggravated by chronic pain. Some socioeconomic variables are also vulnerable to such cycles: for example, poverty is a risk factor for chronic pain, while chronic pain leads to disability, which contributes to poverty. Sullivan et al[117] provide a comprehensive review of the interaction between mental health and chronic pain. Jensen et al[119] review measurement tools for assessing psychosocial factors relevant to disability and chronic pain. A few tools for assessing psychosocial factors are listed in Table 25.4.[89,107,121-143]

Yellow flags have been defined as psychosocial factors that increase the likelihood that acute pain will progress into chronic pain and disability.[144-146] Although most sources combine all psychosocial factors into the concept of yellow alert flags, Table 25.5 outlines a terminology proposed by Nicholas et al.[144] In this terminology *yellow flags* include beliefs, emotional responses, and pain behavior; *orange flags* represent frank psychiatric symptoms; and *blue flags* reflect the interaction between work and health perceptions. The yellow flags with greatest impact appear to be (1) the belief that pain and activity are harmful, (2) a depressed mood and social withdrawal, (3) the expectation that passive treatment will help more than active treatment, and (4) low self-efficacy.[147] Other important factors include sickness behavior (e.g., excessive rest), history of pain or disability, poor job satisfaction, overprotective family or lack of support, and problems with claims or compensation.[146] Psychosocial issues should not be reduced into a single factor affecting pain. Each person is different and each psychosocial factor reflects a complex interaction among all components of the ICF model: environmental and personal factors affect activity, participation, and even body function and the health condition.[145] Psychosocial issues should be considered individually for each patient, because interventions addressing specific psychosocial factors are more successful than interventions that do not.[145] However, the presence of psychological factors should not invalidate the patient's pain complaint and

Table 25.4 Psychosocial Assessment Tools by Construct

Construct	Tool	Description	References/Websites*
Catastrophizing	Pain Catastrophizing Scale (see Appendix 25.A)	13 items on 3 subscales: rumination, magnification, helplessness; norms available	Sullivan and Pivik [131] http://sullivan-painresearch.mcgill.ca/pcs.php [online access; Appendix in User's Manual]
Coping	Chronic Pain Coping Inventory™ (CPCI™)	Short form has 8 or 16 questions with 8 categories	Hadjistavropoulos et al[133] www4.parinc.com/Products/ [fee required for access] Available in Jensen et al[136]
Coping	Coping Strategies Questionnaire (CSQ) for Pain-Related Coping	Short form has 7 or 14 items with 7 categories: 6 cognitive and one behavioral	Hadjistavropoulos et al[133] http://parqol.com/ Available in Jensen et al[136]
Depression	Center for Epidemiologic Studies Depression Scale (CES-D)	20 items validated for use in chronic pain	Radloff et al[124] www.chcr.brown.edu/pcoc/cesdscale.pdf [online access]
Depression	Primary Care Evaluation of Mental Disorders (Prime-MD)	2 questions	Arroll et al, Whooley et al[125,126] www.psy-world.com/prime-md_print1.htm [online access]
Depression	Patient Health Questionnaire-2 (PHQ-2) PHQ-9	2 questions 9 questions	Brody et al, Spitzer et al, Haggman et al[127,129,143] www.phqscreeners.com [online access]
Fear-avoidance	Tampa Scale of Kinesiophobia	17-question scale with subscales of somatic focus and activity avoidance	Vlaeyen et al, Roelofs et al[122,123] www.tac.vic.gov.au/upload/tampa_scale_kinesiophobia.pdf [online access]
Fear-avoidance	Fear-Avoidance Beliefs Questionnaire (FABQ)	16 questions with subscales for work (FABQ-W) and physical activity (FABQ-PA) Originally for low back pain but modified for general musculoskeletal pain	George and Stryker, Waddell et al[89,121] www.qcomp.com.au/media/29364/fear—avoidance-beliefs-questionnaire%5B1%5D.pdf [online access]
Pain beliefs	Pain Beliefs and Perceptions Inventory	16 items with 4 subscales: pain as mystery, as constant, as permanent, self-blame 8-item short form	Williams and Thorn, Jensen et al[135,136] www.tac.vic.gov.au [online access]
Pain self-efficacy	Pain Self-Efficacy Questionnaire (PSEQ)	10 questions	Nicholas[134] www.tac.vic.gov.au [online access]
Perceived injustice	Injustice Experience Questionnaire	12 questions with subscales of blame and severity	Sullivan et al[132] http://sullivan-painresearch.mcgill.ca/ieq.php [online access]
Post-traumatic stress disorder (PTSD)	Primary Care Post-Traumatic Stress Disorder Screen (see Appendix 25.B)	4 questions, score >2 suggests PTSD	Prins et al[130] www.ptsd.va.gov/professional/pages/assessments/pc-ptsd.asp [online access]

Continued

Table 25.4	Psychosocial Assessment Tools by Construct—cont'd		
Construct	Tool	Description	References/Websites*
Post-traumatic stress disorder	Post-traumatic Stress Disorder (PTSD) Checklist	17 questions	Allen and Annells[142] www.mirecc.va.gov/docs/visn6/3_PTSD_CheckList_and_Scoring.pdf [online access]
Readiness to change	Pain Stages of Change Questionnaire (PSOCQ)	30 item self-report	Kerns et al[140,141] www.painpoints.com/patients/downloads/patient_questionnaire.pdf [online access]
Readiness to change	Multidimensional Pain Readiness to Change Questionnaire (MPRCQ2)	69 Q: 9 change domains: exercise, task persistence, relaxation, cognitive control, pacing, avoid pain, contingent rest, assertive communication, body mechanics	Questionnaire available in Nielson et al[139] www.ncbi.nlm.nih.gov/pubmed/18337183 [online access through PubMed]
Sleep	Pittsburgh Sleep Quality Index (PSQI)	23 questions	Buysse et al[107] www.wsna.org/Topics/Fatigue/documents/PSQI.pdf [online access]
Sleep	Medical Outcomes Study (MOS) Sleep Scale Survey Instrument	12 items	Hays et al[138] www.rand.org/health/surveys_tools/mos/mos_sleep.html [online access]
Stress	Perceived Stress Scale	4-, 10-, and 14-item scales	Cohen et al[137] www.psy.cmu.edu/~scohen/[online access]

*Selected scales are available at the websites indicated; some require a fee for access.

Table 25.5	Alert Flags for Chronic Pain[144]	
Flag Color	Type of Problem	Examples
Red	Serious physical pathology	Cauda equina syndrome, fracture, tumor.
Orange	Psychiatric symptoms	Clinical depression, post-traumatic stress disorder, personality disorder.
Yellow	Beliefs, appraisals, and judgments	Negative pain beliefs. Expectation of poor outcome.
	Emotional responses	Fear, anxiety, catastrophization, distress.
	Pain behavior, including pain coping strategies	Fear-avoidance behavior, dependence on passive interventions.
Blue	Perceptions about relationship between work and pain	Belief that work will cause further injury and pain. Belief that supervisor and co-workers are unsupportive.
Black	System or contextual obstacles	No modified duty options at work. Legislation restricting return to work options. Lack of insurance coverage. Overly solicitous family or health providers.

should not interfere with attempts to identify and address physical sources that cause or exacerbate pain.[16]

Pain Beliefs and Coping

Pain-related beliefs include people's understanding about what is causing their pain, the meaning of their pain, and expectations regarding the impact pain has on their present and future lives. Beliefs associated with better outcomes include having control over pain, global self-efficacy, pain self-efficacy, control over life, and internal pain control. Beliefs associated with poor outcomes include the following: pain indicates injury/damage and should be avoided, pain will be constant, pain is disabling, emotions influence pain, and that other people should be solicitous because of the pain, helplessness, and external locus of control (the belief that pain is controlled by someone other than the individual in pain).[119] Some people with chronic pain believe that someone is to blame for their pain and that their pain is unfair; such feelings of injustice can interfere with rehabilitation.[132]

Coping is the way in which people manage stress. Some coping mechanisms are beneficial, or adaptive, whereas others are destructive, or maladaptive. Beneficial coping responses include activities to distract oneself from the pain, task persistence, exercise, ignoring pain, coping self-statements, and acceptance of the condition. Detrimental coping responses include guarding, resting, venting emotions, passive coping (avoidance), and asking for assistance.[119,148]

Anxiety and Fear Avoidance

Anxiety is a normal response to acute pain and can be an adaptive response encouraging people to stop activities causing tissue damage. However, if the cause of pain cannot be found, anxiety is replaced by frustration that the cause cannot be found, hostility that other people do not believe the pain is real, fear that the pain will not go away, and discouragement because nothing helps.[149] Anxiety is a common co-morbidity with chronic pain,[150] and evidence suggests that anxiety may be a risk factor for acute pain becoming chronic.[16,150] Anxiety is more highly correlated with chronic pain than depression. Post-traumatic stress disorder, a special case of anxiety disorder, is particularly common in chronic pain.[150]

An adaptive anxiety response in acute pain can become a maladaptive fear response in chronic pain. The *Fear-Avoidance Model* of pain proposes that some people have an exaggerated fear that movement will cause reinjury and/or increase pain.[151,152] Fear of pain can even become more disabling than the actual pain. People with pain either confront or avoid these fears; those who confront will increase activity and will generally have improved functional outcomes and decreased pain. Fear-induced avoidance of activity leads to hypervigilance, inaccurate predictions about pain, misinterpretation of body sensations, muscular reactivity, and physical deconditioning.[151,152] Figure 25.3 shows how these factors result in increased pain and increased disability for a given level of pain. Maladaptive beliefs are reinforced as people expect activity to increase pain and expect pain to lead to disability.[16,120,151] Decreased activity due to fear results in deconditioning impaired motor control due to disuse, both of which increase likelihood of increased pain.[16,151,153]

Catastrophizing

Catastrophizing includes pessimism, helplessness to control symptoms, magnification (threat exaggeration), and rumination (excessive focus on pain sensations).

Figure 25.3 The fear-avoidance model shows how the pain experience can resolve in the absence of fear or become a vicious cycle in the presence of pain-related fear. Negative affect and poor coping skills cause the pain experience to be perceived as a threat; pain catastrophizing increases pain-related fear, hypervigilance, and avoidance. Activity avoidance leads to secondary problems such as deconditioning, depression, and additional disability, which further exacerbate the negative aspects of the pain experience. On the other hand, individuals who do not perceive pain as a threat are more likely to progress back into activities that had been painful, leading to recovery.

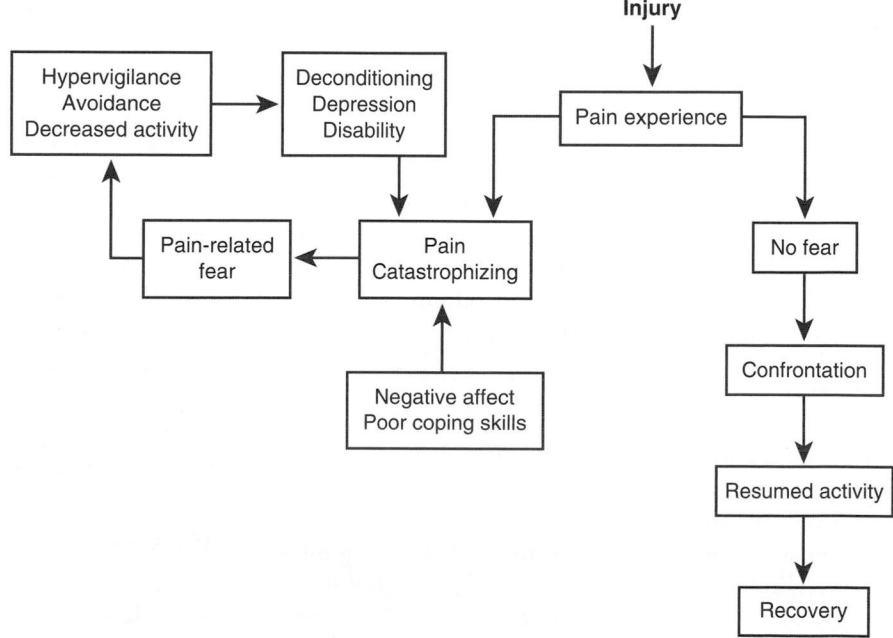

Catastrophizing involves both cognitive appraisal and beliefs or attitudes; however, it can also be described as a (maladaptive) coping mechanism.[29,31,117,119,154] It appears to be an interaction between inherited temperament and personal history and experience.[29] Examples of catastrophizing self-statements might include the following: "this pain has destroyed my life," "I know there is something terribly wrong with me," "I can't stop thinking about how much it hurts," or "I can't stand this anymore." Appendix 25.A contains the *Pain Catastrophizing Scale*.[131] Catastrophizing is the strongest and most consistent psychosocial factor affecting both pain intensity and function.[119,120,154] Interestingly, catastrophizing activates the same portions of the brain activated with suffering.[29]

Depression and Grieving

Depression is a very common co-morbidity with chronic pain, ranging between 13% and 85% of patients depending on the population,[16,73,155,156] suggesting that depression can both cause and be caused by pain.[31] Depression is associated with increased catastrophizing, fear of pain, and perceived disability,[157] as well as increased pain complaints and poorer rehabilitation outcomes.[155] Depression is a strong predictor for the development of chronic pain and disability following acute LBP.[6,92] Physiologically, depression is associated with increased activity in portions of the brain that mediate the affective component of pain.[158]

People in severe pain are unable to fulfill social roles such as maintain a job, sustain family relationships, or satisfy personal needs for growth and recreation. As a result, people with chronic pain may suffer and grieve for their loss of identity, job, relationships, or hobbies. They may feel guilt for their failure to perform life roles. Family and friends may also feel loss.[159-161] These experiences may lead to depression or grieving. The traditional model of grief proposed by Kübler-Ross posits that people go through five stages in the grieving process: *denial, anger, bargaining, depression*, and *acceptance*.[162] However, the stages of grieving model has been challenged when applied to chronic illness as an oversimplification of a more complex narrative.[163] A recent model of grieving associated with chronic pain proposes a process of adaptation and relearning the world, associated with four processes occurring along a continuum: despair to hope, lack of understanding to insight, meaning disruption to meaning, bodily discomfort to reintegrated body.[160,164]

Stress

The body's short-term response to acute stress allows the organism to respond to the threat. Acute stress may produce analgesia, as is sometimes seen in soldiers or athletes. Stress-induced analgesia works through both opiate- and non–opiate-mediated mechanisms via descending inhibition.[48] Prolonged psychological or physiological stress, however, leads to a dysfunctional response with excessive

immune system suppression, muscle atrophy, compromised tissue growth and repair, autonomic dysfunction, cognitive changes, and structural changes in the brain.[48,50,149] Stress-related mechanisms appear to be important in a number of chronic pain syndromes such as chronic headaches, fibromyalgia, and TMJ disorders, as well as other central sensitization conditions such as chronic fatigue and irritable bowel, PTSD, anxiety, and depression.[48,50] Appendix 25.B includes the four-question *Primary Care Post-Traumatic Stress Disorder Screen*.[130] Stress-mediated peripheral and central sensitization involves activation of the autonomic nervous system and the HPA axis.[48,50,165] Chronic pain also aggravates stress when patients feel blamed or labeled as complainers, when multiple tests do not identify a source of the pain, when treatment is ineffective, and when they are unable to work or perform activities of daily living (ADL), sleep, or maintain relationships.[149]

Nonorganic Findings

Waddell et al[166] first presented the concept of nonorganic findings to identify patients who would benefit from further psychological testing. The original implication was that these patients had findings not consistent with an organic basis for their pain, hence psychological sources needed to be considered. The five components of Waddell and colleagues' nonorganic testing are superficial or nonanatomical tenderness, pain in response to simulation tests, inconsistent responses to distraction, regional sensory and strength impairments, and overreaction (sometimes referred to as *Waddell signs*). Positive findings in three or more of these categories are considered a *positive nonorganic test*.[166,167]

Research confirms that having multiple positive Waddell signs is correlated with increased psychological distress, pain severity, and perceived disability.[144,168] Although Waddell signs appear to have value in identifying people at risk for poor response to treatment, they should not be considered as truly "nonorganic." Research indicates there is an organic basis for at least some of them; for example, overreaction and superficial tenderness are consistent with allodynia due to central sensitization.[21,168] Although Waddell signs are commonly misinterpreted to indicate malingering, this was not their intended use: evidence does not show an association between Waddell signs and malingering or secondary gain.[169] In summary, assessment of nonorganic findings can be constructive as long as the findings are considered within the context of current knowledge about chronic pain. Chronic pain may exist in the absence of peripheral tissue damage, central sensitization amplifies the pain response, and it is common for people with chronic pain to have psychosocial factors affect their pain.[21,144]

Personality Disorders

Some evidence suggests that personality disorders, such as borderline, histrionic, or obsessive compulsive, are not risk factors for developing chronic pain, but are associated with poorer prognosis. Other research suggests increased prevalence of personality disorders among people who have chronic pain.[19,170] In either case, it does appear that chronic pain may exacerbate personality disorders.[19] The reader is referred to Dersh et al[19] for further discussion of issues and evidence related to personality disorders.

Social Support

Social factors operate at a societal level, at the level of workplace or school, or microlevel of interpersonal relationships and informal help.[171] General social support is one of the ICF environmental factors relevant to chronic pain,[26] and lack of social support is identified as one of many potential barriers to treatment that are difficult to overcome.[16] General or global social support and social reinforcers for wellness behavior tend to be beneficial.[118,119,172] However, the impact of social responses to pain behaviors depends on the nature of the behavior and whether the response is solicitous or punishing. Solicitous behaviors are pain-contingent responses such as sympathy, encouragement to avoid pain and do less, and allowing people to avoid tasks due to pain. Solicitous responses lead to increased pain and decreased function.[119,173] Punishing or negative responses to pain behaviors also lead to increased pain and depression.[154]

■ EXAMINATION OF PAIN

Pain is a purely subjective phenomenon. Unlike range of motion (ROM), strength, or tissue extensibility, pain has no objective or specific measurement tool. However, the measurement of pain has become a vital part of patient examination. The Joint Commission on Accreditation of Healthcare Organizations (JCAHO) has emphasized the importance of pain assessment and treatment by calling pain "the fifth vital sign." Effective examination of chronic pain is more complex than the visual analog or numeric rating scales typically used for acute pain. The psychosocial aspects of chronic pain should be examined and evaluated to better identify psychosocial factors and guide intervention within a biopsychosocial model of care.

A thorough patient examination allows the physical therapist to hypothesize potential sources of the pain (i.e., nociceptive due to peripheral tissue damage, peripheral neurogenic, central neurogenic). Patients with chronic pain disorders may also have acute or subacute conditions superimposed on chronic pain: that is, a person with fibromyalgia may still have rotator cuff impingement, lumbar instability, or carpal tunnel syndrome. Since conditions associated with peripheral tissue injury may exacerbate peripheral or central sensitization, physical therapists need to consider whether to treat the superimposed musculoskeletal conditions and/or the underlying chronic pain.

Pain should be examined both at rest and with movement.[174] Several mnemonics can be used to guide the examination of pain; *PQRST* and *SOCRATES* are shown in Box 25.3.[175-177] The standard tools for quantifying pain severity are the *visual analogue scale (VAS)* and the more commonly used *numeric rating scale (NRS)*. The VAS and NRS correlate well with one another and are equally sensitive whereas the *verbal (categorical) rating scale (VRS)* of mild, moderate, severe is not as accurate. The NRS is easier to understand, faster to score, and more practical than VAS. A variety of *Faces scales* are used for children over 3 years old.[174,178] While severity is the most commonly measured parameter, clinical guidelines for chronic pain management emphasize that single-dimension pain examination such as the VAS or NRS are inadequate for chronic pain and that it is essential to use a multidimensional tool that examines the emotional and cognitive aspects of pain as well. Furthermore, emphasis on pain rating scales encourages attention to and preoccupation with pain, which interferes with effective pain management.[3] Consequently, de-emphasis of pain quantification in chronic pain management may clash with the JCAHO focus on pain measurement.

Body diagrams provide information about pain location, radiation, and character. Pain diagrams require more patient instruction than pain quantification, hence are more time consuming to administer. Patients are instructed to distinguish between aching, burning, stabbing, pins and needles, and numbness; and sometimes sensations such as heaviness, swelling, or other autonomic symptoms. Information about the location and nature of the pain

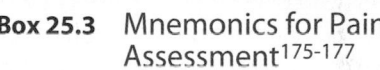

Box 25.3   Mnemonics for Pain Assessment[175-177]

PQRST

- **P**rovoking/precipitating factors
- **Q**uality of pain
- **R**egion and radiation
- **S**everity or associated symptoms
- **T**emporal factors/timing

SOCRATES

- **S**ite: Where is the pain?
- **O**nset: When and how did it start? Sudden or gradual? Trauma, illness, or other possible cause?
- **C**haracter: How does the pain feel? Sharp? Stabbing? Burning? Aching? Other?
- **R**adiation: Does the pain radiate? Where? What causes radiation?
- **A**ssociations: Other symptoms, such as numbness, paresthesias, heaviness, other?
- **T**ime course: How does the pain vary over the day?
- **E**xacerbating/relieving: What aggravates or relieves the pain?
- **S**everity: Intensity rating

can be used to hypothesize about the source of the pain: sclerotomes, referred pain, dermatomes, and peripheral nerve patterns all implicate specific structures whereas symmetrical patterns of autonomic symptoms implicate central neurogenic involvement. Data obtained from body diagrams is more difficult to analyze objectively than data obtained from VAS or other pain tools and observer bias may influence analysis of body diagram data.[179]

Pain Questionnaires and Outcome Measures

A multitude of pain questionnaires and outcome measures exist to measure both nonspecific and disease-specific aspects of pain from a biopsychosocial perspective. For a more comprehensive discussion of pain examination, interested readers are referred to several excellent review articles;[174,180-183] in addition, the website *Pain Treatment Topics* includes brief summaries of many examination tools, as well as links to those tools (see Appendix 25.E). Table 25.6 provides a short list of practical examination instruments appropriate for chronic pain.[178,180,184-198]

The *McGill Pain Questionnaire (MPQ)* and the *Short Form MPQ (SF-MPQ)* examine sensory, affective-emotional, evaluative, and temporal aspects of pain.[174,195,199] The original MPQ was intended to indicate the possible source of pain through descriptors the patient selected. Word category 1 (e.g., "quivering," "beating," or "pounding") suggested vascular origin; categories 2 through 8 suggested neurogenic origin; category 9 suggested musculoskeletal origin; and categories 10 through 20 reflected the emotional content of pain.[195] The SF-MPQ includes fewer verbal descriptors.[199] Other tools also help distinguish the source of the pain. For example, the *Leads Assessment of Neuropathic Symptoms and Signs* (LANSS) distinguishes between neurogenic and nociceptive pain with sensitivity of 80% to 85% and specificity of 80% to 94%.[200] The *Neuropathic Pain Scale* (NPS) also distinguishes between neuropathic and non-neuropathic pain.[201]

Ideally, a comprehensive outcome measure should examine each of the domains within the ICF: body structure or function, activity, and participation.[202]

Table 25.6	Pain Assessment Tools Appropriate for Chronic Pain*		
Pain Scale	**Properties**	**Items**	**References/Websites/ Description**
Body Map	Able to monitor location of pain and other symptoms	Body chart	Margolis et al[184] www.aapmr.org/patients/ conditions/pain/Documents/ paindrawing.pdf [online access]
Body Outline Marking	For children 4–7 years to communicate pain location	Body outline	von Baeyer et al[185] Children mark pain location on a body outline
Brief Pain Inventory (long and short forms)	Multidimensional scale includes body function, activity, and participation	Long form has 32 items Short form has 9 items	Atkinson et al[194] http://pain-topics.org/clinical_ concepts/assess.php [online access]
Checklist of Nonverbal Pain Indicators (CNPI)	For adult patients who are nonverbal or have dementia	5 behaviors	Feldt,[187] Bjoro and Herr[188] http://painconsortium.nih.gov/ pain_scales/ChecklistofNonverbal. pdf [online access]
FACES	For children to rate pain severity	1 item (series of facial expressions illustrating different pain intensities)	Tomlinson et al[178] http://painconsortium.nih.gov/ pain_scales/ChecklistofNonverbal. pdf [online access]
Geriatric Pain Measure (GMP) (regular and short forms)	Multidimensional scale includes body function, activity, and participation	GPM has 24 items GPM-SF has 12 items	Ferrell et al, Blozik et al[196,197] www.palliativecareswo.ca/ Regional/LondonMiddlesex/ Geriatric%20Pain%20Measure% 20GPM.pdf [online access]
Global Pain Scale	Subscales: pain, feelings, clinical outcomes, activities	33 items for full version, 20 items on short form	Gentile et al[186] www.paindoctor.com/global-pain- scale [online access]

Table 25.6   Pain Assessment Tools Appropriate for Chronic Pain*—cont'd

Pain Scale	Properties	Items	References/Websites/Description
Graded Chronic Pain Scale	Assesses ICF domains of impairment, activity, and participation restriction	7 items in original, 2 items in the Two Item Graded Chronic Pain Scale	Von Korff et al[192] Original scale: http://pelvicgirdlepain.com/references/Questionnaire-of-von-Korff-et-al-for-grading-the-severity-of-chronic-pain.pdf Two-Item scale: http://primarycareforall.org/wp-content/uploads/2011/10/Two-Item-Graded-Chronic-Pain-Scale.pdf [online access]
Leeds Assessment of Neuropathic Symptoms and Signs (LANSS)	Score distinguishes between neuropathic and non-neuropathic pain; includes self-report and objective testing	7 self-report and 2 sensory testing items for allodynia and hyperalgesia	Bennett[190] www.painxchange.com.au/AssessmentTools/Appendices/PDF/Apx4_LANSS.pdf [online access]
McGill Pain Scale (PMQ)	Assesses pain intensity, sensory, affective, evaluative, and miscellaneous pain	78 items: 20 pain descriptors (sensory [1–10], affective 11–15], evaluative [16], and miscellaneous [17–20]), 1 pain intensity item	Melzack[195] www.ama-cmeonline.com/pain_mgmt/pdf/mcgill.pdf [online access]
McGill Pain Scale Short Form (SF-MPQ)	Assesses pain intensity, sensory, and affective pain	17 items: 11 sensory descriptors, 4 affective descriptors, 2 pain intensity	Melzack[199] http://prc.coh.org/pdf/McGill%20Short-Form%20Pain%20Questionnaire.pdf [online access]
Pain Disability Index	Impact of pain on life participation	7 items	Tait et al[193] www.prp-sandiego.com/uploads/Pain_Disability_Index.pdf [online access]
Pain Quality Assessment Scale (PQAS)	Distinguishing types of pain and an outcome measure	20 pain descriptor items and 1 temporal pattern; differentiates between nociceptive and neurogenic pain	Victor et al[191] www.mapi-trust.org [online access]
Pain Thermometer	10-unit thermometer for adults with impaired cognition	1 item	Herr et al[198] www.painknowledge.org/physiciantools/Pain_Thermometer/Pain_Thermometer_1_23_08.pdf
Self-report Leeds Assessment of Neuropathic Symptoms and Signs (S-LANSS)	Distinguishes between neuropathic and non-neuropathic pain; S-LANSS is the LANSS without the 2 objective testing questions	7 self-report questions	Bennett et al[189] http://clahrc-gm.nihr.ac.uk/cms/wp-content/uploads/GM-SAT_SLANNS.pdf [online access]
Visual Analog Scale (VAS), Numeric Rating Scale (NRS)	10 cm line or 0–10 scale for pain severity	1 item	Burckhardt[180] Measures pain across a continuum of values (often from *No Pain* to *Worst Possible Pain*)

*Many of these and other pain scales can be found at http://pain-topics.org/clinical_concepts/assess.php.
ICF = International Classification of Functioning, Disability and Health.

The *Brief Pain Inventory (BPI)* examines pain now, worst, least, and average over 24 hours. It rates pain interference with functional activities such as general activity, walking, normal work, relations with other people, mood, sleep, and enjoyment of life. The BPI was initially designed for cancer-related pain, but has since been validated with other sources of pain. [114,174] The *Initiative on Methods, Measurement, and Pain Assessment in Clinical Trials (IMMPACT)* is a multimodal examination tool that includes the domains of (1) pain, (2) physical functioning, (3) emotional functioning, (4) patient ratings of improvement and satisfaction with treatment, (5) other symptoms and adverse events during treatment, and (6) patient demographics. [203]

Some tools have been developed to examine specific types of pain. For example, Jensen et al[181] review several tools specific for neuropathic pain. Some pain assessment tools are condition-specific: for example, the *Western Ontario and McMaster University Osteoarthritis Index (WOMAC)* for osteoarthritis of the knee, the *Oswestry Low Back Pain Disability Questionnaire* for LBP, the *Revised Fibromyalgia Impact Questionnaire (FIQR),* and the *Headache Impact Test.* Some disease- or condition-specific tools (such as the FIQR) examine both pain and other symptoms or activity restrictions relevant to those conditions. Inclusion of nonpain symptoms such as anxiety, depression, sleep quality, balance, and memory provides a more comprehensive picture of the patient's complaints, but may obscure examination of pain.

Because pain is an integration of physical, emotional, and cognitive processes, physical measurements of chronic pain are of limited value. While people experiencing acute pain usually demonstrate physiological arousal (e.g., increased heart rate), such arousal is not typically associated with chronic pain. Box 25.4 lists verbal and nonverbal forms of pain expression that may be useful in acute pain; however, such pain expressions can be misleading in patients with chronic pain owing to multiple factors influencing the pain. [175] Some potential physical measurements of allodynia and central sensitization include *von Frey filaments* for pain threshold, temperature discrimination using test tubes filled with cold and hot (40°C) water for thermal allodynia; cotton, wool, or an artist's brush for mechanical allodynia, and a blunt needle for hyperalgesia; and temporal summation. [174] The LANSS also includes physical assessment of allodynia (brushing the skin) and hyperalgesia (hypersensitivity to pinprick in the locations of pain). [181,190]

Examination of Pain in Special Populations

Children, the elderly, and people with dementia or limited cognitive function pose special challenges to examination of pain. Historically, it was believed that infants had immature nervous systems that were not able to experience pain. This is now known to be incorrect; the necessary neural pathways for pain experience are present

---

Box 25.4　Pain Expression and Factors Affecting Pain Expression[175]

Forms of Pain Expression

- Vocalizations: Verbal pain report, crying, moaning, sighing, screaming.
- Movement and mobility: Decreased motion, rubbing, guarding, splinting, muscle spasm, limping.
- Facial expression: Wincing, grimacing, frowning.
- Mood and behavior: Distress, anxiety, depression, irritability, aggression, quietness, withdrawal, decreased cognition, decreased appetite, sleep deprivation, confusion.

Factors Affecting Pain Expression

- Nature of the pain: Type, intensity, location.
- Cognitive status, mood, sedation.
- Meaning of pain to the individual, learned pain behaviors from family or culture.
- Expectations regarding pain and pain relief, perceived consequences of the pain.
- Acceptable behaviors within the family or culture, other people's responses.
- Situation and environment.

---

and functioning starting at 24 weeks of gestation. Pain experiences in infants or children can cause permanent changes in neural structure and function, leading to increased pain perception later in life. Children experience a range of common pain conditions, including headaches and migraines, back pain, and muscle and joint pain. [44] In some cases, the conditions may present differently than in adults; for example, migraines in children often present as abdominal symptoms without actual headache. [204]

A variety of *faces scales* exist for use with children who are able to articulate their pain, typically used with children over 4 years old. The various faces scales may include from 5 to 10 options of facial expressions representing different severities of pain. [178] Younger children can use the *Pieces of Hurt Scale,* in which they indicate how many poker chips of pain they have, from one to four. [183] For infants and children who are nonverbal, several observational pain assessment tools exist for acute pain; for example, *Crying, Requires increased oxygen administration, Increased vital signs, Expression, Sleeplessness (CRIES)* Pain Scale for infants 0 to 6 months; *Face, Legs, Activity, Cry, Consolability Scale (FLACC)* for infants and children 2 months to 7 years; *COMFORT Pain Scale* for unconscious or ventilated infants, children, or adolescents. [174,205,206] Since behavioral signs are different for acute and chronic pain, these observational scales are probably not valid for chronic pain. [207]

There is no indication that pain sensation diminishes with age as do vision, hearing, and the other special senses.[44,208] However, research suggests that with advancing age there are a higher proportion of C fibers relative to A-δ fibers, resulting in more diffuse, burning pain rather than localized prickling pain among the elderly. Older individuals may report "discomfort" or "aches" rather than "pain," so clinicians should be alert to changes in pain descriptors with age.[209] Several reports review pain assessment tools for elderly individuals with dementia or who are nonverbal; the *Pain Thermometer* is more accurate than the NPS or VAS for elderly persons with cognitive deficits.[188,198] As with the pain assessment tools for infants, these tools were developed for acute pain and it is not clear that these observational tools accurately reflect chronic pain. Bruckenthal et al[209] present a useful summary of issues related to pain assessment in the elderly.

Narrative Examination of Pain

The current emphasis on objective measurement should not overshadow the importance of narrative reasoning approaches to examining patients with chronic pain. During the history taking, narrative reasoning strives to understand the patient's story, illness experience, beliefs, fears, and expectations. The emphasis of narrative reasoning is therefore to understand the patient's experience, beliefs, and feelings rather than to quantify or objectify pain. Narrative information is often obtained verbally during history taking or while talking during interventions; nonverbal information such as weeping or avoidance of eye contact also conveys narrative information. Edwards et al[210] present a comprehensive approach to applying narrative reasoning throughout the patient care process. Given the importance of psychosocial issues in chronic pain, the narrative approach may be particularly valuable in this patient population.[211,212]

■ MEDICAL MANAGEMENT OF CHRONIC PAIN

Medical Diagnostic Testing

There are no general imaging or laboratory tests diagnostic for chronic pain. Furthermore, positive findings on imaging tests do not prove that the identified pathology is related to the patient's pain, as indicated in multiple studies showing positive lumbar imaging findings in people without LBP,[16,213,214] and the mismatch between radiographic findings of OA and pain.[215] Repeated diagnostic testing to search for an undefined physical abnormality is generally not indicated because it encourages patients to focus on physical abnormalities that might not exist (adhering to a biomedical model) rather than looking for strategies to manage the pain using a biopsychosocial model.[216]

Laboratory tests, such as thyroid hormone levels, sedimentation rates, Lyme titers, or general blood screening, can be appropriate to rule out conditions that are treatable. Electrodiagnostic testing, such as needle electromyogram (EMG), is not indicated unless there is suggestion of specific neuropathy. Diagnostic nerve blocks (peripheral or sympathetic), joint blocks (facet or sacroiliac), and provocative discography can help determine whether a given structure is involved; see any of the clinical guidelines on chronic pain for more information on interventional testing.[15,16,18,216] Ultimately, excessive or repeated tests foster patients' obsession with obtaining a pathophysiological diagnosis and may interfere with chronic pain management.[15,16,216]

Pharmacological Management of Chronic Pain

Medications are typically staged, starting with those least likely to cause adverse side effects to those with greatest risk. The various classes of medication are shown in Table 25.7, along with primary indication(s) and adverse effects.[16,217-219] In general, treatment starts with acetaminophen and proceeds to nonsteroidal anti-inflammatory drugs (NSAIDs) and topical medications. NSAIDS are generally beneficial for arthritic pain and LBP, but are believed to be ineffective for neuropathic pain.[220] *Adjuvant medications* (medications whose primary indication is a condition other than pain, but which have demonstrated benefit in pain management) are added next. Muscle relaxants and weak opiates are added if prior medications, physical therapy, and cognitive therapy are unsuccessful. Kroenke et al[218] and Turk et al[220] provide good overviews of the mechanisms and efficacy of various classes of medications for chronic pain.[218,220]

Adjuvant medications include antidepressant, antiseizure, muscle relaxant, and sleep medications. Antidepressants for pain are typically used at much lower dosages than when used to treat depression because the mechanism of action is distinct from treatment of depression. Tricyclic antidepressants (TCAs) have demonstrated benefit for neurogenic pain, fibromyalgia, LBP, headaches, and irritable bowel.[220] Results for selective serotonin reuptake inhibitors (SSRIs) for chronic pain are inconsistent. Serotonin-norepinephrine reuptake inhibitors (SNRIs) appear to have the benefits of TCAs for managing neuropathic pain with fewer side effects.[220] Overall, TCAs and SNRIs are more effective than SSRIs for managing chronic pain.[16,219] Evidence is also strong for some anticonvulsant medications in managing neuropathic pain, including fibromyalgia and lumbar radiculopathy.[220] Medications to treat sleep disturbance can also be beneficial because sleep disturbance frequently exacerbates chronic pain.[219] Benzodiazepines and muscle relaxant medications are generally not recommended for prolonged use in chronic pain because risks are relatively high and there is little evidence of benefit.[16] Cyclobenzaprine, however, has been shown to be effective for fibromyalgia and conditions involving chronic muscle spasm.[220]

Topical medications for chronic pain fall into three broad categories: those creating cooling sensations, those

Table 25.7   Medications for Chronic Pain[218]

Class	Medication	Type of pain	Possible Adverse Effects
Para-aminophenols	Acetaminophen	Most	Liver toxicity
NSAIDs	Naproxen, salsalate, etodolac, ibuprofen, diclofenac	Nociceptive, inflammatory	GI bleeding, nausea, cardiac risk
Topical	Capsaicin, lidocaine, salsalate, NSAID, menthol	Nociceptive, peripheral neurogenic	Skin irritation
Adjuvant: antidepressants (tricyclics, SNRIs)	Amitriptyline, nortriptyline (Tramadol has SNRI effects)	Peripheral or central neurogenic; some nociceptive pain	Hypertension, orthostatic hypotension, arrhythmias, falls in the elderly, dry mouth, constipation, blurry vision, sedation, insomnia; risk of serotonin syndrome
Adjuvant: anticonvulsants	Gabapentin, duloxetine, pregabalin, topiramate	Peripheral or central neurogenic	Dizziness, fatigue, ataxia, peripheral edema, dry mouth, weight gain or loss, liver damage
Muscle relaxant	For spasticity: baclofen, dantrolene, and tizanidine For musculoskeletal conditions: carisoprodol, chlorzoxazone, cyclobenzaprine, metaxalone, methocarbamol, and orphenadrine	Muscle spasm or trigger points: FMS, MPS	Dizziness, drowsiness, fatigue, weakness
Weak opiate	Tramadol	Peripheral or central neurogenic	Nausea, constipation, sedation, dizziness, vomiting, pruritus, sexual dysfunction, sleep disturbance, hyperalgesia, tolerance, addiction; risk of serotonin syndrome
Strong opiate	Codeine, hydrocodone, morphine, oxycodone, methadone, fentanyl patch	Peripheral or central neurogenic, cancer pain	Nausea, constipation, sedation, dizziness, vomiting, pruritus, sexual dysfunction, sleep disturbance and hyperalgesia, tolerance, addiction; risk of serotonin syndrome

FMS = fibromyalgia syndrome; MPS = myofascial pain syndrome; NSAID= Nonsteroidal anti-inflammatory; SNRI = serotonin and norepinephrine reuptake inhibitor.

creating warmth sensations, and those with bioactive agents. Those creating cooling sensation, generally menthol-based, work as a counterirritant probably via the gate control mechanism. Those creating the sensation of warmth are generally capsaicin-based. An important aspect of capsaicin-based topical medications is that the counterirritant effect begins immediately after application but the neurogenic effect requires daily use for 6 to 8 weeks. One proposed explanation for the time required is that repeated use of capsaicin depletes nerve endings of substance P; the actual physiology appears to be more complex.[221,222] A variety of NSAIDs can be

administered via topical rubs. Research shows that medication can be absorbed through the skin into muscle, synovium, and joint tissue.[223] Lidocaine cream or patch can be beneficial for peripheral neurogenic pain.[224] Opiates can also be administered topically, but are less commonly used this way.

The benefits and risks of opiate use in managing nonmalignant (i.e., noncancer) chronic pain remain controversial.[15,16,216,218,220,225,226] Although opiates are frequently prescribed for nonmalignant chronic pain, evidence suggests that decreases in pain are small and improvements in quality of life are limited with less functional improvements than with other analgesic medications.[218,220] Furthermore, evidence suggests that opiate use may encourage focus on pain and illness behavior.[226] The potential for both physiological tolerance and addiction makes opiates even more controversial, and careful screening for addictive history or personality is indicated before initiating opiate medication.[15,16,224] Concern is often raised about the safety of people taking opiate medications while performing tasks such as driving; research suggests that risk of car accidents increases when opiates are initiated or when the dose is increased, but not when doses are stable and appropriate.[216] Opiate-induced hyperalgesia, due to changes in receptors or neural circuits, may undermine pain management.[220,226] The incidence of opiate abuse also remains controversial, with current estimates of abuse among patients receiving opiates between 18% and 41%.[226]

An important consideration with all medications is the potential *placebo effect*, the benefit resulting from the patient's belief that the treatment will be successful. The placebo effect appears to be mediated by the brain's reward system, which also mediates some components of chronic pain. The placebo effect is as high as 20% to 40%, depending on the condition for which the medication is given.[227] Interestingly, placebos are more likely to result in decreased pain if they cause side effects.[220] Recent research suggests that the placebo effect can be effective in managing irritable bowel syndrome (another central sensitization condition) even when the subject knows that the medication is a placebo.[228]

Serotonin syndrome (serotonin toxicity) is a potentially dangerous consequence of polypharmacy (use of multiple drugs to treat the same condition) with medications often used to manage chronic pain. The most likely medications involved are SSRIs, SNRIs, TCAs, some opiates, and triptans (used as an abortive medication for migraines) and less obvious medications such as antibiotics.[15,229] Because the condition is potentially lethal, the physical therapist should remain alert for symptoms of serotonin syndrome: agitation, anxiety, confusion, hypomania, hyperthermia, tachycardia, diaphoresis, flushing, mydriasis (prolonged pupil dilation), hyperreflexia, clonus, myoclonus, shivering, tremor, and hypertonia.[229,230]

Interventional Medicine

Interventional medicine includes injections, surgical procedures, and implantable devices (Table 25.8). Several

Table 25.8 Interventional Procedures for Chronic Pain[18]

Procedure	Description	Indication
Joint block	Injection of anesthetic with our without steroids into facets or sacroiliac (SI) joint	Facet or SI pain
Trigger point injection	Botulinum toxin A (botox) injections into trigger points	Myofascial pain syndrome, which may be associate with various other pain syndromes
Nerve block	Injection of anesthetic with our without steroids into peripheral nerve, celiac plexus, paravertebral sympathectomy, medial branch block, stellate ganglion block, cervical paravertebral sympathectomy	Low back pain (LBP) Complex regional pain syndrome (CRPS)
Epidural, intrathecal injections	Steroid injections with or without local anesthetics; opioid injections into intrathecal space	Neck pain, LBP, radiculopathy, postherpetic neuralgia (PHN)
Ablative techniques	Chemical denervation, cryoneurolysis, cryoablation, thermal intradiscal procedures, radiofrequency ablation	Neuropathic, facet, or musculoskeletal pain
Implanted electrical stimulator	Subcutaneous peripheral nerve stimulation and spinal cord stimulation	Peripheral nerve injuries, neuropathic pain, CRPS, failed low back surgery, phantom limb pain, cauda equina injury, radiculopathy, peripheral vascular disease, visceral pain, multiple sclerosis
Implantable drug delivery	Infusion of medication into spinal cord or specific arteries serving involved structures	Cancer, refractory spasticity due to cerebral or spinal cord injury, intractable pain with objective pathology
Minimally invasive spinal procedure	Vertebroplasty, kyphoplasty, percutaneous disc decompression, nucleoplasty	Osteoporotic compression fracture, radiculopathy

CRPS = complex regional pain syndrome; LBP = low back pain; PHN = postherpetic neuralgia; SI = sacroiliac.

reviews of interventional procedures for chronic pain are available and the evidence for effectiveness is summarized in Appendix 25.C.[15,16,18,216,220,231-238]

Injections are most often to the epidural space, nerves, facet joints, or muscles. Joint and nerve blocks are sometimes used diagnostically, to confirm involvement of specific structures. Surgical options are considered only when all other efforts at pain management have failed and there is ongoing, observed pathology perpetuating the pain. Patients need to be carefully selected for permanent surgical procedures. Psychological evaluation should confirm that pain is not perpetuated by psychosocial factors, because these would persist after surgery and result in failed intervention. When possible, a temporary version of the intervention should be implemented first to determine that the surgery would be successful (e.g., guidelines recommend a 1-week trial before permanent implantation of epidural or intrathecal infusion pumps or spinal cord stimulators).[15,18] Injections into nerve, joint, or muscle should be followed with active rehabilitation to take advantage of the time in which pain is reduced or eliminated.[15,16]

■ PHYSICAL THERAPY EXAMINATION

The Therapeutic Relationship

Patient-centered care requires assessing both the illness and the patient's experience of the illness, understanding the patient as a person, and engaging in shared decision making.[212] Patient-centered care therefore requires effective communication and an effective patient–provider relationship. However, the difficulty of managing chronic pain can place significant strain on both patient and provider.

There is a perception among some clinicians that patients with chronic pain are difficult. Indeed, patients with chronic pain may be angry, abusive, demanding, deceitful, or nonadherent or engage in doctor-shopping.[212,239,240] See Box 25.2 for additional chronic pain syndrome behaviors.[3] Understanding the source of these patient behaviors helps clinicians empathize and improves communication. For example, patients may be defensive or hostile because of previous negative interactions with unsupportive medical professionals.[240] Since chronic pain can lack objective findings of a physical cause for the pain, many patients have struggled with not being believed by health care providers.[212,241] The biomedical model divides conditions into exclusively physical or exclusively psychological; since psychosocial factors often exacerbate chronic pain, prior health care providers may have treated patients as though their pain was not real.[242] In the absence of observable pathology, many people with chronic pain have been considered malingerers, liars, hysterics, drug-seekers, or considered to have a purely psychiatric problem.[20] Having struggled to be believed by past providers, patients may arrive in the physical therapy clinic prepared for another fight. Accepting that the patient's pain experience is real can accomplish a great deal in establishing rapport.

Psychological or socioeconomic challenges, sometimes beyond the patient's immediate control, compound difficulties. For example, depression makes it difficult for patients to adhere to their home program. Anxiety or catastrophization leads them to overreact, appearing to "symptom-magnify." Patients may be in the anger phase of the grieving process, grieving for the past life they have lost. Patients who believe in a purely biomedical model may arrive wanting the problem to be "fixed"; such patients may be passive about their care and unwilling to take an active role in pain management.

The effective clinician develops strategies for identifying and dealing with difficult behavior to enhance patient adherence and reduce the chance of frustration and burnout. Strategies to diffuse anger, relieve anxiety, eliminate ambiguity, and maintain appropriate professional boundaries are as important to clinical practice as the skillful application of any treatment technique.[212,239,240,243] Klyman et al[240] provide a useful mnemonic for working effectively with difficult patients, called *GUT REACTIONS*, described in Box 25.5.

Since a high proportion of people with chronic pain have experienced some form of abuse, physical therapists need to be sensitive to the needs of this population, especially given the importance of touch to physical therapy. Survivors of abuse may have difficulty distinguishing symptoms such as fatigue or hunger from distress or

---

Box 25.5   Mnemonic for Managing Difficult Patients: GUT REACTIONS[240]

- **G**: What is your *Gut reaction* to this patient?
- **U**: What can you *Understand* about the patient's feelings?
- **T**: How can your feelings and understanding guide your *Treatment*?
- **R**: Patients often *Regress* when facing illness, pain, and loss.
- **E**: How does the patient's *Environment* affect the condition or situation?
- **A**: *Anxiety* is important and often contagious to caregivers.
- **C**: *Consistency* and *Continuity* are important for effective care.
- **T**: *Tolerant* means listening to the patient's emotions, with their ambiguity, ambivalence, and conflicts.
- **I**: Attentive listening has an important *Influence* on the patient.
- **O**: The *Original* parent–child relationship may influence the patient–provider relationship.
- **N**: The caregiver's *Needs* should not be neglected.
- **S**: *Symptoms* serve a purpose and may have both physical and psychological causes.

pain; they also may have difficulty distinguishing between physical and emotional pain.[82-85,244] Physical therapists working with this population should know how to ask about and respond to revelations of past or present abuse.[82] An appropriate question would be: "Many people with chronic pain have had frightening or painful experiences, sometimes as a child. Has anything like this ever happened to you?" Since patients expect physical therapists to be asking about physical trauma, it may be necessary to clarify that physical, sexual, or emotional trauma in childhood can all contribute to chronic pain as an adult. The physical therapist's response to a revelation is critical to developing a trusting relationship. It should include an acknowledgement that those traumatic experiences are very difficult and can be stressful to live with, even as an adult, and that it takes great courage to talk about such experiences.

Survivors of sexual abuse often become stressed by physical contact needed in physical therapy and clinicians should be sensitive to their special needs. Physical therapists should be aware of strategies for working with survivors of childhood sexual abuse who may present with hypervigilance, anxiety, disempowerment, distrust, somatization, transference, or dissociative reactions.[82-85] Strategies include the following: ensure two-way communication; observe body language; establish positive rapport and a trusting therapeutic relationship; give the patient control and respect boundaries; obtain consent frequently; keep the patient an active participant; pay attention to physical stressors; recognize and respond to triggers; check in with the patient; and try alternative treatment approaches if the patient is uncomfortable.

Health care providers should also take care of their own emotional well-being. Chronic pain is difficult to treat, often leaving both patients and providers unsatisfied with the results. Clinicians may feel frustrated and inadequate, leading to stress and burnout.[212] Even when patient–provider interactions are constructive, the emotional needs of patients with chronic pain can lead to *empathy fatigue* for the clinician, a state of emotional, mental, and physical exhaustion.[245] Stebnicki[245] offers strategies for avoiding empathy fatigue: provide a support system within the facility where clinicians can discuss the stress of working with difficult patients, provide mentoring for new clinicians, encourage support networks outside the workplace, avoid having one clinician treat many difficult patients at one time, and promote education and wellness programs within the clinic or organization.

Subjective Examination

The subjective examination for a patient with chronic pain is based on the nature of the patient's complaints and presentation. A thorough subjective interview is critical for developing a physical therapy diagnosis, understanding the patient's narrative, and developing rapport with the patient.[210] Box 25.6 outlines the examination elements recommended in the *Guide to Physical Therapist Practice*. Questions about the pain should include a description of the pain (e.g., using the SOCRATES mnemonic described in Box 25.3) as well as addressing the emotional and functional consequences of the pain. Multidimensional pain assessment tools provide quantitative baseline data regarding pain severity and impact. The interview should also ask about nonpain signs and symptoms, including motor, sensory, and autonomic changes.[18] Follow-up questions should address psychosocial issues described above, such as abuse history, anxiety, depression, and so forth. Even if using a depression or anxiety assessment tool, verbal questions about these topics may help the patient appreciate the relevance to pain. Questions about the patient's use or abuse of medications, alcohol, or other drugs are also relevant.

Systems Review

The complex nature of chronic pain means that the systems review component of the patient examination is extremely important. Systems review in the *Guide to Physical Therapist Practice* includes cardiovascular/pulmonary, integumentary, musculoskeletal, neuromuscular, and communication components. Cardiovascular screening of vital signs examines whether there are cardiovascular restrictions to aerobic exercise. While measuring respiratory rate, clinicians should observe the breathing pattern, because overuse of accessory breathing muscles can aggravate pain. The integumentary system should be examined, particularly for old injuries or surgeries that could compromise fascial mobility or lymphatic flow. For patients presenting with widespread musculoskeletal pain, musculoskeletal screening should include the *Brighton Score as part of the Brighton Criteria* (Box 25.7) for hypermobility syndrome (also known as Ehlers-Danlos syndrome, hypermobility type).[246,247] Patients with hypermobility syndrome may present with diagnoses of fibromyalgia, myofascial pain syndrome, chronic headaches, or spinal pain; if the underlying hypermobility is not identified and addressed, treatment is more likely to fail.[248] Neuromuscular screening should include balance, locomotion, and transfers. Testing for clonus, hyperreflexia, and hypertonicity is important if there is any suspicion of serotonin syndrome (see section titled Pharmacological Management of Chronic Pain).[230] The communication, affect, cognition, and learning style component of the systems review is particularly important given the psychosocial aspects of chronic pain. Evidence shows that physical therapists are not accurate in determining the presence of depression[143] or fear avoidance[249] based on observation; consequently, screening tools are appropriate components of the systems review.[126-128]

Chronic pain often involves multiple body systems, such as the gastrointestinal system with irritable bowel syndrome or the urinary tract with chronic pelvic pain.[216] Goodman and Snyder[250] provide a comprehensive discussion of review of systems.

Box 25.6   Examination Elements Relevant to Chronic Pain[24]

Documentation of history may include the following:

- General demographics
- Social history
  - Abuse history
  - Other traumatic experience
- Employment/work (job/school/play)
- Growth and development
- Living environment
  - Support system
- General health status (self-report, family report, caregiver report)
  - Psychological health status may include screening tool for:
    - Anxiety disorder
    - Depression
    - Post-traumatic stress disorder
  - Symptoms other than pain, such as dizziness, fatigue, loss of balance, and so forth
  - Sleep disturbance
- Social/health habits (past and current)
  - Exercise habits
  - Use of alcohol or nonprescription drugs
- Family history
- Medical/surgical history
- Current condition(s)/chief complaint(s)
  - Pain assessment addressing all aspects of the pain experience
- Functional status and activity level
  - Self-report of activity or performance restriction
- Medications
- Other clinical tests

Systems Review

- Cardiovascular/pulmonary
  - Breathing pattern: diaphragmatic or chest breathing
- Integumentary
- Musculoskeletal
  - May include Brighton Criteria for hypermobility syndrome
- Neuromuscular
  - Gross mobility and coordination
- Communication, affect, cognition, learning style
  - Current emotional state

Tests and Measures

(Will vary depending on specific presentation and diagnosis)

- Aerobic capacity and endurance:
  - Physical performance measures such as 6-minute walk, 30 second sit-stand

- Anthropometric characteristics
- Arousal, mentation, and cognition
  - Pain beliefs, fear-avoidance beliefs, pain-related readiness to change
- Assistive and adaptive devices
- Circulation (arterial, venous, lymphatic)
  - Lymphedema
- Cranial and peripheral nerve integrity
  - Nerve tests for neurogenic pain, vestibular tests, sensation, including hyperalgesia and allodynia
- Environmental, home, and work (job/school/play) barriers
- Ergonomics and body mechanics
- Gait, locomotion, and balance
  - Balance, balance confidence, Timed Up and Go
- Integumentary integrity
  - Skin temperature, texture or turgor (for autonomic involvement)
- Joint integrity and mobility
  - Any joint disorder contributing nociceptive input
- Motor function
- Muscle performance
  - Including trigger point assessment
- Neuromotor development and sensory integration
  - Proprioception
- Orthotic, protective, and supportive devices
- Pain
  - Pressure point threshold (using an algometer)
  - Trigger point palpation
- Posture
- Prosthetic requirements
- Range of motion
- Reflex integrity
  - Upper motor neuron screens such as Babinski and Hoffmann
- Self-care and home management
- Sensory integrity
  - Proprioception
- Ventilation, respiration, and gas exchange
  - Respiratory pattern
- Work, community, and leisure integration or reintegration

Box 25.7   The 1998 Brighton Criteria
for Hypermobility Syndrome,
or Ehlers-Danlos Syndrome,
Hypermobility Type[247]

The nine points of the Brighton score are assessed if the:

- Elbows hyperextend past 10° (1 point each side)
- Knees hyperextend past 10° (1 point each side)
- The 5th finger metacarpophalangeal joint extends past 90° (1 point each side)
- Thumb apposes to the forearm (1 point each side)
- Hands can be placed flat on the floor while standing with knees straight

Major Criteria

- Brighton score of 4 or more
- Joint pain in 4 or more joints for longer than 3 months

Minor Criteria

- Brighton score of 1–3 (or even 0 if age over 50)
- Pain in 1–3 joints, or back pain, for longer than 3 months
- Joint dislocation
- 3 or more instances of damage to the soft tissues (lesions)
- Exceptionally tall, slim build with unusually long, slender fingers ("Marfanoid habitus")
- Thin or unusually stretchy skin, stretch marks or scarring from minor cuts
- Drooping eyelids, short-sightedness or slanting eyes
- Varicose veins, hernia, or prolapse of the womb (uterus) or rectum

For a diagnosis of hypermobility syndrome to be confirmed, an individual should have:

- 2 major criteria **or**
- 1 major + 2 minor criteria **or**
- 4 minor criteria **or**
- 2 minor criteria + a first-degree relative (parent, child, brother or sister) with confirmed hypermobility.

Tests and Measurements

Body Structure and Function Measures

The specific body structure and function measures needed will be determined by how the patient presents, because each patient with chronic pain has different structural and functional involvement. If the clinician hypothesizes that a specific neuromusculoskeletal condition may be the cause of nociceptive, inflammatory, or peripheral neurogenic pain, the examination should include specific tests and measures for those conditions. For example, a patient with stroke-related pain may have shoulder instability, a patient with diabetic neuropathy may have carpal tunnel syndrome, or a patient with postconcussion headaches may have cervical instability. Patients with systemic pain conditions, such as MS, could have an acute musculoskeletal injury superimposed on the underlying chronic

pain. Therefore, standard musculoskeletal and neurological tests may be appropriate.

On the other hand, not all positive findings indicate tissue damage relevant to that patient's chronic pain. Diagnostic imaging of the lumbar spine, for example, frequently identifies pathological structures even when no pain is present. Multiple computed tomography (CT) and magnetic resonance imaging (MRI) studies show high rates of disk herniation and spinal stenosis in persons without symptoms.[16,213,214] Furthermore, patients with central sensitization may have a positive response to many pain provocation tests due to hyperalgesia and allodynia. The current discussion will not address all the tests and measurements that could be performed, but will outline how testing might be modified for patients with chronic pain.

Palpation for tenderness may be useful for identifying tissue damage, muscle spasm, trigger points, or hyperalgesia and allodynia. Palpation can be quantified through use of an *algometer*, which measures palpation pressure. *Pressure pain threshold (PPT)* is the point at which pressure changes from comfortable pressure to slightly unpleasant pain.[251] The amount of pressure needed to create slightly unpleasant pain is decreased in involved structures. Changes in PPT may also be noted in remote sites, such as over the tibialis anterior in patients with neck pain. Decreased PPT at remote sites is an indication of hyperalgesia, providing evidence of central sensitization and predicting a poorer outcome.[252,253] Allodynia can be examined with light brushing or by using test tubes filled with cold and hot (40°C) water for thermal allodynia. Mechanical hyperalgesia or temporal summation can be examined with a dull needle or von Frey filaments.[174,181,189]

Many widespread pain complaints are associated with myofascial trigger points.[16,61,254] *Trigger points (TrPs)* are defined as ropelike taut bands within a muscle fiber. Palpation may elicit local tenderness or referral along the pattern specific for that muscle. To elicit the referred pain pattern associated with trigger points, pressure needs to be maintained for at least 10 seconds or only local tenderness will be detected.[255] Palpation of a TrP may elicit a local twitch response, a transient contraction of the muscle fiber, or a *jump response*, which is patient vocalization or withdrawal from the palpation. An *active TrP* exists when the patient reports spontaneous local or referred pain for that TrP. A *latent TrP* exists when local or referred pain is only elicited with palpation.[255,256]

An examination of balance and proprioception is often indicated because the primary injury or disease, deconditioning, and/or fear of movement may compromise balance.[257-265] Chronic pain has been associated with balance impairments and increased risk of falls among the elderly and even near-falls can exacerbate pain conditions by straining muscles. The specific choice of balance test depends on the patient (see Chapter 6, Examination of Coordination and Balance, for a discussion of balance tests). Some patients will have difficulty with a basic Romberg test, whereas others will have no difficulty completing the Berg Balance Scale. Proprioception and motor control deficits perpetuate microtrauma and macrotrauma and pain. For example, post-stroke shoulder pain is associated with impaired proprioception,[261] and cervical joint position sense is compromised in patients with chronic neck pain.[262,263,265] Joint position sense can be examined using traditional tests for proprioceptive awareness (see Chapter 3, Examination of Sensory Function), a goniometer, or a laser pointer.[266,267]

Activity and Participation Measures

Activity limitations can be examined through either self-report or performance measures. Self-report of activity limitations may be nonspecific, disease specific, or customized for the patient. Activities commonly affected by chronic pain include physical functions such as walking, mobility, changing or maintaining body position, toileting, preparing meals, and doing housework. Activity limitation due to chronic pain may also include difficulty focusing attention or handling stress and other psychological demands (see Table 25.1).[23,25-28] Quantification of activity limitations or participation restrictions, independent of symptoms, allows the therapist to develop appropriate goals and outcomes when pain and other symptoms are not likely to resolve with intervention.[16] These tools may also be used to gather information about the impact that secondary problems, such as deconditioning, fatigue, sleep disturbance, or fear of movement, have on a patient's ability to participate in life situations. Many tools include separate sections for symptoms, activity, and participation components. For example, the *Revised Fibromyalgia Impact Questionnaire* (FIQR) has one section for symptoms, one section for activity restrictions, and one for the affective consequences of the illness.[268] Activity and quality-of-life tools should be culturally appropriate; the FIQR, for example, emphasizes housekeeping tasks that are generally less relevant for men. Ideally, tools should examine ability to perform activities without reference to pain, because the belief that activity should be discontinued with increased pain is counterproductive for people with chronic pain. The *Oswestry Low Back Pain Disability Questionnaire,* for example, asks how much each activity is restricted by pain, resulting in an examination of pain more than an examination of function or activity level. The *Patient-Specific Functional Scale (PSFS)* allows patients to identify specific functional activities of personal importance affected by their pain condition.[269] The PSFS is particularly helpful in identifying several key outcomes for a patient whose presentation may otherwise be somewhat overwhelming to the clinician. In some patients, symptoms other than pain can limit activity. For example, impaired balance is common among people with fibromyalgia; the *Activity-Specific Balance Confidence Scale (ABC)* can be used as a self-report tool for balance confidence.[270]

For patients with widespread pain, physical activity measures can assess multiple body regions with one test. For example, the *30-Second Sit-to-Stand Test, Timed Up and Go*, and *10-Meter Walk Test* are efficient ways to assess functional lower extremity (LE) strength and balance. Combined performance tests such as the *Short Physical Performance Battery* (SPPB), which combines sit-to-stand transitions, balance, and walking velocity, reflect activity and predict participation restrictions.[271,272] Although the SPPB was designed for the elderly, it provides an appropriate level of challenge for many adults with chronic pain. Formal functional capacity evaluations can be useful for establishing a person's physical work capability.[215] Chronic pain is often associated with deconditioning, which exacerbates activity and participation restrictions.[273] A 2- or 6-minute walk test can provide valuable information about endurance and willingness to exercise, as well as activity tolerance.

Chronic pain leads to participation restrictions such as impaired family relationships, inability to engage in employment, and compromised intimate relationships.[26] Participation restrictions are often included in self-assessment tools, either the multifactorial pain assessment or the activity assessment tools described above.

■ PHYSICAL THERAPY EVALUATION, DIAGNOSIS, AND PROGNOSIS

Evaluation

According to the *Guide to Physical Therapist Practice*, evaluation is a dynamic process integrating subjective and objective examination data to make clinical judgments.[24] One of the first clinical judgments in the evaluation of a patient with chronic pain is the identification of factors leading to, perpetuating, or exacerbating the pain. The ICF model identifies personal and environmental contextual factors that can affect body function or structure, activity, or participation. Personal factors contributing to chronic pain include age, gender, heredity, past and present experience, occupation, education, personality, coping strategies, and social or cultural background. Personal factors include such traits as anxiety, fear-avoidance, catastrophizing, depression, and low patient motivation. These traits may also be characterized as body function involvement (global psychosocial functions) in the ICF model (see Table 25.1).

Many contributing factors, such as age, gender, and heredity, are nonmodifiable. Personal history factors may also contribute to the patient's complaints; for example, PTSD or a history of childhood abuse is common among people with chronic pain conditions. It is important to realize that traumatic personal history not only contributes to psychological distress and maladaptive behaviors that exacerbate pain, but also changes the CNS to perpetuate chronic pain.[74,78,86,274,275] Just as a myocardial infarction caused by stress is just as real as any other myocardial infarction, chronic pain caused by distress or prior traumatic experiences is just as real as any other chronic pain. Whatever factors may contribute to a given patients' chronic pain, it is important for health care providers to acknowledge that chronic pain has multiple contributing factors and affects the whole patient.[16]

Possible outcomes of the evaluation process may be referral to or consultation with another practitioner either instead of or in combination with physical therapy intervention. Yellow flags, suggesting psychosocial factors, were discussed under Psychosocial Factors Associated with Chronic Pain in a previous section of this chapter. Examples of red flags suggesting systemic involvement include personal or family history of cancer, recent infection, significant weight change without effort, pain unrelieved by rest or change in position, inability to relieve or provoke symptoms during the examination, night pain, pain in a visceral referral pattern, and certain associated signs and symptoms.[250] Readers are referred to Goodman and Snyder's *Differential Diagnosis for Physical Therapists* for an extensive discussion of how to screen for red flags.[250] Each patient's situation should be examined individually because many people with chronic pain have one or more red or yellow flags that may be readily explained, do not require referral, and do not interfere with physical therapy. However, multiple yellow or red flags should lead the physical therapist to consider whether referral to another health care provider is indicated, and whether that referral should occur at the same time as or instead of physical therapy intervention.[250] The judgment about who needs to be referred can be difficult with patients who have chronic pain, because they may have many yellow and red flags. When in doubt, the referring physician should be contacted to discuss these findings.

Chronic pain is often poorly correlated to physical findings; therefore, body structure and function findings are often consequences of chronic pain rather than causes. For example, CRPS is often associated with edema, autonomic signs, atrophy, and weakness resulting from the pain. Edema, in this case, would not be an indicator of local inflammation but related to disuse and sympathetic dysfunction. The physical therapist may therefore identify patient-nonspecific problems such as generalized weakness, decreased ROM, poor cardiovascular fitness, decreased function, and so forth.

Diagnosis

According to the *Guide to Physical Therapist Practice*, diagnosis is the process of integrating examination and evaluation information to develop a prognosis, plan of care, and intervention strategies. There are several different ways in which the physical therapist may need to categorize patients with pain. First, is the pain acute, persistent, or chronic? Is the pain nociceptive, inflammatory, peripheral neurogenic, or central neurogenic? Is the patient's presentation consistent with a defined syndrome? Identifying pathological or anatomical causes for the chronic pain is occasionally helpful, but often is not possible, and should not be the overriding emphasis of the diagnostic process. Acute conditions

superimposed on and aggravating underlying chronic pain can and should be identified.[216]

Chronic pain often occurs in the absence of observed tissue injury or damage or when the amount of pain is not proportional to the observed tissue injury or damage. Acute or persistent pain may become chronic if peripheral or central sensitization occurs. In the case of patients with a 3-month or more history of pain, the physical therapist needs to decide whether the pain is truly chronic in the sense that it occurs in the absence of observed tissue injury or damage, or whether it is persistent but the causes have not been identified or addressed.[216] Persistent causes for acute and subacute pain must therefore be sought and identified. For example, a patient may have daily pain due to lumbar segmental instability, myofascial trigger points, or OA. In cases of persistent peripheral pain without central or peripheral sensitization, evaluation should identify the factors contributing to tissue damage and impeding healing. In lumbar instability, poor motor control is a modifiable contributing factor. The causes of isolated myofascial trigger points may be eliminated through patient education regarding body mechanics and the existing trigger points resolved through exercise or manual therapy. Although the underlying OA cannot be modified by physical therapy, the pain and activity limitations can be managed to minimize the patient's activity and participation restrictions. Persistent pain can be resolved or managed to the extent that the physiological, personal, and environmental contributing factors can be addressed and the tissue can heal.

Neurogenic pain can also be persistent or chronic. In cases where the nerve damage is reversible, neurogenic pain is similar to other forms of persistent pain. For example, mild carpal tunnel syndrome (with neuropraxia) can be managed to the extent that the contributing factors can be addressed and healing facilitated. Other forms of neurogenic pain, such as diabetic neuropathy or that associated with MS, involve permanent damage to neural tissue and, like the example of OA, can be managed to minimize the patient's activity limitations and participation restrictions. In cases where persistent musculoskeletal or neurogenic pain cannot be resolved, many of the intervention strategies for chronic pain can be beneficial.

A second decision the physical therapist needs to make in the diagnostic process is categorization of the type or types of pain: nociceptive, inflammatory, peripheral neurogenic, or central. Knowing the type of pain assists in determining prognosis, plan of care (POC), and intervention. For example, central pain generally has a poorer prognosis because the changes in the CNS are difficult or impossible to reverse and central sensitization is more likely to be self-perpetuated through psychosocial factors that lie outside the physical therapist's control. Patients may have multiple types of pain and the relative intensity of different types of pain may vary from day to day. For example, people with a central pain condition such as migraine often also have myofascial trigger points provoking nociceptive pain. A flare of nociceptive myofascial pain may trigger a migraine and amplify central sensitization, which will further amplify nociceptive pain. Recognizing both components of pain improves the likelihood that intervention will be successful.[16,216] The discussion of common forms of chronic pain, earlier in the chapter, describes the types of pain occurring in various common conditions.

Prognosis

Prognosis determines "the level of optimal improvement that may be attained through intervention and the required amount of time required to reach that level"[24, p S682] Prognosis depends on personal and environmental factors identified in the evaluation process. Table 25.9 shows a variety of factors relevant for chronic pain that affect prognosis.[26-28] For example, yellow flags are associated with poorer prognosis in chronic LBP. Although some of these personal factors will compromise prognosis, others may be beneficial to the patient. For example, medical co-morbidities, anxiety, or a history of sexual abuse compromise prognosis, whereas a record of regular exercise, adequate stress management strategies, and good emotional function lead to an improved prognosis.

Pain readiness to change is a personal characteristic that is also related to prognosis. As with other forms of readiness to change based on the *Transtheoretical Model of Behavior Change*, individuals who are ready to change are more likely to incorporate pain management strategies into their lives, hence their prognosis is better. Patients resistant to change are unlikely to be compliant with rehabilitation and are less likely to benefit.[139,140,276]

Table 25.9	Environmental Contextual Factors Affecting Prognosis, Using ICF Terminology[25-27]
ICF Code	**ICF Category Title**
E355	Health professionals
E410, E425, E430	Attitudes of family, friends, colleagues, community
E450, E455	Attitudes of health and health-related professionals
E460, E570,	Social attitudes, services, and policies
E575	General social support services, systems, and policies
E580	Health services, systems, and policies
E590	Labor and employment services, systems, and policies
E540	Transportation services, systems, and policies
E135	Products and technology for employment
E155	Design and construction of buildings

Two tools for examining pain-related readiness to change are described in Table 25.4. Environmental factors such as having a support system, attitudes of friends and family, or access to comprehensive health care all affect prognosis. Table 25.9 lists a number of environmental factors relevant to chronic pain.[26-28]

Treatment goals for patients with chronic pain should deemphasize pain reduction and instead focus on restoration of activity and participation through self-management. Box 25.8 includes a range of general anticipated goals and expected outcomes for the patient with chronic pain. Studies show that activity and participation restrictions are often related more to fear-avoidance and deconditioning than to pain.[15,16] Functional restoration requires a biopsychosocial treatment approach emphasizing a supportive process for transferring to the patient primary responsibility for his or her physical and emotional well-being; independent long-term management is the primary desired outcome.[15] The Institute for Clinical Systems Improvement (ICSI) Chronic Pain Guidelines recommend five components to the goals: increased function, increased physical activity, stress management, improved sleep, and decreased pain.[16]

■ PHYSICAL THERAPY MANAGEMENT OF CHRONIC PAIN

The Multidisciplinary Pain Management Team

The principles of chronic pain management include a range of physical, psychological, vocational, and medical objectives (Box 25.9). The physical therapist's role in management of chronic pain depends on both the patient and the environment in which the therapist practices. Figure 25.4 shows the general progression of interventions from least invasive (e.g., independent exercise and over-the-counter medications) to most invasive (e.g., surgical interventions such as neuroablation, implanted spinal analgesia or stimulator). The specific order of implementation may vary based on patient preference; for example, some patients may prefer cognitive approaches to physical therapy or may prefer both physical therapy and cognitive-behavioral therapy (CBT) over medication use. A multidisciplinary pain management team may include any of the following health professionals: primary care physician, pain specialist, physiatrist, anesthesiologist, psychiatrist, psychologist, pharmacist, social worker, caseworker, physical therapist, occupational therapist, sleep specialist, or nurse.[2,277] Although multidisciplinary care has been shown to be more effective than monotherapy or standard medical care, the optimal components of multidisciplinary care have not been identified,[277] and the cost-effectiveness has been questioned.[278]

A physical therapist working within a multidisciplinary pain clinic may be able to refer psychological issues

Box 25.8   Anticipated Goals and Expected Outcomes

Impact of pathology/pathophysiology is reduced.

• Patient/client, family, and caregiver knowledge and awareness of the disease, prognosis, and plan of care are enhanced.
• Symptom management is enhanced.
• Risk of secondary impairment is reduced.
• Intensity of care is reduced.

Impact of restrictions due to body structure and function is reduced.

• Balance is improved.
• Endurance is increased.
• Joint integrity and mobility are improved.
• Motor function is improved.
• Muscle performance (strength, power, and endurance) is increased.
• Postural control is improved.
• Quality and quantity of movement between and across body segments are improved.
• Range of motion is improved.
• Relaxation is increased.
• Sensory awareness is increased.
• Pain is decreased.

Activity and participation restrictions are reduced.

• Functional independence in activities of daily living (ADL) and instrumental activities of daily living (IADL) is increased.
• Physical function is improved.
• Disability associated with chronic illnesses is reduced.
• Performance levels in self-care, home management, work (job/school/play), community, or leisure actions, tasks, or activities are improved.

Decision making regarding self-management is enhanced.

• Decision making is enhanced regarding health, wellness, and fitness needs.
• Decision making is enhanced regarding patient/client health and the use of health care resources by patient/client, family, significant others, and caregivers.
• Awareness and use of community resources are improved.
• Behaviors that foster healthy habits, wellness, and prevention are acquired.
• Decision making is enhanced regarding patient/client health and the use of health care resources by patient/client, family, significant others, and caregivers.
• Patient/client knowledge of personal and environmental factors associated with the condition is increased.
• Self-management of symptoms is improved.
• Utilization and cost of health care services are decreased.

Health status and quality of life are improved.

• Health status is improved.
• Risk of recurrence of condition is reduced.
• Safety of patient/client, family, significant others, and caregivers is improved.

Patient/client satisfaction is enhanced.

• Access to and availability of services are acceptable to patient/client and family.
• Quality of rehabilitation services is acceptable to patient/client and family.
• Care is coordinated with patient/client, family, caregivers, and other professionals.
• Patient/client and family feel care is compassionate.

Box 25.9   General Principles of Chronic Pain Management[3]

- Improve ability to cope with pain
- Teach nonpharmacological pain management techniques
- Increase physical strength, endurance, and cardiovascular fitness
- Increase mobility, independence, and functional activity
- Improve sleep
- Teach proper body mechanics
- Increase social and recreational activities
- Improve mood and cognitive function
- Decrease or eliminate dependence on medications
- Decrease overutilization of the health care system
- Improve psychological and emotional well-being
- Enhance vocational potential
- Provide vocational rehabilitation for paid work, volunteer work, and hobbies
- Enhance family communication and function

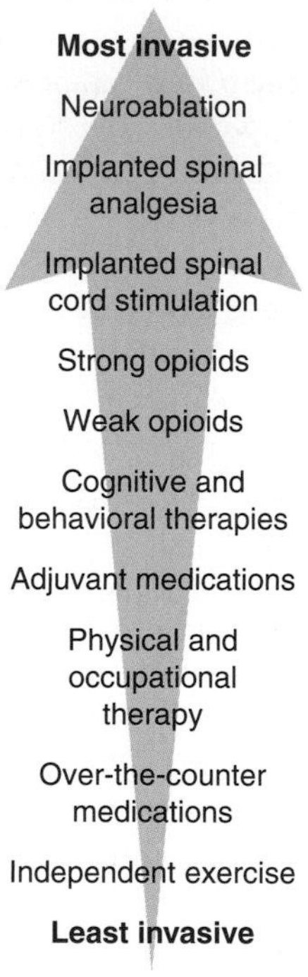

Most invasive

Neuroablation

Implanted spinal analgesia

Implanted spinal cord stimulation

Strong opioids

Weak opioids

Cognitive and behavioral therapies

Adjuvant medications

Physical and occupational therapy

Over-the-counter medications

Independent exercise

Least invasive

Figure 25.4 The pain management continuum starts with independent exercise, progresses to over-the-counter medications, physical or occupational therapy, cognitive-behavioral therapy, prescription medications, and medical (interventional) procedures. The order of intervention may change based on the patient's preference.

---

to the team psychologist and coping skills to the occupational therapist.[35] However, a therapist working in an isolated outpatient clinic might not have access to such collaborations and may need to integrate a broader range of components into the POC while remaining within his or her scope of practice. The following discussion emphasizes what may benefit patients with chronic pain; who provides a given service will depend on the context. In cases when multidisciplinary or specialist care is not available or practical, motivated patients may be able to pursue some aspects of their care independently. Appendix 25.D provides a sample personal care plan for chronic pain self-management.[16] Appendices 25.E and 25.F provide a list of resources for patients interested in taking responsibility for some aspects of their pain management program.

Note that some aspects of pain management, such as relaxation, are applicable to most patients with chronic pain, whereas other approaches are most appropriate for certain pain problems; for example, thermal biofeedback is well suited for migraines whereas stretching is appropriate for myofascial pain. The general principles of chronic pain management need to be adapted to the needs, preferences, and restrictions of any given patient. Appendix 25.C presents a summary of reviews of various chronic pain interventions.

Collaboration, Communication, and Documentation

Patients with chronic pain often have involvement of multiple body systems and may be working with several health care providers. Coordination of care and communication with other providers is essential to a comprehensive, patient-centered approach. It is especially important that the patient receive consistent information from providers regarding such things as the fact that there might not be current tissue damage other than that due to deconditioning, and the need to maintain activity in spite of pain. All providers should be consistent about encouraging functional goals rather than using pain ratings as a guide of treatment success.[216] Patients may need to be referred for consultation with other providers. Some referrals, such as to a psychologist or pain specialist, are obvious. Other potential referrals include a sleep clinic for patients suspected of having a sleep disturbance; occupational therapy for patients with trouble problem solving or managing their medical appointments; relationship counseling for patients whose relationships are stressed by chronic pain; and nutritional counseling, especially for patients whose obesity exacerbates their pain.

Patient/Client-Related Instruction

Patient/client-related instruction is critical when considering chronic pain as a chronic disease that the patient must learn to manage. For the current discussion, the *Guide to Physical Therapist Practice* categories of Functional Training in Self-Care and Home Management and in Work, Community, and Leisure are combined with Patient-Related Instruction because so much of the content overlaps. The physical therapist should identify potential learning barriers such as difficulty concentrating, depression, or refusal to accept a biopsychosocial model of pain, or lack of readiness to change. The family may also require education about chronic pain to both recognize chronic pain as a real disease and to avoid fostering illness behavior in the patient. Box 25.10 identifies several components of patient and family education.

Patients need to understand what types of pain they have to most effectively manage their pain. For example, persistent pain due to OA requires joint protection strategies such as limiting painful activity whereas central sensitization pain requires that patients be encouraged to push through pain. An understanding of the nature of chronic pain and the dissociation between pain and tissue injury or damage helps patients appreciate that (1) hurt does not always mean harm; and (2) there may be no physical damage that surgery or medication can fix.[22,279] Patients need to understand the relationship between mind and body so they do not become defensive about suggestions of psychological management approaches.[216] While some patients will have qualified health providers helping them through the many psychosocial factors associated with chronic pain, many patients will benefit from the many excellent educational resources available.

Box 25.10   Goals of Educational Components of Chronic Pain Management[16]

The goals of patient education are for the patient to:

- Acknowledge that chronic pain is real
- Recognize the complex, biopsychosocial nature of pain, and need for multifaceted management program in which the patient is an active participant
- Understand the impact of pain on sleep, mood, energy, fitness, ability to work, family life, and stress
- Avoid letting pain guide activity or medication use because pain-based treatment encourages pain behavior
- Recognize and utilize wellness behaviors
- Recognize the role of poor posture and body mechanics in perpetuating pain
- Overcome fear of movement through gradual exposure to feared activities
- Learn relaxation strategies
- Actively participate in own management program
- Enlist family support and participation in management program
- Participate in an exercise program, either through physical therapy, independently, or using community resources
- Minimize fear of movement and activity reduction due to fear of movement

---

Appendix 25.F provides a selected list of books to educate patients about issues ranging from pain physiology to maintaining intimacy in the presence of chronic pain. Web-based resources for clinicians, families, and patients with chronic pain can be found in Appendix 25.E.

Self-care training in all environments is critical to effective management of chronic pain (Fig. 25.5).[280] A sample personal care plan is shown in Appendix 25.D. This personal care plan combines goals with patient responsibilities for self-care, including physical therapy, independent exercise, stress management, and sleep hygiene; medications may be included as part of the self-care program. All patients should recognize the role of poor posture and body mechanics in perpetuating pain syndromes.

Since focus on pain and pain reduction causes individuals to become hypervigilant, patients, families, and health care providers need to deemphasize pain severity as a measure of status. Patients should therefore set functional goals that emphasize coping skills and wellness behavior rather than pain-based goals.[35] Graded activity should be performance rather than pain based, reassuring patients that "hurt" does not always lead to "harm" to overcome the fear-avoidance belief.[3,16,22,279] The *Patient-Specific Functional Score* encourages patients to identify and track personally relevant functional goals.[281]

People with chronic pain often need to be encouraged to return to previously enjoyable recreational activities. Some patients feel that they hurt too much to participate in leisure activity or that they should not indulge in pleasurable activities if they are unable to perform "necessary" tasks such as work or home care. Losing pleasurable activities, however, aggravates depression, loss of social life associated with those activities, and deconditioning. Consequently, people with chronic pain may need to schedule leisure and recreational activities and set specific goals including such activities.

Since sleep disturbance is a common occurrence in chronic pain, patients should be educated in proper sleep hygiene. Basic sleep hygiene involves avoiding caffeine, nicotine, alcohol, and medications containing stimulants, especially before bedtime. Sleep hours should be consistent; environmental distractions such as light, noise, and cold should be minimized; stress should be minimized through relaxation or meditation activities. Exercise generally improves quality of sleep, as long as vigorous exercise is avoided within 4 hours of bedtime. Gentle exercises such as stretching, yoga, Qigong, or Tai Chi may improve quality of sleep.[3,50,282-286]

Patients need to understand that stress contributes directly to pain; some patients will be relieved to realize that sympathetic efferents connect directly to nociceptive afferents and the pain-amplifying effects of stress are not all "in their minds."[49] Relaxation can thus decrease pain through reducing nervous system tone, muscle activity, and neuroendocrine reactivity.[14,50] Relaxation techniques include diaphragmatic breathing, biofeedback, progressive

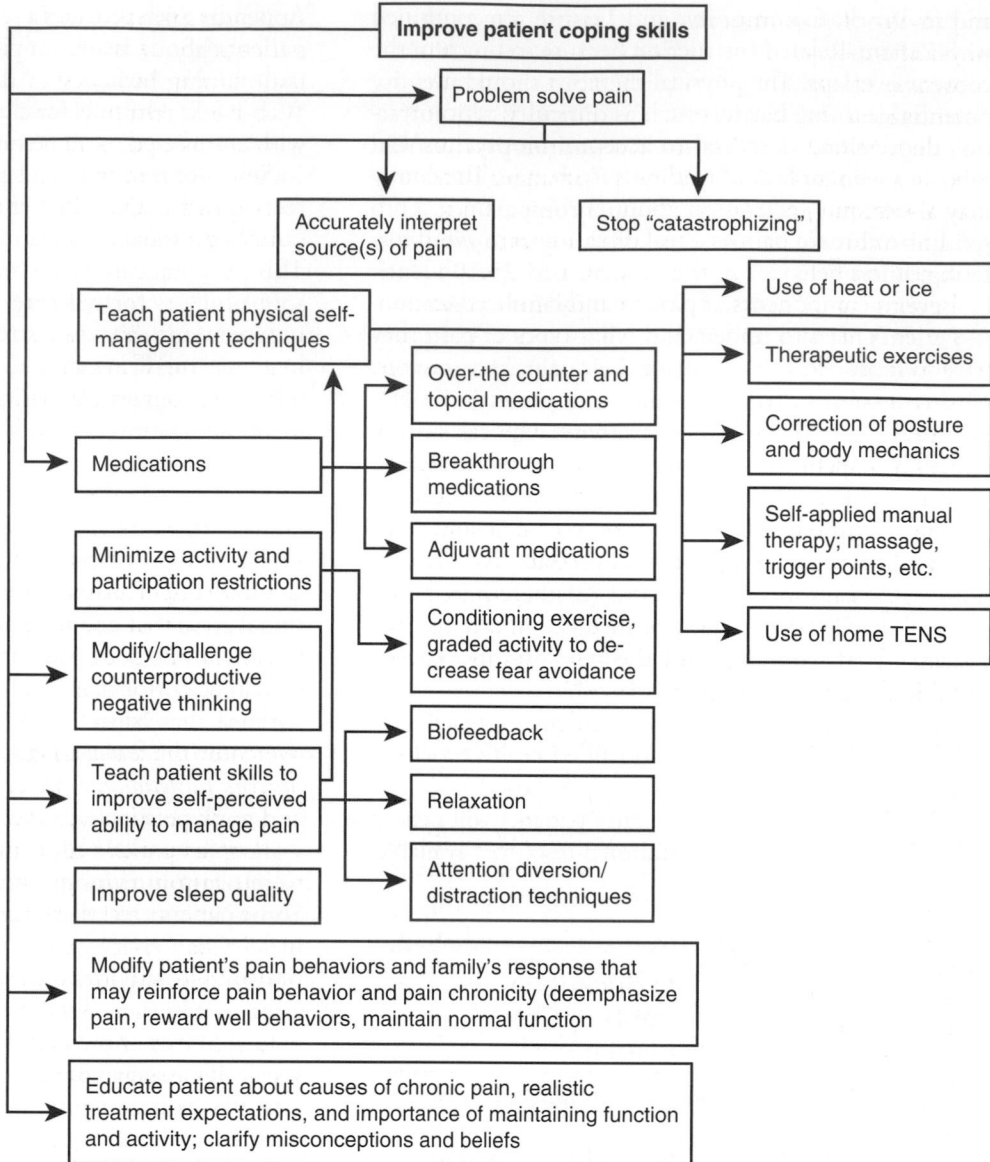

Figure 25.5 Behavioral management of chronic pain. Patients should be educated so that they recognize the various cognitive and behavioral strategies they can use to manage their pain. *Adapted from Mueller, 2000, who proposed a similar model for behavioral management of chronic headaches. Mueller, L: Psychologic aspects of chronic headache. J Am Osteopath Assoc 100(9 Suppl):S14, 2000.*

relaxation, stretching, aerobic exercise, imagery, autogenic training (imagining warmth or heaviness of the limbs), yoga, and meditation.[16] Biofeedback will be discussed below in the section titled Neuromuscular Reeducation under Procedural Interventions. Mindfulness meditation has been successful for managing stress-related diseases such as heart disease and chronic pain. Mindfulness and acceptance-based meditation uses focus on the present moment, attending to thoughts, emotions, sensations, and perceptions without judgment.[16,287-289] The acceptance aspect of mindfulness meditation helps patients differentiate between pain sensations and suffering, hence

improves coping. Appendix 25.E includes several patient resources for learning mindfulness meditation.

Physiological quieting and self-regulation use relaxation training for both physiological and psychological regulation to correct some of the autonomic and neural dysfunctions associated with chronic pain. Although developed for TMJ pain, the principles are generally applicable to other forms of stress-related pain. Self-regulation training includes (1) education and reassurance, (2) strategies to monitor and reduce abnormal muscle function, (3) proprioceptive awareness training, (4) postural relaxation training, (5) diaphragmatic breathing, (6) methods of improving sleep onset, and (7) instruction regarding physical activity, diet, and fluid intake.[14] Hulme[290] recommends a similar self-regulating program for fibromyalgia, emphasizing sleep routine, physiological quieting, nutrition, exercise, medication, positive self-talk, rest/work cycles, pacing/prioritizing, dressing, modalities, and journaling. Hulme's compact disc (CD) guiding individuals through physiological quieting is included in the Resources for Patients in Appendix 25.F.

Patients may benefit from *cognitive-behavioral therapy (CBT)* in which beliefs, attitudes, and behaviors are modified to alter the experience of pain, overcome fear-avoidance, improve function, and minimize disability.[16,35,232,233,291] Beissner et al[291] propose that some CBT techniques lie within the scope of physical therapy practice because therapists already educate patients about relaxation strategies, graded activity, pacing, and identification of counterproductive thought patterns.[14] For therapists working with children, von Baeyer and Tupper[292] present behavioral approaches specifically for working with children. Components of CBT include the following:[14,16,35,291,293]

- Education about the nature of chronic pain, that it might not be associated with damaged tissue, and the importance of self-management.
- Education regarding the impact that cognition (thoughts, beliefs, and behaviors), emotions (fear of pain), and behaviors (activity avoidance due to fear of pain) have on the pain experience. Patients need to accept that self-management includes psychological as well as physical aspects of pain and this does not mean the pain is purely psychological.
- Behavioral activities to improve function, such as activity pacing, pleasurable activity scheduling, relaxation training, diversion, biofeedback, functional restoration, graded activity, and goal setting.
- Cognitive activities to improve responses to pain, such as cognitive restructuring and problem solving. For example, patients could identify and challenge spontaneous thoughts leading to negative emotions and substitute positive coping strategies. Problem solving can overcome barriers such as those associated with regular exercise. Building new narratives based on healthy perceptions can modify abnormal cognitive processes seen in chronic pain and some associated disorders, such as PTSD.[78]
- Development of maintenance strategies to manage pain flares, anticipate future problems, ensure adherence, and progression of exercises and self-care.

Many aspects of CBT are naturally integrated into the POC, such as graded exercise, pacing, problem solving, and functional restoration.[294] For physical therapists unfamiliar with CBT, Rundell and Davenport[293] provide a case report demonstrating the integration of CBT into management of a patient with chronic LBP.

Evidence suggests that CBT strategies can modify several yellow flags associated with disability in chronic pain such as pain beliefs, self-efficacy, and psychological distress.[147,294] Although formal instruction in CBT strategies is preferred, patients may also learn many strategies independently using one of the self-help resources listed in Appendix 25.E. Figure 25.5 shows how a variety of behavioral tools can be integrated into self-management of pain.

Self-care strategies may include a variety of self-applied techniques such as heat, ice, massage, topical rubs, or TENS. Although research into the benefit of TENS for chronic pain remains inconclusive, practice guidelines recommend use of TENS if it increases patient function and activity or decreases need for medications.[15,16,295] Other self-care devices may include home lumbar or cervical traction units, paraffin, or hot tubs. Patients with trigger points may benefit from a trigger point cane or tennis balls in a sock to treat persistent trigger points. Several books listed in Appendix 25.F can be helpful for patients managing multiple and variable trigger points. Patients should understand that the purpose of decreasing pain is to increase function; they should not develop a passive approach limited to pain reduction.

Family and/or caregiver education can be just as important as patient education. Chronic pain affects the whole family through changes in family roles due to the patient's activity and participation restrictions. The family may reinforce the patient's "sick role" in an attempt to be supportive. Both the patient and the family need to understand the importance of maintaining normal activities and participation to minimize disability; patients must not perceive lack of physical assistance as lack of support or concern from family. In contrast, the family may be completely unsupportive, often owing to lack of objective evidence that the pain is real. Family members may be angry with the individual with pain and may blame that individual for financial, personal, or family problems.[3,296]

Personal intimacy is often very difficult with chronic pain, just as it is for other chronic injuries or diseases. Problems may be due to the pain, deconditioning and fatigue, depression, decreased sense of self-worth, or adverse reactions of medications. Distress is often greater for survivors of childhood sexual abuse.[297] It is important that both partners learn about chronic pain so that they understand the reasons for challenges faced. Both partners need to accept that the nature of the intimate relationship can change and not harbor anger, frustration, blame, or guilt. Individuals with chronic pain can improve their self-image through daily exercise, grooming, and cognitive strategies of CBT. Communication is critical so that both partners can contribute suggestions for problem solving. For example, select a time of day with the least amount of pain and fatigue and find positions that minimize stress to the body. Appendix 25.E includes several patient resources for working through the challenges of intimacy with chronic pain.

Procedural Interventions

Therapeutic Exercise

Therapeutic exercise is a key part of chronic pain management.[3,15,16,216] Exercise is associated with decreased pain complaints and protection from future development of pain among individuals with PTSD.[78] Graded exercise directed at decreasing fear-avoidance can overcome the poor prognosis associated with the behavior.[89] Postural exercises to improve posture and body mechanics, as well as to decrease muscular imbalances, help decrease chronic stress on musculoskeletal structures. Aerobic conditioning improves function through counteracting deconditioning that typically occurs as people with chronic pain become sedentary.[3,15,16] Function-based exercises improve tolerance for functional activity. Overall, no one type of exercise (e.g., aerobic, strengthening, stretching, balance, aquatic) is superior to others. Individual patients may tolerate and respond to some forms of exercise better than others. For example, individuals with OA or fibromyalgia are likely to respond well to aquatic therapy in a (warm) therapeutic pool.[15,16]

Since falls and sensory motor problems are more common among individuals with chronic pain,[257-265] balance and proprioceptive training are often important components of the exercise program. A great variety of balance-improving exercises can be integrated into the program. Joint position sense can be both tested and trained using a goniometer or laser pointer.[265-267] For example, in the cervical spine, a laser pointer attached to the patient's eyeglasses or to a plastic hair band can be aimed at a target; patients may practice accurate repositioning or fine motor coordination while tracking shapes. Since proprioceptive information from the cervical spine is integrated with visual and vestibular input, eye and vestibular exercises can be beneficial in conditions involving the cervical spine.[263]

Graded exercise should begin at a level the patient can perform and then gradually increased. Patients need to recognize that some soreness and discomfort is typical and to be expected when beginning an exercise program. They should be reminded that hurt does not always indicate harm or tissue damage. People with chronic pain often have trouble distinguishing psychological distress from physical pain, so they need guidance distinguishing fear of movement from actual pain. Proprioceptive and motor control impairments can affect the ability of people with chronic pain to perform exercises correctly, so repeated feedback during exercise instruction can maximize safety and success. Kinesiophobia can be reduced if early efforts at exercise are successful.[89] Specific performance-based targets can prevent overly enthusiastic patients from overdoing their exercise.

Patients will be most motivated if exercises relate directly to functional goals. For example, a patient who wants to go to the movies with his wife could follow an exercise program designed to overcome his specific obstacles, such as walking from the car to the theater and sitting comfortably through the movie. Exercises with a social component help address isolation often experienced by people with chronic pain; for example, group exercise programs, active family involvement, or dancing can make exercise more enjoyable.

Certain chronic pain conditions respond to specific types of exercise or neuromuscular reeducation. For example, phantom limb, CRPS, dystonia, and stroke are typically associated with changes in sensory and motor mapping in the sensorimotor cortex. In these cases, sensory input through use of a myoelectric prosthesis, virtual reality or mirror training, or sensory discrimination training stimulates cortical reorganization that is generally associated with decreased pain.[216,298,299]

Manual Therapy

Manual therapy may be beneficial in the case of persistent pain with ongoing nociceptive input or in cases where central sensitization is perpetuated by peripheral nociceptive input.[15,16,300] Manual therapy may resolve a transient flare of central sensitization, and thus decrease other symptoms of central sensitization such as hyperalgesia and anxiety.[301] A recent systematic review concluded that manual therapy including manipulation and muscle energy techniques appears to be effective for chronic LBP and knee pain; however, the evidence was weak for other manual therapies (Swedish massage, Feldenkrais, and reflexology) and other sources of chronic pain (fibromyalgia and neck pain).[302] However, this does not confirm that manual therapy is ineffective in other forms of pain.[236] Because manual therapy is unlikely to alleviate the pain completely and there is a risk of patients becoming dependent on it, use of passive manual therapy modalities should be limited. Using massage and trigger point management as maintenance therapy may be part of the patient's self-care program.[15,16]

Neuromuscular Reeducation

Neuromuscular reeducation using EMG biofeedback can teach patients to relax overactive muscles and isolate functional muscles without widespread over-recruitment. Diaphragmatic breathing can also stimulate a relaxation response. Yoga, Tai Chi, or Qigong may be beneficial both through their relaxation effect, proprioceptive training, alleviation of fear-avoidance behavior, and perhaps sleep enhancement, and alleviation of depression and anxiety.[3,50,282-286]

Biofeedback, which uses feedback to the patient to teach modified neural control, can also stimulate a relaxation response and decrease autonomic function associated with stress.[231] A variety of biofeedback devices can be used with chronic pain. Electromyogram works by measuring the intensity of muscle activation. It can be used to teach patients how to relax specific muscles by teaching them to decrease muscle activity. For example, patients with TMJ pain can learn to relax the masseter. Once patients learn to relax the target muscle, they are progressed to maintain or restore that relaxation after adding physical activity such as standing and walking or after visualizing stressful images. Electromyography works well with conditions involving excessive muscle tension or trigger points.[14,282] In some cases, research has identified subgroups more or less likely to benefit; for example, people with cramping phantom limb pain are more likely to benefit from EMG than those with burning pain.[282] Galvanic skin response (GSR) works through controlling the autonomic nervous system and decreasing the stress response. Heart rate variability is a newer form of biofeedback in which autonomic balance is restored by synchronizing breathing with low-frequency patterns.[231,303] Skin temperature can be an effective way to stimulate parasympathetic activity by placing the thermistor (temperature sensor) on the hand and imagining the hands becoming very warm. Temperature biofeedback is also used for migraines, by placing the thermistor directly on the patient's forehead. Respiration rate and heart rate can also be used as biofeedback measures.

Assistive Devices

Patients with persistent activity limitations due to defined physical impairments may benefit from assistive devices to improve function. Patients with joint disorders, such as OA or RA, should consider devices that decrease stress to affected joints. For example, shoe orthotics and knee braces have strong evidence for modest improvements for OA of the knee.[304] Other devices that decrease stress to joints include items such as jar openers and carts for transporting groceries. Conditions associated with focal weakness, such as stroke or MS, may benefit from braces or splints to support weakened structures and decrease muscle length and strength imbalances. Each patient's specific situation needs to be examined and evaluated, because over-reliance on splints and appliances to protect painful regions in the absence of specific pathology can be counterproductive if it reinforces pain and illness behavior.[216]

Physical and Electrotherapeutic Modalities

Evidence for passive physical modalities such as heat, cold, ultrasound, laser, traction, or TENS in the treatment of chronic pain is controversial with weak evidence.[234,305-307] For patients who appear to benefit from such a modality, consideration should be given to whether it can be provided as a self-care strategy such as a home TENS[216] or home traction unit. When instructing a patient in use of a home TENS unit, consideration should be given to use of acupuncture-like parameters (low frequency), which stimulate an endorphin response,

rather than traditional TENS, which stimulates a gate control mechanism.[308]

■ COMPLEMENTARY AND ALTERNATIVE APPROACHES

Complementary and alternative approaches include active therapies such as yoga and Tai Chi, mental therapies such as hypnosis and meditation, manual therapies such as acupuncture and Reiki, devices such as magnets, and herbal and nutritional supplements. Magnets, herbal medicines, and supplements are beyond the scope of this chapter. Since 35% to 63% of people with chronic pain use these approaches,[50,282] physical therapists should be familiar with how they may be integrated into a comprehensive POC.

Movement therapies such as yoga, Tai Chi, and Qigong now have substantial support as forms of exercise for improving flexibility, strength, balance, and proprioception, and decreasing fear of movement.[3,50,282-286] Not only do these activities have physical benefits, they also foster relaxation and independence, both of which are important components of self-management. Furthermore, many of these activities are practiced in a community-based group setting, which addresses issues of isolation and loss of recreational activities.

Manual techniques include acupuncture, chiropractic, massage, Reiki, and therapeutic touch. Insofar as chiropractic includes manual therapy of the spine, it is a potentially effective component of management for spinal pain.[15,16,282] Acupuncture is now practiced in both nontraditional and traditional health settings. Extensive research shows that it can be a beneficial component of pain management, especially when pharmacological options are limited due to co-morbidities or adverse reactions. Various forms of massage have shown temporary benefit for chronic musculoskeletal pain conditions, but long-term benefit occurs only when combined with exercise and patient education.[282] Some of the less common manual approaches, such as Reiki, therapeutic touch, and craniosacral therapy, have inconclusive evidence regarding benefit for chronic pain. It is likely that patients experience a relaxation response with most of these manual approaches; while relaxation is beneficial, active self-directed methods of relaxation are preferable to passive approaches in which patients depend on health care providers.

Mind-body therapies include meditation, mindfulness-based stress reduction, and hypnosis. Biofeedback, CBT, and relaxation training, which were once considered alternative approaches, have now become standard components of pain management. Mindfulness meditation has the longest history of research supporting its beneficial effects for a variety of chronic health conditions.[282,288,289] Hypnosis has been found to be at least as effective as other cognitive and physical interventions for pain; patients are often taught self-hypnosis to facilitate self-management.[173,282,309,310] Mind-body practices appear to work through decreasing stress, anxiety, and dysfunctional thought processes that subsequently decrease autonomic and central arousal, as well as diminish the perception of suffering.[50]

In summary, several complementary and alternative approaches have documented benefit for patients with chronic pain while others do not. In general, side effects are minimal, especially compared to some of the pharmacological and surgical interventions. A few, such as acupuncture or chiropractic manipulation, have specific physical benefits while others, such as the movement and mind-body activities, enhance overall physical fitness and relaxation. Those approaches that foster independent self-management and functional improvements can be appropriate components of a chronic pain self-management plan.

SUMMARY

Chronic pain is a disease process affecting all aspects of the patient's life. The biopsychosocial model integrates physiological, psychological, and social factors, each contributing to the development and experience of chronic pain. Pain may be classified in various ways and the classification can guide selection of interventions. Nociceptive, peripheral neurogenic, and central neurogenic pain each require different intervention approaches, though many chronic pain conditions include a combination of these pain mechanisms. Chronic pain differs from acute pain in that it is not always associated with tissue damage. Peripheral and central sensitization allow pain to be perpetuated even in the absence of peripheral tissue involvement. Intervention therefore needs to address contributing factors and sequelae of chronic pain, such as fear-avoidance, deconditioning, and illness behavior.

Effective management of chronic pain needs to address the whole patient and often also the patient's family. While many interventions can benefit people with chronic pain, the ultimate goal is to help the patient develop a self-management program that maximizes functional activity and minimizes participation restrictions. Although chronic pain is best managed in a multidisciplinary environment, physical therapy can provide significant benefits with or without a pain management team. Physical therapists provide patient education, neuromuscular reeducation, graded exercise, and functional training that are critical to minimize activity and participation restrictions. Although the disease chronic pain cannot be "cured," physical therapy can offer patients hope for an improved quality of life.

Questions for Review

1. Where in the nervous system is pain interpreted?
   a. Substantia gelatinosa
   b. Nociceptors
   c. Limbic system
   d. Cerebral cortex

2. According to the Gate Control Theory, modulation of painful input is achieved through:
   a. Presynaptic inhibition of the transmission cell
   b. Postsynaptic inhibition of the transmission cell
   c. Presynaptic excitation of the transmission cell
   d. Postsynaptic excitation of the transmission cell

3. The Gate Control Theory may explain the analgesic properties of all of the following treatments except:
   a. Conventional transcutaneous electrical nerve stimulation
   b. Acupuncture
   c. Massage
   d. Vibration

4. Contrast the physiology and presentation of acute versus chronic pain.

5. Contrast the biomedical and biopsychosocial models applied to pain.

6. List and propose the mechanism for five risk factors contributing to chronic pain.

7. Explain central sensitization.

8. Outline the components of a physical therapy examination for a patient with chronic pain.

9. Describe several educational and behavioral principles that physical therapists can integrate into the plan of care for patients with chronic pain.

CASE STUDY

HISTORY

The patient is a 28-year-old married female. During the interview, she avoids eye contact, bites her nails, and provides minimal answers to your questions. She does not work outside the home because she has been unable to keep a job as a result of her headaches (HA) and other pain complaints. Her current primary complaint is of HA, neck pain, and jaw pain, though she also reports low back and left (L) shoulder pain. She has had severe HA since age 12, but they became constant after a motor vehicle accident last year. She is sensitive to light, sound, and perfumes. Her HA are over the forehead, behind her right (R) eye, and over the back of her head. She also has dizziness when she stands up or turns suddenly. She has ringing in her R ear and the sensation that both ears are "stopped up." She reports grinding her teeth at night.

PAST MEDICAL HISTORY

Diagnosed with migraines since age 15 and chronic daily headache after her whiplash injury last year. She reports irritable bowel symptoms of abdominal cramps and frequent diarrhea since age 14. She notes that she does not sleep well and has not since she was a child. She has been diagnosed with depression and post-traumatic stress disorder (PTSD).

DEMOGRAPHICS (INCLUDING PSYCHOLOGICAL, SOCIAL, AND ENVIRONMENTAL FACTORS)

Her husband works construction and does not have work for winter months; consequently, money is always tight and is a source of stress between her and her husband. She is on Medicaid; she has applied for disability but been rejected. She reports that her husband is not supportive of her medical complaints and he tells her she is lazy. During follow-up questioning regarding her PTSD she reluctantly reveals that she was repeatedly sexually abused by neighborhood boys when she was a child (ages 11 to 13); that abuse included both vaginal and oral sex. She has had flashbacks and nightmares about the abuse since she was 11 and continues to be afraid of going to sleep for this reason. She states that she does not have a counselor because she is on Medicaid and there are no available counselors; she has been on a waiting list for psychological services for 2 years. She considers her life very high stress; her only stress management strategy is to watch TV and smoke. She reports smoking one-half pack of cigarettes per day; she denies drinking alcohol or using recreational drugs.

MEDICATIONS

Zoloft 50 mg daily (for depression, anxiety, and PTSD), tramadol 50 mg 3 times/day (for pain), Maxalt nasal spray 5 mg (for migraines) PRN, which she uses 1 or 2 times/day because she has migraines daily.

SYSTEMS REVIEW

- *Cardiovascular/pulmonary*: HR 84, BP 95/68, RR 18/min.
- *Integumentary*: No gross abnormality noted.
- *Musculoskeletal*: Brighton score: B elbow and knee hyperextension, B thumb apposition to forearm; standing trunk flexion: hands flat on floor. No gross asymmetry or weakness. Height 5 ft 4 in, weight 145 lb, endomorphic build.
- *Neuromuscular*: Locomotion and transfers normal; resting tremor in the hands.
- *Communication, affect, cognition, learning style*: Flat affect, withdrawn, anxious. Unable to determine learning style.

TESTS AND MEASURES

Self-Care and Activities of Daily Living

Headache Impact Test HIT-6 score of 72/78 (36 = minimum participation restriction, 78 = maximal participation restriction). Patient-Specific Functional Scale: work 10 hours/week outside the home, current ability to perform = 0/10 (0 = unable, 10 = able to perform normally); able to do 2 hours/day of housework and cooking meals 5 days/week, current ability to perform = 3/10.

Posture

Severe forward head, forward shoulders, flat mid-thoracic spine, increased upper thoracic kyphosis and upper cervical lordosis.

Range of Motion

Neck ROM excessive in all directions, with exacerbation of HA on flexion and extension. Cervical extension demonstrates poor motor control with excessive jutting of the chin. Temporomandibular joint opening restricted to about 50%.

Cranial and Peripheral Nerve Integrity

Upper quadrant neurological screen: Normal myotomes and reflexes. Dermatomes normal for light touch except for hypersensitivity and allodynia to light touch over the posterior scalp.

Cranial nerve testing: Normal except for (1) dizziness and increased HA with eye movement for cranial nerve (CN) III, CN IV, CN VI; (2) hypersensitive with allodynia to light touch over the CN V distribution; (3) increased temporal pain with strength testing of the masseter and temporalis.

Joint Integrity and Mobility

Mild ligamentous laxity noted in the transverse ligament. Unable to assess segmental mobility of cervical vertebrae due to patient guarding. Tender over OA, AA, C2/3, T3–5 facets B.

Cervical joint position error excessive for all cervical motions (normal is less than 4.5°).

Muscle Performance

Deep neck flexor strength decreased with poor motor control and limited endurance. Patient unable to correct motion with cueing.

Muscle palpation: Active trigger points B sternocleidomastoid (SCM), masseter, suboccipitals. Pressure to SCM aggravates frontal and retro-orbital HA and increases tinnitus; pressure to masseter increases pain over the temporomandibular joint and tinnitus. Diffuse spasm and tenderness throughout neck and upper back.

Ventilation, Respiration, and Gas Exchange: Breathing Pattern

Excessive use of accessory breathing muscles, which protrude visibly; patient is unable to perform diaphragmatic breathing even when cued to do so.

Circulation

Vertebral artery test: No symptoms at end range for 15 sec; increased dizziness on return to neutral.

GUIDING QUESTIONS

1. Are the sources of this patient's pain nociceptive, peripheral neurogenic, or central neurogenic?

2. How do psychosocial factors in this case contribute to chronic pain?

3. What psychosocial assessment or screening tools might be appropriate to perform with this patient? How might you apply the results of these tools, recognizing that she currently has limited access to psychology or counseling services?

4. What are the symptoms of serotonin syndrome? What physical tests should you perform if you suspect serotonin syndrome, and what results would raise concern?

5. Does this patient have hypermobility syndrome? If so, how does that contribute to her pain?

6. Identify three anticipated goals and three expected outcomes for this patient.

7. What are three interventions you can do in the clinic to reduce central sensitization? What are three community-based activities you can encourage her to participate in to reduce central sensitization?

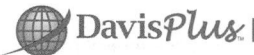 For additional resources, including answers to the questions for review and case study guiding questions, please visit **http://davisplus.fadavis.com**

References

1. Institute of Medicine Committee on Advancing Pain Research, Care, and Education: Relieving Pain in America: A Blueprint for Transforming Prevention, Care, Education, and Research. National Academy of Sciences, Washington, DC, 2011.

2. Mayday Fund Special Committee on Pain and the Practice of Medicine: A Call to Revolutionize Chronic Pain Care in America: An Opportunity in Health Care Reform. Mayday Fund, New York, 2009.

3. Buse, D, Loder, E, and McAlary, P: Chronic pain rehabilitation. Pain Management Rounds 2(6):1–6, 2005.

4. Burgoyne, DS: Prevalence and economic implications of chronic pain. Manage Care 16(2 Suppl 3):2–4, 2007.

5. Turk, DC: Clinical effectiveness and cost-effectiveness of treatments for patients with chronic pain. Clin J Pain 18(6):355–365, 2002.

6. Apkarian, AV, Baliki, MN, and Geha, PY: Towards a theory of chronic pain. Prog Neurobiol 87(2):81–97, 2009.

7. American Pain Foundation: Pain Facts and Statistics, 2009: Retrieved November 2, 2011, from www.painfoundation.org/learn/publications/files/PainFactsandStats.pdf.

8. Reid, KJ, et al: Epidemiology of chronic non-cancer pain in Europe: Narrative review of prevalence, pain treatments and pain impact. Curr Med Res Opin 27(2):449–462, 2011.

9. Harstall, C: How prevalent is chronic pain? Pain Clinical Updates 11(2):1–4, 2003.

10. Centers for Disease Control and Prevention: National Health Interview Survey: Table 53 (page 1 of 5). Joint pain among adults 18 years of age and over, by selected characteristics: United States, selected years 2002–2009. Retrieved November 2, 2011, from www.cdc.gov/nchs/data/hus/2010/053.pdf.

11. International Association for the Study of Pain (IASP): Neuropathic pain. In Charlton, JE (ed): Core curriculum for professional education in pain, ed 3. IASP Press, Seattle, 2005.

12. Fredheim, OM, et al: Chronic non-malignant pain patients report as poor health-related quality of life as palliative cancer patients. Acta Anaesthesiol Scand 52(1):143–148, 2008.

13. International Association for the Study of Pain (IASP): IASP Taxonomy: Pain terms. 2012. Retrieved January 29, 2012, from www.iasp-pain.org/Content/NavigationMenu/GeneralResourceLinks/PainDefinitions/default.htm.

14. Sauer, SE, Burris, JL, and Carlson, CR: New directions in the management of chronic pain: Self-regulation theory as a model for integrative clinical psychology practice. Clin Psychol Rev 30(6):805–814, 2010.

15. California Department of Industrial Relations: Medical Treatment Utilization Schedule (MTUS): Chronic Pain Medical Treatment Guidelines. Department of Industrial Relations, San Francisco, 2009. Retrieved January 31, 2012, from https://www.dir.ca.gov/dwc/DWCPropRegs/MTUS_Regulations/MTUS_Chronic PainMedicalTreatmentGuidelines.pdf.

16. Institute for Clinical Systems Improvement (ICSI): Health Care Guideline: Assessment and Management of Chronic Pain, 2009. Retrieved January 31, 2012, from www.icsi.org/pain_chronic_assessment_and_management_of_14399/pain_chronic_assessment_and_management_of_guideline.html.

17. Sluka, KA: Definitions, concepts, and models of pain. In Sluka, KA (ed): Mechanisms and Management of Pain for the Physical Therapist. IASP Press, Seattle, 2009, pp 3–18.

18. American Society of Anesthesiologists Task Force on Chronic Pain Management: Practice guidelines for chronic pain management. Anesthesiology 112(4):1, 2010.

19. Dersh, J, Polatin, PB, and Gatchel, RJ: Chronic pain and psychopathology: Research findings and theoretical considerations. Psychosom Med 64(5):773–786, 2002.

20. Woolf, CJ: Central sensitization: Implications for the diagnosis and treatment of pain. Pain 152(3 Suppl):S2, 2011.

21. Fishbain, DA, et al: A structured evidence-based review on the meaning of nonorganic physical signs: Waddell signs. Pain Med 4(2):141–181, 2003.

22. Nijs, J, et al: Treatment of central sensitization in patients with "unexplained" chronic pain: What options do we have? Expert Opin Pharmacother 12(7):1087–1098, 2011.

23. World Health Organization: International Classification of Functioning, Disability and Health (ICF). Retrieved September 25, 2011, from www.who.int/classifications/icf/en/.

24. American Physical Therapy Association: Interactive Guide to Physical Therapist Practice. 2003. Retrieved September 15, 2011, from http://guidetoptpractice.apta.org/.

25. World Health Organization: Towards a Common Language for Functioning, Disability and Health. 2002. Retrieved November 2, 2011, from www.who.int/classifications/icf/training/icfbeginners-guide.pdf.

26. Cieza, A, et al: ICF Core Sets for chronic widespread pain. J Rehabil Med 44(Suppl):63–68, 2004.

27. Schwarzkopf, SR, et al: Towards an ICF Core Set for chronic musculoskeletal conditions: Commonalities across ICF Core Sets for osteoarthritis, rheumatoid arthritis, osteoporosis, low back pain and chronic widespread pain. Clin Rheumatol 27(11):1355–1361, 2008.

28. Rundell, SD, Davenport, TE, and Wagner, T: Physical therapist management of acute and chronic low back pain using the World Health Organization's International Classification of Functioning, Disability and Health. Phys Ther 89(1):82–90, 2009.

29. Wade, JB, et al: Role of pain catastrophizing during pain processing in a cohort of patients with chronic and severe arthritic knee pain. Pain 152(2):314–319, 2011.

30. Siddall, PJ, and Cousins, MJ: Persistent pain as a disease entity: Implications for clinical management. Anesth Analg 99(2):510–520, 2004.

31. Dickinson, BD, et al: Maldynia: Pathophysiology and management of neuropathic and maladaptive pain—a report of the AMA council on science and public health. Pain Med 11(11):1635–1653, 2010.

32. Henry, JL: The need for knowledge translation in chronic pain. Pain Res Manage 13(6):465–476, 2008.

33. Argoff, CE, et al: Multimodal analgesia for chronic pain: Rationale and future directions. Pain Med 10 (Suppl 2):S53–S66, 2009.

34. Sluka, KA: Mechanisms and Management of Pain for the Physical Therapist. IASP Press, Seattle, 2009.

35. Flor, H, TD: Chronic Pain: An Integrated Biobehavioral Approach. IASP Press, Seattle, 2011.

36. Ford, B: Pain in Parkinson's disease. Mov Disord 25(Suppl 1):S98–S103, 2010.

37. Sluka, KA: Central mechanisms involved in pain processing. In Sluka, KA (ed): Mechanisms and Management of Pain for the Physical Therapist. IASP Press, Seattle, 2009, pp 41–72.

38. Schnitzler, A, and Ploner, M: Neurophysiology and functional neuroanatomy of pain perception. J Clin Neurophysiol 17(6):592–603, 2000.

39. Melzack, R: From the gate to the neuromatrix. Pain Suppl 6:S121–S126, 1999.

40. Melzack, R: Pain—an overview. Acta Anaesthesiol Scand 43(9):880–884, 1999.

41. Melzack, R: Pain and the neuromatrix in the brain. J Dent Educ 65(12):1378–1382, 2001.

42. Melzack, R, and Wall, PD: Pain mechanisms: A new theory. Science 150(699):971–979, 1965.

43. Ossipov, MH, Dussor, GO, and Porreca, F: Central modulation of pain. J Clin Invest 120(11):3779–3787, 2010.

44. Helms, JE, and Barone, CP: Physiology and treatment of pain. Crit Care Nurse 28(6):38–49, 2008.

45. Baker, K: Recent advances in the neurophysiology of chronic pain. Emerg Med Australas 17(1):65–72, 2005.

46. Sluka, KA: Peripheral mechanisms involved in pain processing. In Sluka, KA (ed): Mechanisms and Management of Pain for the Physical Therapist. IASP Press, Seattle, 2009, pp 19–40.

47. Dubin, AE, and Patapoutian, A: Nociceptors: The sensors of the pain pathway. J Clin Invest 120(11):3760–3772, 2010.

48. McEwen, BS, and Kalia, M: The role of corticosteroids and stress in chronic pain conditions. Metabolism 59(Suppl 1):S9–S15, 2010.

49. Bruehl, S: An update on the pathophysiology of complex regional pain syndrome. Anesthesiology 113(3):713–725, 2010.

50. Taylor, AG, et al: Top-down and bottom-up mechanisms in mind-body medicine: Development of an integrative framework for psychophysiological research. Explore J Sci Healing 6(1):29–41, 2010.

51. Staud, R: Future perspectives: Pathogenesis of chronic muscle pain. Best Pract Res Clin Rheumatol 21(3):581–596, 2007.

52. May, A: Chronic pain may change the structure of the brain. Pain 137(1):7–15, 2008.

53. Flor, H: The functional organization of the brain in chronic pain. Prog Brain Res 129:313–322, 2000.

54. May, A: Structural brain imaging: A window into chronic pain. Neuroscientist 17(2):209–220, 2011.

55. Dahl, JB, and Moiniche, S: Pre-emptive analgesia. Br Med Bull 71:13–27, 2004.

56. Ypsilantis, E, and Tang, TY: Pre-emptive analgesia for chronic limb pain after amputation for peripheral vascular disease: A systematic review. Ann Vasc Surg 24(8):1139–1146, 2010.

57. Woolf, CJ: What is this thing called pain? J Clin Invest 120(11):3742–3744, 2010.

58. Smart, KM, et al: Clinical indicators of "nociceptive," "peripheral neuropathic" and "central" mechanisms of musculoskeletal pain. A Delphi survey of expert clinicians. Man Ther 15(1):80–87, 2010.

59. World Health Organization: WHO Steering Group on Pain Guidelines: WHO Treatment Guidelines on Chronic Non-malignant Pain in Adults (Scoping Document). Retrieved January 31, 2012, from www.who.int/medicines/areas/quality_safety/Scoping_WHO Guide_non-malignant_pain_adults.pdf.

60. Murray, GM: Referred pain, allodynia and hyperalgesia. J Am Dent Assoc 140(9):1122–1124, 2009.

61. Staud, R, et al: Enhanced central pain processing of fibromyalgia patients is maintained by muscle afferent input: A randomized, double-blind, placebo-controlled study. Pain 145(1-2):96–104, 2009.

62. DeSantana, JM, and Sluka, KA: Central mechanisms in the maintenance of chronic widespread noninflammatory muscle pain. Curr Pain Headache Rep 12(5):338–343, 2008.

63. Shah, JP, and Gilliams, EA: Uncovering the biochemical milieu of myofascial trigger points using in vivo microdialysis: An application of muscle pain concepts to myofascial pain syndrome. J Bodyw Mov Ther 12(4):371–384, 2008.

64. Mense, S: Muscle pain: Mechanisms and clinical significance. Dtsch Arztebl Int 105(12):214–219, 2008.

65. Nee, RJ, BD: Management of peripheral neuropathic pain: Integrating neurobiology, neurodynamics, and clinical evidence. Phys Ther in Sport 7:36–49, 2006.

66. Lötsch, J, Geisslinger, G, and Tegeder, I: Genetic modulation of the pharmacological treatment of pain. Pharmacol Ther 124(2):168–184, 2009.

67. Norbury, TA, et al: Heritability of responses to painful stimuli in women: A classical twin study. Brain 130:3041–3049, 2007.

68. Fillingim, RB, et al: Genetic contributions to pain: A review of findings in humans. Oral Dis 14(8):673–682, 2008.

69. Wright, LJ, et al: Chronic pain, overweight, and obesity: Findings from a community-based twin registry. J Pain 11(7):628–635, 2010.

70. Schur, EA, et al: Feeling bad in more ways than one: Comorbidity patterns of medically unexplained and psychiatric conditions. J Gen Intern Med 22(6):818–821, 2007.

71. Hurley, RW, and Adams, MC: Sex, gender, and pain: An overview of a complex field. Anesth Analg 107(1):309–317, 2008.

72. Mogil, JS, and Bailey, AL: Sex and gender differences in pain and analgesia. Prog Brain Res 186:141–157, 2010.

73. Munce, SE, and Stewart, DE: Gender differences in depression and chronic pain conditions in a national epidemiologic survey. Psychosomatics 48(5):394–399, 2007.

74. Paras, ML, et al: Sexual abuse and lifetime diagnosis of somatic disorders: A systematic review and meta-analysis. JAMA 302(5):550–561, 2009.

75. Cohen, H, et al: Prevalence of post-traumatic stress disorder in fibromyalgia patients: Overlapping syndromes or post-traumatic fibromyalgia syndrome? Semin Arthritis Rheum 32(1):38–50, 2002.

76. Dobie, DJ, et al: Posttraumatic stress disorder in female veterans: Association with self-reported health problems and functional impairment. Arch Intern Med 164(4):394–400, 2004.

77. Tietjen, GE, et al: Childhood maltreatment and migraine (part I). Prevalence and adult revictimization: A multicenter headache clinic survey. Headache 50(1):20–31, 2010.

78. Peres, JF, Goncalves, AL, and Peres, MF: Psychological trauma in chronic pain: Implications of PTSD for fibromyalgia and headache disorders. Curr Pain Headache Rep 13(5):350–357, 2009.

79. Hauser, W, et al: Emotional, physical, and sexual abuse in fibromyalgia syndrome: A systematic review with meta-analysis. Arthritis Care Res 63(6):808–820, 2011.

80. Haviland, MG, et al: Traumatic experiences, major life stressors, and self-reporting a physician-given fibromyalgia diagnosis. Psychiatry Res 177(3):335–341, 2010.

81. Von Korff, M, et al: Childhood psychosocial stressors and adult onset arthritis: Broad spectrum risk factors and allostatic load. Pain 143(1-2):76–83, 2009.

82. Draucker, CB, and Spradlin, D: Women sexually abused as children: Implications for orthopaedic nursing care. Orthop Nurs 20(6):41–48, 2001.

83. Schachter, CL, et al: Women survivors of child sexual abuse. How can health professionals promote healing? Can Fam Physician 50:405–412, 2004.

84. Schachter, CL, Stalker, CA, and Teram, E: Toward sensitive practice: Issues for physical therapists working with survivors of childhood sexual abuse. Phys Ther 79(3):248–261, 1999.

85. Teram, E, and Stalker CA: Opening the doors to disclosure: Childhood sexual abuse survivors reflect on telling physical therapists about their trauma. Physiotherapy 85(2):88–97, 1999.

86. Noll-Hussong, M, et al: Aftermath of sexual abuse history on adult patients suffering from chronic functional pain syndromes: An fMRI pilot study. J Psychosom Res 68(5):483–487, 2010.

87. Ramond, A, et al: Psychosocial risk factors for chronic low back pain in primary care—a systematic review. Fam Pract 28(1): 12–21, 2011.

88. Hallner, D, and Hasenbring, M: Classification of psychosocial risk factors (yellow flags) for the development of chronic low back and leg pain using artificial neural network. Neurosci Lett 361 (1-3):151–154, 2004.

89. George, SZ, and Stryker, SE: Fear-avoidance beliefs and clinical outcomes for patients seeking outpatient physical therapy for musculoskeletal pain conditions. J Orthop Sports Phys Ther 41(4):249–259, 2011.

90. Helmhout, PH, et al: Prognostic factors for perceived recovery or functional improvement in non-specific low back pain: Secondary analyses of three randomized clinical trials. Eur Spine J 19(4): 650–659, 2010.

91. Leyshon, RT: Coping with chronic pain: Current advances and practical information for clinicians. Work 33(3):369–372, 2009.

92. Young Casey, C, et al: Transition from acute to chronic pain and disability: A model including cognitive, affective, and trauma factors. Pain 134(1-2):69–79, 2008.

93. Shi, Y, et al: Smoking and pain: Pathophysiology and clinical implications. Anesthesiology 113(4):977–992, 2010.

94. Shiri, R, et al: The association between smoking and low back pain: A meta-analysis. Am J Med 123(1):87.e7, 2010.

95. Alkherayf, F, and Agbi, C: Cigarette smoking and chronic low back pain in the adult population. Clin Invest Med 32(5): E360–E367, 2009.

96. Latthe, P, et al: Factors predisposing women to chronic pelvic pain: Systematic review. BMJ 332(7544):749–755, 2006.

97. Zvolensky, MJ, et al: Chronic musculoskeletal pain and cigarette smoking among a representative sample of Canadian adolescents and adults. Addict Behav 35(11):1008–1012, 2010.

98. Weingarten, TN, et al: An assessment of the association between smoking status, pain intensity, and functional interference in patients with chronic pain. Pain Physician 11(5):643–653, 2008.

99. Guh, DP, et al: The incidence of co-morbidities related to obesity and overweight: A systematic review and meta-analysis. BMC Public Health 9:88, 2009.

100. Naughton, F, Ashworth, P, and Skevington, SM: Does sleep quality predict pain-related disability in chronic pain patients? The mediating roles of depression and pain severity. Pain 127(3):243–252, 2007.

101. Gupta, A, et al: The role of psychosocial factors in predicting the onset of chronic widespread pain: Results from a prospective population-based study. Rheumatology (Oxford) 46(4):666–671, 2007.

102. Castro, MM, and Daltro, C: Sleep patterns and symptoms of anxiety and depression in patients with chronic pain. Arq Neuropsiquiatr 67(1):25–28, 2009.

103. Moldofsky, H, and Scarisbrick, P: Induction of neurasthenic musculoskeletal pain syndrome by selective sleep stage deprivation. Psychosom Med 38(1):35–44, 1976.

104. Goral, A, Lipsitz, JD, and Gross, R: The relationship of chronic pain with and without comorbid psychiatric disorder to sleep disturbance and health care utilization: Results from the Israel National Health Survey. J Psychosom Res 69(5):449–457, 2010.

105. Onen, SH, et al: The effects of total sleep deprivation, selective sleep interruption and sleep recovery on pain tolerance thresholds in healthy subjects. J Sleep Res 10(1):35–42, 2001.

106. Davies, KA, et al: Restorative sleep predicts the resolution of chronic widespread pain: Results from the EPIFUND study. Rheumatology (Oxford) 47(12):1809–1813, 2008.

107. Buysse, DJ, et al: The Pittsburgh Sleep Quality Index: A new instrument for psychiatric practice and research. Psychiatry Res 28(2):193–213, 1989.

108. Turner, MK, et al: Prevalence and clinical correlates of vitamin D inadequacy among patients with chronic pain. Pain Med 9(8):979–984, 2008.

109. Leavitt, SB: Vitamin D—a neglected "analgesic" for chronic musculoskeletal pain. Pain Treatment Topics, June 2008. Retrieved September 15, 2011, from http://Pain-Topics.org/VitaminD.

110. McBeth, J, et al: Musculoskeletal pain is associated with very low levels of vitamin D in men: Results from the European male ageing study. Ann Rheum Dis 69(8):1448–1452, 2010.

111. Plotnikoff, GA, and Quigley, JM: Prevalence of severe hypovitaminosis D in patients with persistent, nonspecific musculoskeletal pain. Mayo Clin Proc 78(12):1463–1470, 2003.

112. Straube, S, et al: Vitamin D for the treatment of chronic painful conditions in adults. Cochrane Database of Systematic Reviews 2010, Issue 1. Art. No.: CD007771. DDD: 10.1002/14651858. CD007771.pub2.

113. Astin, JA, et al: Mind-body medicine: State of the science, implications for practice. J Am Board Fam Pract 16(2):131–147, 2003.

114. Astin, JA: Mind-body therapies for the management of pain. Clin J Pain 20(1):27–32, 2004.

115. Szirony, GM: A psychophysiological view of pain: Mind-body interaction in the rehabilitation of injury and illness. Work 15(1):55–60, 2000.

116. McCaffrey, R, Frock, TL, and Garguilo, H: Understanding chronic pain and the mind-body connection. Holist Nurs Pract 17(6):281–287, 2003.

117. Sullivan, M, Gauthier, N, and Tremblay, I: Mental health outcomes of chronic pain. In Wittink, H, and Carr, D (eds): Pain Management: Evidence, Outcomes, and Quality of Life. Elsevier, New York, 2008.

118. Jensen, MP: Psychosocial approaches to pain management: An organizational framework. Pain 152(4):717–725, 2011.

119. Jensen, MP, et al: Psychosocial factors and adjustment to chronic pain in persons with physical disabilities: A systematic review. Arch Phys Med Rehabil 92(1):146–160, 2011.

120. Raichle, KA, Osborne, TL, and Jensen, MP: Psychosocial factors in chronic pain in the dysvascular and diabetic patient. Phys Med Rehabil Clin North Am 20(4):705–717, 2009.

121. Waddell, G, et al: A Fear-Avoidance Beliefs Questionnaire (FABQ) and the role of fear-avoidance beliefs in chronic low back pain and disability. Pain 52(2):157–168, 1993.

122. Vlaeyen, JW, et al: Fear of movement/(re)injury in chronic low back pain and its relation to behavioral performance. Pain 62(3):363–372, 1995.

123. Roelofs, J, et al: The Tampa Scale for Kinesiophobia: Further examination of psychometric properties in patients with chronic low back pain and fibromyalgia. Eur J Pain 8(5):495–502, 2004.

124. Radloff, L: The CES-D scale: A self-report depression scale for research in the general population. Appl Psychol Meas 1:385–401, 1977.

125. Arroll, B, Khin, N, and Kerse, N: Screening for depression in primary care with two verbally asked questions: Cross sectional study. BMJ 327(7424):1144–1146, 2003.

126. Whooley, MA, et al: Case-finding instruments for depression. Two questions are as good as many. J Gen Intern Med 12(7):439–445, 1997.

127. Brody, DS, et al: Identifying patients with depression in the primary care setting: A more efficient method. Arch Intern Med 158(22):2469–2475, 1998.

128. Arroll, B, et al: Validation of PHQ-2 and PHQ-9 to screen for major depression in the primary care population. Ann Fam Med 8(4):348–353, 2010.

129. Spitzer, RL, et al: Utility of a new procedure for diagnosing mental disorders in primary care. The PRIME-MD 1000 study. JAMA 272(22):1749–1756, 1994.

130. Prins, A, et al: The Primary Care PTSD screen (PC-PTSD): Development and operating characteristics. Primary Care Psychiatry 9:9–14, 2003.

131. Sullivan, MJL, and Pivik, J: The Pain Catastrophizing Scale: Development and validation. Psychol Assess 7:524–532, 1995.

132. Sullivan, MJ, et al: The role of perceived injustice in the experience of chronic pain and disability: Scale development and validation. J Occup Rehabil 18(3):249–261, 2008.

133. Hadjistavropoulos, HD, MacLeod, FK, and Asmundson, GJ: Validation of the Chronic Pain Coping Inventory. Pain 80(3):471–481, 1999.

134. Nicholas, MK: The Pain Self-efficacy Questionnaire: Taking pain into account. Eur J Pain 11(2):153–163, 2007.

135. Williams, DA, and Thorn, BE: An empirical assessment of pain beliefs. Pain 36(3):351–358, 1989.

136. Jensen, MP, et al: One- and two-item measures of pain beliefs and coping strategies. Pain 104(3):453–469, 2003.

137. Cohen, S, Kamarck, T, and Mermelstein, R: A global measure of perceived stress. J Health Soc Behav 24(4):385–396, 1983.

138. Hays, RD, et al: Psychometric properties of the Medical Outcomes Study sleep measure. Sleep Med 6(1):41–44, 2005.

139. Nielson, WR, et al: Further development of the Multidimensional Pain Readiness to Change Questionnaire: The MPRCQ2. J Pain 9(6):552–565, 2008.

140. Kerns, RD, et al: Identification of subgroups of persons with chronic pain based on profiles on the Pain Stages of Change Questionnaire. Pain 116(3):302–310, 2005.

141. Kerns, RD, et al: Readiness to adopt a self-management approach to chronic pain: The Pain Stages of Change Questionnaire (PSOCQ). Pain 72(1-2):227–234, 1997.

142. Allen, J, and Annells, M: A literature review of the application of the Geriatric Depression Scale, Depression Anxiety Stress Scales and Post-Traumatic Stress Disorder Checklist to community nursing cohorts. J Clin Nurs 18(7):949–959, 2009.

143. Haggman, S, Maher, CG, and Refshauge, KM: Screening for symptoms of depression by physical therapists managing low back pain. Phys Ther 84(12):1157–1166, 2004.

144. Nicholas, MK, et al: Early identification and management of psychological risk factors ("yellow flags") in patients with low back pain: A reappraisal. Phys Ther 91(5):737–753, 2011.

145. Stewart, J, Kempenaar, L, and Lauchlan, D: Rethinking yellow flags. Man Ther 16(2):196–198, 2011.

146. New Zealand Guidelines Group: Accident Compensation Corporation (ACC): New Zealand Acute Low Back Pain Guide. Wellington, New Zealand Guidelines Group, New Zealand, 2004.

147. Sowden, M, Gray, SE, and Coombs, J: Can four key psychosocial risk factors for chronic pain and disability (yellow flags) be modified by a pain management programme? A pilot study. Physiother 92:43–49, 2006.

148. Molton, IR, et al: Psychosocial factors and adjustment to chronic pain in spinal cord injury: Replication and cross-validation. J Rehabil Res Dev 46(1):31–42, 2009.

149. Gatchel, RJ, et al: The biopsychosocial approach to chronic pain: Scientific advances and future directions. Psychol Bull 133(4):581–624, 2007.

150. Roy-Byrne, PP, et al: Anxiety disorders and comorbid medical illness. Gen Hosp Psychiatry 30(3):208–225, 2008.

151. Vlaeyen, JW, and Linton, SJ: Fear-avoidance and its consequences in chronic musculoskeletal pain: A state of the art. Pain 85(3):317–332, 2000.

152. Turk, DC, and Wilson, HD: Fear of pain as a prognostic factor in chronic pain: Conceptual models, assessment, and treatment implications. Curr Pain Headache Rep 14(2):88–95, 2010.

153. Nijs, J, and Van Houdenhove, B: From acute musculoskeletal pain to chronic widespread pain and fibromyalgia: Application of pain neurophysiology in manual therapy practice. Man Ther 14(1):3–12, 2009.

154. Buenaver, LF, Edwards, RR, and Haythornthwaite, JA: Pain-related catastrophizing and perceived social responses: Inter-relationships in the context of chronic pain. Pain 127(3):234–242, 2007.

155. George, SZ, et al: Depressive symptoms, anatomical region, and clinical outcomes for patients seeking outpatient physical therapy for musculoskeletal pain. Phys Ther 91(3):358–372, 2011.

156. Bair, MJ, et al: Depression and pain comorbidity: A literature review. Arch Intern Med 163(20):2433–2445, 2003.

157. Ruehlman, LS, Karoly, P, and Pugliese, J: Psychosocial correlates of chronic pain and depression in young adults: Further evidence of the utility of the Profile of Chronic Pain: Screen (PCP:S) and the Profile of Chronic Pain: Extended Assessment (PCP:EA) battery. Pain Med 11(10):1546–1553, 2010.

158. Giesecke, T, et al: The relationship between depression, clinical pain, and experimental pain in a chronic pain cohort. Arthritis Rheum 52(5):1577–1584, 2005.

159. Sagula, D, and Rice, K: The effectiveness of mindfulness training on the grieving process and emotional well-being of chronic pain patients. Journal of Clinical Psychology in Medical Settings 11(4):333–342, 2004.

160. Furnes, B, and Dysvik, E: Dealing with grief related to loss by death and chronic pain: An integrated theoretical framework. Part 1. Patient Prefer Adherence 4:135–140, 2010.

161. Chapman, CR, and Gavrin, J: Suffering: The contributions of persistent pain. Lancet 353(9171):2233–2237, 1999.

162. Kübler-Ross, E: On Grief and Grieving: Finding the Meaning of Grief through the Five Stages of Loss. Simon & Schuster, New York, 2005.

163. Telford, K, Kralik, D, and Koch, T: Acceptance and denial: Implications for people adapting to chronic illness: Literature review. J Adv Nurs 55(4):457–464, 2006.

164. Dysvik, E, and Furnes, B: Dealing with grief related to loss by death and chronic pain: Suggestions for practice. Part 2. Patient Prefer Adherence 4:163–170, 2010.

165. Martinez-Lavin, M: Biology and therapy of fibromyalgia. Stress, the stress response system, and fibromyalgia. Arthritis Res Ther 9(4):216, 2007.

166. Waddell, G, et al: Nonorganic physical signs in low-back pain. Spine 5(2):117–125, 1980.

167. Scalzitti, DA: Screening for psychological factors in patients with low back problems: Waddell's nonorganic signs. Phys Ther 77(3):306–312, 1997.

168. Carleton, RN, et al: Waddell's symptoms as correlates of vulnerabilities associated with fear-anxiety-avoidance models of pain: Pain-related anxiety, catastrophic thinking, perceived disability, and treatment outcome. J Occup Rehabil 19(4):364–374, 2009.

169. Fishbain, DA, et al: Is there a relationship between nonorganic physical findings (Waddell signs) and secondary gain/malingering? Clin J Pain 20(6):399–408, 2004.

170. Conrad, R, et al: Temperament and character personality profiles and personality disorders in chronic pain patients. Pain 133 (1-3):197–209, 2007.

171. Blyth, FM, Macfarlane, GJ, and Nicholas, MK: The contribution of psychosocial factors to the development of chronic pain: The key to better outcomes for patients? Pain 129(1-2):8–11, 2007.

172. Rusu, AC, and Hasenbring, M: Multidimensional Pain Inventory derived classifications of chronic pain: Evidence for maladaptive pain-related coping within the dysfunctional group. Pain 134 (1-2):80–90, 2008.

173. Jensen, MP, et al: A comparison of self-hypnosis versus progressive muscle relaxation in patients with multiple sclerosis and chronic pain. Int J Clin Exp Hypn 57(2):198–221, 2009.

174. Breivik, H, et al: Assessment of pain. Br J Anaesth 101(1):17–24, 2008.

175. Briggs, E: Assessment and expression of pain. Nurs Stand 25(2):35–38, 2010.

176. Clayton, HA, et al: A novel program to assess and manage pain. Medsurg Nurs 9(6):318–321, 317, 2000.

177. Kernicki, JG: Differentiating chest pain: Advanced assessment techniques. Dimens Crit Care Nurs 12(2):66–76, 1993.

178. Tomlinson, D, et al: A systematic review of Faces scales for the self-report of pain intensity in children. Pediatrics 126(5): e1168–e1198, 2010.

179. Reigo, T, Tropp, H, and Timpka, T: Pain drawing evaluation—the problem with the clinically biased surgeon. Intra- and inter-observer agreement in 50 cases related to clinical bias. Acta Orthop Scand 69(4):408–411, 1998.

180. Burckhardt, CS: Adult measures of pain. Arthritis and Rheumatism (Arthritis Care and Research) 49(5S):S96–S104, 2003.

181. Jensen, MP: Review of measures of neuropathic pain. Curr Pain Headache Rep 10(3):159–166, 2006.

182. Vetter, TR: A primer on health-related quality of life in chronic pain medicine. Anesth Analg 104(3):703–718, 2007.

183. von Baeyer, CL: Children's self-reports of pain intensity: Scale selection, limitations and interpretation. Pain Res Manage 11(3):157–162, 2006.

184. Margolis, RB, Chibnall, JT, and Tait, RC: Test–retest reliability of the pain drawing instrument. Pain 33(1):49–51, 1988.

185. von Baeyer, CL, et al: Pain charts (body maps or manikins) in assessment of the location of pediatric pain. Pain Manage 1(1): 61–68, 2011.

186. Gentile, DA, et al: Reliability and validity of the Global Pain Scale with chronic pain sufferers. Pain Physician 14(1):61–70, 2011.

187. Feldt, KS: The Checklist of Nonverbal Pain Indicators (CNPI). Pain Manage Nurs 1(1):13–21, 2000.

188. Bjoro, K, and Herr, K: Assessment of pain in the nonverbal or cognitively impaired older adult. Clin Geriatr Med 24(2): 237–262, vi, 2008.

189. Bennett, MI, et al: The S-LANSS score for identifying pain of predominantly neuropathic origin: Validation for use in clinical and postal research. J Pain 6(3):149–158, 2005.

190. Bennett, M: The LANSS pain scale: The Leeds assessment of neuropathic symptoms and signs. Pain 92(1-2):147–157, 2001.

191. Victor, TW, et al: The dimensions of pain quality: Factor analysis of the Pain Quality Assessment Scale. Clin J Pain 24(6):550–555, 2008.

192. Von Korff, M, et al: Grading the severity of chronic pain. Pain 50(2):133–149, 1992.

193. Tait, RC, Chibnall, JT, and Krause, S: The Pain Disability Index: Psychometric properties. Pain 40(2):171–182, 1990.

194. Atkinson, TM, et al: Using confirmatory factor analysis to evaluate construct validity of the Brief Pain Inventory (BPI). J Pain Symptom Manage 41(3):558–565, 2011.

195. Melzack, R: The McGill Pain Questionnaire: Major properties and scoring methods. Pain 1(3):277–299, 1975.

196. Ferrell, BA, Stein, WM, and Beck, JC: The Geriatric Pain Measure: Validity, reliability and factor analysis. J Am Geriatr Soc 48(12):1669–1673, 2000.

197. Blozik, E, et al: Geriatric Pain Measure short form: Development and initial evaluation. J Am Geriatr Soc 55(12):2045–2050, 2007.

198. Herr, K, Bjoro, K, and Decker, S: Tools for assessment of pain in nonverbal older adults with dementia: A state-of-the-science review. J Pain Symptom Manage 31(2):170–192, 2006.

199. Melzack, R: The short-form McGill Pain Questionnaire. Pain 30(2):191–197, 1987.

200. Bennett, MI, et al: Using screening tools to identify neuropathic pain. Pain 127(3):199–203, 2007.

201. Fishbain, DA, et al: Can the Neuropathic Pain Scale discriminate between non-neuropathic and neuropathic pain? Pain Med 9(2):149–160, 2008.

202. Dixon, D, Pollard, B, and Johnston, M: What does the Chronic Pain Grade Questionnaire measure? Pain 130(3):249–253, 2007.

203. Turk, DC, et al: Analyzing multiple endpoints in clinical trials of pain treatments: IMMPACT recommendations. Initiative on methods, measurement, and pain assessment in clinical trials. Pain 139(3):485–493, 2008.

204. Carson, L, et al: Abdominal migraine: An under-diagnosed cause of recurrent abdominal pain in children. Headache 51(5):707–712, 2011.

205. Krechel, SW, and Bildner, J: Cries: A new neonatal postoperative pain measurement score. Initial testing of validity and reliability. Paediatr Anaesth 5(1):53–61, 1995.

206. Franck, LS, et al: A comparison of pain measures in newborn infants after cardiac surgery. Pain 152(8):1758–1765, 2011.

207. von Baeyer, CL, and Spagrud, LJ: Systematic review of observational (behavioral) measures of pain for children and adolescents aged 3 to 18 years. Pain 127(1-2):140–150, 2007.

208. Malleson, P, and Clinch, J: Pain syndromes in children. Curr Opin Rheumatol 15(5):572–580, 2003.

209. Bruckenthal, P, Reid, MC, and Reisner, L: Special issues in the management of chronic pain in older adults. Pain Med 10(Suppl 2):S67–S78, 2009.

210. Edwards, I, et al: Clinical reasoning strategies in physical therapy. Phys Ther 84(4):312–330, 2004.

211. Kelley, P, and Clifford, P: Coping with chronic pain: Assessing narrative approaches. Soc Work 42(3):266–277, 1997.

212. Matthias, MS, et al: The patient-provider relationship in chronic pain care: Providers' perspectives. Pain Med 11(11):1688–1697, 2010.

213. Chiodo, A, et al: Needle EMG has a lower false positive rate than MRI in asymptomatic older adults being evaluated for lumbar spinal stenosis. Clin Neurophysiol 118(4):751–756, 2007.

214. Haig, AJ, et al: Spinal stenosis, back pain, or no symptoms at all? A masked study comparing radiologic and electrodiagnostic diagnoses to the clinical impression. Arch Phys Med Rehabil 87(7):897–903, 2006.

215. Bedson, J, and Croft, PR: The discordance between clinical and radiographic knee osteoarthritis: A systematic search and summary of the literature. BMC Musculoskelet Disord 9:116, 2008.

216. American College of Occupational and Environmental Medicine (ACOEM): Chronic pain. In Occupational Medicine Practice Guidelines: Evaluation and Management of Common Health Problems and Functional Recovery in Workers. ACOEM, Elk Grove Village, IL, 2008, pp 73–502.

217. Ang, DC, et al: Predictors of pain outcomes in patients with chronic musculoskeletal pain co-morbid with depression: Results from a randomized controlled trial. Pain Med 11(4):482–491, 2010.

218. Kroenke, K, Krebs, EE, and Bair, MJ: Pharmacotherapy of chronic pain: A synthesis of recommendations from systematic reviews. Gen Hosp Psychiatry 31(3):206–219, 2009.

219. Park, HJ, and Moon, DE: Pharmacologic management of chronic pain. Korean J Pain 23(2):99–108, 2010.

220. Turk, DC, Wilson, HD, and Cahana, A: Treatment of chronic non-cancer pain. Lancet 377(9784):2226–2235, 2011.

221. Chrubasik, S, Weiser, T, and Beime, B: Effectiveness and safety of topical capsaicin cream in the treatment of chronic soft tissue pain. Phytother Res 24(12):1877–1885, 2010.

222. Knotkova, H, Pappagallo, M, and Szallasi, A: Capsaicin (TRPV1 agonist) therapy for pain relief: Farewell or revival? Clin J Pain 24(2):142–154, 2008.

223. Haroutiunian, S, Drennan, DA, and Lipman, AG: Topical NSAID therapy for musculoskeletal pain. Pain Med 11(4):535–549, 2010.

224. O'Connor, AB, and Dworkin, RH: Treatment of neuropathic pain: An overview of recent guidelines. Am J Med 122(10 Suppl):S22–S32, 2009.

225. Manchikanti, L, et al: Effectiveness of long-term opioid therapy for chronic non-cancer pain. Pain Physician 14(2):E133–E156, 2011.

226. Manchikanti, L, et al: Opioids in chronic noncancer pain. Expert Rev Neurother 10(5):775–789, 2010.

227. Enck, P, Benedetti, F, and Schedlowski, M: New insights into the placebo and nocebo responses. Neuron 59(2):195–206, 2008.

228. Kaptchuk, TJ, et al: Placebos without deception: A randomized controlled trial in irritable bowel syndrome. PLoS One 5(12):e15591, 2010.

229. Isbister, GK, Buckley, NA, and Whyte, IM: Serotonin toxicity: A practical approach to diagnosis and treatment. Med J Aust 187(6):361–365, 2007.

230. Attar-Herzberg, D, et al: The serotonin syndrome: Initial misdiagnosis. Isr Med Assoc J 11(6):367–370, 2009.

231. McKee, MG: Biofeedback: An overview in the context of heart-brain medicine. Cleve Clin J Med 75 Suppl 2:S31–S34, 2008.

232. Henschke, N, et al: Behavioural treatment for chronic low-back pain. Cochrane Database of Systematic Reviews 2010, Issue 7. Art. No.: CD002014. DDD: 10.1002/14651858.CD002014. pub3.

233. Eccleston, C, et al: Psychological therapies for the management of chronic and recurrent pain in children and adolescents. Cochrane Database of Systematic Reviews 2009, Issue 2. Art. No.: CD003968. DDD: 10.1002/14651858.CD003968.pub2.

234. Nnoaham, KE, and Kumbang, J: Transcutaneous electrical nerve stimulation (TENS) for chronic pain. Cochrane Database of Systematic Reviews 2008, Issue 3. Art. No.: CD003222. DDD: 10.1002/14651858.CD003222.pub2.

235. Staal, JB, et al: Injection therapy for subacute and chronic low back pain: An updated Cochrane review. Spine 34(1):49–59, 2009.

236. Rubinstein, SM, et al: Spinal manipulative therapy for chronic low-back pain: An update of a Cochrane review. Spine 36(13):E825–E846, 2011.

237. Nicolaidis, S: Neurosurgical treatments of intractable pain. Metabolism 59(Suppl 1):S27–S31, 2010.

238. Nocom, G, Ho, KY, and Perumal, M: Interventional management of chronic pain. Ann Acad Med Singapore 38(2):150–155, 2009.

239. Saper, JR: "Are you talking to me?" Confronting behavioral disturbances in patients with headache. Headache 46(Suppl 3):S151–S156, 2006.

240. Klyman, CM, et al: A workshop model for educating medical practitioners about optimal treatment of difficult-to-manage patients: Utilization of transference-countertransference. J Am Acad Psychoanal Dyn Psychiatry 36(4):661–676, 2008.

241. Werner, A, and Malterud, K: It is hard work behaving as a credible patient: Encounters between women with chronic pain and their doctors. Soc Sci Med 57(8):1409–1419, 2003.

242. Haugli, L, Strand, E, and Finset, A: How do patients with rheumatic disease experience their relationship with their doctors? A qualitative study of experiences of stress and support in the doctor-patient relationship. Patient Educ Couns 52(2):169–174, 2004.

243. Purtillo, R, HA: Health professional and patient interaction, ed 7. WB Saunders, Philadelphia, 2007.

244. Draucker, CB, et al: Healing from childhood sexual abuse: A theoretical model. J Child Sex Abus 20(4):435–466, 2011.

245. Stebnicki, MA: Stress and grief reactions among rehabilitation professionals: Dealing effectively with empathy fatigue. J Rehabil 66(1):23–29, 2000.

246. Tinkle, BT, et al: The lack of clinical distinction between the hypermobility type of Ehlers-Danlos syndrome and the joint hypermobility syndrome (a.k.a. hypermobility syndrome). Am J Med Genet A 149A(11):2368–2370, 2009.

247. Grahame, R, Bird, HA, and Child, A: The revised (Brighton 1998) criteria for the diagnosis of benign joint hypermobility syndrome (BJHS). J Rheumatol 27(7):1777–1779, 2000.

248. Keer, RGR: Hypermobility syndrome: Diagnosis and management for physiotherapists, ed 1. Butterworth-Heinemann, Maryland Heights, MO, 2003.

249. Calley, DQ, et al: Identifying patient fear-avoidance beliefs by physical therapists managing patients with low back pain. J Orthop Sports Phys Ther 40(12):774–783, 2010.

250. Goodman, C, and Snyder, T: Differential Diagnosis for Physical Therapists, ed 4. Saunders Elsevier, St. Louis, 2007.

251. Walton, DM, et al: Reliability, standard error, and minimum detectable change of clinical pressure pain threshold testing in people with and without acute neck pain. J Orthop Sports Phys Ther 41(9):644–650, 2011.

252. Walton, DM, et al: A descriptive study of pressure pain threshold at 2 standardized sites in people with acute or subacute neck pain. J Orthop Sports Phys Ther 41(9):651–657, 2011.

253. Walton, DM, et al: Pressure pain threshold testing demonstrates predictive ability in people with acute whiplash. J Orthop Sports Phys Ther 41(9):658–665, 2011.

254. Staud, R: Chronic widespread pain and fibromyalgia: Two sides of the same coin? Curr Rheumatol Rep 11(6):433–436, 2009.

255. Travell, JG, and Simons, DG: Myofascial Pain and Dysfunction: The Trigger Point Manual. Lippincott Williams & Wilkins, Baltimore, 2007.

256. Myburgh, C, Larsen, AH, and Hartvigsen, J: A systematic, critical review of manual palpation for identifying myofascial trigger points: Evidence and clinical significance. Arch Phys Med Rehabil 89(6):1169–1176, 2008.

257. Leveille, SG, et al: Chronic musculoskeletal pain and the occurrence of falls in an older population. JAMA 302(20):2214–2221, 2009.

258. Russek, LN, and Fulk, GD: Pilot study assessing balance in women with fibromyalgia syndrome. Physiother Theory Pract 25(8):555–565, 2009.

259. Jones, KD, et al: Fibromyalgia is associated with impaired balance and falls. J Clin Rheumatol 15(1):16–21, 2009.

260. Humphreys, BK: Cervical outcome measures: Testing for postural stability and balance. J Manipulative Physiol Ther 31(7):540–546, 2008.

261. Niessen, MH, et al: Relationship among shoulder proprioception, kinematics, and pain after stroke. Arch Phys Med Rehabil 90(9):1557–1564, 2009.

262. Woodhouse, A, and Vasseljen, O: Altered motor control patterns in whiplash and chronic neck pain. BMC Musculoskelet Disord 9:90, 2008.

263. Kristjansson, E, and Treleaven, J: Sensorimotor function and dizziness in neck pain: Implications for assessment and management. J Orthop Sports Phys Ther 39(5):364–377, 2009.

264. Gill, KP, and Callaghan, MJ: The measurement of lumbar proprioception in individuals with and without low back pain. Spine 23(3):371–377, 1998.

265. Vuillerme, N, and Pinsault, N: Experimental neck muscle pain impairs standing balance in humans. Exp Brain Res 192(4):723–729, 2009.

266. Pinsault, N, et al: Test–retest reliability of cervicocephalic relocation test to neutral head position. Physiother Theory Pract 24(5):380–391, 2008.

267. Balke, M, et al: The laser-pointer assisted angle reproduction test for evaluation of proprioceptive shoulder function in patients with instability. Arch Orthop Trauma Surg 131(8):1077–1084, 2011.

268. Bennett, RM, et al: The Revised Fibromyalgia Impact Questionnaire (FIQR): Validation and psychometric properties. Arthritis Res Ther 11(4):R120, 2009.

269. Chatman, AB, et al: The Patient-Specific Functional Scale: Measurement properties in patients with knee dysfunction. Phys Ther 77(8):820–829, 1997.

270. Myers, AM, et al: Discriminative and evaluative properties of the Activities-specific Balance Confidence (ABC) scale. J Gerontol A Biol Sci Med Sci 53(4):M287–M294, 1998.

271. Eggermont, LH, et al: Comparing pain severity versus pain location in the mobilize Boston study: Chronic pain and lower extremity function. J Gerontol A Biol Sci Med Sci 64(7):763–770, 2009.

272. Vasunilashorn, S, et al: Use of the Short Physical Performance Battery score to predict loss of ability to walk 400 meters: Analysis from the InCHIANTI study. J Gerontol A Biol Sci Med Sci 64(2):223–229, 2009.

273. van Wilgen, CP, et al: Chronic pain and severe disuse syndrome: Long-term outcome of an inpatient multidisciplinary cognitive behavioural programme. J Rehabil Med 41(3):122–128, 2009.

274. Nicolson, NA, et al: Childhood maltreatment and diurnal cortisol patterns in women with chronic pain. Psychosom Med 72(5):471–480, 2010.

275. Bauer, ME, et al: Interplay between neuroimmunoendocrine systems during post-traumatic stress disorder: A minireview. Neuroimmunomodulation 17(3):192–195, 2010.

276. Molton, I, et al: Coping with chronic pain among younger, middle-aged, and older adults living with neurological injury and disease. J Aging Health 20(8):972–996, 2008.

277. Scascighini, L, et al: Multidisciplinary treatment for chronic pain: A systematic review of interventions and outcomes. Rheumatology (Oxford) 47(5):670–678, 2008.

278. Smeets, RJ, et al: More is not always better: Cost-effectiveness analysis of combined, single behavioral and single physical rehabilitation programs for chronic low back pain. Eur J Pain 13(1):71–81, 2009.

279. Nijs, J, et al: How to explain central sensitization to patients with "unexplained" chronic musculoskeletal pain: Practice guidelines. Man Ther 16(5):413–418, 2011.

280. Mueller, L: Psychologic aspects of chronic headache. J Am Osteopath Assoc 100(9 Suppl):S14–S21, 2000.

281. Maughan, EF, and Lewis, JS: Outcome measures in chronic low back pain. Eur Spine J 19(9):1484–1494, 2010.

282. Tan, G, et al: Efficacy of selected complementary and alternative medicine interventions for chronic pain. J Rehabil Res Dev 44(2):195–222, 2007.

283. Lu, WA, and Kuo, CD: The effect of Tai Chi Chuan on the autonomic nervous modulation in older persons. Med Sci Sports Exerc 35(12):1972–1976, 2003.

284. Tsang, WW, and Hui-Chan, CW: Effects of Tai Chi on joint proprioception and stability limits in elderly subjects. Med Sci Sports Exerc 35(12):1962–1971, 2003.

285. Rogers, CE, Larkey, LK, and Keller, C: A review of clinical trials of Tai Chi and Qigong in older adults. West J Nurs Res 31(2):245–279, 2009.

286. Kuramoto, AM: Therapeutic benefits of Tai Chi exercise: Research review. WMJ 105(7):42–46, 2006.

287. Veehof, MM, et al: Acceptance-based interventions for the treatment of chronic pain: A systematic review and meta-analysis. Pain 152(3):533–542, 2011.

288. Ludwig, DS, and Kabat-Zinn, J: Mindfulness in medicine. JAMA 300(11):1350–1352, 2008.

289. Davidson, RJ, et al: Alterations in brain and immune function produced by mindfulness meditation. Psychosom Med 65(4):564–570, 2003.

290. Hulme, JA: Fibromyalgia: A handbook for self-care and treatment, ed 3. Phoenix Publishing, Missoula, MO, 2001.

291. Beissner, K, et al: Physical therapists' use of cognitive-behavioral therapy for older adults with chronic pain: A nationwide survey. Phys Ther 89(5):456–469, 2009.

292. von Baeyer, CL, and Tupper, SM: Procedural pain management for children receiving physiotherapy. Physiother Can 62(4):327–337, 2010.

293. Rundell, SD, and Davenport, TE: Patient education based on principles of cognitive behavioral therapy for a patient with persistent low back pain: A case report. J Orthop Sports Phys Ther 40(8):494–501, 2010.

294. Nicholas, MK, and George, SZ: Psychologically informed interventions for low back pain: An update for physical therapists. Phys Ther 91(5):765–776, 2011.

295. Allen, RJ: Physical agents used in the management of chronic pain by physical therapists. Phys Med Rehabil Clin North Am 17(2):315–345, 2006.

296. Margolis, RB, et al: Evaluating patients with chronic pain and their families: How you can recognize maladaptive patterns. Can Fam Physician 37:429–435, 1991.

297. Smith, AA: Intimacy and family relationships of women with chronic pain. Pain Manage Nurs 4(3):134–142, 2003.

298. Flor, H: Maladaptive plasticity, memory for pain and phantom limb pain: Review and suggestions for new therapies. Expert Rev Neurother 8(5):809–818, 2008.

299. Flor, H, and Diers, M: Sensorimotor training and cortical reorganization. NeuroRehabilitation 25(1):19–27, 2009.

300. Nijs, J, Van Oosterwijck, J, and De Hertogh, W: Rehabilitation of chronic whiplash: Treatment of cervical dysfunctions or chronic pain syndrome? Clin Rheumatol 28(3):243–251, 2009.

301. Castro-Sánchez, AM, et al: Benefits of massage–myofascial release therapy on pain, anxiety, quality of sleep, depression, and quality of life in patients with fibromyalgia. Evid Based Complement Alternat Med 2011:561753, 2011. [Epub December 28, 2010; doi: 10.1155/2011/561753.]

302. Bokarius, AV, and Bokarius, V: Evidence-based review of manual therapy efficacy in treatment of chronic musculoskeletal pain. Pain Pract 10(5):451–458, 2010.

303. Hallman, DM, et al: Effects of heart rate variability biofeedback in subjects with stress-related chronic neck pain: A pilot study. Appl Psychophysiol Biofeedback 36(2):71–80, 2011.

304. Brouwer, RW, et al: Braces and orthoses for treating osteoarthritis of the knee, Cochrane Database of Systematic Reviews 2005, Issue 1. Art. No.: CD004020. DDD: 10.1002/14651858.CD004020.pub2.

305. Philadelphia panel evidence-based clinical practice guidelines on selected rehabilitation interventions for neck pain. Phys Ther 81(10):1701–1717, 2001.

306. Philadelphia panel evidence-based clinical practice guidelines on selected rehabilitation interventions for low back pain. Phys Ther 81(10):1641–1674, 2001.

307. Philadelphia panel evidence-based clinical practice guidelines on selected rehabilitation interventions: Overview and methodology. Phys Ther 81(10):1629–1640, 2001.

308. Leonard, G, Cloutier, C, and Marchand, S: Reduced analgesic effect of acupuncture-like TENS but not conventional TENS in opioid-treated patients. J Pain 12(2):213–221, 2011.

309. Elkins, G, Jensen, MP, and Patterson, DR: Hypnotherapy for the management of chronic pain. Int J Clin Exp Hypn 55(3):275–287, 2007.

310. Stoelb, BL, et al: The efficacy of hypnotic analgesia in adults: A review of the literature. Contemp Hypn 26(1):24–39, 2009.

Supplemental Readings

(Also see Appendices 25.E and 25.F for additional text and web resources.)

Arnstein, P: Clinical Coach for Effective Pain Management. FA Davis, Philadelphia, 2010.

Drench, M, Noonan, A, and Sharby, N: Psychosocial Aspects of Healthcare, ed 3. Prentice Hall, Upper Saddle River, NJ, 2011.

Flor, H, and Turk, D: Chronic Pain: An Integrated Biobehavioral Approach. IASP Press, Seattle, 2011.

Goadsby, P, et al: Chronic Daily Headache for Clinicians. People's Medical Publishing House—USA, Singapore, China, 2005.

Hakim, A, Keer, RJ, and Grahame, R: Hypermobility, Fibromyalgia and Chronic Pain. Churchill Livingstone, New York, 2010.

Jull, G, et al: Whiplash, Headache, and Neck Pain: Research-Based Directions for Physical Therapies. Churchill Livingstone, New York, 2008.

Mense, S, and Gerwin, R: Muscle Pain: Diagnosis and Treatment. Springer, New York, 2010.

Moore, RJ: Biobehavioral Approaches to Pain. Springer, New York, 2009.

Sluka, K: Mechanisms and Management of Pain for the Physical Therapist. IASP Press, Seattle, 2009.

Travell, J, and Simons, DG: Myofascial Pain and Dysfunction: The Trigger Point Manual. Volume 1: Upper Half of Body, ed 2. Lippincott Williams & Wilkins, Baltimore, 1998.

Travell, J, and Simons, DG: Myofascial Pain and Dysfunction: The Trigger Point Manual. Volume 2: The Lower Extremities. Lippincott Williams & Wilkins, Baltimore, 1992.

Van Griensven, H: Pain in Practice: Theory and Treatment Strategies for Manual Therapists. Butterworth-Heinemann, Maryland Heights, MO, 2006.

Wallace, DJ, and Clauw, DJ: Fibromyalgia and Other Central Pain Syndromes. Lippincott Williams & Wilkins, Baltimore, 2005.

Whyte-Ferguson, L, and Gerwin, R: Clinical Mastery in the Treatment of Myofascial Pain. Lippincott Williams & Wilkins, Baltimore, 2004.

Pain Catastrophizing Scale

Everyone experiences painful situations at some point in their lives. Such experiences may include headaches, tooth pain, joint or muscle pain. People are often exposed to situations that may cause pain such as illness, injury, dental procedures or surgery.

Instructions: *We are interested in the types of thoughts and feelings that you have when you are in pain. Listed below are thirteen statements describing different thoughts and feelings that may be associated with pain. Using the following scale, please indicate the degree to which you have these thoughts and feelings when you are experiencing pain*

RATING	0	1	2	3	4
MEANINGE	Not at all	To a slight degree	To a moderate degree	To a great degree	All the time

When I'm in pain ...

Number	Statement	Rating
1	I worry all the time about whether the pain will end.	
2	I feel I can't go on.	
3	It's terrible and I think it's never going to get any better	
4	It's awful and I feel that it overwhelms me.	
5	I feel I can't stand it anymore	
6	I become afraid that the pain will get worse.	
7	I keep thinking of other painful events	
8	I anxiously want the pain to go away	
9	I can't seem to keep it out of my mind	
10	I keep thinking about how much it hurts.	
11	I keep thinking about how badly I want the pain to stop	
12	There's nothing I can do to reduce the intensity of the pain	
13	I wonder whether something serious may happen.	

Source: Sullivan MJL, Bishop S, Pivik J. The pain catastrophizing scale: development Sullivan MJL, Bishop S, Pivik J. The pain catastrophizing scale: and validation. Psychol Assess 7: 524, 1995.

Primary Care Post-Traumatic Stress Disorder Screen

In your life, have you ever had any experience that was so frightening, horrible, or upsetting that, **in the past month**, you:

1. **Have had nightmares about it or thought about it when you did not want to?**
   YES / NO

2. **Tried hard not to think about it or went out of your way to avoid situations that reminded you of it?**
   YES / NO

3. **Were constantly on guard, watchful, or easily startled?**
   YES / NO

4. **Felt numb or detached from others, activities, or your surroundings?**
   YES / NO

Current research suggests that the results of the PC-PTSD should be considered "positive" if a patient answers "yes" to any three items.

A positive response to the screen does not necessarily indicate that a patient has Posttraumatic Stress Disorder. However, a positive response does indicate that a patient *may* have PTSD or trauma-related problems and further investigation of trauma symptoms by a mental-health professional may be warranted.

Prins, A, Ouimette, and Kimerling. The primary care PTSD screen (PC-PTSD): Development and operating characteristics. Prim Care Psych. 9:9, 2003. Reprinted with permission.

Evidence for Various Chronic Pain Interventions Based on Clinical Practice Guidelines, Cochrane Reviews, Meta-analyses (15, 16, 18, 216, 220, 231-238)

Treatment	Strength of Evidence	Decision	Sources
Approach or Model of Care			
• Plan of care using biopsychosocial model	A,D	+	ICSI (16), CDIR (15), ACOEM (216)
• Multidisciplinary pain rehabilitation	D,M,R	+	ICSI (16), CDIR (15), ASA (18), ACOEM (216)
• Patient education	A,D	+	CDIR (15), ACOEM (216)
Physical Rehabilitation			
• Fitness/exercise program	A,M,R	+	ICSI (16), CDIR (15), ASA (18), ACOEM (216)
• Mobilization and manipulation	A,C,R	+	ICSI (16), CDIR (15), CR, ACOEM (216)
• Massage	A	+±	ICSI (16), CDIR (15)
• Biofeedback	M,R	+	ICSI (16), ASA (18), CDIR (15), McKee (231)
• TENS	A	+	ASA (18)
• Other passive modalities	R	-	ICSI (16), Nnoaham et al (234), ACOEM (216)
Psychosocial Management			
• Cognitive-Behavioral Therapy	A,D,M,R	+	ICSI (16), ASA (18), CDIR (15), ACOEM (216), Eccleston, et al (233), Henschke, et al (232)
• Mindfulness-Based Stress Reduction	D	+	ICSI (16)
• Hypnosis	M,R	+	ICSI (16)
Pharmacologic Management			
• Acetaminophen	R	+	CDIR (15), ACOEM (216)
• NSAIDs	A,R	+	ICSI (16), ASA (18), CDIR (15), ACOEM (216)
• Opioids	A,C,D,M,R	+, ±	ICSI (16), ASA (18), CDIR (15), ACOEM (216)
• Antidepressants: TCAs, SSRIs and SNRIs	A,M	+	ICSI (16), ASA (18), CDIR (15), ACOEM (216)
• Anticonvulsants	A,M	+	ICSI (16), ASA (18), CDIR (15), ACOEM (216)
• Topical agents	A,D,M	+	ICSI (16), ASA (18), CDIR (15)
• Muscle relaxants	M,R	+, ±	ICSI (16), CDIR (15), ACOEM (216)
• Anxiolytics	D	+-	ICSI (16), ASA (18), CDIR (15)
• Drugs for insomnia	A,M		ICSI (16)

Continued

Treatment	Strength of Evidence	Decision	Sources
Intervention Management			
• Diagnostic procedure	C,R	+±	ICSI (16), ACOEM (216), ASA (18)
• Therapeutic procedure	A,M,R	+	ICSI (16), ASA (18), CDIR (15)
• Trigger point injection	B,D	+, ±,-	ASA (18), CDIR (15), ACOEM (216)
Complementary Management			
• Acupuncture	A,C,M,R	+, ±	ICSI (16), ASA (18)
• Herbal products	A,D,M,R	±	ICSI (16)
Surgical management	C,M,R	+, ±,-	ICSI (16), ASA (18), CDIR (15)
Palliative Interventions			
• Nucleoplasty	D	+±-	ICSI (16), ASA (18), CDIR (15)
• Spinal cord stimulation	M	±	ICSI (16), ACOEM (216)
• Intrathecal medication delivery	B	+	ICSI (16), ASA (18), CDIR (15)

Class A: Randomized, controlled trial
Class B: Cohort study
Class C: Non-randomized trial, case control, sensitivity and specificity
   assessment, population-based descriptive study
Class D: Cross-sectional study, case series, case reports
Class M: Meta-analysis, systematic review, decision analysis,
   cost-effectiveness analysis
Class R: Consensus statement, consensus report, narrative review
Class X: Medical opinion
Decision: + = positive for effectiveness; ± = uncertain; -= negative for
   effectiveness
TENS = transcutaneous electroneural stimulation
NSAID = non-steroidal anti-inflammatory drug
TCA = tricyclic antidepressant
SSRI = selective serotonin re-uptake inhibitor
SNRI = serotonin-norepinephrine re-uptake inhibitor
ICSI = Institute for Clinical Systems Improvements (16)
CDIR = California Department of Industrial Relations (15)
ASA = American Society of Anesthesiologists, (18)
ACOEM = American College of Occupational and Environmental
   Medicine ACOEM (216)

Personal Care Plan for Chronic Pain

Appendix D - Personal Care Plan for Chronic Pain

This tool has not been validated for research; however, work group consensus was to include it as an example of a patient tool for establishing a plan of care.

1. Set Personal Goals

☐ Improve Functional Ability Score by _____ points by: Date _____
☐ Return to specific activities, tasks, hobbies, sports...by: Date _____
   1. _____
   2. _____
   3. _____
☐ Return to   ☐ limited work/or   ☐ normal work by: Date _____

2. Improve Sleep (Goal: ____ hours/night, Current: ____ hours/night)

☐ Follow basic sleep plan
   1. Eliminate caffeine and naps, relaxation before bed, go to bed at target bedtime _____
☐ Take nighttime medications
   1. _____
   2. _____
   3. _____

3. Increase Physical Activity

☐ Attend physical therapy (days/week _____)
☐ Complete daily stretching (_____ times/day, for _____ minutes)
☐ Complete aerobic exercise/endurance exercise
   1. Walking (_____ times/day, for _____ minutes) or pedometer (_____ steps/day)
   2. Treadmill, bike, rower, elliptical trainer (_____ times/week, for _____ minutes)
   3. Target heart rate goal with exercise _____ bpm
   Strengthening
   1. Elastic, hand weights, weight machines (_____ minutes/day, _____ days/week)

4. Manage Stress – list main stressors _____

☐ Formal interventions (counseling or classes, support group or therapy group)
   1. _____
☐ Daily practice of relaxation techniques, meditation, yoga, creative activity, service activity, etc.
   1. _____
   2. _____
☐ Medications
   1. _____
   2. _____

5. Decrease Pain (best pain level in past week: ____ /10, worst pain level in past week: ____ /10)

☐ Non-medication treatments
   1. Ice Heat _____
   2. _____
☐ Medication
   1. _____
   2. _____
   3. _____
   4. _____
☐ Other treatments _____

Physician name: _____ Date: _____

Web-Based Resources for Clinicians, Families, and Individuals with Chronic Pain

Organization/Purpose	Website
American Academy of Pain Medicine. Professional organization for physicians has some patient educational material.	www.painmed.org
American Chronic Pain Association. Provides education and peer support for patients and families.	www.theacpa.org
American Headache Society Committee for Headache Education (ACHE). Resources for individuals with headaches.	www.achenet.org
American Pain Foundation. Educational material for patients and families, including material specifically for military & veterans with chronic pain. Instructions for 6-week yoga class for chronic pain.	www.painfoundation.org
Australian *Transport Accident Commission* has an extensive selection of physical and psychosocial outcome measures.	http://www.tac.vic.gov.au Go to Provider Resources, Clinical Resources, then Outcome Measures
Change Pain: A modular approach to understanding pain and its management. Educational resources for clinicians.	http://www.change-pain.co.uk/
Fibromyalgia Network. Educational resources for individuals with fibromyalgia.	www.fmnetnews.com
International Association for the Study of Pain (IASP). Professional organization for researchers, clinicians and educators. Has some public education resources.	www.iasp-pain.org
Mayday Pain Project. Educational information for providers, patients, and specific sections for caregivers.	www.painandhealth.org
National Fibromyalgia Association. Educational material for individuals with fibromyalgia.	www.fma.org
Pain Treatment Topics. Educational material for clinicians, patients and families. Links to resources on many other sites. Comprehensive section on pain assessment tools.	www.pain-topics.org
Pain.com. Educational modules and articles for clinicians.	www.pain.com
PainAction. Educational material for patients. Includes self-management tools. Integrated with clinician educational site PainEDU.edu	www.painaction.com
PainDoctor.com. Educational material for patients and families.	www.paindoctor.com
PainEDU.org. Educational material for clinicians and educators. Includes downloadable PowerPoint lectures. Integrated with patient education site PainAction.	www.painedu.org

Web Resources with Clinical Treatment Guidelines for Chronic Pain

Agency for Healthcare Research and Quality Has multiple clinical practice guidelines on chronic pain (and many other conditions) (16, 18, 216)	http://www.guideline.gov/index.aspx Search for Chronic Pain
American Society of Anesthesiologists: Practice Guidelines for Chronic Pain Management (18)	http://www.guideline.gov/index.aspx Search for Chronic Pain http://journals.lww.com/anesthesiology/ Fulltext/2010/04000/Practice_Guidelines_ for_Chronic_Pain_Management_.13.asp
California Department of Industrial Relations, Division of Worker Relations (15)	https://www.dir.ca.gov/dwc/DWCPropRegs/ MTUS_Regulations/MTUS_ChronicPain MedicalTreatmentGuidelines.pdf
Institute for Clinical Systems Improvement Clinical Practice Guideline: Assessment and Management of Chronic Pain ((16)	http://www.icsi.org/guidelines_and_more/ Select Musculo-Skeletal Disorders, then Pain, Chronic *
World Health Organization (WHO) treatment guidelines on pain.	http://www.who.int/medicines/areas/ quality_safety/guide_on_pain/en/

- Angier P, Merryman-Means M, Marie-Sargent J, and Gibson W. The Joy of Comfortable Sex: A Guide for Couples with Back or Neck Pain, Excelsior Books, Albany, NY, 2007.
- Block SH, and Block CB. Mind-Body Workbook for PTSD: A 10-Week Program for Healing After Trauma. New Harbinger Publications, Oakland, CA, 2010.
- Branch R, and Willson R. Cognitive Behavioural Therapy Workbook For Dummies. For Dummies, Hoboken, NJ, 2008.
- Branch R, and Willson R. Cognitive Behavioural Therapy For Dummies, ed 2. John Wiley and Sons, Hoboken, NJ, 2010.
- Butler D, and Moseley L. Explain Pain. Orthopedic Physical Therapy Products, Minneapolis, MN, 2003.
- Caudill MA, Benson H. Managing Pain Before It Manages You, ed 3. Guilford Press, New York, NY, 2008.
- Davies C. The Trigger Point Therapy Workbook: Your Self-Treatment Guide for Pain Relief, ed 2. New Harbinger Publications, Oakland, CA, 2004.
- Davis M, Eshelman ER, and McKay M. The Relaxation & Stress Reduction Workbook, ed 6. New Harbinger Publications, Oakland, CA, 2008.
- Gardner-Nix J. The Mindfulness Solution to Pain: Step-by-Step Techniques for Chronic Pain Management, The PTSD Workbook **2009.**
- Hebert LA. Sex and Back Pain: Advice on Restoring Comfortable Sex Lost to Back Pain. Impacc USA, Greenville, ME, 1997.
- Hulme J. Physiological Quieting (CD), Phoenix Core Solutions, Missoula, MT, 2006.
- Kabat-Zinn J. Full Catastrophe Living: Using the Wisdom of Your Body and Mind to Face Stress, Pain, and Illness. Delta, Brooklyn, NY, 1990.
- Kabat-Zinn J. Mindfulness for Beginners (CD), Sounds True, Louisville, CO, 2006.
- Kabat-Zinn J. Mindfulness Meditation for Pain Relief: Guided Practices for Reclaiming Your Body and Your Life (CD), Sounds True, Louisville, CO, 2009.
- Kassan SK, Vierck CJ, and Vierck E. Chronic Pain for Dummies. For Dummies, Hoboken, NJ, 2008.
- Kaufman M, Silverberg C, and Odette F. The Ultimate Guide to Sex and Disability, ed 2. Cleis Press, Berkely, CA, 2007.
- Otis JD. Managing Chronic Pain: A Cognitive-Behavioral Therapy Approach Workbook. Oxford University Press, New York, NY, 2007.
- Schiraldi G. The Post-Traumatic Stress Disorder Sourcebook, ed 2. McGraw-Hill, Columbus, OH, 2009.
- Tinkle B. Issues and Management of Joint Hypermobility. Left Paw Press, Greens Fork, IN, 2008.
- Tinkle B. Joint Hypermobility Handbook. Left Paw Press, Greens Fork, IN, 2010.
- Turk DC, and Winter F. The Pain Survival Guide: How to Reclaim Your Life. American Psychological Association, Washington, DC, 2005.
- Williams WB, and Poijula S. The PTSD Workbook: Simple, Effective Techniques for Overcoming Traumatic Stress Symptoms. New Harbinger Publications, Oakland, CA, 2002.

Psychosocial Disorders

Pat Precin, MS, OTR/L, LP · Chapter **26**

Psychosocial factors pertain to the psychological development of an individual in relation to his or her social environment.[1] Psychosocial factors are numerous, as a person's psyche is affected by countless events in the internal and external environments. This chapter focuses on the psychosocial factors that may influence the direction of physical therapy intervention. Some examples of psychosocial factors include premorbid status or mental illnesses, personality styles, **coping strategies**, defense mechanisms, and emotional reactions to disability. Others include spirituality, values, environment, adjustment, cognitive abilities, **motivation**, family, social supports, **life roles**, and educational level. All of these factors can affect patients and treatment outcomes.

This chapter (1) identifies and describes how psychosocial factors can influence rehabilitation; (2) demonstrates how to address such factors during physical therapy intervention; and (3) provides indications for referral to psychosocial rehabilitation specialists. Psychosocial factors profoundly affect a patient's ability to recover. Patients who are emotionally upset will have difficulty concentrating on physical therapy goals until emotional issues are addressed. If a patient is motivated to participate in rehabilitation, but his or her family members do not support the patient's rehabilitation goals, the patient will be unlikely to progress on returning home. Mental health status has been shown to be one of the most important predictors of physical health.[2] Wickramasekera et al[3] found that more than 50% of all visits to primary care doctors involved somatic complaints resulting from psychosocial problems. Patients with physical disabilities may fail to respond to treatment if a prominent psychosocial issue is affecting them as well.

Treatment outcomes will be influenced by patients' perceptions of their role in the rehabilitation process. Patients who believe that they possess control regarding their treatment and feel respected by staff tend to experience better **health** outcomes.[4,5] Empowerment, education, inclusion in goal setting, and a high level of engagement are important factors that positively influence **recovery**.

The mind and the body are highly connected.[6] Because of their reciprocal influence, psychosocial and physical issues should be addressed simultaneously to best facilitate recovery. A slow recovery may cause or prolong **depression**, which may in turn further delay the rehabilitation period. Watts[7] believes that mental health interventions should be provided to all rehabilitation patients, because health outcomes tend to be poor and prolonged when psychosocial problems remain unaddressed.

Physical therapists regularly encounter patients who have psychiatric illnesses. Psychiatric conditions occur with some frequency in the general population (Table 26.1), but occur at an even higher rate in rehabilitation settings.[8] For instance, **panic disorder** occurs in 10% to 30% of patients treated in cardiovascular, respiratory, and neurological rehabilitation units, and in 60% of

Table 26.1	Lifetime World Prevalence of the Most Common Psychiatric and Personality Disorders[9]
Major Psychiatric or Personality Disorder	**Lifetime World Prevalence (%)**
Alzheimer's (85+ years old)	16–25
Alcohol abuse or dependence	15
Major depression	10
Marijuana abuse or dependence	5
Schizotypal personality disorder	3
Dependent personality disorder	3
Obsessive-compulsive disorder	2.5
Histrionic personality disorder	2.3
Borderline personality disorder	2
Antisocial personality disorder	2
Panic disorder	1–2
Schizophrenia	1

those treated in cardiology clinics (compared to 1% to 2% in the general population).[9] **Conversion disorder** has been reported to occur at a rate of up to 14% in general medical or surgical inpatient units (compared to 0.5% in the general population).[10] Friedland and McColl[11] found the prevalence of depression and substance abuse to be significantly higher among people with disabilities than in the general population, as did Turner and Beiser,[12] who documented the rate to be three times higher regardless of gender and age. Seventeen percent of senior adults with disabilities also had a diagnosis of major depression, and 14% had mild depression that interfered with daily activities.[13] Twenty-seven percent of patients with stroke were found to be depressed—a finding that correlated with poorer rehabilitation outcomes.[14] Patients with traumatic brain injury (TBI), spinal cord injury (SCI), and Parkinson's disease also reported higher levels of depression compared to the general public.[15,16]

If a patient does not have a preexisting psychosocial illness, he or she is more likely to develop one after the onset of physical illness. Anxiety disorders can result from endocrine (e.g., hyperthyroidism and hypothyroidism, pheochromocytoma, hypoglycemia, and hyperadrenocorticism), cardiovascular (e.g., congestive heart failure, pulmonary embolism, and arrhythmia), respiratory (e.g., chronic obstructive pulmonary disease, pneumonia, and **hyperventilation**), metabolic (e.g., vitamin B_{12} deficiency and porphyria), and neurological conditions (e.g., vestibular dysfunctions, encephalitis, and neoplasm).[9] The onset of depression has also been linked to the presence of an existing physical disability.[11,12] There is evidence for the converse as well; the longer one possesses some form of mental health concern, the greater the risk for developing a physical illness. Depression is a risk factor for heart disease and post-stroke mortality.[17,18] Heinemann et al[19] found that alcohol-related automobile accidents are responsible for a significant number of SCIs, and Zegans[20] reported that psychological problems could be exacerbated by physical illness or injuries. Anxiety can also increase the risk of cardiovascular disease and **hypertension**.[21]

Although the co-occurrence of physical disabilities and mental illness is high, the rate of treatment for mental illness among people with disabilities is low. In 1997, only 23% of adults with depression, 38% with **anxiety** disorders, and 47% with serious mental illness received treatment.[13]

A thorough examination of the patient's **psychological** and **social functioning** can contribute significantly to a better understanding of needs, fears, anxieties, and capabilities, as well as furnish essential information about the patient's emotional adjustment to disability, assets and liabilities, personality structure, and cognitive functioning. These can then be used to better understand the patient's emotional barriers and behavioral difficulties that can impede recovery. Although not inclusive, Box 26.1 highlights the major areas of consideration in a mental health examination.

Whether physical therapists should address psychosocial issues during treatment or refer psychologically impaired patients to other professionals depends on several variables: (1) the severity of the patient's psychosocial

---

Box 26.1 Elements of a Mental Health Examination

Client Demographics

- Gender, age, culture, ethnicity, education, economic status, primary (and secondary) language(s)
- Living environment (past, present, and projected future) and environmental supports
- Family history of psychiatric diagnoses/interventions
- Current complaints
- Psychiatric medication (past and current)
- Roles (past, present, and projected future)
- Occupation (past, present, and projected future)
- Social supports (past, present, and projected future)
- Leisure interests (past, present, and projected future)
- Goals (past, present, and projected future)
- Values (past, present, and projected future)
- History of psychiatric hospitalizations, substance abuse detoxifications, and/or rehabilitation stays

Systems Review

- Psychosocial

Examination

Chosen to measure or identify the following:

- Cognitive status (orientation, memory [short-term, long-term, working memory], executive functioning, judgment, calculations, attention, processing, meta-cognition, use of cognitive strategies), volition, self-awareness, mental status, degree of organicity and cognitive disability and its relationship to the patient's rehabilitative capacity. *Primary impairments*: disorientation, amnesia, word-finding difficulty, impaired memory, poor judgment, executive functioning deficits, thought blocking, poor use of cognitive strategies and/or meta-cognition, lack of motivation, impaired self-awareness of limitations, impairments in mental status.
- Emotional status. *Primary impairments*: anxiety, depression, mania, hypomania, grief, mourning, shock, anger, suicidal ideation, emotional numbness, overwhelmed, paranoia, agitated, low self-esteem, regression, delusions, poor reality testing, inappropriate affect, blunted affect, hypervigilance or hypovigilance, anhedonia (inability to experience pleasure), mood swings.
- Defense mechanisms. *Primary impairments*: The use of predominantly primitive defense mechanisms (such as splitting, acting out, denial, devaluation, dissociation, idealization, isolation of affect, projection) as opposed to more mature defenses (sublimation, humor, rationalization, omnipotence, altruism, autistic fantasy). Defense mechanisms are rigid enough to impair ego functioning.
- Personality types. *Primary impairments*: personality disorders (paranoid, antisocial, dependent, borderline, histrionic, narcissistic, avoidant, obsessive-compulsive, schizoid, schizotypal).
- Coping styles. *Primary impairments*: external locus of control, self-blame, substance abuse, and non direct passive and escape/avoidance modes of coping.

Continued

Box 26.1 Elements of a Mental Health Examination—cont'd

- Determination of suicidal tendencies, decompensation, and other risks. *Primary impairments*: history of suicide attempts in self or family members, current suicidal ideation, suicide note, plan for suicide, emotional and/or behavioral regression, substance abuse, feelings of hopelessness and/or helplessness, birthdays or anniversaries of deaths of loved ones, holidays, anniversaries of traumatic events.
- Symbolic meaning of the disability and loss, and the compensatory reserves that can be elicited. *Primary impairments*: Poor compensatory reserves or use of compensatory strategies. The meaning of the disability is both negative and fixed/rigid (e.g., the disability is karmic or a curse that is deserved).
- Levels of pain, stress, tolerance, and secondary gain. *Primary impairments*: Low frustration tolerance coupled with high levels of pain and/or stress. The secondary gain of the impairment is high (important) enough to cause a fixation at a lower than expected level of functioning, result in malingering, or interfere with rehabilitation.
- Sexual practices. *Primary impairments*: sexual dysfunction, impotence secondary to psychiatric medication, unprotected sex, impulsive sexual behavior, sexual abuse, perversions, hypersexuality, sexual addictions.
- Current functional capacities. *Primary impairments*: Problems with basic activities of daily living or instrumental activities of daily living, inability to perform in current roles and occupations, decreased community mobility, inability to live independently.

issue; (2) the level of comfort with which the physical therapist can address psychosocial problems; and (3) the patient's ability to progress in rehabilitation if existing psychosocial issues are not addressed. Professionals to whom referrals may be made for additional psychosocial intervention include but are not limited to psychiatrists, **psychologists, psychiatric nurses, occupational therapists,** social workers, creative arts therapists, vocational counselors, **rehabilitation counselors, substance abuse professionals,** and **pastoral counselors.**

■ PSYCHOSOCIAL ADAPTATION

The combination of intense psychological stress, uncertain prognosis, prolonged treatment, and interference with daily activities can greatly affect the rehabilitation of patients with disabilities and chronic illnesses. **Disability** is loss of or diminished ability to perform specific social roles normally expected of the patient. **Psychosocial adaptation** to disability and chronic illness is an ongoing, dynamic, evolving process through which a patient strives to attain an optimal state of function within his or her environment.[22] Successful psychosocial adaptation may be characterized by (1) a sense of personal mastery; (2) participation in social, recreational, or vocational pursuits; (3) successful negotiation of the environment; and (4) a realistic awareness of one's current strengths, deficits, and functional capacities.[23] Adjustment is the final phase in adaptation and includes striving to achieve life goals, feeling self-confident and having positive self-esteem, possessing a positive attitude toward one's disability, forming emotional connections to others, and establishing a community member role.[24]

The processes of **adaptation** and adjustment are influenced by whether or not a chronic illness or disability is congenital or adventitious, of sudden onset or gradually progressive, and stable or unstable. Patients born with a physical disability and those who acquire them as a result of accident or disease later in life have substantial psychological differences.[25] Children born with a physical disability have only experienced life with their impairment; the development of their self-identity commonly mirrors that of children without disabilities.

In contrast, patients with adventitious disabilities often experience acute loss and grief. Patients with gradually progressive diseases or disabilities of sudden onset often experience anxiety and **shock** when first becoming aware of their condition. Such anxiety and shock is often followed by anger and depression, as patients realize the magnitude and consequences of their diagnosis.[22] Disabilities of sudden onset (e.g., injuries or accidents) are usually experienced as crises that will change the lives of patients and their families for all time.

Grief, Mourning, and Sorrow

Grief is a psychological state of distress resulting from a significant loss. In reaction to a disability, grief may emerge from lost function, broken relationships, the loss of one's familiar self-identity, and disrupted roles. Grief is characterized by preoccupation with loss and feelings of worthlessness or helplessness. Specific symptoms include feelings of tightness of the throat, muscular weakness, emptiness in the abdomen, anxiety that is described as painful, shortness of breath and choking, and periodic waves of physical distress lasting up to an hour. Other symptoms may include forgetfulness, poor concentration, dissociation, insomnia, loss of appetite, compulsive behavior, an inability to manage time in a productive manner, disorganized cognitive functioning, social **withdrawal,** guilt, decreased ability to make decisions, excessive speech, and hostility.[26] Severe, prolonged cases of grief can compromise the immune system.[27] The grief–mourning period is unpredictable, lasting anywhere from 6 months to 2 or more years. According to Donatelle and Davis, the grieving process consists of

10 stages: (1) frozen feelings; (2) emotional release; (3) loneliness; (4) physical symptoms; (5) guilt; (6) panic; (7) hostility; (8) selective memory; (9) struggle for a new life pattern; and (10) a sense that life is okay.[26] It is important to note that such stages do not always occur in a progressive linear fashion, and some stages may occur simultaneously.

Grief is a natural experience necessary to regain or adapt to one's losses and construct a new self-concept. New coping skills are learned as patients adjust to unfamiliar challenges. There may be a difference between people grieving over loss from a disability and those grieving over other types of losses.[27] When grief occurs as a result of disability, it may become prolonged, as the patient must continuously strive to accept the disability and his or her altered self. Burke et al[28] described the grief of people with disabilities as "chronic sorrow," or a grief regarding the loss of normality. Lindgren et al[29] defined chronic sorrow as (1) progressive sadness that often increases after the initial loss; (2) prolonged periods of sorrow with no predictable end; and (3) recurrent or cyclic in nature as the sadness is continuously triggered by internal or external events that reawaken loss. Patients with chronic sorrow can eventually experience adaptation to their losses if they are highly motivated to rebuild their lives and find meaning in their experience. Conversely, patients with pathological grief often experience prolonged feelings of guilt, anger, and sadness that inhibit function and adaptation.

It is important to recognize that grief can be an all-encompassing experience that can take time and energy away from rehabilitation, thereby affecting the process of rehabilitation and its outcomes. Physical therapists must understand grieving, mourning, and sorrow so that a patient's lack of progress or motivation is not misinterpreted as **malingering**.

Phase Models of Psychosocial Adaptation

The literature regarding psychosocial adaptation to chronic disability and illness falls into two opposing theories of adaptation—one in which adaptation occurs as a set of nonsequential and independent patterns of behavior, and the other in which adaptation occurs progressively through a series of phases.

Phase models suggest that a patient's reaction to chronic disability or illness follows a stable sequence of phases, or stages, that are hierarchically and temporally ordered. This progression is gradual, linear, and involves the psychological assimilation of changes to one's body image and self-concept. The most frequently identified phases in the adaptation to chronic disability and disease are shock, anxiety, denial, depression, internalized anger, externalized hostility, acknowledgment, and final adjustment.[22]

Shock

Shock usually occurs as the initial reaction to a psychological trauma or severe and sudden physical injury. It results from an overwhelming experience and may include the inability to move or speak, psychic numbness, decreased cognitive skills, disorganization, and depersonalization.

During a traumatic event, an individual will respond primarily at the physiological level; emotional reactions are commonly delayed until the event is over and the individual is medically stable. Likewise, the medical emergency team will first implement immediate lifesaving attempts before addressing accompanying psychological issues.

During a perceived or real catastrophic event, an organism would most likely respond with what Selye termed the **general adaptation syndrome** (GAS).[30] Selye described GAS as an organism's defensive adaptation attempt, which expresses itself through physiological and emotional responses aimed at dealing with such emergencies. During GAS, there is a physiochemical chain reaction, whereby a peptide called corticotropin-releasing factor (CRF) is secreted to stimulate the release of adrenocorticotropic hormone (ACTH). ACTH sets into motion an increase of specific physiological activity designed to maximize the body's defense capacity while minimizing the utilization of nonessential physiological activities. Although an increase in CRF serves the person's self-defensive strategies, its inhibitory effect on other body functions—such as the production of insulin and calcium—is undesirable in the long run.

Studies have shown that injection of a CRF antagonist reduces anxiety in stressful situations.[31] When the inhibitory effects of CRF are prolonged, however, the additional undesirable effects of hypertension, digestive problems, and interference with the immune system result. Selye[30] documented the devastating effect that a prolonged GAS response has on human mental and physical functioning.[30] Theorell et al[32] documented the occurrence of resultant illnesses long after the stress-producing event had ended.

Anxiety

Once the magnitude of the traumatic event is comprehended, anxiety in the form of a panic-stricken reaction commonly occurs and is marked by compulsive activity, confusion, elevated pulse rate, difficulty breathing, and cognitive flooding (e.g., when emotions such as anxiety preclude logical thought). Situations that activate the sympathetic nervous system through repeated alarm or chronic stress may alter synaptic transmission and lead to depression and malfunction of normal body systems.

It should be noted that the physiological and psychological reactions to stress are not limited to catastrophic conditions. An extensive body of research shows **stress reactions** to be present in individuals under conditions that may not be traumatic but nevertheless persistent and disruptive. Everyday life frustrations, internal and external conflicts, and changes in life conditions are major causes of the stress reaction that, over time, have a deleterious effect on a person's function and health. Physical therapists should be cognizant that even though a patient's emergency situation is over, a stress reaction may continue to be present.

Denial

Denial is often used as a defense mechanism to alleviate the anxiety and pain associated with a disability or illness. Denial occurs as a specific phase early in the adaptation process and protects the person from having to confront the overwhelming implications of illness or injury all at once. Instead, denial allows a gradual assimilation of one's altered reality. Breznitz[33] identified seven types of denial:

1. Denial of threatening information (using selective inattention and partial awareness)
2. Denial of vulnerability (exerting control and maximizing personal strengths)
3. Denial of urgency (using methods to see the situation as less pressing than it is)
4. Denial of affect (reduction of emotional impact)
5. Denial of affect relevance (diverting attention to other issues and believing that an emotion is coming from an unrelated cause)
6. Denial of personal relevance (attributing difficulties to a benign cause and blaming others when involvement was one's own)
7. Denial of all information (creating a barrier between external reality and one's psyche resulting in total disbelief of having an illness or disability)

Patients in the stage of denial may selectively attend to the environment, choose facts that support their beliefs about themselves and their condition, and ignore facts that remind them of their new challenges. They may have unrealistic and wishful goals for recovery and may be seen as indifferent and aloof.

Depression

The phase of depression occurs as denial lessens, allowing a greater awareness of one's losses. **Depression** is a reactive response of bereavement for impending death, suffering, or the loss of body function. Neurochemical and biological changes resulting from disability or disease, **premorbid** personality and family history, and reactions to stress have all been identified as risk factors for depression.[34,35]

Internalized Anger

Anger occurs in reaction to anxiety, misperception, threats of abandonment, feelings of helplessness, or fear of losing control. Characteristics of anger include hostility, resentment, or hatred. **Anger** is a response to loss and if not expressed is termed **internalized anger**. Internalized anger is associated with self-blame and is a manifestation of self-directed bitterness and resentment. Signs of internalized anger include manipulation, sabotage, and

passive-aggressive behavior. Sometimes anger emerges when a patient attributes his or her own behaviors to the onset of disability or disease. In such cases, internalized anger can result in depression, suicidal tendencies, or **psychosomatic** complaints—particularly in people who have a chronic condition.[36]

There are many reasons why patients may not express anger: fear of losing loved ones or social isolation, **cultural restraints**, lack of awareness, fear of losing control, or belief that expressing anger is inappropriate or dangerous. Repressed anger not only affects a patient's psychological well-being, but may also slow rehabilitation. It is important for physical therapists to encourage expression of angry feelings by providing a safe environment for patients to verbalize their anger in appropriate ways. Therapists might state that anger is a normal emotion—especially under the patient's circumstances—offer reasons why it is important to express anger, and provide anger management techniques (e.g., effective coping strategies). It is equally important for therapists to understand that although a patient's anger may be directed at the therapist, such anger more often reflects the patient's own projected feelings regarding his or her disability.

Externalized Hostility

Externalized hostility is anger directed toward other people or objects in the environment and is an attempt to retaliate against activity limitations. Challenges encountered during rehabilitation may trigger externalized hostility. As time from the onset of the disability passes, externalized hostility tends to become more apparent.[37] Signs include passive-aggressive behaviors that obstruct rehabilitation, aggressive acts, hypercriticism, demanding or antagonistic behaviors, falsely blaming others, and abusive accusations. Patients who express anger aggressively through physical or verbal abuse, sarcasm, or controlling behaviors need the help of the entire team to redirect their anger into productive therapeutic activities that further their rehabilitation goals.

Acknowledgment

Acknowledgment is the first sign that the patient has accepted or recognized the permanency of the condition and its future implications. The patient begins to integrate activity limitations into his or her self-concept. During this phase, the patient accepts himself or herself as a person with a disability, develops a new self-concept, reassesses values, and searches for new goals and meaning.

Adjustment

Adjustment is the final phase in adaptation and involves the development of new ways of interacting successfully with others and one's environment. The person is now adjusted to the outside world after having fully assimilated his or her activity limitations from disability into a new, cohesive self. In this phase, the person regains self-worth, understands that new potentials are possible, pursues vocational and social goals, and overcomes obstacles that arise in the attainment of goals.

There is evidence that the phase model of adjustment to chronic disability or illness is nonlinear, multidimensional, and progressive. Phase models tend to have 10 common assumptions:[22]

1. People may skip one or more phases or may **regress** to an earlier phase, but adaptation is not usually reversible.
2. The pace and structure of adaptation can be influenced by external events or interventions (e.g., environmental changes or counseling) yet are mainly determined by internal processes.
3. Not everyone achieves adjustment; some fixate at earlier phases.
4. Adaptation is an unfolding, dynamic process that gradually shifts from initial experiences of distress to assimilation of loss and reconciliation.
5. The adaptation process is initiated by significant and permanent changes in the body's functional capacities and appearance, which are usually followed by alteration of self-concept and body image.
6. The amount of time spent in each phase varies and may be determined by a combination of the following factors: social support, financial and human resources, past exposure to crises, age at onset, severity, nature of the disability or illness, and premorbid personality.
7. Psychological maturity and growth occur as the patient progresses through the phases.
8. Psychological re-equilibrium occurs through gradual adaptation and integration of the perceived misfortune.
9. Human variability and uniqueness have a strong influence on the temporal ordering of phases—the sequence of phases is not universal.
10. Occasionally, phases may overlap, be nondiscrete, or fluctuate, causing patients to experience more than one reaction at a time.

Chronic Illness and Disability: Differences in Adaptation

There are marked differences in the way that people adapt psychosocially to a disability associated with a traumatic event—such as TBI—versus a chronic illness—such as multiple sclerosis (MS). The onset of disability in a traumatic event is sudden, and medical stability may be achieved shortly after. The onset of a chronic illness is usually insidious and gradual; its course is often uncertain and marked by states of remission and deterioration.[38] In chronic illness each onset of symptoms can be experienced as a new illness.

Shock may not be experienced by people with gradually deteriorating medical conditions (e.g., Parkinson's disease, rheumatoid arthritis, or diabetes mellitus), but

is usually experienced following a trauma (e.g., TBI, myocardial infarction, amputation, or SCI). The phases of anxiety and depression relate more to the past, such as grieving over the loss of premorbid functioning. Shock may be present but not as strong in people with life-threatening or end-stage diseases (e.g., AIDS, cancer, or amyotrophic lateral sclerosis). In a chronic illness, anxiety and depression relate more to the future (e.g., fear of death, feelings of hopelessness, and fear of the unknown).[39] The acknowledgment and adjustment phases may be more difficult to achieve in chronic, life-threatening conditions that require the internalization of and acceptance that the condition may worsen and result in death.

Post-traumatic Rehabilitation

The post-traumatic period may include phases of anxiety, depression, denial, internalized anger, and externalized hostility mentioned earlier, and is usually the time during which much, if not most, of the rehabilitative intervention takes place. It is also the period during which the psychological effects of the traumatic experience are more strongly felt by the patient. It seems as if the psychological defenses and reactions that became secondary during the initial traumatic period (shock phase) begin emerging as the physical injury is dealt with. These repressed reactions seem to interact with a growing awareness of the effects of the disability creating fears, anxieties, and behaviors that the rehabilitation team must address.

Regardless of which phase the patient is in, physical therapists need to be aware of each patient's **psychological needs**. During the initial phases of adaptation, patients may experience an awareness of their injuries that facilitates panic and fear of total dependence. Patients may also experience anxiety as a result of anticipating painful medical treatment. Some patients react to these feelings by desperately seeking control over their rehabilitation. Others experience shock regarding their losses and become overly dependent. Patients may idealize the past and have unrealistic expectations about the duration of their recovery.

During these early stages, physical therapists should praise small gains and work with caregivers so they can offer hope and support to the patient. Therapists should be supportive but careful not to make unrealistic predictions about the expected degree of recovery, because this may lead to disappointment, resentment, and depression.[40] One of the first approaches physical therapists can use to help patients regain self-control is **diaphragmatic breathing**, which may decrease pain and anxiety through the **relaxation response**.[41]

During the middle stages, physical therapists may need to educate patients about medical precautions, contraindicated movements or activities, how the patient's body has adapted to disability, and how to reformulate expectations. Psychosocial instruction should be integrated with information about activities of daily living

(ADL), mobility, strengthening, and endurance. The transition from the patient role to an independent adult member of society is a difficult adjustment and can result in anxiety, depression, and poor social integration.[22,42] Physical therapists should help patients prepare psychologically for discharge and reintegration into society. Some of the issues that patients may fear include negative reactions to their disability, feelings of inadequacy, having to identify new social supports, receiving help in the home environment, and adjusting to a new body image.

Body image includes judgment about one's appearance, an awareness of boundaries and personal space, judgment about one's bodily responses, perception of one's body parts and their movement, and an awareness of physical pleasure and pain. Body image is intimately related to self-concept and self-esteem. It affects a person's functional abilities, cognition, perceptions, attitudes, and emotions, as well as the reactions of others to oneself. Because body image changes throughout life, it is thought to be both dynamic and developmentally based. Difficulties brought on by a disability—such as activity limitations and pain and disfigurement—alter body image and threaten its stability. Patients must then reconstruct their body image and self-perception to adapt to this physical change.[22]

Biordi[43] has identified the following patterns in patients who experienced shifts in body image after disability: (1) denying the existence of one's body; (2) fantasizing about a lost or damaged body part being magically replaced or healthy; (3) concentrating solely on noninjured body parts in order to deny impairment of the affected area; and (4) experiencing a period of defensiveness followed by gradual acceptance and assimilation of their altered body.[43] The physical therapist's comfort level with the patient's physical disability and the therapist's attention to the affected body part may help the patient feel less ashamed about body changes.

■ PERSONALITY AND COPING STYLES

The more a patient has evolved socially and psychologically, the better he or she will be at using adaptive methods to deal with crises. Hence, a patient with a healthy premorbid personality but a severe physical disability may do better in rehabilitation than one with a less severe disability and a pathological premorbid personality.[44] When aware of their patients' personality styles, physical therapists will be more adept at strategizing interventions, developing a plan of care (POC), and motivating and guiding patients through rehabilitation.

Personality Types

Although each personality is unique, personalities have been categorized into different types, such as *type A, perfectionistic, authoritative,* and *passive-aggressive.* These personality types are nonpathological and develop in response to one's environment when young.

Individuals with type A personalities have a compulsive need to be achievers in all aspects of life. They are extremely independent and productive. These qualities also serve as defenses against low self-esteem and interpersonal conflicts. These people usually derive satisfaction from being strong individuals who can help others. If they can no longer participate in this role, they may become depressed because of a perceived inability to confirm their worth through altruistic activities. Physical therapists can use these qualities in patients with type A personalities to motivate their interest in rehabilitation. Because they are often self-starters and take initiative for their own learning, they can usually be depended on to independently practice home exercise programs (HEPs).

Individuals with perfectionistic personalities uphold high standards in order to maintain self-esteem. These individuals judge themselves by inflexible and possibly unachievable criteria and may not be able to tolerate slow progress during rehabilitation. Physical therapists may aid these patients by helping them derive pleasure from simple things, such as a meal, a sunset, a new shirt, or interesting information. Helping them discover value in these things offers them sources of self-esteem other than meeting impossibly high standards.

Individuals with authoritative personalities need to be in control and need things to be done in a particular way because of rigid perceptions regarding values, rules, and the manner in which others should behave. They are often concerned with status, tend to be judgmental, and have difficulty empathizing with others. During rehabilitation, these patients may try to dictate their treatment and engage in a power struggle with their physical therapists. Patients with authoritative personalities have difficulty adapting to disability, which often requires acceptance and compromise. They may require alternative strategies to solve what may have been perceived as an unsolvable problem. Physical therapists should engage patients in problem solving to generate strategies to meet their goals.

Individuals with passive-aggressive personalities express hostility by using passive techniques such as procrastination, **resistance**, stubbornness, and intentional inefficiency. These personalities react to authority negatively and have difficulty working with others. Physical therapists may work more efficiently with passive-aggressive patients by placing the responsibility for progress onto them. Patients can be instructed to make decisions about their treatment whenever possible and then summarize their progress after each session. This deemphasizes the physical therapist's **role** as an authority figure, and therefore the need for a passive-aggressive response.

Personality Disorders

When an individual's personality style deviates from cultural norms over a long period of time, is inflexible or pervasive, causes **distress** to oneself and others, and leads to activity limitations, that personality style is considered to be dysfunctional.[9] Personality disorders have been thoroughly classified. They include paranoid, antisocial (also referred to as sociopath or psychopath), borderline, histrionic, narcissistic, avoidant, dependent, obsessive-compulsive, schizoid, and schizotypal personalities. Freidman and Booth-Kewley[45] state that disability exacerbates preexisting pathology, meaning that the stress of dealing with a physical illness can make personality disorders even more pronounced.

Patients with paranoid personality disorder interpret the motives of others as malevolent when they may not be. This results from a pattern of suspiciousness and distrust. These patients believe that others are trying to exploit, deceive, or harm them. Because of such mistrust, they may discharge themselves from treatment. Physical therapists should look for behaviors that indicate paranoid thoughts such as hostile reactions, guardedness, argumentation, and stubbornness, and encourage patients to express their thoughts at that moment. If the patient seems paranoid, the physical therapist should help him or her to better understand the reality of a specific situation. For instance, if the patient complains about being forced to participate in an elaborate intervention so that, in his or her view, the therapist can make more money, the therapist should review the pros and cons of various treatments and discuss the clinical reasoning involved.

Literature can be very convincing since it does not come directly from the therapist.

Patients with antisocial personality frequently engage in deceit and manipulation. In rehabilitation, they may use an alias, lie to the staff, or malinger. They are irresponsible and often fail to comply with self-care procedures such as hygiene and home maintenance. They seek out and take advantage of weaker staff members, often using wit and charm. When they do not receive what they want, they commonly become irritable and violent, especially when staff members attempt to impose restrictions. They frequently cause disruption to others in rehabilitation. These patients require a cohesive **team approach** with immediate and strong intercommunication to minimize disruptive behaviors and refocus on rehabilitation goals.

Patients with borderline personality disorder have instability in emotions, relationships, and self-image; are impulsive; use primitive defense mechanisms such as splitting (Box 26.2) and devaluation; and tend to engage in self-destructive behaviors such as abusing drugs or **self-mutilation**. On the surface, they may appear critical of others but these are signs of deep vulnerability and should be treated as such. Therapists should respond with understanding and empathy instead of anger, and should emphasize strengths and strategies for ongoing work. Self-mutilating behaviors, such as repetitive cutting with razor blades, pinpricking, or cigarette burning, should be immediately reported to a doctor and referral made to a **psychiatrist**.

Box 26.2 Common Defense Mechanisms

Acting Out

Instead of expressing feelings verbally, the patient uses actions to release stress. For example, a patient is angry with the insurance company for not funding an athletic wheelchair, so refuses to use the standard wheelchair. Acting out occurs because certain feelings such as anger and hurt are too difficult to express verbally. Unexpressed feelings build anxiety until they are released through action.

The therapist should identify the feeling behind the acting out behavior by asking the patient why he or she behaved in that way. For instance, the therapist would ask the patient above about using the wheelchair. The patient's responses will eventually trace back to the original unexpressed feeling. Through questioning, the therapist brings to the patient's awareness the link between the feeling and the action. The patient can now verbalize and discuss the feeling. In the case above, the patient may be more willing to use the wheelchair. A patient who does not have difficulty verbalizing feelings tends not to act out.

Altruism

The patient becomes dedicated to helping others in order to manage his or her own stress. An altruistic patient may stop treatment to help everyone else in the treatment room, including the therapist. Such a patient receives gratification through these actions, and hence decreases his or her stress.

Autistic Fantasy

The patient engages in excessive daydreaming instead of pursuing human relationships in order to decrease stress. The patient may have difficulty following directions, may appear to be in another world, but happily so, and may become emotional and tense when returned to reality. If asked what he or she is thinking about, the patient may describe his or her fantasies, which can be a rich source of wishes and desires that can be used by the therapist to motivate the patient to work on short-term goals. For instance, a male patient relates a fantasy of dating his favorite teen idol. However, in order to engage in dating, he must first develop interpersonal skills and practice them in simulated and real-life settings.

Continued

Box 26.2   Common Defense Mechanisms—cont'd

Denial

Denial protects the ego from being overwhelmed by pain through an unrelenting process of disbelief. In the case of disability, denial may be used to protect the patient from reminders of an altered external reality and the resultant sense of loss. Therefore, the patient may refuse to acknowledge an emotionally painful condition or situation that is apparent to others. The patient often denies the severity of a new disability, believing he or she can return to previous jobs or roles, despite reality testing from the therapist. The patient may refuse rehabilitation, claiming that he or she just wants to leave the hospital in order to care for his or her children.

It is important to help the patient work through denial slowly in order to avoid depression, which may occur if the patient becomes aware of his or her reality before psychologically ready to accept it. If the patient's denial is so great that treatment cannot proceed, he or she should be referred to a psychologist to explore what disability means to his or her future life.

Devaluation

The patient is overly critical of others and of himself or herself and may insult therapists and other personnel. The therapist should not take such insults personally, but should offer empathy and kindness, which usually decrease devaluation and build rapport. Once a patient trusts the therapist, he or she may discuss insecurities and fears instead of defending against them through criticism. If the therapist becomes angry with the patient, the insults usually become worse and a power struggle may ensue.

Displacement

The patient transfers a response to, or feeling about, one object onto a less threatening object to minimize stress. For example, a patient may be angry with a spouse for driving the car recklessly and having an accident but takes the anger out on the physical therapist. In this situation, it may not be safe or helpful for the patient to express anger directly to the spouse, who may be the patient's only emotional support.

The therapist should help the patient transfer the misplaced feeling back to the object for which it was originally intended. The therapist might accomplish this by asking the patient a series of questions concerning the origin of the anger.

Dissociation

The patient deals with stress through a breakdown in memory, perception, consciousness, or sensorimotor behavior. The patient becomes detached from what is happening in the moment because it is too painful. The patient may stop speaking or participating in therapy and stare blankly into space for up to several minutes without responding to the environment. Afterward, the patient may not be aware of his or her dissociated state, or if he or she is, the patient may state that he or she "just spaced out." The patient who uses dissociation usually relies on it often; a physical therapist may note its occurrence several times during a session. It is important to notice what happened just before the dissociation to identify the painful thoughts, feelings, or actions that upset the patient.

Help-Rejecting

The patient deals with the stress of having covert hostile feelings toward caregivers by frequently asking for help and then rejecting every suggestion. Working with a patient who uses help-rejecting as a defense mechanism can be very frustrating. Such patients seem to sincerely seek help but reject all advice as ineffectual. In these cases, it may be helpful to point out to the patient that efforts to help have been thwarted. The patient is usually not aware that he or she has rejected all solutions and may then come up with a solution or be more open to one that has already been proposed.

Humor

Humor can be used to minimize stress by highlighting the ironic or amusing aspects of a stressful situation. For instance, a patient states that he is going to open up a hardware store since he has so much hardware (meaning surgically placed pins and plates) in his leg. A patient who uses humor as a defense mechanism usually feels better if the physical therapist laughs at his or her jokes and participates in joking behavior. It is a safe way for the patient to recognize the difficulty of his or her situation.

Idealization

A patient endows another individual with overly positive attributes to enhance an otherwise negative situation. This other individual may be the therapist, in which case the therapeutic relationship is often strengthened. Or it could be a spouse, in which case problems could arise if he or she is not such a positive support to the patient. It is important to uncover the reality of the situation so necessary treatment and discharge plans can be made.

Box 26.2   Common Defense Mechanisms—cont'd

Intellectualization

A patient uses intellectual reasoning rather than expressing emotions in order to avoid painful feelings. For example, the patient describes neurotransmitters and synapses when asked about a head injury. Therapists can relate to such patients by intellectualizing with them. For example, the therapist may speak about the patient's head injury in terms of science and facts instead of emotions.

Isolation of Affect

A patient separates feelings from ideas when thinking about and discussing an upsetting event to minimize negative feelings associated with it. He or she speaks of the details regarding the recent accident that caused a disability without mentioning any feelings associated with the event to avoid reexperiencing them. Therapists should help the patient integrate feelings about an event into his or her memory of it. This can be achieved by asking the patient how he or she feels about certain aspects of the event while talking about it.

Omnipotence

A patient feels or acts as if he or she is better than others to guard against feelings of inadequacy. For instance, a patient looks down on other patients with disabilities because he does not want to see himself as disabled. A therapist might observe criticism and devaluation of external objects, bragging about accomplishments or skills, conceit, and grandiosity. The therapist could use this defense mechanism to motivate the patient to get better in order to avoid feeling inferior.

Projection

A patient transfers his or her own unacceptable feelings, thoughts, and beliefs onto another person and becomes certain that the other person really feels, thinks, and believes that way. A patient cannot tolerate the idea of having unacceptable feelings such as anger, but expresses them by projecting them onto another person, remaining relatively guilt free. For example, a patient says that his therapist is annoyed with him when in fact the patient is annoyed with his therapist.

Rationalization

A patient uses elaborate explanations to reassure him or her that personal actions are driven by sound motives, when he or she may truly be unsure. A family member caring for a relative with congestive heart failure asks for a do not resuscitate (DNR) status, citing extensive research studies. The family member states that the relative will die soon anyway, thereby concealing the real and less acceptable reason for seeking the DNR status—to relieve himself or herself from caregiving responsibilities.

Repression

A patient unconsciously erases negative experiences, wishes, or thoughts from consciousness in order to decrease stress. For example, a patient finds an endearing letter to a spouse from a student and forgets to mention it because the possibility of the spouse having an affair is painful. Repressed material can be dangerous because it remains in the unconscious. Encouraging the patient to express his or her feelings, both good and bad, helps free him or her of these feelings and any possible negative urges to act on them.

Splitting

A patient views a person or event through a positive or negative lens at any given point in time. Later, the patient may flip his or her feelings to the opposite end of the spectrum regarding the same person or situation, acting in this manner because he or she has difficulty integrating ambivalent feelings. Some patients will often attempt to split staff, identifying one staff member with unrealistic positive attributes, while identifying another staff member with unrealistic negative qualities. The staff member who has been identified as negative has usually denied some desire the patient requested. The patient may approach the positively identified therapist and complain that the first therapist is insensitive and does not understand his or her needs. The patient may express that only the positively identified therapist understands his or her problems. However, when the positively identified therapist also denies the patient's request, the patient then vilifies that therapist as well. The therapist may help the patient to integrate the opposite poles of his or her emotions by bringing both positive and negative emotions into consciousness. The patient then may be able to see the reality of his or her situation.

Sublimation

Sublimation occurs when patients transform unacceptable emotions or desires into socially acceptable actions. For example, a patient who is angry about a recent divorce may be unable to consciously express those feelings for fear of losing the affection of his or her children. Instead of expressing the anger he or she may sublimate those emotions into a more socially acceptable action, such as working out in the gym and eventually training for marathons. By participating in an activity that is valued and admired in the society, he or she gains the positive support of others.

Continued

Box 26.2 Common Defense Mechanisms—cont'd

Suppression

A patient intentionally avoids thoughts of disturbing feelings, situations, experiences, or problems in order to reduce stress. When refusing to talk to his or her therapist about the accident that brought him or her to rehabilitation, the patient suppresses disturbing thoughts. Therapists can refer patients to creative arts therapists (e.g., dance, music, art, drama, or poetry therapists) to facilitate the expression of disturbing thoughts, because such emotions accrue over time if not expressed.

Undoing

A patient uses behavior or words to negate unacceptable actions, thoughts, or feelings. For example, one who is frequently bullied by another patient during rehabilitation feels rage against the aggressor, but invites him or her to lunch.

Note: In both undoing and suppression, disturbing feelings are intentionally avoided. In suppression, the feelings are avoided and nothing else happens. Feelings are avoided and concealed through opposing words or actions. Both undoing and suppression differ from repression in that repression is an unconscious act.

Patients with histrionic personality disorder seek attention via excessive emotionality. Since these patients respond well to audiences, therapists should provide situations in which patients can gain positive attention from doing well in rehabilitation. Physical therapists should set boundaries to help patients achieve a balance between their need to express themselves and their need to focus on therapeutic interventions. A calm and logical approach to rehabilitation helps settle intense emotions. Patients who have difficulty verbalizing their feelings can be referred to a **creative arts therapist** to facilitate expression through nonverbal means—such as music, dance or art.

Patients with narcissistic personality disorder are condescending and have a need for admiration and feelings of superiority. If an illness causes a reduction in this image, they will require help from their physical therapists to identify strengths and feel acceptable.

Patients with schizoid personality disorder have a **flat affect**, or limited range of emotional expression, and are detached from social interactions. The therapist should attend to the patient's rehabilitation without trying to engage him or her in a great deal of social interaction. If the disorder has been long-standing, the patient will likely feel uncomfortable socializing.

Patients with schizotypal personality disorder have eccentric behavior, perceptual or **cognitive distortions**, and marked distress in social relationships. The social intimacy and physical restriction of a rehabilitation environment may cause anxiety. Slow, unforced integration into the therapeutic setting may be required. Asking patients whether their views of reality are accurate may help them remain focused on achieving rehabilitation goals.

Patients with avoidant personality disorder suffer from social inhibition, feelings of inadequacy, and hypersensitivity to criticism. Physical therapists should reassure these patients that they are doing well and emphasize their strengths.

Patients with dependent personality disorder exhibit clinging behavior, need others to care for them, and are submissive. They may fail to function independently in their life roles even after physical functioning has returned, continuing the pattern of dependency. They fear abandonment and require constant reassurances that staff members understand their condition and care about them. Some respond to clear explanations and feedback about their progress and treatment plans. The therapist should reinforce independent behavior through attention and positive feedback while extinguishing dependent behavior by ignoring or redirecting it.

Patients with obsessive-compulsive personality disorder have a long-standing preoccupation with control and order and are often perfectionists. Their self-esteem may suffer if they perceive a loss of control, and they may react by becoming more obstinate, demanding, and inflexible. Those who publicly express their anger may become ashamed. These patients require greater predictability in treatment than usual, dislike change, and do well when given an established routine to follow. The therapist should provide rehabilitative activities that promote a sense of control and predictability, and consider allowing patients to set treatment goals, and then monitor their daily progress.

Coping Styles

Coping styles are ways that people deal with stress and include behavioral, emotional, and cognitive efforts to cope with internal and external challenges that strain ordinary resources.[46] Theories of coping suggest that it is not what happens to people that is important, but rather how they react.[47] Various coping strategies have been identified in the literature and summarized by Livneh and Antonak.[22] They include planning, problem solving, wishful thinking, avoiding, minimizing, seeking social support, searching for meaning, emoting feelings, blaming, accepting, negotiating, disengaging, and turning to religion. These and others can be categorized into three different types of coping: (1) seeking versus avoiding control and information; (2) expressing versus repressing emotional reactions; and (3) seeking versus withdrawing from social interactions and networks.

Coping strategies have been found to be of great importance in rehabilitation. Patients with higher-level coping skills can more easily identify and report symptoms, make treatment decisions, comply with intervention, and accept support. Patients with good problem solving skills and positive attitudes have been found to make more positive adjustments to their disabilities than patients with low self-esteem and poor self-concept.[48] Coping styles often determine whether or not patients seek medical help and follow advice.[46]

Social influences, psychological characteristics, and health beliefs have been shown to modify the impact of disability and disease on an individual. Social activism, positive self-acceptance, and information seeking have predicted better ability to cope with a disability.[49] Krause and Rohe[50] studied the relationship between adjustment and personality following SCI and found that positive values, emotions, actions, and warmth correlated with superior outcomes. Adaptive coping styles that result in positive outcomes for people with disabilities utilize positive, direct, and active problem solving, social support seeking, and information seeking. Maladaptive coping styles that lead to unfavorable adaptation outcomes include self-blame; non-direct, passive, and escape/avoidance modes of coping; and substance abuse.

Locus of control is a belief about one's ability to control life conditions and events.[51] Patients with an *external locus of control* believe that other people or outside factors determine outcomes. Patients with an *internal locus of control* take responsibility for change because they believe they can affect their own circumstances. The latter leads to goal-directed activity and active coping.

The ability to intentionally change the relative importance of events that occur in one's life requires constant practice.[52] It has been shown that patients with external loci of control experience stress and anxiety in rehabilitation, whereas patients with internal loci of control have quicker recoveries, better motivation, more hope, and more energy.

Coping styles can be examined through interviews, observations, self-report surveys, checklists, and information from the family. Treatment considerations based on these findings should include emphasis on previous ways of successfully coping and expanding the range of coping strategies, such as maintaining a journal to increase self-expression. Taking care of a pet or using animal assistance can lend help, comfort, and companionship, as well as increase motivation. Group treatment can also be used to increase social networks.[53,54]

Many people with disabilities who have risk factors for emotional problems, such as lower education, less income, and social isolation, still do well in life because of a certain resilience defined as successful adaptation to stressful situations or events.[55] Researchers of resilience identify protective factors that safeguard people from adverse consequences. Protective factors can arise from the individual, family, and society and are concerned with how these strengths and supports provide security, safety, and positive opportunities.

Turning points are important experiences and realizations that enable people to find new direction, purpose, or meaning in life. King et al[56] reported four protective factors: determination, perseverance, spiritual beliefs, and social support. Seven protective processes were also identified: transcending, self-understanding, accommodating, receiving a diagnosis that helps explain a patient's experiences, believing in oneself, using anger as motivation, and setting goals. These protective factors and processes help people with disabilities during turning points in their lives. Analysis of turning points revealed three major ways that patients maintained meaning in their lives: through doing, belonging, and understanding themselves in relationship to the world. Doing involves participating in activities that are fulfilling and facilitate competency. Belonging involves perceived acceptance by others or membership in a valued group. Understanding oneself in relationship to the larger world provides a sense of identity and sometimes purpose.

■ COMMON DEFENSE REACTIONS TO DISABILITY

Defense mechanisms are coping styles that people use to defend against internal and external stressors. They happen automatically and unconsciously. Some individuals use many different defense mechanisms throughout their lives, but most tend to utilize only one or two. The goal is not to change or modify these defense mechanisms, but to identify them in order to understand the patient's psychological processes that underlie certain behaviors and resistance. Understanding these behaviors can help physical therapists to motivate or redirect patients during difficult times in their rehabilitation. The defense mechanisms described in Box 26.2 are common reactions to disability and can be further explored in the *Diagnostic and Statistical Manual of Mental Disorders.*[9]

Anxiety

Anxiety is the apprehensive anticipation of future danger or misfortune accompanied by feelings of tension and agitation. The anticipated danger may be real or imagined, but is experienced both psychologically and physiologically.[57] The experience of **anxiety** varies in different patients. When someone is nervous (indicating a moderate level of anxiety), he or she may experience an upset stomach or headache. When someone is experiencing a panic attack (indicating a high level of anxiety), he or she may feel impending doom and terror. A symptom of anxiety in one patient may be heart palpitations, while in another it may be shortness of breath. What is anxiety producing to one patient may cause little to no anxiety in another. Given these variables, the following definitions may facilitate physical therapists' understanding of their patients' conditions.

A **panic attack** is a sudden onset of intense, overwhelming fear that may include feelings of imminent danger or impending doom. These attacks are marked by symptoms of palpitations, chest pain, smothering or choking sensations, shortness of breath, and fear of losing control, dying, or going crazy. Panic attacks may be unexpected (occurring without an internal or external trigger) or situational. It is unclear what kind of physiological change in the brain may trigger such a severe response. A **phobia** is an anxiety disorder characterized by intense anxiety resulting from thoughts of, or exposure to, a specific feared situation or object (such as heights, spiders, or elevators) leading to avoidance of that object or situation. **Generalized anxiety disorder** is defined as excessive worry and anxiety without an apparent source persisting for at least 6 months.[9]

Causes of Anxiety

Twenty to 30 million Americans suffer from anxiety.[26] Some signs and symptoms of anxiety are listed in Table 26.2, and behaviors that may result from anxiety are provided in Table 26.3. Much of the literature on stress and coping has identified major life events as stressors. Life events refer to major changes in lifestyle, status, role, or situation. This view is consistent with the notion that stress, though individually mediated, is to some degree environmentally based and/or exacerbated by environmental and social conditions. Various life event measures have been developed and are used in examining potential environmental stress. One of the more well-known and used instruments is the **Holmes-Rahe Social Readjustment Rating Scale** (Appendix 26.A), which quantifies the effects of life changes on stress and health.[58] Such measures of life events assume a relatively global impact, and take into account only those items listed. Although there is justified validity in such an approach, there exist potentially more sensitive and valid measures, one of which is the Hassles Scale.

The **Hassles Scale** (Appendix 26.B), developed by Kanner et al,[59] requires subjects to identify the irritating and frustrating demands of everyday transactions with the environment. This approach takes into account the individual's perception of events believed to pose a threat. It is consistent with the theoretical assumption that chronic struggle may tax coping abilities and lead to greater difficulty in the management of daily life events. Considering the enormous changes in a person's function when disability occurs, patients are more likely to expect an increase in daily hassles and stressors. Dealing with life becomes more taxing when disabling circumstances block one's coping style, causing a gap between the person and his or her fit within the world. Repeat occurrences of stress and the continual need to adjust to new situations can result in repetition of the fight-or-flight response, which can, over time, result in high blood pressure leading to heart attack or stroke.[21]

Anxiety and Rehabilitation

Different levels of anxiety have different effects on patients. If anxiety is completely absent, patients may

Table 26.2	Signs and Symptoms Associated with Low, Moderate, and High Levels of Anxiety	
Low-Level Anxiety	**Moderate-Level Anxiety**	**High-Level Anxiety**
Agitation	Abdominal distress	Chest pains
Apprehension	Aches	Depersonalization
Distress	Chills	De-realization (feeling unreal)
Irritability	Decreased concentration	Difficulty sleeping
Motor restlessness	Diarrhea	Dizziness
Muscle tension	Fear	Dread
Nervousness	Feeling light-headed, unsteady, or faint	Helplessness
Worry	Fever	Horror
	Heart palpitations	Hypervigilance
	Hot flashes	Increased sensitivity to pain
	Increased heart rate	Nausea
	Misperception	Paresthesia
	Shaking or trembling	
	Shortness of breath	
	Sweating	

Table 26.3	Behaviors Associated with Low, Moderate, and High Levels of Anxiety	
Low-Level Anxiety	**Moderate-Level Anxiety**	**High-Level Anxiety**
Avoiding stressful situations	Going to the bathroom frequently	Holding hand over heart
Biting lips	Incessant talking	Reacting to irrelevant cues
Drumming fingers on a tabletop	Mumbling	Throwing up
Fidgeting	Overactivity	
Nail biting	Staring blankly	
Pacing	Verbalizing somatic preoccupations	
Pulling or twirling hair		
Rubbing an object such as worry beads		
Shaking legs		
Sighing heavily		
Tapping feet		

not be motivated to achieve treatment goals. Mild anxiety can be motivating if directed toward rehabilitation. Severe anxiety can escalate quickly and impair all aspects of the patient's life, including rehabilitation outcomes, by intensifying the perception of pain, inhibiting immunosuppression, and prolonging recovery time.[60,61] Patients who had difficulty managing anxiety before physical illness will probably have more difficulty managing stress brought on by disability.

When a patient is anxious, thought and energy often become focused on the anxiety instead of physical therapy, resulting in decreased concentration. Decreased learning may be observed when a patient is unable to concentrate on the therapist's instructions. The patient may be unable to perform motor tasks that require multiple-step directions. Poor concentration can also result in safety risks as the patient's attention may be alternating between the anxiety and the demands of rehabilitation. To appear functional, the patient may try to perform a task having heard only part of the therapist's instructions. Such a patient may fail to understand directions given by the therapist and may not realize that he or she missed important information. Steps may be skipped and a patient may jump ahead too quickly, resulting in injuries to the patient or others.

If patients become fearful because of anxiety, they may avoid certain behaviors in an attempt to decrease their fear. Fearful, anxious patients are reluctant to try new things. They may refuse treatment, remain in their rooms, request a bedpan when they are capable of using the commode, or be reluctant to progress to the next step in therapy. Such patients will commonly make statements such as, "I can't. I don't feel well. I'm too tired. Leave me alone. Not now, I'll do it later. I'm afraid. You can't help me. You don't look strong enough. I'm going to fall."

Patients who express anxiety through overactivity may attempt to progress too quickly through rehabilitation.

They often want to achieve everything at once and appear impatient. They tend to rush through a treatment activity without mastering each step. Such patients frequently talk of discharge before it is an option. They may make rash decisions regarding major life changes, such as purchasing new cars or planning vacations when neither would be in their best interest. Such behaviors may provide immediate relief from anxiety for both patients and their families yet cause more distress in the long run.

When anxiety causes misperception, patients may perceive their level of dysfunction and improvement differently than do their therapists. They often leave therapy sessions with an unrealistic opinion concerning any progress or gains made. Such patients may believe they performed at a higher level than they actually did.

Watching a patient experience a panic attack for the first time can be frightening. It may not be immediately evident to either the patient or physical therapist if the patient has never experienced one before. Patients experiencing a panic attack usually report fear of immediate death. They may start to hyperventilate, then suffer shortness of breath. Sometimes they believe they are having a heart attack as a result of chest pain, heart palpitations, and increased heart rate. Terror and panic ensue, and the therapist may call a code or, if in an outpatient setting, initiate emergency transport of the patient to the hospital.

How to Address Anxiety

Physical therapists need to help patients control anxiety so they can proceed with treatment. Some patients may find it beneficial to discuss their fears and concerns with their physical therapists. In such cases the therapist should initiate a dialogue with the patient, asking, "How are you feeling?" "What is your greatest concern?" "What is the worst thing you believe may happen?" and so forth. Physical therapists can work with patients to help defuse anxiety by using **cognitive restructuring**— or the reshaping of the patient's thoughts and beliefs regarding the feared event. For example, a therapist might help the patient to engage in reality testing by assisting the patient to understand that the occurrence of the feared event is unlikely.

Patients with real and imminent crises may benefit from assistance with problem solving, should their worst-case scenario occur. Such problem solving can help patients to believe that they can survive and live meaningful lives despite the occurrence of feared events. After patients have expressed their feelings, therapists can help them segue into treatment and redirect their emotion into physical activity.

It should be noted that patients who are verbose and cannot stop talking about their fears should not be encouraged to dwell on them during physical therapy sessions. Encouraging patients to verbalize their anxieties is also contraindicated with patients whose psychosomatic complaints are fueled by conversation regarding their anxieties. For patients who are very anxious, it may help to conduct treatment in a setting that is familiar, calm, and comfortable. An unfamiliar setting, too much stimulation in the environment, too many people, or too much noise can increase anxiety levels. It may be helpful to reorient patients to the therapy room and to treatment expectations—each session—to allow them to feel a greater sense of control.

Physical therapists should choose a purposeful activity with the patient's anxiety in mind. Some anxious patients have been known to respond to activities that consist of one repetitive motor action, as rhythmic motion helps to calm them.[62] Gross motor movements help decrease the physical symptoms of anxiety such as muscle aches, agitation, and restlessness. Therapists should begin by involving patients in a therapeutic activity that is easily performed and then increase the complexity of the task once the patient has gained confidence.

Anxious patients who may interrupt the physical therapist while he or she is with other patients may be reassured that they will be seen on a certain date and time. Physical therapists should ignore, without anger, all subsequent intrusions. Setting limits in this fashion helps patients improve their frustration tolerance. Very anxious people often welcome clear boundaries set by therapists because they have difficulty setting limits for themselves.

Stress management techniques are useful before and after a session. Techniques such as meditation, **imagery**, relaxation, stretching, stress management diaries, identifying stressors, biofeedback, nutrition, prioritizing, problem solving, decision making, anger management, Reiki (a Japanese technique for decreasing stress that involves the transfer of healing energy from the practitioner to the patient), music therapy, therapeutic massage, and prayer have been shown to improve both physical and emotional wellbeing.[63-65] Some of these

techniques work more effectively for some patients than others. Choosing one depends on the patient's preference, amount of time available, and materials required.

Relaxation Response

Whichever stress management technique is selected, the overall goal is to teach patients how to experience the **relaxation response** and replicate it independently during stressful situations.[66] After studying the relaxation response for 20 years, Dr. Herbert Benson identified two essential components that elicit the response: (1) repetition of a sound, word, phrase, prayer, or muscular activity; and (2) disregarding distracting thoughts and returning to the repetition. Benson[21] suggests that patients use the following techniques:

1. Choose a phrase, word, or prayer that is part of your belief system.
2. Sit comfortably and quietly.
3. Close your eyes.
4. Relax your muscles beginning with your feet and working your way up your body.
5. Breathe naturally and slowly. Say your phrase, word, or prayer silently as you exhale.
6. Rid yourself of all distracting thoughts by letting them flow in and out of your mind like waves on the ocean, always returning to your phrase, word, or prayer.
7. Continue for up to 20 minutes.
8. Sit quietly for a minute, allowing your thoughts to return before opening your eyes. Sit for another minute before standing.
9. Practice this technique daily on an empty stomach if possible.

The relaxation response has proven to be effective in treating headaches, hypertension, anxiety, cardiac rhythm irregularities, mild and moderate depression, and premenstrual syndrome. The relaxation response works by decreasing heart rate, rate of breathing, metabolism rate, oxygen consumption, and carbon dioxide elimination, and returning the body to a healthier balance.[21,66,67] When within-subject comparisons were made between blood pressure before and after meditation using the nine aforementioned steps above for several weeks, the average systolic blood pressure for the 36 subjects dropped from 146 to 137 mm Hg, and diastolic pressure dropped from 93.5 to 88.9 mm Hg; both are statistically significant changes.[21] The relaxation response seems to decrease blood pressure through counteracting the activity of the sympathetic nervous system—the same mechanism underlying the action of antihypertensive drugs. Lower blood pressure leads to lower risk for atherosclerosis and related diseases.

Guided Imagery

Another intervention is guided imagery, frequently used as a standard of care to improve rehabilitation through relaxation. Guided imagery is said to work by decreasing the levels of cortisol that can inhibit the immune system and slow tissue repair.[68] As in eliciting the relaxation response, the patient should be guided to a state in which the mind is silent and calm. Through use of an audiotape, videotape, or therapy guide, the patient is asked to imagine a special place (e.g., the ocean, a forest, a sunset) and focus on vivid details using the five senses. By focusing on this location for increasing lengths of time, patients learn to gain relief from constant worry by releasing concerns for a period of time and returning to a place of relaxation and peace. Guided imagery enhances the mind–body–spirit connection through the induction of an altered state in which the mind communicates more effectively with the body.[60]

The use of guided imagery has achieved improved outcomes of care through significant reductions in pain, blood pressure, stress, side effects of treatments, headaches, uncertainty, depression, insomnia, blood glucose levels, and histamine response to allergies. Significant enhancement of the immune system and wound and bone healing has also been noted.[69] Because music may trigger emotional responses by influencing the limbic system when used with imagery, music used with guided imagery has been shown to decrease pain through increasing endorphin release.[70,71] Guided imagery with music has also been found to reduce the need for large doses of medication and reduce recovery time.[60]

Desensitization

Phobias severe enough to interfere with daily functioning have been reported by one out of every eight American adults.[26] Patients suffering from phobias that interfere with treatment may require desensitization techniques, also called **situational exposure exercises.** For example, wheelchair users with a fear of elevators who always used stairs before injury now require help in coping with their fears. In a comfortable, calm treatment environment far from an elevator, the physical therapist can have the patient begin to talk about benign aspects of elevators (e.g., what they look like, where they are located, and how many floors are in the building). While the patient is answering these questions, the physical therapist should determine the patient's level of anxiety. What specific issue regarding the elevator is the patient discussing when his or her anxiety increases? If the patient has not as yet become too anxious, the therapist may ask more anxiety-producing questions, such as, "How high is the elevator's ceiling?" "Is there an emergency phone?" "Are you more fearful of taking an elevator by yourself or with a crowd of people and why?" "Have you ever taken an elevator before and if so, what happened?" The therapist should continue to examine the patient's level of anxiety during questioning, stopping just before the patient's anxiety reaches a point at which the patient cannot easily be calmed.

This process, called desensitization, allows the patient to discuss his or her fear in a safe environment where he or she does not feel overwhelmingly anxious. The physical therapist slowly increases the level of anxiety by asking more difficult questions, but only to a tolerable degree. The patient is then asked to visually imagine that he or she is in an elevator, while practicing relaxation techniques. The patient continues to practice this visualization, over time, until he or she can do so without experiencing fear. When the patient can visualize himself or herself in an elevator without experiencing fear, therapy progresses to the real-life experience of riding in an elevator with the therapist. Relaxation techniques continue to be used during such real-life practice. The activity of riding in an elevator with the therapist using relaxation techniques continues until the patient can do so without fear. The final step would be for the patient to practice riding in an elevator alone while using self-induced relaxation techniques. Desensitization therapy has a high rate of effectiveness in the treatment of phobias.

Cognitive-Behavioral Therapy

Cognitive-behavioral therapy (or **cognitive restructuring**) can help decrease anxiety by changing **maladaptive thought patterns** and modifying unhealthy behaviors.[72] Before unhealthy behaviors can be modified, they must first be identified and classified. Because many patients are not conscious of their anxiety, an initial step when using cognitive-behavioral therapy is to help patients recognize anxiety. Determine what the patient's first signs of stress tend to be. Many will reply that they react severely to stress, stating "I throw up," or "I cannot breathe." In these cases, therapists should ask about the existence of less severe signs, such as nail biting or leg shaking.

Next, patients should count how many times a day they experience stress, recording these in a journal. Physical therapists should help patients look for patterns in their anxiety. Are patients more anxious in the morning or evening, when they attend therapy, or when family members visit? The more patients can identify patterns of anxiety, the more they can anticipate it and prepare for anxiety before it occurs. Therapists should encourage patients to use stress management techniques as soon as they experience the first sign of stress so that their anxiety does not escalate. Keeping a stress management journal can give patients insight into how their thoughts affect their behavior. Research has shown that cognitive-behavioral therapy can be as effective as medication.[73-77] Box 26.3 Evidence Summary presents a summary of research data examining the effects of cognitive therapy versus use of antidepressants for depression.

Treatment for Panic Attacks

If the therapist knows that a patient has a history of panic attacks, the following techniques can be helpful.

Box 26.3 Evidence Summary   Research Examining the Effects of Cognitive Therapy versus Antidepressants for Depression—cont'd

Reference	Subjects	Design/Intervention	Duration	Results	Comments
Blackburn and Moorhead[73] (2000)	Depressed (non-bipolar and nonpsychotic) or dysthymic outpatients 64% female; mean age = 43.7	Randomized treatment-outcome study comparing two groups: cognitive therapy (N = 22) and antidepressant treatment (amitriptyline or clomipramine) (N = 20)	12.9 weeks of therapy or medication in a hospital.	21% of the cognitive group became depressed again during a 2-year period following intervention vs. 78% of the antidepressant group, a significant (p < .05) difference.	Cognitive therapy for patients with mild to moderate depression should be considered before referral to a psychiatrist for antidepressants.
Butler et al[74] (2006)	Subjects came from different studies and had a variety of psychiatric diagnoses: unipolar depression, generalized anxiety disorder, panic disorder, social phobia, post-traumatic stress disorder, childhood depressive and anxiety disorders, childhood somatic disorders, adult depression, obsessive-compulsive disorder, bulimia nervosa, schizophrenia, and chronic pain	Meta-analysis of 16 meta-analytic studies examining the efficacy of cognitive behavioral treatment vs. psychopharmacology on psychiatric clients	Duration varied with studies.	Effect sizes for cognitive behavioral therapy in the treatment of generalized anxiety disorder, unipolar depression, panic disorder, post-traumatic stress disorder, panic disorder, and childhood anxiety and depressive disorders were large. Moderate effect sizes were reported for cognitive behavioral therapy in the treatment of chronic pain, marital distress, childhood somatic disorders, and anger. For adults with depression, cognitive-behavioral therapy was more effective than antidepressants. Venlafaxine (Effexor) demonstrated the highest rates of remission compared to SSRIs but other therapies such as cognitive were also necessary for a high percentage of patients to achieve full remission from depression.	Limitations due to a meta-analysis are present in this study; it is difficult to compare studies that use different lengths of treatment and assessments. However, the findings in this review of meta-analytic studies support other studies on the effectiveness of cognitive-behavioral therapy.

Box 26.3 Evidence Summary   Research Examining the Effects of Cognitive Therapy versus Antidepressants for Depression—cont'd

Reference	Subjects	Design/Intervention	Duration	Results	Comments
Lam and Sidney[75] (2004)	A total of 31,368 depressed subjects throughout different studies	Meta-analysis of 16 meta-analyses (227 RCTs and 19 studies of other rigor) examining the efficacy of antidepressants vs. psychotherapies in achieving and sustaining remission from depression	Longitudinal studies	MANOVAs revealed no significant difference between different types of psychotherapy and their effect on decreasing depression regardless of the disorder; however, clients (regardless of disorder) treated with psychotherapy (regardless of the type) showed significant improvement at the end of therapy and at follow-up compared to those in the control group.	The combination of antidepressants and psychological therapy resulted in 70% of the patients sustaining remission from depression over extended periods of time.
Leichsenring et al[76] (2004)	Major depression, maternal depression, post-traumatic stress disorder, bulimia nervosa, anorexia nervosa, opiate dependence, cocaine dependence, cluster C personality disorders, somatoform pain disorder, borderline personality disorder, social phobia, and chronic functional dyspepsia	Meta-analysis of 17 RCTs that examined the effects of various short-term psychotherapies (including cognitive) on depression	Intervention ranged from 7 to 40 sessions. Mean length of follow-up was 1 year.	Patients who received combined intervention made significantly greater improvements than those who received antidepressants alone (OR, 1.86; 95% CI, 1.38–2.52). Medication nonresponders and dropout rates were not significantly different between the two groups (OR, 0.86; 95% CI, 0.60–1.24). Combined intervention was significantly more effective than drug intervention alone in studies where intervention lasted longer than 12 weeks (OR, 2.21; 95% CI, 1.22–4.03), with a significant decrease in dropouts when compared with nonresponders (OR, 0.59; 95% CI, 0.39–0.88).	Not all of the studies in this meta-analysis used cognitive therapy, nor did the meta-analysis identify which elements of the different short-term psychotherapies were effective in reducing depression and preventing relapse.

Continued

Box 26.3 Evidence Summary   Research Examining the Effects of Cognitive Therapy versus Antidepressants for Depression—cont'd

Reference	Subjects	Design/Intervention	Duration	Results	Comments
Pampallona et al[77] (2004)	Control group consisted of wait-listed patients, 16 trials of 910 depressed patients randomized to pharmacotherapy combined with psychotherapy and 932 to pharmacotherapy alone	Systematic review of RCTs that examined the relationships between efficacy of and adherence with psychological intervention plus antidepressant drugs vs. psychopharmacology alone	Duration of intervention varied according to the particular study.		Antidepressants combined with psychotherapy was more effective in the treatment of depression than antidepressants alone.

CI = confidence interval; MANOVAs = multivariate analyses of variance; OR = odds ratio; RCTs = randomized controlled trials; SSRIs = selective serotonin reuptake inhibitors.

Have the patient describe the first signs of discomfort during the attack. Immediately help him or her to breathe long, deep, and slow breaths. This may require the use of a brown paper bag held by the patient over the mouth while breathing into it to slow the inhalation rate. It is beneficial to acknowledge that a panic attack is occurring and that the patient will be all right if he or she continues to focus on breathing slowly and deeply. The panic attack can become severe within minutes and pass just as quickly. The patient most likely will be seated or lying down throughout the panic attack, as it may render him or her incapable of doing anything else.

Patients are usually embarrassed after an attack and may avoid all situations in which they believe one may occur. They may sit on the end of the aisle while watching a movie, may avoid crowds, or, in extreme cases, stop leaving their homes entirely (referred to as **agoraphobia**). Therapists can help patients who experience panic attacks to achieve a more productive life by teaching them techniques to control the attacks before they become severe. Families and patients should be educated to understand that panic attacks involve a real physiological reaction, tend to last only several minutes, and often recur without further intervention. Patients with severe, continuous panic attacks should be referred to a psychiatrist for possible medication management.

When to Make a Referral for Anxiety

Multiple referrals may be necessary. Patients who have panic attacks should be referred to a psychiatrist for a medication consultation. Generalized anxiety can be treated with medication; hence, a referral to a psychiatrist would be appropriate if the anxiety lasts more than a week and interferes with the patient's performance in rehabilitation. Those who continue to experience anxiety from phobias despite desensitization therapy and medication should be referred to a psychologist for a more in-depth exploration of their fears. A referral to a psychologist is indicated if the anxiety seems to be a deeply rooted characteristic of the patient's personality. A social work referral can be helpful if the patient's anxiety results from a lack of necessary resources or involves family members.

In many cases, medication does not fully alleviate patients' anxiety. However, it may decrease it sufficiently enough for patients to begin expressing their fears and implementing strategies to decrease stress. Sometimes a patient may not be forthcoming about his or her anxiety and a formal diagnosis may not be present in the chart. If this is the case, the physical therapist may become aware of an anxiety disorder through the type of medication prescribed. By becoming familiar with the names of different antianxiety medications, physical therapists can identify patients suffering from anxiety. The names, effects, and adverse side effects of commonly prescribed antianxiety medications are presented in Table 26.4.

ACUTE STRESS DISORDER AND POST-TRAUMATIC STRESS DISORDER

People who were disabled as a result of a traumatic event (e.g., a violent crime, abuse, an accident, a natural disaster, or war) or individuals who have witnessed such are

Table 26.4 Effects and Adverse Side Effects of Commonly Prescribed Antianxiety Medications

Medication	Summary of Effects	Adverse Side Effects
Alprazolam (Xanax)	Decrease anxiety, seizures, sleep disorders, alcohol abuse, catatonic schizophrenia	Sedation, potential for abuse, difficult to taper (gradual dose reduction)
Buspirone hydrochloride (BuSpar)	Decrease depression, anxiety, addictions, ADHD	Tremors, decreased appetite, insomnia, restlessness
Chlordiazepoxide (Librium, Mitran, Reposans-10)	Decrease anxiety, seizures, sleep disorders, alcohol abuse, catatonic schizophrenia	Sedation, potential for abuse, difficult to taper
Clorazepate dipotassium (Tranxene, Gen-Xene)	Decrease anxiety, seizures, sleep disorders, alcohol abuse, catatonic schizophrenia	Sedation, potential for abuse, difficult to taper
Diazepam (Diastat, Valium)	Decrease anxiety, seizures, sleep disorders, alcohol abuse, catatonic schizophrenia	Sedation, potential for abuse, difficult to taper
Estazolam (Prosom)	Decrease insomnia	Cognitive impairments, dizziness, daytime sleepiness, anxiety, uncoordinated motor movements, intoxication, drug accumulation
Flurazepam hydrochloride (Dalmane)	Decrease insomnia	Cognitive impairments, dizziness, daytime sleepiness, anxiety, uncoordinated motor movements, intoxication, drug accumulation
Hydroxyzine hydrochloride (Vistaril)	Decrease insomnia, tremors, weight gain, anxiety	Dizziness, sedation, constipation, cotton mouth, weight gain, urinary retention, blurred vision, hypotension, confusion
Lithium carbonate (Eskalith, Lithobid)	Decrease mania and suicidal ideation, stabilizes mood	Toxicity can be lethal, increase weight, nausea, acne, sedation, psoriasis, diarrhea, polydipsia, tremors, edema, uncoordinated motor movements
Lorazepam (Ativan)	Decrease anxiety, seizures, sleep disorders, alcohol abuse, catatonic schizophrenia	Sedation, potential for abuse, difficult to taper
Oxazepam (Serax)	Decrease anxiety, seizures, sleep disorders, alcohol abuse, catatonic schizophrenia	Sedation, potential for abuse, difficult to taper
Temazepam (Restoril)	Decrease insomnia	Cognitive impairments, dizziness, daytime sleepiness, anxiety, uncoordinated motor movements, intoxication, drug accumulation
Triazolam (Halcion)	Decrease insomnia	Cognitive impairments, dizziness, daytime sleepiness, anxiety, uncoordinated motor movements, intoxication, drug accumulation
Zaleplon (Sonata)	Decrease insomnia	Dizziness, drowsiness
Zolpidem tartrate (Ambien)	Decrease insomnia	Dizziness, drowsiness

Note: Brand names are shown in parentheses.
ADHD = attention deficit–hyperactivity disorder.

at risk for **post-traumatic stress disorder** (PTSD) or **acute stress disorder** (ASD). Both are specific forms or subsets of anxiety disorders. The *Diagnostic and Statistical Manual of Mental Disorders* differentiates between both disorders in terms of the duration of the disorder and its symptoms.[9] ASD involves symptoms that must range in duration between 2 days to a maximum of 4 weeks. If symptoms of ASD persist longer than 4 weeks, the diagnosis of ASD is discontinued and changed to PTSD. Post-traumatic stress disorder is differentiated as *acute* PTSD if symptoms last more than 4 weeks but less than 3 months and as *chronic* PTSD if symptoms last 3 months or longer. Both ASD and PTSD, however, must result from exposure to a traumatic event, and PTSD can be qualified with the term "with delayed onset" if symptoms first occur at least half a year after the traumatic event. Research notes that PTSD is an expected outcome for a certain percentage of patients experiencing even mild traumas.[78,79]

Among the symptoms exhibited are one or more of the following: reexperiencing the traumatic event; **numbing** of responsiveness to, or reduced involvement with, the external world; and/or a variety of autonomic, dysphoric, or cognitive symptoms. The reexperiencing of the event is described as recurrent, painful, and consisting of intrusive recollections, dreams and nightmares, and, on rare occasions, dissociative states during which the individual may act as if reliving the actual traumatic event. This may last only several minutes or occur for hours or even days. The numbing of responsiveness, also called *psychic numbing* or *emotional anesthesia*, is expressed by complaints of feeling detached or estranged from others, a loss of ability or interest in previously enjoyable activities, or the lack of any emotions or feelings. Cognitive symptoms may include impairment of memory, concentration, and task completion ability. Patients may experience excessive autonomic arousal resulting in hyperalertness, anticipatory anxiety, an exaggerated startle response, constant scanning of the environment, the perception of people and objects that are not real (i.e., **hallucinations**), or difficulty falling and remaining asleep.[80] Following this state of hypervigilance, the patient may experience a denial reaction marked by a diminution of responsiveness to the environment. Survival guilt may be present in those cases in which others were harmed or killed during a catastrophic event.

Additional associated features that should alert the physical therapist to the presence of PTSD are increased irritability, hostile behavior, constant tension, chronic **free-floating anxiety**, muscle tension, sexual and social difficulties, and somatic stress symptoms. Box 26.4 summarizes some of the prominent behavioral features of PTSD.

Box 26.4 Behavioral Features (Warning Signs) of Possible Post-Traumatic Stress Disorder (PTSD)

Any one of the following behaviors:

- Recurrent, intrusive recollection of traumatic event
- Intrusive and distressing dreams of event
- Dissociative states (behaving as if reliving event; can last for several seconds or minutes)
- Amnesia of events

More than one of the following behaviors:

- Psychic numbing (lack of interest in social or physical environment or activities; significantly lowered participation in social or physical environment)
- Unable to feel emotions (e.g., intimacy, love, sexuality, anger)
- Disturbed sleep patterns
- Hypervigilance
- Exaggerated startle response
- Ongoing level of irritability
- Heightened difficulty with concentration

Not everyone who experiences trauma develops PTSD. The triple vulnerability model postulates that three vulnerabilities need to be present to develop an anxiety disorder: (1) a biological vulnerability; (2) a generalized psychological vulnerability (existing from past experiences of lost control over unpredictable events); and (3) a specific psychological vulnerability that links anxiety to specific situations.[81] Keane and Barlow[82] have proposed an explanation for how PTSD develops based on the triple vulnerability model. They suggest that during a traumatic event, a person experiences alarm and other intense emotions. The person is more likely to develop PTSD if the event and resultant emotions are perceived to be unpredictable and beyond the person's control. If the event is perceived to be predictable and within the person's control, it is less likely that PTSD will occur.

Chronic pain frequently occurs concurrently with PTSD, and the occurrence of both disorders tends to negatively affect the treatment outcome for each.[83] Similar processes, such as avoidance, fear, anxiety, oversensitivity, and catastrophizing (i.e., interpreting an experience as overly threatening), may act to maintain both conditions. Given the high co-morbidity of PTSD and chronic pain, physical therapists should examine patients with PTSD for the existence of chronic pain. The Yale Multidimensional Pain Inventory or the McGill Pain Questionnaire can be administered.[84,85] PTSD may be examined using the Clinician Administered PTSD Scale Revised or the

Posttraumatic Stress Disorder Checklist.[86,87] Examination should also include the patient's beliefs, self-efficacy, level of anxiety, sensitivity, coping style, expectations, and degree of behavioral and cognitive avoidance in order to understand the mechanisms that may maintain these conditions. See Chapter 25, Chronic Pain, for a more detailed discussion of instruments designed to measure pain.

The main desired outcome of treatment for PTSD should be engagement in healthy, satisfying, necessary activities. The physical therapist can help patients to build positive self-efficacy through **cognitive restructuring**, development of healthy coping skills, and learning to use the relaxation response—all in a predictable, safe environment. Techniques used to help decrease catastrophizing and avoidance include situational exposure exercises (mentioned earlier) and **interoceptive exposure exercises** (such as running in place or spinning in a chair).[88] Interoceptive exposure exercises help patients cope with uncomfortable physiological sensations that may prevent participation in activities. Finally, the therapist should provide the patient education regarding how PTSD and pain can facilitate each other and result in avoidance. As participation in healthy activities increases, co-occurring disorders—such as depression, anxiety, panic, and substance abuse—may decrease, and a higher quality of life may ensue for the patient with PTSD.

Depression

Depression refers to feelings of despair and hopelessness, negative shifts in perception, and decreased interest in activities that once provided pleasure. A person may have a depressed personality (referred to as *dysthymia*) and therefore experience sadness throughout his or her entire life. As in most cases of depression, a person may have one or more episodes of depression, before and after which a normal mood exists. A certain degree of depression is normal in response to life's events, but when depression lasts 2 or more weeks and affects occupational and social functioning, it is considered to be **major depression**. Depression may occur as a biochemical imbalance in the brain, which may be triggered by stress, or in response to internal conflicts or life events. For example, the rate of depression in people with SCI is five times higher than that of the general population.[89]

Women with disabilities are more prone to depression (30%)[90] than women without disabilities (10% to 25%),[9] men with disabilities (26%),[90] and the general population (10%).[9] Other researchers support the finding that women with disabilities tend to experience depression more commonly than their male counterparts. In their analysis of 443 women with disabilities, Hughes et al[91] found depression to be a frequently occurring secondary condition (51% of the sample scored in the mildly depressed range or higher on the Beck Depression Inventory–II [BDI-II]). Fifty-nine percent of women with SCI were found to be clinically depressed, compared to a rate of 4.5% to 9.3% of women in the United States at any given time.[92] This high rate of depression among disabled women may be due to the combination of being a woman and having a disability, since both are risk factors for depression. Women are more than twice as likely to have a depressive episode than men due to economic, social, psychological, and biological factors.[93] Female socialization experiences and gender-based roles may also increase their vulnerability to depression. Depression in women has been linked to experiences of abuse and poverty, lack of social support, reduced mobility, chronic pain, lower educational levels, and lower levels of perceived control.[94]

If untreated, depression can spiral into greater severity and may result in suicide; 15% of people who are depressed commit suicide each year.[18] Depression may begin with loss, such as the onset of a physical disability, divorce, death, or the departure of a close friend. As a result of such losses, patients may become appropriately sad and mournful. If patients reach out to friends and express their feelings, they can alleviate feelings of loneliness and isolation that commonly occur in response to loss. However, if patients do not take steps to express their feelings, the downward spiral of depression may continue. Over time, patients may lose interest in activities and remain at home. They may lack the energy or motivation to attend to their responsibilities, and feelings of guilt may ensue. A decrease in role participation usually leads to diminished self-esteem and feelings of worthlessness. Eventually, people stop caring about their hygiene. They may avoid social contact and become increasingly lonely. At this point, staying in bed becomes a welcome alternative to dealing with the outside world and the painful feelings it may incur.

Depression and Rehabilitation

Given the signs and symptoms of depression (Table 26.5) and its associated behaviors (Table 26.6), depression may negatively affect the outcome of treatment. Depressed patients may have difficulty getting out of bed and may not be motivated to attend therapy. If they do attend treatment, they may display **psychomotor retardation** and lack energy and interest; they may also verbalize self-deprecating remarks, feel criticized, and believe that they are progressing inadequately. It may be difficult for physical therapists to leave depressed patients unattended while working with others because the depressed patient may not engage in the prescribed exercises. Patients may feel guilty that they are in the hospital instead of taking care of their children, working to earn money for their family, or engaging in other life roles.

Table 26.5 Signs and Symptoms Associated with Mild, Moderate, and Severe Depression

Mild Depression	Moderate Depression	Severe Depression
Anger	Decreased self-esteem	Anguish
Anxiety	Despair	Change in appetite and weight
Decreased concentration	Despondence	Decreased sex drive
Depressed mood	Excessive guilt	Desperation
Indecisiveness	Fearfulness	Feeling overwhelmed
Intrusive thoughts	Inadequacy	Helplessness
Irritability	Sensitivity	Hopelessness
Lethargy		Insomnia or excessive sleep
Loneliness		Recurrent thoughts of suicide
Neediness		Worthlessness
Sadness		

Table 26.6 Behaviors Associated with Mild, Moderate, and Severe Depression

Mild Depression	Moderate Depression	Severe Depression
Being easily frustrated	Crying	Decreased interest in all activities
Difficulty planning ahead	Feeling pessimistic about the future	Lack of personal hygiene
Obsessing about tasks	Having difficulty making decisions	Staying in bed all day
Sitting alone	Making frequent self-deprecating remarks	Suicide (or suicide attempt)
	Overdependence	
	Reacting strongly to criticism	
	Reporting psychosomatic symptoms	
	Ruminating about problems	
	Ruminating about the past	
	Social withdrawal	

Depression usually affects performance negatively. Depressed patients may not want to make gains in rehabilitation because of decreased motivation and lack of pleasure in life. They may believe that they are unable to progress in rehabilitation as a result of low self-esteem or feelings of hopelessness. Such patients may also have difficulty asserting themselves because of feelings of worthlessness and an inability to express anger. When people feel worthless or have low self-esteem, they may feel unworthy of having or voicing an opinion. Depression may result from anger turned inward. Instead of expressing anger in the moment, depressed patients may turn their anger against themselves or repress it. People who experience this type of depression may not have been allowed to express hostility in the past.

Depressed patients often become immobilized because they have difficulty making decisions. They may

weigh the pros and cons of each choice and become overwhelmed. They may be unable to concentrate on one thought long enough to make decisions. Sometimes depressed patients experience the opposite; when they attempt to execute a decision they may have no thoughts at all (referred to as **thought blocking**). Consequently, they may need 1 to 2 minutes to think about and answer questions.

Treating Patients with Depression

Depressed patients require assistance with motivation. Physical therapists can facilitate motivation by providing encouragement, emphasizing strengths, offering positive feedback, addressing values, and mobilizing guilt into goal acquisition. Empowering patients by providing activities that offer opportunities for self-control and success have been shown to decrease depression.[95,96]

Depressed patients experience a narrowing of perception. They have difficulty seeing alternate solutions to problems or simple tasks and often feel there is no solution to obstacles. They may perceive their condition as terminal when there is no justification for such a belief. Because of these distortions, it is important to offer reality checks—such as pointing out their strengths when they feel worthless. Cognitive therapy can be used to correct ongoing pessimism by challenging negative thought patterns.

If given choices about their treatment, depressed patients may become ambivalent and unable to decide on a course of action. As a result, they may do nothing. Physical therapists should choose treatment that provides the patient with opportunities for progressive success experiences, avoiding feelings of failure. When reluctant patients perceive that they can succeed in therapy instead of giving up, their chances of continuing treatment increase. Progress made in physical rehabilitation can alleviate depression, as patients report feeling better after having succeeded in an activity they believed they could not accomplish.

Perhaps the most valuable information that a physical therapist can offer depressed patients is that depression will not last forever. Patients will eventually become better through the combination of therapy and possible medication management. Depression can cause an activity or life role that once seemed effortless—such as being a partner in a relationship—to become arduous. It is important for the patient to understand that this does not mean that the relationship caused the depression; more likely, the role of partner has become more difficult to carry out because of depression.

Families often experience a depressed family member as lazy, obstinate, or uncaring, and may not recognize that he or she is suffering from an illness. Depression can be just as disabling as a physical illness. Families need to be educated that depression, like physical disability, causes decreased functioning and requires treatment. Recovery from depression does not have a specific timeline. Each patient's situation is unique, as is the recovery period. Most patients cannot "snap out of it" as many family members desire.

When to Make a Referral for Depression

If depression is suspected, the physical therapist should determine if the patient is currently being treated for depression or has received treatment in the past. If the patient has never been treated for depression and is experiencing suicidal ideation (see section on Suicide below) or symptoms of depression that markedly impair life roles, the therapist should refer the patient to a psychiatrist for possible medication management. Medication can enable patients to attend therapy, more readily discuss problems, and express repressed feelings.

However, some patients are reluctant to inform their physical therapist of their depression out of stoicism or shame. (There is often a negative stigma attached to being depressed because, to the uninformed, it may imply weakness or feeling sorry for one's self.) A diagnosis of depression may not be in the chart and the symptoms may be misinterpreted as fatigue. In these cases, knowledge of the names of medications used to treat depression may help therapists identify patients with depression. The names, effects, and adverse side effects of frequently prescribed antidepressant medications are presented in Table 26.7.

Patients with less severe symptoms who are not suicidal can be referred to a psychologist for verbal therapy. If a patient's depression seems to be caused by family turmoil, a referral to a social worker for family intervention can be made. Patients who have difficulty verbalizing their feelings can be referred to a creative arts therapist to facilitate expression through nonverbal means such as music, dance or art. A referral to an occupational therapist can be made to help patients regain function in daily life roles that have been disrupted by depression.

Suicide

Each year more than 35,000 cases of suicide are reported in the United States, and 65,000 additional cases may go unreported due to complications regarding the cause of death.[26] More people lose their lives to suicide than to any other cause, with the exception of cancer and cardiovascular disease. Suicide is often a result of poor social support, low self-esteem, ineffective coping skills, and the inability to see a solution to difficult situations. Risk factors include serious illness, previous suicide attempts, family history of suicide, alcohol and substance abuse/dependence, loss of a loved one through rejection or death, prolonged depression, and financial difficulties.

Recognizing the warning signs of possible suicide risk is important for its prevention. The most frequent signs of suicide risk include the following:

- Direct comments about suicide, such as, "I just want to die"
- Indirect comments about suicide, such as, "My mother will not have to worry about me anymore"
- A plan to commit suicide
- Writing a suicide note
- Preoccupation with death
- A sudden flight into happiness or relief after a long depression
- Excessive risk taking (e.g., driving while inebriated) and a careless attitude
- Final preparations (e.g., composing a will, giving away personal possessions, repairing broken relationships, or writing revealing letters)
- Self-hatred

Table 26.7   Effects and Adverse Side Effects of Commonly Prescribed Antidepressant Medications

Medication	Summary of Effects	Adverse Side Effects
Amitriptyline hydrochloride (Elavil)	Decrease depression, manage anxiety, insomnia, migraines, and chronic pain.	Adverse side effects: dry mouth, urinary retention, constipation, hypotension, dizziness, tachycardia, blurred vision, impaired memory, and weight gain.
Amoxapine (Asendin)	Decrease depression, manage anxiety, insomnia, migraines, and chronic pain.	Dry mouth, urinary retention, constipation, hypotension, dizziness, tachycardia, blurred vision, impaired memory, and weight gain.
Bupropion (Wellbutrin)	Decrease depression, anxiety, addictions, and ADHD.	Tremors, decreased appetite, insomnia, and restlessness.
Celexa (Lexapro)	Decrease depression and anxiety.	Adverse side effects: nervousness, nausea, headache, diarrhea, sexual dysfunction, insomnia, apathy, sweating, hyponatremia, fatigue, and may cause suicidal ideation in children and teens.
Desipramine hydrochloride (Norpramin)	Decrease depression, manage anxiety, insomnia, migraines, and chronic pain.	Adverse side effects: dry mouth, urinary retention, constipation, hypotension, dizziness, tachycardia, blurred vision, impaired memory, and weight gain.
Doxepin hydrochloride (Sinequan, Zonalon)	Decrease depression, manage anxiety, insomnia, migraines, and chronic pain.	Adverse side effects: dry mouth, urinary retention, constipation, hypotension, dizziness, tachycardia, blurred vision, impaired memory, and weight gain.
Fluoxetine (Prozac, Sarafem)	Decrease depression and anxiety.	Nervousness, nausea, headache, diarrhea, sexual dysfunction, insomnia, apathy, sweating, hyponatremia, fatigue, and may cause suicidal ideation in children and teens.
Fluvoxamine (Luvox)	Decrease depression and anxiety.	Nervousness, nausea, headache, diarrhea, sexual dysfunction, insomnia, apathy, sweating, hyponatremia, fatigue, and may cause suicidal ideation in children and teens.
Imipramine hydrochloride (Tofranil)	Decrease depression, manage anxiety, insomnia, migraines, and chronic pain.	Dry mouth, urinary retention, constipation, hypotension, dizziness, tachycardia, blurred vision, impaired memory, weight gain.
Isocurboxazid (Marplan)	Decrease depression and anxiety; used to treat bipolar depression and treatment-resistant depression.	Dizziness, hypotension, weight gain, sedation, cotton mouth, insomnia, and sexual dysfunction.
Maprotiline (Ludiomil)	Decrease depression and manage anxiety, insomnia, migraines, and chronic pain.	Dry mouth, urinary retention, constipation, hypotension, dizziness, tachycardia, blurred vision, impaired memory, and weight gain.

ADHD = attention deficit–hyperactivity disorder.

- Changes in personal appearance, eating habits, sexual drive, sleep patterns, menstrual cycle, behavior (e.g., inability to concentrate or disinterest in activities), or personality (e.g., withdrawal, anxiousness, sadness, irritability, apathy, indecisiveness, or fatigue)
- A recent loss accompanied by an inability to stop grieving

The most important thing for a physical therapist to do when suspecting that a patient is suicidal is to prevent him or her from carrying out the act. This usually involves obtaining help from a mental health professional, preferably a physician with the knowledge and ability to admit the person to a hospital if needed. It is important not to leave the patient alone while waiting for help. During this period, the following should take place:

- Ask patients if they are thinking of hurting or killing themselves.
- Listen to patients without expressing shock, without discrediting what they say, and without devaluing their feelings; take all suicide threats seriously even if you do not believe them at the time.
- Respond to patients with empathy and understanding; tell them how much you care about them and that you will be available to help them.
- Help patients think of alternatives; offer choices based on your knowledge about the patient's life, rather than generic answers that are easy to offer when under pressure.
- Alert family members, friends, and significant others to the patient's suicide risk; all of these individuals may help prevent the patient from trying to commit suicide; suicidal ideation does not go away in a day; additional help is required from all possible sources over time.

■ SUBSTANCE ABUSE

Substance abuse occurs when an individual demonstrates a dysfunctional pattern of drug and/or alcohol use characterized by recurrent and significant adverse consequences. Substances may include, but are not limited to, alcohol, amphetamines, caffeine, marijuana, cocaine, hallucinogens, inhalants, opioids, or sedatives.[9]

Substance Abuse and Rehabilitation

If clients come to the clinic under the influence of drugs or alcohol, they may be inappropriate, argumentative, irritable, disinhibited, stubborn, illogical, or angry and will have difficulty following treatment plans. They may also disturb other clients, some of who may be in their own substance abuse recovery. For these reasons, intoxicated clients should be escorted out of the treatment area and referred back to their substance abuse programs, with a call to their substance abuse program provider describing the incident that occurred. If they are not currently engaged in a substance abuse program, a referral should be made. Although many drugs have unique and specific consequences, Table 26.8 presents an overview of common physiological, psychological, and behavioral manifestations associated with substance abuse.

If patients are not under the influence during treatment, but are using drugs or alcohol at home, they may miss treatment sessions or may come to rehabilitation tired, hungry, or late. They may have poor concentration and irritable moods resulting from hangovers. They may experience recurring injuries from falls. Often, patients will not comply with treatment and fail to complete their home exercises or forget to take their prescribed medications. When prescribed medications are ingested along with illegal substances, adverse drug reactions can occur. Patients may lack insight about the extent of their abuse and the trouble that it produces in their lives. They may mask feelings such as anger, guilt, anxiety, or depression through the numbing effect of the substance, but try to present themselves as though they are fine.

Patients in denial commonly do not perceive their need for physical rehabilitation, often neglect to follow precautions, and frequently attempt to obtain discharge before completing rehabilitation goals. Their low frustration tolerance causes them to quit treatment easily. Whether they are actively using substances or not, patients who have abused substances may have **cognitive deficits** that inhibit their ability to follow or remember instructions. They may experience family discord and lose family support, thus finding themselves homeless. Patients with a history of chronic alcohol abuse tend to have poor balance resulting from changes in the cerebellum and peripheral nerves.[97] To maintain balance, they develop a stereotypic, wide-based gait. Such factors should be considered during gait examination and training. Despite their gruff demeanor, patients who abuse substances can be overly sensitive, easily hurt, suffer from low self-esteem, and easily stressed once they are no longer abusing substances. These patients tend to have poor boundaries. They can be intrusive, flirtatious, or deal seeking in order to obtain what they want, such as alcohol, cigarettes, or extra medication.

Treating Patients Who Abuse Substances

Physical therapists can help patients in recovery by providing opportunities that allow them to gain control over their lives again. Such assistance may include opportunities to practice setting boundaries, regulating emotions, and tolerating frustration. Physical therapists can emphasize healthy activities that provide pleasure and decrease cravings. Stress management, time management, ADL, and social skills are usually necessary skills to promote recovery.

Education on Substance Abuse

Physical therapists, patients, and patients' family members should be aware that substance abuse is an illness. Like physical or mental illness, it causes a decrease in function, requires skilled intervention for recovery, results in decreased **role performance**, and can affect anyone. Patients with a diagnosis of substance abuse usually cannot stop using drugs and alcohol on their own. They need help, and recovery is a lifelong process that includes developing skills to manage cravings, dealing with stress in healthy ways, expressing feelings, participating in 12-step programs, and engaging in drug-free activities.

Table 26.8 Common Physiological, Psychological, and Behavioral Manifestations Associated with Substance Abuse

Physiological

• Abnormal blood pressure	• Hallucinations	• Reduced perception of pain
• Abnormal pupillary response	• Impaired liver function	• Sensory impairments
• Altered appetite	• Irregular or increased heartbeat	• Shiny ears
• Constipation	• Loss of consciousness	• Sleep disturbances
• Cravings	• Malnutrition	• Tremors (shakiness)
• Dizziness	• Peripheral neuropathy	• Unexplained weight loss or gain
• Drowsiness	• Perspiration	• Visible needle marks (if injecting)
• Enlarged heart	• Psychomotor disturbances	
• Gastrointestinal bleeding	• Red nose or eyes	

Psychological

• Confusion	• Disturbances of perception	• Low self-esteem
• Delusions	• Easily frustrated	• Paranoia
• Denial	• Emotional lability	• Poor concentration
• Depression	• Grandiosity	• Poor memory
• Disturbances in interpersonal behavior	• Intense emotions	• Reduced inhibitions
	• Loneliness	• Thought disturbances

Behavioral

• Anger	• Falling	• Lying
• Associating only with other substance abusers	• Financial irresponsibility	• Mood swings
• Belligerence	• Hyperactivity (restlessness)	• Nervousness
• Cheating	• Impaired judgment	• Poor hygiene
• Compulsive use of drugs	• Impaired or inability to fulfill major life roles	• Possession of drug paraphernalia
• Decreased ability to manage stress	• Impulsivity	• Spending money on drugs
• Decreased ability to manage time	• Inability to control drug use	• Staying up all night (insomnia)
• Difficulty holding a job	• Irritability	• Stealing
• Discontinuation of usual activities	• Isolation	• Violence
• Drug-seeking and drug-using behaviors	• Lack of interest in favorite sport or activity	• Withdrawal

When to Make a Referral for Substance Abuse

If the patient is going through withdrawal, the physical therapist should immediately refer the patient to a physician. Signs of withdrawal can include sweating, impaired sleep, seizures, impaired motor coordination, faulty judgment, anxiety, shaking, slurred speech, fluctuating levels of consciousness, and visual and tactile hallucinations. After stabilizing the patient, the physician may transfer him or her to a **detoxification unit.** If the patient is not experiencing withdrawal and is not already in a substance abuse treatment program, physical therapists can make a referral to an appropriate treatment center. Such treatment centers include **28-day inpatient rehabilitation** programs, long-term (1 to 1.5 years) inpatient therapeutic communities, 12-step programs for community-dwelling outpatients, and **dual diagnosis programs** for patients who have also been diagnosed with mental illness.

Patients who have been abusing substances for long periods of time should be referred to a **nutritionist** for proper dietary regulation. Physical therapy patients who have been abusing substances can be referred to occupational therapists to address regulating emotions, setting and maintaining appropriate boundaries, tolerating frustration, managing time, obtaining social skills, and regaining necessary ADL. Occupational therapists also can help patients learn that healthy activities can be pleasurable, through task groups in which patients choose, engage in, and discuss healthy activities. A social work referral can be made if the patient requires **community integration,** family intervention, or social supports.

■ AGITATION AND VIOLENCE

Physical therapists may not expect patients to demonstrate sexual, aggressive, or violent behaviors, yet most have witnessed such behaviors at least once. Therapists should learn how to predict violence, identify signs of escalation, manage aggressive patients, and verbally respond to threats. Violence is not always predictable, but the more therapists understand its signs, the better equipped they will be to handle a dangerous situation.

An initial step involves recognizing the early signs of agitation. Agitation usually does not diminish by itself. Instead, it may build to a verbal altercation or physical act. Some signs of agitation may include clenching fists, pacing back and forth, making angry facial expressions, grunting, groaning, swearing, tapping a foot, spitting, refusing to engage in therapy, throwing objects, and banging weights or other therapeutic equipment.

After observing signs of agitation, physical therapists should identify the source of the agitation in order to better control it. While many situations can cause agitation, it is important to remember that events that agitate one person may have no effect on another; levels of frustration vary from person to person. People with Alzheimer's disease may become agitated because they cannot recall the names of familiar objects or remember familiar motor plans. They may believe that family members are lying to them, deceiving them, or attempting to place them in a nursing home. People can become agitated as a result of physical pain, memory failure, hunger, fatigue, and dependency on others. Temporal lobe injury, psychosis, and the side effects of certain medications can cause agitation. People with personality disorders who have difficulty managing anger and who have experienced an upsetting event can easily become agitated.

Addressing the underlying circumstance causing the agitation may help to defuse it. If the source of agitation is unknown, the physical therapist should acknowledge to the patient, in a non-accusatory manner, that he or she seems upset. Many people are unaware of their agitation and calm down once it is brought to their attention. The therapist can then encourage the patient to verbally express why he or she feels upset. Therapists can also attempt to redirect patient anger into more productive channels and help alter their perspective regarding the disturbing issue.

Violence also can happen without warning. Many therapists working on inpatient TBI units have been bitten, kicked, punched, or scratched. Patients may feel that they are being forced to participate in therapy they do not need, or that they are being treated like children. They may believe that staff members have assumed control over their lives. To avoid humiliating the patient, therapists can use a client-centered therapy approach in which patients are offered respect and included in goal setting and treatment planning.

If efforts to defuse the patient's agitation do not work and he or she becomes violent, the physical therapist should remove all other patients from the area, then leave and call for help. After an act of violence, members of the rehabilitation team should examine what occurred to learn from the incident, prevent a future recurrence, and provide support and education to those involved. In reviewing the incident, the physical therapist should address the following questions:

- What was the patient's potential for aggression?
- What were the signs of escalating anger?
- Did the patient have a history of violence? If yes, under what circumstances did it occur?
- How did therapists and patients respond to the aggressor before, during, and after the act?
- What could have been done differently during the incident?

In addition to managing an agitated or violent patient, physical therapists need to recognize when a patient is undergoing abuse. It is estimated that 10% of women with disabilities experience sexual, physical, or disability-related violence.[98] Abuse has been related to decreased social support, increased social isolation, and elevated levels of depression and stress.[97] Women with disabilities may be even more susceptible to abuse, due to their dual minority status as people with disabilities and as women. As compared to women without disabilities, women having disabilities experienced longer periods of abuse and abuse from a greater number of perpetrators.[99] Nosek et al[100] have identified several factors that predict with 80% accuracy whether or not a woman has experienced abuse within the past year. These include decreased mobility, social isolation, depression, and a lack of education. Examination for abuse should be considered for women with disabilities.[100] Nosek et al developed a four-item screening tool, the Abuse Assessment Screen—Disability (AAS-D), that examines sexual, physical, and disability-related abuse in the past year.

■ HYPERSEXUALITY

Hypersexuality is a state of heightened sexual arousal that may be accompanied by verbal or physical aggression. These behaviors can be caused by mania, childhood sexual abuse, or brain damage. Patients may desire attention, or want to provoke or exert power over others, to impress others, or to show off. Verbal signs of hypersexuality can include whistling; verbalizing sexual desires; or asking for physical closeness, phone numbers, or dates. Physical behaviors include staring, pinching, brushing up against another's body, touching, kissing, exposing genitalia, masturbating, and blocking another's exit from a room.

There are several ways to proceed when a patient exhibits hypersexual behavior. If the therapist feels threatened, he or she should leave the area and obtain assistance. If the patient's hypersexual behavior is a newly observed behavior, the therapist can describe the behavior to the patient and firmly state that it is inappropriate and will not be tolerated. If the therapist believes that the patient is exhibiting symptoms of mania or hypomania, referral should be immediately made to a psychiatrist. Holding a **multidisciplinary team conference** may help the patient understand that hypersexual behaviors are not tolerated in the clinic.

PSYCHOSOCIAL WELLNESS

According to Jacobs and Jacobs[101] and Donatelle and Davis,[26] wellness is a dynamic process in which people attempt to fully develop their emotional, social, environmental, physical, spiritual, and intellectual health. Donatelle and Davis describe a well individual as someone who can forgive himself or herself and others, learn from mistakes, appreciate all things both grand and small, develop a realistic sense of self and the environment, achieve a balance in life roles and daily activities, respect others and maintain healthy relationships, feel a sense of life satisfaction, understand one's needs and express emotions appropriately, and function in his or her community. Achieving this definition of wellness may require substantial effort for someone with a disability who may experience multiple barriers to wellness.

Barriers to Wellness for People with Disabilities

Healthy People 2020 identified gaps and disparities in the health and wellness of Americans with disabilities.[90] It reported that people with disabilities exhibited more symptoms of psychological distress and tended to not engage in as many physical activities as people without disabilities. Objectives to overcome these barriers included to "Increase the proportion of people with disabilities who participate in social, spiritual, recreational, community and civic activities to the degree that they wish" (DH-13) and "Reduce the proportion of people with disabilities who report serious psychological distress" (DH-18).

More specifically, research has found that women with disabilities experience higher levels of stress than do males with disabilities, possibly owing to higher incidences of poverty, violence, abuse, chronic health problems, and social isolation.[93] Economic disadvantage may be due to stress-inducing factors such as earning a lower income, having less access to disability benefits from public programs, having less education than their male counterparts with disabilities, and having a higher likelihood of being unemployed or unmarried.[102] People with SCI report a higher level of perceived stress than the general population, and women with SCI tend to have a higher level of perceived stress than men with SCI.[103]

Social Support

Social support is critical in maintaining or achieving psychosocial wellness. **Social support** is defined as the availability of other persons in the environment who can offer emotional support, financial or material help, a listening ear, guidance, or encouragement. Social support has been associated with increased self-esteem, coping, and adjustment for individuals with disabilities. Evidence suggests that social support plays a strong preventative and palliative role in a wide range of physical and medical conditions. Rintala et al[104] found that the amount of social support was directly related to a sense of life satisfaction and well-being in patients with SCI. Hardy et al[105] and Kaplan[106] found that high social support was predictive of a return to vocational functioning after rehabilitation.

Researchers have suggested that failure to recover from depression stemming from disability may correlate to a lack of adequate social support. Social isolation is a frequently encountered condition associated with disability. Physical restrictions such as pain and mobility limitations may discourage connections with others. The combination of diminished social opportunities, negative societal perceptions, and multiple environmental barriers may result in isolation and a lack of emotional intimacy.

Social support can be used to enhance treatment and promote patient adherence. The physical therapist plays an important role in guiding patient education, including access to resources and instruction in use of adaptive equipment and environmental devices designed to improve a patient's access to social networks and socialization. Appendix 26.C provides Web-based resources for patients, families, and caregivers. It provides resources for improving community accessibility (independent living centers), depression, substance abuse, anxiety, and PTSD.

WELLNESS IN REHABILITATION

Psychosocial wellness requires that patients experience success in both rehabilitation activities and long-term relationships and roles. Rehabilitation activities focus on improving functional outcomes, involvement in meaningful events that foster socialization (e.g., playing wheelchair basketball with other patients), and community reintegration. Long-term relationships and roles include being a spouse, parent, worker, and friend. Psychologists, **social workers**, and occupational therapists can facilitate readjustment to these long-term roles. Both rehabilitation activities and long-term relationships and roles should provide a sense of contentment, happiness, and well-being. Physical therapists can promote and provide opportunities for patients to choose and engage in meaningful activities that promote psychosocial wellness.

Patients who spend a great deal of time dwelling on the past and worrying about the future are unable to be fully cognizant of the present moment. The ability to become absorbed in the present moment can decrease anxiety concerning the past or future—the patient's emotional energy is focused on his or her immediate activities. Each instance in which a patient can focus on the present offers him or her the power to change, to break through old habits, to view circumstances differently, and to recognize available choices. Physical therapists can help patients remain focused on the present moment by selecting activities that are both meaningful to and congruent with the patient's goals for rehabilitation.

Having a daily balance of work, leisure, and social activities is important to sustain psychosocial wellness. Any psychological or physical impairment can disrupt this balance. In a study of the relationship between depression and leisure participation in people with SCI, Loy et al[107] found that patients without depression had wider repertoires and higher levels of leisure activity than patients with depression. Therapists can help patients engage in leisure activities through the use of activity interest surveys and schedules. Activity interest surveys are used to gather information about the types of leisure pursuits patients previously engaged in, which leisure pursuits they currently hold interest in, and which leisure activities they would like to pursue in the future.

A negative outlook inhibits psychosocial wellness. Physical therapists can help patients with negative perspectives to positively alter their expectations through goal setting, identifying optimistic options, using cognitive-behavioral techniques that challenge the validity of negative perceptions, or referring the patient to a psychologist for longer-term intervention.

INTEGRATING PSYCHOSOCIAL FACTORS INTO REHABILITATION: CASE EXAMPLE

Bill, a 19-year-old who was training to be an Olympic gymnast, sustained an SCI in a motorcycle accident. Bill had developed a strong social support system and participated in a variety of extracurricular activities. He was engaged and planning to be married, participated on his college's gymnastic team, and worked as an athletic counselor in the summer camp he had attended since age 7. The SCI he sustained caused a loss of function from his chest down.

All of Bill's energy is now focused on getting through each day. He does not view himself as able to work or attend school. The accident has changed his expectations for the future, his outlook on life, his environmental challenges, and his social support system. His depression was compounded by his broken marriage engagement,

and Bill no longer meets his friends for social events; in fact, he rarely leaves his home other than to attend rehabilitation. Just when he was becoming independent of his parents, Bill has now become dependent on them again. He observes his younger sisters and brothers progressing in their lives and feels stagnant, angry, depressed, and ashamed. His self-esteem, which was once high, is now severely diminished and he has lost his familiar identity.

As part of his rehabilitation, the therapist should provide a safe way for Bill to express his anger; referral to a psychologist is also warranted. The therapist can help him to better understand his physical limitations and capabilities. Based on Bill's strengths and limitations, the therapist should help him to redefine interests that could emerge into new roles and a new identity. For instance, it might be helpful if Bill could identify a meaningful activity that could take the place of his athletic training (such as coaching a children's gymnastic team). Information about college and distance learning could also be beneficial. The therapist also can assist Bill and his family in the understanding of SCI and reasonable expectations for the future.

SUGGESTIONS FOR REHABILITATIVE INTERVENTION

Table 26.9 offers a list of behaviors that suggest inappropriate and pathological response patterns to disability. This list is not meant to be fully inclusive, but rather indicates areas requiring further consideration. It is important to understand that even mild expressions of pathological response patterns can become chronic and worsen in severity over time. Table 26.10 identifies patient behaviors that warrant a mental health consultation.

Box 26.5[108] gives examples of general goals and outcomes for patients with psychosocial issues, and Box 26.6 provides instruments typically used to measure these outcomes organized by the *International Classification of Functioning, Disability, and Health* (ICF) Categories.[109] However, human reactions, response patterns, and the adaptation process are variable and individualistic. Each patient must be approached uniquely and treatment goals should incorporate the patient's individual personality characteristics, responses, and needs. An important component of rehabilitation is the patient–practitioner relationship. Physical therapists can establish a therapeutic atmosphere of communication, understanding, and cooperation with patients, which can serve as the foundation necessary to produce positive rehabilitation outcomes. Therapists can sometimes forget the powerful influence they have in setting the tone of this interaction. The very structure and atmosphere of service delivery and the personality and type of communication provided by the practitioner

Table 26.9   Behaviors Suggesting Pathological Response Patterns

Grieving	Depression	Damaged Self-Esteem	Heightened Possibility for Suicide	Heightened Possibility for Violence
Grieving for actual or perceived impairment of functioning or actual loss is normal and expected, but the following might serve as clues to a more severe reaction: Denial of problem or its severity Exaggeration or idealizing the loss Obsession with the past or the pre-loss state Obsession with guilt related to loss Regression Difficulty with concentration Loss of interest in activities and events Lability of mood Inability to discuss loss Fear of being left alone Acting out behaviors (tantrums, suicidal gestures, promiscuity) Angry stance	Flat affect (showing little emotion) Very low energy levels Manic energy and behavior Psychomotor retardation (slowing down of movement and action) Ruminating about negative thoughts Change in eating and sleeping patterns (insomnia or hypersomnia) Regression Social withdrawal Self-destructive behaviors Loss of interest in environment, people, and events Self-blame and self-criticism	Isolation from social sphere Self-destructive behavior Inability to sustain eye contact Inability to accept praise Judgmental attitude Self-deprecating and self-critical Unwarranted pessimism Unconcern for appearance Unconcern for personal safety	Depression Giving away possessions Hoarding/hiding medications or potential weapons Writing suicide note Updating will Verbalizing loneliness or hopelessness Statements regarding benefit of release of pain, absence, and so forth Intrusiveness of such thoughts	Low threshold for anger Depression High-anxiety state Motoric agitation Self-mutilation Oversensitive Argumentative Inability to express feelings Fears of abandonment Highly dependent Dissociative states

exert a strong influence on patient participation and response to rehabilitation efforts.

Optimizing Patient Involvement

Patients should be involved as fully as possible in their own treatment. This includes involvement in goal setting and treatment planning, as well as in the ongoing evaluation of progress. Patient cooperation is also dependent on the therapist's clear explanation of the patient's situation, anticipated goals and expected outcomes, and interventions. Relating to the patient as a partner in therapy can engender cooperation and trust in the therapeutic relationship. When patients feel a heightened sense of control and ability (i.e., locus of control), feelings of despair and helplessness can be mitigated.

Therapists should also maintain a receptive ear to patient concerns and encourage communication. Listening carefully to patients in a nonjudgmental manner will allow them to reveal concerns and issues they may otherwise feel uncomfortable discussing. Clear and articulate communication, however, can be disrupted by emotion, uncertainty, or power discrepancies that exist when patients become passive recipients of service. Although it may sometimes appear easier to do for patients than to witness their struggle—particularly when patients assume a passive role in rehabilitation—promoting self-reliance and independence fosters patients' engagement and responsibility in their recovery. Allowing patients to maintain a passive role fosters helplessness, encourages dependency, and slows progress in the long term.

Use of Jargon and Labels

Patient–therapist communication should be characterized by simple and easy to understand language that matches the cognitive level of the patient. The use of scientific jargon and labels should be avoided when speaking with patients, because it impedes patient understanding and emotionally distances patients from therapists. Similarly, when patients hear therapists referring to fellow patients by their diagnosis, they receive the message that patients are nothing more than disabilities. Such practice should be avoided and, instead, therapists should use language

Table 26.10	Patient Behaviors Warranting a Mental Health Consultation
Regression	Regression involves reverting to earlier, more immature patterns of functioning. This may be more commonly observed in children but might be observed in adults as well. For example, children may revert back to sucking their thumb, or may appear to have lost their toilet training skills. Regression in adults may generally be seen in lost skills and abilities and/or even in the extreme behavior of reverting to taking a fetal position.
Disorientation	Disorientation is confusion as to time, place, activity, self-identity, or identity of others. Occasional, transient disorientation is not wholly uncommon in the average person, yet persistence in frequency or duration of occurrence is cause for examination and intervention. Any more extreme confused behaviors and thought processes need to be carefully examined.
Delusional thinking	Delusional thinking refers to faulty and mistaken beliefs and, although related to inaccurate interpretation of environment, is distinguished by the persistence of this belief system. This can run the gamut from delusions of grandeur or of persecution, to delusions about the nature and scope of a disability. These delusions hold up and persist in the face of contrary information.
Inaccurate interpretation of environment	This is the broadest category in this list, but fortunately is also the most readily understood category. Clearly, when a patient significantly misinterprets and misunderstands the objective situation and reality about him or her, it is probably most readily noted by non–mental health practitioners in its many expressions. This should draw attention and intervention, not only in its extreme form of a psychotic break, but also in its minor form of small, repeated episodes of misinterpretations.
Inappropriate affect	Affect refers to the mood state displayed by the patient, where feelings such as joy, sadness, fear, and so forth are reflected in body language, facial expression, and verbalizations. Inappropriate affect can be seen in an affective expression alien to the situation; for example, demonstrating and expressing joy on hearing bad news. It also refers to a split between displayed affect and verbalization; for example, the verbal expression of mourning and condolence offered while smiling brightly and jumping for joy.
Hypovigilance or hypervigilance	Hypovigilance can be noted in a patient being oblivious to his or her surroundings and the events around the patient, socially, as well as physically. Hypervigilance refers to an intense focus and alertness to social and physical surrounds. Each of these has different ramifications and meaning to the mental health team. A consultation is suggested as either extreme is approached.
Mood swings	We all experience changes in mood, yet most of the time these changes are relatively appropriate reactions to external determinants, such as the receipt of news and information or to changing occurrences and circumstances in our environment. Although changeable, moods are generally persistent and stable. When mood shifts either to extremes and/or with some frequency, it suggests either instability or that mood is being driven predominantly by internal rather than external factors.
Self-destructive behaviors	Any self-destructive behavior, particularly ones that persist, are cause for serious concern. Self-destructive behaviors can run the gamut from subtle, difficult to detect signs to very clear and frightening overt signs. Subtle signs can include non-adherence with treatment regimen, poor self-maintenance activities such as not eating, overeating, diminishment of personal care and hygiene, or carelessness in negotiating the environment. Clearer signs can include self-inflicted wounds and suicidal ideation and expressions.
Normal behaviors taken to extremes	Normal human behavior enjoys a wide latitude of response repertoire before drawing attention as being out of expected bounds. This latitude must usually be extended further when dealing with someone undergoing a more extreme, traumatic, or stressful experience. Individuals confronted with a disability would be expected to naturally focus their attention, concerns, and anxiety around this issue. The level of focus on a left leg given by someone preparing to have that leg amputated would be considered obsessive in a healthy ambulatory person, yet normal here. Care in judgment is required by the clinician when determining behavior expressions. That said, issues such as obsessiveness, extreme distractibility, immobilization in the face of routine decisions, and unexpected egocentricity or self-denigration may require a consultation. An overly adherent patient, an extremely calm patient, as well as an overly contentious, argumentative, or extremely anxious or hysterical patient also promotes concern. Any response (verbal or behavioral) that appears unwarranted to the stimuli should draw attention. Overreactions in opposite directions or any behavior that appears to be at an extreme, using reasonable judgment, deserves attention.

Box 26.5 Examples of General Goals and Outcomes for Patients with Psychosocial Issues Adapted from the *Guide to Physical Therapist Practice*[108]

Impact of pathology is reduced.
• Patient/client, family, and caregiver knowledge and awareness of the disease, prognosis, and plan of care is enhanced.
• Symptom management is enhanced.
• Changes associated with recovery are monitored.
• Risk of secondary impairments and reoccurrence of condition is reduced.
• Intensity of care is decreased.

Impact of impairments is reduced.
• Cognitive function is improved.
• Communication is improved.
• Ability to participate in rehabilitation is improved.

Ability to perform physical actions, tasks, or activities is improved.
• Independence in ADL is increased.
• Problem solving and decision making skills are improved.
• Safety of client, family, and caregivers is intact.

Disability associated with chronic illness is reduced.
• Ability to assume/resume self-care and home management is improved.
• Ability to assume roles such as participation in work activities (job/school/play) and community leisure roles is improved.
• Awareness and use of community resources are improved.

Health status and quality of life are improved.
• Sense of well-being is enhanced.
• Stressors are reduced and/or the ability to manage them is improved.
• Insight, self-confidence, and self-management skills are improved.
• Health and wellness are improved.

Client satisfaction is enhanced.
• Access to and availability of services are acceptable to client and family.
• Quality of rehabilitation services is acceptable to client and family.
• Care is coordinated with client, family, caregivers, and other professionals.
• Discharge placement needs are determined.

Box 26.6 Outcome Measures for Psychosocial Issues Organized by the *International Classification of Functioning, Disability, and Health* (ICF) Categories[109]

Body Structure and Function Measures

Holmes-Rahe Social Readjustment Scale (see Appendix 26.A)

• Holmes, T, and Rahe, R: The Social Readjustment Scale. J Psychosom Res 11:213, 1967.

The Hassles Scale (see Appendix 26.B)

• Kanner, AD, et al: Comparison of two modes of stress management: Daily hassles and uplifts versus major life events. J Behav Med 4:1, 1981.

Contextual Memory Test

• Toglia, JP: Contextual Memory Test. Therapy Skill Builders, San Antonio, TX, 1993.

Beck Depression Inventory

• Beck, AT, Steer, RA, and Brown, GK: Beck Depression Inventory–II Manual. The Psychological Corporation, San Antonio, Texas, 1987.

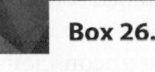

Box 26.6   Outcome Measures for Psychosocial Issues Organized by the *International Classification of Functioning, Disability, and Health* (ICF) Categories[109]—cont'd

Stroop Color and Word Test

• Golden, CJ, and Freshwater, SM: The Stroop Color and Word Test: A Manual for Clinical and Experimental Uses. Stoelting Co, Wood Dale, IL, 2002.

Neurobehavioral Cognitive Status Examination

• Kiernan, RJ, Mueller, J, and Langston, JW: The Neurobehavioral Cognitive Status Examination (COGNISTAT). Northern California Neurobehavioral Group, Inc., San Francisco, 2001.

Generalized Expectancy for Success Scale

• Fibel, B, and Hale, WD: The Generalized Expectancy for Success Scale—a new measure. J Consulting Clin Psych 46:924, 1978/1992.

Beck Hopelessness Scale

• Durham, TW: Norms, reliability, and item analysis of the Hopelessness Scale in general psychiatric, forensic psychiatric, and college populations. J Clin Psych 38(5):597, 1982.

Internal-External Locus of Control Scale

• Rotter, JB: Generalized expectancies for internal versus external control of reinforcement. Psych Mono 80:1, 1966.

Self-Efficacy Scale

• Sherer, M, Maddox, JE, Mercandante, B, Prentice-Dunn, S, Jacobs, B, and Rogers, RW: The Self-Efficacy Scale: Construction and validation. Psych Rep 51:663, 1982.

Sentence Completion Attitude Survey

• Bloom, W: Bloom Sentence Completion Attitude Survey. Stoelting Co., Wood Dale, IL. Website: https://www.stoeltingco.com

Mini-Mental State Examination (MMSE)

• Folstein, MF, Folstein, SE, and McHugh, PR: "Mini-mental state." A practical method for grading the cognitive state of patients for the clinician. J Psychiatr Res 12(3):189, 1975.

Activity Measures

Occupational Questionnaire's Balanced Activity Record

• Smith, HR, Kielhofner, G, and Watts, JH: Occupational Questionnaire. Am J Occup Ther 40:278, 1986. Website: www.moho.uic.edu/mohorelatedrsrcs.html

Interest Checklist

• Kielhofner, G, and Neville, A: Interest Checklist. Slack, Thorofare, NJ, 1983.

Participation Measures

Role Checklist

• Oakley, F, Kielhofner, G, Barris, R, and Reichler, RK: The Role Checklist: Development and empirical assessment of reliability. Occup Ther J Res 6(3):157, 1986.

Community Adaptation Schedule

• Roen, S, and Burnes, A: Community Adaptation Schedule [serial online]. Not dated. Available from Mental Measurements Yearbook with Tests in Print, Ipswich, MA. Accessed January 12, 2011.

that reflects respect for the patient's dignity and unique life circumstances.

Rehabilitation Team Members' Self-Awareness

Finally, and perhaps most important, therapists need to be aware of their own feelings, motivations, and responses. Such self-awareness is critical for therapists to understand their own reactions to patients. It is normal for people to respond to others based on conscious or unconscious memories. Sometimes patients can remind therapists of significant others, such as siblings, parents, spouses, or employers. However, when therapists react to patients based on unconscious associations to others, they can misperceive patient needs and respond inappropriately. For example, unconscious reactions to patients can cause therapists to become overprotective or, at the other extreme, become frustrated with patients without recognizing that their own reactions have more to do with other relationships than with the patient at hand.

Generally, when therapists feel a heightened sense of emotion in response to a particular patient it may often serve as a cue that such emotions stem from unconscious associations to others. When this occurs, it is important for therapists to step back and evaluate their own feelings in order to discern the connection between their reactions to the patient and how the patient may be triggering unconscious emotions.

The converse is also true; patients will respond to therapists based on their own unconscious associations with significant others who have similar personality characteristics to those of the therapist. Therapists must be aware of this normal phenomenon and refrain from responding emotionally to the patient's unconscious associations. Rather, the therapist should continue to build a respectful relationship with the patient that, in time, will demonstrate to the patient that his or her first impressions were misperceptions.

SUMMARY

It is important for physical therapists to identify and understand the individual psychosocial factors that enhance or inhibit the rehabilitation of their patients, and intervene accordingly. Successful intervention depends on the following:

- Understanding the psychosocial aspects of each patient, including personality styles and coping skills
- Recognizing and interpreting the common defense mechanisms that patients use in rehabilitation
- Distinguishing the stages of psychosocial adaptation to disability and helping patients' progress in their own adjustment
- Understanding how to identify anxiety, depression, and substance abuse; determining how to address these problems; and recognizing when referral to other team members is warranted
- Integrating a patient/client-centered approach that emphasizes respect, empathy, and compassion
- Empowering patients and families through psychosocial education, and wellness and prevention strategies
- Working together with patients to develop anticipated goals and expected outcomes congruent with their needs, values, and level of functioning
- Collaborating with patients and team members to establish and implement appropriate interventions
- Developing a team approach and providing referrals as necessary

Questions for Review

1. Identify five psychosocial factors and state how each factor may influence rehabilitation.
2. Give examples of interventions for each psychosocial factor identified in question 1.
3. Differentiate among the different mental health professionals who can treat patients with psychosocial issues by describing their roles.
4. What should therapists do to calm an agitated patient?
5. Describe an approach for managing a violent patient and how to analyze an act of violence after it has occurred.
6. What are the manifestations of hypersexuality and how should it be addressed?
7. Identify and describe the phases of psychosocial adaptation to disability.
8. Discuss three coping strategies that have been found to be effective in the psychosocial adaptation to chronic disability and illness.

9. Describe five common defense mechanisms that patients use in response to disability.

10. What are the signs and symptoms of post-traumatic stress disorder?

11. Differentiate between typical reactions to grieving and pathological reactions.

12. Explain several ways to optimize patient involvement in the rehabilitation process and promote self-reliance.

13. Why is patient/client-centered intervention important? What strategies can be used to achieve this type of interaction?

14. Describe the general adaptation syndrome.

CASE STUDY

The patient is a 68-year-old female, admitted to an inpatient unit 2 days after sustaining a right femoral neck fracture from falling down her basement stairs. Hip replacement surgery (arthroplasty) was performed on the same day as the fall. The referring documentation indicates "weight-bearing as tolerated." The patient complains that she "can't do anything" for herself owing to the fall.

Before her fall, she was in fair health but was experiencing declining eyesight, poor short-term memory, and osteoporosis. Her hip fracture has placed her at high risk for further deconditioning and loss of function. The patient's husband had suffered a prolonged illness; the patient cared for him during the last 5 years until he passed away. She has a son whom she rarely sees, because he is married with children and living in another part of the country. A close friend lives several miles from her and the rest of her friends have died. The patient is embarrassed to be seen in public in a wheelchair.

Given the deaths of her husband and friends, and given her recent accident, the patient is now very anxious about her own mortality for the first time in her life. She is preoccupied with her husband's death since he was so much a part of her life. She feels that she has no future and nothing to look forward to. She no longer knows who she is and longs to "be reunited with" her husband.

GUIDING QUESTIONS

1. Identify the psychosocial factors apparent in this case study.

2. What relevant questions about the patient remain unanswered (i.e., what relevant information is missing)?

3. How might the patient's emotional condition affect rehabilitation?

4. Develop a problem list for the patient.

5. Identify the patient's assets.

6. Identify the general goals of physical therapy intervention on which specific anticipated goals and expected outcomes will be based.

7. Identify the general categories of procedural interventions appropriate for this patient.

8. Identify referrals to other professionals or resources.

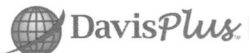 For additional resources, including answers to the questions for review and case study guiding questions, please visit **http://davisplus.fadavis.com**

References

1. Webster's New World Dictionary of American English, ed 2. Prentice-Hall, Upper Saddle River, NJ, 1988.
2. Vaillant, GE: Adaptation to Life. Little, Brown, Boston, 1977.
3. Wickramasekera, I, et al: Applied psychophysiology: A bridge between the biomedical model and the biopsychosocial model in family medicine. Prof Psychol Res Pr 27:221, 1996.
4. Edwards, A, and Elwyn, G: Shared decision-making in health care: Achieving evidence-based patient choice. In Edwards, A, and Elwyn, G (eds): Shared Decision Making in Health Care: Achieving Evidence-Based Patient Choice, ed 2. Oxford University Press, Oxford, UK, 2009, p 3.
5. Siegel, B: Love, Medicine and Miracles. HarperCollins, New York, 1988.
6. Doskoch, P: Happy ever laughter. Psychol Today 29:32, 1996.
7. Watts, R: Trauma counseling and rehabilitation. J Appl Rehab Counseling 28:8, 1997.
8. Gleckman, AD, and Brill, S: The impact of brain injury on family functioning: Implications for subacute rehabilitation programs. Brain Inj 9:385, 1995.
9. American Psychiatric Association: Diagnostic and Statistical Manual of Mental Disorders, ed 4. Text Revision. American Psychiatric Association, Washington, DC, 1994.

10. Moore, D, and Li, L: Substance abuse among applicants for vocational rehabilitation services. J Rehabil 60:48, 1994.
11. Friedland, J, and McColl, M: Disability and depression: Some etiological considerations. Soc Sci Med 34:395, 1992.
12. Turner, RJ, and Beiser, M: Major depression and depressive symptomatology among the physically disabled: Assessing the role of chronic stress. J Nerv Ment Dis 178:343, 1990.
13. Penninx, BWJH, et al: Vitamin B_{12} deficiency and depression in physically disabled older women: Epidemiologic evidence from the Women's Health and Aging Study. Am J Psychiatry 157:715, 2000.
14. Paolucci, S, et al: Post stroke depression and its role in rehabilitation of inpatients. Arch Phys Med Rehabil 80:985, 1999.
15. Kreuter, M, et al: Partner relationships, functioning, mood, and global quality of life in persons with spinal cord injury and traumatic brain injury. Spinal Cord 36:252, 1999.
16. Meara, J, et al: Use of the GDS—Geriatric Depression Scale as a screening instrument for depressive symptomatology in patients with Parkinson's disease and their careers in the community. Age Ageing 28:35, 1999.
17. Denollet, J: Personality and coronary heart disease: The type-D scale-16. Ann Behav Med 20(3):209, 1998.
18. Nemeroff, CB: The neurobiology of depression. Sci Am, p 42, June 1998.
19. Heinemann, A, et al: Substance abuse by persons with recent spinal cord injuries. Rehabil Psychol 35:217, 1990.
20. Zegans, J: The embodied self: Integration in health and illness. Adv J Inst Advance Health 7(3):29, 1991.
21. Benson, H: The Relaxation Response. HarperCollins, New York, 1974.
22. Livneh, H, and Antonak, RF: Psychosocial Adaptation to Chronic Illness and Disability. Aspen, Gaithersburg, MD, 1997.
23. Keany, KC, and Glueckauf, RL: Disability and value changes: An overview and analysis of acceptance of loss theory. Rehabil Psychol 38:199, 1993.
24. Jacobson, AM, et al: Adherence among children and adolescents with insulin-dependent diabetes mellitus over a four-year longitudinal follow-up: I. The influence of patient coping and adjustment. J Pediatr Psychol 15:511, 1990.
25. Grzesiak, RC, and Hicok, DA: A brief history of psychotherapy and physical disability. Am J Psychother 48:240, 1994.
26. Donatelle, RJ, and Davis, LG: Access to Health, ed 6. Allyn & Bacon, Needham Heights, MA, 2000.
27. Strobe, W, and Strobe, MS: Bereavement and Health: The Psychological and Physical Consequences of Partner Loss (The Psychology of Social Issues). Cambridge University Press, New York, 1987.
28. Burke, ML, et al: Current knowledge and research on chronic sorrow: A foundation for inquiry. Death Stud 16:231, 1992.
29. Lindgren, CL, et al: Chronic sorrow: A lifespan concept. Sch Inq Nurs Pract 6:27, 1992.
30. Selye, H: The general adaptation syndrome and the disease of adaptation. J Clin Endocrinol Metab 6:117, 1946.
31. Heinrichs, SC, et al: Anti-stress action of a corticotropin-releasing factor antagonist on behavioral reactivity to stressors of varying type and intensity. Neuropsychopharmacology 11:179, 1994.
32. Theorell, T, et al: "Person Under Train" incidents: Medical consequences for subway drivers. Psychosom Med 54:480, 1992.
33. Breznitz, S: The seven kinds of denial. In Breznitz (ed): The Denial of Stress. International Universities Press, New York, 1983, p 257.
34. Taylor, SE, and Aspinwell, LG: Psychosocial aspects of chronic illness. In Costa, PT, and VandenBox, GR (eds): Psychological Aspects of Serious Illness: Chronic Conditions, Fatal Diseases, and Clinical Care. American Psychological Association, Washington, DC, 1990, p 7.
35. Rodin, G, et al: Depression in the Medically Ill: An Integrated Approach. Brunner/Mazel, New York, 1991.
36. Levin, HS, and Grossman, RG: Behavioral sequelae of closed head injury. Arch Neurol-Chicago 35:720, 1978.
37. Brooks, N: Behavioral abnormalities in head injured patients. Scand J Rehabil Med Suppl 17:41, 1988.
38. Mairs, N: Waist High in the World. Beacon Press, Boston, 1996.
39. Hermann, M, and Wallesch, CW: Depressive changes in stroke patients. Disabil Rehabil 15:55, 1993.
40. Davidhizer, R: Disability does not have to be the grief that never ends: Helping patients adjust. Rehabil Nurs 22(1):32, 1997.
41. Kabat-Zinn, J: Full Catastrophe Living: The Wisdom of Your Body and Mind to Face Stress, Pain, and Illness. Delacorte, New York, 1990.
42. Trieshman, RB: Spinal Cord Injuries: Psychological, Social and Vocational Rehabilitation, ed 2. Demos, New York, 1988.
43. Biordi, DL: Body image. In Larsen, PD, and Lubkin, IM (eds): Chronic Illness: Impact and Intervention, ed 7. Jones & Bartlett, Boston, 2009, p 117.
44. Frank, RG, Rosenthal, M, and Caplan, B (eds): Handbook of Rehabilitation Psychology, ed 2. American Psychological Association, Washington, DC, 2009.
45. Freidman, HS, and Booth-Kewley, S: The "disease-prone personality": A meta-analytic view of the construct. Am Psychol 42:539, 1987.
46. Glanz, K, and Schwartz, MD: Stress, coping, and health behavior. In Glanz, K, Rimer, BK, and Viswanath, K (eds): Health Behavior and Health Education: Theory, Research, and Practice, ed 4. Jossey-Bass, San Francisco, 2008, p 211.
47. McCraty, R, and Tomasino, D: Emotional stress, positive emotions, and coherence. In Arnetz, BB, Ekman, R, and Carlsson, A (eds): Stress in Health and Disease. Wiley-VCH, 2006, p 342.
48. Stone, AA, and Porter, MA: Psychological coping: Its importance for treating medical problems. Mind/Body Med 1(1):46, 1995.
49. Tate, D, et al: Coping with the late effects—differences between depressed and nondepressed polio survivors. Am J Phys Med Rehabil 73:27, 1994.
50. Krause, JS, and Rohe, DE: Personality and life adjustment after spinal cord injury: An exploratory study. Rehabil Psychol 43:118, 1998.
51. Radomski, M: Assessing context: Personal, social, and cultural. In Trombly, CA, and Radomski, M (eds): Occupational Therapy for Physical Dysfunction, ed 5. Lippincott Williams & Wilkins, Baltimore, 2002, p 213.
52. Mpofu, SS: Take Control of Your Health: Master of Your Destiny, Book 1. Author House, Bloomington, IN, 2011.
53. Jorgenson, J: Therapeutic use of companion animals in health care. Image J Nurs Sch 29(3):249, 1997.
54. Webster, G, et al: Relationship and family breakdown following acquired brain injury: The role of the rehabilitation team. Brain Inj 13:593, 1996.
55. Steinhauer, PD: Developing resilience in children from disadvantaged populations. In National Forum on Health Secretariat (eds): Canada Health Action—Building the Legacy. Vol. 1. Determinants of Health: Children and Youth. Éditions MultiMondes, Sainte-Foy, Québec, Canada, 1997, p 51.
56. King, G, et al: Turning points and protective processes in the lives of people with chronic disabilities. Qual Health Res 13(2):184, 2003.
57. Gorman, LM, et al: Psychosocial Nursing Handbook for the Nonpsychiatric Nurse. Williams & Wilkins, Baltimore, 1989, p 51.
58. Holmes, T, and Rahe, R: The Social Readjustment Scale. J Psychosom Res 11:213, 1967.
59. Kanner, AD, et al: Comparison of two modes of stress management: Daily hassles and uplifts versus major life events. J Behav Med 4:1, 1981.
60. Tusek, D: Guided imagery: A powerful tool to decrease length of stay, pain, anxiety, and narcotic consumption. J Invas Cardiol 11:265, 1999.
61. Tiernan, P: Independent nursing interventions: Relaxation and guided imagery in critical care. Crit Care Nurse 14(5):47, 1994.
62. Early, MB: Mental Health Concepts and Techniques for the Occupational Therapy Assistant, ed 3. Lippincott Williams & Wilkins, Baltimore, 2000.
63. Precin, P: Living Skills Recovery Workbook. Butterworth-Heinemann, Woburn, MA, 1999.
64. Walker, LG, and Eremin, O: Psychoneuroimmunology: New fad or the fifth cancer treatment modality? Am J Surg 170:2, 1995.
65. Tusek, D, et al: Effect of guided imagery and length of stay, pain and anxiety in cardiac surgery patients. J Cardiovasc Manage 10:22, 1999.
66. Scheufele, PM: Effects of progressive relaxation and classical music on measurements of attention, relaxation, and stress responses. J Behav Med 23(2):207, 2000.

67. Benson, H, et al: Decreased blood pressure in pharmacologically treated hypertensive patients who regularly elicited the relaxation response. Lancet 1(7852):289, 1974.
68. Rossman, ML: Guided Imagery for Self-Healing: An Essential Resource for Anyone Seeking Wellness. New World Library, Novato, CA, 2000.
69. Dossey, BM: Holistic modalities and healing moments. Am J Nurs 98(6):44, 1998.
70. Eisenman, A, and Cohen, B: Music therapy for patients undergoing regional anesthesia. AORN J 62:947, 1991.
71. White, J: Music therapy: An intervention to reduce anxiety in the myocardial infarction patient. Clin Nurs Specialist 6:58, 1992.
72. Burns, D: The Feeling Good Handbook. Plume, New York, 1999.
73. Blackburn, IM, and Moorhead, S: Update in cognitive therapy for depression. J Cogn Psychother 14(3):305, 2000.
74. Butler, AC, et al: The empirical status of cognitive-behavioral therapy: A review of meta-analyses. Clin Psychol Rev 26(1):17, 2006.
75. Lam, RW, and Sidney, HK: Evidence-based strategies for achieving and sustaining full remission in depression: Focus on meta-analyses. Can J Psychiatry 49:17S, 2004.
76. Leichsenring, F, Rabung, S, and Leibing, E: The efficacy of short-term psychodynamic psychotherapy in specific psychiatric disorders: A meta-analysis. Arch Gen Psychiatry 61(12):1208, 2004.
77. Pampallona, S, et al: Combined pharmacotherapy and psychological treatment for depression: A systematic review. Arch Gen Psychiatry 61(7):714, 2004.
78. Mayou, RA, and Smith, KA: Posttraumatic symptoms following medical illness and treatment. J Psychosom Res 43:121, 1997.
79. Bryant, RA, and Harvey, AG: Avoidant coping style and PTS following motor vehicle accidents. Behav Res Ther 33:631, 1995.
80. Herman, JL: Trauma and Recovery. Basic Books, New York, 1997.
81. Barlow, DH: Unraveling the mysteries of anxiety and its disorders from the perspective of emotion theory. Am Psychol 55:1247, 2000.
82. Keane, TM, and Barlow, DH: Posttraumatic stress disorder. In Barlow, DH (ed): Anxiety and Its Disorders, ed 2. Guilford Press, New York, 2002, p 418.
83. Geisser, ME, et al: The relationship between symptoms of posttraumatic stress disorder and pain, affective disturbance and disability among patients with accident and non-accident related pain. Pain 66:207, 1996.
84. Kerns, RD, et al: West Haven–Yale multidimensional pain inventory (WHYMPI). Pain 23:345, 1985.
85. Melzack, R: McGill Pain Questionnaire: Major properties and scoring methods. Pain 1:277, 1975.
86. Blake, DD, et al: A clinician rating scale for assessing current and lifetime PTSD: The CAPS-1. Behav Ther 13:187, 1990.
87. Weathers, FW, et al: The PTSD Checklist (PCL): Reliability, validity, and diagnostic utility. Annual Meeting of the International Society for Traumatic Stress Studies, San Antonio, TX, 1993.
88. Otis, JD, et al: An examination of the relationship between chronic pain and post-traumatic stress disorder. J Rehabil Res Dev 40(5):397, 2003.
89. Boekamp, JR, et al: Depression following a spinal cord injury. Int J Psychiatr Med 26(3):329, 1996.
90. U.S. Department of Health and Human Services: Healthy People 2020. Understanding and Improving Health, ed 3. US Government Printing Office, Washington, DC, 2010.
91. Hughes, RB, et al: Characteristics of depressed and nondepressed women with physical disabilities. Arch Phys Med Rehabil 86(3):473, 2005.
92. Hughes, RB, et al: Depression and women with spinal cord injury. Top Spinal Cord Inj Rehabil 7(1):16, 2001.
93. McGrath, E, et al: Women and Depression: Risk Factors and Treatment Issues: Final Report of the American Psychological Association's National Task Force on Women and Depression. American Psychological Association, Washington, DC, 1990.
94. Warren, LW, and McEachren, L: Psychosocial correlates of depressive symptomatology in adult women. J Abnormal Psychol 92:151, 1983.
95. Neville, A: The model of human occupation and depressions. Am Occup Ther Assoc Mental Health Special Interest Section Newslett 8(1):1, 1985.
96. Seligman, ME: Helplessness: On Depression, Development and Death. Freeman, San Francisco, 1975.
97. Heinemann, AW: Substance Abuse and Physical Disability. Haworth, New York, 1993.
98. McFarlane, et al: Abuse Assessment Screen–Disability (AAS-D): Measuring frequency, type, and perpetrator of abuse toward women with physical disabilities. J Womens Health Gend Based Med 10:861, 2001.
99. Nosek, MA, et al: National study of women with physical disabilities: Final report. Sex Disabil 19(1):5, 2001.
100. Nosek, MA, et al: Vulnerabilities for abuse among women with disabilities. Sex Disabil 19:177, 2001.
101. Jacobs, K, and Jacobs, L: Quick reference dictionary for occupational therapy. Slack, Thorofare, NJ, 2001.
102. Nosek, MA, and Hughes, RB: Psychosocial issues of women with physical disabilities: The continuing gender debate. RCB 46(4):224, 2003.
103. Rintala, DH, et al: Perceived stress in individuals with spinal cord injury. In Krotoski, DM, Mosek, MA, and Turk, MA (eds): Women with Physical Disabilities: Achieving and Maintaining Health and Well-being. Brookes, Baltimore, 1996, p 223.
104. Rintala, DH, et al: Social support and the well being of persons with spinal cord injury living in the community. Rehabil Psychol 37:155, 1992.
105. Hardy, C, et al: The role of social support in the life stress/injury relationship. Sport Psychologist 5:128, 1991.
106. Kaplan, SP: Psychosocial adjustment three years after traumatic brain injury. Clin Neuropsychol 5:360, 1991.
107. Loy, DP, et al: Dimensions of leisure and depression symptoms after spinal cord injury. Annu Ther Recreat 11:43, 106, 2002.
108. American Physical Therapy Association: Guide to Physical Therapist Practice, ed 2. Phys Ther 81:1, 2001.
109. World Health Organization (WHO): Towards a Common Language for Functioning, Disability and Health ICF. WHO, Geneva, Switzerland, 2002. Retrieved January 1, 2012, from www.who.int/classifications/icf/training/icfbeginnersguide.pdf.

Supplemental Readings

Boersma, K, and Linton, SJ: Screening to identify patients at risk: Profiles of psychological risk factors for early intervention. Clin J Pain 21(1):38, 2005.
Bonder, B: Psychopathology and Function, ed 4. Slack, Thorofare, NJ, 2010.
Brenes, GA, et al: The influence of anxiety on the progression of disability. J Am Geriatr Soc 53(1):34, 2005.
Brown, C, and Stoffel, VC: Occupational Therapy in Mental Health: A Vision for Participation. FA Davis, Philadelphia, 2011.
Drench, ED, et al: Psychosocial Aspects of Health Care. Prentice Hall (Pearson Education, Inc.), Upper Saddle River, NJ, 2003.
Elfstrom, M, et al: Relations between coping strategies and health-related quality of life in patients with spinal cord lesion. J Rehabil Med 37(1):9, 2005.
Falvo, D: Medical and Psychosocial Aspects of Chronic Illness and Disability, ed 3. Jones & Bartlett, Sudbury, MA, 2005.
Hughes, RB, et al: Stress and women with physical disabilities: Identifying correlates. Women Health Issue 15(1):14, 2005.
Kolt, GS, and Anderson, MB (eds): Psychology in the Physical and Manual Therapies. Churchill Livingstone, New York, 2004.
Miller, JF: Coping with Chronic Illness: Overcoming Powerlessness, ed 3. FA Davis, Philadelphia, 2000.

Moldover, JE, et al: Depression after traumatic brain injury: A review of evidence for clinical heterogeneity. Neuropsychol Rev 14(3):143, 2004.

Precin, P (ed): Posttraumatic stress disorder and work. Work: A Journal of Prevention, Assessment and Rehabilitation 38(1), 2011.

Precin, P (ed): Healing 9/11. Haworth Press, Binghamton, NY, 2006.

Precin, P (ed): Surviving 9/11. Haworth Press, Binghamton, NY, 2003.

Precin, P: Client-Centered Reasoning: Narratives of People with Mental Illness. Butterworth-Heinemann, Woburn, MA, 2002.

Precin, P: Living Skills Recovery Workbook. Butterworth-Heinemann, Woburn, MA, 1999.

Rytsala, HJ, et al: Functional and work disability in major depressive disorder. J Nerv Ment Dis Mar 193(3):189, 2005.

Solet, JM: Optimizing personal and social adaptation. In Trombly, CA, and Vining Radomski, M (eds): Occupational Therapy for Physical Dysfunction, ed 5. Lippincott Williams & Wilkins, Baltimore, 2002, p 761.

Yerxa, EJ: The social and psychological experience of having a disability: Implications for occupational therapists. In Pedretti, LW, and Early, MB (eds): Occupational Therapy: Practice Skills for Physical Dysfunction, ed 5. Mosby, St. Louis, 2001, p 470.

Holmes-Rahe Social Readjustment Scale

Rank	Life Event	Mean Value
1	Death of spouse	100
2	Divorce	73
3	Marital separation	65
4	Jail term	63
5	Death of close family member	63
6	Personal injury or illness	53
7	Marriage	50
8	Fired at work	47
9	Marital reconciliation	45
10	Retirement	45
11	Change in health of family member	44
12	Pregnancy	40
13	Sex difficulties	39
14	Gain of new family member	39
15	Business readjustment	39
16	Change in financial state	38
17	Death of close friend	37
18	Change to different line of work	36
19	Change in number of arguments with spouse	35
20	Mortgage over $10,000	31
21	Foreclosure of mortgage or loan	30
22	Change in responsibilities at work	29
23	Son or daughter leaving home	29
24	Trouble with in-laws	29
25	Outstanding personal achievement	28
26	Wife begin or stop work	26
27	Begin or end school	26
28	Change in living conditions	25
29	Revision of personal habits	24
30	Trouble with boss	23
31	Change in work hours or conditions	20
32	Change in residence	20
33	Change in schools	20

Continued

Rank	Life Event	Mean Value
34	Change in recreation	19
35	Change in church activities	19
36	Change in social activities	18
37	Mortgage or loan less than $10,000	17
38	Change in sleeping habits	16
39	Change in number of family get-togethers	15
40	Change in eating habits	15
41	Vacation	13
42	Christmas	12
43	Minor violations of the law	11

From Holmes and Rahe,[58] with permission.

Directions: Hassles are irritants that can range from minor annoyances to fairly major pressures, problems, or difficulties. They can occur few or many times.

Listed on the following pages are a number of ways in which a person can feel hassled. First, circle the hassles that have happened to you *in the past month.* Then look at the numbers on the right of the items you circled. Indicate by circling a 1, 2, or 3 how *severe* each of the *circled* hassles has been for you in the past month. If a hassle did not occur in the last month, do *not* circle it.

		Severity		
Hassles		1. Somewhat Severe	2. Moderately Severe	3. Extremely Severe
(1)	Misplacing or losing things	1	2	3
(2)	Troublesome neighbors	1	2	3
(3)	Social obligations	1	2	3
(4)	Inconsiderate smokers	1	2	3
(5)	Troubling thoughts about your future	1	2	3
(6)	Thoughts about death	1	2	3
(7)	Health of a family member	1	2	3
(8)	Not enough money for clothing	1	2	3
(9)	Not enough money for housing	1	2	3
(10)	Concerns about owing money	1	2	3
(11)	Concerns about getting credit	1	2	3
(12)	Concerns about money for emergencies	1	2	3
(13)	Someone owes you money	1	2	3
(14)	Financial responsibility for someone who does not live with you	1	2	3
(15)	Cutting down on electricity, water, and so forth	1	2	3
(16)	Smoking too much	1	2	3
(17)	Use of alcohol	1	2	3
(18)	Personal use of drugs	1	2	3
(19)	Too many responsibilities	1	2	3
(20)	Decisions about having children	1	2	3
(21)	Non-family members living in your house	1	2	3
(22)	Care for pet	1	2	3
(23)	Planning meals	1	2	3
(24)	Concerned about the meaning of life	1	2	3

Continued

Hassles		Severity		
		1. Somewhat Severe	2. Moderately Severe	3. Extremely Severe
(25)	Trouble relaxing	1	2	3
(26)	Trouble making decisions	1	2	3
(27)	Problems getting along with fellow workers	1	2	3
(28)	Customers or clients give you a hard time	1	2	3
(29)	Home maintenance (inside)	1	2	3
(30)	Concerns about job security	1	2	3
(31)	Concerns about retirement	1	2	3
(32)	Laid-off or out of work	1	2	3
(33)	Do not like current work duties	1	2	3
(34)	Do not like fellow workers	1	2	3
(35)	Not enough money for basic necessities	1	2	3
(36)	Not enough money for food	1	2	3
(37)	Too many interruptions	1	2	3
(38)	Unexpected company	1	2	3
(39)	Too much time on hands	1	2	3
(40)	Having to wait	1	2	3
(41)	Concerns about accidents	1	2	3
(42)	Being lonely	1	2	3
(43)	Not enough money for health care	1	2	3
(44)	Fear of confrontation	1	2	3
(45)	Financial security	1	2	3
(46)	Silly practical mistakes	1	2	3
(47)	Inability to express yourself	1	2	3
(48)	Physical illness	1	2	3
(49)	Side effects of medication	1	2	3
(50)	Concerns about medical treatment	1	2	3
(51)	Physical appearance	1	2	3
(52)	Fear of rejection	1	2	3
(53)	Difficulties with getting pregnant	1	2	3
(54)	Sexual problems that result from physical problems	1	2	3
(55)	Sexual problems other than those resulting from physical problems	1	2	3
(56)	Concerns about health in general	1	2	3
(57)	Not seeing enough people	1	2	3
(58)	Friends or relatives too far away	1	2	3
(59)	Preparing meals	1	2	3
(60)	Wasting time	1	2	3
(61)	Auto maintenance	1	2	3
(62)	Filling out forms	1	2	3

		Severity		
Hassles		**1. Somewhat Severe**	**2. Moderately Severe**	**3. Extremely Severe**
(63)	Neighborhood deterioration	1	2	3
(64)	Financing children's education	1	2	3
(65)	Problems with employees	1	2	3
(66)	Problems on job due to being a woman or man	1	2	3
(67)	Declining physical abilities	1	2	3
(68)	Being exploited	1	2	3
(69)	Concerns about bodily functions	1	2	3
(70)	Rising prices of common goods	1	2	3
(71)	Not getting enough rest	1	2	3
(72)	Not getting enough sleep	1	2	3
(73)	Problems with aging parents	1	2	3
(74)	Problems with your children	1	2	3
(75)	Problems with persons younger than yourself	1	2	3
(76)	Problems with your lover	1	2	3
(77)	Difficulties seeing or hearing	1	2	3
(78)	Overloaded with family responsibilities	1	2	3
(79)	Too many things to do	1	2	3
(80)	Unchallenging work	1	2	3
(81)	Concerns about meeting high standards	1	2	3
(82)	Financial dealings with friends or acquaintances	1	2	3
(83)	Job dissatisfactions	1	2	3
(84)	Worries about decisions to change jobs	1	2	3
(85)	Trouble with reading, writing, or spelling abilities	1	2	3
(86)	Too many meetings	1	2	3
(87)	Problems with divorce or separation	1	2	3
(88)	Trouble with arithmetic skills	1	2	3
(89)	Gossip	1	2	3
(90)	Legal problems	1	2	3
(91)	Concerns about weight	1	2	3
(92)	Not enough time to do the things you need to do	1	2	3
(93)	Television	1	2	3
(94)	Not enough personal energy	1	2	3
(95)	Concerns about inner conflicts	1	2	3
(96)	Feel conflicted over what to do	1	2	3
(97)	Regrets over past decisions	1	2	3
(98)	Menstrual (period) problems	1	2	3
(99)	The weather	1	2	3
(100)	Nightmares	1	2	3

Continued

Hassles		Severity		
		1. Somewhat Severe	2. Moderately Severe	3. Extremely Severe
(101)	Concerns about getting ahead	1	2	3
(102)	Hassles from boss or supervisor	1	2	3
(103)	Difficulties with friends	1	2	3
(104)	Not enough time for family	1	2	3
(105)	Transportation problems	1	2	3
(106)	Not enough money for transportation	1	2	3
(107)	Not enough money for entertainment and recreation	1	2	3
(108)	Shopping	1	2	3
(109)	Prejudice and discrimination from others	1	2	3
(110)	Property, investments, or taxes	1	2	3
(111)	Not enough time for entertainment and recreation	1	2	3
(112)	Yard work or outside home maintenance	1	2	3
(113)	Concerns about news events	1	2	3
(114)	Noise	1	2	3
(115)	Crime	1	2	3
(116)	Traffic	1	2	3
(117)	Pollution			
	HAVE WE MISSED ANY OF YOUR HASSLES? IF SO, WRITE THEM IN BELOW.			
(118)	_____			
	ONE MORE THING: HAS THERE BEEN A CHANGE IN YOUR LIFE THAT AFFECTED HOW YOU ANSWERED THIS SCALE? IF SO, TELL US WHAT IT WAS.			

From Kanner et al,[59] with permission.

Web-Based Resources for Patients, Families, and Caregivers

Improving Community Accessibility

Independent Living Centers:
www.senioroutlook.com
Searches over 40,000 apartment communities for people with disabilities. Includes virtual tours, searches by distance, photographs, and floor plans. Contains information on insurance, storage, home mortgages, moving, types of housing facilities, and a glossary of housing terms. Updated weekly.
Links to Centers for Independent Living:
www.abledata.com
Includes information on and links to periodicals and research on disability, assistive technology, and lists of health care professionals.
The Design Link:
www.designlinc.com/centers3.htm
Provides product information and design tips for families, consumers, and therapists designing for people with disabilities.

Depression Resources

*Web*MD Depression Guide:
www.webmd.com/depression/guide/depression_support_resources
All About Depression:
www.allaboutdepression.com
Internet Mental Health:
www.mentalhealth.com/p71.html

Substance Abuse Resources

National Institutes of Health, National Institute on Drug Abuse, Science of Drug Abuse Addiction:
www.nida.nih.gov/nidahome.html
The Substance Abuse and Mental Health Services Administration:
www.samhsa.gov
National Substance Abuse Index—Directory of Substance Abuse Resources:
www.nationalsubstanceabuseindex.org

Anxiety Resources

HealthCentralAnxietyConnection.com:
www.healthcentral.com/anxiety/websites.html
MedlinePlus—Anxiety:
www.nlm.nih.gov/medlineplus/anxiety.html

Post-Traumatic Stress Disorder (PTSD) Resources

2010 Best Posttraumatic Stress Disorder Resources for Trauma Survivors:
http://thirdofalifetime.wordpress.com/2010-best-ptsd-resources-for-trauma-survivors-pt-1
Department of Defense—Resources for Military Vets with Posttraumatic Stress Disorder:
United States Department of Veterans Affairs
Veterans and Military—Web Resource Links:
www.ptsd.va.gov/public/web-resources/web-military-resources.asp
National Center for Posttraumatic Stress Disorder:
www.ptsd.va.gov/

Chapter 27

Cognitive and Perceptual Dysfunction

Carolyn A. Unsworth, OTR, PhD

LEARNING OBJECTIVES

1. Identify the signs of cognitive and perceptual deficits.
2. Describe how cognitive and perceptual deficits affect a patient's ability to participate in rehabilitation.
3. Explain how a patient can be assisted to compensate for body scheme and/or body image disorders.
4. Describe how spatial relations impairments can affect the patient's ability to follow directions.
5. Compare and contrast the effect of the various agnosias on the patient's ability to recognize stimuli in the environment.
6. Differentiate between ideomotor and ideational apraxia. Describe how a patient with apraxia might behave in response to different instructional sets commonly employed in rehabilitation.
7. Identify how the psychological and emotional status of a patient with cognitive and perceptual deficits may affect participation in rehabilitation.
8. Analyze and interpret patient data, formulate realistic anticipated goals and expected outcomes, and identify appropriate interventions when presented with a clinical case study.

CHAPTER OUTLINE

Cognitive and perceptual deficits are among the chief causes of poor rehabilitation progress for patients who have sustained brain damage, even among those whose motor skills have returned. Cognitive and perceptual deficits are some of the most puzzling and disabling difficulties that a person can experience. Thinking, remembering, reasoning, and making sense of the world around us is fundamental to carrying out daily living activities. When individuals experience problems with these capacities, it can have a devastating effect on their lives and the lives of their family. These people may not be able to live alone, fulfill the responsibilities of paid employment, or sustain a family life and relationships.[1] Thus, effective treatment of many patients with brain damage depends on understanding perception and cognition.

The brain may be damaged through several mechanisms, including infections, such as encephalitis; anoxia, as may occur following near-drowning, cardiopulmonary arrest, or carbon monoxide poisoning; tumors that are benign or malignant; trauma resulting from motor vehicle accidents, falls, or violent incidents (e.g., traumatic sports-related injury, gunshot wound); toxins such as alcohol or substance abuse; and vascular disease, which may produce an infarct or hemorrhagic stroke. The largest two groups of people who acquire cognitive and perceptual impairments following brain damage are persons who experienced stroke and traumatic brain injury (TBI).[1] The physical rehabilitation of these patient groups is addressed in Chapter 15, Stroke, and Chapter 19, Traumatic Brain Injury.

The patient who has sustained an initial cerebral vascular accident (CVA) is thought to have focal or localized damage to discrete areas of the brain, often resulting in discrete cognitive or perceptual deficits. In contrast, patients who have sustained a TBI are presumed to have generalized brain damage resulting in cognitive impairment with generalized deficits in attention, memory, learning, and so forth, rather than specific difficulties in discrete cognitive or perceptual functions. However, elements of both perceptual and cognitive dysfunction may occur in brain damage owing to either CVA or trauma. The distinctions between the two groups of patients become particularly blurred when one considers the patient who has suffered multiple strokes; this patient may in fact present with combined elements of both focal and generalized brain damage. Throughout this chapter, the patient with hemiplegia in whom brain damage has occurred as a result of a stroke will be the focus. The overriding goal of this chapter is to introduce the reader to concepts relating to cognitive and perceptual dysfunction following brain damage.

An important focus for the physical therapist should be an understanding of how a particular cognitive or perceptual impairment might be manifested clinically, and how examination and treatment of movement disorders might be adjusted to capitalize on the abilities and minimize the cognitive or perceptual limitations of the patient. Deficits in the cognitive or perceptual domain must be considered to accurately determine the patient's true residual abilities. Using sets of directions that would confuse a patient with apraxia during a specific examination procedure may paint a picture of a greater or different motor disability than that which actually exists. Often the first clue to a cognitive or perceptual problem appears during initial sensorimotor testing. Awareness of the possibility and nature of cognitive or perceptual deficits will signal the therapist to redirect the method of testing, particularly the instructional sets and cues.

■ COGNITION AND PERCEPTION

The perceptual–motor process is a chain of events through which the individual selects, integrates, and interprets stimuli from the body and the surrounding environment. Cognition can be conceived of as the method used by the central nervous system (CNS) to process information. Cognitive processes include knowing, understanding, awareness, judgment, and decision making.[2] The difficulty of separating perceptual and cognitive deficits is readily apparent, both in patient behavior and in contradictory conceptualizations of these two domains of function. In a review of the literature, Katz[3] found that to some authors, *cognition* is conceived of as a general term that includes perception, attention, thinking, and memory; to other authors, *perception* is an umbrella term that encompasses both cognition and visual perception as subcomponents. At this time, there is insufficient evidence to suggest which approach most

accurately reflects the way we think about and perceive information. What is clear is that normally functioning perceptual and cognitive systems are a necessary key to successful interaction with the environment. Because the majority of work in this field does distinguish between cognition and perception[1] and because it is probably easier to learn about these processes individually, they are defined and addressed separately in this chapter.

Cognitive and perceptual capacities are clearly prerequisites for learning,[4] and rehabilitation is largely a learning process.[2] Thus, it is not surprising that patients with cognitive and perceptual disorders are limited in their ability to learn self-care and activities of daily living (ADL) skills; hence, as a group, they are more limited in their potential for achieving independence.[5] In any rehabilitation program geared toward achievement of maximum independence, there is a compelling need for therapists to learn to recognize behavior related to perceptual deficits. The therapist's modification of examination and treatment approaches in light of these deficits will ensure that patients receive the full benefit of these services.

Cognition and Higher-Order Cognition

Cognition is the act or process of knowing, including awareness, reasoning, judgment, intuition, and memory. **Executive functions** are sometimes included under this heading as well. Executive functions include the capacity to plan, manipulate information, initiate and terminate activities, recognize errors, problem solve, and think abstractly. Commonly, executive functions are categorized as *higher-order cognitive functions*[6] or *metacognitive functions*.[7,8]

Perception

Lezak[4] defines **perception** as the integration of sensory impressions into information that is psychologically meaningful. Thus, perception is the ability to select those stimuli that require attention and action, to integrate those stimuli with each other and with prior information, and finally to interpret them. The resulting awareness of objects and experiences within the environment enables the individual to make sense out of a complex and constantly changing internal and external sensory environment.[9]

The terms *perception* and **sensation** are often confused with each other. Sensation may be defined as the appreciation (awareness) of stimuli through the organs of special sense (e.g., eyes, ears, nose, and so forth), the peripheral cutaneous sensory system (e.g., temperature, taste, touch, and so forth), or internal receptors (e.g., deep receptors in muscles and joints).[9] Perception cannot be viewed as independent of sensation. However, the quality of perception is far more complex than the recognition of the individual sensation.[9] Perceptual deficits do not lie in the sensory ability itself, but rather with the individual's ability to interpret the sensation accurately, and therefore respond appropriately.[1]

RESPONSIBILITIES OF THE PHYSICAL THERAPIST AND THE OCCUPATIONAL THERAPIST

Occupational therapists are the members of the rehabilitation team who are specially trained to examine and treat cognitive and perceptual deficits in relation to functional adaptation. They are responsible for the selection and administration of an appropriate constellation of tests and measures, accurate interpretation of results, and formulation of an overall plan of care (POC) for cognitive and perceptual rehabilitation. If appropriate, the occupational therapist may refer a patient to a neuropsychologist for specific intellectual testing.

In the hospital setting, the physical therapist is often the first member of the rehabilitation team to see a patient with brain injury. The physical therapist must understand the nature of cognitive and perceptual dysfunction and recognize that individuals in certain diagnostic categories, such as those with stroke or TBI, are likely to behave in ways that indicate the presence of particular cognitive or perceptual deficits.[10] When this occurs, the physical therapist should refer the patient to occupational therapy for evaluation and treatment.

The tests and measures described in this chapter are included to assist the reader in understanding the nature of the different cognitive and perceptual disabilities and to guide decision making about referral to another practitioner. They are not a substitute for an intensive evaluation by a trained occupational therapist when referral is deemed necessary.

An understanding of cognitive and perceptual dysfunction may go a long way toward alleviating much of the potential frustration that often accompanies treatment of a patient with brain damage, most of which is the result of inappropriate expectations on the part of team members, the patient, and the family. By collaborating with the occupational therapist, other members of the rehabilitation team, and the family, consistent treatment strategies may be developed and carried out, with obvious benefits to the patient.

CLINICAL INDICATORS

Cognitive and perceptual deficits ought to be ruled out as a cause of diminished functioning in all patients who have experienced brain damage. Such problems are particularly likely culprits in cases in which the patient seems unable to participate fully in self-care tasks and has difficulty participating in physical therapy for reasons that cannot be accounted for by lack of motor ability, sensation, comprehension, or motivation. Cognitive and perceptual dysfunction resulting from acquired brain damage must be differentiated from premorbid cognitive perceptual deficits (from previous trauma, illness, congenital abnormality, or dementing process) and from the general confusion and emotional sequelae that often accompany stroke and brain injury.[4]

Often, patients with cognitive and perceptual difficulties may display the following characteristics: inability to do simple tasks independently or safely, difficulty in initiating or completing a task, difficulty in switching from one task to the next, and a diminished capacity to locate visually or to identify objects that seem obviously necessary for task completion. In addition, they may be unable to follow simple one-step commands, despite apparently good comprehension. They may make the same mistakes over and over. Activities may take an inordinately long time to complete, or they may be done impulsively. Patients may hesitate many times, appear distracted and frustrated, and exhibit poor planning. They are frequently inattentive to one side of the body and extrapersonal space, and may deny the presence or extent of their disability. These characteristics, all or some of which may be present, often make participation in daily living activities and therapy seem an insurmountable problem. These clinical features are explained and expanded on throughout this chapter.

Two typical scenarios are presented to give the reader an idea of when to suspect perceptual dysfunction. The first case involves a patient with a right hemisphere stroke who presents clinically with a left hemiparesis and good speech. Upon observation in the nursing unit, the patient appears to have functional strength in the unaffected right extremities and fair return on the affected left side. Yet the patient seems to have difficulty with simple range of motion (ROM) activities, even in the intact extremities, appearing confused and unable to move the arm up or down on command. The patient cannot seem to follow instructions for walking with a quad cane, constantly confuses the proper step sequence, and is unable to maneuver a wheelchair around the corner without crashing into the wall.

This patient should not be dismissed as uncooperative, intellectually inferior, or confused. In this instance, the patient is likely experiencing difficulty in spatial relations, right–left discrimination, and vertical disorientation, or perhaps left-sided unilateral neglect. Further observation and examination should reveal the precise cause of the difficulties.

The second case involves a patient with left hemisphere damage and a resulting right hemiparesis and mild **aphasia**. The patient can respond reliably to "yes/no" questions and is able to follow simple one-step commands such as, "Put the pencil on the table," or "Give me the cup." However, if asked to point to the arm, or asked to imitate the therapist's movements during an active ROM test even with the unaffected limbs, the patient does not respond and appears totally uncooperative. During therapy, the same patient is on a mat table. The therapist explains and then demonstrates the proper techniques for rolling to one side. The patient does not move. However, a moment later when his wife arrives, the patient quickly initiates rolling in an attempt to sit up to greet his wife. The astute therapist will realize that this patient may not be confused, stubborn, or uncooperative, as indeed he may appear. Rather, he may be suffering from a lack of awareness of body structure and relationship of body parts (somatagnosia), as evidenced by the ROM test incident, and an inability to perform a task on command or to imitate gestures (**ideomotor apraxia**), as demonstrated in the rolling episode.

■ HOSPITALIZATION FOLLOWING BRAIN DAMAGE

The brain that has been damaged functions as a whole, just as it does in individuals without brain damage. When one part is damaged, the behavior observed is not merely the result of the brain operating precisely as in the intact individual minus the function of the area that was subject to anoxia. Rather, it is an outward manifestation of the reorganization of the entire CNS, at multiple levels, working to compensate for the loss.[11]

Because of the brain damage, the patient must cope with a nervous system operating without normal sensory input at all levels, both cortical and subcortical.[11] Normal responses to environmental stimuli are difficult to obtain when the input on which they have to act is deranged or incomplete. Recovery of function can be attributed to structural reorganization of the CNS into a new dynamic system widely dispersed within the cerebral cortex and lower segments.[12,13]

A significant contributor to the clinical picture of a patient after a CVA is the response to hospitalization. From a cognitive and perceptual perspective, when a patient is hospitalized (with or without brain damage), the inputs imposed on that patient's nervous system are radically different from the ones normally received. On the one hand, the environment is sensorially impoverished. There is no variation in temperature and lighting, and familiar background noises (e.g., telephones, airplanes, dogs, buses, and so forth) are missing. On the other hand, an enormous array of unfamiliar noise is present: nurses talking, loudspeakers, and the whir of machines. Strange and different smells, and unfamiliar, unavoidable, and unpleasant sights abound. Often, because of motor impairment, the patient cannot move around to seek or to escape inputs; therefore, a multiplicity of sensory inputs bombards the nervous system. Even if orienting responses are preserved, there is a profound sense of loss of control. This sensory derangement compounds the problems faced by the patient with brain damage, because those very abilities that enable the individual to select, filter out, and integrate incoming sensations to organize the self for appropriate action often fail in this sensorially bizarre environment.

To gain insight into the experience of the patient under such circumstances, it is enlightening to browse through the biographical and autographical reports of some noted neurologists and neuropsychologists, themselves victims or relatives of victims of CVAs. Particularly instructive are the reports of Bach-y-Rita,[14] Brodal,[15] and Gardner.[16]

■ THEORETICAL FRAMEWORKS

The theoretical bases of five approaches to therapy are examined in this section together with the examination procedures and treatment approaches consistent with the theoretical model. It is important to note that treatment approaches are not mutually exclusive. Many therapists use a combination of approaches, guiding selection by their clinical expertise and the patient's response to the interventions. Specific applications of these approaches will be presented following the description of individual cognitive and perceptual deficits in the final section of this chapter. Further information on a variety of theoretical approaches used by occupational therapists when working with patients who have cognitive and perceptual problems can be found in Averbuch and Katz[17] and Unsworth.[1]

The Retraining Approach

Averbuch and Katz[17] described this approach, which focuses on the remediation of underlying skills the patient has lost. Sometimes this approach is referred to as the *transfer-of-training approach*. The approach is based on the assumption that a disruption in one brain region can have a negative impact on brain functioning as a whole. An underlying assumption is that skills learned for one task can generalize to others. In other words, transfer-of-training is assumed. The premise is that practice in one task with particular cognitive or perceptual requirements will enhance performance in other tasks with similar perceptual demands.[1,18,19] Thus, doing specifically selected perceptual exercises, such as pegboard (a board with a regular pattern of small holes for pegs) activities, or parquetry blocks (inlaid blocks of different woods arranged in a geometric pattern) and puzzles, will result in improving the perceptual skills required to perform those functional tasks. For example, Young et al[20] demonstrated that training patients with left hemiplegia in block design (constructing shapes using blocks to match a two-dimensional pattern), in addition to *visual scanning* (using the eyes to follow a target) and *visual cancellation tasks* (placing a line through a specific number, letter, or word embedded randomly among other numbers, letters, or words), resulted in improvements in reading and writing, although no specific training in these areas was offered. Because all tasks require the use of multiple perceptual skills, it is difficult to ascertain precisely which perceptual skills are being trained during any one session.[21]

To date, research has not unequivocally demonstrated a generalization from perceptual–motor training to functional skills.[18,21] Neistadt[19] suggests that the patient's capacity to learn must be evaluated and that learning capacity is the key to a patient's ability to generalize material learned in one situation to others.

If transfer-of-training does occur, then strategies to enhance this can be incorporated into other components of the treatment program such as those aimed at maintaining sitting or standing balance, weight-bearing exercises, or functional use of the more involved extremities.

The Sensory Integrative Approach

Ayres developed the theory of **sensory integration (SI)** in an effort to explain the relationship between neural functioning and the behavior of children with sensorimotor or learning problems.[22] The theory, strongly influenced by the neurobehavioral literature, describes normal sensory integrative development and functioning, defines patterns of sensory integrative dysfunction, and suggests treatment techniques.[22] *Sensory integration* can be defined as the organization of sensation for use.[23,24]

Integration of basic sensorimotor functions (tactile, proprioceptive, and vestibular) proceeds in a developmental sequence in the normal child within the context of goal-directed, meaningful activity. It is assumed that the production of an adaptive response (desired motor response) facilitates sensory integration, which in turn enhances the ability to produce higher-level adaptive behaviors. Sensory integration is thought to occur at all levels of the nervous system.

The underlying assumption for treatment is that, by offering opportunities for controlled sensory input, the therapist can promote normal CNS processing of sensory information and thus elicit specific desired motor responses.[25] The performance of these adaptive responses, in turn, influences the way in which the brain organizes and processes sensation, thus enhancing the ability to learn.

Some of the treatment modalities employed include rubbing or icing to provide sensory input, resistance and weight-bearing to impart proprioceptive input, and the use of spinning or rocking to provide vestibular input. Following the controlled sensory input, an adaptive motor response is required by the patient to integrate the sensations provided by the therapist. In young children, the use of compensatory or **splinter skills** (skills acquired in a manner inconsistent with, or incapable of being integrated with, those already present) is avoided in favor of remediating underlying deficits. For more detailed information the reader is referred to the work of Ayres.[23,24]

Zoltan[2] argues that elderly patients, who comprise the majority of the stroke population, experience sensory integrative dysfunction similar to that of children with learning disabilities because of age-related physiological changes together with environmentally induced sensory deprivation. The limitations in mobility caused by a stroke further prevent the patient from receiving and thus processing adequate sensory input.

The application of this theory to the adult post-stroke population, however, is open to serious debate. Bundy et al[22] argue that the theory explains mild to moderate learning and behavioral problems resulting from a central deficit in processing sensations but are not specifically associated with frank brain damage. Further, there are a number of problems with the application of this approach to adult populations, even if it is theoretically tenable.

The treatment process is ordinarily quite lengthy. In addition, specific tests and measures and treatment approaches have been developed for and standardized on children, who presumably have sufficiently plastic nervous systems to be influenced by this form of therapy. The neurophysiological literature is replete with examples of skills that children can gain using this approach that would not be possible with mature individuals with similar lesions.[26-28] Furthermore, a mature adult with diffuse cerebral damage may have other complicating medical concerns and deficits in mobility that actually contraindicate the use of the equipment that is essential to the treatment process.[22] It is likely that many of the treatment regimens described as sensory integration are best described as a *sensorimotor approach*, which utilizes handling or directed sensory stimulation to elicit a specific motor response.[22]

The Neurofunctional Approach

The *neurofunctional approach* was first described by Giles and Wilson in 1992[29] and is based on learning theory. In contrast to the retraining approach, which assumes that transfer-of-training can occur, the authors of the neurofunctional approach assume that patients with acquired brain injury must practice every activity in its true context in order to recover function. Hence, the focus of this approach is on retraining real-world skills rather than on retraining specific cognitive and perceptual processes.[30] Giles[30] argues that remediation approaches (which include the idea of transfer-of-training) are largely unproven, and thus may result in little functional improvement for the patient. He also suggests that compensatory skills or techniques are taught to a patient without considering if the gains made in terms of quality of life justify the considerable effort required.

The Rehabilitative/Compensatory (Functional) Approach

Probably the most widely used approach in treating perceptual deficits is the *rehabilitative/compensatory approach*[31-33] (also referred to as the *functional approach*), which offers a great deal of practical support for the physical therapist. The basic assumptions underlying this approach are that adults with brain trauma will have difficulty generalizing and learning from dissimilar tasks.[34] Direct repetitive practice of specific functional skills that are impaired is an efficient means of enhancing the patient's independence in those specific tasks. More recently, Fisher[35] extended the work of Trombly[31] by

(1) articulating more explicitly assumptions made about people within the rehabilitative/compensatory model; (2) generalizing this model beyond persons with physical disabilities to those with developmental, cognitive, or psychosocial disabilities; and (3) adding collaborative consultation to education and adaptation as strategies used to effect change.

The proponents of this approach favor addressing the functional problem over and above the treatment of its underlying cause when working with an adult post-stroke population. For example, a patient with difficulty in depth and distance perception, who is therefore unable to navigate a flight of stairs, would be made aware of the deficit, would be provided with external cues to compensate for the perceptual disorder, and would repetitively practice adapted techniques for safe stair climbing. The more closely the therapeutic practice situation resembles the home situation in terms of stair depth and height, amount of traffic, lighting, and so forth, the less generalizing is required and the more success the patient is likely to have when he or she returns home. However, problems might still be displayed in depth and distance perception in other areas of daily function.

In this functional approach, therapy is viewed as learning that takes into consideration the unique strengths and limitations of the individual patient. It is composed of two complementary components: compensation and adaptation.[1] *Compensation* refers to the changes that need to be made in the patient's approach to tasks. *Adaptation* refers to the alterations that need to be made in the human/social and physical environment in order to facilitate relearning of skills. In relation to the human/social environment, the therapist is concerned with altering the actions of others' functioning in the environment to enhance the patient's performance.

To compensate for the disability, the patient first has to be made aware of deficiencies (*cognitive awareness*) and must then be taught how to circumvent them using intact sensations and perceptual skills. The patient should be instructed in specific techniques and assisted in developing successful functional habits. The patient will need to be taught to attend to cues from the environment to enhance skill performance. The therapist helps the patient identify and then call on these new cues. For example, if the patient has a visual field cut, the therapist should explain that because of a visual problem, the patient is seeing only one half of the environment. The patient should then be shown how to turn the head to compensate for the deficit. Environmental scanning (moving head, and therefore eyes, from side-to-side to view surroundings) could be incorporated into general therapy sessions as well.

General suggestions when teaching compensatory techniques include the following: (1) use simple directions; (2) establish and carry out a routine; (3) do each activity in a consistent manner; and (4) employ repetition as much as necessary.

Adaptation refers to the alteration not of the patient's strategy, but of the environment. For example, if the patient cannot differentiate between right and left, or tends to neglect the left side of the body, a piece of red tape on the left shoe during gait training will allow the patient to attend more easily to the left side and thus to follow the therapist's instructions more accurately. The therapist can use this functional approach to assist patients in improving specific motor skills related to treatment goals.

There are several inherent benefits to the rehabilitation/compensatory (functional) approach. First, in the current managed care environment there is a limited amount of time for inpatient rehabilitation.[36] Therefore, therapists need to concentrate on outcome-directed, real-life functional activities because independent performance of these activities at home is the ultimate goal of therapeutic intervention. Interventions directed toward specific functional outcomes are typically reimbursable.[31] In addition, the activities are age appropriate, specific, and clearly relevant to the patient's concerns. For this reason, they tend to be the most motivating. The tasks can also be incorporated into a daily hospital routine. Dressing can be reinforced at bedside by the nursing staff, and eating skills can be reinforced at each mealtime.

The major limitation of this approach is that the methods learned in one task are not typically generalized to the performance of another task. The functional approach has been criticized as the teaching of splinter skills, in which the causes of the dysfunction are not addressed.

Cognitive Rehabilitation and the Quadraphonic Approach

Cognitive rehabilitation focuses on training individuals with brain injury to structure and organize information.[37] It addresses memory, high language disorders, and perceptual dysfunction under one umbrella.[38] Information processing, problem solving, awareness, judgment, and decision making are among the areas included. The therapist using a cognitive remediation approach might be concerned with the patient's perceptual style, including perceptual strategy, response to different types of cues, and rate and consistency of task performance.[39] Diller and Gordon[40] provide a review of the literature pertaining to intervention strategies for cognitive deficits.

Research has demonstrated that even in a non–brain-injured population, skills learned in one task do not automatically transfer to other tasks.[41] Hence, cognitive strategies can be used to facilitate the carryover of skills learned in therapy to functional activities. In her multicontext treatment approach to cognition, Toglia[41] proposes that learning can be conceptualized as a dynamic interplay between characteristics of the patient, characteristics of the task, and the environment in which it is performed. This has also been termed a *dynamic interactional approach*.[42] Characteristics of the individual patient that might affect learning include information processing strategies, metacognition (including awareness of one's own performance), and prior experience, attitudes, and emotions. Task-related variables that are proposed to affect learning include the nature of the task itself (familiarity with the task, spatial arrangements, instruction set, and movement and postural requirements), and the criteria that are used to determine the learner's abilities. Environmental variables include the social and cultural environment in which treatment occurs, as well as the physical context.

The *cognitive rehabilitation approach* to treatment proposes a number of strategies relevant to physical therapist practice. These treatment strategies include the following[41]:

- Analyzing the characteristics of the task to establish criteria to determine if transfer of learning in fact took place.
- Providing interventions to increase patient awareness of abilities, the level of difficulty of the task, and promote self-examination of performance.
- Relating new information or skills to previously learned ones.
- Using multiple environments in which to carry out the training activity to enhance transfer of learning.

Although these treatment strategies are well known within the field of cognitive–perceptual rehabilitation, the efficacy of the techniques remains to be established with the post-stroke population. For a comprehensive understanding and practical guidelines to the evaluation and treatment of patients with cognitive impairments

from a dynamic perspective, the reader is referred to Toglia[42] and Abreu.[43]

Abreu[44] has further developed these treatment strategies as the *quadraphonic approach*. The quadraphonic approach is an interactive rehabilitation approach that provides a holistic perspective for the management of stroke, TBI, brain tumors, cerebral palsy (CP), and other neurological conditions. The quadraphonic approach is based around the idea that the therapist can apply both micro (reductionistic) and a macro (holistic) perspectives for evaluation and treatment, which is an assumption shared by many occupational therapists who work in this field. Diagrammatic presentations of the components of the four key areas of the micro and four key areas of the macro perspectives (hence the term *quadraphonic*) are provided in Figures 27.1 and 27.2, and explained in the text. The *macro* perspective is holistic or humanistic and provides guidelines for the management of functional performance and real-life occupations. In other words, this component of the quadraphonic approach is functional or top-down in focus. When viewing Figure 27.1, the reader can see that the outer square is composed of four characteristics of a client (*lifestyle, lifestage, health*, and *disadvantage status*) that the therapist can explore though interviews and asking the clients to tell their stories. The therapist can then use this information in order to explain and predict the client's behavior and performance. An evaluation then needs to be made of the client's will (volition) and goals, opportunity, and capacity for action as depicted in the triangle. From there the therapist is able to develop a therapy plan with the client (and significant others such as family) that is unique to that client.

In contrast, the *micro* perspective is more remedial in focus and provides guidelines for the management of

The Quadraphonic Approach

Macro perspective

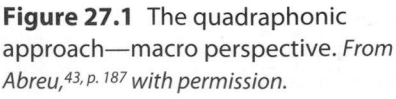

Figure 27.1 The quadraphonic approach—macro perspective. *From Abreu,[43, p. 187] with permission.*

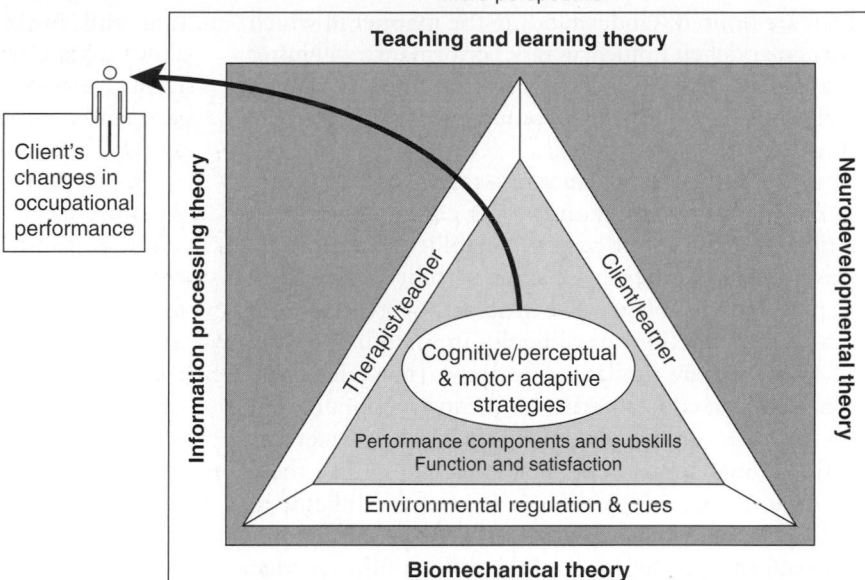

Figure 27.2 The quadraphonic approach—micro perspective. *From Abreu,*[43, p. 185] *with permission.*

performance components or sub-skills that include attention, visual perception, memory, motor planning, postural control, and problem solving. Evaluation and treatment of these performance components is based on a frame of reference that incorporates four theories: (1) information processing; (2) teaching/learning; (3) neurodevelopmental; and (4) biomechanical. These theories are listed in the outer square of Figure 27.2. This figure then presents an inner triangle that depicts how changes in the client's condition are further influenced by three dominant factors, which are the therapist (teacher), the environment in which therapy takes place, and what the client brings to therapy as well. The therapist and client work together to develop cognitive, perceptual, and motor strategies to enhance the client's performance and improve life satisfaction (as shown in the central circle of Fig. 27.1). Hence, the micro perspective is bottom-up or remedial in its focus. An example of a therapist using this approach when working with a patient who has memory and learning problems may be found in Abreu.[43]

■ EXAMINATION OF COGNITIVE AND PERCEPTUAL DEFICITS

The use of systematic data collection provides the scientific basis for guiding intervention. Its importance cannot be overemphasized with respect to all facets of therapeutic intervention, including remediation of cognitive and perceptual dysfunction. **Task analysis** is the breakdown of an activity or task into its component parts together with a delineation of the specific motor, perceptual, and cognitive abilities necessary to perform each component. Task analysis is another tool critical to appropriate therapeutic intervention. For example, the

strength, ROM, and balance abilities necessary to accomplish bed mobility and ambulation activities can be clearly defined by the physical therapist. However, the specific perceptual and cognitive requirements of each step needed to perform these two tasks may not be known. Without knowledge of the perceptual and cognitive requirements for successful completion of a task, the therapist cannot simplify the task for the patient and progressively upgrade it.

Purpose of the Examination

The presence of cognitive and perceptual dysfunction must be confirmed if it is suspected to be interfering with the patient's ability to carry out functional activities.[1] Perceptual performance is positively correlated with ability to perform ADL; however, it is often difficult to correlate specific perceptual deficits gleaned from testing with specific elements of functional ability and loss.[1,45] Thus, formal testing is indicated when there is a functional loss unexplained by motor or sensory impairments, or deficient comprehension. It should be noted that not all areas of functional loss are typically detected within the hospital setting. It is not uncommon for the patient to perform adequately in self-care skills after therapy in the hospital but to fail on the same tasks in other environmental contexts, such as the home. Higher-level tasks, such as driving, banking, or planning a meal, may only emerge as areas of difficulty once the patient is discharged home. When appropriate, the patient's competence in these areas should be considered within the context of an examination of instrumental activities of daily living (IADL) with the occupational therapist while the patient is still hospitalized.

The purpose of patient examination is to determine which cognitive and perceptual abilities are intact and which are limited. Understanding the manner in which a particular deficit influences task performance will foster the application of a therapeutic strategy in which intact capabilities may be used to compensate for or to overcome deficits.[1]

Failure in the performance of a task may result from any number of processes underlying cognition and perception. For example, a patient's inability to complete a jigsaw puzzle may result from an inability to organize the pieces or problem solve where they go (disorder of executive function) or difficulty in attending to one half of the picture (unilateral neglect). The patient may be incapable of concentrating on the instructions (attention deficit), unable to know what the pieces are for (ideational apraxia), or unable to manipulate them (ideomotor apraxia). Although it is often difficult to implicate reliably one or another of these problem areas, the therapist must be aware of the different deficits that may produce similar patterns of behavior.[1,5]

A fascinating study conducted by Galski et al[46] concerning the prediction of driving ability following brain injury (including stroke) in 35 patients underscores the critical nature of carefully selected perceptual and cognitive tests. In this study, 64% of actual behind-the-wheel driving performances were predicted by performance on a selected battery of neuropsychological tests that measured visual perception. Examination of individual test results uncovered the reasons for unsafe driving (such as problems with visual perception, visuomotor coordination, and visuoconstructive abilities), enabling instructors to focus on remediating these specific deficits in preparation for safe driving.

Patient examination is not an end in itself. Careful examination paves the way for realistic and cost-effective intervention.[47] Continuous monitoring of the patient's cognitive and perceptual status will ensure the use of appropriate treatment strategies and their modification when necessary.

Factors Influencing Patient Examination

Psychological and emotional status plays an important role in the patient's ability to cope with disability and with the testing situation. The therapist needs to be aware of behaviors that reflect a patient's psychological response to illness rather than particular cognitive or perceptual abilities. Psychological adjustment to disability depends on many factors, including age, vocational status, education, economic situation, attitude toward the reactions of others, family support, and feelings of competence before the onset of disease (see Chapter 26, Psychosocial Disorders).[45,48,49]

When examining psychological and emotional status the following should be noted: whether the patient is confused; the level of comprehension for verbal instructions (written and spoken); whether communication is enhanced through the use of visual cues and demonstration; the ability to recognize errors; the level of cooperation and initiative (whether the patient is realistic about capabilities and goals); and emotional stability.[50] Disturbances of emotional response are evidenced by rapid and frequent mood changes and low frustration tolerance. Difficult tasks may cause a catastrophic reaction.[45]

The patient's ability to detect relevant cues from the environment or to discriminate between relevant and irrelevant stimuli (necessary for cognitive and perceptual competence) may be adversely influenced by poor judgment, fatigue, and prior expectations. Poor judgment is a major contributor to accidents in patients with hemiplegia. This is related in part to the diminished awareness by these patients as to their altered capabilities. The ambiguity of having one set of functional limbs and one set that is not functional may lead the patient to rely on solutions to the problems of daily living that are familiar but now inappropriate.[45]

Anxiety over capabilities may inhibit optimal performance during examination and treatment. The patient's capacity to perform optimally on testing and to learn is enhanced if anxiety can be reduced.[45] Motivation is influenced by many factors, among them premorbid personality. It is of utmost importance for the therapist to structure the therapeutic environment so that the patient will be positively motivated to learn to his or her maximum ability.[45] To this end, therapeutic tasks should be structured to ensure success, thereby diminishing frustration.

Other factors that may limit a patient's performance on cognitive and perceptual tests include reduced receptive and expressive communication skills, depression, and fatigue. Before a formal examination, the therapist should consider the patient's language skills, and confirm these observations with the speech-language pathologist. The therapist should also be aware of any medications the patient is taking and how these may affect performance. For example, many medications produce drowsiness as a side effect that would affect patient performance during testing.[1] Following stroke, 30% to 50%[12] of people are said to experience depression, the symptoms of which can easily be mistaken for cognitive or perceptual problems. Finally, a determination should be made of the patient's level of fatigue before any examination procedure.

The patient's behavior should not be misinterpreted because of a cultural bias, such as a lack of experience in taking tests. Premorbid intellectual ability should be ascertained from an interview with family or friends, because intellectual abilities may affect performance on some of the tests and measurements, as well as affect behavior in general. Premorbid memory should also be determined.

Finally, it is very important to conduct a sensory examination *before* cognitive or perceptual testing to establish whether the patient has sufficient sensory abilities to proceed with testing (this includes visual screening as well). Distinguishing between sensory and cognitive or perceptual problems is explored in more detail in the next section of this chapter. Each of these problems may adversely influence performance and may also reduce the patient's performance in treatment and capacity to learn from treatment. The therapist should be aware of the potential for these problems arising, and seek to minimize their impact.

Distinguishing between Sensory and Cognitive and Perceptual Deficits

Cognitive and perceptual dysfunction must be differentiated from sensory loss, language impairment, hearing loss, motor loss (weakness, spasticity, incoordination), visual disturbances (poor eyesight, homonymous **hemianopia**), disorientation, and lack of comprehension. The therapist must rule out pure sensory impairments before testing for cognitive and perceptual deficits, otherwise the therapist may incorrectly attribute poor performance to perceptual problems and design treatment accordingly when in fact the problem has a sensory base and should be treated quite differently. The therapist should conduct tests of deep (proprioceptive) sensations (kinesthesia, position sense, vibration), superficial sensations (pain, temperature, light touch, and pressure), and combined cortical sensations (stereognosis, tactile localization two-point discrimination, barognosis, graphesthesia, and recognition of texture) using methods described in Chapter 3, Examination of Sensory Function. The patient's hearing also requires testing. For example, if the patient does not seem to understand what the therapist is saying, hearing problems should be ruled out before more extensive language and cognitive tests are conducted. The therapist may need to confirm with the family if the patient wears a hearing aid and ensure its availability during therapy. If in doubt, the therapist may need to request testing by the speech-language pathologist or audiologist.

The therapist must also determine if the patient has visual impairments because they can easily be mistaken for perceptual problems. Given the prevalence of sensory-based visual problems, the following section focuses on identification of these impairments and the importance of distinguishing between visual and perceptual origins for treatment purposes.

Visual Impairments

Visual impairments are one of the most common forms of sensory loss affecting the patient with hemiplegia.[51,52] The lesion resulting from a stroke may affect the eye, optic radiation, or visual cortex and subsequently the reception, transmission, and appreciation of any visual array. Visual impairments commonly encountered by patients with hemiplegia include poor eyesight, diplopia, homonymous hemianopia, damage to the visual cortex, and retinal damage. Awareness of the presence of these deficits is important so as not to confuse them with

visual perceptual deficiencies, and to ensure their consideration during treatment planning and therapeutic intervention.

The critical nature of the basic visual skills (i.e., acuity, oculomotor control, and intact visual fields) in forming a basis for higher-level visual perception is highlighted by Warren[53,54] in a hierarchical model for the evaluation and treatment of visual perceptual dysfunction. In this developmental model, the basic visual skills enumerated above form the foundation for the next level of visual skills, which include *visual attention* (focusing on one aspect of the environment while ignoring others), *visual scanning* (using eyes to follow a target), and *pattern recognition* (recognition of structures that make a recognizable whole). These skills, along with memory, are required to facilitate the highest-level visual skill termed *visual cognition*.[53,54] This model has implications for the evaluation and treatment of visual perceptual disorders in a bottom-up sequence[54] (i.e., working from the "bottom" initially focusing on underlying skills that will then promote recovery of the next level of skills).

Impairments of oculomotor control (control of eye movements) are a common occurrence following a CVA. Poor visual acuity is another frequent finding following stroke or brain injury, even in the absence of other visual problems.[55] Therefore, it is recommended that the patient receive a comprehensive eye examination and have his or her eyeglass prescription checked.

Diplopia, or double vision, is often present following brain damage. The patient sees two of the entire environment (horizontally, vertically, or diagonally). Diplopia is usually the result of defective function of extraocular muscles in which both eyes are used but not in focus. Treatment usually consists of exercises for the eye muscles. In addition, the patient usually is instructed to wear a patch on alternate eyes until the condition clears. If the condition does not clear, the optometrist may recommend prisms.

Visual field deficit is probably the most common visual deficit affecting patients with hemiplegia[56] and occurs most frequently following damage to the middle cerebral artery near the internal capsule.[9] The diagnostic term for this deficit is *homonymous hemianopia*. The frequency of hemianopia following a right-hemisphere stroke is around 17%.[12] In addition, there is a significant correlation between the presence of visual field deficits and visual neglect.[57] Most important, the presence of a visual field deficit is a significant prognostic sign, predicting both a higher death rate following stroke and poorer performance in ADL, even following rehabilitation.[12,58]

Figure 27.3 demonstrates the normal functioning of the visual fields, in which the left side of the environment (the tree) is perceived by the nasal retina of the left eye and the temporal retina of the right eye, and the right side of the environment (the car) is perceived by the nasal retina of the right eye and the temporal retina of the left eye.

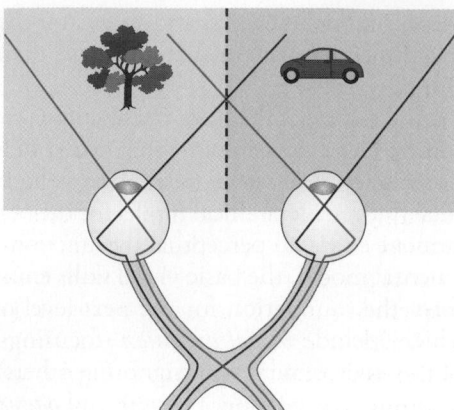

Figure 27.3 Normally functioning visual system; right and left visual fields. See text for explanation.

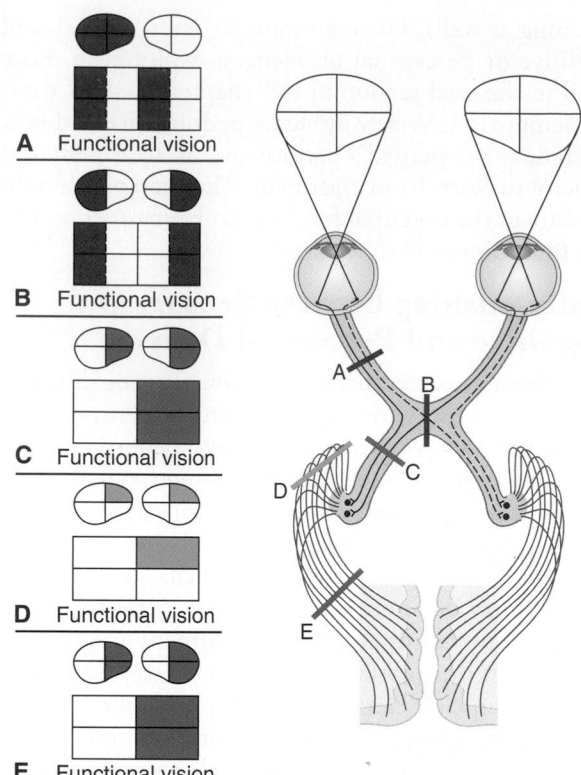

A Functional vision

B Functional vision

C Functional vision

D Functional vision

E Functional vision

Figure 27.4 Visual field deficits (with functional loss) and associated lesions. Vision is shown as clear and visual loss is colored in examples **A–E,** which denote **(A)** blindness in one eye; **(B)** bitemporal hemianopia (tunnel vision); **(C)** homonymous hemianopia; **(D)** quadrantanopia; and **(E)** homonymous hemianopia.

The lesion producing homonymous hemianopia interrupts inflow to the optic pathways on one side of the brain. This produces a loss of the outer half of the visual field from one eye and the inner half of the visual field of the other eye. The result is a loss of incoming information from half of the visual environment (left or right) contralateral to the side of the lesion. Thus, the loss of the left half of the visual field accompanies left hemiplegia and loss of the right visual field accompanies right hemiplegia. Zhang et al[59] suggested that this is a common condition following stroke, and noted a spontaneous recovery rate in less than 40% of cases. Figure 27.4 illustrates visual field deficits associated with a number of lesions to the visual system.

The presence of a visual field cut may inhibit performance in many daily activities. The patient is usually unaware of the condition and does not automatically compensate by turning the head unless specifically instructed. One of the dangers in this condition is street crossing (Fig. 27.5). Another example of the effects of a visual field cut is illustrated in Figure 27.6. When presented with a newspaper, a patient with right homonymous hemianopia may attend to one half of the newspaper page, either to or from the midline.

Because of its prevalence, it is essential for the therapist to determine whether homonymous hemianopia is present or not. A number of testing procedures are currently employed. In the confrontation method, the patient sits opposite the therapist and is instructed to maintain his or her gaze on the therapist's nose (Fig. 27.7). The therapist slowly brings a target, such as the therapists' finger or a pen, into the patient's field of view simultaneously or alternately from the right or left. The patient is instructed to indicate when and where he or she sees the targets.

To help the patient compensate for the visual field deficit, the patient can first be made aware of the deficit and then be instructed to turn the head to the affected side. Patients usually require constant reminders at first,

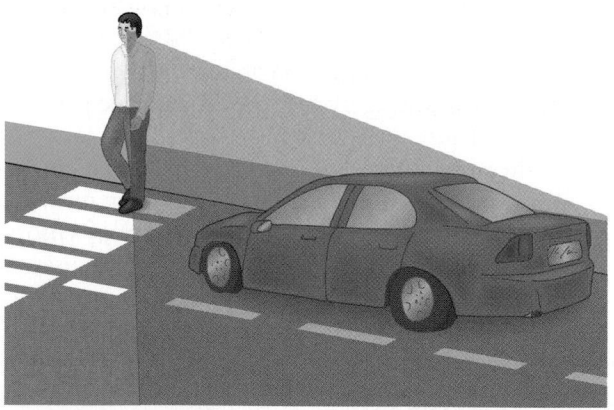

Figure 27.5 The functional significance of hemianopia—it may lead to accidents.

which may be tapered off with time and practice. Early in therapy, items (e.g., eating utensils, writing implements) should be placed where the patient is most apt to see them (on the less affected side). They can be moved progressively to the midline and then to the more affected side, when appropriate. The nursing staff should be made

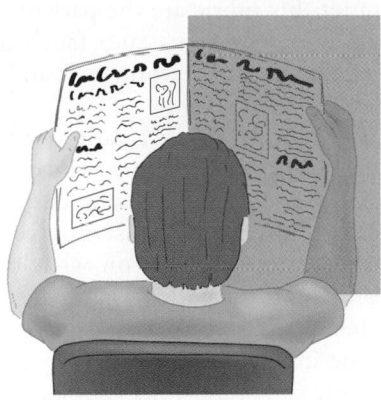

Figure 27.6 A newspaper as it might appear to a patient with right homonymous hemianopia following a stroke. The shading indicates that the patient may be unable to read the right side page.

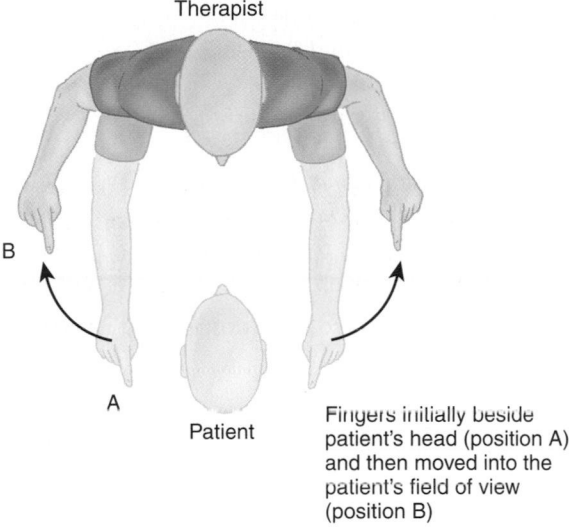

Therapist

B

A

Patient

Fingers initially beside patient's head (position A) and then moved into the patient's field of view (position B)

Figure 27.7 Method for testing hemianopia.

aware of the condition and be requested to place the patient's essential bedside needs such as telephone, tissues, and so forth within the intact visual field. The therapist initially should sit on the patient's less involved side when instructing or giving demonstrations and should alternate this with the more affected side so that the patient receives maximum stimulation. Of course, the patient will have to be reminded to turn the head at first. External cues can be employed as well. For reading, a red line can be drawn on the side of the page that is not seen. Red tape can be placed on the floor, mat, or parallel bars to attract the patient to scan to the side of the environment that is not seen. The patient should be taught to look for these cues. These external cues can be slowly tapered off over time. Patients can be instructed and encouraged to devise their own cues to clue them into the unseen side of the environment in situations that have not been addressed per se in therapy. Exercises that require motor crossing of the midline can be used to reinforce visual crossing of the midline and turning of the head.[60,61]

Oculomotor impairment is another area of deficit in basic visual skills that is common in patients who have had a stroke. Eye movements, which are controlled by the extraocular muscles, are used to detect, identify, and derive meaning from objects and the environment. They allow a person to become oriented to and explore the critical visual aspects of the environment.[11] Two types of eye movements are important to examine: (1) **visual fixation**, which allows the patient to maintain focus on an object as it is brought nearer or farther away; and (2) **ocular pursuits**, which enable the eyes to follow a moving object and visually scan the environment. Often the eyes will not follow a moving object visually, although the patient seems aware of the presence of that object and can locate it if asked. The patient is visually hypoactive. Oculomotor dysfunction often accompanies visual–perceptual dysfunction[62] and is frequently related to attention deficits.[63]

Visual scanning can be tested as follows. Sit opposite the patient. Hold up a pencil with a colorful pencil topper 18 in (45.7 cm) in front of the patient's eyes. Slowly move the pencil horizontally, then vertically, then diagonally. Repeat each direction two to three times. Note the smoothness of eye movements, the presence of a midline jerk or jump, and whether the eyes move together.[2,62]

Aside from the visual sensory impairments outlined above, many patients suffer from visual–perceptual impairment. Damage to areas of the cortex on which visual information converges with information from other senses may interfere with the recognition and interpretation of visual information, even though the visual stimuli may have arrived at the visual cortex uninterrupted. A total failure to appreciate incoming visual sensory information owing to a lesion in the cortex is referred to as **cortical blindness**.[62] There is no statistical correspondence between the presence of visual field cuts and the presence of visual–perceptual disorders.[64] Similarly, there is no correspondence between aphasia, age, and time since infarct, and measures of visual–perceptual dysfunction.[64] However, within the realm of visual–perceptual impairments, there is a significant difference between the performances of patients with right hemiplegia and those with left hemiplegia. Patients with left hemiplegia have frequently been found to perform more poorly on measures of visual–perceptual dysfunction than patients with right hemiplegia. Thus, therapists should be aware of the possibility of visual–perceptual deficits, particularly in the population with left hemiplegia.

Standardized Cognitive and Perceptual Tests

A standardized test is one that has a uniform procedure to administer and score, provides operational definitions for all terms, is norm-referenced,[65] and information is available concerning its reliability and validity, which is essential for correct interpretation of results.[66] Results from standardized tests of cognition and perception can be communicated to other therapists who will share an understanding of the patient's capacities or abilities. Standardized tests can be administered both at admission and at discharge to provide the therapist with a reliable and valid measure of the outcome of therapy.

When conducting a standardized test, the patient should be sitting comfortably and wearing glasses and/or a hearing aid if needed. Ideally, the room should be quiet and free of distraction. The therapist should be positioned opposite or next to the patient. Since the performance of a patient who has had a stroke may vary from day to day, a single testing session may be unreliable.[67] A number of short sessions scheduled on successive days may be preferable. To enhance its practical value, perceptual testing must be done in conjunction with observation in self-care and ADL skills, where the patient's judgment and discriminative abilities with regard to real-life tasks can be determined. It is not uncommon for patients to test poorly for visual–perceptual skills but to perform adequately in ADL with minimal effort or assistance.[63]

The quality of the patient's response to the test media (e.g., how the task is approached, how and why the error is made) is as important to note as the success or failure in completing the selected task. Some aspects of response in the testing situation or during ADL can be referred to as the patient's individual *perceptual style*.

Included under this rubric are the patient's perceptual strategy, response to various cues (such as auditory, visual, and tactile), rate of performance, and consistency of performance.[37]

Occupational therapists use a variety of standardized tests to determine the presence of cognitive and perceptual impairments and resulting disabilities. When selecting a standardized test the therapist must consider many factors. The selection depends on what the therapist wants to learn about the patient, and what the test can potentially reveal.[1] In many cases a single test will not provide all the information required by a therapist to plan treatment, so several tests may be administered (Table 27.1).[5,68-82] In addition to those presented in Table 27.1, other instruments used to measure more global outcomes of rehabilitation include the following:

- *Medical Outcomes Study (MOS), Short Form Health Survey (SF-36)*[83]
- *Australian Therapy Outcome Measures—Occupational Therapy (AusTOMS-OT)*[84]
- *Canadian Occupational Performance Measure (COPM)*[85]
- *Rivermead Rehabilitation Centre Life Goals Questionnaire*[86]
- *Reintegration to Normal Living Index (RNL)*[87]
- *Functional Independence Measure (FIM$_{MR}$^{SM})*[88]

Some of these instruments also incorporate items that measure cognition and perception. For example, the FIM$_{MR}$^{SM} includes three cognition-related items (social

Table 27.1	Summary of Standardized Tests
Test	Description
Arnadottir OT-ADL Neurobehavioral Evaluation (A-ONE)[5]	This test was developed to measure a patient's neurobehavior through daily living tasks (dressing, grooming, hygiene, transfer and mobility, feeding, and communication). Occupational therapists must undertake a 5-day training and certification course to qualify to administer this test. A wide variety of cognitive and perceptual impairments can be detected with this instrument.
Structured Observational Test of Function (SOTOF)[68]	The SOTOF was designed to examine older persons' level of occupational performance and neuropsychological functioning following neurological damage of cortical origin.[69] The instrument consists of a screening test, neuropsychological checklist, and four ADL scales (eating from a bowl, pouring a drink and drinking, putting on an upper body garment, and washing and drying hands). After analyzing observational data, a wide variety of neuropsychological deficits are extrapolated.[68]
Allen Cognitive Level Test (ACL)[70,71]	The ACL is used as a screening tool to estimate a person's cognitive level. Although originally developed for use with clients who have psychiatric problems, this test is also used with people who have acquired brain damage, or experience a dementing illness such as Alzheimer's disease. Following an interview to gain information concerning the client's educational and work background, the client is observed performing the visuomotor task of leather lacing. It is assumed that the client's cognitive functioning is reflected through his or her motor actions.[1]
Chessington Occupational Therapy Neurological Assessment Battery (COTNAB)[72]	The COTNAB was designed to examine cognitive and perceptual deficits in patients 16 years of age and older following stroke or head injury. The battery consists of 12 tests divided into four sections examining visual perception, constructional ability, sensory-motor ability, and ability to follow instructions. Further information about this instrument may be found in Stanley et al[73] and Sloan et al.[74]

Table 27.1	Summary of Standardized Tests—cont'd
Test	**Description**
Loewenstein Occupational Therapy Cognitive Assessment (LOTCA)[75]	The LOTCA is a battery-style test lasting 35 to 40 minutes and composed of 20 subtests that examine four areas: orientation, visual and spatial perception, visuomotor organization, and thinking operations. The instrument was developed for use with people who have experienced stroke, traumatic brain injury, or tumor.
The Behavioural Inattention Test (BIT)[77]	The BIT was developed to examine clients for the presence of unilateral visual neglect and to provide the therapist with information concerning how the neglect affects the client's ability to perform everyday occupations.[78] The BIT consists of nine activity-based subtests and six pen-and-paper subtests. Many of these test items have been used in the past in a nonstandardized way to examine for the presence of neglect.
Rivermead Perceptual Assessment Battery (RPAB)[79]	This instrument was designed to examine visual perceptual impairments in patients following head injury or stroke. The RPAB is a battery consisting of 16 performance tests that examine form discrimination, color constancy, sequencing, object completion, figure–ground discrimination, body image, inattention, and spatial awareness. The test can be completed in approximately 1 hour. For further information on the RPAB, the reader is referred to Jesshope et al.[80]
Rivermead Behavioural Memory Test (RBMT)[81]	This battery was designed to examine everyday memory abilities. It offers the therapist an initial determination of the client's memory function, an indication of appropriate areas for treatment, and enables the therapist to monitor memory skills throughout the treatment program. The RBMT can be administered in approximately 30 minutes by occupational therapists, speech-language pathologists, and psychologists. For further information on the RBMT, the reader is referred to Baddeley at al.[81] and Wilson et al.[82]

interaction, problem solving, and memory). The tests described in the section on specific cognitive and perceptual deficits are used widely in the clinic. Although some of the instruments presented are not standardized, they are still useful, particularly for examining the quality of response to the test stimuli.

■ INTERVENTION

Treatment Approaches

Five major approaches to cognitive and perceptual rehabilitation are commonly employed by occupational therapists. They are the *retraining approach*, the *sensory integrative approach*, the *neurofunctional approach*, the *rehabilitation/compensatory approach*, and the *cognitive rehabilitation/quadraphonic approach*. These approaches were described earlier in the chapter. Although research directly comparing the efficacy of the various approaches has been sparse, attempts have been made recently to empirically define and test the methodologies.[21,25,34,89] Issues to consider in examining the approaches are the availability of standardized measures of change in functional status and ADL, group versus individual treatment, specific stimulus properties, format, length and frequency of feedback, and individual information processing styles.[21]

Neistadt[25,34] described these treatments dichotomously as either remedial or adaptive/compensatory. The remedial approach encompasses the retraining approach, the sensory integrative approach, and the cognitive approach.[1] The neurofunctional approach and

the rehabilitation/compensatory approach are described as adaptive or compensatory. The quadraphonic approach brings together aspects of both the remedial and compensatory approaches. A description of the key components of these two main approaches is presented below. A discussion on education is also provided because no intervention program would be complete without the provision of education to both the patient and the caregivers. Finally, a discussion is provided on integrating these three elements within a rehabilitation program.

The Remedial Approach

Remedial approaches focus on the patient's deficits and attempt to improve functional ability by retraining specific perceptual components of behavior.[25] The assumption uniting this set of tactics is that facilitation of, or training in, underlying skills will enhance the recovery or reorganization of deficient CNS functioning.[21,25] This, in turn, will automatically translate into improvement in functional skills. Remedial approaches are also referred to as bottom-up approaches. These approaches work from the bottom, which is the recovery of underlying skills, and assume that the patient will be able to generalize skills to occupational performance, which is at a higher level.[1,47]

The Adaptive/Compensatory Approach

The adaptive or compensatory approach mandates direct training in the functional skills that are deficient. It does not assume automatic carryover from tasks that are not obviously similar to the functional task to be learned, and thus minimizes the need for generalization. In an adaptive or "top-down" approach, the therapist works with the patient on specific tasks that are required, or those that the patient wants to achieve. In other words, the therapist starts at the top, which is the desired functional outcome, rather than working with the patient on the underlying performance components.[35] Table 27.2 presents a comparison of the assumptions underlying the remedial and adaptive approaches.

Patient, Family, and Caregiver Education

Education for the patient, family, and caregivers is essential for continuity of care. Appendix 27.A includes Web-based resources for clinicians, families, and patients with cognitive and perceptual deficits. The patient and caregivers should understand why it is inadvisable or impossible for

the patient to do some things safely or independently, and why other things must be done in a specific way. Explaining the reasons why the patient behaves in a particular way reduces the likelihood of inappropriate expectations from those without the background to know that brain damage affects not only how the patient moves but also how he or she experiences and thus responds to the world.

Feedback is essential to the patient's learning. The patient's own feedback may be inaccurate owing to perceptual and cognitive dysfunctions. Thus, the individual may be unaware that a task has not been accomplished or that it has not been performed in the safest or most efficient manner. Feedback should be provided in the form of **knowledge of results (KR)** and **knowledge of performance (KP)**. Knowledge of results is information regarding whether or not the patient attained the correct outcome. Knowledge of performance is information regarding the manner in which the task was accomplished.[90]

The form in which this feedback is delivered depends on the specific limitations and strengths of the patient. For example, the physical therapy goal for a patient with left hemiplegia and visual perceptual involvement might be to walk to the end of the parallel bars. KR would consist of a verbal confirmation by the therapist as to whether or not the patient reached the end of the parallel bars. KP might include comments by the therapist concerning the adequacy of the patient's visual scanning, positioning of the lower extremities (LEs), correct posture, and appropriate use of the upper limbs. For the patient with communication impairments, feedback would need to be visual. Tactile input also can be used effectively to cue patients with either right or left hemiplegia. A combination of inputs, using a number of sensory modalities, often facilitates patient success at a given task.

When involving the patient in education sessions, the patient must be addressed as a competent adult, and not patronized. He or she must be regarded as the principal participant in the rehabilitation process. In situations in which the perceptual deficit does not interfere with assimilation of information, the patient should have the major role in the decision making process regarding the goals of therapy.

Table 27.2	Common Assumptions of Adaptive and Remedial Approaches	
Adaptive Approach	**Remedial Approach**
The adult brain has limited potential to repair and reorganize itself after injury.	The adult brain can repair and reorganize itself after injury.
Intact behaviors can be used to compensate for ones that are impaired.	Repair and reorganization is influenced by environmental stimuli.
Adaptive retraining can facilitate the substitution of intact behaviors for impaired ones.	Cognitive, perceptual, and sensorimotor exercises can promote brain recovery and reorganization.
Adaptive activities of daily living provide training in functional behaviors.	Cognitive, perceptual, and sensorimotor exercises provide training in the cognitive and perceptual skills needed for those exercises.
Training in specific, essential activities of daily living tasks is necessary because adults with brain injury have difficulty generalizing learning.	Remedial training in cognitive and perceptual skills will be generalized across all activities requiring those skills.
Functional activities require cognitive and perceptual skills.	Functional activities require cognitive and perceptual skills.
Adaptation and compensation will lead to improved functional performance.	Cognitive and perceptual remediation will lead to improved functional performance.

Refocusing Intervention

Many clinicians begin an intervention program by adopting remedial strategies. In these circumstances, therapists are aiming to maximize recovery of function and educate their patients about the problems experienced and ways that can improve their function. However, some patients may not make much progress. In some cases, the patient may have inadequate language skills to be able to work with the therapist, or may have limited insight to his or her problems and therefore will not work with the therapist. In other cases still, improvements simply do not seem to occur for a variety of reasons that the therapist may not be able to pinpoint. Finally, in the current climate of managed care, the therapist may not have very much time allocated to work with the patient using remedial techniques. The patient's discharge may be imminent, and yet he or she may not be independent or safe enough to be discharged. In such cases, the therapist may switch from a remedial approach to a compensatory one.

When using an adaptive compensatory approach, the therapist will address education of the caregivers as well as the patient. Intervention strategies will focus on changing the environment or the strategy for task completion so that the patient can be safe and independent as quickly as possible. In many instances, therapists use a three-point approach to intervention where they educate patients and caregivers, begin the program using remedial techniques, and then switch to compensation techniques when the patient's improvements have plateaued and/or discharge is imminent.

The Impact of Managed Care

The introduction of managed care in the United States health care system has many implications for treatment of patients with cognitive and perceptual deficits. The most striking of these is the reduction in time allocated for inpatient evaluation and treatment.[36] Cognitive and perceptual problems are not readily visible and are therefore more easily overlooked than physical problems. Hence, pressure to discharge patients quickly, possibly before the full extent of cognitive and perceptual deficits has been revealed, means that patients may be discharged to potentially hazardous situations at home. Therapists need to do an initial screening of all patients with brain damage to determine potential problems as early as possible, and ensure that patients are discharged to a safe environment. Although inpatient rehabilitation time is reduced, there is opportunity for outpatient services conducted in the clinic or in the patient's home.[91] The advantage of home care is that therapists have an opportunity to work with the patient in his or her own environment, and tailor therapy to the patient's current circumstances. Patients with cognitive and perceptual deficits often perform better in their own familiar environments.

The major disadvantage of reduced inpatient treatment time for many patients, including those with cognitive and perceptual deficits, is that a home discharge may not be safe after only limited inpatient rehabilitation. The situation is complicated by having to discharge a patient who does not have family support to another type of institutional care (possibly a nursing home or skilled nursing facility) when in the long term this level of care may not be necessary. It is distressing for patients who are confused owing to cognitive and perceptual problems to be moved, particularly when they may believe the move is permanent.

■ DISCHARGE PLANNING

Discharge planning begins as soon as the patient is admitted for rehabilitation.[92] The most important question to be answered during this stage is where the patient will live after discharge. There are two major types of housing available to persons with disabilities: community-based accommodation and supported accommodation. Community-based accommodation includes private homes, retirement villages, and hotels or rooming houses. Supported accommodation may be defined as any accommodation that provides personal care and medical services on a consistent, continual, or per need basis, and includes nursing homes, skilled nursing facilities, assisted living centers, and sheltered or group housing.[93,94]

The key to discharge planning is to consider the match between the patient's skills and the demands of the environment, and then factor in the support systems available from a spouse, friends, or family to assist with tasks that the patient cannot manage.[94,95] This approach works well when patients and their families have insight and an understanding of the patient's problems. However, cognitive and perceptual deficits are often not very visible and it may be difficult for the family and the patient to understand the functional impact of these deficits. For example, a patient may regain full motor function following a stroke, but experience ongoing difficulties with unilateral neglect. This problem is not readily apparent to the untrained onlooker. However, this patient cannot drive and may be in danger when simply crossing the road. These problems have major lifestyle implications for the patient.

Interventions that facilitate a patient's return to community-based housing usually center on enabling the patient to carry out ADL skills in an acceptable and safe manner. If this cannot be achieved and the patient does not have a live-in caregiver, supported housing such as a nursing home may be the only alternative. Research examining the discharge process for a sample of 62 patients following stroke revealed that the majority were reluctant to consider alternatives to returning home despite having significant self-care deficits.[95] Our housing is central to who we are as individuals and it is very difficult for patients, particularly those with limited insight, to understand and accept that they can no longer live in the community.

■ OVERVIEW OF COGNITIVE AND PERCEPTUAL DEFICITS

This section is divided into seven parts: *attention deficits, memory impairments, impairments of executive function, body scheme and body image impairments, spatial relations impairments, agnosia,* and *apraxia* (Table 27.3). Each category encompasses a constellation of deficits, which are grouped together for ease of understanding. Information pertaining to each deficit will be organized identically as follows:

1. Definition(s)
2. Clinical Examples
3. Lesion Area
4. Testing
5. Treatment Suggestions

Table 27.3	Summary of Cognitive and Perceptual Impairments
Area of Deficit	**Specific Impairments**
Cognition	
Attention deficits	Sustained attention
	Selective attention
	Divided attention
	Alternating attention
Memory impairments	Immediate recall
	Short-term memory
	Long-term memory
Higher-order cognition	
Impairment of executive functions	Volition
	Planning
	Purposive action
	Effective performance
Perception	
Body scheme/body image impairments	Unilateral neglect
	Anosognosia
	Somatoagnosia
	Right–left discrimination
	Finger agnosia
Spatial relation impairments (complex perception)	Figure–ground discrimination
	Form discrimination
	Spatial relations
	Position in space
	Topographical disorientation
	Depth and distance perception
	Vertical disorientation
Agnosias	Visual object agnosia
	Auditory agnosia
	Tactile agnosia
Apraxia	Ideomotor apraxia
	Ideational apraxia
	Buccofacial apraxia

The value of dwelling on probable areas of cortical damage is controversial. The indication of cortical loci is an attempt to relate the study of neuroanatomy to actual patient behavior involving cognitive and perceptual dysfunction. An examination of cortical loci will give the reader a sense of which cognitive and perceptual deficits are likely to be seen together.

As therapists, we are required to assist the patient to bridge the gap between maladaptive behavior and independent function in ADL skills. Whether or not the area of the brain purported to produce a particular dysfunction appears damaged on a computed tomography (CT) scan or other neurological or radiological test is not a key determinant of the rehabilitative approach to therapy. The patient's approach to task performance and the relative strengths or weaknesses of the patient (motor,

cognitive, and perceptual), which the therapist ascertains through thorough observation and testing, are much more pertinent to the selection of appropriate therapeutic strategies than the locus of the lesion.

Testing tools are described for each cognitive or perceptual deficit to enhance the reader's awareness of the complexity of behavior ascribed to perceptual deficiencies. Familiarity with the tools used to examine cognitive or perceptual deficits can serve as an aid in communication between physical and occupational therapists engaged in the treatment of the same patient.

The following section also includes specific treatment suggestions from the sensorimotor, transfer of training, and functional approaches described. The intervention strategies most relevant to physical therapist practice are those dealing with the functional approach and adaptation of the environment. In these sections, examples are given of how to facilitate the patient's success within a treatment session. Information is provided on how the therapist might gear language, demonstrations, feedback, and the use of media and the environment to the individual needs of the cognitively or perceptually impaired patient. The evidence base for treatment is not strong for many of these treatment techniques, and further research is required to support their efficacy.

Attention Deficits

1. *Definitions.* The inability of many patients with hemiplegia to maintain attention during therapy is a frequent complaint of therapists. **Attention** is the ability to select and attend to a specific stimulus while simultaneously suppressing extraneous stimuli.[96] A patient who is inattentive or distractible will have difficulty in processing and assimilating new information or techniques.[97] Often, patients who have suffered a CVA will have low arousal levels, and require a great deal of sensory input to be alerted to the environment. Low arousal thus must be considered as a cause for seeming inattention.

   Four different kinds of attention are generally discussed in the literature. These are sustained attention, focused or selective attention, alternating attention, and divided attention. **Sustained attention** is a capacity to attend to relevant information during activity. Sustained attention implies that a person can maintain a consistent response during a continuous activity. **Focused** or **selective attention** is the capacity to attend to a task despite environmental visual or auditory stimuli. **Alternating attention** is the capacity to move flexibly between tasks and respond appropriately to the demands of each task. **Divided attention** is the capacity to respond simultaneously to two or more tasks or stimuli when all stimuli are relevant.[1]

2. *Clinical Examples.* The patient with a disorder of sustained attention may report that he or she starts to watch a TV program and then "just drifts off."

A patient who has to stop a dressing activity to talk to the therapist may be demonstrating difficulties with focused attention. Patients who are easily disturbed by music or other forms of background noise may also be experiencing problems with focused attention.

A problem with focused attention is often referred to as distractibility. Divided attention is required when more than one response is needed or more than one stimuli needs to be monitored.[98] Selective attention is required when certain stimuli need to be ignored.[99] Patients who have difficulty with divided and alternating attention may have great difficulties with more complex daily living activities such as cooking a meal or driving.

3. *Lesion Areas.* Multiple brain regions are thought to be responsible for producing attention. These include the reticular formation (which regulates arousal), the various sensory systems that deliver and code relevant sensory information, and the limbic and frontal regions that underlie the drive and affective components of concentration.[99]

4. *Testing.* General screening tests such as the *Loewenstein Occupational Therapy Cognitive Assessment*[75] or *Chessington Occupational Therapy Neurological Assessment Battery (COTNAB)*[72] include subtests that examine attentional abilities. To investigate problems of attention, neuropsychologists generally administer the *Stroop Test*,[100] the *Paced Auditory Serial Attention Test (PASAT)*,[101] and the *Trail Making Test.*[102]

5. *Treatment Suggestions.* The purpose of therapy is to increase the patient's attention to appropriate stimuli, and disregard inappropriate stimuli.

a. *Remedial Approach.* Clinically, the ability to attend to a task has implications for the therapeutic process. Patients should be instructed to scan the visual environment in a slow and systematic manner. In the presence of right hemiplegia, the patient should be spoken to more slowly to afford an opportunity to process verbal information and be taught to use visualization techniques to facilitate attendance to verbal tasks. In addition, patients with left hemiplegia should be encouraged to use verbalization to improve performance in visual tasks. A randomized clinical trial (RCT) with 12 patients investigating the effect of training on divided attention skills reported positive outcomes as measured on a rating scale of attentional behavior.[103] Patients were trained to do two computer-based or pen and paper tasks simultaneously. However, there was no generalization from this training to nontarget tasks. In other words, the benefits of this training were not transferred to patient activities of daily living.

Some additional tools that may be used for the remediation of attentional deficits and distractibility are setting time or speed limits, amplification of critical stimuli, and making the crucial stimuli salient (noticeable) to the patient.[63] The environment can be graded by having the patient initially perform some aspects of therapy in a nondistracting setting (closed environment) and then slowly increasing potentially distracting elements, both visual and auditory, as patient tolerance improves (progressing to a more open environment).[1]

b. *Compensatory Approach.* For many patients, the inability to attend to significant stimuli is compounded by distraction due to extraneous stimuli in the environment. Often noise is the most distracting stimulus, causing irritability and diminished concentration. Ponsford et al[104] provide further ideas for working with patients who have limited attention.

A Cochrane review titled *Cognitive Rehabilitation for Attention Deficits following Stroke*[105] revealed a small number controlled trials of attention training in patients with stroke. The results of these studies suggested that training improved alertness and sustained attention on measures of these capacities, but there was no evidence to support or refute the use of cognitive rehabilitation for attention deficits to improve functional independence.

Memory Impairments

Memory can be defined as a "mental process that allows the individual to store experiences and perceptions for recall at a later time."[97, p. 78] All memory is not localized in one particular place in the nervous system; rather, many and perhaps all regions of the brain may contain neurons with adequate plasticity for memory storage.[106] Memory comprises acquisition or learning, storage or retention, and retrieval or recall.[107] Learning is a crucial element of rehabilitation. If the patient is unable to learn, time in rehabilitation may not be well spent. Hence, it is very important for the therapist to take steps to evaluate the patient's memory before beginning physical rehabilitation programs. Three levels of memory will be examined: immediate recall, short-term memory, and long-term memory.

Immediate Recall and Short-Term Memory

1. *Definitions.* **Immediate recall** involves retention of information that has been stored for a few seconds. **Short-term memory** mediates retention of events or learning that has taken place within a few minutes, hours, or days.[4]

2. *Clinical Examples.* A patient with immediate recall difficulties may not be able to remember the instructions given only seconds before by the therapist for what the patient is to do. A patient with a short-term memory problem may not come back to the physical therapy department, even though the therapist asked him or her to return in an hour. Alternatively, the

therapist may teach the patient a new transfer technique, and on the following day find that the patient has not retained any of the steps involved. Patients with severe short-term memory problems may not even be able to hold a simple conversation.[1]

3. *Lesion Areas.* Memory is a complex capacity involving many brain regions including four of the major structures of the cerebral cortex (the frontal, parietal, temporal, and occipital lobes) and the limbic system.[4]

4. *Testing.* The *Rivermead Behavioural Memory Test (RBMT)*[81] can be used to examine memory function. Alternatively, the adequacy of memory functions can be ascertained by having the patient recall lists or collections of objects that have just been presented (immediate recall) or by teaching the patient a new verbal or visual task and asking him or her to recall it a few hours or a day later (short-term memory). Frequently there is a loss of short-term memory following stroke, and this particularly interferes with the patient's ability to benefit from rehabilitation, especially from those activities involving the use of new and heretofore unfamiliar techniques.[45]

5. *Treatment Suggestions.* The purpose of memory retraining is to enable the patient to effectively encode and recall information so that learning can occur.

   a. *Remedial Approach.* Because good attention skills are vital for memory, the therapist must ensure that attention problems are addressed and improvements are noted before initiating work on memory retraining.[1,43] A primary focus of this approach is working with the patient to effectively encode information so it can be more easily retrieved when appropriate. This may include organizing material to be remembered and making logical associations. A determination should be made of how the patient used to remember information and build on these past strategies. There is very little evidence to suggest that drills, computer games, or memory tests such as recalling a list of items that have been covered over have any effect on retraining memory. On the other hand, if the therapist assists the patient to develop memory strategies when playing these games, then these strategies may be generalized to everyday activities. In a Cochrane review,[108] the authors drew on findings from two studies and reported that there was insufficient evidence to support or refute the effectiveness of memory retraining on functional outcomes or measures of memory, and called for further robust trials in this area.

   b. *Compensatory Approach.* The use of a diary or notebook system (memory log) can help many patients to manage their daily living activities. However, the patient needs to have sufficient memory to use this system. Environmental prompts such as a beeper or a wall calendar can be useful to assist patients to remember their routine or to look at their diary. When external aids are used, the patient needs to be taught how to use them. Guidelines for the use of such devices may be found in Sohlberg and Mateer[109] and McKerracher et al.[110]

Long-Term Memory

1. *Definition.* **Long-term memory** consists of early experiences and information acquired over a period of years. Patients who do not have long-term memory are often described as having amnesia.[45]

2. *Clinical Examples.* Patients who experience long-term memory problems may have difficulty recalling events from many years ago such as a child's birth, or their own work experiences. Long-term memory problems are common following brain injury and in Alzheimer's disease, but are not commonly seen following stroke.[45]

3. *Lesion Areas.* As described, memory is a complex capacity involving many brain regions. For a detailed discussion, the reader is referred to Fuster[111] and Lezak.[4]

4. *Testing.* The adequacy of memory functions can be determined by having the patient recall personal historical events. The *Rivermead Behavioural Memory Test (RBMT)*[81] can be used to test memory in a standardized way. It is advisable to question the patient's family as to premorbid memory, because many patients in the stroke-prone age group have already begun to experience declining memory as part of the aging process.

5. *Treatment Suggestions.* Treatments for assisting patients overcome long-term memory impairments are similar to those outlined above for immediate recall and short-term memory impairments. Further information on the management of memory impairments may be found in Wilson and Moffat.[112]

Although the literature contains many studies exploring a variety of memory treatments, few of these were designed as randomized controlled trials (RCTs). A Cochrane review[113] found only one controlled trial in which at least 75% of participants had a stroke. The study reviewed was conducted by Doornheim and De Haan[114] and showed that memory training had no significant effect on memory impairment or subjective memory complaints. The Cochrane reviewers concluded that there is currently insufficient evidence to support or refute the effectiveness of cognitive rehabilitation for memory problems after stroke.

Impairments of Executive Functions

1. *Definition.* As defined by Lezak, "executive functions consist of those capacities that enable a person to engage successfully in independent,

purposive, self-serving behavior."[4] Lezak goes on to describe executive functions as consisting of four overlapping components: volition, planning, purposive action, and effective performance.

Volition is the capacity to determine what one needs and wants to do. It also encompasses a future realization of one's needs and wants. Volition encompasses goal planning and task initiation, self-awareness, awareness of the environment, and social awareness. *Planning* is "the identification and organization of the steps and elements (e.g., skills, material, other persons) needed to carry out an intention or achieve a goal."[4, p. 653] Planning involves weighing alternatives and making choices. *Purposive action* includes productivity and self-regulation, which encompasses the ability to initiate, maintain, switch, and stop complex action sequences in an orderly manner to realize a goal. *Effective performance* is the capacity for quality control, including the ability to self-monitor and self-correct one's behavior. Problems with effective performance are associated with ineffective self-monitoring and difficulty with self-correction; for example, patients may not even perceive their mistakes, whereas others may identify them but take no action to correct them.[115]

2. *Clinical Examples.* Although some patients with executive function disorders are unable to formulate realistic goals or intentions (volition) or plan, others may be able to formulate goals and initiate goal-directed task performance, but owing to defective planning are not able to realize their goals. Patients with planning problems may say or intend one thing, but do another.[4] Family and hospital staff may complain of the patient's apparent apathy, poor or unreliable judgment, inappropriate behavior, difficulty adapting to new situations, and/or lack of attention to the needs and feelings of others.[115]

3. *Lesion Area.* Executive functions have traditionally been associated with the frontal and prefrontal cortex,[6] but the current view is that these capacities are mediated by reciprocal connections with other cortical and subcortical regions via the dorsolateral prefrontal–subcortical circuit.[116]

4. *Testing.* Tests of executive functions include the *Behavioural Assessment of the Dysexecutive Syndrome (BADS),*[117] the *Executive Functions Assessment,*[118] and the *Good Samaritan Hospital for Cognitive Rehabilitation's Executive Functions Behavioural Rating Scale.*[119]

5. *Treatment Suggestions.* The combination of impulsiveness, poor judgment, poor planning ability, and lack of foresight, which is particularly problematic in patients with left hemiplegia, does not bode well for independent functioning. The severity of these impairments may diminish somewhat over time.[9]

Although some general remedial and adaptive treatment suggestions are described here, for more specific details refer to Ponsford et al[104] and Duran and Fisher.[115]

a. *Remedial Approach.* By providing structure, feedback, and routine, a person's performance can be enhanced (e.g., providing structure by giving the patient steps to follow, assisting the task to become routine by repeated practice, or providing immediate feedback about the patient's behavior and the effect it has on others). The therapist initially acts as the patient's frontal lobes, and gradually transfers these responsibilities to the patient. Unless the patient has some awareness of the problems, a remedial approach will not be particularly successful.[104] Honda[120] reported a study with three patients over a 6-month period who were provided with self-instructional training, a problem-solving procedure, and physical-set changing exercises described as moving the four extremities and trunk in time to a metronome. In this study, "Patients were instructed to follow a videotape for 20 minutes. In the tape, a physical therapist moves four extremities and his trunk in time to a metronome. He changes activities every 2 or 3 minutes. The patients were trained with these methods for a total of 6 months. In the self-instructional procedure and problem-solving training phase, psychologists guided and trained patients 1 hour per day twice a week. In the physical set changing exercise phase, patients were advised to practice twice a day watching the instruction videotape. Each training phase lasted 6 weeks."[120, p. 18] While two of the subjects revealed improvements on the neuropsychological test used as an outcome measure, all subjects improved in basic and instrumental ADL. Of course, a limitation of this study is the small sample size and lack of control subjects, since it could be expected that these patients would make spontaneous recovery over the 6-month study period.

Hewitt el al[121] proposed that people with TBI have difficulty with planning because they are not spontaneously using autobiographic memories. The authors asked a control and experimental group of 15 subjects to describe how they would plan common activities. The experimental group underwent a 30-minute training session aimed at prompting retrieval of specific memories to support planning. This intervention was found to be effective in increasing specific memories that could aid planning.

b. *Compensatory Approach.* The therapist can assist the patient to compensate for poor abilities by utilizing other intact cognitive functions and/or modifying the environment. For example, the therapist might ask the patient to perform a task in a room with minimal distractions, or change the demands of the patient's work, home, or community to diminish the need to employ executive functions. A beeper or alarm clock may be used to help a patient overcome poor initiation.

Body Scheme and Body Image Impairments

Body image is defined as a visual and mental image of one's body that includes feelings about one's body, especially in relation to health and disease.[122] The term **body scheme** refers to a postural model of the body, including the relationship of body parts to each other and the relationship of the body to the environment. Commonly, body scheme and body image problems are termed *difficulties with body awareness*. Body awareness is derived from the integration of tactile, proprioceptive, and interoceptive (visceral) sensations, in addition to the individual's subjective feelings about the body.[122] An awareness of body scheme is considered one of the essential foundations for the performance of all purposeful motor behavior.[122] The terms *body awareness*, *body image*, and *body scheme* are often used interchangeably; therefore, when researching this topic, close attention should be paid to the particular definition put forth by each individual author. Specific impairments of body image and body scheme are unilateral neglect, somatoagnosia, right–left discrimination, finger agnosia, and anosognosia.

Unilateral Neglect

1. *Definition.* **Unilateral neglect** is the inability to register and integrate stimuli and perceptions from one side of the body (*body neglect*) and the environment or **hemispace** (*spatial neglect* of the area surrounding one side of the body), which is not due to a sensory loss. Unilateral neglect is also referred to as unilateral spatial neglect, hemi-inattention, hemineglect, and unilateral visual inattention.[123] It is important for the therapist to be familiar with this disorder because it is a frequent clinical finding. Neglect following right cerebral infarction has been reported in between 12% and 95% of patients.[124] The reporting rates vary enormously due to differences in time selected for reporting and techniques used to detect the neglect. However, this disorder is commonly seen in the clinic as having a functional impact on about 20% of patients. Unilateral neglect usually, although not always, affects the left side of the body or hemispace, and for purposes of this discussion, we will assume that it is the left. If a patient has unilateral neglect, he or she seems to ignore the left side of the body and stimuli occurring in the left personal space. This may occur despite intact visual fields, or concomitantly with right or left homonymous hemianopia; however, it is not caused by homonymous hemianopia.[125]

When working with a patient who has unilateral neglect, the therapist should also determine which sensory modalities are affected, including visual, tactile, and auditory. Input from one or all of these modalities may be neglected. Neglect can also be understood in terms of the area of space that is neglected. For example, unilateral neglect may express itself as a disorder of attention and goal-directed behavior in:

- Contralesional personal space (defined as pertaining to the body) such as shaving only the right half of the face, or failing to wash the left side of the body, or
- Contralesional peripersonal space (that area of space within arm distance), for example, failing to use objects on the contralesional side of the meal tray, or
- Contralesional extrapersonal space (that area of space beyond arm length) such as failing to negotiate obstacles, doorways, and so forth during locomotion.[50,123]

Unilateral neglect is also demonstrated by an impaired ability to attend to either the object or the environment as a whole. It is possible that while some patients may neglect half of the environment, others may neglect half of objects in the total environment. In the first case, the patient may neglect most elements of the left side of the entire visual scene (Fig. 27.8). In the second case, a patient may neglect the left side of an object, regardless of its absolute position in the visual display. For example, the patient may neglect the left side of a cup even though it is on his or her right side or omit the left side of objects when drawing items such as an umbrella, picnic basket, and bucket and spade as depicted in Figure 27.9.

Frequently, a patient with unilateral neglect has sensory loss on the more affected side, which compounds the problem. Although a patient with left-sided hemianopia has actual loss of vision from the left visual field of both eyes, he or she may be aware of the problem and compensate automatically or learn to compensate by turning the head. A patient with visual neglect has intact vision but seems unaware of the problem and does not attempt to compensate spontaneously by turning the

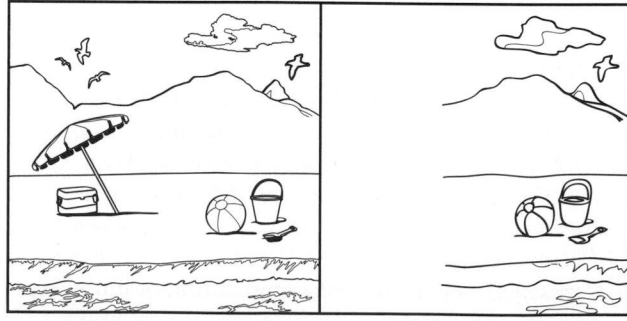

Figure 27.8 Example of a drawing by a patient with unilateral neglect. Therapist's drawing of a beach scene **(left).** Impaired copying by a patient with unilateral neglect—environment neglect following a stroke **(right).**

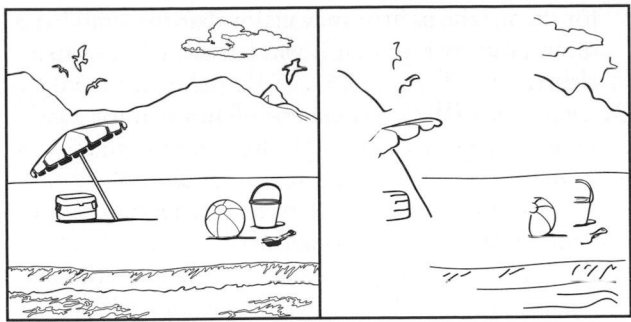

Figure 27.9 Example of a drawing by a patient with unilateral neglect. Therapist's drawing of a beach scene **(left).** Impaired copying by a patient with unilateral neglect—object neglect following a stroke **(right).**

head. In extreme cases the patient appears totally indifferent to the left side of the body and environment, and may deny that the left extremities belong to him or her.[126] More time seems to be required to learn to compensate for this impairment than for hemianopia. There is great difficulty in integrating all stimuli from the left half of the body and personal space for use in ADL skills. As with hemianopia, the patient with visual unilateral neglect often avoids crossing the midline visually or motorically.[61]

2. *Clinical Examples.* The patient may ignore the left half of the body when dressing and forget to put on the left sleeve or left pants leg. Often a male patient will forget to shave the left half of his face. A woman may neglect to put makeup on the left side of her face.[127] The patient may neglect to eat from the left half of a plate and will start reading a newspaper from the middle of the line. Typically, the patient bumps into objects on the left side or tends to veer toward the right when walking or propelling a wheelchair.

3. *Lesion Area.* It has been suggested that lesions involving the inferior–posterior regions of the right parietal lobe are significant determinants of neglect.[125,128]

4. *Testing.* A variety of techniques are useful. No single test is adequate to identify unilateral neglect in all patients because the impairment may be manifested differently in each patient.
   a. The *Behavioural Inattention Test (BIT)*[77] can be used to examine unilateral neglect (see Table 27.1). The patient may also be observed during basic activities of daily living (BADL) such as dressing, or an IADL such as preparing a meal. The therapist observes performance and observes changes in the patient's behavior in response to cueing.
   b. The purpose of therapy is to increase awareness of the left side of the body and space. Current beliefs concerning the mechanisms underlying unilateral neglect guide the majority of treatment

approaches. Rizzolatti and Berti[129] combine the popular attentional and representational models in their premotor theory of neglect. The basis of this theory is that spatial attention is dependent on several independent neural circuits. Attention, and therefore perception of stimuli, is enhanced as a direct result of activation of motor circuits, as occurs when a person moves. Hence, activating motor circuits of the ipsilesional hemisphere (via voluntary movements of the left upper or lower limbs) may facilitate associated sensory circuits. Such movement may in turn lead to improvements in the processing of stimuli from the contralesional (left) side.[123]

5. *Treatment Suggestions.*
   a. *Remedial Approach.* Capitalizing on the rationale of the premotor theory of neglect, the following suggestions are proposed. Stimuli that are specialized for the right side of the brain, such as shapes and blocks, should be used to enhance right brain activation. At the same time, the presence of stimuli that are known to activate the left side of the brain, such as letters and numbers, should be minimized. Use of verbal instructions should be minimized. Simple verbal instructions should be used to encourage the patient to turn the head to the left to anchor his or her attention to that side of space.[126] In addition, research suggests that conducting motor activities with the left body side, such as simply clenching and unclenching the fist, can improve attention to the left body side and hemispace. Robertson et al[130] conducted a study with six individuals with hemiplegia who were asked to walk through a doorway. Each of the subject's walking trajectory (pathway) was measured, and it was found that all trajectories were significantly deviated to the right of center. The subjects were then asked to clench and unclench their left hands before, and during, walking through the doorway. The researchers found that this procedure significantly assisted subjects to center their walking trajectories. Other techniques that have been used to treat patients with unilateral neglect include eye-patching, optokinetic stimulation and prism glasses, neck vibration,[131] and trunk rotation. A review of these treatment techniques may be found in Luauté et al.[132] A review of the effectiveness of a range of these therapies is included in Box 27.1 Evidence Summary.[133-141]
   b. *Compensatory Approach.* The patient is initially educated about the condition, and then strategies to assist managing everyday activities are devised. For example, when reading a book or newspaper, a red ribbon may be placed on the left margin and the patient is taught to scan back to this point after completing each line. The environment may

also be adapted within this approach. The patient is addressed and given demonstrations from the less affected side. The nursing staff should place the patient's call button, telephone, and other essential items on the less affected side. A bold red line may be drawn on the side of the page that is neglected.[122] A mirror may be placed in front of the patient while he or she is dressing or ambulating to draw attention to the neglected side.

c. Several Cochrane reviews have been conducted concerning the effectiveness of cognitive and perceptual rehabilitation. An overview of findings from small Cochrane reviews in the areas of attention and memory rehabilitation was presented earlier. A more extensive Cochrane review[133] was conducted concerning the effectiveness of therapy for unilateral neglect, because there has been an abundance of studies and trials conducted on this puzzling disorder over the past 20 years. Box 27.1 Evidence Summary contains a summary of selected controlled trials included in the Cochrane review[133] and a small number of studies published after the review. Cochrane reviews only include controlled trials and each trial is rated (A, B, or C) on the quality of its randomization process. "A" studies are considered adequate, "B" unclear, and "C" inadequate. Of the 12 studies included in the Cochrane review, the Evidence Summary Box contains all the studies with an A classification (Fanthome et al,[134] Jacquin-Courtois et al,[135] Kalra et al,[136] and Tsang et al[137]) and two randomly selected studies rated as B (Watanabe and Amimoto[138] and Wiart et al[141]). As a result of conducting this review, Bowen and Lincoln[133] concluded that there is some evidence that cognitive rehabilitation for patients with unilateral neglect improves performance on some impairment-based tests. However, the effects of cognitive rehabilitation on reducing activity limitations are unclear. Additional well-designed RCTs and more basic research are required to develop outcome measures in the field.

Anosognosia

1. *Definition.* **Anosognosia** is a severe condition including denial and lack of awareness of the presence or severity of one's paralysis.[50] Anosognosia is defined as a lack of awareness, or denial, of a paretic extremity as belonging to the person, or a lack of insight concerning, or denial of, paralysis.[50] Presence of this disability may compromise rehabilitation potential greatly, because it limits the patient's ability to recognize the need for, and thus to use, compensatory techniques.
2. *Clinical Examples.* Typically, the patient maintains that there is nothing wrong and may disown the paralyzed limbs and refuse to accept responsibility for them. The patient may claim that the limb has a mind of its own or that it was left at home, or in a closet.
3. *Lesion Area.* The pathogenesis of anosognosia remains unclear,[50] although the region of the supramarginal gyrus has been proposed.[142]
4. *Testing.* Anosognosia is identified by talking to the patient. The patient is asked what happened to the arm or leg, whether he or she is paralyzed, how the limb feels, and why it cannot be moved. A patient with anosognosia may deny the paralysis, say that it is of no concern, and fabricate reasons why a limb does not move the way it should.
5. *Treatment Suggestions.* Anosognosia often resolves spontaneously in the first 3 months following stroke.[143] Maeshima et al[143] also noted that until the condition resolves, it seriously hampers rehabilitation. It is extremely difficult to compensate for the condition if it persists long term. Safety is of paramount importance in the treatment and discharge planning for patients suffering from anosognosia, because they typically do not acknowledge their disability and will therefore refuse to be careful.[9]

Somatoagnosia

1. *Definition.* **Somatoagnosia**, or impairment in body scheme, is a lack of awareness of the body structure and the relationship of body parts to oneself or to others. Somatoagnosia is also referred to as *autopagnosia* or simply *body agnosia*.[144] Patients with this deficit may display difficulty following instructions that require distinguishing body parts and may be unable to imitate movements of the therapist.[67] Often patients report that the more affected arm or leg feels unduly heavy. Lack of proprioception may underlie or compound this disorder.[145]
2. *Clinical Examples.* The patient may have difficulty performing transfer activities because he or she does not perceive the meaning of terms related to body parts; for example, "Pivot on your leg and reach for the armrest with your hand." In addition, a patient with a body scheme disorder will have difficulty dressing. Patients may have a hard time participating in exercises that require some body parts to be moved in relation to other body parts; for example, "Bring your arm across your chest and touch your shoulder."
3. *Lesion Area.* The lesion site is often the dominant parietal lobe.[142] Therefore, this disorder is seen primarily with right hemiplegia. However, impairment in body scheme may also occur with left hemiplegia.
4. *Testing.*
   a. The patient is requested to point to body parts named by the therapist, on himself or herself, on the therapist, and on a picture or puzzle of a human figure. Zoltan[2] provides details of these testing procedures. An example of verbal directives from these

(Text continues on page 1249)

Box 27.1 Evidence Summary   Evidence Addressing the Use of Cognitive Rehabilitation Techniques to Increase Activity in Patients with Unilateral Neglect Following Stroke

Reference	Subjects	Design/Intervention	Duration	Results	Comments
Fanthome et al[134] (1995)	Patients with recent RH stroke E = 9; C = 9 Gender (M/F): E = 6/3 C = 6/3 Time post-onset (months): E = 1.0; C = 0.6 IC = <80 years age, no history of dementia or psychiatric problems, not unwell, R handed, score > 6 on Abbreviated Mental Test, score <130 on BIT	RCT Blinded examiner E = Ss wear specially modified glasses which provide a reminder beep if patient fails to move eyes to the L in a 15-second interval C = No treatment for visual inattention	4 wk E = Treatment 2 hr 40 min/wk C = No treatment	After 4 wk, no significant difference between groups in either eye movements or BIT scores.	E and C appeared adequately matched on demographic and clinical data although C slightly older than E; no baseline BIT data.
Jacquin-Courtois et al[135] (2010)	22 Ss, 12 with RH stroke and 10 healthy Ss. IC for stroke Ss = no previous neurological damage; L neglect as detected using line cancellation, line bisection and a copy drawing task; L ear extinction; adequate hearing; R handedness. 11 Ss randomly assigned each to E or C groups. No differences between E and C Ss at baseline for age, or time between stroke and entry to the study	Random allocation of Ss to E and C but randomization not blind and not fully reported. Sought to determine if prism adaptation effects generalize to those neglect symptoms not directly linked to visuo-manual adaptation. Hence, auditory extinction was assessed in neglect Ss before and after treatment with prism glasses. E = wore prism glasses with a 10° shift to the R. C = wore neutral glasses. Outcome measures included a verbal dichotic listening task including 60 pairs of stimuli administered to the R and L ears simultaneously	E = 50 pointing responses to visual targets presented 10° to the R or L of midline lasting approximately 8 min. Dichotic listening test presented 3 times; before prisms, after prisms, and 2 hr later. C = neutral glasses and same dichotic listening test	Prism adaptation found to improve L sided auditory dichotic listening tasks immediately after prism adaptation, and when measured 2 hr later.	The findings suggest that visual adaptation may also affect performance in other sensory modalities (audition) and suggests prism adaptation may have broader treatment effects than for vision alone.

Continued

Box 27.1 Evidence Summary Evidence Addressing the Use of Cognitive Rehabilitation Techniques to Increase Activity in Patients with Unilateral Neglect Following Stroke—cont'd

Reference	Subjects	Design/Intervention	Duration	Results	Comments
Kalra et al[136] (1997)	Patients 2–14 days post-stroke with VN E = 24; C = 23 Mean age (SD): E = 78 (9) C = 76 (10) Median time post-onset: 6 days (2–14 range) EC = TIAs, reversible neurological deficits, hemianopia, or severe dysphasia	RCT (blinded examiner) E = Spatiomotor cueing based on *attentional–motor integration* model; early emphasis on restoration of function; C = Conventional therapy focusing on restoration of tone, movement pattern, and motor activity before addressing skilled functional activity	12 wk Initial baseline measures and following the 12 wk; mean therapy time = 47.7 hr	6 types of outcome data collected: (1) mortality; (2) BI; (3) discharge destination; (4) length of hospital stay; (5) duration of therapy input; and (6) RPAB (cancellation subtest and discharge home). Patients with VN have similar discharge destination despite lower BI scores (compared to patients without VN); spatiomotor cueing improves ($p < .05$) outcome in patients with VN.	Principle behind approach: Movements of affected limb in the deficit hemispace led to summation of activation of affected receptive fields of 2 distinct but linked spatial systems for personal and extrapersonal space; this resulted in improvements in attentional skills and appreciation of spatial relationships on the affected side.
Tsang et al[137] (2009)	35 Ss recruited over 6 months with 1 dropout. Gender M/F (21/13). IC = initially, clients required BIT <129, then other IC applied if R CVA on CT or MRI, with L sided neurological involvement, evidence of visual field inattention, right handed, within 8 wk post-stroke and Glasgow Coma Scale = 15. EC = severe dysphagia, transient TIA or	Single-blind RCT, with pre-test, post-test. E = 17 Ss wore R half-field eye-patching glasses throughout OT treatment. C = 17 Ss with no eye patching. All Ss measured on admission and at 4 wk	E = 4 wk of conventional OT with eye-patching, C = 4 wk of conventional OT	E group had significantly higher BIT scores compared to C at 4 wk, but no difference between group on FIM scores.	Eye patching leads to a reduction in impairment as measured on the BIT but the potential benefits in terms of function were not confirmed in this study. However, FIM may not be the best measure to pick up any functional gains. Also, power analysis revealed that a sample of 59 Ss in each group needed to show statistical significance.

Box 27.1 Evidence Summary		Evidence Addressing the Use of Cognitive Rehabilitation Techniques to Increase Activity in Patients with Unilateral Neglect Following Stroke—cont'd			
Reference	Subjects	Design/Intervention	Duration	Results	Comments
	reversible neurological deficit, significant impairment in visual acuity (e.g., as caused by cataracts); history of other neurological disease, psychiatric disorder or alcoholism. No difference at baseline between E and C for age, sex, stroke type, lesion site, time since onset, past history of stroke, and educational level.				
Watanabe and Amimoto[138] (2010)	10 Ss with unilateral neglect. IC = R-handed with R hemisphere lesion sustained within past 40 days, and capable of driving a wheelchair for 7 m (23 ft) without assistance. EC = unable to distinguish symbols due to visual impairment, who could not understand the research tasks, and if accomplishing the task would be physically difficult. Ss then further screened with Japanese edition of the BIT and were below the cutoff score in at least one of the subtests	Prospective cohort design, with staff blinded to purpose of the research. E = Ss wore fitted prism glasses, displacing Ss visual field by 7° to R. Ss then reached 50 times in front of them in quick succession with R hand for a target. Ss were then blindfolded and measured in 10 trials of pointing straight ahead, and then a wheelchair driving task. Ss timed as they drove 7 m to reach a cone target.	Same day pre-test post-test	10 Ss completed all tasks. Significant shifts between pre-test and post-test in straightening of pointing and in reaching the target faster in the wheelchair.	Findings suggest generalization of prism adaptation on both a pointing task and the ADL task of driving a wheelchair. Study would benefit from use of a control group.

Continued

Box 27.1 Evidence Summary Evidence Addressing the Use of Cognitive Rehabilitation Techniques to Increase Activity in Patients with Unilateral Neglect Following Stroke—cont'd

Reference	Subjects	Design/Intervention	Duration	Results	Comments
Serino et al[139] (2009)	20 R handed Ss with L neglect were divided into matched groups based on neglect severity. IC = scores on the BIT. EC = widespread mental deterioration using MMSE or psychiatric disorders. E = 10, C = 10. Gender (M/F): E = 8/2; C = 6/4. No differences reported between mean age (E = 62, C = 61), education, or time since stroke	Matched pairs, comparison design. Prism glasses that shifted the field of view 10° to the R were worn by Ss in E group. Neglect measured before and after each treatment and 1 month after the end of treatment. During intervention, patients repeatedly point at visual target with R index finger	E and C = 90 trials each weekday (lasting approximately 30 min) for 2 wk	Both groups improved; however, E showed statistically significant improvement over C. Effects confirmed 1 month after treatment ceased.	Design could be strengthened by random allocation to E and C with a larger sample to control for neglect severity. Further research to understand the mechanism by which prism adaptation may be working is required.
Turton et al[140] (2010)	34 Ss post-stroke with L neglect E = 16; C = 18 Mean age: E = 72; C = 71 Gender (M/F): E 8/8, C 11/7 Time post-onset (mean days): E = 45; C = 47 IC = RH stroke at least 20 days before study; self-care problems identified by OT, ability to sit and point with the unaffected hand, and ability to follow instructions	RCT E = repeated touching of target with index finger on a box screen while wearing prism glasses; glasses were 10 diopter prisms that shifted the field of view 6° to the R; C = same task while wearing neutral glasses	E and C = 90 trials each weekday (lasting approximately 30 min) for 2 wk	Data collected: 4 days after finishing treatment, at follow-up 4 wks later. Measures: the CBS and pen-and-paper tests from the BIT. E = showed increased leftward bias in pointing to targets, but no effect of treatment on BIT.	Study appeared to control for bias and compared well-matched groups. Authors suggested differences may not have shown since outcomes were measured 4 days after treatment ended, and previous literature suggests that treatment effect may be immediate and short lived. Authors also suggested that although the current study used prisms that shifted the field of view 6° to R, other studies have used 10° and 15° prisms, and research is needed to determine optimum prism strength and frequency of treatment sessions.

Box 27.1 Evidence Summary   Evidence Addressing the Use of Cognitive Rehabilitation Techniques to Increase Activity in Patients with Unilateral Neglect Following Stroke—cont'd

Reference	Subjects	Design/Intervention	Duration	Results	Comments
Wiart et al[141] (1997)	22 patients post-stroke with severe L neglect (positive findings for neglect on 3 tests); E = 11; C = 11 Mean age: E = 66; C = 72 Gender (M/F): E 6/5, C 6/5 Time post-onset (mean days): E = 35; C = 30 EC = history of stroke; alteration of general status; cognitive difficulties incompatible with rehabilitation	RCT E = experimental treatment is Bon Saint Come (one of the author's) method; thoracolumbar vest worn with attached metal pointer above head; patient points to target on mobile panel; audible and luminous signals provide biofeedback when targets are touched; therapist participates actively during the session, stimulating, guiding, and correcting; C = 3–4 hr traditional rehabilitation per day	E = 1 hr/day (20 days) of experimental treatment followed by traditional rehabilitation (physical therapy for 1–2 hr and 1 hr of occupational therapy); C = 3–4 hr of traditional rehabilitation per day	Two types of outcome data collected: (1) quantitative scoring of neglect (line bisection, line cancellation, bell cancellation); (2) autonomy (FIM). Data collected: day 0, day 30 (after therapy), and day 60. All quantitative and FIM scores improved significantly more in E than in C.	E was younger and had a higher initial FIM score than the C; C had more, but not significantly so, omissions on line cancellation (C = 16; E = 14) and R deviations on line bisection (C = 53%; E = 50%) at baseline compared with E; the Bon Saint Come method shows promise and should be further tested.

BI = Barthel Index; BIT = Behavioural Inattention Test; C = control group; CBS = Catherine Bergego Scale; CT = computed tomography; CVA = cerebrovascular accident; E = experimental group; EC = exclusion criteria; FIM = Functional Independence Measure; HFVS = Harrington Flocks Visual Field Screener; HHA = homonymous hemianopia; IC = inclusion criteria; L = left; MMSE = Mini-Mental Status Examination; MRI = magnetic resonance imaging; MVPT = Motor-Free Visual Perceptual Test; OT = occupational therapist/therapy; R = right; RCT = randomized controlled trial; ReyCFT = Rey Complex Figure Test; RH = right hemisphere; RPAB = Rivermead Perceptual Assessment Battery; S, Ss = subject, subjects; TIA = transient ischemic attack; UK = United Kingdom; VN = visual neglect; WAIS-R = Wechsler Adult Intelligence Scale—Revised.

tests is, "Show me your feet. Show me your chin. Point to your back." The words "right" and "left" should not be used because they may lead to an inaccurate diagnosis in patients who have difficulty with right–left discrimination. Aphasia should be ruled out as a cause of poor performance.

b. The patient is asked to imitate movements of the therapist. For example, the therapist touches his or her cheek, arm, leg, and so forth. A mirror-image response is acceptable.[2]

c. The patient is requested to answer questions about the relationship of body parts. For example, "Are your knees below your head? Which is on top of your head, your hair or your feet?" For patients with aphasia, questions should be phrased to require a yes or no, or true or false response. Patients with intact function in this area should respond correctly most of the time and within a reasonable period of time. Those patients with receptive aphasia are particularly likely to do poorly on tests for somatagnosia.[144]

5. *Treatment Suggestions.* Using a remedial approach, the therapist aims for the patient to associate sen-

sory input with an adaptive motor response.[2] Facilitation of body awareness is accomplished through sensory stimulation to the body part affected. For example, the patient is asked to rub the appropriate body part with a rough cloth as the therapist names it or points to it.[22] Alternatively, the patient verbally identifies body parts, or points to pictures of them as the therapist touches them.

Right–Left Discrimination

1. *Definition.* A **right–left discrimination disorder** is the inability to identify the right and left sides of one's own body or of that of the examiner.[125] This includes the inability to execute movements in response to verbal commands that include the terms "right" and "left." Patients are often unable to imitate movements.[125]

2. *Clinical Examples.* The patient cannot tell the therapist which is the right arm and which is the left. The right shoe cannot be discerned from the left shoe, and the patient is unable to follow instructions using the concept of right–left, such as "turn right at the corner." The patient cannot

distinguish the right from the left side of the therapist.

3. *Lesion Area.* The lesion site is the parietal lobe of either hemisphere.[125] A close relationship between aphasia (usually owing to left hemisphere damage) and deficits in right–left discrimination has been reported. In patients without aphasia (usually those with right hemisphere damage), a relationship has been reported between general mental impairment and right–left discrimination disorder.[144]

4. *Testing.* The patient is asked to point to body parts on command, such as right ear, left foot, right arm, and so forth. Six responses should be elicited on either the patient's own body, on that of the therapist, or on a model or picture of the human body.[144] To rule out somatoagnosia, the patient should be tested first without using the words "right" and "left."

5. *Treatment Suggestions.* If using a compensatory approach, when giving instructions to the patient, the words "right" and "left" should be avoided. Instead, pointing or providing cues using distinguishing features of the limb may be more effective (e.g., "the arm with the watch"). These guidelines are particularly salient for the therapist teaching locomotion or transfers, where confusing instructions may have dangerous consequences. The right side of all common objects such as shoes and clothing should be marked with red tape or seam binding.

Finger Agnosia

1. *Definition.* **Finger agnosia** can be defined as the inability to identify the fingers of one's own hands or of the hands of the examiner.[125]

2. *Clinical Examples.* The disorder is characterized by difficulty in naming the fingers on command, identifying which finger was touched, and, by some definitions, mimicking finger movements. This deficit usually occurs bilaterally and is more common in the middle three fingers.[146] Finger agnosia correlates highly with poor dexterity in tasks that require movements of individual fingers in relation to each other,[1] such as buttoning, tying laces, and typing.

3. *Lesion Area.* Finger agnosia may be the result of a lesion located in either parietal lobe,[147] often in the region of the angular gyrus of the left hemisphere. It is often found in conjunction with an aphasic disorder,[144] or with general mental impairment.[125,144] Bilateral finger agnosia along with right–left discrimination problems, **agraphia**, and *acalculia* is termed *Gerstmann's syndrome.*[125] Gerstmann's syndrome usually is associated with a focal lesion of the dominant hemisphere in the region of the angular gyrus.[142]

4. *Testing.* A portion of *Sauguet's test*[2,144] is recommended. Sauguet's test includes asking the patient to move or point to his or her finger when named by the therapist to determine if finger agnosia is

present. Between five and ten commands from the therapist is adequate. The test is not standardized.

a. The patient is asked to name the fingers touched by the therapist, with the eyes open (five times) and if successful, with vision occluded (five times).

b. The patient is asked to point to the fingers named by the therapist on the patient's own hands (10 times), on the therapist's hands (10 times), and on a schematic model (10 times).

c. The patient is asked to point to the equivalent finger on a life-sized picture when the therapist touches each finger.

d. The patient is asked to imitate finger movements; for example, curl the index finger, touch the thumb to the middle finger.

5. *Treatment Suggestions.* There is very limited evidence to support the efficacy of treatment techniques for finger agnosia. When using a remedial approach, the patient's discriminative tactile systems (touch and pressure) are stimulated. A rough cloth can be used to rub the dorsal surface of the more affected arm, hand, and fingers, and the ventral surface of the more affected fingers. Pressure can be applied to the ventral surface of the hand. For additional details the reader is referred to Zoltan.[2]

Spatial Relations Disorders (Complex Perception)

Spatial relations disorders encompass a constellation of impairments that have in common a difficulty in perceiving the relationship between the self and two or more objects.[148] Research suggests that the right parietal lobe plays a primary role in space perception. Thus, a spatial relations impairment most frequently occurs in patients with right-sided lesions with resulting left hemiparesis.[148]

Spatial relations disorders include impairments of figure–ground discrimination, form discrimination, spatial relations, position in space, and topographical disorientation. Additional visuospatial impairments, such as depth and distance perception and vertical disorientation, will also be discussed in this section. In a study comparing the effectiveness of the cognitive remediation (sometimes referred to as the *transfer-of-training technique*) versus the functional approach, Edmans et al[149] found that both approaches were equally successful in treating perceptual impairments. However, since this study did not control for the effects of spontaneous recovery in both groups, further research is required.

Figure–Ground Discrimination

1. *Definition.* An impairment in visual figure–ground discrimination is the inability to visually distinguish a figure from the background in which it is embedded.[5] Functionally, it interferes with the patient's ability to locate important objects that are not prominent in a visual array. The patient has difficulty ignoring irrelevant visual stimuli and cannot

select the appropriate cue to which to respond.[5] This may lead to distractibility, resulting in a shortened attention span,[150] frustration, and decreased independent and safe functioning.[67]

2. *Clinical Examples.* The patient cannot locate items in a pocketbook or drawer, locate buttons on a shirt, or distinguish the armhole from the remainder of a solid-colored shirt. The patient may not be able to tell when one step ends and another begins on a flight of stairs, especially when descending.

3. *Lesion Area.* Parieto-occipital lesions of the right hemisphere and less frequently the left hemisphere commonly produce this disorder.[151]

4. *Testing.*

   a. The *Ayres Figure–Ground Test* (subtest of the *Southern California Sensory Integration Tests*)[152] requires the subject to distinguish the three objects in an embedded test picture, from a possible selection of six items. This test was standardized on children but may be useful as a clinical tool in identifying perceptual disorders in adults with brain damage.[4] Normative data have been generated for normal adult males.[153] Many other tests have since used a similar approach to test figure–ground perception by showing the patient overlapping line drawings of everyday objects and asking clients to name these as illustrated in Figure 27.10.

   b. *Function-based Tests.* A white towel can be placed on a white sheet, and the patient is asked to find the towel. The patient can be asked to point out the sleeve, buttons, and collar of a white shirt, or to pick out a spoon from an unsorted array of eating utensils. It is necessary to rule out poor eyesight, hemianopia, visual agnosia, and poor

comprehension to improve the validity of these testing techniques.

5. *Treatment Suggestions.*

   a. *Remedial Approach.* The therapist should arrange for practice in visually locating objects in a simple array (such as three very different objects), and progress to more difficult ones (four or five dissimilar objects and three similar ones).

   b. *Compensatory Approach.* The patient is taught to become aware of the existence and nature of the deficit. The patient should be cautioned to examine groups of objects slowly and systematically and should be instructed to use other, intact senses (e.g., touch) when searching for items such as clothing or silverware. When learning to lock a wheelchair, the patient should be advised to locate the brake levers by touch rather than by searching for them visually. Red tape may be placed over the hook-and-loop closure of the shoe or orthosis to aid the patient in locating it. Few items should be placed in the patient's drawers or nightstand, and they should be replaced in the same location each time. Brightly colored tape can be used to mark the edges on stairs. Repetition is a key element of this approach and repeated practice is used in each specific area of difficulty. The same procedure should be employed during each practice session, incorporating verbal cues and touch as adjuncts to vision.

Form Discrimination

1. *Definition.* Impairment in **form discrimination** is the inability to perceive or attend to subtle differences in form and shape. The patient is likely to confuse objects of similar shape or not to recognize an object placed in an unusual position.

2. *Clinical Examples.* The patient may confuse a pen with a toothbrush, a vase with a water pitcher, a cane with a crutch, and so forth.

3. *Lesion Area.* The lesion site is the parieto-temporo-occipital region (posterior association areas) of the nondominant lobe.[4]

4. *Testing.* A number of items similar in shape and different in size are gathered. The patient is asked to identify them. One set of items might be a pencil, pen, straw, toothbrush, and watch, and the other might be a key, paper clip, coins, and ring. Each object is presented several times in different positions (e.g., upside down). Visual object agnosia must be ruled out as a cause for poor performance by first presenting objects separately and asking the patient to identify them or to demonstrate how they are used (see Visual Agnosias below).

5. *Treatment Suggestions.*

   a. *Remedial Approach.* The patient should practice describing, identifying, and demonstrating the use of similarly shaped and sized objects. The

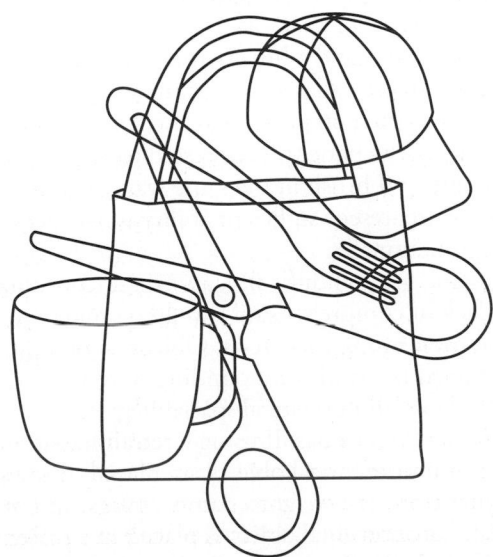

Figure 27.10 An example of a figure–ground perception test.

patient should sort like objects and should be assisted to focus on differentiating object cues.

b. *Compensatory Approach.* The patient must be made aware of the specific deficit. If the patient can read, frequently used and confused objects can be labeled. The patient should be encouraged to use vision, touch, and self-verbalization in combination when objects are confused.

Spatial Relations

1. *Definition.* A **spatial relations disorder**, or spatial disorientation, is the inability to perceive the relationship of one object in space to another object, or to oneself. This may lead to, or compound, problems in constructional tasks and dressing.[5] Crossing the midline may be a problem for patients with spatial relations deficits.[148] Spatial relations skills are required to manage most ADL.

2. *Clinical Examples.* The patient might find it difficult to place the cutlery, plate, and spoon in the proper position when setting the table. The patient may be unable to tell the time from a clock because of difficulty in perceiving the relative positions of the hands.[2,29] The patient may have difficulty learning to position his or her arms, legs, and trunk in relation to the wheelchair to prepare for transferring.

3. *Lesion Area.* The lesion site is predominantly the inferior parietal lobe or parieto-occipital-temporal junction, usually of the right side.[5] Arnadottir and Gudrun[148] explain how a patient with perceptual deficits may have difficulty putting on a shirt. This is illustrated in Figure 27.11. Since the CNS works in a holistic way, the task of putting on a shirt requires visual, tactile, and auditory information as well as attentional and memory capacities and motor output. Figure 27.11 suggests that while damage in a variety of brain areas may affect visuospatial processing, the most common lesion site is the right inferior parietal lobe.

4. *Testing.* Recommended tests include the *Rivermead Perceptual Assessment Battery (RPAB)*[79] and the *Arnadottir OT-ADL Neurobehavioural Evaluation (A-ONE).*[5] To improve the validity of these tests, unilateral neglect and hemianopia should be ruled out as the causes of poor performance. If these impairments are present, the stimulus array should be positioned appropriately.

5. *Treatment Suggestions.* When using a remedial approach, patient ability to orient to other objects can be improved by giving the patient instructions to position himself or herself in relation to the therapist or another object. The therapist might say, "Sit next to me," "Go behind the table," or "Step over the line." In addition, the therapist can set up a maze of furniture (obstacle course). Having the patient copy block or matchstick designs of increasing difficulty will increase awareness of the relationship between one object (block or matchstick) and the next. If the patient avoids crossing the midline, activities that require crossing the midline both motorically and visually can be incorporated into other therapeutic activities (e.g., proprioceptive neuromuscular facilitation [PNF] chop patterns). One specific activity is to have the patient hold a dowel in front with both hands. The therapist guides it from the less involved side to the more involved side. Later, the patient can progress to manipulating the dowel with only verbal or visual cues, and finally to guiding it independently.[154]

Position in Space

1. *Definition.* **Position in space impairment** is the inability to perceive and to interpret spatial concepts such as up, down, under, over, in, out, in front of, and behind.

2. *Clinical Examples.* If a patient is asked to raise the arm "above" the head during ROM activities or is asked to place the feet "on" the footrests, the patient may behave as if he or she does not know what to do.

3. *Lesion Area.* The lesion is usually located in the nondominant parietal lobe.[151]

4. *Testing.* To test function, two objects are used, such as a shoe and a shoebox. The patient is asked to place the shoe in different positions in relation to the shoebox; for example, in the box, on top of the box, or next to the box. Alternatively, the patient is presented with two objects and asked to describe their relationship. For example, a toothbrush can be placed in a cup, under a cup, and so forth, and the patient is then asked to indicate the location of the toothbrush.

Another mode of testing is to have the patient copy the therapist's manipulations with an identical set of objects. For example, the therapist hands the patient a comb and a brush. The therapist then takes an identical set and places them in a particular relationship to each other, such as the comb on top of the brush. The patient is requested to arrange his or her comb and brush in the same way. Success in this task may represent sufficient ability to use position in space functionally.

Figure–ground difficulty, apraxia, incoordination, and lack of comprehension should be ruled out when performing these tests. Objects should be positioned to avoid compounding of results with hemianopia and unilateral spatial neglect.

5. *Treatment Suggestions.* If using a retraining approach, three or four identical objects are placed in the same orientation (wrist weights, combs, mugs, and so forth). An additional object is placed in a different orientation. The patient is asked to identify the odd one, and then to place it in the same orientation as the other objects.

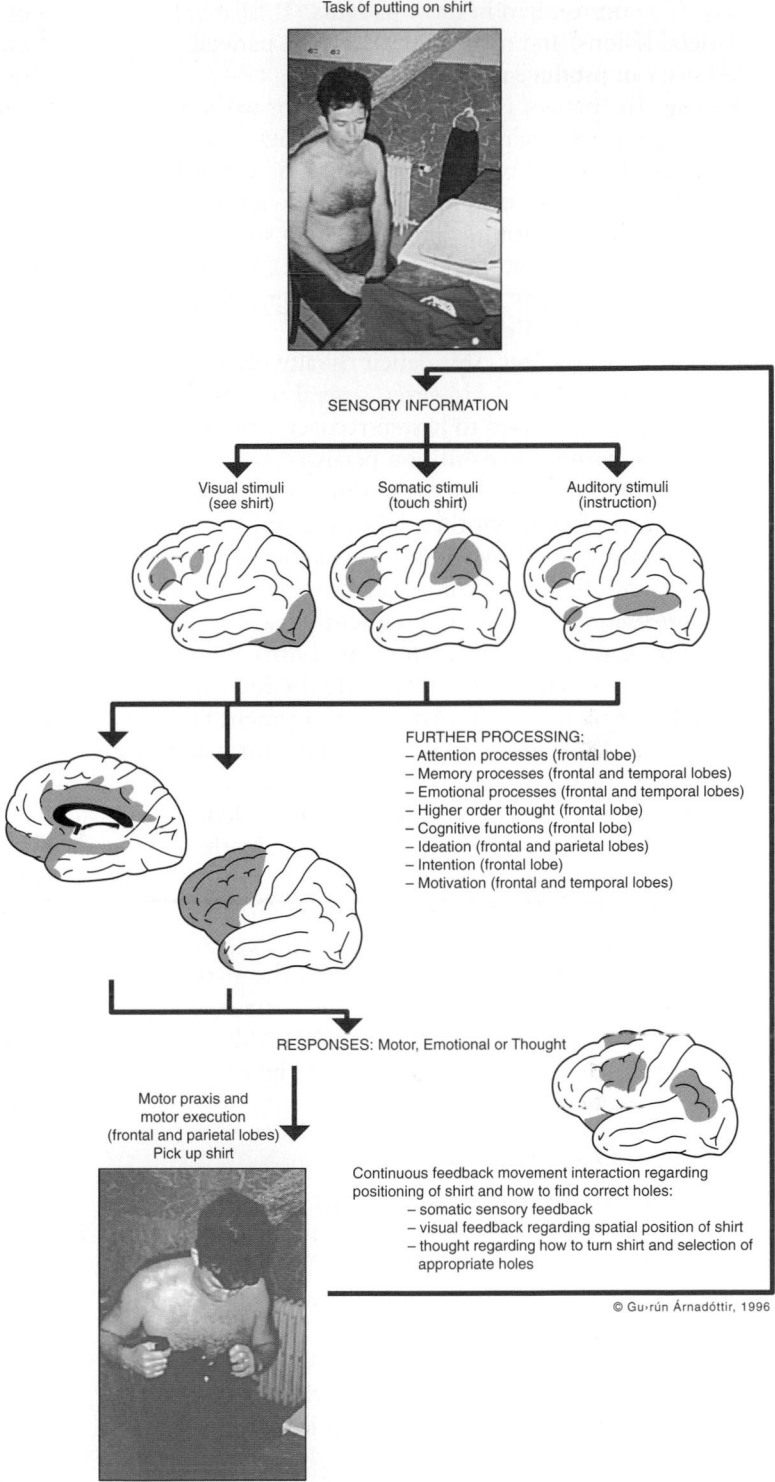

Figure 27.11 Spatial relation processing as a man puts on a shirt. *From Arnadottir and Gudrun,[148, p. 405] with permission.*

Topographical Disorientation

1. *Definition.* Topographical disorientation refers to difficulty in understanding and remembering the relationship of one location to another.[155] As a result, the patient is unable to get from one place to another, with or without a map. This disorder is frequently seen in conjunction with other difficulties in spatial relations.[45]

2. *Clinical Examples.* The patient cannot find the way from his or her room to the physical therapy clinic, despite being shown repeatedly. The patient cannot describe the spatial characteristics of familiar surroundings, such as the layout of his or her bedroom at home.[151]

3. *Lesion Areas.* The majority of cases involve damage to the right retrosplenial cortex, with Brodmann's

area 30 compromised in most patients.[155] Bilateral parietal lesions, and more rarely, left-side parietal lesions, can produce this problem.[151]

4. *Testing.* The patient is asked to describe or to draw a familiar route, such as the block on which he or she lives, the layout of his or her house, or a major neighborhood intersection.[145] A patient with topographical disorientation will be unable to succeed in this task. However, the therapist must differentiate between memory problems and topographical orientation difficulties.

5. *Treatment Suggestions.* This deficit usually resolves 8 weeks after onset.[155] However, several treatment techniques can be used to hasten recovery, or to assist long term if the condition persists.
   a. *Remedial Approach.* The patient practices going from one place to another, following verbal instructions. Initially, simple routes should be used, and then more complicated ones.[2]
   b. *Compensatory Approach.* Frequently traveled routes can be marked with colored dots. The spaces between the dots are gradually increased and eventually eliminated as improvement takes place.[2] This is an example of taking a normally right-hemisphere task and (because there is right-sided damage) converting it into a left-hemisphere task. In this instance we take the spatial task of remembering routes (right-hemisphere task) and substitute sequential landmarks (sequencing is typically a left-hemisphere strength) to accomplish the goal of getting from place to place. The patient should be reminded not to leave the clinic, room, or home unattended, because he or she may get lost.

Depth and Distance Perception

1. *Definition.* The patient with a disorder of depth and distance perception experiences inaccurate judgment of direction, distance, and depth. Spatial disorientation may be a contributing factor in faulty distance perception.

2. *Clinical Examples.* The patient may have difficulty navigating stairs, may miss the chair when attempting to sit, or may continue pouring juice once a glass is filled.[150]

3. *Lesion Areas.* This impairment may occur with a lesion in the posterior right hemisphere in the superior visual association cortices; it may be evident with right-sided or bilateral lesions.[151]

4. *Testing.*
   a. For a functional test of distance perception, the patient is asked to take or to grasp an object that has been placed on a table. The object may also be held in front of the patient, in the air, and the patient is again asked to grasp it. The patient with impaired distance perception will overshoot

or undershoot.[2] However, the movements look purposeful and smooth, which distinguishes this problem from a coordination deficit.
   b. To determine depth perception functionally, the patient can be asked to fill a glass of water.[2] A patient with a depth perception deficit may continue pouring once the glass is filled.

5. *Treatment Suggestions.* The patient should be assisted in becoming aware of the deficit (education to increase cognitive awareness). Emphasis should be placed on the importance of walking carefully on uneven surfaces, particularly the stairs.
   a. *Remedial Approach.* The patient is requested to place the feet on designated spots during gait training.[55] Also, blocks can be arranged in piles 2 to 8 in (5 to 8 cm) high. The patient is asked to touch the top of the piles with the foot. This is done to reestablish a sense of depth and distance.[154]
   b. *Compensatory Approach.* Practice in compensating for disturbances in depth and distance perception occurs intrinsically in many ADL skills, both those involving moving through space and those that involve manipulation. For example, the patient can hold the armrests of a chair to assist with sitting squarely.

Vertical Disorientation

1. *Definition.* **Vertical disorientation** refers to a distorted perception of what is vertical. Displacement of the vertical position can contribute to disturbance of motor performance, both in posture and in gait. Early in recovery, most patients post-CVA demonstrate some impairment in the sense of verticality.[156] This is not associated with or affected by the presence of homonymous hemianopia.[67] Scores on one test for visual perception of the vertical position were found to correlate with differences in walking ability.[67]

2. *Clinical Example.* A person with distorted verticality views the world differently and this may affect upright posture as depicted in Figure 27.12.

3. *Lesion Area.* The lesion site is in the nondominant parietal lobe.

4. *Testing.* The therapist holds a cane vertically and then turns it sideways to a horizontal plane. Researchers use a luminous rod with patients seated in a darkened room.[156] The patient is handed the cane and asked to turn it back to the original position. If the patient's perception of the vertical position is distorted, the cane will most likely be placed at an angle, representing the patient's conception of the world around himself or herself.

5. *Treatment Suggestions.* The patient must be made aware of the deficit. The patient should be instructed to compensate by using touch (tactile cues) for proper self-orientation, especially when going through doorways, in and out of elevators, and on the stairs.

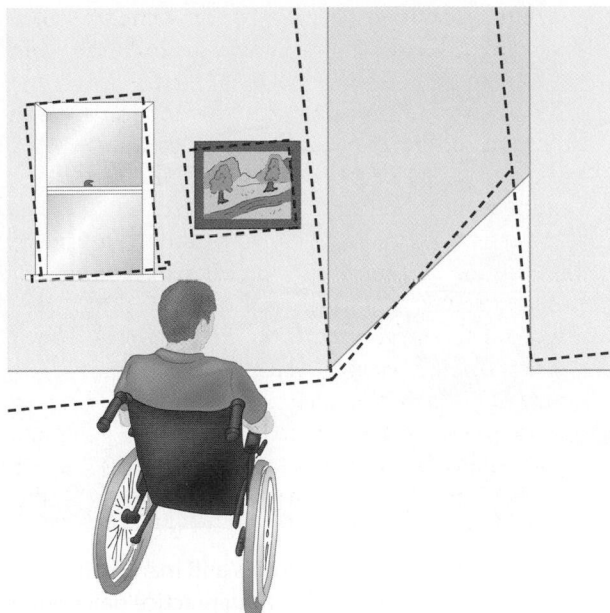

Figure 27.12 Vertical disorientation may contribute to disturbances of posture and gait.

Agnosias (Simple Perception)

Agnosia is the inability to recognize or make sense of incoming information despite intact sensory capacities. Although this condition is relatively rare (as listed by the National Institutes of Health Office of Rare Diseases), it can affect any sensory modality (e.g., vision, audition, touch, taste) and anything (e.g., faces, sounds, colors, familiar or less familiar objects). Although there is an inability to recognize familiar objects using one or two of the sensory modalities, the ability to recognize the same object using other sensory modalities is usually present.[142,157]

Visual Agnosias

1. *Definition.* **Visual object agnosia** is the most common form of agnosia.[4] It is defined as the inability to recognize familiar objects despite normal function of the eyes and optic tracts.[157]

2. *Clinical Examples.* One remarkable aspect of this disorder is the readiness with which the patient can identify an object once it is handled (i.e., information is received from another sensory modality).[158] The patient may not recognize people, possessions, and common objects. Specific types of visual agnosia include **simultanagnosia**, **prosopagnosia**, and color agnosia.

   a. *Simultanagnosia,* also known as Balint's syndrome,[4] is the inability to perceive a visual stimulus as a whole. The patient perceives an entire array one part at a time. The lesion is usually in the dominant occipital lobe.

   b. *Prosopagnosia* was traditionally considered to be the inability to recognize familiar faces. Current thought suggests this phenomenon is related to any visually ambiguous stimulus, the recognition of which depends on evoking a memory context, such as different species of birds or different makes of cars. Prosopagnosia is usually accompanied by visual field impairments. Bilaterally symmetrical occipital lesions are thought to be responsible for this impairment.[15,50,159]

   c. *Color agnosia* is the inability to recognize colors; it is not color blindness. The patient is unable to identify or name colors on command, although color chips can be correctly paired.[50] However, the meaning of color is lost so that the patient no longer associates a duckling as yellow or the sea as blue.[157] Color agnosia is frequently associated with facial or other visual object agnosias.[4,151] It is usually the result of a dominant hemisphere lesion.[4] The simultaneous occurrence of left-sided hemianopia, alexia (inability to read; word blindness), and color agnosia is a classic occipital lobe syndrome.[4]

3. *Lesion Area.* The lesions associated with visual object agnosias are thought to occur in the occipito-temporo-parietal association areas of either hemisphere. These areas are responsible for the integration of visual stimuli with respect to memory.[142] Recent evidence suggests visual object agnosias may result from damage in the medial structures of the ventral occipito-temporal cortex.[160]

4. *Testing.* To test for this deficit, several common objects are placed in front of the patient. The patient is asked to name the objects, to point to an object named by the therapist, or to demonstrate its use. It is important to rule out aphasia and apraxia, although this is not easily done. Details of other nonstandardized and standardized testing procedures are provided in Laver and Unsworth.[157]

5. *Treatment Suggestions.*

   a. *Remedial Approach.* Drills can be used to practice discrimination between faces that are important to the patient (using photographs) and discrimination between colors and common objects. The therapist should assist the patient in picking out salient visual cues for relating names to faces.

      Note: Another tool for treating visual agnosia, as well as many other cognitive and perceptual deficits, is the Easy Street Environment®. These environments have been incorporated into rehabilitation centers in the United States for almost 20 years. The Easy Street Environment® is a modular "world" of life-size streets (with a variety of ambulation surfaces, stairs, curbs, and so forth), vehicles, shops, and offices, which are constructed in a dedicated area within the rehabilitation setting. The Easy Street Environment® has many advantages since it allows occupational therapists, physical therapists, and speech-language pathologists to work with a patient in a safe, private, and comfortable environment where the patient can try out relearned or new skills. The therapist can also save considerable time by taking the patient down the corridor to the Easy Street Environment® rather than to their own local community, although ultimately such an outing to the local community may be undertaken. Figure 27.13 shows a patient with a visual object agnosia learning to use the Easy Street Environment® Automatic Teller Machine (ATM). This patient may also learn new strategies to identify groceries and therefore be able to practice shopping in the Easy Street Environment® Market Place (Fig. 27.14). Behrmann et al[161] have also presented a case study of a 24-year-old male and reported that the patient improved in identifying novel and common objects through recognition training. Positive results were not found for face identification.

   b. *Compensatory Approach.* The patient is instructed to use intact sensory modalities, such as touch or audition, to distinguish people and objects.

Auditory Agnosia

1. *Definition.* **Auditory agnosia** refers to the inability to recognize nonspeech sounds or to discriminate between them. This rarely occurs in the absence of other communication disorders.[4]
2. *Clinical Examples.* The patient with auditory agnosia cannot tell, for example, the difference between the ring of a doorbell and that of a telephone, or between a dog barking and thunder.
3. *Lesion Area.* The lesion is located in the dominant temporal lobe.[4]
4. *Testing.* Testing is usually carried out by a speech-language pathologist. The patient is asked to close

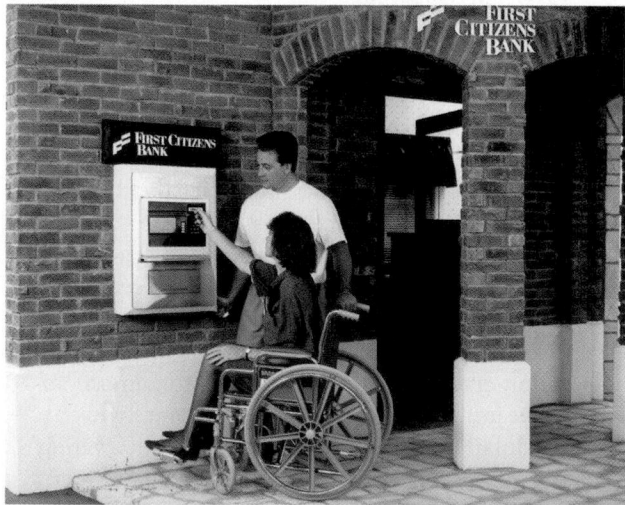

Figure 27.13 A client with an agnosia learns to use an ATM with help from a therapist in the Easy Street Environment®. *Courtesy of Easy Street Environments,® Scottsdale, AZ 85260.*

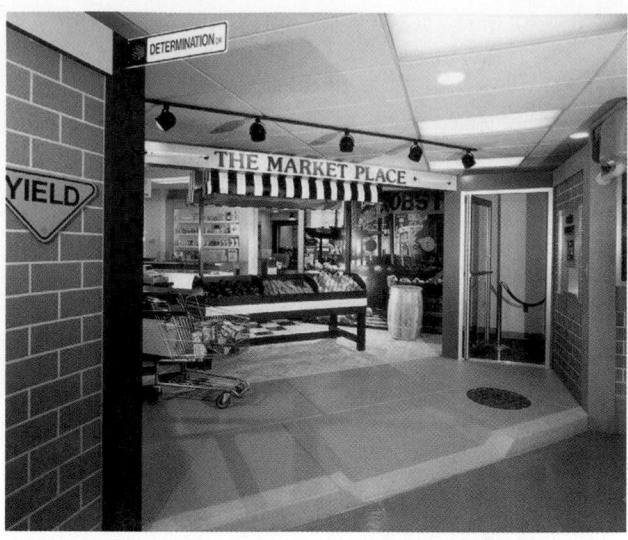

Figure 27.14 Clients with agnosias and many other cognitive and perceptual deficits can practice daily living skills in the controlled Easy Street Environment® such as provided in the Market Store. *Courtesy of Easy Street Environments,® Scottsdale, AZ 85260.*

the eyes and to identify the source of various sounds. The therapist rings a bell, honks a horn, rings a telephone, and so forth, and asks the patient to identify the sound (verbally or by pointing to a picture).
5. *Treatment Suggestions.* Treatment generally consists of drilling the patient on sounds, but this has not been found to be particularly effective.[1,2]

Tactile Agnosia or Astereognosis

1. *Definition.* Tactile agnosia, or *astereognosis,* is the inability to recognize forms by handling them, although tactile, proprioceptive, and thermal sensations may be intact. This impairment commonly causes difficulties in ADL skills, inasmuch as many self-care activities that are normally done in the absence of constant visual monitoring require the manipulation of objects. If tactile agnosia is present in combination with unilateral neglect or other sensory loss, performance in ADL skills may be severely hampered.[67]
2. *Clinical Examples.* If a patient is handed a familiar object (key, comb, safety pin) with vision occluded, the patient will fail to recognize it.
3. *Lesion Area.* The lesion is in the parieto-temporo-occipital lobe (posterior association areas) of either hemisphere.[4]
4. *Testing.* The patient is asked to identify objects placed in the hand by examining them manually without visual cues.
5. *Treatment Suggestions.*
   a. *Remedial Approach.* The patient practices feeling various common objects, shapes, and textures with vision occluded. The patient is instructed to

immediately look at the object for visual feedback and note special characteristics of the object.

b. *Compensatory Approach.* To improve cognitive awareness, the patient is educated concerning the nature of the deficit and is instructed in visual compensation.

Apraxia

Apraxia is an impairment of voluntary skilled learned movement. It is characterized by an inability to perform purposeful movements, which cannot be accounted for by inadequate strength, loss of coordination, impaired sensation, attentional difficulties, abnormal tone, movement disorders, intellectual deterioration, poor comprehension, or uncooperativeness.[162-164] Many patients with apraxia also present with aphasia, and the two deficits are sometimes difficult to distinguish.[4] Donkervoot et al[165] report the prevalence of apraxia among patients with first left hemisphere stroke in rehabilitation as around 28%. The two main forms of apraxia discussed in the literature are *ideomotor* and *ideational apraxia.* Ideomotor and ideational apraxias are generally thought to be the result of dominant hemisphere lesions and may be particularly difficult to test in the patient with aphasia. Although aphasia and apraxia often occur together, there is not a strong correlation between the severity of the aphasia and the severity of the apraxia. A third form of apraxia, *buccofacial apraxia,* is actually a type of ideomotor apraxia and is characterized by difficulties with performing the purposeful movements that involve facial muscles related to the mouth. This may include responding to the command "pretend to blow out a candle," or producing an orderly sequence of phonemes to produce speech. Hence, apraxia is a disorder of skilled movement and not a language disorder.[50] Some rehabilitation texts also describe constructional and dressing apraxias. However, it is generally believed that these are not true apraxias, but rather are difficulties in the application of cognitive and perceptual skill to these tasks. In other words, they are terms used to describe specific difficulties with a construction or drawing task or dressing. Both these problems are more frequently associated with right hemisphere lesions.[166]

Ideomotor Apraxia

1. *Definition.* Ideomotor apraxia refers to a breakdown between concept and performance. There is a disconnection between the idea of a movement and its motor execution. It appears that the information cannot be transferred from the areas of the brain that conceptualize to the centers for motor execution. Thus, the patient with ideomotor apraxia is able to carry out habitual tasks automatically and describe how they are done but is unable to imitate gestures or perform on command.[167,168] Patients with this form of apraxia often **perseverate;**[142] that is, they repeat an activity or a segment of a task over and over, even if it is no longer necessary or

appropriate. This makes it difficult for them to finish one task and go on to the next. Patients with ideomotor apraxia appear most impaired when requested to perform tasks that require use of many implements and that have many steps. This form of apraxia can be demonstrated separately in the facial areas, upper extremity (UE), lower extremity (LE), and for total body movements.[169] Patients with apraxia are often observed to be clumsy in their actual handling of objects. Impairment is often suspected when observing the patient during ADL or during a routine motor examination.

2. *Clinical Examples.* Several examples of ideomotor apraxia follow. The patient is unable to "blow" on command. However, if presented with a bubble wand, the patient will spontaneously blow bubbles. The patient may fail to walk if requested to in a traditional manner. However, if a cup of coffee is placed on a table at the other end of the room and the patient is told, "Please have coffee," the patient is likely to traverse the room to get it.[145] A male patient is asked to comb his hair. He may be able to identify the comb and even tell you what it is used for; however, he will not actually use the comb appropriately when it is handed to him. Despite this observation in the clinic, his wife reports that he combs his hair spontaneously every morning. A female patient is asked to squeeze a dynamometer. She appears not to know what to do with it, although her comprehension is adequate, the task has just been demonstrated, and it is clear that she has adequate strength.

3. *Lesion Area.* Apraxia results most frequently from lesions in the left, dominant hemisphere. There is evidence that both frontal lesions and posterior parietal lesions can result in apraxia.[170]

4. *Testing.* The *Goodglass and Kaplan*[169] test for apraxia is composed of universally known movements, such as blowing, brushing teeth, hammering, shaving, and so forth. It is based on what the authors consider a hierarchy of difficulty for patients with apraxia. First the patient is asked, "Show me how you would bang a nail with a hammer." If the patient fails to do this or uses his or her fist as if it were a hammer, the patient is told, "Pretend to hold the hammer." If the patient fails following this instruction, the therapist demonstrates the act and asks the patient to imitate it. The patient with apraxia typically will not improve after demonstration but will improve with use of the actual implements.[4] The ability to correct oneself on following verbal cueing is considered not indicative of apraxia. Additional apraxia tests may be found in Butler[166] and the work of van Heugten et al,[171] who have adapted the Arnadottir OT-ADL Neurobehavioural Evaluation (A-ONE)[5] as an observational method of testing for apraxia.

5. *Treatment Suggestions.*
   a. *Remedial Approach.* In the remediation of apraxias, it is advised that the therapist speak slowly and use the shortest possible sentences. One command should be given at a time, and the second command should not be given until the first task is completed. When teaching a new task, it should be broken down into its component parts. One component is taught at a time, physically guiding the patient through the task if necessary. It should be completed in precisely the same manner each time.[166] When all the individual units are mastered, an attempt to combine them should be made. A great deal of repetition may be necessary.[67] Family members must be advised to use the exact approach found to be successful in the clinic. Performing activities in as normal an environment as possible is also helpful. Butler[166] provides a case example of a young woman relearning how to drink from a cup using this technique. Using the sensorimotor approach, multiple sensory inputs are used on the affected body parts to enhance the production of appropriate motor responses. The reader is referred to the work of Okoye[172] for additional details on this approach.
   b. *Compensatory Approach.* Donkervoot et al[173] report an RCT that showed the effectiveness of an occupational therapy treatment program including "strategy training" over regular occupational therapy. Strategy training involves teaching the patient compensatory techniques to overcome the apraxia such as use of pictures in the correct sequence to support ADL skills. This approach has been developed further and is now widely used to help patients overcome apraxia. Further studies to support this approach have also come from a group of occupational therapists in the Netherlands and include trials by Donkervoort et al[174] and Geusgens and colleagues.[175,176]

Ideational Apraxia

1. *Definition.* Ideational apraxia is a failure in the conceptualization of the task. It is an inability to perform a purposeful motor act, either automatically or on command, because the patient no longer understands the overall concept of the act, cannot retain the idea of the task, or cannot formulate the motor patterns required. Often the patient can perform isolated components of a task but cannot combine them into a complete act. Furthermore, the patient cannot verbally describe the process of performing an activity, describe the function of objects, or use them appropriately.[177,178]
2. *Clinical Examples.* When presented in the clinic with a toothbrush and toothpaste and told to brush the teeth, the patient may put the tube of toothpaste in the mouth, or try to put toothpaste on the toothbrush without removing the cap. Further, the patient may be unable to describe verbally how tooth brushing is done. Similar phenomena may be evident in all aspects of ADL (washing, meal preparation, and so forth) and so may limit the safety and potential independence of the patient.[5] It has been shown that patients with ideational apraxia who test poorly in the clinical situation appear more able to perform ADL skills at the appropriate time and in a familiar setting.[172]
3. *Lesion Area.* The lesion causing ideational apraxia is thought to be in the dominant parietal lobe. This deficit also may be seen in conjunction with diffuse brain damage, such as cerebral arteriosclerosis.[142]
4. *Testing.* The tests for ideational apraxia are similar to those for ideomotor apraxia. The major expected response difference is that the patient with ideomotor apraxia can perform a motor act spontaneously and automatically at the appropriate time, but the patient with ideational apraxia is unable to do so. Refer to Butler[166] for full testing protocols.
5. *Treatment Suggestions.* The treatment techniques are the same as those for ideomotor apraxia.

Buccofacial Apraxia

1. *Definition.* Buccofacial or oral apraxia involves difficulties with performing purposeful movements with the lips, tongue, cheeks, larynx, and pharynx on command. An unusual condition, Pedersen et al[179] report the prevalence rate in patients with acute stroke as around 6%.
2. *Clinical Examples.* A patient may have difficulty responding to the command "pretend to blow out a candle" or "blow a kiss." However, in a normal context where the patient may perform these actions automatically, performance is not impaired. In addition, while patients may be able to produce the individual phonemes required for speech, the patient may have difficulty in producing an orderly sequence of phonemes. Formulaic speech (common, routine phrases) or automatic expressions such as "have a nice day" may be preserved.[180]
3. *Lesion Area.* Difficulties with buccofacial apraxia seem associated with lesions in the frontal and central opercula, anterior insula, and a small area of the first temporal gyrus (adjacent to the frontal and central opercula). Although buccofacial apraxia often coexists with Broca's aphasia, the two may be seen independently.[180]
4. *Testing.* The patient should be examined by a speech-language pathologist.
5. *Treatment Suggestions.* The speech-language pathologist can advise the health care team on strategies to communicate with patients who have buccofacial apraxia.

SUMMARY

Cognition and perception, the processes by which an individual thinks and selects, integrates, and interprets stimuli from the body and surrounding environment, are critical to the normal functioning of each human being. The patient with brain damage may be lacking in those abilities that allow one to make sense of and to respond appropriately to the outside world. It is essential for the therapy team to work together to be able to recognize when a patient is experiencing some type of cognitive or perceptual dysfunction and to have the requisite tools to understand the causes of the behavior. The team can then determine the best interventions and consistently deliver these. Although it is often the occupational therapist, neuropsychologist, and speech-language pathologist who will guide the selection and implementation of evaluations and interventions for patients with cognitive and perceptual problems, it is essential that the physical therapist understands how these cognitive and perceptual impairments affect the patient's performance and the strategies that improve performance.

This chapter provided an overview of cognitive and perceptual deficits that may occur following brain damage, particularly those resulting from a stroke, and how such deficits can affect the functioning of the patient, especially within the context of the rehabilitation setting. The importance of differentiating cognitive and perceptual deficits from problems related to lack of motor ability, inadequate sensation, poor language skills, and simple uncooperativeness has been emphasized. Although alluded to in a very abbreviated fashion, activity analysis and systematic data collection remain two of the most powerful tools at the disposal of the therapist attempting to develop a firm rationale for, and to empirically justify the efficacy of, any treatment selected. Treatment in the form of adaptation of the physical environment and instructional sets and the teaching of compensatory techniques has been singled out as one of the most effective avenues for intervention.

Questions for Review

1. Patients with cognitive and perceptual deficits display what general characteristics during execution of a task?

2. Identify the underlying premise of the *transfer-of-training approach* to treatment.

3. What is the underlying assumption of the *sensory integrative approach* to treatment? Provide examples of the treatment modalities employed with this approach.

4. How is the performance of specific functional skills enhanced using the *functional approach* to treatment? What are the inherent benefits of using the functional approach?

5. Describe general suggestions for optimizing teaching/learning strategies when using compensatory techniques.

6. Identify the four treatment strategies included in the *cognitive approach* to treatment.

7. What potential influencing factors must be considered when examining a patient with cognitive and perceptual deficits?

8. What examination procedures will assist the therapist in distinguishing between sensory and cognitive or perceptual problems?

9. Differentiate between feedback provided in the form of knowledge of results (KR) versus knowledge of performance (KP).

10. Identify and define the four different types of attention.

11. What is the purpose of memory retraining? Compare and contrast the focus of the *remedial approach* and the *compensatory approach* to memory retraining.

12. Define the following terms: *unilateral neglect, anosognosia, somatoagnosia, finger agnosia,* and *right–left discrimination.*

13. Identify five spatial relations deficits. What general clinical manifestation do these disorders have in common? Define each of the deficits identified and provide an example of how each would influence patient performance of a task.

14. Provide examples of the functional implications of a visual *figure–ground discrimination deficit.* What is the most common lesion site producing this disorder?

15. What is the characteristic feature of apraxia? Define the three types of apraxias and provide examples of task performance characteristics associated with each type of apraxia.

CASE STUDY

The patient is a 72-year-old woman who has just been admitted to a rehabilitation facility following a stroke. The patient experienced a right parietal hemorrhagic stroke. A CT scan revealed a 1.5 in (4 cm) hemorrhage that was subsequently drained. She will be able to stay in the rehabilitation facility for 20 days. Although the patient has some physical problems, the emphasis of this case study is on cognitive and perceptual tests and interventions. The occupational therapist and the physical therapist are collaboratively using a combination of cognitive retraining and the functional approach in therapy.

PAST MEDICAL HISTORY

The patient's past medical history includes insulin-dependent diabetes and mild rheumatoid arthritis in her right shoulder and both hands causing some morning pain and stiffness.

SOCIAL

The patient lives alone in her own home. Supportive friends and family, her two children, and their families live nearby. A local health maintenance organization (HMO) provides her insurance. She is retired from the police force and enjoys gardening, reading, and watching television. She previously drove an automobile with an automatic transmission.

PHYSICAL THERAPY EXAMINATION

When the patient was approached from the left, she seemed to ignore the physical therapist and did not respond to greetings. However, when the therapist sat in the chair on the patient's right side, she seemed to have no problems talking to the therapist.

Range of Motion, Muscle Tone, and Balance

Examination revealed functional ROM, reduced strength in the left upper extremity (UE) with strength generally within the Fair (3/5) range; difficulty manipulating small objects with left hand; and some reduced dynamic standing balance reactions.

Sensation

The physical therapist tested sensation and noted normal sensation in all areas (sharp/dull, light touch, temperature, proprioceptive sensations, cortical sensations) on the right side. However, the patient seemed to have difficulties on the left side and her performance in detecting stimuli seemed inconsistent. Because the physical therapist suspected cognitive and perceptual deficits, a complete sensory test was deferred until the occupational therapist could fully examine the patient.

Functional Status

The physical therapist examined the patient's transfer abilities and instructed her in a safer way to get in and out of bed. The therapist scored the patient on the *Functional Independence Measure (FIM)*[88] and found the following:

Self-Care:
- Eating: FIM level = 4
- Grooming: FIM level = 5
- Bathing: FIM level = 3
- Dressing—upper body: FIM level = 5
- Dressing—lower body: FIM level = 4
- Toileting: FIM level = 6

Transfers:
- Bed, chair, wheelchair: FIM level = 5
- Toilet: FIM level = 5
- Tub: FIM level = 4

Locomotion:
- Walk: FIM level = 5

The physical therapist asked about her family and she was able to provide many details. However, she seemed puzzled about where she was and expressed concern that she was not looking her best and needed to do her hair. The therapist suggested that she might like to brush her hair. The brush was on the table on the patient's left side, and she said she did not have one. The physical therapist cued her to check her bedside table, but on checking she maintained she did not have a brush. At the end of the session (which lasted about 40 minutes) the therapist asked her to demonstrate the bed transfer technique again that she had been taught at the beginning of the session. She seemed confused and could not do what the physical therapist had taught her.

OCCUPATIONAL THERAPY EXAMINATION: COGNITION AND PERCEPTION

The occupational therapist conducted two standardized tests: the *Rivermead Behavioural Memory Test (RBMT)*[81] because the patient demonstrates memory impairments, and the *Arnadottir OT-ADL Neurobehavioral Evaluation (A-ONE)*[5] to examine the impact of the patient's problems on her daily living activities. The occupational therapist also reasoned that further tests of the patient's IADL, including home and driving abilities, would need to be conducted closer to her discharge. The patient's FIM scores for the Social Cognition Items were as follows:

Social Cognition FIM
- Social interaction: FIM level = 6
- Problem solving: FIM level = 6
- Memory: FIM level = 3

GUIDING QUESTIONS

1. What are some of the functional difficulties the patient is having and what cognitive and perceptual deficits might be causing these? Note that there may be more than one deficit affecting the functional problems noted.

2. Develop a clinical asset and problem list.

3. Identify anticipated goals and expected outcomes appropriate for this patient.

4. Identify two treatment strategies to improve spontaneous use of left upper extremity and decrease unilateral neglect.

5. Identify two treatment strategies to improve the patient's memory.

6. How can the success of the patient's rehabilitation program be measured?

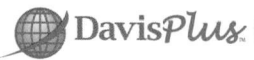 For additional resources, including answers to the questions for review and case study guiding questions, please visit **http://davisplus.fadavis.com**

References

1. Unsworth, C: Cognitive and Perceptual Dysfunction: A Clinical Reasoning Approach to Evaluation and Intervention. FA Davis, Philadelphia, 1999.
2. Zoltan, B: Vision, Perception and Cognition: A Manual for Evaluation and Treatment of the Neurologically Impaired Adult, ed 3 rev. Charles B. Slack, Thorofare, NJ, 1996.
3. Katz, N, et al: Lowenstein Occupational Therapy Cognitive Assessment (LOTCA) battery for brain injured patients: Reliability and validity. Am J Occup Ther 43:184, 1989.
4. Lezak, MD: Neuropsychological Assessment, ed 4. Oxford University Press, New York, 2004.
5. Arnadottir, G: The Brain and Behavior: Assessing Cortical Dysfunction through Activities of Daily Living. Mosby, St. Louis, 1990.
6. Glosser, G, and Goodglass, H: Disorders of executive control functions among aphasic and other brain-damaged patients. J Clin Exp Neuropsychol 12:485, 1990.
7. Katz, N, and Hartman-Maeir, A: Occupational performance and metacognition. Can J Occup Ther 64:53, 1997.
8. Winegardner, J: Executive functions. In Cohen, H (ed): Neuroscience for Rehabilitation. Lippincott, Philadelphia, 1993, p 346.
9. Sharpless, JW: Mossman's A Problem Oriented Approach to Stroke Rehabilitation, ed 2. Charles C Thomas, Springfield, IL, 1982.
10. Edwards, S: Neurological Physiotherapy: A Problem Solving Approach, ed 2. Churchill Livingstone, New York, 2002.
11. Luria, AR: Higher Cortical Functions in Man, ed 2. Basic Books, New York, 1980.
12. Pak, R, and Dombrovy, ML: Stroke. In Good, DC, and Couch, JR (eds): Handbook of Neurorehabilitation. Marcel Dekker, New York, 1994, p 461.
13. Meir, M, et al: Individual differences in neuropsychological recovery: An overview. In Meier, M, et al (eds): Neuropsychological Rehabilitation. Churchill Livingstone, London, 1987, p 71.
14. Bach-y-Rita, P: Brain plasticity as a basis for therapeutic procedures. In Bach-y-Rita, P (ed): Recovery of Function: Theoretical Considerations for Brain Injury Rehabilitation. University Park Press, Baltimore, 1980, p 225.
15. Brodal, A: Self-observations and neuro-anatomical considerations after a stroke. Brain 76:675, 1973.
16. Gardner, H: The Shattered Mind: The Person after Brain Damage. Alfred A. Knopf, New York, 1975.
17. Averbuch, S, and Katz, N: Cognitive rehabilitation: A retraining approach for brain-injured adults. In Katz, N (ed): Cognitive Rehabilitation: Models for Intervention in Occupational Therapy. Andover Medical, Boston, 1992, p 219.
18. Neistadt, ME: The neurobiology of learning: Implications for treatment of adults with brain injury. Am J Occup Ther 48:421, 1994.
19. Neistadt, ME: Assessing learning capabilities during cognitive and perceptual evaluations for adults with traumatic brain injury. Occup Ther Health Care 9:3, 1995.
20. Young, GC, Collins, D, and Hren, M: Effect of pairing scanning training with block design training in the remediation of perceptual problems in left hemiplegics. J Clin Neuropsychol 42:312, 1983.
21. Neistadt, ME: Occupational therapy for adults with perceptual deficits. Am J Occup Ther 42:434, 1988.
22. Bundy, AC, Lane, SJ, and Murray, EA (eds): Sensory Integration: Theory and Practice, ed 2. FA Davis, Philadelphia, 2002.
23. Ayres, JA: Sensory Integration and Learning Disorders. Western Psychological Service, Los Angeles, 1972.
24. Ayres, JA: Sensory Integration and the Child. Western Psychological Services, Los Angeles, 1980.
25. Neistadt, ME: A critical analysis of occupational therapy approaches for perceptual deficits in adults with brain injury. Am J Occup Ther 44:299, 1990.
26. Moore, J: Neuroanatomical considerations relating to recovery of function following brain injury. In Bach-y-Rita, P (ed): Recovery of Function: Theoretical Consideration for Brain Injury Rehabilitation. University Park Press, Baltimore, 1980, p 9.
27. Finger, S, and Stein, DG: Brain Damage and Recovery: Research and Clinical Perspectives. Academic Press, New York, 1982.
28. Braziz, PW, Masdeu, J, and Biller, J: Localization in Clinical Neurology, ed 6. Lippincott Williams & Wilkins, 2011.

29. Giles, GM, and Wilson, JC: Occupational Therapy for the Brain Injured Adult: A Neurofunctional Approach. Chapman & Hall, London, 1992.
30. Giles, GM: A neurofunctional approach to rehabilitation following severe brain injury. In Katz, N (ed): Cognitive Rehabilitation: Models for Intervention in Occupational Therapy. Andover Medical, Boston, 1992, p 195.
31. Trombly, CA (ed): Occupational Therapy for Physical Dysfunction, ed 6. Williams & Wilkins, Baltimore, 2008.
32. Trombly, CA: Conceptual foundations for practice. In Trombly, CA (ed): Occupational Therapy for Physical Dysfunction, ed 5. Lippincott Williams & Wilkins, Baltimore, 2002, p 1.
33. Trombly, CA: Restoring the role of independent person. In Trombly, CA (ed): Occupational Therapy for Physical Dysfunction, ed 5. Lippincott Williams & Wilkins, Baltimore, 2002, p 629.
34. Neistadt, ME: Occupational therapy treatment for constructional deficits. Am J Occup Ther 46:141, 1992.
35. Fisher, AG: An expanded rehabilitative model of practice. In Fisher, AG (ed): Assessment of Motor and Process Skills, ed 2. Three Star Press, Fort Collins, CO, 1997, p 73.
36. Trivedi, AN, et al: Trends in the quality of care and racial disparities in Medicare managed care. N Engl J Med 353:7, 692–700, 2005.
37. Toglia, J, and Abreu, BC: Cognitive Rehabilitation Supplement to Workshop: Management of Cognitive–Perceptual Dysfunction in the Brain-Damaged Adult. Sponsored by Braintree Hospital, Braintree, MA, and Cognitive Rehabilitation Associates, New York, May, 1987.
38. Giantusos, R: What is cognitive rehabilitation? J Rehabil 46:36, 1980.
39. Abreu, BC, and Toglia, JP: Cognitive rehabilitation: A model for occupational therapy. Am J Occup Ther 41:439, 1987.
40. Diller, L, and Gordon, WA: Intervention strategies for cognitive deficits in brain-injured adults. J Consult Clin Psychol 49:822, 1981.
41. Toglia, JP: Generalization of treatment: A multicontext approach to cognitive perceptual impairment in adults with brain injury. Am J Occup Ther 45:505, 1991.
42. Toglia, JP: A dynamic interactional model to cognitive rehabilitation. In Katz, N (ed): Cognition and Occupation across the Lifespan, ed 3. American Occupational Therapy Association, Bethesda, MD, 2011, p 105.
43. Abreu, BC: Evaluation and intervention with memory and learning impairment. In Unsworth, CA (ed): Cognitive and Perceptual Dysfunction: A Clinical Reasoning Approach to Evaluation and Intervention. FA Davis, Philadelphia, 1999, p 163.
44. Abreu, BC: The quadraphonic approach: Holistic rehabilitation for brain injury. In Katz, N (ed): Cognition and Occupation in Rehabilitation: Cognitive Models for Intervention in Occupational Therapy. American Occupational Therapy Association, Bethesda, MD, 1998, p 51.
45. Wilcock, AA: Occupational Therapy Approaches to Stroke. Churchill Livingstone, Melbourne, 1986.
46. Galski, T, Beuno, RL, and Ehle, HT: Driving after cerebral damage: A model with implications for evaluation. Am J Occup Ther 46:324, 1992.
47. Vining Radomski, M, and Schold Davis, E: Optimizing cognitive abilities. In Vining Radomski, M, and Trombly Latham, CA (eds): Occupational Therapy for Physical Dysfunction, ed 6. Lippincott Williams & Wilkins, Baltimore, 2008, p 609.
48. Gainotti, G: Emotional and psychosocial problems after brain injury. Neuropsychol Rehab 3:259, 1993.
49. Bronstein, KS, Popovich, JM, and Stewart-Amidei, C: Promoting Stroke Recovery. Mosby, St. Louis, 1991.
50. Bradshaw, JL, and Mattingley, JB: Clinical Neuropsychology: Behavioral and Brain Science. Academic Press, San Diego, 1995.
51. Cate, Y, and Richards, L: Relationship between performance on tests of basic visual functions and visual-perceptual processing in persons after brain injury. Am J Occup Ther 54:326, 2000.
52. Dirette, DK, and Hinojosa, J: The effects of a compensatory intervention on processing deficits in adults with acquired brain damage. Occup Ther J Res 19:223, 1999.
53. Warren, M: A hierarchical model for evaluation and treatment of visual perceptual dysfunction in adult acquired brain injury, I. Am J Occup Ther 47:42, 1993.
54. Warren, M: A hierarchical model for evaluation and treatment of visual perceptual dysfunction in adult acquired brain injury, II. Am J Occup Ther 47:55, 1993.
55. Sandin, KJ, and Mason, KD: Manual of Stroke Rehabilitation. Butterworth-Heinemann, Boston, 1996.
56. Gresham, GE, et al: Post-Stroke Rehabilitation. Diane Publishing, Darby, PA, 2004.
57. Hier, DB, Mondlock, J, and Caplan, LR: Recovery of behavioral abnormalities after right hemisphere stroke. Neurology 33:345, 1983.
58. Haerer, AF: Visual field defects and the prognosis of stroke patients. Stroke 4:163, 1977.
59. Zhang, X, et al: Natural history of homonymous hemianopia. Neurology 66(6):901, 2006.
60. Pedretti, LW: Evaluation of sensation, perception and cognition. In Pendleton, H, and Schultz-Krohn, W (eds): Pedretti's Occupational Therapy: Practice Skills for Physical Dysfunction, ed 6. Mosby, St. Louis, 2006, p 110.
61. Stilwell, JM: The meaning of manual midline crossing. Sens Integr Q 21:1, 1994.
62. Chaikin, LE: Disorders of vision and visual perceptual dysfunction. In Umphred, DA (ed): Neurological Rehabilitation, ed 5. Mosby, St. Louis, 2006, p 821.
63. Diller, L, and Weinberg, J: Differential aspects of attention in brain-damaged persons. Percept Motor Skills 35:71, 1972.
64. Van Ravensberg, CD, et al: Visual perception in hemiplegic patients. Arch Phys Med Rehabil 65:304, 1984.
65. Anastasi, A, and Urbina, S: Psychological Testing, ed 7. Prentice Hall, New York, 1996.
66. de Clive-Lowe, S: Outcome measurement, cost-effectiveness and clinical audit: The importance of standardised assessment to occupational therapists in meeting these new demands. Br J Occup Ther 59:357, 1996.
67. Wall, N: Stroke rehabilitation. In Logigian, MK (ed): Adult Rehabilitation: A Team Approach for Therapists. Little, Brown, Boston, 1982, p 225.
68. Laver, AJ, and Powell, GE: The Structured Observational Test of Function (SOTOF). NFER-Nelson, Windsor, England, 1995.
69. Laver, AJ: The structured observational test of function. Gerontol Spec Int Sect Newsl 17:1, 1994.
70. Allen, CK: Allen cognitive level test manual. S&S/Worldwide, Colchester, 1990.
71. Allen, CK, Earhart, CA, and Blue, T: Occupational Therapy Treatment Goals for the Physically and Cognitively Disabled. American Occupational Therapy Association, Rockville, MD, 1992.
72. Tyerman, R, et al: COTNAB-Chessington Occupational Therapy Neurological Assessment Battery Introductory Manual. Nottingham Rehab Limited, Nottingham, 1986.
73. Stanley, M, et al: Chessington Occupational Therapy Neurological Assessment Battery: Comparison of performance of people aged 50–65 years with people aged 66 and over. Austral Occup Ther J 42:55, 1995.
74. Sloan, RL, et al: Routine screening of brain damaged patients: A comparison of the Rivermead Perceptual Assessment Battery and the Chessington Occupational Therapy Neurological Assessment Battery. Clin Rehab 5:265, 1991.
75. Itzkovich, M, et al: The Loewenstein Occupational Therapy Assessment (LOTCA) manual. Maddak, Inc., Pequanock, NJ, 1990.
76. Cooke, DM, McKenna, K, and Fleming, J: Development of a standardized occupational therapy screening tool for visual perception in adults. Scand J Occup Ther 12(2):59, 2005.
77. Wilson, B, et al: Behavioural Inattention Test. Thames Valley Test Company, Bury St. Edmunds, 1987.
78. Wilson, B, Cockburn, J, and Halligan, P: Development of a behavioural test of visuospatial neglect. Arch Phys Med Rehabil 68:98, 1987.
79. Whiting, S, et al: RPAB-Rivermead Perceptual Assessment Battery. NFER-Nelson, Windsor, 1985.
80. Jesshope, HJ, Clark, MS, and Smith, DS: The RPAB: Its application to stroke-patients and relationship with function. Clin Rehabil 5:115, 1991.
81. Baddeley, A, et al: RBMT—the Rivermead Behavioural Memory Test, ed 3. Pearson Psychorp, London, 2008.
82. Wilson, B, et al: Development and validation of a test battery for detecting and monitoring everyday memory problems. J Clin Exp Neuropsychol 11:885, 1989.
83. Ware, JJ, and Sherbourne, CD: The MOS 36-item short-form health survey (SF-36): I. Conceptual framework and item selection. Med Care 30:473, 1992.
84. Unsworth, C, and Duncombe, D: Australian Therapy Outcome Measures for Occupational Therapy (AusTOMs). La Trobe University, Melbourne, 2007.

85. Law, M, et al: Canadian Occupational Performance Measure. Canadian Association of Occupational Therapists, Toronto, Ontario, 1991.

86. Davis, A, et al: First steps towards an interdisciplinary approach to rehabilitation. Clin Rehabil 6:237, 1992.

87. Wood-Dauphinee, SL, et al: Assessment of global function: The Reintegration to Normal Living Index. Arch Phys Med 69:583, 1988.

88. Guide for the Uniform Data Set for Medical Rehabilitation (Adult FIM SM): Version 5.0. State University of New York at Buffalo, Buffalo, 1999.

89. Jongbloed, L, et al: Stroke rehabilitation: Sensory integrative treatment versus functional treatment. Am J Occup Ther 43:391, 1989.

90. Gentile, AM: A working model of skill acquisition with special reference to teaching. Quest Monograph 17:61, 1972.

91. Lohman, H and Lamb, A: Payment for services in the United States. In Crepeau, EB, Cohn, ES, and Schell, BAB (eds): Willard and Spackman's Occupational Therapy, ed 11. Lippincott Williams & Wilkins, Philadelphia, 2008, p 494.

92. McKeehan, KM: Conceptual framework for discharge planning. In McKeehan, KM (ed): Continuing Care: A Multidisciplinary Approach to Discharge Planning. Mosby, Toronto, 1981, p 3.

93. Unsworth, CA, and Thomas, SA: Information use in discharge accommodation recommendations for stroke patients. Clin Rehabil 7:181, 1993.

94. Unsworth, CA, Thomas, SA, and Greenwood, KM: Rehabilitation team decisions concerning discharge housing for stroke patients. Arch Phys Med Rehabil 76:331, 1995.

95. Unsworth, CA: Clients' perceptions of discharge housing decisions following stroke rehabilitation. Am J Occup Ther 50:207, 1996.

96. Stringer, AY: A Guide to Adult Neurological Diagnosis. FA Davis, Philadelphia, 1996.

97. Strub, RL, and Black, FW: The Mental Status Examination in Neurology, ed 4. FA Davis, Philadelphia, 2000.

98. Mateer, CA, Kerns, KA, and Eso, KL: Management of attention and memory disorders following traumatic brain injury. J Learn Disabil 29:618, 1996.

99. van Zomeren, AH, and Brouwer, WH: The Clinical Neuropsychology of Attention. Oxford University Press, New York, 1994.

100. Stroop, JR: Studies of inference in serial verbal reactions. J Exp Psychol 18:643, 1935.

101. Gronwall, D: Paced auditory serial addition task: A measure of recovery from concussion. Percept Motor Skills 44:367, 1977.

102. US Army: Army Individual Test Battery. Manual of Directions and Scoring. Adjutant General's Office, 1944.

103. Couillet, J, et al: Rehabilitation of divided attention after severe traumatic brain injury: A randomized trial. Neuropsychol Rehabil 20 (3): 321, 2010.

104. Ponsford, J, Sloan, S, and Snow, P: Traumatic brain injury: Rehabilitation for everyday adaptive living. Lawrence Erlbaum, Hove, 1995.

105. Lincoln, NB, et al: Cognitive rehabilitation for attention deficits following stroke (Cochrane review). In The Cochrane Library, 4, CD002842, 2006.

106. Kepferman, I: Learning and memory. In Kandel, ER, Schwartz, JH, and Jessell, TM (eds): Principles of Neuroscience, ed 4. McGraw Hill, New York, 2000, p 887.

107. Scott Terry, W: Learning and Memory: Basic Principles, Processes and Procedures. Allyn & Bacon, Boston, 2008.

108. Nair, RD, and Lincoln, N: Effectiveness of memory retraining after stroke (Cochrane review). In The Cochrane Database, 3, CD002293, 2007.

109. Sohlberg, MM, and Mateer, CA: Introduction to cognitive rehabilitation: Theory and practice. The Guilford Press, New York, 1989.

110. McKerracher, G, et al: A single case experimental design comparing two notebook formats for a man with memory problems caused by traumatic brain injury. Neuropsychol Rehabil 15(2):115, 2005.

111. Fuster, JM: Memory in the Cerebral Cortex: An Empirical Approach to Neural Networks in the Human and Nonhuman Primate. MIT Press, Cambridge, MA, 1995.

112. Wilson, BA, and Moffat, N: Clinical Management of Memory Problems. Chapman & Hall, London, 1992.

113. Majid, MJ, et al: Cognitive rehabilitation for memory deficits following stroke (Cochrane review). In The Cochrane Library, Issue 3. Update Software, Oxford, 2002.

114. Doornheim, K, and De Haan, EHF: Cognitive training for memory deficits in stroke patients. Neuropsychol Rehabil 8:393, 1998.

115. Duran, L, and Fisher, AG: Evaluation and intervention with executive functions impairment. In Unsworth, CA: Cognitive and Perceptual Dysfunction: A Clinical Reasoning Approach to Evaluation and Intervention. FA Davis, Philadelphia, 1999, p 209.

116. Cummins, JL: Anatomic and behavioral aspects of frontal-subcortical circuits. In Grafman, J, et al (eds): Annals of the New York Academy of Sciences: Structure and Function of the Human Prefrontal Cortex, Vol. 769. New York Academy of Sciences, New York, 1995, p 1.

117. Wilson, BA, et al: Behavioural Assessment of the Dysexecutive Syndrome. Thames Valley Test Co., Bury St. Edmunds, UK, 1996.

118. Pollens, R, et al: Beyond cognition: Executive functions in closed head injury. Cogn Rehabil 65:23, 1988.

119. Sohlberg, MM, Mateer, CA, and Stuss, DT: Contemporary approaches to the management of executive control dysfunction. J Head Trauma Rehabil 8:45, 1993.

120. Honda, T: Rehabilitation of executive function impairment after stroke. Top Stroke Rehabil 6(1):15, 1999.

121. Hewitt, J, et al: Theory driven rehabilitation of executive function: Improving planning skills in people with traumatic brain injury through the use of an autobiographical episodic memory cueing procedure. Neuropsychologia 44(8):1468, 2006.

122. Van Deusen, J: Body Image and Perceptual Dysfunction in Adults. WB Saunders, Philadelphia, 1993.

123. Corben, L, and Unsworth, CA: Evaluation and intervention with unilateral neglect. In Unsworth, CA (ed): Cognitive and Perceptual Dysfunction: A Clinical Reasoning Approach to Evaluation and Intervention. FA Davis, Philadelphia, 1999, p 357.

124. Robertson, IH, and Halligan, PW: Spatial Neglect: A Clinical Handbook for Diagnosis and Treatment. Psychology Press, Hove, 1999.

125. Heilman KM, Watson, RT, and Valenstein, E: Neglect and related disorders. In Heilman, KM, and Valenstein, E (eds): Clinical Neuropsychology, ed 5. Oxford University Press, New York, 2011, p 296.

126. Herman, EWM: Spatial neglect: New issues and their implications for occupational therapy practice. Am J Occup Ther 46:207, 1992.

127. Gordon, WA, et al: Perceptual remediation in patients with right brain damage: A comprehensive program. Arch Phys Med Rehabil 66:353, 1985.

128. Vallar, G: The anatomical basis of spatial hemineglect in humans. In Robertson, IH, and Marshall, JC (eds): Unilateral Neglect: Clinical and Experimental Studies. Lawrence Erlbaum, Hove, 1993, p 27.

129. Rizzolatti, G, and Berti, A: Neural mechanisms of spatial neglect. In Robertson, IH and Marshall, JC (eds): Unilateral Neglect: Clinical and Experimental Studies. Lawrence Erlbaum, Hove, 1993, p 87.

130. Robertson, IH, et al: Walking trajectory and hand movements in unilateral left neglect: A vestibular hypothesis. Neuropsychologia 32:1495, 1994.

131. Saevarsson, S, Kristjánsson, Á, and Halsband, U: Strength in numbers: Combining neck vibration and prism adaptation produces additive therapeutic effects in unilateral neglect. Neuropsychol Rehabil 20(5):704, 2010.

132. Luauté, J, et al: Visuo-spatial neglect: A systematic review of current interventions and their effectiveness. Neurosci Biobehav Rev 30(7):961, 2006.

133. Bowen, A, and Lincoln, N: Cognitive rehabilitation for spatial neglect following stroke (Cochrane review). In The Cochrane Library, Issue 2, 2007. Art. No.: CD 003586.

134. Fanthome, Y, et al: The treatment of visual neglect using feedback of eye movements: A pilot study. Disabil Rehabil 17:413, 1995.

135. Jacquin-Courtois, S, et al: Effect of prism adaptation on left dichotic listening deficit in neglect patients: Glasses to hear better? Brain 133(3): 895, 2010.

136. Kalra, L, et al: The influence of visual neglect on stroke rehabilitation. Stroke 28:1386, 1997.

137. Tsang, MHM, Sze, KH, and Fong, KNK: Occupational therapy treatment with right half-field eye-patching for patients with subacute stroke and unilateral neglect: A randomized controlled trial. Disabil Rehabil 31:630, 2009.

138. Watanabe, S, and Amimoto, K: Generalization of prism adaptation for wheelchair driving tasks in patients with unilateral spatial neglect. Arch Phys Med Rehabil 91:443, 2010.

139. Serino, A, et al: Effectiveness of prism adaptation in neglect reha-bilitation: A controlled trial study. Stroke 40(4):1392, 2009.

140. Turton, AJ, et al: A single blinded randomised controlled pilot trial of prism adaptation for improving self-care in stroke patients with neglect. Neuropsychol Rehabil 20(2):180, 2010.

141. Wiart, L, et al: Unilateral neglect syndrome rehabilitation by trunk rotation and scanning training. Arch Phys Med Rehabil 78:424, 1997.

142. Waxman, S, and deGroot, J: Correlative Neuroanatomy and Functional Neurology, ed 22. Appleton, Los Altos, CA, 1995.

143. Maeshima, S, et al: Rehabilitation of patients with anosognosia for hemiplegia due to intracerebral haemorrhage. Brain Inj 11:691, 1997.

144. Sauguet, J, et al: Disturbances of the body scheme in relation to language impairment and hemispheric locus of lesion. J Neurol Neurosurg Psychiatry 34:496, 1971.

145. Johnstone, M: Restoration of Motor Function in the Stroke Patient, ed 3. Churchill Livingstone, New York, 1987.

146. Hecaen, H, et al: The syndrome of apractagnosia due to lesions of the minor vertebral hemisphere. Arch Neurol Psychiatry 75:400, 1956.

147. Gainotti, G: Emotional behaviour and hemispheric side of the lesion. Cortex 8:41, 1972.

148. Arnadottir, G, and Gudrun, A: Evaluation and intervention with complex perceptual disorder. In Unsworth, CA (ed): Cognitive and Perceptual Dysfunction: A Clinical Reasoning Approach to Evaluation and Intervention. FA Davis, Philadelphia, 1999, p 393.

149. Edmans, JA, Webster, J, and Lincoln, NB: A comparison of two approaches in the treatment of perceptual problems after stroke. Clin Rehabil 14:230, 2000.

150. Halperin, E, and Cohen, BS: Perceptual-motor dysfunction. Stumbling block to rehabilitation. Md Med J 20:139, 1971.

151. Farah, MJ, and Epstein, RA: Disorders of visual-spatial percep-tion and cognition. In Heilman, KM, and Valenstein, E (eds): Clinical Neuropsychology, ed 5. Oxford University Press, New York, 2011, p 152.

152. Ayres, JA: Southern California Sensory Integration Tests. Western Psychological Services, Los Angeles, 1972.

153. Peterson, P, and Wikoff, RL: The performance of adult males on the Southern California figure-ground visual perception test. Am J Occup Ther 37:554, 1983.

154. Anderson, E, and Choy, E: Parietal lobe syndromes in hemiple-gia: A program for treatment. Am J Occup Ther 24:13, 1970.

155. Maguire, EA: The retrosplenial contribution to human naviga-tion: A review of lesion and neuroimaging findings. Scand J Psychol 42:225, 2001.

156. Yelnik, AP, et al: Perception of verticality after recent cerebral hemispheric stroke. Stroke 33:2247, 2002.

157. Laver, AJ, and Unsworth, CA: Evaluation and intervention with simple perceptual impairment (agnosias). In Unsworth, CA (ed): Cognitive and Perceptual Dysfunction: A Clinical Reasoning Approach to Evaluation and Intervention. FA Davis, Philadelphia, 1999, p 299.

158. Bauer, RM: Agnosia. In Heilman, KM, and Valenstein, E (eds): Clinical Neuropsychology, ed 5. Oxford University Press, New York, 2011, p 238.

159. Damasio, AR, Damasio, H, and van Hoesen, GW: Prosopag-nosia: Anatomical basis and behavioral mechanism. Neurology 32:331, 1982.

160. Karnath, HO, et al: The anatomy of object recognition—visual form agnosia caused by medial occipitotemporal stroke. J Neurosci 29(1):5854, 2009.

161. Behrmann, M, et al: Behavioral change and its neural correlates in visual agnosia after expertise training. J Cogn Neurosci 17(4):554, 2005.

162. Croce, R: A review of the neural basis of apractic disorders with implications for remediation. Adapt Phys Act Q 10:173, 1993.

163. Tate, R, and McDonald, S: What is apraxia? The clinician's dilemma. Neuropsychol Rehabil 5:273, 1995.

164. Heilman, KM, and Gonzalez Rothi, LJ: Apraxia. In Heilman, KM, and Valenstein, E (eds): Clinical Neuropsychology, ed 5. Oxford University Press, New York, 2011, p 214.

165. Donkervoot, M, et al: Prevalence of apraxia among patients with a first left hemisphere stroke in rehabilitation centres and nursing homes. Clin Rehabil 14:130, 2000.

166. Butler, J: Evaluation and intervention with apraxia. In Unsworth, CA (ed): Cognitive and Perceptual Dysfunction: A Clinical Reasoning Approach to Evaluation and Intervention. FA Davis, Philadelphia, 1999, p 257.

167. Raade, AS, Roth, LJ, and Heilman, KM: The relationship between buccofacial and limb apraxia. Brain Cognition 16:130, 1991.

168. Mozaz, M, et al: Apraxia in a patient with lesion located in right sub-cortical area: Analysis of errors. Cortex 26:651, 1990.

169. Goodglass, H, et al: The Assessment of Aphasia and Related Dis-orders, ed 3. Lippincott Williams & Wilkins, Philadelphia, 2001.

170. Halsband, U, et al: The role of the pre-motor and the supplemen-tary motor area in the temporal control of movement in man. Brain 116:243, 1993.

171. Van Heugten, CM, et al: Assessment of disabilities in stroke patients with apraxia: Internal consistency and inter-observer reliability. Occup Ther J Res 19:55, 1999.

172. Okoye, R: The apraxias. In Abreu, BC (ed): Physical Disabilities Manual. Raven Press, New York, 1981, p 241.

173. Donkervoot, M, et al: Efficacy of strategy training in left hemi-sphere stroke patients with apraxia: A randomized clinical trial. Neuropsychol Rehabil 11:549, 2001.

174. Donkervoort, M, Dekker J, and Deelman, B: The course of apraxia and ADL functioning in left hemisphere stroke patients treated in rehabilitation centres and nursing homes. Clin Rehabil 20(12):1085, 2006.

175. Geusgens, C, et al: Transfer of training effects in stroke patients with apraxia: An exploratory study. Neuropsychol Rehabil 16(2): 213, 2006.

176. Geusgens, C, et al: Transfer effects of a cognitive strategy training for stroke patients with apraxia. J Clin Exp Neuropsychol 29(8):831, 2007.

177. De Renzi, E, and Lucchelli, F: Ideational apraxia. Brain 111:1173, 1988.

178. Mayer, NH, et al: Buttering a hot cup of coffee: An approach to the study of errors of action in patients with brain damage. In Tupper, DE, and Cicerone, KD (eds): The Neuropsychology of Everyday Life: Assessment and Basic Competencies. Kluwer, London, 1990, p 259.

179. Pedersen, PM, et al: Manual and oral apraxia in acute stroke, frequency and influence on functional outcome. Am J Phys Med Rehabil 80:685, 2001.

180. Heilman, KM, and Valenstein, E (eds): Clinical Neuropsychology, ed 5. Oxford University Press, New York, 2011.

Supplemental Readings

Banich, MT, and Compton, RJ: Cognitive Neuroscience and Neuropsychology, ed 3. Houghton Mifflin, Boston, 2011.

Gravell, R, and Johnson, R (eds): Head Injury Rehabilitation: A Community Team Perspective. Whurr Publishers, London, 2002.

Heilman, KM, and Valenstein, E (eds): Clinical Neuropsychology, ed 5. Oxford University Press, New York, 2011.

Lundy-Eckman, L: Neuroscience: Fundamentals for Rehabilitation, ed 3. Elsevier, New York, 2007.

Mateer, CA, and Sohlberg, MM: Cognitive Rehabilitation: An integrative neuropsychological approach. Guilford Press, New York, 2001.

Ponsford, J (ed): Cognitive and Behavioral Rehabilitation: From Neurobiology to Clinical Practice. Guilford Press, New York, 2004.

Sacks, O: The Man Who Mistook his Wife for a Hat. Harper & Row, New York, 1985.

Strub, RL, and Black, FW: The Mental Status Examination in Neurology, ed 4. FA Davis, Philadelphia, 2000.

Unsworth, C (ed): Cognitive and Perceptual Dysfunction: A Clinical Reasoning Approach to Evaluation and Intervention. FA Davis, Philadelphia, 1999.

Wilson, BA: Memory Rehabilitation: Integrating Theory and Practice. Guilford Press, New York, 2009.

Social Psychology Network from Wesleyan University	www.socialpsychology.org/cognition.htm
Yale Perception and Cognition Laboratory	www.yale.edu/perception/
Better Medicine	www.bettermedicine.com/article/cognitive-impairment
Book chapter on Cognitive Impairment following Traumatic Brain Injury	www.ncbi.nlm.nih.gov/books/NBK2521/
Brain Injury Centre, Australia	www.braininjurycentre.com.au/aus/
Brain Injury Association of America	www.biausa.org/
Brain Injury Resource Center	www.headinjury.com/
The Stroke Association—Cognitive problems after stroke	www.stroke.org.uk/document.rm?id=829
MIT open course on the brain and cognition	http://ocw.mit.edu/courses/brain-and-cognitive-sciences/
University of California, San Diego, Center for Brain and Cognition	http://cbc.ucsd.edu/index.html
The Transitional Learning Center, Galveston, Texas	http://tlcrehab.org/
National Institute of Neurological Disorders and Stroke	www.ninds.nih.gov/news_and_events/proceedings/execsumm07_19_05.htm
International Brain Injury Association Guidelines for Cognitive Rehabilitation	www.internationalbrain.org/

Chapter 28

Neurogenic Disorders of Speech and Language

Martha Taylor Sarno, MA, MD (hon) CCC-SLP, BC-ANCDS
Jessica Galgano, PhD, CCC-SLP

LEARNING OBJECTIVES

1. Differentiate the organization of language with respect to the role of phonological, lexical, syntactic, and semantic systems.
2. Understand the role of the motor speech system in the speech production process.
3. Discuss and characterize the classic aphasic syndromes.
4. Identify and explain the critical factors in the evaluation of recovery and rehabilitation of aphasia.
5. Identify and describe general approaches to aphasia rehabilitation and some specific treatment methods.
6. Identify etiologies of cognitive-communication disorders.
7. Compare and contrast deficits in executive function, pragmatic language, and motor speech in persons with cognitive-communication disorders.
8. Describe the primary types of dysarthria and rationales for dysarthria treatment.
9. Describe apraxia of speech and its treatment.
10. Gain an understanding of swallowing disorders.
11. Describe the goals and rationales for the use of augmentative communication systems.

CHAPTER OUTLINE

Most people take the ability to produce and understand speech for granted and pay little attention to the nature and function of the processes involved in communication. Yet speech, like tool making, sets us apart from animals and is one of our most human behaviors. Even in primitive societies, humans have used the oral–motor speech code to share experiences, ideas, and feelings. Not all communities have developed writing and reading systems.

The use of speech for communication contributes to our identity as human beings and to the perception of "self." As a result, disruptions in the ability to communicate, whether caused by structural abnormalities (e.g., cleft palate), neurological conditions (e.g., stroke, Parkinson's disease), or nonorganic conditions (e.g., nonorganic articulatory disorders) may affect a person's daily life in important ways. For some, the acquisition of a communication disorder may have sufficient impact to cause an individual to withdraw from the workforce. For those whose communication disorders have persisted since childhood, the disorder may represent a significant vocational handicap. In other cases, a disorder that does not impede an individual's vocational life nonetheless interferes with everyday socialization. Communication disorders are complex, multifaceted behavioral impairments often associated so closely with a person's self-image as to threaten the quality of his or her life.

The term **communication** encompasses all of the behaviors, including speech, that human beings use to perceive and transmit information and interact with others. Speech comprises a delicate and rapid sequence of sensory and motor events requiring the coordinated activity of several parts of the body. The use of speech for communication involves many levels of human activity, ranging from the fine motor coordination of components of the oral–motor system to the subtle shades of meaning that occur at the cognitive/semantic level. Gestures, pantomime, and other nonverbal *pragmatic language* behaviors, such as turn taking, are also essential elements of communication.

Among unimpaired speakers, speech behavior varies greatly, yet the oral–motor system is efficient for the exchange of even complicated information. The range of variability is so wide that individuals generally produce different sound waves with different characteristics even when producing the same word. But listeners do not rely solely on information derived from speech waves. We also depend on cues, which are components of what is referred to as *context*. Context includes aspects of a communicative exchange such as the purpose of the activity, the location of the exchange, the knowledge of the participants, the roles of each participant, and the level of formality required by the situation.

This chapter addresses the neurogenic disorders of communication, a category of communication disorders represented by the majority of patients receiving speech-language pathology services in rehabilitation programs. The most common of these disorders are **aphasia**, a language (cerebral) disorder, **dysarthria**, a motor–speech disorder, and cognitive-communication disorders.

The field of speech-language pathology, which came into being in 1925 with the establishment of the American Speech-Language-Hearing Association (ASHA), is dedicated to the diagnosis and treatment of individuals with congenital or acquired communication disorders. Communication disorders in children and adults are estimated to have prevalence in the United States of 5% to 10% and a cost to the economy of $154 billion to $186 billion per year. The number of persons in the United States with communication disorders is estimated at 14 million.[1,2] These statistics have increased by the addition of a large number of military personnel returning from active duty who may manifest a host of communication disorders, including hearing loss, speech-language disorders, and/or cognitive-communication disorders. A significant number of returning military personnel have cognitive-communication disorders secondary to traumatic brain injury (TBI), which include deficits in discourse, pragmatic language, and social communication.[3-6]

The National Institute on Deafness and Other Communication Disorders (NIDCD) reports that 6 to 8 million people in the United States have an acquired or developmental language disorder. It is estimated that about 100,000 persons acquire aphasia annually, and approximately 1 million people currently have aphasia.[7] In addition, approximately 7.5 million people in the United States have voice disorders. The prevalence of articulation or speech sound disorders in children up to 6 or 7 years of age is estimated at 8% to 9%. By age 6 or 7, about 5% of children continue to present with speech disorders. It is also estimated that over 3 million Americans stutter.[2]

Approximately 28 million Americans have a hearing loss. Fifty-five percent of those with hearing impairments are older than 65 years of age, and 12 out of every 1,000 children younger than 18 have a hearing impairment.[8,9] New technology has succeeded in providing the development of cochlear implants (CIs) for persons with profound hearing loss, which have been implanted in children as young as 6 months of age. CIs stimulate the surviving dendrites, spiral ganglion cells, and vestibulocochlear-nerve fibers in the inner ear, making auditory sensations available. Immediate benefits are reported following CI activation, including improvement in speaking, which generally increases over time.[10]

The speech-language pathologist (SLP) profession has grown rapidly. Affiliates (members and certificate holders) in the ASHA increased from 1,623 to 140,000 between 1950 and 2010. Speech-language pathology is a master's degree entry field. As of 2009, 47 states required a license to practice. The ASHA awards the Certificate of Clinical Competence (CCC) to SLPs who meet specified academic and clinical experience requirements, which includes a Clinical Fellowship Year (CFY), a 9-month period of supervision and mentoring by a speech and language pathologist holding ASHA certification. Fifty-seven percent of SLPs work in educational organizations, 37% in residential health care facilities, and approximately 15% in home health, private practice, and speech and hearing centers.[11] The term *SLP* is the official designation of professionals in the field who hold the CCC. The term *speech therapist,* although no longer considered professionally appropriate, is a term that is often used informally.

In order for the presence and degree of speech or language pathology as it is manifest in a given person to be identified and measured, performance must be compared with a standard of "normal." One may choose as the standard (1) the language common to the cultural community of unimpaired persons in which the person lives, in which case an individual's verbal function would be compared with that of others in the same community of similar age, gender, education, and achievement, or (2) the person's verbal behavior before the onset of illness or trauma. The latter will vary from individual to individual and is based on premorbid educational achievement, specific cultural characteristics, personality, and other factors such as cognitive functioning. A person is verbally impaired when he or she deviates in any parameter of language and/or speech processing from the "normal" communication behavior of the community in which he or she functioned premorbidly.

A "normal" standard is implied in the terms *impairment, disability,* and *handicap.* This chapter uses the current World Health Organization (WHO) classification schema, in which the term *disability* is defined as the nature and extent of functioning, and the term *handicap* is defined as a person's involvement in life situations.[12,13]

■ THE ORGANIZATION OF LANGUAGE

When an individual generates an idea that he or she wishes to express, it is transformed into words and sentences by calling into play certain physiological and acoustic events. The message is converted into linguistic form. The listener, in turn, fits the auditory information into a sequence of words and sentences that are ultimately understood.

We refer to the system of symbols that are strung together into sentences expressing our thoughts and the understanding of those messages as *language.* In the first few years of life, infants and children gain a great deal of practice and experience in the use of language, until it becomes habitual and is used with different levels of conscious awareness.

Phonology refers to the study of the sound system of language. Words are made up of speech sounds or *phonemes,* which are generally classified as either *vowels* or *consonants.* Phonemes in and of themselves do not symbolize ideas or objects, but when put together they are the basic linguistic units that make words. Words comprise the *lexicon,* or vocabulary, of a language. English is comprised of 16 vowels and 22 consonants, which are combined into larger units called *syllables.*

A syllable usually consists of a vowel as a central phoneme surrounded by one or more consonants. There are between 1,000 and 2,000 syllables in English. Most languages have their own rules about how phonemes may be combined into larger units. For example, in English, syllables never start with the *ng* phoneme. The most frequently used words in English are sequences of from two to five phonemes. Some have as many as 10 phonemes or as few as one. In general, the most frequently used words have few phonemes. Even though only a small number of phoneme combinations are possible, new words are added to the English language every day. Although there are several hundred thousand English words, we use a repertoire of only about 5,000 to 10,000 words 95% of the time.

The grammar, or *syntax,* of a language determines the sequence of words that are acceptable in the formation of sentences. In English, for example, it is possible to say "The black box is on the table," but the sequence "Box black table on the" is unacceptable. Another example is "The old radio played well," which is syntactically correct, but "Old the well played radio" is not. The sentence "The boy walked to the store" is meaningful, but the sentence "The book walked to the store" is not. The language system that refers to the meanings of words is called *semantics.*

In addition to the phonological (sounds), lexical (vocabulary), syntactical (grammar), and semantic (meaning) language systems, we also utilize *prosody* (stress and intonation) to help make distinctions between questions, statements, expressions of emotional feelings, shock, exclamations, and so forth.

■ SPEECH PRODUCTION

The speech organs consist of the lungs, trachea, larynx (which contains the vocal cords), pharynx, nose, and mouth. When considered together, these organs comprise a "tube" referred to as the *vocal tract,* which extends from the lungs to the lips. Moving the tongue, lips, and any other parts of the tract varies vocal tract shape. Changes in the configuration of the vocal tract act to modify the aerodynamic qualities of the air stream during speech (Fig. 28.1).

The primary function of the vocal organs relates to basic life-sustaining functions such as breathing and swallowing. These organs not only take on different roles

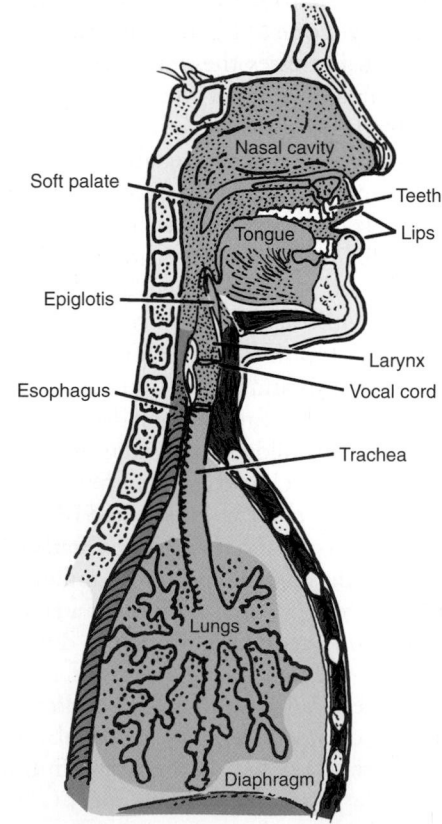

Figure 28.1 The human vocal organ.

for speech, but also function differently when engaged in speech production. For example, breathing for life-sustaining purposes is far more rapid than for speech production. A full cycle of inhalation/exhalation takes approximately 5 seconds, whereas while speaking we control the breathing rate according to the demands of the words and sentences we are producing, sometimes reducing the rate of breathing to as little as 15% devoted to inhalation. This is dictated in part by the fact that, when speaking, we generally take in enough air to vocalize a complete thought and we exhale the air gradually during the production of the thought.

The steady stream of air exhaled from the lungs is the source of energy for speech production, which is made audible by the rapid vibration of the vocal cords. During speech, we continuously alter the shape of the vocal tract by moving the tongue, lips, and other parts of the system. By moving parts of the vocal tract, thereby modifying its acoustic properties, we are able to produce different sounds. That is, by altering the shape of the vocal tract during *phonation*, we transform the air stream into a resonance chamber (Figs. 28.2 and 28.3).

The *larynx* acts as a barrier to prevent food from entering the trachea and lungs by closing automatically during the act of swallowing, which is also helped by the action of the epiglottis. By opening and closing the flow of air from the lungs, the larynx acts as a valve between the lungs and the mouth. The laryngeal valve also acts to lock air into the lungs, which we do automatically when we perform heavy work using our upper extremities. The larynx is not a fixed, rigid organ, but because

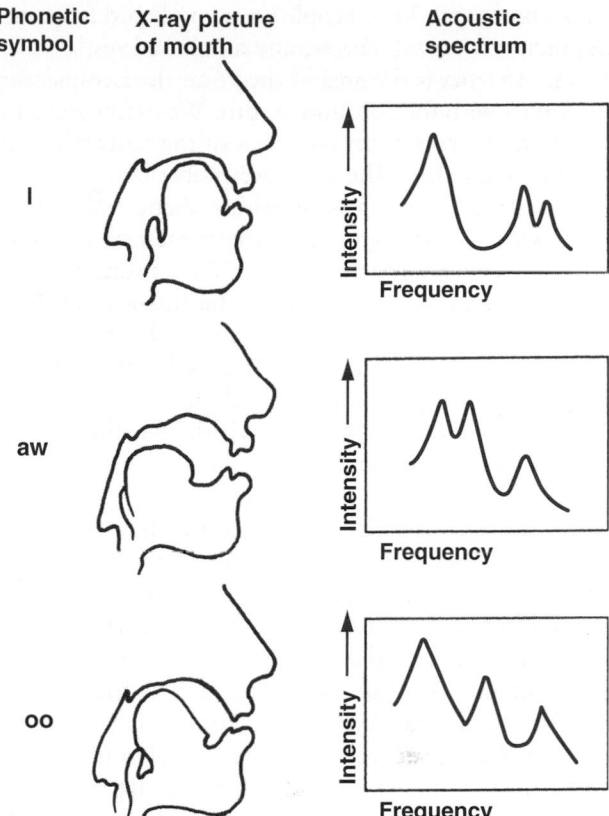

Phonetic symbol   **X-ray picture of mouth**   **Acoustic spectrum**

Figure 28.3 Vocal tract configuration and corresponding spectra for three different vowels. The peaks of the spectra represent vocal tract resonances. The vertical lines for individual harmonics are not shown.

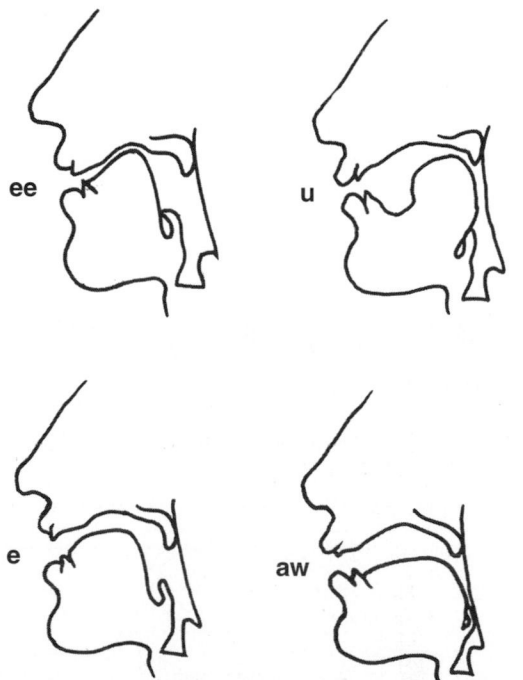

Figure 28.2 Outlines of the vocal tract during articulation of various vowels.

of its cartilaginous construction and corresponding connecting muscles and ligaments moves up and down during both swallowing and speaking.

The *vocal cords,* which create the sounds of speech, are located on either side of the larynx from the Adam's apple at the front to the arytenoid cartilages at the back. Recent neuroimaging research has reported findings that reflect the complexity of motor planning and control of vocal cord movement for voice production, showing that subcortical and cortical interactions control the movement of the vocal cords.[14] We refer to the space between the vocal cords as the *glottis.* When the cords are pressed together, the passage of air is sealed off and the valve is shut. Because the cords are held together at the front where they articulate with the Adam's apple, the open glottis is V-shaped, opening only at the back. When we speak, we vibrate the vocal cords in a rhythmic fashion, opening and closing the air passage from the lungs to the oral/nasal cavities.

The frequency of sound produced by the vocal cords is directly related to their mass, tension, and length. The tension and length of the vocal cords is continuously altered while speaking. In normal speech, the range of vocal cord frequencies is from about 60 to 350 cycles per second (cps). Most people use a vocal cord frequency range that covers about one and a half octaves.

The *pharynx* is the area of the vocal tract connecting the larynx with the nose and mouth. We isolate the nasal cavity from the pharynx and back of the mouth by raising the soft palate. The most adjustable component of the vocal tract is the mouth, whose shape and size can be modified more than any other organ of the oral–motor system by changing the relative position of the palate, tongue, lips, and teeth. The lips are rounded, spread, or closed to alter the shape and length of the vocal tract or to stop airflow. The teeth and their relationship to the lips or tongue tip change the airflow. An important component of the teeth ridge is the *alveolus*, which is the area covered by the gums.

The term *articulation* refers to the articulating, or "meeting," of the various organs of the oral-pharyngeal cavity to produce the sounds of speech. Speech *intelligibility* refers to the adequacy of the acoustic signal produced by a speaker and represents a significant factor in understanding a speaker. A number of factors can influence judgments of intelligibility, such as the presence or absence of visual cues or of extraneous movements (i.e., tremor). The precision of the production of consonant sounds is one of the primary factors that contribute to speech intelligibility. Consonants are described by specifying their place and manner of articulation and whether they are voiced or unvoiced (Table 28.1). The "places" of articulation are the lips (labial), teeth, gums (alveolar), palate, and glottis. The *manner of articulation* refers to the plosive, fricative, nasal, liquid, and semivowel categories.

Plosive sounds, sometimes referred to as "stop" sounds, are those produced by building up air pressure in the oral cavity and suddenly releasing it (e.g., *p, t*). The blockage can occur by pressing the lips together or by pressing the tongue against either the gums or soft palate. There are plosive consonants that are labial, alveolar, or velar (consonants articulated with the back part of the tongue).

Fricatives are produced by making the air turbulent (e.g., *f, v*). Most consonants are produced with the soft palate raised, thereby closing off the flow of air to the nasal cavity, except for the *nasals* (e.g., *m, n, ng*), which are made by lowering the soft palate and blocking the oral cavity somewhere along its length. *Liquids* are sounds made with the soft palate raised: /r/, /l/.

Semivowels refer to those sounds produced by maintaining the vocal tract in a vowel-like position, then changing the position rapidly for the vowel that follows (e.g., *w, y*).

Speech sounds are affected by their *context,* that is, the sounds that immediately precede or follow. A speech sound wave is a continuous event rather than a sequence of discrete segments. The identification of a speech sound depends on relating acoustic features of the sound wave at different points in time.

A standard reference for the quality of vowels is the eight cardinal vowels (Fig. 28.4). This schema of the positions of the tongue for the production of the vowels of the language helps us visualize the tongue's movements during speech. It is, in a sense, a map of the tongue positions for vowel production. Tongue placement is described by specifying the location of the main body of the tongue at its highest point. For example, for the sound /ee/ as in the word *beat,* the tongue tip is pointed in a high frontal configuration, whereas for the sound /ah/ as in the word *father,* the highest point of the tongue is low and posterior in the oral cavity.

All vowel sounds and some consonant sounds are *voiced.* That is, the vocal cords vibrate during their production. When a sound is produced without vocal cord vibration, we say that it is *unvoiced* or voiceless (e.g., *p, s*). Table 28.1 shows that many consonant sounds are articulated in the same manner, and differ only with respect to voicing (e.g., *p-b; s-z; f-v; k-g*).

Speech behavior comprises a complex motor event that goes well beyond the skilled movements required of the oral–motor system. Yet we produce speech without thinking about it even while simultaneously involved in

Table 28.1	Classification of English Consonants by Place and Manner of Articulation				
	Manner of Articulation				
Place of Articulation	Plosive	Fricative	Semivowel	Liquids (including laterals)	Nasal
Labial	p b	—	w	—	m
Labiodental	—	f v	—	—	—
Dental	—	_ th	—	—	—
Alveolar	t d	s z	y	l r	n
Palatal	—	sh zh	—	—	—
Velar	k g	—	—	—	ng
Glottal	—	h	—	—	—

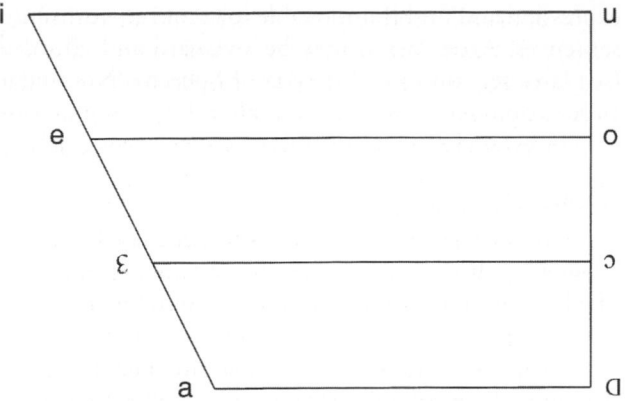

Figure 28.4 The cardinal vowels represented as a vowel quadrilateral. The cardinal vowels are extremely placed reference points for vowel articulation. Vowels on the same horizontal line are believed to have an equally high tongue height while vowels in the left–right position are assumed to be equally backed and fronted. *Adapted from Ladefoged, P: A Course in Phonetics. Harcourt Brace Jovanovich, New York, 1975, with permission.*

other activities. However, to transform thought into speech takes some voluntary, conscious behavior that allows us to take information stored in memory and translate it into a coherent production of words and utterances that follow certain grammatical rules.

In addition to its linguistic aspects, neurogenic communication disorders often involve coexisting mild to severe cognitive deficits that may not only aggravate the communication disorder but also make it difficult to differentiate cognitive from communication deficits. The communication disorder manifest in persons with right brain damage, which is addressed in this chapter, is an example of a disorder in which the cognitive component is a major issue.

The importance of the communication process and its underlying systems becomes apparent when we consider the two most common neurogenic communication disorders: *aphasia* and *dysarthria*. This chapter focuses primarily on aphasia and dysarthria but also considers verbal apraxia, dysphagia, cognitive-communication disorders, and the use of augmentative/alternate systems of communication.

■ APHASIA

An increase in the population of individuals with aphasia is anticipated by the projection that by 2050, 21% to 22% of the U.S. population will be over age 65.[15] It has been estimated that there are over 1 million individuals with aphasia in the United States alone.[2,16,17] In a survey of 850 patients in the first month post-stroke, aphasia was present in 177 patients.[18] It is further estimated that there are more than 100,000 new patients with aphasia each year.[11,19] The majority are currently older than 65 years of age and acquired aphasia as a result of a

stroke. A smaller number are the result of head trauma and neoplasms. Aphasia is also often present in the early stages of Alzheimer's disease.[20] Ellis et al[19] report that the incidence of aphasia and its demographic characteristics has been generally consistent in the United States from 1997 to 2006.

Classification and Nomenclature

In this chapter, the term **aphasia** refers to the acquired communication disorder that is manifest in individuals who were previously capable of using language appropriately. It does not refer to developmental language disorders that may be present in individuals who never developed normal language and for whom the ability to use language may never reach age-appropriate performance levels.

In acquired aphasia, central nervous system (CNS) disease or trauma compromises certain structures in a focal rather than generalized fashion. The study of the neuroanatomical correlates of the aphasias has engaged neurologists since the late 19th century, and the correlation between aphasic syndromes and cerebral localization is relatively consistent. Recent advances in neuroradiological technology have provided many new methods for studying the neural substrates of language and language impairment.[21,22]

Aphasiologists generally agree that there are distinct major aphasic syndromes that adhere to specific profiles of impairment. This is not surprising, because the lesions that produce aphasia, particularly in the patient with cerebrovascular disease, tend to be located in brain loci that are especially vulnerable. It is not always possible, however, to classify patients according to these syndromes. Estimates of the proportion of cases that can be unambiguously classified range from 30% to 80%.[23]

The characteristics of an individual's speech production are used to determine aphasia classification. Speech output that is characterized as hesitant, awkward, interrupted, and produced with effort is referred to as *nonfluent aphasia* in contrast to speech output that is facile in articulation, produced at a normal rate, with preserved flow and melody, and is referred to as *fluent aphasia*. Fluency judgments are made during extended conversation with a patient and are defined as follows.

Fluent Aphasia

Fluent aphasia is characterized by impaired auditory comprehension and fluent speech that is of normal rate and melody. Fluent aphasia is usually associated with a lesion in the vicinity of the posterior portion of the first temporal gyrus of the left hemisphere. When fluent aphasia is severe, word and sound substitutions may be of such magnitude and frequency that speech may be rendered meaningless. Patients with fluent aphasia tend to have greatest difficulty in retrieving those words that are substantive (nouns and verbs). Since their lesions are located in the posterior portion of the brain, distant from motor areas, they also tend to have some degree of impaired awareness and are rarely physically disabled. There are several types of syndromes subsumed under the fluent aphasia classification (Table 28.2).

The most common type of fluent aphasia is *Wernicke's aphasia* (also referred to as *sensory aphasia* and/or *receptive aphasia*). Wernicke's aphasia is usually the result of a lesion in the posterior portion of the first temporal gyrus of the left hemisphere. It is characterized by impaired auditory comprehension and fluently articulated speech marked by word substitutions. Reading and writing are usually severely impaired as well. Although patients with Wernicke's aphasia may produce what seem like complete utterances and use complex verb tenses, they often add a word or phrase and "augment" speech production. Speech is often produced at a rate greater than normal. Although the production of speech sounds is generally precise, patients with Wernicke's aphasia may reverse phonemes and/or syllables (hopspipal/trevilision) and may produce *neologisms* (nonsense words).

In the course of recovery Wernicke's aphasia may evolve into anomic aphasia. *Anomic aphasia* is characterized by a significant word-finding difficulty in the context of fluent, grammatically well-formed speech. Auditory comprehension is generally impaired, especially when listening to complex and/or rapid speech. Speech output may be somewhat vague and the patient may be proficient in producing *circumlocutions* to skirt the lack of specificity of language use.

Nonfluent Aphasia

Nonfluent aphasia is characterized by limited vocabulary, slow, hesitant speech, some awkward articulation, and restricted use of grammar in the presence of relatively preserved auditory comprehension. Nonfluent aphasia is associated with anterior lesions usually involving the third frontal convolution of the left hemisphere. Patients with nonfluent aphasia tend to express themselves in vocabulary that is substantive (nouns, verbs) and lack the ability to retrieve less substantive parts of speech (prepositions, conjunctions, pronouns). Patients with nonfluent aphasia tend to have good awareness of their deficit and usually have impaired motor function on the right side (right hemiplegia–paresis).

Broca's aphasia is a nonfluent type of aphasia also sometimes referred to as *expressive aphasia*, *motor aphasia*, and/or *verbal aphasia*. Broca's aphasia is the result of a lesion involving the third frontal convolution of the left hemisphere, the subcortical white matter, and extending posteriorly to the inferior portion of the motor strip (precentral gyrus). It is characterized by awkward articulation, restricted vocabulary, and restriction to simple grammatical forms in the presence of a relative preservation of auditory comprehension. Writing skills generally mirror the pattern of speech and reading may be less impaired than speech and writing. The patient may be limited to one- and two-word productions for expression and find it impossible to combine words into sentences. Articulation may be awkward and effortful (see later section titled Apraxia of Speech). Nonfluent Broca's aphasia is less common after TBI. Anomic disturbances predominate in aphasia secondary to TBI.

Global Aphasia

A severe aphasia with marked dysfunction across all language modalities and with severely limited residual use of all communication modes for oral–aural interactions is referred to as *global aphasia*. Global aphasia is not a type of aphasia but rather a designation of severity. The patient with global aphasia generally has extensive damage, which may be anywhere in the left hemisphere, and is sometimes bilateral.[24] Global aphasia has been cited as among the most common types of aphasia in patients referred for speech rehabilitation services.[25,26]

Acquired Aphasia

Acquired aphasia in children as a result of cerebral damage caused by head injury, tumor, or stroke results in the same syndromes manifest in adults with aphasia.[27-30] In children with aphasia secondary to TBI, anomic disturbances predominate and there is generally a reduction of output with hesitancy, difficulty initiating speech, and sometimes mutism.[31] Follow-up studies report that a significant number of children with acquired aphasia are slow to develop language and academic skills. Since cerebral plasticity decreases across the developmental spectrum, the age of aphasia onset is a factor in determining the extent of recovery.[30]

Primary Progressive Aphasia

Primary progressive aphasia (PPA), a condition that was first described in 1982, is now a recognized diagnostic category.[32,33] PPA is a slowly progressive isolated aphasia not due to stroke, trauma, tumor, or infection, which does not fit neatly into existing aphasia classification schemes. It can exist in the absence or relative absence of generalized intellectual and behavioral disturbances or cognitive impairment generally associated with dementia. Activities of daily living, judgment, insight, and behavior are usually preserved for at least 2 years and may remain unimpaired and isolated from the language impairment for as long as 20 years.[34] About half of those with PPA eventually develop symptoms of a more pervasive dementia. Spontaneous recovery does not occur.

In its initial presentation, PPA is commonly reported and observed as being a speech or articulation disorder or difficulty in naming. PPA progresses at different rates and in its most severe form can result in the inability to speak. In these cases comprehension usually remains relatively preserved. However, in other cases initial difficulties with and a progressive decline in word retrieval skills and comprehension with relatively preserved speech production abilities is noted.[35] The longer the

Table 28.2 Classification by Aphasia Syndromes

	Wernicke's Aphasia	Broca's Aphasia	Global Aphasia	Conduction Aphasia	Anomic Aphasia	Transcortical Motor Aphasia	Pure Word Deafness
Area of infarction	Posterior portion of temporal gyrus	Third frontal convolution	Third frontal convolution and posterior portion of superior temporal gyrus	Parietal operculum or posterior superior temporal gyrus	Angular gyrus	Supplementary motor areas	Both Heschl's gyri or connection between Heschl's gyrus and posterior superior temporal gyrus
Spontaneous speech	Fluent	Nonfluent	Nonfluent	Fluent or nonfluent	Fluent	Nonfluent	Fluent
Comprehension	Poor	Good	Poor	Good	Good	Good	Poor
Repetition	Poor	Poor (but may be better than spontaneous speech)	Poor	Very poor	Good	Excellent	Poor
Naming	Poor	Poor (but may be better than spontaneous speech)	Poor	Poor	Very poor	Poor	Good
Reading comprehension	Poor	Good	Poor	Good to poor	Good to poor	Good	Good
Writing	Poor	Poor	Poor	Poor	Good to poor	Poor	Good

duration of aphasia as an isolated symptom, the less likely that other signs of dementia will develop.

Historical Perspective

Language disturbances were recorded as early as 3500 BC, and attempts to "retrain" individuals with aphasia have been recorded throughout history.[36] Some of the first documented cases of both natural recovery and intervention were the patients of Nicolo Massa and Francisco Arceo in 1558.[37]

In a landmark paper in the late 19th century, "Du siège de la faculté du langage articulé," Paul Broca was one of the first to discuss the possibility of retraining in aphasia.[38] Dr. Charles K. Mills was the first to address recovery and rehabilitation in aphasia in an English-language publication. He reported the training of a patient with post-stroke aphasia whom he and Donald Broadbent treated, using methods largely determined by

the patient, who began by systematically repeating letters, words, and phrases.[39,40] Mills' observations and approach to aphasia rehabilitation, published over a century ago, are remarkably similar to much present-day practice and thought. Mills noted that not all patients benefit from retraining to the same degree and acknowledged that spontaneous recovery might have an influence on the course and extent of recovery.

World War I and its brain-injured combat survivors led to the establishment of treatment centers where patients with post-traumatic aphasia were treated, especially in Europe. Reports of aphasia rehabilitation experiences during and after the war in England and the United States were also published.[41,42] One of the most comprehensive descriptions of the systematic treatment of a large number of patients with aphasia secondary to head trauma, of whom 90 to 100 were followed for a 10-year period, was provided by Kurt Goldstein in Frankfurt during the Second World War.[43]

Until World War II, reports of retraining civilians with post-stroke aphasia were rare. The aphasia literature was based almost exclusively on post-traumatic aphasia. In 1933, Singer and Low[44] reported the case of a 39-year-old woman who suffered an apparent vascular infarct after a full-term delivery and showed continuous language improvement with consistent training over a 10-year period.

In a landmark 5-year study supported by the Commonwealth Fund, Weisenburg and McBride[45] addressed the general topic of aphasia and commented on the effectiveness of reeducation. The study concerned 60 patients who were younger than 60 years of age, a majority of whom had suffered strokes, and concluded that reeducation increased the rate of recovery, assisted in facilitating the use of compensatory means of communication, and improved morale. Their work also documented the psychotherapeutic benefits of treatment.

Before World War II, aphasia and its concomitant neurological deficits in the patient with stroke were generally viewed as natural and necessary components of the aging process. The treatment of aphasia in the civilian population was not an option.

Many variables had an influence on making the treatment of aphasia the common practice that it is today. The advent of speech and language pathology as a health profession, the emergence of rehabilitation medicine as a medical specialty, the mass media explosion, a larger and more affluent middle class, an increase in the life span, the number of stroke and brain injury survivors, and public expectations of medicine in the age of technology are among them. The last has been particularly true in the industrialized world, where it is widely believed that there is a treatment for every human ill.[46]

Journals devoted to brain/language issues have become indispensable information sources for aphasiologists (e.g., *Journal of Medical Speech and Language Pathology, Aphasiology, Brain and Language,* and *Cortex*). The Academy of Aphasia, a scholarly society dedicated to the study of aphasia, was established in 1962. The National Aphasia Association (NAA) was founded in the United States in 1987 for the purpose of providing information to the public about aphasia, advocating for the aphasia community, and encouraging the establishment of a network of support groups called Aphasia Community Groups (ACGs).[47]

Several informational publications designed for use by the families and friends of patients with aphasia also appeared in the period following World War II.[48-53] One of these, "Understanding Aphasia: A Guide for Family and Friends," is still widely read and has been published in 12 languages.[53]

Aphasia Measures

Many measures of aphasia and related disorders have been developed for use in both clinical and research settings. In an inpatient setting, patients with aphasia are generally screened at bedside. The purpose of a bedside screening is to obtain a general idea of a patient's profile of deficits and preserved areas of language function as a basis for recommendations for more comprehensive testing and possible rehabilitation. However, a comprehensive examination is required to provide a baseline measure against which to gauge progress in the course of rehabilitation.

Comprehensive language tests designed to measure aphasic impairment generally contain specific domains of performance. In addition to the general requirements for the construction of tests, such as reliability, standardization, and demonstrated validity, certain factors are important in the design of tests intended to identify and measure aphasia. These include range of item difficulty, efficacy in measuring recovery, and ability to contribute to diagnostic classification.[2,54] Aphasia tests are generally based on examinations of linguistic task performance and at a minimum include tasks of visual confrontation *naming;* a spontaneous or conversational *speech sample* that is analyzed for fluency of output, effort, articulation, phrase length, prosody, word substitutions, and omissions; *repetition* of digits, single words, multisyllable words, and sentences of increasing length and complexity; *comprehension of spoken language* of single words, of sentences that require only yes/no responses, and pointing on command; *word retrieval* (word finding) measuring the ability to generate words beginning with a particular letter of the alphabet or in a particular semantic category (animals); *reading;* and *writing* from dictation and spontaneously. Some widely used aphasia measures include the *Boston Diagnostic Aphasia Examination (BDAE),*[23] the *Neurosensory Center Comprehensive Examination for Aphasia (NCCEA),*[55] and the *Western Aphasia Battery.*[56]

In addition to measuring performance on specific linguistic tasks, an aphasia evaluation also requires an examination of *functional communication*. This is necessary because an individual's actual use of language in everyday life may not correspond to the degree of pathology measured by specific language task performance.[57,58] Functional communication measures are generally rating scales with high interrater reliability. The *Functional Communication Profile (FCP),*[59,60] *Communicative Activities of Daily Living (CADL),*[61] *Communicative Effectiveness Index,*[62] and ASHA's *Functional Assessment of Communication Skills (ASHA FACS),*[63] which have high interrater reliability, are measures used for this purpose.

In addition to measures of language and functional communication, new tools have been developed to determine the impact of impaired communication skills on quality of life. The scope of SLP practice now encompasses all of the components and factors specified in the WHO framework.[13,65-68] Specifically, concern for the effect of aphasia on family, social, and community life is the basis for more recently designed measures (e.g., Burden of Stroke Scale [BOSS], Functional Life Scale [FLS], Aphasic Depression Rating Scale [ADRS], Frenchay Activities Index, and Stroke and Aphasia Quality of Life Scale–39 [SAQOL-39]).[68-75]

Recovery

If complete recovery from aphasia is to occur, it usually happens within a matter of hours or days following onset. Once aphasia has persisted for several weeks or months, a complete return to a premorbid state is usually the exception. It is the general consensus that language gains in aphasia take place earlier rather than later, and that time since onset is an important recovery variable.[76-81]

Most patients do not consider themselves recovered unless they have fully recovered to previous levels of language performance.[46,82] When unrecovered patients are satisfied with their level of competence and consider themselves recovered, this is a psychological perception and should not be confused with an objective evaluation of communication abilities. For individuals with aphasia, the true test of rehabilitation outcome is their perception of the quality of their life. Measures of life function that include activity levels, socialization, mobility, and community reintegration can be used for this purpose.[83,84]

It is useful to distinguish between two separate recovery dimensions in aphasia: one that is objective and attempts to quantify the extent to which a person has regained language abilities; and another, which measures the recovery of functional communication.

The concept of a functional dimension of communication behavior emerged logically from the experience of treating patients with aphasia in rehabilitation medicine settings. Historically, rehabilitation medicine has acknowledged that the ability of patients to function in daily life (activities of daily living [ADL]) does not necessarily correlate with the degree of physical disability. Similarly, improvement in quantitative measures of language performance does not necessarily correlate with improvement in functional communication.[46]

The majority of patients experience a degree of natural recovery with or without intervention in the period immediately following onset. However, there is a lack of consensus about the duration of the *spontaneous recovery* period.[85-87] Culton[88] reported rapid spontaneous language recovery in the first month following the onset of aphasia, and a number of studies have concluded that the greatest improvement occurs in the first 2 to 3 months after onset.[89-93] Of 850 patients surveyed in the first month following stroke, 177 presented with aphasia. In the 4 to 12 weeks following the stroke, aphasia improved in 74% of the patients and cleared in 44%.[18] Butfield and Zangwill,[94] Sands et al,[95] and Vignolo[89] reported that the recovery rate dropped significantly after 6 months. Others have found that spontaneous recovery occurs up to 6 months[96] or 1 year.[88,90]

Sarno and Levita[97] reported that the greater change took place within a 3-month rather than a 6-month post-onset period in a sample of patients with severe aphasia seen up to 6 months after stroke.

Recovery from aphasia after stroke is difficult to predict, especially during the early recovery stages.[98] Severity and location of lesion have been reported as predictors of language recovery.[99-102] However, these factors are very variable, making it difficult to generate a prognosis for individual patients.[103]

Most investigators have concluded that factors such as age, gender, and handedness do not affect recovery from aphasia.[98,103-105] Although age has been reported as a significant prognostic factor,[89,106-108] many do not support this view.[90,104,109-113] These wide discrepancies regarding the influence of age may relate to differences in sampling and methodology. In a study that compared aphasia recovery in the first post-stroke year between a middle-aged (50 to 64 years old) and older (65 to 80 years old) group, age did not emerge as a significant factor.[83] In addition, educational level or occupational status before illness does not always correlate with recovery. However, Sarno and Levita[97] reported that individuals with aphasia who were employed at the time of stroke recovered more than those who were unemployed. In the healthy aged, language performance declines significantly between the sixth and eighth decades.[106,114,115] Gender does not appear to have an important influence on outcome,[76,104,116] whereas handedness may have an effect.[117]

It is generally agreed that posttraumatic aphasia has a better prognosis than aphasia secondary to vascular lesions.[89,94] In fact, some cases of aphasia secondary to TBI have been reported to recover completely.[91,118] The finding that traumatic aphasia carries a better prognosis than vascular aphasia may be influenced by the fact that patients involved in traumatic events are generally neurologically healthy whereas patients who have had strokes may have widespread vascular involvement.[104]

Both type and severity of aphasia appear to carry predictive value, with global aphasia having the poorest prognosis.[76,119-121] Basso[104] reported that when patients with fluent and nonfluent aphasia of the same severity were compared, there were no differences in degree of recovery. In 881 consecutive acute stroke admissions to a community-based hospital, it was possible to make valid prognoses within 1 to 4 weeks after stroke depending on the initial severity of aphasia.[104]

Not surprisingly, most studies report that patients with severe aphasia do not recover as much as those with mild aphasia.[91,95,120-122] Sarno and Levita[76] found that people with fluent aphasia reached the highest level of functional communication, whereas patients with nonfluent and global aphasia made smaller gains in the 8- to 52-week post-stroke period. Global aphasia sometimes evolves to severe Broca's aphasia when there is significantly improved comprehension. Broca's aphasia may become *anomic aphasia,* and Wernicke's aphasia may evolve to anomic or *conduction aphasia.*[76,91,120-124] When persons with aphasia recover a great deal of language function they are usually left with residual *anomia.*

Patients whose computed tomography (CT) scans show large dominant hemisphere lesions, many small lesions, or bilateral lesions are less likely to recover than those with smaller or fewer lesions.[82,120] Lesions in Wernicke's area or those that extend more posteriorly tend to lead to severe and persistent aphasia. The neuroradiological correlates of aphasia recovery have been addressed by some investigators.[93,125] Yarnell et al[82] reported little prognostic value in angiographic and radioscintigram findings. Similarly, CT scans did not help in predicting who might profit from language retraining in a Norwegian study.[86]

More recent functional imaging studies of aphasia secondary to stroke have suggested that language recovery is dependent on several factors. The neuroplastic changes that are needed during recovery are thought to depend more heavily on left hemispheric changes in activity that slowly manifest over time.[22] Following damage to the left hemisphere, rapid changes have been observed in temporal and frontal areas within the right hemisphere but may reflect maladaptive compensatory activity versus functional reorganization or recovery.[126-135]

Comprehension tends to recover to a greater degree than expression.[26,89,133-136] Although recovery of auditory comprehension involves bilateral temporal lobe activation, there does not seem to be a correlation between the activity of each hemisphere during this process.[126,137-139] As technology advances and research continues, new insights into the mechanisms of recovery and treatment will emerge.[140]

The presence of depression, anxiety, and paranoia have been cited as negative factors in recovery,[141-143] and premorbid personality traits have been identified as important prognostic factors. Eisenson and Herrmann felt that patients with outgoing personalities had a better prognosis than those with introverted, dependent, or rigid personalities.[144-146]

Efficacy of Treatment in Post-Stroke Aphasia

Many methodological problems have limited the number of studies that examine the efficacy of aphasia rehabilitation.[147-153] Nevertheless, treatment accountability issues are compelling and a focus of professional concern.

Studies that investigate treatment effects, specific techniques, and approaches have been reported since the late 1950s.[154] Vignolo,[89] Hagen,[155] and Basso et al[90,119] utilized untreated control and treated groups and showed a positive treatment effect. Edmonds et al[156] and Poeck et al[157] also yielded positive treatment effects with treated and untreated groups. In addition, several reviews and examinations have revealed significant

treatment effects (i.e., improvements in communicative ability) with intense intervention provided over a short period of time.[158-160] Variables such as spontaneous recovery,[91,161,162] age,[109,163] duration, treatment intensity,[122,158-160] and timing of treatment[164] and specific treatment techniques[165-167] have been studied.

Although studies have varied in method and research focus, there have been strong indications for positive treatment effects.[154] Some have maintained that single case studies rather than randomized, controlled trials are the most appropriate method for addressing treatment efficacy.[168,169] Current research utilizing a standard approach to analyze data from single-subject designs are improving the ability to quantify treatment outcomes.[96] A single case approach to the study of aphasia treatment efficacy has not escaped criticism but is far less frequent than criticism of studies based on groups of people with aphasia.[96] Negative views of the group study model are based primarily on the view that individuals are unique, especially with respect to communication behavior.

The Academy of Neurologic Communication Disorders and Sciences (ANCDS) has issued evidence-based practice guidelines for neurogenic communication disorders.[153,170,171] Until now, SLPs have depended on meta-analyses of efficacy studies reported for 45 studies published between 1946 and 1988 and for 55 studies that support better clinical outcome for patients who receive early, intensive treatment.[152,172]

Psychological and Related Factors

It has been observed that the variability of patients' psychological reactions is rarely determined by the type or location of their lesions but is an expression of the whole life experience of the person who has had a stroke.[83,104,143,173,174]

Depression, anxiety, premorbid personality, fatigue, and paranoia are often cited as deterrents to recovery and communication. The social isolation experienced by people with aphasia and their families has a profound impact on quality of life.[83,151] The effect of aphasia on an individual's sense of "self" can be extremely negative, leading to a loss of self-esteem and feelings of helplessness. Also, the opportunity for "healing conversation," so essential to individuals who have suffered losses, is often unavailable to those with aphasia, which may be the result of inadequate social support.

In a study of patients with aphasia participating in a group psychotherapy program, Friedman[175] investigated the nature of psychological regression with impaired reality testing in aphasia. Beyond the communication difficulties posed by aphasia, he observed that patients remained psychologically isolated. They did not maintain a consistent level of group participation and expressed intense feelings that they were very different from other people. Both withdrawal and projection were apparent as each patient acted in isolation and yet complained of these characteristic in others.

Treatment of Aphasia

Aphasia treatment is rarely the same in any two settings. Literally hundreds of specific speech and language treatment techniques are cited in the aphasia literature. The lack of therapeutic uniformity has undoubtedly impeded an adequate number of carefully controlled studies on the effects of language retraining. Most methods derive essentially from traditional pedagogic practices, relying heavily on repetition.[176]

In general, treatment methods can be categorized as those that are largely *indirect stimulation-facilitation* and those that are essentially *direct structured-pedagogic*.[78,118,141,177-180] The two principles that underlie most treatment methods reflect contrasting views of aphasia as either impaired access to language or a "loss" of language. The stimulation methods generally follow an impaired access model and pedagogic approaches are based on a theory of aphasia as a language loss.

In practice, however, much of aphasia treatment addresses the *performance* aspect of language in which repeated practice and "teaching" strategies are assumed to help restore impaired skills through a "task-oriented" approach (i.e., naming practice). One of the commonly used techniques involves self-cueing and repetition exercises that manipulate components of grammar and vocabulary. Another approach involves "stimulating" the patient to use residual language by encouraging conversation in a permissive setting where a patient's responses are unconditionally accepted and topics are of personal interest.[179]

The primary assumption that drives the treatment of aphasia is that language in the brain is not "erased," but that retrieval of its individual units has been impaired. Approaches to aphasia therapy have generally followed one of two models: a *substitute skill model* or a *direct treatment model*, both of which are based on the assumption that the processes that subserve normal performance need to be understood if treatment is to succeed.[180] An example of the substitute skill model can be found in deaf individuals, some of whom use speech reading, a visual input rather than an auditory input, as an aid to comprehend spoken language. If a direct treatment model is followed, specific exercises individually designed to ameliorate specific linguistic deficits are the basis of treatment.

Significant progress and improvements of language and communication performance have been reported in those with aphasia who have received intensive and/or extended periods of language therapy.[153,157,181,182] More recent reports of intensive treatment programs have shown significant improvement of communication abilities several years post-stroke, when aphasia is in the chronic stage.[167,182-184] Some benefits may also be received from

pharmacological treatment with and without speech therapy.[185-192] In addition, improvements have also been documented with the use of transcranial magnetic stimulation,[193] functional magnetic resonance imaging,[194] and transcranial direct current stimulation.[195]

Visual communication therapy (VIC) is an experimental technique designed for persons with global aphasia.[196-200] It employs an index card system of arbitrary symbols representing syntactic and lexical components that patients learn to manipulate so as to (1) respond to a command and (2) express needs, wishes, or other emotions. The system attempts to circumvent the use of natural oral language, which is severely impaired and often unavailable to the patient with global aphasia. An adaptation and application of the VIC system, *Computer-Aided Visual Communication system (C-VIC)*, was developed by Steele et al.[198,199] Weinrich et al[201] demonstrated that C-VIC training can lead to improved spoken language. Investigators conclude that the evidence supports the view that some patients who have severe aphasia can master the basics of an artificial language and that some of the cognitive operations entailed in natural language are preserved despite the severity of the impairment.

Visual Action Therapy (VAT) developed at the Boston Veterans Administration Medical Center by Helm-Estabrooks et al[202,203] was designed to train people with global aphasia to use symbolic gestures representing visually absent objects. The tasks leading to this goal include associating pictured forms with specific objects, manipulating real objects appropriately, and finally producing symbolic gestures that represent the objects used (e.g., cup, hammer, razor).

In an attempt to utilize systematized gestural language to facilitate oral production, American Indian sign language has been modified in a method that combines common gestural sign with oral speech production (Amerind) for selected cases.[204-206]

Melodic Intonation Therapy (MIT) is based on the observation that language may not be available in spontaneous speech but can sometimes be provided in association with known melody, as the therapist gradually introduces spoken material with a melodic rhythm. The patient is encouraged to participate in the process.[207-209]

In the *functional communication treatment (FCT)* method developed by Aten et al,[210,211] emphasis is placed on restoration of communication in the broadest sense. Treatment is designed to improve information processing in the activities necessary to conducting ADL, social interactions, and self-expression of both physical and psychological needs.[210,211]

Promoting Aphasics' Communicative Effectiveness (PACE), a technique intended to reshape structured interaction between clinicians and patients into more natural communicative exchanges, includes several pragmatic components common to natural conversation.[212,213]

Contextualized, constraint-induced language therapy (CILT) is an intensive form of language therapy that is usually administered over a short period of time. Treatment is conducted by an SLP in small groups of two to three persons with aphasia who are required to use and practice only those verbal skills that are difficult or impaired. Forms of communication that can be effective in total communication but are not verbal, including gesturing, drawing, or writing, are constrained.[167,214,215]

Maher et al[215] compared PACE and CILT on the same schedule of intensity and found that both groups made significant improvements but differed in the types of communication behaviors that improved. Those who received CILT performed better on measures examining verbal behaviors and those who received PACE improved on nonverbal behaviors.

Some investigators have reported the use of writing[216] or drawing as a potential means of communication.[217-220] Others have developed interactive approaches to aphasia treatment. Examples include the *communication partners* approach of Lyon,[217-219] a treatment plan designed to enhance communication and well-being in settings where the person with aphasia and the caregiver live; the *supported conversation* approach introduced by Kagan and colleagues,[221-225] in which volunteers are trained as conversation partners to facilitate conversation by using all available modalities, thereby revealing the individual's competence and permitting a communicative interaction; and the *social model of aphasia* approach introduced by Simmons-Mackie,[226-234] which focuses on the fulfillment of social needs and the encouragement of a greater conversational burden on the part of communication partners. Partners are trained to facilitate interaction by modifying some of their interactive behavior.

If an individual is unable to make himself or herself understood and has residual writing and spelling skills, aids that use the alphabet can provide a means of communication (e.g., an alphabet board). A communication book may consist of pictures or words arranged according to topics (e.g., foods, family members) in a notebook for easy access. The same type of material has also been adapted for computerized access in the form of tablet devices (e.g., iPad). Microcomputers were the basis for an approach that Seron et al[235] found effective in treating patients with writing disorders associated with aphasia. With continued exposure to training, improvement in accuracy and recognition time in reading commonly used words[236] and improvement in auditory comprehension were noted in a patient with aphasia who, when followed up at a later date, showed additional gains.[237,238] Computer-generated phonemic cues were effective in improving naming in five patients with Broca's aphasia.[239] An augmentative system was developed for a patient with Broca's aphasia;[240] a word retrieval facilitation program was developed for individuals with aphasia;[241] and Steele et al[199] and Weinrich et al[242]

replicated and extended the findings of Gardner et al[196] and Baker et al[243] by training those with aphasia to use a computerized version of the VIC system.

Use of telecommunications, virtual clinicians, and computer-assisted treatments may lead to improvements in language and communication, especially when utilized as an adjunct to clinical therapy. Data suggest that these types of therapies may be effective for patients in various stages of recovery.[244-249]

Management of the Patient with Aphasia

The unfortunate reality is that once the condition of aphasia has stabilized, very few patients recover normal communication function, with or without speech therapy. Accordingly, aphasia rehabilitation should be viewed as a process of patient management in the broadest sense of the term. That is, the task is primarily one of helping the patient and his or her intimates adjust to the alterations and limitations imposed by the disability. Effective aphasia rehabilitation management requires the participation of several disciplines, including medicine, psychology, physical therapy, occupational therapy, social work, vocational counseling, and, most critically, aphasia therapy.

The selective and discriminating use of speech and language therapy to stimulate and support the patient through the various stages of recovery is an effective management tool.[87,250,251] Experienced aphasia therapists recognize that while working on aphasic deficits, they are simultaneously dealing psychotherapeutically with a readjusting personality.[143] Speech therapy, therefore, serves different purposes at different points along the way. Sometimes it allows patients to "borrow time," as Baretz and Stephenson[252] have aptly stated. Occasionally depression lifts after speech therapy has been initiated, reflecting the supportive and nurturing nature of the therapeutic relationship rather than an objective improvement in recovery of speech and language.[251]

Aphasia recovery can be viewed as a dynamic process consisting of a series of stages like the stages of mourning described by Kübler-Ross,[253] through which the majority of patients evolve. Some, of course, never emerge from a state of severe depression.[254,255] Kübler-Ross[253] and other authors have suggested that the stages through which someone with aphasia passes—including denial, rage, bargaining, and acceptance—could be characterized as attempts to overcome the sense of loss.

By directly addressing a patient's linguistic deficits and channeling attention and energies toward constructive goals, speech therapy may produce a noticeable reduction in depression. Therapy tasks in this instance act as an equivalent for work, which has long been recognized as an antidote for depression.

There is a great tendency to overestimate the capacity of individuals with aphasia to return to work, particularly if the verbal deficits are mild. Premature attempts to return to work can have a negative psychological impact. Professional rehabilitation counselors are best equipped to explore and evaluate a patient's vocational potential and carry out the long and arduous process of evaluating work performance and job requirements.

Experienced aphasia clinicians stress the importance of the patient's family in the rehabilitation process. Some of the potentially negative reactions of the family include overprotectiveness, hostility, anger, unrealistic expectations, overzealousness, lack of knowledge of the dimensions of the disorder, and inability to cope with practical difficulties. The apparently natural tendency of family members to minimize the patient's communication impairment, particularly in the early stages of recovery, requires understanding and tactful management.[143]

The quality of premorbid relationships generally tends to be intensified after a catastrophic event; those that were problematic may deteriorate further, whereas the bond between a loving couple may become stronger. The reversal of roles, changes in levels of dependency, and a changed economic situation, so often a consequence of chronic disability, can have a critical negative impact on the patient and his or her family.[174]

In a positive family milieu, patients are encouraged to develop regular daily routines as close to premorbid patterns as possible and are treated as contributing members of the family. Patients need to be allowed some sense of control. Including the patient in rehabilitation planning promotes restoration of feelings of self-worth. In this regard, the emphasis on function rather than complete recovery, pointing out success rather than performance failure, adds to a patient's sense of self. It is essential to listen to patients, particularly to their expressions of loss. Commiseration is often more comforting than optimistic prognostic statements.

Group speech therapy, stroke clubs, and other social groups that are frequently used resources can be effective tools in the management of some patients with chronic aphasia. The National Aphasia Association (NAA) was founded in the United States in 1987, following the lead of existing advocacy organizations established in Finland (1971), Germany (1978), the United Kingdom (1980), and Sweden (1981). The NAA provides an extensive array of educational and resource information appropriate for patients, families, and professionals on its website (www.aphasia.org). Knowledge that one is not alone often helps to reduce depression and loneliness.[86,141]

Group therapy with peers also provides a comfortable atmosphere in which patients can meet new friends and share feelings, although not all individuals with aphasia find it beneficial. A positive effect seems to be related to level of comprehension, time since onset, and personality factors. Although group therapy generally plays an important role in aphasia rehabilitation, it should be noted that much of its effectiveness depends on the skill and experience of the group leader.[256,257]

Aphasia rehabilitation remains eclectic and specifically tailored to the individual patient. Fundamental to this therapeutic philosophy is the acknowledgement and appreciation of the uniqueness of the individual. No two persons with aphasia are exactly alike in pathology, personality, linguistic deficits, reactions to catastrophic illness, life experience, spiritual values, or a host of other factors. The influence of these factors carries different weight and strength at different stages of recovery and they are all related to recovery outcome.

Those who manage the rehabilitation of patients with aphasia face many ethical–moral dilemmas. One of the principal issues is a result of the necessity in many settings to select those individuals who will receive treatment. Rehabilitation medicine services are not only scarce in many situations, but they are also not considered to be a right or entitlement. Services are usually provided on a selective basis to those individuals believed to have the potential to benefit. This process assumes that we know who can benefit.[16,258-261] Many who are experienced in aphasia rehabilitation management hold the view that all people should be given a trial treatment period to determine their candidacy for further treatment and that trials should be provided at different points in the recovery course. Goal setting, the patient's right to self-determination, and the criteria appropriate in determining the termination of therapy are also important ethical issues.[143,261]

■ COGNITIVE-COMMUNICATION DISORDERS

When the neural regions responsible for the cognitive processes that support communicative function are damaged, a broad spectrum of deficits can result. Many conditions can cause cognitive-communication disorders, including TBI, stroke (especially right hemisphere damage), dementia, brain tumors, aging, degenerative neurological disease, alcohol/drug abuse, and medications. Impairments of executive function, including difficulties with attention and memory, may interfere with a person's ability to transform thoughts and ideas into spoken and/or written language.[262-265] Impaired memory can also affect word retrieval, topic maintenance, a person's ability to recall and integrate information, and the speed of processing information. In addition, organizing information, interpreting visual information, deficits in abstract reasoning, and decreased orientation to person, place, and time are common symptoms. Impairments in speech production, including reduced fluency and prosodic speech features (i.e., rate and rhythm of speech, stress within words to indicate meaning and within sentences to express variations of intent or meaning), are also common.[266] Given the nature of these deficits, participating in social situations can be especially difficult.[267] The difficulties may affect all modes of communication, including understanding, nonverbal and verbal expression, reading, and writing. These impairments can be debilitating and socially isolating, because they impair a person's ability to establish and maintain relationships with others.[268,269]

Impirements of certain aspects of pragmatic language (i.e., language use) and nonverbal communication (including difficulty in initiating, maintaining, and ending conversations), which may result in difficulties maintaining a topic and taking turns in discourse; being concise;[270] understanding and expressing feeling through facial expressions; comprehending nonverbal methods of communication (i.e., gesturing); maintaining eye contact; engaging in conversation or narrative production that is self-focused; interpreting and expressing emotions appropriately; and reduced ability in understanding humor.

Examination of Cognitive-Communication Disorders

Many factors, including the heterogeneity of individuals, limitations of available standardized testing measures, performance differences in structured versus unstructured contexts, and environmental and personal factors, have made the examination of cognitive-communication disorders a challenging area in need of further study.[271,272] A standardized test battery for the identification and measurement of cognitive-communication disorders does not exist and depends entirely on the knowledge, experience, and expertise of the examiner.

Treatment of Cognitive-Communication Disorders

Intervention depends on the type and severity of the cognitive-communication disorder and is usually based on a combination of behavioral, meta-cognitive, and counseling approaches. Patients with cognitive-communication disorders are especially challenging since they often have reduced insight and/or denial.[269,273] The importance of providing speech-language pathology treatment using a team approach has been highlighted as an important element in the rehabilitation process. Such collaborative methods take into account each person's social network (e.g., family, friends, caregivers, and so forth.).[263,264,274,275]

The management of patients with cognitive-communication disorders begins with determining what environmental factors, if any, can be modified to provide the least visual or auditory distraction. Steps also need to be taken to establish a structured routine or daily schedule. These efforts help to reduce communication breakdowns and facilitate communicative success.[274,275] The later stages of intervention emphasize the carryover of skills acquired in therapy to a variety of daily activities and contexts.[263] Box 28.1 provides several suggested strategies to improve communication for patients with cognitive-communication disorders.

Box 28.1 Strategies for Improving Communication in the Presence of Cognitive-Communication Disorder

- Use visual materials/aids to help orient the person to time (e.g., clocks and calendars)
- Break long, complicated tasks into shorter tasks that are easier to follow
- Establish eye contact to initiate and maintain conversation
- When giving verbal directions, use simple sentences and repetitions as necessary
- Accommodate the presence of visual field deficits by helping the person find compensatory means for reading and writing
- Gently state when the topic in a conversation changes prematurely

---

◼ DYSARTHRIA

The term **dysarthria** (sometimes called a *motor speech disorder*) refers to an impairment of speech production resulting from damage to the central or peripheral nervous system, which causes weakness, paralysis, or incoordination of the motor–speech system. Any one or all of the components of the motor–speech system (respiration, phonation, articulation, resonance, and prosody) may by compromised by neural damage. The type and degree of dysarthria depends on the underlying etiology, degree of neuropathology, coexistence of other disabilities, and the individual response of the patient to the condition. It is not unusual for dysarthria to coexist with aphasia in patients who have suffered cerebrovascular accident (CVA) or TBI. The severity of dysarthria may range from the production of occasionally imprecise consonant sounds to speech that is rendered totally unintelligible by the degree of impairment to the underlying systems. When patients are totally unintelligible as the result of severe motor–speech system impairment, they exhibit **anarthria**.

The incidence of dysarthria in the population of individuals with neurogenic disorders is approximately 46%, representing a significant proportion of the patients with communication impairments seen in medical settings.[276] It is difficult to estimate the total number of people affected by dysarthria, because the condition results from a wide range of etiologies (e.g., progressive neurological diseases, TBI, and stroke). For example, approximately 1% of the population older than 60 suffers from Parkinson's disease,[277] and about 89% of those with Parkinson's disease develop a motor speech disorder as the disease progresses.[278]

Dysarthria is generally reflected in deficits occurring in multiple motor–speech systems, but may sometimes occur in a single system (e.g., an impairment of soft palate movement resulting in hypernasality). It is most notably prevalent in cerebral palsy, TBI, CVA, demyelinating diseases (e.g., multiple sclerosis), neoplasm, and progressive neurodegenerative diseases, such as Parkinson's disease, Huntington's chorea, and amyotrophic lateral sclerosis.

There are five primary types of dysarthria: *spastic, flaccid, ataxic, hypokinetic,* and *hyperkinetic.* When two or more types coexist, the term *mixed dysarthria* is used. Coexisting physical disabilities are present in a majority of patients who manifest dysarthria.

Classification and Nomenclature

Spastic dysarthria is characterized by imprecise articulation, slow labored articulation, hypernasality, harsh to strained phonation, and monotonous pitch. Syllables may be given equal stress and inflection. There is often reduced control of exhalation, with shallow inhalations and slow breaths. Spastic dysarthria is the result of bilateral pyramidal system damage involving the corticobulbar tracts (upper motor neurons). The pathology may cause weakness and paresis of the face and tongue musculature on the side opposite to the lesion. There is a high incidence of spastic dysarthria among those with cerebral palsy.[276]

Flaccid dysarthria is characterized by slow/labored articulation, hypernasality, and hoarse, breathy phonation. Phrases may be short, inhalation is shallow, and the control of exhalation may be reduced. There is often a reduction in the variation of pitch and loudness with audible inspirations. Most of these deviant speech characteristics are related to muscular weakness and reduced muscle tone, which affects speech accuracy.

Ataxic dysarthria is characterized by disturbances of timing, movement, range, control, and coordination of the muscles of speech and respiration. Speech is imprecise, slow, and irregular. There may be intermittent periods of explosive inflection, syllable stress, and loudness patterns. Phonemes may be prolonged; pitch and loudness are monotonous. The lesions producing ataxic dysarthria are bilateral, generalized lesions involving the deep midline nuclei and pathways of the cerebellum. Patients with multiple sclerosis and TBI with cerebellar damage often manifest ataxic dysarthria.

Hypokinetic dysarthria is characterized by variable articulatory precision, slow rate of speech, harsh, hoarse voice quality, excessive and overly long pauses, prolonged syllables, and reduced phonation. Patients with Parkinson's disease, Parkinson's-plus syndromes, or parkinsonian-like symptoms often manifest hypokinetic dysarthria, usually caused by lesions of the substantia nigra.

Hyperkinetic dysarthria is characterized by variable articulatory precision, vocal harshness, prolonged sounds and intervals between words, monotonous pitch, and loudness. It is manifest in patients with Huntington's chorea, caused by lesions of the basal ganglia and/or their extrapyramidal projections.

Treatment of Dysarthria

Dysarthria treatment must be individually designed to account for the profile of impairment, as well as the variability of its disabling effects. The performance of components of the motor–speech system does not necessarily result in changes to the disabling effects of dysarthria, that is, the intelligibility or comprehensibility of speech.[258,279] Goals that relate to the level of disability rather than normal speech are generally more realistic because they do not focus on normalcy, which is usually an unachievable goal, or improvement in the performance of a single component of the motor speech system, which may not, in the overall picture, be functionally important.

The ANCDS's initiative to develop evidence-based practice guidelines for neurogenic communication disorders[170,171] has resulted in meta-analyses of efficacy and effectiveness reported for 51 studies published between 1966 and 2004.[280] The focus of dysarthria treatment is sometimes based on an approach that emphasizes compensatory skills. These techniques tend to encourage the patient to minimize the overall disability by using strategies that may actually deviate from normal (i.e., slowing down the rate of speech production to increase intelligibility of consonant production).

Moreover, the overall aim of dysarthria treatment is to improve communicative effectiveness, which can be negatively affected if the speaker is in a noisy place. Patients and communication partners must be trained to seek the most optimal situations for communication interactions. One type of approach is to focus on one of the subsystems of speech production, such as velopharyngeal function.[281] Other approaches include utilizing an approach that results in a spreading of effects and is centered around improving coordination of the subsystems of respiration, phonation, articulation, and resonance.[282] Loudness, speaking rate, and prosodic features of speech (i.e., stress, intonation, rate, and rhythm of speech) have been investigated for their effectiveness in treating dysarthria.

Increasing the loudness of speech is a common target in the treatment of some types of dysarthria, especially Parkinson's disease. The majority of studies that have focused on loudness have examined the short- and long-term efficacy of the Lee Silverman Voice Therapy program (LSVT®/LOUD) for individuals with dysarthria due to Parkinson's disease. Treatment delivery is intensive and focused on high-effort speech and voice exercises to increase loudness, as well as a readjustment of the patient's perception of his or her own loudness levels when speaking.[283,284] Exercise has been reported to stimulate the production of dopamine, thereby reducing symptom presentation.[285] The program is based on several proposed exercise physiology principles that drive neuroplastic changes, including intensive practice, movement complexity, emotional saliency of tasks, timing of treatment (i.e., the earlier, the better), and continuous/daily exercise to slow disease progression.[284] Studies that have examined this treatment method have also reported improvement in swallowing, articulation, and facial expression[286-289] and have demonstrated its success in individuals with dysarthria due to stroke, TBI,[291] multiple sclerosis,[292] cerebral palsy,[293] and Down syndrome.[294]

In addition to focusing on improving loudness, a variety of strategies are used to manipulate speech rate. Speakers tend to be more intelligible when they speak more slowly.[295] The ANCDS review of studies that investigated the effectiveness of rate control techniques concluded that they are dependent on the type and severity of dysarthria and the specific intervention strategies employed. Further study is still needed to delineate an individual's candidacy for this type of technique, as well as what the carryover can be to the natural communication environment.[280]

A third focus of dysarthria treatment is the improvement of the prosodic aspects of speech (i.e., stress patterns within words and sentences, intonation to express meaning, and rate-rhythm interactions). A variety of strategies that target prosody have been implemented, including those using biofeedback and behavioral instruction. Few conclusions can be drawn about the effectiveness of prosody training because of the small number of examinations and wide range of subject characteristics and techniques used.[280]

A limited number of studies have also reported outcomes of therapy focused on providing people with feedback about speech clarity or instructing people with dysarthria to use "clear speech." A meta-analysis of investigations in this area reports a lack of evidence supporting the effectiveness of this approach.[280]

Many persons with motor–speech impairments have been able to increase their communicative effectiveness using augmentative and alternative communication aids (ACA). Low-tech aids, which only require batteries and electricity, include devices such as telephones and communication books. High-tech aids include specially adapted computers and switching systems, as well as speech-generating programs that are available on mobile devices such as laptop or tablet computers and a variety of smartphones.

Recommendations of ACA for persons with dysarthria depend on the severity of the communication disorder and the projected course of the disease and must be carefully selected and managed by the speech-language pathologist.

■ APRAXIA OF SPEECH

Some patients with nonfluent (Broca's) aphasia present with articulatory difficulty characterized by speech sound errors, slow speech rate, slow transitions between sounds, syllables, and words, and impaired prosody in the absence of impaired strength or coordination of the motor speech system.[296-299] This profile of difficulty speaking is referred to as *apraxia of speech* (AOS) (or *speech dyspraxia, verbal apraxia, cortical dysarthria,* or *phonetic disintegration*). Additional behaviors that may be present in persons with AOS include difficulty initiating speech, articulatory struggling, periods of error-free speech production, and a greater number of sound production errors as utterance length increases. These characteristics may be so severe that the patient is barely intelligible but appears to be independent of difficulty in language processing. Unlike dysarthric speakers, individuals with AOS do not generally have deficits in performing nonspeech movements of the oral musculature. The possible independence of this deficit from the language disorder of Broca's aphasia remains controversial.

The disorder of articulation referred to as AOS is seldom, if ever, manifested in the absence of a coexisting Broca's aphasia, however mild. The speech dyspraxia component of this multifaceted communication disorder appears to be especially amenable to direct therapeutic intervention using approaches adapted primarily from traditional articulation therapy techniques, including stress and intonation drills. These approaches, designed to improve phonetic placement accuracy, typically depend on imitation, stress, and gradually shaping sounds currently available to patient until a desired sound is approximated, which is then drilled using kinesthetic, visual, and auditory cues. Generally, the stimuli used as the bases for these exercises are selected in a presumed order of difficulty, beginning with non-oral imitation, followed by sounds, words, phrases, and finally utterances.

Treatment of Apraxia of Speech

In an attempt to synthesize and assess available evidence from the literature, 59 studies were summarized and rated by the ANCDS. The most commonly used approaches are referred to as *articulatory kinematic.* These techniques aim to improve articulatory movements: modeling, imitation, repetition, shaping, electromagnetic articulography, and multimodal and articulatory placement cueing.[299-308]

Integral stimulation, a method originally introduced by Milisen,[309] is a commonly used articulatory kinematic technique that involves imitation and emphasizes the importance of helping the patient focus his or her attention on auditory and visual models of speech. Rosenbek et al[302] developed an eight-step continuum based on this approach that employs a hierarchy of cues in which the timing between the stimulus provided by the clinician and the response produced by the patient is varied.[302]

Sound production treatment, a five-step program based on the Rosenbek et al[302] eight-step continuum, incorporates principles of motor learning such as repeated practice and verbal feedback and is an approach that has been systematically investigated more than any other AOS treatment.[308,310-312]

Visual spectrographic, and *verbal feedback* utilize different sensory modalities to facilitate speech production.[304,306,307,313,314] The effect of the frequency and timing at which feedback is provided has been investigated and found to be important in the treatment of AOS.[306,315]

Rate and rhythm strategies are employed to improve speech sound accuracy by controlling the rate of speech and stress patterns within words and sentences.[316] External devices such as computer-generated pulses or programs, metronomes, pacing boards, and finger tapping are used to manipulate the rate of speech.[317-323]

The long-term nature of recovery of phonemic production in patients with verbal apraxia was confirmed in a study of a patient with Broca's aphasia who received speech therapy for 10 years. The errors that prevailed in the first post-stroke year were compared with performance at 10 years. The features of place and manner of production had improved; although voicing and addition errors (the addition of sounds) persisted, omission errors (the omission of sounds) were virtually eliminated.[324]

Alternative communication aid approaches are often recommended for persons with AOS. In most cases, the use of multiple communication modalities, such as writing, drawing, gesturing, and signing, is suggested as a facilitatory technique to enhance or substitute for impaired speech.[325-328]

Intersystemic facilitation or *reorganization approaches* use intact systems or preserved strengths or abilities of the patient to facilitate and improve accurate speech production.[329] These approaches employ and combine strategies that can be included in more than one category, such as iconic or rhythmic gestures, vibrotactile stimulation, imitation, modeling, and ACA.[330-333]

◼ DYSPHAGIA

The swallowing process is composed of a number of complex neuromuscular events. Normal swallowing requires that an individual be able to move food or liquid from the mouth (*oral phase of swallowing*), through the pharynx (*pharyngeal phase of swallowing*), and into the esophagus. In the oral swallow phase, food is collected in the oral cavity in a single mass, or bolus, which is then propelled into the pharynx and further propelled under pressure into the esophagus. During the oral phase of swallowing, the bolus is first held between the tongue and palate and then propelled by the tongue from the front to the back of the oral cavity. The bolus moves over the back of the tongue into the pharynx, triggering the pharyngeal swallow and the neuromuscular events that propel the bolus into the esophagus. Velopharyngeal closure, tongue base posterior motion, pharyngeal contraction, laryngeal elevation and closure, and upper esophageal opening occur to allow bolus passage into the esophagus. Airway protection involves closure of the airway entrance and airway. The vocal folds close and the epiglottis moves downward to prevent food from entering the trachea during this process.

Dysphagia is defined as a condition in which an individual has had an interruption in either eating function or the maintenance of nutrition and hydration.[334] Many patients with neurogenic communication disorders also manifest deficits in swallowing (dysphagia). From 25% to 50% of individuals who have suffered strokes may have swallowing deficits ranging from mild to severe.[176,335-342] In some cases dysphagia is only present in the acute phase with rapid recovery of swallowing function taking place in the first 3 weeks post-stroke.[343] Swallowing deficits in post-stroke patients are often due to a combination of weakness and incoordination of the oral, pharyngeal, and laryngeal musculature, resulting in inefficient propulsion of a food bolus or liquid through the oral cavity, pharynx, and into the esophagus. Delayed triggering of swallowing is common after stroke.[334] Oral or pharyngeal transit times may be slow. Reduced elevation or closure of the larynx may result in material being misdirected into the airway (aspiration). Dysphagia is also often present in patients with Parkinson's disease,[344] Huntington's disease,[345] the dystonias and dyskinesias,[346,347] amyotrophic lateral sclerosis,[348] multiple sclerosis,[349] neoplasm,[350] dementia,[351] Alzheimer's disease,[352] and other degenerative neurological conditions, as well as cerebral palsy.[353] In addition, dysphagia is often present in TBI.[354]

A dysphagia examination usually begins at bedside and is followed by more objective, instrumental techniques if a pharyngeal phase swallowing disorder is suspected. The most frequently used instrumental technique to view swallowing physiology in a dysphagia examination is the modified barium swallow because it provides a radiographic view of the entire oropharyngeal swallow, including structural movement and bolus flow. Precise physiological swallowing disorders can be identified. In addition, the effects of therapeutic strategies on swallow physiology, safety, and efficiency can be examined. Another useful examination procedure is videoendoscopy. In most settings, the swallowing evaluation is carried out by the SLP.[343]

Treatment of Dysphagia

Dysphagia treatment is designed to improve swallowing efficiency for nutritional purposes and to increase swallowing safety. This can be accomplished by compensatory strategies and/or techniques designed to change swallowing physiology and reduce the risk of aspiration. Compensatory strategies include postural changes that affect the way food passes through the mouth and pharynx, dietary management, and placing food in the mouth in optimal positions. Postural techniques may also be introduced to reduce the possibility of aspiration.[338,355] Specific exercises (and maneuvers) are used to increase the coordination, range of motion, strength, and sensory input of the muscles and structures involved in the oral and pharyngeal phases of swallowing.

These exercises are designed to improve initiation of tongue movement, lingual propulsion, laryngeal elevation, closure, and tongue base approximation to the posterior pharyngeal wall.[356-359]

The physical therapist can play an important role in positioning the patient for optimum swallowing and providing treatment to reduce muscle spasticity, improve muscle strength and coordination, and prevent primitive reflex patterns from interfering with swallowing.[360-364] Box 28.2 provides an overview of implications for the physical therapist when treating patients with communication disorders. Table 28.3 presents Web-based resources for patients, families, and caregivers.

Box 28.2 Communication Disorders: Implications for the Physical Therapist

- Physical therapists often work in settings where they may be the first to become aware of a patient's communication disorder. In such situations, a referral should be made to a speech-language pathologist (SLP) for evaluation. The physical therapist can contribute to the patient's improvement in communication function in two important ways: by providing physiological support for speech functions, and by stimulating and facilitating communication through successful, fulfilling interaction with the patient. In either case, the physical therapist will want to work closely with the SLP to ensure that their treatment goals and interventions are compatible.

- The provision of physiological support for speech functions is especially relevant to the patient with pathology of the oral–motor system (e.g., dysarthria). The physical therapist will want to explore the influence of physiological support on the patient's speech in determining a comprehensive plan of care. Proper posture, for example, can help to inhibit reflexes that may trigger primitive movements. When overflow movements influence a patient's speech function, stabilization techniques may be indicated.

- Control of respiration is essential to the improvement of vocalization and the phrasing of speech. The muscles of respiration can be strengthened along with exercises designed to increase head control, stability, and sitting balance. Proper posture and eye contact enhance the possibility that speech will be audible and clear.

- When a patient is prescribed a communication board, the physical therapist contributes by determining a patient's sitting balance and tolerance, upper extremity motor control, and the best method for responding (e.g., pointing).

- Strengthening exercises to increase the speech and range of motion of the tongue, lips, and general facial musculature and to improve coordination of the oral–motor system also increase the probability of intelligible speech and help the patient with dysarthria and dysphagia. Strategies to improve postural control are especially important for patients with dysphagia, who require individual treatment programs designed to facilitate swallowing and prevent aspiration.

- Communication is a social activity and the physical therapy setting is a natural context for social interaction. The setting can be supportive by providing an atmosphere that is conducive to conversation and allows the patient to engage in a successful verbal interaction.

- Patients who are neurologically compromised often have difficulty processing information in a distracting setting. Excessive noise, competing voices, and the presence of other stimuli can make communication particularly difficult. When possible, the physical therapist should strive to work with patients who are communicatively impaired in a closed environment that is free of distractions. Patients with communication impairments do best when they are positioned in such a way that face-to-face communication is possible, including the visualization of gestures and facial expressions. For this reason, room lighting needs to be sufficient.

- Patients who manifest neurogenic speech-language disorders, especially those with aphasia, pose a considerable challenge to effective communication. The individual nature of each manifestation of aphasia argues for a close working relationship with the speech-language pathologist. This will ensure that the most effective communication strategies are used with each individual patient.

- One of the greatest difficulties in addressing the needs of patients with acquired aphasia has to do with determining and accounting for the patient's level of auditory comprehension. Virtually all patients with aphasia have some degree of difficulty in comprehending spoken language. Physical therapists need to become skilled at recognizing and addressing auditory comprehension deficits because they can be a major deterrent to successful rehabilitation.

- Misconceptions of the auditory comprehension level of a patient with aphasia can range from the assumption that a patient understands everything to the assumption that the patient comprehends nothing and must be excluded from conversation. A guiding principle to keep in mind is that auditory comprehension can vary greatly, depending on the context and complexity of the task at hand. Switching topics quickly, speaking too quickly, background noises, talking while a patient is engaged in physical activity, and conversing with more than one person at a time can impede the individual's ability to process auditory information. Sentences should be short and concise and the patient should be given sufficient time to process the information and formulate a response. Open-ended questions that require elaborate answers, such as *"Tell me about your vacation"* or *"What do you think about the latest news?"*

Box 28.2   Communication Disorders: Implications for the Physical Therapist—cont'd

are generally difficult for patients with aphasia to answer. It is best to ask questions that can be answered with "yes," "no," or another single word. Physical cues to comprehension such as gestures, facial expression, and voice inflection can facilitate and enhance a patient's understanding. It is important for the physical therapist to know that patients with aphasia often find it easier to respond to whole-body or axial commands ("stand up," "sit down") than distal commands ("point," "pick up").

- It can be tempting to try to remedy a laborious communication situation by "talking down" to a patient with aphasia as if speaking to a child, or raising one's voice as if speaking to someone with impaired hearing. The best strategy is to speak a little more slowly, using language that is not too complex, and remaining consistent in giving instructions. This can be particularly important in the physical therapy setting, where verbal commands are a fundamental element in the patient–therapist interaction. At times, it may be necessary to repeat a sentence to be understood.
- Rehabilitation team members almost universally overestimate the degree to which a person with aphasia understands spoken language. Physical therapists, when possible, should consult with the SLP for an indication of the patient's preserved auditory comprehension. It may be necessary to rephrase questions and supplement with body language to ensure comprehension.
- The use of accompanying visual cues, such as gestures and facial expressions, can be extremely helpful for some patients. Others may understand best if a message is supplemented by written cues. Sometimes one can assist by asking questions that can be answered by *yes* or *no* in a "20 questions" format. When someone with aphasia is having trouble with verbal expression it usually helps to allow the patient extra time to speak. If the patient becomes visibly frustrated, it is desirable to remain calm and suggest that the patient wait and try again later.
- During physical therapy interventions, patients with aphasia can be encouraged to produce single-word, repetitive speech that coincides with physical movements as a means of providing supplemental speech practice. Examples of this strategy include activities such as counting movements in series one to ten, and using words like *up*, *down*, *left*, and *right* while performing physical movements. The physical therapist, however, should always remain sensitive to the possibility of making speech demands that are beyond a patient's level of preserved communicative skill.

Table 28.3   Speech and Language Disorder Web-based Resources for Patients, Families, and Caregivers

Organization	Website Address
The American Speech-Language-Hearing Association (ASHA)	www.asha.org
The Academy for Neurologic Communication Disorders and Sciences (ANCDS)	www.ancds.org
National Aphasia Association (NAA)	www.aphasia.org

SUMMARY

Ever since World War II, SLPs have played an important role on the rehabilitation team in the management of patients with neurogenic speech-language disorders, especially aphasia and dysarthria. For the physical therapist, an understanding of normal and pathological communication behaviors can not only make this population of patients more interesting to work with, but can also enhance the quality of treatment he or she provides.

Communication using speech is a complex, species-specific behavior that consists of the coordinated interaction of cognitive, motor, sensory, psychological, and social skills. The neurogenic disorders of speech and language, specifically aphasia and dysarthria, dominate the population of patients with communication impairments in the rehabilitation setting. Viewed as a group, patients with neurogenic communication disorders comprise a relatively severely impaired segment of the disabled population.

The impact of neurogenic speech-language disorders on the self, family, community life, and vocational options makes these disorders especially challenging. The close relationship of one's verbal characteristics to personality and identity may cause even the mildest neurogenic communication disorder to affect the psychosocial domain. Current research is investigating the interaction of linguistic, cognitive, and psychosocial variables and their influence on the outcome of recovery and rehabilitation.

Questions for Review

1. Define *aphasia*.

2. Describe the differences that distinguish nonfluent from fluent aphasic syndromes.

3. Discuss the components of a comprehensive language test designed to measure aphasic impairment.

4. Describe some critical factors that influence recovery from aphasia.

5. Describe the psychological sequelae that may have a negative effect on the outcome of aphasia rehabilitation.

6. List several causes of cognitive-communication impairments.

7. Define *dysarthria*.

8. What neurological conditions are generally associated with dysphagia?

9. Describe augmentative communication systems and some specific techniques/devices that may enhance the treatment of aphasia.

10. How can the physical therapist contribute to the physiological support for speech?

CASE STUDY

The patient is a 62-year-old man who teaches high school. He sustained a right hemiplegia and difficulty communicating as the result of a hemorrhagic stroke, which occurred 8 months ago. At this time, except for dressing, he is independent in basic activities of daily living (BADL) and ambulates with a cane.

At 1 month post-stroke, the patient was limited to yes or no responses and a vocabulary ranging from 30 to 50 nouns and verbs, as well as everyday greetings (hello, goodbye). In the course of a communicative interaction, he often resorted to writing a letter or word or gesturing to help in his communication efforts. He appeared to understand most of what was said, especially when the topic was familiar. He received rehabilitation services during the acute post-stroke phase while hospitalized and received 20 sessions of speech-language pathology services as an outpatient.

At 8 months post-stroke, the patient's communication disorder is marked by a slow, hesitant production of one- and two-word utterances; easily produced automatic speech (i.e., everyday greetings); difficulty expressing complex information; awkward and labored articulation, which causes occasional articulatory imprecision; impaired writing; and some difficulty reading lengthy or complex material. Although the majority of his speaking vocabulary consists of nouns and verbs, adverbs and adjectives are now used with greater frequency. There is a persistent lack of conjunctions, articles, and prepositions in speech, which causes him to have impaired grammar. The patient has no apparent difficulty understanding spoken language except when it is rapid, complex, and/or unfamiliar.

Both the patient and his caregiver report that the frequency of social interactions in his current life has been curtailed dramatically. He continues to see close family members on a regular basis but he rarely sees friends or work companions. The family reports that he is frustrated and depressed over this and feels isolated from the community much of the time. They also indicate that there has been a gradual but noticeable increase in his speaking vocabulary, ability to write, and reading skill. He has recently joined a local stroke group where he hopes to meet others with similar communication difficulties.

GUIDING QUESTIONS

1. A team conference is scheduled the day after you assume treatment responsibilities for the patient. What types of information would you obtain in consultation with the SLP?

2. What communication strategies are generally useful with patients who have sustained a stroke?

3. What approach might you use if the patient became frustrated trying to express himself during a physical therapy treatment?

4. As a physical therapist, what might you do to decrease the patient's sense of isolation and enhance his emotional well-being?

5. In what ways can physical therapy treatment sessions serve to reinforce communication behavior?

DavisPlus | For additional resources, including answers to the questions for review and case study guiding questions, please visit **http://davisplus.fadavis.com**

References

1. Ruben, RJ: Redefining the survival of the fittest: Communication disorders in the 21st century. Laryngoscope 110:241, 2000.
2. National Institutes of Health: National Institute on Deafness and Other Communication Disorders: Statistics and Epidemiology—Statistics on Voice, Speech, and Language. Retrieved January 3, 2011, from www.nidcd.nih.gov/health/statistics/vsl.asp.
3. Parrish, C, et al: Assessment of cognitive-communicative disorders of mild traumatic brain injury sustained in combat. Perspect Neurophysiol Neurogenic Speech Lang Disord 19:47, 2009.
4. Ylvisaker, M, Turkstra, LS, and Coelho, C: Behavioral and social interventions for individuals with traumatic brain injury: A summary of the research with clinical implications. Semin Speech Lang 26(4):256, 2005.
5. Coelho, CA: Discourse production deficits following traumatic brain injury: A critical review of the recent literature. Aphasiology 9:409, 1995.
6. Coelho, CA: Story narratives of adults with closed head injury and non–brain-injured adults: Influence of socioeconomic status, elicitation task, and executive functioning. J Speech Lang Hear Res 45:1232, 2002.
7. Ellis, C, Dismuke, C, and Edwards, K: Longitudinal trends in aphasia in the US. NeuroRehabilitation 27:4, 2010.
8. National Institute on Deafness and Other Communication Disorders (NIDCD): National Strategic Research Plan for Hearing and Hearing Impairments. NIDCD, Bethesda, MD, 1996.
9. Adams, PF, Hendershot, GE, and Marano, MA: Current estimates from the National Health Interview Survey, 1996. Centers for Disease Control and Prevention/National Center for Health Statistics. Vital Health Stat 200:1, 1999.
10. Cohen, N, Waltzman, S, and Fisher, S: A prospective, randomized study of cochlear implants. N Engl J Med 328:233–237, 1993.
11. American Speech-Language-Hearing Association (ASHA): Highlights and Trends: ASHA Counts for Year End 2010. Rockville, MD, 2010. Retrieved August 2, 2011, from www.asha.org/uploaded-Files/2010-Member-Counts.pdf#search=%22ASHA%22.
12. World Health Organization (WHO): ICIDH-2: International Classification of Impairment, Disabilities and Handicap. WHO, Geneva, Switzerland, 1980.
13. World Health Organization (WHO): International Classification of Functioning, Disability and Health. WHO, Geneva, Switzerland, 2009. Retrieved March 9, 2011, from www.who.int/classification/icf.
14. Galgano, J, and Froud, K: Evidence of the voice-related cortical potential: An electroencephalographic study. NeuroImage 44(1):175, 2009.
15. United States Census Bureau: U.S. Interim Projections by Age, Sex, Race and Hispanic Origin: 2000–2050. 2004. Retrieved June 9, 2011, from www.census.gov/ipc/www/usinterimproj/.
16. National Institutes of Health (NIH): Aphasia: Hope through Research. NIH Publication No. 80-391. NIH, Bethesda, MD, 1979.
17. National Institute on Deafness and Other Communication Disorders: NIDCD Fact Sheet: Aphasia. NIH Publication No. 97-4257. Bethesda, MD, 1997.
18. Brust, JC, et al: Aphasia in acute stroke. Stroke 7:167, 1976.
19. Ellis, C, Dismuke, C, and Edwards, K: Longitudinal trends in aphasia in the US. NeuroRehabilitation 27(4):327, 2010.
20. Cummings, JL, et al: Aphasia in dementia of the Alzheimer type. Neurology 35:394, 1985.
21. Hillis, A: New techniques for identifying the neural substrates of language and language impairments. Aphasiology 16(9):855, 2002.
22. Price, CJ, and Crinion, J: The latest on functional imaging studies of aphasic stroke. Curr Opin Neurol 18:429, 2005.
23. Goodglass, H, et al: The Assessment of Aphasia and Related Disorders, ed 3. Lippincott Williams & Wilkins, Philadelphia, 2001.
24. Damasio, A: Signs of aphasia. In Sarno, MT (ed): Acquired Aphasia, ed 3. Academic Press, New York, 1998, p 25.
25. Sarno, MT: A survey of 100 aphasic Medicare patients in a speech pathology program. J Am Geriatr Soc 18:471, 1970.
26. Prins, R, et al: Recovery from aphasia: Spontaneous speech versus language comprehension. Brain Lang 6:192, 1978.
27. Avila, L, et al: Language and focal brain lesion in childhood. J Child Neurol 25(7):829, 2010.
28. Cranberg, LD, et al: Acquired aphasia in childhood: Clinical and CT investigations. Neurology 37:1165, 1987.
29. van Dongen, HR, et al: Clinical evaluation of conversational speech fluency in the acute phase of acquired childhood aphasia: Does a fluency/nonfluency dichotomy exist? J Child Neurol 16:345, 2001.
30. Rapin, I: Acquired aphasia in children. J Child Neurol 10:267–270, 1995.
31. Levin H, et al: Linguistic recovery in aphasia after closed head injury. Brain Lang 12:360, 1981.
32. Mesulam, MM: Slowly progressive aphasia without generalized dementia. Ann Neurol 11:592, 1982.
33. Kempler, D, et al: Slowly progressive aphasia: Three cases with language, memory, CT and PET data. J Neurol Neurosurg Psychiatry 53:987, 1990.
34. Rogers, MA, and Alarcon, NB: Characteristics and management of primary progressive aphasia. Neurophysiol Neurogenic Speech Language Disord Newsl 9:12, 1999.
35. Mesulam, MM, et al: The core and halo of primary progressive aphasia and semantic dementia. Ann Neurol 54:S11, 2003.
36. Benton, AL: Contributions to aphasia before Broca. Cortex 1:314, 1964.
37. Benton, AL, and Joynt, RJ: Early descriptions of aphasia. Arch Neurol 3:109, 1960.
38. Broca, P: Du siège de la faculté du language articulé. Bull Soc Anthropol 6:377, 1885.
39. Broadbent, D: A case of peculiar affection of speech, with commentary. Brain 1:484, 1879.
40. Mills, CK: Treatment of aphasia by training. JAMA 43:1940, 1904.
41. Head, H: Aphasia and Kindred Disorders of Speech, vols. 1 and 2. Cambridge University Press, Cambridge, UK, 1926.
42. Nielsen, J: Agnosia, Apraxia, Aphasia: Their Value in Cerebral Localization. Hoeber, New York, 1946.
43. Goldstein, K: After Effects of Brain Injuries in War: Their Evaluation and Treatment. Grune & Stratton, New York, 1942.
44. Singer, H, and Low, A: The brain in a case of motor aphasia in which improvement occurred with training. Arch Neurol Psychiatry 29:162, 1933.
45. Weisenburg, T, and McBride, K: Aphasia: A Clinical and Psychological Study. Commonwealth Fund, New York, 1935.
46. Sarno, MT: Recovery and rehabilitation in aphasia. In Sarno, MT (ed): Acquired Aphasia, ed 3. Academic Press, San Diego, 1998, p 595.
47. Klein, K: Community-based resources for persons with aphasia and their families. Top Stroke Rehabil 2:18, 1996.
48. American Heart Association: Aphasia and the Family. Publication EM 359, Dallas, 2001.
49. Backus, O, et al: Aphasia in Adults. University of Michigan Press, Ann Arbor, 1947.
50. Boone, D: An Adult Has Aphasia: For the Family, ed 2. Interstate Printers & Publishers, Danville, IL, 1984.
51. Sarno, JE, and Sarno, MT: Stroke: A Guide for Patients and Their Families, ed 3. McGraw-Hill, New York, 1991.
52. Simonson, J: According to the Aphasic Adult. University of Texas (Southwestern) Medical School, Dallas, 1971.
53. Sarno, MT: Understanding Aphasia: A Guide for Family and Friends. Monograph No. 2, ed 4. Rusk Institute of Rehabilitation Medicine, New York University Medical Center, New York, 2004.
54. Spreen, O, and Risser, AH: Assessment of Aphasia. Oxford University Press, New York, 2000.
55. Spreen, O, and Benton, AL: Neurosensory Center Comprehensive Examination for Aphasia, ed 2. University of Victoria, Department of Psychology, Neuropsychology Laboratory, Victoria, BC, 1977.
56. Kertesz, A: Western Aphasia Battery—Revised. Pro-Ed, Austin, TX, 2006.
57. Sarno, MT: The functional assessment of verbal impairment. In Grimby, G (ed): Recent Advances in Rehabilitation Medicine. Almquist & Wiksell, Stockholm, 1983, p 75.
58. Worrall, LE: A conceptual framework for a functional approach to acquired neurogenic disorders of communication. In Worrall, LE, and Frattali, CM (eds): Neurogenic Communication Disorders: A Functional Approach. Thieme, New York, 2000, p 3.
59. Sarno, MT: A measurement of functional communication in aphasia. Arch Phys Med Rehabil 46:107, 1965.

60. Sarno, MT: The Functional Communication Profile: Manual of Directions (Rehabilitation Monograph No. 42). New York University Medical Center, Rusk Institute of Rehabilitation Medicine, New York, 1969.

61. Holland, AL: Communicative Abilities in Daily Living. University Park Press, Baltimore, 1980.

62. Lomas J, et al: The communicative effectiveness index: development and psychometric evaluation of a functional communication measure for adult aphasia. J Speech Hear Disord 54:113, 1989.

63. Frattali, CM, et al: Functional Assessment of Communication Skills for Adults: Administration and Scoring Manual. American Speech and Hearing Association, Rockville, MD, 2003.

64. Simmons-Mackie, N, Threats, T, and Kagan, A: Outcome assessment in aphasia: A survey. J Commun Disord 38:1, 2005.

65. Ad Hoc Committee on the Scope of Practice in Speech-Language Pathology: Scope of practice in speech-language pathology. American Speech Language Pathology Association, 2007. Retrieved January 11, 2012, from www.asha.org/docs/html/SP2007-00283.html.

66. Worrall, L, et al: The validity of functional assessments of communication and the activity/participation components of the ICIDH-2: Do they reflect what really happens in real-life? J Commun Disord 35:107, 2002.

67. Chapey, R, et al: Life participation approach to aphasia: A statement of values for the future. ASHA Leader 5:4, 2000.

68. Doyle, PJ, et al: The Burden of Stroke Scale (BOSS): Validating patient-reported communication difficulty and associated psychological distress in stroke survivors. Aphasiology 17:291, 2003.

69. Doyle, PJ, et al: The Burden of Stroke Scale (BOSS) provided valid and reliable score estimates of functioning and well-being in stroke survivors with and without communication disorders. J Clin Epidemiol 57:997, 2004.

70. Sarno, JE, Sarno, MT, and Levita, E: The functional life scale. Arch Phys Med Rehabil 54(5):214, 1973.

71. Benaim, C, et al: Validation of the aphasic depression rating scale. Stroke 35:1692, 2004.

72. Wade, DT, Legh-Smith, J, and Langton, HR: Social activities after stroke: Measurement and natural history using the Frenchay Activities Index. Int Rehab Med 7:176, 1985.

73. Piercy M, et al: Inter-rater reliability of the Frenchay Activities Index in patients with stroke and their careers. Clin Rehabil 14:433, 2000.

74. Green, J, Forster, A, and Young, J: A test-retest reliability study of the Barthel Index, the Rivermead Mobility Index, the Nottingham Extended Activities of Daily Living Scale and the Frenchay Activities Index in stroke patients. Disabil Rehabil 23:670, 2001.

75. Hilari, K, et al: Stroke and Aphasia Quality of Life Scale–39 (SAQOL-39): Evaluation of acceptability, reliability, and validity. Stroke 34:1944, 2003.

76. Sarno, MT, and Levita, E: Recovery in treated aphasia in the first year post-stroke. Stroke 10:663, 1979.

77. Marshall, RC, and Phillipps, DS: Prognosis for improved verbal communication in aphasic stroke patients. Arch Phys Med Rehabil 4:597, 1983.

78. Darley, FL, et al: Motor Speech Disorders. WB Saunders, Philadelphia, 1975.

79. Sarno, MT: Aphasia rehabilitation. In Dickson, S (ed): Communication Disorders: Remedial Principles and Practices. Scott Foresman, Glenview, IL, 1974, p 404.

80. Sarno, MT: Disorders of communication in stroke. In Licht, S (ed): Stroke and Its Rehabilitation. Williams & Wilkins, Baltimore, 1975, p 380.

81. Sarno, MT: Language rehabilitation outcome in the elderly aphasic patient. In Obler, LK, and Albert, ML (eds): Language and Communication in the Elderly: Clinical, Therapeutic and Experimental Issues. DC Heath, Lexington, MA, 1980, p 191.

82. Yarnell, P, et al: Aphasia outcome in stroke: A clinical neuroradiological correlation. Stroke 7:514, 1976.

83. Sarno, MT: Quality of life in aphasia in the first poststroke year. Aphasiology 11:665, 1997.

84. Sorin-Peters, R: Viewing couples with aphasia as adult learners: Implications for promoting quality of life. Aphasiology 17(4):405, 2003.

85. Darley, F: Language rehabilitation: Presentation 8. In Benton, A (ed): Behavioral Change in Cerebrovascular Disease. Harper, New York, 1970, p 51.

86. Reinvang, I, and Engvik, E: Language recovery in aphasia from 3–6 months after stroke. In Sarno, MT, and Hook, O (eds): Aphasia: Assessment and Treatment. Almquist & Wiksell, Stockholm, Sweden, 1980, p 79.

87. Sarno, MT: Review of research in aphasia: Recovery and rehabilitation. In Sarno, MT, and Hook, O (eds): Aphasia: Assessment and Treatment. Almquist & Wiksell, Stockholm, Sweden, 1980, p 15.

88. Culton, G: Spontaneous recovery from aphasia. J Speech Hear Res 12:825, 1969.

89. Vignolo, LA: Evolution of aphasia and language rehabilitation: A retrospective exploratory study. Cortex 1:344, 1964.

90. Basso, A, et al: Etude controlée de la reéducation du language dans l'aphasie: Comparaison entre aphasiques traites et non-traites. Rev Neurol (Paris) 131:607, 1975.

91. Levita, E: Effects of speech therapy on aphasics' responses to the Functional Communication Profile. Percept Motor Skills 47:151, 1978.

92. Culton, G: Spontaneous recovery from aphasia. J Speech Hear Res 12:825, 1969.

93. Demeurisse, G, et al: Quantitative study of the rate of recovery from aphasia due to ischemic stroke. Stroke 11:455, 1980.

94. Butfield, E, and Zangwill, O: Re-education in aphasia: A review of 70 cases. J Neurol Neurosurg Psychiatry 9:75, 1946.

95. Sands, E, et al: Long term assessment of language function in aphasia due to stroke. Arch Phys Med Rehabil 50:203, 1969.

96. Basso, A: Aphasia and Its Therapy. Oxford University Press, New York, 2003.

97. Sarno, MT, and Levita, E: Natural course of recovery in severe aphasia. Arch Phys Med Rehabil 52:175, 1971.

98. Lazar, RM, and Antoniello, D: Variability in recovery from aphasia. Curr Neurol Neurosci Rep 8:497, 2008.

99. Kertesz, A, and McCabe, P: Recovery patterns and prognosis in aphasia. Brain 100:1, 1977.

100. Pedersen, PM, et al: Aphasia in acute stroke: Incidence, determinants, and recovery. AnnNeurol 38:659, 1995.

101. Pedersen, PM, Vinter, K, and Olsen, TS: Aphasia after stroke: Type, severity and prognosis. The Copenhagen Aphasia Study. Cerebrovasc Dis 17:35, 2004.

102. Wade, DT, et al: Aphasia after stroke: natural history and associated deficits. J Neurol Neurosurg Psychiatry 49:11, 1986.

103. Lazar, RM, et al: Variability in language recovery after first-time stroke. J Neurol Neurosurg Psychiatry 79:530, 2008.

104. Basso, A: Prognostic factors in aphasia. Aphasiology 6:337, 1992.

105. Cappa, S: Spontaneous recovery from aphasia. In Stemmer, B, and Whitaker, HA (eds): Handbook of Neurolinguistics. Academic Press, San Diego, 1998, p 535.

106. Nicholas, M, et al: Empty speech in Alzheimer's disease and fluent aphasia. J Speech Hear Res 28:405, 1985.

107. Nicholas, M, et al: Aging, language, and language disorders. In Sarno, MT (ed): Acquired Aphasia, ed 3. Academic Press, San Diego, 1998, p 413.

108. Holland, AL, et al: Predictors of language restriction following stroke: A multivariate analyses. J Speech Hearing Res 31:232, 1989.

109. Sarno, MT: Final Report. Age, linguistic evolution, and quality of life in aphasia. DHHS Grant No. CMS 5 R01 DC 00432-04. NIDCD, 1997.

110. Kertesz, A: Recovery from aphasia. Adv Neurol 42:23, 1984.

111. Wertz, RT, and Dronkers, NF: Effects of age on aphasia. Proceedings of the Research Symposium on Communication Sciences and Disorders and Aging. ASHA Reports, 19:88, 1990.

112. Pedersen, M, et al: Aphasia in acute stroke: Incidence, determinants, and recovery. Ann Recov 38:659, 1995.

113. Sarno, MT: Preliminary findings: Age, linguistic evolution and quality of life in recovery from aphasia. Scand J Rehabil Med Suppl 26:43, 1992.

114. Bayles, KA, and Kaszniak, AW: Communication and Cognition in Normal Aging and Dementia. Little, Brown, Boston, 1987.

115. Obler, LK, et al: On comprehension across the adult life span. Cortex 21:273, 1985.

116. Sarno, MT, et al: Gender and recovery from aphasia after stroke. J Nerv Ment Dis 173:605, 1985.

117. Borod, J, et al: Long term language recovery in left handed aphasic patients. Aphasiology 78:301, 1990.

118. Kertesz, A: Aphasia and Associated Disorders: Taxonomy, Localization and Recovery. Grune & Stratton, New York, 1979.

119. Shewan, C, and Kertesz, A: Effects of speech and language treatment on recovery from aphasia. Brain Lang 23:272, 1984.

120. Schuell, H, et al: Aphasia in Adults. Harper, New York, 1964.

121. Selnes, OA, et al: Recovery of single-word comprehension CT scan correlates. Brain Lang 21:72, 1984.

122. Wertz, RT, et al: Comparison of clinic, home, and deferred language treatment for aphasia: A VA cooperative study. Arch Neurol 43:653, 1986.

123. Pashek, GV, and Holland, AL: Evolution of aphasia in the first year post onset. Cortex 24:411, 1988.

124. Kertesz, A: Evolution of aphasic syndromes. Top Lang Disord 1:15, 1981.

125. Goldenberg, G, and Scott, J: Influence of size and site of cerebral lesions on spontaneous recovery of aphasia and success of language therapy. Brain Lang 47:684, 1994.

126. Fernandez B, et al: Functional MRI follow-up study of language processes in healthy subjects and during recovery in a case of aphasia. Stroke 35:2171, 2004.

127. Xu, XJ, et al: Cortical language activation in aphasia: A functional MRI study. Chin Med J (Engl) 117:1011, 2004.

128. Abo, M, et al: Language-related brain function during word repetition in post-stroke aphasics. Neuroreport 15:1891, 2004.

129. Peck, KK, et al: Functional magnetic resonance imaging before and after aphasia therapy: Shifts in hemodynamic time to peak during an overt language task. Stroke 35:554, 2004.

130. Rosen, HJ, et al: Neural correlates of recovery from aphasia after damage to left inferior frontal cortex. Neurology 55:1883, 2000.

131. Blank, SC, et al: Speech production after stroke: The role of the right pars opercularis. Ann Neurol 54:310, 2003.

132. Heiss, WD, et al: Speech-induced cerebral metabolic activation reflects recovery from aphasia. J Neurol Sci 145:213, 1997.

133. Lomas, A, and Kertesz, A: Patterns of spontaneous recovery in aphasic groups: A study of adult stroke patients. Brain Lang 5:388, 1978.

134. Kenin, M, and Swisher, L: A study of pattern of recovery in aphasia. Cortex 8:56, 1972.

135. Lebrun, Y: Recovery in polyglot aphasics. In Lebrun, Y, and Hoops, R (eds): Recovery in Aphasics. Neurolinguistics, vol. 4. Swets & Zeitlinger BV, Amsterdam, 1976, p 96.

136. Basso, A, et al: Sex differences in recovery from aphasia. Cortex 18:469, 1982.

137. Sharp, DJ, Scott, SK, and Wise, RJ: Monitoring and the controlled processing of meaning: Distinct prefrontal systems. Cereb Cortex 14:1, 2004.

138. Zahn, R, et al: Recovery of semantic word processing in global aphasia: A functional MRI study. Brain Res Cogn Brain Res 18:322, 2004.

139. Breier, JI, et al: Spatiotemporal patterns of language-specific brain activity in patients with chronic aphasia after stroke using magnetoencephalography. NeuroImage 23:1308, 2004.

140. Crosson, B, et al: Functional MRI of language in aphasia: A review of the literature and the methodological challenges. Neuropsychol Rev 17:157, 2007.

141. Benson, DF: Aphasia, Alexia, and Agraphia. Churchill Livingstone, New York, 1979.

142. Damasio, AR: Aphasia. N Engl J Med 336:531, 1992.

143. Sarno, MT: Aphasia rehabilitation: Psychosocial and ethical considerations. Aphasiology 7:321, 1993.

144. Eisenson, J: Adult Aphasia: Assessment and Treatment. Prentice-Hall, Englewood Cliffs, NJ, 1973.

145. Herrmann, M, et al: The impact of aphasia on the patient and family in the first year post-stroke. Top Stroke Rehabil 2:5, 1995.

146. Eisenson, J: Aphasia: A point of view as to the nature of the disorder and factors that determine prognosis and recovery. Int J Neurol 4:287, 1964.

147. Darley, F: The efficacy of language rehabilitation in aphasia. J Speech Hear Disord 37:3, 1972.

148. Prins, R, et al: Efficacy of two different types of speech therapy for aphasic stroke patients. Appl Psycholing 10:85, 1989.

149. Wertz, RT, et al: Veterans Administration cooperative study on aphasia: A comparison of individual and group treatment. J Speech Hear Disord 24:580, 1981.

150. Wertz, RT: Language treatment for aphasia is efficacious, but for whom? Top Lang Disord 8:1, 1987.

151. Sarno, MT: Recovery and rehabilitation in aphasia. In Sarno, MT (ed): Acquired Aphasia, ed 3. Academic Press, San Diego, 1998, p 595.

152. Robey, RR: A meta-analysis of clinical outcomes in the treatment of aphasia. J Speech Lang Hear Res 41:172, 1998.

153. Beeson, PM, and Robey, RR: Evaluating single-subject treatment research: Lessons learned from the aphasia literature. Neuropsychol Rev 16(4):161, 2006.

154. Marks, M, et al: Rehabilitation of the aphasic patient: A survey of three years experience in a rehabilitation setting. Neurology 7:837, 1957.

155. Hagen, C: Communication abilities in hemiplegia: Effect of speech therapy. Arch Phys Med Rehabil 54:545, 1973.

156. Edmonds, L, Nadeau, S, and Kiran, S: Effect of Verb Network Strengthening Treatment (VNeST) on lexical retrieval of content words in sentences in persons with aphasia. Aphasiology 23(3):402, 2009.

157. Poeck, K, et al: Outcome of intensive language treatment in aphasia. J Speech Hear Disord 54:471, 1989.

158. Bhogal, SK, Teasell, R, and Speechley, M: Intensity of aphasia therapy, impact on recovery. Stroke 34:987, 2003.

159. Hinckley, JJ, and Craig, HK: Influence of rate of treatment on the naming abilities of adults with chronic aphasia. Aphasiology 12:989, 1998.

160. Hinckley, JJ, and Carr, TH: Comparing the outcomes of intensive and non-intensive context-based aphasia treatment. Aphasiology 19(10–11):965, 2005.

161. Levita, E: Effects of speech therapy on aphasics' responses to the Functional Communication Profile. Percept Motor Skills 47:151, 1978.

162. Shewan, CM: Expressive language recovery in aphasia using the Shewan Spontaneous Language Analysis (SSLA) System. J Commun Disord 17:175, 1988.

163. Eslinger, P, and Damasio, A: Age and type of aphasia in patients with stroke. J Neurol Neurosurg Psychiatry 44:377, 1981.

164. Holland, A, and Fridriksson, J: Aphasia management during the early phases of recovery following stroke. Am J Speech Lang Pathol 10:19–28, 2011.

165. Helm-Estabrooks, N, and Ramsberger, G: Treatment of agrammatism in long-term Broca's aphasia. Br J Disord Commun 21:39, 1986.

166. Glindemann, R, et al: The efficacy of modeling in PACE-therapy. Aphasiology 5:425, 1991.

167. Pulvermuller, F, et al: Constraint-induced therapy of chronic aphasia after stroke. Stroke 32:1621, 2001.

168. Howard, D: Beyond randomized controlled trials: The case for effective studies of the effects of treatment in aphasia. Br J Dis Commun 21:89, 1986.

169. Byng, S: Hypothesis testing and aphasia therapy. In Holland, AL, and Forbes, M (eds): Aphasia Treatment. World Perspectives. San Diego, 1993, p 115.

170. Golper, L, et al: Evidence-based practice guidelines for the management of communication disorders in neurologically impaired individuals: Project Introduction. Academy of Neurologic Communication Disorders and Sciences, Minneapolis, MN, 2001. Retrieved June 11, 2011, from www.ancds.duq.edu/guidelines.html.

171. Frattali, C, et al: Development of evidence-based practice guidelines: Committee update. J Med Speech-Lang Pathol 11(3):ix, 2003.

172. Whurr, R, et al: A meta-analysis of studies carried out between 1946 and 1988 concerned with the efficacy of speech and language therapy treatment for aphasic patients. Eur J Commun 27:1, 1992.

173. Ullman, M: Behavioral Changes in Patients following Strokes. Charles C. Thomas, Springfield, IL, 1962.

174. Wahrborg, P: Assessment and Management of Emotional and Psychosocial Reactions to Brain Damage and Aphasia. Singular Publishing Group, San Diego, CA, 1991.

175. Friedman, M: On the nature of regression. Arch Gen Psychiatry 3:17, 1961.

176. Sarno, MT: Language rehabilitation outcome in the elderly aphasic patient. In Obler, LK, and Albert, ML (eds): Language and Communication in the Elderly: Clinical, Therapeutic and Experimental Issues. DC Heath, Lexington, MA, 1980, p 191.

177. Sarno, MT: Disorders of communication in stroke. In Licht, S (ed): Stroke and Its Rehabilitation. Williams & Wilkins, Baltimore, 1975, p 380.

178. Burns, MS, and Halper, AS: Speech/Language Treatment of the Aphasias: An Integrated Clinical Approach. Aspen, Rockville, MD, 1988.

179. Sarno, MT: Management of aphasia. In Bornstein, RA, and Brown, GG (eds): Neurobehavioral Aspects of Cerebrovascular Disease. Oxford University Press, New York, 1990, p 314.

180. Goodglass, H: Neurolinguistic principles and aphasia therapy. In Meier, M, et al (ed): Neuropsychological Rehabilitation. Guilford Press, New York, 1987.

181. Denes, G, et al: Intensive versus regular speech therapy in global aphasia: A controlled study. Aphasiology 10:385, 1996.

182. Meinzer, M, et al: Intensive language training enhances brain plasticity in chronic aphasia. BMC Biology, 2:1, 2004.

183. Meinzer, M, et al: Long-term stability of improved language function in chronic aphasia after constraint-induced aphasia therapy. Stroke 63(7):1462, 2005.

184. Tangeman, PT, Banaitis, DA, and Williams, AK: Rehabilitation of chronic stroke patients: Changes in functional performances. Arch Phys Med Rehabil 71:876, 1990.

185. Bragoni, M, et al: Bromocriptine and speech therapy in non-fluent chronic aphasia after stroke. Neurol Sci 21:19, 2000.

186. Walker-Batson D, et al: A double-blind, placebo-controlled study of the use of amphetamine in the treatment of aphasia. Stroke 32:2093, 2001.

187. Berthier, ML, et al: A randomized, placebo-controlled study of donepezil in post-stroke aphasia. Neurology 67:1687, 2006.

188. Seniow, J, et al: New approach to the rehabilitation of post-stroke focal cognitive syndrome: Effect of levodopa combined with speech and language therapy on functional recovery from aphasia. J Neurol Sci 283:214, 2009.

189. Gupta, SR, and Mlcoch, AG: Bromocriptine treatment of nonfluent aphasia. Arch Phys Med Rehabil 73:373, 1992.

190. Raymer, AM, Bandy, D, and Adair, JC: Effects of bromocriptine in a patient with crossed nonfluent aphasia: A case report. Arch Phys Med Rehabil 82:139, 2001.

191. Sabe, L, Leiguarda, R, and Starkstein, SE: An open-label trial of bromocriptine in nonfluent aphasia. Neurology 42:1637, 1992.

192. Sabe, L, et al: A randomized, double-blind, placebo controlled study of bromocriptine in nonfluent aphasia. Neurology 45:2272, 1995.

193. Martin, P, et al: Research with transcranial magnetic stimulation in the treatment of aphasia. Curr Neurol Neurosci Rep 9(6):451, 2009.

194. Naeser, MA, et al: Overt propositional speech in chronic nonfluent aphasia studied with the dynamic susceptibility contrast fMRI method. Neuroimage 22:29, 2004.

195. Monti, A, et al: Improved naming after transcranial direct current stimulation in aphasia. J Neurol Neurosurg Psychiatry 79:451, 2008.

196. Gardner, H, et al: Visual communication in aphasia. Neuropsychologia 14:275, 1976.

197. Weinrich, MP, et al: Implementation of a visual communicative system for aphasic patients on a microcomputer. Ann Neurol 18:148, 1985.

198. Steele, RD, et al: Evaluating performance of severely aphasic patients on a computer-aided visual communication system. In Brookshire, RH (ed): Clinical Aphasiology: Conference Proceedings. BRK Publications, Minneapolis, 1987, p 46.

199. Steele, RD, et al: Computer-based visual communication in aphasia. Neuropsychologia 27:409, 1999.

200. Weinrich, M: Computerized visual communication as an alternative communication system and therapeutic tool. J Neurolinguistics, 6:159, 1991.

201. Weinrich, M, et al: Training on an iconic communication system for severe aphasia can improve natural language production. Aphasiology 9:343, 1995.

202. Helm, N, and Benson, DF: Visual action therapy for global aphasia. Presentation at the 16th Annual Meeting of the Academy of Aphasia, Chicago, 1978.

203. Helm-Estabrooks, N, et al: Visual action therapy for aphasia. J Speech Hear Disord 47:385, 1982.

204. Skelly, M, et al: American Indian sign (AMERIND) as a facilitator of verbalization for the oral verbal apraxic. J Speech Hear Disord 39:445, 1974.

205. Rao, P, and Horner, J: Gesture as a deblocking modality in a severe aphasic patient. In Brookshire, RH (ed): Clinical Aphasiology: Conference Proceedings. BRK Publications, Minneapolis, 1978, p 180.

206. Rao, P, et al: The use of American-Indian Code by severe aphasic adults. In Chapey, R (ed): Language Intervention Strategies in Aphasia and Related Neurogenic Communication Disorders, ed 4. Lippincott Williams & Wilkins, Baltimore, 2001, p 688.

207. Sparks, R, Helm, N, and Albert, M: Aphasia rehabilitation resulting from melodic intonation therapy. Cortex 10:303, 1997.

208. Belin, P, et al: Recovery from nonfluent aphasia after melodic intonation therapy: A PET study. Neurology 47:1504, 1996.

209. Schlaug, G, Marchina, S, and Norton, A: Evidence for plasticity in white-matter tracts of patients with chronic Broca's aphasia undergoing intense intonation-based speech therapy. Ann N Y Acad Sci 1169:385, 2009.

210. Aten, JL: Adult Aphasia Rehabilitation: Applied Pragmatics. College Hill Press, San Diego, CA, 1985.

211. Aten, JL, et al: The efficacy of functional communication therapy for chronic aphasic patients. J Speech Hear Disord 47:93, 1982.

212. Davis, G, and Wilcox, M: Promoting aphasics' communicative effectiveness. Paper presented to the American Speech-Language-Hearing Association, San Francisco, 1978.

213. Pulvermüller, F, and Roth, VM: Communicative aphasia treatment as a further development of PACE therapy. Aphasiology 5:39, 1991.

214. Pulvermüller, F, and Berthier, ML: Aphasia therapy on a neuroscience basis. Aphasiology 22:563, 2008.

215. Maher, LM, et al: Constraint induced language therapy for chronic aphasia: Preliminary findings. J Int Neuropsychol Soc 9:192, 2003.

216. Beeson, PM, Hirsch, FM, and Rewega, MA: Successful single-word writing treatment: Experimental analysis of four cases. Aphasiology 16:473, 2002.

217. Lyon, JG: Drawing: Its value as a communication aid for adults with aphasia. Aphasiology 9:33, 1995.

218. Lyon, JG: Coping with Aphasia. Singular Publishing Group, San Diego, CA, 1997.

219. Lyon, JG: Communication use and participation in life for adults with aphasia in natural settings: The scope of the problem. Am J Speech Lang Pathol 1:7, 1992.

220. Rao, PR: Drawing and gesture as communication options in a person with severe aphasia. Top Stroke Rehabil 2:49, 1995.

221. Kagan, A, and Gailey, GF: Functional is not enough: Training conversation partners for aphasic adults. In Holland, A, and Forbes, MM (eds): Aphasia Treatment: World Perspectives. Singular Publishing Group, San Diego, 1993, p 199.

222. Kagan, A: Revealing the competence of aphasic adults through conversation: A challenge to health professionals. Top Stroke Rehabil 2:15, 1995.

223. Kagan, A, et al: Training volunteers as conversation partners using "supported conversation for adults with aphasia": A controlled trial. J Speech Lang Hear Res 44:624, 2001.

224. Kagan, A: Supported Conversation for Adults with Aphasia: Methods and Evaluation. Institute of Medical Science, University of Toronto, 1999. Retrieved June 11, 2011, from www.collectionscanada.gc.ca/obj/s4/f2/dsk1/tape9/PQDD_0015/NQ45755.pdf.

225. Kagan, A, Winckel, J, and Shumway, E: Supported Conversation for Aphasic Adults: Increasing Communicative Access (Video). Pat Arato Aphasia Centre, North York, Ontario, Canada, 1996. Available from Aphasia Institute (www.aphasia.ca/).

226. Simmons-Mackie, N: A solution to the discharge dilemma in aphasia: Social approaches to aphasia management: Clinical forum. Aphasiology 12:231, 1998.

227. Simmons-Mackie, N: In support of supported communication for adults with aphasia: Clinical forum. Aphasiology 12:831, 1998.

228. Simmons-Mackie, N: An Ethnographic Investigation of Compensatory Strategies in Aphasia. Unpublished doctoral dissertation. Louisiana State University, Baton Rouge, 1993.

229. Byng, S, and Duchan, J: Social model philosophies and principles: Their applications to therapies for aphasia. Aphasiology 19:906, 2005.

230. Simmons-Mackie, N: Social approaches to the management of aphasia. In Worrall, L, and Frattali, C (eds): Neurogenic Communication Disorders: A Functional Approach. Thieme, New York, 2000, p 162.

231. Pound, C, et al: Beyond aphasia: Therapies for Living with Communication Disability. Speechmark, Bicester, UK, 2000.

232. Simmons-Mackie, N, and Damico, JS: Communicative competence in aphasia: Evidence from compensatory strategies. In Lemme, ML (ed): Clinical Aphasiology (Vol. 23). Pro-Ed, Austin, TX, 1995, p 95.

233. Simmons-Mackie, N, and Damico, J: Reformulating the definition of compensatory strategies in aphasia. Aphasiology 11:761, 1997.

234. Simmons-Mackie, N, and Damico, J: Social role negotiation in aphasia therapy: Competence, incompetence and conflict. In Kovarsky, D, Duchan, J, and Maxwell, M (eds): Constructing (In)Competence: Disabling Evaluations in Clinical and Social Interaction. Erlbaum, Hillsdale, NJ, 1999, p 313.

235. Seron, X, et al: A computer-based therapy for the treatment of aphasic subjects with writing disorders. J Speech Hear Disord 45:45, 1980.

236. Katz, RC, and Nagy, V: A computerized approach for improving word recognition in chronic aphasic patients. In Brookshire, RH (ed): Clinical Aphasiology: Conference Proceedings. BRK Publishers, Minneapolis, 1983.

237. Mills, RH: Microcomputerized auditory comprehension training. In Brookshire, RH (ed): Clinical Aphasiology: Conference Proceedings. BRK Publishers, Minneapolis, 1982, p 147.

238. Mills, RH, and Hoffer, P: Computers and caring: An integrative approach to the treatment of aphasia and head injury. In Marshall, RC (ed): Case Studies in Aphasia Rehabilitation. University Park Press, Baltimore, 1985.

239. Bruce, C, and Howard, D: Computer-generated phonemic cues: An effective aid for naming in aphasia. Br J Disord Commun 22:191, 1987.

240. Garrett, K, et al: A comprehensive augmentative communication system for an adult with Broca's aphasia. Augment Altern Commun 5:55, 1989.

241. Hunnicutt, S: Access: A lexical access program. Proceedings of RESNA 12th Annual Conference, New Orleans, LA, 1989, p 284.

242. Weinrich, MP, et al: Processing of visual syntax in a globally aphasic patient. Brain Lang 36:391, 1989.

243. Baker, E, et al: Can linguistic competence be dissociated from natural language functions? Nature 254:609, 1975.

244. Manheim, LM, Halper, AS, and Cherney, L: Patient-reported changes in communication after computer-based script training for aphasia. Arch Phys Med Rehabil, 90(4):623, 2009.

245. Mortley J, et al: Effectiveness of computerized rehabilitation for long-term aphasia: A case series study. Br J Gen Pract 54:856, 2004.

246. Laganaro, M, Di Pietro, M, and Schnider, A: Computerised treatment of anomia in chronic and acute aphasia: An exploratory study. Aphasiology 17(8):709, 2003.

247. Raymer, AM, Kohen, FP, and Saffell, D: Computerized training for impairments of word comprehension and retrieval in aphasia. Aphasiology 20:257, 2006.

248. Cherney, LR, et al: Computerized script training for aphasia: Preliminary results. Am J Speech Lang Pathol 17:19, 2008.

249. Thompson, C, et al: Sentactics®: Computer-automated treatment of underlying forms. Aphasiology 24(10):1242, 2010.

250. Brumfitt, S, and Clarke, P: An application of psychotherapeutic techniques to the management of aphasia. Paper presented at Summer Conference: Aphasia Therapy. Cardiff, England, July 19, 1980.

251. Tanner, D: Loss and grief: Implications for the speech-language pathologist and audiologist. J Am Speech Hear Assoc 22:916, 1980.

252. Baretz, R, and Stephenson, G: Unrealistic patient. N Y State J Med 76:54, 1976.

253. Kübler-Ross, E: On Death and Dying. Macmillan, New York, 1969.

254. Espmark, S: Stroke before fifty: A follow-up study of vocational and psychological adjustment. Scand J Rehab Med (Suppl) 2:1, 1973.

255. Kauhanen, M, et al: Aphasia, depression, and non-verbal cognitive impairment in ischaemic stroke. Cerebrovasc Dis 10:455, 2000.

256. Kearns, KJ: Group therapy for aphasia: Theoretical and practical considerations. In Chapey, R (ed): Language Intervention Strategies in Adult Aphasia, ed 2. Williams & Wilkins, Baltimore, 1986, p 304.

257. Bollinger, R, et al: A study of group communication intervention with chronic aphasic persons. Aphasiology 7:301, 1993.

258. Caplan, AL, et al: Ethical and policy issues in rehabilitation medicine. Hastings Center (Special Supplement), Briarcliff Manor, NY, 1987.

259. Hass, J, et al: Case studies in ethics and rehabilitation. Hastings Center, Briarcliff Manor, NY, 1988.

260. Sarno, MT: The case of Mr. M: The selection and treatment of aphasic patients. Case studies in ethics and rehabilitation medicine. Hastings Center, Briarcliff Manor, NY, 1988, p 24.

261. Sarno, MT: The silent minority: The patient with aphasia. Hemphill Lecture. Rehabilitation Institute of Chicago, Chicago, 1986.

262. Holland, AL: When is aphasia aphasia? The Problem of closed head injury. In Clinical Aphasiology Conference Proceedings (Oshkosh, WI, June 6–10, 1982). BRK Publishers, Minneapolis, 1982, p 345.

263. Ylvisaker, M, Hanks, R, and Johnson-Green, D: Rehabilitation of children and adults with cognitive-communication disorders after brain injury. ASHA 23(Suppl):59, 2003.

264. Cicerone, K, et al: Evidence-based cognitive rehabilitation: Recommendations for clinical practice. Arch Phys Med Rehabil 81:1596, 2000.

265. Tompkins, CA: Right Hemisphere Communication Disorders: Theory and Management. Singular, San Diego, 1995.

266. Milton, SB, Prutting, CA, and Binder, GM: Appraisal of communicative competence in head injured adults. In Brookshire, RH (ed): Clinical Aphasiology Conference Proceedings. BRK Publishers, Minneapolis, 1984, p 114.

267. Godfrey, HPD, et al: Social interaction and speed of information processing following very severe head injury. Psychol Med 19:175, 1989.

268. Ponsford J, et al: Long-term adjustment of families following traumatic brain injury where comprehensive rehabilitation has been provided. Brain Inj 17(6):453, 2003.

269. Hartley LL: Cognitive-Communication Abilities following Brain Injury. A Functional Approach. Singular, San Diego, 1995.

270. Penn, C, and Cleary, J: Compensatory strategies in the language of closed head injured patients. Brain Inj 2(1):3, 1988.

271. Turkstra, L, Coelho, C, and Ylvisaker, M: The use of standardized tests for individuals with cognitive-communication disorders. Semin Speech Lang 26:215, 2005.

272. Klonoff, PS, et al: Rehabilitation and outcome of right-hemisphere stroke patients: Challenges to traditional diagnostic and treatment methods. Neuropsychology 4:147, 1990.

273. Cherney, LR, and Halper, AS: A conceptual framework for the evaluation and treatment of communication problems associated with right hemisphere damage. In Halper, A, Cherney, L, and Burns, M (eds): Clinical Management of Right Hemisphere Dysfunction, ed 2. Aspen, Gaithersburg, MD, 1996, p 21.

274. Kennedy, MR, et al: Evidence-based practice guidelines for cognitive-communication disorders after traumatic brain injury: Initial committee report. J Med Speech Lang Pathol 10(2), 2002.

275. Ylvisaker, M, et al: Reflections on evidence-based practice and rational clinical decision making. J Med Speech Lang Pathol 10(3), 2002.

276. Duffy, JR: Motor Speech Disorders. Mosby, St. Louis, 1995.

277. Samii, A, Nutt, JG, and Ranson, BR: Parkinson's disease. Lancet 363(9423):1783, 2004.

278. Trail, M, et al: Speech treatment for Parkinson's disease. NeuroRehabilitation 20(3):205, 2005.

279. Yorkston, K, Strand, E, and Kennedy, M: Comprehensibility of dysarthric speech: Implications for assessment and treatment planning. Am J Speech Lang Pathol 5(1):55, 1996.

280. Yorkston, KM, et al: Evidence for effectiveness of treatment of loudness, rate or prosody in dysarthria: A systematic review. J Med Speech Lang Pathol 15(2), 2007.

281. Yorkston, KM, et al: Evidence-based practice guidelines for dysarthria: Management of velopharyngeal function. J Med Speech Lang Pathol 9(4):257, 2001.

282. Dromey, C, and Ramig, LO: Intentional changes in sound pressure and rate: Their impact on measures of respiration, phonation, and articulation. J Speech Lang Hear Res 41(5):1003, 1988.

283. Ramig, L, Pawlas, A, and Countryman, S: The Lee Silverman Voice Treatment: A Practical Guide for Treating the Voice and Speech Disorders in Parkinson Disease. National Center for Voice and Speech, University of Iowa, Iowa City, 1995.

284. Fox, CM, et al: The science and practice of LSVT/LOUD: Neural plasticity–principled approach to treating individuals with Parkinson's disease and other neurological disorders. Semin Speech Lang 27:283, 2006.

285. Sutoo, D, and Akiyama, K: Regulation of brain function by exercise. Neurobiol Dis 13:1, 2003.

286. Dromey, C, Ramig, L, and Johnson, A: Phonatory and articulatory changes associated with increased vocal intensity in Parkinson disease: A case study. J Speech Hear Res 38:751, 1995.

287. Wenke, R, Cornwell, P, and Theodoros, D: Changes to articulation following LSVT® and traditional dysarthria therapy in nonprogressive dysarthria. Int J Speech Lang Pathol 12(3):203, 2010.

288. El Sharkawi, A, et al: Swallowing and voice effects of Lee Silverman Voice Treatment: A pilot study. J Neurol Neurosurg Psychiatry 72:31, 2002.

289. Spielman, J, Borod, J, and Ramig L: Effects of intensive voice treatment (LSVT) on facial expressiveness in Parkinson's disease: Preliminary data. Cogn Behav Neurol 16:177, 2003.

290. Will, L, Ramig, LO, and Spielman, JL: Application of Lee Silverman Voice Treatment (LSVT) to individuals with multiple sclerosis, ataxic dysarthria and stroke. In Proceedings International Conference on Spoken Language Processing, September 16–20, 2002, Denver, CO, p 2497.

291. Wenke, R, Theodoros, D, and Cornwell, P: The short- and long-term effectiveness of the LSVT® for dysarthria following TBI and stroke. Brain Inj 22(4):339, 2008.

292. Sapir, S, et al: Phonatory and articulatory changes in ataxic dysarthria following intensive voice therapy with the LSVT1: A single subject study. Am J Speech Lang Pathol 12:387, 2003.

293. Fox, C: Intensive voice treatment for children with spastic cerebral palsy [Unpublished doctoral dissertation]. University of Arizona, Tucson, AZ, 2002.

294. Petska, J, et al: LSVT1 and children with Down syndrome: A pilot study. Poster session presented at the 13th Biennial Conference on Motor Speech, Austin, TX, March 2006.

295. Yorkston, KM, et al: Management of motor speech disorders in children and adults. Pro-Ed, Austin, TX, 1999.

296. Croot, K: Diagnosis of AOS: Definition and criteria. Semin Speech Lang 23(4):267, 2002.

297. McNeil, MR, Robin, DA, and Schmidt, RA: Apraxia of speech: Definition, differentiation, and treatment. In McNeil, MR (ed): Clinical Management of Sensorimotor Speech Disorders. Thieme, New York, 1997, p 311.

298. McNeil, MR: Clinical characteristics of apraxia of speech: Model/behavior coherence. In Shriberg, LD, and Campbell, TF (eds): Proceedings of the 2002 Childhood Apraxia of Speech Research Symposium. Hendrix Foundation, Carlsbad, CA, 2003, p 13.

299. McNeil, MR, et al: Effects of on-line kinematic feedback treatment for apraxia of speech. Brain Lang 103:223, 2007.

300. Katz, W, et al: Visual augmented knowledge of performance: Treating place-of-articulation errors in apraxia of speech using EMA. Brain Lang 83:187, 2002.

301. Katz, WF, et al: Treatment of an individual with aphasia and apraxia of speech using EMA visually-augmented feedback. Brain and Lang 103:213, 2007.

302. Rosenbek, JC, et al: A treatment for apraxia of speech in adults. J Speech Hear Disord 38:462, 1973.

303. Cherney, LR: Efficacy of oral reading in the treatment of two patients with chronic Broca's aphasia. Top Stroke Rehabil 2(1):57, 1995.

304. Knock, TR, et al: Influence of order of stimulus presentation on speech motor learning: A principled approach to treatment for apraxia of speech. Aphasiology 14(5/6):653, 2000.

305. LaPointe, LL: Sequential treatment of split lists: A case report. In Rosenbek, J, McNeil, M, and Aronson, A (eds): Apraxia of Speech: Physiology, Acoustics, Linguistics, Management. College-Hill Press, San Diego, 1984, p 277.

306. Maas, E, et al: Treatment of sound errors in aphasia and apraxia of speech: Effects of phonological complexity. Aphasiology 16(4/5/6):609, 2002.

307. Raymer, AM, Haley, MA, and Kendall, DL: Overgeneralization in treatment for severe apraxia of speech: A case study. J Med Speech Lang Pathol 10(4):313, 2002.

308. Wambaugh, JL, et al: Effects of treatment for sound errors in apraxia of speech and aphasia. J Speech Lang Hear Res 41:725, 1998.

309. Milisen, R: A rationale for articulation disorders. J Speech Hear Disord (Monograph Suppl) 4:6, 1954.

310. Wambaugh, JL: Stimulus generalization effects of Sound Production Treatment for apraxia of speech. J Med Speech Lang Pathol 12(2), 2004, p 77.

311. Wambaugh, JL, and Nessler, C: Modification of Sound Production Treatment for aphasia: Generalization effects. Aphasiology 18:407, 2004.

312. Wambaugh, JL, and Mauszycki, SC: Sound Production Treatment: Application with severe apraxia of speech. Aphasiology 24(6-8):814, 2010.

313. Ballard, KJ, Maas, E, and Robin, DA: Treating control of voicing in apraxia of speech with variable practice. Aphasiology 21(12):1195, 2007.

314. Maas, E: Conditions of practice and feedback in treatment for apraxia of speech. Perspect Neurophysiol Neurogenic Speech Lang Disord 20:80, 2010.

315. Austermann Hula, SN, et al: Effects of feedback frequency and timing on acquisition, retention, and transfer of speech skills in acquired apraxia of speech. J Speech Lang Hear Res 51:1088, 2008.

316. Wambaugh, JL: Treatment guidelines for acquired apraxia of speech: A synthesis and evaluation of the evidence. J Med Speech Lang Pathol 14(2):xv, 2006.

317. Mauszycki, SC, and Wambaugh, JL: The effects of rate control treatment on consonant production accuracy in mild apraxia of speech. Aphasiology 22(7-8):906, 2008.

318. Brendel, B, and Ziegler, W: Effectiveness of metrical pacing in the treatment of apraxia of speech. Aphasiology 22(1):77, 2008.

319. Brendel, B, Ziegler, W, and Deger, K: The synchronization paradigm in the treatment of apraxia of speech. J Neurolinguistics 13:241, 2000.

320. Dworkin, JP, and Abkarian, GG: Treatment of phonation in a patient with apraxia and dysarthria secondary to severe closed head injury. J Med Speech Lang Pathol 2:105, 1996.

321. McHenry, M, and Wilson, R: The challenge of unintelligible speech following traumatic brain injury. Brain Inj 8(4):363, 1994.

322. Tjaden, K: Exploration of a treatment technique for prosodic disturbance following stroke. Clin Linguist Phon 14(8):619, 2000.

323. Wambaugh, JL, and Martinez, AL: Effects of rate and rhythm control treatment on consonant production accuracy in apraxia of speech. Aphasiology 14(8):851, 2000.

324. Sands, E, et al: Progressive changes in articulatory patterns in verbal apraxia: A longitudinal case study. Brain Lang 6:97, 1978.

325. Fawcus, M, and Fawcus, R: Information transfer in four cases of severe articulatory dyspraxia. Aphasiology 4(2):207, 1990.

326. Lasker, JP, et al: Using motor learning guided theory and augmentative and alternative communication to improve speech production in profound apraxia: A case example. J Med Speech Lang Pathol 16(4):225, 2008.

327. Lustig, AP, and Tompkins, CA: A written communication strategy for a speaker with aphasia and apraxia of speech: Treatment outcomes and social validity. Aphasiology 16(4/5/6):507, 2002.

328. Yorkston, KM, and Waugh, PF: Use of augmentative communication devices with apractic individuals. In Square-Storer, P (ed): Acquired Apraxia of Speech in Aphasic Adults. Lawrence Erlbaum, London, 1989, p 267.

329. Rosenbek, JC, Collins, M, and Wertz, RT: Intersystemic reorganization for apraxia of speech. Clinical aphasiology conference proceedings. In Brookshire, RH (ed): Clinical Aphasiology Conference Proceedings. BRK Publishers, Minneapolis, 1976, p 255.

330. Code, C, and Gaunt, C: Treating severe speech and limb apraxia in a case of aphasia. Br J Disord Commun 21(1):11, 1986.

331. Raymer, AM, and Thompson, CK: Effects of verbal plus gestural treatment in a patient with aphasia and severe apraxia of speech. In Prescott, TE (ed): Clinical Aphasiology (Vol 20). Pro-Ed, Austin, TX, 1991, p 285.

332. Rubow, RT, et al: Vibrotactile stimulation for intersystemic reorganization in the treatment of apraxia of speech. Arch Phys Med Rehabil 63:150, 1982.

333. Lasker, JP, and Bedrosian, JL: Promoting acceptance of augmentative and alternative communication by adults with acquired communication disorders. AAC: Augment Altern Commun 17(3):141, 2001.

334. Buchholz, D: Editorial: What is dysphagia? Dysphagia 11:23, 1996.

335. Groher, MD, and Bukulman, R: The presence of swallowing disorders in two teaching hospitals. Dysphagia 1:3–6, 1986.

336. Veis, S, and Logemann, J: The nature of swallowing disorders in CVA patients. Arch Phys Med Rehabil 66:372, 1985.

337. Wade, DT, and Hewer, RL: Motor loss and swallowing difficulty after stroke: Frequency, recovery, and prognosis. Acta Neurol Scand 76:50, 1987.

338. Low, M, Olsson, L, and Ekberg, O: Videomanometric analysis of supraglottic swallow, effortful swallow, and chin tuck in patients with pharyngeal dysfunction. Dysphagia 16(3):190, 2001.

339. Gordon, C, Langton-Hewer, RL, and Wade, DT: Dysphagia in acute stroke. BMJ 295:411, 1987.

340. Barer, DH: The natural history and functional consequences of dysphagia after hemispheric stroke. J Neurol Neurosurg Psychiatry 52:236, 1989.

341. Horner, J, Brazer, SR, and Massey, EW: Aspiration in bilateral stroke patients: A validation study. Neurology 43(2):430, 1993.

342. Smithard, D: Complications and outcome after acute stroke: Does dysphagia matter? Stroke 27:1200, 1996.

343. Logemann, JA: Evaluation and Treatment of Swallowing Disorders, ed 2. Pro-Ed, Austin, TX, 1998.

344. Miller, N, et al: Hard to swallow: Dysphagia in Parkinson's disease. Age Ageing 35:614, 2006.

345. Walker, FO: Huntington's disease. Lancet 369:218, 2007.

346. Ertekin, C, et al: Oropharyngeal swallowing in craniocervical dystonia. J Neurol Neurosurg Psychiatry 73(4):406, 2002.

347. Hayashi, T, et al: Life-threatening dysphagia following prolonged neuroleptic therapy. Clin Neuropharmacol 20(1):77, 1997.

348. Ertekin, C, et al: Pathophysiological mechanisms of oropharyngeal dysphagia in amyotrophic lateral sclerosis. Brain 123:125, 2000.

349. Thomas, FJ, and Wiles, CM: Dysphagia and nutritional status in multiple sclerosis. J Neurol 246:677, 1999.

350. Mussak, EN, Jiangling, JT, and Voigt, EP: Malignant solitary fibrous tumor of the hypopharynx with dysphagia. Otolaryngol Head Neck Surg 133:805, 2005.

351. Chouinard, J, Lavigne, E, and Villeneuve, C: Weight loss, dysphagia and outcome in advanced dementia. Dysphagia 13:151, 1998.

352. Kalia, M: Dysphagia and aspiration pneumonia in patients with Alzheimer's disease. Metabolism 52(Suppl 2):36, 2003.

353. Bottos, M, et al: Functional status of adults with cerebral palsy and implications for treatment of children. Dev Med Child Neurol 43:516, 2001.

354. Cherney, LR, and Halper, AS: Swallowing problems in adults with traumatic brain injury. Semin Neurol 16:349, 1996.

355. Cherney, LR: Dysphagia in adults with neurologic disorders: An overview. In Cherney, LR, (ed): Clinical Management of Dysphagia in Adults and Children. Aspen, Gaithersburg, MD, 1994, p 1.

356. Logemann, JA, and Kahrilas, P: Relearning to swallow post CVA: Application of maneuvers and indirect biofeedback: A case study. Neurology 40:1136, 1990.

357. Rosenbek, JC: Efficacy in dysphagia. Dysphagia 10:263, 1995.

358. Kasprisin, AT, Clumeck, H, and Nino-Murcia, M: The efficacy of rehabilitative management of dysphagia. Dysphagia 4(1):48, 1989.

359. Lazarus, C, and Logemann, J: Swallowing disorders in closed head trauma patients. Arch Phys Med Rehabil 68:79, 1987.

360. Lazarus, CL, et al: Effects of bolus volume, viscosity, and repeated swallows in nonstroke subjects and stroke patients. Arch Phys Med Rehabil 74:1066, 1993.

361. Lazzara, G, Lazarus, C, and Logemann, JA: Impact of thermal stimulation on the triggering of swallowing reflex. Dysphagia 1:73, 1986.

362. Logemann, JA, et al: Closure mechanisms of laryngeal vestibule during swallowing. Am J Physiol 262(2 pt 1):G338, 1992.

363. Martin, BJW, et al: Normal laryngeal valving patterns during three breath-hold maneuvers: A pilot investigation. Dysphagia 8:11, 1993.

364. Kahrilas, PJ, et al: Volitional augmentation of upper esophageal sphincter opening during swallowing. Am J Physiol 260(3 pt 1): G45, 1991.

Promoting Health and Wellness

Beth Black, PT, DSc
Janet R. Bezner, PT, PhD

Chapter **29**

◼ THE IMPORTANCE OF HEALTH PROMOTION AND WELLNESS INITIATIVES

Despite being among the wealthiest countries in the world,[1] and spending more than $2.3 trillion a year in health care,[2] the United States is ranked only 31st in healthy life expectancy by the World Health Organization (WHO).[3] Some researchers have predicted that after years of increasing life expectancy, life expectancy in the United States will level off or even decline.[4] Researchers and health professionals are struggling to understand this apparent discrepancy between health care expenditures and healthy life expectancy by examining and addressing the determinants of health in the U.S. population. An individual's health is determined by the interaction of numerous factors, including biology and genetics, social and physical environments, health services, and individual behaviors.[5] The relative contribution of individual behaviors to levels of mortality and morbidity in the United States was first demonstrated in a landmark study published in 1993 by McGinnis and Foege.[6] Tobacco use was estimated to be implicated in 19% of deaths, and poor diet and physical inactivity levels contributed to 14% of deaths in the United States in 1990. Mokdad et al[7] later conducted a similar study to determine the behavioral contributors to premature death in the United States in 2000. Tobacco use was responsible for 18.1% of deaths, and poor diet and physical inactivity were estimated to be responsible for 16.6% of deaths.

Recent studies of the U.S. population have shown that these key behaviors of smoking, poor diet, and insufficient physical activity continue at high levels in the population. The Behavioral Risk Factor Surveillance System (BRFSS), the largest telephone survey in the world, tracks the health behaviors and health status of over 200,000 adults in the United States annually.[8] The results of the BRFSS show that obesity levels in the country are climbing at an alarming rate (Fig. 29.1).[9]

According to the 2009 BRFSS, 36.2% of the adult population in the United States is overweight, and an additional 27.2% is obese.[10] A majority of the U.S. adult population does not consume the currently recommended five or more servings per day of fruits and vegetables[11] (Fig. 29.2). Almost half of adults in the United States report that they do not engage in recommended levels of physical activity[12] (Fig. 29.3) Given the strong relationship between these key health behaviors and health status, it is clear that the current health-related behaviors of adults in the United States are adversely affecting healthy life expectancy, and efforts to support healthier behaviors are essential.

The nation's current health promotion and disease prevention agenda is articulated in *Healthy People 2020*, a set of national health objectives developed through a wide-reaching collaborative consensus process and published by the U.S. Department of Health and Human Services.[5] Public health experts, government agencies, professional organizations such as the American Physical Therapy Association (APTA), and members of the public all provided input into this important document. The overall framework for *Healthy People 2020* is outlined in Table 29.1.

Given the broad range of factors that contribute to the health of the population, an **ecological approach** will be required to meet the *Healthy People 2020* goals and

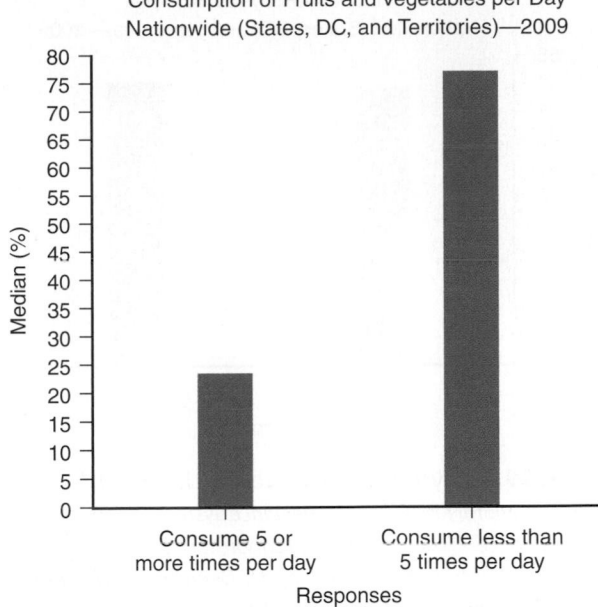

Figure 29.2 Fruit and vegetable consumption by U.S. adults in 2009. *From Behavioral Risk Factor Surveillance System, 2009. Office of Surveillance, Epidemiology, and Laboratory Services, Centers for Disease Control and Prevention, U.S. Department of Health and Human Services, Atlanta, GA. Retrieved July 6, 2011, from http://apps.nccd.cdc.gov/BRFSS/display.asp?cat=FV&yr=2009&qkey=4415&state=US.*

objectives. Interventions must be delivered not only at the level of the individual, but also at community, organizational, environmental, and policy levels (Fig. 29.4).

A number of topic areas requiring particular attention have been identified in *Healthy People 2020*, and for each of these 42 topic areas there is a set of specific objectives. For example, within the topic area of physical activity, there are 15 objectives (Table 29.2) accompanied by specific targets to be achieved within the next 10 years. The ecological approach to addressing the topic areas is clear

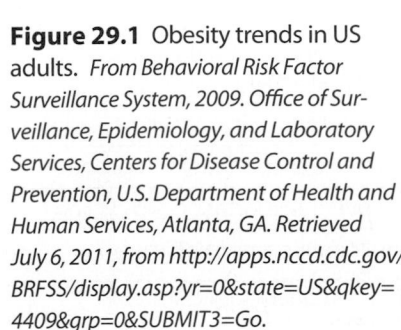

Figure 29.1 Obesity trends in US adults. *From Behavioral Risk Factor Surveillance System, 2009. Office of Surveillance, Epidemiology, and Laboratory Services, Centers for Disease Control and Prevention, U.S. Department of Health and Human Services, Atlanta, GA. Retrieved July 6, 2011, from http://apps.nccd.cdc.gov/BRFSS/display.asp?yr=0&state=US&qkey=4409&grp=0&SUBMIT3=Go.*

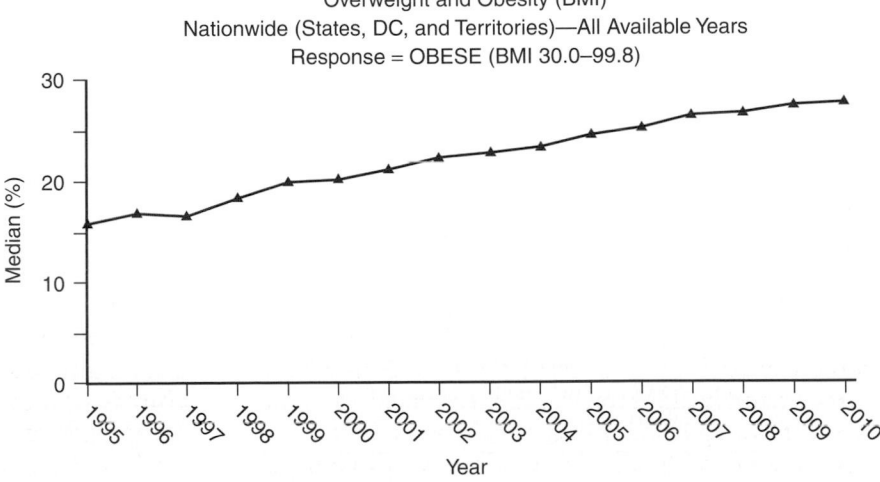

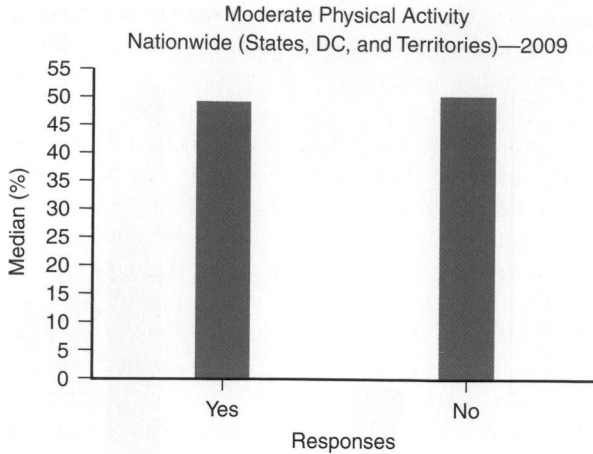

Figure 29.3 Physical activity levels of U.S. adults in 2009. *From Behavioral Risk Factor Surveillance System, 2009. Office of Surveillance, Epidemiology, and Laboratory Services, Centers for Disease Control and Prevention, U.S. Department of Health and Human Services, Atlanta, GA. Retrieved July 6, 2011, from http://apps.nccd.cdc.gov/BRFSS/display.asp?cat=PA&yr=2009 &qkey=4418&state=US.*

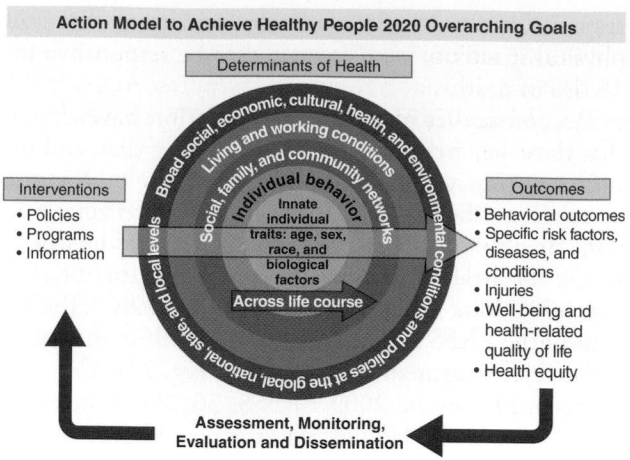

Figure 29.4 Ecological approach to achieve the goals of *Healthy People 2020.*

Table 29.1	*Healthy People 2020* Framework
Vision	A society in which all people live long, healthy lives
Mission	Identify nationwide health improvement priorities Increase public awareness and understanding of the determinants of health, disease, and disability and the opportunities for progress Provide measurable objectives and goals that are applicable at the national, state, and local levels Engage multiple sectors to take actions to strengthen policies and improve practices that are driven by the best available evidence and knowledge Identify critical research, evaluation, and data collection needs
Overarching Goals	Attain high-quality, longer lives free of preventable disease, disability, injury, and premature death Achieve health equity, eliminate disparities, and improve the health of all groups Create social and physical environments that promote good health for all Promote quality of life, healthy development, and healthy behaviors across all life stages

From http://healthypeople.gov/2020/Consortium/HP2020Framework.pdf.

Table 29.2	*Healthy People 2020* Physical Activity Objectives
Healthy People 2020 Physical Activity (PA) Objectives	**Topic Area (Objective Short Title)**
PA-1	Leisure-time physical activity
PA-2	Adult aerobic physical activity and muscle-strengthening activity
PA-3	Adolescent aerobic physical activity and muscle-strengthening activity
PA-4	Daily physical education in schools
PA-5	Adolescent participation in daily school physical education
PA-6	Regularly scheduled recess
PA-7	Time for recess
PA-8	Child and adolescent screen time
PA-9	Physical activity policies in child care settings
PA-10	Access to school physical activity facilities
PA-11	Physician counseling about physical activity
PA-12	Worksite physical activity
PA-13	Active transportation—walking
PA-14	Active transportation—bicycling
PA-15	Built environment policies

From http://healthypeople.gov/2020/topicsobjectives2020/
objectiveslist.aspx?topicId=33.

from the breadth of the objectives established for each of these 42 topic areas. For example, in the topic area of physical activity, one objective is to increase individuals' levels of leisure-time physical activity (Physical Activity Objective–1), whereas Physical Activity Objective–15 identifies the need for legislative policies to address environmental factors to support increased levels of physical activity in a community. Progress toward the objectives and specific targets established for *Healthy People 2020* will be tracked by measuring general health status, health behaviors, health-related quality of life and well-being, determinants of health, and measures of health disparities.

■ THE ROLE OF PHYSICAL THERAPISTS IN HEALTH PROMOTION

Interventions at individual, community, state, and national levels by a broad coalition of public health organizations, health professionals, educators, and government agencies will be required to achieve the objectives outlined in *Healthy People 2020*. All health professionals, regardless of their site or area of practice, have a key role to play in health promotion, either as individual practitioners or as members of an interprofessional health care team.[13] Physical therapists are participating in health promotion initiatives in a variety of ways, from examining what their role should be to providing individual and community-level interventions and programs.[14-17] A number of professional publications describe the important role for physical therapists in the area of health promotion and wellness.[18-21]

The *Guide to Physical Therapist Practice* clearly identifies health promotion and prevention as being within the scope of physical therapist practice.[18] It states, "Physical therapists provide prevention services that forestall or prevent functional decline and the need for more intense care. Through timely and appropriate screening, examination, evaluation, diagnosis, prognosis, and intervention, physical therapists frequently reduce or eliminate the need for costlier forms of care and also may shorten or even eliminate institutional stays. Physical therapists also are involved in promoting health, wellness, and fitness initiatives, including education and service provision that stimulate the public to engage in healthy behaviors."[18, p. S32] The patient history portion of the examination should include information about the client's health status and health habits, a systems review, and tests and measures as indicated to screen for potential problems that could affect current or future health status, such as hypertension, obesity, impaired balance, or poor fitness levels. Interventions that physical therapists can utilize to promote health and prevent or minimize impairments, activity limitations, and disabilities are extensive and can include such diverse activities as education in

healthy lifestyle choices and healthy behaviors, physical activity and aerobic conditioning programs, fall prevention programs, or consultation in workplace redesign. Referrals to other professionals or special programs (e.g., smoking cessation or nutritional counseling) may also be indicated. The principles of evidence-based practice should be considered as physical therapists expand their practices to include not only rehabilitation, but also health promotion. Decisions regarding appropriate programs to institute should be based on evidence of effectiveness of the intervention, the knowledge and skill level of the physical therapist, and the appropriateness of that particular intervention for the individual client given his or her unique needs, preferences, and circumstances.

In the document titled *Professionalism in Physical Therapy: Core Values*, physical therapist behaviors believed to represent the behaviors of a doctoring profession include the following:[21, pp. 1-3]

- Participating in the achievement of health goals of patients/clients and society
- Focusing on achieving the greatest well-being and the highest potential for a patient/client
- Facilitating each individual's achievement of goals for function, health, and wellness
- Participating in achievement of societal health goals

These behaviors indicate a broad role and responsibility for physical therapists in health promotion and suggest the need for physical therapists to participate not only at the individual client level, but also at a societal level. Physical therapists are participating in discussions at a national level regarding public policy, health care reform, and major health initiatives, and are also involved in advocacy efforts to support the objectives articulated in *Healthy People 2020*.[22]

At the Physical Therapy and Society Summit (PASS) meeting, future roles for physical therapists were discussed relative to the evolving health care needs of society.[23] At this conference, the opportunity for physical therapists to take a leadership role in the area of prevention, health, and wellness was emphasized. There has also been a suggestion that physical therapists should be "birth to death" health practitioners, providing regular consultations on exercise and physical activity using a practice model that is similar to the dental model and geared toward prevention and health promotion.[24]

Given the tremendous need for health promotion, and the unique knowledge base and skill set of physical therapists, it is the professional responsibility of all physical therapists to engage in health promotion practice regardless of their practice setting. As physical therapists begin to integrate health promotion interventions into their clinical practice, they should become familiar with the various terms and definitions used in the field of health promotion.

KEY TERMS IN HEALTH PROMOTION

Health and Disease

Different terms are used in the field of health promotion to define **health**. Although health may be seen as pertaining to the physical domain only, most currently used definitions of health conceptualize and describe health as a multidimensional construct involving more than the physical domain. In 1948, the WHO defined health as "a state of complete physical, mental and social well-being and not merely the absence of disease," the definition of health still used by the WHO today.[25] Health has also been described as "a dynamic balance of physical, emotional, social, spiritual, and intellectual health."[26, p. iv] **Disease**, often considered the opposite of health, is defined as a pathological condition affecting the body.[18]

Wellness and Illness

The term **wellness** is also used in the field of health promotion. In 1959, Dunn discussed the relationship between body, mind, and spirit, and defined wellness as "a complex state made up of overlapping levels of wellness."[27, p. 786] Adams et al[28] defined wellness as an individual's sense of growth and balance across the physical, spiritual, emotional, intellectual, social, and psychological domains (Fig. 29.5). These two wellness definitions are worded in such a way that individuals with chronic disease could still be considered "well."

Corbin and Pangrazi describe wellness as "a multidimensional state of being describing the existence of positive health in an individual as exemplified by quality of life and a sense of well-being."[29, p. 1] Some current definitions of health appear similar to definitions of wellness, particularly those definitions of health that include more than the physical domain. Some in the health promotion field conceptualize wellness as a process versus a state.[30] Taken together, these various definitions of wellness indicate that wellness is multidimensional, that **salutogenic** or "health-causing" variables play a key role in well-being, and that the concept of wellness is specific to each individual. **Illness** is the opposite of wellness, is multidimensional, and has been defined as a social construct where individuals are not achieving balance in their lives and are unable to create a higher quality of life.[31]

Quality of Life

There are a number of different definitions for **quality of life**. The Centers for Disease Control and Prevention (CDC) describes health-related quality of life as an individual's or group's perceived physical and mental health over time.[32] Green and Kreuter describe quality of life as "the perception of individuals or groups that their needs are being satisfied and that they are not being denied opportunities to achieve happiness or fulfillment."[33, p. 508]

Health Promotion Models

Primary, Secondary, and Tertiary Prevention

Various health promotion models are used to identify needs and plan health promotion interventions. One such model is the health protection/disease prevention model. Within this model, health is conceptualized as the absence of disease/pathology, and health promotion is therefore aimed at preventing disease. Interventions in this model are categorized as primary, secondary, or tertiary prevention[34] (Fig. 29.6).

Primary prevention includes activities designed to prevent injury or the onset of illness or disease. The use of bicycle helmets and seat belts, water fluoridation, and immunizations are all examples of primary prevention. Physical therapists practice primary prevention when they conduct preseason evaluation and conditioning programs for high school athletes or teach back injury prevention programs at orientation programs for workers in a factory.

Secondary prevention interventions take place following the development of pathology and are intended

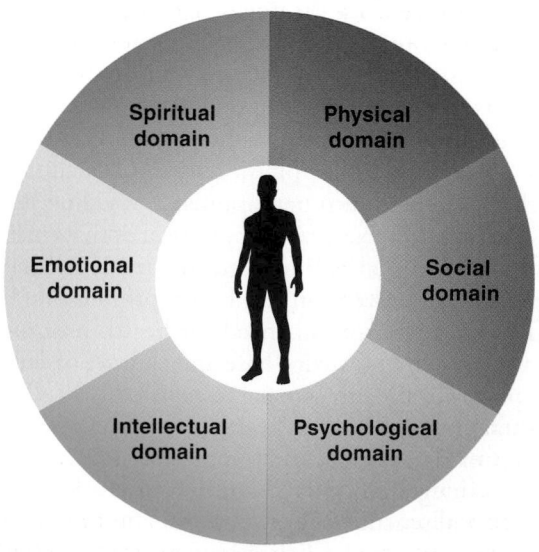

Figure 29.5 Domains of wellness.

Prepathology	Pathology Present	
Goals: Protect health Prevent disease Promote health	Goal: Early diagnosis and intervention to limit impairment and disability	Goal: Rehabilitation following significant impairment or disability
Primary prevention	Secondary prevention	Tertiary prevention

Figure 29.6 Primary, secondary, and tertiary prevention.

to identify and provide treatment for individuals in the early stages of disease in order to minimize the severity of the disease. Screening programs for breast cancer, high blood pressure, and osteoporosis are designed to identify and treat pathology in its earliest stages. Physical therapists engage in secondary prevention when they treat a patient/client with a recent injury or who has been recently diagnosed in the early stages of a chronic condition or disease.

Tertiary prevention activities are designed to slow progression of the disease and improve quality of life. Physical therapists engage in tertiary prevention when they work with patients/clients who have chronic disease or have sustained an irreversible injury—for example, with patients/clients who have long-standing rheumatoid arthritis. Physical therapists have traditionally participated primarily in secondary or tertiary prevention, but as they begin to join their fellow health professionals in health promotion practice, they will increasingly add interventions that fall under the category of primary prevention.

Population Health Management Model

A similar model to the health protection/disease prevention model is the population health management model, which is used to describe health promotion and prevention interventions for a population across a continuum of health risk[35] (Fig. 29.7). The population health management approach categorizes individuals based on risk for developing a disease, and then provides the appropriate intervention for the identified risk factor. Individuals at low or very minimal risk for disease receive interventions to keep them from moving across the continuum to a high-risk category or to actual development of disease or pathology.

■ HEALTH PROMOTION AND HEALTH EDUCATION

Green and Kreuter describe **health promotion** as "any planned combination of educational, political, regulatory, and organizational supports for actions and conditions of living conducive to the health of individuals, groups, or communities."[33, p. 506] The WHO defines health promotion as "the process of enabling people to increase control over, and to improve, their health. It moves beyond a focus on individual behaviour towards a wide range of social and environmental interventions."[36] Gorin and Arnold[37] describe health promotion as activities undertaken to encourage well-being that are directed toward actualizing an individual's potential. According to Gorin and Arnold, a health promotion model has a more positive orientation and connotation than the prevention models described above that focus on simply preventing disease. **Health education** is one component of health promotion. Green and Kreuter define health education as "any planned combination of learning experiences designed to predispose, enable, and reinforce voluntary behavior conducive to health in individuals, groups, or communities."[33, p. 506] Health education interventions aim to provide information to individuals and groups about health-causing actions and the impact of negative health behaviors in order to make a connection between voluntary behaviors and health. The first step toward positive health behavior change is awareness about the relationship between behavior and disease and injury.

■ PHYSICAL ACTIVITY AND EXERCISE

The definitions for physical activity and exercise are not synonymous. **Physical activity** is defined as any body movement produced by skeletal muscle contraction that increases energy expenditure above resting level.[38] It includes body movement carried out not only within formal exercise programs, but also in occupational activities, leisure activities, and transportation activities such as walking and bicycling. **Exercise** is defined as a subcategory of physical activity, and is planned, structured activity that is intended to improve or maintain one or more components of physical fitness.[39] This differentiation is important for physical therapists to consider when they work with patients/clients to help them increase their overall levels of physical activity.

■ THE INTERNATIONAL CLASSIFICATION OF FUNCTIONING, DISABILITY, AND HEALTH AND HEALTH PROMOTION

Consistent with the newer multidimensional definitions of health and wellness, there has been a change in the overall framework used to guide evaluation, planning, and interventions to support and promote health. The prevailing model used in 20th century medicine was the **biomedical model**.[40] This model was based on the biological sciences, and health was conceptualized as the absence of disease. The locus of control in the biomedical model was with the health care providers and the patient was provided with the medical care deemed necessary by

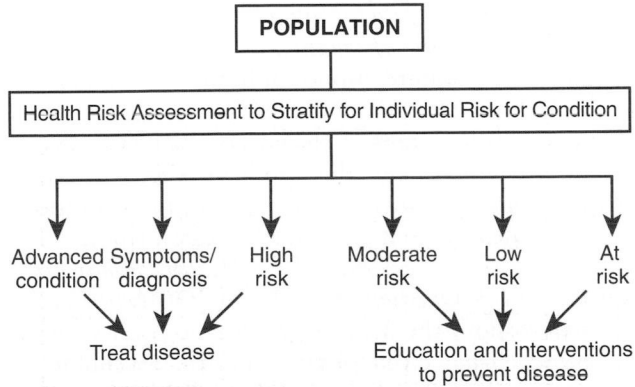

Figure 29.7 Population health management.

health professionals. It was an effective model for managing acute and infectious diseases and illnesses, but proved less effective for managing chronic disease[40] or in addressing the psychological, social, or behavioral dimensions of illness.[41] With its primarily biological focus and external locus of control, it was also less useful in the field of health promotion where patients' decisions, behaviors, and environments are considered important elements in understanding and addressing the multiple determinants of health.[42] As the limitations of using a purely biomedical framework to understand the concept of health became apparent, the **biopsychosocial** model evolved. The various biopsychosocial models used today to explain health and illness incorporate those domains missing from the biomedical model, namely the psychological and social domains. The Nagi disablement model[43] is an example of a biopsychosocial model and was the model used to describe physical therapist practice in the *Guide to Physical Therapist Practice*.[18]

In 2001, the WHO endorsed the International Classification of Functioning, Disability, and Health (ICF) biopsychosocial model.[44] The ICF is intended to provide a common language to describe health, function, and disability to facilitate scientific communication within and across health professions. The APTA has endorsed the use of this model as a framework for physical therapists to use in classifying and describing health, function, and disability.[45] In this model, the complex interrelationships of biological, environmental, and personal factors and the impact of these variables on health, activity, and function are recognized. See discussion of the ICF model in Chapter 1, Clinical Decision Making.

Physical therapists have already begun the process of applying the ICF model to physical therapist practice in rehabilitation.[46-48] A number of health professionals have also started to demonstrate how the ICF can be used in the field of health promotion research and practice.[49-52] Howard et al[50] argue that the ICF, with its acknowledgment of the important contribution of the social and physical environment to an individual's health, supports the ecological approach used in the field of health promotion. The ICF provides both the rationale for physical therapists to look beyond purely biological and physiological factors when examining and evaluating their clients and a framework to guide their plans of care and interventions. Furthermore, the ICF model is consistent with many of the behavior change theories described later in this chapter that are used to plan and implement behavior change interventions.

■ MEASURES OF HEALTH, WELLNESS, QUALITY OF LIFE, AND HEALTH BEHAVIORS

There is no one standard tool for measuring health, wellness, health behaviors, or quality of life. Some tools have been specifically designed to measure the health or health behaviors of a population, whereas other tools are used to measure health and personal health behaviors at the level of the individual patient. A variety of measures of perceived health and quality of life have been developed and can be used at the level of a population, as well as at the level of the individual patient.

Clinical Measures of Health

Clinical measures of health include biometric and physiological measures such as body mass index (BMI), aerobic capacity, or blood pressure. Health risk appraisals (HRAs) are increasingly being used in workforce wellness programs to help assess the level and nature of an individual's current health risks based on history, personal behaviors, and clinical variables. The goal of a health risk appraisal is to provide information about the individual in order to plan and deliver specific interventions targeted to address his or her unique risk factors.[53]

The *Guide to Physical Therapist Practice* recommends that an evaluation of a patient/client's current health status and potential health risks be included in the initial examination through a thorough history and a systems review.[18] Numerous tests and measures can be used by physical therapists during initial examinations to measure patients'/clients' general health status and risk factors.[18]

Self-perceived Health, Wellness, and Quality-of-Life Measures

The importance of adding a measure of an individual's perception of his or her general health to the patient/client examination was demonstrated in a landmark study by Mossey and Shapiro in 1982.[54] In this study of 3,128 noninstitutionalized adults over age 64, self-rated health was the strongest predictor of mortality after age, and was found to be a better predictor of mortality than a number of morbidity and health care utilization measures such as medical diagnosis, number of physician visits, number of hospital admissions, and surgical history. The CDC includes a 14-item perceptual measure of health, the *Healthy Days Measure,* in the annual national BRFSS survey and in the National Health and Nutrition Examination Survey.[55] The National Institutes of Health is developing a *Patient-Reported Outcomes Measurement Information System (PROMIS)* that will be able to capture important health-related quality-of-life information about patients who have chronic diseases and conditions.[56] The goal of the PROMIS initiative is to be able to develop profiles of PROMIS scores across health domains for various chronic conditions that can then be used in clinical research studies. The WHO has developed the *World Health Organization Quality of Life Questionnaire (WHOQOL-100)*[57] and a shorter version, the *WHOQOL-Bref.*[58] Both versions measure self-perceived physical health, psychological health, social relationships, and the individual's perceptions about his or her environment. The WHO tools can be used for the measurement of health at either the population level or the level of the individual patient/client.

Some self-report measures of perceived health, wellness, and quality of life are generic and can be completed by clients with a variety of conditions. One of the most commonly used measures of self-perceived health and quality of life is the *Medical Outcomes Study 36-Item Short-Form Health Survey (SF-36)*.[59] The SF-36 measures self-perceived health and function across eight scales that include physical, psychological, social, and emotional domains. It has been used in general populations and in specific populations, and normative scores for various groups and populations have been documented. Additional measures of self-perceived health used in clinical practice include the *Nottingham Health Profile*,[60] the *Sickness Impact Profile (SIP)*,[61] the *Dartmouth Cooperative Functional Assessment Charts (Dartmouth CO-OP charts)*,[62] and the *Duke Health Profile*.[63] The *Perceived Wellness Survey (PWS)* measures self-perceived wellness across psychological, physical, emotional, spiritual, social, and intellectual domains.[28] The survey consists of 36 statements with six items for each of the six domains. A composite score, a magnitude score, and a balance score can be computed (see Appendix 29.A). This tool has been tested and found to be valid and reliable for use with different populations.[28,64]

Disease-specific Measures of Self-perceived Health, Wellness, and Quality of Life

A number of disease-specific health and wellness measures have been developed for use with specific clinical populations. The items included in these measures may more specifically address issues related to the health and well-being of a particular population than the general measures described above. The *Arthritis Impact Measurement Scale (AIMS)*[65] and *AIMS2*[66] were developed to measure the physical, mental, and social domains of health in persons with rheumatic diseases. The *Child Health Questionnaire (CHQ)* measures the physical and psychosocial well-being of children, and has been found to be a valid and reliable measure of health status across a variety of conditions and disorders.[67] The *Cystic Fibrosis Questionnaire*[68] is a health-related quality-of-life questionnaire that has both parent and child versions to measure the physical, emotional, and social impact of cystic fibrosis on children and their families. Additional disease or condition-specific quality-of-life measures that have been developed include a health and quality-of-life measure for individuals who have had a stroke,[69,70] suffer from acute and chronic facial disorders,[71] and have chronic respiratory disease.[72] The *European Organisation for Research and Treatment of Cancer (EORTC)* has developed a series of questionnaires designed to assess the quality of life of individuals with cancer. The 30-item EORTC quality-of-life measure has been translated and validated into 81 languages, and has disease-specific modules that can be added to it.[73]

Assessing Health Behaviors

Reeves and Rafferty[74] identified four key behaviors as most indicative of a healthy lifestyle: engaging in regular physical activity, eating sufficient daily servings of fruits and vegetables, maintaining a healthy weight, and abstaining from smoking. It is currently recommended that health professionals routinely include an evaluation of these behaviors in their initial assessments of patients/clients.[75,76] The *Guide to Physical Therapist Practice* also recommends that physical therapists include questions regarding health-related behaviors in initial examinations.[18] The health behaviors of engaging in regular physical activity, eating sufficient fruits and vegetables, and abstaining from smoking can be determined through patient interview or through a questionnaire. If the anthropometric measures of height and weight are taken, the client's BMI can be calculated, and the physical therapist can determine whether the patient/client is overweight or obese (Box 29.1).

The *International Physical Activity Questionnaire*,[77] originally developed to track levels of physical activity in populations, has also been used in clinical practice to assess individual patient/client's levels of physical activity.[78] Research is underway to develop a general health behaviors questionnaire that can be used to collect key health behavior information in an efficient manner in the primary care setting.[79]

■ KEY MODIFIABLE PERSONAL HEALTH BEHAVIORS

The CDC's Healthy Living website provides information about numerous behaviors that contribute to a healthy lifestyle.[80] Some of the health behaviors have the support of organizations, agencies, and schools, for example healthy menus in school cafeterias, while others are enforced by local, state, or federal laws, such as seat belt use or nonsmoking environments. Others, though significantly influenced by social, environmental, and economic factors, are primarily the personal responsibility of the individual, such as maintaining a healthy weight, eating a healthy diet, and engaging in physical activity. Some personal health behaviors are considered to be more changeable than others based on clinical research. Behaviors that are more challenging to change

Box 29.1	Body Mass Index (BMI)
BMI	**Weight Status**
Below 18.5	Underweight
18.5 to 24.9	Normal
25.0 to 29.9	Overweight
30 or higher	Obese

are those with an addictive component, those with compulsive elements, and those strongly associated with cultural or family routines, such as diet.[33] The key behaviors of increasing physical activity, increasing fruit and vegetable consumption, and quitting smoking, all included in the objectives of *Healthy People 2020*, have been shown to be modifiable behaviors if the behavior change interventions are appropriately designed and delivered.

The U.S. Preventive Services Task Force (USPSTF) publishes recommendations for various preventative screening measures and health behavior change interventions based on the most current evidence of the effectiveness of interventions in changing or modifying behavior.[81] Clinicians can order a manual with these guidelines from the Agency for Healthcare Research and Quality[82] or can use a website-accessed electronic tool to quickly obtain this information within the clinical setting.[83] Although more research is needed to support the best counseling interventions to increase physical activity, the current evidence-based USPSTF recommendations for physical activity counseling are shown in Box 29.2.

A recent systematic review of the effectiveness of counseling to improve diet and increase physical activity found that behavioral counseling can change these behaviors if the counseling is provided at a sufficient intensity.[84] Given the empirical evidence to support the efficacy of smoking cessation programs, the USPSTF currently recommends that all health care practitioners ask their patients about tobacco use and make appropriate referrals when indicated.[85] There is also evidence to support the relationship between intensive physical activity interventions and decreased risk of falls in older adults.[86] There are, therefore, clinical research studies that support the value of clinicians addressing the modifiable behaviors of tobacco use, unhealthy eating, and inadequate physical activity with their patients/clients. Research in the profession of physical therapy has shown that some physical therapists have already started to address health behaviors with their clients,[14,15,17] but more therapists should be encouraged to engage in these discussions with their patients/clients. It may be necessary to ensure that physical therapists receive additional training in how to counsel patients/clients in behavior change.[87]

■ THEORIES OF BEHAVIOR CHANGE

The decision to engage in or change a health-related behavior is the result of a complex interaction of numerous factors. Just as physical therapists must understand theories of motor control when planning interventions to improve motor function, an understanding of key theories of health behavior change is necessary if physical therapists are going to be effective in helping clients change their behaviors. Various theoretical models of human behavior have been developed and can be categorized as individual models, interpersonal models, and community and group models.[88] Behavior change interventions based on these different theories have been carried out in clinical research trials and have been found to be effective in different situations with different populations.[88]

Health Belief Model

One of the earliest theoretical models developed to explain health behaviors was the *Health Belief Model* (HBM).[89] This individual model of health behavior

---

Box 29.2 U.S. Preventive Services Task Force Recommendations for Physical Activity Counseling

- Regular physical activity helps prevent cardiovascular disease, hypertension, type 2 diabetes, obesity, and osteoporosis. It may also decrease all-cause morbidity and lengthen life span.
- Benefits of physical activity are seen at even modest levels of activity, such as walking or bicycling 30 minutes per day on most days of the week. Benefits increase with increasing levels of activity.
- Whether routine counseling and follow-up by primary care physicians results in increased physical activity among their adult patients is unclear. Existing studies limit the conclusions that can be drawn about efficacy, effectiveness, and feasibility of primary care physical activity counseling. Most studies have tested brief, minimal, and low-intensity primary care interventions, such as 3- to 5-minute counseling sessions in the context of a routine clinical visit.
- Multicomponent interventions combining provider advice with behavioral interventions to facilitate and reinforce healthy levels of physical activity appear to be the most promising. Such interventions often include patient goal setting, written exercise prescriptions, individually tailored physical activity regimens, and mailed or telephone follow-up assistance provided by specially trained staff. Linking primary care patients to community-based physical activity and fitness programs may enhance the effectiveness of primary care clinician counseling.
- Potential harms of physical activity counseling have not been well defined or studied. They may include muscle and fall-related injuries or cardiovascular events. It is unclear whether more extensive patient screening, certain types of physical activity (e.g., moderate vs. vigorous exercise), more gradual increases in exercise, or more intensive counseling and follow-up monitoring will decrease the likelihood of injuries related to physical activity. Existing studies provide insufficient evidence regarding the potential harms of various activity protocols, such as moderate compared with vigorous exercise.

Source: www.uspreventiveservicestaskforce.org/recommendations.htm.

was initially developed and articulated in the 1950s, when social psychologists in the U.S. Public Health Service found that despite public education about the merits of various screening programs, for example, tuberculosis screening, large numbers of adults did not participate in the programs. Over the years, the HBM has been developed and extended to incorporate additional concepts and to explain a variety of health-related behaviors beyond screening. In the HBM, it is hypothesized that an individual's perceptions about his or her susceptibility to and the severity of the disease, along with beliefs about the benefits and barriers of taking the recommended action, will influence the decision to act (Fig. 29.8). Demographic variables, sociopsychological variables, cues to action (internal and/or external factors promoting the behavior change), and *self-efficacy*, defined as the confidence one has that one can successfully execute the action, will also influence the individual's decision to engage in the behavior. Results from numerous research studies conducted with different populations have provided support for this theoretical model,[88] and interventions based on this model have been found to be effective in supporting behavior change.[90-92] If using this model in the clinical setting to promote healthy behaviors, the clinician would first assess the individual's beliefs and perceptions relative to his or her health condition and the recommended health actions. Based on this assessment, the clinician would then provide appropriate interventions, for example, educating the individual about his or her susceptibility to the disease or the effectiveness of a recommended health behavior.

Theory of Reasoned Action and Theory of Planned Behavior

The *Theory of Planned Behavior*, along with its predecessor, the Theory of Reasoned Action, is an individual model of health behavior that emphasizes the importance of and relationship between cognitions (thought processes) and behavioral intention. In 1967 Fishbein proposed the *Theory of Reasoned Action*, in which he hypothesized that an individual's attitudes and beliefs about a particular behavior directly influence the intention to engage in

that behavior, which then leads to the actual behavior.[93] The theory was later expanded to include the construct of perceived behavioral control and renamed the Theory of Planned Behavior[94] (Fig. 29.9).

The key constructs in this theoretical model are attitude toward the behavior, subjective norm, perceived behavioral control, and behavioral intention (Table 29.3). Clinical studies that have examined a variety of health-related behaviors have provided empirical support for the constructs and the relationships articulated in this theory.[88,95-97] A clinician using this theoretical model to design a clinical intervention to change a behavior should begin by assessing the individual's attitude toward the behavior and the individual's perceptions regarding what significant others think about the behavior. The individual's perceived behavioral control can be ascertained by inquiring about any personal, social, or environmental barriers that might limit the ability to successfully engage in the behavior. The clinician can then tailor the intervention to the individual by addressing any areas that were identified. For example, the clinician may need to help the individual problem solve to address a perceived barrier to engaging in the recommended behavior.

Transtheoretical Model (Stages of Change)

The *Transtheoretical Model* (TTM), first articulated by Prochaska in 1979, is categorized as an individual model of health behavior.[98] Key constructs within the TTM includes stages of change, decisional balance, self-efficacy, and processes of change (Table 29.4).

Prochaska[98] hypothesized that there are five stages of change: *precontemplation, contemplation, preparation, action,* and *maintenance* (Box 29.3). A sixth stage called *termination* is occasionally included as the final stage of change, and is defined as the stage when an individual has engaged in the behavior for more than 6 months, is no longer susceptible to temptation, and has high levels of self-efficacy for maintaining the behavior. An individual cycles through the first five stages as he or she makes changes in a particular behavior. Decisional balance and self-efficacy influence an individual's decision to move from one stage to another.

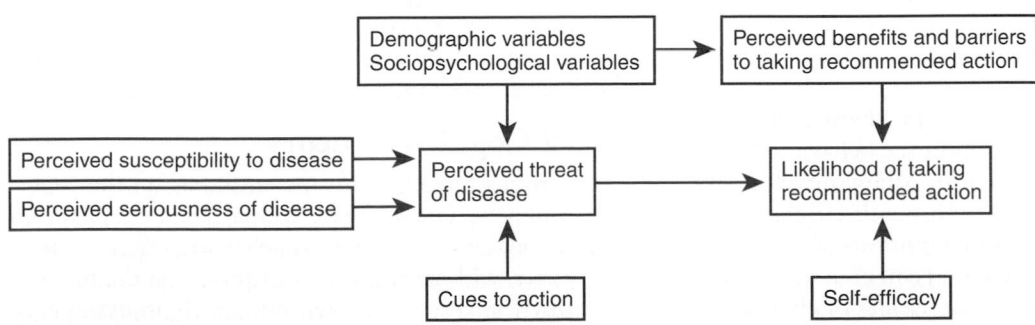

Figure 29.8 Health Belief Model.

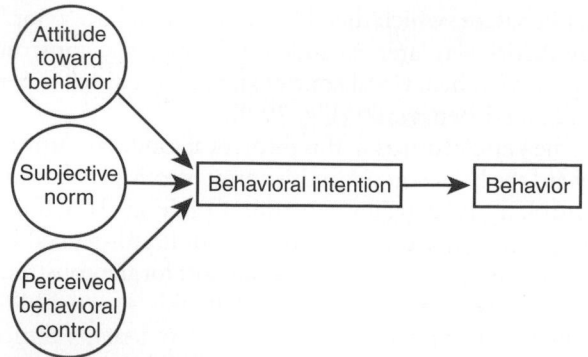

Figure 29.9 Theory of Planned Behavior.

Table 29.3	Key Constructs in the Theory of Planned Behavior[94]
Construct	**Definition**
Attitude toward behavior	Individual's overall attitude toward the behavior
Subjective norm	Individual's beliefs about whether others approve or disapprove of the behavior
Perceived behavioral control	Individual's perception about the level of control he or she has over the behavior
Behavioral intention	Individual's intention to engage in the behavior, the direct precursor to engaging in the behavior

Table 29.4	Key Constructs in the Transtheoretical Model[98]
Construct	**Definition**
Stages of Change	The stages an individual moves through when changing a behavior
Decisional Balance	The process of weighing the pros and cons of changing a behavior
Self-efficacy	The confidence the individual has that he or she can successfully engage in the behavior
Processes of Change	Activities used to support progress through stages

Different strategies (processes of change) are employed at different stages to support the behavior change (Table 29.5). Consciousness raising, dramatic relief, and environmental reevaluation are most useful in the earlier stages of change, whereas counterconditioning, helping relationships, reinforcement management, and stimulus control are most useful in the later stages of change.

Clinical interventions based on this theoretical model have been successful in changing behaviors, particularly

---

Box 29.3   Transtheoretical Model: Stages of Change[88]

Precontemplation

• Individual does not intend to take action within the next 6 months

Contemplation

• Individual intends to take action within the next 6 months

Preparation

• Individual intends to take action within the next 30 days, and has taken some preliminary steps

Action

• Individual has engaged in the behavior for less than 6 months

Maintenance

• Individual has engaged in the behavior for more than 6 months

Termination

• Individual engages in the behavior, has high self-efficacy for the behavior, and is no longer tempted to return to the unhealthy behavior

---

in the areas of smoking, diet, and physical activity.[88] The TTM has also been examined in a study looking specifically at the exercise behaviors of adults with physical disabilities, and the key constructs and relationships hypothesized in this theoretical model of behavior were supported by the researchers' findings.[99] A clinician using this theoretical model to support behavior change in a client should first start with an evaluation of the individual's stage of change for the behavior, as well as an evaluation of the individual's level of self-efficacy for the behavior. See Box 29.4 for a sample stage of change questionnaire and Table 29.6 for a sample self-efficacy questionnaire. Appropriate processes of change can then be selected and implemented by the clinician to match the individual's stage of change and self-efficacy for the behavior (refer to Table 29.5). Low self-efficacy for the behavior can be addressed by discussing how to maintain the behavior even under challenging conditions.

Social Cognitive Theory

The previous models, with the emphasis on the cognitions and behaviors of the individual, can be categorized as individual models of health behavior.[88] *Social Cognitive Theory*, with its additional emphasis on the individual's physical and social environment, is an example of a model of interpersonal health behavior. In a 1962 article on social learning through observation, Bandura[100]

Table 29.5   Transtheoretical Model: Processes of Change[88]

Process of Change	Description	Stage in Which Process of Change Is Used
Consciousness raising	Individual increases level of awareness and acquires information about the behavior	Precontemplation Contemplation
Dramatic relief	Individual experiences negative emotions regarding health risks associated with not changing unhealthy behavior	Precontemplation Contemplation
Environmental reevaluation	Individual evaluates the negative impact on others of continuing the unhealthy behavior	Precontemplation Contemplation
Self-evaluation	Individual considers self-image and examines personal values	Contemplation
Self-liberation	Individual makes a commitment to change behavior	Preparation
Counterconditioning	Individual substitutes healthy behavior for unhealthy behavior	Action Maintenance
Helping relationships	Individual seeks social support for behavior change	Action Maintenance
Reinforcement management	Individual increases rewards for healthy behavior	Action Maintenance
Stimulus control	Individual removes cues for unhealthy behavior, adds cues for healthy behavior	Action Maintenance

---

Box 29.4   Sample Stage of Change Questionnaire

Circle the number before the statement that best describes your current intentions related to walking 150 minutes a week.

1. I currently do not walk 150 minutes a week and have no intentions to start walking 150 minutes a week. (Precontemplation)
2. I currently do not walk 150 minutes a week but plan to start walking 150 minutes a week sometime within the next 6 months. (Contemplation)
3. I currently do not walk 150 minutes a week but I plan to start walking 150 minutes a week sometime within the next month. (Preparation)
4. I walk 150 minutes a week, but have been doing so for less than 6 months. (Action)
5. I walk 150 minutes a week, and have been doing so for 6 months or more. (Maintenance)

---

hypothesized that individuals could learn through watching others' behaviors and rewards. In succeeding years, Bandura[101] further developed the theory, added additional constructs, and changed the name of the theory from Social Learning Theory to Social Cognitive Theory. According to Bandura, an individual's behavior is the result of the constant interaction among the individual's environment, personal factors (including cognitions), and behavior through a process called reciprocal determinism (Fig. 29.10).

Key constructs within the theory include environment, situation, behavioral capability, expectations, expectancies, self-control, observational learning, reinforcement, self-efficacy, and emotional coping responses (Table 29.7). According to Bandura, self-efficacy, the confidence that one can successfully engage in the behavior across different challenging situations, is the single most important prerequisite for behavior change: it affects the individual's level of effort and persistence in engaging in the behavior in the face of difficulty.[102]

A number of clinical trials support the constructs and relationships proposed by this theory.[88,103-109] Interventions incorporating Social Cognitive Theory constructs have been effective in changing health behaviors (see Box 29.5 Evidence Summary). Clinical application of this theoretical model requires attention to the key constructs as they apply for a given behavior and client. For example, the clinician may want to evaluate the individual's physical and social environment to determine what elements in the individual's environment must be changed in order to support the particular health behavior being promoted. If the individual does not have the behavioral capability to carry out a particular behavior, education and training in the skills needed to perform the behavior may be required. The clinician should also use a tool to measure the client's self-efficacy for the behavior and if low levels of self-efficacy are found, specific strategies can be incorporated to build confidence

Table 29.6 Sample Self-Efficacy Questionnaire

Place a checkmark (✓) in the box that corresponds to how confident you are that you could keep up your walking program in the following situations:

Situation	Not at All Confident	Slightly Confident	Moderately Confident	Very Confident	Extremely Confident
When there is bad weather					
When I am tired					
When I am having pain					
When I am away from home					
When I have too much work to do					

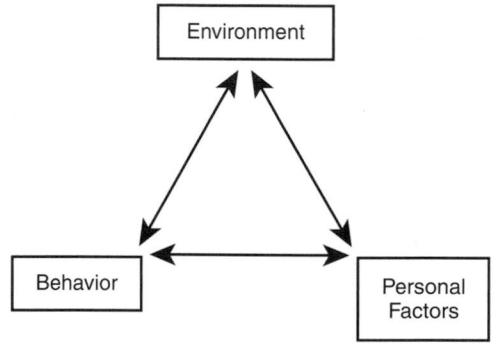

Figure 29.10 Social Cognitive Theory.

(Box 29.6). The role-modeling construct can be incorporated into a behavioral change program by using peer mentors or group leaders.

Physical Activity Model for People with a Disability

The preceding conceptual models can be applied to a variety of health behaviors with diverse populations. The recently proposed *Physical Activity for People with a Disability* (PAD) model has been developed to explain the behavior of physical activity in a population of people with a disability.[110] This model is based on the *Attitude,*

Table 29.7 Key Constructs in Social Cognitive Theory[88]

Construct and Definition	How to Address Construct in Behavioral Change Program
Reciprocal determinism: continuous interaction of individual, behavior, and environment	Consider individual's environment, personal skills, and attitudes when developing strategies to support behavior change
Environment: factors external to the individual that influences behavior	Consider how to incorporate physical and social support for the behavior
Situation: the individual's perception of his or her environment	Correct misperceptions about the environment and the behaviors of others
Behavioral capability: the individual has the knowledge and skills to successfully engage in the behavior	Provide education and skills training
Expectations: the outcomes the individual anticipates from engaging in the behavior	Provide education regarding positive outcomes of the behavior
Expectancies: value the individual places on the outcomes of the behavior	Relate the outcomes to the individual's personal values
Self-control: personal control of the behavior	Incorporate goal-setting and self-monitoring of progress
Observational learning: learning that occurs through watching others successfully engage in the behavior	Consider the use of peers as role models for the behavior
Reinforcement: the positive or negative reinforcement the individual receives after engaging in the behavior	Incorporate self-initiated rewards for meeting goals, and support/encouragement from significant others
Self-efficacy: confidence in ability to successfully perform a specific behavior	Build individual's self-efficacy by breaking the behavior into small achievable steps to ensure success
Emotional coping responses: how the individual copes with emotions	Teach problem solving skills and stress management

Box 29.5 Evidence Summary   Studies Incorporating Social Cognitive Theory Constructs to Promote Changes in Levels of Physical Activity

Reference	Subjects	Design/Intervention	Duration	Results	Comments
Annesi et al[103] (2011)	162 obese, sedentary women	Randomized controlled trial Control group: • Exercise prescription for 3 sessions a week at wellness center • Nutritional and weight loss information • Six 1-hour one-on-one meetings with wellness specialist Intervention group: • Exercise prescription for 3 sessions a week at wellness center • Nutritional and weight loss information • Six 1-hour one-on-one meetings with wellness specialist trained in using "Coach Approach" intervention based on Social Cognitive Theory (SCT): cognitive restructuring, goal setting, behavioral contracting, tailored feedback, instruction in self-regulation	6 months	Exercise session attendance was significantly greater for intervention group $p < .001$ Intervention group had greater improvements in Physical Self-Concept, Exercise Barriers Self-Efficacy, and Body Areas Satisfaction than control group.	Subjects in the control group received similar amount of personal contact time with exercise specialist as subjects in the intervention group to control for potential of bias due to Hawthorne effect. Separate facilities used for control and intervention groups to avoid cross-contamination.
Cramp and Brawley[104] (2006)	57 postnatal women	Randomized controlled trial Control group: • Four-week standard exercise program held twice a week at community fitness facility • Four-week home exercise program Intervention group: • Four-week standard exercise program held twice a week at community fitness facility plus six 20-min SCT-based group cognitive behavioral sessions on setting goals, overcoming barriers to exercise, and self-regulation • Four-week home exercise program with one telephone call from program staff member at end of second week	8 weeks	Intervention group had significantly greater change in frequency and amount of physical activity than control group. Intervention group had higher expectations of achieving positive physical outcomes with exercise, and higher self-efficacy for being able to overcome barriers to exercise.	Investigators ensured both groups had equal contact time with staff (10 hours) by increasing staff contact time for the control group during the 4-week standard exercise time.

Continued

Box 29.5 Evidence Summary Studies Incorporating Social Cognitive Theory Constructs to Promote Changes in Levels of Physical Activity—cont'd

Reference	Subjects	Design/Intervention	Duration	Results	Comments
Ince[105] (2008)	62 university students	Quasi-experimental pre-test/post-test design Intervention: • Two hours/week classroom discussion of health-related fitness, self-assessment and self-regulatory skills, group discussions • Two hours/week: Group gym activities	12 weeks	Significant improvement from baseline in nutrition behavior, health responsibility, social support, exercise behavior, stress management, and overall Adolescent Health Promotion Scale scores. Significant improvement from baseline in moderate, vigorous, and total physical activity levels as measured by the International Physical Activity Questionnaire.	No control group; cannot rule out Hawthorne effect.
Mihalko et al[106] (2006)	79 residents of three independent living communities, mean age 81.6	Randomized controlled trial Control group: • Information flyer advertising physical activity session Intervention group: • Information flyer advertising physical activity session plus brief cognitive-behavioral intervention based on SCT	One 30-minute individual counseling session	Significantly higher percentage of subjects in the intervention group attended the physical activity session.	Cannot rule out Hawthorne effect bias to account for increased attendance by intervention group.
Motl et al[107] (2011)	54 individuals with multiple sclerosis	Randomized controlled trial Control group: • Waitlist (no intervention) Intervention group: • Four multimedia Internet modules that included key elements of SCT: self-efficacy, outcome expectations, addressing barriers, and goal setting • Twice a week Internet chat sessions • Internet discussion forum	3 months	Intervention group significantly increased their physical activity level as measured by Godin Leisure-Time Exercise Questionnaire. No significant change in physical activity for control group. Intervention group significantly increased their goal-setting behaviors as measured by the Exercise Goal Setting Scale. No significant change in goal-setting behaviors for control group.	Subjects were paired at intake for physical activity and disability levels and then randomly assigned to either the control or intervention group to ensure similarity of both groups at baseline. Cannot rule out Hawthorne effect because control group did not receive any intervention.

Box 29.5 Evidence Summary   Studies Incorporating Social Cognitive Theory Constructs to Promote Changes in Levels of Physical Activity—cont'd

Reference	Subjects	Design/Intervention	Duration	Results	Comments
Rogers et al[108] (2009)	41 sedentary women with Stage I, II, or IIIA breast cancer receiving hormonal therapy	Randomized controlled trial Control group: • Received pamphlets about physical activity obtained from the American Cancer Society and were given information about website resources Intervention group: • Multidisciplinary physical activity behavior change program based on key constructs of SCT, and program preferences of subjects • Program components included both group and individual sessions • Six group sessions covered journaling, time management, stress management, dealing with exercise barriers, behavior modification • Twelve individual supervised exercise sessions and three individual counseling sessions with exercise specialists using SCT principles to counsel individuals on exercise and to develop a tailored home exercise program	12 weeks	Statistically significant improvements from baseline levels in physical activity, left handgrip strength, back and leg muscle strength, waist-to-hip ratio, and social well-being in intervention group versus control group.	Sociodemographic characteristics and health-related variables of both groups were similar at start of study. Investigators used an objective measure (accelerometer) for physical activity. Intervention group reported significant increase in joint stiffness.
Wilson et al[109] (2005)	48 underserved adolescents	Quasi-experimental design: Students at intervention school matched for age, gender, race, and percentage of students on free or reduced-price lunch program with students at control school Control school: • Students received four weeks of general health education that did not emphasize physical activity	4 weeks	Students in the intervention group showed a greater increase in time spent in moderate, moderate-vigorous, and vigorous activity from baseline to end of program than students in control group. Students in the intervention group	Groups were similar in sociodemographic variables at baseline. Total research staff/student contact hours were equivalent for both control group and intervention group.

Continued

Box 29.5 Evidence Summary Studies Incorporating Social Cognitive Theory Constructs to Promote Changes in Levels of Physical Activity—cont'd

Reference	Subjects	Design/Intervention	Duration	Results	Comments
		Intervention school: • Two hours after school three times a week • Program included a homework-snack component, a physical activity component, and an SCT-based and Self-Determination Theory–based motivational and behavioral component • SCT elements included skill development in self-monitoring and goal setting, and discussions about strategies for engaging in physical activity with friends and family		showed a greater increase in motivation for physical activity and in positive self-concept than students in the control group.	

Box 29.6 Strategies for Enhancing Self-Efficacy[88,101,102]

1. Break the behavior into small achievable steps
2. Set goals, establish a contract
3. Problem solve potential challenges individual might face
4. Mental practice and imagery
5. Log progress, document achievement of goals
6. Use peer role-modeling
7. Ensure positive reinforcement received from others
8. Ensure the correct interpretation of internal physiological states produced by the behavior

Social Influence, and Self-Efficacy (ASE) model.[111] It integrates behavioral theoretical models with disability models, and uses the ICF framework and terminology. In this model, environmental factors and personal factors interact to influence an individual's intention to engage in physical activity. Environmental factors include such variables as transportation, availability and accessibility of facilities, and assistance from others. Environmental factors also encompass social influence variables such as the opinion of family, friends, or health professionals. Personal factors include attitude, self-efficacy, health condition, and facilitators or barriers such as energy level, time, motivation, and skills. The authors of this model suggest that clinical application can include use of the TTM's stages of change. This new model is promising and could provide a helpful framework for

physical therapists to use to address the physical activity levels of patients/clients with disabilities. Ongoing research on this model should be focused on identifying the important personal and environmental facilitators and barriers of physical activity for individuals with chronic disease or disability.

Community Models

A number of behavior change theoretical models have been developed to explain behavior change at a community level. Although a thorough discussion of community models is beyond the scope of this chapter, physical therapists who are interested in changing the health behaviors of a group or community may want to familiarize themselves with community and group models of health behavior change, ecological models of health behavior, and intervention planning models such as the *PRECEDE-PROCEED planning model.*[88]

■ MOTIVATIONAL INTERVIEWING

Motivational interviewing is a client-centered counseling method designed to facilitate a client's internal motivation to change by identifying dissonance between behaviors and values and resolving ambivalence.[112] This counseling technique, initially developed to support behavior change in the treatment of addiction, is now used with a variety of populations where clients' existing behaviors have adversely affected their health or quality of life. It has been effectively used to encourage adherence to medical recommendations in general practice populations, to resolve behavioral issues with criminal justice populations, and to assist couples undergoing marital counseling.[112] Physical therapists have used motivational interviewing to improve adherence with rehabilitation programs.[113]

The hallmark of this technique is the emphasis on exploring the client's values and having the client recognize discordance between current behaviors and life goals. The clinician begins by asking probing questions to encourage the client to discuss his or her priorities in life and how current behaviors support or do not support those priorities. Encouraging the client to consider the pros and cons of continuing with current unhealthy behaviors versus changing to healthier behaviors may help resolve ambivalence by tipping the balance in favor of behavior change. Reflective listening by the clinician will allow a better understanding of the client's point of view and key contextual information related to potential challenges with behavior change. A clinician who is skilled in the motivational interviewing technique is respectful of personal choice and autonomy, is empathetic, avoids arguments, and provides encouragement to support self-efficacy for behavior change (Box 29.7).

Motivational interviewing has been used in the field of health promotion to encourage change in lifestyle behaviors. Regardless of the underlying theoretical behavior change model being used to structure a health behavior change intervention, motivational interviewing can be incorporated as a technique to engage the client in important collaborative discussions about his or her behaviors. There is some empirical evidence of the effectiveness of this technique in supporting behavior change across a number of health-related behaviors, although more research is needed.[114] It has been shown to be effective in encouraging weight loss,[115] physical activity,[116-119] smoking cessation,[120,121] and fruit and vegetable consumption.[119]

■ HEALTH PROMOTION AND WELLNESS FOR INDIVIDUALS WITH IMPAIRMENTS AND DISABILITIES

There is evidence that physical therapists in the United States are moving beyond their traditional roles in secondary and tertiary prevention, and engaging in primary prevention and health promotion practice in the general population.[14,15,17,87] Physical therapists are engaging in screening programs,[122,123] ergonomic consultations,[124] and sports injury prevention and conditioning programs.[125]

There is, however, a great need for physical therapists to engage in more health promotion activities with individuals with disabilities and chronic diseases. One of the specific goals stated in *Healthy People 2020* is to increase the number of health promotion programs for people with disabilities.[5] Research has shown that this population has lower levels of physical activity,[126-129] higher rates of smoking,[130] and higher levels of overweight and obesity than the age-matched general population.[131,132] Physical therapists have a unique knowledge and skill set that positions them well to be leaders in health promotion and wellness initiatives for individuals with disabilities. Unlike other health professionals, therapists also interact with patients over extended periods of time. This extended period of interaction and level of accessibility allows time to develop a rapport with patients and provides the therapist an opportunity to be influential in advocating for healthy behaviors.[133]

Examination and Evaluation

The patient management model in the *Guide to Physical Therapist Practice* provides a framework for therapists to carry out an examination and evaluation that will identify potential opportunities for prevention and health promotion interventions.[18] During the history, the therapist should look beyond questions related to a specific impairment and ask about perceived health or use a self-perceived health, wellness, or quality-of-life questionnaire as described earlier. The therapist should also inquire about health-related behaviors such as physical activity and current smoking status. A systems review should be carried out to screen for risk factors for disease or injury, and appropriate follow-up by the physical therapist or referral to other health professionals as indicated should occur. For example, physical therapists should routinely take blood pressure before having the patient/client engage in physical activity not only as a component of safe practice, but also to be able to identify and report hypertension. Therapists who

---

Box 29.7   Key Principles of Motivational Interviewing[112]

1. Express empathy
   - Listen respectfully
   - Do not judge
   - Build therapeutic alliance
   - Accept ambivalence
2. Develop discrepancy
   - Help client identify discrepancy between present behavior and personal goals and values
   - Have client present reasons for change
3. Roll with resistance
   - Avoid arguing
   - Acceptance of reluctance to change as natural
   - Turn problem back to client and encourage client to suggest solutions
4. Support self-efficacy
   - Enhance client's confidence in his or her ability to successfully change behavior

notice a mole should ask the client if he or she has discussed this predisposing factor for skin cancer with a physician. Fall risk assessments should be conducted with at-risk populations. Based on their examination and evaluation, physical therapists may identify the need to engage patients in discussions about healthy behaviors and discuss the impact unhealthy behaviors may have on recovery. For example, discussion can focus on the impact of nicotine on tissue healing, or high BMI on joint health and overall health and wellness. Referrals should be made to appropriate programs and health professionals when health issues that fall outside of the scope of practice and qualifications of the physical therapist are identified during the examination.

Interventions

Physical Activity/Exercise

The APTA encourages physical therapists and physical therapist assistants to be promoters and advocates for physical activity/exercise.[134] Individuals with chronic disease and disability report lower levels of physical activity and exercise than the general population.[126-129] The lower levels of physical activity/exercise reported by this population may be due to a host of factors, including limited mobility, chronic pain, fatigue, fear of aggravating their condition, or limited access to fitness facilities that have the necessary equipment and personnel to enable safe and effective physical activity.[135-138] Physical therapists are uniquely qualified to evaluate fitness levels and prescribe fitness programs for individuals with medical conditions. The APTA has identified two priority populations requiring the knowledge and skills of physical therapists in physical fitness prescription.[139] The primary priority population consists of individuals with acute and chronic impairments, activity limitations, and disabilities related to movement, function, and

health, and the secondary priority population consists of individuals with identified risk for impairments, activity limitations, and disabilities related to movement, function, and health.

A physical therapy exercise program developed for a patient/client to prevent or remediate impairments falls under the category of secondary or tertiary prevention, but if therapists are truly engaging in primary prevention and health promotion, a physical activity and exercise program to improve overall fitness to the maximal level possible for that patient should also be considered. Participation in physical activity may reduce secondary health problems, improve levels of function, and improve subjective well-being in individuals with chronic medical conditions.[140] There is evidence that exercise can improve quality of life in individuals who are stroke survivors.[141] The CDC recommends that adults participate in 150 minutes of moderate-intensity or 75 minutes of vigorous-intensity aerobic activity every week and muscle-strengthening activities on 2 or more days a week.[80] Children should engage in 60 minutes or more of physical activity every day[80] (Table 29.8).

However, these physical activity recommendations were developed for the general population and may not be appropriate for patients/clients with disabilities and medical conditions. Physical activity recommendations should be tailored to ensure safety and effectiveness for the patient's unique medical condition. Physical therapists must consider not only the patient's condition, but also any co-morbidities and potential side effects or limitations associated with medical treatments when prescribing a physical activity program. There are excellent research-based resources to help physical therapists safely test fitness and prescribe exercise for patients with medical conditions.[16,142,143] Beyond appropriate content of a physical activity program,

Table 29.8	Physical Activity Guidelines
Adults	Aerobic activity every week: 150 minutes of moderate-intensity aerobic activity (e.g., brisk walking) **OR** 75 minutes of vigorous-intensity aerobic activity (e.g., jogging or running) **OR** an equivalent mix of moderate- and vigorous-intensity aerobic activity **AND** Muscle-strengthening activities on 2 or more days a week that work all major muscle groups (legs, hips, back, abdomen, chest, shoulders, and arms)
Children and Adolescents	Should do 60 minutes of physical activity each day Aerobic activity should make up most of the recommended 60 or more minutes of daily physical activity. Can include moderate-intensity aerobic activity, such as brisk walking, or vigorous activity, such as running, but should include vigorous-intensity aerobic activity on at least 3 days per week **AND** Muscle-strengthening activities, such as gymnastics or push-ups, at least three days a week **AND** Bone-strengthening activities, such as jumping rope or running, at least 3 days per week

Source: www.cdc.gov/HealthyLiving/.

physical therapists should consider the previously mentioned theories of behavior change and motivational interviewing to support patients/clients and optimize their chance for successful behavior change as they begin to increase their level of physical activity. Patients/clients can also be informed about physical activity programs in the community that are geared to specific populations. Physical therapists and patients/clients should refer to the consumer website of the National Center on Physical Activity and Disability (see Appendix 29.B) for education and specific information about exercise, as well as sports and recreational activities recommended for those with disabilities.[144] The benefits of engaging in sports should be discussed with patients/clients; people with disabilities who engage in sports have reported enhanced function, social benefits, and an increased sense of optimism.[52]

Smoking Cessation Counseling

There is strong evidence that even brief counseling of patients can be effective to support smoking cessation.[145,146] Given the strong evidence of the health risks associated with smoking and clinical evidence of the effectiveness of even brief counseling sessions, Bodner and Dean[146] effectively argue that counseling patients about smoking behaviors falls within the role of physical therapists and that physical therapists, given their prolonged contact with patients over the course of treatment, have the opportunity and the rapport necessary to be effective in smoking cessation counseling. In their systematic review, they found that intervention models based on the motivational interviewing technique are effective. The Agency for Healthcare Research and Quality recommends that clinicians include a question about smoking as part of their examination and evaluation and has designed a specific evidence-based program to assist clinicians in helping their clients address smoking behaviors.[147] The 5-A's tobacco cessation approach recommends that clinicians *A*sk their patients about tobacco use, *A*dvise tobacco users to quit, *A*ssess the client's readiness to quit, *A*ssist the client with a quit plan, and *A*rrange follow-up to review progress toward quitting (Box 29.8). Physical therapists should also be familiar with smoking cessation programs in the local area and refer patients/clients as appropriate to these specialized programs.

Healthy Weight and Healthy Eating Counseling

Overweight and obesity are associated with the development of numerous conditions and diseases[148] (Box 29.9). The *Guide to Physical Therapist Practice* recommends that anthropometric measurements be included in initial examinations. The measurement of height and weight will allow physical therapists to calculate the patient's BMI. Calculators and charts are available on the CDC website

---

Box 29.8 Helping Smokers Quit: A Guide for Clinicians

1. Ask about tobacco use.
Implement a system in your clinic that ensures that tobacco-use status is obtained and recorded.
2. Advise all tobacco users to quit.
Use clear, strong, and personalized language. For example, "Quitting tobacco is the most important thing you can do to protect your health."
3. Assess readiness to quit.
Ask every tobacco user if he or she is willing to quit at this time.

- If willing to quit, provide resources and assistance.
- If unwilling to quit at this time, help motivate the patient:
  - Identify reasons to quit in a supportive manner.
  - Build patient's confidence about quitting.

4. Assist tobacco users with a quit plan.
Assist the smoker to:

- Set a quit date, ideally within 2 weeks.
- Remove tobacco products from his or her environment.
- Get support from family, friends, and co-workers.
- Review past quit attempts—what helped, what led to relapse.
- Anticipate challenges, particularly during the critical first few weeks, including nicotine withdrawal.
- Identify reasons for quitting and benefits of quitting.

Give advice on successful quitting:

- Total abstinence is essential—not even a single puff.
- Drinking alcohol is strongly associated with relapse.
- Allowing others to smoke in the household hinders successful quitting.

Encourage use of prescribed medications.
Provide resources:

- Recommend toll-free number: 1-800-QUIT NOW (784-8669), the national access number to state-based quitline services.
- Refer to websites for free materials: www.ahrq.gov/path/tobacco.htm, www.smokefree.gov.

5. Arrange follow-up
Schedule follow-up.

- If a relapse occurs, encourage quit attempt.
- Review circumstances that caused relapse. Use relapse as a learning experience.
- Make appropriate referrals.

Adapted from www.ahrq.gov/clinic/tobacco/clinhlpsmksqt.htm.

(see Appendix 29.B) to assist therapists in calculating the patient/client's BMI.[149]

Physical therapists should take the opportunity to educate the patient about the impact excessive weight has on the patient's current condition and future

Box 29.9	Conditions Associated with Overweight and Obesity

Hypertension
Dyslipidemia
Type 2 diabetes
Coronary heart disease
Stroke
Gallbladder disease
Osteoarthritis
Sleep apnea and respiratory problems
Endometrial cancer
Breast cancer
Prostate cancer
Colon cancer

From www.nhlbi.nih.gov/guidelines/obesity/ob_home.htm.

health. As specific nutritional counseling is outside the scope of practice of the physical therapist, therapists should refer patients to qualified health professionals as appropriate. Most weight management programs include physical activity and physical therapists have the knowledge and skills to create and implement physical activity programs for high-risk patients/clients.

HEALTH PROMOTION AND WELLNESS AT THE PROGRAM LEVEL

Patients who are discharged from physical therapy to continue their exercise programs independently often find it challenging to find a facility with the necessary equipment or personnel who are sufficiently trained to address their unique medical challenges. Physical therapists have begun to recognize and address this need for physical activity programming that is specifically tailored to address the needs of patients with chronic conditions or disabilities. Fitness and health promotion programs geared to this population and offered in rehabilitation settings are growing in popularity. For example, physical therapists are providing fitness classes and health promotion programs to individuals with osteoporosis, arthritis, and cancer.[150-152] It is important to remember that these programs should comply with licensing requirements for physical therapists in the state, and that the same standards for physical therapist practice must be maintained whether the physical therapist is providing rehabilitation or health promotion interventions. An excellent resource for physical therapists is the APTA website *Physical Fitness for Special Populations* (see Appendix 29.B).[139] The website provides recommendations for the design of fitness programs tailored to the specific needs of individuals with various medical conditions, such as stroke, type 2 diabetes, and pulmonary pathology. The site also provides valuable information about malpractice and professional liability, Medicare coverage for fitness services, and other helpful resources for physical therapists.

PHYSICAL THERAPISTS AS ADVOCATES

One of the goals stated in *Healthy People 2020* is the need for increased health promotion programming for individuals with disabilities.[5] Physical therapists can make a meaningful contribution to the health of the nation by providing health and wellness to this population within their own practices as described above. In addition, physical therapists should recognize their broader social responsibility, as articulated in the *Core Values* document of the professional association, to advocate for the health and wellness needs of all.[21] Physical therapists, with their unique knowledge base and clinical experience, are extremely cognizant of the needs and challenges faced by individuals with chronic disease and disability, and should participate at both the community and national levels to ensure that this population is provided the same access to health promotion and wellness programming as the rest of the population.

SUMMARY

Physical therapists have the knowledge, the skill set, and the opportunity to engage in health promotion practice across the continuum of care. A population in special need of the guidance and support of physical therapists is the population with medical conditions and disabilities who face unique challenges when trying to incorporate healthy behaviors into their lives. At the Physical Therapy and Society Summit (PASS) meeting, the need for more research to be undertaken to better define physical therapists' role in prevention, health, and wellness, especially with respect to consumers with impairments, was identified.[23] The "Revised Research Agenda for Physical Therapy" identifies specific areas in health promotion requiring more investigation and discussion.[153] These areas include the need to examine the effectiveness of specific health promotion interventions related to the physical activity of clients/patients with movement disorders. As the profession continues to define and develop its role in health promotion and wellness, physical therapists should identify opportunities within their current practice environments to promote optimal levels of health and wellness of their patients/clients.

Questions for Review

1. What factors contribute to the health of an individual?
2. What is *Healthy People 2020*?
3. How does the World Health Organization define *health*?
4. Identify the different domains of wellness.
5. Define *primary*, *secondary*, and *tertiary* prevention.
6. Where in the continuum of primary, secondary, and tertiary prevention have physical therapists traditionally practiced?
7. Differentiate between the terms *health promotion* and *health education*.
8. What is the difference between the terms *exercise* and *physical activity*?
9. What tools could a physical therapist use to measure a patient/client's self-perceived health, wellness, or quality of life?
10. What health-related behaviors should physical therapists inquire about during initial examinations of patients/clients?
11. Describe the following four theories of behavior change: Health Belief Model, Transtheoretical Model and Stages of Change, Theory of Planned Behavior, and Social Cognitive Theory.
12. What is the purpose of motivational interviewing?
13. What are the five steps of the 5-A's tobacco cessation approach?
14. What professional documents support the role of physical therapists in health promotion?

CASE STUDY

Elise Henry is a 72-year-old widow who recently moved into the assisted living center where physical therapy consultation services are provided. The client was referred by a member of the center staff who reports that she is unable to participate in the recreational programs offered by the center due to her physical condition.

PATIENT HISTORY

Mrs. Henry tells the therapist on her initial visit that she is unable to participate in many of the center activities owing to her increasing problems with leg pain. She relates that she was diagnosed with peripheral artery disease 10 years ago. She was not prescribed any medication, but found that if she limited her walking, she could prevent the pain from occurring.

SOCIAL HISTORY

Her former friends live too far away to visit her at the assisted living center. She misses her weekly bridge games with them. Her only son and his family live in another city about an hour's drive away. Her son, daughter-in-law, and two granddaughters visit her about once a month. Her son also phones her every Sunday evening.

SYSTEMS REVIEW

- Height: 5 ft 2 in
- Weight: 145 lb
- Resting heart rate: 72
- Resting blood pressure: 135/85
- No skin breakdown

Rubor of dependency test and pedal pulses are consistent with diagnosis of arterial insufficiency.

HEALTH-RELATED BEHAVIORS

- *Smoking*: Smokes 2 to 3 cigarettes/day; the client has smoked for 50 years.
- *Diet and Nutrition*: Does not eat breakfast, but has coffee and muffins delivered to her room mid-morning. Goes to the center dining room for lunch and dinner. Keeps cookies in her room for snacking during the day.
- *Physical Activity*: She currently spends most of her days watching TV in her room. Her only regular physical activity is walking to and from the dining room for lunch and dinner. The distance from her room to the dining room is approximately 50 feet. She has mild pain in both legs and is slightly short of breath at the end of the walk.

GUIDING QUESTIONS

1. Identify additional tests and/or measures that could be used to assess her level of health.

2. Identify additional tests and/or measures that could be used to assess her level of wellness.

3. What domains of wellness may be at lower levels?

4. Which health-related behaviors might be adversely affecting her health and wellness?

5. How should a conversation about her health and wellness be started?

6. If Mrs. Henry asked for help in changing her behaviors, select a theory of behavior change to guide the intervention. Which behaviors should be targeted?

7. What level of physical activity should Mrs. Henry strive to achieve for health-related benefits?

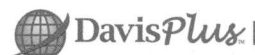 | For additional resources, including answers to the questions for review and case study guiding questions, please visit **http://davisplus.fadavis.com**

References

1. World Development Indicators database: Data and Statistics. World Bank. Retrieved September 1, 2011, from http://sitere-sources.worldbank,org/DATASTATISTICS/resources?gdp.pdf.
2. National Health Expenditure Data. US Department of Health and Human Services. Centers for Medicare and Medical Services. Retrieved July 11, 2011, from www.cms.hhs.gov/NationalHealth ExpendData/downloads/highlights.pdf.
3. World Health Organization: World Health Statistics 2009. Retrieved September 4, 2011, from www.who.int/whosis/whostat/EN_WHS09_Table1pdf.
4. Olshansky, SJ, et al: A potential decline in life expectancy in the United States in the 21st century. N Engl J Med 352:1138, 2005.
5. Healthy People 2020. US Department of Health and Human Services. Retrieved July 6, 2011, from www.healthypeople.gov/2020/about/default.aspx.
6. McGinnis, JM, and Foege, WH: Actual causes of death in the United States. JAMA 270:2207, 1993.
7. Mokdad, AH, et al: Actual causes of death in the United States, 2000. JAMA 291(10):1238, 2004.
8. Behavioral Risk Factor Surveillance System. Office of Surveillance, Epidemiology, and Laboratory Services, Centers for Disease Control and Prevention, US Department of Health and Human Services, Atlanta, GA. Retrieved September 6, 2011, from www.cdc.gov/BRFSS/.
9. Behavioral Risk Factor Surveillance System, 2009. Office of Surveillance, Epidemiology, and Laboratory Services, Centers for Disease Control and Prevention, US Department of Health and Human Services, Atlanta, GA. Retrieved July 6, 2011, from http://apps.nccd.cdc.gov/BRFSS/display.asp?yr=0&state=US&qkey=4409&grp=0&SUBMIT3=Go.
10. Behavioral Risk Factor Surveillance System, 2009. Office of Surveillance, Epidemiology, and Laboratory Services, Centers for Disease Control and Prevention, US Department of Health and Human Services, Atlanta, GA. Retrieved July 6, 2011, from http://apps.nccd.cdc.gov/BRFSS/display.asp?cat=OB&yr=2009&qkey=4409&state=US.
11. Behavioral Risk Factor Surveillance System, 2009. Office of Surveillance, Epidemiology, and Laboratory Services, Centers for Disease Control and Prevention, US Department of Health and

Human Services, Atlanta, GA. Retrieved July 6, 2011, from http://apps.nccd.cdc.gov/BRFSS/display.asp?cat=FV&yr=2009&qkey=4415&state=US.
12. Behavioral Risk Factor Surveillance System, 2009. Office of Surveillance, Epidemiology, and Laboratory Services, Centers for Disease Control and Prevention, US Department of Health and Human Services, Atlanta, GA. Retrieved July 6, 2011, from http://apps.nccd.cdc.gov/BRFSS/display.asp?cat=PA&yr=2009&qkey=4418&state=US.
13. Zenzano, T, et al: The roles of healthcare professionals in implementing clinical prevention and population health. Am J Prev Med 40(2):261, 2011.
14. Shirley, D, van der Ploeg, HP, and Bauman, AE: Physical activity promotion in the physical therapy setting: Perspectives from practitioners and students. Phys Ther 90(9):1311, 2010.
15. Goodgold, S: Wellness promotion beliefs and practices of pediatric physical therapists. Pediatr Phys Ther 17:148, 2005.
16. Jewell, D: The role of fitness in physical therapy patient management: Applications across the continuum of care. Cardiopulm Phys Ther J 17(2):47, 2006.
17. Rea, BL, et al: The role of health promotion in physical therapy in California, New York, and Tennessee. Phys Ther 84(6):510, 2004.
18. American Physical Therapy Association: Guide to Physical Therapist Practice, ed 2. Phys Ther 81:1, 2001.
19. Evaluative Criteria PT Programs. Accreditation Handbook. Commission on Accreditation in Physical Therapy Education, April 2011. Retrieved July 6, 2011, from www.capteonline.org/upload-edFiles/CAPTEorg/About_CAPTE/Resources/Accreditation_Handbook/EvaluativeCriteria_PT.pdf.
20. The Model Practice Act for Physical Therapy. A Tool for Public Protection and Legislative Change, ed 4. Federation of State Boards of Physical Therapy, Alexandria, VA, 2006. Retrieved July 6, 2011, from www.fsbpt.org/download/MPA2006.pdf.
21. Professionalism in Physical Therapy: Core Values. American Physical Therapy Association, Alexandria, VA, 2009. Retrieved Sept 7, 2011, from www.apta.org/uploadedFiles/APTAorg/About_Us/Policies/BOD/Judicial/ProfessionalisminPT.pdf#search=%22core values%22.

22. Advocacy. American Physical Therapy Association, Alexandria, VA. Retrieved September 7, 2011, from www.apta.org/Advocacy/.

23. Kigin, CM, Rodgers, MM, and Wolf, SL: The Physical Therapy and Society Summit (PASS) meeting: Observations and opportunities. Phys Ther 90(11):1555, 2010.

24. Sahrmann, S: Ask an expert. Today in PT 2:20, 2009.

25. What is the WHO Definition of Health? World Health Organization, 2011. Retrieved September 6, 2011, from www.who.int/suggestions/faq/en/.

26. O'Donnell, MP: Definition of health promotion 2.0: Embracing passion, enhancing motivation, recognizing dynamic balance, and creating opportunities. Am J Health Promot 24(1):iv, 2009.

27. Dunn, HL: High-level wellness for man and society. Am J Public Health 49(6):786, 1959.

28. Adams, T, Bezner, J, and Steinhardt, M: The conceptualization and measurement of perceived wellness: Integrating balance across and within dimensions. Am J Health Promot 11(3):208, 1997.

29. Corbin, CB, and Pangrazi, RP: Toward a uniform definition of wellness: A commentary. President's Council on Physical Fitness and Sports Research Digest Series 3, no.15, December 2001.

30. Neilson, E: Health values: Achieving high level wellness: Origin, philosophy, purpose. Health Values 12(3):5, 1988.

31. Edelman, CL, and Mandle, CL: Health Promotion throughout the Lifespan, ed 5. Mosby, St. Louis, 2002.

32. Health-Related Quality of Life. Centers for Disease Control and Prevention, US Department of Health and Human Services, Atlanta, GA. Retrieved March 10, 2011, from www.cdc.gov/hrqol/methods.htm.

33. Green, LW, and Kreuter, MW: Health Promotion Planning, ed 3. McGraw-Hill, New York, 1999.

34. McKenzie, JF, Neiger, BL, and Smeltzer, JL: Planning, Implementing and Evaluating Health Promotion Programs: A Primer, ed 4. Benjamin Cummings, San Francisco, 2005.

35. A Guide to Population Health. United States Air Force Medical Support Agency. Population Health Support Division. Retrieved September 4, 2011, from www.tricare.mil/PHMMSC/mm_guide/Section3/Item6.pdf.

36. Health Promotion. World Health Organization. Retrieved March 10, 2011, from www.who.int/topics/health_promotion/en/.

37. Gorin, SS, and Arnold, J (eds): Health Promotion in Practice. Jossey-Bass, San Francisco, 2006.

38. Physical Activity Guidelines Advisory Committee Report. US Department of Health and Human Services, 2008. Retrieved September 6, 2011, from www.health.gov/paguidelines/Report/Default.aspx.

39. Casperson, CJ, Powell, KE, and Christenson, GM: Physical activity, exercise, and physical fitness: Definitions and distinctions for health-related research. Public Health Rep 100(2):126, 1985.

40. Callahan, LF, and Pinkus, T: Education, self-care, and outcomes of rheumatic diseases: Further challenges to the "Biomedical Model" paradigm. Arthritis Rheum 10(5):283, 1997.

41. Engel, GL: The need for a new medical model: A challenge for biomedicine. In Caplan, AL, McCartney, JJ, and Sisti, DA (eds): Health, Disease, and Illness: Concepts in Medicine. Georgetown University Press, Washington, DC, 2004, p 51.

42. Bandura, A: The primacy of self-regulation in health promotion. Appl Psychol 54(2):245, 2005.

43. Nagi, S: Disability concepts revisited: Implications for prevention. In Pope, A, and Tarlov, A (eds): Disability in America: Toward a National Agenda for Prevention. Institute of Medicine, National Academy Press, Washington, DC, 1991, p 309.

44. International Classification of Functioning, Disability and Health (ICF). World Health Organization. Retrieved September 10, 2011, from www.who.int/classifications/icf/en/.

45. Physical Therapists and Physical Therapist Assistants as Promoters and Advocates for Physical Activity/Exercise RC-08. American Physical Therapy Association, 64th Annual Session House of Delegates, San Antonio, TX, June 9–11, 2008.

46. Escorpizo, R, et al: Creating an interface between the International Classification of Functioning, Disability and Health and physical therapist practice. Phys Ther 90(7):1053, 2010.

47. Fisher, MI, and Howell, D: The power of empowerment: An ICF-based model to improve self-efficacy and upper extremity function of survivors of breast cancer. Rehabil Oncol 28(3):19, 2010.

48. Rauch, A, et al: Using a case report of a patient with spinal cord injury to illustrate the application of the International Classification of Functioning, Disability and Health during multidisciplinary patient management. Phys Ther 90(7):1039, 2010.

49. Fowler, EG, et al: Promotion of physical fitness and prevention of secondary conditions for children with cerebral palsy: Section on pediatrics research summit proceedings. Phys Ther 87(11):1495, 2007.

50. Howard, D, Nieuwenhuijsen, ER, and Saleeby, P: Health promotion and education: Application of the ICF in the US and Canada using an ecological perspective. Disabil Rehabil 30(12-13):942, 2008.

51. Raggi, A, et al: Obesity-related disability: Key factors identified by the International Classification of Functioning, Disability and Health. Disabil Rehabil 32(24):2028, 2010.

52. Wilhite, B, and Shank, J: In praise of sport: Promoting sport participation as a mechanism of health among persons with a disability. Disabil Health J 2(3):116, 2009.

53. Health Risk Appraisals. Centers for Disease Control and Prevention. Atlanta, Georgia. Retrieved September 6, 2011, from www.cdc.gov/nccdphp/dnpao/hwi/programdesign/health_risk_appraisals.htm.

54. Mossey, JM, and Shapiro, E: Self-rated health: A predictor of mortality among the elderly. Am J Public Health 72(8):800, 1982.

55. Health-Related Quality of Life. Centers for Disease Control and Prevention. Atlanta, GA. Retrieved September 6, 2011, from www.cdc.gov/hrqol/hrqol14_measure.htm.

56. Patient Reported Outcomes Measurement Information System. National Institutes of Health, Bethesda, MD. Retrieved July 7, 2011, from www.nihPROMIS.org.

57. WHOQOL-100. World Health Organization. Geneva, Switzerland. Retrieved August 20, 2011, from www.who.int/mental_health/media/68.pdf.

58. WHOQOL-Bref. World Health Organization. Geneva, Switzerland. Retrieved August 20, 2011, from www.who.int/mental_health/media/en/76.pdf.

59. Ware, JE, et al: SF-36 Health Survey Manual and Interpretation Guide. Health Institute, New England Medical Center, Boston, 1993.

60. Hunt, SM, and McEwan, J: Nottingham Health Profile: The development of a subjective health indicator. Sociol Health Illn 2:231, 1980.

61. Bergner, M: The Sickness Impact Profile: Conceptual formulation and methodology for the development of a health status measure. Int J Health Serv 6:393, 1976.

62. Dartmouth CO-OP Project. Dartmouth Medical School, Hanover, NH. Retrieved September 2, 2011, from www.dartmouthcoop-project.org/coopcharts.html.

63. Duke Health Profile. Department of Community and Family Medicine, Duke University Medical Center, Durham, NC. Retrieved Sept 4, 2011, from http://healthmeasures.mc.duke.edu/images/DukeForm.pdf.

64. Harari, MJ, Waehler, CA, and Rogers, JR: An empirical investigation of a theoretically based measure of perceived wellness. J Couns Psychol 52(1):93, 2005.

65. Meenan, RF: The AIMS approach to health status measurement: Conceptual background and measurement properties. J Rheumatol 9:785,1982.

66. Meenan, RF, et al: AIMS2: The content and properties of a revised and expanded Arthritis Impact Measurement Scales health status questionnaire. Arthritis Rheum 35:1, 1992.

67. Landgraf, JM, Abetz, L, and Ware, JEJ: The Child Health Questionnaire (CHQ): A user's manual. Health Institute, New England Medical Center, Boston, 1996.

68. Quittner, AL, et al: CFQ Cystic Fibrosis Questionnaire: A health-related quality of life measure. User manual. English version 1.0. 2000.

69. van Straten, A, et al: A stroke-adapted 30-item version of the Sickness Impact Profile to assess quality of life (SA-SIP30). Stroke 28:2155, 1997.

70. Duncan, PW, et al: The Stroke Impact Scale Version 2.0 Evaluation of reliability, validity and sensitivity to change. Stroke 30:2131, 1999.

71. VanSwearingen, JM, and Brach, JS: The Facial Disability Index: Reliability and validity of a disability assessment instrument

for disorders of the facial neuromuscular system. Phys Ther 76(12):1288, 1996.

72. Guyatt, GH, et al: A measure of quality of life for clinical trials in chronic lung disease. Thorax 42:773, 1987.

73. EORTC QLQ-30. European Organisation for Research and Treatment of Cancer. Quality of Life Department, Brussels, Belgium. Retrieved June 25, 2011, from http://groups.eortc.be/qol/questionnaires_qlqc30.htm.

74. Reeves, MJ, and Rafferty, AP: Healthy lifestyle characteristics among adults in the United States. Arch Intern Med 165:854, 2005.

75. American College of Sports Medicine: ACSM's Guidelines for Exercise Testing and Prescription, ed 8. Lippincott Williams & Wilkins, Baltimore, 2009.

76. Manson, JE, et al: The escalating pandemics of obesity and sedentary lifestyle. Arch Intern Med 164:249, 2004.

77. Craig, CL, et al: International physical activity questionnaire: 12-country reliability and validity. Med Sci Sports Exerc 35:1381, 2003.

78. Woolf, SH, Jonas S, and Kaplan-Liss, E: Health Promotion and Disease Prevention in Clinical Practice. Lippincott Williams & Wilkins, Philadelphia, 2008.

79. Fernald, DH, et al: Common Measures, Better Outcomes (COMBO). A field test of brief health behavior measures in primary care. Am J Prev Med 35 (5S):S414, 2008.

80. Healthy Living. Centers for Disease Control and Prevention. Atlanta, GA. Retrieved September 6, 2011, from www.cdc.gov/HealthyLiving/.

81. Recommendations. US Preventative Services Task Force, Rockville, MD. Retrieved September 4, 2011, from www.uspreventiveservicestaskforce.org/recommendations.htm.

82. The Guide to Clinical Preventive Services 2010–2011. Recommendations of the US Preventive Services Task Force. Agency for Healthcare Research and Quality, Department of Health and Human Services, Rockville, MD, 2010.

83. Electronic Preventive Services Selector. Agency for Healthcare Research and Quality, Department of Health and Human Services, Rockville, MD. Retrieved September 6, 2011, from http://epss.ahrq.gov/ePSS/index.jsp.

84. Lin, JS, et al: Behavioral counseling to promote physical activity and a healthful diet to prevent cardiovascular disease in adults: A systematic review for the US Preventive Services Task Force. Ann Intern Med 153:736, 2010.

85. Counseling and Interventions to Prevent Tobacco Use and Tobacco-Caused Disease in Adults and Pregnant Women. US Preventative Services Task Force, Rockville, MD, 2009. Retrieved September 6, 2011, from www.uspreventiveservicestaskforce.org/uspstf/uspstbac2.htm.

86. Michael, YL, et al: Primary care–relevant interventions to prevent falling in older adults: A systematic evidence review for the US Preventative Services Task Force. Ann Intern Med 153(12):815, 2010.

87. Bodner, ME, et al: Smoking cessation and counseling: Knowledge and views of Canadian physical therapists. Phys Ther 91(7):1051, 2011.

88. Glanz, K, Rimer, BK and Lewis, FM (eds): Health Behavior and Health Education, ed 3. Jossey-Bass, San Francisco, 2002.

89. Rosenstock, IM: Historical origins of the Health Belief Model. Health Educ Monogr 2:328–335, 1974.

90. Campbell, HM, et al: Relationship between diet, exercise habits, and health status among patients with diabetes. Res Social Adm Pharm 7(2):151, 2011.

91. Haines, TP, et al: Patient education to prevent falls among older hospital inpatients: A randomized controlled trial. Arch Intern Med 171(6):516, 2011.

92. Katz, DA, et al: Health beliefs toward cardiovascular risk reduction in patients admitted to chest pain observation units. Acad Emerg Med 16(5):379, 2009.

93. Fishbein, M (ed): Readings in Attitude Theory and Measurement. Wiley, New York, 1967.

94. Ajzen, I: The theory of planned behavior. Organ Behav Hum Decis Process 50:179, 1991.

95. Godin, G, and Kik, G: The theory of planned behavior: A review of its applications to health-related behaviors. Am J Health Promot 11(2):87, 1996.

96. Armitage, CJ, and Conner, M: Efficacy of the theory of planned behavior. Br J Soc Psychol 40(4):471, 2001.

97. Norman, P, and Conner, M: The theory of planned behavior and exercise: Evidence for the mediating and moderating roles of planning on intention-behavior relationships. J Sport Exerc Psychol 27(4):488, 2005.

98. Prochaska, JO: Systems of Psychotherapy: A Transtheoretical Analysis. Brooks-Cole, Pacific Grove, CA, 1979.

99. Cardinal, BJ, Kosma, M, and McCubbin, JA: Factors influencing the exercise behavior of adults with physical disabilities. Med Sci Sports Exerc 36(5):868, 2004.

100. Bandura, A: Social learning through imitation. In Jones, MR (ed): Nebraska Symposium on Motivation. University of Nebraska Press, Lincoln, NE, 1962, p 211.

101. Bandura, A: Social cognitive theory of self-regulation. Organ Behav Hum Decis Process 50:248, 1991.

102. Bandura, A. Self-Efficacy: The Exercise of Control. WH Freeman, New York, 1997.

103. Annesi, JJ, et al: Effects of the coach approach intervention on adherence to exercise in obese women: Assessing mediation of social cognitive theory factors. Res Q Exerc Sport 82(1):99, 2011.

104. Cramp, AG, and Brawley, LR: Moms in motion: A group-mediated cognitive-behavioral physical activity intervention. Int J Behav Nutr Phys Act 3:23, 2006.

105. Ince, ML: Use of social cognitive theory–based physical activity intervention on health-promoting behaviors of university students. Percept Mot Skills 107:833, 2008.

106. Mihalko, SL, Wickley, KL, and Sharpe, BL: Promoting physical activity in independent living communities. Med Sci Sports Exerc 38(1):112, 2006.

107. Motl, RW, et al: Internet intervention for increasing physical activity in persons with multiple sclerosis. Mult Scler 17(1):116, 2011.

108. Rogers, LQ, et al: A randomized trial to increase physical activity in breast cancer survivors. Med Sci Sports Exerc 41(4):935, 2009.

109. Wilson, DK, et al: A preliminary test of a student-centered intervention on increasing physical activity in underserved adolescents. Ann Behav Med 30(2):119, 2005.

110. van der Ploeg, HP, et al: Physical activity for people with a disability: A conceptual model. Sports Med 34(10):639, 2004.

111. De Vries, H, Dijkstra, M, and Kuhlman, P: Self-efficacy: The third factor besides attitude and subjective norm as a predictor of behavioral intentions. Health Educ Res 3:273, 1988.

112. Miller, WR, and Rollnick, S: Motivational Interviewing ed 2. Guilford Press, New York, 2002.

113. Vong, SK, et al: Motivational enhancement therapy in addition to physical therapy improves motivational factors and treatment outcomes in people with low back pain: A randomized controlled trial. Arch Phys Med Rehabil 92(2):176, 2011.

114. Rubak, S: Motivational interviewing: A systematic review and meta-analysis. Br J Gen Pract 55(513):305, 2005.

115. Greaves, CJ, et al: Motivational interviewing for modifying diabetes risk: A randomised controlled trial. Br J Gen Pract 58(553):535, 2008.

116. Bennett, JA, et al: Motivational interviewing to increase physical activity in long-term cancer survivors: A randomized controlled trial. Nurs Res 56(1):18, 2007.

117. Brodie, DA, and Inoue, A. Motivational interviewing to promote physical activity for people with chronic heart failure. J Adv Nurs 50(5):518, 2005.

118. Lohmann, H, Siersma, V, and Olivarius, NF: Fitness consultations in routine care of patients with type 2 diabetes in general practice: An 18-month non-randomised intervention study. BMC Fam Pract 11:83, 2010.

119. Van Keulen, HM, et al: Tailored print communication and telephone motivational interviewing are equally successful in improving multiple lifestyle behaviors in a randomized controlled trial. Ann Behav Med 41(1):104, 2011.

120. Lai, DTC, et al: Motivational interviewing for smoking cessation. Cochrane Database of Systematic Reviews 2010, Issue 1. Art. No.: CD006936. DOI: 10.1002/14651858.CD006936.pub2.

121. Soria, R, et al: A randomised controlled trial of motivational interviewing for smoking cessation. Br J Gen Pract 56(531):768, 2006.

122. Meeks, S: The role of the physical therapist in the recognition, assessment, and exercise intervention in persons with, or at risk for, osteoporosis. Top Geriatr Rehabil 21(1):42, 2005.

123. Dibble, L, and Lange, M: Predicting falls in individuals with Parkinson disease: A reconsideration of clinical balance measures. J Neurol Phys Ther 30(2):60, 2006.

124. DeWeese, C: How multiple interventions reduced injuries and costs in one plant. Work 26(3):251, 2006.

125. Gilchrist, J: A randomized controlled trial to prevent noncontact anterior cruciate ligament injury in female collegiate soccer players. Am J Sports Med 36(8):1476, 2008.

126. Boslaugh, SE, and Andresen, EM: Correlates of physical activity for adults with disability. Prev Chronic Dis 3(3):1, 2006.

127. Buchholz, AC, McGillivray, CF, and Pencharz, PB: Physical activity levels are low in free-living adults with chronic paraplegia. Obes Res 11:563, 2003.

128. Hootman, JM, et al: Physical activity levels among the general US adult population and in adults with and without arthritis. Arthritis Care Res 49(1):129, 2003.

129. Zhao, G, et al: Physical activity in US older adults with diabetes mellitus: Prevalence and correlates of meeting physical activity recommendations. J Am Geriatr Soc 59(1):132, 2011.

130. Armour, BS, et al: State-level prevalence of cigarette smoking and treatment advice, by disability status, United States, 2004. Prev Chronic Dis 4(4):A86, 2007.

131. Rimmer, R, Rowland, JL, and Yamaki, K: Obesity and secondary conditions in adolescents with disabilities: Addressing the needs of an underserved population. J Adolesc Health 41(3):224, 2007.

132. Rimmer, JH, and Wang, E: Obesity prevalence among a group of Chicago residents with disabilities. Arch Phys Med Rehab 86(7):1461, 2005.

133. Perreault, K: Linking health promotion with physiotherapy for low back pain: A review. J Rehabil Med 40:401, 2008.

134. American Physical Therapy Association: Physical therapists and physical therapist assistants as promoters and advocates for physical activity/exercise. House of Delegates P06-08-07-08.

135. Junker, L, and Carlberg, EB: Factors that affect exercise participation among people with physical disabilities. Adv Physiother 13(1):18, 2011.

136. Petursdottir, U, Arnadottir, SA, and Halldorsdottir, S: Facilitators and barriers to exercising among people with osteoarthritis: A phenomenological study. Phys Ther 90(7):1014, 2010.

137. Rimmer, JH, et al: Physical activity participation among persons with disabilities: Barriers and facilitators. Am J Prev Med 26(5):419, 2004.

138. Rogers, LQ, et al: Exploring social cognitive theory constructs for promoting exercise among breast cancer patients. Cancer Nurs 27(6):462, 2004.

139. Physical Fitness for Special Populations. American Physical Therapy Association, Alexandria, VA. Retrieved September 1, 2011, from www.apta.org/PFSP/.

140. Physical Activity among Adults with a Disability—United States, 2005. Morbidity and Mortality Weekly Report, Centers for Disease Control and Prevention, 2007.Retrieved September 2, 2011, from www.cdc.gov/mmwr/preview/mmwrhtml/mm5639a2.htm.

141. Chen, MD, and Rimmer, JH: Effects of exercise on quality of life in stroke survivors: A meta-analysis. Stroke 42(3):832, 2011.

142. Goodman, C, and Helgeson, K: Exercise Prescription for Medical Conditions. FA Davis, Philadelphia, 2011.

143. Durstine, JL, et al: ACSM's Exercise Management for Persons with Chronic Diseases and Disabilities, ed 3. Human Kinetics, Champaign, IL, 2009.

144. The National Center on Physical Activity and Disability. University of Illinois at Chicago, Department of Disability and Human Development, College of Applied Health Sciences, Chicago, IL. Retrieved September 6, 2011, from www.ncpad.org/.

145. Quinn, VP, et al: Effectiveness of the 5-As tobacco cessation treatments in nine HMOs. J Gen Intern Med 24(2):149, 2009.

146. Bodner, ME, and Dean, E: Advice as a smoking cessation strategy: A systematic review and implications for physical therapists. Physiother Theory Pract 25(5-6):369, 2009.

147. Helping Smokers Quit: A Guide for Clinicians. Revised May 2008. Agency for Healthcare Research and Quality. Rockville, MD. Retrieved September 2, 2011, from www.ahrq.gov/clinic/tobacco/clinhlpsmksqt.htm.

148. Clinical Guidelines on the Identification, Evaluation, and Treatment of Overweight and Obesity in Adults. National Heart, Lung and Blood Institute, Department of Health and Human Services, National Institutes for Health, Bethesda, MD. Retrieved September 2, 2011, from www.nhlbi.nih.gov/guidelines/obesity/ob_home.htm.

149. Body Mass Index. Centers for Disease Control and Prevention, Atlanta, GA. Retrieved July 6, 2011, from www.cdc.gov/healthyweight/assessing/bmi/index.html.

150. Shipp, KM: Exercise for people with osteoporosis: Translating the science into clinical practice. Curr Osteoporos Rep 4(4):129, 2006.

151. Breedland, I, et al: Effects of a group-based exercise and educational program on physical performance and disease self-management in rheumatoid arthritis: A randomized controlled study. Phys Ther 91(6):879, 2011.

152. Adamsen, L, et al: Effect of a multimodal high-intensity exercise intervention in cancer patients undergoing chemotherapy: Randomised controlled trial. BMJ 339:b3410, 2009.

153. Goldstein, MS, et al: The revised research agenda for physical therapy. Phys Ther 91(2):165, 2011.

The following statements are designed to provide information about your wellness perceptions. Please carefully and thoughtfully consider each statement, then select the *one* response option with which you *most* agree.

	Very Strongly Disagree					Very Strongly Agree
1. I am always optimistic about my future.	1	2	3	4	5	6
2. There have been times when I felt inferior to most of the people I knew.	1	2	3	4	5	6
3. Members of my family come to me for support.	1	2	3	4	5	6
4. My physical health has restricted me in the past.	1	2	3	4	5	6
5. I believe there is a real purpose for my life.	1	2	3	4	5	6
6. I will always seek out activities that challenge me to think and reason.	1	2	3	4	5	6
7. I rarely count on good things happening to me.	1	2	3	4	5	6
8. In general, I feel confident about my abilities.	1	2	3	4	5	6
9. Sometimes I wonder if my family will really be there for me when I am in need.	1	2	3	4	5	6
10. My body seems to resist physical illness very well.	1	2	3	4	5	6
11. Life does not hold much future promise for me.	1	2	3	4	5	6
12. I avoid activities that require me to concentrate.	1	2	3	4	5	6
13. I always look on the bright side of things.	1	2	3	4	5	6
14. I sometimes think I am a worthless individual.	1	2	3	4	5	6
15. My friends know they can always confide in me and ask me for advice.	1	2	3	4	5	6
16. My physical health is excellent.	1	2	3	4	5	6
17. Sometimes I don't understand what life is all about.	1	2	3	4	5	6
18. Generally, I feel pleased with the amount of intellectual stimulation I receive in my daily life.	1	2	3	4	5	6
19. In the past, I have expected the best.	1	2	3	4	5	6
20. I am uncertain about my ability to do things well in the future.	1	2	3	4	5	6
21. My family has been available to support me in the past.	1	2	3	4	5	6
22. Compared to people I know, my past physical health has been excellent.	1	2	3	4	5	6
23. I feel a sense of mission about my future.	1	2	3	4	5	6
24. The amount of information that I process in a typical day is just about right for me (i.e., not too much and not too little).	1	2	3	4	5	6
25. In the past, I hardly ever expected things to go my way.	1	2	3	4	5	6
26. I will always be secure with who I am.	1	2	3	4	5	6
27. In the past, I have not always had friends with whom I could share my joys and sorrows.	1	2	3	4	5	6

		Very Strongly Disagree					Very Strongly Agree
28.	I expect to always be physically healthy.	1	2	3	4	5	6
29.	I have felt in the past that my life was meaningless.	1	2	3	4	5	6
30.	In the past, I have generally found intellectual challenges to be vital to my overall well-being.	1	2	3	4	5	6
31.	Things will not work out the way I want them to in the future.	1	2	3	4	5	6
32.	In the past, I have felt sure of myself among strangers.	1	2	3	4	5	6
33.	My friends will be there for me when I need help.	1	2	3	4	5	6
34.	I expect my physical health to get worse.	1	2	3	4	5	6
35.	It seems that my life has always had purpose.	1	2	3	4	5	6
36.	My life has often seemed void of positive mental stimulation.	1	2	3	4	5	6

PWS Scoring Sheet for Use with Individual Clients

Instructions: Record your score from the PWS instrument for each numbered item below. Note the * items indicating reverse scoring. Add the numbers in each column and divide by 6 to determine each subscale score.
*Reverse Score (e.g., 1 = 6, 2 = 5, 3 = 4, 4 = 3, 5 = 2, and 6 = 1)

Psychological

Item Number	Score
1.	
*7.	
13.	
19.	
*25.	
*31.	
Total =	
Divided by 6 =	

Physical

Item Number	Score
*4.	
10.	
16.	
22.	
28.	
*34.	
Total =	
Divided by 6 =	

Emotional

Item Number	Score
*2.	
8.	
*14.	
*20.	
26.	
32.	
Total =	
Divided by 6 =	

Spiritual

Item Number	Score
5.	
*11.	
*17.	
23.	
*29.	
35.	
Total =	
Divided by 6 =	

Continued

Social		Intellectual	
Item Number	*Score*	*Item Number*	*Score*
3.		6.	
*9.		*12.	
15.		18.	
21.		24.	
*27.		30.	
33.		*36.	
Total =		Total =	
Divided by 6 =		Divided by 6 =	

Agency for Healthcare Research and Quality: Health Promotion/Disease Prevention	www.ahrq.gov/browse/hpdp.htm
American Physical Therapy Association: Physical Fitness for Special Populations	www.apta.org/PFSP/
CDC: Behavioral Risk Factor Surveillance System	www.cdc.gov/brfss/
CDC: Healthy Living	www.cdc.gov/healthyliving/
CDC: Body mass index calculator	www.cdc.gov/healthyweight/assessing/bmi/
CDC: Youth Risk Behavior Surveillance System	www.cdc.gov/HealthyYouth/yrbs/index.htm
Healthy People 2020	www.healthypeople.gov/2020/default.aspx
National Center on Physical Activity and Disability	www.ncpad.org/
U.S. Preventive Services Task Force	www.uspreventiveservicestaskforce.org/index.html

CDC = Centers for Disease Control and Prevention.

Orthotics, Prosthetics, and Prescriptive Wheelchairs

Orthotics

Joan E. Edelstein, PT, MA, FISPO, CPed
Christopher Kevin Wong, PT, PhD, OCS

Chapter **30**

LEARNING OBJECTIVES

1. Relate the major parts of the shoe to the requirements of individuals fitted with lower extremity orthoses.
2. Compare the characteristics, advantages, and disadvantages of plastics, metals, and other materials used in orthoses.
3. Describe the components of contemporary foot, ankle-foot, knee-ankle-foot, hip-knee-ankle-foot, trunk-hip-knee-ankle-foot, and trunk orthoses.
4. Explain the orthotic options available for patients with paraplegia.
5. Identify the features of lower extremity and trunk orthoses that are considered during the examination process.
6. Outline the physical therapist's role in management of patients fitted with lower extremity and trunk orthoses.
7. Analyze and interpret patient data, formulate realistic goals and outcomes, and develop a plan of care when presented with a clinical case study.

CHAPTER OUTLINE

An **orthosis** is an external appliance worn to restrict or assist motion or to transfer load from one area of the body to another. The older term, *brace*, is a synonym. A splint connotes an orthosis intended for temporary use. An **orthotist** is the health care professional who designs, fabricates, and fits orthoses for the limbs and trunk, and a **pedorthist** is the health care professional who designs, fabricates, and fits only shoes and foot orthoses. The term *orthotic* is an adjective, although some use the word as a noun. Archaeological evidence indicates

1325

that orthoses have been used at least since the fifth Egyptian dynasty (2750 to 2625 BC).[1] The term *orthosis* appears to have been coined in the mid-20th century.

This chapter presents the most frequently prescribed orthoses for the lower extremity (LE) and the trunk, as well as new developments in the field. Key elements in preparing patients to use orthoses are discussed. Focus is placed on orthotic design characteristics, their biomechanical rationale, merits of specific materials, and criteria for judging the adequacy of orthotic fit, function, and construction. Although every attempt is made to use evidence-based research to guide clinical practice, the heterogeneity within the population of orthotic users and within orthotic designs confounds this effort.[2]

■ TERMINOLOGY AND TYPES OF ORTHOSES

Generic terminology is superseding the traditional use of eponyms (surname of developer). Naming orthoses by the joints they encompass and the type of motion control facilitates communication among clinicians and consumers. Thus, *foot orthoses* (FOs) are appliances applied to the foot and placed inside or outside the shoe, such as metatarsal pads and heel lifts. *Ankle-foot orthoses* (AFOs) encompass the shoe and terminate below the knee. The *knee-ankle-foot orthosis* (KAFO) extends from the shoe to the thigh. A *hip-knee-ankle-foot orthosis* (HKAFO) is a KAFO with a pelvic band that surrounds the lower trunk. A *trunk-hip-knee-ankle-foot orthosis* (THKAFO) covers part of the thorax as well as the lower extremities (LEs). *Knee orthosis* (KO) and *hip orthosis* (HO) are other applications of the same system of nomenclature.

■ LOWER EXTREMITY ORTHOSES

Lower extremity orthoses range from shoes used for clinical purposes to THKAFOs. Characteristics and functions of the principal FOs, AFOs, KAFOs, HKAFOs, and THKAFOs, and trunk orthoses, together with the clinically important attributes of shoes, will be described. Although physical therapists also encounter KOs, HOs, and orthoses for special purposes, such as management of Legg-Calvé-Perthes disease, these

orthoses are not included because they are used less frequently than the appliances that do appear in this chapter. Similarly, orthoses for the upper limb are omitted from this chapter because they are less commonly prescribed and in most instances are used only for a brief duration.

Shoes

The shoe is the foundation for most LE orthoses. Each part of the shoe contributes to the efficacy of orthotic management and offers many options for selection. Shoes transfer body weight to the ground and protect the wearer from the terrain and the weather. The ideal shoe should distribute bearing forces so as to provide optimum comfort, function, and appearance of the foot. For the individual with an orthopedic disorder, footwear can serve two additional purposes: (1) it reduces pressure on sensitive deformed structures by redistributing force toward pain-free areas; and (2) it serves as the foundation for AFOs and more extensive bracing. Unless the shoe is correctly fitted and appropriately modified, the alignment of the orthosis will not provide the designed pattern of weight-bearing. The major parts of the shoe are the upper, sole, heel, and reinforcements. These features are found in both the dress leather shoe (Fig. 30.1A) and the athletic shoe (Fig. 30.1B).

Upper

The portion of the shoe over the dorsum of the foot is the *upper*. It consists of an anterior component called the *vamp* and the posterior part, the *quarter*. If the shoe is to be used with an AFO having an insert as its foundation, then the vamp should extend to the proximal portion of the dorsum to secure the shoe and thereby the rest of the orthosis onto the foot. In a laced shoe, the vamp contains the lace stays, which have eyelets for shoelaces (Fig. 30.2). Laces provide more precise adjustment over the entire opening than do strap closures. The latter, however, enable individuals with limited manual dexterity to manage the shoe more easily. For most orthotic purposes, a *Blucher* lace stay is preferable; it is distinguished by the separation between the anterior margins of the lace stays and the vamp. The alternate design is the *Bal,* or *Balmoral,*

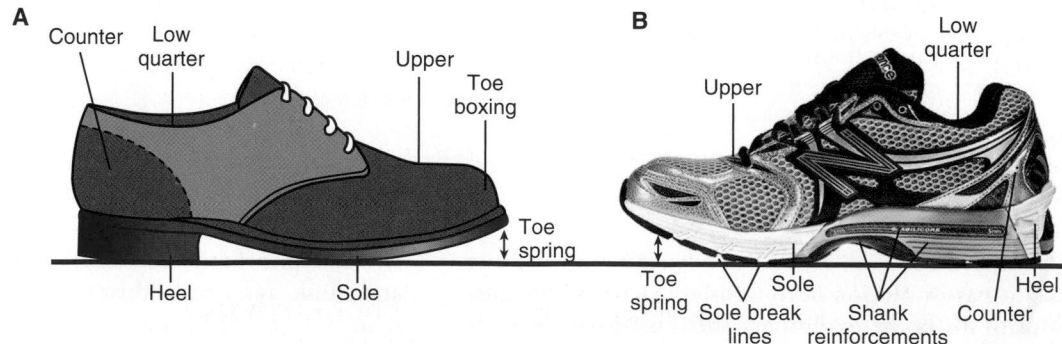

Figure 30.1 (A) Parts of a low quarter shoe with a Blucher lace stay. Note that the counter and toe boxing are internal reinforcing structures of the shoe. **(B)** Parts of a low-quarter running shoe.

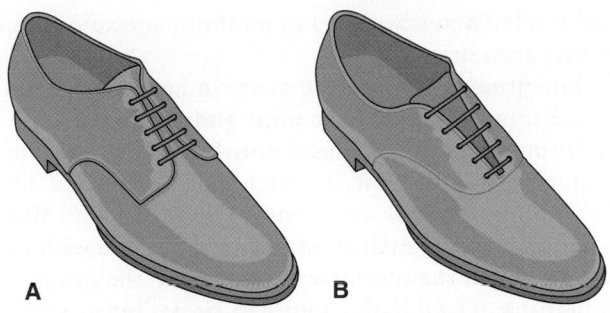

Figure 30.2 Low-quarter shoes: **(A)** Blucher (open lace) and **(B)** Bal (Balmoral) (closed lace). The Blucher lace stay is generally preferred for orthotic use owing to ease in donning (provides greater foot entry space to accommodate orthosis) and adjustability.

lace stay, in which the lace stay is continuous with the vamp. The Blucher opening permits substantial adjustability, an important feature for the patient with edema. It also offers a large inlet into the shoe, so that one can determine whether paralyzed toes lie flat within the shoe. An *extra-depth shoe* is one having an upper contoured with additional vertical space. The shoe is manufactured with a second inner sole that can be removed to accommodate an insert or thick surgical dressing.

Quarter height is another consideration in shoe prescription. The low-quarter terminates below the malleoli and is satisfactory for most clinical purposes. This style does not restrict foot or ankle motion. If the patient will be wearing a plastic orthosis molded about the ankle, it is not necessary to go to the additional expense of providing a high-quarter shoe for ankle support. A high-quarter shoe, covering the malleoli, is indicated to cover the foot having rigid **pes equinus**. It is also appropriate to augment foot stability in the absence of an AFO. The high-quarter shoe, however, is more difficult to don and more expensive than a comparable low-quarter one.

Sole

The *sole* is the bottom portion of the shoe. For use with a riveted metal attachment between shoe and orthosis, the sole should have an outer and an inner sole. Between the two lies a metal reinforcement that receives the rivets. This type of shoe, however, is heavier than an athletic shoe with a single sole. Leather soles absorb little impact shock and provide minimal traction as compared to natural or synthetic rubber soles. To absorb shock, the shoe may have a resilient outer sole, inner sole, or insert. Older people should wear shoes with firm, slip-resistant outsoles to reduce the risk of falling.[3,4]

Regardless of material, the outer sole should not contact the floor at the distal end; the slight rise of the sole is known as *toe spring* (see Fig. 30.1), which allows a rocker effect at late stance. If a lift is added to the sole to compensate for leg length discrepancy, the lift should be beveled to achieve toe spring.

Heel

The *heel* is the portion of the shoe adjacent to the outer sole, under the anatomical heel. A broad, low heel provides greatest stability and distributes force between the back and front of the foot most evenly. For adults, a 1-in (2.5-cm) heel tilts the center of gravity slightly forward to aid transition through stance phase, but does not disturb normal knee and hip alignment significantly. Slight heel lifts increase the contraction of the medial gastrocnemius and the tibialis anterior.[5] A higher heel places the ankle in greater plantarflexion range and forces the tibia forward. The wearer compensates either by retaining slight knee and hip flexion or by extending the knee and exaggerating lumbar lordosis. The high heel transmits more stress to the metatarsals[6] and knee.[7] Nevertheless, transferring load anteriorly may be desirable if the patient has heel pain. The higher heel also reduces tension on the Achilles tendon and other posterior structures and accommodates rigid pes equinus. Although most heels are made of firm material with a rubber plantar surface, a low resilient heel is indicated to permit slight plantarflexion if the ankle cannot move because of orthotic or anatomical limitation.

Reinforcements

Reinforcements located at strategic points preserve the shape of the shoe. *Toe boxing* in the vamp protects the toes from stubbing and vertical trauma; it should be high enough to accommodate hammer toes or similar deformity. The *shank* piece is a longitudinal plate that reinforces the sole between the anterior border of the heel and the widest part of the sole at the metatarsal heads. A corrugated steel shank is necessary if an orthotic attachment is to be riveted to the shoe. The *counter* stiffens the quarter and generally terminates at the anterior border of the heel. The patient with pes valgus, however, should have a shoe with a long medial counter that provides reinforcement along the medial border of the foot to the head of the first metatarsal, thus resisting the tendency of the foot to collapse medially.

Last

The *last* is the model over which the shoe is made. The last, whether of traditional wood, custom-made plaster, or computer-generated design, remains with the manufacturer; the shoe shape duplicates the last's contour. A given shoe size may be achieved with many lasts, each transmitting different forces to the foot. Consequently, the physical therapist should ascertain that the shoe shape fits the foot satisfactorily, rather than relying on a particular shoe size. The patient with a markedly deformed foot requires a shoe made over a special last, either a factory- or custom-made one.

Foot Orthoses

Foot orthoses are appliances that apply forces to the foot. These may be an insert placed in the shoe, an internal modification affixed inside the shoe, or an external modification attached to the sole or heel of the shoe. They can enhance function by relieving pain. This may be accomplished by transferring weight-bearing stresses to pressure-tolerant sites, protecting painful areas from contact with the shoe, correcting alignment of a flexible segment, or accommodating a fixed deformity. Inserts can also improve the wearer's transition during stance phase, by altering the rollover point in late stance and by equalizing foot and leg lengths on both limbs. In many instances, a particular therapeutic aim can be achieved by a variety of devices.

Internal Modifications

Generally, the closer the modification is to the foot, the more effective it is. Biomechanically, inserts and internal modifications are identical. Both inserts and internal modifications reduce shoe volume, so proper shoe fit must be judged with these components in place. An insert permits the patient to transfer the orthosis from shoe to shoe, if the shoes have the same heel height; otherwise, a rigid insert may rock in the shoe. Most inserts terminate just behind the metatarsal heads; thus, they may slip forward, particularly if the shoe has a relatively high heel. Some inserts extend the full length of the sole, preventing slippage, but occupying the often limited space in the anterior portion of the shoe. Internal modifications are fixed to the shoe's interior, guaranteeing the desired placement, but limiting the patient to the single pair of modified shoes.

Inserts made of resilient materials, such as the rubber, viscoelastic plastics (e.g., Sorbothane and Viscolas), or polyethylene foam, reduce impact shock and shear, thus protecting painful or insensitive feet.[8] Inserts are also constructed of semirigid or rigid plastics and metal, often with a resilient overlay. A full-length insert tends to reduce gait unsteadiness by improving proprioception from the increased foot contact area.[9] A heel-spur insert orthosis (Fig. 30.3), for example, may be made of viscoelastic plastic or rubber.[10] The orthosis slopes anteriorly to reduce load on the painful heel. In addition, the

orthosis has a concave relief to minimize pressure on the tender area.

Longitudinal arch supports are intended to prevent depression of the subtalar joint and flattening of the arch (pes planovalgus, **pes planus**). The orthosis may include a wedge (post) to alter foot alignment. The minimum support is a resilient *scaphoid pad* (Fig. 30.4) positioned at the medial border of the insole with the apex between the sustentaculum tali and the navicular tuberosity. Flexible flat foot can be realigned with a semirigid plastic *University of California Biomechanics Laboratory (UCBL) insert.*[11] It is molded over a plaster model of the foot, taken with the foot in maximum correction. It controls hindfoot valgus and limits subtalar motion. The insert encompasses the heel and midfoot. Corrective alignment includes a three-point counterpressure system and force couple for control of calcaneal eversion; forefoot abduction is controlled by a second three-point counterpressure system (Fig. 30.5).[12] A full-length insert reduces motion at the first metatarsophalangeal joint, resulting in pain reduction.[13,14] Wearing arch supports is associated with increased activation of the tibialis anterior and peroneus longus.[15] With regard to the effect of inserts on proximal joints, the evidence is equivocal; some investigations show that orthoses alter the onset of erector spinae and gluteus medius activity[16] and support the positive effect of FOs on reducing knee pain,[17-21] whereas others show little or no effect.[22,23] Some adults with plantar fasciitis also respond favorably to foot orthoses.[24-28] Children with pes planus may also benefit from wearing longitudinal arch supports, although the evidence is weak.[29,30]

Insert orthoses are also used to relieve pain and activity limitation associated with pes cavus.[31-33] The *metatarsal pad* (Fig. 30.6) is a convex component that may be incorporated in an insert or may be a resilient domed piece glued to the inner sole so that its apex is under the metatarsal shafts. The pad transfers stress from the metatarsal heads to the metatarsal shafts and is

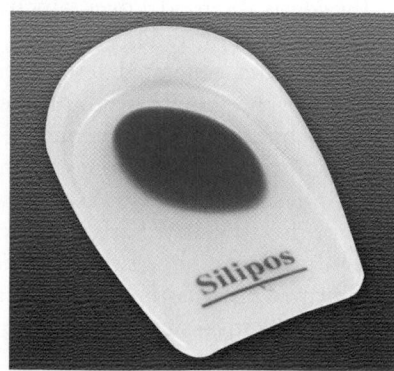
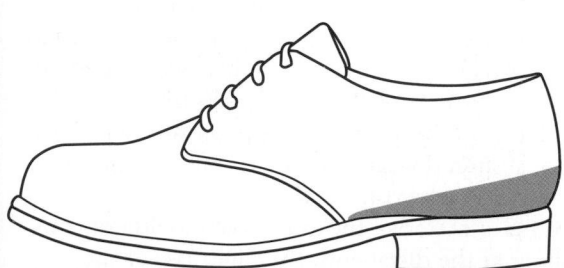

Figure 30.3 (*Left*) Plastic tapered heel spur cushion with concave relief to reduce pressure (available in multiple densities as well as with a removable central plug). *Courtesy of Silipos, Inc., Niagara Falls, NY 14304-3731.* (*Right*) The shaded area of the shoe on the right indicates the relative position of the heel spur cushion when placed in a shoe.

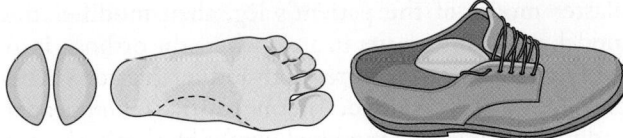

Figure 30.4 Scaphoid pads (*left*) are available with self-adhesive backing. They are positioned (*middle*) medial and plantar to the longitudinal arch; scaphoid pad (*right*) positioned inside of shoe.

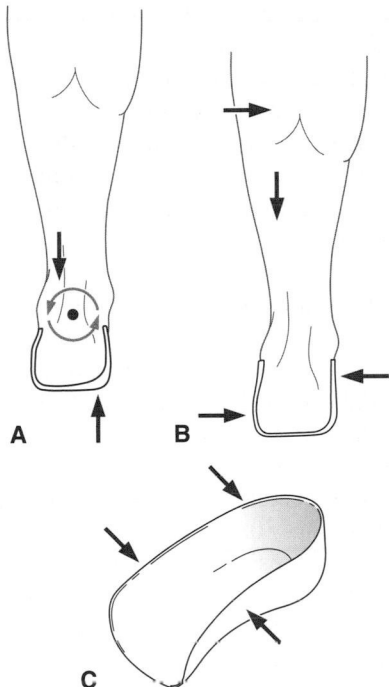

Figure 30.5 University of California Biomechanics Laboratory (UCBL) foot orthosis exerts control at the subtalar joint via a force couple **(A)** and three-point counterforces to control calcaneal eversion **(B)**. A second counterforce system **(C)** restricts forefoot abduction. *From May and Lockard,[12, p. 239] with permission.*

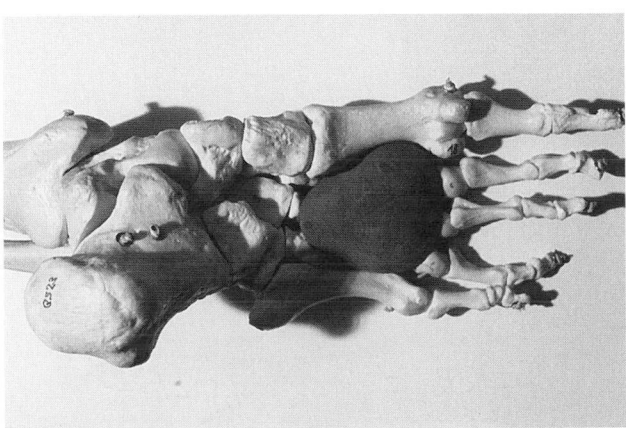

Figure 30.6 Rubber metatarsal pad. Whether used as an internal modification or as part of an insert, the pad should be oriented as shown on the skeletal model.

effective in reducing plantar pressure particularly in patients with diabetic neuropathy.[34-36]

Occasionally, modifications are sandwiched between the inner and outer soles; for example, the patient with marked arthritic changes in the front of the foot probably will be more comfortable if the shoe has a steel band between the soles to eliminate motion at the painful joints. The same effect can be achieved with a rigid insert.

External Modifications

An external modification ensures that the patient wears the appropriate shoes and does not reduce shoe volume, but will erode as the individual walks and is somewhat conspicuous. In addition, the client is limited to wearing the modified shoe, rather than being able to choose from a wide selection of shoes.

A *heel wedge* (Fig. 30.7) is a frequently prescribed external modification. It alters alignment of the rearfoot. A medial heel wedge, by applying laterally directed force, can aid in realigning flexible **pes valgus** or can accommodate rigid **pes varus** by filling the void between the sole and the floor on the medial side. A medial wedge is incorporated in a *Thomas heel*, intended for flexible pes valgus (Fig. 30.8 [middle]). The anterior border of the Thomas heel extends forward on the medial side to augment the effect of the medial wedge in supporting the longitudinal arch. A cushion heel is made of resilient material to absorb shock at heel contact. Because it provides slight plantarflexion, the cushion heel is indicated when the patient wears an orthosis with a rigid ankle. Sole wedges alter medial–lateral forefoot alignment. A lateral wedge shifts weight-bearing to the medial side of the front of the foot. It compensates for fixed forefoot valgus, allowing the entire distal foot to contact the floor.

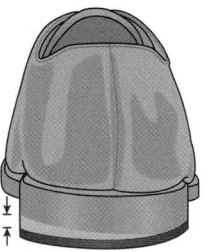

Figure 30.7 Medial heel wedge.

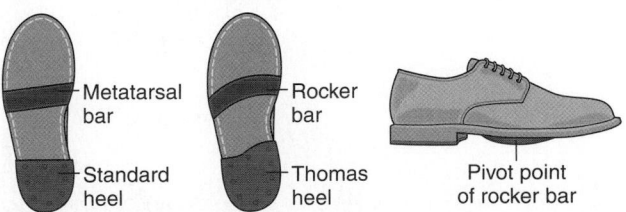

Figure 30.8 Illustrated here are (*left*) a metatarsal bar and standard heel, (*middle*) a rocker bar with a Thomas heel (note the medial extension), and (*right*) pivot point of rocker bar.

A *metatarsal bar* (see Fig. 30.8 [left]) is a flat strip of firm material placed posterior to the metatarsal heads. At late stance, the bar transfers stress from the metatarsophalangeal joints to the metatarsal shafts. A *rocker bar* (see Fig. 30.8 [middle and right]) is a convex transverse band affixed to the sole proximal to the metatarsal heads. It reduces the distance the wearer must travel during stance phase, improving late stance, as well as shifting load from the metatarsophalangeal joints to the metatarsal shafts.[37,38]

The patient with leg length discrepancy of more than 1/2 in (1 cm) will walk better with a shoe lift made of cork or other lightweight material. Approximately 3/8 in (0.8 cm) of the elevation can be accommodated on the insole at the heel of a low-quarter shoe.

Ankle-Foot Orthoses

The AFO is composed of a foundation, ankle control, foot control, and a superstructure.

Foundation

The foundation of the orthosis consists of the shoe and a plastic or metal component.

Insert

A plastic or metal insert or foot plate foundation (Fig. 30.9) has several advantages. Because internal modifications can be incorporated in it, the insert provides good control of the foot. It must be worn with a shoe that closes high on the dorsum of the foot to retain the orthosis. The insert facilitates donning the orthosis because the shoe can be separated from the rest of the brace. The insert also permits interchanging shoes, assuming that all shoes have been made on the same last. Less expensive shoes, such as sneakers, can be worn, because the foundation does not need to be riveted to the shoe. Because the insert is usually made of a thermoplastic material, such as polyethylene or polypropylene, the orthosis with an insert is relatively lightweight. The orthotist creates a plaster model of the patient's leg, then modifies the model, removing plaster in areas where the orthosis is to apply substantial pressure, and adding plaster where pressure relief is required. Thermoplastic is then heated and molded over the modified plaster model.

An insert foundation, however, is inappropriate if the patient cannot be relied on to wear the orthosis with a shoe of proper heel height. If the orthosis is placed in a shoe with too low a heel, the uprights would incline posteriorly, increasing the tendency of the wearer's knee to extend. Conversely, if the orthosis is worn with a higher heeled shoe, the patient might experience knee instability. The insert reduces interior shoe volume, and thus must be used with suitably spacious shoes. Custom-molded foot plates may be more expensive than other types of foundations. If the orthosis is to be used by a very obese or exceptionally active individual, a plastic foot plate may not provide adequate support.

Stirrup

An older foundation for the AFO is the steel stirrup, a U-shaped fixture, the center portion of which is riveted to the shoe through the shank. The arms of the stirrup join the brace uprights at the level of the anatomical ankle, providing congruency between orthotic and anatomical joints. The *solid stirrup* (Fig. 30.10) is a one-piece attachment that provides maximum stability of the orthosis on the shoe. The *split stirrup* (Fig. 30.11) has three segments. The central portion has a transverse rectangular opening. Medial and lateral angled side pieces fit into the opening. The *split stirrup* simplifies donning the orthosis because the wearer can detach the uprights from the shoe. If a central piece is riveted to another shoe, the shoes can be interchanged. The

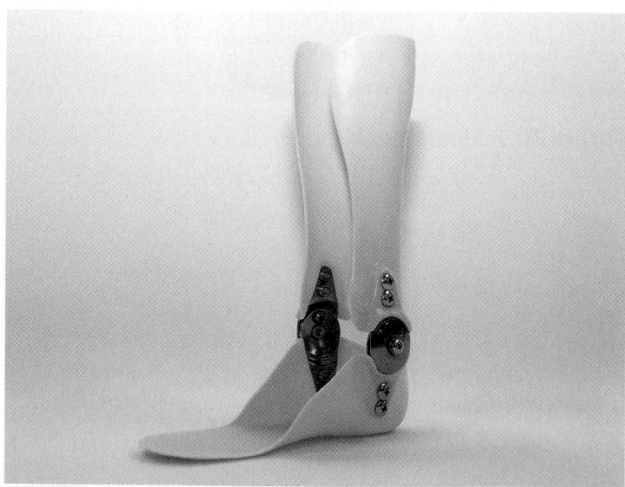

Figure 30.9 AFO with plastic insert.

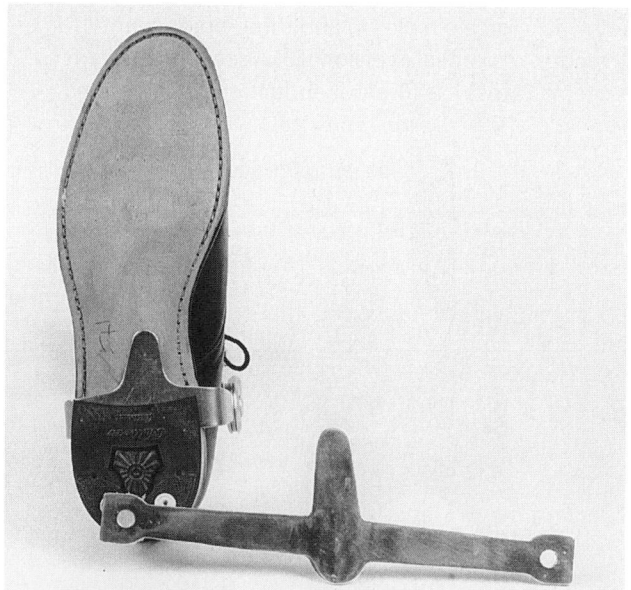

Figure 30.10 Solid stirrup. The stirrup in the foreground is as it comes from the manufacturer before it is U-shaped and fitted to the patient and shoe.

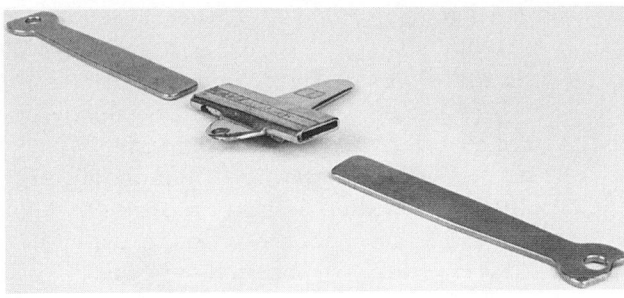

Figure 30.11 Split stirrup.

extremely active client may dislodge a side piece from its receptacle unintentionally. The split stirrup is bulkier and heavier than a solid stirrup.

Ankle Control

Most AFOs are prescribed to control ankle motion by limiting plantarflexion and/or dorsiflexion, or by assisting motion. The patient with dorsiflexor weakness or paralysis risks dragging the toe during swing phase. Dorsiflexion assistance can be provided by a *posterior leaf spring* that arises from a plastic *insert* (Fig. 30.12). During early stance, as the patient applies force to the braced foot, the upright bends backward slightly. When the patient progresses into swing phase, the plastic recoils forward to lift the foot. Thinner, narrower plastic permits relatively greater motion. Motion assistance can also be achieved with a steel dorsiflexion spring assist (Klenzak joint) (Fig. 30.13) incorporated into each stirrup. The coiled spring compresses in stance and rebounds during swing. The tightness of the coil can be adjusted. An orthosis with a dorsiflexion spring assist is noticeably bulkier than the posterior leaf spring model. Both types of spring assists yield slightly into plantarflexion at heel contact, affording the wearer protection against inadvertent knee flexion. Other AFO designs

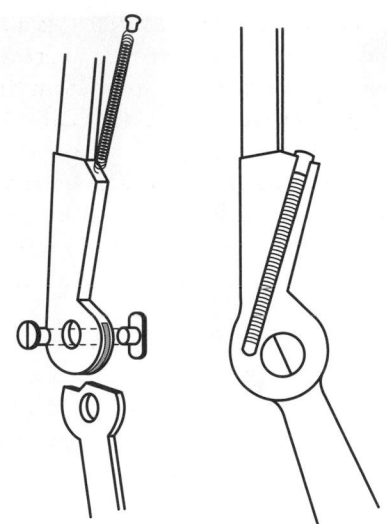

Figure 30.13 Steel dorsiflexion spring assist.

which control toe drag are presented in Figures 30.14 and 30.15. Healthy subjects wearing a posterior leaf spring AFO exhibited less hip extension and ankle plantarflexion during the transition from stance to swing phase.[39] AFOs with flexible ankle control altered the stance phase transition between rear- and forefoot among nondisabled adults.[40]

The alternate approach to prevent toe drag is plantarflexion resistance, which stops the ankle from plantarflexing so that the patient with weak dorsiflexors will not catch the toes and stumble during swing phase. A

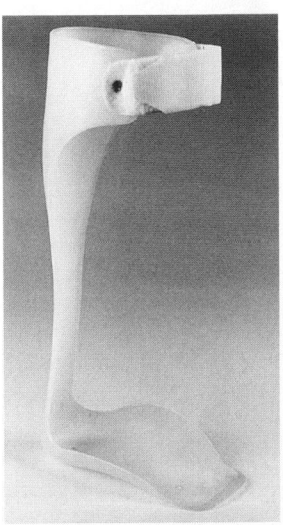

Figure 30.12 Plastic insert on posterior leaf spring AFO.

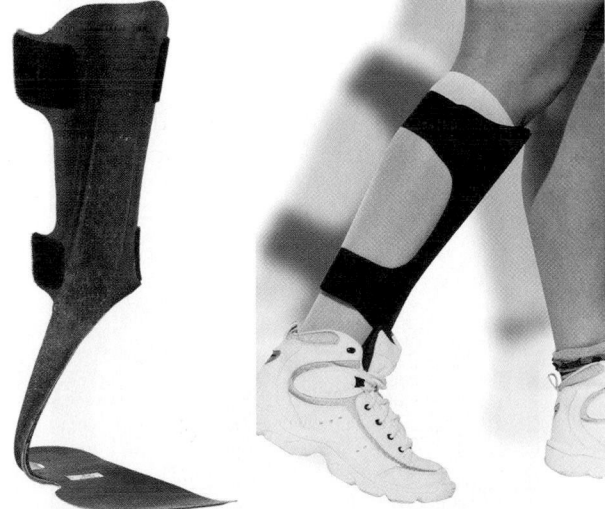

Figure 30.14 ToeOFF® ankle-foot orthosis. This fiber glass, carbon fiber, and Kevlar orthosis is designed to provide dorsiflexion assistance in the presence of mild to severe foot drop accompanied by mild to moderate ankle instability. This orthosis is contraindicated in the presence of moderate to severe spasticity or edema. *Courtesy of CAMP Scandinavia AB. SE 254 67 Helsingborg, Sweden.*

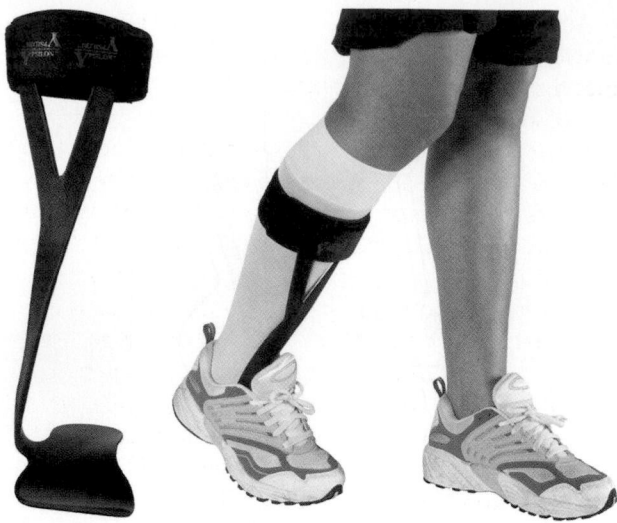

Figure 30.15 Ypsilon™ ankle-foot orthosis. This carbon composite AFO is designed to provide dorsiflexion assistance in the presence of mild to moderate isolated drop foot. It promotes free ankle movements (medial, lateral, and rotational movement). The proximal Y-shape provides tibia crest clearance. This orthosis is contraindicated for an unstable ankle joint or in the presence of moderate to severe spasticity or edema. *Courtesy of CAMP Scandinavia AB. SE 254 67 Helsingborg, Sweden.*

joint placed in a plastic hinged AFO (Fig. 30.16) or a steel posterior stop (Fig. 30.17) can be incorporated in the stirrup. The posterior stop also imposes a flexion force at the knee during early stance, preventing the knee from hyperextending. Healthy adults walking with the ankle fixed in plantarflexion consumed more oxygen than when walking with AFOs which kept the foot in neutral position.[41]

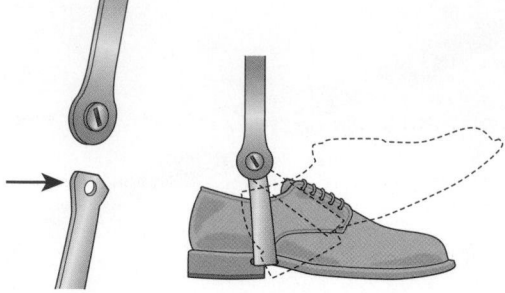

Figure 30.17 Steel stirrup (*left*) with posterior stop at its proximal end (*arrow*). Posterior stop (*right*) incorporated into a stirrup. A posterior stop is designed to allow dorsiflexion and prevent or stop plantarflexion.

An anterior ankle stop limits dorsiflexion, aiding the individual with paralysis of the triceps surae to achieve propulsion during late stance.

Limiting all foot and ankle motion can be done with a plastic *solid ankle-foot orthosis* (Fig. 30.18); its trimlines are anterior to the malleoli. Able-bodied adults fitted with solid ankle AFOs descended stairs more slowly than when walking without orthoses.[42] The solid ankle orthosis may be divided transversely at the ankle, with the two sections hinged, creating the *hinged ankle-foot orthosis* (see Fig. 30.16). It permits slight sagittal motion, facilitating progression to the foot-flat position in early stance. The joint at the hinge may be a plastic overlap or a flexible plastic rod. A versatile option is a pair of metal hinges that can be adjusted to alter the excursion of ankle motion. An alternative to the plastic solid ankle AFO is a metal joint that resists both plantarflexion and dorsiflexion, known as a limited motion joint. One type of limited motion joint is a pair of *bi-channel adjustable ankle locks (BiCAALs)* (Fig. 30.19) that consist of a pair of joints, each of which has an anterior and a posterior

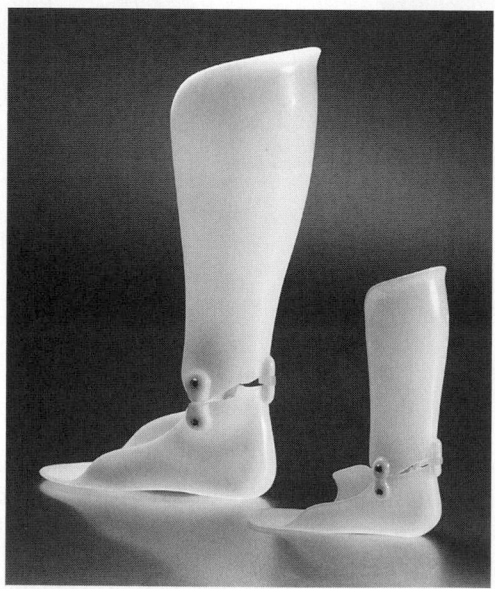

Figure 30.16 Plastic hinged ankle-foot orthoses. *Courtesy of Otto Bock, Minneapolis, MN 55447.*

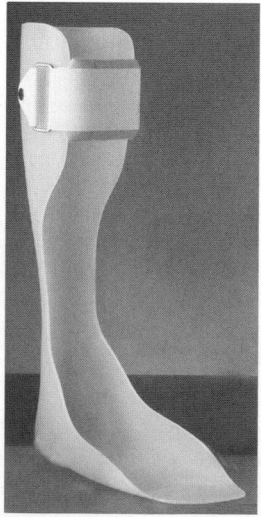

Figure 30.18 Plastic solid AFO. *Courtesy of Otto Bock, Minneapolis, MN 55447.*

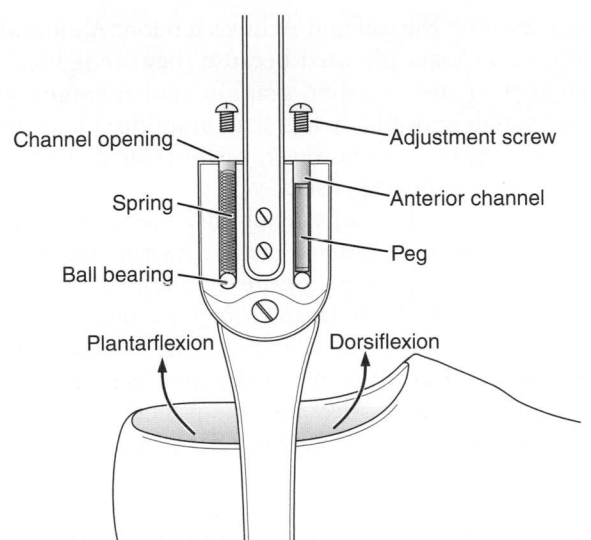

Figure 30.19 Bi-channel adjustable ankle locks (BiCAALs). Note that this ankle joint includes two channels. A spring placed in the posterior channel (shown) provides a dorsiflexion assist. A peg (or pin) placed in the anterior channel (shown) provides a dorsiflexion stop. A peg placed in the posterior channel creates a plantarflexion stop. *From May and Lockard[12, p. 254] with permission.*

spring. The springs may be replaced by metal pegs (or pins), the lengths of which determine the amount of motion provided by the orthosis. To compensate for lack of plantarflexion in early stance, the shoe worn with the solid AFO or the orthosis with a limited motion stop should have a resilient heel. Similarly, to facilitate rollover in late stance, the shoe sole should have a rocker bar. Hinged AFOs reduced frontal plane motion during ramp descent exhibited by subjects who have subtalar osteoarthritis.[43]

Adults with hemiplegia who wore AFOs demonstrated increased cadence, walking speed, step length, and ankle dorsiflexion,[44] and the AFO enabled some patients to walk with increased stride length and cadence.[45-50] Other subjects with stroke improved their scores on the Berg Balance Scale when wearing AFOs[51] and improved weight transfer during stance phase.[52] Balance improvement was also achieved by those wearing an anterior AFO,[53,54] while other subjects demonstrated better function with a posterior leaf spring AFO.[55] Orthoses may either contribute to improved compensatory functions of the nonparetic limb,[56] or may be less important during swing phase of the paretic limb as compared with pelvic obliquity.[57]

A hinged AFO with full-length insert and posterior stop improves early stance stability for subjects with hemiplegia.[58] The alignment of a solid AFO should be individualized to achieve optimal function.[59]

Limited investigation of energy expenditure of adults with hemiplegia wearing AFOs suggests that wearing orthoses results in more efficient gait.[60-62]

Adults with hemiplegia complicated by plantarflexor contracture walk with less plantarflexion and greater knee flexion when wearing either an AFO with posterior stop or a solid AFO.[63]

Functional electric stimulation is an alternative to an AFO for some adults with stroke and other central neuropathies. Various commercially available systems all incorporate a cuff on the proximal leg; the interior of the cuff contains a skin electrode over the peroneal nerve. The electrode is stimulated by a self-contained electrical unit. As compared to walking with an AFO, subjects report more positive results, particularly during swing phase.[64-68]

Children with hemiplegic cerebral palsy improved weight-bearing on the paretic limb while wearing either a posterior leaf spring AFO or a hinged AFO with plantarflexion stop.[69] Other children with similar disability showed slight gait improvement.[70-72] Energy expenditure lessened when children wore a hinged AFO.[73-76] Other investigators found that hinged AFOs were preferable to other designs for level walking[77,78] and stair climbing.[79]

Some young patients with excessive knee flexion achieved better gait when wearing AFOs with anterior band (floor reaction orthosis).[80-82] The desirable effect occurred only if the child did not have knee flexion contracture.

Foot Control

Medial–lateral motion can be controlled with a solid ankle AFO. The rigidity of the orthosis can be increased by using thicker or stiffer plastic, corrugating the plastic, forming the edges with a rolled contour, or embedding carbon fiber reinforcements. A solid ankle AFO (see Fig. 30.18) or a hinged solid ankle AFO (see Fig. 30.16) also controls frontal and transverse plane foot motion of children with cerebral palsy to a limited extent.[83] Less effective is a metal and leather orthosis to which a leather valgus (or varus) correction strap is attached. The valgus correction strap (Fig. 30.20) is sewn to the medial portion of the shoe upper near the sole, and buckles around the lateral upright, exerting a laterally directed force to restrain pronation. The varus correction strap has opposite attachments and force application. Either strap, although adjustable, complicates donning.

Superstructure

The proximal portion of the orthosis, the superstructure, consists of one or two uprights, and a shell, band, or brim. Plastic AFOs usually have a single upright or shell. Both the solid ankle and the hinged solid ankle AFOs have a posterior shell extending from the medial to the lateral midline of the leg, thus providing excellent medial-lateral control and a broad surface to minimize pressure. The posterior leaf spring AFO (see Fig. 30.12) has a single posterior upright that does not contribute to frontal or transverse plane control.

The *spiral AFO* (Fig. 30.21) is a design in which a single upright spirals from the foot plate around the leg,

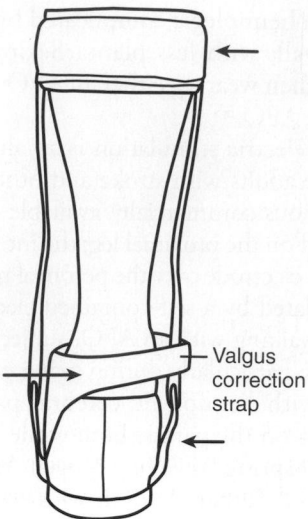

Figure 30.20 Valgus correction strap (also called a "T-strap"). Arrows indicate the three-point pressure system created by the corrective forces (right lower extremity).

Valgus correction strap

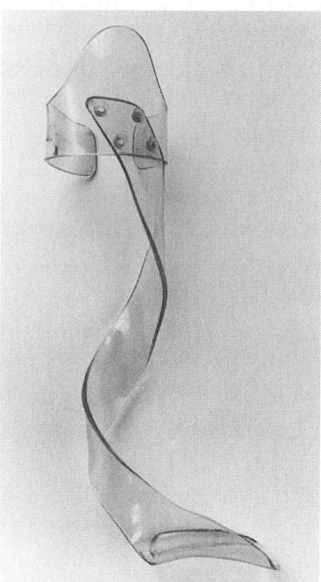

Figure 30.21 Spiral AFO.

terminating in a proximal band. It may be made of polypropylene, nylon acrylic, or carbon fiber. The spiral orthosis controls, but does not eliminate, motion in all planes. Orthoses with plastic shells or uprights are molded over a cast of the patient's leg and are designed to fit snugly for maximal control and minimal conspicuousness. Such AFOs are contraindicated for the individual whose leg volume fluctuates markedly, because the orthoses cannot be adjusted readily.

Metal and leather orthoses usually have medial and lateral uprights to maximize structural stability. Occasionally, a single side upright will suffice when the patient insists on a less conspicuous orthosis and the person is not expected to exert undue force. Some AFOs have an anterior upright, thereby avoiding pressure and

shear stress on the calf and Achilles tendon. Aluminum uprights are typically used because they are lighter in weight than steel. Carbon graphite and titanium uprights weigh appreciably less than aluminum and rival the strength of steel; however, orthoses made of these materials are more expensive.

Most orthoses have a posterior calf band made of rigid plastic or leather-upholstered metal. The band has an anterior buckled or pressure closure strap (Fig. 30.22). The farther the band is from the ankle joint, the more effective the leverage of the orthosis; however, the band must not impinge on the peroneal nerve. An anterior band that is part of a solid ankle AFO imposes posteriorly directed force near the knee, enabling the AFO to resist knee flexion. Such an orthosis is known as a *floor reaction orthosis* (Fig. 30.23). In fact, all LE orthoses are influenced by the floor reaction when the wearer stands or is in the stance phase of gait. If the AFO is to reduce the amount of weight transmitted through the foot, it may have a *patellar-tendon-bearing brim* (Fig. 30.24), resembling a transtibial (below-knee) prosthetic socket. The plastic brim has a slight indentation over the patellar tendon, and is hinged to facilitate donning. The brim must be used with a plastic solid ankle or a steel limited-motion ankle joint.

Knee-Ankle-Foot Orthoses

Individuals with more extensive paralysis or limb deformity may benefit from KAFOs, which consist of a shoe, foundation, ankle control, knee control, and superstructure. KAFOs often include foot control. The shoe, foundation, ankle control, and foot control of the KAFO may be selected from the components already described. Patients with poliomyelitis who wore carbon-composite KAFOs walked better than with leather/metal or plastic/metal KAFOs.[84-86] Donning a plastic and metal KAFO

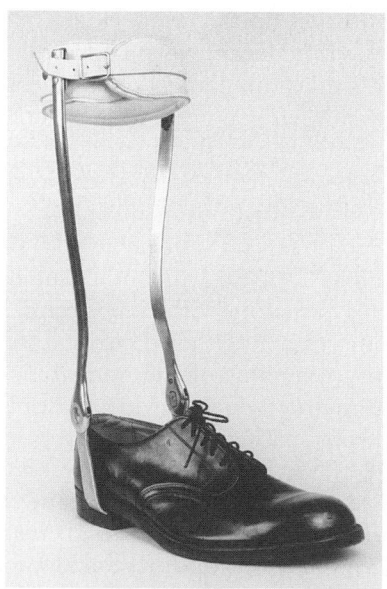

Figure 30.22 Conventional AFO with stirrup attachment, limited motion ankle joints, bilateral uprights, and upholstered metal calf band.

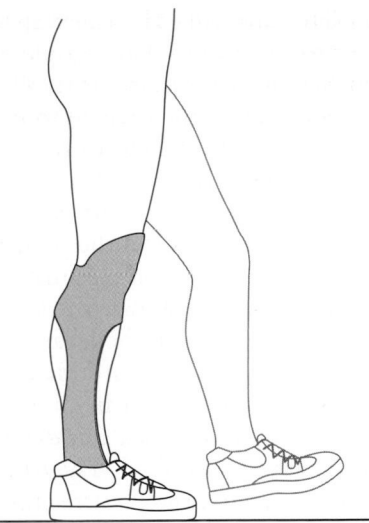

Figure 30.23 Floor reaction AFO with anterior band provides a knee extension moment in stance without preventing flexion during swing. *From May and Lockard,*[12, p. 276] *with permission.*

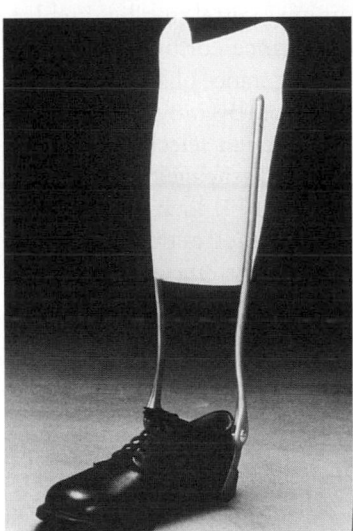 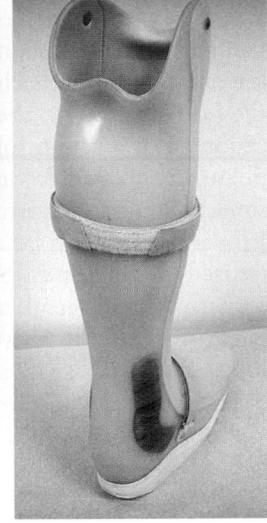

Figure 30.24 (*Left*) AFO with stirrup, hinged ankle joint, steel uprights, and plastic patellar-tendon-bearing brim. (*Right*) Plastic AFO with patellar-tendon-bearing brim to reduce weight-bearing on foot. *Courtesy of Ortho-Bionics Laboratory, Inc., South Ozone Park, NY 11420.*

is appreciably faster than putting on a metal and leather orthosis because the shoe can be separated from the rest of the orthosis.

Knee Control

The simplest knee joint is a hinge. Because most KAFOs include a pair of uprights, the orthosis has a pair of knee hinges that provide medial–lateral and hyperextension restriction while permitting knee flexion.

The *offset joint* (Fig. 30.25 [left and middle]) is a hinge placed posterior to the midline of the leg. When the wearer stands and walks on a level surface, the individual's

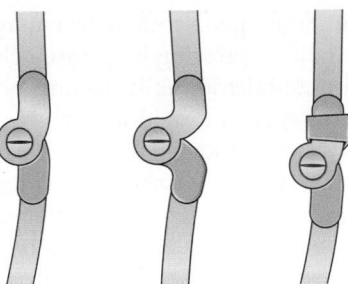

Figure 30.25 Two examples of offset knee joints (*left and middle*) and one of a drop ring lock (*right*).

weight line falls anterior to the offset joint, stabilizing the knee in extension during the early stance phase of gait. The offset joint does not hamper knee flexion during swing or sitting. The joint may, however, flex inadvertently when the wearer walks on ramps.

The most common knee control is the drop ring lock (Fig. 30.25 [right]). When the client stands with the knee fully extended, the ring drops, preventing the uprights from bending. Although both medial and lateral joints should be locked for maximum stability, manipulating a pair of drop ring locks is inconvenient, unless each upright is equipped with a spring-loaded *retention button*. The button permits the wearer to unlock one upright, then attend to the other one without having the first lock drop. The buttons also enable the physical therapist to give the patient a trial period of walking with the knee joints unlocked.

The *pawl lock with bail release* (Fig. 30.26) provides simultaneous locking of both uprights. The pawl is a spring-loaded projection that fits into a notched disk. The patient unlocks the brace by pulling upward on the

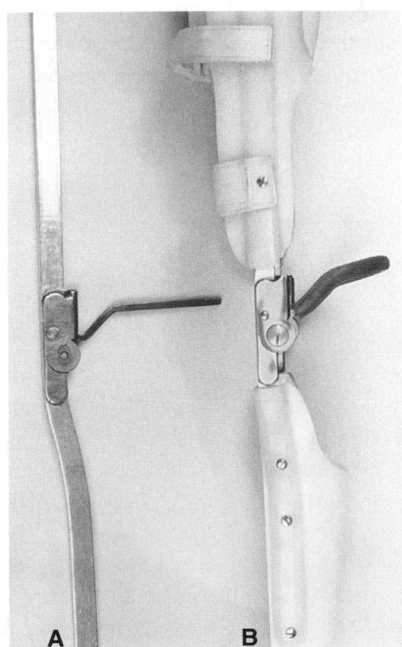

Figure 30.26 Knee joint hinge with pawl lock: basic component (**A**) and pawl lock installed in KAFO with bail shaped to curve posteriorly (**B**).

posterior bail. Some people are agile enough to be able to nudge the bail by pressing it against a chair. The bail is bulky and may release the locks unexpectedly if the wearer is jostled against a rigid object.

The offset joint and knee joints with basic drop ring or pawl locks are contraindicated in the presence of knee flexion contracture. If one cannot achieve full passive knee extension, an adjustable knee joint such as the fan lock, serrated lock (Fig. 30.27), or ratchet lock is required. Such joints usually have a drop ring lock for stability in the partially flexed attitude.

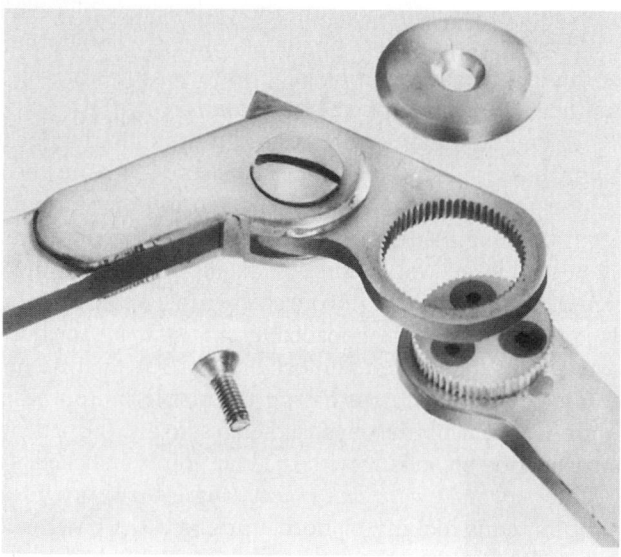

Figure 30.27 Knee joint hinge with serrated knee lock. Note the location of the knee hinge and the serrated disk. *From Fishman, S, et al: Lower extremity orthoses. In American Academy of Orthopaedic Surgeons: Atlas of Orthotics, ed 2. Mosby, St. Louis, 1985, p 213, with permission.*

Sagittal stability is augmented by a kneecap (Fig. 30.28A) or an anterior band or strap that completes the three-point pressure system necessary for stability. The cap or band applies a posteriorly directed force to complement the anteriorly directed forces from the back of the shoe and the thigh band. The leather knee cap has four straps buckled to both uprights above and below the knee. The knee cap requires the patient to buckle two straps when donning the orthosis. When the straps are tight enough to stabilize the knee, the cap is likely to restrict flexion when the wearer sits. A more practical alternative is a rigid anterior band, either a pretibial band or a suprapatellar band, both of which apply posteriorly directed force, but do not interfere with sitting and are easier to don. The bands generally are molded of plastic and thus not readily adjustable. The prepatellar band rests over the bony proximal portion of the leg and requires careful contouring to be comfortable. The suprapatellar band fits over the fleshy anterodistal thigh. Examples of combined metal and plastic KAFOs are presented in Fig. 30.28 (B and C).

Another means of obtaining sagittal stability involves a KAFO with an electronic stance control mechanism that prevents knee flexion during stance phase and permits knee flexion during swing phase. By moving a lever on the side of the joint, the patient can select the mode of action: (1) stance control that is disengaged during swing phase, (2) no stance control, and (3) lock in full extension. Preliminary investigation indicates that adults with LE paralysis walked faster and more efficiently, with increased cadence and step length, and fewer compensatory trunk movements, as compared with use of a locked KAFO.[87-95] KAFOs with computer-controlled knee joints are also available[96] (Fig. 30.29). A KAFO with electronic knee control enables some patients with stroke and other neuropathies to walk[97] (Fig. 30.30).

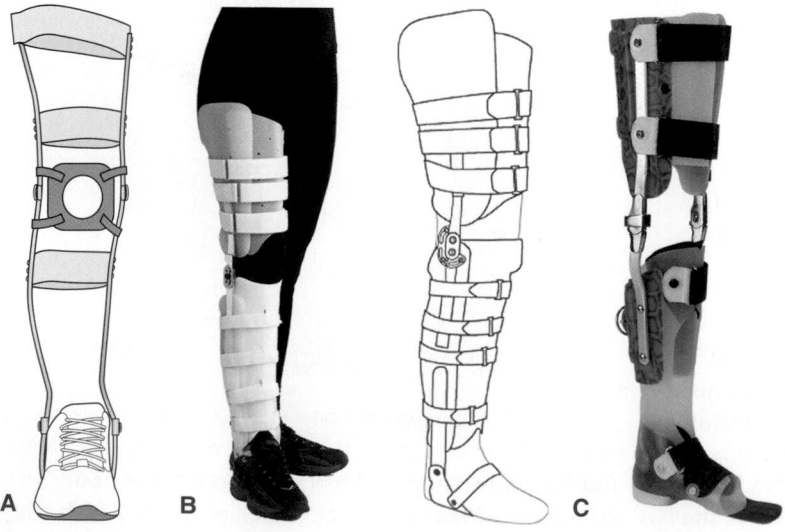

Figure 30.28 **(A)** Conventional KAFO with knee cap. **(B)** Plastic KAFO pictured on a subject together with schematic of same orthosis. *Courtesy of Orthomerica Products, Inc., Orlando, FL 32810.* **(C)** This orthosis allows conversion between an AFO and KAFO based on patient requirements. The knee component that provides more proximal alignment and stability is detachable to create an AFO. *Courtesy of Orthomerica Products, Inc., Orlando, FL 32810.*

A   B   C

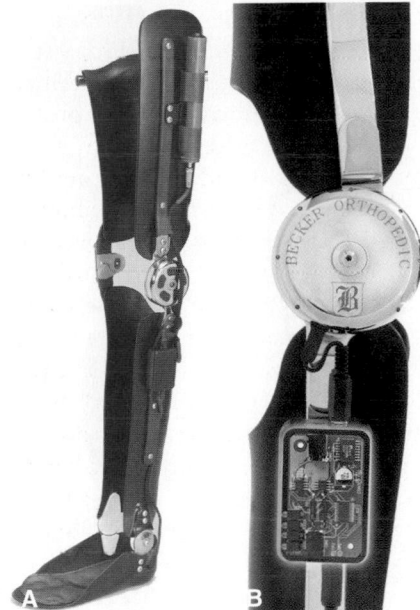

Figure 30.29 (A) Computer-controlled KAFO. **(B)** Close-up of knee joint. The E-Knee™ pictured here is a force-activated, computer-controlled knee unit powered by a lithium battery. The pressure-sensitive footplate signals the microprocessor to lock knee when pressure is applied and to unlock in the absence of pressure. The unit is recharged using a standard electrical outlet. *Becker E-Knee, Becker Orthopedic, Troy, MI 48083.*

Frontal plane control may be achieved with plastic calf shells shaped to apply corrective force for **genu valgum** or **genu varum**. To reduce genu valgum, the medial portion of the shell extends proximally in order to apply laterally directed force at the knee. The semi-rigid shell is more effective than a valgum correction strap, which is a knee cap with a fifth strap designed to be buckled around the lateral upright. The opposite force application is indicated for the patient who has genu varum. The shell does not require time in donning and applies force over a broad area without impinging on the popliteal fossa.

Superstructure

Thigh bands provide structural stability to the orthosis. If the distal portion of the limb cannot tolerate full weight-bearing, then the proximal thigh band may be shaped to form a weight-bearing brim. To eliminate all weight-bearing through the lower extremity, the orthosis must include a weight-bearing brim, a locked knee joint, and a *patten* bottom. The patten is a distal extension that keeps the foot on the braced side off the floor (Fig. 30.31). To maintain a level pelvis, the patient must also wear a lift on the opposite shoe; the height of the lift should equal the height of the patten.

Hip-Knee-Ankle-Foot Orthoses

Addition of a pelvic band and hip joints converts the KAFO to an HKAFO.

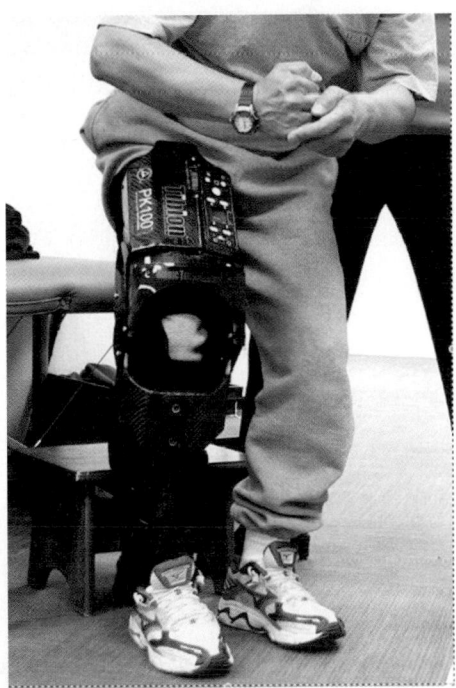

Figure 30.30 Patient moving from sit-to-stand wearing the Tibion Bionic Leg (Tibion Corporation, Sunnyvale, CA 94085). This is a KAFO with electronic knee control designed to support the rehabilitation process. A computer allows the therapist to program the amount of support the orthosis is providing during various tasks.

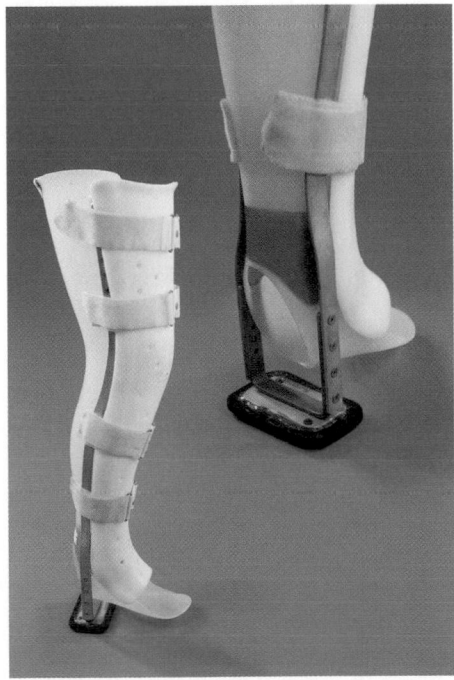

Figure 30.31 The patten bottom is the distal component of an orthosis designed to eliminate weight-bearing from the limb. The patten bottom prevents the foot from contacting the floor.

Hip Joint

The usual hip joint is a metal hinge (Fig. 30.32) that connects the lateral upright of the KAFO to a pelvic band. The joint prevents abduction and adduction, as well as hip rotation. If the patient requires only control of hip rotation, a simpler alternative to the hip joint and pelvic band is a webbing strap. To reduce internal rotation, the strap resembles a Silesian belt on a prosthesis. The center of the strap is riveted to the rear of a waist belt. Each end of the strap is attached to the proximal end of the lateral upright. To reduce external rotation, a strap joins the lateral uprights of the KAFOs, passing anteriorly at the level of the groin. If flexion control is required, a drop ring lock is added to the hip joint. A two-position lock stabilizes the patient in hip extension for standing and walking, and at 90 degrees of hip flexion for sitting.

Pelvic Band

An upholstered metal band (Fig. 30.33) anchors the HKAFO to the trunk. The band is designed to lodge between the greater trochanter and the iliac crest on each side. HKAFOs are not used very often because they are much more awkward to don than KAFOs, and, if the hip joints are locked, they restrict gait to the swing-to or swing-through pattern. The pelvic band may be uncomfortable when the wearer sits.

Trunk-Hip-Knee-Ankle-Foot Orthoses

Patients who require more stability than provided by HKAFOs may be fitted with THKAFOs (Fig. 30.34), which incorporate a lumbosacral orthosis attached to

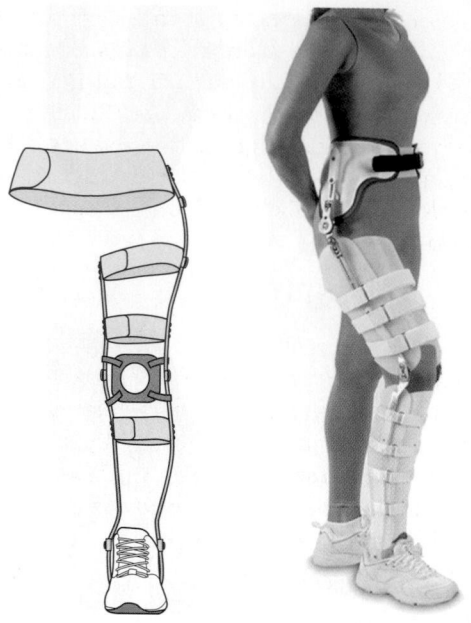

Figure 30.33 (*Left*) Conventional HKAFO with stirrup; uprights; hinged ankle, knee, and hip joints; drop ring locks at the knee and hip; and pelvic band. (*Right*) Plastic and metal HKAFO with hip and knee joints unlocked. *Courtesy of Orthomerica Products, Inc., Orlando, FL 32810.*

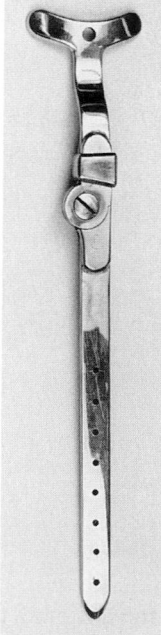

Figure 30.32 Hip joint with drop ring lock.

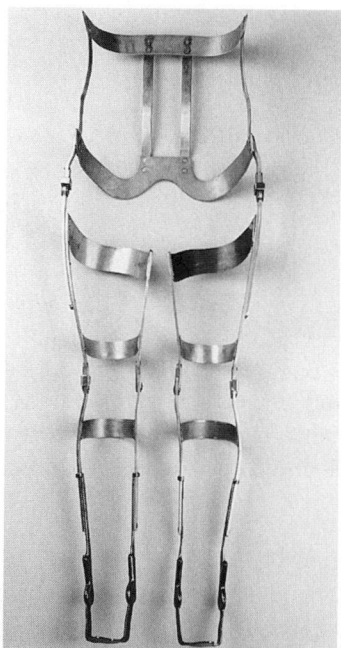

Figure 30.34 Conventional THKAFO without upholstery. This image illustrations the foundational structure of these cumbersome orthoses. To this large heavy metal frame, the additional weight of the upholstery, needed straps and pads, and shoes was added. Patients once leaving the rehabilitation setting often discarded such extensive bracing.

KAFOs. The pelvic band of the trunk orthosis serves as the pelvic band used on HKAFOs. Because the THKAFO is very difficult to don and is heavy and cumbersome, it is seldom worn after the client is discharged from the rehabilitation program. Alternative orthoses providing standing stability, with or without provision for walking, are available for some individuals with paraplegia.

Orthotic Options for Patients with Paraplegia

Orthoses are often prescribed for patients with spina bifida, spinal cord injury, or other disorders that result in paraplegia. The functional goals for such people include standing to maintain skeletal, renal, respiratory, circulatory, and gastrointestinal function and some form of ambulation. Upright posture also affords the individual important psychological benefits.

Mass-Produced Orthoses

Several appliances are marketed for children who have spina bifida or other disorders resulting in paraplegia. The mass-produced orthoses provide the youngster with considerable function and are less expensive and easier to don than many custom-made devices. The stabilizing points on these orthoses are the same, namely a means of securing the shoes to the base, an anterior knee band, posterior dorsolumbar band, and an anterior chest band. The orthoses permit the wearer to stand without crutch support, freeing the hands for play or vocational activities.

Standing Frame and Swivel Walker

The *standing frame* (Fig. 30.35) consists of a broad base, posterior nonarticulated uprights extending from a flat base to a midtorso chest band, and a posterior thoracolumbar band. Anterior leg bands contribute to stability. A similar orthosis is the *swivel walker*, which is made in both child and adult sizes. The major difference is the base. The swivel walker has two distal plates that rock slightly to enable a swiveling gait. Standing frames offering a variety of features are commercially available (Fig. 30.36).

Parapodium

The *parapodium* (Fig. 30.37) is manufactured in child sizes, and permits the wearer to sit. The base is flat. One version of parapodium has a provision for keeping the knees locked while the child unlocks the hips in order to lean forward to pick up objects from the floor. With some of these devices, the child can move from place to place by rotating the upper torso to shift weight, causing the frame to rock and rotate alternately on one edge then the other. For walking longer distances, the youngster uses crutches or a walker in the swing-to or swing-through pattern. The appliances are worn on the outside

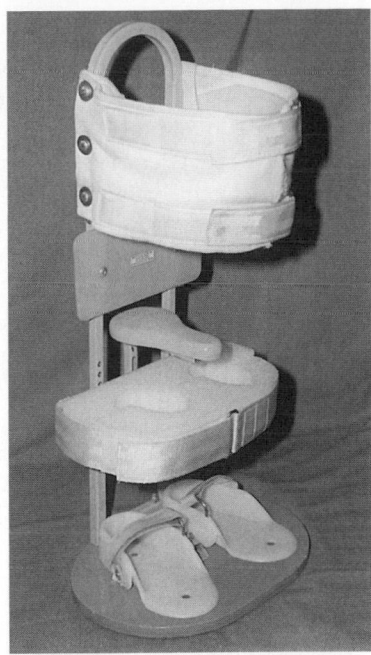

Figure 30.35 Standing frame. *Courtesy of Variety Village, Electro Limb Production Centre, Scarborough (Toronto), Ontario, Canada.*

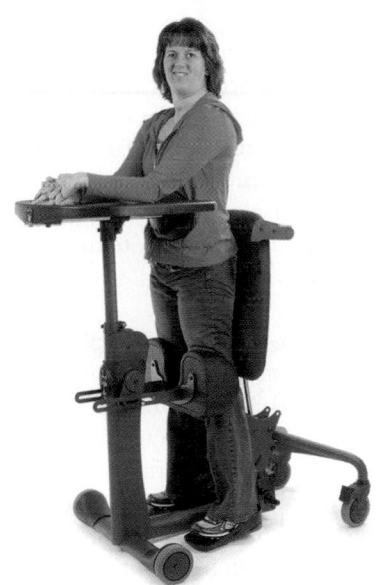

Figure 30.36 Adult standing frame. *Courtesy of Altimate Medical, Inc., Morton, MN 56270.*

of clothing, which school-age children eventually find cosmetically objectionable.

Custom-Made Orthoses

Although the mass-produced devices afford considerable function to their users, many individuals seek more streamlined orthoses. Custom-made AFOs, KAFOs, and THKAFOs provide sufficient rigidity, either by metal

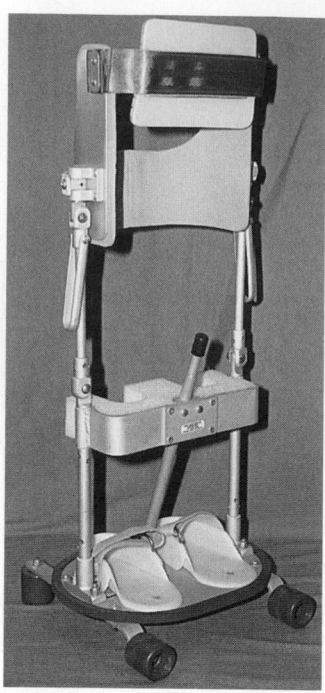

Figure 30.37 Parapodium. *Courtesy of Variety Village, Electro Limb Production Centre, Scarborough (Toronto), Ontario, Canada.*

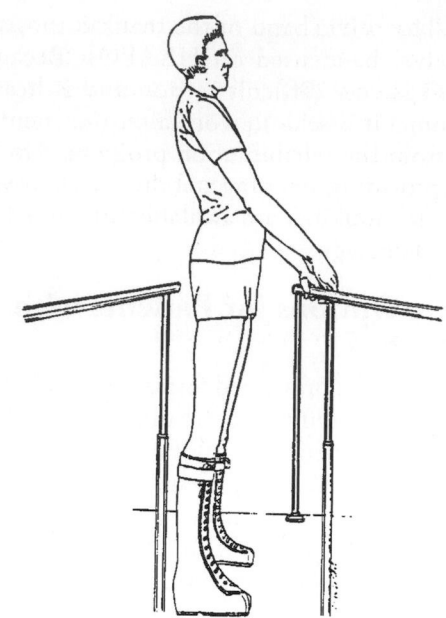

Figure 30.38 Stabilizing boots. *From Kent, HO: Vannini-Rizzoli stabilizing orthosis (boot): Preliminary report on a new ambulatory aid for spinal cord injury. Arch Phys Med Rehabil 73: 302, 1992, p 304, with permission.*

joints or orthotic alignment, to enable selected individuals to stand. Ambulation requires crutches or similar aids, together with well-coordinated use of the trunk and upper limbs. Some patients may not realize the extent of the physical conditioning program required to prepare them for ambulation. Consequently, a trial period is advisable using mass-produced, adjustable, temporary orthoses.

Stabilizing Boots

AFOs designed for adults with paraplegia include a pair of stabilizing boots molded to conform to the patient's legs and feet (Fig. 30.38). The foot plate is angled at approximately 15° plantarflexion to shift the wearer's center of gravity anterior to the ankles. The plastic component is inserted into leather boots which have flat soles. The legs are thus inclined posteriorly to keep the knees extended. The patient maintains standing stability by leaning backward, with the iliofemoral ligaments resisting a backward fall. A pair of crutches or a walker is needed for two- or four-point gait. Ambulation requires shifting the upper torso diagonally forward to allow one leg to swing ahead. The orthoses are easy to don and do not restrict sitting. The candidate must not have any hip or knee flexion contractures, and must be able to extend the hips and lumbar spine by trunk motion.

Craig-Scott KAFOS

A pair of *Craig-Scott KAFOs* (Fig. 30.39) may be prescribed for adults with paraplegia. Each orthosis includes either a shoe reinforced with transverse and longitudinal plates and BiCAAL ankle joints set in slight dorsiflexion

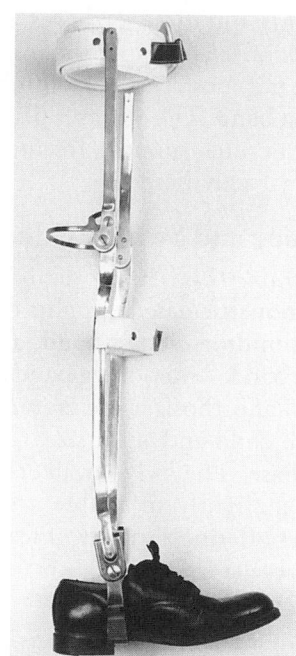

Figure 30.39 Craig-Scott KAFOs.

or a plastic solid ankle section, as well as a pretibial band, a pawl knee lock with bail release, and a single thigh band. The orthoses enable the patient to stand with sufficient backward lean so as to prevent untoward hip or trunk flexion. The gait pattern usually is swing-to or swing-through, with the aid of crutches or a walker. Although the orthoses do not restrict hip motion, the patient with thoracic spinal injury cannot control the hips, and the orthosis has no mechanism to aid single-leg progression. Some individuals perform a two- or four-point gait by shifting the trunk enough to allow the leg to swing forward in a pendular manner.

The *Walkabout orthosis* consists of a pair of KAFOs with a hinge mechanism joining the medial uprights of the two orthoses. The mechanism permits hip flexion and extension, but restricts hip abduction, adduction, and rotation.

Reciprocating Gait Orthoses

Children and adults can be fitted with a *reciprocating gait orthosis (RGO)* (Figs. 30.40 and 30.41). The RGO is a THKAFO in which the orthotic hip joints are connected by one or two metal cables or rods. The knees are stabilized with knee locks, and the feet are encased in solid ankle orthoses. To walk, the wearer follows

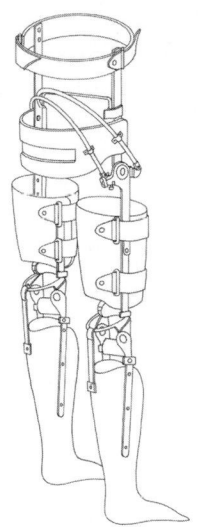

Figure 30.40 Reciprocating gait orthosis. *Courtesy of Fillauer Companies, Inc., Chattanooga, TN 37406.*

a four-stage procedure: (1) shift weight to the right leg, (2) tuck the pelvis by extending the upper thorax, (3) press on the crutches, and (4) allow the left leg to swing through. For the next step, one shifts to the left leg, tucks, presses, and then allows the right leg to swing. The steel cable(s) or rods prevent inadvertent hip flexion on the supporting leg. Reciprocal four- or two-point gait is stable, because one foot is always on the floor, but the pace is slow. For sitting, the wearer releases the cable(s) to enable both hips to flex. RGOs require substantial energy expenditure on the part of the wearer.[98-101]

Alternatives for patients with thoracic level spinal cord injury are the ParaWalker and the ParaStep. The ParaWalker is a THKAFO with massive hip joints. The clinician can limit the flexion and extension excursion of the hip joints. Gait is similar to that with an RGO. Subjects who wore the ParaWalker had fewer pressure sores and no fractures.[102] The ParaStep is a system combining AFOs with skin electrodes over the quadriceps and glutei maximus. Energy expenditure with either device is very high.[103]

■ TRUNK ORTHOSES

Trunk orthoses may be used in association with LE orthoses or may be worn to reduce disabilities caused by low-back pain, neck sprain, scoliosis, or other skeletal or neuromuscular disorders. By supporting the trunk, the orthosis assists in controlling spinal motion; however, forces that the orthosis exerts are modified by the skin, subcutaneous tissue, and musculature that surround the vertebral column, and, in the case of higher orthoses, by the thoracic cage. Patients with spinal cord injury benefit from trunk orthoses in two ways: (1) the orthoses control motion of the lumbar region, with or without thoracic control, and (2) they compress the abdomen to improve respiration. Individuals with cervical lesions may need to wear an orthosis that restrains neck motion until stability is achieved by surgery or other means. A

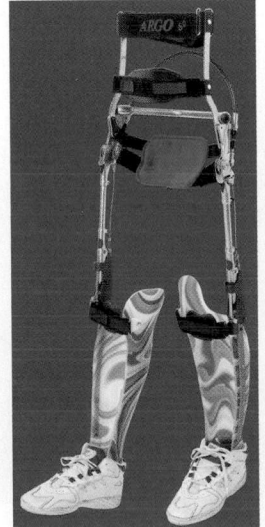
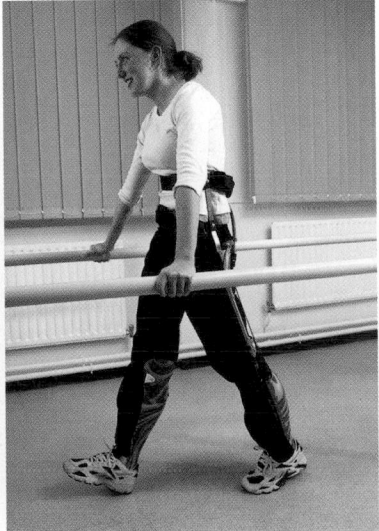

Figure 30.41 ARGO reciprocating gait orthosis. This system includes pneumatic struts at the knee that extend the knees and ensure locks are engaged on standing. *Courtesy of RSL Steeper, Rochester Kent ME2 4DP, United Kingdom.*

special group of trunk orthoses is intended for children and adolescents with scoliosis.

Corsets

If abdominal compression is the sole goal, a corset (Fig. 30.42) will suffice. It is a fabric orthosis that has no horizontal rigid structures, although many have vertical rigid reinforcements. The corset may cover only the lumbar and sacral regions, or may extend superiorly as a thoracolumbosacral corset. The primary effect of a corset is to increase intraabdominal pressure, although the orthosis does reduce frontal movement.[104]

Some individuals with low back disorders find that corsets relieve pain.[105] The efficacy of orthotic intervention to reduce or prevent low back pain remains controversial.[106] The increase in intraabdominal pressure reduces stress on posterior spinal musculature, thus diminishing the load on the lumbar intervertebral disks. Although temporary reduction of abdominal and erector spinae muscular activity is therapeutic, long-term reliance on a corset can promote muscular atrophy[107-109] and contracture, as well as psychological dependence on the appliance.

Rigid Orthoses

Most lumbosacral and thoracolumbosacral orthoses include a corset or a fabric abdominal front to compress the abdomen. Rigid orthoses are distinguished by the presence of horizontal, as well as vertical, rigid plastic or metal components. Motion limitation is accomplished by a series of three-point pressure systems, in which force in one direction is counteracted by two forces in the opposite direction.

Lumbosacral Flexion, Extension, Lateral Control Orthoses

A typical example of a rigid trunk orthosis is the *lumbosacral flexion, extension, lateral control (LS FEL) orthosis* (Fig. 30.43), also known as a *Knight spinal orthosis*. This appliance includes a pelvic band, which should provide firm anchorage over the midsection of the buttocks, and a thoracic band, intended to lie horizontally over the lower thorax without impinging on the scapulae. The bands, which may be foam-lined rigid plastic or leather-upholstered metal, are joined by a pair of posterior uprights on either side of the vertebral spines, and a pair of lateral uprights placed at the right and left lateral midlines of the torso. A corset or abdominal front completes the LS FEL orthosis. The orthosis restrains flexion by a three-point system consisting of posteriorly directed force from the top and bottom of the abdominal front or corset and an anteriorly directed force from the

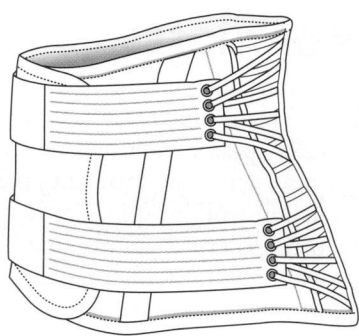

Figure 30.42 Lumbosacral corset (cotton/elastic polymer) with front hook-and-loop closure.

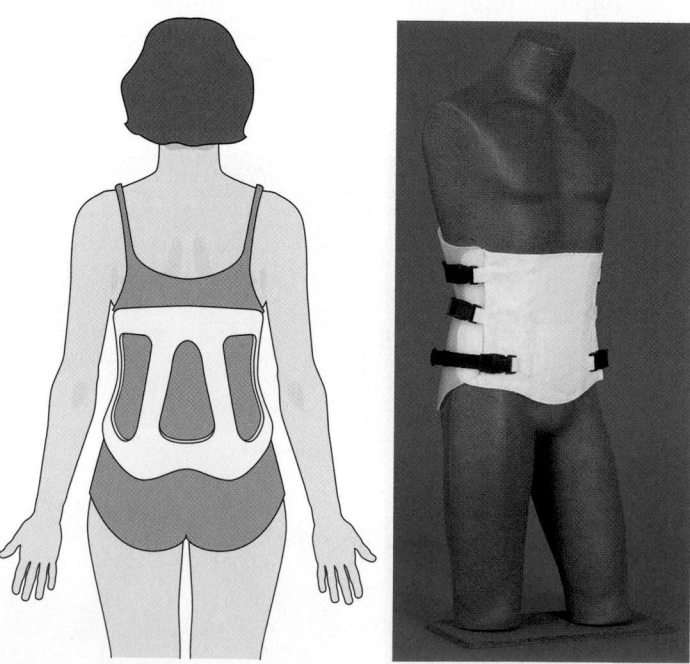

Figure 30.43 (*Left*) Conventional lumbosacral flexion, extension, lateral (LS FEL) control orthosis, and (*right*) custom-fabricated plastic LS FEL control orthosis with corset front. *Courtesy of Orthomerica Products, Inc., Orlando, FL 32810.*

posterior midportion of the orthosis. Extension is controlled by posteriorly directed force from the midsection of the abdominal front or corset and anteriorly directed force from the upper and lower posterior segments. The lateral aspects resist lateral flexion. Other rigid lumbosacral (LS) orthosis are made entirely of polyethylene with removable replaceable liners (Fig. 30.44).

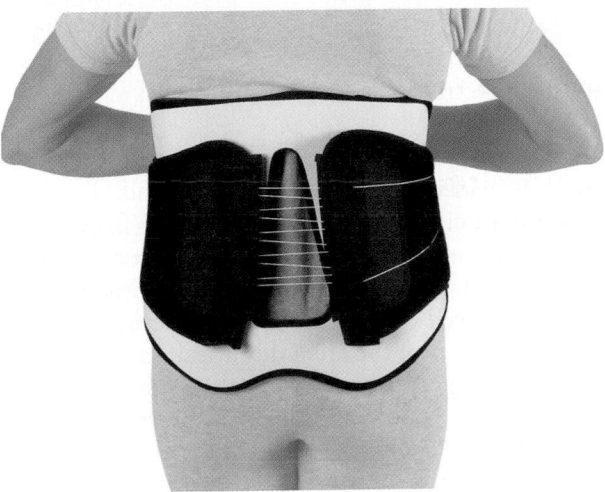

Figure 30.44 Prefabricated, adjustable lumbosacral flexion, extension, lateral control orthosis. *Courtesy of Orthomerica Products, Inc., Orlando, FL 32810.*

Thoracolumbosacral Flexion, Extension Control Orthoses

Also called a *Taylor brace*, the *thoracolumbosacral flexion, extension control (TLS FE) orthosis* consists of a pelvic band, posterior uprights terminating at midscapular level, an abdominal front or corset, and axillary straps attached to an interscapular band. This orthosis reduces flexion by a three-point system consisting of posteriorly directed force from the axillary straps and the bottom of the abdominal front or corset, and anteriorly directed force from the midportion of the posterior uprights. Extension resistance is provided by posteriorly directed force from the midsection of the abdominal front or corset and anteriorly directed force from the pelvic and interscapular bands. Addition of lateral uprights converts the orthosis to a TLS FEL *Knight Taylor* orthosis (Fig. 30.45). Although TLSOs reduce segmental and gross spinal movements, the amount of movement reduction varies greatly from one person to another.[110] Trunk movement restriction is evident when the wearer walks.[111] A plastic *thoracolumbosacral jacket* limits trunk motion in the frontal, sagittal, and transverse planes providing maximum support.

Cervical Orthoses

Cervical orthoses are classified according to design characteristics. Minimal motion control is provided by collars (Fig. 30.46) that encircle the neck with fabric,

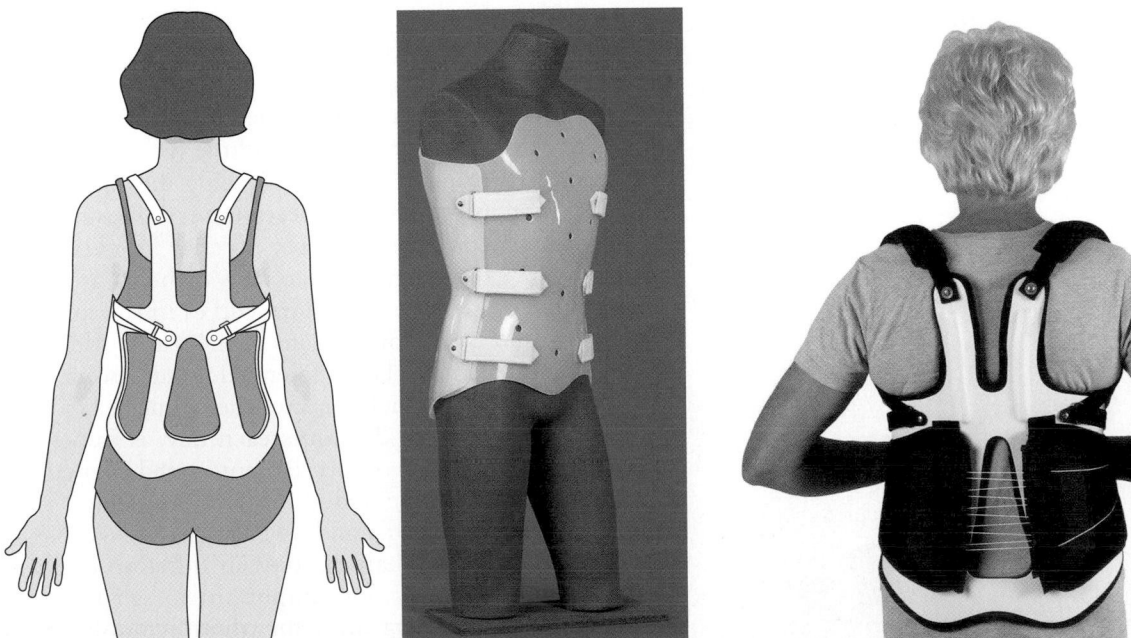

Figure 30.45 *(Left)* Conventional thoracolumbosacral flexion, extension, lateral control orthosis (TLS FEL). *(Middle)* Custom-fabricated plastic TLS FEL. *Courtesy of Orthomerica Products, Inc., Orlando, FL 32810. (Right)* Prefabricated, adjustable TLS FEL.

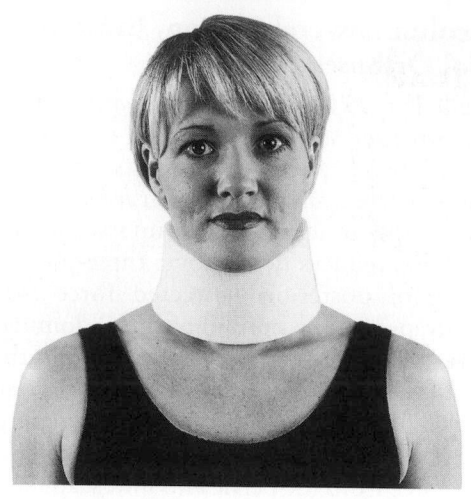

Figure 30.46 Soft foam rubber collar. *Courtesy of Camp Healthcare Corporation, Jackson, MI 49204.*

resilient foam, or rigid plastic. The therapeutic benefit of collars remains controversial.[112,113] The *Philadelphia collar* (Fig. 30.47) has mandibular and occipital extensions and a rigid anterior strut; it is sometimes used for upper cervical injuries.[114-117] For moderate control, a *four-post orthosis* (Fig. 30.48) is used. Usually it has two anterior adjustable posts joining a sternal plate to a mandibular plate and two posterior uprights connecting a thoracic plate to an occipital plate. The sternal plate is strapped to the thoracic plate and the occipital plate is strapped to the mandibular plate. If the cervical orthosis does not fit properly, motion restriction is compromised.[118]

Maximum orthotic control of the neck may be achieved either with a *Minerva* or a *halo orthosis* (Fig. 30.49). The Minerva orthosis is a noninvasive appliance that has a rigid plastic posterior section extending from the head to the midtrunk; the superior

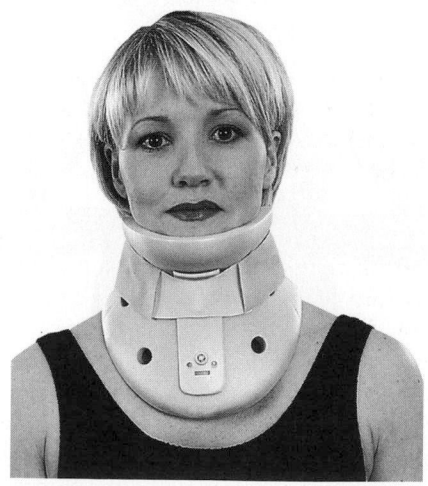

Figure 30.47 Philadelphia collar. *Courtesy of Camp Healthcare Corporation, Jackson, MI 49204.*

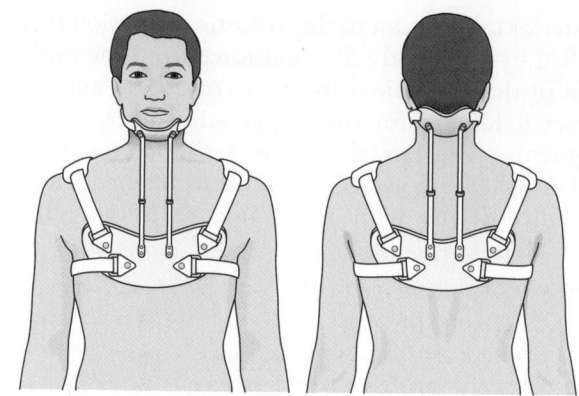

Figure 30.48 Four-post cervical orthosis.

portion is held in place by a forehead band. The halo orthosis has a circular band of metal that is fixed to the skull by four tiny screws. Uprights connect the halo to a thoracic vest. Recent investigations confirm that the halo vest allowed cervical fractures to heal,[119,120] particularly fractures of the second cervical vertebra.[121-123] By limiting upper trunk motion, this orthosis reduces stride length,[124] and results in temporary atrophy of neck muscles.[125]

Scoliosis Orthoses

Children and adolescents with kyphoses or thoracic, thoracolumbar, or lumbar scolioses may be fitted with a TLSO that applies distraction, derotation, and bending forces to realign the vertebral column and thoracic cage.[126-128] Brace effectiveness depends on the flexibility of the patient's torso[129] and snugness of contact with the wearer's trunk.[130] Although substantial improvement is evident when the orthosis is worn, long-term follow-up indicates that the major achievement is that the orthosis prevents the curve from increasing beyond its original contour. Bracing diminishes the likelihood of surgical correction of scoliosis.[131,132] Orthotic management is most effective for curves less than 35° Cobb angle.[133] Scoliosis orthoses are most effective on patients who have curves in the midthoracic or more inferior portions of the trunk. Although part-time wearing is better tolerated by adolescents, the classic protocol, which requires the youngster to wear the orthosis snugly 23 hours each day, is associated with more favorable results. Patients with larger curves achieve some curve reduction from bracing.[134,135] Braces do not impair standing balance.[136] Psychological factors, rather than the type or duration of brace wear, appear to be more important in self-reported quality of life among those for whom scoliosis braces are prescribed.[137,138] Adults with scoliosis do not benefit from orthoses.[139]

The Milwaukee orthosis (Fig. 30.50), the oldest of contemporary scoliosis orthoses, is still prescribed. It consists of a frame composed of a pelvic girdle, two

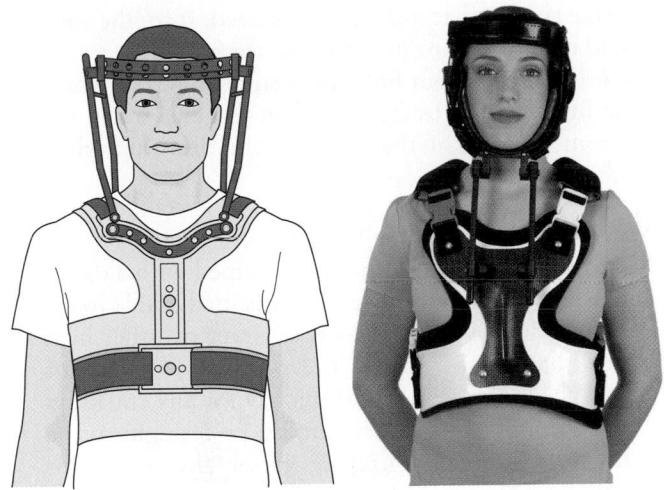

Figure 30.49 (*Left*) The halo cervical orthosis provides maximum stabilization of the head and cervical spine. The graphite ring (halo) allows placement of titanium pins into outer table of skull. (*Right*) Noninvasive halo devices are also available. They are effectively used as transitional bracing after removal of a halo cervical orthosis. Pictured here is the Lerman Non-invasive Halo. *Courtesy of Trulife USA, Jackson, MI 49203.*

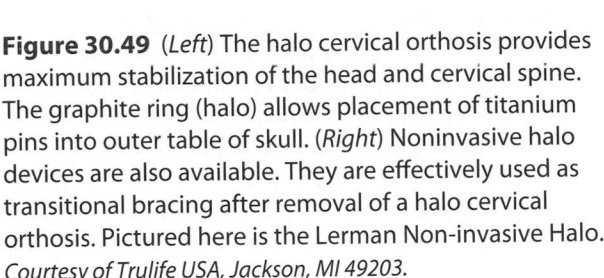

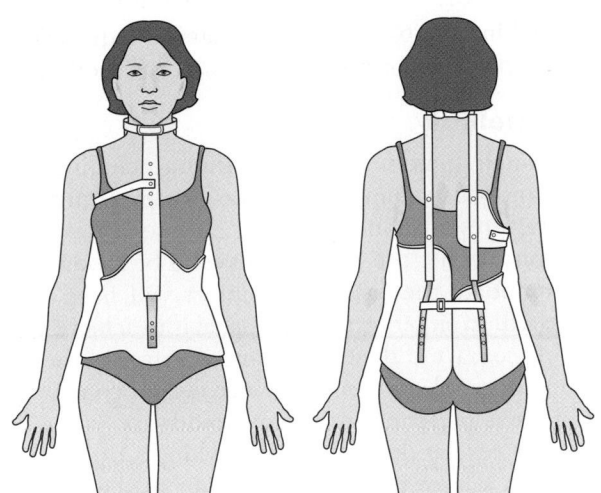

Figure 30.50 Milwaukee orthosis (plastic and metal).

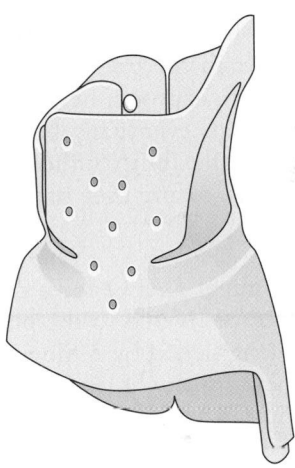

Figure 30.51 Boston thoracolumbosacral orthosis.

posterior uprights, an anterior upright, and a superior ring that can be hidden by clothing. Various pads are strapped to the frame to apply corrective forces. The Boston orthosis (Fig. 30.51) usually does not extend as high as the Milwaukee orthosis; its foundation is a mass-produced plastic module that the orthotist alters to fit the individual patient. Effectiveness is enhanced by snugly strapping the interior pads to the torso.[140] Long-term results are favorable,[141] with patients preferring it to surgery.[142] The Wilmington orthosis is another option; it is a custom-made thoracolumbosacral jacket intended to guide the trunk to straighter alignment.

Night bracing is an alternate approach to scoliosis management. When the patient is in bed the effects of gravity are minimized allowing substantial corrective forces to be applied.[143] Nevertheless there is a higher risk of progression.[144] Both the Charleston bending brace and the Providence brace provide overcorrection of the spinal curve on the recumbent patient.[145,146]

Scoliosis orthoses are also used for adolescents with hyperkyphosis.[147]

■ ORTHOTIC MAINTENANCE

To obtain the best service from orthoses, the patient should observe basic routine inspection and care procedures. Written instructions help reinforce the recommendations of the orthotist and therapist.

Shoes

Whether or not the shoe is attached directly to the orthosis, it is important that footwear be kept in good condition, with replacement of the sole and heel as soon as moderate wear is evident. The replacements should include whatever wedges, bars, or elevations were originally prescribed. The patient who tends to strike on the toe may need metal toe plates to preserve the sole. Shoes that are outgrown or distorted will not afford the wearer optimal function from the orthosis. If a stirrup is attached to the shoe, the patient should inspect the rivets to make certain that none has separated; if so, the shoe should be returned to the orthotist for repair.

Clean hose without holes or mends should be worn. In addition, long hosiery or cotton leggings shield the leg from pressure at the edges of the brace uprights, bands, and shells.

Shells, Bands, and Straps

Plastic bands and shells should be wiped with a damp cloth to remove any surface soil. It is inadvisable to try to hasten drying by using a hair dryer or other heat source that might soften the plastic. The patient should check the plastic periodically for any cracking; if any is noted, the orthosis should be brought to the orthotist for immediate repair. Hook-and-pile straps eventually become infiltrated with lint, which interferes with the hook-and-loop closing action; the straps should be inspected to determine if they should be replaced. Leather bands require periodic cleaning and can be washed with mild saddle soap. If the original leather deteriorates to the point that portions of the underlying metal are exposed, new leatherwork is required. Leather straps eventually become brittle and may break. A loss of flexibility indicates that it is time to replace the straps, before they break.

Uprights

In a plastic and metal KAFO for a child, the metal upright is screwed or riveted to the plastic shell. The orthosis can be lengthened by removing the fasteners and inserting them in new holes drilled farther up on the calf shell and farther down on the thigh shell. In a metal and leather AFO or KAFO for a child, the uprights are overlapped and secured with screws. The orthosis is lengthened by removing all screws, setting the uprights at the appropriate distance, and reinserting the screws.

Joints and Locks

Metal components should be kept away from sand, liquids, and similar substances. If the joints do not move smoothly or become noisy or if the locks do not engage properly, cleaning and lubrication may remedy the problem. Otherwise, professional attention is required.

■ PHYSICAL THERAPY MANAGEMENT

Physical therapists participate in management of the wearer of an orthosis (1) before orthotic prescription, (2) at orthotic prescription, (3) on delivery of the orthosis, and (4) during training to facilitate proper use and care of the orthosis. In the ideal situation, the therapist is a member of an orthotic clinic team, working directly with the physician and orthotist to develop the orthotic prescription and examine the patient and orthosis before and after training. The physical therapist is also responsible for training the patient. Whether or not the hospital or rehabilitation center has a clinic team, the physical therapist is expected to accomplish the following.

Preorthotic Examination

The purposes of the preorthotic examination are to:

- Contribute to the orthotic prescription (analyze potential of orthotic components to remediate impairment, activity limitations, or disability).
- Examine the prescribed orthosis through analysis of (1) effects and benefits in terms of improved function, (2) movement while patient wears the device, (3) practicality and ease of use, (4) alignment and fit, and (5) safety during use of device.
- Facilitate orthotic acceptance.
- Train the patient to don, use, and maintain the orthosis.

Matching the patient's biomechanical requirements to the appropriate orthosis requires careful examination.

Joint Mobility

A thorough goniometric examination, including both active and passive range of motion, is a prerequisite to orthotic prescription. If the patient has a fixed foot deformity, either the shoe will have to be modified to accommodate the foot, or an insert will have to be fabricated. In either instance, the goal is to achieve comfortable contact of the entire plantar surface of the foot on the inner sole of the shoe. Knee flexion contracture necessitates prescription of accommodative joints, because the regular drop ring and pawl locks can be used only with a knee that can be brought to the fully extended position. Hip flexion contracture precludes the prescription of orthoses that depend on alignment for stability, such as the offset knee joint, stabilizing boots, or Craig-Scott KAFOs.

Limb Length

The therapist should ascertain whether leg lengths are equal. If the patient can stand, one can check the pelvis to determine if it is level. For the recumbent individual, one can measure each LE from the anterior superior iliac spine to the medial malleolus. A difference of more than 1/2 in (1 cm) should be compensated by a shoe elevation. For the patient with weakness in one limb, a 1/2-in (1 cm) lift on the contralateral shoe will aid clearance of the involved LE during swing phase.

Muscle Function

The manual muscle test (MMT) should be augmented by an examination of functional activities to determine what substitutions the patient makes to accomplish standing and walking. Although the muscle test may reveal marked weakness, if the patient can manage without an orthosis, it is unlikely that it will be accepted. For example, the person with dorsiflexor weakness who can ambulate by exaggerating hip flexion during swing phase may not agree to an AFO with a posterior stop. An important consideration in examination of muscle function is that traditional MMTs may be inappropriate in the presence of marked spasticity. In such instances, functional tests of motor performance are essential.

Sensation

The clinician should record the extent of any sensory loss. Intimately fitted plastic orthoses are satisfactory for individuals with sensory loss if the edges of the orthosis are smooth and the orthosis does not pinch the patient's flesh. Proprioceptive loss may indicate the need for orthotic stabilization, such as a solid ankle AFO to control a Charcot neuropathic ankle. Patients should be taught to inspect the skin (including presence of volume changes) regularly and instructed to bring any changes to the attention of the physical therapist.

Upper Limbs

Although the patient is being considered as a candidate for LE or trunk orthoses, the therapist must determine the mobility and muscle power of the upper limbs. Significant weakness, stiffness, or deformity will interfere with donning the orthosis. Substitution of hook-and-loop closures for leather buckles may suffice. If the individual cannot ambulate without canes or crutches, the therapist should determine whether standard aids will be satisfactory or whether modification of the hand pieces is required. If the upper limbs are very weak, the patient will not be able to use the LE orthoses for walking. Alternate standing arrangements may be preferable, such as the use of a standing frame, standing table, or standing wheelchair to provide weight-bearing stress.

Psychological Status

Realistic orthotic prescription requires ascertaining that the patient is willing to wear the orthosis. The patient with a recent spinal cord injury may still deny the permanence of paralysis and thus oppose wearing orthoses that are visible reminders of disability. The adolescent with spina bifida may prefer to sit unbraced in a wheelchair rather than struggle with donning orthoses and walking slowly, in a manner very different from the individual's peers. The patient with spinal cord injury must be prepared to work vigorously to increase upper limb and trunk strength and aerobic capacity. The person who has sustained a cerebral vascular accident resulting in severe perceptual deficits may not be able to walk, even with orthotic assistance, because the environment now seems unfamiliar. An orthosis for prevention of contractures may be prescribed, rather than one that is designed to aid gait.

The therapist should determine the extent to which the patient is likely to comply with instructions pertaining to orthotic use and care. For example, if it is doubtful that the individual will wear appropriate shoes with an insert orthosis, then the prescription should specify stirrup attachment to suitable shoes.

Orthotic Prescription

Lower extremity orthoses benefit individuals with a wide variety of musculoskeletal and neurological disorders. The particular diagnosis is less important in formulating the prescription than consideration of the patient's impairments and activity limitations. Prognosis also influences prescription. The person who is likely to recover partial or full function should have an orthosis that can be adjusted to accommodate the changing status. An individual with recent hemiplegia, for example, may exhibit marked spasticity, indicating a need for limiting motion at the ankle. As the person regains voluntary control and spasticity decreases, the orthotic ankle joint can be adjusted to permit more movement.

Lifestyle has a bearing on orthotic selection. A very active patient requires an orthosis made of exceptionally sturdy materials. Split stirrups, for example, may not be appropriate because they can spring loose from the receptacle on the shoe if excessive medial–lateral or rotational stress is applied. The patient's concern with appearance is another practical consideration; it may dictate use of a shoe insert so that reasonably fashionable shoes may be worn. Similarly, plastic shells are less bulky than metal uprights and calf bands, and do not present a shiny metal appearance. Although most people want the orthosis to be as inconspicuous as possible, some children and adults opt for bright colors, which can be achieved with various plastics.

Ankle-Foot Orthoses

The primary candidates for AFOs are those with peripheral neuropathy, especially peroneal lesions, and hemiplegia. Those with foot drag can be fitted with an AFO with a posterior stop; this design, however, tends to cause the knee to flex excessively in early stance when controlled plantarflexion is normally achieved. In the absence of plantarflexion, the patient may flex the knee to effect a foot-flat position. The alternative is a resilient shoe heel, or an AFO with a plastic posterior leaf spring or a metal dorsiflexion spring assist, both of which permit controlled plantarflexion early in stance to reduce knee stress.

Orthotic management of a patient with hemiplegia depends on the extent of spasticity and paralysis. If the motor loss is confined to poor dorsiflexion, the posterior leaf spring AFO suffices. An even simpler and less expensive option is a 1/2-in (1-cm) lift on the heel and sole of the contralateral shoe to provide clearance for the paretic limb during swing phase. Those with medial–lateral and sagittal plane instability require an AFO with limited-motion ankle joints or a plastic spiral AFO. With pain or severe instability, a solid ankle AFO is required. In the presence of severe spasticity, a spring assist for joint motion is contraindicated because the spring action may serve to increase spasticity.

Knee-Ankle-Foot and Other Lower Extremity Orthoses

A KAFO may be used to compensate for paralysis of the entire LE. The physical therapist should allow the patient the use a temporary orthosis in order to proceed more confidently with prescription of an expensive, custom-made orthosis. Several versions of temporary orthoses are manufactured and prove exceedingly useful in demonstrating whether the patient is likely to benefit from orthotic knee control.

Stabilizing AFOs, Craig-Scott KAFOs, HKAFOs, and the reciprocating gait orthosis are some options for patients with paraplegia. For the child, the orthotic program should start with a simple standing frame and progress to the parapodium before involving the child in the greater expense and donning difficulty of form-fitting bracing. Older children and adults may begin with a swivel walker or lightweight modular frames.

Trunk Orthoses

A corset may be adequate to increase intraabdominal pressure and thereby may reduce the discomfort of low back pain. Where greater motion restriction is indicated, such as for the individual with trunk paralysis, the LS FEL, TLS FE, or TLS FEL orthosis provides substantial support. Plastic lumbosacral or thoracolumbosacral jackets offer maximum support. Cervical orthoses, whether collars or post devices, restrain motion and remind the wearer not to move the head in an abrupt manner. Collars also retain body heat, which may prove therapeutic. For maximum neck control, a halo orthosis is required.

Many orthoses are available for management of patients with scoliosis. These include the Milwaukee orthosis, which covers the greatest body area, as well as the Boston and Wilmington orthoses. The Providence and Charleston braces are designed for nighttime use only.

Orthotic Examination

Examination is an essential element of orthotic management. The physical therapist should be certain that the orthosis fits and functions properly before attempting to train the patient to use it. Analysis may be conducted under the aegis of a formal orthotic clinic team. If so, when the orthosis is delivered, the team should determine the adequacy of the orthosis as pass, provisional pass, or fail. Pass indicates that the orthosis is altogether satisfactory and the patient is ready for training. Provisional pass means that minor faults exist, generally having to do with the cosmetic finishing of the appliance; the patient can wear the orthosis in the training program without harmful effect. Failure signifies that the orthosis has a major defect that would interfere with training; for example, shoes that are too tight for

the patient. The problem must be resolved before training can begin. If the orthosis is not prescribed by a clinic team, the physical therapist should use the evaluation procedure to ensure that the orthosis meets the patient's needs. Final evaluation is performed at the conclusion of training to judge the fit and function of the orthosis and the patient's skill in using it.

Lower Extremity Orthotic Examination

Orthotic examination includes both static and dynamic elements. The *static* component examines the orthosis on the patient while standing and sitting, as well as examination of the device off the individual. The *dynamic* component of the examination addresses analysis of the wearer's gait. An LE orthotic examination form is provided in Appendix 30.A, and a trunk orthotic examination form is provided in Appendix 30.B.

Static Examination

The orthosis is inspected as the wearer stands and sits. The patient's skin and the construction of the orthosis are checked with the orthosis off the patient. The orthosis should be compared with the prescription. Departures from the original specifications must be approved by the individual who approved the prescription.

The patient should stand in parallel bars, or other secure environment, and should attempt to bear equal weight on both feet. The shoe should fit satisfactorily, particularly in length, width, and snugness of the counter. Whether or not wedges or lifts have been added to the shoe, the sole and heel should rest flat on the floor, except for the distal portion, which should curve upward slightly to aid in late stance. The orthotic ankle joint should be at the distal tip of the medial malleolus to be congruent with the anatomical ankle and avoid vertical motion of the orthosis on the leg during gait.

The calf band should terminate below the fibular head to avoid impingement on the peroneal nerve. If a patellar-tendon-bearing brim is used, it should have a concave relief to limit pressure on the fibular head. This component does not eliminate distal weight-bearing; however, one should judge to see that the shoe heel is somewhat unloaded. This can be estimated by placing a ribbon in the shoe before the patient dons the shoe. One end of the ribbon hangs out the back of the shoe. When the patient stands with the shoe and orthosis on, the therapist should be able to pull the ribbon out of the shoe. The calf shell, band, or patellar-tendon-bearing brim should not intrude on the popliteal fossa; if so, the patient would have difficulty flexing the knee when sitting. Donning ease is affected by the type of closure of both the shoe and band.

The mechanical knee joints should be congruent with the anatomical knee; for the adult, the usual placement is approximately 3/4 in (2 cm) above the medial tibial plateau. The knee lock should function properly, because use of a lock is often the major reason for wearing a KAFO. The medial upright should terminate approximately 1.5 in (4 cm) below the perineum. The calf and distal thigh shells or bands should be equidistant so that when the orthosis is flexed, as in sitting, the plastic or metal parts will contact one another, rather than pinch the back of the wearer's leg.

If the KAFO has a quadrilateral brim to reduce weight-bearing through the skeleton, the brim should have adequate relief for the sensitive adductor longus tendon and should provide a sufficient seat for the ischial tuberosity.

The hip joint is set slightly above and anterior to the greater trochanter to compensate for the usual angulation of the femoral neck; setting the joint anterior to the trochanter takes into account the medial rotation of the femur. The pelvic band should conform to the contours of the wearer's torso, without edge pressure.

When the brace is off, the therapist should inspect the patient's skin to detect any irritations attributable to the orthosis. One should move the orthotic joints slowly to check range of motion. Binding refers to tilting of the distal portion of the joint in relation to the proximal member so as to interfere with movement. If the medial and lateral stops do not contact their respective stops at the same time, the stop that contacts first will erode more rapidly and may contribute to twisting of the orthosis.

Dynamic Examination

The gait pattern exhibited by the person who wears an orthosis reflects both the contribution of the wearer's general health status and orthotic motion control and assistance. Table 30.1 relates orthotic and anatomical causes of the most commonly observed gait deviations.

During early stance, the patient may exhibit foot slap, striking with toes first, or flat-foot contact, indicating inability to restrain plantarflexion or failure of the orthosis to support the foot and ankle. Excessive medial or

Table 30.1	Orthotic Gait Analysis	
Deviation	**Orthotic Causes**	**Anatomical Causes**
Early Stance		
1. Foot slap: forefoot slaps the ground	Inadequate dorsiflexion assist Inadequate plantarflexion stop	Weak dorsiflexors
2. Toes first: tiptoe posture may or may not be maintained throughout stance	Inadequate heel lift Inadequate dorsiflexion assist Inadequate plantarflexion stop Inadequate relief of heel pain	Short LE Pes equinus Extensor spasticity Heel pain
3. Flat foot contact: entire foot contacts ground initially	Inadequate traction from sole Requires walking aid (e.g., cane) Inadequate dorsiflexion stop	Poor balance Pes calcaneus
4. Excessive medial (or lateral) foot contact: medial (or lateral) border contacts floor	Transverse plane malalignment	Weak invertors (evertors) Pes valgus (varus) Genu valgum (varum)
5. Excessive knee flexion: knee collapses when foot contacts ground	Inadequate knee lock Inadequate dorsiflexion stop Plantarflexion restriction (stop) Inadequate contralateral shoe lift	Weak quadriceps Short contralateral LE Knee pain Knee and/or hip flexion contracture Flexor synergy Pes calcaneus
6. Hyperextended knee: knee hyperextends as weight is transferred to LE	Genu recurvatum inadequately controlled by plantarflexion stop Excessively concave (deep) calf band Pes equinus uncompensated by contralateral shoe lift Inadequate knee lock	Weak quadriceps Lax knee ligaments Extensor synergy Pes equinus Short contralateral LE Contralateral knee and/or hip flexion contracture
7. Anterior trunk bending: patient leans forward as weight is transferred to LE	Inadequate knee lock	Weak quadriceps Hip flexion contracture Knee flexion contracture

Continued

Table 30.1   Orthotic Gait Analysis—cont'd

Deviation	Orthotic Causes	Anatomical Causes
8. Posterior trunk bending: patient leans backward as weight is transferred to LE	Inadequate hip lock Knee lock	Weak gluteus maximus Knee ankylosis
9. Lateral trunk bending: patient leans toward stance leg as weight is transferred to LE	Excessive height of medial upright of KAFO Excessive abduction of hip joint of HKAFO Requires walking aid (e.g., cane) Insufficient shoe lift	Weak gluteus medius Abduction contracture Dislocated hip Hip pain Poor balance Short leg
10. Wide walking base: heel centers more than 4 in (10 cm) apart	Excessive height of medial upright of KAFO Excessive abduction of hip joint of HKAFO Insufficient lift on contralateral shoe Knee lock Requires walking aid (e.g., cane)	Abduction contracture Poor balance Short contralateral LE
11. Internal (or external) rotation: LE internally (or externally) rotated	Uprights incorrectly aligned in transverse plane Requires orthotic control (e.g., rotation control straps, pelvic band)	Internal (or external) hip rotators spastic External (or internal) hip rotators weak Anteversion (retroversion) Weak quadriceps: external rotation
Late Stance		
1. Inadequate transition: delayed or absent transfer of weight over the forefoot	Plantarflexion stop Inadequate dorsiflexion stop	Weak plantarflexors Achilles tendon sprain or rupture Pes calcaneus Forefoot pain
Swing		
1. Toe drag: toes maintain contact with ground	Inadequate dorsiflexion assist Inadequate plantarflexion stop	Weak dorsiflexors Plantarflexor spasticity Pes equinus Weak hip flexors
2. Circumduction: LE swings outward in a semicircular arc	Knee lock Inadequate dorsiflexion assist Inadequate plantarflexion stop	Weak hip flexors Extensor synergy Knee and/or ankle ankylosis Weak dorsiflexors Pes equinus
3. Hip hiking: LE elevated at pelvis to enable the limb to swing forward	Knee lock Inadequate dorsiflexion assist Inadequate plantarflexion stop	Short contralateral LE Contralateral knee and/or hip flexion contracture Weak hip flexors Extensor synergy Knee and/or ankle ankylosis Weak dorsiflexors Pes equinus

Table 30.1 Orthotic Gait Analysis—cont'd

Deviation	Orthotic Causes	Anatomical Causes
4. Vaulting: exaggerated plantarflexion of contralateral LE to enable the limb to swing forward	Knee lock Inadequate dorsiflexion assist Inadequate plantarflexion stop	Weak hip flexors Extensor spasticity Pes equinus Short contralateral LE Contralateral knee and/or hip flexion contracture Knee and/or ankle ankylosis Weak dorsiflexors

LE = lower extremity.

lateral contact may indicate that the orthosis does not track the way the patient's limb does. Knee hyperextension or excessive flexion indicates that the orthosis is not applying adequate control. A posterior stop on the AFO should prevent the lax knee from hyperextending. If the patient wears a KAFO and has knee hyperextension, the stops in the knee joint are set improperly or have eroded, or the calf and thigh shells or bands are too deep. Anterior and posterior trunk bending are seen at early stance when the patient attempts to control a weak knee or hip. If the quadriceps are weak, the patient will bend forward. The person who fears that the knee may collapse may benefit from an AFO with a solid ankle and an anterior band, or a KAFO with a knee lock. If the gluteus maximus is weak, the individual is apt to lean backward. Lordosis indicates hip flexion contracture or a KAFO that does not fit properly. Lateral trunk bending in early stance phase may result from hip abductor weakness or hip instability; however, uncompensated shortness of the limb will also give rise to this problem, as will a medial upright on a KAFO that is too high, or an abducted pelvic joint on an HKAFO. A wide walking base may be the patient's compensation for a medial upright or shell that impinges into the perineum.

The client may have difficulty during late stance either delaying weight transfer or being unable to transfer weight over the affected foot. The problem can be mitigated with an anterior stop and a rocker bar. One should be certain that the trimlines of the solid ankle AFO or the stops on the stirrup function properly.

During swing phase, the patient must be able to clear the floor with the braced leg. Hip hiking (pelvic elevation) occurs when the hip flexors are weak, as well as when the limb is functionally longer than the contralateral limb. Increased length may be produced by a faulty posterior stop that no longer limits plantarflexion, or by a locked knee joint. The problem should be anticipated and, for the unilateral KAFO wearer, can be prevented by adding a 1/2 in (1 cm) lift to the contralateral shoe. Internal or external hip rotation may be caused by

imbalance between medial and lateral musculature; the orthotic causes relate to malalignment of the brace. Similarly, excessive medial or lateral foot contact may indicate that the orthosis does not track the way the patient's limb does. A walking base that is abnormally wide can be caused by a limb that is longer than that on the opposite side. Vaulting refers to exaggerated plantarflexion on the contralateral limb during swing phase of the affected side. Vaulting occurs because the braced leg is functionally too long, possibly because the posterior ankle stop has eroded or a knee lock is used. The less agile patient may obtain foot clearance by hip hiking, that is, elevating the pelvis on the swing side.

Trunk Orthosis Static Examination

Lumbosacral and thoracolumbosacral orthoses usually include thoracic and pelvic bands, which should fit flat against the trunk without edge pressure. Uprights should not press against bony prominences, particularly when the patient sits. The abdominal front should extend from just below the xiphoid process to just above the pubic symphysis. The cervical orthosis should hold the head in the best tolerated position. Rigid components, such as a mandibular plate, occipital plate, sternal plate, or thoracic plate, should be shaped to apply maximum area to the body segment.

Facilitating Orthotic Acceptance

Clinic team management is valuable in fostering acceptance of the orthosis by the patient. The team also enables clinicians to join efforts to help the client achieve the maximum benefit from orthotic rehabilitation. Bringing the new wearer of an orthosis in contact with other users in the physical therapy department can help the new patient recognize that orthotic use is not a strange occurrence. Peer support groups for patients and their families are helpful for sharing concerns and anxieties and reaching workable solutions to common problems. Support groups usually are organized for people having particular disabilities, such as paraplegia or hemiplegia; many clients will have orthoses as part of their rehabilitation. The physical therapist can guide some meetings of the group. The therapist works most closely with the patient, usually on a daily basis, and thus is able to identify those individuals whose response to disability is sufficiently aberrant as to require psychological attention. Appendix 30.C provides website-based orthotic resources for clinicians, families, and patients.

Orthotic Instruction and Training

Orthoses are designed to provide the individual with a maximum of function with a minimum of discomfort and effort. No single training program suits every orthosis wearer because of the wide range of disorders for which orthotic management is indicated. To the extent possible, however, the physical therapist should instruct the patient in the correct manner of donning the orthosis, developing standing balance, walking safely, and performing other ambulatory activities.

Optimal performance depends on the favorable interaction of many factors. Foremost is the extent of skeletal and neuromuscular involvement. The mobility, strength, and coordination of all body segments, especially in the LEs and trunk, are important, as are the individual's muscle tone, cardiovascular and pulmonary health, body weight, psychological status, and chronological age. The quality of the orthosis also influences the client's achievements.

Most orthosis wearers have chronic conditions, such as rheumatoid arthritis, or permanent sequelae from trauma, such as paraplegia following spinal cord injury. Orthotic management enhances function without necessarily influencing the underlying pathology. Training people with chronic disorders prepares the patient for lifelong activity with an orthosis. Persons with reversible disorders, such as peroneal nerve injury, often benefit from temporary use of an orthosis. Such individuals should learn proper use of the orthosis to prevent secondary disorders and should receive reexamination so that the orthosis may be altered as the condition changes. Patients with progressive disorders, such as muscular dystrophy and multiple sclerosis, require vigilant reexamination so that the extent of physical deterioration may be reflected in orthotic changes, as well as continual training to cope with altered functional abilities. For all situations, an individually devised exercise and activity program should enable the patient to manage efficiently for maximum independence.

Donning Orthoses

Regardless of type of LE orthosis, the patient should wear clean, properly fitting hose. The AFO with shoe insert is most easily donned by applying the orthosis to the foot and leg, before placing the braced limb in the shoe. If the AFO has a split stirrup, the shoe should be donned first; then the orthosis should be fitted into the box caliper on the shoe. If the AFO has a solid stirrup, the patient will have to insert the foot into the shoe, then fasten the calf band.

The same general procedures are useful with KAFOs. The patient may find donning easier if the brace is applied while lying on a bed or a mat table. If the KAFO is donned while the patient sits, the therapist should check the tightness of the orthotic knee cap, if this component is part of the orthosis. A kneecap that is comfortable for sitting will probably be too loose for effective knee control when the wearer stands. Donning HKAFOs and THKAFOs is much more arduous. The beginner should lie on a mat table alongside the orthosis. By rolling to one side, the patient should be able to pull the brace under the legs so as to permit lying in it. Then the patient sits with knees extended to don shoes and fasten straps.

Lumbosacral and thoracolumbosacral corsets and rigid orthoses should be donned while the patient is supine to achieve maximum compression of the abdomen. The orthosis should be fastened from the bottom upward.

Standing Balance

The problem of standing safely is most difficult for the individual who wears a pair of KAFOs or more extensive bracing. In ordinary standing, all weight passes through the feet, whereas when standing and walking with orthoses and crutches, the patient must learn to distribute weight partly on the hands and partly on the feet. With orthoses, the line of gravity falls within a tripod bounded by the hands and feet. The tripod is a compromise between leaning too far forward on the hands, to increase stability at the price of fatiguing the arms, and leaning too far backward, which reduces arm strain but makes balance precarious. As balance improves, the patient uses the hands only for balance, rather than for substantial weight-bearing.

The person who wears bilateral KAFOs will need crutches or other aids for independent gait. A prerequisite for crutch ambulation is the ability to shift weight. Shifting weight to the heels takes pressure off the hands so they can be moved. Using parallel bars, the beginner shifts all weight to the feet and raises and lowers one hand, then the other hand. The goal is to be able to lift both hands simultaneously, as may be done with crutches when performing a drag-to or similar gait. Once the patient is able to shift weight from the feet to the hands and back to the feet confidently, the same exercise should be done with crutches. Advanced skills, such as moving the hands and eventually the crutches, behind the body, should be practiced. Those who will walk in reciprocal fashion, alternating footsteps, need to practice diagonal weight shifting.

Gait Training

The various crutch gaits differ in the sequence of crutch and footsteps. Patterns vary in speed, safety, and amount of energy required. The patient should learn as many gaits as possible, so as to modify walking in crowds, over long distances, and in situations in which speed is desired. In addition to walking forward, the client needs to be able to walk sideward, turn corners, and maneuver on different surfaces, such as rugs, gravel, grass, and through doors. A repertoire of gaits permits the client to adjust to environmental requirements. Gait selection depends on the individual's functional ability, including the following areas:

- *Step ability*: Can the patient take steps with either one or both LEs?
- *Weight-bearing and balance ability*: Can the patient bear weight and remain balanced on one or both LEs?
- *Upper-limb power*: Can the patient push the body off the floor by pressing down on the hands?

Reciprocal Gaits

The four- and two-point gaits require that one move the LEs alternately by hip flexion or pelvic elevation. The patient shifts weight as each LE is moved. The four-point sequence is (1) right hand, (2) left foot, (3) left hand, and (4) right foot. The two-point sequence requires greater balance and coordination, but is a faster mode of walking: (1) right hand and left leg; (2) left hand and right leg. The patterns also are useful when one is confronted with crowds or slippery surfaces. These gaits are suited to persons who lack the coordination and balance needed for simultaneous gaits.

Simultaneous Gaits

If both LEs are moved simultaneously, the patient places considerable stress on the upper limbs. The series includes the drag-to, swing-to, and swing-through patterns. Although the swing-through gait can be performed rapidly, simultaneous gaits generally are slow and very fatiguing, because the upper limbs are poorly adapted for ambulatory function; a sizable amount of nonfunctioning bodily structure must be controlled by a smaller muscular apparatus. The weight of the orthoses and, in the case of a patient with spinal cord lesion, absence of peripheral sensation aggravate the problem of using a simultaneous gait pattern.

The drag-to gait is the most elementary of the group, but it is very slow. The sequence is (1) advance both hands, then (2) push on the crutches enough to drag the feet forward. The feet do not pass ahead of the hands. The swing-to pattern is more rapid, because the patient swings rather than drags the LEs. Swinging is accomplished by extending the elbows and depressing the shoulder girdle to elevate the trunk and LEs. The swing-through gait is the most advanced pattern, requiring much balance, strength, and coordination of the upper limbs, because the patient swings the LEs beyond the hands, or crutch tips. The sequence is (1) advance both hands, (2) swing both LEs to a point in front of the hands to reverse the basic tripod position, and (3) advance both hands to the starting position. The swing-through gait requires extensive preliminary training, including push-ups to strengthen the arms. The gait is rapid but requires more floor space than the other patterns, to permit alternate swinging of LEs and crutches.

The ultimate test of walking proficiency is the ability to conduct a conversation while ambulating, an activity pattern that indicates some degree of automatic functioning. Practice in the clinical setting should be extended to walking on varied terrain, indoors and outdoors.

Related Activities

The patient should learn as many activities as physical condition permits. Daily life often involves negotiating stairs, curbs, and ramps, as well as transferring from the chair to the upright position, and into an automobile. Instruction in driving a suitably equipped car is an important part of rehabilitation. Not all individuals who wear orthoses achieve the full range of ambulatory activities, yet they benefit from partial independence in accomplishing tasks, at least from the psychological and physiological values attendant to ambulation.

Final Examination and Follow-up Care

Before discharge, the orthosis wearer and the brace should be examined to make certain that fit, function, appearance, and use are acceptable. The patient should return to the hospital or rehabilitation center at regular intervals so that the clinic team can monitor the individual's function and the orthosis, and can spot incipient abrasions or other signs of misfit or disrepair. The follow-up visit also enables the physical therapist to reinforce skills taught in the intensive program and address any new problems the patient may present.

Functional Capacities

The patient's ambulatory ability and capacity for other physical activities reflect both orthotic and anatomical factors. Energy measurement is a valuable guide to functional capacity. Energy cost is calculated from the amount of oxygen consumed as the subject performs. Consumption may be determined either per unit of distance traversed or per unit of time. Everyone tends to select a walking speed that requires the least energy per unit of distance. If the energy cost is too high, the patient will realize that ambulation is not practical. Sometimes, high energy cost is tolerable for short distances, as in household ambulation. Community ambulation, however, demands sustained effort for longer distances, plus the ability to maneuver over curbs and other irregularities in the walking surface and cross the street within the time allowed by the traffic light. Many energy studies have been conducted with the two largest groups of individuals who wear orthoses, namely those with paraplegia and those with hemiplegia.[148]

Paraplegia

The level of spinal cord damage is a critical determinant of functional capacity. Investigators generally conclude that functional ambulation is not feasible for those with lesions above the T11 segment of the spinal cord. Children wearing the reciprocating gait orthosis while performing the swing-through crutch gait have approximately the same energy expenditure as when propelling a wheelchair. Adults with thoracic injuries consume nine times the energy expended by nondisabled individuals per meter, and those with lumbar lesions require triple the normal amount of oxygen when walking at self-selected speeds. Those with high-level paraplegia use three times their own basal oxygen rate ambulating with Craig-Scott KAFOs; they choose a very slow walking pace. Subjects with lesions between T11 and L2 wearing bilateral KAFOs select walking speeds less than half that of nondisabled persons, with oxygen uptake six times normal. Wheelchair propulsion by the same group increases oxygen uptake less than 10% more than normal, at a considerably faster speed. The very high energy cost may be accounted for by the fact that the LE paralysis requires that the individual move by upper limb and thoracic action, usually in a swing-to or swing-through gait. This pattern is extremely strenuous, taxing nondisabled adults by at least 75% more energy than normal walking.

Of less significance in determining functional capacity is the type of orthosis. Restraining both plantarflexion and dorsiflexion, as provided by Craig-Scott KAFOs, reduces energy demand very slightly. Ankle restraint, however, makes no appreciable difference in the energy required to negotiate stairs and ramps. Performance is somewhat more efficient with molded plastic KAFOs, which weigh slightly less than traditional metal and leather braces. Most subjects fitted with a reciprocating gait orthosis preferred it primarily because of its appearance and perception of stability.

One should not lose sight of the principal purpose of ambulation, namely to get from one place to another, rather than to execute an exhausting physical stunt. The nearly universal abandonment of orthoses by individuals with thoracic spinal cord injury after discharge from the rehabilitation center attests to the fact that most decide that accomplishing vocational and recreational tasks is more important than struggling with brace donning and energy-costly ambulation.

Hemiplegia

Although the increased energy demand occasioned by hemiplegic ambulation is not nearly as dramatic as that for paraplegic gait, the cost should be considered in planning reasonable goals. Energy cost rises in proportion to the amount of spasticity. The increase ranges from no appreciable difference for persons with hemiplegia to a 100% increase for relatively inexperienced walkers. On average, comfortable gait is approximately half the speed of that for nondisabled individuals.

The type of orthosis does not appear to make much difference in functional capacity, although patients with hemiplegia perform more efficiently with some form of AFO than without any bracing. Investigation of the factors that influence energy expenditure, especially physical status, helps the clinician plan the most appropriate rehabilitation program and forecast long-term performance.

SUMMARY

This chapter has focused on lower extremity and trunk orthoses. The most frequently prescribed orthoses and orthotic components have been presented. In addition, the responsibilities of the physical therapist in orthotic management have been emphasized.

Ideally, an orthosis is prescribed by an orthotic clinic team composed of a physician, physical therapist, and orthotist. The prescription should be based on a thorough examination, with particular attention to the specific factors discussed in this chapter. Input from the patient and all team members during the decision making process is critical. This approach will ensure an optimum match between the patient's biomechanical and psychological requirements and an appropriate orthosis capable of performing its intended function. Once the orthosis has been prescribed, it should be evaluated to ensure satisfactory fit, function, and construction, and the patient should have the benefit of a suitable training program for donning the orthosis and using it effectively.

Questions for Review

1. Discuss the purpose of a correctly fitted shoe in orthotic management.

2. Describe the purpose (function) of the following external shoe modifications: heel wedge, sole wedge, metatarsal bar, and rocker bar.

3. What are the advantages of a plastic orthotic shoe insert as compared with the solid stirrup?

4. For the patient with dorsiflexor weakness or paralysis, explain how a posterior leaf spring AFO imparts its function during early stance and swing phases of gait.

5. What is the function of the proximal anterior band on a floor reaction AFO?

6. How do tone-inhibiting AFOs improve the patient's function?

7. Indicate the clinical use of an AFO with a patellar-tendon-bearing brim.

8. What strategies can be used to increase the rigidity of plastic orthoses?

9. What is the function of an offset knee joint on a knee-ankle-foot orthosis (KAFO)?

10. Describe the three-point system in a lumbosacral flexion, extension, control orthosis.

11. What data should be gathered before formulating an orthotic prescription?

12. Compare and contrast the orthotic options for a patient with hemiplegia.

13. What are the purposes of the preorthotic examination?

14. What features of the AFO are considered during the static evaluation?

15. What are the anatomical and orthotic causes of vaulting?

CASE STUDY

PATIENT HISTORY AND CURRENT PROBLEM

The patient is a 65-year-old woman who had poliomyelitis at age 3. She sustained complete paralysis of the right LE and left foot and ankle. During childhood she wore bilateral knee-ankle-foot (KAFO) orthoses and ambulated with a four-point gait with the aid of a pair of axillary crutches. When she was 18, she had a left ankle and subtalar fusion. She was fitted with a right KAFO, which included a stirrup foundation, posterior ankle stop, drop ring knee lock, knee pad, and leather-covered calf and thigh bands. For the next 40 years, she wore the same brace, and had the leather and shoe replaced whenever they became worn. She used a cane in the left hand when she walked outdoors. She returned to the rehabilitation department today complaining of pain in the right knee and fatigue. She also said that her brace tears her stockings at the knee. She is curious about new orthotic developments.

PAST MEDICAL HISTORY

Except for poliomyelitis, she enjoyed good health although her endurance was always less than that of her friends.

SOCIAL HISTORY

The patient is a reference librarian who lives with her husband. She enjoys visiting her grandchildren, attending the theater, and participating in political campaigns.

PHYSICAL THERAPY EXAMINATION FINDINGS

- *Cognitive status*: Alert, oriented, memory intact
- *Endurance*: Limited, primarily restricted by discomfort in her right knee. She can walk for three city blocks before having to rest.
- *Vision*: Intact with corrective lens
- *Blood pressure*: 136/74
- *Respiratory rate*: Within functional limits (WFL)

Range of Motion Examination

Motion	Right	Left
Hip flexion	WFL	WFL
Hip extension	WFL	WFL
Hip abduction	WFL	WFL
Hip adduction	WFL	WFL
Hip external rotation	WFL	WFL
Hip internal rotation	WFL	WFL
Knee	25°–0°–120°*	WFL
Ankle dorsiflexion	0°–5°	0° (no motion)
Plantarflexion	0°–40°	0° (no motion)
Inversion	0°–10°	0° (no motion)
Eversion	0°–5°	0° (no motion)

*Right knee exhibits 25° of hyperextension.
WFL = within functional limits.

Sensation
- All modalities WFL bilaterally in both limbs
- Sensation in both upper limbs WFL

Strength: Manual Muscle Test (MMT) Grades

Motion	Right	Left
Hip flexion	2–/5	4/5
Hip extension	0	4/5
Hip abduction	0	4/5
Hip adduction	0	4/5
Hip internal rotation	0	4/5
Hip external rotation	0	3+/5
Knee flexion	0	4–/5
Extension	0	3+/5
Ankle dorsiflexion	0	N/A
Plantarflexion	0	N/A
Inversion	0	N/A
Eversion	0	N/A
Upper limb strength	WFL	WFL

N/A = not applicable owing to fusion; WFL = within functional limits.

Orthotic Examination
Uprights malaligned permitting 20° knee hyperextension. Posterior ankle stop worn, permitting 10° plantarflexion. Leather on calf and thigh bands is worn.

Balance
Standing
- *Static*: Good; able to maintain static position for unlimited period.
- *Dynamic*: Good on level surface. Not tested on ramp; patient reports that balance on ramps is precarious.

Sitting
- WFL

Gait
Patient walks slowly with a right KAFO with considerable trunk bending to the right. Bending reduces when she uses a cane in the left hand. She reports that she has great difficulty ascending and descending ramps. Additional findings include the following:
- Overall decrease in speed of movement
- Broad walking base
- Circumducts right leg
- Right knee hyperextends within the orthosis
- Right ankle plantarflexion limited by orthosis
- Left foot and ankle immobile

Functional Status
- Independent in transfers: sit-to-stand; floor-to-stand transfer
- Independent in all basic activities of daily living (BADL)
- Independent in approximately 85% of instrumental activities of daily living (IADL) (limitations imposed by pain, fatigue, and low ambulatory tolerance)

PATIENT-DESIRED OUTCOME AND GOALS
- Walk without knee pain.
- Improve endurance.
- Improve appearance.
- Reduce frequency of torn stockings in the vicinity of the knee.

GUIDING QUESTIONS
1. Formulate a clinical problem list.
2. Formulate a patient asset list.
3. Establish anticipated goals and expected outcomes of physical therapy.
4. Formulate a physical therapy plan of care.

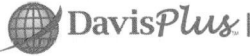 **DavisPlus** | For additional resources, including answers to the questions for review and case study guiding questions, please visit **http://davisplus.fadavis.com**

References

1. American Academy of Orthopaedic Surgeons: Orthopaedic Appliances Atlas, Vol 1. JW Edwards, Ann Arbor, MI, 1952.
2. Fatone, S: Challenges in lower extremity orthotic research. Prosthet Orthot Int 34:235, 2010.
3. Menant, JC, et al: Optimizing footwear for older people at risk of falls. J Rehabil Res Dev 45:1167, 2008.
4. Hijmans, JM, et al: A systematic review of the effects of shoes and other ankle or foot appliances on balance in older people and people with peripheral nervous system disorders. Gait Posture 25:316, 2007.
5. Johanson, MA, et al: Effect of heel lifts on plantarflexor and dorsiflexors activity during gait. Foot Ankle Int 31:1014, 2010.
6. Hong, WH, et al: Influence of heel height and shoe insert on comfort perception and biomechanical performance of young female adults during walking. Foot Ankle Int 26:1042, 2005.
7. Kerrigan, DC, et al: Moderate-heeled shoe and knee joint torques relevant to the development and progression of knee osteoarthritis. Arch Phys Med Rehabil 86:871, 2005.
8. Mohamed, O, et al: The effects of Plastazote and Aliplast/Plastazote orthoses on plantar pressures in elderly persons with diabetic neuropathy. J Prosthet Orthot 16:55, 2004.
9. Wrobel, JS, et al: A proof-of-concept study for measuring gait speed, steadiness, and dynamic balance under various footwear conditions outside of the gait laboratory. J Am Podiatr Med Assoc 100:242, 2010.
10. Seligman, DA, and Dawson, DR: Customized heel pads and soft orthotics to treat heel pain and plantar fasciitis. Arch Phys Med Rehabil 84:1564, 2003.
11. Leung, AKL, et al: Biomechanical gait evaluation of the immediate effect of orthotic treatment for flexible flat foot. Prosthet Orthot Int 22:25, 1998.
12. May, BJ, and Lockard, MA: Prosthetics and Orthotics in Clinical Practice. FA Davis, Philadelphia, 2011.
13. Rao, S, et al: Orthoses alter in vivo segmental foot kinematics during walking in patients with midfoot arthritis. Arch Phys Med Rehabil 91:608, 2010.
14. Welsh, BJ, et al: A case-series study to explore the efficacy of foot orthoses in treating first metatarsophalangeal joint pain. J Foot Ankle Res 27:3, 2010.
15. Murley, GS, Landorf, KB, and Menz, HB: Do foot orthoses change lower limb muscle activity in flat-arched feet toward a pattern observed in normal-arched feet? Clin Biomech (Bristol, Avon) 25:728, 2010.
16. Bird, AR, Bendrups, AP, and Payne, CB: The effect of foot wedging on electromyographic activity in the erector spinae and gluteus medius muscles during walking. Gait Posture 18:81, 2003.
17. Gelis, A, et al: Is there an evidence-based efficacy for the use of foot orthotics in knee and hip osteoarthritis? Elaboration of French clinical practice guidelines. Joint Bone Spine 75:714, 2008.
18. Gross, MT, and Foxworth, JL: The role of foot orthoses as an intervention for patellofemoral pain. J Orthop Sports Phys Ther 33:661, 2003.
19. Saxena, A, and Haddad, J: The effect of foot orthoses on patellofemoral pain syndrome. J Am Podiatr Med Assoc 93:264, 2003.
20. Butler, RJ, et al: Effect of laterally wedged foot orthoses on rearfoot and hip mechanics in patients with medial knee osteoarthritis. Prosthet Orthot Int 33:107, 2009.
21. Van Raaij, TM, et al: Medial knee osteoarthritis treated by insoles or braces: A randomized trial. Clin Orthop Relat Res 468:1926, 2010.

22. Nawoczenski, DA, and Ludewig, PM: The effect of forefoot and arch posting orthotic designs on first metatarsophalangeal joint kinematics during gait. J Orthop Sports Phys Ther 34:317, 2004.

23. Houssain, M, et al: Foot orthoses for patellofemoral pain in adults. Cochrane Database Syst Rev CD008402, 2011.

24. Roos, E, Engstrom, M, and Soderberg, B: Foot orthoses for the treatment of plantar fasciitis. Foot Ankle Int 27:606, 2006.

25. Landorf, KB, Keenan, AM, and Herbert, RD: Effectiveness of foot orthoses to treat plantar fasciitis. Arch Intern Med 166:1305, 2006.

26. Baldassin, V, Gomes, CR, and Beraldo, PS: Effectiveness of prefabricated and customized foot orthoses made from low-cost foam for noncomplicated plantar fasciitis: A randomized controlled trial. Arch Phys Med Rehabil 90:701, 2009.

27. Hume, P, et al: Effectiveness of foot orthoses for treatment and prevention of lower limb injuries: A review. Sports Med 38:759, 2008.

28. Richter, RR, Austin, TM, and Reinking, MF: Foot orthoses in lower limb overuse conditions: A systematic review and meta-analysis: Critical appraisal and commentary. J Athl Train 46:103, 2011.

29. Rome, K, Ashford, RL, and Evans, A: Non-surgical interventions for paediatric pes planus. Cochrane Database Syst Rev CD006311, 2010.

30. Powell, M, Seid, M, and Szer, IS: Efficacy of custom foot orthotics in improving pain and functional status in children with juvenile idiopathic arthritis: A randomized trial. J Rheumatol 32:943, 2005.

31. Burns, J, et al: Interventions for the prevention and treatment of pes cavus. Cochrane Database Syst Rev CD006154, 2007.

32. Burns, J, et al: Effective orthotic therapy for the painful cavus foot: A randomized controlled trial. J Am Podiatr Med Assoc 96:205, 2006.

33. Hawke, F, et al: Custom-made foot orthoses for the treatment of foot pain. Cochrane Database System Rev CD006801, 2008.

34. Hastings, MK, et al: Effect of metatarsal pad placement on plantar pressure in people with diabetes mellitus and peripheral neuropathy. Foot Ankle Int 28:84, 2007.

35. Lott, DJ, et al: Effect of footwear and orthotic devices on stress reduction and soft tissue strain of the neuropathic foot. Clin Biomech (Bristol, Avon) 22:352, 2007.

36. Brodtkorb, TH, Kogler GF, and Arndt, A: The influence of metatarsal support height and longitudinal axis position on plantar foot loading. Clin Biomech (Bristol, Avon) 23:640, 2008.

37. Wang, CC, and Hansen, AH: Response of able-bodied persons to changes in shoe rocker radius during walking: Changes in ankle kinematics to maintain a consistent roll-over shape. J Biomech 43:2288, 2010.

38. Hutchins, S, et al: The biomechanics and clinical efficacy of footwear adapted with rocker profiles—evidence in the literature. Foot (Edinb) 19:165, 2009.

39. Nair, PM, et al: Stepping in an ankle foot orthosis re-examined: A mechanical perspective for clinical decision making. Clin Biomech (Bristol, Avon) 25:618, 2010.

40. Guillebastre, B, Calmels, P, and Rougier, P: Effects of rigid and dynamic ankle-foot orthoses on normal gait. Foot Ankle Int 30:51, 2009.

41. Herndon, SK, et al: Center of mass motion and the effects of ankle bracing on metabolic cost during submaximal walking trials. J Orthop Res 24:2170, 2006.

42. Radtka, SA, et al: The kinematic and kinetic effects of solid, hinged, and no ankle-foot orthoses on stair locomotion in healthy adults. Gait Posture 24:211, 2006.

43. Huang, YC, et al: Effects of ankle-foot orthoses on ankle and foot kinematics in patients with subtalar osteoarthritis. Arch Phys Med Rehabil 87:1131, 2006.

44. Gok, H, et al: Effects of ankle-foot orthoses on hemiparetic gait. Clin Rehabil 17:137, 2003.

45. Tyson, SF, and Thornton, HA: The effect of a hinged ankle foot orthosis on hemiplegic gait: Objective measures and users' opinions. Clin Rehabil 15:53, 2001.

46. Bregman, DJJ, et al: Polypropylene ankle foot orthoses to overcome drop-foot gait in central neurological patients: A mechanical and functional evaluation. Prosthet Orthot Int 34:293, 2010.

47. Erel, S, et al: The effects of dynamic ankle-foot orthoses in chronic stroke patients at three-month follow-up: A randomized controlled trial. Clin Rehabil 25:1, 2011.

48. Esquenazi, A, et al: The effect of an ankle-foot orthosis on temporal spatial parameters and asymmetry of gait in hemiparetic patients. PM R 1:1014, 2009.

49. Wang, RY, et al: Gait and balance performance improvements attributable to ankle-foot orthosis in subjects with hemiparesis. Am J Phys Med Rehabil 86:556, 2007.

50. Abe, H, et al: Improving gait stability in stroke hemiplegic patients with a plastic ankle-foot orthosis. Tohoku J Exp Med 18:193, 2009.

51. Cakar, E, et al: The ankle-foot orthosis improves balance and reduces fall risk of chronic spastic hemiparetic patients. Eur J Phys Rehabil Med 46:363, 2010.

52. Nolan, KJ, and Yarossi, M: Weight transfer analysis in adults with hemiplegia using ankle foot orthosis. Prosthet Orthot Int 35:45, 2011.

53. Hung, JW, et al: Long-term effect of an anterior ankle-foot orthosis on functional walking ability of chronic stroke patients. Am J Phys Med Rehabil 90:8, 2011.

54. Chen, CK, et al: Effects of an anterior ankle-foot orthosis on postural stability in stroke patients with hemiplegia. Am J Phys Med Rehabil 87:815, 2008.

55. Chen, CC, et al: Kinematic features of rear-foot motion using anterior and posterior ankle-foot orthoses in stroke patients with hemiplegic gait. Arch Phys Med Rehabil 91:1862, 2010.

56. Simons, CD, et al: Ankle-foot orthoses in stroke: Effects on functional balance, weight-bearing asymmetry and the contribution of each lower limb to balance control. Clin Biomech (Bristol, Avon) 24:769, 2009.

57. Cruz, TH, and Dhaher, YY: Impact of ankle-foot-orthosis on frontal plane behaviors post-stroke. Gait Posture 30:312, 2009.

58. Fatone, S, Gard, SA, and Malas, BS: Effect of ankle-foot orthosis alignment and foot-plate length on the gait of adults with poststroke hemiplegia. Arch Phys Med Rehabil 90:810, 2009.

59. Jagadamma, KC, et al: The effects of tuning an Ankle-Foot Orthosis Footwear Combination on kinematics and kinetics of the knee joint of an adult with hemiplegia. Prosthet Orthot Int 34:270, 2010.

60. Danielsson, A, and Sunnerhagen, KS: Energy expenditure in stroke subjects walking with a carbon composite ankle foot orthosis. J Rehabil Med 36:165, 2004.

61. Bregman, DJJ, et al: Polypropylene ankle foot orthosis to overcome drop-foot in central neurological patients: A mechanical and functional evaluation. Prosthet Orthot Int 34:293, 2010.

62. Franceschini, M, et al: Effects of an ankle-foot orthosis on spatiotemporal parameters and energy cost of hemiparetic gait. Clin Rehabil 17:368, 2003.

63. Mulroy, SJ, et al: Effect of AFO design on walking after stroke: Impact of ankle plantar flexion contracture. Prosthet Orthot Int 34:277, 2010.

64. Ring, H, et al: Neuroprosthesis for footdrop compared with an ankle-foot orthosis: Effects on postural control during walking. J Stroke Cerebrovasc Dis 18:41, 2009.

65. van Swigchem, R, et al: Is transcutaneous peroneal stimulation beneficial to patients with chronic stroke using an ankle-foot orthosis? A within-subjects study of patients' satisfaction, walking speed and physical activity level. J Rehabil Med 42:117, 2010.

66. Kasar, TM, et al: Novel patterns of functional electrical stimulation have an immediate effect on dorsiflexor muscle function during gait for people poststroke. Phys Ther 90:55, 2010.

67. Sheffler, LR, et al: Peroneal nerve stimulation versus an ankle foot orthosis for correction of footdrop in stroke: Impact on functional ambulation. Neurorehabil Neural Repair 20:355, 2006.

68. Sheffler, LR, Bailey, SN, and Chae, J: Spatiotemporal and kinematic effect of peroneal nerve stimulation versus an ankle-foot orthosis in patients with multiple sclerosis: A case series. PM R 1:604, 2009.

69. O'Reilly, T, et al: Effects of ankle-foot orthoses for children with hemiplegia on weight-bearing and functional ability. Pediatr Phys Ther 21:225, 2009.

70. Desloovere, K, et al: How can push-off be preserved during use of an ankle foot orthosis in children with hemiplegia? A prospective controlled study. Gait Posture 24:142, 2006.

71. Romkes, J, Hell, AK, and Brunner, R: Changes in muscle activity in children with hemiplegic cerebral palsy while walking with and without ankle-foot orthoses. Gait Posture 24:467, 2006.

72. Van Gestel, L, et al: Effect of dynamic orthoses on gait: A retrospective control study in children with hemiplegia. Dev Med Child Neurol 50:63, 2008.

73. Brehm, MA, Harlaar, J, and Schwartz, M: Effect of ankle-foot orthoses on walking efficiency and gait in children with cerebral palsy. J Rehabil Med 40:529, 2008.

74. Maltais, D, et al: Use of orthoses lowers the O₂ cost of walking in children with spastic cerebral palsy. Med Sci Sports Exerc 33:320, 2001.

75. Balaban, B, et al: The effect of hinged ankle-foot orthosis on gait and energy expenditure in spastic hemiplegic cerebral palsy. Disabil Rehabil 29:139, 2007.

76. Smiley, SJ, et al: A comparison of the effects of solid, articulated, and posterior leaf-spring ankle-foot orthoses and shoes alone on gait and energy expenditure in children with spastic diplegic cerebral palsy. Orthopedics 25:411, 2002.

77. Radtka, SA, Skinner, SR, and Johanson, ME: A comparison of gait with solid and hinged ankle-foot orthoses in children with spastic diplegic cerebral palsy. Gait Posture 21:303, 2005.

78. Buckon, CE, et al: Comparison of three ankle-foot orthosis configurations for children with spastic diplegia. Dev Med Child Neurol 46:590, 2004.

79. Sienko-Thomas, S, et al: Stair locomotion in children with spastic hemiplegia: The impact of three different ankle foot orthosis (AFO) configurations. Gait Posture 16:180, 2002.

80. Rogozinski, BM, et al: The efficacy of the floor-reaction ankle-foot orthosis in children with cerebral palsy. J Bone Joint Surg Am 91:2440, 2009.

81. Lucareli, PR, et al: Changes in joint kinematics in children with cerebral palsy while walking with and without a floor reaction ankle-foot orthosis. Clinics (Sao Paulo) 62:63, 2007.

82. Kane, K, and Barden, J: Comparison of ground reaction and articulated ankle-foot orthoses in a child with lumbosacral myelomeningocele and tibial torsion. J Prosthet Orthot 22:222, 2010.

83. Westberry, DE, et al: Impact of ankle-foot orthoses on static foot alignment in children with cerebral palsy. J Bone Joint Surg Am 89:806, 2007.

84. Hachisuka, K, et al: Clinical application of carbon fibre reinforced plastic leg orthosis for polio survivors and its advantages and disadvantages. Prosthet Orthot Int 30:129, 2006.

85. Brehm, MA, et al: Effect of carbon-composite knee-ankle-foot orthoses on walking efficiency and gait in former polio patients. J Rehabil Med 39:651, 2007.

86. Hachisuka, K, et al: Oxygen consumption, oxygen cost and physiological cost index in polio survivors: A comparison of walking without orthosis, with an ordinary or a carbon-fibre reinforced plastic knee-ankle-foot orthosis. J Rehabil Med 39:646, 2007.

87. Hebert, JS, and Liggins, AB: Gait evaluation of an automatic stance-control knee orthosis in a patient with postpoliomyelitis. Arch Phys Med Rehabil 86:1676, 2005.

88. Irby, SE, Bernhardt, KA, and Kaufman, KR: Gait of stance control orthosis users: The dynamic knee brace system. Prosthet Orthot Int 29:269, 2005.

89. Irby, SE, Bernhardt, KA, and Kaufman, KR: Gait changes over time in stance control orthosis users. Prosthetic Orthot Int 31:353, 2007.

90. Yakimovich, T, Lemaire, ED, and Kofman, J: Preliminary kinematic evaluation of a new stance-control knee-ankle-foot orthosis. Clin Biomech (Bristol, Avon) 21:1081, 2006.

91. Yakimovich, T, Lemaire, ED, and Kofman, J: Engineering design review of stance-control knee-ankle-foot orthoses. J Rehabil Res Dev 46:257, 2009.

92. Davis, PC, Bach, TM, and Pereira, DM: The effect of stance control orthoses on gait characteristics and energy expenditure in knee-ankle-foot orthosis users. Prosthet Orthot Int 34:206, 2010.

93. McMillan, AG, et al: Preliminary evidence for effectiveness of a stance control orthosis. J Prosthet Orthot 16:6, 2004.

94. Zissimopoulos, A, Fatone, S, and Gard, SA: Biomechanical and energetic effects of a stance-control orthotic knee joint. J Rehabil Res Dev 44:503, 2007.

95. Bernhardt, KA, Irby, SE, and Kaufman, KR: Consumer opinions of a stance control knee orthosis. Prosthet Orthot Int 30:246, 2006.

96. Hwang, S, et al: Biomechanical effect of electromechanical knee-ankle-foot orthosis on knee joint control in patients with poliomyelitis. Med Biol Eng Comput 46:541, 2008.

97. Horst, RW: A bio-robotic leg orthosis for rehabilitation and mobility enhancement. Conf Proc IEEE Eng Med Biol Soc 2009-5090-3, 2009.

98. Johnson, WB, Fatone, S, and Gard, SA: Walking mechanics of persons who use reciprocating gait orthoses. J Rehabil Res Dev 46:435, 2009.

99. Leung, AK, et al: The Physiological Cost Index of walking with an isocentric reciprocating gait orthosis among patients with T(12)–L(1) spinal cord injury. Prosthet Orthot Int 33:61, 2009.

100. Merati, G, et al: Paraplegic adaptation to assisted-walking: Energy expenditure during wheelchair versus orthosis use. Spinal Cord 38:37, 2000.

101. Plassat, R, et al: Gait orthosis in patients with complete thoracic paraplegia: Review of 43 patients. Ann Readapt Med Phys 48:240, 2005.

102. Roussos, N, et al: A long-term review of severely disabled spina bifida patients using a reciprocal walking system. Disabil Rehabil 23:239, 2001.

103. Spadone, R, et al: Energy consumption of locomotion with orthosis versus Parastep-assisted gait: A single case study. Spinal Cord 41:97, 2003.

104. Vogt, L, et al: Lumbar corsets: Their effect on three-dimensional kinematics of the pelvis. J Rehabil Res Dev 37:495, 2000.

105. Van Duijvenbode, IC, et al: Lumbar supports for prevention and treatment of low back pain. Cochrane Database Syst Rev 16:CD001823, 2008.

106. Jellema, P, et al: Lumbar supports for prevention and treatment of low back pain: A systematic review within the framework of the Cochrane Back Review Group. Spine 26:377, 2001.

107. Cholewicki, J, et al: Lumbosacral orthoses reduce trunk muscle activity in a postural control task. J Biomech 40:1731, 2007.

108. Cholewicki, J, et al: The effects of a three-week use of lumbosacral orthoses on trunk muscle activity and on the muscular response to trunk perturbations. BMC Musculoskelet Disord 11:154, 2010.

109. Fayolle-Minon, I, and Calmeis, P: Effect of wearing a lumbar orthosis on trunk muscles: Study of the muscle strength after 21 days of use on healthy subjects. Joint Bone Spine 75:58, 2008.

110. van Leeuwen, PJ, et al: Assessment of spinal movement reduction by thoraco-lumbar-sacral orthoses. J Rehabil Res Dev 37:395, 2000.

111. Konz, R, Fatone, S, and Gard, S: Effect of restricted spinal motion on gait. J Rehabil Res Dev 43:161, 2006.

112. Kongsted, A, et al: Neck collar, "act-as-usual" or active mobilization for whiplash injury? A randomized parallel-group trial. Spine 332:618, 2007.

113. Kuijper, B, et al: Cervical collar or physiotherapy versus wait and see policy for recent onset cervical radiculopathy: Randomised trial. BMJ 339, 2009.

114. Gavin, TM, et al: Biomechanical analysis of cervical orthoses in flexion and extension: A comparison of cervical collars and cervical thoracic orthoses. J Rehabil Res Dev 40:527, 2003.

115. Tescher, AN, et al: Range-of-motion restriction and craniofacial tissue-interface pressure from four cervical collars. J Trauma 63:112, 2007.

116. Zhang, S, et al: Evaluation of efficacy and 3D kinematic characteristics of cervical orthoses. Clin Biomech (Bristol, Avon) 20:264, 2005.

117. Cosan, TE, et al: Indications of Philadelphia collar in the treatment of upper cervical injuries. Eur J Emerg Med 8:33, 2001.

118. Bell, KM, et al: Assessing range of motion to evaluate the adverse effects of ill-fitting cervical orthoses. Spine J 9:225, 2009.

119. Sawers, A, DiPaola, CP, and Rechtine, GR 2nd: Suitability of the noninvasive halo for cervical spine injuries: A retrospective analysis of outcomes. Spine J 9:216, 2009.

120. Ivanocic, PC, Beauchman, NN, and Tweardy, L: Effect of halo-vest components on stabilizing the injured cervical spine. Spine 34:167, 2009.

121. Platzer, P, et al: Nonoperative management of odontoid fractures using a halothoracic vest. Neurosurgery 61:522, 2007.

122. German, JW, Hart, BL, and Benzel, ED: Nonoperative management of vertical C2 body fractures. Neurosurgery 56:516, 2005.

123. Koech, F, et al: Nonoperative management of type II odontoid fractures in the elderly. Spine 33:2881, 2008.

124. Ohnishi, K, et al: Effects of wearing halo vest on gait: Three-dimensional analysis in healthy subjects. Spine 30:750, 2005.

125. Ono, A, et al: Muscle atrophy after treatment with Halovest. Spine 30:E8, 2005.

126. Fayssoux, RS, Cho, RH, and Herman, MJ: A history of bracing for idiopathic scoliosis in North America. Clin Orthop Relat Res 468:654, 2010.

127. Sponseller, PD: Bracing for adolescent idiopathic scoliosis in practice today. J Pediatr Orthop 31:S53, 2011.

128. Kotwicki, T, and Cheneau, J: Passive and active mechanisms of correction of thoracic idiopathic scoliosis with a rigid brace. Stud Health Technol Inform 136:320, 2008.

129. Clin, J, et al: Correlation between immediate in-brace correction and biomechanical effectiveness of brace treatment in adolescent idiopathic scoliosis. Spine 35:1706, 2010.

130. Lou, E, et al: Correlation between quantity and quality of orthosis wear and treatment outcomes in adolescent idiopathic scoliosis. Prosthet Orthot Int 28:49, 2004.

131. Negrini, S, et al: Braces for idiopathic scoliosis in adolescents. Spine (Phila) 35:1285, 2010.

132. Dolan, LA, and Weinstein, SL: Surgical rates after observation and bracing for adolescent idiopathic scoliosis: An evidence-based review. Spine 32:S91, 2007.

133. Maruyama, T, Grivas, TB, and Kaspiris, A: Effectiveness and outcomes of brace treatment: A systematic review. Physiother Theory Pract 27:26: 2011.

134. Katz, DE, and Durani, AA: Factors that influence outcome in bracing large curves in patients with adolescent idiopathic scoliosis. Spine 26:2354, 2001.

135. Negrini, S, et al: Idiopathic scoliosis patients with curves more than 45 Cobb degrees refusing surgery can be effectively treated through bracing with curve improvements. Spine J 36:1, 2011.

136. Sadeghi, H, et al: Bracing has no effect on standing balance in females with adolescent idiopathic scoliosis. Med Sci Monit 14:CR293, 2008.

137. Rivett, L, et al: The relationship between quality of life and compliance to a brace protocol in adolescents with idiopathic scoliosis: A comparative study. BMC Musculoskelet Disord 10:5, 2009.

138. Vasiliadis, E, et al: The influence of brace on quality of life of adolescents with idiopathic scoliosis. Stud Health Technol Inform 123:352, 2006.

139. Glassman, SD, et al: The costs and benefits of nonoperative management for adult scoliosis. Spine 35:578, 2010.

140. Mac-Thiong, JM, et al: Biomechanical evaluation of the Boston brace system for the treatment of adolescent idiopathic scoliosis: Relationship between strap tension and brace interface forces. Spine 29:26, 2004.

141. Lange, JE, Steen, H, and Brox, JI: Long-term results after Boston brace treatment in adolescent idiopathic scoliosis. Scoliosis 4:17, 2009.

142. Bunge, EM, et al: Patients' preferences for scoliosis brace treatment: A discrete choice experiment. Spine 35:57, 2010.

143. Clin, J, et al: A biomechanical study of the Charleston brace for the treatment of scoliosis. Spine 35:E940, 2010.

144. Gepstein, R, et al: Effectiveness of the Charleston bending brace in the treatment of single-curve idiopathic scoliosis. J Pediatr Orthop 22:84, 2002.

145. D'Amato, CR, Griggs, S, and McCoy, B: Nighttime bracing with the Providence brace in adolescent girls with idiopathic scoliosis. Spine 26:2006, 2001.

146. Seifert, J, and Selle, A: Is night-time bracing still appropriate in the treatment of idiopathic scoliosis? Orthopade 38:146, 2009.

147. Zaina, F, et al: Review of rehabilitation and orthopedic conservative approach to sagittal plane diseases during growth: Hyperkyphosis, junctional kyphosis, and Scheuermann disease. Eur J Phys Rehabil Med 45:595, 2009.

148. Gonzalez, E, and Edelstein, J: Energy expenditure in ambulation: In Gonzalez, E, et al (eds): Downey and Darling's Physiological Basis of Rehabilitation Medicine, ed 3. Butterworth-Heinemann, Boston, 2001, p 417.

Supplemental Readings

Edelstein, JE, and Bruckner, J: Orthotics: A Comprehensive Clinical Approach. Slack, Thorofare, NJ, 2002.

Edelstein, JE, and Moroz, A: Lower extremity Prosthetics and Orthotics: Clinical Essentials. Slack, Thorofare, NJ, 2011.

Farris, RJ, Quintero, HA, and Goldfarb, M: Preliminary Evaluation of a Powered Lower Limb Orthosis to Aid Walking in Paraplegic Individuals. IEEE Trans Neural Syst Rehabil Eng 19:(6)652, 2011.

Hsu, JD, Michael, JW, and Fisk, JR, (eds): Atlas of Orthoses and Assistive Devices, ed 4. Mosby Elsevier, Philadelphia, 2008.

Ibuki, A, et al: The effect of tone-reducing orthotic devices on soleus muscle reflex excitability while standing in patients with spasticity following stroke. Prosthet Orthot Int 34:(1)46, 2010.

Lusardi, MM, and Nielsen, CC: Orthotics and Prosthetics in Rehabilitation, ed 2. Saunders, St. Louis, 2007.

May, BJ, and Lockard, MA: Prosthetics and Orthotics in Clinical Practice. FA Davis, Philadelphia, 2011.

Nawoczenski, DA, and Epler, ME: Orthotics in Functional Rehabilitation of the Lower Limb. WB Saunders, Philadelphia, 1997.

Neville, C, and Houck, J: Choosing among 3 ankle-foot orthoses for a patient with stage II posterior tibial tendon dysfunction. J Orthop Sports Phys Ther 39(11):816, 2009.

Oosterwaal, M, et al: Generation of subject-specific, dynamic, multisegment ankle and foot models to improve orthotic design: A feasibility study. BMC Musculoskelet Disord 12:256, 2011.

Seymour, R: Prosthetics and Orthotics: Lower Limb and Spinal. Lippincott Williams & Wilkins, Philadelphia, 2002.

Lower Extremity Orthotic Examination

1. Is the orthosis as prescribed?
2. Can the client don the orthosis easily?

Standing

3. Is the shoe satisfactory and does it fit properly?
4. Are the sole and heel of the shoe flat on the floor?
5. If a shoe insert is used, is there minimal rocking between insert and shoe?

Ankle

6. Do the mechanical ankle joints coincide with the anatomical ankle (anatomical ankle joint axis is approximated by a horizontal line between the malleoli at level of the distal tip of the medial malleolus)?
7. Is there adequate clearance between the anatomical ankle and the mechanical ankle joints?
8. Does the valgus or varus correction strap control the foot position?

Knee

9. Does the mechanical knee joint(s) coincide with the anatomical knee (0.5–0.75 in [1.2–1.9 cm]) above medial tibial plateau?
10. Is there adequate clearance between the anatomical knee and the mechanical knee joint?
11. Is the knee lock secure and easy to operate?

Shells, Bands, Cuffs, and Uprights

12. Do the shells, bands, cuffs, and uprights conform to the contours of the leg and thigh?
13. Is there adequate clearance between the top of the calf shell or band and the head of the fibula?
14. Is there adequate clearance between the orthosis and the perineum?
15. Is the orthosis below the greater trochanter but at least 1 in (2.5 cm) higher than the medial shell or upright?
16. Are the uprights at the midline of the leg and thigh?
17. Do the shells, bands, and cuffs conform to the contours of the leg and thigh?
18. Is any flesh roll above the shell or band minimal?
19. Are the bottom of the thigh shell or distal thigh band and the top of the calf shell or band equidistant from the knee?

20. In a child's orthosis, is there adequate provision for lengthening the orthosis?

Weight-Relieving Components

21. In a patellar-tendon-bearing brim, is there adequate relief for the head of the fibula?
22. With a quadrilateral brim, is the client free from excessive pressure in the anteromedial and medial aspect of the brim?
23. With a quadrilateral brim, does the ischial tuberosity rest on the ischial seat?
24. With a patellar-tendon-bearing brim, is there adequate reduction in weight-bearing through the orthosis?

Hip

25. Is the center of the pelvic joint slightly above and ahead of greater trochanter?
26. Is the hip lock secure and easy to operate?
27. Does the pelvic band fit the torso accurately?

Stability

28. Does the orthosis provide adequate stability to the client?

Sitting

29. Can the patient sit comfortably with hips and knees flexed 90°?
30. Can the patient lean forward to touch the shoes?

Walking

31. Is the patient's performance in level walking satisfactory?
32. Is the patient's performance on stairs and ramps satisfactory?
33. Is the orthosis sufficiently rigid?
34. Does the varus or valgus correction strap provide adequate support?
35. Does the orthosis operate quietly?
36. Does the patient consider the orthosis satisfactory as to comfort, function, and appearance?

Orthosis Off the Patient

37. Is the skin free of abrasions or other discolorations attributable to the orthosis?
38. Is the construction satisfactory?
39. Do all components function satisfactorily?

1. Is the orthosis as prescribed?
2. Can the client don the orthosis easily?

Standing

Pelvic Band

3. Does the pelvic band lie flat on the trunk below the posterior superior iliac spines?
4. Does the pelvic band pass between the trochanters and iliac crests?

Thoracic Band

5. Does the thoracic band lie flat on the trunk below the scapulae?
6. Does the thoracic band lie horizontally on the trunk?

Uprights

7. Do the posterior uprights avoid pressure on bony prominences, such as the vertebral spines or scapulae?
8. Do the lateral uprights extend along the lateral midlines of the trunk?

Abdominal Front

9. Is the abdominal front of adequate size?

Cervical Orthosis

10. Is the head in the prescribed position?
11. Do all rigid components fit properly?

Sitting

12. Can the patient sit comfortably with the hips and knees flexed 90°?
13. Does the patient consider the orthosis satisfactory as to comfort, function, and appearance?

Orthosis Off the Patient

14. Is the skin free of abrasions or other discolorations attributable to the orthosis?
15. Is the construction satisfactory?
16. Do all components function satisfactorily?

Web-Based Orthotic Resources for Clinicians, Families, and Patients

Organization/Resource	Website
American Academy of Orthotists and Prosthetists	www.oandp.org
American Orthotic and Prosthetic Association	www.aopanet.org
Digital Resource Foundation for the Orthotics and Prosthetics Community	www.drfop.org
Orthotic and Prosthetic Activities Foundation	http://opfund.org/programs/initiatives.asp
Orthotic and Prosthetic Education and Research Foundation	www.operf.org/research
Resource for Orthotics and Prosthetics Information	www.oandp.com

Prosthetics

Chapter 31

Joan E. Edelstein, PT, MA, FISPO, CPed
Christopher Kevin Wong, PT, PhD, OCS

LEARNING OBJECTIVES

1. Describe the components of transtibial and transfemoral prostheses, including advantages and disadvantages of alternative components and materials.
2. Explain the distinctive features of partial foot, Syme's, knee and hip disarticulation prostheses, and bilateral prostheses.
3. Outline the maintenance program for prosthetic components.
4. Conduct static and dynamic evaluation of transtibial and transfemoral prostheses.
5. Summarize the physical therapist's role in management of individuals with lower-limb amputation.
6. Analyze and interpret patient data, formulate realistic goals and outcomes, and develop a plan of care when presented with a clinical case study.

CHAPTER OUTLINE

Physical therapists are concerned with the care of individuals with lower- and upper-limb amputations. Patients are often fitted with a *prosthesis* to replace the absent part of the leg or arm. In the broadest sense, prostheses also include dentures, titanium femoral heads, and plastic heart valves. A *prosthetist* is a health care professional who designs, fabricates, and fits limb prostheses.

The major causes of amputation are peripheral vascular disease, trauma, malignancy, and congenital deficiency. In the United States, vascular disease accounts for most leg amputations, particularly among patients with diabetes.[1] Individuals older than 60 constitute the largest group of people with amputation. Trauma is responsible for the majority of amputations in younger adults and adolescents. Men are more likely to sustain amputation because of trauma and vascular disease. Bone and soft tissue tumors are sometimes treated by amputation, with adolescence the period of peak incidence. Congenital deficiency refers to the absence or abnormality of a limb evident at birth.

This chapter focuses on the lower extremity (LE) because many more people have lost a portion of the LE, as compared with the upper extremity (UE). Physical therapists are key members of the rehabilitation team, working with prosthetists, physicians, occupational therapists, and others to foster the patient's welfare. For individuals with LE amputation, physical therapists have the major role in assisting the person to regain function. Lower extremity prostheses will be described, together with a program for training patients in their use. For patients with UE amputation, physical therapists may play a lesser role, cooperating with occupational therapists, depending on the administrative organization of the health care facility.

Historic records confirm that the concept of replacing a missing limb is very old. A forked stick that formed a peg leg to support a transtibial (below-knee) amputation limb was known in antiquity. Today, most individuals with LE amputation are provided with a prosthesis because function with one LE is very different from maneuvering with two.

The principal LE prostheses are partial foot, Syme's, transtibial, and transfemoral, as well as knee and hip disarticulation. The physical therapist should be familiar with their characteristics and maintenance, as well as the rehabilitation of patients fitted with these devices.

■ PARTIAL FOOT AND SYME'S PROSTHESES

The purposes of partial foot prostheses are to (1) restore, as much as possible, foot function, particularly in walking; and (2) simulate the shape of the missing foot segment. The patient who has lost one or more toes may simply pad the toe section of the shoe to improve the appearance of the upper portion of the shoe. Standing will not be affected, assuming the metatarsal heads remain. When the individual walks, late stance will be less forceful, particularly if both phalanges of the great toe are absent. An arch support foot orthosis helps to maintain alignment of the amputated foot, especially if one or more proximal phalanges have been amputated.[2]

Transmetatarsal amputation disturbs foot appearance more noticeably. A prosthesis prevents the shoe from developing an unnatural crease in the forefoot area. The patient bears most weight on the heel and reduces the amount of time spent on the affected foot during walking. A particularly useful prosthesis consists of a plastic socket for the remainder of the foot. The socket is affixed to a rigid plate that extends the full length of the inner sole of the shoe. The plate has a cosmetic toe filler. The socket protects the amputated ends of the metatarsals, and the rigid plate restores foot length so that the person can spend more time during the stance phase of gait on the affected side than would otherwise be the case. To aid late stance, the bottom of the prosthesis or the sole of the shoe may have a convex rocker bar.[3]

Amputation or disarticulation through the tarsals, such as Lisfranc and Chopart disarticulations,[4] poses the additional problem of retaining the small foot segment in the shoe during swing phase. Foot length is apt to be diminished further by an equinus deformity of the amputated limb, resulting from unbalanced contraction of the triceps surae. Consequently, the prosthesis described for the transmetatarsal amputation may be augmented with a plastic calf shell, which is strapped around the leg.[5,6]

Syme's amputation involves surgical sectioning through the distal tibia and fibula, removal of the entire foot, and preservation of the calcaneal fat pad. The patient can usually bear significant weight through the distal end of the amputation limb.[7,8] The socket (Fig. 31.1) trimlines (edges) are located in the proximal portion of the lower leg. The socket has a relief (concavity) for the tibial crest. If the distal end of the Syme's limb is markedly bulbous, the lower part of the medial wall can be made removable; the patient dons the socket, and then fastens the wall section in place. The socket for an amputation limb having relatively vertical contours

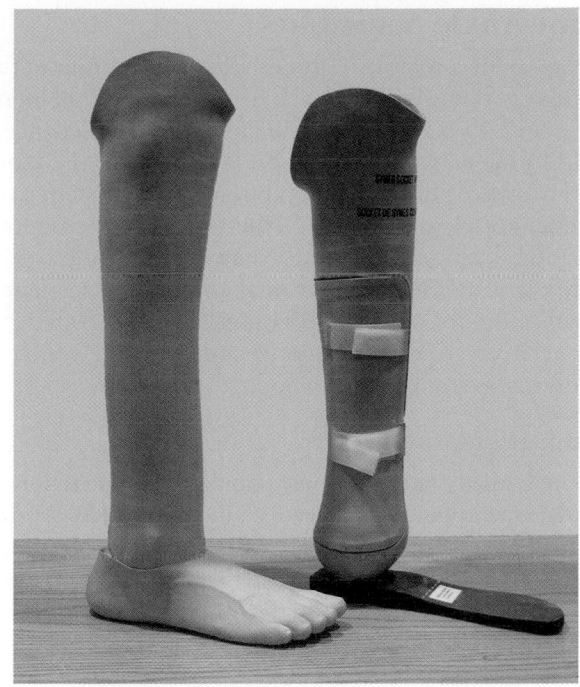

Figure 31.1 Syme's prostheses. (*Left*) Socket with continuous walls. (*Right*) Socket with medial opening.

does not need a removable section; this design has a resilient liner that assists entry of the bulbous distal end of the amputated limb, enabling the wearer to don the prosthesis easily. The prosthesis includes a foot specifically designed to accommodate the long socket (Fig. 31.2). The Syme's prosthesis is suspended by the contour of its brims and socket walls, ordinarily without any other suspension mechanism.

■ TRANSTIBIAL PROSTHESES

The transtibial level, formerly known as below-knee, refers to an amputation in which the tibia and fibula are transected. The patient retains the anatomical knee with its motor and sensory functions. This is the predominant site of amputation, particularly for individuals with vascular disease.[9] Prostheses for transtibial amputations include a foot-ankle assembly, shank (lower leg), socket, and suspension component.

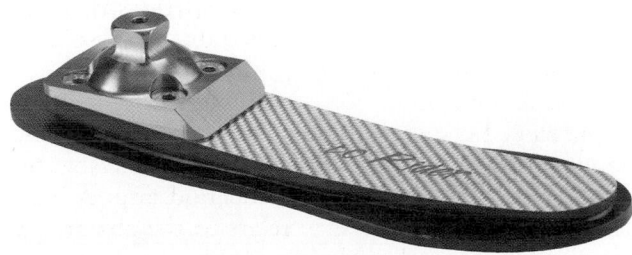

Figure 31.2 Lo Rider foot for Syme's prosthesis. *Courtesy of Otto Bock, Minneapolis, MN 55447.*

Foot-Ankle Assemblies

A foot-ankle assembly restores the general contour of the patient's foot, absorbs shock at heel contact, plantarflexes in early stance, and simulates metatarsophalangeal (MTP) hyperextension (toe-break action) in the latter part of stance phase; patients appear to prefer a foot with a relatively rigid forefoot.[10] The foot is in the neutral position during swing phase. Many assemblies also provide slight motion in the frontal and transverse planes, attempting to mimic physiological foot action.[11-16] Newer feet are often made of carbon fiber, which is lighter and stronger than wood.

Nonarticulated Feet

In the United States, the most popular foot type is nonarticulated, without a space between the foot and lower portion of the shank. As compared with articulated feet, nonarticulated components are lighter in weight and more durable; some versions are made to suit high-heeled shoes.

SACH Foot

The nonarticulated *solid ankle cushion heel (SACH)* assembly is commonly prescribed (Fig. 31.3A). The longitudinal portion is a wooden or metal *keel*, which terminates at a point corresponding to the metatarsophalangeal joints. The keel is covered with rubber; the posterior portion is resilient, to absorb shock and permit plantarflexion in early stance. Anteriorly, the junction of the keel and the rubber toe sections allows the foot to hyperextend in late stance. The SACH foot is manufactured in a wide range of sizes to accommodate infants, adolescents, and adults. It is available with heel cushions of varying degrees of compressibility for those who strike the heel with different amounts of force. SACH feet can be ordered in several plantarflexion angles to fit shoes with diverse heel heights. The heel cushion allows a very small amount of medial–lateral and transverse motion.

Other Nonarticulated Feet

A newer version of the SACH foot is the *stationary attachment flexible endoskeleton (SAFE)* foot (Fig. 31.3B). It has a rigid ankle block joined to the posterior portion of the keel at a 45° angle, which is comparable to that of the anatomical subtalar joint. The junction permits the wearer to maintain contact with moderately uneven terrain, because of the relatively great range of medial–lateral motion permitted in the rear foot. The SAFE foot,

however, is somewhat heavier and more expensive than the SACH foot.

Feet that have a springy sole store energy in early and midstance as the wearer moves over the foot, bending it slightly. In late stance, as the wearer transfers loading to the opposite foot, the spring in the prosthetic foot recoils, returning some of the stored energy. Such feet are described as energy storing/energy releasing, or dynamic.[11] Both the *Flex-Foot* and the *Springlite foot* (Fig. 31.4) include a long band of carbon fiber, extending from the toe to the proximal shank, as well as a posterior heel section. The long band acts as a leaf spring, enabling the foot to store considerable energy in early and midstance, and then to release energy at the end of stance phase. Active wearers, such as those who play basketball or run, utilize the energy-storing and energy-releasing capacity of these feet. The C-Walk® (Fig. 31.5) is another example of an energy-storing foot. Other energy storing prosthetic feet are shown in Figure 31.6. They are more expensive than SACH feet. Many of these

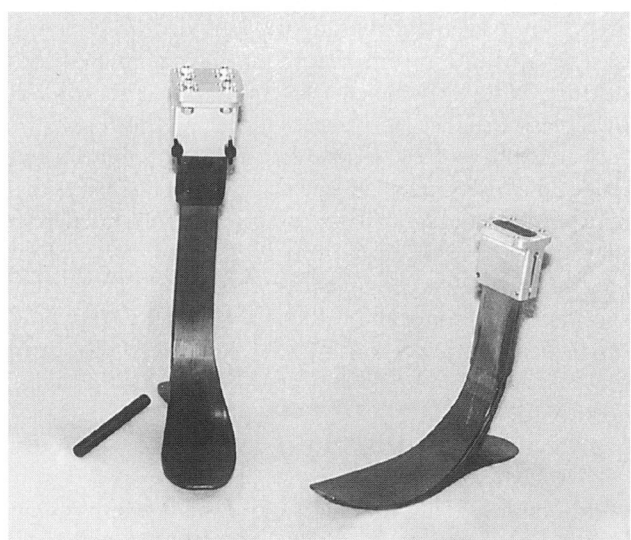

Figure 31.4 Springlite foot.

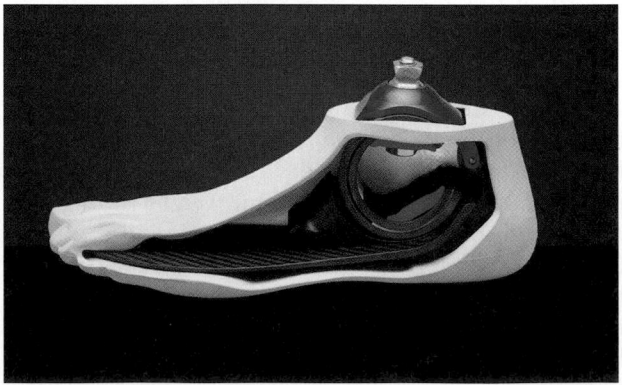

Figure 31.5 C-Walk foot. *Courtesy of Otto Bock, Minneapolis, MN 55447.*

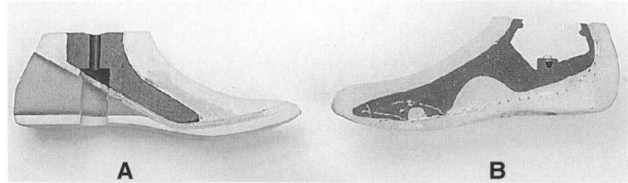

Figure 31.3 Cross section of nonarticulated foot-ankle assemblies. **(A)** SACH. **(B)** SAFE.

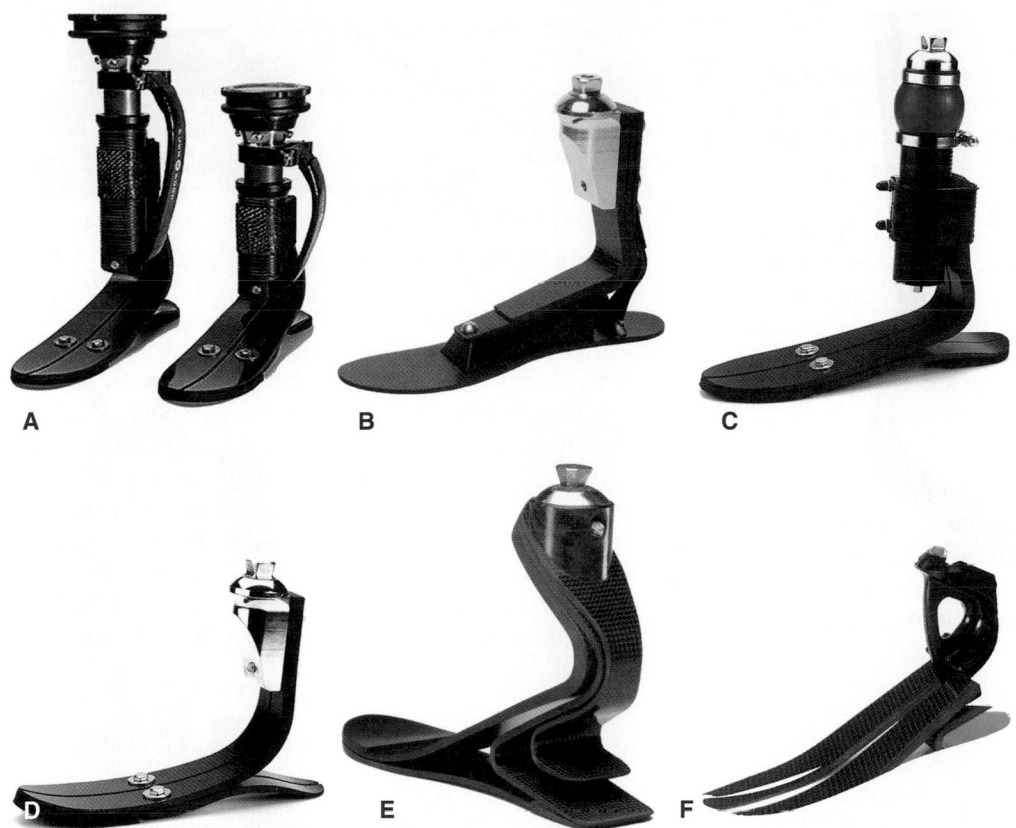

Figure 31.6 Nonarticulated energy-storing prosthetic feet. **(A)** Re-Flex VSP® and Re-Flex VSP Low Profile®, **(B)** Talux®, **(C)** Ceterus®, **(D)** Vari-Flex®. *Courtesy of Ossur, Aliso Viejo, CA, 92656.* **(E)** Renegade. *Courtesy of Freedom Innovations, Fayette, UT 84630.* **(F)** ELITE 2®. *Courtesy of Endolite, Miamisburg, OH 45342.*

feet can be sheathed in a cosmetic cover (Fig. 31.7). Athletes may opt to interchange the basic prosthetic foot for one designed for sprinting (Fig. 31.8).

Articulated Feet

Manufactured with separate foot and lower shank sections, articulated feet have the sections joined by a metal

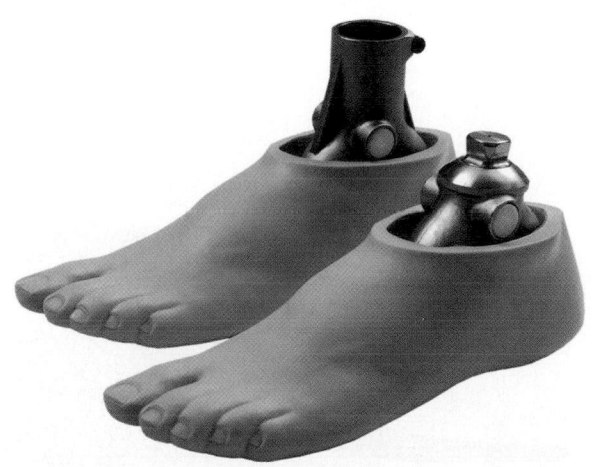

Figure 31.7 Cosmetic foot covers. *Courtesy of Ossur, Aliso Viejo, CA 92656.*

bolt or cable. Rubber bumpers usually control the ease of foot motion. Articulated feet are subject to eventual loosening, which may be signaled by a squeaking noise.

Single-Axis Feet

The most common example of an articulated foot is the *single-axis foot* (Fig. 31.9). A rear bumper absorbs shock and controls plantarflexion excursion; it is easy for the prosthetist to substitute a firmer or softer bumper, depending on the force that the patient applies in early stance. A heavy or very active client requires a firm bumper, whereas a frail individual needs a bumper that is soft enough to permit the foot to plantarflex with minimal loading. At early stance, bearing-weight on the heel causes the foot to plantarflex, ensuring that the wearer achieves the stable foot-flat position. Anterior to the ankle bolt is firmer rubber or similar material, the dorsiflexion stop, which resists dorsiflexion as the wearer transfers weight forward over the foot. The single-axis foot does not allow medial–lateral or transverse motion. Some people prefer this simplicity of control.

Multiple-Axis Feet

These components move slightly in all planes to aid the wearer in maintaining maximum contact with the

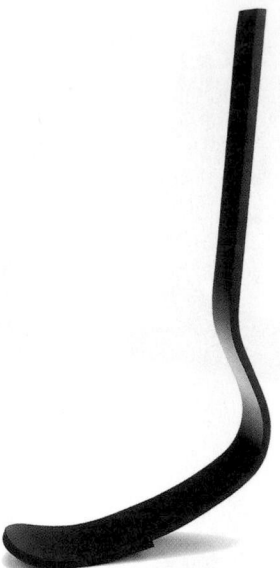

Figure 31.8 Flex-foot Cheetah® foot. *Courtesy of Ossur, Aliso Viejo, CA 92656.*

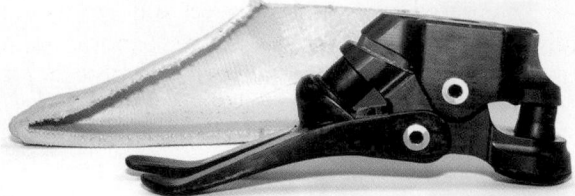

Figure 31.10 Multiple-axis foot.

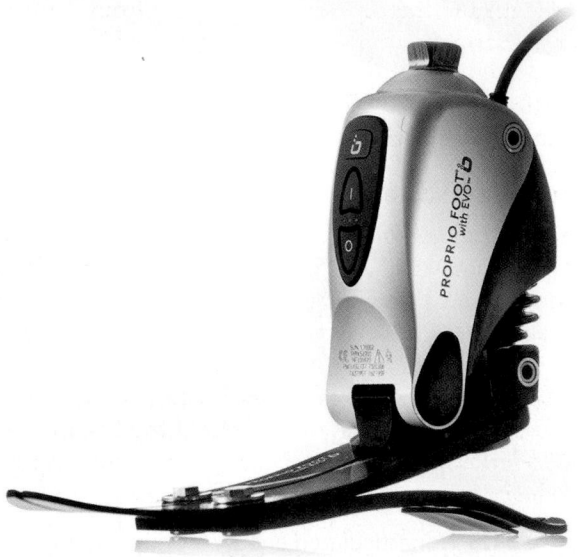

Figure 31.11 ProprioFoot®. *Courtesy of Ossur, Aliso Viejo, CA 92656.*

walking surface, even if the surface slopes or has slight irregularities (Fig. 31.10). A recent version of the multiple-axis foot is the ProprioFoot® (Fig. 31.11), which includes electronic sensors to detect when the wearer needs dorsiflexion; it also provides greater ankle excursion than other foot-ankle assemblies and reduces pressure on the amputation limb.[17,18] Multiple-axis feet are heavier and less durable than single-axis or nonarticulated feet.

Selection of the appropriate foot is based on the needs of the individual, considering the wearer's activity level, weight, and level of amputation, as well as the length and shape of the residual limb. The patient may also benefit from a rotator and a vertical shock absorber.

Rotators and Shock Absorbers

A rotator is a component placed above the prosthetic foot to absorb shear stress in the transverse plane. A shock absorber reduces vertical impact. These components protect the user from skin chafing, which would otherwise occur if the socket were permitted to slide against the skin.[19-21] Rotators and shock absorbers are

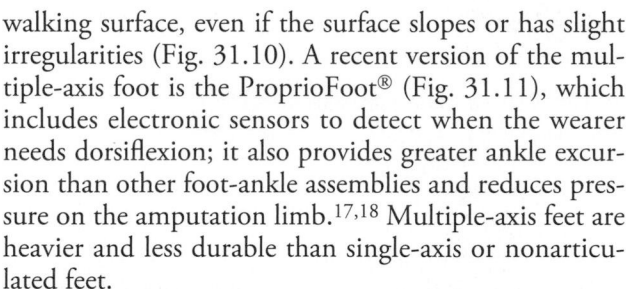

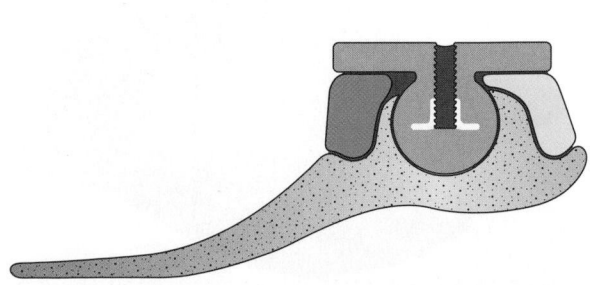

Figure 31.9 (*Left*) Single-axis foot. (*Right*) Cross section: anterior bumper controls dorsiflexion, posterior bumper controls plantarflexion.

most often used with single-axis feet and by very active individuals, especially those with transfemoral amputations. A rotator with or without a shock absorber may be contained within a prosthetic foot, such as Ceterus® (Fig. 31.6C), or may be installed in the shank, such as the Delta Twist® (Otto Bock, Minneapolis, MN 55447) (Fig. 31.12).

Shank

The shank is the substitute for the human leg, restoring leg length and transmitting body weight from the socket to the prosthetic foot. The shank is located between the foot-ankle assembly (or rotator) and the socket in a transtibial prosthesis. The two types of shank are *exoskeletal* and *endoskeletal*.

Exoskeletal Shank

The *exoskeletal shank* (Fig. 31.13 [*left*]), sometimes called *crustacean*, is typically made of rigid plastic (older versions are made of wood). The rigid exterior is shaped to simulate the contour of the anatomical leg. Although the shank is usually finished with plastic tinted to match the wearer's skin color, some individuals opt for a multicolored or patterned shank. The exoskeletal shank is very durable and, with the plastic finish, is impervious to liquids. Because they are less lifelike and do not permit changes in alignment of the prosthesis, exoskeletal shanks are less frequently prescribed.

Endoskeletal Shank

The *endoskeletal shank* (Fig 31.13 [*right*] and Fig. 31.14), or *modular shank*, consists of a central aluminum or rigid plastic tube (called a *pylon*) usually covered with foam rubber and a sturdy stocking or similar finish. With its cover, the endoskeletal shank is more natural in

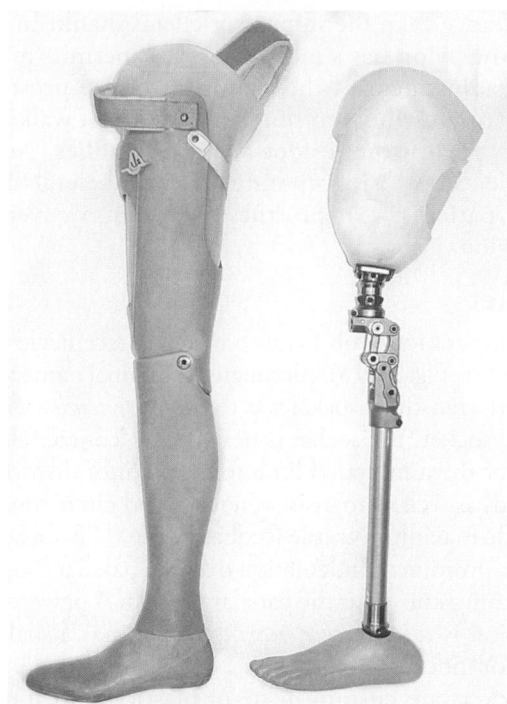

Figure 31.13 (*Left*) Exoskeletal transfemoral prosthesis. (*Right*) Endoskeletal transfemoral prosthesis with cosmetic cover removed.

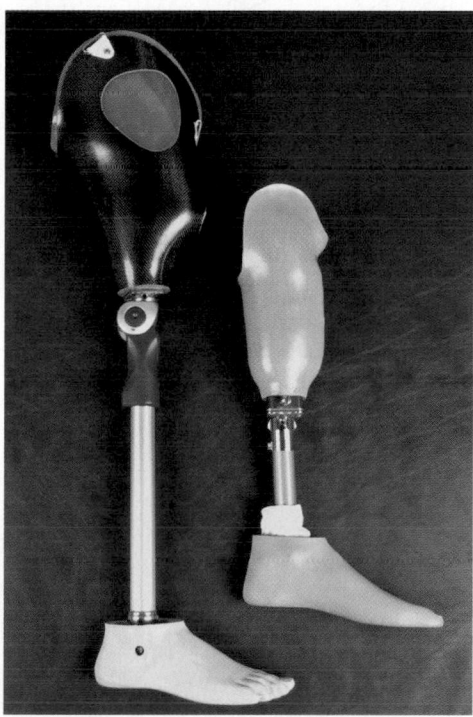

Figure 31.14 Endoskeletal (modular) shank on (*left*) transfemoral prosthesis and on (*right*) transtibial prosthesis. *From Roy, SH, Wolf, SL, and Scalzitti, DA: The Rehabilitation Specialist's Handbook, ed 4. FA Davis, Philadelphia, 2013, p 953, with permission.*

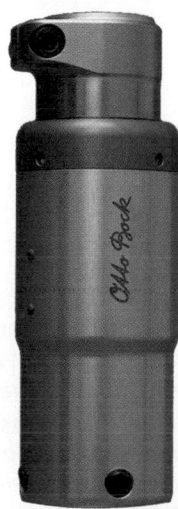

Figure 31.12 Rotator/shock absorber intended to be installed in pylon. *Delta Twist®, Courtesy of Otto Bock, Minneapolis, MN 55447.*

appearance than the shiny exoskeletal shank. In addition, the pylon has a mechanism that permits making slight adjustment of the alignment of the prosthesis; this may contribute to comfort and ease of walking. A variety of prosthetic foot-ankle assemblies, such as the Flex Foot®, incorporate an endoskeletal shank. Some patients wear prostheses without a cover over the pylon.

Socket

The amputation limb fits into a plastic receptacle called the socket (Fig. 31.15). Although the original name for the modern transtibial socket was the *patellar-tendon-bearing (PTB)* socket, the socket is designed to contact all portions of the amputated limb for maximum distribution of load, as well as to assist venous blood circulation and provide maximum tactile feedback. The PTB socket features a prominent indentation over the patellar ligament, sometimes known as the patellar tendon. A newer socket variation is *total surface bearing*, which has a shallower anterior indentation.[22]

Sockets are custom made of plastic molded over a model of the patient's amputation limb. The model may be produced from a plaster cast of the amputation limb or by *computer-aided design/computer-aided manufacture (CAD-CAM)*. The latter involves an electronic sensor, which transmits a detailed map of the limb to a computerized program consisting of socket-shape variations; the prosthetist selects the appropriate shape, which is transmitted to an electronic carver that creates the model over which the plastic is shaped. Whether the model is made by hand or by computer, it provides *reliefs*, concavities in the socket over areas contacting sensitive structures, such as bony prominences; reliefs are located over the fibular head, tibial crest, tibial condyles, and anterior–distal tibia. The posterior brim is shaped to provide adequate room for the medial and lateral hamstring tendons, so that the patient is comfortable when sitting. *Build-ups* are convexities in the socket over areas contacting pressure-tolerant tissues, such as the belly of the gastrocnemius; patellar ligament; proximomedial tibia, corresponding to the pes anserinus; and the tibial and fibular shafts (see Fig. 31.15).

When viewed from above, the socket resembles a triangle, the apex of which is formed by the relief for the tibial tubercle and crest, and the base angles of which are the hamstring reliefs. The anterior wall terminates at the mid-patella, or above. The medial and lateral walls extend at least to the femoral condyles. The posterior wall lies across the popliteal fossa.

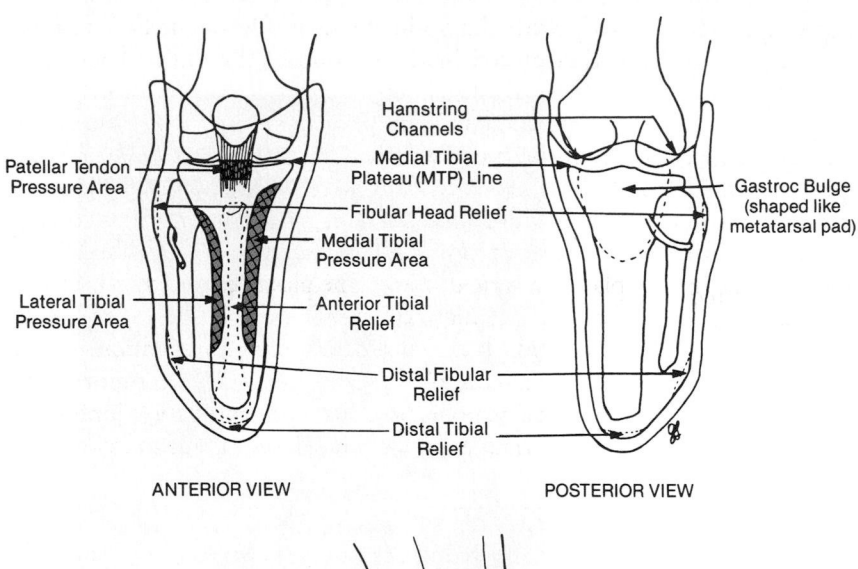

Patellar Tendon Pressure Area

Hamstring Channels

Medial Tibial Plateau (MTP) Line

Fibular Head Relief

Medial Tibial Pressure Area

Gastroc Bulge (shaped like metatarsal pad)

Lateral Tibial Pressure Area

Anterior Tibial Relief

Distal Fibular Relief

Distal Tibial Relief

ANTERIOR VIEW　　　　POSTERIOR VIEW

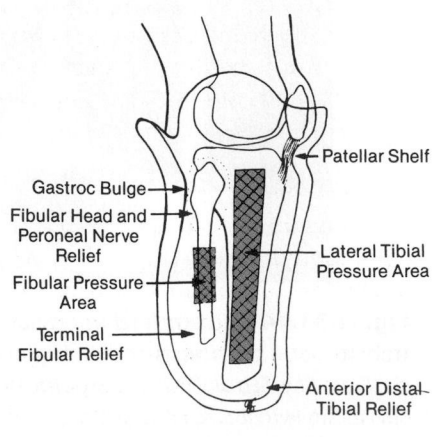

Patellar Shelf

Gastroc Bulge

Fibular Head and Peroneal Nerve Relief

Fibular Pressure Area

Lateral Tibial Pressure Area

Terminal Fibular Relief

Anterior Distal Tibial Relief

LATERAL VIEW

Figure 31.15 Transtibial patellar-tendon-bearing socket. Areas of relief (also called *channels*) over pressure-sensitive tissues. Build-ups (also called *bulges*) contact pressure-tolerant tissues. *From Sanders, GT: Lower Limb Amputations: A Guide to Rehabilitation. FA Davis, Philadelphia, 1986, p 176, with permission.*

The socket is aligned on the shank in slight flexion to enhance loading on the patellar ligament, prevent genu recurvatum, and resist the tendency of the amputation limb to slide too deeply into the socket. Flexion also facilitates contraction of the quadriceps muscle. The socket is also aligned with a slight lateral tilt to reduce loading on the fibular head.[23,24]

Lined Socket

The transtibial socket generally includes a resilient liner, made of polyethylene foam,[25] polyurethane,[26] silicone,[27] or similar materials. In addition to cushioning the amputation limb, the removable liner facilitates alteration of socket size; the prosthetist can add material to the outside of the liner, reducing the volume of the socket while preserving smooth interior contours. The liner, however, adds to the bulk of the prosthesis and is a heat insulator, which the wearer may find uncomfortable in hot weather. Individuals with Syme's and transtibial amputations usually wear cotton, wool, or synthetic fabric socks to ensure a snug socket fit. An alternative to the polyethylene liner is a sheath made of silicone or similar material, which fits so snugly that the wearer has little risk of abrasion between the socket and skin.

Socks, Sheaths, and Liners

All individuals with LE amputations, except those wearing transfemoral prostheses suspended by total suction or those using a sheath, require a supply of clean socks of appropriate material, size, and shape. It is expeditious to order at least a dozen socks at the time the prosthesis is prescribed, so that third-party payment may cover this relatively inexpensive but important accessory.

Fabric socks are woven in various thicknesses, referred to as *ply*, designating the number of threads knitted together. Cotton socks absorb perspiration readily and are the least allergenic; they are made in two-, three-, and five-ply, the last being the thickest. Wool socks provide good cushioning, woven in three-, five-, and six-ply; they are expensive and must be laundered carefully. Orlon/Lycra socks are manufactured in two- and three-ply thicknesses. They can be washed easily without shrinking. This synthetic fabric combination affords considerable resilience, but does not absorb much perspiration.

A nylon sheath creates a smooth surface over the skin, thereby reducing the risk of chafing, especially in hot weather and among those with much scarring. Some transtibial prosthesis wearers are able to use a woman's knee-high nylon stocking if the amputated limb is slender. Because nylon does not absorb sweat, liquid passes through the weave to be absorbed by an outer sock of cotton or wool. Silicone, urethane, and other synthetic sheaths provide excellent shock absorption and abrasion resistance; they also can aid in suspending the socket on the patient's limb, and are designed to be worn next to the skin. They are, however, more expensive than fabric socks or sheaths.

It is common practice to add more socks as the amputation limb volume reduces. Nevertheless, when the patient requires a total of 15-ply of socks to achieve snug fit, the socket should be altered or replaced by the prosthetist. Excessive sock padding distorts the weight-bearing characteristics of the socket, losing the effect of strategically placed build-ups and reliefs.

Regardless of material, the shape of the sock or sheath is important for comfort. An interface of proper size fits smoothly without wrinkling or undue stretching. The sock or sheath should be long enough to terminate above the most proximal part of the socket.

Silicone gel suspension liners are another form of socket-residual limb interface. These liners cushion the residual limb as well as function as a primary or secondary suspension system. Some include a nylon outer cover, with liner thickness tapering distally, and may be indicated for particularly active users and those with fragile or sensitive residual limbs. They are available in locking, custom, and seal-in designs (Fig. 31.16).

Unlined Socket

Although the unlined socket is sometimes referred to as a hard socket, that term is a misnomer, because the wearer has a soft interface provided by socks or a sheath worn with the unlined socket. Occasionally, a resilient pad is placed in the bottom of the unlined socket to cushion the distal end of the amputation limb. The unlined socket is a more satisfactory choice for the person whose limb has stabilized in volume, because it is easier to clean; however, it is more difficult to alter the shape of the unlined socket in comparison to the lined socket.

A newer type of unlined socket is made of thin thermoplastic in a rigid frame. The plastic can be spot-heated to facilitate alteration of socket fit. It adheres to the skin better than rigid plastic, thereby improving suspension. It contributes to comfort by dissipating body heat more effectively and responds to changes in amputation limb shape as the patient contracts and relaxes various muscles.

Suspension

During the swing phase of walking, or whenever the wearer is not standing on the prosthesis, such as when climbing stairs or jumping, the prosthesis requires some form of suspension to hold it in place.

Cuff Variants

The modern transtibial prosthesis originated with a supracondylar cuff (Fig. 31.17 [*left*]), which is still widely used. The cuff may be a leather, flexible plastic, or fabric-webbing strap. It encircles the thigh immediately above the femoral condyles, and permits the user to adjust the snugness of suspension easily. Some individuals, however, object to the profile of the distal thigh created by the cuff. Others who have severely arthritic

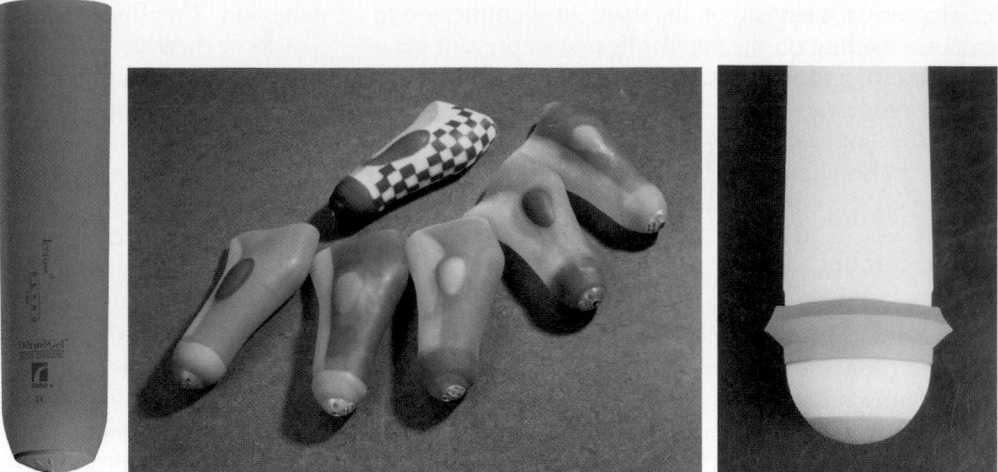

Figure 31.16 Silicone liners: (*Left*) Iceross® Dermo locking silicone gel liner. *Courtesy of Ossur, Aliso Viejo, CA 92656.* (*Middle*) Custom liners with fibular head padding. *Courtesy of Otto Bock, Minneapolis, MN 55447.* (*Right*) Seal-in designs. *From Roy, SH, Wolf, SL, and Scalzitti, DA: The Rehabilitation Specialist's Handbook, ed 4. FA Davis, Philadelphia, 2013, p 977, with permission.*

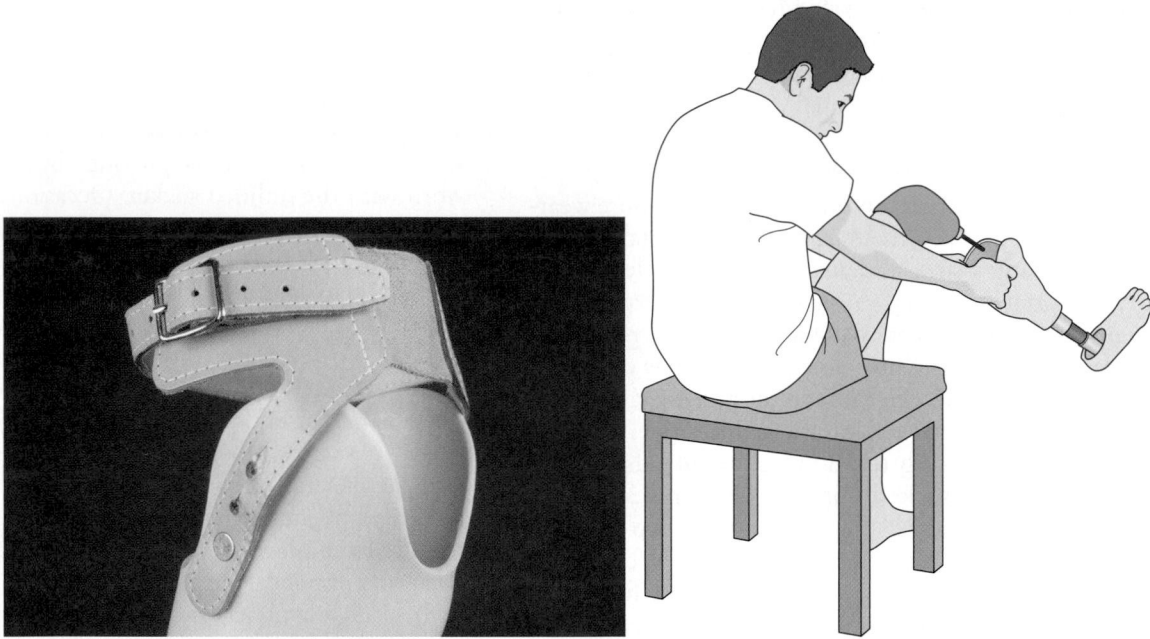

Figure 31.17 (*Left*) Supracondylar cuff suspension for transtibial prostheses. *From Roy, SH, Wolf, SL, and Scalzitti, DA: The Rehabilitation Specialist's Handbook, ed 4. FA Davis, Philadelphia, 2013, p 977, with permission.* (*Right*) Patient donning a transtibial prosthesis using a roll-on sleeve that includes a pin and shuttle lock assembly.

hands or limited vision have difficulty engaging the buckle or pressure hook-and-loop closure on the cuff.

A fork strap and waist belt may be used to augment the cuff. The elastic fork strap extends from the outside of the anterior portion of the socket to a waist belt. The fork strap and waist belt may be indicated for individuals who climb ladders or engage in other activities during which the prosthesis is unsupported by the ground for long periods. Alternatives to the cuff

include a rubber sleeve, a tubular component that covers the proximal socket and the distal thigh; or a sleeve that includes a distal pin to create a shuttle lock (Fig. 31.17 [*right*]), described in the following section titled Distal Attachments. The sleeve provides excellent suspension and a streamlined silhouette when the wearer sits. Donning the sleeve, however, requires two strong hands and a thigh that does not have excessive subcutaneous tissue.

Distal Attachments

Very secure suspension is achieved with the use of a silicone sheath with a distal metal pin (Fig. 31.18; see Fig 31.17 [*right*]). The sheath clings to the skin. The user inserts the sheathed limb into the prosthesis, guiding the attached pin into a receptacle, also called a shuttle lock, in the socket. During swing phase, the pin mechanism prevents the prosthesis from slipping.

Vacuum-assisted suspension is another alternative mode of suspension. The system (Fig. 31.19) combines a pump, liner, and sleeve to achieve elevated vacuum in an airtight environment. Vacuum promotes fluid exchange, reduces moisture buildup, regulates volume fluctuations, and increases proprioceptive awareness of the limb's position in space.

A surgical approach to distal attachment is known as *osseointegration*[28] in which the surgeon implants a metal post in the distal bone. The post protrudes through the skin and locks into a mechanism in the prosthesis. Osseointegration eliminates the need for other suspension apparatus; however, fluid drainage and infection at the skin/post interface are sometimes troublesome. The procedure was developed in Europe and is not yet readily available in North America.

Brim Variants

The socket walls may be extended proximally to suspend the prosthesis. With *supracondylar (SC) suspension* (Fig. 31.20 [*left*]), the medial and lateral walls extend above the femoral condyles. Some SC suspension designs include a plastic wedge on the medial wall (Fig. 31.20 [*middle*]). When donning the prosthesis, the client removes the wedge, places the amputation limb in the socket, and then places the wedge between the socket and the medial condyle to retain the prosthesis on the limb. Alternatively, the wedge can be incorporated in a

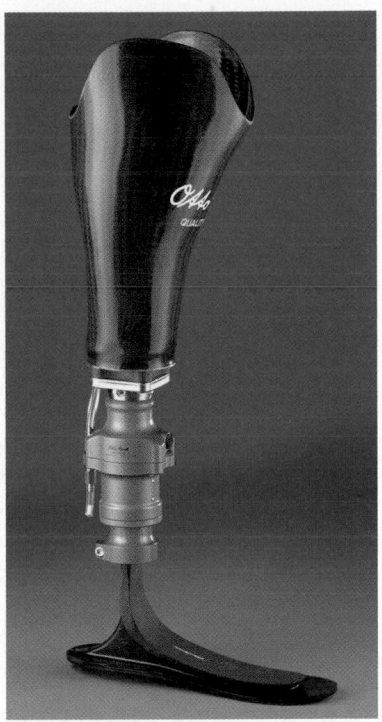

Figure 31.19 Harmony® Volume Management System. *Courtesy of Otto Bock, Minneapolis, MN 55447.*

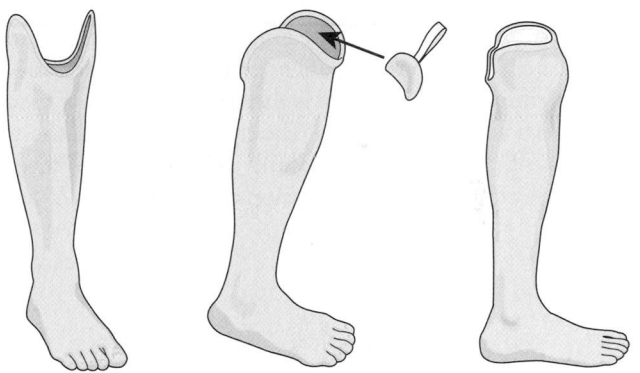

Figure 31.20 (*Left*) Transtibial prosthesis with supracondylar (SC) suspension. (*Middle*) SC suspension using wedge insert. (*Right*) Transtibial socket with supracondylar/suprapatellar (SC/SP) suspension.

liner; for donning, the patient applies the liner, and then inserts the limb, with liner, into the socket. Supracondylar suspension increases medial–lateral stability of the prosthesis, presents a pleasing contour at the knee, and eliminates the need to engage a buckle or hook-and-loop closure on a cuff. It is more difficult to fabricate (and, hence, more expensive), and it is not readily adjustable.

Presenting a contour of medial and lateral walls similar to the supracondylar suspension, the supracondylar/suprapatellar (SC/SP) suspension (Fig. 31.20 [*right*]) also features an anterior wall that terminates above the patella.

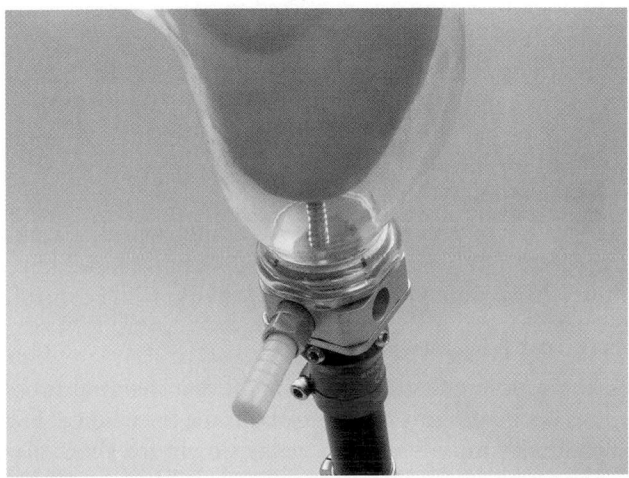

Figure 31.18 Transtibial distal pin attachment. The pin fits into a receptacle in the socket bottom and is then tightened into place.

The short amputated limb is well accommodated by SC/SP suspension. The high anterior wall may interfere with kneeling and presents a conspicuous contour when the wearer sits.

Thigh Corset

Some individuals with very sensitive skin may benefit from thigh corset suspension (Fig. 31.21). Metal hinges attach distally to the medial and lateral aspects of the socket and proximally to a flexible plastic corset. Corset heights vary and may reach the ischial tuberosity for maximum weight relief on the amputation limb. The hinges increase frontal plane stability, and the corset increases area for weight-bearing load distribution. The resulting prosthesis, however, is heavier and apt to foster piston action because the hinges have a single pivot joint that does not articulate collinearly with the anatomical knee. Prolonged use of a thigh corset produces pressure atrophy of the thigh. A prosthesis with corset suspension is more difficult to don because the wearer must fasten a series of pressure closure hook-and-loop straps.

■ TRANSFEMORAL PROSTHESES

Individuals with amputation between the femoral condyles and greater trochanter are fitted with transfemoral (above-knee) prostheses. Those whose limbs retain the distal part of the femur can wear a knee disarticulation prosthesis, which differs from the transfemoral prosthesis in the type of knee unit and socket. If the amputation is proximal to the greater trochanter, the patient cannot retain or control a transfemoral prosthesis and is therefore a candidate for a hip disarticulation prosthesis. The transfemoral prosthesis consists of (1) foot-ankle assembly; (2) shank; (3) knee unit; (4) socket; and (5) suspension device.

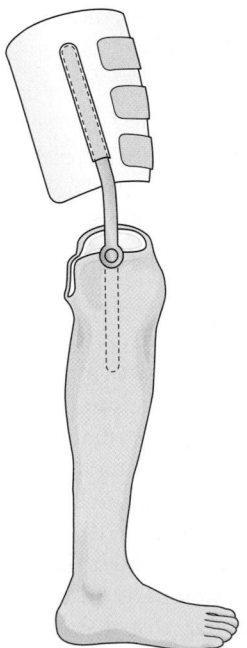

Figure 31.21 Transtibial thigh corset suspension.

Foot-Ankle Assemblies and Shanks

Although the SACH foot is often prescribed for transfemoral prostheses, the single-axis foot is more frequently used for transfemoral than for transtibial prostheses. The single-axis foot reaches the foot-flat position with minimal application of weight-bearing load. Nevertheless, almost any foot, including the energy storing/releasing designs, can be incorporated in a transfemoral prosthesis. As compared with wearers of transtibial prostheses, however, most wearers of transfemoral prostheses do not load the prosthesis as vigorously. Consequently, less energy would be stored and released in a dynamic response foot.

Either the sturdy exoskeletal shank or the more attractive endoskeletal shank may be used. The latter creates a more pleasing appearance, particularly in the knee area, is adjustable in alignment, and is lighter than an exoskeletal shank. Limited research is inconclusive regarding the merit of minimizing prosthetic weight.[29] Problems of durability remain, particularly at the knee, where constant bending of the joint, especially when the wearer is kneeling, accelerates deterioration of the rubber cover. A rotator with or without a shock absorber incorporated in the shank diminishes shear stress on the amputation limb.[30]

Knee Units

The prosthetic knee enables the user to bend the knee when sitting or kneeling and, in most instances, also permits knee flexion during the latter portion of the stance phase and throughout the swing phase of walking. Commercial knee units may be described according to four features: (1) axis; (2) friction mechanism; (3) extension aid; and (4) mechanical stabilizer. Many combinations of features are available; not every knee unit has all four components.

Axis System

The thigh piece can be connected to the shank either by a *single-axis hinge*, which is a common arrangement, or by *polycentric linkage*. Polycentric systems (Fig. 31.22) have pivoting bars and provide greater stability to the knee, inasmuch as the momentary center of knee rotation is posterior to the wearer's weight line during most of stance phase.[31] The polycentric knee provides mechanical swing control that allows a single optimal walking speed. For variable cadence, some polycentric knee units incorporate pneumatic or hydraulic swing control.

Friction Mechanisms

In the simplest sense, the leg of the transfemoral prosthesis is a pendulum swinging about the knee hinge. For the elderly individual who walks slowly for short distances, a basic pendulum is adequate. More energetic walkers, however, benefit from adjustable friction mechanisms that modify the pendulum action of the leg to reduce the asymmetry between the motions of the sound

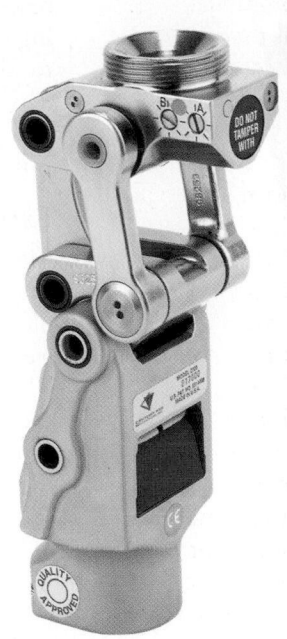
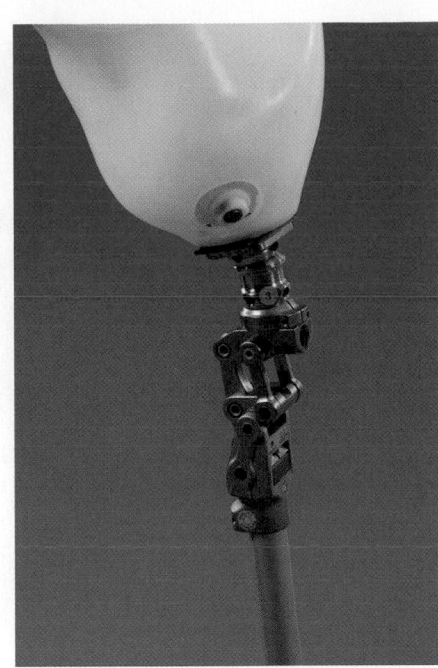

Figure 31.22 (*Left*) Polycentric knee unit designed to provide stability during stance. *Courtesy of Ossur, Aliso Viejo, CA 92656.* (*Right*) Polycentric knee unit in place on a transfemoral prosthesis.

and prosthetic limbs. If the prosthetic knee does not have sufficient friction to retard its natural pendulum action, the person who walks rapidly experiences excessive knee flexion (high heel rise) at the beginning of swing phase and abrupt, often noisy, knee extension at the end of swing phase (terminal swing impact). Friction mechanisms change the leg swing by modifying knee motion during various parts of swing phase and by affecting knee swing according to walking speed. Two interrelated issues involved in friction mechanisms are the time during swing phase when friction affects the knee unit and the medium through which the mechanism operates.

Constant and Variable

The most commonly prescribed knee unit has *constant friction* (Fig. 31.23), generally a pair of clamps that grasp the knee bolt. The clamps resist shank motion throughout swing phase time, providing a constant amount of friction. The clamps are easy to loosen or tighten to change the ease of knee motion. A more sophisticated device applies *variable friction*, in which the amount of

friction changes during a given portion of swing phase. At early swing, high friction is applied to retard excessive knee flexion; during midswing, friction diminishes to permit the knee to swing easily; at late swing, friction increases to dampen impact.

Medium

The medium through which friction is applied influences performance. The usual medium is *sliding friction,* contact of one solid structure on another. A clamp sliding about the knee bolt is simple and inexpensive, but it does not accommodate automatically to changes in walking speed. A more complex approach is *fluid friction,* either oil (*hydraulic friction*) (Fig. 31.24) or air (*pneumatic friction*). Unlike sliding friction, fluid friction varies directly with velocity. Thus with a hydraulic or pneumatic unit, if the wearer walks faster, the knee increases friction instantly to prevent excessive knee flexion and abrupt extension. Consequently, the movements of the prosthetic and sound limbs are less asymmetrical than would be the case with sliding friction. Oil or air is contained in a cylinder in the knee unit. A piston descends in the cylinder during early swing, causing the knee to flex. The speed of piston descent depends on the type of fluid and the walking speed. Later, the piston ascends, extending the knee. Hydraulic units provide more friction than do pneumatic devices. Both types are more expensive than the simpler sliding friction designs.

Microprocessor-controlled hydraulic units, such as the C-Leg® (Fig. 31.25), utilize electronic sensors, which detect the rate and range of shank movement 50 or more times per second, providing almost instant friction adjustment to changes in the gait pattern.[32-41] Units are programmed with a computer, and may provide stumble

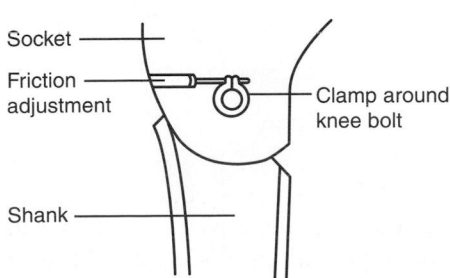

Figure 31.23 Constant-friction knee unit with clamp that encircles the knee bolt.

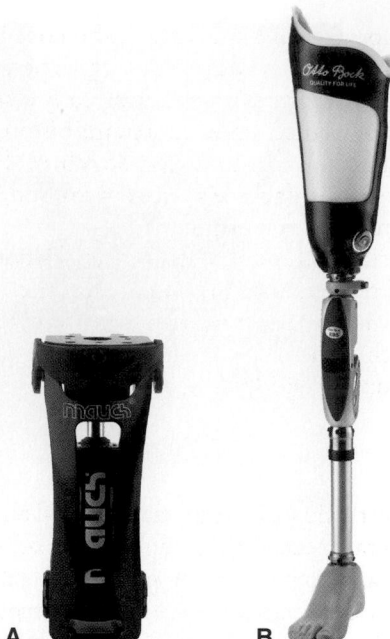

Figure 31.24 (A) Mauch® (SNS®) single-axis hydraulic knee unit with swing and stance control. *Courtesy of Ossur, Aliso Viejo, CA 92656.* **(B)** The 3R60 Ergonomically Balanced Stride (EBS) hydraulic system controls the knee during swing allowing greater ease in initiating swing and a greater range of walking speeds. Note that this prosthesis includes a flexible socket supported within a rigid frame. *Courtesy of Otto Bock, Minneapolis, MN 55447.*

recovery, locking option, and accommodation to walking on various terrain and bicycle riding. An alternative to oil-filled hydraulic units is the Rheo® knee (Ossur, Aliso Viejo, CA 92656), which has magnetized fluid and sensors that detect knee action in much smaller time units.[42]

Extension Aids

Many knee units include a mechanism to assist knee extension during the latter part of swing phase. The simplest type is an *external extension aid*, consisting of elastic webbing in front of the knee axis. The elastic stretches when the knee flexes in early swing and recoils to extend the knee in late swing. Webbing tension is easily adjusted, but tends to pull the knee into extension when the wearer sits. The *internal extension aid* is an elastic strap or coiled spring within the knee unit. It functions identically to the external aid during walking, but unlike the external aid, the internal type keeps the knee flexed when the individual sits. Acute knee flexion causes the strap or spring to pass behind the knee axis, maintaining the flexed attitude. Fluid-controlled knee units incorporate an internal extension aid.

Although most extension aids affect the wearer's performance during late swing and early stance phases, the Power Knee® (Fig. 31.26) also assists the user to ascend stairs step-over-step as well as to rise from a chair. The unit incorporates accelerometers, gyroscopes, a torque sensor, and an on-board computer.

Stabilizers

Most knee units do not have a special device to increase stability. The patient controls prosthetic knee action by hip motion, aided by the alignment of the knee in relation

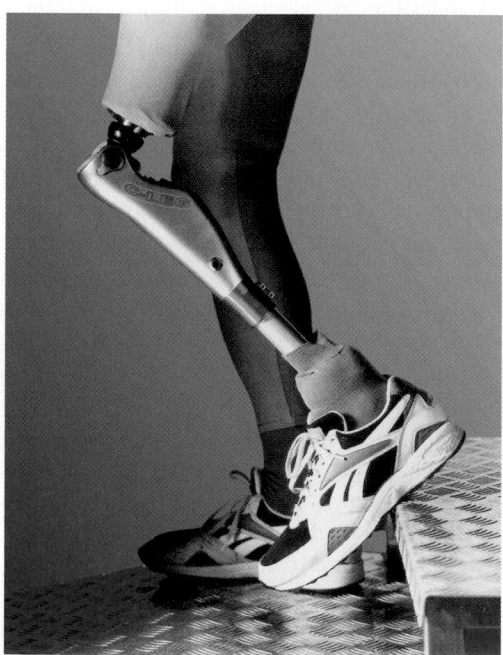

Figure 31.25 C-Leg®. *Courtesy of Otto Bock, Minneapolis, MN 55447.*

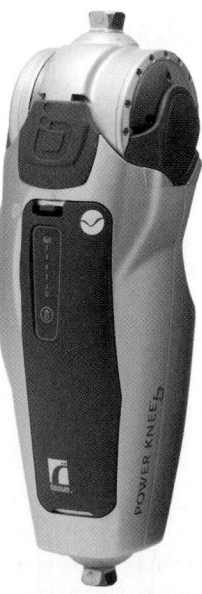

Figure 31.26 Power Knee®. *Courtesy of Ossur, Aliso Viejo, CA 92656.*

to other components of the prosthesis. The knee axis is usually aligned posterior to a line extending from the greater trochanter to the ankle (trochanter-knee-ankle [TKA] line). The patient who has excellent balance and muscular control may have the knee bolt placed on the line, thus creating TKA alignment. Some hydraulic knee units are aligned with the knee axis anterior to the trochanter-ankle line. Elderly or debilitated patients may benefit from a stabilizing mechanism, as do some people who walk on very rough terrain, such as hunters.

Manual Lock

The simplest mechanical stabilizer is a manual lock (Fig. 31.27), in which a rod lodges in a receptacle and is released only when the wearer manipulates an unlocking lever. When engaged, the manual lock prevents knee flexion. The user is secure not only during early stance when stability is desired, but also throughout the entire gait cycle. To compensate for difficulty in advancing the locked prosthesis, the shank should be shortened approximately 1/2 in (1 cm). The manual lock must be disengaged when the wearer sits. Nevertheless, some people with impaired balance prefer the stability of the locked knee.[43]

Friction Brake

A more elaborate stabilizing system, the *friction brake*, provides very high friction during early stance as the wearer bears weight on the prosthesis, resisting the tendency of the knee to flex.[44] One design, incorporated in a sliding friction unit, involves the mating of a wedge

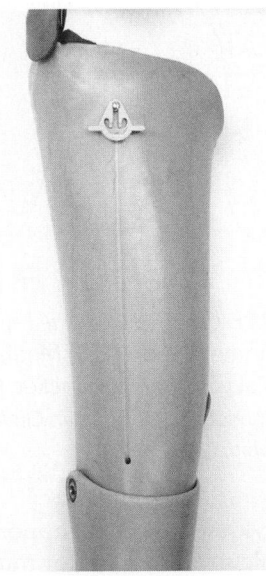

Figure 31.27 Single-axis knee unit with manual lock. Note that this configuration has a proximal release attached by a high-density plastic wire to the knee. For patients with impaired balance, the proximal release eliminates the need to flex forward and reach down to the knee unit for unlocking.

and groove upon loading, assuming the knee is flexed less than 25 degrees. Another version of friction brake is found in some hydraulic units; during early stance, additional fluid resistance markedly retards piston descent within the fluid cylinder and thus stabilizes the knee. Microprocessor units include stance control and, in most instances, a manual lock option.

From midstance through heel contact, friction brakes do not interfere with knee motion. In addition, they do not impede the patient who transfers from sitting to standing. Such devices add to the cost of the prosthesis and, if improperly used, may not protect the patient from falling.

Sockets

As with all prosthetic sockets, the transfemoral one should be a total-contact receptacle to distribute load over the maximum area, thereby reducing pressure. Total-contact fitting also provides counterpressure to assist venous return and prevent distal edema, and enhances sensory feedback to foster better control of the prosthesis.

Most transfemoral sockets are made of a flexible thermoplastic socket encased in a rigid frame. The frame enables the wearer to transmit weight through the distal components of the prosthesis to the ground. The flexible socket provides sensory input from external objects, such as chairs; it also dissipates body heat and facilitates alterations in socket fit. A polyester laminate socket is entirely rigid.

Transfemoral sockets are designed to emphasize loading on pressure-tolerant structures, such as the gluteal musculature, sides of the thigh, and, to a lesser extent, distal end of the amputated limb. The socket must avoid excessive pressure on the pubic symphysis and perineum.

Quadrilateral Socket

The basic transfemoral socket shape is quadrilateral when viewed from above (Fig. 31.28). The socket features a horizontal posterior shelf for the ischial tuberosity and gluteal musculature, a medial brim at the same level as the posterior shelf, an anterior wall 2.5 to 3 in (6 to 8 cm) higher to apply a posteriorly directed force to the thigh to retain the ischial tuberosity on its shelf, and a lateral wall the same height as the anterior wall to aid in medial–lateral stabilization. Concave reliefs are (1) anteromedial, for the pressure-sensitive adductor longus tendon and obturator nerve; (2) posteromedial, for the sensitive hamstring tendons and sciatic nerve; (3) posterolateral, to permit the gluteus maximus to contract and bulge without being crowded; and (4) anterolateral, to allow adequate room for the rectus femoris. The anterior wall has a convexity, Scarpa's bulge, to maximize pressure distribution in the vicinity of the femoral (Scarpa's) triangle. The lateral wall may have reliefs for the greater trochanter and the distal end of the femur.

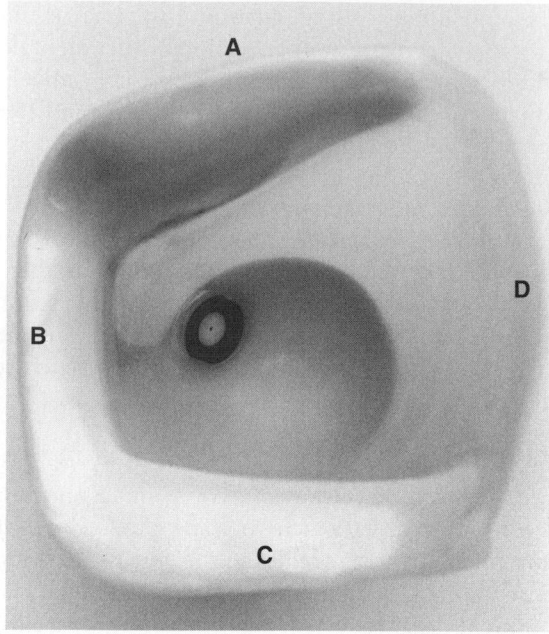

Figure 31.28 Quadrilateral socket viewed from above. **(A)** Anterior wall. **(B)** Medial wall. **(C)** Posterior wall. **(D)** Lateral wall.

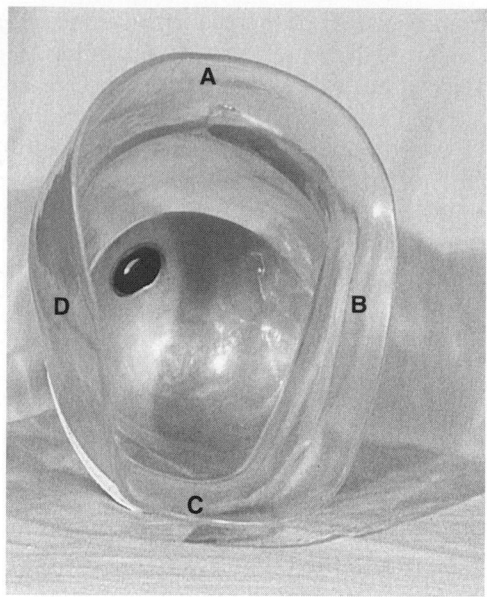

Figure 31.29 Ischial containment flexible transfemoral socket. **(A)** Anterior brim. **(B)** Medial brim. **(C)** Posterior brim. **(D)** Lateral brim.

Ischial Containment Socket

An alternate design type is the ischial containment socket (Fig. 31.29), sometimes called the *contoured adducted trochanter-controlled alignment method.*[45,46] Its walls cover the ischial tuberosity and part of the ischiopubic ramus to augment socket stability. To increase frontal plane stability and minimize bulk between the thighs, the mediolateral width of the socket is narrower than that of the quadrilateral socket. The anterior wall is lower than in the quadrilateral socket, whereas the lateral wall covers the greater trochanter. Weight-bearing occurs on the sides and bottom of the amputated limb.

Slight socket flexion is desirable for the following reasons: (1) to facilitate contraction of the hip extensors; (2) to reduce lumbar lordosis; and (3) to provide a zone through which the thigh may be extended to permit the wearer to take steps of approximately equal length. For wearers of quadrilateral sockets, socket flexion also enhances positioning of the ischial tuberosity on the posterior brim. Figure 31.30 presents a schematic of pelvic position within the ischial containment socket.

ComfortFlex™ Socket

The ComfortFlex™ (Hanger, Inc., Oklahoma City, OK 73118) is a soft flexible socket (plastic and silicone materials) placed in a carbon graphic frame (Fig. 31.31). This sockets design is available for various-level amputations (e.g., transfemoral, transtibial, hip disarticulation, hemipelvectomy). The carbon

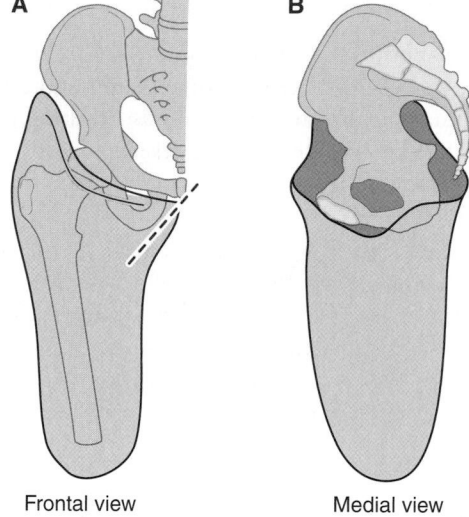

Frontal view   Medial view

Figure 31.30 (A) Frontal view of the femur and pelvis in the ischial containment socket. **(B)** Medial view of the pelvis in the ischial containment socket. *From May, BJ, and Lockard, MA: Prosthetics and Orthotics in Clinical Practice. FA Davis, Philadelphia, 2011, p 95.*

fiber frame provides structural support while the intimately fit flexible socket allows for muscle contraction and improved control of the prosthesis. The transfemoral socket is designed to "lock" the ischium and pubic ramus into the socket improving anterior/posterior and lateral stability and reducing socket rotation. The sockets are contoured to accommodate bone and soft tissue structures (e.g., muscles, tendons, nerves, vascular structures).

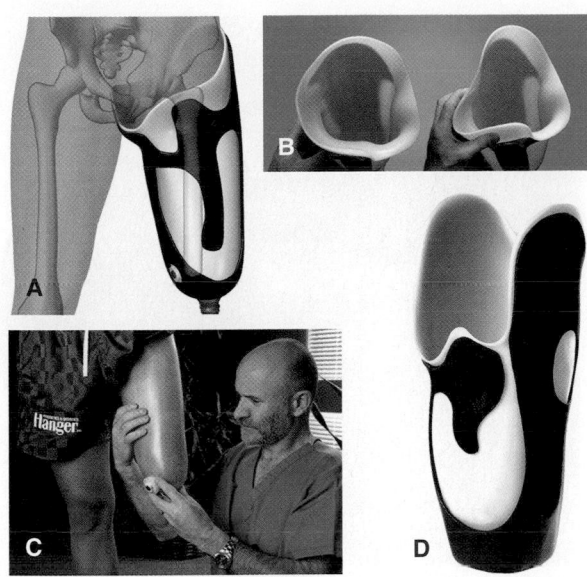

Figure 31.31 ComfortFlex™ socket design. **(A)** Anatomical orientation of transfemoral socket. **(B)** Overhead view of transfemoral socket (thumb and finger pressure illustrating socket flexibility). **(C)** Socket without carbon graphic frame. **(D)** Transtibial socket design. *Courtesy of Hanger, Inc., Oklahoma City, OK 73118.*

Suspensions

Three means are used to suspend the transfemoral prosthesis: (1) total suction, (2) partial suction, and (3) no suction (require auxiliary suspension).

Suspension Suspension

Suction refers to the difference between pressure inside and outside the socket. With suction suspension, internal socket pressure is less than external pressure; consequently, atmospheric pressure causes the socket to remain on the thigh. A one-way air-release valve located at the bottom of the socket enables residual air to be expelled.

Total Suction

Maximum control of the prosthesis, without any encumbering auxiliary suspension can be achieved only when the socket brim fits very snugly. Some people add a transfemoral suspension sleeve (Fig. 31.32), especially when engaging in vigorous activities. If the patient experiences reduction in amputation limb volume, suction will be lost and an auxiliary suspension will be required.

Partial Suction

A socket that is slightly loose may provide partial suction suspension combined with auxiliary suspension; the socket has a valve. The patient wears one or more socks, or a synthetic liner. Because air enters the space between the sock's fibers, auxiliary suspension is needed, either a fabric Silesian belt (Fig. 31.33), or a rigid plastic or metal hip joint and pelvic band. These aids encircle the pelvis. The Silesian belt also controls the transverse plane

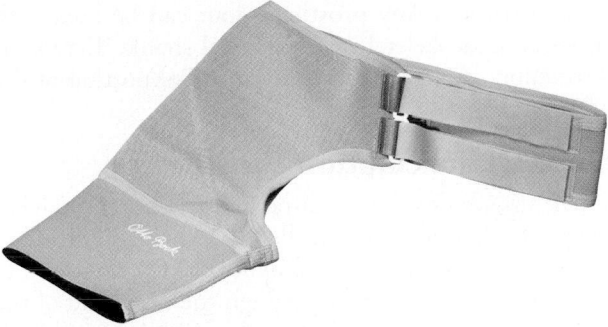

Figure 31.32 Transfemoral suspension sleeve. *Courtesy of Otto Bock, Minneapolis, MN 55447.*

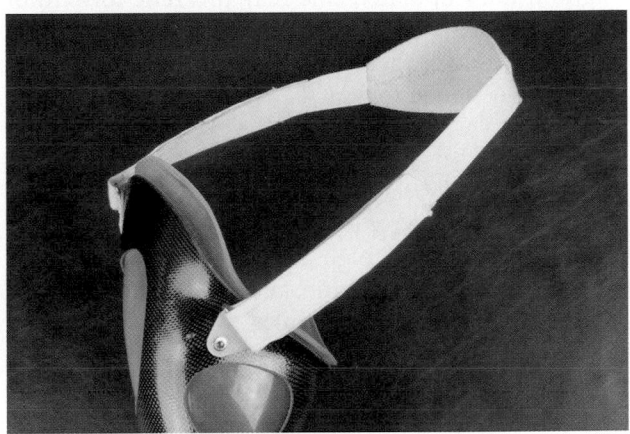

Figure 31.33 Silesian belt. *From Roy, SH, Wolf, SL, and Scalzitti, DA: The Rehabilitation Specialist's Handbook, ed 4. FA Davis, Philadelphia, 2013, p 977, with permission).*

orientation of the prosthesis on the thigh, while the hip joint restricts transverse and frontal motion at the hip. The pelvic band adds weight to the prosthesis and may impose uncomfortable pressure against the torso when the wearer sits.

No Suction

If the socket has a distal hole without a valve, then no pressure difference exists between the inside and the outside of the socket. The client wears one or more socks and requires a pelvic band. The pelvic band has a rigid metal or nylon single-axis hip joint attached to a leather belt, which encircles the pelvis. The relatively loose socket makes donning easy, but hinders control of the prosthesis and may make sitting uncomfortable.

Osseous integration is another less common suspension alternative. A metal post implanted in the femur locks into a fixture embedded in the distal portion of the socket.[45]

■ DISARTICULATION PROSTHESES

Individuals with knee or hip disarticulation wear prostheses that include the same distal components as prostheses for lower levels. Any prosthetic foot can be used with either an endoskeletal or exoskeletal shank. The major distinction, therefore, is in the proximal portion of the prostheses.

Knee Disarticulation Prostheses

When amputation is at or distal to the femoral condyles, the patient should have excellent prosthetic control because (1) thigh leverage is maximum; (2) most of the body weight can be borne through the distal end of the femur; and (3) the broad condyles provide rotational stability.[46,47] The problem presented by knee disarticulation is primarily cosmetic; when the individual sits, the thigh on the amputated side may protrude forward of the sound knee. The knee disarticulation prosthesis has a streamlined knee that minimizes protrusion, as well as a specially designed socket.

Knee Units

Several units are specifically manufactured for knee disarticulation. All have a thin proximal attachment plate to minimize added thigh length. One may choose among hydraulic, pneumatic, and sliding friction units, with or without polycentric linkage. Even with a special knee unit, the thigh will be slightly longer. Consequently, the shank is shortened equivalently, so that when the person stands, the pelvis is level. When the individual sits, the thigh on the prosthetic side will project slightly.

Sockets

Two types of sockets are currently in use. Both are made of plastic and usually terminate below the ischial tuberosity. Generally, no additional suspension aids are needed. One version features an anterior opening to accommodate a bulbous amputation limb. After the limb is inserted, the wearer closes the socket with lacing or hook-and-loop closure. The other design has no anterior opening and is suitable for limbs that are not bulbous.

Hip Disarticulation Prostheses

A hip disarticulation prosthesis[48,49] (Fig. 31.34) is fitted to a person with amputation above the greater trochanter (very short transfemoral), removal of the femoral head from the acetabulum (hip disarticulation), or removal of the femur and any portion of the pelvis (transpelvic amputation, also known as hemipelvectomy). The modern prosthesis was developed in Toronto and is sometimes called the *Canadian Hip Disarticulation Prosthesis*. Prostheses for proximal levels share common hip, knee, and foot assemblies, but differ with regard to socket design. The endoskeletal thigh and shank predominate because they save appreciable weight in these massive prostheses. The prosthesis may be shortened slightly, to aid clearance during swing phase, encourage the wearer to apply maximum weight to the prosthesis, and increase stability.

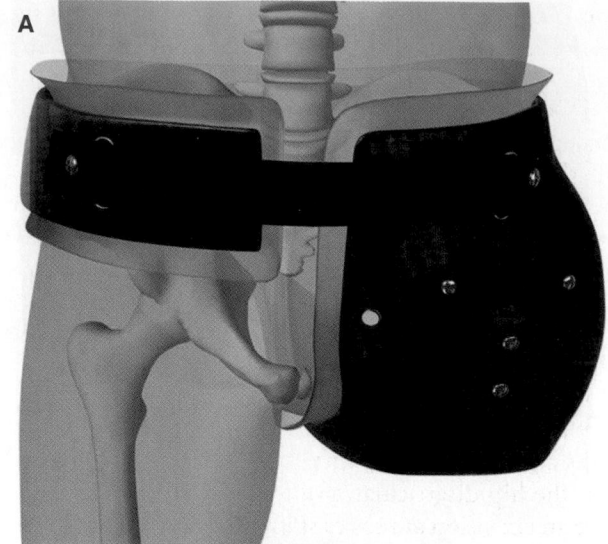

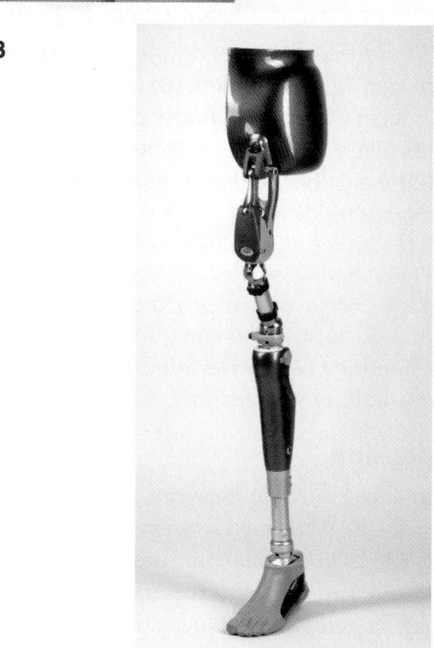

Figure 31.34 (A) Anatomical orientation of the Comfort-Flex™ hip disarticulation socket; additional components of the completed prosthesis included a hip joint, rotator, knee unit, pylon, and foot. Note that the socket covers the amputated side and wraps around the pelvis and is secured with anterior fasteners. *Courtesy of Hanger, Inc., Oklahoma City, OK 73118.* **(B)** Hip disarticulation prosthesis with Helix 3D® hip joint. *Courtesy of Otto Bock, Minneapolis, MN 55447.*

Sockets

The basic socket is plastic molded to provide weight-bearing on the ipsilateral ischial tuberosity and buttock (gluteal musculature). The person with transpelvic amputation who does not retain the ipsilateral tuberosity or iliac crest has a socket with a higher proximal trimline, sometimes encompassing the lower thorax.

This individual supports weight on the remainder of the pelvis, on the abdomen, and perhaps on the lower ribs.

Hip Units

The prosthetic hip joint has an extension aid to bias the prosthesis toward the stable neutral position. Positioning the mechanical hip anterior to a point corresponding to the anatomical hip also contributes to hip stability. The joint is set below the normal hip, so that when the wearer sits, the prosthetic thigh will not protrude unattractively. All hip joints provide hip flexion; some also allow transverse rotation.[50,51]

Knee Units

Although virtually any knee unit can be incorporated into the hip disarticulation prosthesis, the unit should have an extension aid to resist knee flexion during stance phase. The prosthetic knee is aligned relatively posteriorly to contribute to stability.

■ BILATERAL PROSTHESES

Bilateral amputations occur either simultaneously, as in the case of trauma or congenital limb deficiency, or sequentially, as is seen with peripheral vascular disease. In the latter instance, previous experience with a unilateral prosthesis is invaluable in determining whether the patient will benefit from a pair of prostheses.

Bilateral Syme's and Transtibial Prostheses[52]

Any foot design can be worn, although both prosthetic feet must be the same design from the same manufacturer to reduce the likelihood of gait asymmetry. Ideally, foot and shoe size should be shorter than the person's preamputation size to facilitate transition through stance phase; wider feet contribute to stability. Shanks, sockets, and suspensions need not match; each component should suit the characteristics of the individual amputation limb.

Bilateral Transfemoral Prostheses[53,54]

Other than matching prosthetic foot design and size, each amputation limb is fitted on an individual basis. The patient will perform activities in a manner similar to someone with unilateral transfemoral amputation.

The patient may be fitted with short, nonarticulated prostheses. The lower center of gravity provides the individual with more stability. Gait is awkward, with exaggerated trunk rotation; crutches or canes need to be adjusted to suit the person's short stature. Transferring into an adult-size chair, as well as climbing stairs, is more difficult than with longer prostheses. Patients who object to the markedly altered appearance created by these short prostheses may refuse to wear them.

Longer prostheses should include a matched pair of feet. Endoskeletal shanks are highly desirable to reduce prosthetic weight and enable minute changes in alignment; typically the shanks are shortened by several inches to reduce the effort required to walk with the prostheses. Any type of knee unit may be worn; they need not be the same on both prostheses. Nevertheless, one should avoid a pair of manually locked knee units because they would make chair transfers and stair maneuvering very difficult. Sockets do not have to match; however, a pair of ischial containment sockets will minimize the walking base because the sockets have a relatively narrow mediolateral dimension, as compared with quadrilateral sockets. Any type of suspension may be worn.

■ PROSTHETIC MAINTENANCE

Optimal function depends on proper care of socks or sheaths, prosthesis, amputation limb, and intact limb, as well as general health maintenance. Guidelines for personal hygiene are presented in Chapter 22, Amputation. In addition to ensuring cleanliness, the individual should wear a well-fitting sock and shoe on the sound foot. It must be the mate to the shoe on the prosthesis. Both shoes should be in excellent condition.

As with any appliance, the prosthesis benefits from simple regular maintenance, which generally avoids costly, time-consuming repairs. Printed instructions pertaining to the prosthesis and socks or sheath are helpful for patient education.

Foot-Ankle Assemblies

One should avoid getting the prosthetic foot wet, especially if the foot is an articulated model. If this happens, the shoe and sock should be removed to allow the foot to dry completely, away from direct heat. The wearer should also avoid stepping into sand and similar materials that might enter the cleft between the foot and shank section and restrict the excursion of the foot. The prosthetist will have to disassemble the foot to clean it.

The client should inspect the foot periodically to spot cracking at the toe-break or tip of the keel; such a crack will curl the toes and prevent smooth transition during late stance. A deteriorated heel cushion or plantar bumper will cause one to appear to be walking in a hole. Although most feet are now molded to simulate toes, the patient should not walk without a shoe because the sole of the prosthetic foot is not intended to resist much abrasion.

Foot socks wear much more quickly on the prosthetic side, because the hard foot-ankle assembly and shank rub against the fabric. Stair risers also scuff the sock. Some people find that wearing two socks helps cushion the outer one against premature formation of holes.

The individual must be instructed regarding wearing shoes of the same heel height as was the case when the prosthesis was aligned. Too low a heel interrupts late stance; an unduly high heel makes the knee less stable. If the prosthesis has the usual foot designed for low-heeled shoes, and the wearer wishes to wear flat-heeled shoes, a 1/2 in (1 cm) shim (a thin tapered wedge) should be placed inside both shoes at the heel. High-heeled shoes require that the foot be changed, either by unbolting it and replacing it with a foot with an appropriate plantarflexion angle, or by adjusting the heel-height feature found in certain models of feet (e.g., Runway® [Freedom Innovations, Fayette, UT 84630]; Elation® [Ossur, Aliso Viejo, CA 92656]). Boots and other footwear with stiff upper sections restrict the action of any foot assembly that is designed to provide substantial dorsiflexion and plantarflexion.

Removing the shoe is easier if the prosthesis is not worn. With the shoe unlaced completely, one grasps the rear of the shoe, then pulls the shoe off the back of the foot. Finally, the shoe is moved upward off the forefoot. The shoe should be put on the prosthetic foot with the aid of a shoehorn.

Shanks

The usual finish of exoskeletal shanks is polyester laminate, which is impervious to most liquids. It needs to be wiped only periodically with a cloth dampened with dilute detergent to remove surface soil. Marks can be gently removed with kitchen cleanser; excessive abrasion will dull the finish.

The soft foam cover of the endoskeletal prosthesis requires reasonable caution against exposure to direct heat, penetrating objects, and solvents. The outer covering will need replacement whenever it becomes unacceptably soiled or torn. The transfemoral version tends to deteriorate at the knee, especially if the wearer kneels a great deal.

Knee Units

Sliding friction mechanisms tend to loosen with walking and thus require periodic tightening to retain the original adjustment. The frequency of tightening depends on how much the wearer walks. Most units have a pair of screws in front or in the rear of the knee unit that can be turned clockwise with an Allen wrench (small L-shaped metal bar with hexagonal head at each end) or common screwdriver. After turning each screw a quarter turn, the client should walk for at least 5 minutes to ascertain the effectiveness of the adjustment.

Squeaking at the knee or articulated ankle usually indicates the need for oil. The rubber or felt extension bumper in the knee unit will erode after prolonged vigorous use, and the wearer will then notice that the knee begins to hyperextend. The bumper, visible when the knee is flexed, must be replaced by the prosthetist.

The external extension aid eventually loses its elasticity. The user will then experience high heel rise in early swing and slow knee extension at the end of swing phase. The simplest approach is to tighten the strap through its buckle. Eventually, the prosthetist will need to replace the elastic webbing. Internal elastic extension aids are not subject to rubbing from the trouser leg or skirt and thus do not lose elasticity as readily. Steel spring internal

aids usually retain their effectiveness for the life of the prosthesis.

Pneumatic and hydraulic units must be protected against tears of the rubber shield protecting the piston. The piston must not be scratched, because this would allow air and debris to enter the cylinder. Air bubbles in the unit will cause a spongy feeling, and possibly noise with walking. At night, the prosthesis should be stored upright, with the knee extended to exclude air from the cylinder.

Electronic units must not be immersed or used in a particle-filled environment, such as a commercial bakery or lumberyard (sawdust).

Sockets and Suspensions

Plastic sockets should be washed with a cloth dampened in warm water that has a very small amount of mild soap dissolved in it. The socket is then wiped with a damp, soap-free cloth, and dried with a fresh towel. In warm climates, the socket should be washed every evening so that it will be completely dry when the patient dresses the following morning. Socket liners made of polyethylene foam can be washed by hand in tepid water with mild soap, rinsed, and air-dried overnight. They should not be subjected to direct sunlight when removed from the prosthesis. Other sheaths and liners should be maintained according to the manufacturer's instructions.

Leather corsets should be kept dry. Use of saddle soap will keep leather clean. If the patient is incontinent, the thigh corset should be made of flexible *polyester laminate* or polypropylene, which are impervious to urine.

The transfemoral suction valve should be brushed daily to remove talcum and lint, which might clog the tiny aperture. The valve should be inserted and removed only with one's fingers, because tools are apt to damage the internal mechanism or outer threads.

■ PHYSICAL THERAPY MANAGEMENT

Physical therapists participate in the management of patients with amputation at several key stages: (1) preoperative; (2) postoperative–preprosthetic; (3) prosthetic prescription; (4) prosthetic examination; and (5) prosthetic training.

The first two stages are described in Chapter 22, Amputation. The following discussion emphasizes the responsibilities of the physical therapist with regard to the patient and prosthesis. Ideally, the therapist works as a member of a clinic team, together with the physician and prosthetist. Others, such as a social worker, vocational counselor, and psychologist may participate in the team on a regular basis or as needed. The clinic team provides the best environment for exchange of information and viewpoints regarding the patient and fostering efficient treatment;[55,56] the team meets to formulate the prosthetic prescription, examine the newly delivered prosthesis, and reexamine the patient and prosthesis upon completion of prosthetic training. The therapist, therefore, has an integral part to play in these critical points in rehabilitation, as well as conducting prosthetic training. If a formal clinic team is not established in the therapist's work setting, one must coordinate the recommendations of the physician and prosthetist.

With either administrative situation, the physical therapist:

- Addresses nonprosthetic considerations
- Contributes to prosthetic prescription
- Examines the prosthesis
- Facilitates prosthetic acceptance
- Instructs the patient in donning, use, and maintenance of the prosthesis

Preprescription Considerations

Successful prosthetic rehabilitation depends on matching the individual's physical and psychosocial characteristics to a prosthesis composed of carefully selected components. Although everyone who wears a prosthesis has an amputation or comparable limb deficiency, the reverse is not true. That is, some people with amputations are not candidates for prostheses or prefer not to use prostheses. Prostheses are contraindicated for patients with severe dementia or depression or advanced cardiopulmonary disease. If the person displays significant changes associated with organic brain syndrome, prosthetic fitting is contraindicated. Individuals with bilateral amputations who are unable to transfer independently or don underwear by themselves are unlikely to benefit from definitive prostheses. Similarly, a patient with bilateral amputations who had sustained unilateral amputation previously and was unable to don and walk with a unilateral prosthesis is not a candidate for a pair of prostheses. Some people with high amputations, especially hip disarticulation, find that a prosthesis is unduly cumbersome; they prefer to ambulate with a pair of crutches or depend on a wheelchair. Several sports, particularly swimming, are generally easier to perform without a prosthesis.

Physical Examination

The physical therapist should examine joint mobility and active and passive range of motion of all joints on both LEs. Knee and hip flexion contractures compromise prosthetic alignment and appearance. A knee lock may be needed in a transfemoral prosthesis. A patient with knee contracture requires an alternative transtibial socket design. Severe contractures may contraindicate provision of a prosthesis. The deleterious effects of contractures are especially serious with bilateral amputations.

The length of the amputation limb should be measured. The individual with a short transtibial amputation may require SC/SP suspension. Every attempt should be made to fit the patient with a short transfemoral amputation with suction or partial-suction suspension to retain the prosthesis on the thigh.

Strength of all limb and trunk muscles should be examined. Frequently, the elderly patient with vascular disease experiences reduced physical activity as LE pain and foot ulceration develop. Such an individual may present with marked debility, which would interfere with prosthetic use or necessitate use of a unit with a knee lock.

The therapist should inspect the skin, noting the status of the incision and any other lesions. The patient may require a nylon or silicone sheath to provide a smooth interface between socket and skin to avoid irritating tender or grafted skin.

An examination of sensory function should be performed. For example, someone with impaired proprioception at the knee will need extra prosthetic stability in the form of higher medial and lateral socket walls, or side joints attached to a thigh corset, on the transtibial prosthesis. Blindness does not preclude fitting, but it does pose problems with regard to selecting components that are easy to don, as well as altering the training program. If the patient complains of a neuroma, the problem must be addressed surgically or conservatively (e.g., cortisone injection) before fitting can proceed.

The therapist should examine the patient's ability to learn and retain new information, including both short- and long-term memory. Neurological conditions, such as cerebrovascular accident, complicate fitting and training. Ipsilateral hemiplegia is not as detrimental to prosthetic rehabilitation as contralateral paralysis. In both instances, the prosthesis should be designed for maximum stability. Patients with mild neurological impairments often respond favorably to altered training strategies, which the therapist designs on an individualized basis.

The circulation and anthropometric dimensions of the amputation and sound limbs require careful scrutiny. The physical therapist should teach the patient to inspect the intact foot, using a hand mirror to visualize the plantar surface. Inspection aims to identify skin lesions and incipient areas of abrasion so that corrective measures may be instituted before ulceration or infection ensues. In addition, the patient should be taught to keep the sound foot clean and should wear clean socks or stockings and a well-fitting shoe (see Chapter 14, Vascular, Lymphatic, and Integumentary Disorders, for additional guidelines for managing the patient with peripheral vascular disease). Sequential measurements of amputation limb circumference as well as palpation will indicate whether the individual has edema. Measures should be instituted to stabilize limb volume so that the patient can retain the fit of the prosthetic socket. The patient with vascular impairment may benefit from prosthetic fitting, which transfers some stress from the contralateral limb. In addition, should the person come to bilateral amputation, previous experience with donning and controlling a unilateral prosthesis is invaluable in adjusting to a pair of prostheses.

Prosthetic prescription is also based on the patient's aerobic capacity and endurance. The clinic team must formulate realistic goals based on the individual's physical capacity, particularly related to exercise tolerance and level of deconditioning. The person who is not expected to walk rapidly is an unlikely candidate for an energy-storing/releasing foot or a fluid-controlled knee unit. Nevertheless, a fluid-controlled knee unit that incorporates a braking mechanism is appropriate for selected patients with generalized weakness.

Obesity is another factor to be considered in the preprescription examination. The obese individual is more apt to fluctuate in body weight, necessitating provision of socket liners and several socks to compensate for changing limb circumference. Similarly, those who have renal disease, especially if requiring dialysis, experience volume changes that need prosthetic accommodation.

Arthritis affects prosthesis prescription. Diminished LE mobility or deformity may compromise prosthetic alignment. Patients with hip or knee arthroplasty, however, function quite well with a prosthesis. Hand and wrist function affects the mode of donning; a laced corset should be avoided. Canes and crutches may require modification.

Functional examination is an essential component of physical therapy management (see Chapter 8, Examination of Function). Among the most useful examination procedures involves observing the patient's ability to transfer from sit-to-stand and bed-to-wheelchair. To accomplish these maneuvers, the individual must have reasonable strength, balance, and coordination, as well as adequate comprehension.

Psychosocial Considerations

Ordinarily, the physical therapist treats the patient more frequently than any other member of the clinic team and thus is more likely to be attuned to changes in the individual's psychosocial status. Ample evidence supports the psychological, as well as physical, benefit of clinic team management.[55,56] Many people with amputation confront psychosocial issues, which should be recognized and addressed.[57-64] For example, the patient who is excessively fearful may be served best by prosthetic rehabilitation beginning with a *temporary (provisional) prosthesis.*

Temporary Prostheses
Transtibial Temporary Prosthesis

Most transtibial temporary prostheses have sockets made of thermoplastic material that becomes malleable at temperatures low enough to permit forming directly on the patient. One can also obtain mass-produced adjustable sockets; it may be necessary to pad the socket bottom so that the amputation limb does not develop distal edema. Some temporary prostheses have a plaster socket molded to the amputated limb. Plaster is inexpensive, readily available, and easy to use. The resulting socket, however, is rather heavy and bulky. Suspension is usually by a cuff or thigh corset. The pylon can be an aluminum

component manufactured for this purpose; such a pylon has a proximal fixture that permits small changes in prosthetic alignment. A simpler pylon can be made with polyvinylchloride piping, such as used for plumbing. The pipe is lightweight and can be spot-heated to enable slight alteration in alignment. A SACH foot is customarily used on temporary prostheses.

Transfemoral Temporary Prosthesis

The easiest approach is to use a polypropylene socket (Fig. 31.35), which is manufactured in several sizes and has straps for circumferential adjustment. The socket can be suspended with a Silesian bandage or pelvic band, and is mounted on a knee unit, which may include a manual lock. Alternatively, a custom-fabricated socket of plaster or low-temperature thermoplastic can be used. Some individuals with bilateral transfemoral amputations use a pair of short prostheses. These are nonarticulated prostheses; the sockets are mounted on short platforms, drastically reducing the wearer's height in order to increase balance stability. The platforms each have a rearward projection to protect the patient from a backward fall.

Motivation is a cardinal determinant of prosthetic outcome. Again, strong motivation demonstrated through use of a temporary prosthesis and adherence with other elements of the rehabilitation program is a reliable predictor of prosthetic success. One should guard against unrealistic expectations. Involving the patient and family in group situations with other persons with amputation in the physical therapy department and

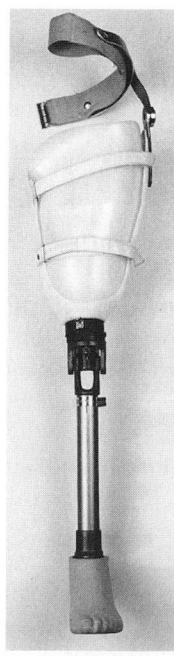

Figure 31.35 Transfemoral temporary prosthesis with adjustable polypropylene socket, pelvic band, knee unit with manual lock, and adjustable shank with SACH foot.

in social environments fosters constructive attitudes. The therapist should also weigh the likelihood that the individual will be able to care for complex prosthetic mechanisms and have the financial resources to obtain prosthetic servicing, especially of less durable components, such as the foam rubber covering of the endoskeletal shank.

Prosthetic Prescription

No prosthetic component is ideal for all clients. It is necessary to select components that are most apt to meet each individual's needs. Alternatives to every element of the prosthesis have advantages and disadvantages. The task of the physical therapist, in conjunction with other team members, is to judge the relative merits of various feet, shanks, and other components in light of objective and subjective information pertaining to the prosthetic candidate. In 1995, Medicare identified functional levels applicable to individuals with unilateral transtibial and transfemoral prostheses:[65]

- K0: Not a candidate
- K1: Household ambulation
- K2: Limited community ambulation
- K3: Community ambulation and the ability to vary cadence with vocational, therapeutic, or exercise needs
- K4: High levels of activity such as demonstrated by active adults and athletes

These levels determine the medical necessity of knee and ankle-foot units.

Some people can be expected to function best with a sophisticated prosthesis that enhances the wearer's ability to engage in vigorous walking and athletics. Others are well served by simple, inexpensive devices. The most accurate predictor of future function is the patient's performance with a previous prosthesis. For the wearer who seeks a replacement prosthesis, the clinic team should consider the extent of use of the previous limb, together with any changes in the patient's health status and lifestyle. For example, if the person fitted with one prosthesis now returns with bilateral amputation, never having used the original prosthesis, that patient is a very poor candidate for bilateral prosthetic fitting. In contrast, another person who had been fitted with a simple transfemoral prosthesis expresses the wish to participate in sports. By demonstrating good use of the original prosthesis, that individual is likely to derive considerable benefit from a new prosthesis with a fluid-controlled knee unit and an energy-storing/releasing foot.

Prescription for the new patient is more difficult. Depending on the interval between amputation surgery and prescription, the amputation limb may not have stabilized in volume; the patient may not have achieved the maximum benefit from the preprosthetic program. The best criterion for prosthetic prescription in such an instance is performance with a temporary (provisional) prosthesis. As mentioned earlier, this appliance includes a well-fitting socket, suitable suspension, pylon, and foot; the transfemoral model usually has a knee unit. The temporary prosthesis allows preliminary gait and activities training. The major difference between the temporary and definitive (permanent) prosthesis is appearance. The temporary socket is designed for easy alteration to accommodate change in amputation limb volume. Ordinarily, little attention is paid to the color and exterior shape of the temporary prosthesis.

Prosthetic Examination/Evaluation

The prosthesis should be examined before the patient engages in prosthetic training and should be reexamined at the conclusion of training. The procedure is intended to determine the adequacy of prosthetic fit and function, as well as the wearer's opinion of appearance and overall satisfaction. This process typically follows a sequence of examining the prosthesis while the patient stands (static analysis), examining the patient's gait (dynamic analysis), and finally examining the prosthesis off the patient (additional static analysis). In many institutions, the physical therapist examines the prosthesis and presents a summary of findings to the clinic team. The team makes the final determination regarding the acceptability of the prosthesis.

No special materials are needed to examine the prosthesis, except for a checklist, a straight (armless) chair, a few sheets of paper, a ruler, lift blocks, and colored chalk. For final evaluation, stairs and a ramp are needed. The checklists referred to in the following sections can be found in Appendices 31.A and 31.B.

At initial evaluation, the team has three options: (1) pass, (2) provisional pass, or (3) fail. Pass indicates that no changes are needed in the prosthesis and the patient can proceed to training. Provisional pass signals that one or more minor problems require correction, none of which would interfere with training. Failure is the team's judgment that the prosthesis has a major fault that should be corrected to the team's satisfaction before commencement of prosthetic training. For example, poor finishing of the prosthetic foot merits a provisional pass, whereas a socket that abrades the amputation limb should be graded as fail. If the therapist intends to provide treatment to a patient who is not managed by a formal clinic team, it is especially critical that one examine the prosthesis before initiating instruction and training to discover any problems that would interfere with the future program. At the final evaluation, two ratings are available: *pass* indicates that no problems exist and the patient uses the prosthesis in a manner commensurate with that individual's physical capacity; *fail* means that major or minor problems remain.

Transtibial Examination

Most items on the checklist in Appendix 31.A are self-explanatory. Each contributes to forming an accurate judgment of the adequacy of the prosthesis.

Static Analysis

The prosthesis is examined while the wearer stands and sits. In addition, the amputation limb and details of the prosthesis are examined. The prosthesis should be compared with the prescription. The individual who authorized the prescription must approve departures from the original specifications.

The new wearer should stand in the parallel bars or other secure environment, attempting to bear equal weight on both feet. The therapist should solicit subjective comments about comfort. Estimates of anteroposterior and mediolateral alignment are aided by slipping a sheet of paper under various parts of the shoe. Ideally, the patient should stand with both heels and soles flat on the floor. Misalignment, indicated by excessive weight-bearing on one portion of the shoe, may be confirmed by subsequent analysis of gait.

Most prostheses are constructed so that when the individual stands, the pelvis is level;[36] if the pelvis tilts, the therapist should place lifts under the foot on the shorter side to restore a level pelvis. If the total lift measures 1/2 in (1 cm) or less, no attention is needed. For greater discrepancy, one should seek causative factors. An amputation limb that sinks too far into the socket will make the prosthetic side appear short, and the wearer will probably complain of discomfort.

Piston action refers to vertical motion of the socket when the patient elevates the pelvis. Slippage can be determined by chalk marking the sock at the posterior margin of the socket, and then having the patient elevate the ipsilateral pelvis. The socket should slip less than 1/4 in (0.5 cm). Looseness, inadequate suspension, or both cause socket slippage. Socket walls should fit snugly, as should the thigh corset if it is part of the prosthesis.

Comfortable sitting is a primary need for all people. The posterior brim should not impinge into the popliteal fossa, and hamstring reliefs should be adequate, especially on the medial side where the semitendinosus and semimembranosus insert relatively distally. Placement of the tabs of the cuff or the joints of the corset also influences sitting comfort.

Dynamic Analysis

Analysis of the gait pattern and performance of other ambulatory activities is an essential part of rehabilitation. For most patients, a major reason for prosthetic fitting is to resume walking. Nevertheless, no prosthesis eradicates entirely the anatomical and physiological changes produced by amputation. When walking, the person who wears a prosthesis compensates for anatomical and prosthetic deficiencies.[66-71] Some are inherent to amputation; others are abnormalities of the body or the prosthesis. Because virtually all people walk with a prosthesis in a manner different from the nondisabled walking pattern, prosthetic gait represents compensation for the patient's altered locomotor apparatus. The term *gait compensation* may be a more accurate descriptor than the more commonly used *gait deviation* inasmuch as the patient with amputation is most unlikely ever to walk exactly like a nondisabled person.

No prosthesis restores sensation, skeletal continuity, muscle integrity, or full body weight. Anatomical deficiencies are aggravated in the presence of pain, contracture, weakness, instability, or incoordination. Similarly, prosthetic components do not replace every function of the missing limb. For example, prosthetic feet do not move through the full excursion of the human counterpart. Inadequacies in the prosthesis compel the wearer to adopt gait compensations. Such problems include a poorly fitted socket, prosthetic misalignment, malfunctioning components, and improper height of the prosthesis. Compounding the problem are incorrect donning of the prosthesis and wearing inappropriate shoes. The physical therapist must determine when gait compensation exists and the potential causes so that remedial action may be taken. Otherwise, the patient is compelled to expend more energy walking and to exhibit a more conspicuously abnormal gait. The new wearer will have had brief experience walking in the prosthesis during the course of prosthetic fabrication. Although a smooth gait is unlikely on the day of the initial examination, gross departure from the usual gait exhibited by others with similar prostheses should be noted and causes sought.

Transtibial analysis focuses on action of the knee on the amputated side during stance phase. Both knees should flex in a controlled manner during their respective early and late stance phases. Excessive flexion of the knee on the amputated side indicates that the socket is aligned too far anterior in relation to the foot or is excessively flexed; this deviation may cause the patient to fall. If the knee flexes too much only during early stance, the cause may be a heel cushion that is too firm for that wearer. Conversely, insufficient knee flexion results from posterior displacement of the socket or inadequate socket tilt. When viewed in the frontal plane, the socket brim should maintain reasonable contact with the leg; excessive lateral thrust of the prosthetic brim suggests that the prosthetic foot has been positioned too far medially. Table 31.1 summarizes the prosthetic and anatomical causes of transtibial gait compensations/deviations.

At the initial evaluation, performance on stairs and inclines may be omitted because the patient has not had training in these activities.

Inspection of the Prosthesis Off the Patient

The posterior wall should be approximately at the same level as the build-up for the patellar *ligament* (tendon) when the patient stands. To check this, the prosthesis is stood upright on a table; one end of a ruler is then placed on the anterior socket bulge and the opposite end on the posterior brim. In a well-constructed prosthesis, the ruler will slant upward toward the rear, indicating that when the individual stands in the prosthesis and compresses

Table 31.1   Transtibial Prosthetic Gait Analysis

Compensation/Deviation	Prosthetic Causes	Anatomical Causes
Early Stance		
1. Excessive knee flexion	High shoe heel Insufficient plantarflexion Stiff heel cushion Socket too far anterior Socket excessively flexed Cuff tabs too posterior	Flexion contracture Weak quadriceps
2. Insufficient knee flexion	Low shoe heel Excessive plantarflexion Soft heel cushion Socket too far posterior Socket insufficiently flexed	Extensor spasticity Weak quadriceps Anterior-distal pain Arthritis
Midstance		
1. Lateral thrust	Excessive foot inset	
2. Medial thrust	Excessive foot outset	
Late Stance		
1. Early knee flexion: also referred to as "drop off"	High shoe heel Insufficient plantarflexion Keel too short Dorsiflexion stop too soft Socket too far anterior Socket excessively flexed Cuff tabs too posterior	Flexion contracture
2. Delayed knee flexion: perception of walking uphill	Low shoe heel Excessive plantarflexion Keel too long Dorsiflexion stop too stiff Socket too far posterior Socket insufficiently flexed	Extensor spasticity

the heel cushion, the posterior wall will be at the proper height.

The amputation limb should be examined for signs of proper loading with respect to the type of prosthesis worn. Any straps or cuff should provide reasonable adjustability. Construction is a guide to future durability, as well as contributing to acceptable appearance of the prosthesis.

Transfemoral Examination

A similar checklist is used to evaluate the transfemoral prosthesis (Appendix 31.B). It is important to recognize that seldom is one item of major significance. The therapist and entire team should look for patterns that might herald future difficulty. For example, misalignment detected in static analysis should be confirmed during gait.

Static Analysis

The patient who has a flesh roll above the socket either did not don the socket properly or has a thigh that is larger than that for which the socket was made. Perineal pressure results from sharpness of the medial brim or insufficiency of the adductor longus relief in a quadrilateral socket.

The knee unit should be stable enough to withstand a blow delivered by the therapist to the posterior aspect of the unit when the patient stands. Stability is influenced by the *alignment* of the knee in relation to the hip and prosthetic ankle. The farther posterior the knee bolt, the more stable the knee will be. Polycentric linkage and mechanical stabilizers also contribute to stability. If the socket is opaque, the only way to judge its snugness is by palpating tissue protruding through the valve hole when the valve is removed.

The checklist is designed to help the clinician determine the fit of the socket, regardless of shape or material. If the prosthesis has a quadrilateral socket, proper location of the adductor longus tendon and ischial tuberosity ensures that the patient has donned the socket correctly. A horizontal posterior brim allows weight to be borne on the gluteal musculature as well as the ischial tuberosity. The ischial containment socket is intended to cover the ischial tuberosity, yet allows the client to move the hip in all directions comfortably, without socket gapping.

The lateral attachment of the Silesian belt should be superior and posterior to the greater trochanter for best control of prosthetic rotation. Anteriorly, the attachment should be at the level of the ischial tuberosity, or slightly below, to aid in adducting the prosthesis.

The pelvic joint and band should fit the torso snugly for optimum control of the prosthesis and to minimize bulkiness. The joint axis should be superior and anterior to the greater trochanter.

The patient should be able to sit comfortably with the prosthesis. Posterior discomfort may indicate inadequate hamstring relief, or a sharp or thick posterior brim.

Dynamic Analysis

Gait analysis gives the clinic team members the opportunity to determine the adequacy of socket fit and of prosthesis alignment and adjustment. The patient also influences the walking pattern by the timing and force of muscular contraction and the presence or absence of contractures. The goal of walking with a transfemoral prosthesis is a comfortable, safe, efficient gait, rather than duplicating the gait of someone wearing a transtibial prosthesis or one who does not have amputation.[72] Table 31.2 summarizes the prosthetic and anatomical causes of transfemoral gait compensations/deviations.

Compensations/Deviations Best Viewed from Behind

Many individuals with transfemoral amputation abduct the prosthesis to improve frontal plane balance (*abducted gait*). Hip abduction contracture predisposes patients to this deviation, which is seen in stance phase. Inadequate socket adduction, socket looseness, or medial discomfort also causes the fault. *Circumduction* is a displacement exhibited in swing phase if the prosthesis is too long or if the patient is reluctant to allow the knee unit to bend. Socket looseness also may result in circumduction. The patient may shift the trunk excessively. *Lateral trunk bending* toward the prosthetic side during stance phase generally accompanies abducted gait. It should be noted, however, that all individuals with transfemoral amputation have an incomplete abductor mechanism, and tend to compensate by bending toward the prosthetic side, especially when fatigued. Although the anatomical hip and gluteus medius are usually in good condition, lack of skeletal continuity to the ground (imposed by the amputation) compromises the effectiveness of abductor contraction. If the prosthesis is too long, the patient will abduct; if it is too short, the patient will bend the trunk laterally.

Whips refer to medial or lateral rotation of the heel at late stance. If the socket does not fit well, contraction with bulging of the thigh musculature will cause the

Table 31.2 Transfemoral Prosthetic Gait Analysis

Compensation/Deviation	Prosthetic Causes	Anatomical Causes
Lateral Displacements		
1. Abduction: stance	Long prosthesis Abducted hip joint Inadequate lateral wall adduction Sharp or high medial wall	Abduction contracture Weak abductors Lateral/distal pain Adductor redundancy instability
2. Circumduction: swing	Long prosthesis Locked knee unit Loose friction Inadequate suspension Small socket Loose socket Foot plantarflexed	Abduction contracture Poor knee control
Trunk Shifts		
1. Lateral bend: stance	Short prosthesis Inadequate lateral wall adduction Sharp or high medial wall	Abduction contracture Weak abductors Hip pain Instability Short amputation limb
2. Forward flexion: stance	Unstable knee unit Short walker or crutches	Instability
3. Lordosis: stance	Inadequate socket flexion	Hip flexion contracture Weak extensors

Table 31.2 Transfemoral Prosthetic Gait Analysis—cont'd

Compensation/Deviation	Prosthetic Causes	Anatomical Causes
Rotations		
1. Medial (or lateral) whip: heel off	Faulty socket contour Knee bolt externally (or internally) rotated Foot malrotated Prosthesis donned in malrotation	With sliding friction unit, fast pace
2. Foot rotation at heel contact	Stiff heel cushion Malrotated foot	
Excessive Knee Motion		
1. High heel rise: early swing	Inadequate friction Slack extension aid	
2. Terminal impact: late swing	Inadequate friction Taut extension aid	Forceful hip flexion
Reduced Knee Motion		
1. Vault: swing	See above: circumduction	With sliding friction unit, fast pace
2. Hip hike: swing	See above: circumduction	Weak dorsiflexors Plantarflexor spasticity Pes equinus Weak hip flexors
Uneven Step Length	Uncomfortable socket Insufficient socket flexion	Hip flexion contracture Instability

prosthesis to rotate abruptly as it is being unloaded at the end of stance phase. Although less likely, malrotation of the knee unit or foot-ankle assembly may contribute to whipping. *Rotation of the foot on heel contact* is a much more serious deviation. It indicates inadequate compression of the heel cushion or plantar bumper and can result in a fall.

Compensations/Deviations Best Viewed from the Side

Forward trunk shifting in stance phase is a compensation that some patients use to cope with knee instability. If the walker or crutches are too short, the individual will lean forward. Lumbar *lordosis* results from inadequate socket flexion and is aggravated by a hip flexion contracture.

Improper adjustment of the knee unit gives rise to *uneven heel rise* (excessive knee flexion) and *terminal swing impact* (abrupt knee extension). If both deviations are present, the probable cause is insufficient friction. If the knee exhibits impact without undue heel rise, it is more likely that the extension aid is too tight.

To compensate for reduced knee motion, the vigorous walker may demonstrate *vaulting* by excessively plantarflexing the sound ankle to afford extra room to clear the prosthesis during prosthetic swing phase. A less strenuous compensation for excessive actual or functional prosthesis length is *hip hiking*, when the patient elevates the pelvis on the prosthetic side.

Unequal step length will be evident if the patient has a hip flexion contracture or inadequate balance. A longer step taken with the prosthesis gives the person more time on the sound limb. A flexion contracture or insufficient socket flexion (limiting hip extension range) prevents the sound limb from passing the prosthetic side during swing phase on the sound side (i.e., shorter step length on the sound side).

Inspection of the Prosthesis Off the Patient

Following the static evaluation, the therapist should examine the prosthesis and amputation limb as indicated on the checklist. A resilient back pad (placed externally on the posterior wall) enables the patient to sit quietly without undue trouser or skirt abrasion. The pad is unnecessary with a flexible socket.

Facilitating Prosthetic Acceptance

Amputation generally is regarded as a grievous occurrence, with its visibility a constant reminder of the individual's abnormality. The physical therapist can help the patient and family accept the reality of amputation and the prosthesis by verbal and nonverbal communication. One's calm respect for the patient as a worthy human being, regardless of limb condition, should set a model for the attitudes of others. Clinic team management accords not only the benefits of better prosthetic provision but also brings the individual in contact with clinicians who convey experience and confidence in dealing with problems that the person may have considered unique.

As soon as possible, the hospitalized patient should be treated in the physical therapy department, rather than at bedside. The bustle of the department should help dispel despondency. Although postoperative mourning is expected, prolonged depression is not constructive. Peer support groups are often very effective in aiding acceptance of the prosthesis and in learning special procedures for accomplishing activities. Observation and eventual participation in specially designed sports programs is another way people learn to cope and gain the most from rehabilitation. The physical therapist, by virtue of close daily contact with the patient, is also in a position to recommend to the clinic those who might profit from psychological counseling or psychiatric services, particularly when pain is an issue. Appendix 31.C provides website-based prosthetic resources for clinicians, families, and patients.

Prosthetic Training

Learning to use a prosthesis effectively involves being able to don it correctly, develop good balance and coordination, walk in a safe and reasonably symmetrical manner, and perform other ambulatory and self-care activities. Anticipated goals and expected outcomes depend on the patient's physical and psychological status, preprosthetic experience, and quality of prosthesis. Using the prosthesis only to assist in transferring from the wheelchair to the toilet may be an appropriate outcome for an elderly person with multiple disabilities, whereas the program for the youngster with traumatic amputation might extend to a full range of sports.

Donning

Correct application of the prosthesis and frequent inspection of the amputation limb are very important, especially for the beginner and those with poor circulation. Patients with partial foot, Syme's, and transtibial amputations can don the prosthesis while seated, after having applied the correct number and sequence of socks or sheath. Then, in most instances, the individual simply inserts the amputation limb into the socket. With SC/SP suspension, one applies the liner to the amputation limb, then inserts the limb and liner into the socket. The initial entry into the socket with corset suspension may be made while sitting; however, final tightening of laces or straps should be done in the standing position to ensure that the limb is lodged suitably in the socket.

Those with transfemoral amputation also can begin the donning process while seated. Total suction wearers may use either a pulling or pushing method. To pull oneself into the socket, the patient applies a light dusting of talcum powder to the thigh to reduce friction. Then

one applies a pulling sock, a tubular cotton stockinet approximately 30 in (76 cm) long, a roll of elastic bandage wound around the thigh, or a nylon stocking. Whatever the donning aid, it should be placed high in the groin to pull in proximal tissues. After placing the sock-encased thigh into the socket, one draws the distal end of the aid through the valve hole. Although it is possible to complete the donning process while seated, most people prefer to stand while pulling the sock or other aid out through the valve hole. By leaning forward, the body's weight line will prevent the prosthetic knee from flexing inadvertently. The patient alternately flexes and extends the sound hip and knee while tugging downward on the donning aid until it slips out from the prosthesis. Finally, one inserts the valve. Another approach to donning is to coat the thigh with lubricating lotion, push it into the socket, and then install the valve.

Patients who use partial suction apply a sock, making certain the proximal margin of the sock extends to the inguinal ligament. The patient then introduces the amputation limb into the socket, taking care that the thigh is correctly oriented; pulls the distal end of the sock down through the valve hole enough to ensure that the skin is smooth; tucks the sock back into the socket; and inserts the valve. Finally, one secures the pelvic band or Silesian belt. If suction is not used, donning is similar to the method used with partial suction, except that there is no valve.

Balance and Coordination

Exercises are similar for all patients with LE amputations, although the individual with a transfemoral or hip disarticulation prosthesis may be expected to encounter more difficulty controlling the mechanical knee, as compared to those with two anatomical knees. All must learn to balance on the amputated side.[73-77] A graduated program for increasing prosthetic tolerance minimizes the danger of skin abrasion, particularly if the amputation limb presents skin grafts, poor circulation, or diminished sensation. The patient should alternately exercise and rest, with cardiopulmonary monitoring a routine part of the program, especially for high-risk individuals.

Some clinicians eschew parallel bars because the fearful patient pulls on them, which will be fruitless when progressing to a cane. When bars are used, the therapist should encourage the patient to rest the open hand on the bar for support, rather than using a viselike grip. A plinth or sturdy table offers the dual advantages of providing good support on only one side, ordinarily the contralateral side, and unidirectional control, because the patient can only push, never pull, for balance.

Static erect balance reintroduces the novice to bipedal posture. The patient should strive for level pelvis and shoulders, vertical trunk without excessive lordosis, and equal weight-bearing. The therapist should guard and assist the patient as necessary. When the physical therapist stands near the prosthesis, this encourages the patient to shift his or her weight onto it. To suggest symmetrical performance, refer to the limbs as "right" and "left," or "sound" and "prosthetic," rather than discouraging the patient with "good" and "bad." The client must learn to use proximal sensory receptors to maintain balance and perceive the position of the prosthesis without looking at the floor. Some patients respond well to increased use of visual feedback (e.g., using a mirror).

Dynamic exercises improve medial–lateral, sagittal, and rotary control. The patient learns that hip flexion causes the knee to bend, and hip extension stabilizes the knee during stance phase. Placing the sound foot ahead of the prosthesis makes the prosthetic knee more stable. Patients should be instructed in weight shifting in both symmetrical and stride positions and in stepping movements. Stepping on a low stool or step platform with the sound foot obliges the patient to shift weight onto the prosthesis and increases stance phase duration on the prosthesis. Having all exercises performed rhythmically with both the right and left LEs fosters symmetrical performance.

Gait Training

Walking is a natural progression from dynamic balance exercises as the patient takes successive steps. Patients tend to place greater load and exert more propulsive force on the intact side; consequently, gait training should emphasize symmetrical performance.[67-73] Inasmuch as hamstrings become the main muscles of propulsion, strengthening exercises are indicated. Some people respond well to proprioceptive neuromuscular facilitation.[74] Rhythmic counting and walking in time with music in 2/4 time also improves gait symmetry and speed. In the physical therapy department, an apparatus that includes a suspension harness (partial body weight support) provides a protected environment for the patient to learn gradual weight-bearing on the prosthesis. A balance apparatus (e.g., Balance Master®) providing electronic feedback with or without emphasis on psychological awareness of bodily position is another training option.

Either a cane or pair of forearm crutches is an appropriate aid for the client who is unable to achieve a safe gait without undue fatigue. Sometimes the cane is used only outdoors to aid in negotiating curbs and other ground irregularities and to signal oncoming traffic. Ordinarily the cane is used on the contralateral side to enhance frontal plane balance. If bilateral assistance is required, a pair of forearm crutches is preferable to two canes. The crutches remain clasped around the forearms when the user opens a door. Axillary crutches tempt the patient to lean on the axillary bars, risking impingement of the radial nerves; they are also inconvenient when climbing stairs. An aluminum walker provides maximum stability, which is particularly useful for patients with generalized weakness. The walker should be adjusted so that the user does not lean too far forward.

Patients with transtibial amputation walk faster with a two-wheeled walker as compared with a four-footed walker.[75] Fear of falling can undermine walking and social activity participation. Improving the patient's balance confidence is essential to lessen this concern.[76,77]

Functional Training

The prosthesis wearer who is learning to walk also should gain experience in performing a wide variety of functional mobility skills. Activities such as transferring to various chairs add interest to the program and, for some patients, may be more important than long-distance ambulation.

The training program for vigorous individuals includes stair climbing, negotiating ramps, retrieving objects from the floor, kneeling, sitting on the floor, running, driving a car, and engaging in sports. The fundamental difference between these activities and walking is the way each LE is used. Walking implies symmetrical usage, but the other activities are done asymmetrically, with greater reliance on the strength, agility, and sensory control of the sound limb.

Generally, the patient should have the opportunity to analyze each new situation and arrive at a solution to the problem, rather than depending on directions from the therapist. Most tasks can be accomplished safely in several ways. The learner profits from practice in clinical decision making and observing other prosthesis wearers as well as from professional instruction.

Transfers

Rising from different chairs, the toilet, and car are primary skills even for people who are elderly or debilitated. Most patients enter the physical therapy department in a wheelchair. Initially, the patient can park the chair at the parallel bars or at a plinth. After locking the wheelchair and raising the footrests, the patient should sit forward and transfer weight to the intact leg, then push down on the armrests. The individual will find that placing the sound foot close to the chair enables rising by extending the knee and hip on the sound side. Sitting is accomplished by placing the sound foot close to the chair and lowering oneself by controlled hip and knee flexion on the sound side.

For both standing and sitting, the beginner should have the advantage of a chair with armrests that enables use of the hands to control and assist trunk movement. Later the person should practice sitting in deep upholstered sofas and low chairs, as well as benches, the toilet, and other seats that do not have armrests. Transfer into an automobile should be an integral part of the training activities; otherwise, the patient faces a gloomy future, confined to home or dependent on special transportation systems. To enter the right (passenger) side of an automobile, the prosthetic wearer faces toward the front of the car. The person with a right prosthesis puts the right hand on the door post and the left hand on the back of the front seat, then swings the left leg into the car, slides onto the car seat, and finally places the prosthesis in the car. The individual with a left prosthesis may find that sitting sideways with both feet out the car door is easiest. One then pivots on the seat while swinging the prosthesis into the car, then puts the intact right foot inside the car.

Climbing Stairs, Ramps, and Curbs

Patients with Syme's and transtibial amputations generally ascend and descend stairs and inclines with steps of equal length in step-over-step progression.[78-80] Those with unilateral transfemoral amputation, in contrast, usually ascend by leading with the sound foot and learn to descend by first placing the prosthesis on the lower step. A few individuals with transfemoral amputation subsequently learn to control prosthetic knee flexion in order to descend step-over-step. Those fitted with the Power Knee® may be able to ascend stairs step-over-step.

Curbs present a slightly different problem, because there is no handrail. The techniques are basically the same, however.

Ramps may be difficult if the prosthetic foot does not have sufficient anteroposterior excursion.[81,82] With steep stairs, ramps, and curbs, the individual may climb diagonally or sidestep with the prosthesis kept on the downhill side. Patients should also learn how to maneuver over obstacles on the walking surface.[83]

Final Evaluation and Follow-up Care

Economic strictures may compel the therapist to conclude the training program after the patient is able to walk and to negotiate basic transfers and stair climbing but before the full range of training activities is completed. Before discharge, the patient and prosthesis should be reexamined to make certain that socket fit, prosthetic appearance, and function are acceptable. The checklist used for initial evaluation can be used. The physical therapist should instruct the patient with regard to the patient's responsibility for reporting skin redness and any loose or missing parts from the prosthesis.

The new prosthesis wearer should return to the training site at regular intervals so that the clinic team may examine socket fit. Most will require major socket revision or replacement during the first year to accommodate amputation limb volume reduction. Follow-up visits are good opportunities to augment training and to encourage the individual to engage in the widest possible range of activities.

Functional Capacities

Functional capacities refer to the individual's ability to walk, transfer from chairs, climb stairs, and perform other ambulatory activities, including recreational endeavors. A primary responsibility of the clinic team is to predict the probable function of the person with a new amputation, to determine whether the individual would benefit from a prosthesis, and what degree of activity is likely. Because many people with LE amputation are elderly with several medical problems, the need for accurate forecasting and ongoing monitoring is especially critical.

Walking with a prosthesis increases energy cost.[84-88] Compared with those people with two sound limbs, the individual with a unilateral transtibial prosthesis requires slightly more oxygen when walking at a comfortable speed;[89,90] the person wearing a transfemoral prosthesis consumes nearly 50% more oxygen than normal,[91] although selection of prosthetic feet and knee units usually modifies the energy demand.[92-95] The prosthesis wearer chooses a comfortable pace, because at a speed that is natural for the individual, the energy cost per minute is similar to that of the person who does not require a prosthesis, although speed is slower. The lower the amputation level, the less the metabolic disadvantage. Among persons with transtibial amputations older than 40, those with long amputation limbs average minimal increase in energy, but persons with shorter limbs work harder. Those with bilateral transtibial amputations expend less energy than those with unilateral transfemoral amputations. Individuals whose amputation was traumatic perform more efficiently than those whose amputation was caused by vascular disease at every amputation level. People who sustained trauma walk faster and use less oxygen than their dysvascular counterparts.

The increased metabolic expenditure results in part from the socket, which surrounds semifluid tissue, giving imperfect anchorage imposing challenges to limb control. The foot-ankle assembly transmits no plantar tactile or proprioceptive sensation, does not move through as large an excursion as the anatomical foot, and does not initiate the dynamic propulsion characteristic of normal gait. The transfemoral prosthesis also incorporates a knee unit that provides no proprioception to the wearer. The problem is aggravated by the fact that a prosthesis is operated by remotely located muscles that contract longer and more forcefully than in normal gait. With transfemoral amputation, for example, the wearer positions the prosthetic foot by hip motion. The resulting alteration of motion is reflected in asymmetry of timing, further disturbing gait smoothness. Individuals with prostheses walk with greater vertical movement, inasmuch as the knee, whether mechanical for the transfemoral prosthesis wearer or anatomical in the transtibial wearer, does not flex as much as the contralateral knee during stance phase.

Use of a hip disarticulation prosthesis demands considerable energy expenditure.[96]

People wearing bilateral prostheses consume even more oxygen and walk more slowly than those with unilateral amputation at a given level.[97]

With the exception of patients on beta-blockers, heart rate response is an important indication of the metabolic cost of prosthetic use for most individuals. Overall, strength, balance ability, etiology of amputation, and level of amputation predict the extent of impairment.[98]

Other measures of functional capacities include utilization of prostheses[99-102] and quality-of-life surveys.[103-116] Return to work[117-118] and ability to drive an automobile[119,120] are other indicators of rehabilitation success.

Sports participation (Fig. 31.36) is an excellent extension of rehabilitation for patients of all ages.[121-134] Older adults may enjoy fishing, golfing, dancing, Tai Chi Chuan, and shuffleboard, and younger people may add basketball, tennis, archery, and track events to their range of activities. Most sports do not require any adaptation to the prosthesis. Horseback riding is a superb activity that fosters trunk control and seated balance. The hiker should pack extra amputation limb socks or a sheath to protect the skin; a well-fitting, comfortable hiking boot is essential. Bowling and participating in shot put are facilitated by emphasizing balance on the intact LE. For sports that involve running, an energy-storing/releasing foot is most suitable. The socket should fit snugly with very secure suspension to minimize abrasion of the amputation limb. Clients with Syme's or transtibial amputations usually run with reasonably symmetrical step lengths, although they will favor the sound limb, which has greater propulsive ability.[7] Those with a knee disarticulation or transfemoral amputation will derive most of the propulsive force from the sound leg and use the prosthesis as a momentary prop. Many marathon competitions have a category for people with disabilities. Jumping, as in basketball, requires the athlete to generate a substantial upward force with the sound leg; landing is more comfortable on the sound leg, particularly for those who wear transfemoral prostheses. Some activities are facilitated by minor modification of the equipment, such as a toe loop on a bicycle pedal or an adapted prosthesis.

Other activities are generally performed without a prosthesis, such as swimming and skiing. The skier will

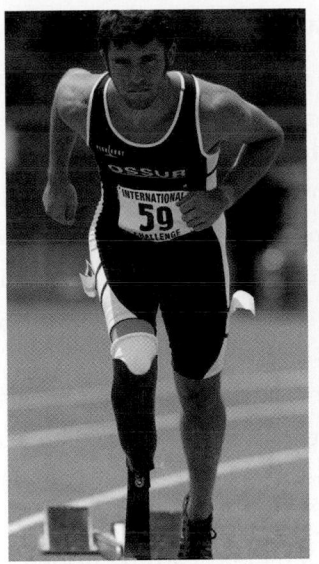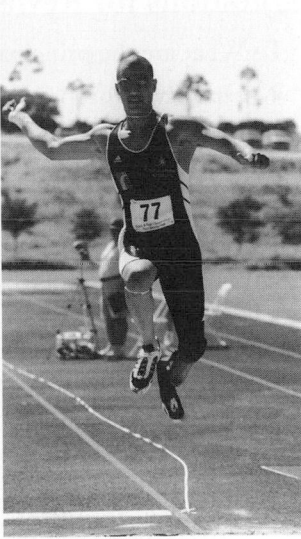

Figure 31.36 Participants in a distance run (*left*) and long jump (*right*) event. *Courtesy of Ossur, Aliso Viejo, CA 92656.*

probably use ski poles equipped with small rudders, in a "three-track" manner. Soccer is usually played without a prosthesis, with the player using a pair of crutches. Some individuals enjoy playing tennis and field events in a wheelchair. Equipment and techniques developed for individuals with paraplegia usually can be adapted for people with amputations.

Recreational programs designed for adults with amputations help the participants to return to active lifestyles. The physical therapist should be able to refer patients to convenient recreational clubs and sporting events. The desired outcome is to maximize each person's functional capacity and quality of life.

SUMMARY

This chapter has focused on the prosthetic management of adults with lower-limb amputations. Characteristics and function of the principal lower-limb prostheses and prosthetic components have been discussed. In addition, the responsibilities of the physical therapist in prosthetic management have been emphasized. Successful prosthetic rehabilitation depends on close collaboration among the patient, physical therapist, physician, prosthetist, and other team members. This will provide an environment for information exchange and foster coordinated management. The result will be an optimum match between the patient's physical and psychosocial characteristics and a prosthesis capable of fulfilling its intended purposes.

Questions for Review

1. What are the principal causes of amputation in the elderly? In the young?

2. Describe appropriate prostheses for individuals with the following partial foot amputations: phalangeal, transmetatarsal, and Syme's.

3. Distinguish between the Syme's and the transtibial amputation limbs and prostheses.

4. What prosthetic feet are especially suitable for elderly patients? Why?

5. Name the reliefs and build-ups in the transtibial socket.

6. Contrast the modes of suspension for the transtibial prosthesis. Which suspension is indicated for an individual with a very short amputation limb?

7. Classify knee units according to friction mechanisms.

8. Compare the quadrilateral and the ischial containment transfemoral sockets.

9. Describe the modes of suspension of the transfemoral prosthesis. In which type(s) does the client wear a sock?

10. How is the wearer of a hip disarticulation prosthesis prevented from inadvertently flexing the prosthetic hip and knee?

11. Outline a maintenance program for a transfemoral prosthesis with hydraulic knee unit and endoskeletal shank.

12. What factors should be considered before formulating a prosthetic prescription?

13. How can the physical therapist determine and improve the patient's psychological status?

14. What features of the transtibial prosthesis are considered in static evaluation? In dynamic evaluation?

15. Delineate the training program for a patient with a transfemoral prosthesis.

CASE STUDY

The patient is a 67-year-old man with diabetic arteriosclerosis. He sustained a right transtibial amputation 5 months ago. He was treated in the inpatient physical therapy department for 3 weeks. The wound healed satisfactorily. His physical therapist taught him to transfer independently and ambulate using a temporary prosthesis and a walker. He was discharged with a home program consisting of exercises to promote strength, joint mobility, and endurance. He was also told to keep an elastic shrinker sock on his amputation limb whenever he was not wearing the temporary prosthesis. In addition, the physical therapist instructed the patient in care of the left foot, including thorough foot washing every evening; inspecting all surfaces of the foot, using a mirror; wearing a clean sock and well-fitting shoe each day; and careful nail trimming. He was fitted with a permanent prosthesis 3 months after surgery. The prosthesis consisted of a SACH foot, endoskeletal shank, total contact socket, and cuff suspension. He returned to the rehabilitation department today complaining of difficulty keeping his balance on the irregular terrain on the golf course where he had gone for the first time since his surgery. He also mentioned that his golf score was poorer than it had ever been.

PAST MEDICAL HISTORY

The patient was in fairly good health until 6 months ago, when he went on a long-awaited trip to Europe. On the trip he did much more walking than usual, even though he had to stop every 50 feet because of cramping pain in his legs. His wife noticed that the hallux and second toe on his right foot were discolored. The discolored area became painful. After his return home, he was examined by his primary care physician and was diagnosed with gangrene and adult-onset diabetes. Despite aggressive wound care, the gangrene progressed to involve the entire foot. An amputation was required. His diabetes is now stabilized with diet and medication.

SOCIAL HISTORY

The patient is a retired accountant who lives with his wife. For years, he played golf on vacations. Upon retirement last year, he had looked forward to more frequent golfing.

PHYSICAL THERAPY EXAMINATION FINDINGS

- *Cognitive status*: Alert, oriented, memory intact
- *Vision*: Intact with corrective lens
- *Cardiopulmonary*:
  - Vital signs seated at rest: Blood pressure 140/86, heart rate 84, respiration within normal limits (WNL)
  - Endurance: Fair, tolerance to activity is approximately 30 minutes (with some fluctuation); occasional rest periods required
- *Integumentary*: Incision well healed without adherent scar
- *Neuromuscular*:
  - Sensation: Both upper and lower extremities: sharp/dull, light touch, temperature, and proprioception all WNL bilaterally
  - Reflexes: WNL

Range of Motion

- Goniometric examination of both LEs: WNL

Observational Gait Analysis (General Findings)

- Overall decrease in speed of movement
- Diminished, awkward weight transfer

Hip/Pelvis (Bilateral)

- Decreased pelvic rotation
- Diminished hip flexion

Knee

- Diminished right knee flexion

Foot/Ankle

- Minimal medial–lateral motion of the right prosthetic foot

Gait

The patient is a functional ambulator using a transtibial prosthesis. Gait is slow, with longer steps on the right side; without the cane he leans to the right side. When outdoors he uses a cane in the left hand. He can climb stairs slowly, using the handrail. On uneven surfaces, he widens his walking base and walks slowly.

Strength

Manual Muscle Test (MMT) Grades		Right	Left
Hip	Flexion	4/5	4/5
	Extension	4/5	4/5
	Abduction	4/5	4/5
	Adduction	4/5	4/5
	Internal rotation	4–/5	4–/5
	External rotation	4–/5	4–/5
Knee	Flexion	4–/5	4/5
	Extension	3+/5	4–/5
Foot/ankle	Dorsiflexion	N/A	4/5
	Plantar flexion	N/A	4/5
	Inversion	N/A	4/5
	Eversion	N/A	4/5
Upper limb	WFL	WFL	WFL

N/A = not applicable owing to amputation; WFL = within functional limits.

Prosthetic Examination
- Socket is loose, as indicated by piston action

Balance

Standing
- Static: Good; able to maintain static position for unlimited period
- Dynamic: Fair +; difficulty maintaining balance on uneven terrain

Sitting
- WFL

Examination of Function
- Patient independent in transfers: bed, chair (FIM level = 7); requires minimal assistance in floor-to-stand transfers.
- Patient is independent in all basic activities of daily living (BADL).
- Patient is independent in approximately 80% of instrumental activities of daily living (IADL) (limitations imposed by fatigue and low ambulatory tolerance).

PATIENT DESIRED OUTCOMES
- Play golf at previous level of proficiency
- Walk without depending on cane when outdoors
- Improve endurance

GUIDING QUESTIONS

1. Formulate a clinical problem list, including impairments, activity limitations, and participation restrictions.

2. Formulate a patient asset list.

3. Establish anticipated short-term goals and expected long-term outcomes, with regard to impact on:
   - Impairments
   - Activity limitations
   - Participation restrictions
   - Risk reduction/prevention
   - Health, wellness, and fitness
   - Patient/client satisfaction

4. Formulate a plan of care, with reference to *Guide to Physical Therapist Practice*.

5. Identify three impairments to address initially to improve this patient's activity limitations and participation restrictions.

6. Describe three treatment interventions focused on functional outcomes that could be used during the first weeks of therapy, indicating how you could progress each intervention.

7. What important safety precautions should be observed during treatment of this patient?

8. Describe strategies that can be used to develop self-management skills and promote self-efficacy in achieving goals and outcomes.

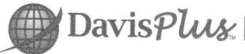 For additional resources, including answers to the questions for review and case study guiding questions, please visit **http://davisplus.fadavis.com**

References

1. Ziegler-Graham, K, et al: Estimating the prevalence of limb loss in the United States: 2005 to 2050. Arch Phys Med Rehabil 89:422, 2008.
2. Rommers, GM, et al: Shoe adaptation after amputation of the II–V phalangeal bones of the foot. Prosthet Orthot Int 30:324, 2006.
3. Dudkiewicz, I, et al: Trans-metatarsal amputation in patients with a diabetic foot: Reviewing 10 years' experience. Foot 19:201, 2009.
4. Dillon, MP, and Barker, TM: Comparison of gait of persons with partial foot amputation wearing prosthesis to matched control group: Observational study. J Rehabil Res Dev 45:1317, 2008.
5. Burger, H, et al: Biomechanics of walking with silicone prosthesis after midtarsal (Chopart) disarticulation. Clin Biomech (Bristol, Avon) 24:510, 2009.
6. Berke, GM, et al: Biomechanics of ambulation following partial foot amputation: A prosthetic perspective. J Prosthet Orthot 19:85, 2007.
7. Yu, GV, et al: Syme's amputation: A retrospective review of 10 cases. Clin Podiatri Med Surg 22:395, 2005.
8. Frykberg, RG, et al: Syme amputation for limb salvage: Early experience with 26 cases. J Foot Ankle Surg 46:93, 2007.
9. Johannsson, A, Larsson, GU, and Ramstrand, N: Incidence of lower-limb amputation in the diabetic and nondiabetic general population: A 10-year population-based cohort study of initial unilateral and contralateral amputations and reamputations. Diabetes Care 32:275, 2009.
10. Klodd, E, et al: Effects of prosthetic foot forefoot flexibility on oxygen cost and subjective preference rankings of unilateral transtibial prosthesis users. J Rehabil Res Dev 47:543, 2010.

11. Czerniecki, JM: Research and clinical selection of foot-ankle systems. J Prosthet Orthot 17:S35, 2005.
12. Versluys, R, et al: Prosthetic foot: State-of-the-art review and the importance of mimicking human ankle-foot biomechanics. Disabil Rehabil Assist Technol 4:65, 2009.
13. Hsu, MJ, et al: The effects of prosthetic foot design on physiologic measurements, self-selected walking velocity, and physical activity in people with transtibial amputation. Arch Phys Med Rehabil 87: 123, 2006.
14. Zmitrewicz, RJ, et al: The effect of foot and ankle prosthetic components on braking and propulsive impulses during transtibial amputee gait. Arch Phys Med Rehabil 87:1334, 2006.
15. Zmitrewicz, RJ, Neptune, RR, and Sasaki, K: Mechanical energetic contributions from individual muscles and elastic prosthetic feet during symmetric unilateral transtibial amputees walking: A theoretical study. J Biomech 40:1824, 2007.
16. Agrawal, V, et al: Symmetry in external work (SEW): A novel method of quantifying gait differences between prosthetic feet. Prosthet Orthot Int 33:146, 2009.
17. Wolf, SI, et al: Pressure characteristics at the stump/socket interface in transtibial amputees using an adaptive prosthetic foot. Clin Biomech (Bristol, Avon) 24:860, 2009.
18. Alimusaj, M, et al: Kinematics and kinetics with an adaptive ankle foot system during stair ambulation of transtibial amputees. Gait Posture 30:356, 2009.
19. Berge, JS, Czerniecki, JM, and Klute, GK: Efficacy of shock-absorbing versus rigid pylons for impact reduction in transtibial amputees based on laboratory, field, and outcome metrics. J Rehabil Res Dev 42:795, 2005.
20. Adderson, JA, et al: Effect of a shock-absorbing pylon on transmission of heel strike forces during the gait of people with unilateral transtibial amputations: A pilot study. Prosthet Orthot Int 31:384, 2007.
21. Ross, J, et al: Study of telescopic pylon on lower limb amputees. Orthopad Technik 3:1, 2003.
22. Selles, RW, et al: A randomized controlled trial comparing functional outcome and cost efficiency of a total surface-bearing socket versus a conventional patellar tendon-bearing socket in transtibial amputees. Arch Phys Med Rehabil 86:154, 2005.
23. Chow, DH, et al: The effect of prosthesis alignment on the symmetry of gait in subjects with unilateral transtibial amputation. Prosthet Orthot Int 30:114, 2006.
24. Jia, X, et al: Effects of alignment on interface pressure for transtibial amputees during walking. Disabil Rehabil Assist Technol 3:339, 2008.
25. Klute, GK, Glaister, BC, and Berge, JS: Prosthetic liners for lower limb amputees: A review of the literature. Prosthet Orthot Int 34: 146, 2010.
26. Kristinsson, O: The ICEROSS concept: A discussion of philosophy. Prosthet Orthot Int 17:49, 1993.
27. Astrom, I, and Stenstrom, A: Effect on gait and socket comfort in unilateral trans-tibial amputees after exchange to a polyurethane concept. Prosthet Orthot Int 28:28, 2004.
28. Brånemark, R, et al: Osseointegration in skeletal reconstruction and rehabilitation. J Rehabil Res Dev 38:175, 2001.
29. Meikle, B, et al: Does increased prosthetic weight affect gait speed and patient preference in dysvascular transfemoral amputees? Arch Phys Med Rehabil 84:1657, 2003.
30. Van der Linden, ML, Twiste, N, and Rithalia, SV: The biomechanical effects of the inclusion of a torque absorber on transfemoral amputee gait. Prosthet Orthot Int 26:35, 2002.
31. Radcliffe, CW: Four-bar linkage prosthetic knee mechanisms: Kinematics, alignment and prescription criteria. Prosthet Orthot Int 18:159, 1994.
32. Sapin, E, et al: Functional gait analysis of trans-femoral amputees using two different single-axis prosthetic knees with hydraulic swing-phase control: Kinematic and kinetic comparison of two prosthetic knees. Prosthet Orthot Int 32:201, 2008.
33. Chin, T, et al: Successful prosthetic fitting of elderly trans-femoral amputees with Intelligent Prosthesis (IP): A clinical study. Prosthet Orthot Int 31:271, 2007.
34. Jepson, F, et al: A comparative evaluation of the Adaptive knee and Catech® knee joints: A preliminary study. Prosthet Orthot Int 32: 84, 2008.
35. Swanson, E, Stube, J, and Edman, P: Function and body image levels in individuals with transfemoral amputations using the C-Leg®. J Prosthet Orthot 17:80, 2005.
36. Orendurff, M, et al: Gait efficiency using the C-Leg. J Rehabil Res Dev 43:239, 2006.
37. Segal, AD, et al: Kinematic and kinetic comparisons of trans-femoral amputee gait using C-Leg and Mauch SNS prosthetic knees. J Rehabil Res Dev 43:857, 2006.
38. Seymour, R, et al: Comparison between the C-Leg microprocessor-controlled prosthetic knee and nonmicroprocessor-controlled prosthetic knees: A preliminary study of energy expenditure, obstacle course performance and quality of life survey. Prosthet Orthot Int 31:51, 2007.
39. Kahle, JT, Highsmith, MJ, and Hubbard, SL: Comparison of non-microprocessor knee mechanism versus C-Leg on Prosthesis Evaluation questionnaire, stumbles, falls, walking tests, stair descent, and knee preference. J Rehabil Res Dev 45:1, 2008.
40. Brodtkorb, TH, et al: Cost-effectiveness of C-leg compared with non-microprocessor-controlled knees: A modeling approach. Arch Phys Med Rehabil 89:24, 2008.
41. Highsmith, MJ, et al: Safety, energy efficiency, and cost efficacy of the C-Leg for transfemoral amputees: A review of the literature. Prosthet Orthot Int 34:362, 2010.
42. Johansson, JL, et al: A clinical comparison of variable-damping and mechanically passive prosthetic knee devices. Am J Phys Med Rehabil 84:563, 2005.
43. Devlin, M, et al: Patient preference and gait efficiency in a geriatric population with transfemoral amputation using a free-swinging versus a locked prosthetic knee joint. Arch Phys Med Rehabil 83:246, 2002.
44. Lythgo, N, Marmaras, B, and Connor, H: Physical function, gait, and dynamic balance of transfemoral amputees using two mechanical passive prosthetic knee devices. Arch Phys Med Rehabil 91:1565, 2010.
45. Hagberg, K, and Brånemark, R: One hundred patients treated with osseointegrated transfemoral amputation prosthesis: Rehabilitation perspective. J Rehabil Res Dev 46:331, 2009.
46. Morse, BC, et al: Through-knee amputation in patients with peripheral arterial disease: A review of 50 cases. J Vasc Surg 48:638, 2008.
47. Ten Duis, K, et al: Knee disarticulation: Survival, wound healing, and ambulation: A historic cohort study. Prosthet Orthot Int 33:52, 2009.
48. Fernandez, A, and Formigo, J: Are Canadian prostheses used? A long-term experience. Prosthet Orthot Int 29:177, 2005.
49. Yari, P, Dijkstra, P, and Geertzen, J: Functional outcome of hip disarticulation and hemipelvectomy: A cross-sectional national descriptive study in the Netherlands. Clin Rehabil 22:1127, 2008.
50. Ludwigs, E, et al: Biomechanical differences between two exoprosthetic hip joint systems during level walking. Prosthet Orthot Int 34:449, 2010.
51. Nelson, LM, and Carbone, NT: Functional outcome measurements of a veteran with a hip disarticulation using a Helix 3D hip joint: A case report. J Prosthet Orthot 23:21, 2011.
52. Su, PF, et al: Differences in gait characteristics between persons with bilateral transtibial amputations, due to peripheral vascular disease and trauma, and able-bodied ambulators. Arch Phys Med Rehabil 89:1386, 2008.
53. Traballesi, M, et al: Prognostic factors in prosthetic rehabilitation of bilateral dysvascular above-knee amputees: Is the stump condition an influencing factor? Eura Medicophys 43:1, 2007.
54. McNealy, LL, and Gard, SA: Effect of prosthetic ankle units on the gait of persons with bilateral transfemoral amputations. Prosthet Orthot Int 32:111, 2008.
55. Potter, BK, and Scoville, CR: Amputation is not isolated: An overview of the US Army Amputee Patient Care Program and associated amputee injuries. J Am Acad Orthop Surg 14:S188, 2008.
56. Granville, R, and Menetrez, J: Rehabilitation of the lower-extremity war-injured at the center for the intrepid. Foot Ankle Clin 15:187, 2010.
57. Highsmith, MJ: Barriers to the provision of prosthetic services in the geriatric population. Top Geriatr Rehabil 24:325, 2008.
58. O'Neill, BF, and Evans, JJ: Memory and executive function predict mobility rehabilitation outcome after lower-limb amputation. Disabil Rehabil 11:1, 2009.
59. Atherton, R, and Robertson, N: Psychological adjustment to lower limb amputation amongst prosthesis users. Disabil Rehabil 28:1201, 2006.

60. Coffey, L, et al: Psychosocial adjustment to diabetes-related lower limb amputation. Diabet Med 26:1063, 2009.

61. Mayer, A, et al: Body schema and body awareness of amputees. Prosthet Orthot Int 32:363, 2008.

62. Desmond, D, et al: Pain and psychosocial adjustment to lower limb amputation amongst prosthesis users. Prosthet Orthot Int 32:244, 2008.

63. Callaghan, B, Condie, E, and Johnston, M: Using the common sense self-regulation model to determine psychological predictors of prosthetic use and activity limitation in lower limb amputees. Prosthet Orthot Int 32:324, 2008.

64. Wegener, ST, et al: Self-management improves outcomes in persons with limb loss. Arch Phys Med Rehabil 90:373, 2009.

65. Centers for Medicare and Medicaid Services: Medicare and You 2011. Department of Health and Human Services, Baltimore, MD, 2011. Retrieved May 26, 2011, from www.medicare.gov/publications/pubs/pdf/10050.pdf.

66. Vrieling, AH, et al: Gait initiation in lower limb amputees. Gait Posture 27:423, 2008.

67. Vrieling, AH, et al: Gait termination in lower limb amputees. Gait Posture 27:82, 2008.

68. Fraisse, N, et al: Muscles of the below-knee amputees. Ann Readapt Med Phys 51:281, 2008.

69. Silverman, AK, et al: Compensatory mechanisms in below-knee amputee gait in response to increasing steady-state walking speeds. Gait Posture 28:602, 2008.

70. Vanicek, N, et al: Gait patterns in transtibial amputee fallers vs. non-fallers: Biomechanical differences during level walking. Gait Posture 29:415, 2009.

71. Nolan, L, and Lees, A: The functional demands on the intact limb during walking for active trans-femoral and trans-tibial amputees. Prosthet Orthot Int 24:117, 2000.

72. van Keeken, HG, et al: Controlling propulsive forces in gait initiation in transfemoral amputees. J Biomech Eng 130:011002, 2008.

73. Matjacic, Z, and Burger, H: Dynamic balance training during standing in people with trans-tibial amputation: A pilot study. Prosthet Orthot Int 27:214, 2003.

74. Miller, WC, et al: The influence of falling, fear of falling, and balance confidence on prosthetic mobility and social activity among individuals with lower extremity amputation. Arch Phys Med Rehabil 82:1238, 2001.

75. Sjodahl, C, et al: Gait improvement in unilateral transfemoral amputees by a combined psychological and physiotherapeutic treatment. J Rehabil Med 33:114, 2001.

76. Yigiter, K, et al: A comparison of traditional prosthetic training versus proprioceptive neuromuscular facilitation resistive gait training with trans-femoral amputees. Prosthet Orthot Int 26:213, 2002.

77. Tsai, HA, et al: Aided gait of people with lower-limb amputations: Comparison of 4-footed and 2-wheeled walkers. Arch Phys Med Rehabil 84:584, 2003.

78. Ramstrand, N, and Nilsson, KA: A comparison of foot placement strategies of transtibial amputees and able-bodied subjects during stair ambulation. Prosthet Orthot Int 33:348, 2009.

79. Schmalz, T, Blumentritt, S, and Marx, B: Biomechanical analysis of stair ambulation in lower limb amputees. Gait Posture 25:267, 2007.

80. Vrieling, AH, et al: Uphill and downhill walking in unilateral lower limb amputees. Gait Posture 28:235, 2008.

81. Fradet, L, et al: Biomechanical analysis of ramp ambulation of transtibial amputees with an adaptive ankle foot system. Gait Posture 32:191, 2010.

82. Vickers, DR, et al: Elderly unilateral transtibial amputee gait on an inclined walkway: A biomechanical analysis. Gait Posture 27:518, 2008.

83. Vrieling, AH, et al: Obstacle crossing in lower limb amputees. Gait Posture 26:587, 2007.

84. Gonzalez, E, and Edelstein, J: Energy expenditure in ambulation. In Gonzalez, E, et al (eds): Downey and Darling's Physiological Basis of Rehabilitation Medicine, ed 3. Butterworth-Heinemann, Boston, 2001, p 417.

85. Goktepe, AS, et al: Energy expenditure of walking with prostheses: Comparison of three amputation levels. Prosthet Orthot Int 34:31, 2010.

86. Schmalz, T, Blumentritt, S, and Jarasch, R: Energy expenditure and biomechanical characteristics of lower limb amputee gait: The influence of prosthetic alignment and different prosthetic components. Gait Posture 16:255, 2002.

87. Genin, JJ, et al: Effect of speed on the energy cost of walking in unilateral traumatic lower limb amputees. Eur J Appl Physiol 103:655, 2008.

88. Detrembleur, C, et al: Relationship between energy cost, gait speed, vertical displacement of centre of body mass and efficiency of pendulum-like mechanism in unilateral amputee gait. Gait Posture 21:333, 2005.

89. Houdijk, H, et al: The energy cost for the step-to-step transition in amputee walking. Gait Posture 30:35, 2009.

90. Bussmann, JB, et al: Daily physical activity and heart rate response in people with a unilateral transtibial amputation for vascular disease. Arch Phys Med Rehabil 85:240, 2004.

91. Huang, GF, Chou, YL, and Su, FC: Gait analysis and energy consumption of below-knee amputees wearing three different prosthetic feet. Gait Posture 12:162, 2000.

92. Graham, LE, et al: A comparative study of oxygen consumption for conventional and energy-storing prosthetic feet in transfemoral amputees. Clin Rehabil 22:896, 2008.

93. Kaufman, KR, et al: Energy expenditure and activity of transfemoral amputees using mechanical and microprocessor-controlled prosthetic knees. Arch Phys Med Rehabil 89:1380, 2008.

94. Chin, T, et al: Comparison of different microprocessor controlled knee joints on the energy consumption during walking in transfemoral amputees: Intelligent knee prosthesis (IP) versus C-Leg. Prosthet Orthot Int 30: 73, 2006.

95. Datta, D, et al: A comparative evaluation of oxygen consumption and gait pattern in amputees using intelligent prostheses and conventionally damped knee swing-phase control. Clin Rehabil 19:398, 2005.

96. Chin, T, et al: Energy expenditure during walking in amputees after disarticulation of the hip: A microprocessor-controlled swing-phase control knee versus a mechanical-controlled stance-phase control knee. J Bone Joint Surg 87B:117, 2005.

97. Wright, DA, Marks, L, and Payne, RC: A comparative study of the physiological costs of walking in ten bilateral amputees. Prosthet Orthot Int 32:57, 2008.

98. Raya, MA, et al: Impairment variables predicting activity limitation in individuals with lower limb amputation. Prosthet Orthot Int 34:73, 2010.

99. Raichle, KA, et al: Prosthesis use in persons with lower- and upper-limb amputation. J Rehabil Res Dev 45:961, 2008.

100. Gailey, R, et al: Unilateral lower-limb loss: Prosthetic device use and functional outcomes in service members from Vietnam war and OIF/OEF conflicts. J Rehabil Res Dev 47:317, 2010.

101. Pezzin, LE, et al: Use and satisfaction with prosthetic limb devices and related services. Arch Phys Med Rehabil 85:723, 2004.

102. Karmarkar, AM, et al: Prosthesis and wheelchair use in veterans with lower-limb amputation. J Rehabil Res Dev 46:567, 2009.

103. Epstein, RA, Heinemann, AW, and McFarland, LV: Quality of life for veterans and service members with major traumatic limb loss from Vietnam and OIF/OEF conflicts. J Rehabil Res Dev 47:373, 2010.

104. Zidarov, D, Swaine, B, and Gauthier-Gagnon, C: Quality of life of persons with lower-limb amputation during rehabilitation and at 3-month follow-up. Arch Phys Med Rehabil 90:634, 2009.

105. Asano, M, et al: Predictors of quality of life among individuals who have a lower limb amputation. Prosthet Orthot Int 32:231, 2008.

106. Bosmans, JC, et al: Survival of participating and nonparticipating limb amputees in prospective study: Consequences for research. J Rehabil Res Dev 47:457, 2010.

107. Johannesson, A, Larsson, GU, and Oberg, T: From major amputation to prosthetic outcome: A prospective study of 190 patients in a defined population. Prosthet Orthot Int 28:9, 2004.

108. Davies, B, and Datta, D: Mobility outcome following unilateral lower limb amputation. Prosthet Orthot Int 27:186, 2003.

109. Deans, SA, McFadyen, AK, and Rowe, PJ: Physical activity and quality of life: A study of a lower-limb amputee population. Prosthet Orthot Int 32:186, 2008.

110. Remes, L, et al: Predictors for institutionalization and prosthetic ambulation after major lower extremity amputation during an eight-year follow-up. Aging Clin Exp Res 21:129, 2009.

111. Taylor, SM, et al: "Successful outcome" after below-knee amputation: An objective definition and influence of clinical variables. Am Surg 74:607, 2008.

112. Ebrahimzadeh, MH, and Hariri, S: Long-term outcomes of unilateral transtibial amputations. Mil Med 174:593, 2009.

113. Hagberg, K, and Brånemark, R: Consequences of non-vascular transfemoral amputation: A survey of quality of life, prosthetic use and problems. Prosthet Orthot Int 25:186, 2001.

114. MacNeill, HL, et al: Long-term outcomes and survival of patients with bilateral transtibial amputation after rehabilitation. Am J Phys Med Rehabil 87:189, 2008.

115. Bilodeau, S, et al: Lower limb prosthetics utilization by elderly amputees. Prosthet Orthot Int 24:124, 2000.

116. Dillingham, TR, Pezzin, LE, and Mackenzie, EJ: Discharge destination after dysvascular lower-limb amputations. Arch Phys Med Rehabil 84:1662, 2003.

117. Burger, H, and Marincek, C: Return to work after lower limb amputation. Disabil Rehabil 29:1323, 2007.

118. Bruins, M, et al: Vocational reintegration after a lower limb amputation: A qualitative study. Prosthet Orthot Int 27:4, 2003.

119. Boulias, C, et al: Return to driving after lower-extremity amputation. Arch Phys Med Rehabil 87:1183, 2006.

120. Meikle, B, Devlin, M, and Pauley, T: Driving pedal reaction times after right transtibial amputation. Arch Phys Med Rehabil 87:390, 2006.

121. Legro, MW, et al: Recreational activities of lower-limb amputees with prostheses. J Rehabil Res Dev 38:319, 2001.

122. Fergason, JR, and Boone, DA: Custom design in lower limb prosthetics for athletic activity. Phys Med Rehabil Clin North Am 11:681, 2000.

123. Yazicioglu, K, et al: Effect of playing football (soccer) on balance, strength, and quality of life in unilateral below-knee amputees. Am J Phys Med Rehabil 86:800, 2007.

124. Farley, R, Mitchell, F, and Griffiths, M: Custom skiing and trekking adaptations for a trans-tibial and trans-radial quadrilateral amputee. Prosthet Orthot Int 28:60, 2004.

125. Kars, C, et al: Participation in sports by lower limb amputees in the Province of Drenthe, The Netherlands. Prosthet Orthot Int 33:356, 2009.

126. Nolan, L: Lower limb strength in sports-active transtibial amputees. Prosthet Orthot Int 33:230, 2009.

127. Brown, MB, Millard-Stafford, ML, and Allison, AR: Running-specific prostheses permit energy cost similar to nonamputees. Med Sci Sports Exerc 41:1080, 2009.

128. Weyand, PG, et al: The fastest runner on artificial legs: Different limbs, similar function? J Appl Physiol 107:903, 2009.

129. Pailler, D, et al: Evolution in prostheses for sprinters with lower-limb amputation. Ann Readapt Med Phys 47:374, 2004.

130. Gailey, R, and Harsch, P: Introduction to triathlon for the lower limb amputee triathlete. Prosthet Orthot Int 33:242, 2009.

131. Nolan, L, and Lees, A: The influence of lower-limb amputation level on the approach in the amputee long jump. J Sports Sci 25:393, 2007.

132. Nolan, L, Patritti, BL, and Simpson, KJ: A biomechanical analysis of the long-jump technique of elite female amputee athletes. Med Sci Sports Exerc 38:1829, 2006.

133. Nolan, L, and Patritti, BL: The take-off phase in transtibial amputee high jump. Prosthet Ortho Int 32:160, 2008.

134. Minnoye, SL, and Plettenburg, DH: Design, fabrication, and preliminary results of a novel below-knee prosthesis for snowboarding: A case report. Prosthet Orthot Int 33:272, 2009.

Supplemental Reading

Carroll, K, and Edelstein, J (eds): Prosthetics and Patient Management: A Comprehensive Clinical Approach. Slack, Thorofare, NJ, 2006.

Edelstein, J, and Moroz, A: Lower-Limb Prosthetics and Orthotics: Clinical Concepts. Slack, Thorofare, NJ, 2011.

Fitzlaff, G, and Heim, S: Lower Limb Prosthetic Components: Design, Function and Biomechanical Properties. Verlag Orthopadie Technik, Dortmund, Germany, 2002.

Lusardi, MM, and Nielsen, CC: Orthotics and Prosthetics in Rehabilitation, ed 2. Butterworth Heinemann, Boston, 2006.

May, BJ, and Lockard, MA: Prosthetics and Orthotics in Clinical Practice. FA Davis, Philadelphia, 2011.

Parker, JN, and Parker, PM (eds): Amputation: A Medical Dictionary, Bibliography and Annotated Research Guide to Internet References. ICON Health Publications, San Diego, CA, 2003.

Rehabilitation Institute of Chicago: Lower Extremity Amputation: A Guide to Functional Outcomes in Physical Therapy Management. Pro-Ed, Austin, TX, 2005.

Seymour, R: Prosthetics and Orthotics: Lower Limb and Spinal. Lippincott Williams & Wilkins, Philadelphia, 2002.

Smith, DG, et al (eds): Atlas of Amputations and Limb Deficiencies, ed 3. American Academy of Orthopaedic Surgeons, Chicago, 2004.

Transtibial (Below-Knee) Prosthetic Examination

1. Is the prosthesis as prescribed?
2. Can the client don the prosthesis easily?

Standing

3. Is the client comfortable when standing with the heel midlines 6 in (15 cm) apart?
4. Is the anterior–posterior alignment satisfactory?
5. Is the medial–lateral alignment satisfactory?
6. Do the contours and color of the prosthesis match the opposite limb?
7. Is the prosthesis the correct length?
8. Is piston action minimal?
9. Does the socket contact the amputation limb without pinching or gapping?

Suspension

10. Does the suspension component fit the amputation limb properly?
11. Does the cuff, fork strap, or thigh corset have adequate provision for adjustment?

Sitting

12. Can the client sit comfortably with hips and knees flexed 90°?

Walking

13. Is the client's performance in level walking satisfactory?
14. Is the client's performance on stairs and ramps satisfactory?
15. Can the client kneel satisfactorily?
16. Does the suspension function properly?
17. Does the prosthesis operate quietly?
18. Does the client consider the prosthesis satisfactory as to comfort, function, and appearance?

Prosthesis Off the Client

19. Is the skin free of abrasions or other discolorations attributable to this prosthesis?
20. Is the socket interior smooth?
21. Is the posterior wall of the socket of adequate height?
22. Is the construction satisfactory?
23. Do all components function satisfactorily?

Transfemoral (Above-Knee) Prosthetic Examination

1. Is the prosthesis as prescribed?
2. Can the client don the prosthesis easily?

Standing

3. Is the client comfortable when standing with the heel midlines 6 in (15 cm) apart?
4. Is any flesh roll above the socket minimal?
5. Is the client free from vertical pressure in the perineum?
6. Do the contours and color of the prosthesis match the opposite limb?
7. Is the prosthesis the correct length?
8. Is the knee stable?
9. When the socket valve is removed, is the distal tissue firm?

Quadrilateral Socket

10. Does the ischial tuberosity rest on the posterior brim?
11. Is the posterior brim approximately parallel to the floor?
12. Is the adductor longus tendon located in the anterior–medial corner?

Ischial Containment Socket

13. Does the posterior–medial corner of the socket cover the ischial tuberosity?
14. Can the client hyperextend the hip on the amputated side comfortably?
15. Can the client flex the hip 90° comfortably, without socket gapping?
16. Can the client abduct the hip on the amputated side comfortably, without socket gapping?

Suspension

17. Does the Silesian bandage control prosthetic rotation and adduction adequately?
18. Does the pelvic band conform to the torso?

Sitting

19. Can the client sit comfortably with hips and knees flexed 90°?
20. Does the socket remain securely on the thigh, without gapping or rotating?
21. Are both thighs approximately the same length and height from the floor?
22. Can the client lean forward to touch the shoes?

Walking

23. Is the client's performance in level walking satisfactory?
24. Is the client's performance on stairs and ramps satisfactory?
25. Does the suspension function properly?
26. Does the prosthesis operate quietly?
27. Does the client consider the prosthesis satisfactory as to comfort, function, and appearance?

Prosthesis Off the Client

28. Is the skin free of abrasions or other discolorations attributable to this prosthesis?
29. Is the socket interior smooth?
30. With the prosthesis fully flexed on a table, can the thigh piece be brought to at least the vertical position?
31. If the socket is totally rigid, is a back pad attached?
32. Is the construction satisfactory?
33. Do all components function satisfactorily?

Organization/Resource	Website
Achilles International—Achilles Track Club	www.achillestrackclub.org
Active Amputee	www.activeamp.org
American Academy of Orthotists and Prosthetists	www.oandp.org
American Amputee Soccer Association	www.ampsoccer.org
American Orthotic and Prosthetic Association	www.aopanet.org
Amputee Coalition of America	www.amputee-coalition.org
Disabled Sport USA	www.dsusa.org
Hemipelvectomy and Hip-Disarticulation Help	http://hphdhelp.org
Limbs for Life Foundation	www.limbsforlife.org
National Amputee Foundation	www.nationalamputation.org
National Amputee Golf Association	www.nagagolf.org
Prosthetics Outreach Foundation	www.pofsea.org
Resource for Orthotics and Prosthetics Information	www.oandp.com

Faith Saftler Savage, PT, ATP

LEARNING OBJECTIVES

1. Describe the components of the examination process for prescribing a wheelchair.
2. Discuss the relationship between elements of patient history and the wheelchair prescription.
3. Describe the optimal sitting posture for an individual using a seating system.
4. Explain the different methods of seating simulation and the expected outcomes.
5. Describe factors that affect determination of seat and back support features.
6. Discuss the benefits and contraindications of various seating system features.
7. Recognize the components of a problem solving model and describe each component when presented with a clinical case study.

CHAPTER OUTLINE

P hysical and occupational therapists are often called on to prescribe a wheelchair. A properly prescribed wheelchair can be a useful device in reintegrating a person with a disability into the community, whereas a poorly prescribed one can actually exacerbate the problems associated with activity limitations and disability. This chapter presents a systematic approach to determining the appropriate components of a prescriptive wheelchair, beginning with a thorough examination and culminating with a plan of care (POC) that includes the proper seating system and wheeled mobility base. The seating system and mobility base combine to create a prescriptive wheelchair, a seated environment from which the patient can achieve maximum function.

Optimal fit of a wheelchair is important to assist the person in improving mobility, posture, and function. Properly fitted wheelchairs assist with preventing problems associated with poor posture, including pressure sores, respiratory difficulties, discomfort, and abandonment of equipment. Cosmetics (appearance), durability, weight, and intended use need to be considered when determining the most appropriate wheelchair system.

Determining the appropriate wheelchair and seating system requires a thorough examination to ensure optimal equipment is obtained. Too often, a basic commercial system is provided, but this is frequently not the best solution. The solution must consider multiple patient-, environmental-, and diagnosis-related factors and requires a comprehensive examination by the professional team. The examination is time consuming and may require several sessions to complete. However, additional time provided "up front" will

The editors acknowledge the contributions of Adrienne Falk Bergen, PT, ATP, to earlier versions of this work.

decrease errors and future costs associated with the mistakes created by data obtained from a less than optimal examination.

Wheelchairs are not just mobility devices but are also *seating support devices*. If inappropriate seating supports are provided, the end user (i.e., the patient) may be unable to propel a manual wheelchair, operate a power wheelchair, or achieve effective positioning at a table for meals. All relevant aspects of a person's lifestyle should be considered to ensure safety and optimal function.

The entire team contributes to the wheelchair prescription decision making. It is important that all those concerned with the person's present and future function be a part of this team. The team may include the wheelchair user, therapists, family members, caregivers, nurses, physicians, educators, vocational counselors, and a qualified rehabilitation technology supplier. To ensure that the most suitable device is obtained, the team must have a clear idea of who will be using it, what functional level is expected, and where the chair will be used. Team members contribute to the examination reports and letter of medical necessity, which must be prepared to secure funding. Once the chair is supplied, the appropriate team members are responsible for adjusting and fitting the final device, as well as teaching the patient and any caregivers how to use and maintain the unit to ensure optimal long-term performance.

A prescriptive wheelchair is a combination of a postural support system and a mobility base that are joined to create a dynamic seated environment (Fig. 32.1). The *postural support system* is made up of the surfaces that contact the user's body directly. This includes the seat, back, and foot supports, as well as any additional components needed to maintain postural alignment. Maintenance of postural alignment may require such additions as a head support; lateral supports for the trunk, hips, and knees; medial support for the knees; and upper extremity (UE) support surfaces, as well as straps (e.g., anterior chest or pelvis) needed to keep the user interfaced with the support surfaces. The *mobility base* consists of the tubular frame, armrests, foot supports, and wheels. Once the decisions are made about the type of support system needed, the team must then decide what type of mobility base best suits the user's functional level and environmental needs. Clear information will be needed to ensure that the postural support system and the mobility base interface properly. For users who utilize more than one mobility base (e.g., power and manual), the most cost-effective approach is to have one support system interface with all the mobility bases. This is not always practical, and sometimes it is best to have the full-support system on the chair used most frequently, and forgo optimal postural support in the backup system used to facilitate transport for short trips.

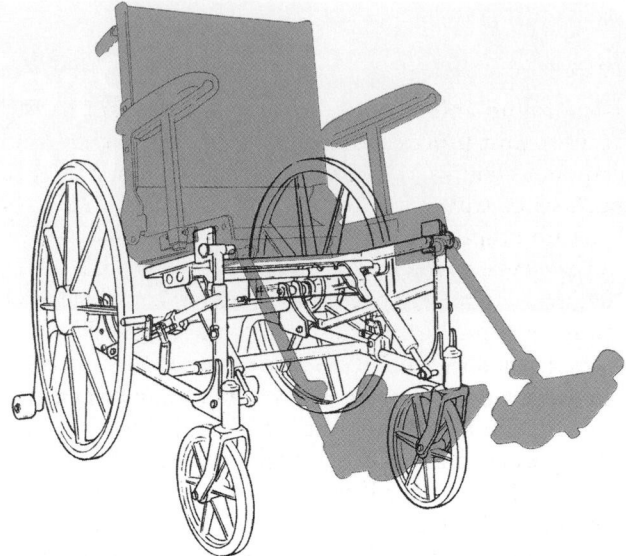

Figure 32.1 A prescriptive wheelchair consists of the postural support system and a mobility base.

Creating a dynamic seating system involves several important steps:

- Gathering background information, including diagnosis, prognosis, functional skills, anticipated goals, and expected outcomes
- Performing a comprehensive examination
- Conducting seating simulations (testing linear and angular dimensions determined from the mat examination in a seating device with the ability to add postural supports to assist in determining optimal seating supports) and equipment trials (testing manual wheelchairs, power wheelchairs, and/or seating supports and cushions before ordering equipment)
- Developing a POC that includes appropriate recommendations and product choices

As noted, the overall desired outcome is to create a dynamic seating system that provides a comfortable base from which the user can attain maximum function. Before the examination, team member expectations should be discussed. A great deal can be learned at this point about what the various team members hope the system will be able to do for the patient. It is extremely important that all issues are identified and openly discussed before the process is begun. Patients, family members, or caregivers may assume that the wheelchair and seating system can achieve unrealistic goals (e.g., normalize posture, provide total pain relief, allow independent transfers). When these unlikely goals are not met, these individuals are often so disappointed that they cannot see the other benefits of the system. Early, open discussion is critical to the decision making process.

■ EXAMINATION

History Taking

Background information is an essential part of the examination process. During the history taking, one can determine what seating and mobility options have been successful in the past, as well as those that have been unsatisfactory; initial goals and concerns related to the new equipment can also be identified. All areas (patient, environmental, and diagnosis related) that require compatibility or interface with the mobility and seating support system should be discussed. For instance, if someone uses a van for transportation, door opening size and seat setup should be discussed. Moving from one style of chair to another might prevent easily getting through the van door if the individual is sitting taller in the new chair or experience difficulty turning the chair once inside the van owing to increased length of the new wheelchair.

Of considerable importance is knowledge of how positioning of one body part affects another. Impairments of a single joint or body segment can directly affect sitting position and alignment. For example, if there is inadequate hip flexion, what happens to the body when in a seated position? Is there any chance that limited range of motion (ROM) will change over time? Can adjustability be built into the seating system to accommodate changes? Should other positioning programs be instituted in addition to seating to assist with improving ROM?

Information about past and future surgeries should be gathered to have a better understanding of current seating needs as well as to gain insight into future requirements. For example, a person who has undergone a spinal fusion may have a pelvic obliquity that cannot be corrected and requires accommodation in the seating system. A person who has had hip surgery (e.g., femoral osteotomy, total hip replacement) may have a leg length difference and the seat cushion needs to accommodate the difference in leg lengths. A person with hip pain may require a seating design to accommodate ROM limitations that may be the cause of the pain. After completing the mat assessment but before completing the seating assessment, it may be necessary to consult with the physician regarding tone management, pain management, or other surgical intervention that may be necessary. A person with multiple sclerosis (MS) with increased lower extremity tone may have significant knee ROM limitations that need to be addressed before seating in a wheelchair. A baclofen pump may be necessary to control tone and assist with increasing ROM before completing the assessment for the seating system. A person with cerebral palsy (CP) may have significant hip ROM limitations that require surgical intervention to improve sitting posture.

Overview: Tests and Measures

Strength and Endurance

Gross and fine motor skills are examined to determine the amount of support a person needs for seating. Strength, endurance, and their impact on function should be addressed within the context of the person's day. A person might function well for 1 hour in the morning and need minimal support during that time but may need more support in the afternoon owing to poor endurance and fatigue. This may make a difference in the ability to perform functional activities throughout the day.

Sensation and Skin Integrity

Individuals who use a wheelchair for locomotion have an increased chance of developing pressure sores from prolonged sitting. The ability to change position or to request positioning changes (if unable to perform independently) based either on a timed interval or due to discomfort is important in the prevention of pressure sores. Individuals with decreased sensation (e.g., spinal cord injury [SCI]) are unable to perceive discomfort from prolonged positioning. In such situations, positioning changes should occur at timed intervals and be incorporated into the daily schedule.

Location and size of old wounds should be noted to ensure appropriate pressure-relieving strategies are provided. Location of new wounds must be investigated to determine the cause (e.g., faulty bed or wheelchair positioning). The proposed seat cushion and back support should be examined and evaluated to determine their potential for promoting healing of any current pressure sores and preventing development of new pressure sores. Pressure mapping is accomplished using a special piece of material with sensors combined with computer software that shows high- and low-pressure areas when sitting on a specific cushion. This map can be used to assist in determining an appropriate seat cushion and is beneficial as a teaching tool when providing instruction in using a tilt-in-space feature, a recline feature, and any adjustments to the seat cushion. When using the tilt feature and recline feature, the pressure on the map changes and areas of high pressure will diminish, assisting individuals in understanding the need for changing their position. Various cushions can also be tested to assist the examiner and individual in choosing the most appropriate seat cushion based on pressure distribution.[1-3]

Vision and Hearing

Vision affects ability to drive a power wheelchair and to maneuver a manual wheelchair. Visual impairments may be more apparent outdoors rather than indoors. It is important to determine how visual problems affect mobility and to determine if the person can learn compensatory techniques to be independent and safe.

Hearing deficits can also pose safety concerns. If driving outdoors, a person with a hearing impairment may not hear a car horn or someone calling to them to stop. Various headrests may diminish the ability to hear well. Determining optimal equipment to compensate for hearing loss is important for safety and independence.

Health Status

Poor positioning of the pelvis and trunk can increase the risk of developing urinary tract and respiratory infections. Complete bladder emptying is more difficult if a person sits in a posterior pelvic tilt. Other risk factors for urinary tract infections include poor technique during intermittent catheterization or changing of indwelling catheter. If a person sits with a kyphotic or scoliotic spine, breathing is compromised and clearing lungs of secretions is more difficult, which increases the risk for respiratory infections.[4,5]

Nutrition has a direct impact on overall health. Poor nutrition can increase healing time, increase risk of developing pressure sores and infections, and create weight management problems. Impaired swallowing will also affect nutrition. Weight gain and loss either from food intake, gastrointestinal tube placement, or medications should be discussed to make informed decisions about seat width of the wheelchair.

Functional Abilities

Toileting

Bathroom issues should be addressed to determine if the person uses a toilet, urinal, catheter, or protective undergarments. If using the toilet, the ability to transfer from the wheelchair to and from the toilet will be important. The effect of the seat height on transfers and the ability to swing away the footrests to approach the toilet must be considered. If using a urinal, the seat style needs to be discussed to prevent accidental tipping of the urinal. If using a catheter and the person empties the urine collection bag into the toilet, access to the toilet needs to be discussed. If the person frequently experiences urinary accidents, a waterproof cover on the seat cushion may be considered.

Bathing and Washing

Accessing the bathroom sink, bathtub, and shower is more difficult when sitting in a wheelchair. Many bathrooms are small and it can be difficult or impossible to maneuver in this space. Concerns include seat height for transfers, style of footrests for transfers, and access to sink for washing. Bathroom modifications may be needed for safety and improved access (see Chapter 9, Examination of the Environment).

Dressing

Some individuals find it easier to don clothing when in their wheelchair. Footrest and armrest style and durability need to be considered to ensure the system will accommodate the extra weight placed on both these components during dressing activities. Use of tilt-in-space seating or a reclining back system may benefit the person who dresses in the wheelchair.

Eating

The seat and armrest height of the wheelchair may preclude positioning the wheelchair at some tables or desks. The style of table or desk may also interfere with access (e.g., number and arrangement of legs, height of working surface, presence of drawers). If a person needs assistance during mealtime, caregivers need to have ease of access. Positioning of head/neck and trunk alignment is important while eating to ensure a safe environment, optimize swallowing, and minimize choking potential.[6] Power seat elevators can increase access to tables of varying heights.

Communication

Some patients require alternative forms of communication. Consultation with the speech-language pathologist is important to determine the type of communication device being used and the method of mounting the device to the wheelchair. This may include a tray to support the device or a separate mounting system attached to the wheelchair. Switches may be used to operate the device; mounting of switches will need to be determined to ensure optimal access and ease of use.

Transfers

The type of transfer used is another important consideration when prescribing a wheelchair. The patient's transfer performance (e.g., complete independence, supervision, moderate assistance) will affect selection of wheelchair features. Armrest style, footrest style, trunk support style, and seat height can all influence safety, as well as the type and amount of assistance required.

Ambulation

Although a person requires a wheelchair for long-distance travel, he or she still may be able to ambulate short distances. The person needs to be able to stand up from the wheelchair and access the assistive device. The seat height, footrest style, and armrest style are important to ensure safe standing and seating to and from the wheelchair. An assistive device (e.g., cane, crutches, walker) may need to be attached to the wheelchair via a special holder and the optimal method of access determined.

Wheelchair Mobility—Manual and Power

Wheel position is important for independent manual mobility. If the feet are used to propel the chair, seat height is important to ensure that the feet reach the floor and to prevent the person from sliding down in the wheelchair. Hand control position is important for independent power mobility. If unable to use a standard hand control, other drive controls are available; strategic placement of alternative controls will assist in providing independent power mobility. If the person is dependent and caregivers are moving the wheelchair, the style of push handles and wheel locks is important.

Environmental Issues and Transportation

Many issues affect a person's ability to access his or her environment. Stairs interfere with access, as do narrow doorways. Small elevators will affect a person's ability to move safely in and out of the elevator, as well as access the push buttons to reach various floors. Transportation also affects access.[7] Wheelchairs may need to be folded for car transport. Van transportation can be difficult as well. The doorway opening and tie-down system inside the van can affect safety. Although it is safer to have a wheelchair facing forward, some vans are equipped with tie-down systems for the wheelchair to be oriented sideward. This can make it more difficult for a person to maintain a safe sitting position. Wheelchair frames and wheels are not designed to withstand the forces generated in a crash when a chair is oriented sideward. There is inadequate support to the individual when oriented sideways and there is a greater tendency to fall/tip sideways causing injury. The person may transfer into a regular seat once inside the van; safe storage of the wheelchair is then a consideration. Steep or stone driveways, dirt roads, potholes, and lack of beveled curbs will all adversely affect a person's ability to safely access the community.

Cognitive and Behavioral Issues

Cognitive and behavioral issues can affect the type of equipment provided to a person with disabilities. The person may be extremely rough on equipment and/or may use equipment as a weapon to hurt others. When providing various types of equipment, safety should always be considered first. Large rehabilitation centers often have programs in place to address these types of issues.

■ SEATING PRINCIPLES

Seating principles provide important general guidelines for patient positioning in a seating device. The overarching intent of the principles is to maximize function by promoting comfort, stability, and optimal interaction with the environment.

Principle 1: Stabilize Proximally to Promote Improved Distal Mobility and Function

This principle is a basic underlying strategy and commonly used by therapists treating individuals with neuromuscular involvement. Stabilizing proximally provides a foundation for distal movement. When eating, stabilizing an elbow on a table and then stabilizing a wrist may promote independence during meals. To improve trunk posture, stabilizing the pelvis is important. In sitting, pelvic stability should be addressed first because it is the foundation for the rest of the body. When assessing how much or where stability is needed, start with the pelvis and move down, then up, and reassess at each level to determine where active control and skill development is needed, as well as the amount of support needed to maintain good posture.

Principle 2: Achieve and Maintain Pelvic Alignment

The pelvis should be positioned in a neutral to slight anterior tilt and optimally be level (not oblique or rotated). This position allows for maintaining the normal lumbar curve, provides weight-bearing on the ischial tuberosities, and promotes active trunk ROM and co-contraction of trunk muscles. Weight-bearing on the ischial tuberosities also promotes symmetry and provides a more stable upright position (rather than sitting on the sacrum or coccyx). Promoting flexion at the hips and extension in the low back can be effective in decreasing abnormal tonal patterns. A level pelvis allows for equal weight-bearing and even pressure distribution and improves alignment in body areas above and below the pelvis. To achieve good pelvic alignment, ROM limitations must be accommodated, as well as all linear dimensions (e.g., thigh and calf length, trunk and hip width). To maintain this alignment, pelvic positioning devices may need to be considered. A pelvic positioning device is a flexible strap or rigid bar that assists in controlling pelvic movement. A flexible strap should lie just below the anterior superior iliac spines (ASISs), be very snug, and be at a 45° to 90° angle to the seat surface. This angle of pull is dependent on how the person moves the pelvis. Key considerations for the pelvic flexible strap positioning device include placement or angle, size, method of cinching, direction of pull, and location of buckle. A rigid device should lie just below the ASISs (also called a sub-ASIS bar) with the bar attached to metal brackets that mount to the seat or frame of the chair. This device prevents pelvic movement and may be beneficial for an individual with excessive pelvic shifting.[8] Another method to maintain pelvic position is to use knee blocks. The knee blocks provide anterior support to the knees and prevent the individual from sliding forward in the wheelchair.

Principle 3: Facilitate Optimal Postural Alignment in all Body Segments, Accommodating for Impairments in Range of Motion

Once the pelvis is stabilized, attention is directed toward alignment of other body segments. Good alignment promotes improved balance, stability, comfort, and function; helps prevent deformity from habitual asymmetrical posturing; and prevents skin breakdown from uneven pressure. To achieve optimal alignment, it must be determined if improved alignment can be achieved passively on a mat table and then in the seated position. If good alignment can be achieved, it must be determined whether the person can maintain alignment using muscular effort or if external supports are required. Time must be allocated to practice motor skills and movements within the context of improved postural alignment, especially if dramatic alignment changes have ensued. For joints and/or body segments that are not amenable to passive alignment, accommodation is needed (e.g., fixed contractures). For example, accommodation would be needed for a person who presents with long-standing hip ROM limitations from prolonged sitting in a *windswept lower extremity (LE) posture* (one hip in abduction and external rotation and the opposite in adduction and internal rotation). Attempts at aligning the LEs would cause pelvic rotation and trunk rotation. The LEs must be positioned in the windswept posture. Alignment of the pelvis takes priority over alignment of other body segments. Providing optimal pelvic and trunk alignment is most important.

Principle 4: Limit Abnormal Movement and Improve Function

Seating equipment can be designed to inhibit abnormal tone, postures, and movements and to improve health, comfort, and function. Abnormal movements should be discouraged or blocked (controlled) based on anticipated goals and expected outcomes. Observation and analysis of abnormal movements will provide clues to what triggers the response. Determining initiating triggers will inform decisions about seating strategies that may contribute to inhibiting unwanted movement. This requires good problem solving skills. Determining the source of the problem may allow decreased use of support blocks.

Principle 5: Provide the Minimum Support Necessary to Achieve Anticipated Goals and Expected Outcomes

The patient is provided the least restrictive supports required to facilitate the acquisition of new skills and foster independence rather than create unnecessary dependence on equipment. This is especially important to the younger person who is growing and changing, as well as the person who has not had the opportunity to improve function owing to poor positioning and excessive equipment use. Supports can be used intermittently throughout the day to provide learning opportunities (acquisition of new skills) over time. Using a minimum of supports can improve cosmetic appearance and self-esteem. Other equipment may need to be used for specific activities or for opportunities to improve strength and skills.

Principle 6: Provide Comfort

Seating equipment should be comfortable. Discomfort leads to increased abnormal tone and movement, postural asymmetry, and fatigue; decreased endurance,

attentiveness, and concentration; and finally disuse of equipment. Critical to the provision of equipment is involvement of the user who should participate in the process and be allowed an opportunity to express likes and dislikes of the system. A poorly fitting system only creates more problems for a person who is already making lifestyle changes to accommodate his or her activity limitations.

■ WHEELCHAIR PRESCRIPTION

The physical therapy data collection for a prescriptive wheelchair includes determining level of function and posture in existing equipment, performing various measures on a mat table, and performing a seating simulation. If significant changes are being made to a seating system, the simulation will provide the patient an opportunity to "test" and provide feedback about the seating recommendations.

It is important to take time at the beginning of the examination process to explain to the patient and caregivers what will be happening, what information will be gathered, and why the information is important. Everyone should be made to feel that his or her input is necessary and valuable. Time should be allocated during data collection for comments or questions from the patient, caregivers, and other team members. Before each stage of the process, the patient should be asked if it is acceptable to proceed. For example, "I would like to put my hands on your pelvis, is that okay?" It is important to move slowly and speak calmly, because quick movements or loud speech may increase anxiety. For some patients, this may increase muscle tone, interfering with data collection. It is important to explain what is being observed or measured so that patients and caregivers can understand information exchanged among team members, and so they can fully comprehend the team's findings and the subsequent recommendations.

Although time consuming, it is absolutely critical that the physical examination be complete and accurate because changes may be difficult to make later. Accurate recording provides a permanent record of why certain decisions were made. During the ordering or manufacturing process, additional decisions concerning modifications may be needed. If accurate measurements are on file, decisions can often be made without recalling the person to the clinic.

Function and Posture in Existing Equipment

Observing the patient in his or her existing wheelchair provides a great deal of information. The patient should be in the best or most commonly assumed position, with supports and straps in place. Questions should include how the patient and/or caregiver perceive the device is working; has it always worked like this, or has its function decreased over time? If it worked well initially, but does not work well now, is this because of patient change (weight gain or loss, growth, functional gain or loss) or equipment change (broken or missing parts, decreased reliability)? Information can be gathered during this portion of the examination about patient and caregiver attitudes and technology savvy, as well as their physical use of the equipment. Throughout the initial visit, team members should continuously observe the existing equipment, the patient, the caregivers, and their physical and psychosocial interactions.

The team should gather data about the patient's postural alignment at the head, shoulders, trunk, pelvis, and LEs using both visual observation and palpation. Pelvic alignment is examined by palpation along the pelvis crests and on the ASISs. The position of the pelvis (e.g., rotation, posterior or anterior tilt) should be carefully documented.

With the patient's shirt removed or at least lifted to nipple level, trunk posture can be observed directly. A combination of visual observation and palpation will allow determination of alignment (for example, abdominal wrinkles usually mean a rounded spine). In the presence of abnormal alignment, the therapist should determine (1) if alignment can be corrected using gentle pressure; and (2) what factors may be interfering with good postural alignment.

The patient should transfer onto a mat table. Observation of the specific transfer method used and level of assistance required will avoid creating a new system that interferes with this function.

Mat Table Measures

Supine Position

The supine examination provides an opportunity to learn about the person's strength and range of available movement, as well as how movement of one body part affects tone, comfort, position, control, and performance in other body segments. The goal is to preserve spinal alignment whenever possible, maintaining the natural lumbar curve whenever it can be produced. The person should be examined in a gravity-minimized position (supine [preferred] or side-lying) to determine if ROM limitations exist. This position also allows preliminary linear measurements, including thigh length, calf length, trunk width, and hip width.

The supine examination usually requires more than one examiner. The patient should be positioned supine on a firm surface (a mat table or carpeted floor works well; a bed may not be firm enough). The range of available pelvic and hip movements as they relate to spinal and pelvic alignment should be determined. The purpose is to determine the maximum ROM available before spinal and pelvic alignment is disturbed.

Range of Motion

Hip flexion, knee extension with hips flexed, and ankle dorsiflexion with knees flexed are the most important LE ROM values to obtain.[9,10] A complete ROM examination

of both UEs and LEs, head/neck, trunk, and pelvis is needed since limitations in these areas will affect a person's ability to propel the wheelchair, position the head for safe eating, and sit with good upright alignment.

Hip flexion is measured with the person in the supine position (Fig. 32.2). Knees should be flexed to decrease the influence of the hamstring muscles. The pelvis should be in a neutral to slight anterior tilt position. Both hips should be flexed slowly keeping one hand flat under the lumbar/sacral area of the person's spine until posterior movement of the pelvis (out of a slight anterior tilt) is felt. The end of hip flexion ROM for seating is defined as the angle of hip flexion just before the pelvis moves posteriorly.

Goniometric values for hip abduction, adduction, and internal and external rotation should also be obtained. If the pelvis is oblique or rotated, it may be necessary to allow the LEs to assume the windswept position, or be abducted before measuring hip flexion. The goal is to achieve neutral pelvis alignment before measuring and to ensure that the pelvis does not shift into a posterior pelvic tilt, obliquity, or rotated position during the examination.

Knee extension is measured with the person in the supine position with both hips flexed to the optimal angle determined (above) and the knees initially flexed (Fig. 32.3). While maintaining the hip angle and keeping one hand under the lumbar/sacral area of the spine, the knees are extended slowly toward the ceiling until

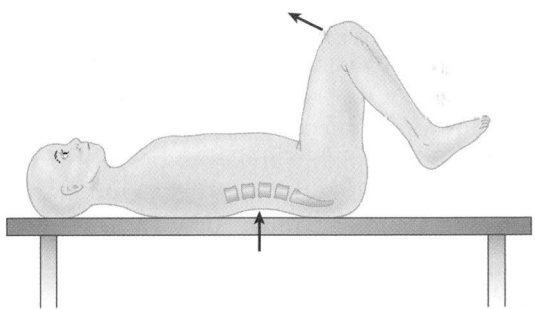

Figure 32.2 The examiner must monitor the lumbar curve as the hips are flexed.

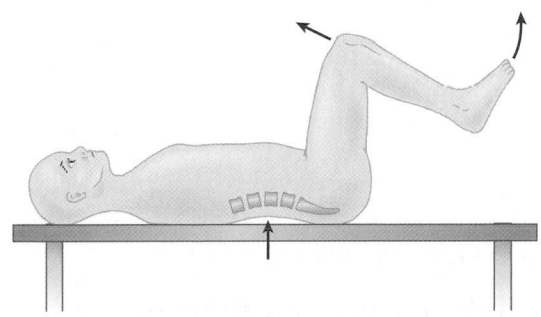

Figure 32.3 The examiner must monitor the lumbar curve and hamstring tightness behind the knees as the knees are extended.

the pelvis begins to move or excessive tightness/tension is felt in the hamstrings. It is especially important to maintain the appropriate hip position while extending the knees since the hamstring muscles are a two-joint muscle and the amount of range achieved is dependent on the position of the hips.[11] When the hips are extended, knee extension range tends to be increased and when the hips are flexed, knee extension range tends to be decreased due to hamstring muscle tightness.

Ankle dorsiflexion ROM is also measured in the supine position. Hips and knees should be positioned in available hip flexion and knee extension alignment (as determined above). The ankle should be maintained in a neutral inversion/eversion position and an attempt made to achieve neutral dorsiflexion/plantarflexion position at the ankle. The gastrocnemius muscle is a two-joint muscle and ROM at the ankle is affected by the position at the knee. If the knee is extended and muscle tightness is present, decreased dorsiflexion is noted. With the knee flexed, increased dorsiflexion is achieved. Although it is important to measure ROM with knee extended (bed positioning, standing, and ambulation), this is an assessment for seating and muscle tightness limitations must be addressed in a simulated position on the mat to better understand posture achieved in sitting.

Range of motion of the spine, head/neck, and UEs should be examined to determine the impact of limitations on posture. If significant scoliosis exists, decisions will need to be made regarding method to support the scoliosis and obtain optimal trunk position because this will affect pelvic position. Contractures in the neck region affect head position. Attempts to align the head with a lateral flexion contracture may cause the trunk to shift to the side. Once the trunk shifts, the pelvis and LE positions will be affected. The UE position becomes critical when determining ability to propel the wheelchair or if specific UE positioning (e.g., support surface) is required to maintain current ROM.

Other measurements needed when the person is supine include thigh length, calf length, and pelvic width. These will be starting point measurements for testing in a seated position.

Thigh length measures are taken in supine on a mat table or other firm surface with the hips and knees in the optimal position determined above. The measure is taken from the mat surface to just before the popliteal fossa (Fig. 32.4). Accuracy is important in measuring thigh length. If the measurement is too long, it will be difficult to get the hips fully back on the seat and properly supported in the wheelchair; this will create problems over time. If the person has a windswept or abducted lower extremity posture, measure on a straight line to the shortest side. If needed, use a clipboard or other firm surface to act like the seat surface for more accurate measuring. Leg (calf) length should be taken when the person is supine on a mat table. The hip, knee, and ankle should be positioned as previously deter-

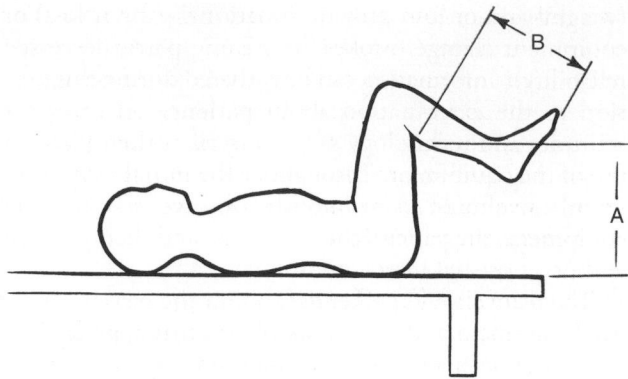

Figure 32.4 **(A)** In the supine position with the hips and knees flexed the examiner can measure the undersurface of the thigh from the popliteal fossa to a firm support surface **(B)**. Note that this position can also be used to measure leg length from the popliteal fossa to the heel.

mined. Measure from the popliteal fossa to the bottom of the heel to determine leg length. For increased accuracy, remeasure in the sitting position with appropriate footwear. Preliminary measurement for pelvic width should be taken in the supine position. This is the widest portion of the hips from one greater trochanter to the other. Final measurement needs to be completed in the sitting position owing to soft tissue spread.

Seat to Back Support Angle

Measuring hip flexion will assist in determining the trunk to thigh angle and ultimately the seat to back support angle[12,13] (Fig. 32.5). If hip flexion is to 75°, the trunk to thigh angle is 105°. In addition to the trunk to thigh angle, other data needed to determine the final seat to back support angle include the center of mass of head and trunk over the sitting base, body contours, tone, movement patterns, and comfort. The combined information guides determination of the final seat to back support angle. For example, if hip flexion is to 95°, the trunk to thigh angle is 85° (Fig. 32.6A). However, this position may not provide good stability, resulting

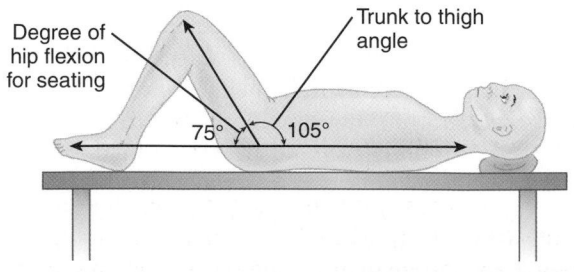

Figure 32.5 The amount of hip flexion determines the trunk to thigh angle. If the degree of hip flexion for seating is 75°, the trunk to thigh angle is 105°.

in trunk flexion and making it more difficult to maintain an upright sitting posture (Fig. 32.6B). In this example, the patient may need a final seat to back support angle of 100° to address center of mass, body contour, and comfort issues (Fig. 32.6C). Many times the trunk to thigh angle will be the seat to back support angle, but tone, movement, and comfort should not be overlooked when finalizing this angle.

Seat to Leg Support Angle

Knee extension ROM assists in determining thigh to leg angle (Fig. 32.7). The final seat to leg support angle is determined by considering the thigh to leg angle, abnormal tone, movement patterns, and comfort[12,13] (Fig. 32.8). Hamstring muscle tightness must be accommodated to prevent the pelvis from shifting into a posterior pelvic tilt. Many people will require a seat to

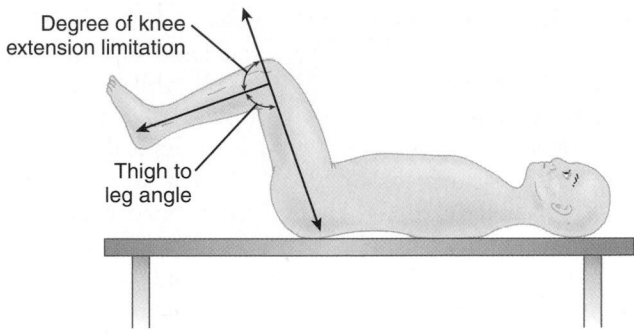

Figure 32.7 Thigh to leg angle is determined during mat examination and is based on the degree of knee extension limitation when the hip is positioned in available ROM.

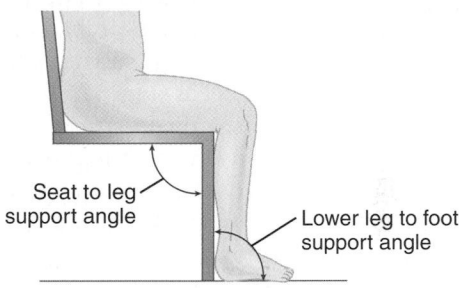

Figure 32.8 Seat to leg support angle and lower leg to foot support angle are final seating angles determined during seating simulation accommodating range of motion, tone, and comfort at the knees and ankles.

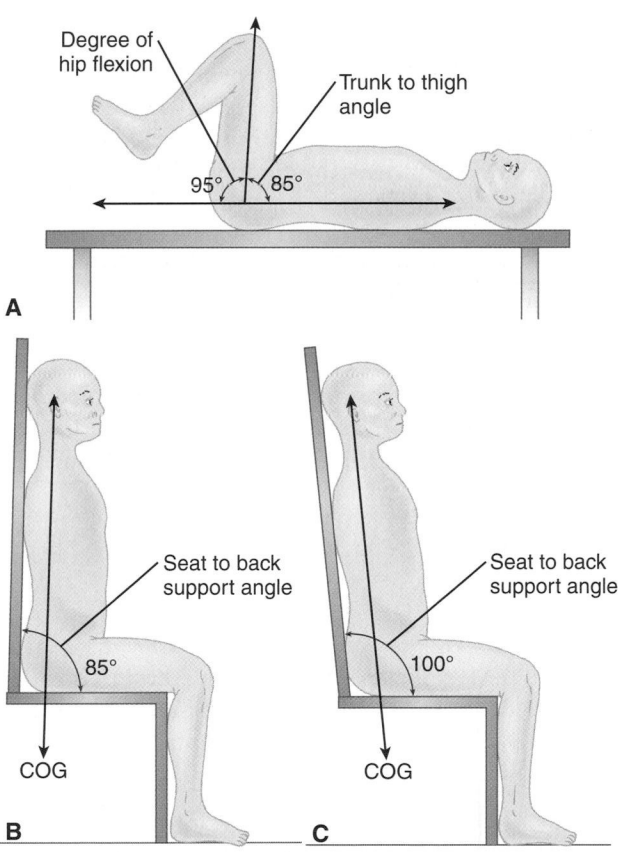

Figure 32.6 **(A)** If the degree of hip flexion for seating is to 95°, the trunk to thigh angle is 85°. **(B)** Seat to back support angle does not always correlate with trunk to thigh angle. In this example, if the seat to back support angle is set at 85°, tolerance to sitting in this position may be poor and cause the person to fall forward or constantly be working to hold himself or herself upright. Body shape, center of mass, and sitting tolerance must be addressed. **(C)** Opening the seat to back support angle to 100° better accommodates body shape and center of mass and tolerance to sitting upright improves.

leg support angle of 90° or less to accommodate hamstring tightness or fixed knee flexion contractures to maintain a neutral pelvic tilt position.

Lower Leg Support to Foot Support Angle

Ankle dorsiflexion ROM assists in determining lower leg to foot support angle (Fig. 32.9). The final lower leg to foot support angle is determined by considering ankle ROM and deformities and abnormal tone and movement patterns[12,13] (see Fig 32.8). The use of ankle-foot orthoses (AFOs) will also affect the final lower leg support to foot support angle.

Seated Examination

Seated examination using a simulator allows testing of hypotheses generated during the supine examination and provides an opportunity to determine patient tolerance to the recommended angles and to check if the thigh length is accurate.[14] The ideal simulator chair has an adjustable seat to back support angle, seat to leg support angle, and lower leg to foot support angle and the ability to adjust seat depth, calf length, and trunk length. Other features of an optimal simulator include the ability to add lateral trunk supports, lateral knee supports, medial knee supports, arm supports, head

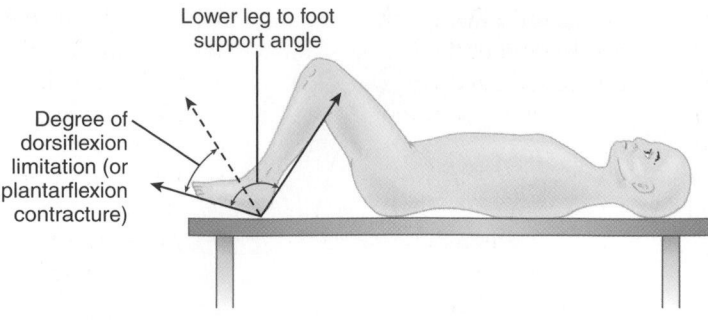

Figure 32.9 Lower leg to foot support angle is determined during mat examination and is based on ankle range of motion.

supports, and other support surfaces to determine optimal positioning. An adjustable chair provides the evaluator with the ability to use the chair for a variety of people to determine optimal sitting posture. The ability to tilt the wheelchair assists in assessing the effect of gravity on the patient.[15] A planar seating simulation chair is available commercially specifically for assisting therapists in determining positioning needs (Fig. 32.10). If unable to obtain this specific chair, a tilt-in-space and recliner wheelchair can be used for testing, but care should be taken to obtain the necessary seat to back support angle, thigh length, and wheelchair width if using this type of system for seating simulation.

Seating simulation provides the opportunity to observe tone and movement, alignment, and function. Supports may be added and subtracted to assist in determining if a person tolerates more or less support. Changing the amount of tilt influences the impact of gravity on a person's ability to sit upright. Finally, asking the person how he or she feels and working together assists in improving posture, comfort, and function.

Some aspects of seating simulation can also be performed while seated on a mat table. The examiner's hands are used to determine amount of support and location of supports. Trunk strength and balance can be assessed while sitting on the mat table, but if the person has significant physical involvement, it is very difficult to accurately determine seating supports needed in this position (Fig. 32.11).

Using a simulation chair in the supported sitting position, all angular dimensions should be finalized, including seat to back, seat to leg, and lower leg to foot support angles. The linear dimensions need to be finalized as well (Fig. 32.12.) The examiner should remeasure the sitting depth from behind the buttocks to the popliteal fossa (Fig. 32.12A). This may differ from the supine measurement, and careful examination should reveal whether the difference is secondary to correctable postural difficulties or simply variable flesh distribution in sitting versus supine. Leg measurement (Fig. 32.12B), from the popliteal fossa to the heel with customary footwear in place, will be needed to determine footrest length on the wheelchair. The sitting knee flexion angle

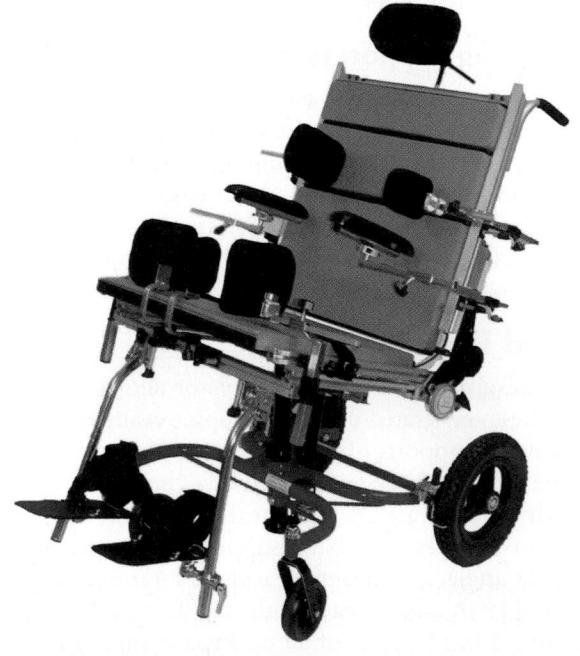

Figure 32.10 Planar seating simulation chair. *Courtesy of Prairie Seating Corporation, Skokie, IL 60077.*

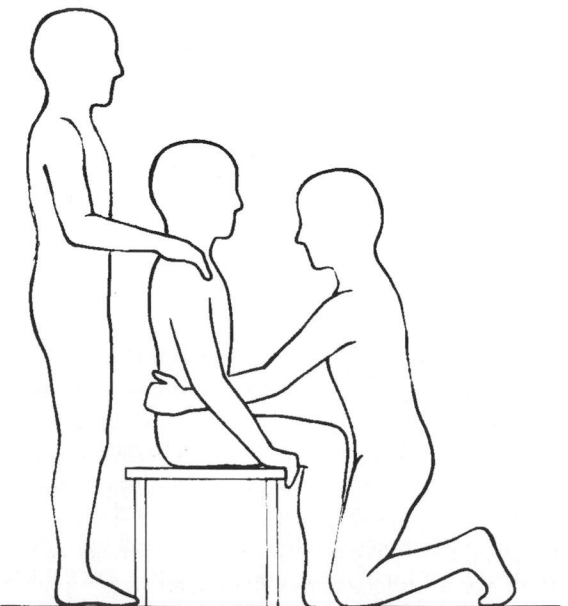

Figure 32.11 The sitting position can be used to determine the amount and location of required support.

should also be documented (Fig. 32.12C). Measurement of back height should be taken from the sitting surface to the posterior superior iliac crests (Fig. 32.12D), lower scapula (Fig. 32.12E), top of the shoulder (Fig. 32.12F), occiput (Fig. 32.12G), and crown of the head (Fig. 32.12H). These measurements will provide a detailed record should decisions regarding wheelchair back height be needed once the examination is completed. Measurement of the *hanging elbow* (Fig. 32.12I) is needed to determine proper armrest height. With the person in a corrected sitting position, the UE is positioned at the side of the body with 90° of elbow flexion and the shoulder in a neutral position. A measurement is taken from the bottom of the elbow or forearm to the sitting surface.

During the seated examination, measurements should be taken of width (Fig. 32.12J) and depth (Fig. 32.12K) of the trunk and width (Fig. 32.12L) of the hips for decisions regarding support accessories and width of the seating system and the mobility base. If the patient is seated

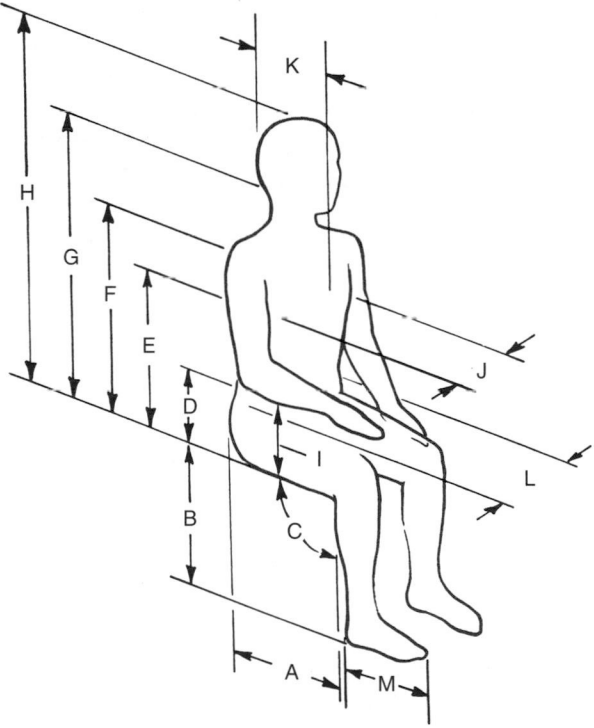

Figure 32.12 The following measurements are added to those taken in the supine position. **(A)** Sitting depth from behind the buttocks to popliteal fossa (right and left side); **(B)** leg measured from popliteal fossa to heel (right and left side); **(C)** knee flexion angle; **(D)** back height from sitting surface to posterior superior iliac crest, **(E)** from sitting surface to lower scapula, **(F)** from sitting surface to top of shoulder, **(G)** from sitting surface to occiput, and **(H)** from sitting surface to crown of head; **(I)** hanging elbow from sitting surface to the elbow or forearm; **(J)** width and **(K)** depth of trunk; **(L)** width of hips; and **(M)** measurement of foot length.

asymmetrically, it will be necessary to measure across the widest span of the patient's seated body (e.g., outside hip on the adducted side to outside knee of the abducted leg). A measurement of foot length (Fig. 32.12M) should also be taken. To ensure accurate recommendations it is important to consider orthoses, clothing, and recent weight loss or gain, as well as the patient's potential for growth, when recording these measurements. If it takes more than a few months to secure funding it may be necessary to remeasure the client before placing the order.

Wheelchair Testing

Once optimal positioning is determined, discussion can then follow regarding functional needs of the wheelchair user that need to be addressed, such as eating, communication, computer access, switch access, manual and/or power mobility, or transfers.

Time should be allocated for testing trial equipment in the clinic setting. This provides an opportunity for the patient to determine personal tolerance to the recommended changes. If possible, testing of trial equipment should be done in the patient's home environment and community to allow the patient to practice using the equipment and ensure that the equipment meets the expected outcomes.

■ INTERVENTION

The data gathered during the physical examination, seating simulation, and wheelchair testing are now analyzed to determine equipment parameters based on specific client-centered goals. Discussion ensues to determine if the client is functioning at highest potential or if additional support would help to improve function of distal body parts.[16,17] Each piece of equipment provided needs to be justified; for example, justification for lateral knee supports might be the need to maintain neutral alignment of the LEs or the need to prevent excessive active hip abduction. For each component required for postural support, mounting location, method of stabilization, strength, and durability must be finalized. For example, lateral trunk supports might be needed for postural support but will interfere with a sliding board transfer. Swing-away hardware will move the support out of the way, but the specific hardware to use is dependent on the ability of the client or caregiver to access the hardware and shift it out of the way. Testing of these details is important to ensure that maximal independence is achieved with the new equipment.

Problem Solving Model

A problem solving approach can guide selection of needed seating features by using a sequence of (1) identification of equipment-related clinical problems; (2) establishing objectives for equipment intervention; (3) making equipment property recommendations; and (4) identification of equipment specifications.[18,19] Box 32.1 provides an example of this strategy.

Box 32.1   Example of Problem Solving Model Grid

Clinical Problems	Objectives for Equipment Intervention	Equipment Property Recommendations	Product Specifications
Diagnosis of cerebral palsy (CP); fluctuating muscle tone with wide excursion, ataxic tremors on active movement, poor grading of movement, and poor ability to isolate muscle groups	Increase stability through pelvis, trunk, and lower extremities (LEs) to improve upper extremity (UE) function	Molded surfaces that provide maximal contact and control to increase body stability Stabilizing bar for left UE to improve function in right UE	Determine specific molding system Determine final location for stabilizing bar and type of bar to use for maximal durability
Range of motion (ROM) limitations: hip flexion: 0–80°; knee extension with hip flex: 0–100°, ankle dorsiflexion with knee flexed: 0–0° (no motion), able to achieve good pelvic position, mild trunk scoliosis, good UE ROM	Accommodate ROM limitations with seat to back support angle of 100°, seat to lower leg support angle of 80°, and lower leg to foot support angle of 90° to assist in maintaining pelvis in slight anterior tilt, level and not rotated and maintain symmetrical trunk alignment	Adjustable-angle back hardware to accommodate hip ROM limitation Swing-away footrest system with angle-adjustable footplates to accommodate knee and ankle ROM Foot stabilizers to assist with maintaining stability and posture	Adjustable-angle backposts Adjustable-angle footplates Shoe holders with hook-and-loop or D-ring closure for independence
Poor posture in current manual wheelchair, sits in posterior pelvic tilt, spine is kyphotic with mild scoliosis	Achieve and maintain slight anterior pelvic tilt, level and not rotated Accommodate for mild scoliosis and maintain symmetrical trunk alignment Increase trunk elongation	Medial knee support, pelvic positioning strap to stabilize pelvis, molded seat and back system for optimal control, support, and postural correction	Medial knee support separate from molded seat for transfers Push-button pelvic positioning strap 1.5 in (3.8 cm) wide with flat mount (no grommets) Molded seat and back system
Propels manual wheelchair slowly for short distances only with wide excursion of movement and increased energy expenditure	Increase independence in mobility by providing power mobility. Decrease energy expenditure and decrease wide excursion of movement	Power wheelchair system with parameters that can be adjusted for ataxic movement, decreased movement control, speed, and acceleration Power base that provides increased foot/caster clearance	Test various power wheelchairs to determine optimal base for driving and positioning Determine if able to achieve good posture throughout the day with one set position or if needs a tilt-in-space seating system
Requires supervision for transfers in and out of wheelchair	Improve independence in ability to transfer in and out of wheelchair	Accommodate leg length and ROM at knee and ankle Keep seat as low to floor as possible but maintain caster clearance Swing-away footrest system Flat seat surface for ease in getting on and off seat Flip-down medial knee support Adjustable-height armrests	Swing-away footrests with angle-adjustable footplates ensuring access and independence with swing-away feature Flip-down medial knee support ensuring ability to move support out of way independently Adjustable-height armrests

Box 32.1   Example of Problem Solving Model Grid—cont'd

Clinical Problems	Objectives for Equipment Intervention	Equipment Property Recommendations	Product Specifications
Uses keyboard for computer independence	Maintain independence in computer keyboard access	Swing-away joystick mount to ensure access to tables	Swing-away joystick mount ensuring ability to independently move it out of the way.
Uses urinal for independence in bathroom	Maintain independence in bathroom	Flip-down medial knee support	Flip-down medial knee support ensuring independence

It can assist in guiding the thought process and ensuring that all issues are addressed. This allows thoroughness and improves the ability to articulate reasons for choosing specific wheelchair components. The process is patient centered rather than product centered and will assist in obtaining optimal equipment.

Clinical Problems, Objectives, Property Recommendations, and Product Specifications

Clinical Problems

Information needed in this area includes data obtained from history, preliminary examination, supine and seated examinations, and determination of functional abilities to preserve and functional abilities to attain.

Objectives

Goals should be set related to positioning and alignment, motor control, health, function, environmental issues, and social/emotion issues. Goals can be general (e.g., improve skin integrity) but will need to become more specific (e.g., reduce pressure under left ischial tuberosity to prevent pressure sores in this area) to determine equipment properties.

Property Recommendations

Consideration is given to the different surfaces and features of the equipment. *Properties* are the specific details of the final product. The surface shape and flexibility, dimensions, placement, and attachment features should be included in this section. Careful consideration of properties will ensure a final product that promotes optimal independence.

Product Specifications

The list of property recommendations will be reviewed to determine the final product. If no commercial option is available with the needed properties, determination of a method to customize is needed. The supplier should be knowledgeable and be able to assist the therapist in obtaining the most appropriate equipment to address all needs.

The benefit of using this decision making process is to help keep the process client centered rather than product driven. It promotes problem solving and improves accuracy when choosing final product components.

When using this process, the person's diagnosis assists in determining specific properties of final equipment, as well as the priority of the properties. If working with someone with an SCI with previous pressure sore problems on the buttocks, the properties of the seat cushion become important. If working with someone with progressive MS, the ability to modify the equipment over time will be important. When considering the patient's medical diagnosis, it is important to determine if the condition is stable and if not, the type of changes that are expected. If the medical condition is stable but the person is newly injured (e.g., SCI), changes to equipment may be needed over time as the person adjusts to using a wheelchair for primary mobility purposes. If working with someone who is stable and has always done things one way, it is important to provide him or her with other options and determine if poor habits can be changed.

A well-planned seating system may be able to normalize tone, decrease pathological reflex activity, improve postural symmetry, enhance ROM, maintain and/or improve skin condition, increase comfort and sitting tolerance, decrease fatigue, and improve function of the autonomic nervous system. In addition, the base of the seating system can allow for changes in orientation in space (recline and tilt). A properly prescribed mobility base will improve access to the physical environment (both manual and power-activated), whether alone or with a caregiver. It should be effective for accomplishing all home, school, work, and recreational activities and, where necessary, assist the caregiver with patient management.

When setting priorities, it is important that clinical team members do not overload the patient with their professional opinions. Clinical teams may not be fully aware of the barriers facing the individual using a wheelchair in his or her physical environment. Clinicians may observe a patient ambulating in the clinic and feel that with added practice he or she could ambulate full time. This clinician may consider recommending crutches and a simple manual wheelchair. In the patient's real environment, however, long distances may need to be traversed to independently shop, attend community activities, and function at school or work. Walking to these activities would require extraordinary effort, and propelling a standard manual wheelchair may not offer much additional assistance. A motorized scooter or wheelchair may be more effective as a supplement for environmental mobility.

Postural Support System

The components of the system that will directly affect comfort and maintenance of posture are the seat surface, back surface, pelvic positioner, UE surface, and LE surfaces. These areas should be addressed together as the postural support system. Increased contact between the user and the support surfaces increases comfort and control and decreases pressure over bony prominences.[20-23] The continuum of available support surfaces runs from firm *planar surfaces* (wood, firm foam) (Fig. 32.13), through *deformable surfaces* (knit-covered foam) (Figs. 32.14 and 32.15), and *contoured surfaces* (Fig. 32.16), up to and including *custom-molded surfaces* (Fig. 32.17).

Angular relationships between the surfaces at the hip and knee joints (thigh and back surfaces, thigh and leg surfaces) previously determined during seating simulation must be included in final setup of postural support surfaces. This information will allow the planned intervention to accommodate limitations in ROM, ensure proper alignment of body segments, and minimize pressure distal to the joint. Changes of

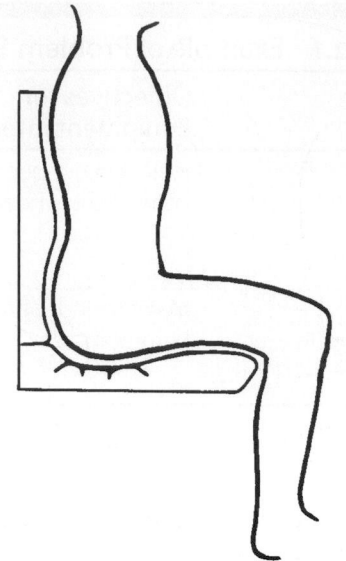

Figure 32.14 Some types of foam will contour as a response to body weight.

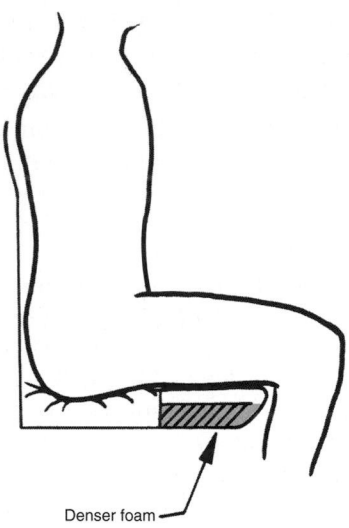

Denser foam

Figure 32.15 An option for creating contoured seats is use of varying density (firmness) of foam.

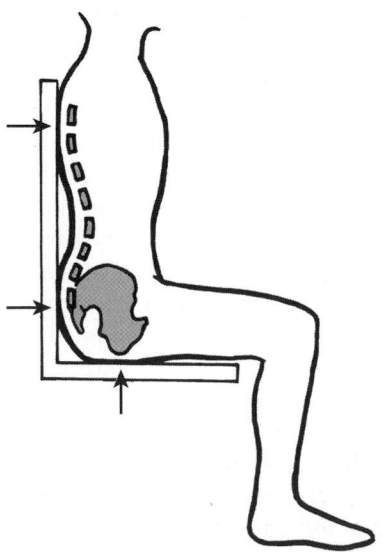

Figure 32.13 Patients seated on planar surfaces may show increased pressure over bony prominences.

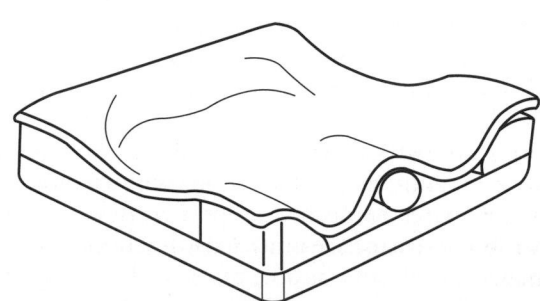

Figure 32.16 Firmer foam shapes can be placed under a more flexible foam to create a contoured cushion.

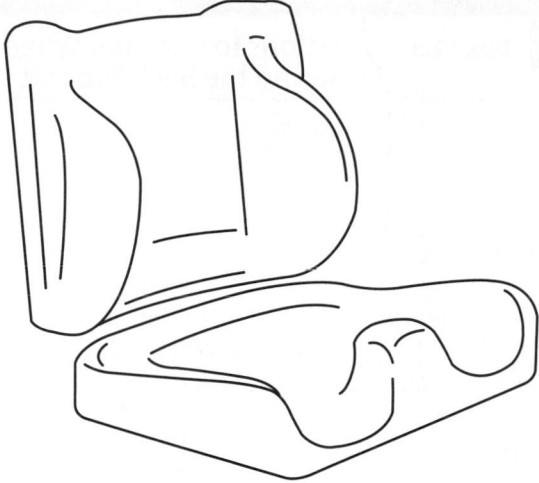

Figure 32.17 Custom-molded cushions match the patient's body contours.

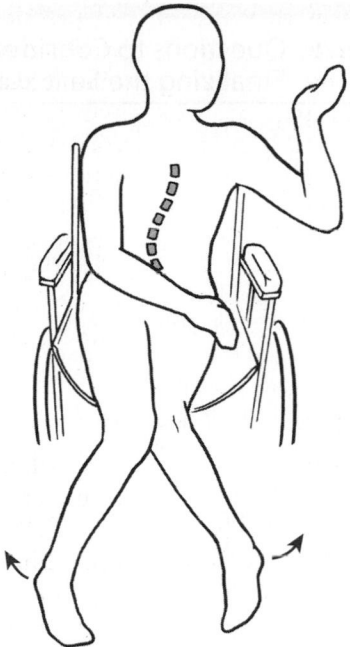

Figure 32.18 Overall poor sitting posture and asymmetries created by a sling seat.

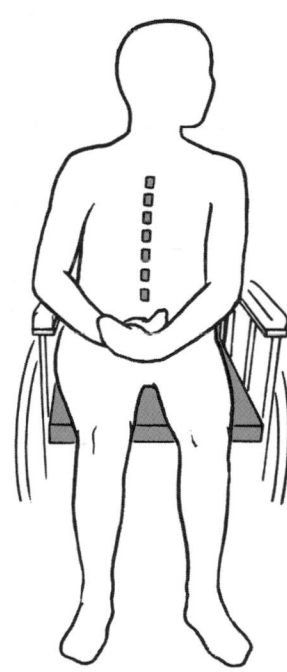

Figure 32.19 A firm sitting surface enhances sitting posture and provides a stable base of support.

orientation in space (fixed or dynamic) affect the user's comfort level, pressure over skin surfaces, fatigue, and ability to work in gravity-minimized and gravity-influenced positions. Attention to these features will help ensure the success of the seating intervention. Appendix 32.A provides an overview of features of the wheelchair postural support system.

Seat Support

The seat support is the surface under the buttocks and thighs. A firm seat support is critical in creating good LE alignment, good pressure distribution, and improved comfort. Many basic manual wheelchairs come with sling upholstery. Over time, this type of surface creates poor pelvic positioning (Fig. 32.18). The hips tend to slide forward and the thighs tend to shift into hip adduction and internal rotation. Sling upholstery is used to increase the ease of folding the wheelchair. However, if the system is needed for more than transportation, a firm seat support should be added to the wheelchair. A solid seat board can be placed under the cover of a seat cushion to provide the firm base of support or a special seat pan (solid seat of metal or plastic that mounts directly to the seat frame or with attaching hardware to seat frame) can be added to the wheelchair once the upholstery is removed (Fig. 32.19).

Different seat supports have different properties. Foam, air, gel, combination types, and custom-shaped cushions are used to promote improved positioning, improved stability for UE activities, improved pressure relief, and improved comfort.[24] The person should test various seat cushions to determine what system is optimal.

Properties of the seat that need to be considered include the surface shape, firmness, flexibility, dimensions, placement, and attachment features. The most critical dimensions include the seat depth and seat width. If the seat depth is too long, it promotes a posterior pelvic tilt and kyphotic spine posture. If the seat width is too wide, it will make propelling the wheelchair more difficult and if too narrow, increase pressure on the hips from the armrests and footrest system.

Box 32.2 provides a list of questions that should be considered when finalizing the seat support.

> **Box 32.2   Questions to Consider When Finalizing the Seat Support**
>
> - Does the seat provide adequate support to promote good sitting posture?
> - Will the pressure distribution on the seat prevent pressure sores?
> - Is the shape of the seat cushion appropriate for the patient's body contours?
> - Does the person need a custom shape to accommodate deformities and maximize support?
> - Is pressure relief provided if the person is unable to complete weight shifts independently using UEs or through a tilt or recline option?
> - Is the seat depth an appropriate length?
> - Is the seat width appropriate for propelling the wheelchair and for comfortable positioning?
> - Is the seat surface appropriate for safe transfers into and out of the wheelchair?
> - Are special combinations of foam, air, or gel seat cushions needed to maximize comfort and pressure relief?

> **Box 32.3   Questions to Consider When Finalizing the Back Support**
>
> - Is the back support in an appropriate position for upright trunk posture (seat to back support angle, orientation in space)?
> - Is the back support an appropriate shape to fit the patient's body contours? (If using a commercially available back support with contour it should be examined to ensure the support will fit the person. At times, the patient's hips may be too wide to fit between the fixed lateral supports of a commercial back.)
> - Does the patient require a custom shape to provide full contact and support?
> - Does the back support provide adequate control for muscle weakness and trunk asymmetries?
> - Is the back comfortable when used in a tilted or reclined position?
> - Does the back support allow performance of functional activities (propelling, reaching, transfers)?
> - Is pressure distribution/relief adequate for a person with a bony spine, protruding sacrum, or to prevent pressure sores?
> - Are special combinations of foam, air, or gel needed to maximize comfort and pressure relief?

Back Support

The back support is the surface behind the trunk. A firm back support is critical to promote good trunk posture and, in conjunction with lateral trunk supports, contributes to maintaining midline posture. Many basic manual wheelchairs have sling upholstery and this promotes poor trunk posture. There is an increased risk of a kyphotic spine and posterior pelvic tilt. The back support height can be varied depending on the needs of the individual. A shorter back may be appropriate for a person propelling the wheelchair with a taller back needed for a person who uses the tilt-in-space feature. A shorter back is more appropriate for a person with good trunk control and the ability to maintain good alignment without using lateral trunk supports. Back height is determined based on the person's trunk control, functional abilities, and comfort.

Different back supports have different properties. Foam, air, gel, combination types, and custom-shaped cushions are used to promote improved positioning, pressure relief, and comfort. The person should test various back cushions to determine what system is optimal.

Properties of the back that need to be considered include the surface shape, firmness and flexibility, dimensions, placement, and attachment features. The most critical dimensions include the back height and back width. Box 32.3 presents questions that should be considered when finalizing the back support.

In addition to the seat and back support, other supports might be necessary to ensure optimal positioning, pressure relief, and comfort, including lateral trunk and hip supports, lateral and medial knee supports, head and foot support, anterior chest and UE support, and pelvic support.[25] When determining the need for the support, consideration should be given to surface shape, firmness and flexibility, dimensions, placement, and type of attachment.

Pelvic Positioner

A belt or more rigid pelvic positioner may be needed to maintain good pelvic position (prevent the hips from sliding) and/or for safety.[26] The direction, angle of pull, and number of anchor points of the belt is important.[27] For example, if one hip tends to pull forward consistently, it may be useful to have the belt tighten by pulling it down toward that hip. The angle of pull to the seating surface should normally be 45° to 60° (Fig. 32.20).[26] Some patients respond well to belts that form a 90° angle with the sitting surface. This pull discourages patients who tend to extend in their wheelchairs as a result of increases in tone. This 90° placement also leaves the pelvis free for anterior tilting, an assist for those patients who can use this mobility for added function (Fig. 32.21). Some patients can benefit from multiple angles of pull. For these clients, a four-point belt might be most appropriate. A four-point belt provides four places to anchor the belt. The top two anchors assist in pulling the pelvis back against the back support

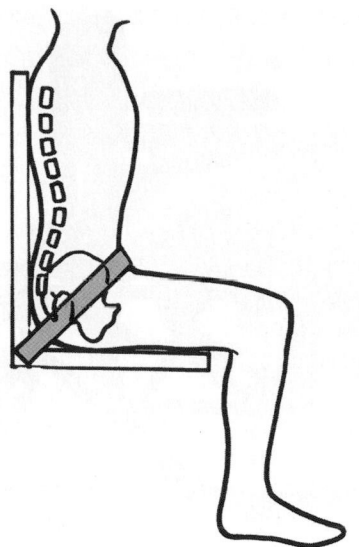

Figure 32.20 The pelvic belt should cross the pelvic-femoral junction at approximately a 45° to 60° angle to the seating surface.

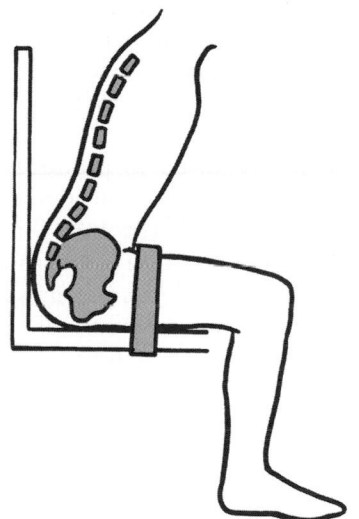

Figure 32.21 A belt placed over the upper thigh (at a 90° angle to the sitting surface) will free the pelvis for natural anterior tilting.

and the bottom two anchors assist in preventing the pelvis from shifting forward and up. Other pelvic positioners are available as discussed in Seating Principle 2: Achieve and Maintain Pelvic Alignment.

Upper Extremity Supports

Wheelchair armrests have many important functions. They provide a support surface for arms as well as a surface for pushing up to standing and a mechanism for ischial pressure relief (sitting pushups). The armrests are also used to support trays for UE support or communication devices. The height, length, and width of the armrests are important measurements to ensure

independence and comfort. If the armrests are too high, undue stress can be placed on the shoulders and if too low, slumping to reach the support frequently occurs. If the armrests are too wide, it may interfere with lifting the armrest for transfers or affect the ability to propel the wheelchair. If too narrow, the arms may slip off rendering the armrests ineffective in assisting with trunk posture.

For some individuals, the armrests will be used to mount an *upper extremity support surface (UESS)* such as a tray or trough. These surfaces provide several important functions. They can be used to achieve symmetrical positioning of the UEs, maintain corrected alignment of the glenohumeral joint and scapula, and serve as a work or communication surface. They also can act as an adjunct to the postural control system by supporting the weight of the upper limbs and decreasing pull on the shoulders and trunk.

Lower Extremity Supports

Style and position are important considerations when selecting foot support systems. Placement of the foot support system will directly affect the position of the entire lower body, affecting tone and posture in the trunk, head, and arms. Adequate hip flexion will help keep the pelvis well positioned on the sitting surface. Appropriate foot support height and style are required for maintenance of this position. Foot supports that are too low will result in lower knees, placing the hips in a more open angle and encouraging forward sliding of the pelvis. Foot supports that are too high may unload the thighs, placing increased weight on the ischial tuberosities. Elevating leg rests even in their lowered position may place excessive stretch on tight hamstrings, pulling the pelvis into a posterior tilt (Fig. 32.22). Any limitation of motion imposed by the hamstrings will directly influence the choice of foot positioners. To achieve maximum comfortable hip flexion, it may be necessary to flex the knees more than 90°, requiring special intervention on the foot supports. Decisions regarding straps and foot positioners must be made early, based on available ROM, to ensure caster (front wheel) clearance on the final unit.

Secondary Support Surfaces

Other supports may be needed to improve trunk alignment, LE alignment, and head position. These supports are added to the main support surfaces and include, but are not limited to, lateral trunk supports, medial and lateral knee supports, lateral thigh supports, headrest, and anterior chest supports. When determining the need for these supports, a specific goal should be identified to justify each item.

The Wheeled Mobility Base

The wheeled base forms the mobility structure for the seating system. Mobility bases include manual systems

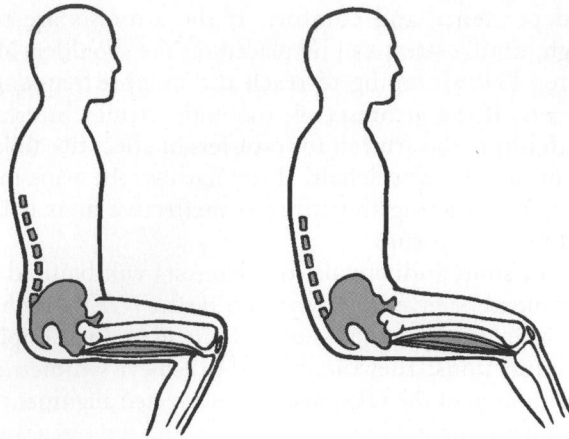

Figure 32.22 Sitting alignment with the hamstrings on slack and the knees flexed (*left*) and positioning assumed with feet resting on elevating foot rests (*right*) causing tension on the hamstring that pulls the pelvis into a posterior tilt.

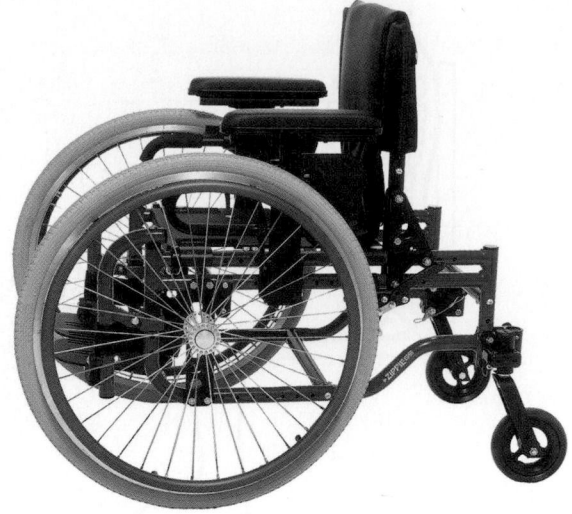

Figure 32.23 Wheelchairs with large front wheels and small rear casters may be easier for some patients to push, but are more difficult to use outdoors. *Courtesy of Sunrise Medical, Carlsbad, CA 92008.*

and power systems. Manual systems can be set up for independent use where the user is able to propel the wheelchair or dependent use where a caregiver moves the chair.

Manual Mobility Systems

Dependent manual systems include strollers, pushchairs, and some manual wheelchairs. These systems typically have small wheels that are not intended for self-propulsion. They may also be set up for increased ease of folding for transportation.

Four different methods of self-propulsion are available in the independent manual mobility category. Independent manual propulsion using both hands is indicated for those with good UE function and strength and is the most common. This system is usually set up with large rear wheels. However, the large wheels can be positioned in the center of the base (mainly used with children) or in the front of the base (Fig. 32.23). Positioning the wheels in different configurations can improve the ability to reach and propel the wheelchair. This is especially critical when considering the possible implications for long-term function of the shoulder girdle.

Research indicates that patients who use manual wheelchairs, especially if they are not properly fitted to their bodies and functional level, are in danger of UE damage from *repetitive strain injuries* (RSIs). Repetitive strain injuries can result in damage to soft tissue (tendons, ligaments, nerves) or bony structures secondary to frequent repeated motions such as wheelchair push strokes. The damage can include inflammation, compression, and/or tears in the shoulder joint and surrounding structures, resulting in pain and decreased function.[28,29]

Repetitive strain injuries have been identified in the shoulders, wrists, and hands of wheelchair users. Even patients without documented RSI report increased pain in these joints with prolonged wheelchair use.[30,31] Small muscles are required to produce large forces repeatedly to move the chair through space. These same muscles are typically required for a variety of activities of daily living (ADL) tasks, thus increasing the demands placed on the same muscles with the potential of causing trauma. Muscles are used in atypical positions, and become overstretched and overused. Stress on the muscles and joints increases with increased wheelchair weight, increased user weight, and environmental factors. Many symptoms are not felt until the condition is well advanced. Rotator cuff injuries and instability of the glenohumeral joint are common at the shoulder. Since a number of muscles cross the wrist and elbow, problems occurring at the wrist often create pain at the elbow. Medial epicondylitis and carpal tunnel syndrome (CTS) are common. See Box 32.4 Evidence Summary for a summary of studies addressing UE pain associated with wheelchair propulsion.

When prescribing wheelchairs and features for patients who are able to self-propel, consideration must be given to preventing RSI whenever possible. An important prevention strategy is careful positioning of the UE to allow the most efficient stroke during propulsion, reducing the amount of force needed per stroke and reducing the number of strokes required to move the chair. It is also critical to observe wrist alignment and make any needed recommendations to minimize trauma and the chance of impingement leading to CTS.[32-34] Other criteria that should be

Box 32.4 Evidence Summary   Studies Addressing Pain Associated with Wheelchair Propulsion

Reference	Purpose	Subjects/Design	Results	Conclusions/Comments
Sie et al[28] (1992)	To document the prevalence of UE pain according to specific UE regions, and the relationship of UE pain to time since injury in Ss with SCI.	Nonrandomized cohort study; questionnaire sent to 239 Ss > 1 year post-SCI; mean age 37.4 years. Ss interviewed for presence of UE pain (shoulders, upper arms, elbows, lower arms, wrists, and hands), screened for CTS.	55% of Ss with tetraplegia (quadriplegia) reported pain in at least one region of UE, 40% in more than one region. 64% of Ss with paraplegia reported UE pain, 32% in more than one region. 59% of all Ss reported some UE pain, 30% reported pain requiring medication, limiting function, or causing pain with ADL. Ss with paraplegia reported less significant pain than those with tetraplegia. 41% of all Ss reported shoulder pain.	Shoulder region was the most common painful area in Ss with tetraplegia, and second most common in Ss with paraplegia. There was a general trend indicating that UE pain increased with time past since injury, up to 20 years. There was a steady increase in frequency of CTS-related complaints with time since injury up to 19 years, in Ss with paraplegia.
Fullerton et al (2003)[a]	To compare the onset and prevalence of shoulder pain in the athletic and nonathletic W/C user populations.	Cohort study; 20-item questionnaire, mailed to a randomized group of 500 individuals through the Virginia SCI Registry, 257 Ss were obtained, 86% had SCI. Patients were considered athletic if (1) trained at least 3 hours/week, (2) involved in at least 3 competitions per year, (3) had a W/C modified for sports. 172 of the Ss were identified as athletes.	48% of all Ss reported shoulder pain, 70% of these Ss sought treatment for pain, and 92% had pain with ADL. 66% of nonathletes reported pain, only 39% of athletes reported pain. Pain and athletic status were not significantly related to onset of shoulder pain. There was no significant difference between Ss with tetraplegia and Ss with paraplegia. Age had a strong effect for both pain and athletic status. Nonathletic Ss were found to be more than twice as susceptible to shoulder pain as athletes independent of age, SCI level, and number of years in W/C.	A limitation of this study is that one question remains unanswered: Do nonathletes have more pain because they are not athletic, or are they not athletic because of shoulder pain? There is a possibility of sampling bias because many of the questionnaires were hand-distributed.

Continued

Box 32.4 Evidence Summary   Studies Addressing Pain Associated with Wheelchair Propulsion—cont'd

Reference	Purpose	Subjects/Design	Results	Conclusions/Comments
Curtis et al (1999)[b]	To compare the prevalence and intensity of shoulder pain experienced during daily functional activities in W/C users with tetraplegia and paraplegia.	Nonrandomized cohort study; self-report survey; 55 women and 140 men; 92 Ss with tetraplegia (mean age 32.9 years) and 103 Ss with paraplegia (mean age 34.4 years). Ss used manual wheelchair for 3 hours per week and had at least 1 year since onset of SCI. Groups were partitioned according to age, level of daily activity, and years of W/C use.	There was no significant difference between Ss with tetraplegia and with paraplegia in terms of age, years of wheelchair use, and weekly hours of activity. Ss with paraplegia performed more transfers per week and spent more hours per week using W/C (both significant). Less than 15% of all Ss experienced shoulder pain before becoming W/C users, 78% with tetraplegia and 59% with paraplegia had felt shoulder pain since they started using the W/C. There was significantly higher prevalence of previous, bilateral, and current shoulder pain in Ss with tetraplegia than those with paraplegia. Both groups had most severe shoulder pain when pushing the W/C up an incline, pushing for more than 10 minutes, and while sleeping.	This study documents a strong influence of shoulder pain on the performance of functional activities after SCI. Ss with tetraplegia, increased age, and duration of W/C use were associated with avoiding strenuous functional activities.
Veeger et al (2002)[c]	To examine the mechanical load on the glenohumeral joint and on the shoulder muscles during W/C propulsion at everyday intensities.	Nonrandomized cohort study; three experienced male W/C users, ages 22, 27, and 38. Weight 180, 176, and 209 lb (81.5, 80, and 95 kg), respectively. All participated in W/C sports on a weekly basis. Each underwent four, 4-minute W/C exercise tests at two target resistances (10 and 20 N), and target speeds (0.83 and 1.39 m.s[−1]), during which data were collected for construction of a musculoskeletal model of the UE. Anthropometric parameters of the model based on data from two cadaver studies. Individual muscle performance estimates based on this model.	Push time shortened significantly when velocity increased, while recovery time was reduced considerably with an increase power output. The muscle that produced the largest force during the push phase was the subscapularis. Supraspinatus and infraspinatus were also highly active. Pectoralis major produced a moderate internal rotational force. Biceps produced more force than triceps during push phase. During recovery phase, the scapular part of the deltoid produced more force than all other muscles. The supraspinatus was by far the most taxed muscle when force output is considered relative to maximal force.	Peak glenohumeral contact forces varied between 800 and 1400 N. The supraspinatus and infraspinatus may be responsible for an external rotation compensatory moment for the deltoid (excessive internal rotation may cause the greater tubercle to move directly under the acromion, thus increasing probability for impingement). Despite the relatively low contact forces, the peak forces and peak stresses in the rotator cuff muscles (particularly supraspinatus) appear high. These high peak stresses might cause overuse injuries.

Box 32.4 Evidence Summary   Studies Addressing Pain Associated with Wheelchair Propulsion—cont'd

Reference	Purpose	Subjects/Design	Results	Conclusions/Comments
			Also highly active were the forearms (pronators and the supinating effect of the biceps).	
Boninger et al (2001)[d]	To investigate MRI and radiographic abnormalities in individuals with paraplegia who were W/C users.	Nonrandomized cohort study; 28 Ss with paraplegia, 19 male and 9 female (mean age 35 yr), with a traumatic SCI at the 4th thoracic level or below, occurring more than 1 year before the start of the study. Ss used manual W/C full-time for mobility. Each subject completed a standardized questionnaire, had a uniform physical examination focusing on the shoulder, and underwent imaging studies (radiographic and MRI). BMI was calculated.	5 Ss displayed osteolysis of the distal clavicle, 11 displayed subacromial spur, and 8 displayed AC DJD. Only nine Ss had radiographs that were read as entirely normal. One subject was found to have a rotator cuff tear. Distal clavicular edema was the most common abnormality found in MRI (20 subjects), 18 Ss displayed AC DJD, CA ligament problems were common as well. Ss with a high BMI had a greater degree of abnormality.	It is hypothesized that shoulder injuries are due to the repetitive loading that occurs during transfers and W/C propulsion. BMI alone was not related to abnormalities, which may suggest that taller subjects who weigh more have musculoskeletal systems that are better able to handle increased stresses.
Samuelsson et al (2004)[e]	To describe the consequences of shoulder pain on activity and participation in Ss with paraplegia who use a W/C, and describe the prevalence and type of shoulder pain.	Nonrandomized cohort study; 56 potential Ss with paraplegia due to SCI (12 women, 44 men, mean age 49 years), more than 1 year before study were screened for participation via questionnaire; 21 (37.5%) of those responding had shoulder pain. 13 of these Ss were used to delineate the type and consequence of shoulder pain. The CMS, WUSPI, KBADLI, and COPM were used to describe the impact of shoulder pain on activity.	The highest pain intensity was found for loading a wheelchair into a car, followed by pushing up inclines outdoors and usual ADL at work and school. 54% of Ss presented with problems related to self-care activities; 23% productivity; 23% leisure activities. The most common problem was transferring in and out of a car (62%) and W/C propulsion (46%).	Sitting posture may be related to shoulder pain in this population. W/C users with SCI tend to adopt a kyphotic posture, which causes an abnormal rotation of the scapula. This could contribute to entrapment of the greater tubercle beneath the acromion. The most defined problems related to shoulder pain were associated with W/C use.

Evidence Summary Box prepared by Stephen A. Caronia.

[a]Fullerton, HD, et al: Shoulder pain: A comparison of wheelchair athletes and nonathletic wheelchair users. Med Sci Sports Exerc 35(12):1958, 2003.

[b]Curtis, KA, et al: Shoulder pain in wheelchair users with tetraplegia and paraplegia. Arch Phys Med Rehabil 80(4):453, 1999.

[c]Veeger, HEJ, et al: Load on the shoulder in low intensity wheelchair propulsion. Clin Biomech 17(3):211, 2002.

[d]Boninger, MI, et al: Shoulder imaging abnormalities in individuals with paraplegia. J Rehabil Res Dev 38(4):401, 2001.

[e]Samuelsson, KAM, Tropp, H, and Gerdle, B: Shoulder pain and its consequences in paraplegic spinal cord–injured, wheelchair users. Spinal Cord 42(1):41, 2004.

AC = acromio-clavicular (joint); ADL = activities of daily living; BMI = body mass index; CA = coraco-acromial (ligament); CMS = Constant Murley Scale; COPM = Canadian Occupational Performance Measure; CTS = carpal tunnel syndrome; DJD = degenerative joint disease; KBADLI = Klien and Bell ADL Index; MRI = magnetic resonance imaging; NI = not indicated; SCI = spinal cord injury; Sh = shoulder; Ss = subjects; UE = upper extremity; WUSPI = Wheelchair Users Shoulder Pain Index; W/C = wheelchair.

considered in prescribing a self-propelled wheelchair include selecting a chair that

- Has the lightest weight possible
- Has a stable frame for most efficient movement
- Is well manufactured, with high-quality bearings (increased ease of motion for moving parts) for less roll resistance when push forces are applied, and secure nonmoving parts
- Provides optimal wheel size and type consistent with patient size and function
- Provides the best possible combination for ease of propulsion and stability

Many features must be considered when determining the optimal manual wheelchair setup for a person who is able to self-propel. Many bases are available, each with small differences that can increase or decrease the person's functional skills A rigid frame is lighter weight than a folding frame but may be more difficult to transport for some individuals. The ability to adjust the front and rear seat height by changing casters, fork lengths, and rear wheel size can assist a person with balance issues. The ability to change the seat back angle and the frame angle can assist a person with postural issues.

The second method of self-propulsion is using a one-arm drive system. This is appropriate for a person who is only able to functionally use one UE. In this case, there are two rims on the side being used to propel the wheelchair. The outer rim enables the chair to turn in one direction, the inner rim to turn in the other direction, and engaging both rims enables the chair to move forward (Fig. 32.24).

The third method of self-propulsion is using one or both feet. When using this method, care should be taken to ensure that the seat is low enough to the floor so the person continues to have good positioning and does not risk sliding out of the wheelchair.

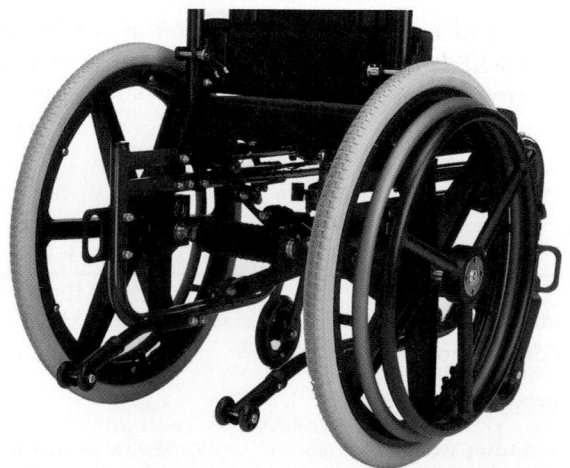

Figure 32.24 A double handrim on one side allows the user to drive a one-arm drive wheelchair with one hand. *Courtesy of Sunrise Medical, Carlsbad, CA 92008.*

The final method that can be used for self-propulsion is a combination of one arm and one leg. In this case, care must be taken to have the seat low enough to the floor, as well as have the rear wheel an appropriate size and position to use for functional mobility.

Power Mobility Systems

A power mobility system (Fig. 32.25) consists of a base or frame, a seating system, and electronics (batteries, motors, control module, and driver control).

If a person is unable to mobilize a manual wheelchair and is cognitively aware of surroundings, power mobility should be considered.[35-38] It should also be considered for wheelchair riders who are marginal self-propellers in manual wheelchairs. They may be able to move around indoors, and on level surfaces outdoors, but cannot move around in the community environment without unduly stressing muscles and joints, creating postural problems, and/or imposing cardiovascular strain. Long-term overuse injury of muscles and joints and the possibility of skeletal deformity must be discussed with the patient and caregiver as part of the examination process. Patients must face the possibility that injury may create problems significant enough to impede function in critical areas such as transfers and ADL.[28-34,39-43]

An examination of the patient's full environment must be made to determine if power mobility will be helpful and usable (see Chapter 9, Examination of the Environment). Architectural barriers such as steps might preclude the use of power mobility or require that the patient have both a power and manual system for use at different times. In addition, attention should be given to how the chair will be transported, and the level of technology tolerance of both the consumer and caregiver. For patients whose condition is changing, a long-term plan must be established to guide decision making when choosing products. When considering power mobility for individuals who may have cognitive impairments, the rule of thumb is that the driver is aware of safety for himself or herself and others. In most cases, the ability to stop and to judge when to stop is more difficult to teach than driving itself. Awareness, reliable movement, motivation, and good response time are all important factors in wheelchair use.

Control Options

A variety of control options are available for powered mobility, including hand control, head array systems, sip 'n' puff breath control system, single switch systems, and scanning array systems.

Hand Controls

The most efficient method for driving a power wheelchair is with a hand. Joystick controls are used to control the direction and speed of the wheelchair. The final placement of the joystick is important to ensure that the person can reach the control without difficulty and without putting excessive stress on the wrist, elbow, or

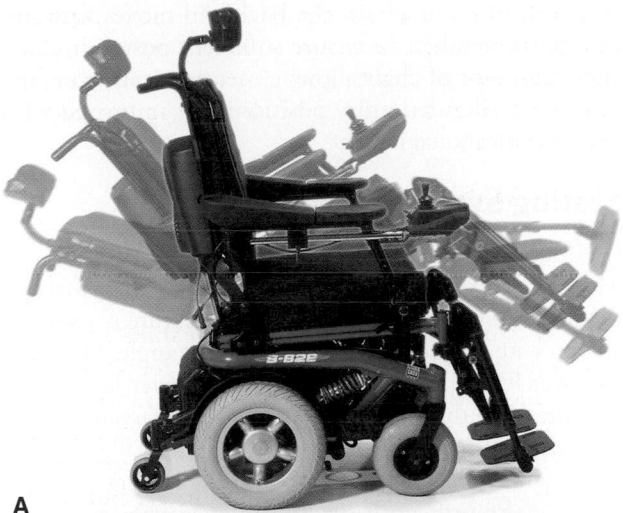

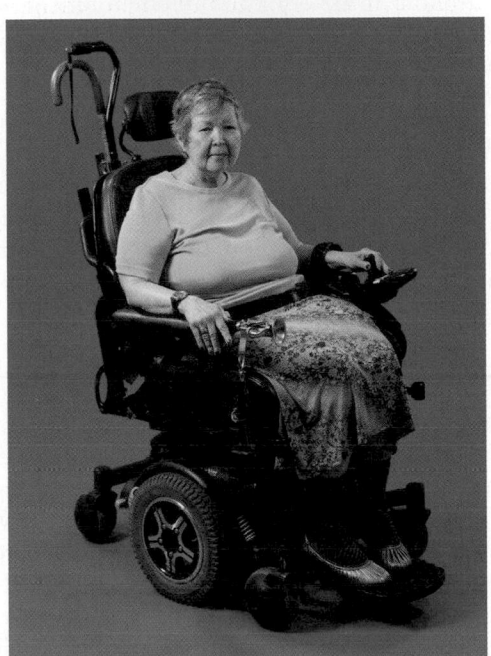

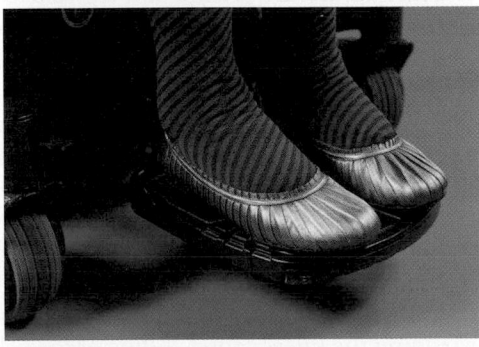

Figure 32.25 (A) Motorized wheelchairs offer patients with poor coordination, weakness, or paralysis an opportunity to move around in their environment. This chair is also equipped with a power-operated seating system. *Courtesy of Sunrise Medical, Carlsbad, CA 92008.* **(B)** Patient seated in a motorized chair; note that this chair includes a storage space for canes behind seat back. **(C)** Close-up of platform flip-up footrest.

shoulder. Access to on/off switch, mode switch, and/or speed dial must be assessed to ensure independent control and prevent accidental hitting when driving.

Head Array Systems

Some individuals are unable to use their hand to mobilize the wheelchair but have good head control. A head array system can be used for driving. A simple system consists of three switches. The switch behind the head allows the chair to move forward, the one to the left side of the head turns the chair left, and the one to the right side of the head turns the chair to the right. Hitting a combination of the switches allows the user to maneuver the chair with increased ease. A fourth switch can be used for reverse or to toggle the system so the rear pad on the head array becomes reverse. This fourth switch can also be used to change the speeds and operate other wheelchair functions. Good head control is needed to operate this type of system.

Sip 'n' Puff System/Breath Control System

The sip 'n' puff system is used with breath control. A straw is used in the mouth. A hard puff allows the chair to move forward, a hard sip for reverse, a soft puff is right, and a soft sip is left. The air control is from the mouth rather than from the lungs. Systems can be calibrated for easier or harder puffs and sips. The system can be set up in latch mode (forward is locked after a hard puff) so the person is not required to constantly be puffing into the straw to keep the chair moving forward. Once in latch mode, small puffs or sips provide steer correction. A hard sip stops the chair. When using this type of system, it is important to have good lip closure without leakage through the mouth or nose for optimal efficiency. A combination of sip 'n' puff and switches can be used for driving a wheelchair if a person has difficulty differentiating the hard and soft puffs and sips.

Single Switch Systems

A variety of single switches can be set up for driving a power wheelchair. If a person is unable to use a head array or sip 'n' puff system, single switches can be set up at any area with even minimal active movement (e.g., hand, elbow, head, chin, knee, foot, and so forth) to control the wheelchair. A tray can be used with good gross movement of the UE to activate a series of switches with each one assigned a different function. The switches can be different styles, sizes, and colors to differentiate function. Four switch placements are needed to operate a wheelchair using this method.

Scanning Array System

A scanning array is available for a person who only has one switch placement site available. A light scans around a display highlighting different directions. When the light hits the direction of travel, activation of the switch moves the chair in that direction. Once the contact is removed from the switch, the scanner light continues to move around the display in a preset fashion. Although this type of system can be slow and tedious, the ability to drive independently is extremely rewarding for the motivated person.

Other Systems

Foot, arm, and chin control systems are available for driving a power wheelchair. A variety of switch options are available that include proximity switches, zero touch switches, and infrared switches for driving a power wheelchair. Testing of the recommended equipment is essential to ensure that the person can drive safely and efficiently both indoors and outdoors.

Power Wheelchair Bases

Four types of power wheelchair bases are available for mobility, and each system has its own set of benefits. Every person is different and many people can only drive one type of power base. Testing is needed for both new users and experienced users who may want to change the type of chair they have been driving.

Scooters

This style chair can be three or four wheeled and operates with a hand control lever system (see Chapter 9, Examination of the Environment). The seat options tend to be limited in sizes and supports. Many individuals like scooters for the ability to maneuver in small places, the ability to rotate the seat for transfers, and in some cases, the ability to elevate the seat for improved reach. These can be easier to disassemble for transport but might not have the power or electronic capabilities needed for driving outdoors. Although scooters tend to be less costly, consideration of a person's disability, changing needs, and environmental issues need to discussed before moving forward with purchasing a scooter.

Rear Wheel Drive Bases

A rear wheel drive wheelchair has the fixed drive wheels in the rear of the chair and the casters are in the front. Individuals driving this type of base see exactly where they are going and are able to watch their feet to ensure they do not hit walls, doors, or other items. Until recently, this was the most commonly used wheel drive base. With improved technology, center wheel drive bases are now the most commonly used base system.

Center Wheel Drive Bases

A center wheel drive wheelchair has the fixed drive wheels in the center of the chair and small casters both in front and in the rear of the chair. The chair turns from the center and care must be taken when turning to know what is behind and in front of the chair. Better LE positioning can be attained owing to improved caster clearance.

Front Wheel Drive Bases

A front wheel drive wheelchair has the fixed drive wheels in the front of the chair and the casters are in the rear. When turning the chair, the back end moves first and care must be taken to ensure sufficient posterior clearance. This type of chair allows closer proximity to tables or sinks. Lower extremity positioning is improved with no caster clearance issues.

Seating System Features
Adjustable Tilt-in-Space Seating Systems

Manual and power wheelchairs can have an adjustable tilt-in-space feature. The tilt-in-space feature is a seating system with a fixed seat to back support angle, fixed seat to lower leg support angle, and fixed lower leg to foot support angle that can be adjusted to tilt rearward or upright depending on the needs of the person (Fig. 32.26). In a manual wheelchair, in most cases, a caregiver needs to change the tilt position. In a power wheelchair, the person can independently adjust the seat tilt with switch access. The tilt feature is beneficial for individuals who have fair to poor trunk control and are unable to sit up straight against gravity for the full day. The tilt provides them with a resting and repositioning position. The tilt also assists with positioning a person in the wheelchair after transfers. The tilt feature can assist in improving balance and head positioning, improving skin integrity by assisting with shifting pressure from buttocks to back, and improving comfort.[44,45]

Adjustable Recline System and Elevating Leg Rest System

Both manual and power wheelchairs can have an adjustable backrest system and an adjustable leg rest system. This allows the person to recline in the wheelchair. This can assist with pressure relief and pressure distribution, bowel and bladder care, orthostatic hypertension, comfort, and ROM.[44] Each of these features can be ordered separately. On a manual wheelchair, a caregiver must adjust the recline and leg rest features. On a power wheelchair, the person can use power recline and power elevating leg rests independently with switch access. If manual elevating leg rests are obtained, the person will be dependent for leg positioning. Care must be taken when determining the need for both these features. In most cases, elevating the leg rests does not decrease edema; the legs need to be raised above the heart to achieve this effect. Hamstring muscle tightness needs to be examined to determine if appropriate sitting posture can be maintained with the legs elevated. Too often, extending the knees causes sliding of the pelvis on the seat surface. This increases the potential of pressure sores under the buttocks and promotes poor trunk posture. If increased muscle tone is present in the LEs, knee extension may cause spasms and pull the knee into flexion, often causing the leg to slip off the elevating leg rests and potentially causing injuries. The recline feature also needs to be examined carefully to ensure that the change in back position does not increase the potential for sliding down in the wheelchair.

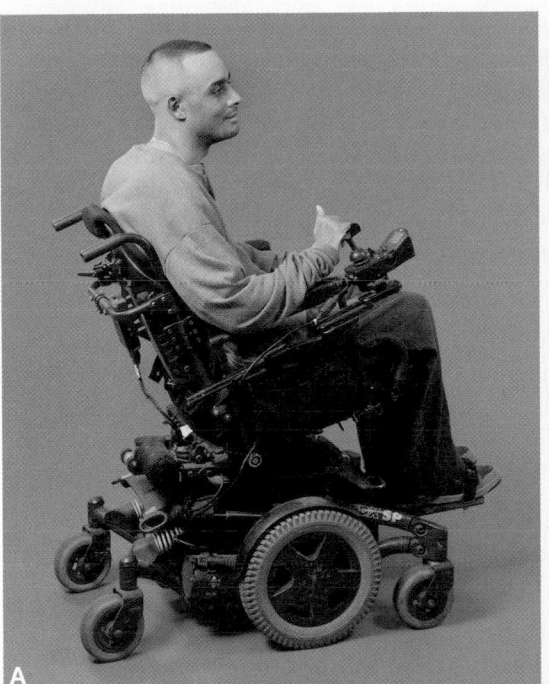
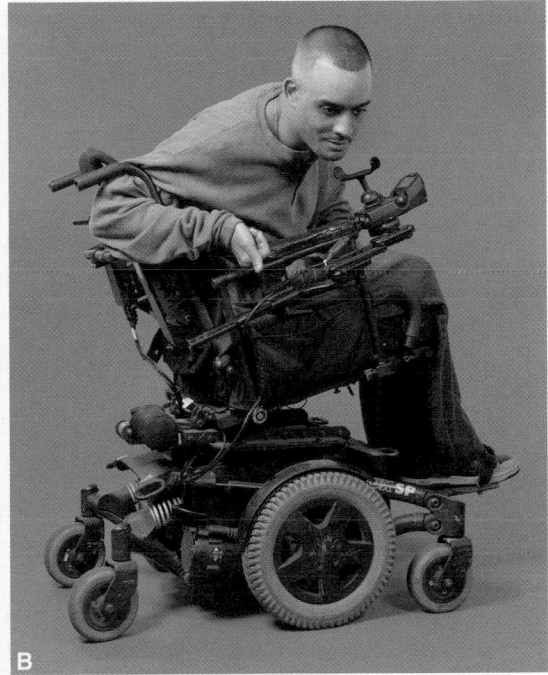
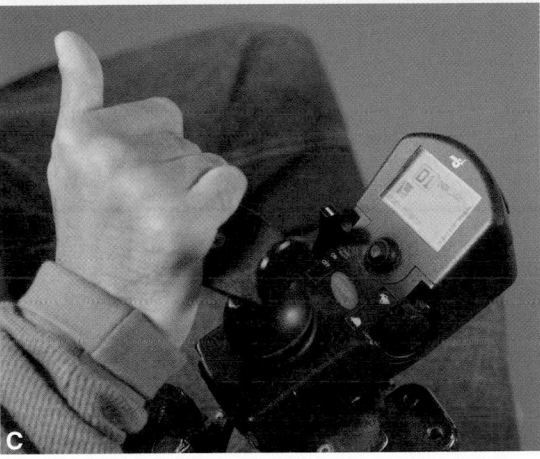

Figure 32.26 **(A)** Tilt-in-space wheelchairs tilt through space with their angles preset. **(B)** Patient performing pressure-relief maneuver in tilt-in-space chair. **(C)** Close-up of goal-post joystick.

Power Seat Elevator

A power seating system may include a power seat elevator feature. This feature allows the seat to be raised or lowered to accommodate for height differences and improve reach. This can improve access to tables, sinks, cabinets, and so forth. The feature can also increase ease for transfers on and off the toilet and bed. In the raised position, it can also provide improved social interaction. The power wheelchair can be driven using this feature, but the speed of the chair is slowed for safety concerns.

Standers

A stander is a device that allows a person to come to standing who ordinarily would be unable to stand without support. The stander can be a stand-alone device with or without wheels. For a person who would like to stand throughout the day without transferring to a different device, a stander is available in a manual wheelchair and a power wheelchair. In the manual wheelchair, the system is set up to raise and lower the person using his or her own arm strength. The added stander portion increases the weight of the chair but allows changing position throughout the day as needed to stand, stretch, reach, and work. In the power system, a switch is used to activate the stander and the same benefits achieved with a manual system can be achieved in the power system.

Power Assist Wheels

Power assist wheels are attached to a manual wheelchair. This provides the person with an assist on each propulsion.[46-49] It increases the ease of pushing a manual wheelchair both indoors and outdoors. This can assist a person who prefers to use a manual wheelchair rather than shifting to a power wheelchair.

Specific Wheelchair Frame Features

Sling Back and Sling Seat Upholstery

Sling back and seat upholstery are standard items on basic manual wheelchairs. This is convenient when a person needs to fold the wheelchair for car transportation. However, sling upholstery can promote poor sitting posture, posterior pelvic tilt, hyperextended neck, and poor LE positioning. The sling upholstery should only be used when the chair is primarily being used for transportation, if the person will only be using it for short periods of time, if the person is able to reposition himself or herself and is not at risk for developing contractures, and if the system needs to be as light as possible for mobility. Sling back upholstery is a standard item on basic power wheelchairs. Caution should be used when recommending this type of back due to the potential for poor trunk posture, increased kyphosis, and increased hyperextended neck posture. If at all possible, sling upholstery should be avoided due to potential for development of poor posture and increased health problems. Firm back and seat supports can be added to the wheelchair and removed for transportation purposes. Figure 32.27 provides an overview of the foundational components of a prescriptive wheelchair.

Back Angle Adjustment

The back angle adjustment is available on some basic manual and power wheelchairs and most tilt-in-space seating systems. The back posts can be angled and bolted in a specific position. Depending on the wheelchair manufacturer and the wheelchair style, various amounts of back angle are available. Some chairs only have 10° of adjustment while others have 30° of adjustment. This feature is beneficial for a person with limited hip flexion, as well as a person who needs a fixed rearward tilt position who does not want a tilt-in-space seating system.

Seat Frame Angle and Height

The manufacturer of manual wheelchairs sets the seat frame angle and height. Some wheelchairs are available with adjustable axle plates and adjustable forks. This provides the ability to alter the wheel size, caster size, and wheel placement to achieve a specific height and specific frame angle (Fig. 32.28). This can help a person with hamstring tightness by improving clearance for feet or assist a person with difficulty sitting upright to be tilted rearward slightly for improved posture and UE control. This can also assist a person with reaching the floor for propulsion using the feet or improve the ease for performing transfers.

Footrest System

The footrest system is made up of hangers, extensions, and footplates. The hangers mount to the wheelchair, and the extensions provide the appropriate length for the calf and footplate support. The hangers swing out of

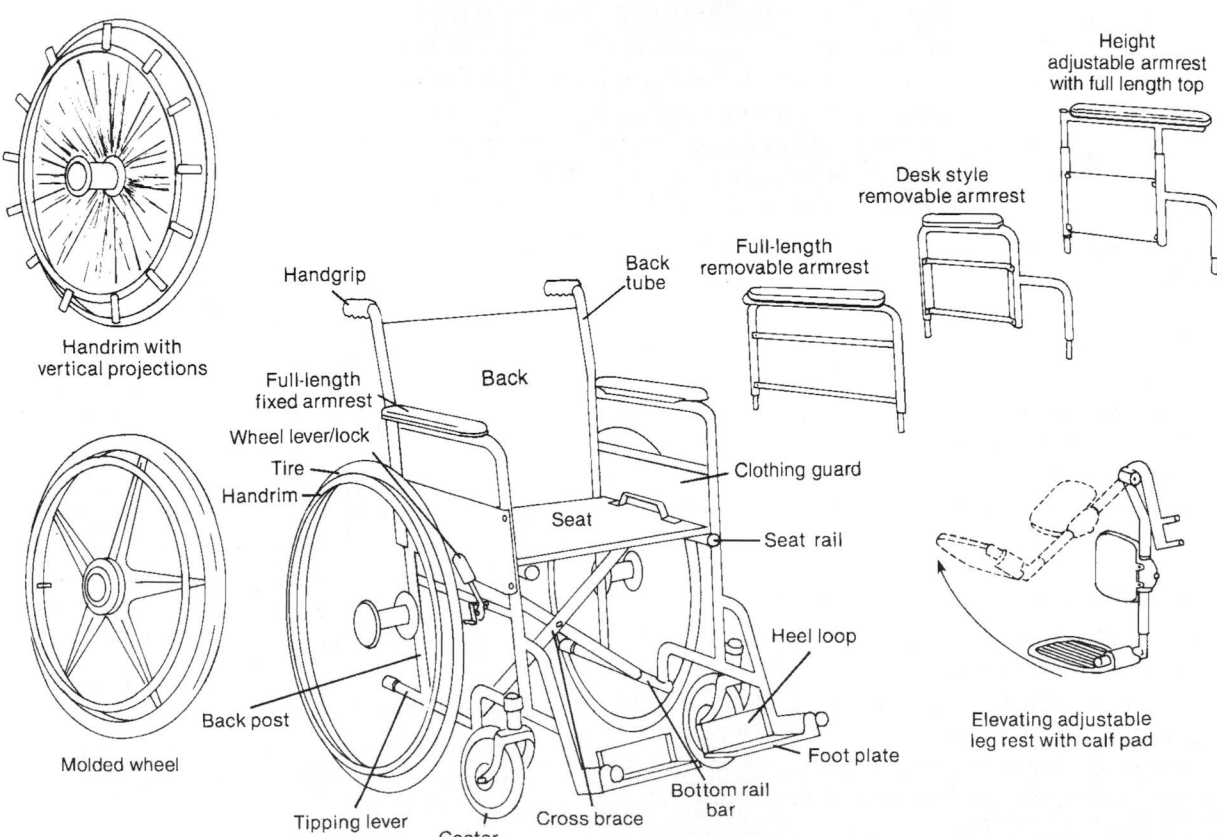

Figure 32.27 Foundation components of a prescriptive wheelchair.

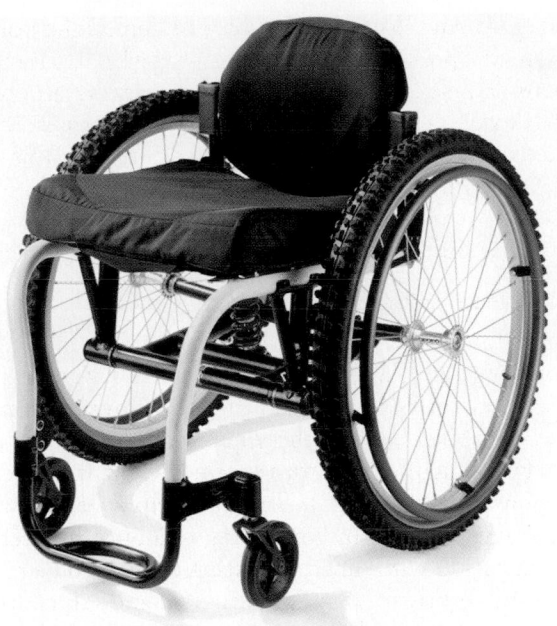

Figure 32.28 Lightweight rigid frame chair with adjustable suspension system, seat back angle, wheel base, and footrest lengths. The chair has knobby tires on spoked wheels. *Courtesy of Sunrise Medical, Carlsbad, CA 92008.*

the way for transfers. If transferring independently, practice trials using the release mechanism will ensure patient skill and safety in their operation. The footplates can be fixed or adjustable. The adjustable footplates (footplate can be moved and, depending on placement and angle, affects the foot and knee position) allow optimal positioning of the foot when tightness is present at the knees (seat to lower leg support angle) or foot (lower leg to foot support angle). This provides increased flexibility for positioning, especially if a person has changing needs.

Armrest System

Armrests come in desk length or full-length styles. They can be fixed height or adjustable height. There are a variety of methods to move the armrests out of the way for access to tables and for transfers. The person's functional skills will determine what system is optimal for independence.

Wheel Options

Rear wheel options on a manual wheelchair are important to ensure independent propulsion. If wheels are too large, excess strain can be put on the shoulders. If wheels are too small, they may be difficult to reach and propel. The type of wheel is important depending on the types of terrain the person will be using. Knobby tires may assist in rough terrain. A variety of wheel rims are available. Aluminum rims can be coated, have projections, or be a smaller size depending on method used for pushing.

Caster size options are numerous. A larger caster (8 in) may interfere with foot clearance depending on positioning needs. A smaller caster may provide improved positioning of feet and greater ease turning the wheelchair. Larger casters may improve ease of traveling over potholes or grates.

Options on a power wheelchair are more limited depending on the style of the wheelchair, but the tires tend to be wider for better traction. More options are available for casters on a rear wheel drive wheelchair and some prefer a larger front caster for improved driving on uneven terrain.

Seat Width and Depth

Manual and power wheelchairs come in a variety of widths and depths. If providing a person with a manual wheelchair, it is important to make sure the chair is not too wide or too narrow since this will affect the ability to propel the wheelchair (Figs. 32.29 and 32.30). Testing of the various chair widths is important to ensure that the shoulders are protected from excessive strain. The seat depth is important to ensure that optimal positioning can be achieved with seating supports.

Power wheelchairs and tilt-in-space seating systems may be available with adjustable seat widths and depths. This feature allows fine-tuning adjustments and attaining optimal sitting posture over time. Often, a range is provided for the adjustable seat width. Care should be taken to choose the most optimal range. For instance, if a width of 20 in (50.8 cm) is needed, a frame may be selected that can be adjusted from 16 to 20 in (40.6 to 50.8 cm) or 20 to 24 in (50.8 to 60.9 cm). If the patient is unlikely to gain weight, the smaller size should be chosen; if the potential for weight gain is evident, the larger size should

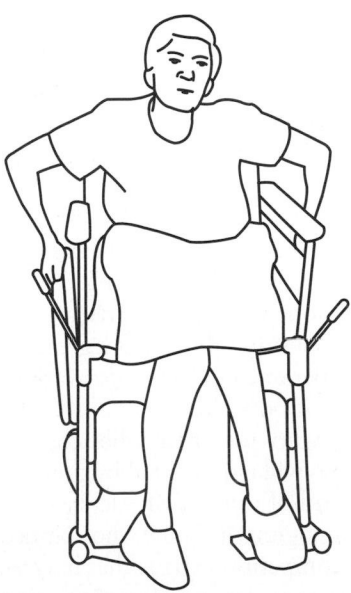

Figure 32.29 A wheelchair that is too wide will make wheel access and propulsion more difficult for the patient.

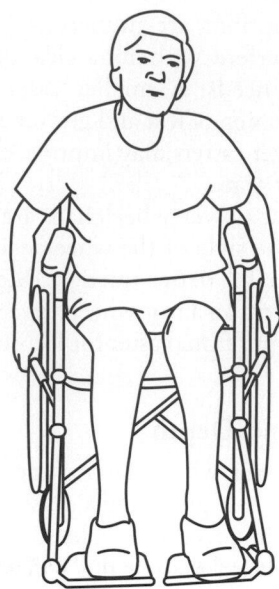

Figure 32.30 A narrower wheelchair allows easier wheel access and propulsion.

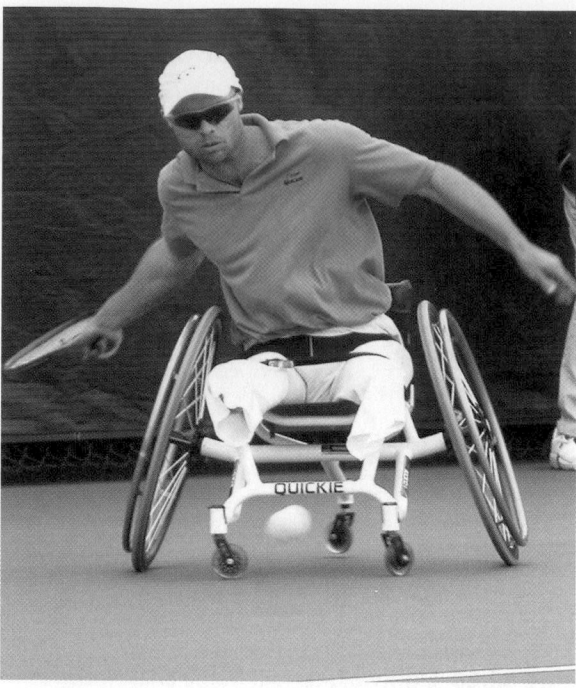

Figure 32.31 This court chair is shown being used for tennis play. It can also be used for basketball. The back is very low to allow free trunk and arm movement. The wheels are radically cambered for stability. *Courtesy of Sunrise Medical, Carlsbad, CA 92008.*

be chosen. The newer power wheelchairs tend to have more seat depth adjustability, but again, care should be taken with the base length of the chair to make sure it will not be too long for maneuvering safely indoors.

■ SPORTS AND RECREATION

Many users are active in recreational and competitive sports, some of which are done from the wheelchair. These patients may need more than one wheelchair: a *street* or *everyday* chair, and a finely tuned *competition chair* or *recreational chair* (Figs. 32.31 to 32.37). For some sports such as archery, discus, shot put, and precision javelin, a more stable chair is an advantage. A wide wheel camber (angle of the wheel, top of the wheel is closer to the user and the bottom of the wheel is further away to provide a more stable system) (Fig. 32.31) can achieve this even on a lightweight frame. For basketball, tennis, and dancing, the chair's responsiveness is critical. Competition chairs are usually of rigid construction, and made of very strong lightweight materials. Wheel and caster placement, tires, axles, and bearings can make a radical difference in chair performance when matched with the user's body weight and configuration. Users who participate in more than one activity may want a chair with a great deal of adjustability to allow parameter changes for various activities or multiple chairs, if possible.

Individuals who use their wheelchairs on off-road, challenging trails will require knobby tires (see Fig. 32.28), because the tread of normal wheelchair tires will tend to get stuck in softer ground. Those who compete in road racing will need competition chairs that have taken many of their design features from racing bicycles: narrow, hard tires; frames made of lightweight alloys, titanium, or carbon; low seats for minimum air resistance; and small

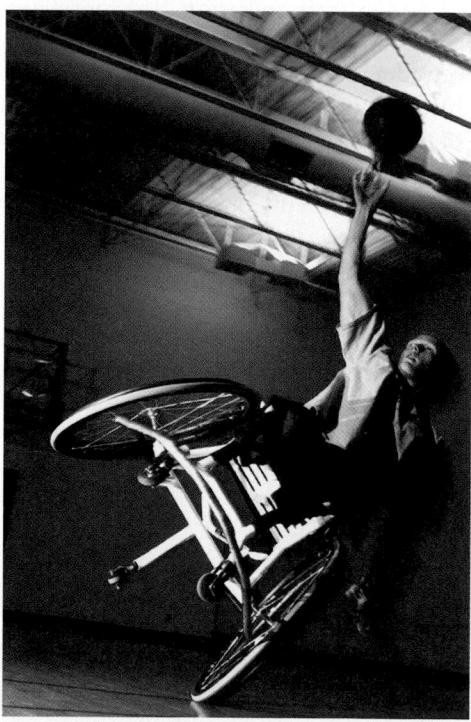

Figure 32.32 This court chair is being used for basketball. *Courtesy of Sunrise Medical, Carlsbad, CA 92008.*

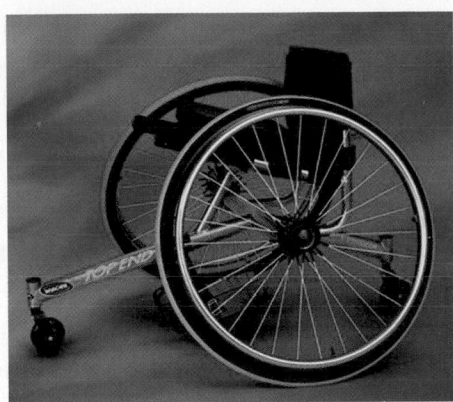

Figure 32.33 This tennis chair has a single front caster and a very low back. *Courtesy of Invacare Corporation, Elyria, OH 44035.*

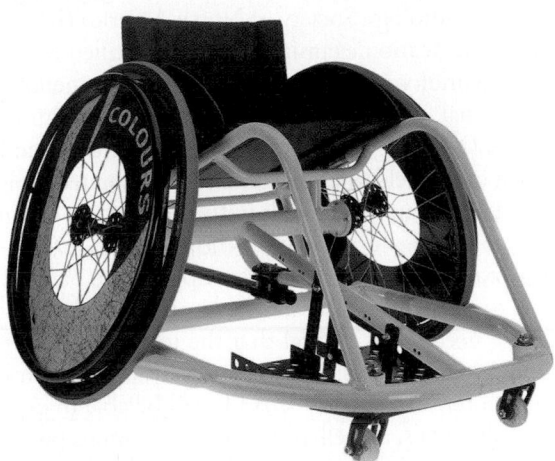

Figure 32.34 Some sports chairs are designed for high-contact sports such as football, rugby, and hockey. This chair has a rigid frame with larger than standard tubing and a very wide front end. *Courtesy of Colours in Motion, Anaheim, CA 92806.*

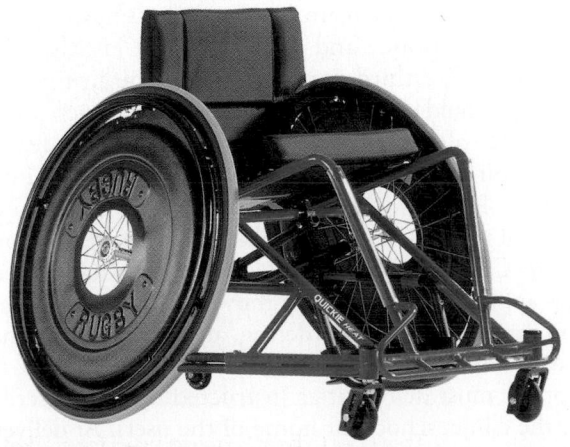

Figure 32.35 This wheelchair has been designed for use in Quad Rugby, which is a high-contact sport. *Courtesy of Sunrise Medical, Carlsbad, CA 92008.*

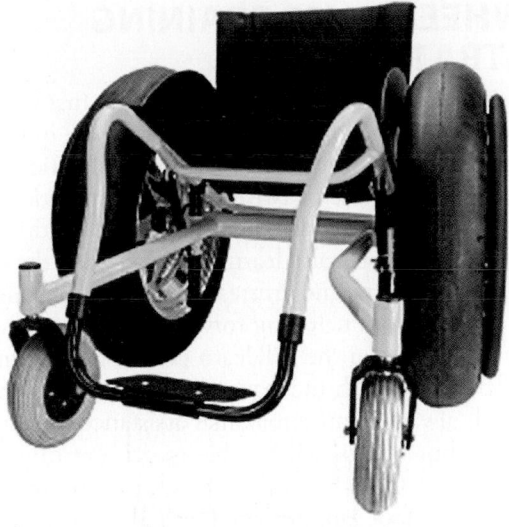

Figure 32.36 This wheelchair and its tires and casters have been designed for use on sand and in the water. *Courtesy of Colours in Motion, Anaheim, CA 92806.*

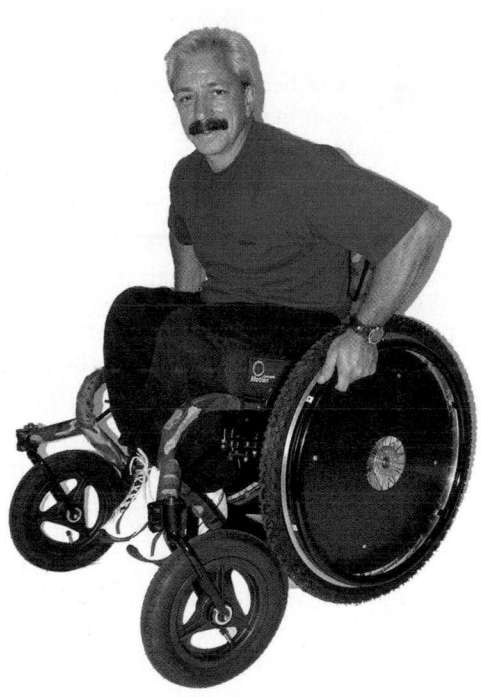

Figure 32.37 This wheelchair is designed for all-terrain use. *Courtesy of Motion Concepts, Concord, Ontario, Canada, L4K3C1.*

push rims for higher gearing. Racers usually sit in a tucked position, with approximately 120° of hip flexion, knees flexed, and legs strapped together to present a very sleek line and minimal wind resistance as the unit (wheelchair and user) moves quickly along the track. For tennis and dance, the chair is trimmed down to its sleekest configuration with all accessories, even wheel locks, removed. Wheel hubs and spoke configurations are designed to hold a tennis ball during competition. The backs are as low as possible to leave the user's upper body free for movement (see Fig. 32.31).

■ WHEELCHAIR TRAINING STRATEGIES

Many individuals using a wheelchair for the first time will require a training period. During this time the individual will learn how to propel the chair in all directions (i.e., using both arms, one or two arms in combination with one or two legs, or one arm using a dual-wheel drive system). He or she must also learn how to operate the wheel locks, foot supports, and armrests, and to use the mechanisms safely without tipping forward or sideways out of the chair seat. He or she will learn how to transfer in and out of the chair with the least possible assistance. Some users will always require maximal assistance for transfer activities, but others will be able to achieve functional independence. Chair features such as removable or swing-away arm and foot supports and lowered seat heights may be important for independence. For patients who perform standing transfers (independent or assisted), special attention should be given to the user's ability to get out of or back into the chair, because the seat height may prove problematic. Most chairs with a cushion allow a user to slide forward and come to standing. Many patients may benefit from adjustable height armrests. In addition to adjusting for arm support needs, these armrests can be raised during sit-to-stand transfers.

Although sidewalk cutouts are now mandated in many areas, patients who are capable of independent community mobility benefit from learning to do *wheelies* to negotiate existing curbs. The chair is balanced on the rear wheels while the front casters are elevated and then propelled forward to mount the curb.

Patients who drive need to practice transfers from the wheelchair to the car seat. The wheelchair is then pulled into the vehicle either behind the seat, or across the person's body into the passenger seat. Alternatively, the individual may transfer into the front passenger seat and then pull the wheelchair into the vehicle. The method selected is very dependent on the chair's folded size and weight, the user's upper body skill and strength, and the internal configuration of the car. Active patients also need to practice controlled falls out of the wheelchair and floor-to-wheelchair transfers that can be utilized in the event of falls.

Power chair training is slightly different, and usually concentrates primarily on driving skill and safety. The initial challenge is to locate a reliable access control site and method (e.g., hand control with a joystick, head control with individual switches). Training then involves working with the user on consistent responses (especially to "stop" commands, or the recognized need to stop based on the user's awareness) and accurate maneuverability. Although switch activation can be judged using a computer program, actual road time is necessary for training and ensuring that the driver knows how to respond to a variety of situations, distractions, and obstacles.

It is also important for wheelchair users to learn how to ask for help and how to direct helpers who might be touching them or the wheelchair. Some rehabilitation facilities have large fleets of sample chairs that can be used with patients for examination and training. If this option is not available, a qualified supplier or manufacturer's representative in the area should be contacted.

■ ROLE OF THE CERTIFIED REHABILITATION TECHNOLOGY SUPPLIER

Traditional home care and/or durable medical equipment companies are qualified to accept basic prescriptive wheelchair information (basic manual wheelchairs only) over the phone. They keep standard-sized items in stock, and can get them to the user quickly, often within 24 hours. More specialized equipment usually requires input to the team from an Assistive Technology Professional (ATP) who has passed the Rehabilitation Engineering and Assistive Technology Society of North America (RESNA) national certification examination or a Certified Rehabilitation Technology Supplier (CRTS) who is a member of the National Registry of Rehabilitation Technology Suppliers (NRRTS) and is also an ATP. He or she is a specialist in the field of complex rehabilitation technology service delivery and can work with the team to design a system that fits the patient's unique needs. Once the team's goals are explained to the supplier, he or she will be able to provide a list of available products that match the user's needs. It is critical that the team hear about all of the options, not just the products available from one manufacturer. The CRTS or ATP will be able to explain the pros and cons, as well as the prices of various products and options, to everyone involved. It may be advisable for the user to actually try several products before a decision is made. The supplier can work with the team to arrange this opportunity.

Once a system has been selected, the clinical team's recommendations (including physical, psychosocial, and cognitive factors if applicable) are compiled into a letter of medical necessity. The letter of medical necessity (with physician and clinic team member signatures), a physician's prescription, and price estimate are then forwarded to the third-party payer(s). The justification package should explain the medical need for each feature requested, along with the anticipated goal the feature will accomplish, and expected outcome from the intervention. Providing measurable functional outcomes is essential to help the payer make an informed decision.

The CRTS or ATP should keep all of the team members apprised as the process moves along from submission through approval, ordering, and receipt of the chair and its components. Once the system is complete, the supplier must deliver it as instructed by the prescriber (to the clinic, school, or home of the user). At delivery, those involved with formulating the prescription should have an opportunity to inspect the system and be sure that it meets the specifications, as well as to observe and assist as the supplier makes final adjustments. The process may require more than one or two visits for complex systems that require interim fittings.

On final delivery, the CRTS or ATP explains to the user and/or caregivers how to use the chair, including use of all safety features (straps, wheel locks, anti-tipping devices), assembly and disassembly for folding, and normal maintenance (including battery maintenance on power wheelchairs and scooters). Once the chair is delivered, the user and/or caregivers should carefully read any manuals provided and mail in all warranty and registration materials. The user and/or caregivers are responsible for all normal cleaning and maintenance. The supplier and the company he or she works for should be located close enough to the user to provide emergency repairs as needed. Warranty repairs are the responsibility of the supplier who provided the chair (most warranties cover the cost of labor for 12 months following purchase and then labor costs become the responsibility of the owner).

SUMMARY

A systematic approach to prescribing a wheelchair has been presented. The individual components of both the postural support and the wheeled mobility base have been described. The primary outcome in developing any prescriptive wheelchair is maximum function and independence. It must be the result of a thorough evaluation using a patient-centered problem solving approach, with attention to the specific factors discussed in this chapter. Input from the user and all team members during the decision making phase is critical. This process will result in an optimally designed chair capable of achieving its intended purpose. Using a patient-centered approach with open communication among team members, rehabilitation technology supplier, and manufacturer will ensure that each prescriptive wheelchair will meet the needs of the individual.

Questions for Review

1. Explain what information or data are gathered during each of the following portions of the examination process:

   a. Background information

   b. Examination of function using existing equipment

   c. Examination in the supine position

   d. Examination in the seated position

2. Discuss the importance of using seating principles when performing seating assessments.

3. Explain the difference between range of motion for a seating assessment and range of motion for a standard physical therapy examination.

4. When determining seat to back support angle, what parameters are used to finalize this angle?

5. What techniques should be used when measuring seat depth?

6. Why should recommended equipment be tested by the intended user? What specific issues need to be tested?

7. When would you recommend a wheelchair with sling seat and back upholstery?

8. When would you recommend the following types of cushions?

   a. Firm seat cushion

   b. Contoured seat cushion

   c. Air seat cushion

   d. Custom-molded seat cushion

9. Why is a pelvic positioner important and what methods can be used to make it more effective?

10. Describe the following wheelchair components; compare and contrast their functional benefits:

   a. Detachable swing-away footrests versus elevating leg rests

   b. Fixed-height armrests versus adjustable-height armrests

   c. Single-axle placement versus multiple-axle placement

   d. Proportional drive versus micro-switch driving

11. Identify four methods of self-propulsion in manual mobility and the benefits of each method.

12. Explain the benefits and contraindications of power mobility.

13. Identify four methods for driving a power wheelchair and discuss the clinical presentation of the patient who will benefit from each system.

14. Describe the various power wheelchair bases available and the benefits of each system.

15. Discuss the pros and cons of a tilt-in-space system versus a recline system with elevating leg rests.

CASE STUDY

Patient is a 56-year-old male with a diagnosis of multiple sclerosis. He currently uses a scooter for mobility and complains of seat discomfort and difficulty getting under tables. He resides in a long-term care facility.

Patient sits in a posterior pelvic tilt with a kyphotic spine in his scooter. He tends to lean to the left side. His hips and knees are in increased flexion due to the seat height being too low. Patient stabilizes himself in the scooter by maintaining his hands on the scooter handles at all times.

Patient is able to drive the scooter safely and independently. He is able to perform his ADL while using the scooter.

Patient has minimal range of motion limitations that affect his seating when assessed in the supine position. Hip flexion is 0 to 80° bilaterally. He lacks 90° of knee extension when hip is flexed to 80° bilaterally. Ankle dorsiflexion is neutral bilaterally when knee is flexed to 90°. Pelvic movement is flexible. Trunk posture is good but patient has the tendency to lean his shoulders to the left side with a shift of his trunk to the right side. Increased tone noted in both lower extremities. Patient has a stage II pressure sore on his right ischial tuberosity.

Patient was positioned in a seating simulation chair. Improved posture noted in trunk and pelvis in comparison to position in scooter. He preferred to be tilted rearward slightly and noted that this position assisted with his balance. The change in posture was significant and he will need a trial with this posture to ensure ability to perform ADL and improve his comfort with postural alignment changes.

Goals for patient include the following:
• Improve sitting posture and comfort
• Improve skin integrity
• Improve access to sink and tables for functional activities
• Improve independence in mobility in facility and out in community

GUIDING QUESTIONS

1. What type of power wheelchair would you have this patient test?

2. What type of electronics should be considered?

3. Based on range of motion limitations, what are the concerns for a seating system?

4. What type of seat cushion would you recommend?

5. What type of back cushion would you recommend?

6. Fill out a problem solving grid and address issues of posture, skin integrity, health/medical issues, functional tasks and abilities, environmental issues, caregiver needs, social and emotional issues, and mobility issues. Use the following four column headings in developing the grid: Problems and Potential Problems, Objectives, Properties, and Product.

🌐 **DavisPlus** | For additional resources, including answers to the questions for review and case study guiding questions, please visit **http://davisplus.fadavis.com**

References

1. Brienza, D, et al: A randomized clinical trial on preventing pressure ulcers with wheelchair seat cushions. J Am Geriatr Soc 58(12):2308, 2010.
2. Janice Eng, J, et al (eds): Spinal Cord Injury Rehabilitation Evidence (SCIRE) Project. Vancouver, BC. Retrieved September 1, 2012, from www.scireproject.com.
3. National Pressure Ulcer Advisory Panel (NPUAP), Washington, DC, 20007. Retrieved September 1, 2012, from www.npuap.org.
4. Barks, L: Therapeutic positioning, wheelchair seating and pulmonary function of children with cerebral palsy: A research synthesis. Rehab Nurs 29(5):146–153, 2004.
5. Nwaobi, OM: Effect of adaptive seating on pulmonary function of children with cerebral palsy. Devel Med Child Neurol 28(3): 351, 1986.
6. Hulme, JB, et al: Effects of adaptive seating devices on the eating and drinking of children. Am J Occup Ther 41(2):81, 1987.
7. Department of Education: Rehabilitation Engineering Research Center (RERC) on Wheelchair Transportation Safety. Department of Education, Washington, DC. Retrieved September 1, 2012, from www.rercwts.org.
8. Reid, DT, et al: Functional impact of a rigid pelvic stabilizer on children with cerebral palsy who use wheelchairs: Users' and caregivers' perceptions. Pediatr Rehabil 3(3):101, 1999.
9. Minkel, JL: Long term rehab: Sitting outside of the box: Clinicians need to let go of the 90/90/90 seating rule to explore more efficacious alternatives. Rehab Manage 14:50–51, 82, 2001.
10. Waugh, K: Measuring the right angle. Rehab Manage 18(1):40, 2005.
11. McCarthy, JJ, et al: The relationship between tight hamstrings and lumbar hypolordosis in children with cerebral palsy. Spine 25(2): 211, 2000.
12. ISO 16840: Wheelchair Seating, Section 1: Vocabulary, reference axis convention and measures for body posture and postural support surfaces. International Organization for Standardization, TC-173, SC-1, WG-11, 2006.
13. ISO 7176-26: Wheelchairs, Part 26: Vocabulary. International Organization for Standardization, TC-173, SC-1, WG-11, 2007.
14. Hundertmark, LH: Evaluating the adult with cerebral palsy for specialized adaptive seating. Phys Ther 65(2):209, 1985.
15. Saftler, F, et al: Use of a positioning chair in conjunction with proper seating principles for a seating evaluation. Proceedings from ICCART, 1988.
16. Curtis, KA, et al: Functional reach in wheelchair users: The effects of trunk and lower extremity stabilization. Arch Phys Med Rehabil 76(4):360, 1995.
17. Troy, BS, et al: An analysis of work postures of manual wheelchair users in the office environment. J Rehabil Res Dev 34(2):151, 1997.
18. Cox, E: Dynamic Positioning Treatment: A New Approach to Customized Therapeutic Equipment for the Developmentally Disabled. Christian Publishing Services, Inc., Tulsa, OK, 1987, pp 93–96.
19. Waugh, K: A Problem Solving Model for Seating Assessment. 27th International Seating Symposium, pp 269–270, 2011.
20. Sprigle, S, Chung, KC, and Brubaker, CE: Reduction of sitting pressures with custom contoured cushions. J Rehabil Res Dev 27(2):135, 1990.
21. Sprigle, S, Chung, KC, and Brubaker, CE: Factors affecting seat contour characteristics. J Rehabil Res Dev 27(2):127, 1990.
22. Hobson, DA: Comparative effects of posture and pressure distribution at the body-seat interface. J Rehabil Res Dev 29(4):21, 1992.
23. Sprigle, S, and Chung, K: The use of contoured foam to reduce seat interface pressures. Proceedings of the 12th Annual Conference of the Rehabilitation Engineering Society of North America (RESNA), New Orleans, LA, June 25–30, 1989. RESNA Press, Washington, DC, 1989.
24. Aissaoui, R, et al: Effect of seat cushion on dynamic stability in sitting during a reaching task in wheelchair users with paraplegia. Arch Phys Med Rehabil 82(2):274, 2001.
25. Holmes, KJ, et al: Management of scoliosis with special seating for the non-ambulant spastic cerebral palsy population—a biomechanical study. Clin Biomech (Bristol, Avon) 18(6):480, 2003.
26. Bergen, AF: A seat belt is a seat belt is a. . . . Assist Technol 1:7, 1989.
27. Margolis, S, et al: The sub-ASIS bar: An effective approach to pelvic stabilization in seated position. Proceedings of the 8th Annual Conference of RESNA, Memphis, TN, June 24–28, 1985. RESNA Press, Washington, DC, 1985.
28. Sie, IH, et al: Upper extremity pain in the post-rehabilitation spinal cord injured patient. Arch Phys Med Rehabil 73:44, 1992.
29. Boninger, ML, et al: Shoulder imaging abnormalities in individuals with paraplegia. J Rehabil Res Dev 38(4):401, 2001.
30. Boninger, ML, et al: Wheelchair pushrim kinetics: Body weight and median nerve function. Arch Phys Med Rehabil 80(8): 910, 1999.
31. Boninger, ML, et al: Shoulder magnetic resonance imaging abnormalities, wheelchair propulsion, and gender. Arch Phys Med Rehabil 84(11):1615, 2003.
32. Brubaker, CE: Wheelchair prescription: An analysis of factors that affect mobility and performance. J Rehabil Res Dev 23(4):19, 1986.
33. Highes, CJ, et al: Biomechanics of wheelchair propulsion as a function of seat position and user-to-chair interface. Arch Phys Med Rehabil 73(3):263, 1992.
34. Masse, LC, Lamontagne, M, and O'Riain, MD: Biomechanical analysis of wheelchair propulsion for various seating positions. J Rehabil Res Dev 29(3):12, 1992.
35. Butler, C: Effects of powered mobility on self-initiated behaviors of very young children with locomotor disability. Dev Med Child Neurol 28:325, 1986.
36. Butler, C, Okamoto, GA, and McKay, TM: Powered mobility for very young disabled children. Dev Med Child Neurol 25: 472, 1983.
37. Lotto, W, and Milner, M: Evaluations and Development of Powered Mobility Aids for 2–5 Year Olds with Neuromuscular Disorders. Ontario Crippled Child Centre, Toronto, Ontario, 1983.
38. Trefler, E, et al: Selected Readings on Powered Mobility for Children and Adults with Severe Physical Disabilities. RESNA Press, Washington, DC, 1986.
39. Wei, SH, et al: Wrist kinematic characterization of wheelchair propulsion in various seating positions: Implication to wrist pain. Clin Biomech (Bristol, Avon) 18(6):S46, 2003.
40. Boninger, ML, et al: Manual wheelchair push rim biomechanics and axle position. Arch Phys Med Rehabil 81(5):608, 2000.
41. Lal, S: Premature degenerative shoulder changes in spinal cord injury patients. Spinal Cord 36(3):186, 1998.
42. van der Woude, LH, et al: Seat height in handrim wheelchair propulsion. J Rehabil Res Dev 26(4):31, 1989.
43. Beaumont-White, S, and Ham, RO: Powered wheelchairs: Are we enabling or disabling? Prosthet Orthot Int 21(1):62, 1997.
44. Lacoste, M, et al: Powered tilt/recline systems: Why and how are they used? Assist Technol 15(1):58, 2003.
45. Angelo, J: Using single-subject design in clinical decision making: The effects of tilt-in-space on head control for a child with cerebral palsy. Assist Technol 5(1):46–49, 1993.
46. Algood, SD, et al: Effect of a pushrim-activated power-assist wheelchair on the functional capabilities of persons with tetraplegia. Arch Phys Med Rehabil 86(3):380, 2005.
47. Cooper, RA, et al: Evaluation of a pushrim-activated, power-assisted wheelchair. Arch Phys Med Rehabil 82(5):702, 2001.
48. Levy, CE, and Chow, JW: Pushrim-activated power-assist wheelchairs: Elegance in motion. Am J Phys Med Rehabil 83(2):166, 2004.
49. Levy, CE, et al: Variable ratio power assist wheelchair eases wheeling over a variety of terrains for elders. Arch Phys Med Rehabil 85(1):104, 2004.

Supplemental Readings

Brienza, D, et al: A randomized clinical trial on preventing pressure ulcers with wheelchair seat cushions. J Am Geriatr Soc 58(12): 2308, 2010.

Cowan, RE, et al: Impact of surface type, wheelchair weight, and axle position on wheelchair propulsion by novice older adults. Arch Phys Med Rehabil 90(7):1076, 2009.

Dieruf, K, Ewer, L, and Boninger, D: The natural-fit handrim: Factors related to improvement in symptoms and function in wheelchair users J Spinal Cord Med 31(5):578, 2008.

Isaacson, M: Best practices by occupational and physical therapists performing seating and mobility evaluations. Assist Technol 23(1):13, 2011.

Jan, Y, et al: Effect of wheelchair tilt-in-space and recline angles on skin perfusion over the ischial tuberosity in people with spinal cord injury. Arch Phys Med Rehabil 91(11):1758, 2010.

Karmarkar, AM, et al: Analyzing wheelchair mobility patterns of community-dwelling older adults. J Rehabil Res Dev 48(9):1077, 2011.

Kloosterman, MGM, et al: Comparison of shoulder load during power-assisted and purely hand-rim wheelchair propulsion. Clin Biomech 27(5):428, 2012.

Mahajan, H, et al: Comparison of virtual wheelchair driving performance of people with TBI using an isometric and a conventional joystick. Arch Phys Med Rehabil 92(8):1298, 2011.

Morrow, MMB, et al: Shoulder demands in manual wheelchair users across a spectrum of activities. J Electromyogr Kinesiol 20(1): 61, 2010.

Rushton, PW, et al: Development and content validation of the Wheelchair Use Confidence Scale: A mixed-methods study. Disabil Rehabil Assist Technol 6(1):57, 2011.

Sonenblum, SE, Sprigle, S, and Lopez, RA: Manual wheelchair use: Bouts of mobility in everyday life. J Am Geriatr Soc 58(12): 2308, 2010.

Vanlandewijck, YC, Verellen, Jo, and Tweedy, S: Towards evidence-based classification in wheelchair sports: Impact of seating position on wheelchair acceleration. J Sports Sci 29(10):1089, 2011.

Vereecken, M, Vanderstraeten, G, and Ilsbroukx, S: From "Wheelchair Circuit" to "Wheelchair Assessment Instrument for People with Multiple Sclerosis": Reliability and validity analysis of a test to assess driving skills in manual wheelchair users with multiple sclerosis. Arch Phys Med Rehabil 93(6):1052, 2012.

	Characteristics	Postural Control Provided (at Impairment Level)	Functional Assistance Provided (at the Activity Limitation/ Disability Level)	Advantages	Disadvantages
Seat Supports					
Solid insert	Padded insert board; reinforcement board inside cushion cover; contoured or flat insert board between cushion and wheelchair upholstery. Can be used with any cushion, custom made or premade, for comfort or pressure relief. Velcro® interface to upholstery. Spans seat rails or mounts to upholstery between seat rails. Works best with cushions that have zip-off cover to allow use of wide strips of Velcro® interfacing to hold cushion securely. Addition of extra Velcro® sewn to upholstery and underside or cover will hold better during sliding transfers.	Creates stable, level base of support. Decreases tendency toward adduction and internal rotation of LEs, posterior pelvic tilt, and slipping forward in the seat.	Good base on which to promote trunk extension and upper body stability. Enhances distal function (head and UEs).	Low cost. Adds minimal weight to frame. Removes easily for chair folding. Wheelchair can still be used if solid insert is lost or forgotten.	Increases seat height. Can shift on seat and produce asymmetrical sitting surface.

Continued

	Characteristics	Postural Control Provided (at Impairment Level)	Functional Assistance Provided (at the Activity Limitation/ Disability Level)	Advantages	Disadvantages
Solid hook-on seat	Seat upholstery is removed and solid seat is installed using hardware to hook to seat rails. Hardware can be fixed level with seat rails or dropped lower than seat rails. Angle and height adjustable; allows changing position of seat surface on frame of new or existing frame.	Improves pelvic position. Creates stable, level base of support. Decreases tendency toward adduction and internal rotation of LEs, posterior pelvic tilt, and slipping forward on the seat. Encourages level pelvis, neutral pelvic tilt, symmetrical spinal alignment. Raising anterior portion of seat can help keep patient back on wheelchair seat. Raising posterior aspect of seat can facilitate trunk co-contraction.	Good base on which to promote trunk extension and upper body stability. Enhances distal function (head and UEs). With forward slope, allows increased ROM in UE for reach and wheel approach.	Can change slope of seat without tilt-in-space chair. Wheelchair cannot be used if seat support is missing; ensures use at all times. Dropped style can reduce effect of thick seat cushion on seat height. Does not shift during transfers. Seat angles can be changed to accommodate limited ROM.	More difficult to remove for folding than Velcro® interface. Adds weight to frame.

Seat Cushions

	Characteristics	Postural Control Provided (at Impairment Level)	Functional Assistance Provided (at the Activity Limitation/ Disability Level)	Advantages	Disadvantages
Comfort cushion (planar/contoured)	Usually planar, but may have slight generic contour. Varying degrees of firmness available for different comfort levels. Can be made of layered foam to mix firmness for postural control and to accommodate limited ROM (e.g., greater flexion in one hip as compared to the other can be accommodated by different firmnesses, or by actually cutting the foam into different shapes).	Increases comfort; facilitates level pelvis; promotes a neutral pelvic position. Provides surface to create stable base of support.	Appropriate for patients with minimal seating needs. Does not interfere with sliding transfers.	Inexpensive. Lightweight. Patient can sit anywhere on cushion without discomfort. Totally flat cushions with one firmness throughout can be rotated to decrease spot wear.	No pressure relief. Minimal support. Minimal postural control.

	Characteristics	Postural Control Provided (at Impairment Level)	Functional Assistance Provided (at the Activity Limitation/ Disability Level)	Advantages	Disadvantages
Pressure-relieving foam (contoured, custom contoured)	Based on principle that increased surface contact results in improved pressure distribution/relief. Custom made or premade contour depends on need to accommodate individual postural asymmetries. Varying degrees of firmness available. Can be made of layered foam to mix firmness for postural control and to accommodate limited ROM. Generic shapes work best with symmetrical individuals.	Shaped to control postural alignment. Increases comfort; facilitates level pelvis; promotes a neutral pelvic position. Provides surface to create stable base of support. Custom-made contour more effective when accommodating asymmetries.	Appropriate for patients with moderate to significant seating needs. Assists with controlling posture and/or accommodating pelvic asymmetries to allow level shoulders and more erect head position. Increases sitting time; decreases problems with pressure over bony prominences; improves postural stability allowing increased upper body function.	Increased surface contact, creating improved pressure distribution. Accommodates moderate to severe postural asymmetry. Easier for caregivers to position and reposition the patient. Low maintenance.	More expensive. May interfere with sliding transfers. Patient may feel "locked in" because movement on cushion surface is restricted.
Pressure-relieving fluid or fluid/ foam combination	Based on the principle that increased surface contact results in improved pressure distribution/relief; generic contour or planar surface with fluid-filled sack. Bony prominences are "immersed" in the fluid, increasing surface contact. Some types have positioning components to accommodate for postural asymmetries and provide improved postural control. Combination units allow the foam base to be cut to accommodate limited ROM. Generic contoured shapes work best with symmetrical individuals.	Provides surface to create stable base of support. Some have add-on pieces to control postural alignment. Increases comfort; facilitates level pelvis; promotes a neutral pelvic position. Increases sitting tolerance for patients who sit with oblique pelvis. Provides appropriate support for pelvis to promote level shoulders and erect head.	Appropriate for patients with moderate to significant seating needs. Assists with controlling posture and/or accommodating pelvic asymmetries to allow level shoulders and more erect head position. Results in increased sitting time; decreased problems with pressure over bony prominences; improved postural stability; and increased upper body function. Gel medium usually increases stability at the pelvis; the pelvis sinks in and is "held" by the foam base, essentially broadening the base of support area.	Increases surface area, contact creates improved pressure distribution. Accommodates moderate to severe postural asymmetry. Increases stability at the pelvis. Easier for caregivers to position and reposition patient.	More expensive. Some maintenance required. Heavier than foam or air. Patient may feel "locked in" because movement on cushion surface is restricted.

Continued

	Characteristics	Postural Control Provided (at Impairment Level)	Functional Assistance Provided (at the Activity Limitation/ Disability Level)	Advantages	Disadvantages
	Firm underbase provides stable support for proper seating alignment.				
Pressure-relieving air	Appears planar, but responds to patient weight. Patient is "immersed" in the cushion based on regulation of the amount of air. Based on principle that increased surface contact results in improved pressure distribution/relief; bony prominences are "floating."	Does not provide a very stable base of support; some users find it too unstable. Individuals with decreased trunk stability tend to keep arms closer to the body for stability, decreasing UE reach distance. Some air cushions are segmented to allow more air into selected segments to improve postural control (it should be noted that segmented cushions are less pressure relieving because the air cannot flow from one segment of the cushion to another). Additional postural accommodation can be provided by placing foam pieces under the cushion.	Indicated for patients with moderate to significant pressure-relieving needs. Results in increased sitting time; decreased problems with pressure over bony prominences.	Very lightweight. Accommodates moderate to severe postural asymmetry. Increases surface contact for improved pressure distribution.	More expensive. Base provided may be too unstable for some users; unstable base may make transfers difficult. Air pressure must be monitored carefully. Continuous maintenance required.

Back Supports

	Characteristics	Postural Control Provided (at Impairment Level)	Functional Assistance Provided (at the Activity Limitation/ Disability Level)	Advantages	Disadvantages
Pita back	Solid board (padded or unpadded) that slips into a pocket in the back upholstery. Provides mild to moderate level of support.	Assists patients who need a reminder to sit with trunk extension. Assists with maintaining a	Provides enough support to encourage trunk extension.	Lightweight. Slips in and out easily for folding.	Only provides slight degree of support. Wheelchair can be used without this back support.

	Characteristics	Postural Control Provided (at Impairment Level)	Functional Assistance Provided (at the Activity Limitation/ Disability Level)	Advantages	Disadvantages
	Useful for patients who need a slight reminder to sit upright.	neutral pelvis and an upright sitting posture.			It can be lost or left behind when the chair is folded.
Solid back insert	Maintains pelvic alignment when correctly interfaced with seat surface (based on ROM examination to determine available hip flexion). If attached to the upholstery by Velcro®, or hung between the back canes, it provides moderate support and will not decrease seat surface depth on the chair. If hung or belted in front of the back canes, will decrease seat surface depth. Will assume the angle of the back canes unless braced across the top. Special foaming can be used to accommodate back contour or provide some postural control.	Maintains pelvic alignment when interfaced with seat surface. Enhances upright sitting, trunk and head alignment. Provides some lateral control if shaped foaming is used.	Enhances trunk control to allow improved distal function.	Removes easily for folding. Assists with postural control. Adds minimal weight to chair.	May not be stable in chair. Wheelchair can be used without this back support. It can be lost or left behind when the chair is folded.
Solid hook-on back	Very stable back support that can be aligned and angled as needed to create appropriate seat/back angle; accommodates for limited ROM. Can hold planar, contoured, or molded back, or air flotation cushion for pressure relief. Can be manufactured or custom made.	Enhances upright sitting; accommodates for limited ROM; accommodates for any degree of deformity; provides support as needed. Maintains client in position deemed appropriate based on examination findings.	Provides support to enhance movement control of the UE and the head. Increases surface area, contact provides improved comfort and pressure relief. Maintains trunk alignment to enhance pelvic positioning.	Solid support structure. Resists extensor thrusting. Accepts planar, contoured, or molded surfaces. Wheelchair cannot be used without this back support in place. Allows attachment of additional supports such as headrests, which work best	Increases weight of wheelchair. Requires manipulation of hardware to remove and fold wheelchair.

Continued

	Characteristics	Postural Control Provided (at Impairment Level)	Functional Assistance Provided (at the Activity Limitation/ Disability Level)	Advantages	Disadvantages
	Allows for provision of maximum support when needed. Mounts using permanent or removable hardware; with use of permanent hardware, can actually strengthen frame.			when back structure is solid and stable.	

Specialized Support Components

	Characteristics	Postural Control Provided (at Impairment Level)	Functional Assistance Provided (at the Activity Limitation/ Disability Level)	Advantages	Disadvantages
Head/neck supports	Provides support for patients with fair, poor, or absent head control. Mounting hardware can be fixed, removable, and/or flip back; hardware can be adjusted in one, two, or multiple planes.	Posterior, lateral, and anterior head or neck controllers available. Promotes maintenance of a neutral cervical spine and head position. Eliminates lateral flexion and rotation, which, when not controlled, can disturb trunk and pelvic alignment.	Supports the head to assist with respiration, visual interaction with environment, feeding, and swallowing. Improves safety during transport on level surfaces and when patient is transported seated in wheelchair placed in a motor vehicle.	Provides support and improves alignment. Improves safety during transport.	May interfere with head movement. May trigger extensor thrust. May cause skin problems in areas of high pressure.
Lateral trunk supports	Indicated in the presence of weak or spastic trunk muscles. Can be straight or contoured for more control. Mounting hardware can be fixed or swing-away for transfers.	Improves trunk stability and alignment (within available range); improves pelvic alignment. Controls lateral trunk flexion.	Improves trunk control; facilitates UE movement and distal control. Improves respiration, feeding, and swallowing.	Improves stability and alignment. Improves head alignment and control. Enhances safety during movement through space.	May interfere with trunk movement. Increases weight of the system. May interfere with attempts to self-propel with UE.
Anterior chest support	Assists with maintenance of upright trunk posture and control of shoulder position. Can be minimally supportive or maximally supportive depending on configuration of features (e.g., straps, padded straps, butterfly, and bib).	Supports trunk along anterior surface of trunk and shoulders, eliminates forward lean. May influence and discourage shoulder protraction.	Trunk support may improve respiration, eating, and swallowing. Stabilizes trunk to allow improved UE function and head control. Shoulder control promotes better head posture.	Supports trunk in upright position. Stabilizes trunk to free arms and head for movement. Improves head position for respiration, eating, swallowing, and visual interaction with environment.	Restricts trunk movement. Overuse limits patient's opportunity to improve trunk control.

	Characteristics	Postural Control Provided (at Impairment Level)	Functional Assistance Provided (at the Activity Limitation/ Disability Level)	Advantages	Disadvantages
Lateral hip guides	Improves pelvic alignment on seat. Assists with maintaining pelvic position on contoured seat.	Improves weight distribution on pelvis. Improves pelvic positioning; enhances alignment of upper and lower body segments; contributes to alignment of entire body. Assists with maintenance of pelvic alignment, which reduces asymmetries in trunk and LEs.	Allows patient to achieve or tolerate better alignment. Increases sitting time.	Improves and maintains alignment. Improves symmetrical weight-bearing through pelvis.	May interfere with transfers if not removable. Patient may feel "locked in" on seat. Increases weight of the system.
Lateral knee guides	May be built into the cushion contours, or fabricated from separate pieces of padded wood or plastic attached to the seat or armrest of the wheelchair; should extend to the end of the knee if maximal control is required.	Helps to maintain LE alignment; reduces excessive abduction and external rotation (e.g., patients who tend to fall into abduction, push into abduction, or whose legs do not come into neutral). Improves neutral alignment of LEs; assists with maintenance of pelvic position. Maintains LE alignment in combination with anterior knee block.	Improves pelvic position. Promotes improved trunk position and UE function. Maintains neutral alignment of LEs. Reduces forward sliding of pelvis on seat.	Maintains LE alignment. Assists with maintenance of pelvic position on seat.	If high enough to provide control, may interfere with transfers unless removable. Adds weight to the seating system.

Continued

	Characteristics	Postural Control Provided (at Impairment Level)	Functional Assistance Provided (at the Activity Limitation/ Disability Level)	Advantages	Disadvantages
Medial knee block	May be built into the cushion contours, or be a separate or removable flip-down block. For maximal control, the medial knee block should be positioned at the distal portion of the limb, between the condyles. The support should never be used to stabilize the pelvis on the seat by pressing into the groin; it also should not be used to stop the user from sliding off the front of the seat.	Prevents LEs from moving into adduction. If wide enough, may decrease spasticity. Maintains LE alignment. When used with windblown position,[a] medial knee block can prevent pelvis from continuing to rotate forward. Use of wider blocks will keep the greater trochanter properly seated in the hip joint.	Helps to maintain a broad, stable base of support; this base improves alignment of the upper body.	Maintains LE alignment. Reduces extensor tone. May help to elongate adductors. Provides broad base of support.	May interfere with transfers. Increases weight of seat.
Anterior knee block	Increases pelvic stability; most effective way to maintain proper pelvic position on the seat. *Note:* If hips are subluxed, dislocated, or not properly formed, approval from an orthopedist should be obtained.	Maintains pelvic alignment; maintains pelvis in neutral; prevents pelvis form moving forward on seat surface. Assists with maintenance of LE alignment when used with medial and lateral knee controls.	Helps to maintain a broad, stable base of support with neutral pelvic alignment; this base will promote improved alignment and functional use of upper body. When used in conjunction with forward-sloped seat, may facilitate trunk co-contraction, extension, and improved UE ROM.	Maintains LE alignment. Reduces extensor tone. Provides broad base of support. Increases stability.	May impose too much pressure at the hips and over the patellas. Patient may feel restricted.

[a]Windblown position: Both LEs oriented to one side with one LE adducted and the other abducted.
LE = lower extremity; ROM = range of motion; UE = upper extremity.

Web-Based Resources for Clinicians, Families, and Patients with Chronic Pulmonary Dysfunction

American Heart Association
http://www.americanheart.org

American Lung Association
http://www.lung usa.org
http://www.lung.org/stop-smoking

National Heart, Lung and Blood Institute
http://www.nhlbi.nih.gov/

Cystic Fibrosis Resources
www.ncbi.nlm.nih.gov/pubmedhealth/PMH0001197/
http://www.cff.org/

COPD Resourccs
www.ncbi.nlm.nih.gov/pubmedhealth/PMH0001153/
http://www.goldcopd.org

Asthma Resources
www.ncbi.nlm.nih.gov/pubmedhealth/PMH0001196/
http://www.ginasthma.org/

Interstitial Pulmonary Fibrosis Resources
http://www.pulmonaryfibrosis.orglipf

Pulmonary Rehabilitation Clinical Practice Guidelines
http://www.guideline.gov/content.aspx?id=10856

St. George's Respiratory Questionnaire
http://healthstatus.sgul.ac.uk/sgrqdownloads

Chronic Respitatory Questionnaire
http://www.flintbox.com/public/project/3192

Web-Based Resources for Clinicians, Families, and Patients with Heart Disease

American Heart Association
www.americanheart.org

National Heart, Lung and Blood Institute
wwwonhlbi.nih.gov/

Heart Disease
www.nlm.nih.gov/medlineplus/heartdiseases.html

Cardiac Rehabilitation
www.nhlbi.nih.gov/health/health-topics/topics/rehab/

American Association of Cardiovascular and Pulmonary Rehabilitation
www.aacvpr.org

World Health Organization
www.who.int/topics/cardiovascular diseases/

Centers for Disease Control and Prevention
www.ccic.gov/heartdiscase/

Clinical Practice Guidelines
www.guidel ine.gov/content.aspx?id=10856

Amcrican Association of Physical Medicine and Rchabilitation
www.aapmr.org

International Brain Injury Association
http://www.internationalbrain.org/

North American Brain Injury Society
http://www.nabis.org/

Brain Injury Association of America (BIA)
http://www.biausa.org/

Brain Injury Special Interest Group of the APTA Neurology Section
http://www.neuropt.org/special-interest-groups/brain-injury

The Academy of Certified Brain Injury Specialists (ACBIS)
http://www.acbis.pro/

Evidence-Based Review of Moderate to Severe Acquired Brain Injury
http://www.abiebr.com/

Rehabilitation Measures Database
http://www.rehabmeasures.org/

Traumatic Brain Injury Model Systems: National Registry
http://www.tbindc.org/regi stry/center.php

The Center for Outcome Measurement in Brain Injury
http://www.tbims.org/combi/

A

Acalculia Inability to perform simple arithmetic operations; inability to calculate.

Acceleration The rate of change of velocity with respect to time.

Accelerometer Device used to measure the vertical, anterior-posterior, and medial-lateral accelerations of the body.

Accessibility The degree to which an environment affords use of its resources with respect to an individual's level of function.

Accessible design Structural plan of buildings or dwellings that meet prescribed standards for accessibility.

Accessory (joint play) motions Motions between adjacent joint surfaces that occur when a bone moves through a range of motion. These motions are not under voluntary control and include glides (slides), distractions, compressions, rolls, and spins.

Acting out Instead of expressing feelings verbally, the patient uses actions to release stress.

Active range of motion (AROM) *See* **Range of motion**.

Activities of daily living (ADL) Daily living skills necessary for an individual to manage his or her life.

Basic ADL (BADL) include skills such as oral hygiene, showering or bathing, dressing, feeding, toilet hygiene, and personal device care (e.g., a splint).

Instrumental ADL (IADL) include housekeeping, preparing meals, shopping, telephoning, and managing finances, as well as work and leisure activities, functional communication and socialization, community mobility, and health maintenance. Often included in IADL are sexual expression, medication routine, and emergency response.

Activity (WHO/ICF) The execution of a task or action by an individual.

Activity limitations (WHO/ICF) The difficulties an individual may have in executing activities.

Acute coronary syndrome (ACS) (ischemic heart disease, coronary artery disease) A spectrum of entities that suddenly impairs blood flow through the coronary arteries, ranging from the least involved condition on the spectrum (unstable angina) to acute myocardial infarction and sudden cardiac death.

Acute pain *See* **Pain**.

Acute stress disorder (ASD) Diagnostic subset of "stress disorders" that generally indicate a sudden onset of relatively short duration. According to DSM-IV-TR criteria, symptoms must range in duration between 2 days and 4 weeks.

Adaptability The ability to adapt and refine a learned skill to changing task and environmental demands.

Adaptation Alteration of a skill or the environment to compensate for dysfunction.

Adaptive equipment Devices or equipment designed and fabricated to improve performance in activities of daily living.

Agility The ability to perform coordinated movements combined with upright standing balance.

Agoraphobia Fear of going outdoors or leaving one's home.

Agraphia Disorder of writing not due to motor difficulties in letter formation.

Akathisia Motor restlessness and intolerance of inactivity.

Akinesia Complete or partial loss of voluntary muscle movement.

Algometer Instrument used to measure sensitivity to pain.

Alignment Position of one component relative to another; refers to both angular and linear positions.

Allodynia An ordinarily painless stimulus, once perceived, is experienced as being painful.

Alternating attention The capacity to move between tasks and respond appropriately to the demands of each task.

Altruism Acting for the benefit of others regardless of the consequences for oneself.

Amyotrophic lateral sclerosis (ALS) A degenerative disease of the nervous system of unknown cause, affecting both upper and lower motor neurons; commonly known as Lou Gehrig's disease.

Analgesia Absence of pain in response to stimulus that would normally be painful.

Anarthria Lack of speech resulting from pathology, particularly in the brainstem, causing severe impairment of the motor–speech system. *See also* **Dysarthria**.

Aneurysm Localized arterial wall weakness with abnormal dilation of a blood vessel owing to a congenital defect.

Anger Strong feeling of hostility or displeasure brought on by a psychological interpretation of having been denied, offended, or wronged followed by the wish for retaliation.

Angina Oppressive pain or pressure in the chest caused by inadequate blood flow and oxygenation of the heart muscle.

Angiogenesis Formation of new blood vessels.

Angular acceleration Rate of change of the angular velocity of a body with respect to time.

Angular velocity Rate of body segment rotation around an axis.

Ankle-brachial index (ABI) Test designed to assess the vascular system; lower extremity blood pressure is divided by upper extremity blood pressure and a ratio or index is calculated. Segmental pressures can also be examined to determine different pressures and levels of vascular flow.

Ankylosis Joint fusion that may be the result of destruction of articular cartilage and subchondral bone, infection, or by surgery.

Anorexia Loss of appetite or aversion to food; emotional disorder marked by obsessive efforts to lose weight.

Anosmia Loss of the sense of smell.

Anosognosia Perceptual impairment including denial, neglect, and lack of awareness of the presence or severity of one's disability.

Anterior cord syndrome A spinal cord injury (SCI) resulting in loss of motor function (corticospinal tract damage) and loss of the sense of pain and temperature (spinothalamic tract damage) below the level of the lesion. Proprioception, light touch, and vibratory sense are generally preserved.

Antibody A substance produced by B lymphocytes in response to a unique antigen.

Antigen Any substance capable of eliciting an immune response or of binding with an antibody.

Anxiety Emotional state consisting of uneasy feelings of anticipation or dread of real or imagined danger; associated with an autonomic response.

Aphasia Communication disorder caused by brain damage and characterized by an impairment of language comprehension, formulation, and use; excludes disorders associated with primary sensory deficits, general mental deterioration, or psychiatric disorders. Partial impairment often is referred to as dysphasia.

Broca's aphasia (expressive or motor aphasia) A type of nonfluent aphasia; characterized by awkward articulation, restricted vocabulary, and restriction of simple grammatical forms with relative preservation of auditory comprehension. Associated with lesions involving the third frontal convolution of the left hemisphere (Broca's area).

Fluent aphasia Characterized by impaired auditory comprehension and fluent speech that is of normal rate and melody.

Global aphasia Severe aphasia with marked dysfunction across all language modalities; severely limited residual use of all communication modes for oral–aural interactions; global is not a type of aphasia but a designation of severity.

Nonfluent aphasia Characterized by limited vocabulary, slow, hesitant speech, some awkward articulation, and restricted use of grammar in the presence of relatively preserved auditory comprehension.

Primary progressive aphasia (PPA) A slowly progressive isolated aphasia not due to stroke, trauma, tumor, or infection, which does not fit neatly into existing aphasia classification schemes. It can exist in the absence or relative absence of generalized intellectual and behavioral disturbances or cognitive impairment generally associated with dementia.

Wernicke's aphasia (sensory aphasia or receptive aphasia) The most common type of fluent aphasia; characterized by impaired ability to understand spoken or written words. Associated with lesions to the Wernicke's area of temporal lobe of dominant hemisphere.

Apnea Absence of respiration, usually temporary in duration.

Apprehension test Test in which a patient's joint is placed in a vulnerable position for subluxation or dislocation; test is positive if the patient becomes apprehensive.

Apraxia An impairment of voluntary learned movement that is characterized by an inability to perform purposeful movements not accounted for by inadequate strength, loss of coordination, impaired sensation, attention deficits, or lack of comprehension.

Ideational apraxia An inability to perform a purposeful motor act, either automatically or on command; the patient no longer understands the overall concept of the task.

Ideomotor apraxia The inability to perform a motor act on command and to imitate gestures, even though the patient understands the concept of the task and is able to carry out habitual tasks automatically.

Apraxia of speech (verbal or speech apraxia) Impairment of volitional articulatory movement secondary to cortical dominant hemisphere lesion; manifested in imprecise and awkward articulation and distortion of phoneme production without commensurate pathology of the motor–speech system.

Arousal Alertness; the state of being prepared to act.

Arrhythmia A disturbance in the electrical activity of the heart that results in impaired electrical impulse formation or conduction.

Arteriole Smallest subunit of the arterial system.

Arteriosclerosis A thickening or hardening and loss of elasticity of arterial walls.

Arteriosclerosis obliterans Arteriosclerosis in which the lumen of the artery is completely occluded.

Arteriovenous malformation (AVM) An abnormality in embryonic development leading to a skein of tangled arteries and veins (usually without an intervening capillary bed); rupture produces hemorrhage.

Arthralgia Pain in one or more joints.

Arthrodesis Surgical immobilization of a joint that allows the bones to fuse.

Arthrokinematics Motion of adjacent joint surfaces that occurs when a bone moves through a range of motion.

Arthroplasty Joint surgery in which the joint components are replaced with artificial components (common examples are the hip and knee).

Associated reactions Automatic responses of the limbs that occur as a result of action occurring in some other part of the body, either by voluntary or reflex stimulation. In hemiplegia, associated reactions are stereotyped and abnormal.

Associative stage Middle of three stages of motor learning (proposed by Fitts) in which establishment of a motor pattern is achieved through continued practice.

Asthenia Generalized muscle weakness, especially in muscular or cerebellar disease.

Asynergia Loss of ability to associate muscles together synergistically for complex movements.

Ataxia Uncoordinated movement that manifests when voluntary movements are attempted; may influence gait, posture, and patterns of movements.

Atherosclerosis A form of arteriosclerosis marked by cholesterol-lipid-calcium deposits in the walls of arteries that may restrict blood flow.

Athetosis Condition in which slow, involuntary, writhing, twisting, "worm-like" movements occur.

Attention Capacity of the brain to process information from the environment or from long-term memory.

Auditory agnosia Inability to recognize nonspeech sounds or to discriminate between sounds.

Auscultation Listening for sounds within the body, especially from the chest, neck, or abdomen.

Auscultatory gap During blood pressure determination, a period of silence during auscultation; may occur in the presence of hypertension or aortic stenosis.

Autolytic débridement Use of the body's endogenous enzymes to digest devitalized tissue and promote formation of granulation tissue.

Autonomic dysreflexia (hyperreflexia) A pathological autonomic reflex seen in patients with spinal cord injuries; typically occurs in lesions above T6 (above sympathetic splanchnic outflow). It is precipitated by a noxious stimulus below the level of the lesion and produces an acute onset of autonomic activity; considered an emergency situation characterized by hypertension, bradycardia, headache, and sweating.

Autonomous stage The final of three stages of motor learning (proposed by Fitts) characterized by motor performance that, after considerable practice, is largely automatic.

Axonotmesis Nerve injury that damages the axon but leaves the neural tube intact; produces Wallerian degeneration distal to a lesion.

B

Baker's Cyst (popliteal cyst) A benign swelling of the semimembranous bursa found behind the knee joint.

Balance (postural stability) The ability to control the center of mass (COM) within the boundaries of the base of support (BOS); a state of equilibrium.

Barognosis Ability to recognize weight.

Basic activities of daily living (BADL) *See* **Activities of daily living**.

Benign paroxysmal positional vertigo (BPPV) Vertigo and nystagmus as a result of otoconia in the semicircular canals, displaced from the utricle.

Beveled Cut in a slanting manner from horizontal to vertical.

Bio-burden Quantity of bacteria in a wound; the quantitative biopsy is the gold standard for determining bio-burden.

Biomedical model Conceptual model of health and illness that is based on biological factors.

Biopsychosocial model A model of illness that uses a combined approach of incorporating biological/physiological, psychological, and social realms.

Blanch To lose color.

Blanch test (blanching test) A test of the integrity of the circulation performed by applying and then quickly releasing pressure, such as pressure to a finger-nail or toenail; the blanched nail normally regains a pink appearance within 2 seconds or less. Failure to do so suggests impaired blood flow to the extremity.

Blast injury When an explosive device detonates it produces a transient shock wave, which can cause traumatic brain injury (TBI).

Blood pressure Amount of pressure within the arteries throughout the cardiac cycle; a product of CO_2 and peripheral vascular resistance.

Diastolic pressure The pressure of the blood during relaxation (diastole) and filling of the ventricles; in health normally about 60 to 79 mm Hg.

Systolic pressure The pressure of the blood during contraction (systole) of the ventricles; in health normally about 100 to 119 mm Hg.

Body functions (WHO/ICF) The physiological functions of body systems, including psychological functions.

Body image A visual and mental image of one's body that includes feelings about one's body, especially in relation to health and disease.

Body mass index (BMI) An index used to control for both height and weight; determined by dividing body weight by standing height.

Body scheme A postural model of one's body, including the relationship of the body parts to each other and the relationship of the body to the environment.

Body structures (WHO/ICF) The anatomical parts of the body, such as organs, limbs, and their components.

Bootstrap technique In statistics, a technique used to establish the boundaries (prediction regions) about the mean curve for healthy control subjects; establishes the limits of normal variability for a given variable.

Bouchard's node A bony enlargement of the proximal interphalangeal (PIP) joint of a finger; commonly associated with osteoarthritis.

Boutonniere deformity Finger position marked by extension of the metacarpophalangeal (MCP) and distal interphalangeal (DIP) joints and flexion of the proximal interphalangeal (PIP) joint; caused by rupture of the extensor tendon of the involved finger. Commonly associated with rheumatoid arthritis.

Bradycardia Slow heartbeat marked by a pulse rate below 60 beats per minute in adults.

Bradykinesia Extreme slowness and difficulty maintaining movement.

Bradyphrenia Slowness of thought and information processing; seen in some forms of dementia and Parkinson's disease.

Bradypnea Abnormally slow respiratory rate consisting of 10 or fewer breaths per minute.

Brainstem herniation Secondary brain damage and neurological deterioration owing to significant edema and elevated intracranial pressures, resulting in contralateral and caudal shifts of brain structures.

Break test Method of applying resistance during manual muscle testing or handheld dynamometry in which the patient holds a joint position usually at end range; patient is instructed not to let the examiner "break" the hold.

Broca's aphasia *See* **Aphasia.**

Brown-Sequard syndrome A spinal cord injury resulting from hemisection of the cord. On the ipsilateral (same) side as the lesion, damage to the lateral corticospinal tract results in paralysis; damage to the dorsal column results in loss of proprioception, light touch, and vibratory sense. On the side contralateral (opposite) to the lesion, damage to the spinothalamic tracts results in loss of sense of pain and temperature.

Bruit An adventitious sound heard in a blood vessel during auscultation that is caused by turbulent flow of blood.

Bunion Lateral deviation of the great toe; hallux valgus.

C

Cachexia State of ill health with an appearance of malnutrition and wasting that is associated with many chronic diseases.

Cadence Number of steps per unit of time.

Calculation ability Competence in foundational mathematical abilities such as addition, subtraction, multiplication, and division.

Caloric test A procedure use to assess vestibular function in patients who complain of dizziness, standing balance disturbances, or unexplained sensorineural hearing loss. With the patient supine, each ear canal is irrigated with warm (44°C [111.2°F]) water for 30 seconds, followed by irrigation with cooler (30°C [86°F]) water. Warm water elicits rotatory nystagmus to the side being irrigated; cooler water produces nystagmus to the opposite side.

Canalithiasis Fragments of otoconia floating freely in the endolymph of the semicircular canal; associated with positional vertigo.

Capacity (WHO-ICF) An individual's ability to execute a task or an action; the highest probable level of functioning in a given domain at a given moment.

Capacity qualifiers An indication of the extent of activity limitation; used to describe an individual's highest probable level of functioning (ability to do the task or action).

Capsular pattern A characteristic pattern of restricted passive osteokinematic motion, usually involving more than one motion at a joint that indicates intra-articular joint inflammation or capsular fibrosis.

Cardiac index (CI) Cardiac output (CO) in relation to the body surface area (BSA), expressed in meters such that CI = CO/BSA.

Cardiac output (CO) The amount of blood discharged from the ventricles per minute, expressed in L/min; the product of heart rate (HR) and stroke volume (SV).

Cardiogenic shock Inadequate cardiac output (CO) and insufficient arterial blood pressure (BP) to perfuse the major organs owing to severe left ventricle (LV) failure.

Cardiomyopathy Any disease that affects the heart muscle, diminishing cardiac performance.

Cardiovascular disease (CVD) Any disease of the heart or blood vessels, including atherosclerosis, cardiomyopathy, coronary artery disease, peripheral vascular disease, and others.

Carpal tunnel syndrome Compression of the median nerve in the carpal tunnel, which results in weakness, pain, and changes in sensation in the hand and fingers.

Causalgia *See* **Complex regional pain syndrome**.

Cauterization Closing of tissue with a caustic chemical agent.

Center of mass (COM) The midpoint of body mass in erect standing posture; the COM is located at the level of the second sacral segment.

Center of pressure (COP) The point of application of the ground reaction force (in a symmetrical bilateral stance, it is located between the feet).

Central cord syndrome A spinal cord injury (SCI) resulting in more severe neurological involvement of the upper extremities (cervical tracts are more centrally located) than of the lower extremities (lumbar and sacral tracts are located more peripherally). Varying degrees of sensory impairment occur but tend to be less severe than motor deficits.

Central pain Pain initiated or caused by a primary lesion or dysfunction in the central nervous system.

Central post-stroke (thalamic) pain Central pain that occurs after infarction involving the spinothalamic system, ventral posterolateral thalamus, or subcortical parietal lobe; pain is described as constant and burning with intermittent sharp pains; exacerbated by noxious stimuli.

Central vestibular lesion A lesion in the vestibular nuclei or pathways carrying vestibular afferent input to the parieto-insular lobe of the cortex.

Cerebral edema An accumulation of excess fluids within the brain that begins within minutes of the insult (brain injury); significant edema can elevate intracranial pressures, leading to intracranial hypertension and brainstem herniation.

Cerebral embolus Bits of matter (blood clot, plaque, and, less commonly, air and fat) formed elsewhere are released into the bloodstream and travel to the cerebral arteries, where they lodge in a vessel, producing occlusion and infarction.

Cerebral hemorrhage (nontraumatic spontaneous hemorrhage) Typically occurs in small blood vessels weakened by atherosclerosis, producing an aneurysm.

Cerebral infarction Ischemia and necrosis of an area of the brain following a reduction of blood flow that falls below the critical level necessary for cell survival.

Cerebral shock Transient hypotonia and motor loss following injury to the brain.

Cerebral thrombosis The formation or development of a blood clot within the cerebral arteries or their branches; also includes extracranial vessels (carotid or vertebral arteries).

Cerebrovascular accident (CVA) *See* **Stroke**.

Cervical vertigo Term used to describe symptoms of dizziness, imbalance, and lightheadedness believed to arise from a cervical pathology.

Charcot joint A progressive, degenerative arthropathy of single or multiple joints caused by underlying neuropathy.

Cheyne-Stokes respiration Breathing pattern characterized by a period of apnea lasting 10 to 60 seconds, followed by gradually increasing depth and frequency of respirations (hyperventilation); occurs with depression of the cerebral hemispheres (e.g., coma), in basal ganglia disease, and occasionally in congestive heart failure.

Chorea A movement disorder characterized by involuntary, rapid, irregular, jerky movements; seen in Huntington's disease (also called choreiform movements).

Choreoathetosis Movement disorder with features of both chorea and athetosis; seen in some forms of cerebral palsy.

Chronic pain *See* **Pain**.

Chronic pain syndrome *See* **Pain**.

Chronic venous insufficiency Venous insufficiency that persists over a long period of time.

Circadian rhythm Biological process that occurs on a regular and predictable 24-hour cycle (e.g., variations in vital sign values).

Circle of Willis Normal anatomical union of the anterior, middle, and posterior cerebral arteries (branches of the carotid and vertebrobasilar arteries) forming an anastomosis at the base of the brain.

Claw toe Contraction of the proximal interphalangeal and distal interphalangeal joints of a toe, usually not the big toe; caused by tightened ligaments and tendons that produce severe pressure and pain.

Clinical reasoning The multidimensional process that involves a wide range of cognitive skills used to process information, reach decisions, and determine actions.

Closed-loop control system A motor control system that employs feedback and a reference for correctness to compute error and initiate subsequent corrections.

Closed skills Skills performed in a stable, predictable (closed) environment.

Closed wound care technique Wound-care approach that involves covering a wound from the outside environment with an appropriate dressing.

Clubbing Bulbous swelling of the distal fingers accompanied by a loss of the normal angle between the nail bed and the skin; associated with diagnoses imposing long-standing hypoxia and cyanosis such as congenital heart defects and pulmonary disorders; may also occur in the toes.

Cluster analysis A statistical technique for classifying patterns (e.g., gait), locomotion by placing subjects in homogeneous groups, or clusters, based on specified input parameters.

Cognition The act or process of knowing, including awareness, reasoning, judgment, intuition, and memory.

Cognitive-behavioral therapy (Cognitive therapy) A psychosocial intervention that helps decrease anxiety by promoting a change in attitudes, values, or beliefs; helps to change negative maladaptive thoughts and beliefs into positive, more adaptive ones.

Cognitive deficits Below average functioning in memory, judgment, construction, attention, sequencing, planning, recognition, or sorting.

Cognitive distortions Misperceptions of thoughts, ideas, or beliefs, or exaggerations.

Cognitive restructuring The cognitive-behavioral therapy technique of reshaping a person's thoughts/beliefs.

Cognitive stage The first of three stages of motor learning (proposed by Fitts), in which the learner develops an overall understanding of the skill (cognitive map); heavily based on cognitive and visual processes.

Cogwheel rigidity *See* **Rigidity**.

Coma A state of unconsciousness from which one cannot be aroused; the patient is unresponsive to stimulation. The patient's eyes are closed, there are no sleep/wake cycles, and the patient is ventilator dependent.

Community integration Introducing or reintroducing a person into a community.

Compensated heart failure Heart failure in which the patient's congestive symptoms can be relieved by medical intervention.

Compensation (1) Making up for a defect, such as hypertrophy of cardiac muscle to offset an impairment in circulatory function; (2) accomplishment of a movement pattern or task in a way that is different than the method used before the injury.

Compensatory intervention (training) *See* **Intervention**.

Complete blood count (CBC) Analysis of blood that includes separate counts for red and white blood cells.

Complete decongestive therapy (CDT) A specialized treatment used primarily for lymphedema consisting of manual lymphatic drainage, lymphedema bandaging, skin care, compression garments, and exercise used to open collateral lymphatics, remove excess fluid from an affected limb, and provide support to the impaired integumentary system until elastic qualities return.

Complete spinal cord injury (ASIA A) No sensory or motor function in the lowest sacral segments (S4 and S5).

Complex regional pain syndrome (CRPS) A complex disorder or group of syndromes that include reflex sympathetic dystrophy (RSD) (type 1) and causalgia (type 2); symptoms include intense burning pain and related sensory abnormalities, abnormal blood flow and sweating, abnormal motor function, and trophic skin changes.

Compression The approximation of joint surfaces.

Compression therapy The use of external compression to provide therapeutic levels of support for the venous and/or lymphatic systems. May be provided with one or a combination of the following: over-the-counter or custom compression garments, bandaging, multiple-layer applications of foam and bandaging, intermittent compression pump.

Computer-aided design/computer-aided manufacture (CAD-CAM) Technique for prosthetic socket construction that involves electronic mapping of the amputated limb, relating the limb shape to socket designs, and automatic carving of a positive model over which plastic is molded to create the socket.

Conduction aphasia A rare form of aphasia, characterized by intact auditory comprehension, fluent speech production, and inability to repeat what is heard.

Congestive heart failure (CHF) Heart failure accompanied by signs and symptoms of edema (i.e., pulmonary and/or peripheral congestion).

Consciousness A state of awareness; implies orientation to person, place, and time.

Contextual factors (WHO/ICF) Represent the entire background of an individual's life and living situation and include the following:

> *Environmental factors* Components of the physical, social, and attitudinal environment in which people live and conduct their lives, including social attitudes, architectural characteristics, and legal and social structures.

> *Personal factors* Characteristics of an individual's life, including gender, age, coping styles, social background, education, profession, past and current experience, overall behavior pattern, character, and other factors that influence how disability is experienced by an individual.

Conversion disorder A psychological disorder expressed by symptoms or deficits in sensory or motor systems that mimic a neurological or general medical disease.

Coordination The ability to execute smooth, accurate, and controlled motor responses.

Coping skills Strategies used to adapt to and manage life's demands and roles, stress, illness, disability, or other life changes.

Coronary artery bypass graft (CABG) Surgical approach that uses a donor vessel to bypass a coronary artery lesion (narrowed lumen) and establish an alternate improved blood supply.

Coronary artery disease (CAD) Also called coronary heart disease (CHD), the pathological process of atherosclerosis specifically affecting the coronary arteries.

Cortical blindness A total failure to appreciate incoming visual sensory information owing to a lesion in the cortex, rather than injury to the eyes.

Crackles (rales) An abnormal auscultatory finding within the lungs characterized by rattling or bubbling sounds that occur because of secretions in the air passages of the respiratory tract; the sound often is compared with that of rustling a cellophane bag.

C-reactive protein (CRP) A protein produced by the liver and found in the blood; used as a measure of disease activity (immune response).

Creative arts therapists Masters'-level therapists who use an artistic modality such as art, drama, music, or dance to sustain or increase patients' functional capacities and psychosocial well-being. They are referred to as art therapists, drama therapists, music therapists, and dance therapists.

Crepitus Crackling or grating feeling or sound under the skin and in the joints; usually indicates damage or wearing of cartilage.

Cultural restraints Taboos within a particular society such as incest or manifesting anger.

Cupulolithiasis Fragments of otoconia attached to the cupula of the semicircular canals; associated with positional vertigo.

Cyanosis Bluish-gray discoloration of the skin and mucous membranes caused by an excess of deoxygenated hemoglobin in the blood; associated with decreased cardiac output, exposure to cold (vasoconstriction), or arterial or venous obstruction.

Central cyanosis Diffuse skin color changes in "central" aspects of the body (e.g., trunk, head), as well as color changes in mucous membranes; indicates marked arterial desaturation and occurs when oxygen saturation is less than 80%. Associated with diseases of the cardiovascular/pulmonary system.

Peripheral cyanosis Color changes in the nail beds and lips owing to decreased cardiac output, exposure to cold (vasoconstriction), or arterial or venous obstruction; frequently transient and is often relieved by warming the area.

Cycle time (stride time) The amount of time required to complete a gait cycle; measured in seconds.

Cyst An abnormal sac with a membranous lining that contains gas, fluid, or a semisolid material.

Cystic fibrosis A potentially fatal autosomal recessive disease that manifests itself in multiple body systems, including the lungs, the pancreas, the urogenital system, the skeleton, and the skin. Causes chronic obstructive pulmonary disease (COPD), frequent lung infections, deficient pancreatic enzymes, osteoporosis, and an abnormally high electrolyte concentration in the sweat.

D

Dakin's solution A diluted sodium hypochlorite solution used to treat skin and tissue infections. The active ingredient is chlorine bleach.

Débridement The removal of foreign material and necrotic or damaged tissue from a wound.

Decerebrate rigidity Sustained contraction and posturing of the trunk and limbs in a position of full extension; seen in the unconscious patient with severe brain injury and a lesion in the brainstem between the superior colliculi and vestibular nucleus.

Decorticate rigidity Sustained contraction and posturing of the trunk and lower limbs in extension, and the upper limbs in flexion, fists clenched; seen in the unconscious patient with severe brain injury and a lesion at the level of the diencephalon (above the superior colliculus).

Deep brain stimulation (DBS) The implantation of electrodes into the brain where they block nerve signals that cause symptoms; pacemaker is implanted within the chest; used in the treatment of Parkinson's disease.

Deep partial-thickness burn Burn injury that extends down into the deep reticular layer of the dermis.

Deep vein thrombosis (DVT) Formation of a blood clot in the deep venous system; occurring most frequently in the lower extremities; clinical manifestations include warmth, pain, and swelling in the affected extremity.

Defense mechanism A psychological means of coping with conflict or anxiety; examples include denial, sublimation, repression, rationalization, conversion, and dissociation.

Degenerative joint disease (DJD) *See* **Osteoarthritis**.

Delirium (acute confusional state) A clouding of consciousness with dulling of cognitive processes and general impairment of alertness; patients may demonstrate confusion, agitation, disorientation, and illusions or hallucinations.

Dementia A broad base of cognitive deficits caused by a progressive organic mental disorder; characterized by confusion, disorientation, memory loss, personality disintegration, and deterioration of intellectual capacity and function.

Demyelination Disruption of the myelin sheath that slows neural transmission and causes nerves to fatigue rapidly; seen in multiple sclerosis.

Denial Refusal to acknowledge the truth or reality of a situation; a defense mechanism used to alleviate the anxiety and pain associated with functional limitation or disability; removes realities from conscious awareness.

Depression A mental state characterized by feelings of despair, hopelessness, and loss of interest or pleasure in living.

Major depression A depressive episode that lasts two or more weeks and affects occupational and social functioning.

Dermatome A band or region of skin supplied by a single sensory nerve.

Desquamation Peeling of the outer layers of the epidermis.

Detoxification unit A 5- to 7-day inpatient unit that treats people who are withdrawing from drugs/alcohol.

Devaluation The patient is overly critical of others and of himself or herself and may insult therapists and other personnel.

Diagnosis (physical therapy) The identification of the impact of a condition on function at the level of the system (especially the movement system) and at the level of the whole person.

Diaphoresis Profuse sweating.

Diaphragmatic breathing Deep inhalations that utilize the lower portion of the lungs and the diaphragm muscle.

Diastole Period of cardiac muscle relaxation, alternating in the cardiac cycle with systole or contraction; cardiac muscle fibers lengthen and the chambers fill with blood.

Diastolic pressure *See* **Blood pressure**.

Diffuse axonal injury (DAI) The predominant mechanism of injury in most individuals with severe to moderate traumatic brain injury (TBI). The mechanism of DAI is microscopic; the acceleration/deceleration forces cause disruption of neurofilaments within the axon leading to axonal degeneration.

Diplopia Double vision; two images are seen that are displaced either horizontally or vertically.

Disability (WHO/ICF) Encompasses dysfunction at one or more of the following levels: impairment, activity limitation, and participation restriction.

Disablement An interaction/complex relationship between a health condition and contextual factors (i.e., environmental and personal factors).

Discourse Conversation; generally refers to written or spoken communication.

Disease A pathological condition of the body or abnormal entity with a characteristic group of signs and symptoms affecting the body; with known or unknown etiology.

Disease-modifying antirheumatic drugs (DMARDs) A classification of antirheumatic agents that can alter the course of disease, as opposed to simply treating symptoms such as inflammation and pain.

Distraction The linear separation of joint surfaces.

Distress A term denoting a negative perception or response to a stressor whereby the stressor becomes immobilizing (overwhelming), initiating a sympathetic physiological stress response on the individual. Also see *stress reaction, eustress.*

Divided attention The capacity to respond simultaneously to two or more tasks or stimuli when all stimuli are relevant.

Dix-Hallpike test *See* **Hallpike-Dix maneuver**.

Dizziness Sensation of lightheadedness, whirling, or feeling a tendency to fall.

Donor site Site from which a skin graft is taken.

Double support time The amount of time spent in the gait cycle when both lower extremities are in contact with the supporting surface; measured in seconds.

Dual-diagnosis programs Long-term treatment interventions designed for people suffering from co-occurring substance abuse and mental illness; focus is on helping individuals become sober, remain abstinent, and manage psychiatric symptoms; typically provided at specialized treatment centers.

Dynamic postural control The ability to maintain postural stability and orientation while superimposing movement (e.g., weight shifting, reaching, stepping).

Dysarthria A category of motor speech disorders caused by impairment in parts of the central or peripheral nervous system that mediate speech production. Respiration, articulation, phonation, resonance, and/or prosody may be affected; volitional and automatic actions (e.g., chewing and swallowing) and movement of the jaw and tongue may also be deviant. It excludes apraxia of speech and functional or central language disorders.

Dysautonomia Dysfunction of the autonomic nervous system, with a wide range of autonomic irregularities; a clinical feature of parkinsonism, Shy-Drager syndrome, and others.

Dyscalculia Impaired ability to perform simple arithmetic operations; difficulty in accomplishing calculations.

Dysdiadochokinesia Impaired ability to perform rapid alternating movements.

Dysequilibrium Impaired balance; sensation that one is off balance.

Dysesthesia An unpleasant abnormal sensation, such as a sense of burning, cutting, numbness, prickling, stinging, or tingling of the skin.

Dyskinesia Impaired ability to execute voluntary movement; characterized by uncontrolled or involuntary movements.

Dysmetria Impaired ability to judge the distance or range of a movement.

Dysphagia Inability to swallow or difficulty swallowing.

Dyspnea Air hunger resulting in difficult or labored breathing; sometimes accompanied by pain. Normally accompanies vigorous exercise.

Dyspraxia A disturbance in the programming, control, and execution of volitional movements.

Dyssynergia (movement decomposition) Impaired coordination of muscular contractions and movement.

Dysthymic disorder Chronic depression and dysphoric mood, resulting in poor appetite or overeating, insomnia or hypersomnia, low energy, low self-esteem, and poor concentration.

Dystonia A movement disorder characterized by disordered tone and involuntary movements involving large portions of the body, typically twisting or writhing motions.

E

Ecological approach A health promotion approach that considers the important influence of the social and physical environments on an individual's behaviors.

Ejection fraction (EF) The relationship between stroke volume (SV) and left ventricular end diastolic volume (LVEDV) such that EF = SV ÷ LVEDV. This value represents the ratio of the volume of blood ejected by the left ventricle (LV) per contraction relative to the volume of blood received by the LV following diastole. Normal EF is approximately 55%–75% (67% ± 8%) and is widely used clinically as an index of contractility.

Electrical burn Injury sustained from the passage of electrical current through the tissues of the body.

Electromyography (EMG) Recording of motor unit activity to evaluate the scope of a neuromuscular disorder by assessing muscle potentials during various stages of contraction and at rest.

Elephantiasis Most severe stage of lymphedema. It results from long-standing, untreated lymphedema.

Enablement A process by which physical or mental capacities are restored or developed by addressing the interaction between the person and the environment.

End-feel The normal tissue resistance experienced by the therapist when excessive pressure is applied at the end of a range of motion or accessory motion.

End-of-dose deterioration (wearing-off state) A worsening of symptoms during the expected timeframe of medication effectiveness; seen with long-term use of L-dopa therapy in patients with Parkinson's disease.

Endogenous Originating or produced within the organism.

Endolymph Fluid within the semicircular canals that contains a high concentration of potassium, with a lower concentration of sodium. It moves freely within each canal in response to the direction of the angular head rotation.

Environmental accessibility Absence or removal of physical barriers from the entrance of and within a building or dwelling to allow use by individuals with disabilities.

Environmental barrier Physical impediments that prevent individuals from functioning optimally in their surroundings, including safety hazards, access problems, and home or workplace design difficulties (e.g., revolving doors, stairways, narrow doorways).

Environmental control unit (ECU) An electrical interface that allows the user to control a variety of electrical appliances and devices; operation is accomplished by use of a central control panel.

Environmental factors (WHO/ICF) The physical, social, and attitudinal environment in which people live and conduct their lives, including social attitudes, architectural characteristics, and legal and social structures.

Enzymatic débridement Removal of necrotic tissue by use of topical ointments, impregnated with enzymes, placed directly in the wound.

Eosinophils A type of white blood cell, usually only accounting for about 5% of all white blood cells.

Episcleritis Irritation and inflammation of the episclera, a thin layer of tissue covering the white part (sclera) of the eye.

Epithelial healing The process of regeneration of the epidermis through epidermal cell migration, proliferation, and differentiation.

Epitope A molecular region on an antigen's surface capable of eliciting an immune response and of combining with the specific antibody produced by such a response.

Erythema Redness of the skin due to capillary dilation. In light-skinned individuals this will appear pink to bright red. In dark-skinned individuals, there is a deepening of normal color or a purple coloration.

Erythrocyte sedimentation rate (ESR) A measure of the rate of sedimentation of red blood cells (RBCs) in an anticoagulated whole blood sample over a specified period of time; an indicator of inflammatory and necrotic processes.

Eschar The dead, necrotic tissue cast off from the surface of the skin, especially after a burn wound; material is often crusty or scabbed.

Escharotomy Midlateral incision of the burned eschar used to relieve pressure in an extremity or on the trunk.

Euphoria An exaggerated feeling of well-being, a sense of optimism incongruent with the patient's incapacitating disability.

Eupnea Normal respiration.

Eustress A term denoting a positive perception or response to a stressor whereby the stressor is seen as, or becomes, enervating or motivating, rather than overwhelming or negative.

Evidence-based clinical practice guidelines (EBCPGs) Systematically developed statements to assist practitioner and patient decisions about appropriate health care for specific clinical circumstances.

Evidence-based practice (EBP) The integration of best research evidence with clinical expertise and the patient's unique values and circumstances.

Exacerbation (relapse) An acute worsening or flare-up of neurological signs and symptoms lasting more than 24 hours but generally of longer duration; seen in multiple sclerosis.

Executive functions (higher-order cognitive functions) Those cognitive abilities that enable a person to engage in purposeful behaviors; includes volition, planning, purposeful action, recognizing errors, problem solving, and thinking abstractly.

Exercise A subcategory of physical activity; consists of planned, structured activity intended to improve or maintain one or more components of physical fitness.

Exercise tolerance test (ETT) (stress test or graded exercise test) An examination of the ability of the cardiovascular system to accommodate increasing metabolic demand with increasing exercise intensities; monitored using electrocardiographic, hemodynamic, and symptomatic responses. Myocardial ischemia, electrical instability, and other exertional intolerance abnormalities are determined.

Exostoses A spur or bony outgrowth from a bone.

Expected outcomes The intended results of patient/client management; the predicted changes in impairments, activity limitations, and participation restrictions along with health, risk reduction and prevention, wellness and fitness, and optimization of patient/client satisfaction expected as a result of implementing the plan of care. Outcomes define the patient's expected level at the conclusion of the episode of care and should be measurable and time limited.

Expiratory reserve volume (ERV) The amount of air that can be exhaled after a tidal exhalation.

Externalized hostility Putting blame on external situations or people instead of taking responsibility for one's undesirable predicaments.

Exteroceptors Sensory receptors that provide information from the external environment.

Extra-articular Occurring outside a joint.

Exudate Fluid, cells, and other materials released from cells or blood vessels through small pores or breaks in cell membranes; usually has a high content of serum proteins, cells, or solid debris (perspiration, pus, serum).

F

Fasciculations Spontaneous potentials seen on EMG with irritation or degeneration of the anterior horn cell, chronic peripheral nerve lesions, nerve root compression, and muscle spasms or cramps.

Fatigue The inability to contract muscle repeatedly over time.

Feedback Response-produced sensory information received during or after movement; used to monitor movement output for corrective actions; may be intrinsic or augmented.

Feedforward control The sending of signals in advance of movement to ready a part of the system for incoming sensory feedback or for a future motor command; allows for anticipatory adjustments in postural activity.

Festinating gait Walking characterized by a progressive increase in speed with a shortening of stride; common in Parkinson's disease.

Fibrillation potentials Small, spontaneous, biphasic EMG spikes, classically indicative of lower motor neuron disorders or myopathies, occurring with a muscle at rest.

Fibrin A whitish-yellow protein formed by the action of thrombin on fibrinogen.

Fibroblasts Cells or corpuscles from which connective tissue is developed; produces collagen, elastin, and reticular protein fibers.

Fibrosis A condition marked by proliferation of fibrous connective tissue; spreads over or replaces normal smooth muscle or other normal organ tissue.

Finger agnosia The inability to identify the fingers on one's own hands or on the hands of the examiner, including difficulty in naming the fingers on command, identifying which finger was touched, and mimicking finger movements.

Fistula An abnormal tube-like passage from a normal cavity or tube to a free surface or to another cavity.

Flail joint An unstable, weakened joint.

Flat affect Displaying little or no emotion.

Fluent aphasia *See* **Aphasia**.

Focused attention *See* **Selective attention**.

Foot angle Angle of foot placement with respect to the line of progression; measured in degrees.

Force plates Load transducers capable of measuring ground reaction forces and the center of pressure.

Form discrimination The ability to perceive or to attend to subtle differences in form and shape.

Free-floating anxiety A psychodynamic construct denoting generalized feelings of anxiety whereby the individual is unable to state or locate the source, cause, or reason for such feelings.

Freezing A sudden episode of immobility or block in movement, seen in Parkinson's disease.

Full-thickness burn Burn involving the entire thickness of the epidermal and dermal skin.

Full-thickness skin graft Graft containing epidermis and full dermal thickness.

Function (APTA/*Guide to Physical Therapist Practice*) Those activities identified by an individual as essential to support physical, social, and psychological well-being and to create a personal sense of meaningful living.

Functional capacities The ability to perform in the following performance components: cognitive, social interactions, frustration tolerance, concentration, ambulation, stress management, time management, activities of daily living, and life roles (work, education, household maintenance, and parenting).

Functional limitation (APTA/ *Guide to Physical Therapist Practice*) The restriction of the ability to perform at the level of the whole person, a physical action, task, or activity in an efficient, typically expected, or competent manner.

Functional maintenance program A rehabilitation program designed to manage the effects of progressive disease; includes strategies to prevent or slow decline of function, and promote regular exercise, good health, and self-management skills.

Functional mobility skills (FMS) Those activity skills that involve movement of the body, including transfers, walking, and lifting or carrying objects.

Functional residual capacity (FRC) The combination of residual volume and expiratory reserve volume.

Functional training The education and training of patients in basic and instrumental activities of daily living (ADL) that are intended to improve the ability to perform physical actions, tasks, or activities in an efficient, typically expected, or competent manner.

Function-induced recovery (use-dependent cortical reorganization) The ability of the nervous system to modify itself in response to changes in activity and the environment; neural reorganization occurs as a result of increased use of involved body segments in behaviorally relevant tasks (e.g., forced use).

Fund of knowledge Mental status screening test that utilizes questions related to the patient's learning history and life experiences.

G

Gangrene Tissue death or necrosis; usually due to impaired or absent blood supply. May be localized or involve an entire extremity or organ.

Gaze A state of looking in one direction; directional gaze is determined by control of different combinations of contractions by the extraocular muscles.

Gaze instability A disturbance of eye conjugate movement in which gaze is deviated or unstable. Patients with gaze instability have difficulty maintaining visual focus during head motion.

General adaptation syndrome (GAS) An organism's immediate reaction to an extreme catastrophe; a defensive adaptation response aimed at dealing with real or perceived emergency situations.

Generalized anxiety disorder Excessive worry, apprehension, and concern persisting for at least 6 months; may be accompanied by irritability, fatigue, and disturbed sleep patterns.

Genu valgum A deformity in which the lower extremities curve inward with knees close together; knock-knees.

Genu varum A deformity in which the lower extremities curve outward with knees wide apart; bow legs.

Glide (slide) The linear (translatory) motion of one surface sliding over another surface; the same point on one surface comes into contact with new points on the other surface.

Gliosis Proliferation of neuroglial tissue within the central nervous system that results in glial scars (plaques); seen in MS.

Global aphasia *See* **Aphasia.**

Goals (anticipated) The intended results of patient/client management; the changes in impairments, activity limitations, and participation restrictions along with health promotion, risk reduction and prevention, wellness and fitness, and optimization of patient/client satisfaction that are expected as a result of implementing the plan of care. Goals define the interim steps that are necessary to achieve expected outcomes and should be measurable and time limited.

Gold standard Accepted, accurate measure of a particular phenomenon that can serve as the normative standard for other measures.

Granulation tissue A matrix of collagen, hyaluronic acid, and fibronectin in a newly formed vascular network.

Graphesthesia (traced figure identification) Recognition of numbers, letters, or symbols traced on the skin with vision occluded.

Grief A psychological state of distress or sadness associated with a significant loss.

Ground (floor) reaction force (GRF) Vertical, anterior-posterior, and medial-lateral forces created as a result of foot contact with the supporting surface; forces are equal in magnitude and opposite in direction to the force applied by the foot to the ground.

Guided movement Involves physically or verbally assisting the learner through the task or activity to be learned; behaviors are limited or controlled to prevent errors.

H

Habituation training Training using repeated movements to reduce symptoms associated with the provocative motion.

Hallpike-Dix maneuver Positional test used to reproduce symptoms of vertigo and nystagmus and diagnose benign positional vertigo.

Hallucination Sensing things that are not tangibly real and believing that they are. When visually hallucinating, people see things that are not really there. During auditory hallucinations, people hear voices and believe that others are talking to them. Tactile hallucinations are sensations of the skin that are not real, such as feeling bugs crawling on one's skin.

Hallux valgus An abnormal deviation of the big toe away from the midline of the body or toward the other toes of the foot.

Hammer toe A deformed claw-shaped toe characterized by hyperextension of the metatarsophalangeal and distal interphalangeal joints and flexion of the proximal interphalangeal joint.

Handheld dynamometer A portable testing device placed between the patient's body part and the therapist's hand that measures mechanical force.

Hassles Scale An instrument measuring the irritating and frustrating demands of everyday transactions experienced by an individual.

Head-shaking–induced nystagmus (HSN) Test used to discern asymmetry of peripheral vestibular input to the central vestibular neurons.

Head tilt Term used to indicate a static lateral flexion of the neck; may indicate utricular dysfunction.

Health A state of complete physical, mental, and social well-being and not merely the absence of diseases and infirmity.

Health condition (WHO/ICF) An umbrella term for disease, disorder, injury, or trauma; may include other circumstances, such as aging, stress, congenital anomaly, or genetic predisposition. It may also include information about pathogeneses and/or etiology.

Health education One component of health promotion, and is any combination of learning experiences designed to encourage, assist, and support individuals to voluntarily engage in health-supporting behaviors.

Health promotion Any planned combination of educational, regulatory, social, and political interventions designed to support the health of individuals or communities.

Heart failure The inability of the heart to circulate blood effectively to meet the body's metabolic needs; caused by impaired ventricle functioning of the heart, as well as dysfunction of other organs, including lungs, kidneys, and liver.

Left-sided heart failure (LHF) Occurs with failure of the left ventricle (LV) to maintain left ventricular output; leads to a backup of fluid into the left atrium (LA) and lungs, producing hallmark pulmonary signs of shortness of breath (SOB) and cough.

Right-sided heart failure (RHF) Occurs with failure of the right ventricle (RV) to maintain right ventricular output; leads to a backup of fluid into the right atrium (RA) and venous vasculature, producing hallmark peripheral signs of jugular venous distention and peripheral edema.

Heart sounds The auscultatory sounds of the cardiac cycle, identified as S1 (lub), which occurs at closure of the mitral (and tricuspid) valve and marks the beginning of systole, and S2 (dub), which occurs at aortic (and pulmonic) valve closure and marks the end of systole.

Heberden's node A bony enlargement of the end joint of a finger (DIP) commonly present with osteoarthritis.

Help-rejecting Patient approach to dealing with the stress of having covert hostile feelings toward caregivers by frequently asking for help and then rejecting every suggestion.

Hemarthrosis A bloody effusion within a joint.

Hemianopia (hemianopsia) Inability to see in one half of the visual field.

Hemiballismus Sudden, jerky, forceful, flailing motions of one side of the body.

Hemiparesis Weakness on one side of the body.

Hemiplegia Paralysis on one side of the body.

Hemispace One half of the spatial field around the body.

Hemorrhagic stroke *See* **Stroke**.

Hemosiderin staining A brownish discoloration of the skin due to a pigment released from hemoglobin following red blood cell lysis.

Hemostasis An arrest of bleeding.

Heterotopic ossification Abnormal bone growth in muscle or other connective tissue; can restrict range of motion and lead to impaired function; also known as ectopic bone formation.

Holistic A treatment approach that values the multifaceted dimensions of a patient's life, including social roles, culture, religion, gender, age, community, ethnicity, personality, social support, and anything else that has influenced or now influences the patient.

Holmes-Rahe Social Readjustment Rating Scale One of the better-known and widely used assessment instruments that quantifies the effects of life changes on stress and health.

Honeycombing A radiological term used to describe the presence of many small, thick-walled, air-filled cysts that result from interstitial pulmonary fibrosis and tissue remodeling.

Hyperalgesia An excessive sensitivity to pain.

Hyperarousal Excessive responsiveness to sensory stimulation; found in traumatic brain injury, post-traumatic stress disorder, alcohol withdrawal, and other conditions.

Hypercapnea Increased levels of carbon dioxide in the blood; caused by inadequate ventilation or large imbalance between ventilation and perfusion of the blood.

Hyperesthesia Increased sensitivity to stimulation, excluding the special senses. Hyperesthesia includes both allodynia and hyperalgesia, but the more specific terms should be used wherever they are applicable.

Hyperinflation An abnormal increase in the amount of air within the thorax at the end of a tidal exhalation.

Hyperkeratosis A local overabundant thickening of skin.

Hyperkinesia (hyperkinesis) A general term used to describe abnormally increased muscle activity or movement; restlessness.

Hypermetria Excessive distance or range of a movement; an overestimation of the required motion needed to reach a target object.

Hypermobility Excessive joint motion.

Hyperpathia A painful syndrome characterized by an abnormally painful reaction to a stimulus, especially a repetitive stimulus, as well as an increased threshold.

Hyperreactivity Increased or excessive activity of any cell, organ, tissue, or organism.

Hyperreflexia Increased reflex responses.

Hypertension Higher than normal blood pressure; systolic blood pressure (SBP) is consistently greater than 140 mm Hg and/or diastolic blood pressure (DBP) is equal to or greater than 90 mm Hg.

Hypertonia Abnormally increased muscle tone.

Hypertrophic scar Scar overgrowth that stays within the boundaries of a wound and is characteristically described as red, raised, and firm.

Hyperventilation Abnormally fast rate and depth of respiration.

Hypocapnia An abnormally low level of carbon dioxide in the blood; associated with hyperventilation.

Hypokinesia A state of diminished ability to move; an overall decrease in motor reaction to stimulus, difficulty initiating movement, and a decrease in the total number and amplitude of movements.

Hypokinetic dysarthria Difficult and defective speech characterized by decreased voice volume, monotone/monopitch speech, imprecise or distorted articulation, and uncontrolled speech rate; common in Parkinson's disease.

Hypometria Shortened distance or range of a movement; an underestimation of the required motion needed to reach a target object.

Hypomimia A reduction in movements and expressiveness of the face.

Hypomobility Restricted joint motion.

Hypotension An abnormally low blood pressure not adequate for normal perfusion and oxygenation of the tissues.

Orthostatic hypotension A sudden drop in blood pressure with movement to an upright position after getting up from a bed or chair.

Hypothermia Core body temperature is below 35°C (95°F).

Hypotonia Muscle tone is reduced below normal resting levels.

Hypoventilation Decrease in the rate and depth of respiration.

Hypovolemia Abnormally low volume of circulating blood in the body.

Hypovolemic shock Shock caused by substantial fluid loss from intravascular space (e.g., loss of blood or electrolyte solution).

Hypoxemia Decreased oxygen concentration in arterial blood; measured by arterial oxygen partial pressures values.

Hypoxia Oxygen deficiency in body tissues.

I

Iatrogenic Any injury or illness that occurs as a result of medical or surgical treatment.

Ideational apraxia *See* **Apraxia**.

Ideomotor apraxia *See* **Apraxia**.

Illness Encompasses the personal behaviors that emerge when the reality of having a disease is internalized and experienced by an individual.

Imagery Visualizing a scene or mentally rehearsing a script for a specific purpose such as relaxation.

Immediate postoperative prosthesis (IPOP) Following lower limb amputation, immediately fitting the residual limb with a prosthetic socket-shaped dressing in surgery.

Immediate recall Retention of information that has been stored for several seconds.

Immune response Response to an antigen that occurs when lymphocytes identify an antigenic molecule as foreign and produce antibodies and lymphocytes capable of reacting with it and rendering it harmless.

Impairment (WHO/ICF) A problem in body function or structure, such as a significant deviation or loss.

Inclinometer A device that uses gravity's effect on pointers or fluid levels to measure joint position and motion.

Incomplete injury (SCI) A spinal cord injury having motor and/or sensory function below the neurological level including sensory and/or motor function at S4 and S5.

Indurated Hardened, as in an area of hardened tissue.

Inhalation injury Injury to the lungs due to breathing hot and/or toxic gases; associated with burns in a closed space.

Inhibitory cutoff The velocity at which inhibition (hyperpolarization) of the vestibular afferents in the contra-rotational labyrinth becomes zero.

Initial contact (gait) The moment in time when the outstretched limb first contacts the ground to initiate stance and a new gait cycle; period of double-limb support.

Initial swing (gait) The first one third of swing; begins when the foot lifts from the ground.

Inspiratory capacity (IC) Tidal volume plus inspiratory reserve volume; the amount of air that can be inhaled from the end of a tidal exhalation.

Inspiratory reserve volume (IRV) The amount of air that can be inspired after a tidal inspiration.

Instrumental activities of daily living (IADL) *See* **Activities of daily living.**

Intention tremor (action tremor) *See* **Tremor.**

Intermittent claudication Severe pain in the lower extremity that occurs with activity but subsides with rest; the result of inadequate arterial blood supply to the exercising muscles.

Internalized anger Anger turned inward instead of expressed outwardly toward a situation or person.

International Classification of Functioning, Disability, and Health (ICF) A meaningful description of the components of health and its relationship to a person with a health condition; from the World Health Organization (WHO).

Interoceptive exposure exercises A desensitization tool often used for post-traumatic stress disorder to help patients cope with uncomfortable physiological sensations.

Interval measure Utilizes a classification scheme in which values are separated by equal intervals, but has no true zero.

Intervention (APTA/*Guide to Physical Therapist Practice*) The purposeful interaction of the physical therapist with the patient/client and, when appropriate, other individuals involved in the care of the patient/client, using various physical therapy procedures and techniques to produce changes in the condition.

Compensatory intervention Treatment directed toward improving the patient's status in terms of impairments, activity limitations, participation restrictions, and recovery of function; directed toward performing the movement pattern or task in a way that is different than the method used prior to the injury. Includes use of adaptive equipment and technology to accomplish the task.

Restorative intervention Treatment directed toward remediating or improving the patient's status in terms of impairments, activity limitations, participation restrictions, and recovery of function; directed toward performing the movement pattern or task in the same manner as was performed premorbidly.

Intracerebral hemorrhage (IH) Rupture of a cerebral blood vessel with subsequent bleeding into the brain.

Intracranial pressure (ICP) Measure of pressure inside the cranium; normal ICP is 5 to 10 mm Hg.

Intrusive recollections The experiencing of dreams and nightmares about disturbing events of the past; often experienced with post-traumatic stress disorder.

Ipsilateral pushing (contraversive pushing, Pusher syndrome) An unusual motor behavior following stroke characterized by active pushing with the stronger extremities toward the hemiparetic side, leading to a lateral postural imbalance and a tendency to fall toward the hemiparetic side.

Ischemia A temporary deficiency in oxygenated blood supply to an organ or tissue.

Ischemic cascade (secondary injury) Brain cell injury and death that progresses rapidly within the core infarction area and over time within the ischemic penumbra (the transitional area surrounding the ischemic core).

Ischemic stroke *See* **Stroke.**

Isokinetic dynamometer A testing and exercise device that controls the velocity of a limb's movement, keeping it at a constant rate while offering accommodating resistance throughout the range of motion.

J

Joint mobilization Passive therapeutic techniques applied specifically to joint structures that utilize arthrokinematic motions to increase or maintain joint play and range of motion or to treat pain.

Joint play (accessory) motions Motions that occur between joint surfaces that accompany osteokinematic motions but are not under voluntary control; includes glides (slides), distractions, compressions, rolls, and spins. Joint play can also refer to the distensibility of the joint capsule and ligaments that allow joint motion to occur.

K

Kinematic analysis A description of the type, amount, and direction of motion; does not include the forces producing the motion.

Kinesthesia The ability to perceive the extent (range) and direction of movement; awareness of movement.

Kinetic analysis The study of the forces that cause motion.

Knowledge of performance (KP) Augmented feedback about the nature or quality of the movement pattern produced; information about movement kinematics.

Knowledge of results (KR) Augmented feedback about the nature of the end result of movement produced in relation to the goal; information about movement outcome.

L

Lacunar infarction *See* **Stroke**.

Lag phenomenon Describes a substantial difference in passive versus active range of motion secondary to tendon damage or muscle weakness.

Lateropulsion Tendency to fall to one side.

Lead pipe rigidity *See* **Rigidity**.

Lead-up tasks Component tasks or activities used to prepare learners for more important and complex functional tasks.

Left-sided heart failure *See* **Heart failure**.

Lexicon The vocabulary of a language, an individual speaker, or group of speakers, or a subject.

Lhermitte's sign A sign of posterior column damage in the spinal cord; flexion of the neck produces an electric shock–like sensation running down the spine and into the lower extremities.

Life roles Areas of responsibility in a person's life, such as father, worker, student, community member, or athlete.

Ligamentous instability test (ligament stress test) A test in which a patient's joint is maneuvered passively to determine the integrity of ligaments and other joint structures.

Lightheadedness Sense of feeling as if about to faint.

Limits of stability (LOS) The maximum distance an individual is able or willing to lean in any direction without loss of balance or changing the base of support (BOS); the midpoint of limits of stability is centered alignment (center of mass [COM] alignment).

Linear velocity The rate at which a body moves in a straight line.

Linear work Force multiplied by distance.

Lipodermatosclerosis The progressive replacement of skin, subcutaneous connective, and adipose tissues by fibrous tissue (sclerosis). This can occur as a result of calf pump failure in chronic venous insufficiency, and as a result of long-standing inflammation or edema in lymphedema.

Loading response (gait) The phase during which body weight is rapidly accepted onto the outstretched limb; the shock associated with loading the limb is absorbed while stability is maintained; period of double limb support.

Locked-in syndrome (LIS) Tetraplegia (complete paralysis) and lower bulbar palsy (anarthria) with preserved consciousness following stroke involving bilateral infarction of the ventral pons.

Locus of control A belief about one's ability to control life conditions and events.

Long-term memory Recall of early experiences and information acquired over a period of years from the distant past.

Lower motor neuron A peripheral motor neuron that originates in the ventral horns of the gray matter of the spinal cord and terminates in skeletal muscles.

Lower motor neuron syndrome Lesions affecting the anterior horn cell or peripheral nerve produce decreased or absent tone, hyporeflexia, weakness or paralysis, muscle fasciculations and fibrillations with denervation, and neurogenic atrophy.

Lymphedema An abnormal accumulation of tissue fluid in the interstitial spaces produced by impairment of normal uptake of tissue fluid by the lymphatic vessels or the excessive production of tissue fluid caused by venous obstruction that increases capillary blood pressure; can be primary (congenital) or secondary (following surgical removal of lymph channels).

Primary lymphedema Lymphedema caused by a condition that is congenital or hereditary with abnormal lymph node or lymph vessel formation.

Secondary lymphedema Lymphedema caused by injury to one or more components of the lymphatic system; some portion of the lymphatic system has been blocked, dissected, fibrosed, or otherwise damaged or altered.

Lymphorrhea Flow of lymph from ruptured lymph vessels to the surface of the skin.

Lymphscintigraphy A test performed using dye and a specialized camera and computer to visualize a variety of lymphatic system functions.

M

Maceration The process of softening a solid (skin) by saturating it with fluid or drainage.

Make test (active resistance test) A method of applying resistance during manual muscle testing in which the patient moves through an arc of motion against the therapist's resistance. In handheld dynamometry, the term also has been used to indicate a patient's performance of a maximal isometric contraction against the therapist's resistance.

Maladaptive thought patterns Repetitive thoughts that inhibit a productive, happy life.

Malignant pain *See* **Pain**.

Malinger To feign illness or symptoms often to support claims made in a lawsuit.

Mallet finger Flexion of the distal phalanx of a finger caused by avulsion of the extensor tendon; also called drop finger or baseball finger.

Manual muscle testing (MMT) A formal examination and grading system that uses arc of motion, gravity, and manually applied resistance to quantify muscle strength on an ordinal scale.

Maximal oxygen uptake (VO_{2max}) The product of maximal cardiac output (L blood·min^{-1}) and arteriovenous oxygen difference (mL O_2 per L blood).

Memory Mental process that allows retention and recall of past experiences, perceptions, knowledge, or thoughts.

Ménière's disease Recurrent group of symptoms including episodic vertigo, tinnitus, sensation of fullness in the ear, and hearing loss.

Mesh graft Process whereby the donor skin is placed through a device that increases the surface area of the graft.

Metabolic equivalents (METs) A rating of energy expenditure for a given activity based on oxygen consumption; one MET represents the basic systemic oxygen requirement at rest, roughly 3.5 mL O_2/kg/min.

Metatarsalgia A cramping burning pain below and between the metatarsal bones.

Micrographia An abnormally small handwriting that is difficult to read; commonly seen in Parkinson's disease.

Micturition Voiding of urine; urination.

Mid stance (gait) The phase during which body weight progresses over a single stable limb.

Mid swing (gait) The phase that occurs during the middle third of swing as the thigh advances forward and the tibia achieves a vertical position.

Milroy's disease The autosomal dominant, congenital form of lymphedema resulting in the aplasia or hypoplasia of lymph vessels.

Minimal clinical important difference (MCID) The smallest difference in a measured variable that signifies an important rather than trivial difference in the patient's condition.

Minimal detectable change (MDC) The smallest amount of change in a measurement which exceeds the measurement error of the instrument.

Minimally conscious state Condition of low arousal in patients with severe traumatic brain injury. There is some, but minimal evidence of self-awareness or environmental awareness. Cognitively mediated behaviors occur inconsistently and are reproducible or sustained such that they can be differentiated from reflexive behaviors.

Moment torque A force that produces rotation; force multiplied by the perpendicular distance from the axis of rotation.

Motivation The internal state that tends to affect or stimulate behavior and direct an individual toward a goal.

Motor ability (capability, aptitude) A relatively stable characteristic or trait that is genetically determined or developed during growth and maturation; largely unmodifiable by practice.

Motor control An area of study dealing with the understanding of the neural, physical, and behavioral aspects of biological (human) movement.

Motor development The evolution of changes in motor behavior occurring as a result of growth, maturation, and experience across the life span.

Motor learning A set of internal processes associated with practice or experience leading to relatively permanent changes in motor skill capability.

Motor level In spinal cord injury, the most caudal segment of the spinal cord with normal motor function bilaterally.

Motor neuron disease A heterogeneous spectrum of inherited or acquired clinical disorders of the upper motor neurons, lower motor neurons, or both.

Motor plan An idea or plan for purposeful movement made up of component motor programs; a complex motor program.

Motor planning Movement preparation including the when, where, and how to initiate movement.

Motor (procedural) memory The memory for movement or motor information.

Motor program An abstract representation that, when initiated, results in the production of a coordinated movement sequence.

Motor unit action potential (MUAP) Depolarization of the motor nerve produces electrical activity that is recorded and displayed graphically as the MUAP; characterized by its amplitude, duration, and shape.

Multidisciplinary team conference A meeting of professionals with different fields of expertise (e.g., medicine, social work, nursing, occupational and physical therapy, speech-language pathology) used to discuss the progress and future plans of patients.

Multi-infarct dementia Deteriorative mental state characterized by reduction in intellectual faculties; the result of multiple small strokes.

Multiple sclerosis (MS) A chronic disease of the central nervous system characterized by inflammation, selective demyelination, and gliosis of neurons of the brain and spinal cord. This results in disruptions in nerve impulse conduction causing symptoms of weakness, loss of coordination, numbness, and disturbances of visual, bowel, bladder, and sexual functions.

Murmur An abnormal sound when listening to the heart or neighboring large blood vessels.

Muscle endurance The ability to sustain forces repeatedly or to generate forces over a period of time.

Muscle performance The capacity of a muscle or group of muscles to generate forces.

Muscle power Work produced per unit of time or the product of strength and speed.

Muscle strength The force exerted by a muscle to overcome resistance in one maximal effort.

Muscle tension State of partial muscle contraction that is characterized by persistent, involuntary contraction of muscle fibers or of a muscle or muscles; can be increased with pain and excessive irritability.

Muscle tone The velocity-dependent resistance to stretch exhibited by muscles.

Musculoskeletal injury Injury to muscular or skeletal system that affects movement.

> *Acute stage* First 48 to 72 hours following the onset of injury; usually characterized by tissue inflammation associated with hyperemia.

> *Chronic stage* Time span beyond 3 to 6 months following the onset of a condition; characterized by the body's attempt at tissue repair.

> *Subacute stage* The time period between the acute and chronic stages of a condition; considered to begin by 72 hours after injury and continuing for as long as 3 to 6 months.

Mutism Inability or unwillingness to speak.

Myocardial infarction (MI) Death of myocardial cells as a result of coronary artery occlusion.

Myocardial oxygen demand (MVO) The amount of oxygen required for the metabolic needs of the myocardium; clinically calculated as the product of heart rate (HR) and systolic blood pressure (SBP), known as the rate pressure product (RPP).

Myodesis Suturing muscle to bone.

Myopathy Primary disease of muscle; may be congenital or acquired.

Myoplasty Plastic surgery of muscles.

Myositis Inflammation of muscle tissue; often produces pain, stiffness, and weakness.

Myxoid Containing or resembling mucus.

N

Necrosis The death of cells, tissues, or organs.

Nerve conduction velocity (NCV) test Involves direct stimulation of motor or sensory nerves to determine the velocity of conduction of an impulse; used to identify blockage or disruption of nerve integrity.

Neurapraxia A temporary impairment in nerve conduction typically caused by local compression or blockage of a peripheral nerve, such as in carpal tunnel syndrome.

Neurological level In spinal cord injury, the most caudal level of the spinal cord with normal motor and sensory function on both the left and right sides of the body.

Neuroma A benign neoplasm composed largely of neurons and nerve fibers usually arising from nerve tissue; associated with radiating pain along the peripheral nerve.

Neuropathy Any disease of nerves; characterized by inflammation or degeneration.

> *Polyneuropathy* Affects multiple nerves and typically results in sensory changes, distal weakness, and hyporeflexia (e.g., diabetic polyneuropathy).

Neuroplasticity The ability of the nervous system to adapt to trauma or disease; the ability of nerve cells to alter their structure and function in response to internal and external factors.

Neurotmesis Nerve injury with complete loss of function of the nerve and disruption of the neural tube.

Neutrophils A common type of white blood cell, making up about 50% to 75% of all white blood cells; these cells increase in response to infection.

Nocebo (nocebo effect) The opposite of a placebo or the placebo effect. A nocebo is an inert treatment or event that increases symptoms because the patient believes it will increase symptoms. The expectation of pain can result in both increased pain from painful stimuli and allodynia, pain from a normally nonpainful stimulus.

Nociceptive pain *See* **Pain**.

Nominal measure Utilizes a classification scheme based on categories without order or rank, the simplest of which are dichotomous response sets such as "present/absent" and "yes/no"; may also have more than two categories.

Noncapsular pattern A restriction of passive osteokinematic motion; not consistent with proportioned restriction of a capsular pattern; indicates a cause other than intra-articular inflammation or capsular fibrosis.

Nonfluent aphasia *See* **Aphasia**.

Numbing or psychic numbing (emotional anesthesia) Feelings of being detached or estranged from others, a loss of ability or interest in previously enjoyable activities, or the lack of any emotions or feelings.

Nutritionist A professional trained to educate and provide patients with appropriate diets based on their individual needs, and to educate them on the benefits of good nutrition.

Nystagmus Involuntary rhythmic or cyclical movements of the eyes in any direction. If due to vestibular asymmetry, it has clearly defined fast and slow components beating in opposite directions.

> *Pendular nystagmus* Nystagmus characterized by movement that is approximately equal in both directions.

> *Positional nystagmus* Nystagmus induced by change in head position.

Spontaneous nystagmus Nystagmus that is present when the head is still. Often due to acute vestibular pathology and generally resolves within 7 days.

O

Obligatory synergies Strongly linked muscles that act together in an abnormal and stereotyped movement pattern; isolated joint movements outside an obligatory synergy are not possible.

Occupational therapist A professional who helps patients maximize functional capacities and performance using a holistic approach and a variety of modalities including group, family, role related activities, individual therapy sessions, and activity analyses and training.

Ocular pursuit The ability of the eyes to follow a moving object.

Ocular tilt reaction (OTR) Triad of ocular signs including skew deviation, ocular torsion, and head tilt.

Ocular torsion The superior poles of the eyes rotate in a clockwise or counterclockwise direction.

On–off phenomenon Abrupt and often unpredictable fluctuations in motor performance and response; common in Parkinson's disease with progression and long-term use of L-dopa therapy.

Open-loop control system A motor control system that employs a control system with preprogrammed instructions (motor program) to a set of effectors; run off virtually without the influence of peripheral feedback or error detection processes.

Open skills Skills that are performed in a changing, unpredictable environment.

Open (wound care) technique Absence of dressings; often used after skin grafting to the face.

Opera-glass hand A deformity of the hand seen in chronic absorptive arthritis; the fingers and wrists are shortened with bone absorption and skin hangs in folds over the joints creating an appearance that the phalanges are retracted telescopically into one another.

Ordinal measure Utilizes a classification scheme that rates observations in terms of the relationship between items (e.g., less than, equal to, or greater than).

Orientation The ability to comprehend and to adjust oneself within an unfamiliar environment with respect to awareness of time, person, and place.

Orthopnea Labored breathing that occurs when lying flat and improves by moving to sitting or standing.

Orthostatic hypotension *See* **Hypotension**.

Oscillopsia A subjective perception that stationary objects in the visual environment are swinging or in motion.

Osteoarthritis (OA) (degenerative joint disease [DJD]) Disease of the cartilage characterized by degenerative and/or hypertrophic changes in the bone and cartilage in one or more joints eventually leading to joint destruction, pain, swelling, and stiffness.

Osteokinematics Gross, angular motions of bones around a joint axis, such as flexion, extension, abduction, adduction, or rotation.

Osteomyelitis Inflammation of the bone marrow and adjacent bone, caused by a pathogenic organism.

Osteophyte A pathological bony outgrowth usually from the joint margin.

Osteoporosis A condition characterized by decrease in bone mass with decreased density and enlargement of bone spaces producing porous and brittle bones.

Osteotomy Surgical excision of a bone usually performed to correct a deformity.

Otolith organs Vestibular organs that detect linear acceleration.

Ototoxicity Toxicity of cranial nerve VIII or the vestibular system; caused by certain antibiotics (aminoglycosides [gentamycin, streptomycin]).

P

Pack-years (smoking) The number of packs of cigarettes smoked per day times the number of years of smoking.

Pain An unpleasant sensory and emotional experience associated with actual or potential tissue damage, (or described in terms of such damage) or psychological origin.

Acute pain Pain that is associated with tissue damage or the threat of such damage that typically resolves once the tissue heals or the threat resolves.

Chronic pain Pain that persists past the healing phase following an injury; impairment is greater than anticipated based on the physical findings or injury and occurs in the absence or observed tissue injury or damage.

Chronic pain syndrome Pain that exists when individuals have developed extensive pain behaviors such as preoccupation with pain, passive approach to health care, significant life disruption, feelings of isolation, doctor shopping, or are demanding or angry.

Malignant pain Pain associated with cancer.

Nociceptive pain Pain that arises from actual or threatened damage to non-neural tissue and is due to the activation of pain receptors, nociceptors.

Psychogenic pain An older term for pain believed to be caused by psychological influences when organic were absent or not severe enough to explain complaint.

Recurrent pain Repeated episodes of acute pain.

Referred pain Spontaneous pain outside the area of injury or source of pain.

Pain neuromatrix A complex network of synaptic links within the central nervous system, initially determined by genetics but modified by psychological and sensory inputs both before and during the pain experience.

Palliative care A care approach for individuals with life-threatening illnesses that focuses on improving quality of life for patients and their families through the management of pain and other physical, psychosocial, and spiritual problems.

Pallor Paleness or absence of color in the skin.

Panic attack Sudden onset of intense apprehension, fear, or discomfort; may include feelings of imminent danger or impending doom.

Panic disorder A disorder in which individuals suffer from recurrent panic attacks.

Pannus Inflammatory granulation tissue seen in rheumatoid arthritis that spreads from the synovial membrane and invades the joint eventually leading to joint ankylosis.

Papilloma Epithelial tumor of skin consisting of hypertrophied papillae covered by a layer of epithelium. Warts and polyps are examples of papillomas.

Papules Red elevated areas on the skin.

Paraplegia Complete paralysis of all or part of the trunk and both lower extremities.

Paresthesia An abnormal sensation, whether spontaneous or evoked.

Paroxysmal nocturnal dyspnea (PND) Labored or difficult breathing (shortness of breath [SOB]) that awakens a person suddenly from sleep.

Partial-thickness burn Burn involving the epidermis and part of the dermis. Subcategories are superficial partial-thickness and deep partial-thickness burns, depending on the amount of dermis involved.

Participation (WHO/ICF) Involvement in a life situation.

Participation restrictions (WHO/ICF) Problems an individual may experience in involvement in life situations.

Passive range of motion (PROM) *See* **Range of motion**.

Pastoral counselors People with a particular religious affiliation trained to counsel others in need; many hospitals are staffed with pastoral counselors available 24 hours a day.

Patellar-tendon-bearing (PTB) Refers to the total-contact transtibial socket that places moderate load on the patellar tendon.

Pendular nystagmus *See* **Nystagmus**.

Perception The process of selection, integration, and interpretation of stimuli from one's own body and the surrounding environment.

Percussion (respiratory technique) A procedure utilized with pulmonary postural drainage to loosen secretions from the bronchial walls; the therapist uses slightly cupped hands to percuss the chest wall.

Percutaneous transluminal coronary angioplasty (PTCA) A procedure in which a catheter is placed within the coronary arteries at the site of a lesion; a balloon is inflated and stent positioned to compress plaque against the arterial wall, thereby increasing the luminal area. The balloon is deflated and removed and the stent remains to hold the lumen open.

Performance The ability to produce a movement; a manner of functioning dependent on an understanding of the nature of the task and practice.

Performance-based test Examination of a particular skill based on observation during the performance of an activity.

Performance curve Used to plot performance trials and determine the average of a subject or group of subjects across a number of practice trials.

Performance qualifiers Indicate the extent of participation restriction (difficulty) in performing tasks or actions in an individual's current real-life environment.

Perfusion The flow of blood to an organ's tissue.

Perilymphatic fistula (PLF) A rupture of the oval or round windows, causing an opening between the middle and inner ear.

Peripheral arterial disease (PAD) Atherosclerotic disease affecting the aortoiliac, axillary, carotid, or femoral arteries; contributes to claudication, ischemic rest pain, amputation, stroke, and other conditions.

Peripheral cyanosis *See* **Cyanosis**.

Peripheral neuropathy Pathological condition of the peripheral nerves; characterized by muscle weakness, paresthesias, impaired reflexes, and autonomic symptoms.

Peripheral vascular disease (PVD) Any condition of the blood vessels that causes partial or complete obstruction of flow of blood to or from the arteries or veins outside the chest.

Peripheral vestibular lesion A lesion of the peripheral vestibular organ or cranial nerve VIII.

Perseveration (perseverate) Abnormal compulsive and inappropriate repetition of words or behaviors; observed in patients with diseases of the frontal lobes of the brain or schizophrenia.

Persistent vegetative state A continuing and unremitting clinical condition of complete unawareness of the environment accompanied by sleep–wake cycles with either complete or partial preservation of hypothalamic and brainstem autonomic functions. The patient may have reflexive movement and the eyes may be open, but there is no awareness of the surroundings or situation. Cognitive and communication function is absent.

Personal factors (WHO/ICF) The particular background of an individual's life, including gender, age, coping styles, social background, education, profession, past and current experience, overall behavior pattern, character, and other factors that influence how disability is experienced by an individual.

Pes equinus A foot deformity in which the heel is elevated and the foot is maintained in plantarflexion.

Pes planus A foot deformity in which the longitudinal arch is flattened; flat foot.

Pes valgus (talipes valgus) A foot deformity in which the heel and foot are turned outward.

Pes varus (talipes varus) A foot deformity in which the heel and foot are turned inward.

Phantom limb pain Any of a series of painful sensations experienced in the limb or part of a limb that has been amputated.

Phantom limb sensation The feeling that a limb or part of a limb is still there after it has been amputated; normal response following amputation that subsides over time.

Phobia An unrelenting, irrational, intense fear of a specific object or situation; associated with a persistent desire to avoid the feared (phobic) stimulus; may interfere with social functioning.

Phoneme The smallest phonetic unit in a language that is capable of conveying a distinction in meaning, as the "m" of mat and the "b" of bat in English.

Phonology The study of how sounds are organized and used in natural languages.

Physical activity Any body movement produced by skeletal muscle contraction that increases energy expenditure above resting level.

Physical function (APTA/*Guide to Physical Therapist Practice*) Fundamental component of health status describing the state of those sensory and motor skills necessary for usual daily activities, including work and recreation.

Piston action (pistoning) Vertical motion of the prosthetic socket on the amputated limb; evident during gait as an up-and-down movement of the prosthesis. Pistoning is caused by looseness of the socket or inadequate suspension, or both.

Pitting edema Peripheral edema particularly evident in gravity-dependent lower extremities by the presence of indentations in the skin when pressure is applied.

Placebo (placebo effect) A placebo is an inert treatment, such as a sugar pill or fake treatment, that is beneficial because the patient believes it will be beneficial.

Plan of care (POC) (APTA/*Guide to Physical Therapist Practice*) An outline of anticipated patient management including anticipated goals and expected outcomes; the predicted level of optimal improvement; specific interventions to be used and proposed duration and frequency of interventions; and anticipated discharge plans.

Polyarthritis Arthritis involving two or more joints.

Polycythemia A greater than usual amount of circulating red blood cells.

Polyethylene Thermoplastic material used for flexible prosthetic sockets; the plastic becomes malleable when heated, permitting its contour to be changed.

Polyneuropathy *See* **Neuropathy**.

Polyphasic potentials Motor unit potentials with more than three phases, typically seen with active contraction in myopathies or with reinnervation.

Positional nystagmus *See* **Nystagmus**.

Position in space impairment The inability to perceive and interpret spatial concepts such as up, down, under, over, in, out, in front of, and behind.

Positive sharp waves Spontaneous, biphasic EMG spike with a sharp initial positive deflection (below baseline) followed by a slow negative phase; typically indicative of motor neuron disorders, denervation, or myopathies.

Post-traumatic amnesia (PTA) Loss of memory for events immediately following a trauma/brain injury.

Post-traumatic stress disorder (PTSD) An anxiety disorder resulting from exposure to a traumatic event or ongoing chronic abuse.

Postural control The ability to control the body's position in space for stability and orientation.

Postural drainage (respiratory technique) Positioning a patient such that the bronchus is perpendicular to the ground and the mucociliary transport of secretions is facilitated.

Postural orientation The control of relative positions of body parts by skeletal muscles with respect to each other and gravity; the ability to maintain normal alignment relationships between the various body segments and between the body and environment.

Postural stress syndrome Postural abnormalities and stress secondary to lack of movement, muscle rigidity, faulty posture, and ligamentous strain.

Postural tremor (static tremor) *See* **Tremor**.

Pragmatic language Refers to the component of communication that goes beyond language in terms of isolated word meaning and grammar; a system of rules that governs the appropriate use of language for the communicative context, especially in interpersonal situations.

Premorbid Occurring before a patient became ill or injured.

Pressure Calculated as the force per unit area; generally expressed as N/cm^2 or kPa.

Pressure ulcer (pressure or bed sore) Damage to the skin or underlying structures as a result of tissue compression and inadequate perfusion; typically occurs on skin areas over bony prominences in patients who are bed or chair bound.

Pre-swing (gait) The phase during which body weight is rapidly unloaded from the reference limb to the contralateral limb that has just made contact with the ground; period of double-limb support.

Prevention (APTA/*Guide to Physical Therapist Practice*) Activities that are directed toward (1) achieving and restoring optimal functional capacity; (2) minimizing impairments, activity limitations, and participation restrictions; (3) maintaining health; and (4) creating appropriate environmental adaptations to enhance independent function.

> *Primary prevention* Prevention of disease in a susceptible or potentially susceptible population through specific measures.

> *Secondary prevention* Efforts to decrease the duration of illness, severity of diseases, and sequelae through early diagnosis and prompt intervention.

> *Tertiary prevention* Efforts to limit the degree of disability and promote rehabilitation and restoration of function in patients/clients with chronic and irreversible diseases.

Primary excision Surgical removal of eschar.

Primary lymphedema *See* **Lymphedema**.

Primary prevention *See* **Prevention**.

Primary progressive aphasia (PPA) *See* **Aphasia**.

Prognosis The predicted optimal level of improvement in function and amount of time needed to reach that level.

Proprioception The awareness of position sense and posture.

Proprioceptors Sensory receptors that respond to pressure, position, or stretch; found in muscles, tendons, ligaments, joints, and fascia.

Prosodic features The rhythmic and intonational elements of speech that are relatively independent of the quality of speech sounds; they are organized into autonomous systems, of which the most important are rate, stress, and intonation.

Prosopagnosia An inability to recognize faces or other visual stimuli as being familiar and distinct from one another.

Protective sensation The level of intact sensation needed to allow an individual to sense trauma to the body part in order to protect the traumatized area.

Protrusio acetabuli An uncommon defect of the acetabulum whereby the acetabulum is too deep and may extend into the pelvis.

Pseudobulbar affect (PBA) (emotional dysregulation syndrome) Unstable or changeable emotional state characterized by sudden and unpredictable episodes of crying, laughing, or other emotional displays inconsistent with mood and context.

Pseudoexacerbation Refers to the temporary worsening of symptoms that typically comes and goes quickly, usually within 24 hours; for example, excess heat in patients with multiple sclerosis.

Pseudolaxity Apparent laxity of a ligament due to joint space narrowing.

Pseudomonas aeruginosa A gram-negative bacteria noted for its resistance to antibiotics.

Psychiatric nurse Nurses who work with clients with psychiatric disorders with specific knowledge and expertise in this area.

Psychiatrist A physician who has completed 4 years of residency (1 year in internal medicine and 3 years in psychiatry) who provides psychiatric treatment using psychotropic medications and/or individual therapy.

Psychoeducation Instruction provided to patients with mental health conditions and/or their family members or caregivers.

Psychogenic pain *See* **Pain**.

Psychological function Ability to use mental and affective resources effectively relative to the requirements of a particular situation.

Psychological needs Emotional requirements that differ among individuals but may include love, attention, peace of mind, nurturance, feeling safe, and social support.

Psychologist A professional with a doctoral degree in psychology trained in research, personality theories, psychopathology, cognition, assessment of psychiatric patients, group therapy, cognitive-behavioral therapy, and other interventions.

Psychomotor retardation Slow movements that result from depression.

Psychosocial adaptation (to a disability or chronic illness) An ongoing, dynamic, evolving process through which a patient strives to attain an optimal state of function within his or her environment.

Psychosomatic Feeling ill without evident physical cause.

Pulmonary edema Pulmonary congestion; may be due to an increase in capillary hydrostatic pressure (e.g., left ventricular dysfunction), decreased plasma oncotic pressure, lymphatic insufficiency, altered alveolar-capillary membrane permeability, or other less common causes.

Pulse pressure The difference between the diastolic and systolic blood pressures.

Purposeful activities Activities used in rehabilitation for the purpose of attaining goals (goal-directed) and that patients find meaningful.

Pursed-lip breathing (respiratory technique)
Breathing through puckered or pursed lips; slows breathing rate and extends exhalation time to make room for the next inhalation; exhalation is actively pushed through a narrowed mouth (or pursed lips).

Pus Viscous fluid mixture of debris, fluid, dead and dying cells, and necrotic tissue components that have accumulated at an injury site.

Pusher syndrome *See* **Ipsilateral pushing**.

Push–pull mechanism Term useful to describe how the brain discerns a direction of rotation by comparing excitatory and inhibitory input from each vestibular system.

Pyrexia Increased body temperature; fever.

Pyrogens Fever-producing substances.

Q

Quality of life (QOL) The sense of total well-being that encompasses both physical and psychosocial aspects of an individual's life.

R

Radiometer A temperature-measuring device designed to measure infrared radiation.

Ramp grade Degree of inclination or slope of a ramp; 1:12, or 1 in of threshold height for every 12 in of ramp length.

Range of motion (ROM) The arc through which movement occurs at a joint or series of joints.

Passive range of motion (PROM) The amount of joint motion available when a joint is moved through the range without assistance from the patient.

Active range of motion (AROM) Amount of joint motion available with unassisted voluntary joint motion.

Rapport The relationship, usually positive, between two people (e.g., between patient and professional staff member).

Rating of Perceived Exertion (Borg RPE Scale) A subjective scale that allows an individual to estimate effort and exertion, breathlessness, and fatigue during physical work; the original 15-grade interval scale with grades ranging from 6 (no exertion at all) to 20 (maximum exertion) was developed by Gunnar Borg.

Rating of shortness of breath (Dyspnea Scale) A subjective assessment of shortness of breath as it relates to exercise intensity.

Ratio measure A classification scheme in which values are separated by equal intervals and have a true zero.

Raynaud's disease A primary vasospastic disease of small arteries and arterioles; there is an exaggerated vasomotor response initiated by exposure to cold or emotion disturbance. Etiology is unknown.

Raynaud's phenomenon Intermittent attacks of pallor or cyanosis of the small arteries and arterioles of the fingers as a result of inadequate arterial blood flow.

Rebound phenomenon When resistance to an isometric contraction is removed suddenly the body segment forcibly moves a short distance in the direction in which effort was focused before "rebounding" in the opposite direction. Absence of this check reflex is associated with cerebellar disease.

Recovery Regaining health, living skills, and well-being after an illness or injury.

Recovery of function The reacquisition of movement skills lost through injury; the motor task is performed in the same manner as it was before the injury.

Recurrent pain *See* **Pain**.

Referred pain *See* **Pain**.

Regression A turning back or return to a former state; a return of symptoms.

Rehabilitation counselors Professionals who help people with disabilities to maximize their level of function and employability.

Relaxation response The sense of calm and well-being attained by using stress management techniques.

Reliability Degree to which an instrument measures a phenomenon dependably, time after time, with accuracy and predictably and without variation. Types of reliability include *intratester* and *intertester*.

Remission The lessening in severity (partial) or an abatement of symptoms (complete).

Removable rigid dressing A rigid postamputation dressing that can be removed as desired.

Residual limb The part of the extremity that remains after amputation.

Residual volume (RV) The volume of air remaining within the lungs when expiratory reserve volume (ERV) has been exhaled.

Resistance (psychological) A patient's reluctance to follow a rehabilitation plan or to discuss certain feelings because of a conscious or unconscious fear.

Resistance exercise Exercise in which a muscle contraction is opposed by an outside force, to increase strength or endurance.

Respiration The exchange of gas within the body. *External respiration* is the exchange of gas between the alveoli and the pulmonary capillaries. *Internal respiration* is the exchange of gas between the capillary and the tissue.

Resting tremor *See* **Tremor**.

Restorative intervention *See* **Intervention**.

Restrictive lung disease A group of pulmonary disorders characterized by difficulty in expanding the lungs and a reduction in total lung volume.

Rete pegs Ridge-like undulations between the contact layers of the epidermis and the dermis.

Retention Refers to the ability of the learner to demonstrate a skill over time and after a period of no practice (retention interval).

Retention interval An interval of no practice between the end of original learning and the retention test.

Retention test A performance test administered after a retention interval for the purposes of assessing learning.

Reticular A delicate network of cells or fibers of connective tissue.

Retinal slip Occurs when visual images fall off the fovea of the retina. Also, a technique used to induce adaptation.

Retractions The moving inward of the soft tissue of the intercostal, subcostal, or subclavicular region during inspiration; a marker of respiratory distress.

Rheumatoid arthritis (RA) A chronic autoimmune disease affecting the synovium characterized especially by pain, stiffness, inflammation, swelling, and sometimes destruction of joints and includes systemic features such as malaise, fever, and organ involvement.

Rheumatoid factors (RFs) Autoantibodies that are present in the blood of many people with rheumatoid arthritis (immunoglobulins) and, when present, suggest greater likelihood of severe disease.

Right–left discrimination disorder The inability to identify the right and left sides of one's own body or that of the examiner.

Right-sided heart failure *See* **Heart failure**.

Rigidity An increase in muscle tone causing resistance to passive motion; stiffness, immovability.

Cogwheel rigidity Jerky, ratchet-like resistance to passive movement as muscles alternately tense and relax; occurs when tremor coexists with rigidity.

Leadpipe rigidity A sustained resistance to passive movement with no fluctuations.

Role A specified cluster of behaviors and expectations attached to each distinct, identified relationship to another person or persons (e.g., parent, teacher, health care provider).

Role performance The ability to carry out responsibilities involved in a particular role (*see* **Role**).

Roll An angular motion between two joint surfaces, similar to the bottom of a rocking chair rolling over the floor. New points on one surface come into contact with new points on the other surface.

Roll-gliding The combination of a roll and glide. As a roll occurs between two joint surfaces, one surface slides on the other.

Romberg's sign Inability to maintain standing balance when eyes are closed and the feet are close together; sign is positive if the patient sways and falls when the eyes are closed. Seen in sensory ataxia.

Sharpened Romberg Inability to maintain standing balance when the eyes are closed and the feet are in a heel-toe (tandem) position.

Rotational work Torque multiplied by the arc of movement.

Rubor Redness of the skin caused by inflammation.

Rule of Nines Estimation used to determine the amount of total body surface area that has been burned. It divides the body into segments that are approximately 9% of the total (adults).

S

Saccade Fast, involuntary eye movements.

Salutogenic Health-causing.

Scanning speech A speech pattern that is slow and may be slurred or hesitant with prolonged syllables and inappropriate pauses; the melodic quality of speech is altered.

Schema A rule, concept, or relationship formed on the basis of experience; the basis of schema theory of motor control.

Schizophrenia A chronic major mental illness involving hallucinations, delusions, avolition (lack of desire), flat affect, and/or alogia (restrictions in the productivity and fluency of speech and thoughts) that result in a progressive decrease in overall functioning.

Scleritis An inflammatory disease associated with rheumatoid arthritis that affects the white outer coating of the eye.

Scleroderma A chronic disease of unknown etiology that causes a sclerosis or hardening of the skin and other internal organs.

Sclerotome Deep somatic tissue such as subchondral bone, periosteum, joint capsule, ligament, muscle, tendon, and fascia corresponding to spinal segments providing their sensory innervation.

Secondary lymphedema *See* **Lymphedema**.

Secondary prevention *See* **Prevention**.

Selective (focused) attention The capacity to attend to a task despite competing environmental visual or auditory stimuli.

Self-mutilation The act of causing physical harm to oneself (e.g., cutting one's own skin, pulling out hair, head banging, biting oneself, burning oneself, and causing infections that may result in amputations). Psychiatrically involved patients may engage in these activities to feel real if they are feeling numb, to externalize internal pain, to relieve intense anxiety, or to get attention.

Self-report A data collection approach where the patient is asked questions directly either by the therapist or a trained interviewer (interviewer report) or through the use of a self-administered reporting instrument.

Semantics The study of meaning that is used by humans to express themselves through language.

Semicircular canals (SCCs) Angular accelerometers of the vestibular system.

Sensation The awareness of conditions inside or outside the body resulting from stimulation of the body's sensory receptors and transmission of the nerve impulse along an afferent fiber to the brain.

Sensitivity The proportion of times that a test correctly identifies an abnormality or condition when that abnormality or condition is actually present.

Sensory conflict theory Predominant explanation for motion sickness; describes sensory inputs of proprioception, vestibular, and visual information not matching stored neural patterns.

Sensory integration The ability of the brain to process and organize disparate information from the different senses and develop meaningful perceptions to guide adaptive responses (cognitive or motor).

Sensory level (SCI) In spinal cord injury, the most caudal segment of the spinal cord with normal sensory function bilaterally.

Shaking (respiratory technique) A bouncing maneuver, created by the therapist's hands, is applied to the rib cage throughout the expiratory phase of breathing to assist the mucociliary transport system; promotes release of secretions.

Sharp débridement (wound care) Use of sterile scissors and forceps to remove eschar.

Sheet graft Autograft that is applied in a single sheet without alteration; may be split-thickness or full-thickness in depth.

Shock (physiological) A clinical syndrome marked by inadequate perfusion and oxygenation of cells, tissues, and organs; usually the result of marginal or markedly lower blood pressure.

Shock (psychological) Response to an unexpected trauma with characteristics of disbelief, disassociation, and inability to focus on reality. Shock is one of the first stages of adaptation and may last for hours, days, or weeks, depending on the individual.

Short-term memory (recent memory) The ability to remember current day-to-day events, learn new information, and retrieve information after an interval of minutes, hours, or days.

Sialorrhea Production of excessive saliva with drooling.

Sigh (respiration) A deep inspiration followed by a prolonged, audible expiration; occasional sighs are normal and function to expand alveoli; frequent sighs are abnormal and may be indicative of emotional stress.

Simultanagnosia The inability to perceive a visual stimulus as a whole; also known as Balint's syndrome.

Situational exposure exercises The cognitive-behavioral therapy technique of desensitization where the patient is slowly exposed to anxiety-producing activities that were previously avoided. This technique is often used in the treatment of anxiety disorders such as post-traumatic stress disorder and phobias.

Skew deviation One eye is superiorly displaced in comparison with the other eye.

Skin substitutes Tissues engineered in a laboratory that are used to restore the essential functions of the skin, provide a barrier to the environment, and control evaporative water loss; used in burn care.

Slough Dead or necrotic tissue separated from living tissue or an ulceration.

Smooth pursuit Volitional eye movement used to follow a moving target; most effective for target velocities less than 60°/sec.

Social function Ability to interact successfully with others in the performance of social roles and obligations; includes social interactions, roles, and networks.

Social support The availability of other persons in the environment who can offer emotional support, financial or material help, a listening ear, guidance, or encouragement.

Social workers Professionals who help patients obtain necessary resources in their communities, such as social security, disability, or unemployment benefits; may also offer individual or family therapy.

Somatoagnosia Impairment in body scheme; a lack of awareness of the body structure and the relationship of body parts of oneself or of others.

Spasticity A motor disorder characterized by velocity-dependent increased muscle tone, exaggerated tendon jerks, and clonus; the result of an upper motor neuron lesion.

Spatial relations disorder A constellation of deficits that have in common a difficulty in perceiving the relationship between objects in space, or the relationship between the self and two or more objects; included are disorders of figure–ground discrimination, form discrimination, spatial relations, position in space perception, and topographical orientation.

Specificity The proportion of times that a test correctly identifies the abnormality as being absent when it truly is absent.

Spin The rotation of a surface around a stationary axis; the same point on the moving surface creates an arc of a circle as the surface moves.

Spinal shock (SCI) Transient period of areflexia and flaccid paralysis immediately following spinal cord injury. There is an absence of reflex activity, impairment of autonomic regulation resulting in hypotension, and loss of control of sweating and piloerection; typically resolves in 2 to 6 weeks after trauma.

Splinter skill A trained or learned skill that is acquired in a manner inconsistent with, or incapable of being integrated with, skills the individual already possesses; not easily generalized to other environments or to variations of the same task.

Split-thickness skin graft Graft containing epidermis and part of the dermis.

Spontaneous nystagmus *See* **Nystagmus**.

Spontaneous recovery Recovery resulting from repair processes occurring within the central nervous system immediately after the insult.

Stability or static postural control Refers to the ability to maintain a posture with orientation of the center of mass over the base of support and the body held steady (e.g., holding in sitting, kneeling, or standing).

Standard precautions Guidelines recommended by the Centers for Disease Control and Prevention (CDC) for reducing the risk of transmission of blood-borne and other pathogens in hospitals. These precautions synthesize the major features of universal precautions designed to reduce the risk of transmission of blood-borne pathogens (e.g., hand washing and wearing personal protective equipment) and body substance isolation measures designed to reduce the risk of pathogens from moist body substances and apply them to all patients receiving care in hospitals regardless of their diagnosis or presumed infection status. Standard precautions apply to (1) blood; (2) all body fluids, secretions, and excretions except sweat, regardless of whether or not they contain blood; (3) broken skin; and (4) mucous membranes.

Staphylococcus aureus A microorganism commonly found on the skin, nasal cavities, and oral cavities. A methicillin-resistant strain is called MRSA and a vancomycin-resistant strain is called VRSA. Life-threatening infections have been connected to both strains.

Stemmer's sign The inability to pick up a fold of skin at the base of the second toe. A positive sign means evidence of lymphedema, but the absence of a positive sign does not mean lymphedema is not present.

Step length (gait) The linear distance between two successive points of contact of the right and left lower extremities; measured in centimeters or meters.

Step time (gait) The amount of time that elapses between consecutive right and left foot contacts (heel strikes); usually measured in seconds.

Step width (gait) Width of the walking base (base of support), measured as the linear distance (in the frontal plane) between one foot and the opposite foot; measured in centimeters or meters.

Stereognosis The ability to recognize the shape of objects by touch.

Stereotactic surgery Surgical lesioning of the brain.

Stertor A snoring sound due to secretions in the trachea and large bronchi (adj. *stertorous*).

Stress reaction The observable consequences of the stressor; accompanied by sympathetic signs and symptoms such as palpitations, cold sweat, faint feelings, dilated pupils, pallor, fear, and a host of other complaints.

Stretching The application of manual or mechanical force to elongate (lengthen) structures that have adaptively shortened and are hypomobile.

Stride length (gait) The linear distance between two successive points of contact of the same foot; generally measured in centimeters or meters.

Stride time (gait) The amount of time that elapses during one stride; usually measured in seconds.

Stridor A harsh, high-pitched crowing sound that occurs with upper airway obstructions caused by narrowing of the glottis or trachea (e.g., tracheal stenosis, presence of a foreign object).

Stroke (cerebrovascular accident [CVA]) Acute onset of neurological dysfunction due to an abnormality in cerebral circulation with signs and symptoms that correspond to involvement of focal areas of the brain.

Hemorrhagic stroke Abnormal bleeding into the extravascular areas of the brain; usually results from rupture of an aneurysm, extremely high blood pressure, brain trauma, or brain tumors.

Ischemic stroke The result of a thrombus, embolism, or conditions that produce low systemic perfusion pressures and loss of cerebral circulation resulting in anoxia and infarction.

Lacunar stroke Blood flow is blocked in very small arterial vessels deep within the cerebral white matter with involvement of the internal capsule; characterized by contralateral pure motor or sensory deficits without visual field, cognitive, or speech deficits.

Thrombotic stroke (atherothrombotic brain infarction [ABI]) Formation of a blood clot or thrombus within the cerebral arteries or their branches or the internal carotid or vertebral arteries, causing an occlusion and cerebral infarction; large vessel thrombosis is the most common and is associated with long-standing atherosclerosis.

Stroke volume (SV) The volume of blood ejected from the left ventricle with each myocardial contraction, expressed in mL/min.

Subarachnoid hemorrhage Rupture and bleeding of a cerebral vessel into the subarachnoid space; may occur spontaneously, the result of an aneurysm or arteriovenous malformation, or secondary to trauma.

Subdural hematoma Extravascular blood mass located beneath the dura mater of the brain.

Subluxation Partial dislocation of bones in a joint.

Subordinate part An element of movement without which the task cannot proceed safely or efficiently.

Substance abuse professionals Individuals specifically trained to work with people with substance abuse/dependence problems. Many substance abuse counselors are in recovery themselves, thus adding to their experience and ability to help others with the same problems, and many are Certified Alcohol and Substance Abuse Counselors (CASACs).

Suffering The affective component of pain that includes both emotional (e.g., anxiety and anger) and cognitive (e.g., thoughts of helplessness) components; may be due to a combination of unpleasantness and catastrophizing (making a "catastrophe" out of minor issues).

Summary (additive) measure Approach to grading a specific series of skills by awarding points for each task or activity; totals the score as a percentage of 100 or as a fraction.

Sustained attention (vigilance) The ability to maintain attention to relevant information; sustained attention implies the ability to maintain consistent performance during a continuous activity.

Swan neck deformity A deformed position of the finger, in which there is flexion of the metacarpophalangeal (MCP) and distal interphalangeal (DIP) joints with hyperextension of the proximal interphalangeal (PIP) joint; results from contracture of intrinsic muscles with dorsal subluxation of lateral extensor tendons.

Swing time (gait) The amount of time during the gait cycle that one foot is off the ground; measured in seconds.

Swollen joint count A component of the clinical assessment used to determine disease activity in rheumatoid arthritis. The swollen joint count is a sum of the number of joints deemed inflamed by the examiner.

Syme's amputation Amputation at the supramalleolar level, in which all foot bones are removed and the calcaneal fat pad is attached distally to cushion the end of the limb.

Synergy (normal) Functionally linked muscles that are constrained by the CNS to act cooperatively to produce an intended motor action; used to simplify control, reduce or constrain the degrees of freedom, and initiate coordinated patterns of movement.

Synovectomy Surgical removal of a synovial membrane.

Synovitis Inflammation of a synovial membrane.

Synovium A thin membrane in synovial joints that lines the joint capsule and secretes synovial fluid.

Systems theory A theory of motor control that describes a process by which various brain and spinal centers work cooperatively to accommodate the demands of intended movements; control of movement is viewed as variable.

Systole Period during which the ventricles of the heart are contracting; the contraction phase of the cardiac cycle.

Systolic pressure *See* **Blood pressure**.

T

Tachycardia An abnormally rapid (high) pulse rate; greater than 100 beats per minute in adults.

Tachypnea An abnormally fast respiratory rate; greater than 24 breaths per minute.

Task analysis The breakdown of an activity or task into its component parts and a delineation of the specific motoric, perceptual, and cognitive abilities that are necessary to perform each component.

Team approach A widely used approach to inpatient rehabilitation in which a group of professionals provide multidisciplinary interventions. Participants are usually a physiatrist (a physician specializing in rehabilitation), physical therapist, occupational therapist, social worker, speech-language pathologist, and nurse.

Tender joint count A component of the clinical assessment used to determine disease activity in rheumatoid arthritis. Tender joint count is determined by patients' pain response to pressure exerted on joints by the clinician.

Tenodesis Attaching tendon to bone.

Tensile strength The maximum amount of stress that a material can be subjected to before it breaks or tears.

Terminal stance (gait) The phase during which body weight completes progression over a single stable limb; the reference limb's heel lifts from the ground and a trailing limb posture is achieved.

Terminal swing (gait) The phase that occurs during the final third of swing as the knee extends in preparation for initial contact and start of the next gait cycle.

Tertiary prevention *See* **Prevention**.

Tetraplegia (quadriplegia) Complete paralysis of all four extremities and trunk, including the respiratory muscles.

Thermistor A temperature-measuring device designed to gauge the contact temperature of the skin.

Thoracic excursion Thoracic movement, from full exhalation to full inspiration, measured using a tape measure around the base of the thorax; normal thoracic movement is approximately 2 to 3 inches.

Thought blocking A symptom, usually of schizophrenia, in which the mind goes blank. An episode can last for a few seconds or be a chronic condition.

Thromboangiitis obliterans Inflammation of the intimal layer of a blood vessel, with clot formation, also referred to as Buerger's disease.

Thrombosis The formation or presence of a blood clot within the vascular system.

Thrombotic stroke (atherothrombotic brain infarction [ABI]) *See* **Stroke.**

Thrombus A blood clot that adheres to the wall of a blood vessel or organ.

Tidal volume (TV) The amount of air inspired and expired during normal resting ventilation.

Tinnitus Phantom noise (ringing, roaring, buzzing) detected in one or both ears.

Topographical disorientation Difficulty understanding and remembering the relationship of one place to another.

Torque Force multiplied by perpendicular distance from the axis of rotation; a force that produces rotation.

Total lung capacity The total amount of air that can be held within the thorax (IRV + TV + ERV + RV).

Transfemoral Above-knee.

Transfer of learning Refers to the gain (or loss) in the capability of task performance as a result of practice or experience on some other task.

Transient ischemic attack (TIA) Temporary interruption of blood supply to the brain; symptoms of neurological deficit may last for only a few minutes or hours but do not last longer than 24 hours. After the attack no evidence of residual brain damage or neurological damage remains.

Transitional mobility Refers to skills that allow movement from one posture to another (e.g., supine-to-sit, sit-to-stand).

Transtibial Below-knee.

Tremor Rhythmic, involuntary movements resulting from alternate contraction and relaxation of opposing muscles.

Essential tremor A benign tremor, usually of the head, chin, hands, and occasionally the voice; not associated with other neurological complications.

Intention (action) tremor Tremor is exhibited or intensified when attempting coordinated voluntary movements; seen in cerebellar disease.

Postural tremor Tremor involves the head and trunk and seen when muscles are used to maintain an upright posture against gravity.

Resting tremor Tremor is present at rest and diminished or suppressed by voluntary movement and disappears with sleep; seen in Parkinson's disease.

Senile tremor A benign essential tremor found in individuals older than 60; marked by rapid, alternating movements of the upper extremities that occur during purposeful movements.

Trigger finger Catching, snapping, or locking of the involved finger flexor tendon when it becomes momentarily stuck in the tendon sheath.

Tunneling Tissue destruction that occurs in the form of a tunnel in the fascial layers along the fascial planes between the muscles under the skin.

Turning points Important experiences and realizations that enable people to find new direction, purpose, or meaning in life.

Two-point discrimination Ability to distinguish two blunt points applied to the skin simultaneously.

U

Ulceration An area of epithelial sloughing associated with damage to underlying tissue and a suppurative or nonhealing lesion on a surface such as skin, cornea, or mucous membrane.

Ulnar drift Ulnar drift (also known as ulnar deviation) is a condition where there is a shift in the direction of the fingers or wrist toward the ulna, usually due, in fingers, to inflammation of the MP joints with displacement and corresponding rupture of tendons.

Undermining When débridement removes skin and subcutaneous tissue damage, the results may leave a shape like a cave, or a hole with a lip around the edge that is referred to as undermining.

Unilateral neglect The inability to register and to integrate visual stimuli and perceptions from one side of the environment (usually the left), not attributable to sensory-based problems. As a result, the patient ignores stimuli occurring in that side of personal space.

Universal design A structural plan for buildings and dwellings that meet the requirements of all people, including those with activity limitations and disability; takes into consideration the needs of a wide range of individuals, as well as the changing needs of human beings across the life span.

Upper motor neurons (UMNs) Neurons within the central nervous system that give rise to the descending motor pathways.

V

Validity The degree to which an instrument or tool measures what it is designed to measure; different types of validity include construct, content, criterion-based, concurrent, and predictive validity.

Valsalva maneuver An attempt to exhale forcibly with the glottis, nose, and mouth closed, causing increased intrathoracic pressure, slowed pulse, decreased return of blood to the heart, and increased venous pressure.

Varicose veins Enlarged, dilated superficial veins. The condition can occur anywhere in the body but is most common in the lower extremities and in the esophagus.

Venous reflux The backflow of blood through a vein that has valvular incompetence.

Ventilation The act of moving air in and out of the lungs.

Venules The smallest subunits of the venous system.

Vertebrobasilar insufficiency (VBI) Ischemia in the area of junction for the vertebral and basilar arteries.

Vertical disorientation A distorted perception of the upright (vertical) position.

Vertigo The sensation of moving around in space or of having objects move about the person; sense of spinning.

Vesicular breath sounds The normal intensity of a breath sound heard during auscultation of the lungs.

Vestibular Schwanomma (acoustic neuroma) A benign tumor from the Schwann cells of the vestibulocochlear cranial nerve.

Vestibulo-ocular reflex (VOR) Reflex responsible for generating compensatory eye movements during head rotation. Enables clear vision while the head is in motion.

Vestibulo-ocular reflex gain Ratio of eye velocity to head velocity.

Vestibulo-ocular reflex phase The phase of the VOR that represents the timing relationship between head motion and eye motion. Ideally, eye position should arrive at a point in time that is equal with the oppositely directed head position.

Vestibulospinal reflex (VSR) Reflex responsible for generating compensatory body movements in order to maintain head and postural stability, thereby preventing falls.

Vibration Mechanical oscillation of an object (e.g., tuning fork used for sensory testing).

Visual fixation The ability to maintain focus on an object as it is brought closer to and farther away from the eyes.

Visual object agnosia The inability to recognize familiar objects despite normal function of the eyes and optic tracts.

Visual or linear analogue scale A measurement scale in which a horizontal or vertical straight line is labeled with descriptive or numeric terms to anchor the extremes of the scale; the individual is asked to bisect the line at a point representing the self-reported position on the scale.

Visual proprioception Detection by the visual system of the relative orientation of body parts and orientation of the body in space; provides a basis for movement control.

Vital capacity (VC) The greatest volume of air that can be exhaled from a full inspiration, or the greatest volume of air that can be inhaled from a full exhalation.

Vocational counselor A professional who assists individuals with disabilities to find and maintain employment.

W

Walking velocity The rate of linear forward motion (displacement) of the body per unit of time in a given direction; measured in meters per minute (or centimeters per second). Walking velocity = distance/time.

Wellness The sense that one is living in a manner that permits growth and balance in the physical, emotional, spiritual, intellectual, social, and psychological domains of human experience.

Wernicke's aphasia See **Aphasia**.

Wheeze A musical adventitious sound heard during lung auscultation when expired air is forced through a narrowed airway.

Withdrawal Symptoms that accompany cessation of alcohol, amphetamines, sedatives, opioids, cocaine, hypnotics, or anxiolytics that have been abused over a period of time. Withdrawal symptoms differ with the substance abused and are usually the opposite of the symptoms of intoxication, but may also include perspiration, agitation, and physical pain.

X–Z

Xenograft (or heterograft) Skin used as a temporary wound cover, which is harvested from another species of animal, usually a pig.

Zone of coagulation In a burn wound, central area of necrotic tissue.

Zone of hyperemia In a burn wound, an area with increased circulation.

Zone of partial preservation (SCI) In a complete spinal cord injury, an area of partial preservation (sparing) of motor and/or sensory function in segments caudal to the neurological level.

Zone of stasis In a burn wound, an area where circulation is diminished and compromised.

Z-plasty Procedure used to surgically lengthen a burn scar or contracture to allow for greater range of motion.

INDEX